- Comprehensive coverage of drug compatibilities - syringe, Y-site, additive, and solution.

- Implications of too-rapid IV medication administration.

- Detailed patient education information for every medication-assumes no previous knowledge about medication education.

- Special dosing considerations in second-color highlight for patients with renal and hepatic impairment.

- Most complete life-span dosing considerations for adult, elderly, pediatric, and neonatal patients.

**Expert nurses rely on this exceptional reference!**

- Alphabetical organization for quick look-ups.

- Pain Assessment Guidelines and Lab Test considerations.

- **Unique coverage of the average wholesale price for 300 top drugs**—especially useful to advanced practice nurses with prescriptive authority as well as home health nurses.

- More new monographs including the latest FDA approvals.

- Monographs of the most popular natural products, including drug-natural product interactions.

- All drug entries are labeled as Rx (prescription) or OTC (over the counter).

- Flavors of syrups and chewable tablets-great for the pediatric nurse and the patient.

- 50 Comprehensive Drug Classes-with natural products in a separate class.

- Extensive table of more than 500 commonly used combination drugs- includes the dosage amount of active generic ingredient.

- FREE access to www.DrugGuide.com. Make it your reliable source for the latest FDA drug releases in full monograph style.

- Full-sized CD-ROM version offers access to more than 350 of the most popular drugs by generic or trade name. Print entire monograph or parts-whatever you need to create fully customized med cards. Enhance safe practice and protect your patients with the Preventing Medication Errors tutorial.

This reference not only provides the pharmacologic profile of what each drug does and how it works but also links essential nursing data, such as which parameters to assess in the patient taking the drug, how to administer the medication, and how to evaluate the drug's effectiveness while incorporating unique information about how to prevent medication errors. The 9th edition meets and fills the drug information needs of every student and practicing nurse, facilitating and emphasizing the nurse's role in safe and effective management of medication therapies.

From THE PUBLISHER.

# EARLY MANAGEMENT OF ANAPHYLACTIC REACTIONS

1. **Discontinue suspected drug.**
   (stop IV, tourniquet IM or subcut site).
2. **Maintain airway.** Aminophylline or other bronchodilators may be required for severe respiratory distress.
3. **Administer *epinephrine*.**
   **Subcut (Adults):** 0.2–0.5 mg, may repeat q 5–15 min
   **Subcut (Children):** 0.01 mg/kg or 0.1 mg may repeat q 5–15 min
   **IV (Adults):** 0.3–0.5 mg over 5 min, may repeat q 15 min or 0.1 mg over 5–10 min *or* 1–4 mcg/min infusion
   **IV (Children):** 0.01 mg/kg/dose or 0.1–0.2 mg over 5 min, may repeat q 30 min or 0.1–1.5 mcg (maxium)/kg/min infusion
4. **Administer *antihistamines*.** May prevent recurrence and decrease intensity of reaction.
   ***diphenyhydramine* (Benadryl)**
   **IM, IV (Adults):** 50–100 mg single dose, may follow with 5 mg/kg/day in divided doses or 50 mg every 6 hr for 1–2 days
   **IM, IV (Children):** 5 mg/kg/day in divided doses q 6–8 hr (not to exceed 300 mg/day), may follow with oral therapy for 1–2 days
   ***cimetidine* (Tagamet)**
   **IV (Adults):** 300 mg q 6 hrs
   **IV (Children):** 25–30 mg/kg/day in 6 divided doses
5. **Support blood pressure.** If necessary use fluids and/or vasopressors. Patients receiving beta blockers may be resistant to the effects of vasopressers.
6. **Administer *corticosteroids*** (may decrease intensity of reaction).
   ***hydrocortisone* (Solu-Cortef)**
   ***IV (Adults and Children):*** 100–1000 mg, may follow with 7 mg/kg/day IV or oral therapy for 1–2 days.
7. **Document reaction** in medical record, inform patient/family to carry identification

# *Davis's*

# DRUG GUIDE

# FOR NURSES

## NINTH EDITION

JUDITH HOPFER DEGLIN, PharmD
University of Connecticut
School of Pharmacy
Storrs, Connecticut

APRIL HAZARD VALLERAND, PhD, RN
Wayne State University
College of Nursing
Detroit, Michigan

 F. A. DAVIS COMPANY • Philadelphia

F. A. Davis Company
1915 Arch Street
Philadelphia, PA 19103
www.fadavis.com

Printed in the United States of America

Last digit indicates print number 10 9 8 7 6 5 4 3 2 1
Publisher, Nursing: Robert Martone
Director of Production: Michael W. Bailey
Managing Editor: Mimi McGinnis
Developmental/XML Editor: Robert Allen
Editorial Consultant: Tracey Hopkins
Project Editor: Michelle Clarke

NOTE: As new scientific information becomes available through basic and clinical research, recommended treatments and drug therapies undergo changes. The authors and publisher have done everything possible to make this book accurate, up to date, and in accord with accepted standards at the time of publication. However, the reader is advised always to check product information (package inserts) for changes and new information regarding dose and contraindications before administering any drug. Caution is especially urged when using new or infrequently ordered drugs.

Deglin, Judith Hopfer, 1950 -
    Davis's drug guide for nurses/Judith Hopfer Deglin, April Hazard Vallerand.-9th ed.
    p.; cm.
    Includes bibliographical references and index.
    ISBN 0-8036-1152-8 (pbk.: w/cd)—ISBN 0-8036-1154-4 (w/o cd)
    1. Drugs—Handbooks, manuals, etc. 2. Nursing—Handbooks, manuals, etc. 3. Clinical pharmacology—Handbooks, manuals, etc.
    [DNLM: 1. Pharmaceutical Preparations—administration & dosage—Handbooks. 2. Drug Therapy—nursing—Handbooks. 3. Pharmacology, Clinical—methods—Handbooks. QV 735 D318 2005] I. Title: Drug guide for nurses. II. Vallerand, April Hazard. III. Title.
    RM301.12.D44 2005
    615'.1'024613-dc22

                                                                        2004043949
                                                                        CIP

## DEDICATION

*In loving memory of my older children, Samantha Ann and Randy Eli, both struck and killed by a drinking driver on January 9, 1997. Their memory remains with us in our hearts forever. The wonder and joy they brought to our lives continues to inspire us.*

*To Stu. for his continued support and love.*

*To my younger children, Hanna Fern and Reuben Seth, for making us a family and filling our days with love and happiness.*

JHD

To my father, Keith Hazard, whose love and support are always there.
To my mother-in-law, Roberta, who is always there when I need her.
To my son, Ben, whose transition from child to young man makes me proud.
To my daughter, Kate, who reminds me what is really important.
To my husband, Warren, my colleague and friend, whose encouragement and love I have always cherished.

AHV

## ACKNOWLEDGMENTS

We offer our thanks to the students and nurses who have used our book over the past 17 years. We hope our book provides you with the current knowledge of pharmacotherapeutics you need to continue to give quality care in our rapidly changing health-care environment.

Judi and April

# CONSULTANTS

Regina S. Cunningham, RN, PhD, AOCN
Chief Nursing Officer/Director of Ambulatory
Services
The Cancer Institute of New Jersey
New Brunswick, New Jersey

Margaret Falahee, MA, MSN, FNP
Clinical Assistant Professor
UMDNJ School of Nursing
Wayne State University College of Nursing
Detroit, Michigan

Linda Felver, Ph.D., RN
Associate Professor
Oregon Health & Science University School of
Nursing
Portland, Oregon

Althea DuBose Hayes, RD
Renal Dietitian
Fresenius Medical Services
Ann Arbor, Michigan

Lynn R. Parker McBride, MA, NP, CNS, RN
Holistic Nurse Practitioner
Drew University
Madison, New Jersey

Oncology Nurse Practitioner
New York University Medical Center
New York, New York

Rosemary C. Polomano, Ph.D, RN, FAAN
Senior Nursing Research Specialist
Center for Evaluation, Research and Informatics
Milton S. Hershey Medical Center
Philadelphia, Pennsylvania

Noel Dougherty Rosner, MSN, RN, ANP-C
Nurse Practitioner
Raritan Bay Medical Center
Department of Infectious Diseases
Perth Amboy, New Jersey

Lisa Velazquez-Marsh, BSN, RN, OCN
North Florida Regional Hospital
Gainesville, Florida

Frances B. Wimbush, PhD, RN
Adjunct Faculty
Wayne State University
College of Nursing
Ocean View, Delaware

## With special contributions by:

Elizabeth A. Duthie, RN, MA
Director of Nursing for Patient Care Systems
New York University Medical Center
New York, New York

Laurie Wilhite, Pharm. D
Clinical Associate Professor
University of Minnesota
College Pharmacy
Minneapolis, Minnesota

# CONTENTS

# HOW TO USE *DAVIS'S DRUG GUIDE FOR NURSES*

*Davis's Drug Guide for Nurses* provides comprehensive, up-to-date drug information in well-organized, nursing-focused monographs. It also includes extensive supplemental material in 18 appendices and the accompanying CD-ROM, thoroughly addresses the issue of safe medication administration, and educates the reader about 50 different therapeutic classes of drugs. Use this book to enhance your competence in implementing and evaluating medication therapies. The following sections describe the organization of *Davis's Drug Guide for Nurses* and explain how to quickly find the information you need.

## Safe Medication Use Articles

Comprising "Medication Errors: Improving Practices and Patient Safety", "Detecting and Managing Adverse Drug Reactions", "Special Dosing Considerations", and "Educating Patients about Medication Use", the safe medication use articles provide an overview of the medication safety issues that confront practitioners and patients. Leading off this series, the medication errors article familiarizes you with the systems issues and clinical situations repeatedly implicated in medication errors and suggests practical means to avoid them. It also teaches you about *high alert* medications, which have a greater potential to cause patient harm than other medications. "Detecting and Managing Adverse Drug Reactions" explains the different types of adverse reactions and provides guidance on how to detect and manage them. "Special Dosing Considerations" identifies the patient populations, such as neonates and patients with renal impairment, who require careful dosage adjustments to ensure optimal therapeutic outcomes. "Educating Patients About Medication Use" reviews the most important teaching points for nurses to discuss with their patients and their families. In addition to these safety articles, other critical information is highlighted in blue throughout the drug monographs. This allows the reader to quickly identify important information and to see how nursing practice, including assessment, implementation, and patient teaching, relates to it.

## Classifications Article

Medications in the same therapeutic class often share similar mechanisms of action, assessment guidelines, precautions, and interactions. The Classifications article provides summaries of the major therapeutic classifications used in *Davis's Drug Guide for Nurses*. It also provides patient teaching information common to all agents within the class and a list of drugs within each class.

## Drug Monographs

Drug monographs are organized in the following manner:

**High Alert Status** Some medications, such as chemotherapeutic agents, anticoagulants, and insulins, have a greater potential for harm than others. These medications have been identified by the *Institute for Safe Medication Practices* as **high alert drugs.** *Davis's Drug Guide for Nurses* includes a high alert tab in the upper right corner of the monograph header in appropriate medications to alert the nurse to the medication's risk. The term high alert is used in other parts of the monograph as well, to help the nurse administer these medications safely.

**Generic/Trade Name:** The generic name appears first, with a pronunciation key, followed by an alphabetical list of trade names. Canadian trade names appear in curly brackets ({}). Common names, abbreviations, and selected foreign names are also included.

**Classification:** The therapeutic classification, which categorizes drugs by the disease state they are used to treat, appears first, followed by the pharmacologic classification, which is based on the drug's mechanism of action.

**Controlled Substance Schedule:** All drugs regulated by federal law are placed into one of five schedules, based on the drug's medicinal value, harmfulness, and potential for abuse or addiction. Schedule I drugs, the most dangerous and having no medicinal value, are not included in *Davis's Drug Guide for Nurses*. (See Appendix N for a description of the Schedule of Controlled Substances and a list of controlled substances found in *Davis's Drug Guide for Nurses*.)

**Pregnancy Category:** Pregnancy categories (A, B, C, D, and X) provide a basis for determining a drug's potential for fetal harm and are included in each monograph. The designation UK is used when the pregnancy category is unknown. (See Appendix L for more information.)

**Indications:** Medications are approved by the FDA (Food and Drug Administration) for specific disease states. This section identifies the diseases or conditions for which the drug is commonly used and includes significant unlabeled uses as well.

**Action:** This section contains a concise description of how the drug produces the desired therapeutic effect.

**Pharmacokinetics:** Pharmacokinetics refers to the way the body processes a medication by absorption, distribution, metabolism, and excretion. This section also includes information on the drug's half-life.

> **Absorption:** Absorption describes the process that follows drug administration and its subsequent delivery to systemic circulation. If only a small fraction is absorbed following oral administration (diminished bioavailability), then the oral dose must be much greater than the parenteral dose. Absorption into systemic circulation also follows other routes of administration such as topical, transdermal, intramuscular, subcutaneous, rectal, and ophthalmic routes. Drugs administered intravenously are usually 100% bioavailable.

> **Distribution:** This section comments on the drug's distribution in body tissues and fluids. Distribution becomes important in choosing one drug over another, as in selecting an antibiotic that will penetrate the central nervous system to treat meningitis or in avoiding drugs that cross the placenta or concentrate in breast milk. Information on protein binding is included for drugs that are >95% bound to plasma proteins, which has implications for drug-drug interactions.

**Metabolism and Excretion:** Drugs are primarily eliminated from the body either by hepatic conversion to inactive compounds (metabolism or biotransformation) and subsequent excretion by the kidneys, or by renal elimination of unchanged drug. Therefore, drug metabolism and excretion information is important in determining dosage regimens and intervals for patients with impaired renal or hepatic function. The creatinine clearance (CCr) helps quantify renal function and guides dosage adjustments. Formulas to estimate CCr are included in Appendix G.

**Half-Life:** The half-life of a drug is the amount of time it takes for the drug level to decrease by 50% and roughly correlates with the duration of action. Half-lives are given for drugs assuming the patient has normal renal or hepatic function. Conditions that alter the half-life are noted.

**Contraindications and Precautions:** Situations in which drug use should be avoided or alternatives strongly considered are listed as contraindications. In general, most drugs are contraindicated in pregnancy or lactation, unless the potential benefits outweigh the possible risks to the mother or baby (e.g., anticonvulsants, antihypertensives, and antiretrovirals). Contraindications may be absolute (i.e., the drug in question should be avoided completely) or relative, in which certain clinical situations may allow cautious use of the drug. The precautions portion includes disease states or clinical situations in which drug use involves particular risks or in which dosage modification may be necessary. Extreme cautions are noted separately to draw attention to conditions under which use of the drug results in serious, potentially life-threatening consequences.

**Adverse Reactions and Side Effects:** Although it is not possible to include all reported reactions, major side effects for all drugs are included. Life-threatening adverse reactions or side effects are **CAPITALIZED**, and the most frequent side effects are underlined. Those underlined generally have an incidence of 10% or greater. Those not underlined occur in fewer than 10% but more than 1% of patients. Although life-threatening reactions may be rare (fewer than 1%), they are included because of their significance.

**Interactions:** As the number of medications a patient receives increases, so does the likelihood of experiencing a drug-drug interaction. The most important drug-drug interactions and their results are provided. Significant drug-food and drug-natural product interactions also are noted. Recommendations for avoiding or minimizing these interactions are also presented.

**Route and Dosage:** Routes of administration are grouped together and include recommended dosages for adults, children, and other more specific age groups (such as geriatric patients). Dosage units are expressed in the terms in which they are usually prescribed. For example, penicillin G dosage is given in units rather than in milligrams. Dosing intervals also are provided in the manner in which they are frequently ordered. If a specific clinical situation (indication) requires a different dosage or interval, this is listed separately for clarity. Specific dosing regimens for hepatic or renal impairment are also included.

**Availability:** This section lists the strengths and concentrations of available dosage forms. Such information is useful in planning more convenient regimens (fewer tablets/capsules, less injection volume) and in determining whether certain dosing forms are available (suppositories, oral concentrates, sustained- or extended-release forms). Flavors of oral liquids and chewable tablets have been included to improve compliance and adherance in pediatric patients. General availability and average wholesale prices of commonly prescribed drugs have also been added as an aid to nurses with prescriptive authority.

**Time/Action Profile:** The time/action profile provides the onset of drug action, its peak effect, and its duration of activity. This can aid in planning administration schedules and allows the reader to appreciate differences in choosing one route over another.

**Nursing Implications:** This section has been developed to help the nurse apply the nursing process to pharmacotherapeutics. It is divided into subsections that give the nurse a step-by-step guide to clinical assessment, implementation, and evaluation as they relate to medication administration.

 **Assessment:** This section includes guidelines for assessing patient history and physical data before and during during drug therapy. The **General** section describes assessment that is pertinent to all patients taking the medication. Assessments specific to the drug's various indications are also included. The **Lab Test Considerations** section provides the nurse with information regarding which laboratory tests to monitor and how the results may be affected by the medication. **Toxicity and Overdose** discusses therapeutic serum drug levels and signs and symptoms of toxicity. The antidote and treatment for toxicity or overdose of appropriate medications also are included.

 **Potential Nursing Diagnoses:** The nursing diagnoses approved by the North American Nursing Diagnoses Association (NANDA) are used. The two or three most pertinent diagnoses that apply to a patient receiving the medication are listed. Following each diagnosis, the location of the information from which the diagnosis has been developed is listed in parentheses to provide a reference for the nursing diagnosis-for instance, Infection, risk for (Indications, Side Effects). Since patient education is fundamental to all nurse-patient interactions, the deficient knowledge diagnosis does not appear but should be assumed to be a nursing diagnosis applicable to all drugs.

 **Implementation:** Guidelines specific for medication administration are discussed in this subsection. **High Alert** information, i.e., information that directly relates to preventing medication errors with inherently dangerous drugs, is included first if applicable. This includes sound-alike look-alike name confusion with high alert drugs. The information listed under the **General** heading applies to all routes of administration and includes timing of administration and details for patient care. If the drug is not a high alert drug, Sound alike-look alike names are contained here in blue type. Other headings in this section provide data regarding routes of administration. **PO** describes when and how to administer the drug, whether tablets may be crushed or capsules opened, and when to administer the medication in relation to food. **IV** provides details for reconstitution and dilution. **Direct IV** (IV Push), **Intermittent Infusion**, and **Continuous Infusion** specify amount and type of further dilution and stability information. **Rate** includes infusion time for each type of administration. **Syringe Compatibility/Incompatibility** identifies compatabile medications when mixed in a syringe. This type of compatibility is usually limited to 15 minutes after mixing. **Y-Site Compatibility/Incompatibility** identifies medications compatible or incompatible with each drug when administered via Y-site injection or 3-way stopcock in IV tubing. **Additive Compatibility/Incompatibility** identifies medications compatible or incompatible when admixed in solution. This type of compatibility is usually limited to 24 hours. **Solution Compatibility/Incompatibility** identifies compatible or incompatible solutions for dilution or administration purposes. Compatibility information is compiled from Trissel's *Handbook of Injectable Drugs*, ed 12. (See Bibliography.)

**Patient/Family Teaching:** This section includes information that should be taught to patients and/or families of patients. Side effects that should be reported, information on minimizing and managing side effects, details on administration, and follow-up requirements are presented. The nurse also should refer to the **Implementation** section for specific information to teach to the patient and family about taking the medication. **Home Care Issues** discusses aspects to be considered for medications taken in the home setting.

**Evaluation:** Outcome criteria for determination of the effectiveness of the medication are provided.

# MEDICATION ERRORS: Improving Practices and Patient Safety

It is widely acknowledged that medication errors result in thousands of adverse drug events and preventable reactions and deaths per year. Nurses, physicians, pharmacists, patient safety organizations, Food and Drug Administration, the pharmaceutical industry, and other parties share in the responsibility for determining how medication errors occur and designing strategies to reduce error.

One impediment to understanding the scope and nature of the problem has been the reactive and proactive "blaming, shaming, training" culture that singled out one individual as the cause of the error. Also historically, medication errors that did not result in patient harm—near-miss situations in which an error could have but didn't happen—or errors that did not result in serious harm were not reported. In contrast, serious errors often instigated a powerful punitive response in which one or a few persons were deemed to be at fault and lost their jobs and sometimes their licenses as a result.

In 1999, the Institute of Medicine published *To Err Is Human: Building a Safer Health System*, which pointed out that excellent healthcare providers do make medication errors, that many of the traditional processes involved in the medication use system were error-prone, and that other factors, notably drug labeling and packaging, contributed to error. Furthermore, the IOM report, in conjunction with other groups such as the United States Pharmacopeia (USP) and the Institute for Safe Medication Practices (ISMP), called for the redesign of error-prone systems to include better processes that anticipated the fallibility of humans working within the system. This initiative is helping shift the way the health care industry addresses medication errors from a single person/bad apple cause to a systems issue.[1]

The National Coordinating Council for Medication Error Reporting and Prevention (NCC-MERP) developed the definition of a medication error that reflects this shift and captures the scope and breadth of the issue:

"A medication error is any preventable event that may cause or lead to inappropriate medication use or patient harm while the medication is in the control of the health care professional, patient, or consumer. Such events may be related to professional practice, health care products, procedures, and systems, including prescribing; order communication; product labeling, packaging, and nomenclature; compounding; dispensing; distribution; administration; education; monitoring; and use."[2]

Inherent in this definition's mention of related factors are the human factors that are part of the medication use system. For example, a nurse or pharmacist may automatically reach into the bin where dobutamine is usually kept, see "do" and "amine" but select dopamine instead of dobutamine. Working amidst distractions, working long hours or shorthanded, and working in a culture where perfection is expected and questioning is discouraged are other examples of the human factors and environmental conditions that contribute to error. The goal for the design of any individual or hospital-wide medication use system is to determine where systems are likely to fail and to build in safeguards that minimize the potential for error.

One way to begin that process is to become familiar with medications or practices that have historically been shown to be involved in serious errors.

## High Alert Medications

Some medications, because of a narrow therapeutic range or inherent toxic nature, have a high risk of causing devastating injury or death if improperly ordered, prepared, stocked, dispensed, administered, or monitored. Although these medications may not be involved in more errors, they require special attention due to the potential for serious, possibly fatal consequences. These have been termed **high-alert medications**, to communicate the need for extra care and safeguards. Many of these drugs are used commonly in the general population or are used frequently in urgent clinical situations. The Joint Commission on Accreditation of Healthcare Organizations (JCAHO) monitors the five most often prescribed high-alert medications: insulin, opiates and narcotics, injectable potassium chloride (or phosphate) concentrate, intravenous anticoagulants (such as heparin); and sodium chloride solutions above 0.9 percent. (See Table 1 for a complete list of the high alert meds found in *Davis's Drug Guide for Nurses*; visit the Institute for Safe Medication Practices at www.ismp.org for more information on high alert drugs).

## Causes of Medication Errors

Many contributing factors and discrete causes of error have been identified, including failed communication, poor drug distribution practices, dose miscalculations, drug packaging and drug-device related problems, incorrect drug administration, and lack of patient education.[3]

**Failed Communication:** Failed communication covers many of the errors made in the ordering phase, and although ordering is performed by the prescriber, the nurse, the clerk and the pharmacist who interpret that order are also involved in the communication process.

- *Poorly handwritten or verbal orders.* Handwriting is a major source of error and has led to inaccurate interpretations of the drug intended, the route of administration, the frequency, and dose. Telephone and verbal orders are likewise prone to misinterpretation.
- *Drugs with similar-sounding or similar-looking names.* Similar sounding trade names, or trade names that look similar when handwritten, are frequently confused. Amiodarone and amrinone (now renamed inamrinone to help prevent confusion), or Zebeta® and Diabeta® are two examples. The United States Pharmacopoeia (USP) has identified over 700 "sound-alike, look-alike" drugs. Mix-ups are more likely when each drug has similar dose ranges and frequencies.
- *Misuse of zeroes in decimal numbers.* Massive, ten-fold overdoses are traceable to not using a leading zero (.2 mg instead of 0.2 mg) or adding an unnecessary trailing zero (2.0 mg instead of 2 mg) in decimal expressions of dose. Similar overdosages are found in decimal expressions in which the decimal point is obscured by poor handwriting, stray marks or lined orders sheets (e.g., reading 3.1 grams as 31 grams). Under-dosing also may occur by the same mechanism and prevent a desired, perhaps life-saving effect.
- *Use of apothecary measures (grains, drams) or package units (amps, vials, tablets) instead of metric measures (grams, milligrams, milliequivalents).* Apothecary measurements are poorly understood and their abbreviations are easily confused with other units of measurement. Use of such measures should be abandoned. Errors also occur when dosage units are used instead of metric weight. For example, orders for 2 tablets, 1½ vials or 2 ampoules can result in overdose or underdose when the medications ordered come in various strengths.
- *Misinterpreted abbreviations.* Abbreviations can be misinterpreted or, when used in the dosage part of the order, can result in incorrect dosage of the correct medication. For example, lower or upper case "U" for units has been read as a zero, making 10 u of insulin look like 100 units when handwritten. The Latin abbreviation "QOD" for every other day has been misinterpreted as QID (4 times per day). See Table 2 for a list of confusing abbreviations and safer alternatives.
- *Ambiguous or incomplete orders.* Orders that do not clearly specify dose, route, frequency, or indication do not communicate complete information and are open to misinterpretation.

**Poor Distribution Practices:** Poor distribution includes error-prone storing practices such as keeping similar looking products next to each other. Dispensing multidose floor stock vials of potentially dangerous drugs instead of unit doses is also associated with error as is allowing non-pharmacists to dispense medications in the absence of the pharmacist.

**Dose Miscalculations:** Dose miscalculations are a prime source of medication error. Also, many medications need to be dose-adjusted for renal or hepatic impairment, age, height and weight, and body composition, (i.e., correct for obesity). Complicated dosing formulas provide many opportunities to introduce error. Often vulnerable populations, such as premature infants, children, the elderly, and those with serious underlying illnesses are at greatest risk.

**Drug Packaging And Drug Delivery Systems:** Similar packaging or poorly designed packaging encourages error. Drug companies may use the same design for different formulations, or fail to highlight information about concentration or strength. Lettering, type size, color, and packaging methods can either help or hinder drug identification. Drug delivery systems include infusion pumps and rate controllers. Some models do not prevent free flow of medication, leading to sudden high dose infusion of what often are potent and dangerous medications. The lack of safeguards preventing free flow and programming errors are among the problems encountered with infusion control devices.

**Incorrect Drug Administration:** Incorrect drug administration covers many problems. Misidentification of a patient, incorrect route of administration, missed doses, or improper drug preparation are types of errors that occur during the administration phase.

**Lack of Patient Education:** Safe medication use is enhanced in the hospital and the home when the patient is well informed. The knowledgeable patient can recognize when something has changed in his or her medication regimen and can question the health care provider. At the same time, many issues related to medication errors, such as ambiguous directions, unfamiliarity with a drug, and confusing packaging, affect the patient as well as the health care provider, underscoring the need for careful education. Patient education also enhances adherence, which is a factor in proper medication use.

### Prevention Strategies

Since medication use systems are complex and involve many steps and people, they are error-prone. On an individual basis, nurses can help reduce the incidence of error by implementing the following strategies:

- Clarify any order that is not obviously and clearly legible. Ask the prescriber to print orders using block style letters.
- Do not accept orders with the abbreviation "u" for units. Clarify the dosage and ask the prescriber to write out the word units.
- Clarify any abbreviated drug name or the abbreviated dosing frequencies q.d., q.o.d., and q.i.d. Suggest abandoning Latin abbreviations in favor of spelling out dosing frequency.
- Do not accept dosages expressed in package units or volume instead of metric weight. Clarify any order written for number of ampoules, vials, or tablets (e.g., calcium, 1 ampoule or epinephrine, 1 Bristojet).
- Decimal point errors can be hard to see. Suspect a missed decimal point and clarify any order if the dose requires more than 3 dosing units.
- If dose ordered requires use of multiple dosage units or very small fractions of a dose unit, review the dosage, have another health care provider check the original order and recalculate formulas and confirm the dosage with the prescriber.

- If taking a verbal order, ask prescriber to spell out the drug name and dosage to avoid sound alike confusion (e.g., hearing Cerebyx for Celebrex, or fifty for fifteen). Read back the order to the prescriber after you have written it in the chart. Confirm and document the indication to further enhance accurate communication.
- Clarify any order that does not include metric weight, dosing frequency, or route of administration.
- Check the nurse's/clerk's transcription against the original order. Make sure stray marks or initials do not obscure the original order.
- Do not start a patient on new medication by borrowing medications from another patient. This action bypasses the double check provided by the pharmacist's review of the order.
- Always check the patient's name band before administering medications. Verbally addressing a patient by name does not provide sufficient identification.
- Use the facility's standard drug administration times to reduce the chance an omission error.
- Be sure to fully understand any drug administration device before using it. This includes infusion pumps, inhalers, and transdermal patches.
- Have a second practitioner independently check original order, dosage calculations and infusion pump settings for high alert medications.
- Realize that the printing on packaging boxes, vials, ampoules, pre-filled syringes or any container in which a medication is stored can be misleading. Be sure to differentiate clearly the medication and the number of milligrams per milliliter versus the total number of milligrams contained within. Massive overdoses have been administered by assuming that the number of milligrams per ml is all that is contained within the vial or ampoule. Read the label when obtaining the medication, before preparing or pouring the medication, and after preparing or pouring the medication.
- Educate patients about the medications they take. Provide verbal and written instruction and ask the patient to restate important points. Refer to Educating Patients about Safe Medication Use on page xxxi for recommendations on what patients should understand about their medications.

As stated previously, errors are a result of problems within the medication use system and cannot be eliminated by the vigilance of any one group of health care providers. System redesign involves strong leadership from administration and all involved departments. Health care facilities should consider the following when addressing the issue of medication errors:

- Do not provide unit stock of critical, high alert medications. If eliminating these medications from floor stock is not feasible, consider reducing the number available and standardizing the concentrations or forms in which the medication is available.
- Create committees that address safety issues.
- Install a computer physician order entry (CPOE) system to help reduce prescribing orders. Link order entry to pertinent lab, allergy, and medication data.
- Implement bar code technology to ensure the right drug reaches the right patient.
- Develop policies that discourage error-prone prescribing practices such as inappropriate use of verbal orders, use of confusing dosing symbols, and use of abbreviations.
- Develop policies that encourage better communication of medication information such as requiring block-style printing of medications, including indication in prescription, and using both the trade and generic name in prescriptions.
- Ensure a reasonable workload for pharmacists and nurses and provide a well-designed work area.
- Limit the availability of varying concentrations of high alert medications.
- Provide standard concentrations and infusion rate tables.
- Supply pharmacy and patient care areas with current reference material.
- Cultivate a culture that does not assign blame when medication errors occur but looks for root causes instead.

■ Encourage staff to participate in the USP-ISMP-MERP error reporting program.

## REFERENCES

1. Kohn, LT, Corrigan, JM, and Donaldson MS (eds); To Err Is Human: Building a Safer Health System. National Academy Press, Washington, DC, 1999.
2. National Coordinating Council for Medication Error Reporting and Prevention. http://www.nccmerp.org/aboutMedErrors.html
3. Cohen, MR. Medication Errors: Causes, Prevention, Risk Management. Jones and Bartlett Publishers, Sudbury, 1999.

### Table 1: High Alert Medications In Davis's Drug Guide For Nurses

| | | |
|---|---|---|
| amiodarone | epinephrine | methotrexate |
| asparaginase | epirubicin | metoprolol |
| bleomycin | eptifibatide | midazolam |
| buprenorphine | esmolol | milrinone |
| busulfan | etoposides | morphine |
| butorphanol | fentanyl (oral/transmucosal) | nalbuphine |
| calcium salts | fentanyl (parenteral) | nesiritide |
| carboplatin | fentanyl (transdermal) | oxycodone |
| carmustine | fluorouracil | oxymorphone |
| chloralhydrate | gemcitabine | pancuronium |
| cisplatin | heparin | potassium supplements |
| codeine | heparins (low molecular weight)/heparinoids | propranolol |
| colchicine | hydrocodone | sodium chloride |
| cyclophosphamide | hydromorphone | thrombolytic agents |
| cytarabine | hypoglycemic agents, oral | tirofiban |
| daunorubicin citrate liposome | imatinib | topotecan |
| daunorubicin hydrochloride | inamrinone | trastuzumab |
| digoxin | insulins | vinblastine |
| dobutamine | labetalol | vincristine |
| docetaxel | lidocaine | vinorelbine |
| dopamine | magnesium sulfate IV | |
| doxorubicin hydrochloride | meperidine | warfarin |
| doxorubicin hydrochloride liposome | methadone | |

### Table 2: Abbreviations and Symbols Associated with Medication Errors

| Abbreviation/Symbol | Intended Meaning | Mistaken For | Recommendation |
|---|---|---|---|
| AZT | Zidovudine | Azithioprine | Use full drug name |
| CPZ | Compazine | Thorazine (chlorpromazine) | Use full drug name |
| HCl | Hydrochloric acid | KCl (potassium chloride) | Use full drug name |
| HCT | Hydrocortisone | hydrochlorthiazide | Use full drug name |
| MgSO$_4$* | Magnesium sulfate | Morphine sulfate | Use full drug name |
| MS, MSO$_4$* | Morphine sulfate | Magnesium sulfate | Use full drug name |
| MTX | Methotrexate | Mitoxantrone | Use full drug name |
| Nitro drip | Nitroprusside | Nitroglycerin | Use full drug name |
| Norflox | Norfloxacin | Norflex | Use full drug name |
| PCA | Procainamide | Patient controlled analgesia | Use full drug name |
| PIT | Pitocin | Pitressin | Use full drug name |

| Abbreviation/Symbol | Intended Meaning | Mistaken For | Recommendation |
|---|---|---|---|
| μg[†] | microgram | Mg (milligram) | Use mcg |
| / (slash mark) | "per" | "1" (numeral one) | Spell out per |
| HS or hs[†] | Half strength or hour of sleep | One mistaken for the other | Spell out half strength or bedtime |
| + | Plus sign | "4" (numeral four) | Spell out and |
| Zero **after** a decimal point (e.g., 1.0 mg)* | 1 mg | 10 mg | DO NOT USE zero after a decimal point |
| No zero **before** a decimal point (e.g.,. 1 mg)* | .1 mg | 1 mg | ALWAYS USE zero before a decimal point |
| u or U* | units | 0 (zero), 4 (four) or cc | Spell out unit |
| I.U.* | International Units | IV or 10 | Spell out unit |
| HS* | Half strength | Hour of sleep | Write out medication strength. |
| q.d or QD* | Every day | q.i.d (4 times per day) | Write out daily |
| q.o.d. or QOD* | Every other day | q.i.d. (4 times per day) or qd (daily) | Write out every other day |
| SC, SQ, sub q[†] | subcutaneously | SC mistaken as SL (sublingual), SQ as "5 every" or "every" | Use subcut or write out subcutaneously |
| AD, AS, AU[†] | Right ear, left ear, each ear | OD, OS, OU (right eye, left eye, each eye) | Spell out right ear, left ear, each ear |
| OD, OS, OU | Right eye, left eye, each eye | AD, AS, AU (right ear, left ear, each ear) | Spell out right eye, left eye, each eye |
| Cc[†] | cubic centimeters | u (units) | Use ml |
| @ | At | 2 | Use at |
| & | And | 2 | Use and |
| + | Plus or and | 4 | Use and |
| ° | hour | Zero (q 1° seen as q 10) | Use hr, h, or hour |
| Drug name and dose run together. Example: Inderal40 mg | Inderal 40 mg | Inderal 140 mg | Leave space between drug name, dose, and unit of measure |
| Numerical dose and unit of measure run together. Example: 10mg | 10 mg | 100 mg | Leave space between drug dose and unit of measure |

*Appears on JCAHO's "Do Not Use" list of abbreviations.

†Appears on JCAHO's list of abbreviations not recommended for use.

Adapted with permission from The Institute for Safe Medication Practices Safety Alert, Vol 8: Issue 24. Nov 27, 2003.

# DETECTING AND MANAGING ADVERSE DRUG REACTIONS

An *adverse drug reaction* (ADR) is any unexpected, undesired, or excessive response to a medication that results in:

■ temporary or permanent serious harm or disability
■ admission to a hospital, transfer to a higher level of care, or prolonged stay
■ death.

Adverse drug reactions are distinguished from adverse drug events, in which causality is uncertain, and side effects, which may be bothersome to the patient and necessitate a change in therapy but are not considered serious.[1] Although some ADRs are the result of medications errors, many are not.

## Types of ADRs

The Food and Drug Administration (FDA) classifies ADRs into 2 broad categories: Type A and Type B.[2] Type A reactions are predictable reactions based on the primary or secondary pharmacologic effect of the drug. Dose-related reactions and drug-drug interactions are examples of Type A reactions. Type B reactions are unpredictable, are not related to dose, and are not the result of the drug's primary or secondary pharmacologic effect. Idiosyncratic and hypersensitivity reactions are examples of Type B reactions.

**Dose-Related Reactions (Toxic Reactions):** In dose related reactions, the dose prescribed for the patient is excessive. Although a variety of mechanisms may interact, reasons for this type of reaction include:

■ renal or hepatic impairment
■ extremes in age (neonates and frail elderly)
■ drug-drug or drug-food interactions
■ underlying illness. Dose-related reactions are often the result of preventable errors in prescribing in which physiologic factors such as age, renal impairment, and weight were not considered sufficiently, or in inadequate therapeutic monitoring. Medications with narrow therapeutic ranges (digoxin, aminoglycosides, antiepileptic drugs) and those that require careful monitoring or laboratory testing (anticoagulants, nephrotoxic drugs) are most frequently implicated in dose-related reactions.[3,4] Dose-related reactions usually are managed successfully by temporarily discontinuing the drug and then reducing the dose or increasing the dosing interval. In some instances, the toxic effects need to be treated with another agent (e.g. digibind for digoxin toxicity or kayexalate for drug induced hyperkalemia). Appropriately timed therapeutic drug level monitoring, review of new drugs added to an existing regimen that may affect the drug level, and frequent assessment of relevant laboratory values are critical to safe medical management and prevention of dose-related reactions.

**Drug-Drug Interactions:** Drug-drug interactions occur when the pharmacokinetic or pharmacodynamic properties of an individual drug affect another drug. Pharmacokinetics refers to the way the body processes a medication (absorption, distribution, metabolism, and elimination). In a drug-drug interaction, the pharmacokinetic properties of one drug can cause a change in drug concentration of another drug and an altered response. For example, one drug may block enzymes that metabolize a second drug. The concentration of the second drug is then increased and may become toxic or cause adverse reactions. Pharmacodynamic drug-drug interactions involve the known effects and side-effects of the drugs. For example, two drugs with similar therapeutic effects may act together in a synergistic way. The increased anticoagulant effects that occur when warfarin and aspirin are taken together, or the increased CNS depression that results when two drugs with CNS depressant effects potentiate each other, are examples of pharmacodymanic drug-drug interactions. Certain classes of drugs are more likely to result in serious drug-drug interactions and patients receiving these agents should be monitored carefully. The medication classes include anticoagulants, oral hypoglycemic agents, nonsteroidal anti-inflammatory agents, MAO inhibitors, antihypertensives, antiepileptics, and antiretrovirals. In addition, specific drugs such as theophylline, cimetidine, lithium, and digoxin may result in serious ADRs.

**Idiosyncratic Reactions:** Idiosyncratic reactions occur without relation to dose and are unpredictable and sporadic. Reactions of this type may manifest in many different ways, including fever, blood dyscrasias, cardiovascular effects, or mental status changes. The time frame between the occurrence of a problem and initiation of therapy is sometimes the only clue linking drug to symptom. Some idiosyncratic reactions may be explained by genetic differences in drug-metabolizing enzymes.

**Hypersensitivity Reactions:** Hypersensitivity reactions are usually allergic responses. Manifestations of hypersensitivity reactions range from mild rashes, to nephritis, pneumonitis, hemolytic anemia, and anaphylaxis. Protein drugs (vaccines, enzymes) are frequently associated with hypersensitivity reactions. In most instances, antibody formation is involved in the process and therefore cross-sensitivity may occur. An example of this is hypersensitivity to penicillin and cross-sensitivity with other penicillins and/or cephalosporins. Documenting drugs to which the patient is allergic and the specific hypersensitivity reaction is very important. If the reaction to an agent is anaphylaxis the nurse should monitor the patient during administration of a cross-hypersensitive agent, especially during the initial dose, and ensure ready access to emergency resuscitative equipment.

### Recognizing an ADR

Adverse drug reactions should be suspected whenever there is a negative change in a patient's condition, particularly when a new drug has been introduced. Strategies that can enhance recognition include knowing the side effect/adverse reaction profile of medications. Nurses should be familiar with a drug's most commonly encountered side effects and adverse reactions before administering it. (In *Davis's Drug Guide for Nurses*, side effects are underlined, and adverse reactions are CAPITALIZED and appear in second color in the **Adverse Reactions and Side Effects** section.) As always, monitoring the patient's response to a medication and ongoing assessment are key nursing actions. Learn to recognize patient findings that suggest an ADR has occurred. These include:

- rash
- change in respiratory rate, heart rate, blood pressure or mental state
- seizure
- anaphylaxis

- diarrhea
- fever.

Any of these findings can suggest an ADR and should be reported and documented promptly so that appropriate interventions, including discontinuation of suspect medications, can occur. Prompt intervention can prevent a mild adverse reaction from escalating into a serious health problem. Other steps taken by the health care team when identifying and treating an ADR include:

1. Determining that the drug ordered was the drug given and intended.
2. Determining that the drug was given in the correct dosage by the correct route.
3. Establishing the chronology of events: time drug was taken and onset of symptoms.
4. Stopping the drug and monitoring patient status for improvement (dechallenge)
5. Restarting the drug, if appropriate, and monitoring closely for adverse reactions (rechallenge).[2]

## Prevention

Healthcare organizations have responded to consumer, regulator and insurer pressures by developing programs that aim to eliminate preventable ADRs. In the inpatient setting, computer systems can display the patient's age, height, weight, and creatinine clearance or serum creatinine level and send an alert to the clinician if a prescribed dose is out of range for any of the displayed parameters. Allergy alerts and drug-drug interactions can be presented to the clinician at the time an order is entered.

In the outpatient setting, strategies that increase the patient's knowledge base and access to pharmacists and nurses may help prevent adverse reactions.[5] Outpatient pharmacy computer systems that are linked within a chain of pharmacies may allow the pharmacist to view the patient's profile if the patient is filling a prescription in a pharmacy other than the usual one. Many pharmacy computers have dose limits and drug-drug reaction verfication to assist pharmacists filling orders.

Such strategies are a valuable auxiliary to but cannot replace conscientious history taking, careful patient assessment, and ongoing monitoring. A thorough medication history including all prescription and non-prescription drugs, all side effects and adverse reactions encountered, allergies, and all pertinent physical data should be available to the prescriber. The prescriber is responsible for reviewing this data, along with current medications, laboratory values and any other variable that affects drug response.

It is not expected that practitioners will remember all relevant information when prescribing. In fact, reliance on memory is error fraught and clinicians need to use available resources to verify drug interactions whenever adding a new drug to the regimen. Setting expectations that clinicians use evidence-based information rather than their memories when prescribing, dispensing, administering or monitoring patients has the potential to reduce the incidence ofpreventable ADRs.

## Food and Drug Administration MedWatch Program

To monitor and assess the incidence of adverse reactions, the Food and Drug Administration (FDA) sponsors MedWatch, a program that allows health care practitioners and consumers the opportunity to report serious adverse reactions or product defects encountered from medications, medical devices, special nutritional products, or other FDA-regulated items. The FDA considers serious those reactions that result in death, life-threatening illness or injury, hospitalization, disability, congenital anomaly, or those that require medical/surgical intervention.

In addition to reporting serious adverse reactions, health care providers should also report problems related to suspected contamination, questionable stability, defective components, or poor packaging/labeling. Reports should be submitted even if there is some uncertainty about the cause/effect relationship or if some details are missing. This reporting form may be accessed at www.fda.gov/medwatch/report/hcp.htm. Reports also may be faxed to the FDA (1-800-FDA-0178).

Reactions to vaccines should be reported to the Vaccine Adverse Event Reporting System (VAERS; 1-800-822-7967). Nurses share with other health care providers an obligation to report adverse reactions to the MedWatch program so that all significant data can be analyzed for opportunities to improve patient care.

## REFERENCES

1. Lehmann, John. "Adverse Events - Adverse Reactions." Drug Intel 2002-2003 http://www.drugintel.com/public/medwatch/adverse_drug_events.htm (accessed 10 July 2003).
2. Goldman S., Kennedy D., Lieberman R., "Clinical Therapeutics and the Recognition of Drug-Induced Disease." FDA MEDWATCH Continuing Education Article (1995) http://www.fda.gov/medwatch/articles/dig/rcontent.htm#toc (accessed 10 July 2003).
3. Daniels C., Calis K., "Clinical Analysis of Adverse Drug Reactions." Pharmacy Update National Institutes of Health. Sept-Oct 2001. http /www.cc.nih.gov/phar/updates/septoct01/01sept-oct.html (accessed 10 July 2003).
4. Winterstein A., et. al. "Identifying Clinically Significant Preventable Adverse Drug Events Through a Hospital's Database of Adverse Drug Reaction Reports." Am J Health-Syst Pharm 59(18):1742-1749, 2002.
5. Ghandi T., Weingart S., Borus J., et. al. "Adverse Drug Events in Ambulatory Care." New England Journal of Medicine. Volume 348:1556-1564. Number 16. April 17, 2003.

# SPECIAL DOSING CONSIDERATIONS

For many patients the average dose range for a given drug can be toxic. The purpose of this section is to describe vulnerable patient populations for which special dosing considerations must be made to protect the patient and improve clinical outcomes.

## The Pediatric Patient

The main reason for adjusting dosages in pediatric patients is body size, which is measured by body weight or body surface area (BSA). Weight-based pediatric drug dosages are expressed in number of milligrams per kilogram of body weight (mg/kg) while dosages calculated on body surface area are expressed in number of milligrams per meter squared (mg/m$^2$). BSA is determined using a BSA nomogram Appendix H) or calculated by using formulas (Appendix G).

The neonate and the premature infant require additional adjustments secondary to immature function of body systems. For example, absorption may be incomplete or altered secondary to differences in gastric pH or motility. Distribution may be altered because of varying amounts of total body water, and metabolism and excretion can be delayed due to immature liver and kidney function. Furthermore, rapid weight changes and progressive maturation of hepatic and renal function require frequent monitoring and careful dosage adjustments in the neonate.

## The Geriatric Patient

Absorption, distribution, metabolism and excretion are altered in adults over 55 years of age, putting the older patient at risk for toxic reactions. Pharmacokinetic properties in the older patient are affected by

- percentage of body fat, lean muscle mass and total body water
- decreased plasma proteins, especially in the malnourished patient, which allows a larger proportion of free or unbound drug to circulate an exert effects
- diminIshed GI motility and blood flow, which delays absorption
- slower hepatic and renal function, which delays excretion.

All of these variables change with age, however, not predictably. Older patients should be prescribed the lowest possible effective dose at the initiation of therapy followed by careful titration of doses as needed. Just as importantly, they should be monitored very carefully for signs and symptoms of adverse drug reactions.

Another concern is that many elderly patients are prescribed multiple drugs. As the number of medications a patient takes increases, so does the risk for an adverse drug reaction. One drug may negate, potentiate, or otherwise alter the effects of another drug (drug-drug interaction) and this situation is compounded by concurrent use of nonprescription drugs and natural products. In general, doses of most medications especially digoxin, sedative/hypnotics, anticoagulants, thrombolytics, nonsteroidal anti-inflammatory agents, and antihypertensives should be decreased in the geriatric population.

## The Patient of Reproductive Age

Both the mother and the fetus must be considered when prescribing medications to the pregnant woman. The placenta protects the fetus only from extremely large molecules. The fetus is particularly vulnerable during the first and the last trimesters of pregnancy. During the first trimester, vital organs are forming and ingestion of teratogenic drugs may lead to fetal malformation or miscarriage. Unfortunately, this is the time when a woman is least likely to know that she is pregnant. In the third trimester, drugs administered to the mother and transferred to the fetus may not be safely metabolized and excreted by the fetus. This is especially true of drugs administered near term. After the infant is delivered, he or she no longer has the placenta to help with drug excretion and drugs administered before delivery may result in toxicity. It is wise to inform all women of childbearing age of potential for harm from medications to the unborn child.

The possibility of a medication altering sperm quality and quantity in a potential father also is an area of concern. Male patients should be informed of this risk when taking any medications known to have this potential.

## Renal Disease

The kidneys are the major organ of drug elimination and failure to account for decreased renal function is a preventable source of adverse drug reactions. Renal function is measured by the creatinine clearance (CCr), which can be approximated in the absence of a 24-hour urine collection (Appendix G). In addition, dosages in the renally impaired patient can be optimized by measuring medication blood levels.

Patients with underlying renal disease, premature infants with immature renal function, and elderly patients with age-related decrease in renal function require careful dose adjustments. Renal function may fluctuate over time and should be re-assessed periodically.

## Liver Disease

The liver is the major organ of drug metabolism. It changes a drug from a relatively fat-soluble compound to a more water-soluble substance, which means that the drug can then be excreted by the kidneys. Liver function is not as easily quantified as renal function and it therefore is difficult to predict the correct dosage for a patient with liver dysfunction based on laboratory tests.

A patient who is severely jaundiced or who has very low serum proteins (particularly albumin) can be expected to have some problems metabolizing drugs. In advanced liver disease, portal vascular congestion also impairs drug absorption. Examples of drugs that should be carefully dosed in patients with liver disease include theophylline, diuretics, phenytoin, and sedatives. Some drugs require the liver for activation (such as sulindac or cyclophosphamide) and should be avoided in patients with severely compromised liver function.

## Congestive Heart Failure

Heart failure results in passive congestion of blood vessels to the GI tract, which impairs drug absorption. Heart failure also slows drug delivery to the liver, delaying metabolism. Renal function is frequently compromised as well, adding to delayed elimination and prolonged drug action. Dosages of drugs metabolized mainly by the liver or excreted mainly by the kidneys should be decreased in patients with congestive heart failure.

## Body Size

Drug dosing is often based on total body weight. However, some drugs selectively penetrate fatty tissues. If the drug does not penetrate fatty tissues (e.g., digoxin, gentamicin), dosages for the obese patient should be determined by ideal body weight or estimated lean body mass. Ideal body weight may be determined from tables of desirable weights or may be estimated using formulas for lean body mass when the patient's height and weight are known (Appendix G). If such adjustments are not made considerable toxicity can result.

Body size is also a factor in patients who are grossly underweight. Elderly patients, chronic alcoholics, patients with AIDS, and patients who are terminally ill from cancer or other debilitating illnesses need careful attention to dosing. Patients who have had a limb amputated also need to have this change in body size taken into account.

## Drug Interactions

Use of multiple drugs, especially those known to interact with other drugs, may necessitate dosage adjustments. Drugs highly bound to plasma proteins, such as warfarin and phenytoin, may be displaced by other highly protein-bound drugs. When this phenomenon occurs, the drug that has been displaced exhibits an increase in its activity because the free or unbound drug is active.

Some drugs decrease the liver's ability to metabolize other drugs. Drugs capable of doing this include cimetidine and chloramphenicol. Concurrently administered drugs that are both highly metabolized by the liver may need to be administered in decreased dosages. Other agents such as phenobarbital, other barbiturates, and rifampin are capable of stimulating the liver to metabolize drugs more rapidly, requiring larger doses to be administered.

Drugs that significantly alter urine pH can affect excretion of drugs for which the excretory process is pH dependent. Alkalinizing the urine will hasten the excretion of acidic drugs. Acidification of the urine will enhance reabsorption of acidic drugs, prolonging and enhancing drug action. In the reverse situation, drugs that acidify the urine will hasten the excretion of alkaline drugs. An example of this is administering sodium bicarbonate in cases of aspirin overdose. Alkalinizing the urine promotes renal excretion of aspirin.

Some drugs compete for enzyme systems with other drugs. Allopurinol inhibits the enzyme involved in uric acid production, but it also inhibits metabolism (inactivation) of 6-mercaptopurine, greatly increasing its toxicity. The dosage of mercaptopurine needs to be significantly reduced when coadministered with allopurinol.

The same potential for interactions exists for some foods. Dietary calcium, found in high concentrations in dairy products, combines with tetracycline and prevents its absorption. Foods high in pyridoxine (vitamin $B_6$) can negate the anti-Parkinson effect of levodopa. Grapefruit juice inhibits the enzyme that breaks down some drugs and concurrent ingestion may significantly increase drug levels and the risk for toxicity. There are no general guidelines for nutritional factors. It is prudent to check whether these problems exist and to make the necessary dosage adjustments.

Many commonly taken natural products interact with pharmaceutical drugs. St. John's Wort, garlic, ephedra and other natural products can interact with medications and cause known or unpredictable reactions. Nurses and prescribers should consult drug references and remember that the average dosing range for drugs is intended for an average patient. However, every patient is an individual with specific drug-handling capabilities. Taking these special dosing considerations into account allows for an individualized drug regimen that promotes the desired therapeutic outcome and minimizes the risk of toxicity.

# EDUCATING PATIENTS ABOUT SAFE MEDICATION USE

Research has shown that patients need information about several medication-related topics, no matter what the medication. A well-informed patient and/or family can help prevent medication errors by hospital staff and is less likely to make medication errors at home. Adherence to the medication regimen is another goal achieved through patient education.

Before beginning any teaching, however, always assess the patient's current knowledge by asking if he or she is familiar with the medication, how it is taken at home, what precautions or follow up care are required and other questions specific to each drug. Based on the patient's current knowledge level and taking into consideration factors such as readiness to learn, environmental and social barriers to learning or adherence, and cultural factors, discuss the following:

1. **Generic and brand names of the medication.** Patients should know both the brand and generic names of each medication for two reasons. It helps them identify their medications when a generic equivalent is substituted for a brand name version and it prevents patients or health care providers from making sound-alike confusion errors when giving or documenting a medication history. An example of this is saying Celebrex but meaning or hearing Cerebyx.

2. **Purpose of the medication.** Patients have a right to know what the therapeutic benefit of the medication will be but also should be told the consequences of not taking the prescribed medication. This may enhance adherence. For example, a patient may be more likely to take blood pressure medication if told lowering high blood pressure will prevent heart attack, kidney disease, or stroke, rather than saying only that it will lower blood pressure.

3. **Dosage and how to take the medication.** To derive benefit and avoid adverse reactions or other poor outcomes, the patient must know how much of the medication to take and when to take it. Refer to dosages in metric weight (i.e., milligram, gram) rather than dosage unit (tablet) or volume (1 teaspoon). The patient must also be informed of the best time to take the medication, for example on an empty or a full stomach, before bedtime, or with or without other medications. If possible, help the patient fit the medication schedule into his or her own schedule so that taking the medication is not difficult or forgotten.

4. **What to do if a dose is missed.** Always explain to patients what to do if a dose is missed. Patients have been reported to take a double dose of medications when a missed dose occurs, putting themselves at risk for side effects and adverse reactions.

5. **Duration of therapy.** It is not uncommon for patients to stop taking a medication when they feel better or to discontinue a medication when they cannot perceive a benefit. For very long term, even lifelong therapy, the patient may need to be reminded that the medication helps maintain the current level of wellness. Patients may need to be reminded to finish short-term courses of medications even though they frequently will feel much better before the prescription runs out. Some medications cannot be discontinued abruptly and patients should be warned to consult a health care professional before discontinuing such agents. Patients will need to know to refill prescriptions several days before running out or to take extra medication if traveling.

6. **Minor side effects and what to do if they occur.** Inform the patient that all medications have potential side effects. Explain the most common side effects associated with the medication and how to avoid or manage them if they occur. An informed patient is less likely to stop taking a medication because of a minor and potentially avoidable side effect.

7. **Serious side effects and what to do if they occur.** Inform the patient of the possibility of serious side effects. Describe signs and symptoms associated with serious side effects and tell the patient to immediately inform a physician or nurse should they occur. Tell the patient to call before the next dose of the medication is scheduled and to not assume that the medication is the source of the symptom and prematurely discontinue it.

8. **Medications to avoid.** Drug-drug interactions can dampen drug effects, enhance drug effects, or cause life-threatening adverse events such as cardiac dysrhythmias, hepatitis, renal failure, or internal bleeding. The patient and family need to know which other medications, including which over-the-counter medications, to avoid.

9. **Foods to avoid and other precautions.** Food-drug interactions are not uncommon and can have effects similar to drug-drug interactions. Excessive sun exposure resulting in severe dermal reactions is not uncommon and represents an environmental-drug interaction. Likewise, the patient should be informed of what activities to avoid, in case the medication affects alertness or coordination, for example.

10. **How to store the medication:** Medications must be stored properly to maintain potency. Most medications should not be stored in the bathroom medicine cabinet because of excess heat and humidity. In addition, thoughtful storage practices, such as separating two family members' medications, can prevent mix-ups and inadvertent accessibility by children (or pets). Review storage with patients and ask about current methods for storing medications.

11. **Follow up care.** Anyone taking medication requires ongoing care to assess effectiveness and appropriateness of medications. Many medications require invasive and noninvasive testing to monitor blood levels; hematopoietic, hepatic or renal function; or other effects on other body systems. Ongoing medical evaluation may result in dosage adjustments, change in medication or discontinuation of medication.

12. **What not to take.** Inform patients not to take expired medications or someone else's medication. Warn them not to self-medicate with older, no longer used prescriptions even if the remaining supply is not expired. Tell patients to keep a current record of all medications taken and to ask health care providers if new medications are meant to replace a current medication.

As you teach, encourage the patient and the family to ask questions. Providing feedback about medication questions will increase their understanding and help you identify areas that need reinforcement. Also, ask patients to repeat what you have said and return demonstrate application or administration techniques.

Stress the importance of concurrent therapies. Medications often are only a part of a recommended therapy. Review with the patient and family other measures that will enhance or maintain health. Always consider the cultural context in which health information is provided and plan accordingly. This might include obtaining a same-gender translator or adjusting dosing times to avoid conflict with traditional rituals.

Finally, provide written instructions in a simple and easy-to-read format. Keep in mind that most health care information is written at a 10th grade reading level, while many patients read at a 5th grade level. Tell patients to keep the written instructions so that they can be reviewed at home, when stress levels are lower and practical difficulties in maintaining the medication plan are known.

# CLASSIFICATIONS

## ■ ANTI-ALZHEIMER'S AGENTS

### PHARMACOLOGIC PROFILE

#### General Use

Management of Alzheimer's dementia.

#### General Action and Information

All agents act by increasing the amount of acetylcholine in the CNS by inhibiting cholinesterase. No agents to date can slow the progression of Alzheimer's dementia. Current agents may temporarily improve cognitive function and therefore improve quality of life.

#### Contraindications

Hypersensitivity. Tacrine should not be used in patients who have had previous hepatic reactions to the drug.

#### Precautions

Use cautiously in patients with a history of 'sick sinus syndrome' or other supraventricular cardiac conduction abnormalities (may cause bradycardia). Cholingeric effects may result in adverse GI effects (nausea, vomiting, diarrhea, weight loss) and may also increase gastric acid secretion resulting in GI bleeding, especially during concurrent NSAID therapy. Other cholinergic effects may include urinary tract obstruction, seizures, or bronchospasm.

#### Interactions

Additive effects with other drugs having cholinergic properties. May exaggerate the effects of succinylcholine-type muscle relaxation during anesthesia. May decrease therapeutic effects of anticholinergics.

### NURSING IMPLICATIONS

#### Assessment

- Assess cognitive function (memory, attention, reasoning, language, ability to perform simple tasks) throughout therapy.
- Monitor nausea, vomiting, anorexia, and weight loss. Notify health care professional if these side effects occur.

#### Potential Nursing Diagnoses

- Thought processes, disturbed (Indications).
- Nutrition, imbalanced: less than body requirements.
- Knowledge, deficient, related to disease processes and medication regimen (Patient/Family Teaching).

#### Patient/Family Teaching

- Instruct patient and caregiver that medication should be taken as directed.
- Advise patient and caregiver to notify health care professional if nausea, vomiting, anorexia, and weight loss occur.

#### Evaluation

**Clinical response to therapy can be evaluated by:** ■ Temporary improvement in cognitive function (memory, attention, reasoning, language, ability to perform simple tasks) in patients with Alzheimer's disease.

**Anti-Alzheimer's agents included in *Davis's Drug Guide for Nurses***

donepezil 338
galantamine 466
memantine 1118

rivastigmine 937
tacrine 989

# ■ ANTIANEMICS

## PHARMACOLOGIC PROFILE

### General Use
Prevention and treatment of anemias.

### General Action and Information
Iron (ferrous fumarate, ferrous gluconate, ferrous sulfate, iron dextran, iron sucrose, polysaccharide-iron complex, sodium ferric gluconate complex) is required for production of hemoglobin, which is necessary for oxygen transport to cells. Cyanocobalamin and hydroxocobalamin (Vitamin $B_{12}$) and folic acid are water-soluble vitamins that are required for red blood cell production. Darbepoetin and epoetin stimulate production of red blood cells. Nandrolone stimulates production of erythropoetin.

### Contraindications
Undiagnosed anemias. Hemochromatosis, hemosiderosis, hemolytic anemia (Iron). Uncontrolled hypertension (Darbepoetin, epoetin).

### Precautions
Use parenteral iron (iron dextran, iron sucrose, sodium ferric gluconate complex) cautiously in patients with history of allergy or hypersensitivity reactions.

### Interactions
Oral iron can decrease the absorption of tetracyclines, fluoroquinolones, or penicillamine Vitamin E may impair the therapeutic response to iron. Phenytoin and other anticonvulsants may decrease the absorption of folic acid Response to Vitamin $B_{12}$ or folic acid may be delayed by chloramphenicol Darbepoetin and epoetin may increase the requirement for heparin during hemodialysis.

## NURSING IMPLICATIONS

### Assessment
- Assess patient's nutritional status and dietary history to determine possible causes for anemia and need for patient teaching.

### Potential Nursing Diagnoses
- Activity intolerance (Indications).
- Nutrition, imbalanced: less than body requirements (Indications).
- Knowledge, deficient, related to disease processes and medication regimen (Patient/Family Teaching).

### Implementation
- Available in combination with many vitamins and minerals (see Appendix B).

### Patient/Family Teaching
- Encourage patients to comply with diet recommendations of health care professional. Explain that the best source of vitamins and minerals is a well-balanced diet with foods from the four basic food groups.

- Patients self-medicating with vitamin and mineral supplements should be cautioned not to exceed RDA. The effectiveness of mega doses for treatment of various medical conditions is unproven and may cause side effects.

## Evaluation

**Clinical response to therapy can be evaluated by:** ■ Resolution of anemia.

## Antianemics included in *Davis's Drug Guide for Nurses*

*hormones*
darbepoetin 270
epoetin 270
nandrolone decanoate 729

*iron supplements*
carbonyl iron 565
ferrous fumarate 565
ferrous gluconate 565
ferrous sulfate 565

iron dextran 565
iron polysaccharide 565
iron sucrose 565
sodium ferric gluconate complex 565

*vitamins*
cyanocobalamin 1087
folic acid 454
hydroxocobalamin 1087

# ■ ANTIANGINALS

## PHARMACOLOGIC PROFILE

### General Use

Nitrates are used to treat and prevent attacks of angina. Only nitrates (sublingual, lingual spray, or intravenous) may be used in the acute treatment of attacks of angina pectoris. Calcium channel blockers and beta blockers are used prophylactically in long-term management of angina.

### General Action and Information

Several different groups of medications are used in the treatment of angina pectoris. The nitrates (isosorbide dinitrate, isosorbide mononitrate, and nitroglycerin) are available as a lingual spray, sublingual tablets, parenterals, transdermal systems, and sustained-release oral dosage forms. Nitrates dilate coronary arteries and cause systemic vasodilation (decreased preload). Calcium channel blockers dilate coronary arteries (some also slow heart rate). Beta blockers decrease myocardial oxygen consumption via a decrease in heart rate. Therapy may be combined if selection is designed to minimize side effects or adverse reactions.

### Contraindications

Hypersensitivity. Avoid use of beta blockers or calcium channel blockers in advanced heart block, cardiogenic shock, or untreated CHF.

### Precautions

Beta blockers should be used cautiously in patients with diabetes mellitus, pulmonary disease, or hypothyroidism.

### Interactions

Nitrates, calcium channel blockers, and beta blockers may cause hypotension with other antihypertensives or acute ingestion of alcohol Verapamil, diltiazem, and beta blockers may have additive myocardial depressant effects when used with other agents that affect cardiac function. Verapamil has a number of other significant drug-drug interactions.

## NURSING IMPLICATIONS

### Assessment

- Assess location, duration, intensity, and precipitating factors of patient's anginal pain.

- Monitor blood pressure and pulse periodically throughout therapy.

**Potential Nursing Diagnoses**

- Pain, acute (Indications).
- Tissue perfusion, ineffective (Indications).
- Knowledge, deficient, related to disease processes and medication regimen (Patient/Family Teaching).

**Implementation**

- Available in various dose forms. See specific drugs for information on administration.

**Patient/Family Teaching**

- Instruct patient on concurrent nitrate therapy and prophylactic antianginals to continue taking both medications as ordered and to use SL nitroglycerin as needed for anginal attacks.
- Advise patient to contact health care professional immediately if chest pain does not improve; worsens after therapy; is accompanied by diaphoresis or shortness of breath; or if severe, persistent headache occurs.
- Caution patient to make position changes slowly to minimize orthostatic hypotension.
- Advise patient to avoid concurrent use of alcohol with these medications.

**Evaluation**

**Effectiveness of therapy can be demonstrated by:** ■ Decrease in frequency and severity of anginal attacks ■ Increase in activity tolerance.

**Antianginals included in *Davis's Drug Guide for Nurses***

*beta blockers*
atenolol 91
carteolol 164
labetalol 587
metoprolol 682
nadolol 720
propranolol 891

*calcium channel blockers*
diltiazem 308

felodipine 412
isradipine 574
nicardipine 747
nifedipine 753
verapamil 1077

*nitrates*
isosorbide dinitrate 572
isosorbide mononitrate 572
nitroglycerin 763

# ■ ANTIANXIETY AGENTS

## PHARMACOLOGIC PROFILE

### General Use

Antianxiety agents are used in the management of various forms of anxiety, including generalized anxiety disorder (GAD). Some agents are more suitable for intermittent or short-term use (benzodiazepines) while others are more useful long-term (buspirone, paroxetine, venlafaxine).

### General Action and Information

Most agents cause generalized CNS depression. Benzodiazepines may produce tolerance with long-term use and have potential for psychological or physical dependence. These agents have NO analgesic properties.

### Contraindications

Hypersensitivity. Should not be used in comatose patients or in those with pre-existing CNS depression. Should not be used in patients with uncontrolled severe pain. Avoid use during pregnancy or lactation.

**C L A S S I F I C A T I O N S**

## Precautions
Use cautiously in patients with hepatic dysfunction, severe renal impairment, or severe underlying pulmonary disease (benzodiazepines only). Use with caution in patients who may be suicidal or who may have had previous drug addictions. Patients may be more sensitive to CNS depressant effects; dosage reduction may be required.

## Interactions
Mainly for benzodiazepines; additive CNS depression with alcohol, antihistamines, some antidepressants, opioid analgesics, or phenothiazines may occur. Most agents should not be used with MAO inhibitors.

## NURSING IMPLICATIONS
### Assessment
- **General Info:** Monitor blood pressure, pulse, and respiratory status frequently throughout IV administration.
- Prolonged high-dose therapy may lead to psychological or physical dependence. Restrict the amount of drug available to patient, especially if patient is depressed, suicidal, or has a history of addiction.
- **Anxiety:** Assess degree of anxiety and level of sedation (ataxia, dizziness, slurred speech) before and periodically throughout therapy.

### Potential Nursing Diagnoses
- Injury, risk for (Side Effects).
- Knowledge, deficient, related to disease processes and medication regimen (Patient/Family Teaching).

### Implementation
- **General:** Patients changing to buspirone from other antianxiety agents should receive gradually decreasing doses. Buspirone will not prevent withdrawal symptoms.

### Patient/Family Teaching
- May cause daytime drowsiness. Caution patient to avoid driving and other activities requiring alertness until response to medication is known.
- Advise patient to avoid the use of alcohol and other CNS depressants concurrently with these medications.
- Advise patient to inform health care professional if pregnancy is planned or suspected.

### Evaluation
**Effectiveness of therapy can be demonstrated by:** ▪ Decrease in anxiety level.

## Antianxiety agents included in *Davis's Drug Guide for Nurses*

*benzodiazepines*
alprazolam 25
chlordiazepoxide 191
diazepam 293
lorazepam 629
midazolam 687
oxazepam 789

*miscellaneous*
buspirone 137
doxepin 343
hydroxyzine 518
meprobamate 1174
paroxetine 813
venlafaxine 1075

**C
L
A
S
S
I
F
I
C
A
T
I
O
N
S**

# ■ ANTIARRHYTHMICS

## PHARMACOLOGIC PROFILE

### General Use
Suppression of cardiac arrhythmias.

### General Action and Information
Correct cardiac arrhythmias by a variety of mechanisms, depending on the group used. The therapeutic goal is decreased symptomatology and increased hemodynamic performance. Choice of agent depends on etiology of arrhythmia and individual patient characteristics. Treatable causes of arrhythmias should be corrected before therapy is initiated (e.g., electrolyte disturbances, other drugs). Antiarrhythmics are generally classified by their effects on cardiac conduction tissue (see the following table). Adenosine, atropine, and digoxin are also used as antiarrhythmics.

## MECHANISM OF ACTION OF MAJOR ANTIARRHYTHMIC DRUGS

| CLASS | DRUGS | MECHANISM |
|---|---|---|
| I | moricizine | Shares properties of IA, IB, and IC agents |
| IA | quinidine, procainamide, disopyramide | Depress Na conductance, increase APD and ERP, decrease membrane responsiveness |
| IB | tocainide, lidocaine, phenytoin, mexiletine | Increase K conductance, decrease APD and ERP |
| IC | flecainide, propafenone | Profound slowing of conduction, markedly depress phase O |
| II | acebutolol, esmolol, propranolol | Interfere with Na conductance, depress cell membrane, decrease automaticity, and increase ERP of the AV node, block excess sympathetic activity |
| III | amiodarone, dofetilide, ibutilide, sotalol | Interfere with norepinephrine, increase APD and ERP |
| IV | diltiazem, verapamil | Increase AV nodal ERP, Ca channel blocker |

APD = action-potential duration; Ca = calcium; ERP = effective refractory period; K = potassium; Na = sodium.

### Contraindications
Differ greatly among various agents. See individual drugs.

### Precautions
Differ greatly among agents used. Appropriate dosage adjustments should be made in elderly patients and those with renal or hepatic impairment, depending on agent chosen. Correctable causes (electrolyte abnormalities, drug toxicity) should be evaluated. See individual drugs.

### Interactions
Differ greatly among agents used. See individual drugs.

## NURSING IMPLICATIONS

### Assessment
■ Monitor ECG, pulse, and blood pressure continuously throughout IV administration and periodically throughout oral administration.

### Potential Nursing Diagnoses
■ Cardiac output, decreased (Indications).
■ Knowledge, deficient, related to disease processes and medication regimen (Patient/Family Teaching).

## Implementation

- Take apical pulse before administration of oral doses. Withhold dose and notify physician or other health care professional if heart rate is <50 bpm.
- Administer oral doses with a full glass of water. Most sustained-release preparations should be swallowed whole. Do not crush, break, or chew tablets or open capsules, unless specifically instructed.

## Patient/Family Teaching

- Instruct patient to take oral doses around the clock, as directed, even if feeling better.
- Instruct patient or family member on how to take pulse. Advise patient to report changes in pulse rate or rhythm to health care professional.
- Caution patient to avoid taking OTC medications without consulting health care professional.
- Advise patient to carry identification describing disease process and medication regimen at all times.
- Emphasize the importance of follow-up exams to monitor progress.

## Evaluation

**Effectiveness of therapy can be demonstrated by:** ■ Resolution of cardiac arrhythmias without detrimental side effects.

## Antiarrhythmics included in *Davis's Drug Guide for Nurses*

*class IA*
disopyramide 322
moricizine 708
procainamide 874
quinidine 906

*class IB*
fosphenytoin 840
lidocaine 613
mexiletine 1174
phenytoin 840
tocainide 1185

*class IC*
flecainide 1169
propafenone 884

*class II*
acebutolol 4

esmolol 388
propranolol 891
sotalol 977

*class III*
amiodarone 41
dofetilide 335
ibutilide 530

*class IV*
diltiazem 308
verapamil 1077

*miscellaneous*
adenosine 13
atropine 95
digoxin 303

# ■ ANTIASTHMATICS

## PHARMACOLOGIC PROFILE

### General Use

Management of acute and chronic episodes of reversible bronchoconstriction. Goal of therapy is to treat acute attacks (short-term control) and to decrease incidence and intensity of future attacks (long-term control). The choice of modalities depends on the continued requirement for short term control agents.

### General Action and Information

Adrenergic bronchodilators and phosphodiesterase inhibitors both work by increasing intracellular levels of cyclic-3', 5'-adenosine monophsphate (cAMP); adrenergics by increasing production and phosphodiesterase inhibitors by decreasing breakdown. Increased levels of cAMP produce bronchodilation. Corticosteroids act by decreasing airway inflammation. Anticholinergics (ipratropium) produce bronchodilation by decreasing intracellular levels of cyclic guanosine monophosphate (cGMP). Leukotriene receptor antagonists and mast cell stabilizers decrease the release of substances that can contribute to bronchospasm.

### Contraindications

Inhaled corticosteroids, long-acting adrenergic agents, and mast cell stabilizers should not be used during acute attacks of asthma.

### Precautions

Adrenergic bronchodilators and anticholinergics should be used cautiously in patients with cardiovascular disease. Chronic use of systemic corticosteroids should be avoided in children or during pregnancy or lactation. Diabetic patients may experience loss of glycemic control during corticosteroid therapy. Corticosteroids should never be abruptly discontinued.

### Interactions

Adrenergic bronchodilators and phosphodiesterase inhibitors may have additive CNS and cardiovascular effects with other adrenergic agents. Cimetidine increases theophylline levels and the risk of toxicity. Coritcosteroids may decrease the effectiveness of antidiabetics Corticosteroids may cause hypokalemia which maybe additive with potassium-losing diuretics and may also increase the risk of digoxin toxicity.

## NURSING IMPLICATIONS

### Assessment

- Assess lung sounds and respiratory function prior to and periodically throughout therapy.
- Assess cardiovascular status of patients taking adrenergic bronchodilators or anticholinergics Monitor for ECG changes and chest pain.

### Potential Nursing Diagnoses

- Airway clearance, ineffective (Indications).
- Knowledge, deficient, related to disease processes and medication regimen (Patient/Family Teaching).
- Noncompliance (Patient/Family Teaching).

### Patient/Family Teaching

- Instruct patient to take antiasthmatics as directed. Do not take more than prescribed or discontinue without discussing with health care professional.
- Advise patient to avoid smoking and other respiratory irritants.
- Instruct patient in correct use of metered-dose inhaler or other administration devices (see Appendix F).
- Advise patient to contact health care professional promptly if the usual dose of medication fails to produce the desired results, if symptoms worsen after treatment, or if toxic effects occur.
- Patients using inhalation medications and bronchodilators should be advised to use the bronchodilator first and allow 5 minutes to elapse before administering other medications, unless otherwise directed by health care professional.

### Evaluation

**Clinical response to therapy can be evaluated by:** - Prevention of and reduction in symptoms of asthma.

## Antiasthmatics included in *Davis's Drug Guide for Nurses*

**bronchodilators**
albuterol 16
epinephrine 366
formoterol 456
levalbuterol 607
metaproterenol 657
pirbuterol 856
salmeterol 950
terbutaline 1003

**corticosteroids**
beclomethasone 235
betamethasone 242
budesonide 235
cortisone 242
dexamethasone 242
flunisolide 235

fluticasone 235
hydrocortisone 242
methylprednisolone 242
prednisolone 242
prednisone 242
triamcinolone 235

**leukotriene antagonists**
zafirlukast 1187

**mast cell stabilizers**
cromolyn 640
nedocromil 640

**monoclonal antibodies**
omalizumab 778

**adrenergics**
epinephrine 366

# ■ ANTICHOLINERGICS

## PHARMACOLOGIC PROFILE

### General Use

**Atropine**—Bradyarrhythmias. **Ipratropium**—bronchospasm (inhalation) and rhinorrhea (intranasal). **Scopolamine**—Nausea and vomiting related to motion sickness and vertigo. **Propantheline and glycopyrrolate**—Decreasing gastric secretory activity and increasing esophageal sphincter tone. Atropine and scopolamine are also used as ophthalmic mydriatics. Benztropine, biperidin, and trihexyphenidyl are used in the management of Parkinson's disease. Oxybutynin and tolterodine are used as urinary tract spasmodics.

### General Action and Information

Competitively inhibit the action of acetylcholine In addition, atropine, glycopyrrolate, propantheline, and scopolamine are antimuscarinic in that they inhibit the action of acetylcholine at sites innervated by postganglionic cholinergic nerves.

### Contraindications

Hypersensitivity, narrow-angle glaucoma, severe hemorrhage, tachycardia (due to thyrotoxicosis or cardiac insufficiency), or myasthenia gravis.

### Precautions

Geriatric and pediatric patients are more susceptible to adverse effects. Use cautiously in patients with urinary tract pathology; those at risk for GI obstruction; and those with chronic renal, hepatic, pulmonary, or cardiac disease.

### Interactions

Additive anticholinergic effects (dry mouth, dry eyes, blurred vision, constipation) with other agents possessing anticholinergic activity, including antihistamines, antidepressants, quinidine, and disopyramide May alter GI absorption of other drugs by inhibiting GI motility and increasing transit time. Antacids may decrease absorption of orally administered anticholinergics.

## NURSING IMPLICATIONS

### Assessment

- Assess vital signs and ECG frequently during IV drug therapy. Report any significant changes in heart rate or blood pressure or increase in ventricular ectopy or angina promptly.
- Monitor intake and output ratios in elderly or surgical patients; may cause urinary retention.
- Assess patient regularly for abdominal distention and auscultate for bowel sounds. Constipation may become a problem. Increasing fluids and adding bulk to the diet may help alleviate constipation.

### Potential Nursing Diagnoses

- Cardiac output, decreased (Indications).
- Oral mucous membrane, impaired (Side Effects).
- Constipation (Side Effects).

### Implementation

- **PO:** Administer oral doses of atropine, glycopyrrolate, propantheline, or scopolamine 30 min before meals.
- Scopolamine transdermal patch should be applied at least 4 hr before travel.

### Patient/Family Teaching

- **General Info:** Instruct patient that frequent rinses, sugarless gum or candy, and good oral hygiene may help relieve dry mouth.
- May cause drowsiness. Caution patient to avoid driving or other activities requiring alertness until response to medication is known.
- **Ophth:** Advise patients that ophthalmic preparations may temporarily blur vision and impair ability to judge distances. Dark glasses may be needed to protect eyes from bright light.

### Evaluation

**Effectiveness of therapy can be demonstrated by:** ■ Increase in heart rate ■ Decrease in nausea and vomiting related to motion sickness or vertigo ■ Dryness of mouth ■ Dilation of pupils ■ Decrease in GI motility ■ Resolution of signs and symptoms of Parkinson's disease.

### Anticholinergics included in *Davis's Drug Guide for Nurses*

atropine 95
benztropine 108
biperiden 115
dicyclomine 299
difenoxin/atropine 318
diphenoxylate/atropine 318
glycopyrrolate 477
hyoscyamine 520

ipratropium 560
oxybutynin 793
propantheline 1180
scopolamine 957
tolterodine 1041
trihexyphenidyl 1186
trimethobenzamide 1187

# ■ ANTICOAGULANTS

## PHARMACOLOGIC PROFILE

### General Use

Prevention and treatment of thromboembolic disorders including deep vein thrombosis, pulmonary embolism, and atrial fibrillation with embolization. Also used in the management of MI sequentially or in combination with thrombolytics and/or antiplatelet agents.

## General Action and Information

Anticoagulants are used to prevent clot extension and formation. They do not dissolve clots. The two types of anticoagulants in common use are parenteral heparins and oral warfarin Therapy is usually initiated with heparin or a heparin-like agent because of rapid onset of action, while maintenance therapy consists of warfarin Warfarin takes several days to produce therapeutic anticoagulation. In serious or severe thromboembolic events, heparin therapy may be preceded by thrombolytic therapy. Low doses of heparin or heparin-like compounds and fondaparinux are mostly used to prevent deep vein thrombosis after certain surgical procedures and in similar situations in which prolonged bedrest increases the risk of thromboembolism. Argatroban and lepirudin are used as anticoagulation in patients who have developed thrombocytopenia during heparin therapy.

## Contraindications

Underlying coagulation disorders, ulcer disease, malignancy, recent surgery, or active bleeding.

## Precautions

Anticoagulation should be undertaken cautiously in any patient with a potential site for bleeding. Pregnant or lactating patients should not receive warfarin Heparin does not cross the placenta. Heparin and heparin-like agents should be used cautiously in patients receiving epidural analgesia.

## Interactions

Warfarin is highly protein bound and may displace or be displaced by other highly protein-bound drugs. The resultant interactions depend on which drug is displaced. Bleeding may be potentiated by aspirin or large doses of penicillins or penicillin-like drugs, cefotetan, cefoperazone, plicamycin, valproic acid, or NSAIDs.

## NURSING IMPLICATIONS

### Assessment

- Assess patient taking anticoagulants for signs of bleeding and hemorrhage (bleeding gums; nosebleed; unusual bruising; tarry, black stools; hematuria; fall in hematocrit or blood pressure; guaiac-positive stools; urine; or NG aspirate).
- Assess patient for evidence of additional or increased thrombosis. Symptoms will depend on area of involvement.
- **Lab Test Considerations:** Monitor prothrombin time (PT) or international normalized ratio (INR) with warfarin therapy, activated partial thromboplastin time (aPTT) with full-dose heparin therapy and hematocrit and other clotting factors frequently during therapy.
- Monitor bleeding time throughout antiplatelet therapy. Prolonged bleeding time, which is time and dose dependent, is expected.
- **Toxicity and Overdose:** If overdose occurs or anticoagulation needs to be immediately reversed, the antidote for heparins is protamine sulfate; for warfarin, the antidote is vitamin K (phytonadione [AquaMEPHYTON]). Administration of whole blood or plasma may also be required in severe bleeding due to warfarin because of the delayed onset of vitamin K.

### Potential Nursing Diagnoses

- Tissue perfusion, ineffective (Indications).
- Injury, risk for (Side Effects).
- Knowledge, deficient, related to disease processes and medication regimen (Patient/Family Teaching).

## Implementation

- Inform all health care professionals caring for patient of anticoagulant therapy. Venipunctures and injection sites require application of pressure to prevent bleeding or hematoma formation.
- Use an infusion pump with continuous infusions to ensure accurate dosage.

## Patient/Family Teaching

- Caution patient to avoid activities leading to injury, to use a soft toothbrush and electric razor, and to report any symptoms of unusual bleeding or bruising to health care professional immediately.
- Instruct patient not to take OTC medications, especially those containing aspirin, NSAIDs, or alcohol, without advice of health care professional.
- Review foods high in vitamin K (see Appendix Q) with patients on warfarin Patient should have consistent limited intake of these foods, as vitamin K is the antidote for warfarin and greatly alternating intake of these foods will cause PT levels to fluctuate.
- Emphasize the importance of frequent lab tests to monitor coagulation factors.
- Instruct patient to carry identification describing medication regimen at all times and to inform all health care professionals caring for patient of anticoagulant therapy before laboratory tests, treatment, or surgery.

## Evaluation

**Clinical response to therapy can be evaluated by:** ■ Prevention of undesired clotting and its sequelae without signs of hemorrhage. Prevention of stroke, MI, and death in patients at risk.

## Anticoagulants included in *Davis's Drug Guide for Nurses*

*antithrombotics*
heparin 492

*coumarins*
warfarin 1097

*thrombin inhibitors*
argatroban 85
bivalirudin 122

desirudin 282
lepirudin (rDNA) 599

*heparins (low molecular weight)/heparinoids*
dalteparin 495
enoxaparin 495
fondaparinux 495
tinzaparin 496

# ■ ANTICONVULSANTS

## PHARMACOLOGIC PROFILE

### General Use

Anticonvulsants are used to decrease the incidence and severity of seizures due various etiologies. Some anticonvulsants are used parenterally in the immediate treatment of seizures. It is not uncommon for patients to require more than one anticonvulsants to control seizures on a long term basis. Many regimens are evaluated with serum level monitoring.

### General Action and Information

Anticonvulsants include a variety of agents, all capable of depressing abnormal neuronal discharges in the CNS that may result in seizures. They may work by preventing the spread of seizure activity, depressing the motor cortex, raising seizure threshold, or altering levels of neurotransmitters, depending on the group. See individual drugs.

### Contraindications

Previous hypersensitivity.

### Precautions

Use cautiously in patients with severe hepatic or renal disease; dosage adjustment may be required. Choose agents carefully in pregnant and lactating women. Fetal hydantoin syndrome may occur in offspring of patients who receive phenytoin during pregnancy.

### Interactions

Barbiturates stimulate the metabolism of other drugs that are metabolized by the liver, decreasing their effectiveness. Hydantoins are highly protein-bound and may displace or be displaced by other highly protein-bound drugs Lamotrigine, tiagabine, and topiramate are capable of interacting with several other anticonvulsants For more specific interactions, see individual drugs. Many drugs are capable of lowering seizure threshold and may decrease the effectiveness of anticonvulsants, including tricyclic antidepressants and phenothiazines.

## NURSING IMPLICATIONS

### Assessment

- Assess location, duration, and characteristics of seizure activity.
- **Toxicity and Overdose:** Monitor serum drug levels routinely throughout anticonvulsant therapy, especially when adding or discontinuing other agents.

### Potential Nursing Diagnoses

- Injury, risk for (Indications, Side Effects).
- Knowledge, deficient, related to disease processes and medication regimen (Patient/Family Teaching).

### Implementation

- Administer anticonvulsants around the clock. Abrupt discontinuation may precipitate status epilepticus.
- Implement seizure precautions.

### Patient/Family Teaching

- Instruct patient to take medication every day, exactly as directed.
- May cause drowsiness. Caution patient to avoid driving or other activities requiring alertness until response to medication is known. Do not resume driving until physician gives clearance based on control of seizures.
- Advise patient to avoid taking alcohol or other CNS depressants concurrently with these medications.
- Advise patient to carry identification describing disease process and medication regimen at all times.

### Evaluation

**Effectiveness of therapy can be demonstrated by:** ■ Decrease or cessation of seizures without excessive sedation.

## Anticonvulsants included in *Davis's Drug Guide for Nurses*

*barbiturates*
pentobarbital 1177
phenobarbital 1135

*benzodiazepines*
clonazepam 210
clorazepate 216
diazepam 293

*hydantoins*
fosphenytoin 840
phenytoin 840

*valproates*
divalproex sodium 1068
valproate sodium 1068
valproic acid 1068

*miscellaneous*
acetazolamide 1158
carbamazepine 155
gabapentin 465
lamotrigine 593
levetiracetam 609

# ■ ANTIDEPRESSANTS

## PHARMACOLOGIC PROFILE

### General Use

Used in the treatment of various forms of endogenous depression, often in conjunction with psychotherapy. Other uses include:Treatment of anxiety (doxepin) Enuresis (imipramine) Chronic pain syndromes (amitriptyline, doxepin, imipramine, and nortriptyline) Smoking cessation (bupropion) Bulimia (fluoxetine) Obsessive-compulsive disorder (fluoxetine, sertraline) Generalized anxiety disorder (venlafaxine, paroxetine).

### General Action and Information

Antidepressant activity is most likely due to preventing the reuptake of dopamine, norepinephrine, and serotonin by presynaptic neurons, resulting in accumulation of these neurotransmitters. The two major classes of antidepressants are the tricyclic antidepressants and the SSRIs Most tricyclic agents possess significant anticholinergic and sedative properties, which explains many of their side effects (amitriptyline, amoxapine, doxepin, imipramine, nortriptyline). The SSRIs are more likely to cause insomnia (fluoxetine, fluvoxamine, paroxetine, sertraline).

### Contraindications

Hypersensitivity. Should not be used in narrow-angle glaucoma. Should not be used in pregnancy or lactation or immediately after MI.

### Precautions

Use cautiously in older patients and those with pre-existing cardiovascular disease. Elderly men with prostatic enlargement may be more susceptible to urinary retention. Anticholinergic side effects of tricyclic antidepressants (dry eyes, dry mouth, blurred vision, and constipation) may require dosage modification or drug discontinuation. Dosage requires slow titration; onset of therapeutic response may be 2-4 wk. May decrease seizure threshold, especially bupropion.

### Interactions

**Tricyclic antidepressants**—May cause hypertension, tachycardia, and convulsions when used with MAO inhibitors. May prevent therapeutic response to some antihypertensives. Additive CNS depression with other CNS depressants. Sympathomimetic activity may be enhanced when used with other sympathomimetics. Additive anticholinergic effects with other drugs possessing anticholinergic properties. **MAO inhibitors**—Hypertensive crisis may occur with concurrent use of MAO inhibitors and amphetamines, methyldopa, levodopa, dopamine, epinephrine, norepinephrine, desipramine, imipramine, guanethidine, reserpine, vasoconstrictors, or ingestion of tyramine-containing foods. Hypertension or hypotension, coma, convulsions, and death may occur with meperidine or other opioid analgesics and MAO inhibitors Additive hypotension with antihypertensives or spinal anesthesia and MAO inhibitors Additive hypoglycemia with insulin or oral hypoglycemic agents and MAO inhibitors SSRIs, bupropion, or venlafaxine should not be used in combination with or within weeks of MAO inhibitors (see individual monographs). Risk of adverse reactions may be increased by almotriptan, frovatriptan, rizatriptan, naratriptan, sumatriptan, or zolmitriptan.

## NURSING IMPLICATIONS

### Assessment

- Monitor mental status and affect. Assess for suicidal tendencies, especially during early therapy. Restrict amount of drug available to patient.
- **Toxicity and Overdose:** Concurrent ingestion of MAO inhibitors and tyramine-containing foods may lead to hypertensive crisis. Symptoms include chest pain, severe headache, nuchal rigidity, nausea and vomiting, photosensitivity, and enlarged pupils. Treatment includes IV phentolamine.

### Potential Nursing Diagnoses

- Coping, ineffective (Indications).
- Injury, risk for (Side Effects).
- Knowledge, deficient, related to disease processes and medication regimen (Patient/Family Teaching).

### Implementation

- Administer drugs that are sedating at bedtime to avoid excessive drowsiness during waking hours, and administer drugs that cause insomnia (fluoxetine, fluvoxamine, paroxetine, sertraline, MAO inhibitors) in the morning.

### Patient/Family Teaching

- Caution patient to avoid alcohol and other CNS depressants. Patients receiving MAO inhibitors should also avoid OTC drugs and foods or beverages containing tyramine (see Appendix Q) during and for at least 2 wk after therapy has been discontinued, as they may precipitate a hypertensive crisis. Health care professional should be contacted immediately if symptoms of hypertensive crisis develop.
- Inform patient that dizziness or drowsiness may occur. Caution patient to avoid driving and other activities requiring alertness until response to the drug is known.
- Caution patient to make position changes slowly to minimize orthostatic hypotension.
- Advise patient to notify health care professional if dry mouth, urinary retention, or constipation occurs. Frequent rinses, good oral hygiene, and sugarless candy or gum may diminish dry mouth. An increase in fluid intake, fiber, and exercise may prevent constipation.
- Advise patient to notify health care professional of medication regimen and any herbal alternative therapies before treatment or surgery. MAO inhibitor therapy usually needs to be withdrawn at least 2 wk before use of anesthetic agents.
- Emphasize the importance of participation in psychotherapy and follow-up exams to evaluate progress.

### Evaluation

**Effectiveness of therapy can be demonstrated by:** ■ Resolution of depression ■ Decrease in anxiety ■ Control of bedwetting in children over 6 yr of age ■ Management of chronic neurogenic pain.

## Antidepressants included in *Davis's Drug Guide for Nurses*

*selective serotonin reuptake inhibitors (SSRIs)*
citalopram 204
escitalopram 387
fluoxetine 446
fluvoxamine 1170
paroxetine 813
sertraline 961

*tetracyclic antidepressants*
mirtazapine 696

*tricyclic antidepressants*
amitriptyline 44
amoxapine 1161
desipramine 279
doxepin 343
imipramine 540
nortriptyline 768

*monamine oxidase (MAO) inhibitors*
phenelzine 704
tranylcypromine 704

# ■ ANTIDIABETICS

## PHARMACOLOGIC PROFILE

### General Use

Insulin is used in the management of type 1 diabetes mellitus. It may also be used in type 2 diabetes mellitus when diet and/or oral medications fail to adequately control blood sugar. The choice of insulin preparation (rapid-acting, intermediate-acting, long-acting) and source (beef, beef/pork, pork, semisynthetic, human recombinant DNA) depend on the degree of control desired, daily blood glucose fluctuations, and history of previous reactions. Oral agents are used primarily in type 2 diabetes mellitus. Oral agents are used when diet therapy alone fails to control blood glucose or symptoms or when patients are not amenable to using insulin Some oral agents may be used with insulin.

### General Action and Information

Insulin, a hormone produced by the pancreas, lowers blood glucose by increasing transport of glucose into cells and promotes the conversion of glucose to glycogen. It also promotes the conversion of amino acids to proteins in muscle, stimulates triglyceride formation, and inhibits the release of free fatty acids. Sulfonylureas, nateglinide, repaglinide, and metformin lower blood glucose by stimulating endogenous insulin secretion by beta cells of the pancreas and by increasing sensitivity to insulin at intracellular receptor sites. Intact pancreatic function is required. Miglitol delays digestion of ingested carbohydrates, thus lowering blood glucose, especially after meals. It may be combined with Sulfonylureas Pioglitizone and rosiglitazone increase insulin sensitivity.

### Contraindications

**Insulin**—Hypoglycemia. **Oral hypoglycemic agents**—Hypersensitivity (cross-sensitivity with other Sulfonylureas and sulfonamides may exist). Hypoglycemia. Type 1 diabetes. Avoid use in patients with severe kidney, liver, thyroid, and other endocrine dysfunction. Should not be used in pregnancy or lactation.

### Precautions

**Insulin**—Infection, stress, or changes in diet may alter requirements. **Oral hypoglycemic agents**—Use cautiously in geriatric patients. Dosage reduction may be necessary. Infection, stress, or changes in diet may alter requirements. Use with Sulfonylureas with caution in patients with a history of cardiovascular disease. Metformin may cause lactic acidosis.

### Interactions

**Insulin**—Additive hypoglycemic effects with oral hypoglycemic agents. **Oral hypoglycemic agents**—Ingestion of alcohol may result in disulfiram-like reaction with some agents. Alcohol, corticosteroids, rifampin, glucagon, and thiazide diuretics may decrease effectiveness. Anabolic steroids, chloramphenicol, clofibrate, MAO inhibitors, most NSAIDs, salicylates, sulfonamides, and warfarin may increase hypoglycemic effect. Beta blockers may produce hypoglycemia and mask signs and symptoms.

## NURSING IMPLICATIONS

### Assessment

- Observe patient for signs and symptoms of hypoglycemic reactions.
- Miglitol and pioglitazone do not cause hypoglycemia when taken alone but may increase the hypoglycemic effect of other hypoglycemic agents.

## Albuterol (Proventil®)

2 mg

4 mg

## Alendronate (Fosamax®)

5 mg

10 mg

35 mg

70 mg

## Alprazolam (Xanax®)

0.25 mg    0.5 mg    1 mg    2 mg

0.5 mg (XR)    1 mg (XR)

2 mg (XR)    3 mg (XR)

## Amitriptyline (Geneva® Brand)

10 mg    25 mg

50 mg    75 mg

100 mg    150 mg

## Amlodipine (Norvasc®)

2.5 mg

5 mg

10 mg

## Amoxicillin (Amoxil®)

200 mg Chewable    400 mg Chewable

250 mg    500 mg

500 mg    875 mg

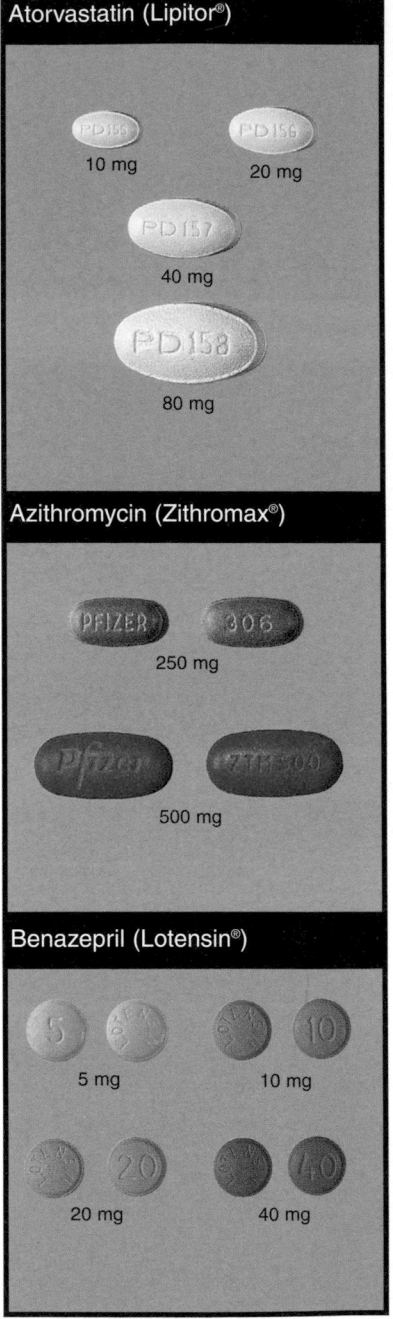

## Amoxicillin (Trimox®)

BRISTOL 7278
250 mg

BRISTOL 7279
500 mg

## Amoxicillin/Clavulanate (Augmentin®)

200 mg amoxicillin /
28.5 mg clavuanate
(chewable tablets)

400 mg amoxicillin /
57 mg clavuanate
(chewable tablets)

250/125

500/125

250 mg amoxicillin /
125 mg clavuanate

500 mg amoxicillin /
125 mg clavuanate

AUGMENTIN 875

875 mg amoxicillin /
125 mg clavuanate

AC 1000/62.5

1000 mg amoxicillin/ 62.5 mg clavuanate
(Augmentin XR)

## Atenolol (Tenormin®)

25 mg

ICI    50s
50 mg

ICI    105
100 mg

## Atorvastatin (Lipitor®)

PD 155
10 mg

PD 156
20 mg

PD 157
40 mg

PD 158
80 mg

## Azithromycin (Zithromax®)

PFIZER    306
250 mg

Pfizer    ZTH 500
500 mg

## Benazepril (Lotensin®)

5
5 mg

10
10 mg

20
20 mg

40
40 mg

## Bupropion (Wellbutrin®)

75 mg    100 mg

100 mg SR

150 mg SR    200 mg SR

150 mg XL    300 mg XL

## Bupropion (Zyban®)

150 mg

## Buspirone (BuSpar®)

5 mg    10 mg

15 mg    30 mg

## Carvedilol (Coreg®)

0.312 mg    0.625 mg

12.5 mg    25 mg

## Cefprozil (Cefzil®)

250 mg

500 mg

## Cefuroxime (Ceftin®)

125 mg    250 mg

500 mg

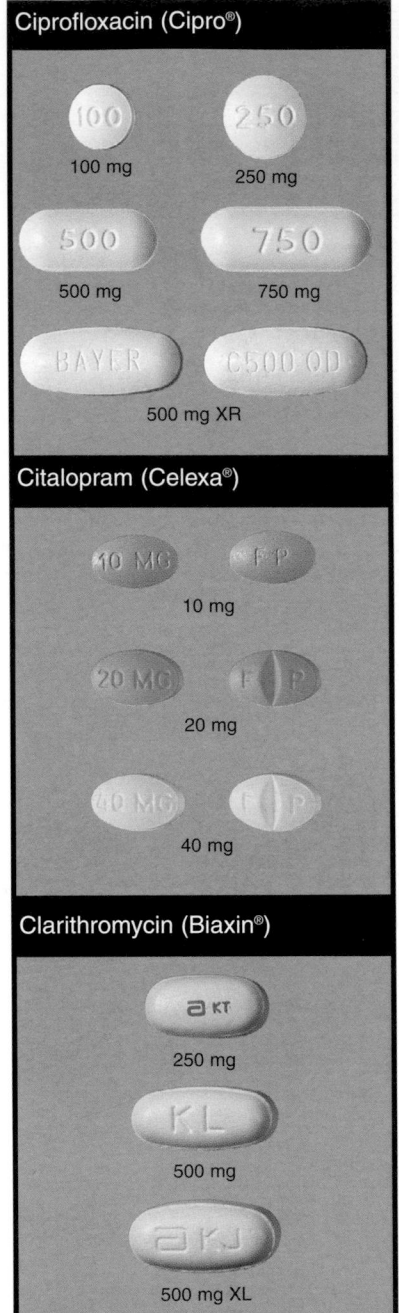

**Celecoxib (Celebrex®)**

100 mg  200 mg

400 mg

**Cephalexin (Keflex®)**

KEFLEX 250 mg
250 mg

KEFLEX 500 mg
500 mg

**Cetirizine (Zyrtec®)**

5 mg

10 mg

**Ciprofloxacin (Cipro®)**

100 mg  250 mg

500 mg  750 mg

500 mg XR

**Citalopram (Celexa®)**

10 mg

20 mg

40 mg

**Clarithromycin (Biaxin®)**

250 mg

500 mg

500 mg XL

## Clonazepam (Klonopin®)

0.5 mg

1 mg

2 mg

## Clopidogrel (Plavix®)

75 mg

## Codeine/Acetaminophen (Tylenol® with Codeine)

15 mg Codeine/
300 mg Acetaminophen
(No. 2)

30 mg Codeine/
300 mg Acetaminophen
(No. 3)

60 mg Codeine/
300 mg Acetaminophen
(No. 4)

## Cyclobenzaprine (Flexeril®)

5 mg

10 mg

## Diazepam (Valium®)

2 mg

5 mg

10 mg

## Digoxin (Lanoxin®)

0.125 mg    0.25 mg

## Digoxin (Lanoxicaps®)

0.05 mg    0.1 mg    0.2 mg

## Diltiazem (Cardizem-CD®)

120 mg    180 mg

240 mg    300 mg

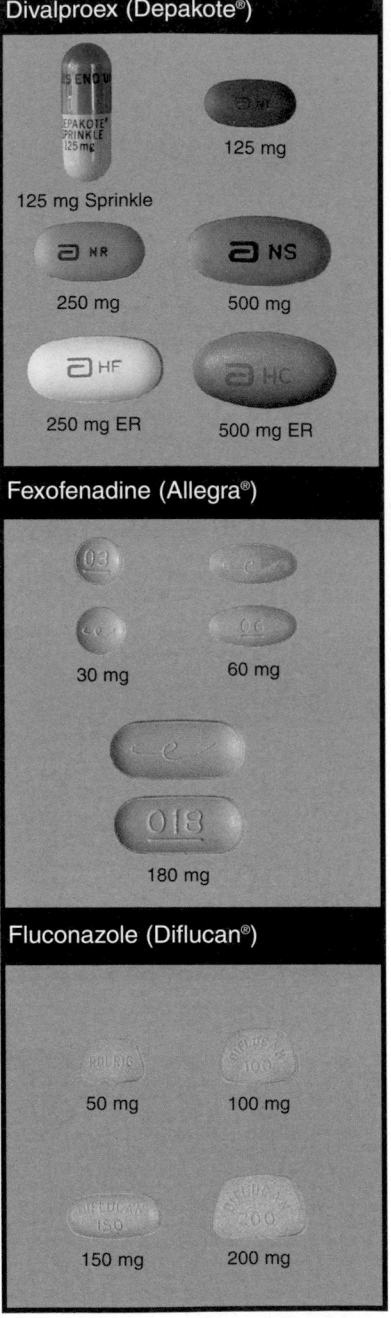

**Doxazosin (Cardura®)**

CARDURA 1 mg — 1 mg
CARDURA 2 mg — 2 mg
CARDURA 4 mg — 4 mg
CARDURA 8 mg — 8 mg

**Enalapril (Vasotec®)**

MSD 14 — 2.5 mg
MSD 712 — 5 mg
MSD 713 — 10 mg
MSD 714 — 20 mg

**Erythromycin (Ery-Tab®)**

EC — 250 mg
EH — 333 mg
EL — 500 mg

**Esomeprazole (Nexium®)**

20 mg — 20 mg
40 mg — 40 mg

**Divalproex (Depakote®)**

DEPAKOTE® SPRINKLE 125 mg — 125 mg Sprinkle
125 mg
a NR — 250 mg
a NS — 500 mg
a HF — 250 mg ER
a HC — 500 mg ER

**Fexofenadine (Allegra®)**

03 — 30 mg
06 — 60 mg
018 — 180 mg

**Fluconazole (Diflucan®)**

50 mg — 50 mg
DIFLUCAN 100 — 100 mg
DIFLUCAN 150 — 150 mg
DIFLUCAN 200 — 200 mg

© 2004, SFI

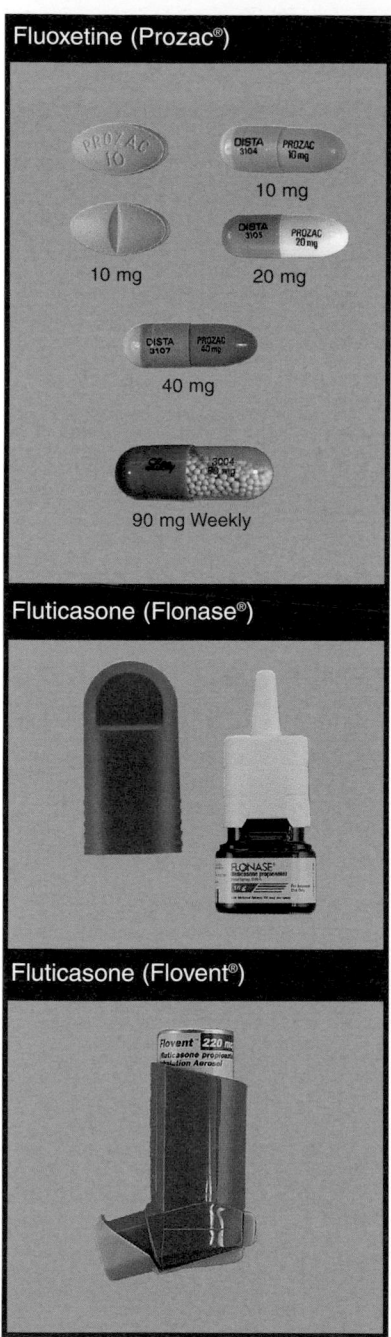

## Fluoxetine (Prozac®)

PROZAC 10 — 10 mg

DISTA 3104 / PROZAC 10 mg — 10 mg

10 mg

DISTA 3105 / PROZAC 20 mg — 20 mg

DISTA 3107 / PROZAC 40 mg — 40 mg

Lilly 3004 90 mg — 90 mg Weekly

## Fluticasone (Flonase®)

FLONASE

## Fluticasone (Flovent®)

Flovent 220 mcg
fluticasone propionate
Inhalation Aerosol

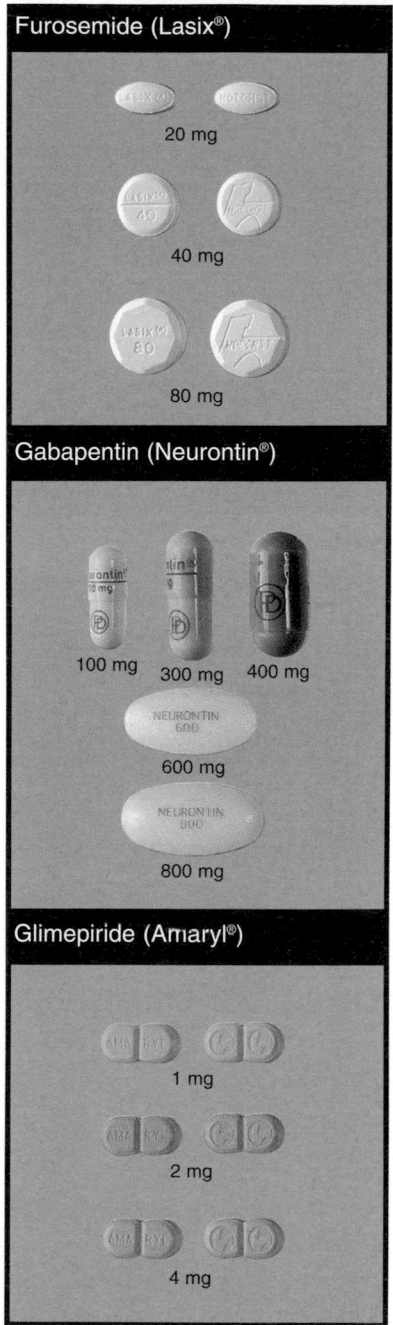

## Furosemide (Lasix®)

LASIX 20 — 20 mg

LASIX 40 — 40 mg

LASIX 80 — 80 mg

## Gabapentin (Neurontin®)

Neurontin 100 mg — 100 mg

Neurontin 300 mg — 300 mg

Neurontin 400 mg — 400 mg

NEURONTIN 600 — 600 mg

NEURONTIN 800 — 800 mg

## Glimepiride (Amaryl®)

AMARYL — 1 mg

AMARYL — 2 mg

AMARYL — 4 mg

## Glipizide (Glucotrol®)

5 mg

10 mg

2.5 mg XL    5 mg XL

10 mg XL

## Glyburide (DiaBeta®)

1.25mg

2.5 mg

5 mg

## Haloperidol (Geneva® Brand)

0.5 mg    1 mg

2 mg    5 mg

10 mg    20 mg

## Hydrocodone/Acetaminophen (Lortab®)

Hydrocodone 2.5 mg/
Acetaminophen 500 mg

Hydrocodone 5 mg/
Acetaminophen 500 mg

Hydrocodone 7.5 mg/
Acetaminophen 500 mg

Hydrocodone 10 mg/
Acetaminophen 500 mg

## Ipratropium (Atrovent®)

## Irbesartan (Avapro®)

75 mg

150 mg

300 mg

## Isosorbide Mononitrate (Imdur®)

30 mg

60 mg

120 mg

## Levofloxacin (Levaquin®)

250 mg

500 mg

750 mg

## Levothyroxine (Levoxyl®)

| 25 mcg | 50 mcg | 75 mcg |
| 88 mcg | 100 mcg | 112 mcg |
| 125 mcg | 137 mcg | 150 mcg |
| 175 mcg | 200 mcg | 300 mcg |

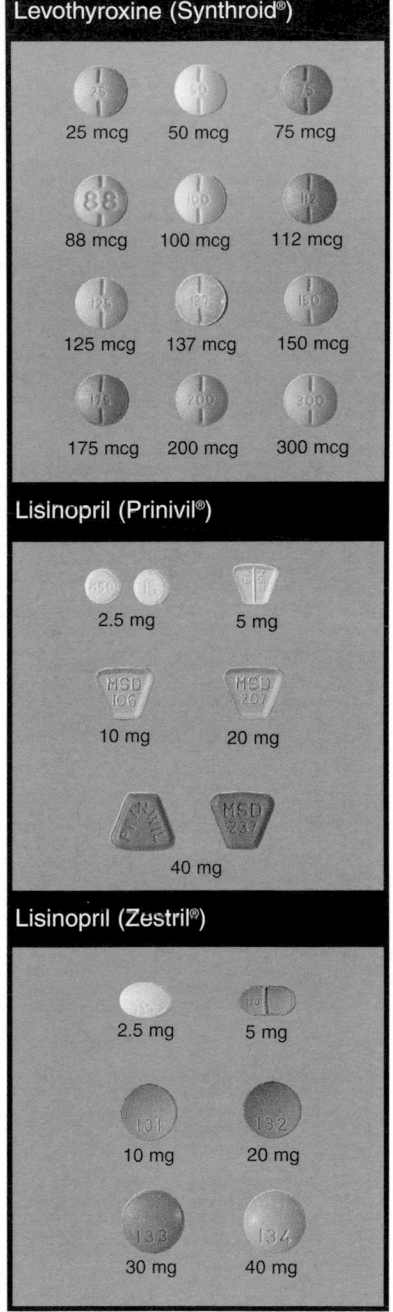

## Levothyroxine (Synthroid®)

| 25 mcg | 50 mcg | 75 mcg |
| 88 mcg | 100 mcg | 112 mcg |
| 125 mcg | 137 mcg | 150 mcg |
| 175 mcg | 200 mcg | 300 mcg |

## Lisinopril (Prinivil®)

2.5 mg

5 mg

10 mg

20 mg

40 mg

## Lisinopril (Zestril®)

2.5 mg

5 mg

10 mg

20 mg

30 mg

40 mg

## Loratadine (Claritin®)

10 mg

10 mg Reditab®

## Lorazepam (Ativan®)

0.5 mg

1 mg

2 mg

## Lovastatin (Mevacor®)

10 mg

20 mg

40 mg

## Medroxyprogesterone (Provera®)

2.5 mg

5 mg

10 mg

## Metformin (Glucophage®)

500 mg          850 mg

1000 mg

500 mg XR          750 mg XR

## Methylphenidate (Concerta®)

alza 18          alza 27
18 mg            27 mg

alza 36          alza 54
36 mg            54 mg

## Methylphenidate (Ritalin®)

5 mg

10 mg

20 mg

20 mg SR

## Metoprolol (Lopressor®)

GEIGY    GEIGY
51 51    71 71
50 mg    100 mg

## Metoprolol (Toprol XL®)

A β     A 100
25 mg     50 mg

A mS     A 100
100 mg     200 mg

## Montelukast (Singulair®)

SINGULAIR     MRK 711
4 mg

SINGULAIR     MRK 275
5 mg

MRK 117
10 mg

## Nabumetone (Relafen®)

RELAFEN     RELAFEN
500     750
500 mg     750 mg

## Nifedipine (Adalat® CC)

ADALAT CC    30
30 mg

ADALAT CC    60
60 mg

ADALAT CC    90
90 mg

## Nifedipine (Procardia-XL®)

PROCARDIA XL 30     60
30 mg     60 mg

90 mg
60 mg

## Nitroglycerin (Nitrostat®)

Nitrostat

## Olanzepine (Zyproxa®)

LILLY 4112     LILLY 4115
2.5 mg     5 mg

LILLY 4116     LILLY 4117
7.5 mg     10 mg

LILLY 4415     LILLY 4420
15 mg     20 mg

## Omeprazole (Prilosec®)

10 mg  20 mg  40 mg

## Ondansetron (Zofran®)

4 mg

8 mg

## Oxycodone/Acetaminophen (Percocet®)

Oxycodone 2.5 mg/
Acetaminophen 325 mg

Oxycodone 5 mg/
Acetaminophen 325 mg

Oxycodone 7.5 mg/
Acetaminophen 500 mg

Oxycodone 10 mg/
Acetaminophen 500 mg

Oxycodone 7.5 mg/
Acetaminophen 325 mg

Oxycodone 10 mg/
Acetaminophen 325 mg

## Pantoprazole (Protonix®)

40 mg

## Paroxetine (Paxil®)

10 mg

20 mg

30 mg

40 mg

12.5 mg CR

25 mg CR

37.5 mg CR

## Penicillin V Potassium (Veetids®)

250 mg

500 mg

## Phenytoin extended (Dilantin® Kapseals)

30 mg

100 mg

## Pioglitazone (Actos®)

15 mg

30 mg

45 mg

## Potassium Chloride (K-Dur®)

10 mEq

20 mEq

## Potassium Chloride (Klor-Con®)

8 mEq

10 mEq

## Pravastatin (Pravachol®)

10 mg

20 mg

40 mg

## Prednisone (Deltasone®)

2.5 mg

5 mg

10 mg

20 mg

50 mg

## Propoxyphene/Acetaminophen (Darvocet-N®)

Propoxyphene napsylate 50 mg/
Acetaminophen 325 mg

Propoxyphene napsylate 100 mg/
Acetaminophen 650 mg

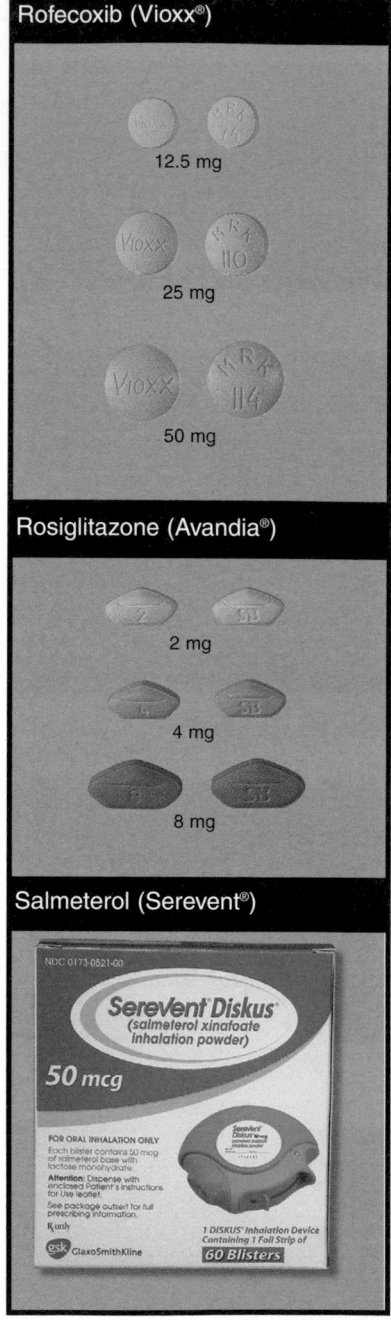

## Quinapril (Accupril®)

PD 527 | 5
5 mg

10
10 mg

PD 532 | 20
20 mg

PD 535 | 40
40 mg

## Raloxifene (Evista®)

LILLY
4165
60 mg

## Risperidone (Risperdal®)

JANSSEN
RIS 0.25
0.25 mg

JANSSEN
RIS 0.5
0.5 mg

JANSSEN
R | 1
1 mg

JANSSEN
R 2
2 mg

JANSSEN
R 3
3 mg

JANSSEN
R 4
4 mg

## Rofecoxib (Vioxx®)

VIOXX | MRK 74
12.5 mg

VIOXX | MRK 110
25 mg

VIOXX | MRK 114
50 mg

## Rosiglitazone (Avandia®)

2 | SB
2 mg

4 | SB
4 mg

8 | SB
8 mg

## Salmeterol (Serevent®)

NDC 0173-0521-00

**SereVent® Diskus®**
(salmeterol xinafoate
inhalation powder)

**50 mcg**

FOR ORAL INHALATION ONLY
Each blister contains 50 mcg
of salmeterol base with
lactose monohydrate.

**Attention:** Dispense with
enclosed Patient's Instructions
for Use leaflet.

See package outsert for full
prescribing information.

$R$ only

**gsk** GlaxoSmithKline

1 DISKUS® Inhalation Device
Containing 1 Foil Strip of
**60 Blisters**

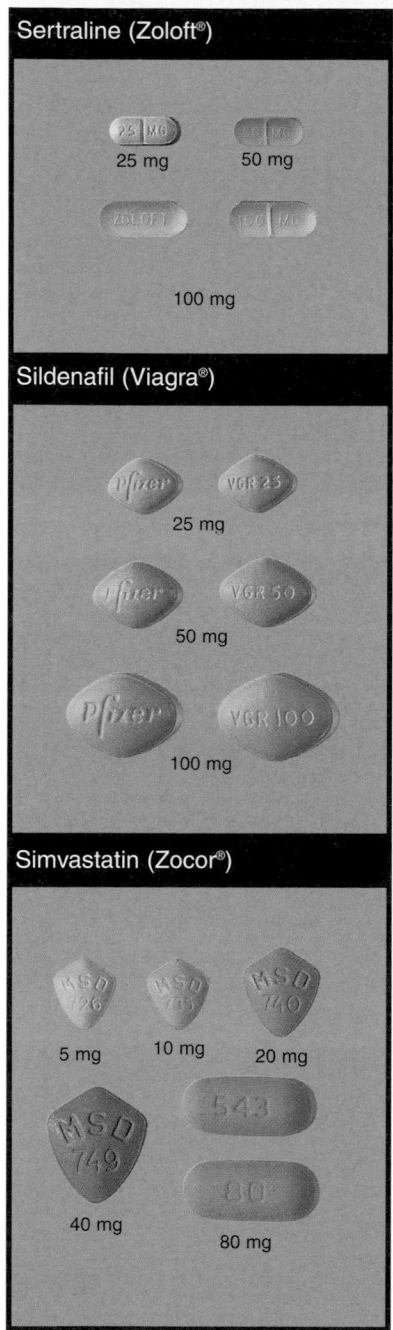

### Sertraline (Zoloft®)

25 mg     50 mg

100 mg

### Sildenafil (Viagra®)

25 mg

50 mg

100 mg

### Simvastatin (Zocor®)

5 mg   10 mg   20 mg

40 mg

80 mg

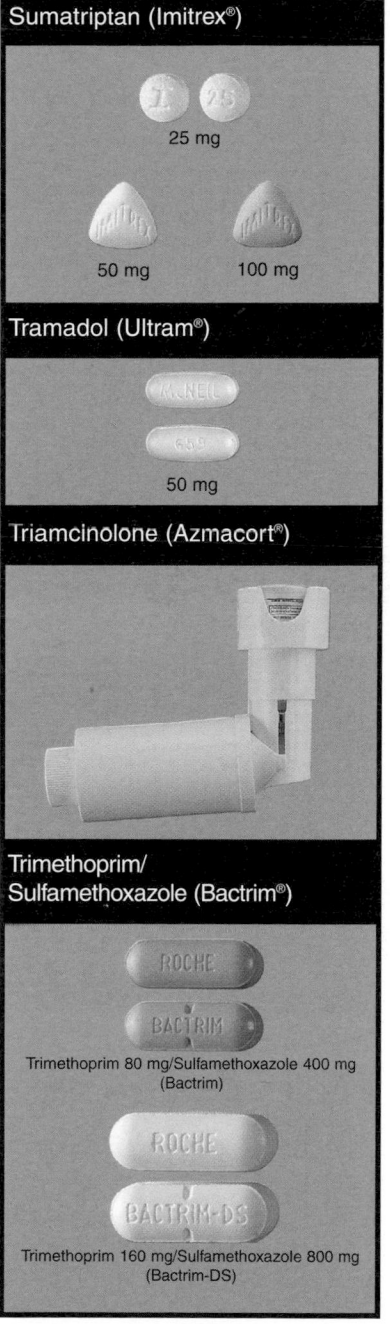

### Sumatriptan (Imitrex®)

25 mg

50 mg     100 mg

### Tramadol (Ultram®)

50 mg

### Triamcinolone (Azmacort®)

### Trimethoprim/ Sulfamethoxazole (Bactrim®)

Trimethoprim 80 mg/Sulfamethoxazole 400 mg
(Bactrim)

Trimethoprim 160 mg/Sulfamethoxazole 800 mg
(Bactrim-DS)

## Venlafaxine (Effexor®)

25 mg    37.5 mg    50 mg

75 mg     100 mg

37.5 mg XR

75 mg XR

150 mg XR

## Verapamil (Calan®)

40 mg    80 mg    120 mg

120 mg SR    180 mg SR

240 mg SR

## Verapamil (Isoptin-SR®)

120 mg SR    180 mg SR

240 mg SR

## Verapamil (Verelan®)

120 mg

180 mg

240 mg

360 mg

## Warfarin (Coumadin®)

1 mg    2 mg    2.5 mg

3 mg    4 mg    5 mg

6 mg    7.5 mg    10 mg

## Zolpidem (Ambien®)

5 mg    10 mg

© 2004, SFI

- Patients who have been well controlled on metformin but develop illness or laboratory abnormalities should be assessed for ketoacidosis or lactic acidosis. Assess serum electrolytes, ketones, glucose, and, if indicated, blood pH, lactate, pyruvate, and metformin levels. If either form of acidosis is present, discontinue metformin immediately and treat acidosis.
- **Lab Test Considerations:** Serum glucose and glycosylated hemoglobin should be monitored periodically throughout therapy to evaluate effectiveness of treatment.

## Potential Nursing Diagnoses

- Nutrition, imbalanced: more than body requirements (Indications).
- Knowledge, deficient, related to medication regimen (Patient/Family Teaching).
- Noncompliance (Patient/Family Teaching).

## Implementation

- **General:** Patients stabilized on a diabetic regimen who are exposed to stress, fever, trauma, infection, or surgery may require sliding scale insulin. Withhold oral hypoglycemic agents and reinstitute after resolution of acute episode.
- Patients switching from daily insulin dose may require gradual conversion to oral hypoglycemics.
- **Insulin:** Available in different types and strengths and from different species. Check type, species, source, dose, and expiration date with another licensed nurse. Do not interchange insulins without physician's order. Use only insulin syringes to draw up dose. Use only U100 syringes to draw up insulin lispro dose.

## Patient/Family Teaching

- **General Info:** Explain to patient that medication controls hyperglycemia but does not cure diabetes. Therapy is long-term.
- Review signs of hypoglycemia and hyperglycemia with patient. If hypoglycemia occurs, advise patient to take a glass of orange juice or 2–3 tsp of sugar, honey, or corn syrup dissolved in water (glucose, not table sugar, if taking miglitol), and notify health care professional.
- Encourage patient to follow prescribed diet, medication, and exercise regimen to prevent hypoglycemic or hyperglycemic episodes.
- Instruct patient in proper testing of serum glucose and ketones.
- Advise patient to notify health care professional if nausea, vomiting, or fever develops; if unable to eat usual diet; or if blood glucose levels are not controlled.
- Advise patient to carry sugar or a form of glucose and identification describing medication regimen at all times.
- Insulin is the recommended method of controlling blood glucose during pregnancy. Counsel female patients to use a form of contraception other than oral contraceptives and to notify health care professional promptly if pregnancy is planned or suspected.
- **Insulin:** Instruct patient on proper technique for administration; include type of insulin, equipment (syringe and cartridge pens), storage, and syringe disposal. Discuss the importance of not changing brands of insulin or syringes, selection and rotation of injection sites, and compliance with therapeutic regimen.
- **Sulfonylureas:** Advise patient that concurrent use of alcohol may cause a disulfiram-like reaction (abdominal cramps, nausea, flushing, headache, and hypoglycemia).
- **Metformin:** Explain to patient the risk of lactic acidosis and the potential need for discontinuation of metformin therapy if a severe infection, dehydration, or severe or continuing diarrhea occurs or if medical tests or surgery is required.

## Evaluation

**Effectiveness of therapy can be demonstrated by:** ■ Control of blood glucose levels without the appearance of hypoglycemic or hyperglycemic episodes.

CLASSIFICATIONS

C L A S S I F I C A T I O N S

**Antidiabetics included in *Davis's Drug Guide for Nurses***

*alpha-glucosidase inhibitors*
acarbose 2
miglitol 693

*biguanides*
metformin 660

*insulins*
concentrated regular insulin 553
insulin aspart, rDNA origin 552
insulin glargine 553
insulin lispro, rDNA origin 553
insulin lispro/protamine insulin lispro mixture, rDNA origin 553
insulin zinc suspension (lente insulin) 553
insulin zinc suspension, extended (ultralente insulin) 553

NPH insulin (isophane insulin suspension) 553
NPH/regular insulin mixtures 553
regular insulin (insulin injection) 553

*meglitinides*
nateglinide 734
repaglinide 917

*sulfonylureas*
glimepiride 522
glipizide 522
glyburide 522

*thiazolidinediones*
pioglitazone 852
rosiglitazone 943

# ■ ANTIDIARRHEALS

## PHARMACOLOGIC PROFILE

### General Use
For the control and symptomatic relief of acute and chronic nonspecific diarrhea.

### General Action and Information
Diphenoxylate/atropine, difenoxin/atropine, and loperamide slow intestinal motility and propulsion. Kaolin/pectin and bismuth subsalicylate affect fluid content of the stool. Bismuth subsalicylate is also used a part of the management of ulcer disease due to *Helicobater pylori* Polycarbophil acts as an antidiarrheal by taking on water within the bowel lumen to create a formed stool. Polycarbophil may also be used to treat constipation. Octreotide is used specifically for diarrhea associated with GI endocrine tumors.

### Contraindications
Previous hypersensitivity. Severe abdominal pain of unknown cause, especially when associated with fever.

### Precautions
Use cautiously in patients with severe liver disease or inflammatory bowel disease. Safety in pregnancy and lactation not established (diphenoxylate/atropine and loperamide). Octreotide may aggravate gallbladder disease.

### Interactions
Kaolin may decrease absorption of digoxin Polycarbophil decreases the absorption of tetracycline Octreotide may alter the response to insulin or oral hypoglycemic agents.

## NURSING IMPLICATIONS

### Assessment
■ Assess the frequency and consistency of stools and bowel sounds before and throughout therapy.
■ Assess patient's fluid and electrolyte status and skin turgor for dehydration.

### Potential Nursing Diagnoses
■ Diarrhea (Indications).

■ Constipation (Side Effects).

■ Knowledge, deficient, related to disease processes and medication regimen (Patient/Family Teaching).

## Implementation

■ Shake liquid preparations before administration.

## Patient/Family Teaching

■ Instruct patient to notify health care professional if diarrhea persists; or if fever, abdominal pain, or palpitations occur.

## Evaluation

**Effectiveness of therapy can be demonstrated by:** ■ Decrease in diarrhea.

## Antidiarrheals included in *Davis's Drug Guide for Nurses*

bismuth subsalicylate 118
difenoxin/atropine 318
diphenoxylate/atropine 318
kaolin/pectin 1173

loperamide 624
octreotide 773
polycarbophil 1178

# ■ ANTIEMETICS

## PHARMACOLOGIC PROFILE

### General Use

Phenothiazines, dolasetron, granisetron, metoclopramide, trimethobenzamide, and ondansetron are used to manage nausea and vomiting of many causes, including surgery, anesthesia, and antineoplastic and radiation therapy. Dimenhydrinate, scopolamine, and meclizine are used almost exclusively to prevent motion sickness.

### General Action and Information

Phenothiazines act on the chemoreceptor trigger zone to inhibit nausea and vomiting. Dimenhydrinate, scopolamine, and meclizine act as antiemetics mainly by diminishing motion sickness. Metoclopramide decreases nausea and vomiting by its effects on gastric emptying. Dolasetron, granisetron, and ondansetron block the effects of serotonin at 5-HT$_3$ receptor sites.

### Contraindications

Previous hypersensitivity.

### Precautions

Use phenothiazines cautiously in children who may have viral illnesses. Choose agents carefully in pregnant patients (no agents are approved for safe use).

### Interactions

Additive CNS depression with other CNS depressants including antidepressants, antihistamines, opioid analgesics, and sedative/hypnotics Phenothiazines may produce hypotension when used with antihypertensives, nitrates, or acute ingestion of alcohol.

## NURSING IMPLICATIONS

### Assessment

■ Assess nausea, vomiting, bowel sounds, and abdominal pain before and following administration.

■ Monitor hydration status and intake and output. Patients with severe nausea and vomiting may require IV fluids in addition to antiemetics.

**Potential Nursing Diagnoses**
- Fluid volume, deficit (Indications).
- Nutrition, imbalanced: less than body requirements (Indications).
- Injury, risk for (Side Effects).

**Implementation**
- For prophylactic administration, follow directions for specific drugs so that peak effect corresponds to time of anticipated nausea.
- Phenothiazines should be discontinued 48 hr before and not resumed for 24 hr following myelography, as they lower seizure threshold.

**Patient/Family Teaching**
- Advise patient and family to use general measures to decrease nausea (begin with sips of liquids and small, nongreasy meals; provide oral hygiene; and remove noxious stimuli from environment).
- May cause drowsiness. Advise patient to call for assistance when ambulating and to avoid driving or other activities requiring alertness until response to medication is known.
- Advise patient to make position changes slowly to minimize orthostatic hypotension.

**Evaluation**
**Effectiveness of therapy can be demonstrated by:** ■ Prevention of, or decrease in, nausea and vomiting.

**Antiemetics included in *Davis's Drug Guide for Nurses***

*5 HT₃ antagonists*
dolasetron 337
granisetron 480
ondansetron 781
palonosetron 805

*phenothiazines*
chlorpromazine 1165
prochlorperazine 876
promethazine 882

thiethylperazine 1184

*miscellaneous*
aprepitant 83
dimenhydrinate 312
meclizine 642
metoclopramide 678
scopolamine 957
trimethobenzamide 1187

# ■ ANTIFUNGALS

## PHARMACOLOGIC PROFILE

### General Use
Treatment of fungal infections. Infections of skin or mucous membranes may be treated with topical or vaginal preparations. Deep-seated or systemic infections require oral or parenteral therapy. New parenteral formulations of amphotericin employ lipid encapsulation technology designed to decrease toxicity.

### General Action and Information
Kill (fungicidal) or stop growth of (fungistatic) susceptible fungi by affecting the permeability of the fungal cell membrane or protein synthesis within the fungal cell itself.

### Contraindications
Previous hypersensitivity.

### Precautions
Because most systemic antifungals may have adverse effects on bone marrow function, use cautiously in patients with depressed bone marrow reserve. Amphotericin B commonly

causes renal impairment. Fluconazole requires dosage adjustment in the presence of renal impairment. Adverse reactions to fluconazole may be more severe in HIV-positive patients.

### Interactions
Differ greatly among various agents. See individual drugs.

## NURSING IMPLICATIONS

### Assessment
■ Assess patient for signs of infection and assess involved areas of skin and mucous membranes before and throughout therapy. Increased skin irritation may indicate need to discontinue medication.

### Potential Nursing Diagnoses
■ Infection, risk for (Indications).
■ Skin integrity, impaired (Indications).
■ Knowledge, deficient, related to disease processes and medication regimen (Patient/Family Teaching).

### Implementation
■ **General:** Available in various dosage forms. Refer to specific drugs for directions for administration.
■ **Topical:** Consult physician or other health care professional for cleansing technique before applying medication. Wear gloves during application. Do not use occlusive dressings unless specified by physician or other health care professional.

### Patient/Family Teaching
■ Instruct patient on proper use of medication form.
■ Instruct patient to continue medication as directed for full course of therapy, even if feeling better.
■ Advise patient to report increased skin irritation or lack of therapeutic response to health care professional.

### Evaluation
**Effectiveness of therapy can be demonstrated by:** ■ Resolution of signs and symptoms of infection. Length of time for complete resolution depends on organism and site of infection. Deep-seated fungal infections may require prolonged therapy (weeks–months). Recurrent fungal infections may be a sign of serious systemic illness.

### Antifungals included in *Davis's Drug Guide for Nurses*

*systemic*
amphotericin B deoxycholate 55
amphotericin B cholesteryl sulfate 55
amphotericin B lipid complex 55
amphotericin B liposome 55
caspofungin 168
fluconazole 429
itraconazole 576
ketoconazole (systemic) 579
terbinafine 1001
voriconazole 1095

*topical/local*
butenafine 78
butoconazole 81
ciclopirox 78

clotrimazole 78
econazole 78
haloprogin 78
ketoconazole 78
miconazole 78
naftifine 78
nystatin 78
oxiconazole 78
sulconazole 78
terbinafine 78
terconazole 81
tioconazole 81
tolnaftate 78

**C
L
A
S
S
I
F
I
C
A
T
I
O
N
S**

# ■ ANTIHISTAMINES

## PHARMACOLOGIC PROFILE

### General Use

Relief of symptoms associated with allergies, including rhinitis, urticaria, and angioedema, and as adjunctive therapy in anaphylactic reactions. Topical and ophthalmic antihistamines may immunize systemic side effects. Some antihistamines are used to treat motion sickness (dimenhydrinate and meclizine), insomnia (diphenhydramine), Parkinson-like reactions (diphenhydramine), and other nonallergic conditions.

### General Action and Information

Antihistamines block the effects of histamine at the $H_1$ receptor. They do not block histamine release, antibody production, or antigen-antibody reactions. Most antihistamines have anticholinergic properties and may cause constipation, dry eyes, dry mouth, and blurred vision. In addition, many antihistamines cause sedation. Some phenothiazines have strong antihistaminic properties (hydroxyzine and promethazine).

### Contraindications

Hypersensitivity and narrow-angle glaucoma. Should not be used in premature or newborn infants.

### Precautions

Elderly patients may be more susceptible to adverse anticholinergic effects of antihistamines Use cautiously in patients with pyloric obstruction, prostatic hypertrophy, hyperthyroidism, cardiovascular disease, or severe liver disease. Use cautiously in pregnancy and lactation.

### Interactions

Additive sedation when used with other CNS depressants, including alcohol, antidepressants, opioid analgesics, and sedative/hypnotics MAO inhibitors prolong and intensify the anticholinergic properties of antihistamines.

## NURSING IMPLICATIONS

### Assessment

- **General Info:** Assess allergy symptoms (rhinitis, conjunctivitis, hives) before and periodically throughout therapy.
- Monitor pulse and blood pressure before initiating and throughout IV therapy.
- Assess lung sounds and character of bronchial secretions. Maintain fluid intake of 1500–2000 ml/day to decrease viscosity of secretions.
- **Nausea and Vomiting:** Assess degree of nausea and frequency and amount of emesis when administering for nausea and vomiting.
- **Anxiety:** Assess mental status, mood, and behavior when administering for anxiety.
- **Pruritus:** Observe the character, location, and size of affected area when administering for pruritic skin conditions.

### Potential Nursing Diagnoses

- Airway clearance, ineffective (Indications).
- Injury, risk for (Adverse Reactions).
- Knowledge, deficient, related to disease processes and medication regimen (Patient/Family Teaching).

### Implementation

- When used for prophylaxis of motion sickness, administer at least 30 min and preferably 1–2 hr before exposure to conditions that may precipitate motion sickness.

- When administering concurrently with opioid analgesics (hydroxyzine, promethazine), supervise ambulation closely to prevent injury secondary to increased sedation.

### Patient/Family Teaching

- Inform patient that drowsiness may occur. Avoid driving or other activities requiring alertness until response to drug is known.
- Caution patient to avoid using concurrent alcohol or CNS depressants.
- Advise patient that good oral hygiene, frequent rinsing of mouth with water, and sugarless gum or candy may help relieve dryness of mouth.
- Instruct patient to contact health care professional if symptoms persist.

### Evaluation

**Effectiveness of therapy can be demonstrated by:** ■ Decrease in allergic symptoms. ■ Prevention or decreased severity of nausea and vomiting ■ Decrease in anxiety. ■ Relief of pruritus. ■ Sedation when used as a hypnotic.

### Antihistamines included in *Davis's Drug Guide for Nurses*

*systemic*
azatadine 1162
brompheniramine 1164
cetirizine 188
promethazine 882
chlorpheniramine 193
cyproheptadine 261
desloratadine 283
dimenhydrinate 312
fexofenadine 424
hydroxyzine 518

loratadine 628
meclizine 642

*ophthalmic antihistamines*
azelastine 1147
emedastine 1147
levocabastine 1147
olopatadine 1147

*topical*
diphenhydramine (oral, parenteral) 316
doxepin 343

## ■ ANTIHYPERTENSIVES

### PHARMACOLOGIC PROFILE

### General Use

Treatment of hypertension of many causes, most commonly essential hypertension. Parenteral products are used in the treatment of hypertensive emergencies. Oral treatment should be initiated as soon as possible and individualized to ensure adherence and compliance for long-term therapy. Therapy is initiated with agents having minimal side effects. When such therapy fails, more potent drugs with different side effects are added in an effort to control blood pressure while causing minimal patient discomfort.

### General Action and Information

As a group, the antihypertensives are used to lower blood pressure to a normal level (<90 mm Hg diastolic) or to the lowest level tolerated. The goal of antihypertensive therapy is prevention of end-organ damage. Antihypertensives are classified into groups according to their site of action. These include peripherally-acting antiadrenergics; centrally-acting alpha-adrenergics; beta blockers; vasodilators; ACE inhibitors; angiotensin II antagonists; calcium channel blockers, and diuretics Hypertensive emergencies may be managed with parenteral agents, such as enalaprilat or fenoldopam.

### Contraindications

Hypersensitivity to individual agents.

### Precautions

Choose agents carefully in pregnancy, during lactation, or in patients receiving digoxin ACE inhibitors and angiotensin II antagonists should be avoided during pregnancy. Alpha-adrenergic agonists and beta blockers should be used only in patients who will comply, because abrupt discontinuation of these agents may result in rapid and excessive rise in blood pressure (rebound phenomenon). Thiazide diuretics may increase the requirement for treatment of diabetics. Vasodilators may cause tachycardia if used alone and are commonly used in combination with beta blockers Some antihypertensives cause sodium and water retention and are usually combined with a diuretic.

### Interactions

Many drugs can negate the therapeutic effectiveness of antihypertensives, including antihistamines, NSAIDs, sympathomimetic bronchodilators, decongestants, appetite suppressants, antidepressants, and MAO inhibitors Hypokalemia from diuretics may increase the risk of digoxin toxicity. Potassium supplements and potassium-sparing diuretics may cause hyperkalemia when used with ACE inhibitors.

### NURSING IMPLICATIONS

### Assessment

- Monitor blood pressure and pulse frequently during dosage adjustment and periodically throughout therapy.
- Monitor intake and output ratios and daily weight.
- Monitor frequency of prescription refills to determine compliance.

### Potential Nursing Diagnoses

- Tissue perfusion, ineffective (Indications).
- Knowledge, deficient, related to disease processes and medication regimen (Patient/Family Teaching).
- Noncompliance (Patient/Family Teaching).

### Implementation

- Many antihypertensives are available as combination products to enhance compliance (see Appendix B).

### Patient/Family Teaching

- Instruct patient to continue taking medication, even if feeling well. Abrupt withdrawal may cause rebound hypertension. Medication controls but does not cure hypertension.
- Encourage patient to comply with additional interventions for hypertension (weight reduction, low-sodium diet, regular exercise, discontinuation of smoking, moderation of alcohol consumption, and stress management).
- Instruct patient and family on proper technique for monitoring blood pressure. Advise them to check blood pressure weekly and report significant changes.
- Caution patient to make position changes slowly to minimize orthostatic hypotension. Advise patient that exercise or hot weather may enhance hypotensive effects.
- Advise patient to consult health care professional before taking any OTC medications, especially cold remedies.
- Advise patient to inform health care professional of medication regimen before treatment or surgery.
- Patients taking ACE inhibitors or angiotensin II antagonists should notify health care professional if pregnancy is planned or suspected.
- Emphasize the importance of follow-up exams to monitor progress.

### Evaluation

**Effectiveness of therapy can be demonstrated by:** ■ Decrease in blood pressure.

### Antihypertensives included in *Davis's Drug Guide for Nurses*

***adrenergics***
clonidine 212

***aldosterone antagonists***
eplerenone 373

***ACE inhibitors***
benazepril 72
captopril 72
enalapril/enalaprilat 72
fosinopril 72
lisinopril 72
moexipril 72
perindopril 72
quinapril 72
ramipril 72
trandolapril 72

***angiotensin II receptor antagonists***
candesartan 69
eprosartan 69
irbesartan 69
losartan 69
olmesartan 69
telmisartan 69
valsartan 69

***beta blockers (nonselective)***
carteolol 164
carvedilol 166
labetalol 587
nadolol 720
penbutolol 819
pindolol 849
propranolol 891
timolol 1034

***beta blockers (selective)***
acebutolol 4
atenolol 91

betaxolol 110
bisoprolol 120
metoprolol 682

***calcium channel blockers***
amlodipine 47
diltiazem 308
felodipine 412
isradipine 574
nicardipine 747
nifedipine 753
nisoldipine 759
verapamil 1077

***centrally acting antiadrenergics***
guanabenz 1171
guanfacine 486
methyldopa 672

***loop diuretics***
torsemide 1047

***peripherally acting antiadrenergics***
doxazosin 342
guanadrel 1172
prazosin 872
terazosin 1000

***thiazide diuretics***
chlorothiazide 326
chlorthalidone (thiazide–like) 326
hydrochlorothiazide 326

***thiazide-like diuretics***
indapamide 545
metolazone 680

***vasodilators***
fenoldopam 416
hydralazine 508
minoxidil (systemic) 1174
nitroprusside 766

## ■ ANTI-INFECTIVES

### PHARMACOLOGIC PROFILE

### General Use

Treatment and prophylaxis of various bacterial infections. See specific drugs for spectrum and indications. Some infections may require additional surgical intervention and supportive therapy.

### General Action and Information

Kill (bactericidal) or inhibit the growth of (bacteriostatic) susceptible pathogenic bacteria. Not active against viruses or fungi. Anti-infectives are subdivided into categories depending on chemical similarities and antimicrobial spectrum.

## Contraindications

Known hypersensitivity to individual agents. Cross-sensitivity among related agents may occur.

## Precautions

Culture and susceptibility testing are desirable to optimize therapy. Dosage modification may be required in patients with hepatic or renal insufficiency. Use cautiously in pregnant and lactating women. Prolonged inappropriate use of broad spectrum anti-infective agents may lead to superinfection with fungi or resistant bacteria.

## Interactions

Penicillins and aminoglycosides chemically inactivate each other and should not be physically admixed. Erythromycins may decrease hepatic metabolism of other drugs. Probenecid increases serum levels of penicillins and related compounds. Highly protein-bound anti-infectives such as sulfonamides may displace or be displaced by other highly bound drugs. See individual drugs. Extended-spectrum penicillins (ticarcillin, piperacillin) and some cephalosporins (cefoperazone, cefotetan) may increase the risk of bleeding with anticoagulants, thrombolytic agents, antiplatelet agents, or NSAIDs Fluoroquinolone absorption is decreased by antacids, bismuth subsalicylate, iron salts, sucralfate, and zinc salts.

## NURSING IMPLICATIONS

### Assessment

- Assess patient for signs and symptoms of infection prior to and throughout therapy.
- Determine previous hypersensitivities in patients receiving penicillins or cephalosporins.
- Obtain specimens for culture and sensitivity prior to initiating therapy. First dose may be given before receiving results.

### Potential Nursing Diagnoses

- Infection, risk for (Indications).
- Knowledge, deficient, related to disease processes and medication regimen (Patient/Family Teaching).
- Noncompliance (Patient/Family Teaching).

### Implementation

- Most anti-infectives should be administered around the clock to maintain therapeutic serum drug levels.

### Patient/Family Teaching

- Instruct patient to continue taking medication around the clock until finished completely, even if feeling better.
- Advise patient to report the signs of superinfection (black, furry overgrowth on the tongue; vaginal itching or discharge; loose or foul-smelling stools) and allergy to health care professional.
- Instruct patient to notify health care professional if fever and diarrhea develop, especially if stool contains pus, blood, or mucus. Advise patient not to treat diarrhea without consulting health care professional.
- Instruct patient to notify health care professional if symptoms do not improve.

### Evaluation

**Effectiveness of therapy can be demonstrated by:** ■ Resolution of the signs and symptoms of infection. Length of time for complete resolution depends on organism and site of infection.

# Anti-infectives included in *Davis's Drug Guide for Nurses*

*aminoglycosides*
amikacin 35
gentamicin 35
kanamycin 35
neomycin 35
netilmicin 35
streptomycin 35
tobramycin 35

*carbapenems*
ertapenem 382
imipenem/cilastatin 538

*first-generation cephalosporins*
cefadroxil 173
cefazolin 173
cephalexin 173
cephapirin 173
cephradine 173

*second-generation cephalosporins*
cefaclor 176
cefmetazole 176
cefonicid 176
cefotetan 176
cefoxitin 176
cefprozil 176
cefuroxime 176
loracarbef 176

*third-generation cephalosporins*
cefdinir 181
cefepime 182
cefoperazone 182
cefotaxime 182
cefpodoxime 182
ceftazidime 182
ceftibuten 182
cefditoren 182
ceftizoxime 182
ceftriaxone 182

*extended spectrum penicillins*
piperacillin 853
piperacillin/tazobactam 853
ticarcillin 1029
ticarcillin/clavulanate 1029

*fluoroquinolones*
alatrofloxacin 435
ciprofloxacin 435
enoxacin 435
gatifloxacin 435
gemifloxacin 435
levofloxacin 435
lomefloxacin 435

moxifloxacin 435
norfloxacin 435
ofloxacin 435
sparfloxacin 435
trovafloxacin 435

*macrolides*
azithromycin 99
clarithromycin 205
erythromycin 384

*penicillins*
amoxicillin 48
amoxicillin/clavulanate 51
ampicillin 59
ampicillin/sulbactam 62
benzathine penicillin G 821
penicillin G 821
penicillin V 821
procaine penicillin G 821
cloxacillin 825
dicloxacillin 825
nafcillin 825
oxacillin 825

*sulfonamides*
trimethoprim/sulfamethoxazole 1058
doxycycline 1010
minocycline 1010
tetracycline 1010

*miscellaneous*
drotrecogin 355
linezolid 619
metronidazole 685
mupirocin 713
nitrofurantoin 761
quinupristin/dalfopristin 911
trimethoprim 1057
vancomycin 1071

# ■ ANTINEOPLASTICS

## PHARMACOLOGIC PROFILE

### General Use

Used in the treatment of various solid tumors, lymphomas, and leukemias. Also used in some autoimmune disorders such as rheumatoid arthritis (cyclophosphamide, methotrexate). Often used in combinations to minimize individual toxicities and increase response. Chemotherapy may be combined with other treatment modalities such as surgery and radiation therapy. Dosages vary greatly, depending on extent of disease, other agents used, and patient's condition. Some new formulations (daunorubicin, doxorubicin) encapsulated in a lipid membrane have less toxicity with greater efficacy.

### General Action and Information

Act by many different mechanisms (see the following table). Many affect DNA synthesis or function; others alter immune function or affect hormonal status of sensitive tumors. Action may not be limited to neoplastic cells.

## MECHANISM OF ACTION OF VARIOUS ANTINEOPLASTICS

| MECHANISM OF ACTION | AGENT | EFFECTS ON CELL CYCLE |
|---|---|---|
| ALKYLATING AGENTS<br>Cause cross-linking of DNA | busulfan<br>carboplatin<br>chlorambucil<br>cisplatin<br>cyclophosphamide<br>ifosfamide<br>mechlorethamine<br>melphalan<br>procarbazine<br>temozolamide | Cell cycle–nonspecific |
| ANTHRACYCLINES<br>Interfere with DNA and RNA synthesis | daunorubicin<br>doxorubicin<br>epirubicin<br>idarubicin | Cell cycle–nonspecific |
| ANTITUMOR ANTIBIOTIC<br>Interfere with DNA and RNA synthesis | bleomycin<br>mitomycin<br>mitoxantrone<br>plicamycin | Cell cycle–nonspecific (except bleomycin) |
| ANTIMETABOLITES<br><br>Take the place of normal proteins | cytarabine<br><br>fluorouracil<br>hydroxyurea<br>methotrexate | Cell cyclespecific, work mostly in S phase (DNA synthesis) |
| ENZYMES<br>Deplete asparagine | asparaginase<br>pegaspargase | Cell-cycle phase–specific |
| ENZYME INHIBITORS<br>Inhibits topoisomerase | irinotecan<br>topotecan | Cell-cycle phase–specific |
| Inhibits kinase | imatinib | Unknown |
| HORMONAL AGENTS<br>Alter hormonal status in tumors that are sensitive | bicalutamide<br>estramustine<br>flutamide<br>leuprolide<br>megestrol<br>nilutamide<br>tamoxifen<br>testosterone<br>  (androgens)<br>triptorelin | Unknown |
| HORMONAL AGENTS–AROMATASE INHIBITORS<br>Inhibit enzyme responsible for activating estrogen | anastrazole<br>letrozole | Unknown |
| IMMUNE MODULATORS | aldesleukin<br>alemtuzumab | Unknown |

| MECHANISM OF ACTION | AGENT | EFFECTS ON CELL CYCLE |
|---|---|---|
| | gemtuzumab | |
| | toremifene | |
| | trastuzumab | |
| PODOPHYLLOTOXIN DERIVATIVES | etoposide | Cell-cycle phase–specific |
| Damages DNA before mitosis | | |
| TAXOIDS | docetaxel | Cell-cycle phase–specific |
| Interupt interphase and mitosis | paclitaxel | |
| VINCA ALKALOIDS | vinblastine | Cell cycle–specific, work during M phase (mitosis) |
| Interfere with mitosis | vincristine | |
| | vinorelbine | |
| MISCELLANEOUS | aldesleukin | Unknown |
| | altretamine | Unknown |

## Contraindications

Previous bone marrow depression or hypersensitivity. Contraindicated in pregnancy and lactation.

## Precautions

Use cautiously in patients with active infections, decreased bone marrow reserve, radiation therapy, or other debilitating illnesses. Use cautiously in patients with childbearing potential.

## Interactions

Allopurinol decreases metabolism of mercaptopurine Toxicity from methotrexate may be increased by other nephrotoxic drugs or larger doses of aspirin or NSAIDs Bone marrow depression is additive. See individual drugs.

## NURSING IMPLICATIONS

### Assessment

- Monitor for bone marrow depression. Assess for bleeding (bleeding gums, bruising, petechiae, guaiac stools, urine, and emesis) and avoid IM injections and rectal temperatures if platelet count is low. Apply pressure to venipuncture sites for 10 min. Assess for signs of infection during neutropenia. Anemia may occur. Monitor for increased fatigue, dyspnea, and orthostatic hypotension.
- Monitor intake and output ratios, appetite, and nutritional intake. Prophylactic antiemetics may be used. Adjusting diet as tolerated may help maintain fluid and electrolyte balance and nutritional status.
- Monitor IV site carefully and ensure patency. Discontinue infusion immediately if discomfort, erythema along vein, or infiltration occurs. Tissue ulceration and necrosis may result from infiltration.
- Monitor for symptoms of gout (increased uric acid, joint pain, and edema). Encourage patient to drink at least 2L of fluid each day. Allopurinol may be given to decrease uric acid levels. Alkalinization of urine may be ordered to increase excretion of uric acid.

### Potential Nursing Diagnoses

- Infection, risk for (Side Effects).
- Nutrition, imbalanced: less than body requirements (Adverse Reactions).
- Knowledge, deficient, related to disease processes and medication regimen (Patient/Family Teaching).

### Implementation

- Solutions for injection should be prepared in a biologic cabinet. Wear gloves, gown, and mask while handling medication. Discard equipment in designated containers (see Appendix M).
- Check dose carefully. Fatalities have resulted from dosing errors.

**CLASSIFICATIONS**

## Patient/Family Teaching

- Caution patient to avoid crowds and persons with known infections. Health care professional should be informed immediately if symptoms of infection occur.
- Instruct patient to report unusual bleeding. Advise patient of thrombocytopenia precautions.
- These drugs may cause gonadal suppression; however, patient should still use birth control, as most antineoplastics are teratogenic. Advise patient to inform health care professional immediately if pregnancy is suspected.
- Discuss with patient the possibility of hair loss. Explore methods of coping.
- Instruct patient to inspect oral mucosa for erythema and ulceration. If ulceration occurs, advise patient to use sponge brush and to rinse mouth with water after eating and drinking. Topical agents may be used if mouth pain interferes with eating. Stomatitis pain may require treatment with opioid analgesics.
- Instruct patient not to receive any vaccinations without advice of health care professional. Antineoplastics may decrease antibody response and increase risk of adverse reactions.
- Advise patient of need for medical follow-up and frequent lab tests.

## Evaluation

**Effectiveness of therapy can be demonstrated by:** ■ Decrease in size and spread of tumor ■ Improvement in hematologic status in patients with leukemia.

## Antineoplastics included in *Davis's Drug Guide for Nurses*

*alkylating agents*
busulfan 139
carboplatin 158
carmustine 162
chlorambucil 1164
cisplatin 201
cyclophosphamide 255
ifosfamide 534
melphalan 648
mechlorethamine 1173
procarbazine 1180
temozolomide 1184

*anthracyclines*
daunorubicin citrate liposome 273
daunorubicin hydrochloride 275
doxorubicin hydrochloride liposome 349
doxorubicin hydrochloride 346
epirubicin 370
idarubicin 532

*antiandrogens*
bicalutamide 113
flutamide 453
nilutamide 756

*antiestrogens*
tamoxifen 993
toremifene 1046

*antimetabolites*
cytarabine 263
fluorouracil 443
hydroxyurea 1172

methotrexate 668
gemcitabine 471

*antitumor antibiotics*
bleomycin 123
mitomycin 699
mitoxantrone 701
plicamycin 860

*aromatase inhibitors*
anastrazole 68
letrozole 601

*enzyme inhibitors*
gefitinib 470
imatinib 536
irinotecan 562
topotecan 1044

*enzymes*
asparaginase 89
pegaspargase 816

*hormones*
goserelin 1171
leuprolide 604
medroxyprogesterone 229
triptorelin 1061

*monoclonal antibodies*
alemtuzumab 1160
gemtuzumab ozogamicin 1170
rituximab 935
trastuzumab 1052

*podophyllotoxin derivatives*
etoposide phosphate 406

# ■ ANTIPARKINSON AGENTS

## PHARMACOLOGIC PROFILE

### General Use

Used in the treatment of parkinsonism of various causes: degenerative, toxic, infective, neoplastic, or drug-induced.

### General Action and Information

Drugs used in the treatment of the parkinsonian syndrome and other dyskinesias are aimed at restoring the natural balance of two major neurotransmitters in the CNS: acetylcholine and dopamine. The imbalance is a deficiency in dopamine that results in excessive cholinergic activity. Drugs used are either anticholinergics (benztropine, biperiden, and trihexyphenidyl) or dopaminergic agonists (bromocriptine, levodopa, and pergolide). Pramipexole and ropinerole are two new nonergot dopamine agonists. Entacapone inhibits the enzyme that breaks down levodopa, thereby enhancing its effects.

### Contraindications

Anticholinergics should be avoided in patients with narrow-angle glaucoma.

### Precautions

Use cautiously in patients with severe cardiac disease, pyloric obstruction, or prostatic enlargement.

### Interactions

Pyridoxine, MAO inhibitors, benzodiazepines, phenytoin, phenothiazines, and haloperidol may antagonize the effects of levodopa Agents that antagonize dopamine (phenothiazines, metoclopramide) may decrease effectiveness of dopamine agonists.

## NURSING IMPLICATIONS

### Assessment

- Assess parkinsonian and extrapyramidal symptoms (akinesia, rigidity, tremors, pill rolling, mask facies, shuffling gait, muscle spasms, twisting motions, and drooling) before and throughout course of therapy. On-off phenomenon may cause symptoms to appear or improve suddenly.
- Monitor blood pressure frequently during therapy. Instruct patient to remain supine during and for several hours after first dose of bromocriptine, as severe hypotension may occur.

### Potential Nursing Diagnoses

- Mobility, impaired physical (Indications).
- Injury, risk for (Indications).
- Knowledge, deficient, related to disease processes and medication regimen (Patient/Family Teaching).

## Implementation

- In the carbidopa/levodopa combination, the number following the drug name represents the milligram of each respective drug.

## Patient/Family Teaching

- May cause drowsiness or dizziness. Advise patient to avoid driving or other activities that require alertness until response to medication is known.
- Caution patient to make position changes slowly to minimize orthostatic hypotension.
- Instruct patient that frequent rinsing of mouth, good oral hygiene, and sugarless gum or candy may decrease dry mouth. Patient should notify health care professional if dryness persists (saliva substitutes may be used). Also notify the dentist if dryness interferes with use of dentures.
- Advise patient to confer with health care professional before taking OTC medications, especially cold remedies, or drinking alcoholic beverages. Patients receiving levodopa should avoid multivitamins. Vitamin $B_6$ (pyridoxine) may interfere with levodopa's action.
- Caution patient that decreased perspiration may occur. Overheating may occur during hot weather. Patients should remain indoors in an air-conditioned environment during hot weather.
- Advise patient to increase activity, bulk, and fluid in diet to minimize constipating effects of medication.
- Advise patient to notify health care professional if confusion, rash, urinary retention, severe constipation, visual changes, or worsening of parkinsonian symptoms occur.

## Evaluation

**Effectiveness of therapy can be demonstrated by:** ■ Resolution of parkinsonian signs and symptoms ■ Resolution of drug-induced extrapyramidal symptoms.

### Antiparkinson agents included in *Davis's Drug Guide for Nurses*

*anticholinergics*
benztropine 108
biperiden 115
trihexyphenidyl 1186

*antiviral*
amantadine 29

*catechol-O-methyltransferase inhibitors*
entacapone 362
tolcapone 1040

*dopamine agonists*
bromocriptine 1163
carbidopa/levodopa 610
levodopa 610
pergolide 832
pramipexole 870
ropinirole 942

*monoamine oxidase type B inhibitors*
selegiline 958

# ■ ANTIPLATELET AGENTS

## PHARMACOLOGIC PROFILE

### General Use

Antiplatelet agents are used to treat and prevent thromboembolic events such as stroke and MI. Dipyridamole is commonly used after cardiac surgery.

### General Action and Information

Inhibit platelet aggregation, prolongs bleeding time, and are used to prevent MI or stroke (aspirin, clopidogrel, dipyridamole, ticlopidine). Eptifibatide and tirofiban are used in the management of various acute coronary syndromes. These agents have been used concurrently/sequentially with anticoagulants and thrombolytics.

## Contraindications
Hypersensitivity, ulcer disease, active bleeding, and recent surgery.

## Precautions
Use cautiously in patients at risk for bleeding (trauma, surgery). History of GI bleeding or ulcer disease. Safety not established in pregnancy, lactation, or children.

## Interactions
Concurrent use with NSAIDs, heparin, thrombolytics, or warfarin may increase the risk of bleeding.

## NURSING IMPLICATIONS

### Assessment
- Assess patient for evidence of additional or increased thrombosis. Symptoms will depend on area of involvement.
- Assess patient taking antiplatelet agents for symptoms of stroke, peripheral vascular disease, or MI periodically throughout therapy.
- **Lab Test Considerations:** Monitor bleeding time throughout antiplatelet therapy. Prolonged bleeding time, which is time- and dose-dependent, is expected.

### Potential Nursing Diagnoses
- Tissue perfusion, ineffective (Indications).
- Injury, risk for (Side Effects).
- Knowledge, deficient, related to disease processes and medication regimen (Patient/Family Teaching).

### Implementation
- Use an infusion pump with continuous infusions to ensure accurate dosage.

### Patient/Family Teaching
- Instruct patient to notify health care professional immediately if any bleeding is noted.

### Evaluation
**Effectiveness of therapy can be demonstrated by:** ■ Prevention of stroke, MI, and vascular death in patients at risk.

### Antiplatelet agents included in *Davis's Drug Guide for Nurses*

*glycoprotein IIb/IIIa inhibitors*
eptifibatide 377
tirofiban 1036

*platelet adhesion inhibitors*
dipyridamole 320

*platelet aggregation inhibitors*
cilostazol 199
clopidogrel 215
ticlopidine 1031

■ **ANTIPSYCHOTICS**

## PHARMACOLOGIC PROFILE

### General Use

Treatment of acute and chronic psychoses, particularly when accompanied by increased psychomotor activity. Use of clozapine is limited to schizophrenia unresponsive to conventional therapy. Selected agents are also used as antihistamines or antiemetics Chlorpromazine is also used in the treatment of intractable hiccups.

### General Action and Information

Block dopamine receptors in the brain; also alter dopamine release and turnover. Peripheral effects include anticholinergic properties and alpha-adrenergic blockade. Most antipsychotics are phenothiazines except for haloperidol, which is a butyrophenone, and clozapine, which is a miscellaneous compound. Newer 'atypical' agents such as olanzapine, quetiapine, and risperidone may have fewer adverse reactions. Phenothiazines differ in their ability to produce sedation (greatest with chlorpromazine and thioridazine), extrapyramidal reactions (greatest with prochlorperazine and trifluoperazine), and anticholinergic effects (greatest with chlorpromazine).

### Contraindications

Hypersensitivity. Cross-sensitivity may exist among phenothiazines Should not be used in narrow-angle glaucoma. Should not be used in patients who have CNS depression.

### Precautions

Safety in pregnancy and lactation not established. Use cautiously in patients with symptomatic cardiac disease. Avoid exposure to extremes in temperature. Use cautiously in severely ill or debilitated patients, diabetic patients, and patients with respiratory insufficiency, prostatic hypertrophy, or intestinal obstruction. May lower seizure threshold. Clozapine may cause agranulocytosis. Most agents are capable of causing neuroleptic malignant syndrome. Should not be used routinely for anxiety or agitation not related to psychoses.

### Interactions

Additive hypotension with acute ingestion of alcohol, antihypertensives, or nitrates Antacids may decrease absorption. Phenobarbital may increase metabolism and decrease effectiveness. Additive CNS depression with other CNS depressants, including alcohol, antihistamines, antidepressants, opioid analgesics, or sedative/hypnotics Lithium may decrease blood levels and effectiveness of phenothiazines May decrease the therapeutic response to levodopa May increase the risk of agranulocytosis with antithyroid agents.

## NURSING IMPLICATIONS

### Assessment

- Assess patient's mental status (orientation, mood, behavior) before and periodically throughout therapy.
- Monitor blood pressure (sitting, standing, lying), pulse, and respiratory rate before and frequently during the period of dosage adjustment.
- Observe patient carefully when administering medication to ensure medication is actually taken and not hoarded.
- Monitor patient for onset of *akathisia*—restlessness or desire to keep moving—and extrapyramidal side effects; *parkinsonian*—difficulty speaking or swallowing, loss of balance control, pill rolling, mask-like face, shuffling gait, rigidity, tremors; and *dystonia*—muscle spasms, twisting motions, twitching, inability to move eyes, weakness of arms or legs—every 2 mo during therapy and 8–12 wk after therapy has been discontinued. Parkinsonian effects are more common in geriatric patients and dystonias are more common

in younger patients. Notify health care professional if these symptoms occur, as reduction in dosage or discontinuation of medication may be necessary. Trihexyphenidyl or diphenhydramine may be used to control these symptoms.

- Monitor for *tardive dyskinesia*—uncontrolled rhythmic movement of mouth, face, and extremities; lip smacking or puckering; puffing of cheeks; uncontrolled chewing; rapid or worm-like movements of tongue. Notify health care professional immediately if these symptoms occur; these side effects may be irreversible.
- Monitor for development of *neuroleptic malignant syndrome*—fever, respiratory distress, tachycardia, convulsions, diaphoresis, hypertension or hypotension, pallor, tiredness, severe muscle stiffness, loss of bladder control. Notify health care professional immediately if these symptoms occur.

## Potential Nursing Diagnoses
- Thought processes, disturbed (Indications).
- Knowledge, deficient, related to disease processes and medication regimen (Patient/Family Teaching).
- Noncompliance (Patient/Family Teaching).

## Implementation
- **General:** Keep patient recumbent for at least 30 min following parenteral administration to minimize hypotensive effects.
- To prevent contact dermatitis, avoid getting solution on hands.
- Phenothiazines should be discontinued 48 hr before and not resumed for 24 hr following myelography, as they lower the seizure threshold.
- **PO:** Administer with food, milk, or a full glass of water to minimize gastric irritation.
- Dilute most concentrates in 120 ml of distilled or acidified tap water or fruit juice just before administration.

## Patient/Family Teaching
- Advise patient to take medication exactly as directed and not to skip doses or double up on missed doses. Abrupt withdrawal may lead to gastritis, nausea, vomiting, dizziness, headache, tachycardia, and insomnia.
- Advise patient to make position changes slowly to minimize orthostatic hypotension.
- Medication may cause drowsiness. Caution patient to avoid driving or other activities requiring alertness until response to the medication is known.
- Caution patient to avoid taking alcohol or other CNS depressants concurrently with this medication.
- Advise patient to use sunscreen and protective clothing when exposed to the sun to prevent photosensitivity reactions. Extremes of temperature should also be avoided, as these drugs impair body temperature regulation.
- Advise patient that increasing activity, bulk, and fluids in the diet helps minimize the constipating effects of this medication.
- Instruct patient to use frequent mouth rinses, good oral hygiene, and sugarless gum or candy to minimize dry mouth.
- Advise patient to notify health care professional of medication regimen before treatment or surgery.
- Emphasize the importance of routine follow-up exams and continued participation in psychotherapy as indicated.

## Evaluation
**Effectiveness of therapy can be demonstrated by:** ■ Decrease in excitable, paranoic, or withdrawn behavior. Relief of nausea and vomiting. Relief of intractable hiccups.

**Antipsychotics included in *Davis's Drug Guide for Nurses***

*phenothiazines*
chlorpromazine 1165
fluphenazine 448
prochlorperazine 876
thioridazine 1015
trifluoperazine 1186
*miscellaneous*
aripiprazole 87

clozapine 218
haloperidol 489
olanzapine 775
quetiapine 905
risperidone 930
ziprasidone 1105

# ■ ANTIPYRETICS

## PHARMACOLOGIC PROFILE

### General Use
Used to lower fever of many causes (infection, inflammation, and neoplasms).

### General Action and Information
Antipyretics lower fever by affecting thermoregulation in the CNS and by inhibiting the action of prostaglandins peripherally. Many antipyretics affect platelet function; of these, aspirin has the most profound effect as compared with other salicylates, ibuprofen, or ketoprofen.

### Contraindications
Avoid aspirin, ibuprofen, or ketoprofen in patients with bleeding disorders (risk of bleeding is less with other salicylates). Aspirin and other salicylates should be avoided in children and adolescents.

### Precautions
Use aspirin, ibuprofen, or ketoprofen cautiously in patients with ulcer disease. Avoid chronic use of large doses of acetaminophen.

### Interactions
Large doses of aspirin may displace other highly protein-bound drugs. Additive GI irritation with aspirin, ibuprofen, ketoprofen, and other NSAIDs or corticosteroids Aspirin, ibuprofen, ketoprofen, or naproxen may increase the risk of bleeding with other agents affecting hemostasis (anticoagulants, thrombolytic agents, antineoplastics, and certain anti-infectives).

## NURSING IMPLICATIONS

### Assessment
- Assess fever; note presence of associated symptoms (diaphoresis, tachycardia, and malaise).

### Potential Nursing Diagnoses
- Body temperature, risk for imbalanced (Indications).
- Knowledge, deficient, related to disease processes and medication regimen (Patient/Family Teaching).

### Implementation
- Administration with food or antacids may minimize GI irritation (aspirin, ibuprofen, ketoprofen, naproxen).
- Available in oral and rectal dosage forms and in combination with other drugs.

## Patient/Family Teaching

- Advise patient to consult health care professional if fever is not relieved by routine doses or if greater than 39.5°C (103°F) or lasts longer than 3 days.
- Centers for Disease Control and Prevention warns against giving aspirin to children or adolescents with varicella (chickenpox) or influenza-like or viral illnesses because of a possible association with Reye's syndrome.

## Evaluation

**Effectiveness of therapy can be demonstrated by:** ■ Reduction of fever.

## Antipyretics included in *Davis's Drug Guide for Nurses*

acetaminophen 6
aspirin 1127
choline and magnesium salicylates 947
choline salicylate 947
ibuprofen 528

ketoprofen 580
magnesium salicylate 947
naproxen 730
salsalate 947
sodium salicylate 947

# ■ ANTIRETROVIRALS

## PHARMACOLOGIC PROFILE

### General Use

The goal of antiretroviral therapy in the management of HIV infection is to improve CD4 cell counts and decrease viral load. If accomplished, this generally results in slowed progression of the disease, improved quality of life, and decreased opportunistic infections. Perinatal use of agents also prevents transmission of the virus to the fetus. Post-exposure prophylaxis with antiretrovirals is also recommended.

### General Action and Information

Because of the rapid emergence of resistance and toxicities of individual agents, HIV infection is almost always managed by a combination of agents. Selections and doses are based on individual toxicities, underlying organ system disease, concurrent drug therapy, and severity of illness. Various combinations are used; up to 4 agents may be used simultaneously. More than 100 agents are currently being tested in addition to those already approved by the FDA.

### Contraindications

Hypersensitivity. Because of highly varying toxicities among agents, see individual monographs for more specific information.

### Precautions

Many agents require modification for renal impairment. Protease inhibitors may cause hyperglycemia and should be used cautiously in patients with diabetes. Hemophiliacs may also be at risk of bleeding when taking protease inhibitors See individual monographs for specific information.

### Interactions

There are many significant and potentially serious drug-drug interactions among the antiretrovirals They are affected by drugs that alter metabolism; some agents themselves affect metabolism. See individual agents.

## NURSING IMPLICATIONS

### Assessment

- Assess patient for change in severity of symptoms of HIV and for symptoms of opportunistic infections throughout therapy.

- **Lab Test Considerations:** Monitor viral load and CD4 counts prior to and periodically during therapy.

## Potential Nursing Diagnoses
- Infection, risk for (Indications).
- Knowledge, deficient, related to disease processes and medication regimen (Patient/Family Teaching).
- Noncompliance (Patient/Family Teaching).

## Implementation
- Administer doses around the clock.

## Patient/Family Teaching
- Instruct patient to take medication exactly as directed, around the clock, even if sleep is interrupted. Emphasize the importance of complying with therapy, not taking more than prescribed amount, and not discontinuing without consulting health care professional. Missed doses should be taken as soon as remembered unless almost time for next dose; patient should not double doses. Inform patient that long-term effects are unknown at this time.
- Instruct patient that antiretrovirals should not be shared with others.
- Inform patient that antiretroviral therapy does not cure HIV and does not reduce the risk of transmission of HIV to others through sexual contact or blood contamination. Caution patient to use a condom during sexual contact and to avoid sharing needles or donating blood to prevent spreading the AIDS virus to others.
- Advise patient to avoid taking any Rx or OTC medications or herbal or alternative therapies without consulting health care professional.
- Emphasize the importance of regular follow-up exams and blood counts to determine progress and monitor for side effects.

## Evaluation
**Effectiveness of therapy can be demonstrated by:** ■ Decrease in viral load and increase in CD4 counts in patients with HIV.

## Antiretrovirals included in *Davis's Drug Guide for Nurses*

***non-nucleoside reverse transcriptase inhibitors***
delavirdine 278
efavirenz 359
nevirapine 743
***nucleoside reverse transcriptase inhibitors***
abacavir 1
didanosine 300
lamivudine 591
stavudine 980

tenofovir disoproxil fumarate 998
zalcitabine 1188
zidovudine 1103

***protease inhibitors***
amprenavir 64
indinavir 546
lopinavir/ritonavir 625
nelfinavir 738
ritonavir 625
saquinavir 952

# ■ ANTIRHEUMATICS

## PHARMACOLOGIC PROFILE

### General Use
Antirheumatics are used to manage symptoms of rheumatoid arthritis (pain, swelling) and in more severe cases to slow down joint destruction and preserve joint function. NSAIDs, aspirin, and other salicylates are used to manage symptoms such as pain and swelling, allowing continued motility and improved quality of life. Corticosteroids are reserved for more ad-

vanced swelling and discomfort, primarily because of their increased side effects, especially with chronic use. They can be used to control acute flares of disease. Neither NSAIDs nor corticosteroids prevent disease progression or joint destruction. Disease-modifying antirheumatics drugs (DMARDs, sometimes called slow-acting agents) slow the progression of rheumatoid arthritis and delay joint destruction. DMARDs are reserved for severe cases because of their toxicity. Several months of therapy may be required before benefit is noted and maintained. Serious and frequent adverse reactions may require discontinuation of therapy, despite initial benefit.

### General Action and Information

Both NSAIDs and corticosteroids have potent anti-inflammatory properties. DMARDs work by a variety of mechanisms. See individual agents, but most work by suppression the auto-immune response thought to be responsible for joint destruction.

### Contraindications

Hypersensitivity. Patients who are allergic to aspirin should not receive other NSAIDs Corticosteroids should not be used in patients with active untreated infections.

### Precautions

NSAIDs and corticosteroids should be used cautiously in patients with a history of GI bleeding. Corticosteroids should be used with caution in diabetic patients. Many DMARDs have immunosuppressive properties and should be avoided in patients for whom immunosuppresion poses a serious risk including patients with active infections, underlying malignancy, and uncontrolled diabetes mellitus.

### Interactions

NSAIDs may diminish the response to diuretics and antihypertensives Corticosteroids may augment hypokalemia from other medications and increase the risk of digoxin toxicity. DMARDs increase the risk of serious immunosuppression with other immunosuppressants.

### NURSING IMPLICATIONS

### Assessment

- Assess patient monthly for pain, swelling, and range of motion.

### Potential Nursing Diagnoses

- Pain, chronic (Indications).
- Knowledge, deficient, related to disease processes and medication regimen.

### Implementation

- Most agents require regular administration to obtain maximum effects.

### Patient/Family Teaching

- Instruct patient to contact health care professional if no improvement is noticed within a few days.

### Evaluation

**Clinical response to therapy can be evaluated by:** ■ Improvement in signs and symptoms of rheumatoid arthritis.

### Antirheumatics included in *Davis's Drug Guide for Nurses*

*corticosteroids*
betamethasone 242
cortisone 242
dexamethasone 242
hydrocortisone 242
methylprednisolone 242

prednisolone 242
prednisone 242
triamcinolone 235

*DMARDs*
anakinra 66
etanercept 400

# ■ ANTITUBERCULARS

## PHARMACOLOGIC PROFILE

### General Use

Used in the treatment and prevention of tuberculosis. Combinations are used in the treatment of active disease tuberculosis to rapidly decrease the infectious state and delay or prevent the emergence of resistant strains. In selected situations, intermittent (twice weekly) regimens may be employed. Streptomycin is also used as an antitubercular. Rifampin is used in the prevention of meningococcal meningitis and *Haemophilus influenzae* type b disease.

### General Action and Information

Kill (tuberculocidal) or inhibit the growth of (tuberculostatic) mycobacteria responsible for causing tuberculosis. Combination therapy with two or more agents is required, unless used as prophylaxis (isoniazid alone).

### Contraindications

Hypersensitivity. Severe liver disease.

### Precautions

Use cautiously in patients with a history of liver disease or in elderly or debilitated patients. Ethambutol requires ophthalmologic follow-up. Safety in pregnancy and lactation not established, although selected agents have been used without adverse effects on the fetus. Compliance is required for optimal response.

### Interactions

Isoniazid inhibits the metabolism of phenytoin Rifampin significantly decreases saquinavir levels (combination should be avoided).

## NURSING IMPLICATIONS

### Assessment

- Mycobacterial studies and susceptibility tests should be performed prior to and periodically throughout therapy to detect possible resistance.
- Assess lung sounds and character and amount of sputum periodically throughout therapy.

### Potential Nursing Diagnoses

- Infection, risk for (Indications).
- Knowledge, deficient, related to disease processes and medication regimen (Patient/Family Teaching).
- Noncompliance (Patient/Family Teaching).

### Implementation

- Most medications can be administered with food or antacids if GI irritation occurs.

## Patient/Family Teaching

- Advise patient of the importance of continuing therapy even after symptoms have subsided.
- Emphasize the importance of regular follow-up exams to monitor progress and check for side effects.
- Inform patients taking rifampin that saliva, sputum, sweat, tears, urine, and feces may become red-orange to red-brown and that soft contact lenses may become permanently discolored.

## Evaluation

**Effectiveness of therapy can be demonstrated by:** ■ Resolution of the signs and symptoms of tuberculosis. Negative sputum cultures.

## Antituberculars included in *Davis's Drug Guide for Nurses*

ethambutol 1168
isoniazid 570
pyrazinamide 1181

rifampin 925
rifapentine 927

# ■ ANTIULCER AGENTS

## PHARMACOLOGIC PROFILE

### General Use

Treatment and prophylaxis of peptic ulcer and gastric hypersecretory conditions such as Zollinger-Ellison syndrome. Histamine $H_2$-receptor antagonists (blockers) and proton pump inhibitors are also used in the management of GERD.

### General Action and Information

Because a great majority of peptic ulcer disease may be traced to GI infection with the organism *Helicobacter pylori*, eradication of the organism decreases symptomatology and recurrence. Anti-infectives with significant activity against the organism include amoxicillin, clarithromycin, metronidazole, and tetracycline Bismuth also has anti-infective activity against *H. pylori* Regimens usually include: a histamine $H_2$-receptor antagonist or a proton pump inhibitor and 2 anti-infectives with or without bismuth subsalicylate for 1-14 days.

Other medications used in the management of gastric/duodenal ulcer disease are aimed at neutralizing gastric acid (antacids), decreasing acid secretion (histamine $H_2$ antagonists, proton pump inhibitors, misoprostol), or protecting the ulcer surface from further damage (misoprostol, sucralfate). Histamine $H_2$-receptor antagonists competitively inhibit the action of histamine at the $H_2$ receptor, located primarily in gastric parietal cells, resulting in inhibition of gastric acid secretion. Misoprostol decreases gastric acid secretion and increases production of protective mucus. Proton pump inhibitors prevent the transport of hydrogen ions into the gastric lumen.

### Contraindications

Hypersensitivity.

### Precautions

Most histamine $H_2$ antagonists require dosage reduction in renal impairment and in elderly patients. Magnesium-containing antacids should be used cautiously in patients with renal impairment. Misoprostol should be used cautiously in women with childbearing potential.

### Interactions

Calcium- and magnesium-containing antacids decrease the absorption of tetracycline and fluoroquinolones. Cimetidine inhibits the ability of the liver to metabolize several drugs, increasing the risk of toxicity from warfarin, tricyclic antidepressants, theophylline, metoprolol, phenytoin, propranolol, and lidocaine. Omeprazole decreases metabolism of phenytoin, diazepam, and warfarin. All agents that increase gastric pH will decrease the absorption of ketoconazole.

## NURSING IMPLICATIONS

### Assessment

- **General Info:** Assess patient routinely for epigastric or abdominal pain and frank or occult blood in the stool, emesis, or gastric aspirate.
- **Antacids:** Assess for heartburn and indigestion as well as the location, duration, character, and precipitating factors of gastric pain.
- **Histamine H$_2$ Antagonists:** Assess elderly and severely ill patients for confusion routinely. Notify physician or other health care professional promptly should this occur.
- **Misoprostol:** Assess women of childbearing age for pregnancy. Medication is usually begun on 2nd or 3rd day of menstrual period following a negative serum pregnancy test within 2 wk of beginning therapy.
- **Lab Test Considerations:** Histamine H$_2$ antagonists antagonize the effects of pentagastrin and histamine during gastric acid secretion test. Avoid administration during the 24 hr preceding the test.
- May cause false-negative results in skin tests using allergen extracts. These drugs should be discontinued 24 hr prior to the test.

### Potential Nursing Diagnoses

- Pain, acute (Indications).
- Knowledge, deficient, related to disease processes and medication regimen (Patient/Family Teaching).

### Implementation

- **Antacids:** Antacids cause premature dissolution and absorption of enteric-coated tablets and may interfere with absorption of other oral medications. Separate administration of antacids and other oral medications by at least 1 hr.
- Shake liquid preparations well before pouring. Follow administration with water to ensure passage to stomach. Liquid and powder dosage forms are considered to be more effective than chewable tablets.
- Chewable tablets must be chewed thoroughly before swallowing. Follow with half a glass of water.
- Administer 1 and 3 hr after meals and at bedtime for maximum antacid effect.
- **Misoprostol:** Administer with meals and at bedtime to reduce the severity of diarrhea.
- **Proton pump inhibitors:** Administer before meals, preferably in the morning. Capsules should be swallowed whole; do not open, crush, or chew.
- May be administered concurrently with antacids.
- **Sucralfate:** Administer on an empty stomach 1 hr before meals and at bedtime. Do not crush or chew tablets. Shake suspension well prior to administration. If nasogastric administration is required, consult pharmacist, as protein-binding properties of sucralfate have resulted in formation of a bezoar when administered with enteral feedings and other medications.

### Patient/Family Teaching

- **General Info:** Instruct patient to take medication as directed for the full course of therapy, even if feeling better. If a dose is missed, it should be taken as soon as remembered but not if almost time for next dose. Do not double doses.
- Advise patient to avoid alcohol, products containing aspirin, NSAIDs, and foods that may cause an increase in GI irritation.
- Advise patient to report onset of black, tarry stools to the physician or other health care professional promptly.

- Inform patient that cessation of smoking may help prevent the recurrence of duodenal ulcers.
- **Antacids:** Caution patient to consult health care professional before taking antacids for more than 2 wk or if problem is recurring. Advise patient to consult health care professional if relief is not obtained or if symptoms of gastric bleeding (black, tarry stools; coffee-ground emesis) occur.
- **Misoprostol:** Emphasize that sharing of this medication may be dangerous.
- Inform patient that misoprostol may cause spontaneous abortion. Women of childbearing age must be informed of this effect through verbal and written information and must use contraception throughout therapy. If pregnancy is suspected, the woman should stop taking misoprostol and immediately notify her health care professional.
- **Sucralfate:** Advise patient to continue with course of therapy for 4–8 wk, even if feeling better, to ensure ulcer healing.
- Advise patient that an increase in fluid intake, dietary bulk, and exercise may prevent drug-induced constipation.

## Evaluation

**Effectiveness of therapy can be demonstrated by:** ■ Decrease in GI pain and irritation. Prevention of gastric irritation and bleeding. Healing of duodenal ulcers can be seen by x-rays or endoscopy. Therapy with histamine $H_2$ antagonists is continued for at least 6 wk after initial episode Decreased symptoms of GERD. Increase in the pH of gastric secretions (antacids). Prevention of gastric ulcers in patients receiving chronic NSAID therapy (misoprostol only).

## Antiulcer agents included in *Davis's Drug Guide for Nurses*

*antacids*
aluminum hydroxide 27
magaldrate 633
magnesium hydroxide/aluminum hydroxide 633

*histamine $H_2$ antagonists*
cimetidine 499
famotidine 499
nizatidine 499
ranitidine bismuth citrate 499
ranitidine 499

*proton-pump inhibitors*
esomeprazole 391

lansoprazole 595
omeprazole 780
rabeprazole 913

*miscellaneous*
amoxicillin 48
bismuth subsalicylate 118
clarithromycin 205
metronidazole 685
misoprostol 697
pantoprazole 812
propantheline 1180
sodium bicarbonate 970
sucralfate 1183

# ■ ANTIVIRALS

## PHARMACOLOGIC PROFILE

### General Use

Acyclovir, famciclovir, and valacylovir are used in the management of herpesvirus infections. Acyclovir also is used in the management of chickenpox. Oseltamivir and zanamivir are used primarily in the prevention of influenza A viral infections. Cidofovir, ganciclovir, valganciclovir, and foscarnet are used in the treatment of cytomegalovirus (CMV) retinitis. Vidarabine is used only to treat ophthalmic viral infections. Penciclovir and docosanol are used in the treatment and prevention of oral-facial herpes simplex.

### General Action and Information

Most agents inhibit viral replication.

**Contraindications**

Previous hypersensitivity.

**Precautions**

All except zanamivir require dosage adjustment in renal impairment. Acyclovir may cause renal impairment. Acyclovir may cause CNS toxicity. Foscarnet increases risk of seizures.

**Interactions**

Acyclovir may have additive CNS and nephrotoxicity with drugs causing similar adverse reactions.

## NURSING IMPLICATIONS

### Assessment

- **General Info:** Assess patient for signs and symptoms of infection before and throughout therapy.
- **Ophth:** Assess eye lesions before and daily during therapy.
- **Topical:** Assess lesions before and daily during therapy.

### Potential Nursing Diagnoses

- Infection, risk for (Indications).
- Skin integrity, impaired (Indications).
- Knowledge, deficient, related to disease processes and medication regimen (Patient/Family Teaching).

### Implementation

- Most systemic antiviral agents should be administered around the clock to maintain therapeutic serum drug levels.

### Patient/Family Teaching

- Instruct patient to continue taking medication around the clock for full course of therapy, even if feeling better.
- Advise patient that antivirals and antiretrovirals do not prevent transmission to others. Precautions should be taken to prevent spread of virus.
- Instruct patient in correct technique for topical or ophthalmic preparations.
- Instruct patient to notify health care professional if symptoms do not improve.

### Evaluation

**Effectiveness of therapy can be demonstrated by:** ■ Prevention or resolution of the signs and symptoms of viral infection. Length of time for complete resolution depends on organism and site of infection.

### Antivirals included in *Davis's Drug Guide for Nurses*

| | |
|---|---|
| acyclovir 8 | lamivudine 591 |
| amantadine 29 | oseltamivir 786 |
| cidofovir 198 | penciclovir 1175 |
| docosanol 1168 | ribavirin 921 |
| famciclovir 411 | valacyclovir 1063 |
| foscarnet 458 | valganciclovir 1066 |
| ganciclovir 468 | zanamivir 1102 |

# ■ BETA BLOCKERS

## PHARMACOLOGIC PROFILE

### General Use

Management of hypertension, angina pectoris, tachyarrhythmias, hypertrophic subaortic stenosis, migraine headache (prophylaxis), MI (prevention), glaucoma (ophthalmic use), CHF (carvedilol and sustained-release metoprolol only) and hyperthyroidism (management of symptoms only).

### General Action and Information

Beta blockers compete with adrenergic (sympathetic) neurotransmitters (epinephrine and norepinephrine) for adrenergic receptor sites. Beta$_1$-adrenergic receptor sites are located chiefly in the heart where stimulation results in increased heart rate, contractility, and AV conduction. Beta$_2$-adrenergic receptors are found mainly in bronchial and vascular smooth muscle and the uterus. Stimulation of beta$_2$-adrenergic receptors produces vasodilation, bronchodilation and uterine relaxation. Blockade of these receptors antagonizes the effects of the neurotransmitters. Beta blockers may be relatively selective for beta$_1$-adrenergic receptors (acebutolol, atenolol, betaxolol, esmolol, and metoprolol) or nonselective (carteolol, carvedilol, labetalol, levobunolol, nadolol, penbutolol, pindolol, propranolol, sotalol, and timolol) blocking both beta$_1$- and beta$_2$-adrenergic receptors. Carvedilol and labetalol have additional alpha-adrenergic blocking properties. Acebutolol, carvedilol, penbutolol, and pindolol possess intrinsic sympathomimetic action (ISA) that may result in less bradycardia than other agents. Ophthalmic beta blockers decrease production of aqueous humor.

### Contraindications

Uncompensated CHF (most beta blockers), acute bronchospasm, some forms of valvular heart disease, bradyarrhythmias, and heart block.

### Precautions

Use cautiously in pregnant and lactating women (may cause fetal bradycardia and hypoglycemia). Use cautiously in any form of lung disease or underlying compensated CHF (most agents). Use with caution in diabetics and patients with severe liver disease. Beta blockers should not be abruptly discontinued in patients with cardiovascular disease.

### Interactions

May cause additive myocardial depression and bradycardia when used with other agents having these effects (digoxin and some antiarrhythmics). May antagonize the therapeutic effects of bronchodilators May alter the requirements for insulin or hypoglyemic agents in diabetics. Cimetidine may decrease the metabolism and increase the effects of some beta blockers.

## NURSING IMPLICATIONS

### Assessment

- **General Info:** Monitor blood pressure and pulse frequently during dosage adjustment and periodically throughout therapy.
- Monitor intake and output ratios and daily weight. Assess patient routinely for signs and symptoms of CHF (dyspnea, rales/crackles, weight gain, peripheral edema, jugular venous distention).
- **Angina:** Assess frequency and severity of episodes of chest pain periodically throughout therapy.
- **Migraine prophylaxis:** Assess frequency and severity of migraine headaches periodically throughout therapy.

### Potential Nursing Diagnoses

- Tissue perfusion, ineffective (Indications).

■ Knowledge, deficient, related to disease processes and medication regimen (Patient/Family Teaching).

■ Noncompliance (Patient/Family Teaching).

## Implementation

■ Take apical pulse prior to administering. If heart rate is <50 bpm or if arrhythmias occur, hold medication and notify health care professional.

■ Many beta blockers are available in combination products to enhance compliance (see Appendix B).

## Patient/Family Teaching

■ **General Info:** Instruct patient to continue taking medication, even if feeling well. Abrupt withdrawal may cause life-threatening arrhythmias, hypertension, or myocardial ischemia. Medication controls but does not cure hypertension.

■ Encourage patient to comply with additional interventions for hypertension (weight reduction, low-sodium diet, regular exercise, smoking cessation, moderation of alcohol consumption, and stress management).

■ Instruct patient and family on proper technique for monitoring blood pressure. Advise them to check blood pressure weekly and report significant changes to health care professional.

■ Caution patient to make position changes slowly to minimize orthostatic hypotension. Advise patient that exercising or hot weather may enhance hypotensive effects.

■ Advise patient to consult health care professional before taking any OTC medications or herbal/alternative therapies, especially cold remedies.

■ Caution patient that these medications may cause increased sensitivity to cold.

■ Diabetics should monitor blood glucose closely, especially if weakness, malaise, irritability, or fatigue occurs.

■ Advise patient to advise health care professional of medication regimen prior to treatment or surgery.

■ Advise patient to carry identification describing disease process and medication regimen at all times.

■ Emphasize the importance of follow-up exams to monitor progress.

■ **Ophth:** Instruct patient in correct technique for administration of ophthalmic preparations.

## Evaluation

**Effectiveness of therapy can be demonstrated by:** ■ Decrease in blood pressure ■ Decrease in frequency and severity of anginal attacks ■ Control of arrhythmias ■ Prevention of myocardial reinfarction ■ Prevention of migraine headaches ■ Decrease in tremors ■ Lowering of intraocular pressure.

## Beta blockers included in *Davis's Drug Guide for Nurses*

*beta blockers (nonselective)*
carteolol 164
carvedilol 166
labetalol 587
nadolol 720
penbutolol 819
pindolol 849
propranolol 891
sotalol 977
timolol 1034

*beta blockers (selective)*
acebutolol 4

atenolol 91
betaxolol 110
bisoprolol 120
esmolol 388
metoprolol 682

*ophthalmic beta blockers*
betaxolol 1150
carteolol 1150
levobetaxolol 1150
levobunolol 1150
metipranolol 1150
timolol 1150

# ■ BONE RESORPTION INHIBITORS

## PHARMACOLOGIC PROFILE

### General Use

Bone resorption inhibitors are primarily used to treat and prevent osteoporosis in postmenopausal women. Other uses include treatment of osteoporosis due to other causes, including corticosteroid therapy, treatment of Paget's disease of the bone, and management of hypercalcemia.

### General Action and Information

Biphosphonates (alendronate, etidronate, risedronate, and tilundronate inhibit resorption of bone by inhibiting hydroxyapatite crystal dissolution and osteoclast activity. Raloxifene binds to estrogen receptors, producing estrogen-like effects on bone including decreased bone resorption and decreased bone turnover.

### Contraindications

Hypersensitivity. Biphosphonates should not be used in patients with hypocalcemia. Raloxifene should not be used in women with child-bearing potential or a history of thromboembolic disease.

### Precautions

Use cautiously in patients with renal impairment; some agents should be avoided in moderate to severe renal impairment.

### Interactions

Calcium supplements decrease absorption of biphosphonates. Tilundronate's effects may be altered by aspirin or other NSAIDs Aspirin may increase GI adverse reactions with alendronate Cholestyramine decreases absorption of raloxifene (concurrent use is contraindicated).

## NURSING IMPLICATIONS

### Assessment

- Assess patients for low bone density before and periodically during therapy.
- Assess for symptoms of Paget's disease (bone pain, headache, decreased visual and auditory acuity, increased skull size).
- **Lab Test Considerations:** Monitor serum calcium in patients with osteoporosis. Monitor alkaline phosphatase in patients with Paget's disease.

### Potential Nursing Diagnoses

- Injury, risk for (Indications).
- Knowledge, deficient, related to disease processes and medication regimen (Patient/Family Teaching).

### Patient/Family Teaching

- Instruct patient to take medication exactly as directed.
- Encourage patient to participate in regular exercise and to modify behaviors that increase the risk of osteoporosis.

### Evaluation

**Clinical response to therapy can be evaluated by:** ■ Prevention of or decrease in the progression of osteoporosis in postmenopausal women. Decrease in the progression of Paget's disease.

**Bone resorption inhibitors included in *Davis's Drug Guide for Nurses***

*biphosphonates*
alendronate 18
etidronate 402
ibandronate 527
pamidronate 806
risedronate 929

tiludronate 1033
zoledronic acid 1108

*selective estrogen receptor modulators*
raloxifene 914

# ■ BRONCHODILATORS

## PHARMACOLOGIC PROFILE

### General Use

Used in the treatment of reversible airway obstruction due to asthma or COPD. Recently revised recommendations for management of asthma recommend that rapid-acting inhaled beta-agonist bronchodilators (not salmeterol) be reserved as acute relievers of bronchospasm; repeated or chronic use indicates the need for additional long-term control agents, including inhaled corticosteroids, mast cell stabilizers, and long-acting bronchodilators (oral theophylline or beta-agonists) and leukotriene modifiers (montelukast, zafirlukast).

### General Action and Information

Beta-adrenergic agonists (albuterol, epinephrine, isoproterenol, metaproterenol, pirbuterol, and terbutaline) produce bronchodilation by stimulating the production of cyclic adenosine monophosphate (cAMP). Newer agents (albuterol, metaproterenol, pirbuterol, and terbutaline) are relatively selective for pulmonary (beta$_2$) receptors, whereas older agents produce cardiac stimulation (beta$_2$-adrenergic effects) in addition to bronchodilation. Onset of action allows use in management of acute attacks except for salmeterol, which has delayed onset. Phosphodiesterase inhibitors (aminophylline and theophylline) inhibit the breakdown of cAMP. Ipratropium is an anticholinergic compound that produces bronchodilation by blocking the action of acetylcholine in the respiratory tract. Montelukast, zafirlukast, and zileuton are leukotriene modifiers Leukotrienes are components of slow-reacting substance of anaphylaxis A (SRS-A), which may be a cause of bronchospasm.

### Contraindications

Hypersensitivity to agents, preservatives (bisulfites), or propellants used in their formulation. Avoid use in uncontrolled cardiac arrhythmias.

### Precautions

Use cautiously in patients with diabetes, cardiovascular disease, or hyperthyroidism.

### Interactions

Therapeutic effectiveness may be antagonized by concurrent use of beta blockers. Additive sympathomimetic effects with other adrenergic (sympathetic) drugs, including vasopressors and decongestants. Cardiovascular effects may be potentiated by antidepressants and MAO inhibitors.

## NURSING IMPLICATIONS

### Assessment

■ Assess blood pressure, pulse, respiration, lung sounds, and character of secretions before and throughout therapy.
■ Patients with a history of cardiovascular problems should be monitored for ECG changes and chest pain.

## Potential Nursing Diagnoses

- Airway clearance, ineffective (Indications).
- Activity intolerance (Indications).
- Knowledge, deficient, related to disease processes and medication regimen (Patient/Family Teaching).

## Implementation

- Administer around the clock to maintain therapeutic plasma levels.

## Patient/Family Teaching

- Emphasize the importance of taking only the prescribed dose at the prescribed time intervals.
- Encourage the patient to drink adequate liquids (2000 ml/day minimum) to decrease the viscosity of the airway secretions.
- Advise patient to avoid OTC cough, cold, or breathing preparations without consulting health care professional and to minimize intake of xanthine-containing foods or beverages (colas, coffee, and chocolate), as these may increase side effects and cause arrhythmias.
- Caution patient to avoid smoking and other respiratory irritants.
- Instruct patient on proper use of metered-dose inhaler (see Appendix F).
- Advise patient to contact health care professional promptly if the usual dose of medication fails to produce the desired results, symptoms worsen after treatment, or toxic effects occur.
- Patients using other inhalation medications and bronchodilators should be advised to use bronchodilator first and allow 5 min to elapse before administering the other medication, unless otherwise directed by health care professional.

## Evaluation

**Effectiveness of therapy can be demonstrated by:** ■ Decreased bronchospasm. Increased ease of breathing.

## Bronchodilators included in *Davis's Drug Guide for Nurses*

*adrenergics*
albuterol 16
epinephrine 366
formoterol 456
levalbuterol 607
metaproterenol 657
pirbuterol 856
salmeterol 950
terbutaline 1003

*anticholinergics*
ipratropium 560
*leukotriene antagonists*
montelukast 706
zafirlukast 1187
zileuton 1188
*xanthines*
aminophylline 126
theophylline 126

# ■ CALCIUM CHANNEL BLOCKERS

## PHARMACOLOGIC PROFILE

### General Use

Used in the treatment of of hypertension (amlodipine, diltiazem, felodipine, isradipine, nicardipine, nifedipine, nisoldipine, verapamil) or in the treatment and prophylaxis of angina pectoris or coronary artery spasm (amlodipine, diltiazem, felodipine, nicardipine, verapamil). Verapamil and diltiazem are also used as antiarrhythmics Nimodipine is used to prevent neurologic damage due to certain types of cerebral vasospasm.

### General Action and Information

Block calcium entry into cells of vascular smooth muscle and myocardium. Dilate coronary arteries in both normal and ischemic myocardium and inhibit coronary artery spasm. Diltiazem and verapamil decrease AV conduction. Nimodipine has a relatively selective effect on cerebral blood vessels.

### Contraindications

Hypersensitivity. Contrainidcated in bradycardia, 2nd- or 3rd-degree heart block, or uncompensated CHF (verapamil).

### Precautions

Safety in pregnancy and lactation not established. Use cautiously in patients with liver disease or uncontrolled arrhythmias.

### Interactions

Additive myocardial depression with beta blockers and disopyramide (diltiazem and verapamil). Effectiveness may be decreased by phenobarbital or phenytoin and increased by propranolol or cimetidine Verapamil and diltiazem may increase serum digoxin levels and cause toxicity.

### NURSING IMPLICATIONS

### Assessment

- **General Info:** Monitor blood pressure and pulse frequently during dosage adjustment and periodically throughout therapy.
- Monitor intake and output ratios and daily weight. Assess patient routinely for signs and symptoms of CHF (dyspnea, rales/crackles, weight gain, peripheral edema, jugular venous distention).
- **Angina:** Assess frequency and severity of episodes of chest pain periodically throughout therapy.
- **Arrhythmias:** ECG should be monitored continuously during IV therapy and periodically during long-term therapy with verapamil.
- **Cerebral vasospasm:** Assess patient's neurological status (level of consciousness, movement) before and periodically during therapy with nimodipine.

### Potential Nursing Diagnoses

- Tissue perfusion, ineffective (Indications).
- Pain, acute (Indications).
- Knowledge, deficient, related to disease processes and medication regimen (Patient/Family Teaching).

### Implementation

- May be administered without regard to meals.
- Do not open, crush, or chew sustained-release capsules.

### Patient/Family Teaching

- **General Info:** Instruct patient to continue taking medication, even if feeling well.
- Caution patient to make position changes slowly to minimize orthostatic hypotension. Advise patient that exercising or hot weather may enhance hypotensive effects.
- Instruct patient on the importance of maintaining good dental hygiene and seeing dentist frequently for teeth cleaning to prevent tenderness, bleeding, and gingival hyperplasia (gum enlargement).
- Advise patient to consult health care professional before taking any OTC medications or herbal/alternative therapies, especially cold remedies.
- Advise patient to advise health care professional of medication regimen prior to treatment or surgery.

- Advise patient to carry identification describing disease process and medication regimen at all times.
- Emphasize the importance of follow-up exams to monitor progress.
- **Angina:** Instruct patients on concurrent nitrate therapy to continue taking both medications as directed and using SL nitroglycerin as needed for anginal attacks. Advise patient to contact health care professional if chest pain worsens or does not improve after therapy, or is accompanied by diaphoresis or shortness or breath, or if severe, persistent headache occurs. Caution patient to discuss exercise precautions with health care professional prior to exertion.
- **Hypertension:** Encourage patient to comply with additional interventions for hypertension (weight reduction, low-sodium diet, regular exercise, smoking cessation, moderation of alcohol consumption, and stress management). Medication controls but does not cure hypertension.
- Instruct patient and family on proper technique for monitoring blood pressure. Advise them to check blood pressure weekly and report significant changes to health care professional.

## Evaluation

**Effectiveness of therapy can be demonstrated by:** ■ Decrease in blood pressure ■ Decrease in frequency and severity of anginal attacks ■ Decrease need for nitrate therapy ■ Increase in activity tolerance and sense of well-being ■ Suppression and prevention of supraventricular tachyarrhythmias ■ Improvement in neurological deficits due to vasospasm following subarachnoid hemorrhage.

### Calcium channel blockers included in *Davis's Drug Guide for Nurses*

amlodipine 47
diltiazem 308
felodipine 412
isradipine 574
nicardipine 747

nifedipine 753
nimodipine 757
nisoldipine 759
verapamil 1077

# ■ CENTRAL NERVOUS SYSTEM STIMULANTS

## PHARMACOLOGIC PROFILE

### General Use
Used in the treatment of narcolepsy and as adjunctive treatment in the management of ADHD.

### General Action and Information
Produce CNS stimulation by increasing levels of neurotransmitters in the CNS. Produce CNS and respiratory stimulation, dilated pupils, increased motor activity and mental alertness, and a diminished sense of fatigue. In children with ADHD these agents decrease restlessness and increase attention span.

### Contraindications
Hypersensitivity. Should not be used in pregnant or lactating women. Should not be used in hyperexcitable states. Avoid using in patients with psychotic personalities or suicidal/homicidal tendencies. Contraindicated in glaucoma and severe cardiovascular disease.

### Precautions
Use cautiously in patients with a history of cardiovascular disease, hypertension, diabetes mellitus, or in elderly or debilitated patients. Continual use may result in psychological dependence or addiction.

## Interactions

Additive sympathomimetic (adrenergic effects). Use with MAO inhibitors can result in hypertensive crises. Alkalinizing the urine (sodium bicarbonate, acetazolamide) decreases excretion and enhances effects of amphetamines Acidification of the urine (ammonium chloride, large doses of ascorbic acid) decreases effect of amphetamines Phenothiazines may also decrease effects. Methylphenidate may decrease the metabolism and increase effects of other drugs (warfarin, anticonvulsants, tricyclic antidepressants).

## NURSING IMPLICATIONS

### Assessment

- **General Info:** Monitor blood pressure, pulse, and respirations before administering and periodically during therapy.
- Monitor weight biweekly and inform health care professional of significant loss.
- Monitor height periodically in children; inform health care professional if growth inhibition occurs.
- May produce false sense of euphoria and well-being. Provide frequent rest periods and observe patient for rebound depression after the effects of the medication have worn off.
- **ADHD:** Assess attention span, impulse control, and interactions with others in children. Therapy may be interrupted at intervals to determine if symptoms are sufficient to warrant continued therapy.
- **Narcolepsy:** Observe and document frequency of episodes.

### Potential Nursing Diagnoses

- Thought processes, disturbed (Side Effects).
- Knowledge, deficient, related to disease processes and medication regimen (Patient/Family Teaching).

### Patient/Family Teaching

- Instruct patient not to alter dose without consulting health care professional. These medications have high dependence and abuse potential. Abrupt cessation with high doses may cause extreme fatigue and mental depression.
- Advise patient to avoid intake of large amounts of caffeine.
- Medication may impair judgment. Caution patient to avoid driving or other activities requiring judgment until response to medication is known.
- Inform patient that periodic holidays from the drug may be used to assess progress and decrease dependence.

### Evaluation

**Clinical response to therapy can be evaluated by:** ■ Decreased frequency of narcoleptic episodes ■ Improved attention span and social interactions.

### Central nervous system stimulants included in *Davis's Drug Guide for Nurses*

amphetamine mixtures 53
dexmethylphenidate 288
dextroamphetamine 290

methylphenidate 675
pemoline 1175

# ■ CORTICOSTEROIDS

## PHARMACOLOGIC PROFILE

### General Use

Used in replacement doses (20 mg of hydrocortisone or equivalent) systemically to treat adrenocortical insufficiency. Larger doses are usually used for their antiinflammatory, immunosuppressive, or antineoplastic activity. Used adjunctively in many other situations, including hypercalcemia and autoimmune diseases. Topical corticosteroids are used in a variety of inflammatory and allergic conditions. Inhalant corticosteroids are used in the chronic management of reversible airway disease (asthma); intranasal and ophthalmic corticosteroids are used in the management of chronic allergic and inflammatory conditions.

### General Action and Information

Produce profound and varied metabolic effects, in addition to modifying the normal immune response and suppressing inflammation. Available in a variety of dosage forms, including oral, injectable, topical, and inhalation. Prolonged used of large amounts of topical or inhaled agent may result in systemic absorption and/or adrenal suppression.

### Contraindications

Serious infections (except for certain forms of meningitis). Do not administer live vaccines to patients on larger doses.

### Precautions

Prolonged treatment will result in adrenal suppression. Do not discontinue abruptly. Additional doses may be needed during stress (surgery and infection). Safety in pregnancy and lactation not established. Long-term use in children will result in decreased growth. May mask signs of infection. Use lowest dose possible for shortest time possible. Alternate-day therapy is preferable during long-term treatment.

### Interactions

Additive hypokalemia with amphotericin B, potassium-losing diuretics, mezlocillin, piperacillin, and ticarcillin Hypokalemia may increase the risk of digoxin toxicity. May increase requirements for insulin or oral hypoglycemic agents Phenytoin, phenobarbital, and rifampin stimulate metabolism and may decrease effectiveness. Oral contraceptives may block metabolism. Cholestyramine and colestipol may decrease absorption.

## NURSING IMPLICATIONS

### Assessment

- These drugs are indicated for many conditions. Assess involved systems prior to and periodically throughout course of therapy.
- Assess patient for signs of adrenal insufficiency (hypotension, weight loss, weakness, nausea, vomiting, anorexia, lethargy, confusion, restlessness) prior to and periodically throughout course of therapy.
- Children should have periodic evaluations of growth.

### Potential Nursing Diagnoses

- Infection, risk for (Side Effects).
- Knowledge, deficient, related to disease processes and medication regimen (Patient/Family Teaching).
- Body image, disturbed (Side Effects).

### Implementation

- **General:** If dose is ordered daily or every other day, administer in the morning to coincide with the body's normal secretion of cortisol.

**CLASSIFICATIONS**

- **PO:** Administer with meals to minimize gastric irritation.

**Patient/Family Teaching**

- Emphasize need to take medication exactly as directed. Review symptoms of adrenal insufficiency that may occur when stopping the medication and that may be life-threatening.
- Encourage patients on long-term therapy to eat a diet high in protein, calcium, and potassium and low in sodium and carbohydrates.
- These drugs cause immunosuppression and may mask symptoms of infection. Instruct patient to avoid people with known contagious illnesses and to report possible infections. Advise patient to consult health care professional before receiving any vaccinations.
- Discuss possible effects on body image. Explore coping mechanisms.
- Advise patient to carry identification in the event of an emergency in which patient cannot relate medical history.

**Evaluation**

**Effectiveness of therapy can be demonstrated by:** ■ Suppression of the inflammatory and immune responses in autoimmune disorders, allergic reactions, and organ transplants ■ Replacement therapy in adrenal insufficiency ■ Resolution of skin inflammation, pruritus, or other dermatologic conditions.

**Corticosteroids included in *Davis's Drug Guide for Nurses***

*corticosteroids, inhalation*
beclomethasone 235
budesonide 235
flunisolide 235
fluticasone 235
triamcinolone 235

*corticosteroids, nasal*
beclomethasone 235
budesonide 235
flunisolide 235
fluticasone 235
mometasone 239
triamcinolone 235

*corticosteroids, ophthalmic*
dexamethasone 1152
flurometholone 1152
loteprednol 1152
medrysone 1152
prednisolone 1152
rimexolone 1152

*corticosteroids, systemic (short-acting)*
cortisone 242
hydrocortisone 242

*corticosteroids, systemic (intermediate-acting)*
methylprednisolone 242
prednisolone 242

prednisone 242
triamcinolone 235

*corticosteroids, systemic (long-acting)*
betamethasone 242
budesonide 235
dexamethasone 242

*corticosteroids, topical/local*
alclometasone 250
amcinonide 250
betamethasone 242
clobetasol 250
clocortolone 250
desonide 235
desoximetasone 250
dexamethasone 242
diflorasone 250
fluocinolone 250
fluocinonide 251
flurandrenolide 251
fluticasone 235
halcinonide 251
halobetasol 251
hydrocortisone 242
methylprednisolone 242
mometasone 239
prednicarbate 251
triamcinolone 235

# ■ DIURETICS

## PHARMACOLOGIC PROFILE

### General Use

Thiazide diuretics and loop diuretics are used alone or in combination in the treatment of hypertension or edema due to CHF or other causes. Potassium-sparing diuretics have weak diuretic and antihypertensive properties and are used mainly to conserve potassium in patients receiving thiazide or loop diuretics. Osmotic diuretics are often used in the management of cerebral edema.

### General Action and Information

Enhance the selective excretion of various electrolytes and water by affecting renal mechanisms for tubular secretion and reabsorption. Groups commonly used are thiazide diuretics and thiazide-like diuretics (chlorothiazide, chlorthalidone, hydrochlorothiazide, indapamide, and metolazone), loop diuretics (bumetanide, furosemide, and toresemide), potassium-sparing diuretics (amiloride, spironolactone, and triamterene), and osmotic diuretics (mannitol). Mechanisms vary, depending on agent.

### Contraindications

Hypersensitivity. Thiazide diuretics may exhibit cross-sensitivity with other sulfonamides.

### Precautions

Use with caution in patients with renal or hepatic disease. Safety in pregnancy and lactation not established.

### Interactions

Additive hypokalemia with corticosteroids, amphotericin B, mezlocillin, piperacillin, or ticarcillin Hypokalemia enhances digitalis glycoside toxicity. Potassium-losing diuretics decrease lithium excretion and may cause toxicity. Additive hypotension with other antihypertensives or nitrates Potassium-sparing diuretics may cause hyperkalemia when used with potassium supplements or ACE inhibitors.

## NURSING IMPLICATIONS

### Assessment

- **General Info:** Assess fluid status throughout therapy. Monitor daily weight, intake and output ratios, amount and location of edema, lung sounds, skin turgor, and mucous membranes.
- Assess patient for anorexia, muscle weakness, numbness, tingling, paresthesia, confusion, and excessive thirst. Notify physician or other health care professional promptly if these signs of electrolyte imbalance occur.
- **Hypertension:** Monitor blood pressure and pulse before and during administration. Monitor frequency of prescription refills to determine compliance in patients treated for hypertension.
- **Increased Intracranial Pressure:** Monitor neurologic status and intracranial pressure readings in patients receiving osmotic diuretics to decrease cerebral edema.
- **Increased Intraocular Pressure:** Monitor for persistent or increased eye pain or decreased visual acuity.
- **Lab Test Considerations:** Monitor electrolytes (especially potassium), blood glucose, BUN, and serum uric acid levels before and periodically throughout course of therapy.
- Thiazide diuretics may cause increased serum cholesterol, low-density lipoprotein (LDL), and triglyceride concentrations.

### Potential Nursing Diagnoses

- Fluid volume, excess (Indications).

- Knowledge, deficient, related to disease processes and medication regimen (Patient/Family Teaching).

## Implementation

- Administer oral diuretics in the morning to prevent disruption of sleep cycle.
- Many diuretics are available in combination with antihypertensives or potassium-sparing diuretics.

## Patient/Family Teaching

- **General Info:** Instruct patient to take medication exactly as directed. Advise patients on antihypertensive regimen to continue taking medication, even if feeling better. Medication controls but does not cure hypertension.
- Caution patient to make position changes slowly to minimize orthostatic hypotension. Caution patient that the use of alcohol, exercise during hot weather, or standing for long periods during therapy may enhance orthostatic hypotension.
- Instruct patient to consult health care professional regarding dietary potassium guidelines.
- Instruct patient to monitor weight weekly and report significant changes.
- Caution patient to use sunscreen and protective clothing to prevent photosensitivity reactions.
- Advise patient to consult health care professional before taking OTC medication concurrently with this therapy.
- Instruct patient to notify health care professional of medication regimen before treatment or surgery.
- Advise patient to contact health care professional immediately if muscle weakness, cramps, nausea, dizziness, or numbness or tingling of extremities occurs.
- Emphasize the importance of routine follow-up.
- **Hypertension:** Reinforce the need to continue additional therapies for hypertension (weight loss, regular exercise, restricted sodium intake, stress reduction, moderation of alcohol consumption, and cessation of smoking).
- Instruct patients with hypertension in the correct technique for monitoring weekly blood pressure.

## Evaluation

**Effectiveness of therapy can be demonstrated by:** ■ Decreased blood pressure ■ Increased urine output ■ Decreased edema ■ Reduced intracranial pressure ■ Prevention of hypokalemia in patients taking diuretics ■ Treatment of hyperaldosteronism.

### Diuretics included in *Davis's Drug Guide for Nurses*

*loop diuretics*
bumetanide 130
furosemide 462
torsemide 1047

*osmotic diuretics*
mannitol 638

*potassium-sparing diuretics*
amiloride 324
spironolactone 324
triamterene 324

*thiazide diuretics*
chlorothiazide 326
chlorthalidone (thiazide–like) 326
hydrochlorothiazide 326

*thiazide-like diuretics*
indapamide 545
metolazone 680

*miscellaneous*
acetazolamide 1158

# ■ HORMONES

## PHARMACOLOGIC PROFILE

### General Use

Used in the treatment of deficiency states including diabetes (insulin), diabetes insipidus (desmopressin), hypothyroidism (thyroid hormones), and menopause (estrogens or estrogens/progestins). Estrogenic and progestational hormones are used as contraceptive agents in various combinations and sequences. Hormones may be used to treat hormonally sensitive tumors (androgens, estrogens) and in other selected situations. See individual drugs.

### General Action and Information

Natural or synthetic substances that have a specific effect on target tissue. Differ greatly in their effects, depending on individual agent and function of target tissue.

### Contraindications

Differ greatly among individual agents; see individual entries.

### Precautions

Differ greatly among individual agents; see individual entries.

### Interactions

Differ greatly among individual agents; see individual entries.

## NURSING IMPLICATIONS

### Assessment

- **General Info:** Monitor patient for symptoms of hormonal excess or insufficiency.
- **Sex Hormones:** Blood pressure and hepatic function tests should be monitored periodically throughout therapy.

### Potential Nursing Diagnoses

- Sexual dysfunction (Indications).
- Body image, disturbed (Indications, Side Effects).
- Knowledge, deficient, related to disease processes and medication regimen (Patient/Family Teaching).

### Implementation

- **Sex Hormones:** During hospitalization, continue to administer according to schedule followed prior to hospitalization.

### Patient/Family Teaching

- **General Info:** Explain dosage schedule (and withdrawal bleeding with female sex hormones).
- Emphasize the importance of follow-up exams to monitor effectiveness of therapy and to ensure proper development of children and early detection of possible side effects.
- **Female Sex Hormones:** Advise patient to report signs and symptoms of fluid retention, thromboembolic disorders, mental depression, or hepatic dysfunction to health care professional.

### Evaluation

**Clinical response to therapy can be evaluated by:** ■ Resolution of clinical symptoms of hormone imbalance including menopause symptoms and contraception ■ Correction of fluid and electrolyte imbalances ■ Control of the spread of advanced metastatic breast or prostate cancer ■ Slowed progression of postmenopausal osteoporosis.

## Hormones included in *Davis's Drug Guide for Nurses*

*hormones*
calcitonin (salmon) 148
danazol 1167
darbepoetin 270
desmopressin 284
epoetin 270
estrogens, conjugated 395
estropipate 398
fludrocortisone 431
glucagon 475
goserelin 1171
insulins 552
leuprolide 604
levothyroxine 1024
liothyronine 1024
liotrix 1024
medroxyprogesterone 229
megestrol 645
nafarelin 723
nandrolone decanoate 729
octreotide 773
oxytocin 800
progesterone 229
somatrem (recombinant) 481
somatropin (recombinant) 481
teriparatide 1005
testosterone 1007
thyroid 1024

triptorelin 1061
vasopressin 1073
*contraceptive hormones*
estradiol cypionate 392
estradiol cypionate/medroxyprogesterone
acetate 229
estradiol transdermal system 392
estradiol vaginal ring 392
estradiol vaginal tablet 392
estradiol valerate 392
ethinyl estradiol/desogestrel 227
ethinyl estradiol/drospirenone 227
ethinyl estradiol/ethynodiol 228
ethinyl estradiol/etonogestrel 229
ethinyl estradiol/levonergestrel 2289
ethinyl estradiol/norelgestromin 229
ethinyl estradiol/norethindrone 228
ethinyl estradiol/norgestimate 228
ethinyl estradiol/norgestrel 228
levonorgestrel 228
levonorgestrel/ethinyl estradiol 229
medroxyprogesterone 229
mestranol/norethindrone 228
norethindrone 228
norethindrone/ethinyl acetate 228
norgestimate/ethinyl estradiol 228
norgestrel 228

# ■ IMMUNOSUPPRESSANTS

## PHARMACOLOGIC PROFILE

### General Use

Azathioprine, basiliximab, cyclosporine, daclizumab, mycophenolate, sirolimus, and tacrolimus are used with corticosteroids in the prevention of transplantation rejection reactions. Muromonab-CD3 is used to manage rejection reactions not controlled by other agents. Azathioprine, cyclophosphamide, and methotrexate are used in the management of selected autoimmune diseases (nephrotic syndrome of childhood and severe rheumatoid arthritis).

### General Action and Information

Inhibit cell-mediated immune responses by different mechanisms. In addition to azathioprine and cyclosporine, which are used primarily for their immunomodulating properties, cyclophosphamide and methotrexate are used to suppress the immune responses in certain disease states (nephrotic syndrome of childhood and severe rheumatoid arthritis). Muromonab-CD3 is a recombinant immunoglobulin antibody that alters T-cell function. Basiliximab and daclizumab are monoclonal antibodies.

### Contraindications

Hypersensitivity to drug or vehicle.

## Precautions

Use cautiously in patients with infections. Safety in pregnancy and lactation not established.

## Interactions

Allopurinol inhibits the metabolism of azathioprine Drugs that alter liver-metabolizing processes may change the effect of cyclosporine The risk to toxicity of methotrexate may be increased by other nephrotoxic drugs, large doses of aspirin, or NSAIDs Muromonab-CD3 has additive immunosuppressive properties; concurrent immunosuppressive doses should be decreased or eliminated.

## NURSING IMPLICATIONS

### Assessment

- **General Info:** Monitor for infection (vital signs, sputum, urine, stool, WBC). Notify physician or other health care professional immediately if symptoms occur.
- **Organ Transplant:** Assess for symptoms of organ rejection throughout therapy.
- **Lab Test Consideration:** Monitor CBC and differential throughout therapy.

### Potential Nursing Diagnoses

- Infection, risk for (Side Effects).
- Knowledge, deficient, related to disease processes and medication regimen (Patient/Family Teaching).

### Implementation

- Protect transplant patients from staff and visitors who may carry infection.
- Maintain protective isolation as indicated.

### Patient/Family Teaching

- Reinforce the need for lifelong therapy to prevent transplant rejection. Review symptoms of rejection for transplanted organ and stress need to notify health care professional immediately if they occur.
- Advise patient to avoid contact with contagious persons and those who have recently taken oral polio virus vaccine. Patients should not receive vaccinations without first consulting with health care professional.
- Emphasize the importance of follow-up exams and lab tests.

### Evaluation

**Effectiveness of therapy can be demonstrated by:** ■ Prevention or reversal of rejection of organ transplants or decrease in symptoms of autoimmune disorders.

### Immunosuppressants included in *Davis's Drug Guide for Nurses*

azathioprine 97
basiliximab 105
chlorambucil 1164
cyclophosphamide 255
cyclosporine 258
daclizumab 267

methotrexate 668
muromonab-CD3 714
mycophenolate 717
sirolimus 967
tacrolimus 990
thalidomide 1184

# ■ LAXATIVES

## PHARMACOLOGIC PROFILE

### General Use
Used to treat or prevent constipation or to prepare the bowel for radiologic or endoscopic procedures.

### General Action and Information
Induce one or more bowel movements per day. Groups include stimulants (bisacodyl, sennosides), saline laxatives (magnesium salts and phosphates), stool softeners (docusate), bulk-forming agents (polycarbophil and psyllium), and osmotic cathartics (lactulose, polyethylene glycol/electrolyte). Increasing fluid intake, exercising, and adding more dietary fiber are also useful in the management of chronic constipation.

### Contraindications
Hypersensitivity. Contraindicated in persistent abdominal pain, nausea, or vomiting of unknown cause, especially if accompanied by fever or other signs of an acute abdomen.

### Precautions
Excessive or prolonged use may lead to dependence. Should not be used in children unless advised by a physician or other health care professional.

### Interactions
Theoretically may decrease the absorption of other orally administered drugs by decreasing transit time.

## NURSING IMPLICATIONS

### Assessment
- Assess patient for abdominal distention, presence of bowel sounds, and usual pattern of bowel function.
- Assess color, consistency, and amount of stool produced.

### Potential Nursing Diagnoses
- Constipation (Indications).
- Knowledge, deficient, related to disease processes and medication regimen (Patient/Family Teaching).

### Implementation
- Many laxatives may be administered at bedtime for morning results.
- Taking oral doses on an empty stomach will usually produce more rapid results.
- Do not crush or chew enteric-coated tablets. Take with a full glass of water or juice.
- Stool softeners and bulk laxatives may take several days for results.

### Patient/Family Teaching
- Advise patients, other than those with spinal cord injuries, that laxatives should be used only for short-term therapy. Long-term therapy may cause electrolyte imbalance and dependence.
- Advise patient to increase fluid intake to a minimum of 1500–2000 ml/day during therapy to prevent dehydration.
- Encourage patients to use other forms of bowel regulation: increasing bulk in the diet, increasing fluid intake, and increasing mobility. Normal bowel habits are individualized and may vary from 3 times/day to 3 times/wk.
- Instruct patients with cardiac disease to avoid straining during bowel movements (Valsalva maneuver).

- Advise patient that laxatives should not be used when constipation is accompanied by abdominal pain, fever, nausea, or vomiting.

### Evaluation

**Effectiveness of therapy can be demonstrated by:** ▪ A soft, formed bowel movement ▪ Evacuation of the colon.

### Laxatives included in *Davis's Drug Guide for Nurses*

*bulk-forming agents*
polycarbophil 1178
psyllium 898

*osmotics*
lactulose 589
polyethylene glycol/electrolyte 863
polyethylene glycol 862

*salines*
magnesium chloride 635
magnesium citrate 635

magnesium gluconate 635
magnesium hydroxide 635
magnesium oxide 635
phosphate/biphosphate 845

*stimulant laxatives*
bisacodyl 116
sennosides 960

*stool softeners*
docusate 333

## ▪ LIPID-LOWERING AGENTS

### PHARMACOLOGIC PROFILE

### General Use

Used as a part of a total plan including diet and exercise to reduce blood lipids in an effort to reduce the morbidity and mortality of atherosclerotic cardiovascular disease and its sequelae.

### General Action and Information

HMG-CoA reductase inhibitors (atorvastatin, fluvastatin, lovastatin, pravastatin, simvastatin) inhibit an enzyme involved in cholesterol synthesis. Bile acid sequestrants (cholestyramine, colestipol, colesevelam) bind cholesterol in the GI tract. Fenofibrate, niacin, and gemfibrozil act by other mechanisms (see individual monographs).

### Contraindications

Hypersensitivity.

### Precautions

Safety in pregnancy, lactation, and children not established. See individual drugs. Dietary therapy should be given a 2–3 mo trial before drug therapy is initiated.

### Interactions

Bile acid sequestrants (cholestyramine and colestipol) may bind lipid-soluble vitamins (A, D, E, and K) and other concurrently administered drugs in the GI tract. The risk of myopathy from HMG-CoA reductase inhibitors is increased by niacin, erythromycin, gemfibrozil, and cyclosporine.

### NURSING IMPLICATIONS

### Assessment

- Obtain a diet history, especially in regard to **fat** and alcohol consumption.
- **Lab Test Considerations:** Serum cholesterol and triglyceride levels should be evaluated before initiating and periodically throughout therapy. Medication should be discontinued if paradoxical increase in cholesterol level occurs.
- Liver function tests should be assessed before and periodically throughout therapy. May cause an increase in levels.

**Potential Nursing Diagnoses**

- Knowledge, deficient, related to disease processes and medication regimen (Patient/Family Teaching).
- Noncompliance (Patient/Family Teaching).

**Implementation**

- See specific medications to determine timing of doses in relation to meals.

**Patient/Family Teaching**

- Advise patient that these medications should be used in conjunction with diet restrictions (fat, cholesterol, carbohydrates, and alcohol), exercise, and cessation of smoking.

**Evaluation**

**Effectiveness of therapy can be demonstrated by:** ■ Decreased serum triglyceride and LDL **cholesterol** levels and improved HDL cholesterol ratios. Therapy is usually discontinued if the clinical response is not evident after 3 mo of therapy.

**Lipid-lowering agents included in *Davis's Drug Guide for Nurses***

*bile acid sequestrants*
cholestyramine 196
colesevelam 225
colestipol 226
*HMG-CoA reductase inhibitors*
atorvastatin 505
fluvastatin 505
lovastatin 505
pravastatin 505

rosuvastatin 505
simvastatin 505
*miscellaneous*
ezetimibe 409
fenofibrate 414
gemfibrozil 474
niacin 745
niacinamide 745

# ■ MINERALS/ELECTROLYTES/pH MODIFIERS

## PHARMACOLOGIC PROFILE

### General Use

Prevention and treatment of deficiencies or excesses of electrolytes and maintenance of optimal acid/base balance for homeostasis. Acidifiers and alkalinizers are also used to promote urinary excretion of substances that accumulate in certain disease states (kidney stones, uric acid).

### General Action and Information

Electrolytes and minerals are necessary for many body processes. Maintenance of electrolyte levels within normal limits is required for many physiological processes such as cardiac, nerve, and muscle function; bone growth and stability and a number of other activities. Minerals and electrolytes may also serve as catalysts in many enzymatic reactions. Acid/base balance allows for normal transfer of substances at the cellular and intracellular level.

### Contraindications

Contraindicated in situations in which replacement would cause excess or when risk factors for retention are present.

### Precautions

Use cautiously in disease states in which electrolyte imbalances are common such as significant hepatic or renal disease, adrenal or pituitary disorders.

## Interactions

Depend on individual agents. Alkalinizers and acidifiers can alter the excretion of drugs for which elimination is pH dependent. See specific entries.

## NURSING IMPLICATIONS

### Assessment

■ Observe patient carefully for evidence of electrolyte excess or insufficiency. Monitor lab values before and periodically throughout therapy.

### Potential Nursing Diagnoses

■ Nutrition, imbalanced: less than body requirements (Indications).
■ Knowledge, deficient, related to medication regimen (Patient/Family Teaching).

### Implementation

■ **Potassium Chloride:** Do not administer potassium chloride undiluted.

### Patient/Family Teaching

■ Review diet modifications with patients with chronic electrolyte disturbances.

### Evaluation

**Clinical response to therapy can be evaluated by:** ■ Return to normal serum electrolyte concentrations and resolution of clinical symptoms of electrolyte imbalance ■ Changes in pH or composition of urine, which prevent formation of renal calculi.

## Minerals/Electrolytes/pH Modifiers included in *Davis's Drug Guide for Nurses*

*alkalinizing agents*
sodium bicarbonate 970
sodium citrate and citric acid 974

*calcium salts*
calcium acetate 150
calcium carbonate 150
calcium chloride 150
calcium citrate 150
calcium gluceptate 150
calcium gluconate 150
calcium lactate 150
tricalcium phosphate 150

*magnesium salts*
magnesium chloride 635
magnesium citrate 635
magnesium gluconate 635
magnesium hydroxide 635
magnesium oxide 635
magnesium sulfate 637

*phosphate supplements*
sodium phosphate 864

*potassium and sodium phosphates*
monobasic potassium phosphate 864
monobasic potassium and sodium phosphates 864

potassium phosphates 864
potassium and sodium phosphates 864

*potassium phosphates*
monobasic potassium phosphate 864
potassium phosphate 864
potassium phosphates 864

*potassium salts*
potassium acetate 866
potassium bicarbonate 866
potassium bicarbonate/potassium chloride 866
potassium bicarbonate/potassium citrate 866
potassium chloride 866
potassium chloride/potassium bicarbonate/ potassium citrate 867
potassium gluconate 867
potassium gluconate/potassium chloride 867
potassium gluconate/potassium citrate 867

*miscellaneous*
sodium chloride 972
sodium phosphate 864
zinc sulfate 1189

# ■ NATURAL/HERBAL PRODUCTS

## PHARMACOLOGIC PROFILE

### General Use

These remedies are used for wide variety of conditions. Prescriptions are not required and consumers have the choice of many products.

### General Action and Information

Usage of these agents is based on historical and sometimes anecdotal evidence. The FDA has little control over these agents, so currently there is little standardization among products.

### Contraindications

Hypersensitivity. Most products are plant extracts that may contain a variety of impurities.

### Precautions

Elderly, pediatric, and pregnant or lactating patients should be aware that these agents carry many of the same risks as prescription medications. Patients with serious chronic medical conditions should consult their health care professional before use.

### Interactions

These agents have the ability to interact with prescription medications and may prevent or augment a desired therapeutic outcome. *St. John's wort* and *kava-kava* have the greatest risk for serious interactions.

## NURSING IMPLICATIONS

### Assessment

■ Assess the condition for which the patient is taking the product.

### Potential Nursing Diagnoses

■ Knowledge, deficient, related to disease processes and medication regimen (Patient/Family Teaching).

### Patient/Family Teaching

■ Discuss with patient the reason for using the product. Encourage patient to choose products with USP label, if possible, to guarantee content and purity of medication.
■ Inform patient of known side effects and interactions with other medications.

### Evaluation

**Clinical response to therapy can be evaluated by:** ■ Improvement in condition for which medication was taken.

### Natural/Herbal Products included in *Davis's Drug Guide for Nurses*

| | |
|---|---|
| arnica 1190 | ginseng 1202 |
| black cohosh 1191 | glucosamine 1203 |
| chondroitin 1193 | hawthorne 1204 |
| dongquai 1194 | kava-kava 1206 |
| echinacea 1195 | milk thistle 1207 |
| feverfew 1196 | SAMe 1209 |
| garlic 1198 | saw palmetto 1210 |
| ginger 1199 | St. John's wort 1211 |
| ginkgo 1200 | valerian 1212 |

# ■ NONOPIOID ANALGESICS

## PHARMACOLOGIC PROFILE

### General Use

Used to control mild to moderate pain and/or fever. Phenazopyridine is used only to treat urinary tract pain, and capsaicin is used topically for a variety of painful syndromes.

### General Action and Information

Most nonopioid analgesics inhibit prostaglandin synthesis peripherally for analgesic effect and centrally for antipyretic effect. Tramadol is a centrally acting agent.

### Contraindications

Hypersensitivity and cross-sensitivity among NSAIDs may occur.

### Precautions

Use cautiously in patients with severe hepatic or renal disease, chronic alcohol use/abuse, or malnutrition. Tramadol has CNS depressant properties.

### Interactions

Long-term use of acetaminophen with NSAIDs may increase the risk of adverse renal effects. Prolonged high-dose acetaminophen may increase the risk of bleeding with warfarin Hepatotoxicity may be additive with other hepatotoxic agents, including alcohol NSAIDs increase the risk of bleeding with warfarin, thrombolytic agents, antiplatelet agents, some cephalosporins, and valproates (effect is greatest with aspirin). NSAIDs may also decrease the effectiveness of diuretics and antihypertensives The risk of CNS depression with tramadol is increased by concurrent use of other CNS depressants, including alcohol, antihistamines, sedative/hypnotics, and some antidepressants.

## NURSING IMPLICATIONS

### Assessment

- **General Info:** Patients who have asthma, allergies, and nasal polyps or who are allergic to tartrazine are at an increased risk for developing hypersensitivity reactions.
- **Pain:** Assess pain and limitation of movement; note type, location, and intensity prior to and at the peak (see Time/Action Profile) following administration.
- **Fever:** Assess fever and note associated signs (diaphoresis, tachycardia, malaise, chills).
- **Lab Test Considerations:** Hepatic, hematologic, and renal function should be evaluated periodically throughout prolonged high-dose therapy. Aspirin and most NSAIDs prolong bleeding time due to suppressed platelet aggregation and, in large doses, may cause prolonged prothrombin time. Monitor hematocrit periodically in prolonged high-dose therapy to assess for GI blood loss.

### Potential Nursing Diagnoses

- Pain, acute (Indications).
- Body temperature, risk for imbalanced (Indications).
- Knowledge, deficient, related to disease processes and medication regimen (Patient/Family Teaching).

### Implementation

- **PO:** Administer salicylates and NSAIDs after meals or with food or an antacid to minimize gastric irritation.

### Patient/Family Teaching

- Instruct patient to take salicylates and NSAIDs with a full glass of water and to remain in an upright position for 15–30 min after administration.

- Adults should not take acetaminophen longer than 10 days and children not longer than 5 days unless directed by health care professional. Short-term doses of acetaminophen with salicylates or NSAIDs should not exceed the recommended daily dose of either drug alone.
- Caution patient to avoid concurrent use of alcohol with this medication to minimize possible gastric irritation; 3 or more glasses of alcohol per day may increase the risk of GI bleeding with salicylates or NSAIDs Caution patient to avoid taking acetaminophen, salicylates, or NSAIDs concurrently for more than a few days, unless directed by health care professional to prevent analgesic nephropathy.
- Advise patients on long-term therapy to inform health care professional of medication regimen prior to surgery. Aspirin, salicylates, and NSAIDs may need to be withheld prior to surgery.

## Evaluation

**Effectiveness of therapy can be demonstrated by:** ■ Relief of mild to moderate discomfort ■ Reduction of fever.

### Nonopioid analgesics included in *Davis's Drug Guide for Nurses*

## ■ NONSTEROIDAL ANTI-INFLAMMATORY AGENTS

### PHARMACOLOGIC PROFILE

#### General Use

NSAIDs are used to control mild to moderate pain, fever, and various inflammatory conditions, such as rheumatoid arthritis and osteoarthritis. Ophthalmic NSAIDs are used to decrease postoperative ocular inflammation, to inhibit perioperative miosis, and to decrease inflammation due to allergies.

#### General Action and Information

NSAIDs have analgesic, antipyretic, and anti-inflammatory properties. Analgesic and anti-inflammatory effects are due to inhibition of prostaglandin synthesis. Antipyretic action is due to vasodilation and inhibition of prostaglandin synthesis in the CNS. COX-2 inhibitors (celecoxib, rofecoxib, valdecoxib) may cause less GI bleeding.

#### Contraindications

Hypersensitivity to aspirin is a contraindication for the whole group of NSAIDs Cross-sensitivity may occur.

## Precautions

Use cautiously in patients with a history of bleeding disorders, GI bleeding, and severe hepatic, renal, or cardiovascular disease. Safe use in pregnancy is not established and, in general, should be avoided during the second half of pregnancy.

## Interactions

NSAIDs prolong bleeding time and potentiate the effect of warfarin, thrombolytic agents, plicamycin, some cephalosporins, antiplatelet agents, and valproates Prolonged use with aspirin may result in increased GI side effects and decreased effectiveness. NSAIDs may also decrease response to diuretics or antihypertensive therapy. Ibuprofen negates the cardioprotective benefits of low-dose aspirin COX-2 inhibitors do not negate the cardioprotective effect of low-dose aspirin.

## NURSING IMPLICATIONS

### Assessment

- **General Info:** Patients who have asthma, allergies, and nasal polyps or who are allergic to tartrazine are at an increased risk for developing hypersensitivity reactions.
- **Pain:** Assess pain and limitation of movement; note type, location, and intensity prior to and at the peak (see Time/Action Profile) following administration.
- **Fever:** Assess fever and note associated signs (diaphoresis, tachycardia, malaise, chills).
- **Lab Test Considerations:** Most NSAIDs prolong bleeding time due to suppressed platelet aggregation and, in large doses, may cause prolonged PT. Monitor periodically in prolonged high-dose therapy to assess for GI blood loss.

### Potential Nursing Diagnoses

- Pain, acute (Indications).
- Body temperature, risk for imbalanced (Indications).
- Knowledge, deficient, related to disease processes and medication regimen (Patient/Family Teaching).

### Implementation

- **PO:** Administer NSAIDs after meals or with food or an antacid to minimize gastric irritation.

### Patient/Family Teaching

- Instruct patient to take NSAIDs with a full glass of water and to remain in an upright position for 15–30 min after administration.
- Caution patient to avoid concurrent use of alcohol with this medication to minimize possible gastric irritation; 3 or more glasses of alcohol per day may increase the risk of GI bleeding with salicylates or NSAIDs Caution patient to avoid taking acetaminophen, salicylates, or NSAIDs concurrently for more than a few days, unless directed by health care professional to prevent analgesic nephropathy.
- Advise patient on long-term therapy to inform health care professional of medication regimen prior to surgery. NSAIDs may need to be withheld prior to surgery.

### Evaluation

**Effectiveness of therapy can be demonstrated by:** ■ Relief of mild to moderate discomfort ■ Reduction of fever.

C

L

A

S

S

I

F

I

C

A

T

I

O

N

S

Nonsteroidal anti-inflammatory agents included in *Davis's Drug Guide for Nurses*

**nonsteroidal anti-inflammatory agents**
celecoxib 171
diclofenac 296
flurbiprofen 1169
ibuprofen 528
indomethacin 548
ketoprofen 580
ketorolac 583
meloxicam 647
nabumetone 719

naproxen 730
oxaprozin 788
piroxicam 858
sulindac 984
tolmetin 1185
valdecoxib 1064
**ophthalmic NSAIDs**
diclofenac 1154
flurbiprofen 1154
ketorolac 1155
suprofen 1155

# ■ OPIOID ANALGESICS

## PHARMACOLOGIC PROFILE

### General Use
Management of moderate to severe pain. Fentanyl is used as a general anesthetic adjunct.

### General Action and Information
Opioids bind to opiate receptors in the CNS, where they act as agonists of endogenously occurring opioid peptides (eukephalins and endorphins). The result is alteration to the perception of and response to pain.

### Contraindications
Hypersensitivity to individual agents.

### Precautions
Use cautiously in patients with undiagnosed abdominal pain, head trauma or pathology, liver disease, or history of addiction to opioids Use smaller doses initially in the elderly and those with respiratory diseases. Prolonged use may result in tolerance and the need for larger doses to relieve pain. Psychological or physical dependence may occur.

### Interactions
Increases the CNS depressant properties of other drugs, including alcohol, antihistamines, antidepressants, sedative/hypnotics, phenothiazines, and MAO inhibitors Use of partial-antagonist opioid analgesics (buprenorphine, butorphanol, nalbuphine, and pentazocine) may precipitate opioid withdrawal in physically dependent patients. Use with MAO inhibitors or procarbazine may result in severe paradoxical reactions (especially with meperidine). Nalbuphine or pentazocine may decrease the analgesic effects of other concurrently administered opioid analgesics.

## NURSING IMPLICATIONS

### Assessment
- Assess type, location, and intensity of pain prior to and at peak following administration. When titrating opioid doses, increases of 25–50% should be administered until there is either a 50% reduction in the patient's pain rating on a numerical or visual analogue scale or the patient reports satisfactory pain relief. A repeat dose can be safely administered at the time of the peak if previous dose is ineffective and side effects are minimal. Patients requiring higher doses of opioid agonist-antagonists should be converted to an opioid agonist.

- Opioid agonist-antagonists are not recommended for prolonged use or as first-line therapy for acute or cancer pain.
- An equianalgesic chart (see Appendix O) should be used when changing routes or when changing from one opioid to another.
- Assess blood pressure, pulse, and respirations before and periodically during administration. If respiratory rate is <10/min, assess level of sedation. Physical stimulation may be sufficient to prevent significant hypoventilation. Dose may need to be decreased by 25–50%. Initial drowsiness will diminish with continued use.
- Assess prior analgesic history. Antagonistic properties of agonist-antagonists may induce withdrawal symptoms (vomiting, restlessness, abdominal cramps, and increased blood pressure and temperature) in patients physically dependent on opioids.
- Prolonged use may lead to physical and psychological dependence and tolerance. This should not prevent patient from receiving adequate analgesia. Most patients who receive opioid analgesics for pain do not develop psychological dependence. Progressively higher doses may be required to relieve pain with chronic therapy.
- Assess bowel function routinely. Prevention of constipation should be instituted with increased intake of fluids and bulk, stool softeners, and laxatives to minimize constipating effects. Stimulant laxatives should be administered routinely if opioid use exceeds 2–3 days, unless contraindicated.
- Monitor intake and output ratios. If significant discrepancies occur, assess for urinary retention and inform physician or other health care professional.
- **Toxicity and Overdose:** If an opioid antagonist is required to reverse respiratory depression or coma, naloxone (Narcan) is the antidote. Dilute the 0.4-mg ampule of naloxone in 10 ml of 0.9% NaCl and administer 0.5 ml (0.02 mg) by direct IV push every 2 min. For children and patients weighing <40 kg, dilute 0.1 mg of naloxone in 10 ml of 0.9% NaCl for a concentration of 10 mcg/ml and administer 0.5 mcg/kg every 1–2 min. Titrate dose to avoid withdrawal, seizures, and severe pain.

## Potential Nursing Diagnoses

- Pain, acute (Indications).
- Sensory perception, disturbed (auditory, visual) (Side Effects).
- Injury, risk for (Side Effects).
- Knowledge, deficient, related to disease processes and medication regimen (Patient/Family Teaching).

## Implementation

- Do not confuse morphine with hydromorphone or meperidine; errors have resulted in fatalities.
- Explain therapeutic value of medication before administration to enhance the analgesic effect.
- Regularly administered doses may be more effective than prn administration. Analgesic is more effective if given before pain becomes severe.
- Coadministration with nonopioid analgesics may have additive analgesic effects and may permit lower doses.
- Medication should be discontinued gradually after long-term use to prevent withdrawal symptoms.

## Patient/Family Teaching

- Instruct patient on how and when to ask for pain medication.
- Medication may cause drowsiness or dizziness. Caution patient to call for assistance when ambulating or smoking and to avoid driving or other activities requiring alertness until response to medication is known.
- Advise patient to make position changes slowly to minimize orthostatic hypotension.

- Caution patient to avoid concurrent use of alcohol or other CNS depressants with this medication.
- Encourage patient to turn, cough, and breathe deeply every 2 hr to prevent atelectasis.

### Evaluation

**Effectiveness of therapy can be demonstrated by:** ■ Decreased severity of pain without a significant alteration in level of consciousness or respiratory status.

### Opioid analgesics included in *Davis's Drug Guide for Nurses*

*opioid agonists/antagonists*
buprenorphine 132
butorphanol 143
pentazocine 1176

*opioid agonists*
codeine 1126
fentanyl (oral transmucosal) 417
fentanyl (parenteral) 419
fentanyl (transdermal) 422

hydrocodone 510
hydromorphone 513
meperidine 650
methadone 662
morphine 709
nalbuphine 724
oxycodone 795
oxymorphone 798
propoxyphene 888

## ■ SEDATIVE/HYPNOTICS

### PHARMACOLOGIC PROFILE

### General Use

Sedatives are used to provide sedation, usually prior to procedures. Hypnotics are used to manage insomnia. Selected agents are useful as anticonvulsants (clorazepate, diazepam, phenobarbital), skeletal muscle relaxants (diazepam), adjuncts in the management of alcohol withdrawal syndrome (chlordiazepoxide, diazepam, oxazepam), as adjuncts in general anesthesia (droperidol) or amnestics (midazolam, diazepam).

### General Action and Information

Cause generalized CNS depression. May produce tolerance with chronic use and have potential for psychological or physical dependence. These agents have NO analgesic properties.

### Contraindications

Hypersensitivity. Should not be used in comatose patients nor in those with pre-existing CNS depression. Should not be used in patients with uncontrolled severe pain. Avoid use during pregnancy or lactation.

### Precautions

Use cautiously in patients with hepatic dysfunction, severe renal impairment, or severe underlying pulmonary disease. Use with caution in patients who may be suicidal or who may have had previous drug addictions. Hypnotic use should be short-term. Geriatric patients may be more sensitive to CNS depressant effects; dosage reduction may be required.

### Interactions

Additive CNS depression with alcohol, antihistamines, some antidepressants, opioid analgesics, or phenothiazines Barbiturates induce hepatic drug-metabolizing enzymes and can decrease the effectiveness of drugs metabolized by the liver, including oral contraceptives. Should not be used with MAO inhibitors.

## NURSING IMPLICATIONS

### Assessment

- **General Info:** Monitor blood pressure, pulse, and respiratory status frequently throughout IV administration. Prolonged high-dose therapy may lead to psychological or physical dependence. Restrict the amount of drug available to patient, especially if patient is depressed, suicidal, or has a history of addiction.
- **Insomnia:** Assess sleep patterns before and periodically throughout course of therapy.
- **Seizures:** Observe and record intensity, duration, and characteristics of seizure activity. Institute seizure precautions.
- **Muscle Spasms:** Assess muscle spasms, associated pain, and limitation of movement before and throughout therapy.
- **Alcohol Withdrawal:** Assess patient experience alcohol withdrawal for tremors, agitation, delirium, and hallucinations. Protect patient from injury.

### Potential Nursing Diagnoses

- Sleep pattern disturbed (Indications).
- Injury, risk for (Side Effects).
- Knowledge, deficient, related to disease processes and medication regimen (Patient/Family Teaching).

### Implementation

- Supervise ambulation and transfer of patients following administration of hypnotic doses. Remove cigarettes. Side rails should be raised and call bell within reach at all times. Keep bed in low position.

### Patient/Family Teaching

- Discuss the importance of preparing the environment for sleep (dark room, quiet, avoidance of nicotine and caffeine). If less effective after a few weeks, consult health care professional; do not increase dose. Gradual withdrawal may be required to prevent reactions following prolonged therapy.
- May cause daytime drowsiness. Caution patient to avoid driving and other activities requiring alertness until response to medication is known.
- Advise patient to avoid the use of alcohol and other CNS depressants concurrently with these medications.
- Advise patient to inform health care professional if pregnancy is planned or suspected.

### Evaluation

**Effectiveness of therapy can be demonstrated by:** ■ Improvement in sleep patterns ■ Control of seizures ■ Decrease in muscle spasms ■ Decreased tremulousness ■ More rational ideation when used for alcohol withdrawal.

### Sedative/hypnotics included in *Davis's Drug Guide for Nurses*

*barbiturates*
phenobarbital 1135

*benzodiazepines*
chlordiazepoxide 191
clorazepate 216
diazepam 293
flurazepam 451
lorazepam 629
midazolam 687
oxazepam 789

temazepam 997
triazolam 1055

*miscellaneous*
droperidol 353
promethazine 882
chloral hydrate 189
dexmedetomidine 287
hydroxyzine 518
zaleplon 1101
zolpidem 1111

# ■ SKELETAL MUSCLE RELAXANTS

## PHARMACOLOGIC PROFILE

### General Use

Two major uses are spasticity associated with spinal cord diseases or lesions (baclofen and dantrolene) or adjunctive therapy in the symptomatic relief of acute painful musculoskeletal conditions (cyclobenzaprine, diazepam, and methocarbamol). IV dantrolene is also used to treat and prevent malignant hyperthermia.

### General Action and Information

Act either centrally (baclofen, carisoprodol, cyclobenzaprine, diazepam, and methocarbamol) or directly (dantrolene).

### Contraindications

Baclofen and oral dantrolene should not be used in patients in whom spasticity is used to maintain posture and balance.

### Precautions

Safety in pregnancy and lactation not established. Use cautiously in patients with a history of previous liver disease.

### Interactions

Additive CNS depression with other CNS depressants, including alcohol, antihistamines, antidepressants, opioid analgesics, and sedative/hypnotics.

## NURSING IMPLICATIONS

### Assessment

■ Assess patient for pain, muscle stiffness, and range of motion before and periodically throughout therapy.

### Potential Nursing Diagnoses

■ Pain, acute (Indications).
■ Mobility, impaired physical (Indications).
■ Injury, risk for (Side Effects).

### Implementation

■ Provide safety measures as indicated. Supervise ambulation and transfer of patients.

### Patient/Family Teaching

■ Encourage patient to comply with additional therapies prescribed for muscle spasm (rest, physical therapy, heat).
■ Medication may cause drowsiness. Caution patient to avoid driving or other activities requiring alertness until response to drug is known.
■ Advise patient to avoid concurrent use of alcohol or other CNS depressants with these medications.

### Evaluation

**Effectiveness of therapy can be demonstrated by:** ■ Decreased musculoskeletal pain ■ Decreased muscle spasticity ■ Increased range of motion ■ Prevention or decrease in temperature and skeletal rigidity in malignant hyperthermia.

### Skeletal muscle relaxants included in *Davis's Drug Guide for Nurses*

*centrally-acting*
diazepam 293
orphenadrine 785
baclofen 103
carisoprodol 160
chlorzoxazone 195

cyclobenzaprine 254
metaxalone 659
methocarbamol 666
*direct-acting*
dantrolene 268

# ■ THROMBOLYTICS

## PHARMACOLOGIC PROFILE

### General Use

Acute management of coronary thrombosis (MI). Streptokinase and urokinase are used in the management of massive pulmonary emboli, deep vein thrombosis, and arterial thromboembolism. Alteplase is used in the management of acute ischemic stroke.

### General Action and Information

Converts plasminogen to plasmin, which then degrades fibrin in clots. Alteplase, reteplase, and urokinase directly activate plasminogen. Anistreplase and streptokinase bind with plasminogen to form activator complexes, which then convert plasminogen to plasmin. Results in lysis of thrombi in coronary arteries, pulmonary emboli, or deep vein thrombosis, or clearing of clots in cannulae/catheters.

### Contraindications

Hypersensitivity. Cross-sensitivity with anistreplase and streptokinase may occur. Contraindicated in active internal bleeding, history of cerebrovascular accident, recent CNS trauma or surgery, neoplasm, or arteriovenous malformation. Severe uncontrolled hypertension and known bleeding tendencies.

### Precautions

Recent (within 10 days) major surgery, trauma, GI or GU bleeding. Severe hepatic or renal disease. Subacute bacterial endocarditis or acute pericarditis. Use cautiously in geriatric patients. Safety not established in pregnancy, lactation, or children.

### Interactions

Concurrent use with aspirin, NSAIDs, warfarin, heparins, abciximab, ticlopidine, or dipyridamole may increase the risk of bleeding, although these agents are frequently used together or in sequence. Risk of bleeding may also be increased by concurrent use with cefotetan, cefoperazone, plicamycin, and valproic acid.

## NURSING IMPLICATIONS

### Assessment

- Begin therapy as soon as possible after the onset of symptoms.
- Monitor vital signs, including temperature, continuously for coronary thrombosis and at least every 4 hr during therapy for other indications. Do not use lower extremities to monitor blood pressure.
- Assess patient carefully for bleeding every 15 min during the 1st hr of therapy, every 15–30 min during the next 8 hr, and at least every 4 hr for the duration of therapy. Frank bleeding may occur from sites of invasive procedures or from body orifices. Internal bleeding may also occur (decreased neurologic status; abdominal pain with coffee-ground emesis or black, tarry stools; hematuria; joint pain). If uncontrolled bleeding occurs, stop medication and notify physician immediately.

- Inquire about previous reaction to anistreplase or streptokinase therapy. Assess patient for hypersensitivity reaction (rash, dyspnea, fever, changes in facial color, swelling around the eyes, wheezing). If these occur, inform physician promptly. Keep epinephrine, an antihistamine, and resuscitation equipment close by in the event of an anaphylactic reaction.
- Inquire about recent streptococcal infection. Anistreplase and streptokinase may be less effective if administered between 5 days and 6 mo of a streptococcal infection.
- Assess neurologic status throughout therapy.
- Altered sensorium or neurologic changes may be indicative of intracranial bleeding.
- **Coronary Thrombosis:** Monitor ECG continuously. Notify physician if significant arrhythmias occur. IV lidocaine or procainamide (Pronestyl) may be ordered prophylactically. Cardiac enzymes should be monitored. Radionuclide myocardial scanning and/or coronary angiography may be ordered 7–10 days following therapy to monitor effectiveness of therapy.
- Monitor heart sounds and breath sounds frequently. Inform physician if signs of CHF occur (rales/crackles, dyspnea, S3 heart sound, jugular venous distention, relieved CVP).
- **Pulmonary Embolism:** Monitor pulse, blood pressure, hemodynamics, and respiratory status (rate, degree of dyspnea, arterial blood gases).
- **Deep Vein Thrombosis/Acute Arterial Occlusion:** Observe extremities and palpate pulses of affected extremities every hour. Notify physician immediately if circulatory impairment occurs. Computed tomography, impedance plethysmography, quantitative Doppler effect determination, and/or angiography or venography may be used to determine restoration of blood flow and duration of therapy; however, repeated venograms are not recommended.
- **Cannula/Catheter Occlusion:** Monitor ability to aspirate blood as indicator of patency. Ensure that patient exhales and holds breath when connecting and disconnecting IV syringe to prevent air embolism.
- **Acute Ischemic Stroke:** Assess neurologic status. Determine time of onset of stroke symptoms. Alteplase must be administered within 3 hr of onset.
- **Lab Test Considerations:** Hematocrit, hemoglobin, platelet count, fibrin/fibrin degradation product (FDP/fdp) titer, fibrinogen concentration, prothrombin time, thrombin time, and activated partial thromboplastin time may be evaluated prior to and frequently throughout therapy. Bleeding time may be assessed prior to therapy if patient has received platelet aggregation inhibitors. Obtain type and cross match and have blood available at all times in case of hemorrhage. Stools should be tested for occult blood loss and urine for hematuria periodically during therapy.
- **Toxicity and Overdose:** If local bleeding occurs, apply pressure to site. If severe or internal bleeding occurs, discontinue infusion. Clotting factors and/or blood volume may be restored through infusions of whole blood, packed RBCs, fresh frozen plasma, or cryoprecipitate. Do not administer dextran, as it has antiplatelet activity. Aminocaproic acid (Amicar) may be used as an antidote.

## Potential Nursing Diagnoses

- Tissue perfusion, ineffective (Indications).
- Injury, risk for (Side Effects).
- Knowledge, deficient, related to disease processes and medication regimen (Patient/Family Teaching).

## Implementation

- This medication should be used only in settings in which hematologic function and clinical response can be adequately monitored.
- Starting two IV lines prior to therapy is recommended: one for the thrombolytic agent, the other for any additional infusions.
- Avoid invasive procedures, such as IM injections or arterial punctures, with this therapy. If such procedures must be performed, apply pressure to all arterial and venous puncture

sites for at least 30 min. Avoid venipunctures at noncompressible sites (jugular vein, subclavian site).

- Systemic anticoagulation with heparin is usually begun several hours after the completion of thrombolytic therapy.
- Acetaminophen may be ordered to control fever.

### Patient/Family Teaching

- Explain purpose of medication and the need for close monitoring to patient and family. Instruct patient to report hypersensitivity reactions (rash, dyspnea) and bleeding or bruising.
- Explain need for bedrest and minimal handling during therapy to avoid injury. Avoid all unnecessary procedures such as shaving and vigorous tooth brushing.

### Evaluation

**Effectiveness of therapy can be demonstrated by:** ■ Lysis of thrombi and restoration of blood flow ■ Prevention of neurologic sequelae in acute ischemic stroke ■ Cannula or catheter patency.

### Thrombolytics included in *Davis's Drug Guide for Nurses*

| | |
|---|---|
| alteplase 1018 | streptokinase 1018 |
| anistreplase 1018 | tenecteplase 1018 |
| reteplase 1018 | urokinase 1018 |

# ■ VACCINES/IMMUNIZING AGENTS

## PHARMACOLOGIC PROFILE

### General Use

Immune globulins provide passive immunization to infectious diseases by providing antibodies. Immunization with vaccines and toxoids containing bacterial or viral antigenic material results in endogenous production of antibodies.

### General Action and Information

Immunity from immune globulins is rapid, but short-lived (up to 3 months). Active immunization with vaccine or toxoids produces prolonged immunity (years).

### Contraindications

Hypersensitivity to product, preservatives, or other additives. Some products contain thimerisol, neomycin, and/or **egg protein.**

### Precautions

Severe bleeding problems (IM injections).

### Interactions

Decreased antibody response to vaccine/toxoids and increased risk of adverse reactions in patients receiving concurrent antineoplastic, immunosuppressive, or radiation therapy.

## NURSING IMPLICATIONS

### Assessment

- Assess previous immunization history and history of hypersensitivity.

### Potential Nursing Diagnoses

- Infection, risk for (Indications).
- Knowledge, deficient, related to disease processes and medication regimen (Patient/Family Teaching).

## Implementation

- Measles, mumps, and rubella vaccine, trivalent oral polio virus vaccine, and diptheria toxoid, tetanus toxoid, and pertussis vaccine may be given concurrently.
- Administer each immunization by appropriate route.

## Patient/Family Teaching

- Inform patient/parent of potential and reportable side effects of immunization. Health care professional should be notified if patient develops fever over 39.4°C (103°F); difficulty breathing; hives; itching; swelling of the eyes, face, or inside of nose; sudden severe tiredness or weakness; or convulsions occur.
- Review next scheduled immunization with parent. Emphasize the importance of keeping a record of immunizations and dates given.

## Evaluation

**Effectiveness of therapy can be demonstrated by:** ■ Prevention of diseases through active immunity.

## Vaccines/immunizing agents included in *Davis's Drug Guide for Nurses*

*immune globulins*

cytomegalovirus immune globulin 1166
$Rh_o(D)$ immune globulin standard dose IM 919

$Rh_o(D)$ globulin IV 919
$Rh_o(D)$ globulin microdose IM 919

# ■ VASCULAR HEADACHE SUPPRESSANTS

## PHARMACOLOGIC PROFILE

### General Use

Used for acute treatment of vascular headaches (migraine, cluster headaches, migraine variants). Other agents such as some beta blockers and some calcum channel blockers are used for suppression of frequently occurring vascular headaches.

### General Action and Information

Ergot derivatives (ergotamine, dihydroergotamine) directly stimulate alpha-adrenergic and serotonergic receptors, producing vascular smooth muscle vasoconstriction. Almotriptan, frovatriptan, naratriptan, rizatriptan, sumatriptan and zolmitriptan produce vasoconstriction by acting as serotonin ($5\text{-}HT_1$) agonists.

### Contraindications

Avoid using these agents in patients with ischemic cardiovascular disease.

### Precautions

Use cautiously in patients with a history of or risk for cardiovascular disease.

### Interactions

Avoid concurrent use of ergot derivative agents with serotonin agonist agents; see also individual agents.

## NURSING IMPLICATIONS

### Assessment

- Assess pain location, intensity, duration, and associated symptoms (photophobia, phonophobia, nausea, vomiting) during migraine attack.

### Potential Nursing Diagnoses

- Pain, acute (Indications).

- Knowledge, deficient, related to disease processes and medication regimen (Patient/Family Teaching).

**Implementation**
- Medication should be administered at the first sign of a headache.

**Patient/Family Teaching**
- Inform patient that medication should be used only during a migraine attack. It is meant to be used for relief of migraine attacks but not to prevent or reduce the number of attacks.
- Advise patient that lying down in a darkened room following medication administration may further help relieve headache.
- May cause dizziness or drowsiness. Caution patient to avoid driving or other activities requiring alertness until response to medication is known.
- Advise patient to avoid alcohol, which aggravates headaches.

**Evaluation**
**Effectiveness of therapy can be demonstrated by:** ■ Relief of migraine attack.

**Vascular headache suppressants included in** *Davis's Drug Guide for Nurses*

*alpha-adrenergic blockers*
dihydroergotamine 380
ergotamine 380

*beta blockers*
propranolol 891
timolol 1034

*5 HT₁ agonists*
almotriptan 24
eletriptan 361

frovatriptan 460
naratriptan 732
rizatriptan 938
sumatriptan 986
zolmitriptan 1109

*miscellaneous*
divalproex sodium 1068
valproate sodium 1068
valproic acid 1068
verapamil 1077

## ■ VITAMINS

### PHARMACOLOGIC PROFILE

### General Use
Used in the prevention and treatment of vitamin deficiencies and as supplements in various metabolic disorders.

### General Action and Information
Serve as components of enzyme systems that catalyze numerous varied metabolic reactions. Necessary for homeostasis. Water-soluble vitamins (B-vitamins and vitamin C) rarely cause toxicity. Fat-soluble vitamins (vitamins D and E) may accumulate and cause toxicity.

### Contraindications
Hypersensitivity to additives, preservatives, or colorants.

### Precautions
Dosage should be adjusted to avoid toxicity, especially for fat-soluble vitamins.

### Interactions
Pyridoxine in large amounts may interfere with the effectiveness of levodopa Cholestyramine, colestipol, and mineral oil decrease absorption of fat-soluble vitamins.

## NURSING IMPLICATIONS

### Assessment
- Assess patient for signs of vitamin deficiency before and periodically throughout therapy.
- Assess nutritional status through 24-hr diet recall. Determine frequency of consumption of vitamin-rich foods.

### Potential Nursing Diagnoses
- Nutrition, imbalanced: less than body requirements (Indications).
- Knowledge, deficient, related to disease processes and medication regimen (Patient/Family Teaching).

### Implementation
- Because of infrequency of single vitamin deficiencies, combinations are commonly administered.

### Patient/Family Teaching
- Encourage patients to comply with diet recommendations of physician or other health care professional. Explain that the best source of vitamins is a well-balanced diet with foods from the four basic food groups.
- Patients self-medicating with vitamin supplements should be cautioned not to exceed RDAs. The effectiveness of megadoses for treatment of various medical conditions is unproved and may cause side effects and toxicity.

### Evaluation
**Effectiveness of therapy can be demonstrated by:** ■ Prevention of or decrease in the symptoms of vitamin deficiencies.

### Vitamins included in *Davis's Drug Guide for Nurses*

*fat-soluble vitamins*
calcifediol 1089
calcitriol 1089
dihydrotachysterol 1089
doxercalciferol 1089
ergocalciferol 1089
paricalcitol 1089
phytonadione 846
vitamin E 1093

*water soluble vitamins*
ascorbic acid 1162

leucovorin calcium 602
folic acid 454
niacin 745
niacinamide 745
pyridoxine 901
riboflavin 1182
thiamine 1014
cyanocobalamin 1087
hydroxocobalamin 1087

# ■ WEIGHT CONTROL AGENTS

## PHARMACOLOGIC PROFILE

### General Use
These agents are used in the management of exogenous obesity as part of a regimen including a reduced-calorie diet. They are especially useful in the presence of other risk factors including hypertension, diabetes or dyslipidemias.

### General Action and Information
Phentermine and sibutramine are anorexiants that are designed to decrease appetite via their action in the CNS. Orlistat is a lipase inhibitor that decreases absorption of dietary fat.

## Contraindications

None of these agents should be used during pregnancy or lactation. Phentermine and sibutramine should not be used in patients with severe hepatic or renal disease, uncontrolled hypertension, known CHF, or cardiovascular disease. Orlistat should not be used in patients with chronic malabsorption.

## Precautions

Phentermine and sibutramine should be used cautiously in patients with a history of seizures, or narrow-angle glaucoma and in geriatric patients.

## Interactions

Phentermine and sibutramine may have additive, adverse effects with CNS stimulants, some vascular headache suppressants, MAO inhibitors, and some opioids (concurrent use should be avoided). Orlistat reduces absorption of some fat-soluble vitamins and beta-carotene.

## NURSING IMPLICATIONS

### Assessment

- Monitor weight and dietary intake prior to and periodically during therapy. Adjust concurrent medications (antihypertensives, antidiabetics, lipid-lowering agents) as needed.

### Potential Nursing Diagnoses

- Body image, disturbed (Indications).
- Nutrition, imbalanced: more than body requirements (Indications).
- Knowledge, deficient, related to medication regimen (Patient/Family Teaching).

### Patient/Family Teaching

- Advise patient that regular physical activity, approved by health care professional, should be used in conjunction with medication and diet.

### Evaluation

**Clinical response to therapy can be evaluated by:** ■ Slow, consistent weight loss when combined with a reduced-calorie diet.

### Weight control agents included in *Davis's Drug Guide for Nurses*

orlistat 1175
phentermine 1178

sibutramine 1182

# abacavir

(ah-**back**-ah-veer)

Ziagen

## CLASSIFICATION(S):

**Therapeutic:** *antiretrovirals*
**Pharmacologic:** *nucleoside reverse transcriptase inhibitors*

**Pregnancy Category C**

## INDICATIONS

■ Management of HIV infection (AIDS) in combination with other antiretrovirals.

## ACTION

■ Converted inside cells to carbovir triphosphate, its active metabolite. Carbovir triphosphate inhibits the activity of HIV-1 reverse transcriptase, which in turn terminates viral DNA growth. **Therapeutic Effects:** ■ Slows the progression of HIV infection and decreases the occurrence of its sequelae ■ Increases CD4 cell counts and decreases viral load.

## PHARMACOKINETICS

**Absorption:** Rapidly and extensively (83%) absorbed.

**Distribution:** Distributes into extravascular space and readily distributes into erythrocytes.

**Metabolism and Excretion:** Mostly metabolized by the liver; 1.2% excreted unchanged in urine.

**Half-life:** 1.5 hr.

## CONTRAINDICATIONS AND PRECAUTIONS

**Contraindicated in:** ■ Hypersensitivity ■ Lactation (breastfeeding not recommended for HIV-infected patients).

**Use Cautiously in:** ■ Pregnancy (safety not established) ■ Children <3 mo (safety not established).

## ADVERSE REACTIONS AND SIDE EFFECTS*

■ **CNS:** headache, insomnia ■ **GI:** HEPATOTOXICITY, diarrhea, nausea, vomiting, anorexia ■ **Derm:** rashes ■ **F and E:** LACTIC ACIDOSIS ■ **Misc:** HYPERSENSITIVITY REACTIONS.

## INTERACTIONS

**Drug-Drug:** ■ **Alcohol** increases blood levels ■ May increase **methadone** metabolism in some patients; slight increase in **methadone** dosing may be needed.

## ROUTE AND DOSAGE

■ **PO (Adults):** 300 mg twice daily.

■ **PO (Children 3 mo–16 yr):** 8 mg/kg twice daily (not to exceed 300 mg twice daily).

## AVAILABILITY

■ **Tablets:** 300 mg$^{Rx}$ ■ *Oral solution (strawberry/banana flavor):* 20 mg/ml in 240-ml bottles$^{Rx}$ ■ lamivudine and zidovudine (Trizivir). See Appendix B.

TIME/ACTION PROFILE (blood levels)

|    | ONSET | PEAK | DURATION |
|----|-------|------|----------|
| PO | unknown | unknown | unknown |

# NURSING IMPLICATIONS

## ASSESSMENT

❑ Assess patient for change in severity of HIV symptoms and for symptoms of opportunistic infections throughout therapy.

❑ Assess patient for signs of hypersensitivity reactions (fever, rash, fatigue, nausea, vomiting, cough, dyspnea, pharyngitis, diarrhea, abdominal pain). May also cause elevated liver function tests, increased creatine phosphokinase or creatinine, and lymphopenia. Discontinue abacavir at the first sign of hypersensitivity reaction. Do not restart abacavir following reaction; more severe symptoms may occur within hours and may include life-threatening hypotension and death. Symptoms usually resolve upon discontinuation.

❑ May cause lactic acidosis and severe hepatomegaly with steatosis. Monitor patient for signs (increased serum lactate levels, elevated liver enzymes, liver enlargement on palpation). Therapy should be suspended if clinical or laboratory signs occur.

{ } = Available in Canada only.
*CAPITALS indicates life-threatening; underlines indicate most frequent.

■ *Lab Test Considerations:* Monitor viral load and CD4 cell count regularly during therapy.

❑ May cause increased serum glucose and tri-glyceride levels.

## POTENTIAL NURSING DIAGNOSES

■ Infection, risk for (Indications).

■ Noncompliance (Patient/Family Teaching).

## IMPLEMENTATION

■ **PO:** May be administered with or without food. Oral solution may be stored at room temperature or refrigerated; do not freeze.

## PATIENT/FAMILY TEACHING

❑ Emphasize the importance of taking abacavir exactly as directed. It must always be used in combination with other antiretroviral drugs. Do not take more than prescribed amount and do not stop taking without consulting health care professional. If a dose is missed, take as soon as remembered; do not double doses.

❑ Instruct patient that abacavir should not be shared with others.

❑ Inform patient that abacavir does not cure AIDS or prevent associated or opportunistic infections. Abacavir does not reduce the risk of transmission of HIV to others through sexual contact or blood contamination. Caution patient to use a condom, and avoid sharing needles or donating blood to prevent spreading the AIDS virus to others. Advise patient that the long-term effects of abacavir are unknown at this time.

❑ Advise patient of potential for hypersensitivity reactions that may result in death. Instruct patient to discontinue abacavir and notify health care professional immediately if symptoms of hypersensitivity occur. Medication guide for patients should be dispensed with prescription. Advise patient to read it thoroughly. A warning card summarizing symptoms of abacavir hypersensitivity should be provided with each prescription; instruct patient to carry card at all times.

❑ Emphasize the importance of regular follow-up exams and blood counts to determine progress and monitor for side effects.

## EVALUATION

**Effectiveness of therapy can be demonstrated by:** ■ Delayed progression of AIDS, and decreased opportunistic infections in patients with HIV ■ Decrease in viral load and increase in CD4 cell counts.

## acarbose
(aye-**kar**-bose)
Precose

### CLASSIFICATION(S):
**Therapeutic:** antidiabetics
**Pharmacologic:** alpha-glucosidase inhibitors

### Pregnancy Category B

## INDICATIONS

■ Management of type 1 diabetes in conjunction with dietary therapy; may be used with insulin or other hypoglycemic agents.

## ACTION

■ Lowers blood glucose by inhibiting the enzyme alpha-glucosidase in the GI tract. Delays and reduces glucose absorption. **Therapeutic Effects:** ■ Lowering of blood glucose in diabetic patients, especially postprandial hyperglycemia.

## PHARMACOKINETICS

**Absorption:** <2% systemically absorbed; action is primarily local (in the GI tract).

**Distribution:** Unknown.

**Metabolism and Excretion:** Minimal amounts absorbed are excreted by the kidneys.

**Half-life:** 2 hr.

## CONTRAINDICATIONS AND PRECAUTIONS

**Contraindicated in:** ■ Hypersensitivity ■ Diabetic ketoacidosis ■ Cirrhosis ■ Serum creatinine >2 mg/dl ■ Pregnancy, lactation, or children.

**Use Cautiously in:** ■ Presence of fever, infection, trauma, stress (may cause hyperglycemia, requiring alternative therapy).

## ADVERSE REACTIONS AND SIDE EFFECTS*

■ **GI:** <u>abdominal pain</u>, <u>diarrhea</u>, <u>flatulence</u>, ↑ transaminases.

## INTERACTIONS

**Drug-Drug:** ■ **Thiazide diuretics** and **loop diuretics, corticosteroids, phenothiazines, thyroid preparations, estrogens, conjugated, progestins, hormonal contraceptives, phenytoin, niacin, sympathomimetics, calcium channel blockers,** and **isoniazid** may ↑ glucose levels in diabetic patients and lead to ↓ control of blood glucose ■ Effects are ↓ by **intestinal adsorbents,** including **activated charcoal** and **digestive enzyme preparations (amylase, pancreatin)**; avoid concurrent use ■ ↑ effects of **sulfonylurea hypoglycemic agents** ■ May ↓ absorption of **digoxin**; may require dosage adjustment.

**Drug-Natural Products:** ■ **Glucosamine** may worsen blood glucose control ■ **Chromium** and **coenzyme Q-10** may ↑ hypoglycemic effects.

## ROUTE AND DOSAGE

■ **PO (Adults):** 25 mg 3 times daily; may be increased q 4–8 wk as needed/tolerated (range 50–100 mg 3 times daily; not to exceed 50 mg 3 times daily in patients ≤60 kg or 100 mg 3 times daily in patients >60 kg).

## AVAILABILITY

■ *Tablets:* 25 mg$^{Rx}$, 50 mg$^{Rx}$, 100 mg$^{Rx}$.

TIME/ACTION PROFILE (effect on blood glucose)

| | ONSET | PEAK | DURATION |
|---|---|---|---|
| PO | unknown | 1 hr | unknown |

# NURSING IMPLICATIONS

## ASSESSMENT

❑ Observe patient for signs and symptoms of hypoglycemia (sweating, hunger, weakness, dizziness, tremor, tachycardia, anxiety), especially when taking concurrently with other oral hypoglycemic agents.

■ *Lab Test Considerations:* Monitor serum glucose and glycosylated hemoglobin periodically during therapy to evaluate effectiveness.

❑ Monitor AST and ALT every 3 mo for the 1st yr and then periodically. Elevated levels may require dosage reduction or discontinuation of acarbose. Elevations occur more commonly in patients taking more than 300 mg/day and in female patients. Levels usually return to normal without other evidence of liver injury after discontinuation.

■ *Toxicity and Overdose:* Symptoms of overdose are transient increase in flatulence, diarrhea, and abdominal discomfort. Acarbose alone does not cause hypoglycemia; however, other concurrently administered hypoglycemic agents may produce hypoglycemia requiring treatment.

## POTENTIAL NURSING DIAGNOSES

■ Nutrition, imbalanced: more than body requirements (Indications).

■ Noncompliance (Patient/Family Teaching).

## IMPLEMENTATION

■ **General:** Patients stabilized on a diabetic regimen who are exposed to stress, fever, trauma, infection, or surgery may require administration of insulin.

❑ Does not cause hypoglycemia when taken while fasting, but may increase hypoglycemic effect of other hypoglycemic agents.

■ **PO:** Administer with first bite of each meal 3 times/day.

## PATIENT/FAMILY TEACHING

❑ Instruct patient to take acarbose at same time each day. If a dose is missed and the meal is completed without taking the dose, skip missed dose and take next dose with the next meal. Do not double doses.

❑ Explain to patient that acarbose controls hyperglycemia but does not cure diabetes. Therapy is longterm.

❑ Review signs of hypoglycemia and hyperglycemia (blurred vision; drowsiness; dry mouth; flushed, dry skin; fruit-like breath odor; increased urination; ketones in urine; loss of appetite; stomachache; nausea or vomiting; tiredness; rapid, deep breathing; unusual thirst; unconsciousness) with patient. If hypoglycemia occurs, advise patient to take a form of oral glucose (e.g., glucose tablets, liquid gel glucose) rather than sugar (absorption of sugar is blocked by acarbose) and notify health care professional.

❑ Encourage patient to follow prescribed diet, medication, and exercise regimen to prevent hypoglycemic or hyperglycemic episodes.

❑ Instruct patient in proper testing of serum glucose and urine ketones. Monitor closely during periods of stress or illness. Notify health care professional if significant changes occur.

❑ Caution patient to avoid using other medications without consulting health care professional.

❑ Advise patient to inform health care professional of medication regimen before treatment or surgery.

❑ Advise patient to carry a form of oral glucose and identification describing disease process and medication regimen at all times.

❑ Emphasize the importance of routine follow-up examinations.

## EVALUATION

**Effectiveness of therapy can be demonstrated by:** ■ Control of blood glucose levels without the appearance of hypoglycemic or hyperglycemic episodes.

---

## acebutolol

(a-se-**byoo**-toe-lole)

{Monitan}, Sectral

### CLASSIFICATION(S):

**Therapeutic:** antiarrhythmics (class II), antihypertensives

**Pharmacologic:** beta blockers

### Pregnancy Category B

---

## INDICATIONS

■ Treatment of hypertension (single agent or with other antihypertensives) ■ Treatment of ventricular tachyarrhythmias. **Unlabeled uses:** ■ Prophylaxis of MI, treatment of angina pectoris, management of anxiety, tremors, thyrotoxicosis, mitral valve prolapse, idiopathic hypertrophic subaortic stenosis.

## ACTION

■ Blocks stimulation of beta$_1$-(myocardial)-adrenergic receptors. Does not usually affect beta$_2$ (pulmonary, vascular, or uterine) receptor sites ■ Mild intrinsic sympathomimetic activity (ISA). **Therapeutic Effects:** ■ Decreased heart rate ■

Decreased AV conduction ■ Decreased blood pressure.

## PHARMACOKINETICS

**Absorption:** Well absorbed following oral administration but rapidly undergoes metabolism.

**Distribution:** Minimal penetration of the CNS. Crosses the placenta and enters breast milk in small amounts.

**Metabolism and Excretion:** Mostly metabolized to diacetolol, which is also a beta blocker.

**Half-life:** 3–4 hr (8–13 hr for diacetolol).

## CONTRAINDICATIONS AND PRECAUTIONS

**Contraindicated in:** ■ Uncompensated CHF ■ Pulmonary edema ■ Cardiogenic shock ■ Bradycardia or heart block ■ Obstructive airway disease including asthma.

**Use Cautiously in:** ■ Renal or hepatic impairment (dosage reduction recommended if CCr <50 ml/min/1.73 m$^2$) ■ Geriatric patients (increased sensitivity) ■ Thyrotoxicosis (may mask symptoms) ■ Diabetes mellitus (may mask symptoms of hypoglycemia) ■ Pregnancy, lactation, or children (safety not established; neonatal bradycardia, hypotension, hypoglycemia, and respiratory depression may occur rarely) ■ History of severe allergic reactions (intensity of reactions may be increased).

## ADVERSE REACTIONS AND SIDE EFFECTS*

■ **CNS:** fatigue, weakness, anxiety, depression, dizziness, drowsiness, insomnia, memory loss, nervousness, nightmares ■ **EENT:** blurred vision, stuffy nose ■ **Resp:** bronchospasm, wheezing ■ **CV:** BRADYCARDIA, CHF, PULMONARY EDEMA, hypotension, peripheral vasoconstriction ■ **GI:** constipation, diarrhea, nausea, vomiting ■ **GU:** impotence, diminished libido, urinary frequency ■ **Derm:** rashes ■ **Endo:** hyperglycemia, hypoglycemia ■ **MS:** arthralgia, joint pain ■ **Misc:** drug-induced lupus syndrome.

## INTERACTIONS

**Drug-Drug:** ■ **General anesthetics, IV phenytoin,** and **verapamil** may cause additive myocardial depression ■ Concurrent use with **digoxin** may increase bradycardia ■ **Antihypertensives,** acute ingestion of **alcohol,** or **nitrates** may cause additive hypotension ■ Use with **epinephrine** may result in unopposed alpha-adrenergic stimulation ■ Concurrent use with **thyroid preparations** may decrease effectiveness ▪ Concurrent use with **insulin** may result in prolonged hypoglycemia ▪ May decrease effectiveness of **theophylline**.

## ROUTE AND DOSAGE

- **PO (Adults):** 400–800 mg/day—single dose or twice daily (up to 1200 mg/day or 800 mg/day in geriatric patients).
- ❏ **Renal Impairment**
- **PO (Adults):** If CCr <50 ml/min/1.73 m², use 50% of normal dose. If CCr <25 ml/min/ 1.73 m², use 25% of normal dose.

## AVAILABILITY (generic available)

▪ *Capsules:* 200 mg$^{Rx}$, 400 mg$^{Rx}$ ▪ Cost: 200 mg $80.25/100, 400 mg $107.03/100 ▪ *Tablets:* {100 mg$^{Rx}$}, {200 mg$^{Rx}$}, {400 mg$^{Rx}$}.

TIME/ACTION PROFILE

|  | ONSET | PEAK | DURATION |
|---|---|---|---|
| PO (effect on BP) | 1–1.5 hr | 2–8 hr | 12–24 hr |
| PO (antiarrhythmic) | 1 hr | 4–6 hr | up to 10 hr |

## NURSING IMPLICATIONS

### ASSESSMENT

- ❏ Monitor blood pressure, ECG, and pulse frequently during dosage adjustment period and periodically throughout therapy.
- ❏ Monitor intake and output ratios and daily weights. Assess routinely for signs and symptoms of CHF (dyspnea, rales/crackles, weight gain, peripheral edema, jugular venous distention).
- ❏ Monitor frequency of prescription refills to determine compliance.
- ▪ *Lab Test Considerations:* May cause increased BUN, serum lipoprotein, potassium, triglyceride, and uric acid levels.
- ❏ May cause increased serum alkaline phosphatase, LDH, AST, and ALT levels.
- ❏ May cause increased ANA titers.
- ❏ May cause increase in blood glucose levels.

### POTENTIAL NURSING DIAGNOSES

- ▪ Cardiac output, decreased (Side Effects).

- ▪ Noncompliance, related to medication regimen (Patient/Family Teaching).

## IMPLEMENTATION

- ▪ **PO:** Take apical pulse prior to administering. If <50 bpm or if arrhythmia occurs, withhold medication and notify physician or other health care professional.
- ❏ May be administered with food or on an empty stomach.

## PATIENT/FAMILY TEACHING

- ▪ **General Info:** Instruct patient to take medication exactly as directed, at the same time each day, even if feeling well; do not skip or double up on missed doses. If a dose is missed, it should be taken as soon as possible up to 4 hr before next dose. Abrupt withdrawal may precipitate life-threatening arrhythmias, hypertension, or myocardial ischemia.
- ❏ Advise patient to make sure enough medication is available for weekends, holidays, and vacations. A written prescription may be kept in wallet in case of emergency.
- ❏ Teach patient and family how to check pulse and blood pressure. Instruct them to check pulse daily and blood pressure biweekly and to report significant changes to health care professional.
- ❏ May cause drowsiness or dizziness. Caution patients to avoid driving or other activities that require alertness until response to the drug is known.
- ❏ Caution patient that this medication may increase sensitivity to cold.
- ❏ Instruct patient to consult health care professional before taking any OTC medications, especially cold preparations, concurrently with this medication.
- ❏ Diabetic patients should closely monitor blood glucose, especially if weakness, malaise, irritability, or fatigue occurs. May mask tachycardia and blood pressure changes as signs of hypoglycemia, but dizziness and sweating may still occur.
- ❏ Advise patient to notify health care professional if slow pulse, difficulty breathing, wheezing, cold hands and feet, dizziness, light-headedness, confusion, depression,

{ } = Available in Canada only.
*CAPITALS indicates life-threatening; <u>underlines</u> indicate most frequent.

rash, fever, sore throat, unusual bleeding, or bruising occurs.

❑ Instruct patient to inform health care professional of medication regimen prior to treatment or surgery.

❑ Advise patient to carry identification describing disease process and medication regimen at all times.

■ **Hypertension:** Reinforce the need to continue additional therapies for hypertension (weight loss, sodium restriction, stress reduction, regular exercise, moderation of alcohol consumption, and smoking cessation). Acebutolol controls but does not cure hypertension.

## EVALUATION

**Effectiveness of therapy can be demonstrated by:** ■ Decrease in blood pressure ■ Control of arrhythmias without appearance of detrimental side effects.

## acetaminophen

(a-seet-a-**min**-oh-fen)

{Abenol}, Acephen, Aceta, Aminofen, Apacet, APAP, {Apo-Acetaminophen}, Aspirin Free Anacin, Aspirin Free Pain Relief, Children's Pain Reliever, Dapacin, Feverall, Extra Strength Dynafed E.X., Extra Strength Dynafed (Billups, P.J.), Genapap, Genebs, Halenol, Infant's Pain Reliever, Liquiprin, Mapap, Maranox, Meda, Neopap, Oraphen-PD, Panadol, paracetamol, Redutemp, Ridenol, Silapap, Tapanol, Tempra, Tylenol, Uni-Ace

### CLASSIFICATION(S):

**Therapeutic:** *antipyretics, non-opioid analgesics*

### Pregnancy Category B

## INDICATIONS

■ Mild pain ■ Fever.

## ACTION

■ Inhibits the synthesis of prostaglandins that may serve as mediators of pain and fever, primarily in the CNS ■ Has no significant anti-inflammatory properties or GI toxicity. **Therapeutic Effects:** ■ Analgesia ■ Antipyresis.

## PHARMACOKINETICS

**Absorption:** Well absorbed following oral administration. Rectal absorption is variable.

**Distribution:** Widely distributed. Crosses the placenta; enters breast milk in low concentrations.

**Metabolism and Excretion:** 85–95% metabolized by the liver. Metabolites may be toxic in overdose situation. Metabolites excreted by the kidneys.

**Half-life:** 1–4 hr.

## CONTRAINDICATIONS AND PRECAUTIONS

**Contraindicated in:** ■ Previous hypersensitivity ■ Products containing alcohol, aspartame, saccharin, sugar, or tartrazine (FDC yellow dye #5) should be avoided in patients who have hypersensitivity or intolerance to these compounds.

**Use Cautiously in:** ■ Hepatic disease/renal disease (lower chronic doses recommended) ■ Chronic alcohol use/abuse ■ Malnutrition.

## ADVERSE REACTIONS AND SIDE EFFECTS*

■ **GI:** HEPATIC FAILURE , HEPATOTOXICITY (overdose)
■ **GU:** renal failure (high doses/chronic use)
■ **Derm:** rash, urticaria.

## INTERACTIONS

**Drug-Drug:** ■ Chronic high-dose acetaminophen (>2 g/day) may increase the risk of bleeding with **warfarin** (PT should be monitored regularly and INR should not exceed 4) ■ Hepatotoxicity is additive with other **hepatotoxic substances,** including **alcohol** ■ Concurrent use of **sulfinpyrazone, isoniazid, rifampin, rifabutin, phenytoin, barbiturates,** and **carbamazepine** may increase the risk of acetaminophen-induced liver damage (limit self-medication); these agents will also decrease therapeutic effects of acetaminophen ■ Combined use with **salicylates** or **NSAIDs** increases the risk of adverse renal effects ■ **Propranolol** decreases metabolism and may increase effects ■ May decrease effects of **lamotrigine, zidovudine,** and **loop diuretics.**

## ROUTE AND DOSAGE

Children ≤12 yr should not receive >5 doses/ 24 hr without notifying physician or other health care professional.

- **PO (Adults):** 325–650 mg q 4–6 hr or 1 g 3–4 times daily or 1300 mg q 8 hr (not to exceed 4 g or 2.5 g/day in patients with hepatic/renal impairment).
- **PO (Children >14 yr):** 650 mg q 4 hr as needed.
- **PO (Children 12–14 yr):** 640 mg q 4 hr.
- **PO (Children 11 yr):** 480 mg q 4 hr as needed.
- **PO (Children 9–10 yr):** 400 mg q 4 hr as needed.
- **PO (Children 6–8 yr):** 320 mg q 4 hr as needed.
- **PO (Children 4–5 yr):** 240 mg q 4 hr as needed.
- **PO (Children 2–3 yr):** 160 mg q 4 hr as needed.
- **PO (Children 1–2 yr):** 120 mg q 4 hr as needed.
- **PO (Children 4–11 mo):** 80 mg q 4 hr as needed.
- **PO (Children 0–3 mo):** 40 mg q 4 hr as needed.
- **Rect (Adults and Children >12 yr):** 650 mg q 4–6 hr as needed.
- **Rect (Children 6–12 yr):** 325 mg q 4–6 hr as needed (not to exceed 2.6 g/24 hr).
- **Rect (Children 3–6 yr):** 120–125 mg q 4–6 hr as needed (not to exceed 720 mg/24 hr).
- **Rect (Children 1–3 yr):** 80 mg q 4 hr as needed.
- **Rect (Children 3–11 mo):** 80 mg q 6 hr as needed.

## AVAILABILITY (generic available)

■ *Chewable tablets (fruit, bubblegum, or grape flavor):* 80 mg$^{OTC}$, 160 mg$^{OTC}$ ■ *Granules:* 80 mg/packet$^{OTC}$ ■ *Oral powder (capsule for sprinkle):* 80 mg$^{OTC}$, 160 mg$^{OTC}$ ■ *Tablets:* 160 mg$^{OTC}$, 325 mg$^{OTC}$, 500 mg$^{OTC}$, 650 mg$^{OTC}$ ■ Cost: 325 mg $1.81/60, 500 mg $1.60/100 ■ *Capsules:* 325 mg$^{OTC}$, 500 mg$^{OTC}$ ■ *Solution (berry, fruit, and grape flavor):* {80 mg/ml$^{OTC}$}, 80 mg/1.66 ml$^{OTC}$, 100 mg/ml$^{OTC}$ ■

*Liquid (mint):* 160 mg/5 ml$^{OTC}$, 500 mg/15 ml$^{OTC}$ ■ *Elixir (grape and cherry flavor):* 80 mg/2.5 ml$^{OTC}$, 80 mg/5 ml$^{OTC}$, 120 mg/5 ml$^{OTC}$, 160 mg/5 ml$^{OTC}$ ■ *Drops:* 80 mg/0.8 ml $^{OTC}$ ■ *Suspension:* {32 mg/ml$^{OTC}$}, {80 mg/ml$^{OTC}$} ■ *Syrup:* 16 mg/ml$^{OTC}$ ■ *Suppositories:* 80 mg$^{OTC}$, 120 mg$^{OTC}$, 300 mg$^{OTC}$, 325 mg$^{OTC}$, 650 mg$^{OTC}$ ■ many other medications. See Appendix B.

**TIME/ACTION PROFILE** (analgesia and antipyresis)

|  | ONSET | PEAK | DURATION |
|---|---|---|---|
| PO | 0.5–1 hr | 1–3 hr | 3–8 hr† |
| Rect | 0.5–1 hr | 1–3 hr | 3–4 hr |

†Depends on dose.

# NURSING IMPLICATIONS

## ASSESSMENT

- **General Info:** Assess overall health status and alcohol usage before administering acetaminophen. Malnourished patients or chronic alcohol abusers are at higher risk of developing hepatotoxicity with chronic use of usual doses of this drug.
- ❑ Assess amount, frequency, and type of drugs taken in patients self-medicating, especially with OTC drugs. Prolonged use of acetaminophen alone or combined with salicylates or NSAIDs increases the risk of adverse renal effects. For short-term use, combined doses of acetaminophen and salicylates should not exceed the recommended dose of either drug given alone.
- **Pain:** Assess type, location, and intensity prior to and 30–60 min following administration.
- **Fever:** Assess fever; note presence of associated signs (diaphoresis, tachycardia, and malaise).
- *Lab Test Considerations:* Hepatic, hematologic, and renal function should be evaluated periodically throughout prolonged, high-dose therapy.
- ❑ May alter results of blood glucose monitoring. May cause falsely decreased values when measured with glucose oxidase/peroxidase method, but probably not with hexokinase/G6PD method. May also cause falsely in-

creased values with certain instruments; see manufacturer's instruction manual.

❑ Increased serum bilirubin, LDH, AST, ALT, and prothrombin time may indicate hepatotoxicity.

■ *Toxicity and Overdose:* If overdose occurs, **acetylcysteine** (Mucomyst) is the antidote.

## POTENTIAL NURSING DIAGNOSES

■ Pain, acute (Indications).

■ Body temperature, risk for imbalanced (Indications).

## IMPLEMENTATION

■ **General:** When combined with opioids do not exceed the maximum recommended daily dose of acetaminophen.

■ **PO:** Administer with a full glass of water.

❑ May be taken with food or on an empty stomach.

## PATIENT/FAMILY TEACHING

❑ Advise patient to take medication exactly as directed and not to take more than the recommended amount. Chronic excessive use of >4 g/day (2 g in patients with chronic alcoholism) may lead to hepatotoxicity, renal, or cardiac damage. Adults should not take acetaminophen longer than 10 days and children not longer than 5 days unless directed by health care professional. Short-term doses of acetaminophen with salicylates or NSAIDs should not exceed the recommended daily dose of either drug alone.

❑ Advise patient to avoid alcohol (3 or more glasses per day increase the risk of liver damage) if taking more than an occasional 1–2 doses and to avoid taking concurrently with salicylates or NSAIDs for more than a few days, unless directed by health care professional.

❑ Advise parents or caregivers to check concentrations of liquid preparations. Errors have resulted in serious liver damage.

❑ Inform patients with diabetes that acetaminophen may alter results of blood glucose monitoring. Advise patient to notify health care professional if changes are noted.

❑ Caution patient to check labels on all OTC products. Advise patients to avoid taking more than one product containing acetaminophen at a time to prevent toxicity.

❑ Advise patient to consult health care professional if discomfort or fever is not relieved by routine doses of this drug or if fever is greater than 39.5°C (103°F) or lasts longer than 3 days.

## EVALUATION

**Effectiveness of therapy can be demonstrated by:** ■ Relief of mild pain ■ Reduction of fever.

# acyclovir
## (ay-**sye**-kloe-veer)
{Avirax}, Zovirax

## CLASSIFICATION(S):
**Therapeutic:** *antivirals*
**Pharmacologic:** *purine analogues*

## Pregnancy Category B (PO, IV), C (topical)

## INDICATIONS

■ **PO:** Recurrent genital herpes infections. Localized cutaneous herpes zoster infections (shingles) and chickenpox (varicella) ■ **IV:** Severe initial episodes of genital herpes in nonimmunosuppressed patients. Mucosal or cutaneous herpes simplex infections or herpes zoster infections (shingles) in immunosuppressed patients. Herpes simplex encephalitis ■ **Topical:** *Cream*—Recurrent herpes labialis (cold sores). *Ointment*—Treatment of limited non–life-threatening herpes simplex infections in immunocompromised patients (systemic treatment is preferred).

## ACTION

■ Interferes with viral DNA synthesis. **Therapeutic Effects:** ■ Inhibition of viral replication, decreased viral shedding, and reduced time for healing of lesions.

## PHARMACOKINETICS

**Absorption:** Despite poor absorption (15–30%), therapeutic blood levels are achieved.
**Distribution:** Widely distributed. CSF concentrations are 50% of plasma. Crosses placenta; enters breast milk.
**Metabolism and Excretion:** >90% eliminated unchanged by kidneys; remainder metabolized by liver.

**Half-life:** 2.1–3.5 hr ( ↑ in renal failure).

## CONTRAINDICATIONS AND PRECAUTIONS

**Contraindicated in:** ■ Hypersensitivity to acyclovir or valacyclovir.

**Use Cautiously in:** ■ Pre-existing serious neurologic, hepatic, pulmonary, or fluid and electrolyte abnormalities ■ Renal impairment (dosage alteration recommended if CCr <50 ml/min) ■ Geriatric patients (due to age related ↓ in renal function) ■ Obese patients (dose should be based on ideal body weight) ■ Pregnancy and lactation (safety not established; topical products not approved for pediatric use).

## ADVERSE REACTIONS AND SIDE EFFECTS*

■ **CNS:** SEIZURES, dizziness, headache, hallucinations, trembling ■ **GI:** diarrhea, nausea, vomiting, abdominal pain, anorexia ■ **GU:** RENAL FAILURE, crystalluria, hematuria ■ **Derm:** acne, hives, skin rashes, unusual sweating ■ **Endo:** changes in menstrual cycle ■ **Hemat:** THROMBOTIC THROMBOCYTOPENIC PURPURA/HEMOLYTIC UREMIC SYNDROME (high doses in immunosuppressed patients) ■ **Local:** pain, phlebitis, local irritation ■ **MS:** joint pain ■ **Misc:** polydipsia.

## INTERACTIONS

**Drug-Drug:** ■ **Probenecid** ↑ blood levels of acyclovir ■ Concurrent use of other **nephrotoxic drugs** ↑ risk of adverse renal effects ■ **Zidovudine** and IT **methotrexate** may ↑ risk of CNS side effects.

## ROUTE AND DOSAGE

❑ **Initial Genital Herpes**

■ **PO (Adults):** 200 mg q 4 hr while awake (5 times/day) for 7–10 days.

■ **IV (Adults):** 5 mg/kg q 8 hr for 5 days.

❑ **Chronic Suppressive Therapy for Recurrent Genital Herpes**

■ **PO (Adults):** 400 mg twice daily or 200 mg 3–5 times/day for up to 12 mo.

❑ **Intermittent Therapy for Recurrent Genital Herpes**

■ **PO (Adults):** 200 mg q 4 hr while awake (5 times/day) for 5 days, start at first sign of symptoms.

❑ **Acute Treatment of Herpes Zoster**

■ **PO (Adults):** 800 mg q 4 hr while awake (5 times/day) for 7–10 days.

❑ **Chickenpox**

■ **PO (Adults and Children):** 20 mg/kg (not to exceed 800 mg/dose) qid for 5 days.

❑ **Mucosal and Cutaneous Herpes Simplex Infections in Immunosuppressed Patients**

■ **IV (Adults and Children >12 yr):** 5 mg/kg q 8 hr for 7 days.

■ **IV (Children <12 yr):** 10 mg/kg q 8 hr for 7 days.

■ **Topical (Adults):** 0.5 in. ribbon of 5% *ointment* for every 4-square-in. area q 3 hr (6 times/day) for 7 days.

❑ **Herpes Simplex Encephalitis**

■ **IV (Adults):** 10 mg/kg q 8 hr for 10 days.

■ **IV (Children 3 mo–12 yr):** 20 mg/kg q 8 hr for 10 days.

■ **IV (Children birth–3 mo):** 10 mg/kg q 8 hr for 10 days.

❑ **Varicella Zoster Infections in Immunosuppressed Patients**

■ **IV (Adults):** 10 mg/kg q 8 hr for 7 days.

■ **IV (Children <12 yr):** 20 mg/kg q 8 hr for 7 days.

❑ **Renal Impairment**

■ **PO, IV (Adults and Children):** *CCr >50 ml/min/1.73 m²*—100% of dose q 8 hr; *CCr 25 –50 ml/min/1.73 m²*—100% of dose q 12 hr; *CCr 10 –25 ml/min/1.73 m²*—100% of dose q 24 hr; *CCr 0–10 ml/min/1.73 m²*—50% of dose q 24 hr.

❑ **Herpes labialis**

■ **Topical (Adults and Children >12 yr):** Apply 5 times/day, start at first symptoms.

## AVAILABILITY (generic available)

■ *Capsules:* 200 mg$^{Rx}$ ■ Cost: $177.32/100 ■ *Tablets:* 200 mg$^{Rx}$, 400 mg$^{Rx}$, 800 mg$^{Rx}$ ■ Cost: 400 mg $253.51/100, 800 mg $492.96/100 ■ *Suspension:* 200 mg/5 ml$^{Rx}$ ■ Cost: $112.57/473 ml ■ *Injection:* 500-mg vials$^{Rx}$, 1000-mg vials$^{Rx}$ ■ *Cream:* 5% in 2 g$^{Rx}$ ■ *Ointment:* 5% 3 and 15g$^{Rx}$ ■Cost: $27.36/5%/3 g.

TIME/ACTION PROFILE (antiviral blood levels)

| | ONSET | PEAK | DURATION |
|---|---|---|---|
| PO | unknown | 1.5–2.5 hr | 4 hr |
| IV | prompt | end of infusion | 8 hr |

## NURSING IMPLICATIONS

### ASSESSMENT

❑ Assess lesions before and daily during therapy.

❑ Monitor neurologic status in patients with herpes encephalitis.

■ *Lab Test Considerations:* Monitor BUN, serum creatinine, and CCr before and during therapy. Increased BUN and serum creatinine levels or decreased CCr may indicate renal failure.

### POTENTIAL NURSING DIAGNOSES

■ Skin integrity, risk for impaired (Indications).

■ Infection, risk for (Patient/Family Teaching).

### IMPLEMENTATION

■ **General:** Acyclovir treatment should be started as soon as possible after herpes simplex symptoms appear and within 24 hr of a herpes zoster outbreak.

■ **PO:** Acyclovir may be administered with food or on an empty stomach, with a full glass of water.

❑ Shake oral suspension well before administration.

■ **IV:** Maintain adequate hydration (2000–3000 ml/day), especially during first 2 hr after IV infusion, to prevent crystalluria.

❑ Observe infusion site for phlebitis. Rotate infusion site to prevent phlebitis.

❑ Acyclovir injectable should not be administered topically, IM, subcut, PO, or in the eye.

■ **Intermittent Infusion:** Reconstitute 500-mg or 1-g vial with 10 ml or 20 ml, respectively, of sterile water for injection for a concentration of 50 mg/ml. Do not reconstitute with bacteriostatic water with benzyl alcohol or parabens. Shake well to dissolve completely. Dilute in at least 100 ml of D5W, D5/0.25% NaCl, D5/0.45% NaCl, D5/0.9% NaCl, 0.9% NaCl, or LR for a concentration not to exceed 7 mg/ml. Use reconstituted solution within 12 hr. Once diluted for infusion, the solution should be used within 24 hr. Refrigeration results in precipitation, which dissolves at room temperature.

■ *Rate:* Administer via infusion pump over at least 1 hr to minimize renal tubular damage.

■ **Y-Site Compatibility:** ◆ allopurinol ◆ amikacin ◆ ampicillin ◆ cefamandole ◆ cefazolin ◆ cefonicid ◆ cefoperazone ◆ cefotaxime ◆ cefoxitin ◆ ceftazidime ◆ ceftizoxime ◆ ceftriaxone ◆ cefuroxime ◆ cephapirin ◆ chloramphenicol ◆ cimetidine ◆ clindamycin ◆ dexamethasone sodium phosphate ◆ dimenhydrinate ◆ diphenhydramine ◆ doxycycline ◆ erythromycin lactobionate ◆ famotidine ◆ filgrastim ◆ fluconazole ◆ gatifloxacin ◆ gentamicin ◆ granisetron ◆ heparin ◆ hydrocortisone sodium succinate ◆ hydromorphone ◆ imipenem/cilastatin ◆ linezolid ◆ lorazepam ◆ magnesium sulfate ◆ melphalan ◆ methylprednisolone sodium succinate ◆ metoclopramide ◆ metronidazole ◆ multivitamin infusion ◆ nafcillin ◆ oxacillin ◆ paclitaxel ◆ penicillin G potassium ◆ pentobarbital ◆ perphenazine ◆ piperacillin ◆ potassium chloride ◆ propofol ◆ ranitidine ◆ sodium bicarbonate ◆ tacrolimus ◆ teniposide ◆ theophylline ◆ thiotepa ◆ ticarcillin ◆ tobramycin ◆ trimethoprim/sulfamethoxazole ◆ vancomycin ◆ zidovudine.

■ **Y-Site Incompatibility:** ◆ amifostine ◆ aztreonam ◆ cefepime ◆ dobutamine ◆ dopamine ◆ fludarabine ◆ foscarnet ◆ idarubicin ◆ levofloxacin ◆ ondansetron ◆ piperacillin/tazobactam ◆ sargramostim ◆ vinorelbine.

■ **Additive Compatibility:** ◆ fluconazole.

■ **Additive Incompatibility:** ◆ blood products ◆ protein-containing solutions.

■ **Topical:** Apply to skin lesions only; do not use in the eye.

### PATIENT/FAMILY TEACHING

■ **General Info:** Advise patient to take medication exactly as directed for the full course of therapy. If a dose is missed, take as soon as possible but not just before next dose is due; do not double doses. Acyclovir should not be used more frequently or longer than prescribed.

❑ Advise patients that the additional use of OTC creams, lotions, and ointments may delay healing and may cause spreading of lesions.

❑ Inform patient that acyclovir is not a cure. The virus lies dormant in the ganglia, and acyclovir will not prevent the spread of infection to others.

❏ Advise patient that condoms should be used during sexual contact and that no sexual contact should be made while lesions are present.

❏ Patient should consult health care professional if symptoms are not relieved after 7 days of topical therapy or if oral acyclovir does not decrease the frequency and severity of recurrences. Immunocompromised patients may require a longer time, usually 2 weeks, for crusting over of lesions.

❏ Instruct women with genital herpes to have yearly Papanicolaou smears because they may be more likely to develop cervical cancer.

■ **Topical:** Instruct patient to apply ointment in sufficient quantity to cover all lesions every 3 hr, 6 times/day for 7 days. 0.5-in. ribbon of ointment covers approximately 4 square in. Use a finger cot or glove when applying to prevent inoculation of other areas or spread to other people. Keep affected areas clean and dry. Loose-fitting clothing should be worn to prevent irritation.

❏ Avoid drug contact in or around eyes. Report any unexplained eye symptoms to health care professional immediately; ocular herpetic infection can lead to blindness.

## EVALUATION
**Effectiveness of therapy can be demonstrated by:** ■ Crusting over and healing of skin lesions ■ Decrease in frequency and severity of recurrences ■ Acceleration of complete healing and cessation of pain in herpes zoster ■ Decrease in intensity of chickenpox.

# adalimumab
(a-da-li-**mu**-mab)
Humira

## CLASSIFICATION(S):
**Therapeutic:** antirheumatics
**Pharmacologic:** DMARDs, monoclonal antibodies

### Pregnancy Category B

## INDICATIONS
■ Treatment of moderately to severely active rheumatoid arthritis in patients who have responded inadequately to other DMARDs; may be used with other DMARDs.

## ACTION
■ Neutralizes and prevents the action of tumor necrosis factor (TNF), resulting in anti-inflammatory and antiproliferative activity. **Therapeutic Effects:** ■ Decreased pain and swelling with decreased rate of joint destruction in patients with rheumatoid arthritis.

## PHARMACOKINETICS
**Absorption:** 64% absorbed after subcut administration.
**Distribution:** Synovial fluid concentrations are 31–96% of serum.
**Metabolism and Excretion:** Unknown.
**Half-life:** 14 days (range 10–20 days).

## CONTRAINDICATIONS AND PRECAUTIONS
**Contraindicated in:** ■ Hypersensitivity ■ Active infection (including chronic or localized) ■ Lactation.
**Use Cautiously in:** ■ History of recurrent infection or underlying illness/treatment predisposing to infection ■ Patients residing, or who have resided, where tuberculosis or histoplasmosis are endemic ■ Pre-existing or recent onset CNS demyelinating disorders ■ History of lymphoma ■ Geriatric patients (higher risk of infection/malignancy) ■ Pregnancy (use only if clearly needed) ■ Children (safety not established).

## ADVERSE REACTIONS AND SIDE EFFECTS*
■ **CNS:** <u>headache</u> ■ **CV:** hypertension ■ **GI:** abdominal pain, nausea ■ **GU:** hematuria ■ **Derm:** <u>rash</u> ■ **Local:** <u>injection site reactions</u> ■ **Metab:** hypercholesterolemia, hyperlipidemia ■ **MS:** back pain ■ **Misc:** allergic reactions including ANAPHYLAXIS, INFECTIONS (including reactivation tuberculosis).

## INTERACTIONS
**Drug-Drug:** ■ **Live vaccinations** should not be given concurrently.

## ROUTE AND DOSAGE

■ **Subcut (Adults):** 40 mg every other week; patients not receiving concurrent methotrexate may receive additional benefit by increasing dose to 40 mg once weekly.

## AVAILABILITY

■ *Solution for subcut injection (prefilled syringes):* 40 mg/0.8 ml.

TIME/ACTION PROFILE (improvement)

|        | ONSET   | PEAK    | DURATION |
|--------|---------|---------|----------|
| Subcut | 8–26 wk | 131 hr* | 2 wk†    |

*Blood level.

†Following discontinuation.

## NURSING IMPLICATIONS

### ASSESSMENT

❑ Assess patient for pain and range of motion before and periodically during therapy.

❑ Assess patient for signs of infection (fever, dyspnea, flu-like symptoms, frequent or painful urination, redness or swelling at the site of a wound) prior to injection. Adalimumab is contraindicated in patients with active infection. New infections should be monitored closely; most common are upper respiratory tract infections, bronchitis, and urinary tract infections. Infections may be fatal, especially in patients taking immunosuppressive therapy.

❑ Monitor for injection site reactions (redness and/or itching, rash, hemorrhage, bruising, pain, or swelling). Rash will usually disappear with in a few days. Application of a towel soaked in cold water may relieve pain or swelling.

❑ Assess patient for latex allergy. Needle cover of syringe contains latex and should not be handled by persons sensitive to latex.

❑ Monitor patient for signs of anaphylaxis (urticaria, dyspnea, facial edema) following injection. Medications (antihistamines, corticosteroids, epinephrine) and equipment should be readily available in the event of a severe reaction.

❑ Assess patient for latent tuberculosis with a tuberculin skin test prior to initiation of therapy. Treatment of latent tuberculosis should be started before therapy with adalimumab.

■ *Lab Test Considerations:* May cause agranulocytosis, granulocytopenia, leukopenia, pancytopenia, and polycythemia.

## POTENTIAL NURSING DIAGNOSES

■ Pain, acute (Indications).

■ Infection, risk for (Side Effects).

## IMPLEMENTATION

■ **General:** Administer initial injection under supervision of a health care professional.

❑ Do not administer solutions that are discolored or contain particulate matter. Discard unused solution.

❑ Other DMARDs should be continued during adalimumab therapy.

■ **Subcut:** Administer at a 45° angle in upper thighs or abdomen, avoiding the 2 inches around the navel. Put pressure on injection site for 10 sec, do not rub. Rotate injection sites; avoid areas that are tender, bruised, hard, or red.

## PATIENT/FAMILY TEACHING

❑ Instruct patient on the correct technique for administering adalimumab. Review patient information sheet, preparation of dose, administration sites and technique, and disposal of equipment into a puncture-resistant container.

❑ Advise patient to use calendar stickers provided to by manufacturer to assist in remembering when dose is due. If a dose is missed, instruct patient to administer as soon as possible, then take next dose according to regular schedule. If more than prescribed dose is taken, caution patient to consult health care professional or the HUMIRA Patient Resource Center at 1–800–4HUMIRA (448–6472).

❑ Caution patient to notify health care professional immediately if signs of infection, severe rash, swollen face, or difficulty breathing occurs while taking adalimumab.

❑ Advise patient to consult health care professional before taking other Rx or OTC medications or herbal products.

❑ Instruct patient to notify health care professional of medication regimen prior to treatment or surgery.

### EVALUATION

**Effectiveness of therapy can be demonstrated by:** ■ Decreased pain and swelling with decreased rate of joint destruction in patients with rheumatoid arthritis.

# adenosine
(a-**den**-oh-seen)
Adenocard, Adenoscan

*CLASSIFICATION(S):*
*Therapeutic: antiarrhythmics*

**Pregnancy Category C**

## INDICATIONS

■ Conversion of paroxysmal supraventricular tachycardia (PSVT) to normal sinus rhythm when vagal maneuvers are unsuccessful ■ As a diagnostic agent (with noninvasive techniques) to assess myocardial perfusion defects occurring as a consequence of coronary artery disease.

## ACTION

■ Restores normal sinus rhythm by interrupting re-entrant pathways in the AV node ■ Slows conduction time through the AV node ■ Also produces coronary artery vasodilation. **Therapeutic Effects:** ■ Restoration of normal sinus rhythm.

## PHARMACOKINETICS

**Absorption:** Following IV administration, absorption is complete.

**Distribution:** Taken up by erythrocytes and vascular endothelium.

**Metabolism and Excretion:** Rapidly converted to inosine and adenosine monophosphate.

**Half-life:** <10 sec.

## CONTRAINDICATIONS AND PRECAUTIONS

**Contraindicated in:** ■ Hypersensitivity ■ 2nd- or 3rd-degree AV block or sick sinus syndrome, unless a functional artificial pacemaker is present.

**Use Cautiously in:** ■ Patients with a history of asthma (may induce bronchospasm) ■ Unstable angina ■ Pregnancy or lactation.

## ADVERSE REACTIONS AND SIDE EFFECTS*

■ **CNS:** apprehension, dizziness, headache, head pressure, light-headedness ■ **EENT:** blurred vision, throat tightness ■ **Resp:** shortness of breath, chest pressure, hyperventilation ■ **CV:** facial flushing, transient arrhythmias, chest pain, hypotension, palpitations ■ **GI:** metallic taste, nausea ■ **Derm:** burning sensation, facial flushing, sweating ■ **MS:** neck and back pain ■ **Neuro:** numbness, tingling ■ **Misc:** heaviness in arms, pressure sensation in groin.

## INTERACTIONS

**Drug-Drug:** ■ **Carbamazepine** may increase the risk of progressive heart block ■ **Dipyridamole** potentiates the effects of adenosine (dosage reduction of adenosine recommended) ■ Effects of adenosine may be decreased by **theophylline** or **caffeine** (larger doses of adenosine may be required) ■ Concurrent use with **digoxin** may increase the risk of ventricular fibrillation.

## ROUTE AND DOSAGE

■ **IV (Adults and Children >50 kg):** *Antiarrhythmic*—6 mg by rapid IV bolus; if no results, repeat 1–2 min later as 12-mg rapid bolus. This dose may be repeated (single dose not to exceed 12 mg). *Diagnostic use*—140 mcg/kg/min for 6 min (0.84 mg/kg total).

■ **IV (Children <50 kg):** *Antiarrhythmic*—0.05–0.1 mg/kg as a rapid bolus, may repeat in 1–2 min; if response is inadequate, may increase by 0.05–0.1 mg/kg until sinus rhythm is established or maximum dose of 0.3 mg/kg is used.

## AVAILABILITY

■ *Injection:* 6 mg/2-ml vial[Rx] (Adenocard), 3 mg/1 ml in 30-ml vial[Rx] (Adenoscan).

TIME/ACTION PROFILE (antiarrhythmic effect)

|  | ONSET | PEAK | DURATION |
|---|---|---|---|
| IV | immediate | unknown | 1–2 min |

{ } = Available in Canada only.
*CAPITALS indicates life-threatening; underlines indicate most frequent.

## NURSING IMPLICATIONS

### ASSESSMENT

❑ Monitor heart rate frequently (every 15–30 sec) and ECG continuously throughout therapy. A short, transient period of 1st-, 2nd-, or 3rd-degree heart block or asystole may occur following injection; usually resolves quickly due to short duration of adenosine. Once conversion to normal sinus rhythm is achieved, transient arrhythmias (premature ventricular contractions, atrial premature contractions, sinus tachycardia, sinus bradycardia, skipped beats, AV nodal block) may occur, but generally last a few seconds.

❑ Monitor blood pressure during therapy.

❑ Assess respiratory status (breath sounds, rate) following administration. Patients with history of asthma may experience bronchospasm.

### POTENTIAL NURSING DIAGNOSES

■ Cardiac output, decreased (Indications).

### IMPLEMENTATION

■ **General:** Do not confuse adenosine (Adenocard) with adenosine phosphate.

❑ Crystals may occur if adenosine is refrigerated. Warm to room temperature to dissolve crystals. Solution must be clear before use. Discard unused portions.

■ **Direct IV:** Administer undiluted.

■ *Rate:* Administer over 1–2 seconds via direct IV or into proximal IV line. Follow with rapid saline flush to ensure injection reaches systemic circulation. Slow administration may cause increased heart rate in response to vasodilation.

■ **Intermittent Infusion:** Administer 30-ml vial undiluted as a peripheral infusion. Do not administer solutions that are discolored or contain particulate matter. Discard unused portion.

■ *Rate:* Administer at a rate of 140 mcg/kg/min over 6 min for a total dose of 0.84 mg/kg. Thallium-201 should be injected as close to the venous access as possible at the midpoint (after 3 min) of the infusion.

■ **Y-Site Compatibility:** ◆ Thallium-201.

### PATIENT/FAMILY TEACHING

❑ Caution patient to change positions slowly to minimize orthostatic hypotension. Doses >12 mg decrease blood pressure by decreasing peripheral vascular resistance.

❑ Instruct patient to report facial flushing, shortness of breath, or dizziness.

### EVALUATION

**Effectiveness of therapy can be demonstrated by:** ■ Conversion of supraventricular tachycardia to normal sinus rhythm ■ Diagnosis of myocardial perfusion defects.

## alatrofloxacin, See FLUOROQUINOLONES.

## albumin (human)

(al-**byoo**-min)

Albuminar, Albutein, Buminate, normal human serum albumin, Plasbumin

### CLASSIFICATION(S):

**Therapeutic:** *volume expanders*
**Pharmacologic:** *blood products, colloids*

### Pregnancy Category C

### INDICATIONS

■ Expansion of plasma volume and maintenance of cardiac output in situations associated with fluid volume deficit, including shock, hemorrhage, and burns ■ Temporary replacement of albumin in diseases associated with low levels of plasma proteins, such as nephrotic syndrome or end-stage liver disease, resulting in relief or reduction of associated edema.

### ACTION

■ Provides colloidal oncotic pressure, which serves to mobilize fluid from extravascular tissues back into the intravascular space ■ Requires concurrent administration of appropriate crystalloid. **Therapeutic Effects:** ■ Increase in intravascular fluid volume.

### PHARMACOKINETICS

**Absorption:** Following IV administration, absorption is essentially complete.

**Distribution:** Confined to the intravascular space, unless capillary permeability is increased.

**Metabolism and Excretion:** Probably degraded by the liver.

**Half-life:** 2–3 wk.

## CONTRAINDICATIONS AND PRECAUTIONS

**Contraindicated in:** ■ Allergic reactions to albumin ■ Severe anemia ■ CHF ■ Normal or increased intravascular volume.

**Use Cautiously in:** ■ Severe hepatic or renal disease ■ Dehydration (additional fluids may be required).

## ADVERSE REACTIONS AND SIDE EFFECTS*

■ **CNS:** headache ■ **CV:** PULMONARY EDEMA, fluid overload, hypertension, hypotension, tachycardia ■ **GI:** increased salivation, nausea, vomiting ■ **Derm:** rash, urticaria ■ **MS:** back pain ■ **Misc:** chills, fever, flushing.

## INTERACTIONS

**Drug-Drug:** ■ None significant.

## ROUTE AND DOSAGE

Dosage is highly individualized and depends on condition being treated.

❑ **Shock—5% Albumin**

■ **IV (Adults):** 500 ml, may be repeated within 30 min.

■ **IV (Children):** 50 ml.

■ **IV (Infants and Neonates):** 10–20 ml/kg as a 5% solution.

❑ **Hypoproteinemia—25% Albumin**

■ **IV (Adults):** 50–75 g.

■ **IV (Children):** 25 g.

❑ **Acute Nephrosis—25% Albumin**

■ **IV (Adults):** 100–200 ml.

## AVAILABILITY

■ *Injection:* 5%Rx, 25%Rx.

TIME/ACTION PROFILE (oncotic effect)

| | ONSET | PEAK | DURATION |
|---|---|---|---|
| IV | 15–30 min | unknown | unknown |

## NURSING IMPLICATIONS

### ASSESSMENT

■ **General Info:** Monitor vital signs, CVP, and intake and output before and frequently throughout therapy. If fever, tachycardia, or hypotension occurs, stop infusion and notify physician immediately. Antihistamines may be required to suppress this hypersensitivity response. Hypotension may also result from infusing too rapidly. May be given without regard to patient's blood group.

❑ Assess for signs of vascular overload (elevated CVP, rales/crackles, dyspnea, hypertension, jugular venous distention) during and after administration.

■ **Surgical Patients:** Assess for increased bleeding after administration caused by increased blood pressure and circulating blood volume. Albumin does not contain clotting factors.

■ *Lab Test Considerations:* Serum albumin levels should increase with albumin therapy.

❑ Monitor serum sodium levels; may cause increased concentrations.

❑ Infusions of normal serum albumin may cause false elevation of alkaline phosphatase levels.

❑ Hemorrhage: Monitor hemoglobin and hematocrit levels. These values may decrease because of hemodilution.

### POTENTIAL NURSING DIAGNOSES

■ Cardiac output, decreased (Indications).

■ Fluid volume, deficit (Indications).

■ Fluid volume, excess (Side Effects).

### IMPLEMENTATION

■ **General:** Follow manufacturer's recommendations for administration. Administer through a large-gauge (at least 20-gauge) needle or catheter. Record lot number in patient record.

❑ Solution should be clear amber; 25% albumin solution is equal to 5 times the osmotic value of plasma. Do not administer solutions that are discolored or contain particulate matter. Each liter of normal serum albumin contains 130–160 mEq of sodium and is thus no longer labeled "salt-poor" albumin.

{ } = Available in Canada only.
*CAPITALS indicates life-threatening; underlines indicate most frequent.

❑ Administration of large quantities of normal serum albumin may need to be supplemented with whole blood to prevent anemia. If more than 1000 ml of 5% normal serum albumin is given or if hemorrhage has occurred, the administration of whole blood or packed RBCs may be needed. Hydration status should be monitored and maintained with additional fluids.

■ **Intermittent Infusion:** Administer 5% normal serum albumin undiluted. Normal serum albumin 25% may be administered undiluted or diluted in 0.9% NaCl, D5W, or sodium lactate injection; do not dilute in plain sterile water. Infusion must be completed within 4 hr.

■ *Rate:* Rate of administration is determined by concentration of solution, blood volume, indication, and patient response. In patients with normal blood volume, rate of 5% and 25% solutions should not to exceed 2–4 ml/min and 1 ml/min, respectively. The rate for children is usually 25–50% the adult rate.

❑ *Hypovolemia:* 5% or 25% normal serum albumin may be administered as rapidly as tolerated and repeated in 15–30 min if necessary.

❑ *Burns:* Rate after the first 24 hr should be set to maintain a plasma albumin level of 2.5 g/100 ml or a total serum protein level of 5.2 g/100 ml.

❑ *Hypoproteinemia:* Normal serum albumin 25% is the preferred solution because of the increased concentration of protein. The rate should not exceed 2–3 ml/min of 25% or 5–10 ml/min of 5% solution to prevent circulatory overload and pulmonary edema. This treatment provides a temporary rise in plasma protein until the hypoproteinemia is corrected.

■ **Y-Site Compatibility:** ◆ diltiazem.

■ **Y-Site Incompatibility:** ◆ vancomycin ◆ verapamil.

■ **Solution Compatibility:** 0.9% NaCl, D5W, D5/0.9% NaCl, D5/0.45% NaCl, sodium lactate ⅙ M, D5/LR, and LR.

### PATIENT/FAMILY TEACHING

❑ Explain the purpose of this solution to the patient.

❑ Instruct patient to report signs and symptoms of hypersensitivity reaction.

### EVALUATION

**Effectiveness of therapy can be demonstrated by:** ■ Increase in blood pressure and blood volume when used to treat shock and burns ■ Increased urinary output reflects the mobilization of fluid from extravascular tissues ■ Elevated serum plasma protein in patients with hypoproteinemia.

# albuterol

### (al-**byoo**-ter-ole)

AccuNeb, Airet, {Gen-Salbutamol}, {Novo-Salmol}, Proventil, Proventil HFA, salbutamol, Ventodisk, Ventolin, Ventolin HFA, Volmax, VoSpira ER

### CLASSIFICATION(S):

*Therapeutic: bronchodilators*
*Pharmacologic: adrenergics*

### Pregnancy Category C

### INDICATIONS

■ Used as a bronchodilator to control and prevent reversible airway obstruction caused by asthma or COPD ■ **Inhaln:** Used as a quick-relief agent for acute bronchospasm and for prevention of exercise-induced bronchospasm ■ **PO:** Used as a long-term control agent in patients with chronic/persistent bronchospasm.

### ACTION

■ Binds to beta$_2$-adrenergic receptors in airway smooth muscle, leading to activation of adenyl cyclase and increased levels of cyclic-3′, 5′-adenosine monophosphate (cAMP). Increases in cAMP activate kinases, which inhibit the phosphorylation of myosin and decrease intracellular calcium. Decreased intracellular calcium relaxes smooth muscle airways ■ Relaxation of airway smooth muscle with subsequent bronchodilation ■ Relatively selective for beta$_2$ (pulmonary) receptors. **Therapeutic Effects:** ■ Bronchodilation.

### PHARMACOKINETICS

**Absorption:** Well absorbed after oral administration but rapidly undergoes extensive metabolism.

**Distribution:** Small amounts appear in breast milk.

**Metabolism and Excretion:** Extensively metabolized by the liver and other tissues.
**Half-life:** 3.8 hr.

## CONTRAINDICATIONS AND PRECAUTIONS

**Contraindicated in:** ■ Hypersensitivity to adrenergic amines ■ Hypersensitivity to fluorocarbons (some inhalers).

**Use Cautiously in:** ■ Cardiac disease ■ Hypertension ■ Hyperthyroidism ■ Diabetes ■ Glaucoma ■ Geriatric patients ( ↑ risk adverse reactions; may require dosage reduction) ■ Pregnancy (near term), lactation, and children <2 yr (safety not established) ■ Excess inhaler use may lead to tolerance and paradoxical bronchospasm.

## ADVERSE REACTIONS AND SIDE EFFECTS*

■ **CNS:** <u>nervousness</u>, <u>restlessness</u>, <u>tremor</u>, headache, insomnia ■ **CV:** <u>chest pain</u>, <u>palpitations</u>, angina, arrhythmias, hypertension ■ **GI:** nausea, vomiting ■ **Endo:** hyperglycemia ■ **F and E:** hypokalemia ■ **Neuro:** tremor.

## INTERACTIONS

**Drug-Drug:** ■ Concurrent use with other **adrenergic agents** will have ↑ adrenergic side effects ■ Use with **MAO inhibitors** may lead to hypertensive crisis ■ **Beta blockers** may negate therapeutic effect ■ Risk of hypokalemia ↑ concurrent use of **potassium-losing diuretics** ■ Hypokalemia ↑ the risk of **digoxin** toxicity.

**Drug-Natural Products:** ■ Use with caffeine-containing herbs (**cola nut, guarana, tea, coffee**) ↑ stimulant effect.

## ROUTE AND DOSAGE

■ **PO (Adults and Children ≥12 yr):** 2–4 mg 3–4 times daily (not to exceed 32 mg/day) or 4–8 mg of extended-release tablets twice daily.

■ **PO (Geriatric Patients):** Initial dose should not exceed 2 mg 3–4 times daily, may be increased carefully (up to 32 mg/day).

■ **PO (Children 6–12 yr):** 2 mg 3–4 times daily or 4 mg as extended-release tablets twice daily; may be carefully increased as needed (not to exceed 24 mg/day).

■ **PO (Children 2–6 yr):** 0.1 mg/kg 3 times daily (not to exceed 2 mg 3 times daily initially); may be carefully increased to 0.2 mg/kg 3 times daily (not to exceed 4 mg 3 times daily).

■ **Inhaln (Adults and Children ≥4 yr):** *Via metered-dose inhaler*—2 inhalations q 4–6 hr or 2 inhalations 15 min before exercise (90 mcg/spray); some patients may respond to 1 inhalation.

■ **Inhaln (Adults and Children >12 yr):** *Via nebulization or IPPB*—2.5 mg 3–4 times daily.

■ **Inhaln (Children 2–12 yr):** *Via nebulization or IPPB*—0.1–0.15 mg/kg/dose 3–4 times daily *or* 1.25 mg 3–4 times daily for children 10–15 kg *or* 2.5 mg 3–4 times daily for children >15 kg.

■ **Inhaln (Adults and Children ≥4 yr):** *Via Rotahaler inhalation device*— 200 mcg (as Ventolin Rotacaps) q 4–6 hr (up to 400 mcg q 4–6 hr). May also be given 15 min before exercise.

## AVAILABILITY (generic available)

■ *Tablets:* 2 mg[Rx], 4 mg[Rx] ■ Cost: 2 mg $31.00/60, 4 mg $90.24/100 ■ *Extended-release tablets:* 4 mg[Rx], 8 mg[Rx] ■Cost: 4 mg $/100 ■ *Oral solution (strawberry-flavored syrup):* 2 mg/5 ml[Rx] ■ Cost: 2 mg/5 ml $11.07/118 ml ■ *Metered-dose aerosol:* 90 mcg/spray[Rx], {100 mcg/spray[Rx]}, {80 inhalations/canister[Rx]}, {200 inhalations/canister[Rx]} ■ Cost: 90 mcg/spray $17.66/6.8 g, $35.06/17 g, $32.02/17 g refill ■ *Inhalation solution:* 0.63 mg/3ml[Rx], 1.25 mg/3 ml[Rx], 0.5 mg/ml[Rx], 0.83 mg/ml in vials and 3 ml unit dose[Rx], {1 mg/ml[Rx]}, {2 mg/ml[Rx]}, 5 mg/ml[Rx] ■Cost: 0.5 mg/ml $21.20/20 ml; 0.83 mg/ml $45.34/3ml 25's ■ *Powder for inhalation (Rotacaps):* 200 mcg[Rx] ■Cost: 200 mcg $37.92/100 ■ *Powder for inhalation (Ventodisk):* {200 mcg[Rx]}, {400 mcg[Rx]} ■ ipratropium (Combivent, DuonNeb). See Appendix B.

TIME/ACTION PROFILE (bronchodilation)

|  | ONSET | PEAK | DURATION |
|---|---|---|---|
| PO | 15–30 min | 2–3 hr | 8 hr or more |
| PO–ER | 30 min | 2–3 hr | 12 hr |
| Inhaln | 5–15 min | 60–90 min | 3–6 hr |

{ } = Available in Canada only.
*CAPITALS indicates life-threatening; <u>underlines</u> indicate most frequent.

## NURSING IMPLICATIONS

### ASSESSMENT

❑ Assess lung sounds, pulse, and blood pressure before administration and during peak of medication. Note amount, color, and character of sputum produced.

❑ Monitor pulmonary function tests before initiating therapy and periodically during therapy to determine effectiveness of medication.

❑ Observe for paradoxical bronchospasm (wheezing). If condition occurs, withhold medication and notify physician or other health care professional immediately.

■ **Lab Test Considerations:** May cause transient ↓ in serum potassium concentrations with nebulization or higher-than-recommended doses.

### POTENTIAL NURSING DIAGNOSES

■ Airway clearance, ineffective (Indications).

### IMPLEMENTATION

■ **General:** Do not confuse Salbutamol (albuterol) with Salmeterol.

■ **PO:** Administer oral medication with meals to minimize gastric irritation.

❑ Extended-release tablets should be swallowed whole; do not break, crush, or chew. **Inhaln:** Allow at least 1 min between inhalations of aerosol medication.

❑ For nebulization or IPPB, the 0.5- 0.83-, 1-, and 2-mg/ml solutions do not require dilution before administration. The 5 mg/ml solution must be diluted with 2.5 ml of 0.9% NaCl for inhalation. Diluted solutions are stable for 24 hr at room temperature or 48 hr if refrigerated.

❑ For nebulizer, compressed air or oxygen flow should be 6–10 L/min; a single treatment of 3 ml lasts about 10 min.

❑ IPPB usually lasts 5–20 min.

### PATIENT/FAMILY TEACHING

■ **General Info:** Instruct patient to take albuterol exactly as directed. If on a scheduled dosing regimen, take missed dose as soon as remembered, spacing remaining doses at regular intervals. Do not double doses or increase the dose or frequency of doses. Caution patient not to exceed recommended dose; may cause adverse effects, paradoxical bronchospasm (more likely with first dose

from new cannister), or loss of effectiveness of medication.

❑ Instruct patient to contact health care professional immediately if shortness of breath is not relieved by medication or is accompanied by diaphoresis, dizziness, palpitations, or chest pain.

❑ Instruct patient to prime unit with 4 sprays before using and to discard cannister after 200 sprays. Actuators should not be changed among products.

❑ Inform patient that these products contain hydrofluoralkane (HFA) and the propellant and are described as non-CFC or CFC-free (contain no chlorofluorocarbons).

❑ Advise patient to consult health care professional before taking any OTC medications, natural/herbal products, or alcohol concurrently with this therapy. Caution patient also to avoid smoking and other respiratory irritants.

❑ Inform patient that albuterol may cause an unusual or bad taste.

■ **Inhaln:** Instruct patient in the proper use of the metered-dose inhaler, Rotahaler, or nebulizer (see Appendix F).

❑ Advise patients to use albuterol first if using other inhalation medications and allow 5 min to elapse before administering other inhalant medications unless otherwise directed.

❑ Advise patient to rinse mouth with water after each inhalation dose to minimize dry mouth.

❑ Instruct patient to notify health care professional if no response to the usual dose of albuterol or if contents of one canister are used in less than 2 wk.

### EVALUATION

**Effectiveness of therapy can be demonstrated by:** ■ Prevention or relief of bronchospasm.

---

## alclometasone, See CORTICOSTEROIDS (TOPICAL/LOCAL).

---

## alendronate

(a-**len**-drone-ate)
Fosamax

**CLASSIFICATION(S):**
**Therapeutic:** *bone resorption inhibitors*
**Pharmacologic:** *biphosphonates*
**Pregnancy Category C**

## INDICATIONS

■ Treatment and prevention of postmenopausal osteoporosis ■ Treatment of osteoporosis in men ■ Treatment of Paget's disease of the bone ■ Treatment of corticosteroid-induced osteoporosis in patients (men and women) who are receiving ≥7.5 mg of prednisone/day (or equivalent) with evidence of decreased bone mineral density.

## ACTION

■ Inhibits resorption of bone by inhibiting osteoclast activity. **Therapeutic Effects:** ■ Reversal of the progression of osteoporosis with decreased fractures ■ Decreased progression of Paget's disease.

## PHARMACOKINETICS

**Absorption:** Poorly absorbed (0.6–0.8%) after oral administration.
**Distribution:** Transiently distributes to soft tissue, then distributes to bone.
**Metabolism and Excretion:** Excreted in urine.
**Half-life:** 10 yr (reflects release of drug from skeleton).

## CONTRAINDICATIONS AND PRECAUTIONS

**Contraindicated in:** ■ Renal insufficiency (CCr <35 ml/min) ■ Pregnancy or lactation.
**Use Cautiously in:** ■ Patients with active GI pathology (dysphagia, esophageal disease, gastritis, duodenitis, ulcers) ■ Pre-existing hypocalcemia or vitamin D deficiency.

## ADVERSE REACTIONS AND SIDE EFFECTS*

■ **CNS:** headache ■ **EENT:** blurred vision, conjunctivitis, eye pain/inflammation ■ **GI:** abdominal distention, abdominal pain, acid regurgitation, constipation, diarrhea, dyspepsia, dysphagia, esophageal ulcer, flatulence, gastritis, nausea, taste perversion, vomiting ■ **Derm:** erythema, photosensitivity, rash ■ **MS:** musculoskeletal pain.

## INTERACTIONS

**Drug-Drug:** ■ **Calcium supplements, antacids,** and **other oral medications** ↓ the absorption of alendronate ■ Doses >10 mg/day ↑ risk of adverse GI events when used with **NSAIDs** ■ **IV ranitidine** ↑ blood levels.
**Drug-Food:** ■ **Food** significantly ↓ absorption. **Caffeine (coffee, tea, cola), mineral water,** and **orange juice** also ↓ absorption.

## ROUTE AND DOSAGE

■ **PO (Adults):** *Treatment of osteoporosis—* 10 mg once daily or 70 mg once weekly. *Prevention of osteoporosis—* 5 mg once daily or 35 mg once weekly. *Paget's disease—* 40 mg once daily for 6 mo. Retreatment may be considered for patients who relapse. *Treatment of corticosteroid-induced osteoporosis in men and premenopausal women—* 5 mg once daily. *Treatment of corticosteroid-induced osteoporosis in postmenopausal women not receiving estrogen—* 10 mg once daily.

## AVAILABILITY (generic available)

■ *Tablets:* 5 mg$^{Rx}$, 10 mg$^{Rx}$, 35 mg$^{Rx}$, 40 mg$^{Rx}$, 70 mg$^{Rx}$ ■ Cost: 5 mg $66.61/30, 10 mg $66.61/30, 40 mg $159.01/30.

TIME/ACTION PROFILE (inhibition of bone resorption)

| | ONSET | PEAK | DURATION |
|---|---|---|---|
| PO | 1 mo | 3–6 mo | 3 wk–7 mo† |

†After discontinuation of alendronate.

# NURSING IMPLICATIONS

## ASSESSMENT

■ **Osteoporosis:** Assess patients for low bone mass before and periodically during therapy.
■ **Paget's Disease:** Assess for symptoms of Paget's disease (bone pain, headache, decreased visual and auditory acuity, increased skull size).
■ *Lab Test Considerations: Osteoporosis:* Assess serum calcium before and periodical-

ly during therapy. Hypocalcemia and vitamin D deficiency should be treated before initiating alendronate therapy. May cause mild, transient elevations of calcium and phosphate.

❑ *Paget's Disease:* Monitor alkaline phosphatase before and periodically during therapy. Alendronate is indicated for patients with alkaline phosphatase twice the upper limit of normal.

## POTENTIAL NURSING DIAGNOSES

■ Injury, risk for (Indications).

## IMPLEMENTATION

■ **General:** Do not confuse Fosamax (alendronate) with Flomax (tamsulosin).

■ **PO:** Administer first thing in the morning with 6–8 oz plain water 30 min before other medications, beverages, or food.

## PATIENT/FAMILY TEACHING

❑ Instruct patient on the importance of taking exactly as directed, first thing in the morning, 30 min before other medications, beverages, or food. Waiting longer than 30 min will improve absorption. Alendronate should be taken with 6–8 oz plain water (mineral water, orange juice, coffee, and other beverages decrease absorption). If a dose is missed, skip dose and resume the next morning; do not double doses or take later in the day. If a weekly dose is missed, take the morning after remembered and resume the following week on the chosed say. Do not take 2 tablets on the same day. Do not discontinue without consulting health care professional.

❑ Caution patient to remain upright for 30 min following dose to facilitate passage to stomach and minimize risk of esophageal irritation. Advise patient to discontinue alendronate and notify health care provider if pain or difficulty swallowing, retrosternal pain or new/worsening heartburn occur.

❑ Advise patient to eat a balanced diet and consult health care professional about the need for supplemental calcium and vitamin D.

❑ Encourage patient to participate in regular exercise and to modify behaviors that increase the risk of osteoporosis (stop smoking, reduce alcohol consumption).

❑ Caution patient to use sunscreen and protective clothing to prevent photosensitivity reactions.

❑ Advise patient to notify health care professional if blurred vision, eye pain or inflammation occur.

❑ Advise female patient to notify health care professional if pregnancy is planned or suspected or if she is breastfeeding.

## EVALUATION

**Effectiveness of therapy can be demonstrated by:** ■ Prevention of or decrease in the progression of osteoporosis in postmenopausal women ■ Treatment of osteoporosis in men ■ Decrease in the progression of Paget's disease ■ Treatment of corticosteroid-induced osteoporosis.

# alfuzosin

(al-**fyoo**-zo-sin)

Uroxatral

## CLASSIFICATION(S):

**Therapeutic:** *urinary tract antispasmodics*
**Pharmacologic:** *peripherally acting antiadrenergics*

### Pregnancy Category B

## INDICATIONS

■ Management of symptomatic benign prostatic hypertrophy (BPH).

## ACTION

■ Selectively blocks alpha$_1$– adrenergic receptors in the lower urinary tract to relax smooth muscle in the bladder neck and prostate. **Therapeutic Effects:** ■ Increased urine flow and decreased symptoms of BPH.

## PHARMACOKINETICS

**Absorption:** 49% absorbed following oral administration, food enhances absorption.
**Distribution:** Unknown.
**Metabolism and Excretion:** Mostly metabolized by the liver (CYP3A4 enzyme system); 69% eliminated in feces, 24% in urine.
**Half-life:** 10 hr.

## CONTRAINDICATIONS AND PRECAUTIONS

**Contraindicated in:** ■ Hypersensitivity ■ Moderate to severe hepatic impairment ■ Potent inhibitors of the CYP3A4 enzyme system ■ Concurrent use of other alpha-adrenergic blocking agents ■ Severe renal impairment ■ Women or children.

**Use Cautiously in:** ■ Congenital or acquired QTc prolongation or concurrent use of other drugs know to prolong QTc ■ Geriatric patients (consider age-related changes in body mass, cardiac, renal and hepatic function) ■ Mild hepatic impairment.

## ADVERSE REACTIONS AND SIDE EFFECTS*

■ **CNS:** dizziness, fatigue, headache ■ **Resp:** bronchitis, sinusitis, pharyngitis ■ **CV:** postural hypotension ■ **GI:** abdominal pain, constipation, dyspepsia, nausea ■ **GU:** impotence.

## INTERACTIONS

**Drug-Drug:** ■ **Ketoconazole, itraconazole,** and **ritonavir** ↓ metabolism and significantly ↑ levels and effects (concurrent use in contraindicated) ■ Levels are also ↑ by **cimetidine, atenolol,** and **diltiazem** ■ Alfuzosin ↑ levels and may ↑ effects of **atenolol** and **diltiazem** (monitor blood pressure and heart rate) ■ ↑ risk of hypotension with **antihypertensives, nitrates,** and acute ingestion of **alcohol**.

## ROUTE AND DOSAGE

■ **PO (Adults):** 10 mg once daily.

## AVAILABILITY

■ *Extended-release tablets:* 10 mg^Rx.

TIME/ACTION PROFILE

| | ONSET | PEAK | DURATION |
|---|---|---|---|
| PO-ER | within hr | 8 hr | 24 hr |

# NURSING IMPLICATIONS

## ASSESSMENT

❑ Assess patient for symptoms of benign prostatic hypertrophy (urinary hesitancy, feeling of incomplete bladder emptying, interruption of urinary stream, impairment of size and force of urinary stream, terminal urinary dribbling, straining to start flow, dysuria, ur-

gency) before and periodically during therapy.

❑ Assess patient for orthostatic reaction and syncope. Monitor BP (lying and standing) and pulse frequently during initial dose adjustment and periodically thereafter. May occur within a few hrs after initial doses and occasionally thereafter.

❑ Rule out prostatic carcinoma before therapy; symptoms are similar.

## POTENTIAL NURSING DIAGNOSES

■ Injury, risk for (Side Effects).
■ Noncompliance (Patient/Family Teaching).

## IMPLEMENTATION

■ **PO:** Administer with food at the same meal each day. Tablets must be swallowed whole; do not crush, break, or chew.

## PATIENT/FAMILY TEACHING

❑ Instruct patient to take medication with the same meal each day. Take missed doses as soon as remembered. If not remembered until next day, omit; do not double doses.

❑ May cause dizziness or drowsiness. Advise patient to avoid driving or other activities requiring alertness until response to the medication is known.

❑ Caution patient to avoid sudden changes in position to decrease orthostatic hypotension.

❑ Advise patient to consult health care professional before taking any cough, cold, or allergy remedies.

❑ Instruct patient to notify health care professional of medication regimen before any surgery.

❑ Advise patient to notify health care professional if frequent dizziness or fainting occurs.

❑ Emphasize the importance of follow-up exams to evaluate effectiveness of medication.

## EVALUATION

**Effectiveness of therapy can be demonstrated by:** ■ Decreased symptoms of benign prostatic hypertrophy.

{ } = Available in Canada only.
*CAPITALS indicates life-threatening; underlines indicate most frequent.

# allopurinol

(al-oh-**pure**-i-nole)

Alloprim, {Apo-Allopurinol}, Lopurin, {Purinol}, Zyloprim

## CLASSIFICATION(S):

**Therapeutic:** antigout agents, antihyperuricemics
**Pharmacologic:** xanthine oxidase inhibitors

## Pregnancy Category C

## INDICATIONS

■ **PO:** Prevention of attack of gouty arthritis and nephropathy ■ **PO, IV:** Treatment of secondary hyperuricemia, which may occur during treatment of tumors or leukemias.

## ACTION

■ Inhibits the production of uric acid. **Therapeutic Effects:** ■ Lowering of serum uric acid levels.

## PHARMACOKINETICS

**Absorption:** Well absorbed (80%) following oral administration.

**Distribution:** Widely distributed in tissue water.

**Metabolism and Excretion:** Metabolized to oxypurinol, an active compound with a long half-life. 12% excreted unchanged, 76% excreted as oxypurinol.

**Half-life:** 2–3 hr (oxypurinol 24 hr).

## CONTRAINDICATIONS AND PRECAUTIONS

**Contraindicated in:** ■ Hypersensitivity ■ Pregnancy or lactation.

**Use Cautiously in:** ■ Acute attacks of gout ■ Renal insufficiency (dosage reduction required if CCr <20 ml/min) ■ Dehydration (adequate hydration necessary).

## ADVERSE REACTIONS AND SIDE EFFECTS*

■ **CNS:** drowsiness ■ **GI:** diarrhea, hepatitis, nausea, vomiting ■ **GU:** renal failure ■ **Derm:** rash, urticaria ■ **Hemat:** bone marrow depression ■ **Misc:** hypersensitivity reactions.

## INTERACTIONS

**Drug-Drug:** ■ Use with **mercaptopurine** and **azathioprine** increases bone marrow depressant properties—dosages of these drugs should be reduced ■ Use with **ampicillin** or **amoxicillin** increases the risk of rash ■ Use with **oral hypoglycemic agents** and **warfarin** increases the effects of these drugs ■ Use with **thiazide diuretics** or **ACE inhibitors** increases the risk of hypersensitivity reactions ■ Large doses of allopurinol may increase the risk of **theophylline** toxicity.

## ROUTE AND DOSAGE

❏ **Management of Gout**

■ **PO (Adults):** *Initially*—100 mg/day; increase at weekly intervals based on serum uric acid (not to exceed 800 mg/day). Doses >300 mg/day should be given in divided doses. *Maintenance dose*—100–200 mg 2–3 times daily. Doses of ≤300 mg may be given as a single daily dose.

❏ **Management of Secondary Hyperuricemia**

■ **PO (Adults):** 600–800 mg/day in divided doses starting 12 hr–3 days before chemotherapy or radiation.

■ **PO (Children 6–10 yr):** 300 mg daily.

■ **PO (Children <6 yr):** 150 mg daily.

■ **IV (Adults):** 200–400 mg/m²/day (up to 600 mg/day) as a single daily dose or in divided doses q 6–12 hr.

■ **IV (Children):** 200 mg/m²/day initially as a single daily dose or in divided doses q 6–12 hr.

❏ **Renal Impairment**

■ **PO (Adults):** *CCr 60 ml/min*—200 mg/day; *CCr 40 ml/min*—150 mg/day; *CCr 20 ml/min*—100 mg/day; *CCr 10 ml/min*—100 mg/day every other day; *CCr <10 ml/min*—100 mg 3 times weekly.

■ **IV (Adults):** *CCr 10–20 ml/min*—200 mg/day; *CCr 3–10 ml/min*—100 mg/day; *CCr <3 ml/min*—100 mg/day at extended intervals.

## AVAILABILITY (generic available)

■ *Tablets:* 100 mg$^{Rx}$, 300 mg$^{Rx}$ ■ Cost: 100 mg $18.50/100, 300 mg $11.75/90 ■ *Injection:* 500 mg/vial$^{Rx}$.

TIME/ACTION PROFILE (hypouricemic effect)

| | ONSET | PEAK | DURATION† |
|---|---|---|---|
| PO, IV | 2–3 days | 1–3 wk | 1–2 wk |

†Duration after discontinuation of allopurinol.

## NURSING IMPLICATIONS

### ASSESSMENT

- **General Info:** Monitor intake and output ratios. Decreased kidney function can cause drug accumulation and toxic effects. Ensure that patient maintains adequate fluid intake (minimum 2500–3000 ml/day) to minimize risk of kidney stone formation.
- ❑ Assess patient for rash or more severe hypersensitivity reactions. Discontinue allopurinol immediately if rash occurs. Therapy should be discontinued permanently if reaction is severe. Therapy may be reinstated after a mild reaction has subsided, at a lower dose (50 mg/day with very gradual titration). If skin rash recurs, discontinue permanently.
- **Gout:** Monitor for joint pain and swelling. Addition of colchicine or NSAIDs may be necessary for acute attacks. Prophylactic doses of colchicine or an NSAID should be administered concurrently during the first 3–6 mo of therapy because of an increased frequency of acute attacks of gouty arthritis during early therapy.
- **Lab Test Considerations:** Serum and urine uric acid levels usually begin to decrease 2–3 days after initiation of oral therapy.
- ❑ Monitor blood glucose in patients receiving oral hypoglycemic agents. May cause hypoglycemia.
- ❑ Hematologic, renal, and liver function tests should be monitored before and periodically throughout therapy, especially during the first few months. May cause elevation of serum alkaline phosphatase, bilirubin, AST, and ALT levels. Decreased CBC and platelets may indicate bone marrow depression. Elevated BUN, serum creatinine, and CCr may indicate nephrotoxicity. These are usually reversed with discontinuation of therapy.

### POTENTIAL NURSING DIAGNOSES

- Pain, acute (Indications).

## IMPLEMENTATION

- **PO:** May be administered with milk or meals to minimize gastric irritation. May be crushed and given with fluid or mixed with food for patients who have difficulty swallowing.
- **Intermittent Infusion:** Reconstitute each 30-ml vial with 25 ml of sterile water for injection. Solution should be clear and almost colorless with only slight opalescence. Dilute to desired concentration with 0.9% NaCl or D5W for a final concentration of not >6 mg/ml. Administer within 10 hr of reconstitution; do not refrigerate. Do not administer solutions that are discolored or contain particulate matter.
- *Rate:* Infusion should be initiated 24–48 hr before start of chemotherapy known to cause tumor cell lysis. Rate of infusion depends on volume of infusate. May be administered as a single infusion or equally divided infusions at 6-, 8-, or 12-hr intervals at a concentration of not >6 mg/ml.
- **Additive Incompatibility:** ◆ amikacin ◆ amphotericin B ◆ carmustine ◆ cefotaxime ◆ chlorpromazine ◆ cimetidine ◆ clindamycin ◆ cytarabine ◆ dacarbazine ◆ daunorubicin ◆ diphenhydramine ◆ doxorubicin ◆ doxycycline ◆ droperidol ◆ floxuridine ◆ gentamicin ◆ haloperidol ◆ idarubicin ◆ imipenem/cilastatin ◆ mechlorethamine ◆ meperidine ◆ metoclopramide ◆ methylprednisolone sodium succinate ◆ minocycline ◆ nalbuphine ◆ netilmicin ◆ ondansetron ◆ prochlorperazine ◆ promethazine ◆ sodium bicarbonate ◆ streptozocin ◆ tobramycin ◆ vinblastine.

## PATIENT/FAMILY TEACHING

- ❑ Instruct patient to take allopurinol exactly as directed. If a dose is missed, take as soon as remembered. If dosing schedule is once daily, do not take if remembered the next day. If dosing schedule is more than once a day, take up to 300 mg for the next dose.
- ❑ Instruct patient to continue taking allopurinol along with an NSAID or colchicine during an acute attack of gout. Allopurinol helps prevent but does not relieve acute gout attacks.

❑ Alkaline diet may be ordered. Urinary acidification with large doses of vitamin C or other acids may increase kidney stone formation (see Appendix Q). Advise patient of need for increased fluid intake.

❑ May occasionally cause drowsiness. Caution patient to avoid driving or other activities requiring alertness until response to drug is known.

❑ Instruct patient to report skin rash or influenza symptoms (chills, fever, muscle aches and pains, nausea, or vomiting) occurring with or shortly after skin rash to health care professional immediately; may indicate hypersensitivity.

❑ Advise patient that large amounts of alcohol increase uric acid concentrations and may decrease the effectiveness of allopurinol.

❑ Emphasize the importance of follow-up exams to monitor effectiveness and side effects.

### EVALUATION

**Effectiveness of therapy can be demonstrated by:** ■ Decreased serum and urinary uric acid levels. May take 2–6 wk to observe clinical improvement in patients treated for gout.

## almotriptan

(al-moe-**trip**-tan)

Axert

### CLASSIFICATION(S):

**Therapeutic:** vascular headache suppressants

**Pharmacologic:** 5 $HT_1$ agonists

### Pregnancy Category C

### INDICATIONS

■ Acute treatment of migraine headache.

### ACTION

■ Acts as an agonist at specific 5-$HT_1$ receptor sites in intracranial blood vessels and sensory trigeminal nerves. **Therapeutic Effects:** ■ Cranial vessel vasoconstriction with associated decrease in release of neuropetides and resultant decrease in migraine headache.

### PHARMACOKINETICS

**Absorption:** Well absorbed following oral administration (70%).

**Distribution:** Unknown.

**Metabolism and Excretion:** 40% excreted unchanged in urine; 27% metabolized by monoamine oxidase-A (MAO-A); 12% metabolized by cytochrome P450 hepatic enzymes (3A4 and 2D6); 13% excreted in feces as unchanged and metabolized drug.

**Half-life:** 3–4 hr

### CONTRAINDICATIONS AND PRECAUTIONS

**Contraindicated in:** ■ Hypersensitivity ■ Ischemic cardiovascular, cerebrovascular, or peripheral vascular syndromes ■ History of significant cardiovascular disease ■ Uncontrolled hypertension ■ Should not be used within 24 hr of other 5-$HT_1$ agonists or ergot-type compounds (dihydroergotamine) ■ Basilar or hemiplegic migraine ■ Concurrent MAO-A inhibitor therapy or within 2 wk of discontinuing MAO-A inhibitor therapy.

**Use Cautiously in:** ■ Cardiovascular risk factors (hypertension, hypercholesterolemia, cigarette smoking, obesity, diabetes, strong family history, menopausal women or men >40 yr); use only if cardiovascular status has been evaluated and determined to be safe and first dose is administered under supervision ■ Impaired hepatic or renal function ■ Pregnancy, lactation, or children <18 yr (safety not established).

### ADVERSE REACTIONS AND SIDE EFFECTS*

■ **CNS:** drowsiness, headache ■ **CV:** CORONARY ARTERY VASOSPASM, MI, myocardial ischemia, VENTRICULAR FIBRILLATION, VENTRICULAR TACHYCARDIA ■ **GI:** dry mouth, nausea ■ **Neuro:** paresthesia.

### INTERACTIONS

**Drug-Drug:** ■ Concurrent use with **MAO-A inhibitors** increases blood levels and the risk of adverse reactions (concurrent use or use within 2 wk or MAO inhibitor is contraindicated) ■ Concurrent use with other **5-$HT_1$ agonists** or **ergot-type compounds (dihydroergotamine)** may result in additive vasoactive properties (avoid use within 24 hr of each other) ■ Concurrent use with **SSRI antidepressants** may result in weakness, hyperreflexia, and incoordination ■ Blood levels and effects may be increased by **ketoconazole, itra-**

conazole, ritonavir, and **erythromycin** (inhibitors of CYP 3A4 enzymes).

## ROUTE AND DOSAGE

- **PO (Adults):** 6.25–12.5 mg initially, may repeat in 2 hr; not to exceed 2 doses per 24-hr period.
- ❏ Hepatic/Renal Impairment
- **PO (Adults):** 6.25 mg initially, may repeat in 2 hr; not to exceed 2 doses per 24–hr period.

## AVAILABILITY

- *Tablets:* 6.25 mg$^{Rx}$, 12.5 mg$^{Rx}$.

TIME/ACTION PROFILE (Blood levels)

| | ONSET | PEAK | DURATION |
|---|---|---|---|
| PO | unknown | 1–3 hr | unknown |

## NURSING IMPLICATIONS

### ASSESSMENT

- ❏ Assess pain location, character, intensity, and duration and associated symptoms (photophobia, phonophobia, nausea, vomiting) during migraine attack.

### POTENTIAL NURSING DIAGNOSES

- Pain, acute (Indications).

### IMPLEMENTATION

- **PO:** Tablets should be swallowed whole with liquid.

### PATIENT/FAMILY TEACHING

- ❏ Inform patient that almotriptan should only be used during a migraine attack. It is meant to be used for relief of migraine attacks but not to prevent or reduce the number of attacks.
- ❏ Instruct patient to administer almotriptan as soon as symptoms of a migraine attack appear, but it may be administered any time during an attack. If migraine symptoms return, a second dose may be used. Allow at least 2 hr between doses, and do not use more than 2 doses in any 24-hr period.
- ❏ If first dose does not relieve headache, additional almotriptan doses are not likely to be effective; notify health care professional.

- ❏ Caution patient not to take almotriptan within 24 hr of another vascular headache suppressant.
- ❏ Advise patient that lying down in a darkened room following almotriptan administration may further help relieve headache.
- ❏ Caution patient not to use almotriptan if she is pregnant, suspects she is pregnant, plans to become pregnant, or is breastfeeding. Adequate contraception should be used during therapy.
- ❏ Advise patient to notify health care professional prior to next dose of almotriptan if pain or tightness in the chest occurs during use. If pain is severe or does not subside, notify health care professional immediately. If feelings of tingling, heat, flushing, heaviness, pressure, drowsiness, dizziness, tiredness, or sickness develop discuss with health care professional at next visit.
- ❏ May cause dizziness or drowsiness. Caution patient to avoid driving or other activities requiring alertness until response to medication is known.
- ❏ Advise patient to avoid alcohol, which aggravates headaches, during almotriptan use.
- ❏ Instruct patient to consult health care professional before taking other prescription or OTC or herbal/alternative preparations.

### EVALUATION

**Effectiveness of therapy can be demonstrated by:** ■ Relief of migraine attack.

### alprazolam
(al-**pray**-zoe-lam)
{Apo-Alpraz}, {Novo-Alprazol}, {Nu-Alpraz}, Xanax, Xanax XR

**CLASSIFICATION(S):**
*Therapeutic: antianxiety agents*
*Pharmacologic: benzodiazepines*

Schedule IV

Pregnancy Category D

## INDICATIONS

■ Treatment of anxiety ■ Management of panic attacks. **Unlabeled uses:** ■ Management of symptoms of premenstrual syndrome (PMS).

## ACTION

■ Acts at many levels in the CNS to produce anxiolytic effect ■ May produce CNS depression ■ Effects may be mediated by GABA, an inhibitory neurotransmitter. **Therapeutic Effects:** ■ Relief of anxiety.

## PHARMACOKINETICS

**Absorption:** Well absorbed (90%) from the GI tract; absorption is slower with extended–release tablets.

**Distribution:** Widely distributed, crosses blood-brain barrier. Probably crosses the placenta and enters breast milk. Accumulation is minimal.

**Metabolism and Excretion:** Metabolized by the liver (CYP3A4 enzyme system) to an active compound that is subsequently rapidly metabolized.

**Half-life:** 12–15 hr.

## CONTRAINDICATIONS AND PRECAUTIONS

**Contraindicated in:** ■ Hypersensitivity ■ Cross-sensitivity with other benzodiazepines may exist ■ Patients with pre-existing CNS depression ■ Severe uncontrolled pain ■ Narrow-angle glaucoma ■ Pregnancy and lactation ■ Concurrent itraconazole or ketoconazole.

**Use Cautiously in:** ■ Hepatic dysfunction ( ↓ dose required) ■ Concurrent use of nefazodone, fluvoxamine, cimetidine ( ↓ dose recommended) ■ Concurrent use with fluoxetine, hormonal contraceptives, propoxyphene, diltiazem, isoniazid, erythromycin, clarithromycin, grapefruit juice ( ↓ dose may be necessary) ■ History of suicide attempt or drug dependence ■ Elderly or debilitated patients ( ↓ dose required).

## ADVERSE REACTIONS AND SIDE EFFECTS*

■ **CNS:** dizziness, drowsiness, lethargy, confusion, hangover, headache, mental depression, paradoxical excitation ■ **EENT:** blurred vision ■ **GI:** constipation, diarrhea, nausea, vomiting ■ **Derm:** rashes ■ **Misc:** physical dependence, psychological dependence, tolerance.

## INTERACTIONS

**Drug-Drug:** ■ **Alcohol, antidepressants, other benzodiazepines, antihistamines, and opioid analgesics**—concurrent use results in ↑ CNS depression ■ **Hormonal contraceptives, disulfiram, fluoxetine, isoniazid, metoprolol, propoxyphene, propranolol, valproic acid, CYP3A4 inhibitors (erythromycin, ketoconazole, itraconazole, fluvoxamine, cimetidine, nefazodone)** ↓ metabolism of alprazolam, ↑ blood levels and ↑ its actions (dosage adjustments may be necessary) ■ May ↓ efficacy of **levodopa** ■ **CYP3A4 inducers (rifampin, carbamazepine, or barbiturates)** ↑ metabolism and ↓ effects of alprazolam ■ Sedative effects may be ↓ by **theophylline** ■ **Cigarette smoking** ↓ blood levels and effects.

**Drug-Natural Products:** ■ **Kava, valerian, chamomile,** or **hops** can ↑ CNS depression.

**Drug-Food:** ■ Concurrent ingestion of **grapefruit juice** ↑ blood levels.

## ROUTE AND DOSAGE

❑ **Anxiety**

■ **PO (Adults):** 0.25–0.5 mg 2–3 times daily (not >4 mg/day; begin with 0.25 mg 2–3 times daily in geriatric/debilitated patients).

❑ **Panic Attacks**

■ **PO (Adults):** 0.5 mg 3 times daily; may be increased as needed (not >10 mg/day). *Extended–release tablets (Xanax XR)*—0.5–1 mg once daily in the morning, may be increased every 3–4 days by not more than 1 mg/day; up to 10 mg/day (usual range 3–6 mg/day).

## AVAILABILITY (generic available)

■ *Tablets:* 0.25 mg[Rx], 0.5 mg[Rx], 1 mg[Rx], 2 mg[Rx] ■ Cost: 0.25 mg $98.21/100, 0.5 mg $122.35/100, 1 mg $163.25/100, 2 mg $277.56/100 ■ *Extended-release tablets:* 0.5 mg[Rx], 1 mg[Rx], 2 mg[Rx], 3 mg[Rx].

TIME/ACTION PROFILE (sedation)

|  | ONSET | PEAK | DURATION |
|---|---|---|---|
| PO | 1–2 hr | 1–2 hr | up to 24 hr |

# NURSING IMPLICATIONS

## ASSESSMENT

- Assess degree and manifestations of anxiety and mental status prior to and periodically during therapy.
- Assess patient for drowsiness, light-headedness, and dizziness. These symptoms usually disappear as therapy progresses. Dose should be reduced if these symptoms persist.
- Prolonged high-dose therapy may lead to psychological or physical dependence. Risk is greater in patients taking >4 mg/day. Restrict the amount of drug available to patient.
- **Lab Test Considerations:** Monitor CBC and liver and renal function periodically during long-term therapy. May cause ↓ hematocrit and neutropenia.

## POTENTIAL NURSING DIAGNOSES

- Anxiety (Indications).
- Injury, risk for (Side Effects).

## IMPLEMENTATION

- **General:** Do not confuse Xanax (alprazolam) with Zantac (ranitidine).
- If early morning anxiety or anxiety between doses occurs, the same total daily dose should be divided into more frequent intervals.
- **PO:** May be administered with food if GI upset occurs.
- Tablets may be crushed and taken with food or fluids if patient has difficulty swallowing. Do not crush, break, or chew extended-release tablets.

## PATIENT/FAMILY TEACHING

- Instruct patient to take medication exactly as directed; do not skip or double up on missed doses. If a dose is missed, take within 1 hr; otherwise, skip the dose and return to regular schedule. If medication is less effective after a few weeks, check with health care professional; do not increase dose. Abrupt withdrawal may cause sweating, vomiting, muscle cramps, tremors, and seizures.
- May cause drowsiness or dizziness. Caution patient to avoid driving and other activities requiring alertness until response to the medication is known.

- Advise patient to avoid the use of alcohol or other CNS depressants concurrently with alprazolam. Instruct patient to consult health care professional before taking OTC medications or natural/herbal products concurrently with this medication.

## EVALUATION

**Effectiveness of therapy can be demonstrated by:** ■ Decreased sense of anxiety ▫ Increased ability to cope ■ Decreased frequency and severity of panic attacks. Treatment with this medication should not exceed 4 mo without re-evaluation of the patient's need for the drug ■ Decreased symptoms of premenstrual syndrome.

---

# alteplase, See THROMBOLYTIC AGENTS.

---

# aluminum hydroxide

AlternaGEL, Alu-Cap, {Alugel}, Aluminet, Alu-Tab, Amphojel, Basalgel, Dialume

## CLASSIFICATION(S):

**Therapeutic:** antiulcer agents, hypophosphatemics
**Pharmacologic:** antacids, phosphate binders

### Pregnancy Category UK

## INDICATIONS

■ Lowering of phosphate levels in patients with chronic renal failure ■ Adjunctive therapy in the treatment of peptic, duodenal, and gastric ulcers ■ Hyperacidity, indigestion, reflux esophagitis.

## ACTION

■ Binds phosphate in the GI tract ■ Neutralizes gastric acid and inactivates pepsin. **Therapeutic Effects:** ■ Lowering of serum phosphate levels ■ Healing of ulcers and decreased pain associated with ulcers or gastric hyperacidity ■ Constipation limits use alone in the treatment of ulcer disease ■ Frequently found in combination with magnesium-containing compounds.

## PHARMACOKINETICS

**Absorption:** With chronic use, small amounts of aluminum are systemically absorbed.

**Distribution:** If absorbed, aluminum distributes widely, crosses the placenta, and enters breast milk. Concentrates in the CNS with chronic use.

**Metabolism and Excretion:** Mostly excreted in feces. Small amounts absorbed are excreted by the kidneys.

**Half-life:** Unknown.

## CONTRAINDICATIONS AND PRECAUTIONS

**Contraindicated in:** ■ Severe abdominal pain of unknown cause.

**Use Cautiously in:** ■ Hypercalcemia ■ Hypophosphatemia ■ Pregnancy (generally considered safe; chronic high-dose therapy should be avoided).

## ADVERSE REACTIONS AND SIDE EFFECTS*

■ **GI:** constipation ■ **F and E:** hypophosphatemia.

## INTERACTIONS

**Drug-Drug:** ■ Absorption of **tetracyclines, chlorpromazine, iron salts, isoniazid, digoxin,** or **fluoroquinolones** may be decreased ■ **Salicylate** blood levels may be decreased ■ **Quinidine, mexiletine,** and **amphetamine** levels may be increased if enough antacid is ingested such that urine pH is increased.

## ROUTE AND DOSAGE

❑ **Hypophosphatemia**

■ **PO (Adults):** 1.9–4.8 g (30–40 ml of regular suspension or 15–20 ml of concentrated suspension) 3–4 times daily.

■ **PO (Children):** 50–150 mg/kg/24 hr in 4–6 divided doses; titrate to normal serum phosphate levels.

❑ **Antacid**

■ **PO (Adults):** 500–1500 mg (5–30 ml) 3–6 times daily.

## AVAILABILITY (generic available)

■ *Capsules:* 475 mg^OTC, 500 mg^OTC ■ *Tablets:* 300 mg^OTC, 500 mg^OTC, 600 mg^OTC ■ *Suspen-*

*sion:* 320 mg/5 ml^OTC, 450 mg/5 ml^OTC, 600 mg/5 ml^OTC, 675 mg/5 ml^OTC ■ magnesium carbonate, calcium carbonate, simethicone, and mineral oil. See Appendix B.

### TIME/ACTION PROFILE

|  | ONSET | PEAK | DURATION |
|---|---|---|---|
| PO† | hr–days | days–wk | days |
| PO‡ | 15–30 min | 30 min | 30 min–3 hr |

†Hypophosphatemic effect.
‡Antacid effect.

# NURSING IMPLICATIONS

## ASSESSMENT

❑ Assess location, duration, character, and precipitating factors of gastric pain.

■ *Lab Test Considerations:* Monitor serum phosphate and calcium levels periodically during chronic use of aluminum hydroxide.

❑ May cause increased serum gastrin and decreased serum phosphate concentrations.

❑ In treatment of severe ulcer disease, guaiac stools and emesis and monitor pH of gastric secretions.

## POTENTIAL NURSING DIAGNOSES

■ Pain, acute (Indications).

■ Constipation (Side Effects).

## IMPLEMENTATION

■ **General:** Antacids cause premature dissolution and absorption of enteric-coated tablets and may interfere with absorption of other oral medications. Separate administration of aluminum hydroxide and oral medications by at least 1–2 hr.

❑ Tablets must be chewed thoroughly before swallowing to prevent their entering small intestine in undissolved form. Follow with a glass of water.

❑ Shake liquid preparations well before pouring. Follow administration with water to ensure passage into stomach.

❑ Liquid dosage forms are considered more effective than tablets.

■ **Hypophosphatemic:** For phosphate lowering, follow dose with full glass of water or fruit juice.

■ **Antacid:** May be given in conjunction with magnesium-containing antacids to minimize constipation, except in patients with renal failure. Administer 1 and 3 hr after meals and at bedtime for maximum antacid effect.

❑ For treatment of peptic ulcer, aluminum hydroxide may be administered every 1–2 hr while the patient is awake or diluted with 2–3 parts water and administered intragastrically every 30 min for 12 or more hr per day. Physician may order NG tube clamped after administration.

❑ For reflux esophagitis, administer 15 ml 20–40 min after meals and at bedtime.

### PATIENT/FAMILY TEACHING

■ **General Info:** Instruct patient to take aluminum hydroxide exactly as directed. If on a regular dosing schedule and a dose is missed, take as soon as remembered if not almost time for next dose; do not double doses.

❑ Advise patient not to take aluminum hydroxide within 1–2 hr of other medications without consulting health care professional.

❑ Advise patients to check label for sodium content. Patients with CHF or hypertension, or those on sodium restriction, should use low-sodium preparations.

❑ Inform patients of potential for constipation from aluminum hydroxide.

■ **Hypophosphatemia:** Patients taking aluminum hydroxide for hyperphosphatemia should be taught the importance of a low-phosphate diet.

■ **Antacid:** Caution patient to consult health care professional before taking antacids for more than 2 wk if problem is recurring, if taking other medications, if relief is not obtained, or if symptoms of gastric bleeding (black tarry stools, coffee-ground emesis) occur.

### EVALUATION

**Effectiveness of therapy can be demonstrated by:** ■ Decrease in serum phosphate levels ■ Decrease in GI pain and irritation ❑ Increase in the pH of gastric secretions. In treatment of peptic ulcer, antacid therapy should be continued for at least 4–6 wk after symptoms have disappeared because there is no correlation between disappearance of symptoms and healing of ulcers.

# amantadine

(a-**man**-ta-deen)

Symmetrel

### CLASSIFICATION(S):

**Therapeutic:** antiparkinson agents, antivirals

**Pregnancy Category C**

### INDICATIONS

■ Symptomatic initial and adjunct treatment of Parkinson's disease ■ Prophylaxis and treatment of influenza A viral infections.

### ACTION

■ Potentiates the action of dopamine in the CNS ■ Prevents penetration of influenza A virus into host cell. **Therapeutic Effects:** ■ Relief of parkinsonian symptoms ■ Prevention and decreased symptoms of influenza A viral infection.

### PHARMACOKINETICS

**Absorption:** Well absorbed from the GI tract.

**Distribution:** Distributed to various body tissues and fluids. Crosses blood-brain barrier and enters breast milk.

**Metabolism and Excretion:** Excreted unchanged in the urine.

**Half-life:** 24 hr.

### CONTRAINDICATIONS AND PRECAUTIONS

**Contraindicated in:** ■ Hypersensitivity.

**Use Cautiously in:** ■ Seizure disorders ■ Liver disease ■ Psychiatric problems ■ Cardiac disease ■ Renal impairment (dosage reduction/increased dosing interval required if CCr ≤50 ml/min) ■ May increase susceptibility to rubella infections ■ Geriatric patients ■ Pregnancy and lactation (safety not established).

### ADVERSE REACTIONS AND SIDE EFFECTS*

■ **CNS:** <u>ataxia</u>, <u>dizziness</u>, <u>insomnia</u>, anxiety, confusion, depression, drowsiness, psychosis, seizures ■ **EENT:** blurred vision, dry mouth ■ **Resp:** dyspnea ■ **CV:** <u>hypotension</u>, CHF, edema ■ **GU:** urinary retention ■ **Derm:** <u>mottling</u>, live-

---

{ } = Available in Canada only.

*CAPITALS indicates life-threatening; <u>underlines</u> indicate most frequent.

do reticularis, rashes ■ **Hemat:** leukopenia, neutropenia.

## INTERACTIONS

**Drug-Drug:** ■ Concurrent use of **antihistamines, phenothiazines, quinidine, disopyramide,** and **tricyclic antidepressants** may increase anticholinergic effects (dry mouth, blurred vision, constipation) ■ Increased risk of adverse CNS reactions with **alcohol** ■ Increased risk of CNS stimulation with other **CNS stimulants.**

## ROUTE AND DOSAGE

❑ **Parkinson's Disease**

■ **PO (Adults):** 100 mg 1–2 times daily (up to 400 mg/day).

❑ **Influenza A Viral Infection**

■ **PO (Adults and Children >12 yr):** 200 mg/day as a single dose or 100 mg bid (not >100 mg/day in geriatric patients).

■ **PO (Children 9–12 yr):** 100 mg q 12 hr *or* 2.2 mg/kg q 12 hr for children ≥10 yr weighing <45 kg.

■ **PO (Children 1–9 yr):** 1.5–3 mg/kg q 8 hr or 2.2–4.4 mg/kg q 12 hr (doses as low as 1.5 mg/kg q 12 hr have been used; not to exceed 150 mg/day).

❑ **Renal Impairment**

■ **PO (Adults):** *CCr 30–50 ml/min*—200 mg on the first day, then 100 mg once daily; *CCr 15–29 ml/min*—200 mg on the first day, then 100 mg every other day; *<15 ml/min or hemodialysis patients*—200 mg once every 7 days.

## AVAILABILITY (generic available)

■ *Liquid-filled capsules:* 100 mg^Rx ■ *Tablets:* 100 mg^Rx ■ Cost: $15.72/100 ■ *Syrup (raspberry flavor):* 50 mg/5 ml^Rx ■ Cost: $31.48/480 ml.

TIME/ACTION PROFILE (antiparkinson effect)

| | ONSET | PEAK | DURATION |
|---|---|---|---|
| PO | within 48 hr | up to 2 wk | unknown |

## NURSING IMPLICATIONS

### ASSESSMENT

■ **General Info:** Monitor blood pressure periodically. Assess patient for drug-induced orthostatic hypotension.

❑ Monitor intake and output closely in geriatric patients. May cause urinary retention. Report significant discrepancy or bladder distention.

❑ Monitor vital signs and mental status periodically during first few days of dosage adjustment in patients receiving >200 mg daily; side effects are more likely.

❑ Assess for CHF (peripheral edema, weight gain, dyspnea, rales/crackles, jugular venous distention), especially in patients on chronic therapy or with a history of CHF.

❑ Assess patient for the appearance of a diffuse red mottling of the skin (livedo reticularis), especially in the lower extremities or on exposure to cold. Disappears with continued therapy but may not completely resolve until 2–12 wk after therapy has been discontinued.

■ **Parkinson's Disease:** Assess akinesia, rigidity, tremors, and gait disturbances before and throughout therapy.

■ **Influenza Prophylaxis or Treatment:** Monitor respiratory status (rate, breath sounds, sputum) and temperature periodically. Supportive treatment is indicated if symptoms occur.

■ *Toxicity and Overdose:* Symptoms of toxicity include CNS stimulation (confusion, mood changes, tremors, seizures, arrhythmias, and hypotension). There is no specific antidote, although physostigmine has been used to reverse CNS effects.

## POTENTIAL NURSING DIAGNOSES

■ Mobility, impaired physical.
■ Infection, risk for (Indications).

## IMPLEMENTATION

■ **General:** Do not confuse amantadine with rimantidine or ranitidine.

■ **PO:** Do not administer last dose of medication near bedtime; may produce insomnia in some patients.

❑ Administering amantadine in divided doses may decrease CNS side effects.

❑ The contents of capsules may be mixed with food or fluids if the patient has difficulty swallowing.

■ **Antiviral Prophylaxis:** Treatment should be started in anticipation of contact or as soon as possible after exposure and continue for at least 10 days following exposure. Infectious period is just before onset of symptoms to up to 1 wk after. If vaccine is unavailable or contraindicated, may be administered up to 90 days to protect from repeated exposures.

❏ May be used with inactivated influenza A virus vaccine until protective antibody response develops. Administer for 2–3 wk after vaccine has been given.

■ **Antiviral Treatment:** Administer as soon as possible after onset of symptoms and continue for 24–48 hr after symptoms disappear.

## PATIENT/FAMILY TEACHING

■ **General Info:** Advise patient to take medication around the clock as directed and not to skip doses or double up on missed doses. If a dose is missed, do not take within 4 hr of the next dose.

❏ May cause dizziness or blurred vision. Advise patient to avoid driving or other activities that require alertness until response to the drug is known.

❏ Advise patient to make position changes slowly to minimize orthostatic hypotension.

❏ Inform patient that frequent mouth rinses, good oral hygiene, and sugarless gum or candy may decrease dry mouth. Consult health care professional if dry mouth persists for >2 wk.

❏ Advise patient to confer with health care professional before taking OTC medications, especially cold remedies, or drinking alcoholic beverages.

❏ Instruct patient to notify health care professional if confusion, mood changes, difficulty with urination, edema and shortness of breath, or worsening of Parkinson's disease symptoms occurs.

■ **Antiviral:** Instruct patient and family to notify health care professional if influenza symptoms occur when amantadine is used as prophylaxis or if symptoms do not improve in a few days when product is used for treatment.

■ **Parkinson's Disease:** Advise patient that up to 2 wk of therapy may be needed for full benefit of medication. Notify health care professional if medication gradually loses its effectiveness. Amantadine should be tapered gradually; abrupt withdrawal may precipitate a parkinsonian crisis.

## EVALUATION

**Effectiveness of therapy can be demonstrated by:** ■ Decrease in akinesia and rigidity. Full therapeutic effects may require 2 wk of therapy ■ Absence or reduction of influenza A symptoms.

# amcinonide, See CORTICOSTEROIDS (TOPICAL/LOCAL).

# amifostine
(a-mi-**fos**-teen)
Ethyol

*CLASSIFICATION(S):*
*Therapeutic:* cytoprotective agents

**Pregnancy Category C**

## INDICATIONS

■ Reduces renal toxicity from cisplatin ■ Reduces the incidence of moderate to severe xerostomia from postoperative radiation for head and neck cancer in which the radiation port includes a large portion of the parotid glands.

## ACTION

■ Converted by alkaline phosphatase in tissue to a free thiol compound that binds and detoxifies damaging metabolites of cisplatin and reactive oxygen species generated by radiation. **Therapeutic Effects:** ■ Decreased renal damage from cisplatin ■ Decreased severity of xerostomia following radiation for head and neck cancer.

## PHARMACOKINETICS

**Absorption:** IV administration results in complete bioavailability.

**Distribution:** Unknown.

**Metabolism and Excretion:** Rapidly cleared from plasma; converted to cytoprotective compounds by alkaline phosphatase in tissues.

**Half-life:** 8 min.

## CONTRAINDICATIONS AND PRECAUTIONS

**Contraindicated in:** ■ Known sensitivity to aminothiol compounds ■ Hypotension or dehydration ■ Lactation ■ Concurrent antineoplastic therapy for other tumors (especially malignancies of germ cell origin).

**Use Cautiously in:** ■ Geriatric patients or patients with cardiovascular disease (risk of adverse reactions may be increased) ■ Pregnancy or children (safety not established).

## ADVERSE REACTIONS AND SIDE EFFECTS*

■ **CNS:** dizziness, somnolence ■ **EENT:** sneezing ■ **CV:** hypotension ■ **GI:** hiccups, nausea, vomiting ■ **Derm:** flushing ■ **F and E:** hypocalcemia ■ **Misc:** allergic reactions including ANAPHYALXIS, STEVENS-JOHNSON SYNDROME, TOXIC EPIDERMAL NECROLYSIS, TOXODERMA, ERYTHEMA MULTIFORME, EXFOLIATIVE DERMATITIS (↑ when used as a radioprotectant), chills.

## INTERACTIONS

**Drug-Drug:** ■ Concurrent use of **antihypertensives** ↑ risk of hypotension.

## ROUTE AND DOSAGE

❑ **Reduction of Renal Damage with Cisplatin**

■ **IV (Adults):** 910 mg/m² once daily, within 30 min before chemotherapy; if full dose is poorly tolerated, subsequent doses should be decreased to 740 mg/m².

❑ **Reduction of Xerostomia from Radiation**

■ **IV (Adults):** 200 mg/m² once daily, as a 3-minute infusion starting 15–30 min before standard fraction radiation therapy.

## AVAILABILITY

■ *Powder for injection:* 500 mg/vial^Rx.

TIME/ACTION PROFILE

| | ONSET | PEAK | DURATION |
|---|---|---|---|
| IV | unknown | unknown | unknown |

# NURSING IMPLICATIONS

## ASSESSMENT

❑ Monitor blood pressure before and every 5 min during infusion. Antihypertensives should be discontinued 24 hr prior to treatment. If significant hypotension requiring interruption of therapy occurs, place patient in Trendelenburg position and administer an infusion of 0.9% NaCl using a separate IV line. If blood pressure returns to normal in 5 min and patient is asymptomatic, infusion may be resumed so that full dose may be given.

❑ Assess fluid status before administration. Correct dehydration before instituting therapy. Nausea and vomiting are frequent and may be severe. Prophylactic antiemetics including dexamethasone 20 mg IV and a serotonin-antagonist antiemetic (ondansetron, dolasetron, granisetron) should be administered before and during infusion. Monitor fluid status closely.

❑ Observe patient for signs and symptoms of anaphylaxis (rash, pruritus, laryngeal edema, wheezing). Discontinue the drug and notify physician or other health care professional immediately if these problems occur. Keep epinephrine, an antihistamine, and resuscitation equipment close by in case of an anaphylactic reaction.

■ **Xerostomia:** Assess patient for dry mouth and mouth sores periodically during therapy.

■ *Lab Test Considerations:* Monitor serum calcium concentrations before and periodically during therapy. May cause hypocalcemia. Calcium supplements may be necessary.

## POTENTIAL NURSING DIAGNOSES

■ Injury, risk for (Indications).

## IMPLEMENTATION

■ **Intermittent Infusion:** Reconstitute with 9.7 ml of sterile 0.9% NaCl. Dilute further with 0.9% NaCl for a concentration of 5–40 mg/ml. Do not administer solutions that are discolored or contain particulate matter. Solution is stable for 5 hr at room temperature or 24 hr if refrigerated.

■ *Rate: For renal toxicity:* Administer over 15 min within 30 min of chemotherapy administration. Longer infusion times are not as well tolerated. *For xerostomia:* Administer over 3 min starting 15–30 min prior to radiation therapy.

■ **Y-Site Compatibility:** ◆ amikacin ◆ aminophylline ◆ ampicillin ◆ ampicillin/sulbactam ◆ aztreonam ◆ bleomycin ◆ bumetanide ◆ buprenorphine ◆ butorphanol ◆ calcium gluconate ◆ carboplatin ◆ carmustine ◆ cefazolin ◆

cefonicid ✦ cefotaxime ✦ cefotetan ✦ cefoxitin ✦ ceftazidime ✦ ceftizoxime ✦ ceftriaxone ✦ cefuroxime ✦ cimetidine ✦ ciprofloxacin ✦ clindamycin ✦ cyclophosphamide ✦ cytarabine ✦ dacarbazine ✦ dactinomycin ✦ daunorubicin ✦ diphenhydramine ✦ dobutamine ✦ docetaxel ✦ dopamine ✦ doxorubicin ✦ doxycycline ✦ droperidol ✦ enalaprilat ✦ etoposide ✦ famotidine ✦ floxuridine ✦ fluconazole ✦ fludarabine ✦ fluorouracil ✦ furosemide ✦ gentamicin ✦ gemcitabine ✦ granisetron ✦ haloperidol ✦ heparin ✦ hydrocortisone ✦ hydromorphone ✦ idarubicin ✦ ifosfamide ✦ imipenem/cilastatin ✦ leucovorin ✦ lorazepam ✦ magnesium sulfate ✦ mannitol ✦ mechlorethamine ✦ meperidine ✦ mesna ✦ methotrexate ✦ methylprednisolone ✦ metoclopramide ✦ metronidazole ✦ mitomycin ✦ mitoxantrone ✦ morphine ✦ nalbuphine ✦ netilmicin ✦ ondansetron ✦ piperacillin ✦ plicamycin ✦ potassium chloride ✦ promethazine ✦ ranitidine ✦ sodium bicarbonate ✦ streptozocin ✦ teniposide ✦ thiotepa ✦ ticarcillin ✦ ticarcillin/clavulanate ✦ tobramycin ✦ trimethoprim/sulfamethoxazole ✦ trimetrexate ✦ vancomycin ✦ vinblastine ✦ vincristine ✦ zidovudine.

■ **Y-Site Incompatibility:** ✦ acyclovir ✦ amphotericin B ✦ cefoperazone ✦ chlorpromazine ✦ cisplatin ✦ ganciclovir ✦ minocycline ✦ prochlorperazine.

■ **Additive Incompatibility:** Do not mix with other solutions or medications.

## PATIENT/FAMILY TEACHING

❑ Explain the purpose of amifostine infusion to patient.

❑ Inform patient that amifostine may cause hypotension, nausea, vomiting, flushing, chills, dizziness, somnolence, hiccups, and sneezing.

## EVALUATION

**Effectiveness of therapy can be demonstrated by:** ■ Prevention of renal toxicity associated with repeated administration of cisplatin in patients with ovarian cancer ■ Decreased severity of xerostomia from radiation treatment of head and neck cancer.

## amikacin, See AMINOGLYCOSIDES.

## amiloride, See DIURETICS (POTASSIUM-SPARING).

# aminocaproic acid

(a-mee-noe-ka-**pro**-ik)

Amicar, epsilon aminocaproic acid

**CLASSIFICATION(S):**

**Therapeutic:** *hemostatic agents*

**Pharmacologic:** *fibrinolysis inhibitors*

**Pregnancy Category C**

## INDICATIONS

■ Management of acute, life-threatening hemorrhage due to systemic hyperfibrinolysis or urinary fibrinolysis. **Unlabeled uses:** ■ Prevention of recurrent subarachnoid hemorrhage ■ Prevention of bleeding following oral surgery in hemophiliacs ■ Management of severe hemorrhage caused by thrombolytic agents.

## ACTION

■ Inhibits activation of plasminogen. **Therapeutic Effects:** ■ Inhibition of fibrinolysis ■ Stabilization of clot formation.

## PHARMACOKINETICS

**Absorption:** Rapidly absorbed following oral administration.

**Distribution:** Widely distributed.

**Metabolism and Excretion:** Mostly eliminated unchanged by the kidneys.

**Half-life:** Unknown.

## CONTRAINDICATIONS AND PRECAUTIONS

**Contraindicated in:** ■ Active intravascular clotting.

**Use Cautiously in:** ■ Upper urinary tract bleeding ■ Cardiac, renal, or liver disease (dosage reduction may be required) ■ Pregnancy

---

{ } = Available in Canada only.
*CAPITALS indicates life-threatening; underlines indicate most frequent.

and lactation (safety not established) ∎ Disseminated intravascular coagulation (should be used concurrently with heparin) ∎ Products containing benzyl alcohol should be avoided in neonates.

## ADVERSE REACTIONS AND SIDE EFFECTS*

∎ **CNS:** dizziness, malaise ∎ **EENT:** nasal stuffiness, tinnitus ∎ **CV:** arrhythmias, hypotension (IV only) ∎ **GI:** anorexia, bloating, cramping, diarrhea, nausea ∎ **GU:** diuresis, renal failure ∎ **MS:** myopathy.

## INTERACTIONS

**Drug-Drug:** ∎ Concurrent use with **estrogens, conjugated** may result in a hypercoagulable state ∎ Concurrent use with **clotting factors** may increase the risk of thromboses.

## ROUTE AND DOSAGE

❏ **Acute Bleeding Syndromes due to Elevated Fibrinolytic Activity**

∎ **PO (Adults):** 5 g 1st hr, followed by 1–1.25 g q hr for 8 hr or until hemorrhage is controlled; or 6 g over 24 hr after prostate surgery (not >30 g/day).

∎ **IV (Adults):** 4–5 g over 1st hr, followed by 1 g/hr for 8 hr or until hemorrhage is controlled; or 6 g over 24 hr after prostate surgery (not >30 g/day).

∎ **PO, IV (Children):** 100 mg/kg or 3 g/m² over 1st hr, followed by continuous infusion of 33.3 mg/kg/hr; or 1 g/m²/hr (total dosage not >18 g/m²/24 hr).

❏ **Subarachnoid Hemorrhage**

∎ **PO (Adults):** *To follow IV*—3 g q 2 hr (36 g/day). If no surgery is performed, continue for 21 days after bleeding stops, then decrease to 2 g q 2 hr (24 g/day) for 3 days, then 1 g q 2 hr (12 g/day) for 3 days.

∎ **IV (Adults):** 36 g/day for 10 days followed by PO.

❏ **Prevention of Bleeding following Oral Surgery in Hemophiliacs**

∎ **PO (Adults):** 75 mg/kg (up to 6 g) immediately after procedure, then q 6 hr for 7–10 days; syrup may also be used as an oral rinse of 1.25 g (5 ml) 4 times a day for 7–10 days.

∎ **IV, PO (Children):** *Also for epistaxis*—50 to 100 mg/kg/dose administered IV every 6 hr for 2 to 3 days starting 4 hr before the procedure. After completion of IV therapy, aminocaproic acid should be given as 50 to 100 mg/kg/dose orally every 6 hr for 5 to 7 days.

## AVAILABILITY

∎ *Tablets:* 500 mg<sup>Rx</sup> ∎ *Syrup (raspberry flavor):* 1.25 g/5 ml<sup>Rx</sup> ∎ *Injection:* 250 mg/ml<sup>Rx</sup>.

TIME/ACTION PROFILE (peak blood levels)

|  | ONSET | PEAK | DURATION |
|---|---|---|---|
| PO | unknown | 2 hr | N/A |
| IV | unknown | 2 hr | N/A |

# NURSING IMPLICATIONS

## ASSESSMENT

❏ Monitor blood pressure, pulse, and respiratory status as indicated by severity of bleeding.

❏ Monitor for overt bleeding every 15–30 min.

❏ Monitor neurologic status (pupils, level of consciousness, motor activity) in patients with subarachnoid hemorrhage.

❏ Monitor intake and output ratios frequently; notify physician if significant discrepancies occur.

❏ Assess for thromboembolic complications (especially in patients with history). Notify physician of positive Homans' sign, leg pain and edema, hemoptysis, dyspnea, or chest pain.

∎ *Lab Test Considerations:* Monitor platelet count and clotting factors prior to and periodically throughout therapy in patients with systemic fibrinolysis

❏ Increased CPK, AST, and serum aldolase may indicate myopathy

❏ May elevate serum potassium.

## POTENTIAL NURSING DIAGNOSES

∎ Tissue perfusion, ineffective (Indications).

∎ Injury, risk for (Indications, Side Effects).

## IMPLEMENTATION

∎ **General:** Do not confuse Amicar (aminocaproic acid) with Amikin (amikacin).

∎ **PO:** Syrup may be used as an oral rinse, swished for 30 sec 4 times/day for 7–10 days for the control of bleeding during dental and oral surgery in hemophilic patients. Small amounts may be swallowed, except during

1st and 2nd trimesters of pregnancy. Syrup may be applied with an applicator in children or unconscious patients.

- **IV:** Stabilize IV catheter to minimize thrombophlebitis. Monitor site closely.
- **Intermittent Infusion:** Do not administer undiluted. Dilute initial 4–5 g dose in 250 ml of sterile water for injection, 0.9% NaCl, D5W, or LR. Do not dilute with sterile water in patients with subarachnoid hemorrhage.
- *Rate:* Administer over 1 hr. Rapid infusion rate may cause hypotension, bradycardia, or other arrhythmias.
- **Continuous Infusion:** Initial dose may be followed by a continuous infusion of 1 g/hr in 50–100 ml of diluent.
- *Rate:* Administer IV solution using infusion pump to ensure accurate dose. Administer via slow IV infusion.
- **Additive Incompatibility:** Do not admix with other medications.

### PATIENT/FAMILY TEACHING

- **General Info:** Instruct patient to notify the nurse immediately if bleeding recurs or if thromboembolic symptoms develop.
- **IV:** Caution patient to make position changes slowly to avoid orthostatic hypotension.

### EVALUATION

**Effectiveness of therapy can be demonstrated by:** ■ Cessation of bleeding ■ Prevention of rebleeding in subarachnoid hemorrhage without occurrence of undesired clotting.

## AMINOGLYCOSIDES

**amikacin**

(am-i-**kay**-sin)

Amikin

**gentamicin†**

(jen-ta-**mye**-sin)

{Cidomycin}, Garamycin, G-Mycin, Jenamicin

**kanamycin**

(kan-a-**mye**-sin)

Kantrex

**neomycin**

(neo-oh-**mye**-sin)

Mycifradin, Myciguent

**netilmicin**

(ne-til-**mye**-sin)

Netromycin

**streptomycin**

(strep-toe-**mye**-sin)

**tobramycin†**

(toe-bra-**mye**-sin)

Nebcin, TOBI

*CLASSIFICATION(S):*
**Therapeutic:** *anti-infectives*
**Pharmacologic:** *aminoglycosides*

**Pregnancy Category C (gentamicin, topical use of others), D (amikacin, kanamycin, netilmicin, streptomycin, tobramycin)**

†See Appendix C for ophthalmic use.

### INDICATIONS

■ **Amikacin, gentamicin, kanamycin, netilmicin, and tobramycin:** Treatment of serious gram-negative bacillary infections and infections caused by staphylococci when penicillins or other less toxic drugs are contraindicated ■ **Streptomycin:** In combination with other agents in the management of active tuberculosis ■ **Kanamycin, neomycin:** Used orally to prepare the GI tract for surgery, to decrease the number of ammonia-producing bacteria in the gut as part of the management of hepatic encephalopathy, and to treat some forms of infectious diarrhea ■ **Tobramycin by inhalation:** Management of *Pseudomonas aeruginosa* in cystic fibrosis patients ■ **Gentamicin, streptomycin:** In combination with other agents in the management of serious enterococcal infections ■ **Gentamicin IM, IV:** Part of endocarditis prophylaxis. **Unlabeled uses:** ■ **Amikacin:** In combination with other agents in the management of *Mycobacterium avium* complex infections.

## ACTION

■ Inhibits protein synthesis in bacteria at level of 30S ribosome. **Therapeutic Effects:** ■ Bactericidal action. **Spectrum:** ■ Most aminoglycosides notable for activity against: ❑ *P. aeruginosa* ❑ *Klebsiella pneumoniae* ❑ *Escherichia coli* ❑ *Proteus* ❑ *Serratia* ❑ *Acinetobacter* ❑ *Staphylococcus aureus* ■ In treatment of enterococcal infections, synergy with a penicillin is required ■ Streptomycin and amikacin also active against *Mycobacterium*.

## PHARMACOKINETICS

**Absorption:** Well absorbed after IM administration. IV administration results in complete bioavailability. Some absorption follows administration by other routes.

**Distribution:** Widely distributed throughout extracellular fluid; crosses the placenta; small amounts enter breast milk. Poor penetration into CSF.

**Metabolism and Excretion:** Excretion is >90% renal.

**Half-life:** 2–4 hr (increased in renal impairment).

## CONTRAINDICATIONS AND PRECAUTIONS

**Contraindicated in:** ■ Hypersensitivity ■ Most parenteral products contain bisulfites and should be avoided in patients with known intolerance ■ Products containing benzyl alcohol should be avoided in neonates ■ Cross-sensitivity among aminoglycosides may occur.

**Use Cautiously in:** ■ Renal impairment (dosage adjustments necessary; blood level monitoring useful in preventing ototoxicity and nephrotoxicity) ■ Hearing impairment ■ Geriatric patients and premature infants (difficulty in assessing auditory and vestibular function; age-related renal impairment) ■ Neuromuscular diseases such as myasthenia gravis ■ Obese patients (dosage should be based on ideal body weight) ■ Pregnancy (tobramycin and streptomycin may cause congenital deafness) ■ Neonates (increased risk of neuromuscular blockade; difficulty in assessing auditory and vestibular function; immature renal function) ■ Lactation, infants, and neonates (safety not established).

## ADVERSE REACTIONS AND SIDE EFFECTS*

■ **EENT:** ototoxicity (vestibular and cochlear) ■ **GU:** nephrotoxicity ■ **F and E:** hypomagnesemia ■ **MS:** muscle paralysis (high parenteral doses) ■ **Misc:** hypersensitivity reactions.

## INTERACTIONS

**Drug-Drug:** ■ Inactivated by **penicillins** and **cephalosporins** when coadministered to patients with renal insufficiency ■ Possible respiratory paralysis after **inhalation anesthetics** or **neuromuscular blocking agents** ■ Increased incidence of ototoxicity with **loop diuretics** ■ Increased incidence of nephrotoxicity with other **nephrotoxic drugs**.

## ROUTE AND DOSAGE

### ❑ Amikacin

■ **IM, IV (Adults and Children and Older Infants):** 5 mg/kg q 8 hr or 7.5 mg/kg q 12 hr. *Urinary tract infections in adults*—250 mg q 12 hr.
■ **IM, IV (Infants):** 10 mg/kg initially, then 7.5 mg/kg q 12 hr.
■ **IM, IV (Neonates):** 10 mg/kg initially, 7.5 mg/kg every 12 hr; *premature neonates*— 10 mg/kg initially, then 7.5 mg/kg q 18–24 hr.

### ❑ Renal Impairment

■ **IM, IV (Adults):** 7.5 mg/kg, further doses and intervals determined on the basis of blood level monitoring and renal function assessment.

### ❑ Gentamicin

Many regimens are used; most involve dosing adjusted on the basis of blood level monitoring and assessment of renal function. For endocarditis prophylaxis regimen.

■ **IM, IV (Adults):** 1 mg/kg q 8 hr (up to 5 mg/kg/day in 3–4 divided doses); *Once-daily dosing (unlabeled)*—4–7 mg/kg q 24 hr.
■ **IM, IV (Children):** 2–2.5 mg/kg q 8 hr.
■ **IM, IV (Infants and Neonates >1 wk):** 2.5 mg/kg q 8 hr.
■ **IM, IV (Infants and Premature Neonates ≤1 wk):** 2.5 mg/kg q 12 hr.

### ❑ Renal Impairment

■ **IM, IV (Adults):** Initial dose of 1–1.7 mg/ kg. subsequent doses/intervals dependent on blood level monitoring and renal function assessment.

□ **Kanamycin**

■ **IM, IV (Adults and Children and Infants):** 5 mg/kg q 8 hr *or* 7.5 mg/kg q 12 hr (not to exceed 1.5 g/day in adults or 30 mg/kg/day in children).

■ **PO (Adults):** *Preoperative intestinal antisepsis*—1 g q hr for 4 doses, then 1 g q 6 hr for 36–72 hr; *hepatic encephalopathy*—2–3 g q 6 hr.

■ **Inhaln (Adults):** 250 mg 4 times daily.

□ **Renal Impairment**

■ **IM, IV (Adults):** 7.5 mg/kg; further dosing and intervals determined by blood level monitoring and assessment of renal function.

□ **Neomycin**

■ **PO (Adults):** *Preoperative intestinal antisepsis*—1 g q hr for 4 doses, then 1 g q 4 hr for 24 hr *or* 1 g 19 hr, 18 hr, and 9 hr before surgery; *hepatic encephalopathy* 4–12 g/day in divided doses.

■ **PO (Children):** *Preoperative intestinal antisepsis*—14.7 mg/kg (417 mg/m²) q 4 hr for 3 days; *hepatic encephalopathy*—50–100 mg/kg/day in divided doses.

■ **Topical (Adults and Children):** Apply cream or ointment 1–5 times daily.

□ **Netilmicin**

■ **IM, IV (Adults):** *Most infections*—1.3–2.2 mg/kg q 8 hr *or* 2–3.25 mg/kg q 12 hr (up to 7 mg/kg/day or 12 mg/kg/day in cystic fibrosis patients); *complicated urinary tract infections*—1.5–2 mg/kg q 12 hr. *Once-daily dosing* 4–8 mg/kg q 24 hr (unlabeled).

■ **IM, IV (Infants and Children 6 wk–12 yr):** 1.83–2.67 mg/kg q 8 hr *or* 2.75–4 mg/kg q 12 hr.

■ **IM, IV (Infants <6 wk):** 2–3.25 mg/kg q 12 hr.

□ **Renal Impairment**

■ **IM, IV (Adults):** Initial dose of 1.3–2.2 mg/kg. Subsequent doses/intervals dependent on blood level monitoring and renal function assessment.

□ **Streptomycin**

■ **IM (Adults):** *Tuberculosis*—1 g/day initially, decreased to 1 g 2–3 times weekly; *other*

*infections*—250 mg–1 g q 6 hr *or* 500 mg–2 g q 12 hr.

■ **IM (Children):** *Tuberculosis*—20 mg/kg/day (not to exceed 1 g/day); *other infections*—5–10 mg/kg q 6 hr *or* 10–20 mg/kg q 12 hr.

□ **Renal Impairment**

■ **IM (Adults):** 1 g initially, further dosing determined by blood level monitoring and assessment of renal function.

□ **Tobramycin**

■ **IM, IV (Adults):** 0.75–1.25 mg/kg q 6 hr *or* 1–1.75 mg/kg q 8 hr (up to 8 mg/kg/day in cystic fibrosis patients).

■ **IM, IV (Children and Older Infants):** 1.5–1.9 mg/kg q 6 hr *or* 2–2.5 mg/kg q 8–16 hr, up to 10 mg/kg/day in cystic fibrosis patients (dosing interval may vary from q 4 hr–q 24 hr, depending on clinical situation).

■ **IM, IV (Infants <1 wk):** Up to 2 mg/kg q 12–24 hr.

■ **Inhaln (Adults and Children ≥6 yr):** 300 mg twice daily for 28 days, then off for 28 days, then repeat cycle.

□ **Renal Impairment**

■ **IM, IV (Adults):** 1 mg/kg initially, further dosing determined by blood level monitoring and assessment of renal function.

**AVAILABILITY**

□ **Amikacin**

■ *Injection:* 50 mg/ml^Rx, 250 mg/ml^Rx.

□ **Gentamicin**

■ *Injection:* 10 mg/ml^Rx, 40 mg/ml^Rx ■ Cost: 40 mg/ml $5.30/2 ml ■ *Premixed injection:* 40 mg/50 ml^Rx, 40 mg/100 ml^Rx, 60 mg/50 ml^Rx, 60 mg/100 ml^Rx, 70 mg/50 ml^Rx, 80 mg/50 ml^Rx, 80 mg/100 ml^Rx, 90 mg/100 ml^Rx, 100 mg/50 ml^Rx, 100 mg/100 ml^Rx, 120 mg/100 ml^Rx, 160 mg/100 ml^Rx, 180 mg/100 ml^Rx.

□ **Kanamycin**

■ *Injection:* 37.5 mg/ml^Rx, 250 mg/ml^Rx, 333.3 mg/ml^Rx ■ *Capsules:* 500 mg^Rx.

□ **Neomycin**

■ *Oral solution:* 125 mg/5 ml^Rx ■ *Tablets:* 500 mg^Rx ■ *Cream:* 0.5%^Rx, ^OTC ■ *Ointment:* 0.5%^Rx, ^OTC ■ other topical antibiotics or anti-inflammatory agents for skin, ear, and eye infections. See Appendix B.

❑ **Netilmicin**

■ *Injection:* 25 mg/ml[Rx], 50 mg/ml[Rx], 100 mg/ml[Rx].

❑ **Streptomycin**

■ *Injection:* {500 mg/ml[Rx]}, 1 g[Rx].

❑ **Tobramycin**

■ *Injection:* 10 mg/ml[Rx], 40 mg/ml[Rx], 1.2-g vial[Rx] ■ *Nebulizer solution:* 300 mg/5 ml in 5-ml ampules[Rx].

TIME/ACTION PROFILE (blood levels*)

|    | ONSET | PEAK | DURATION |
|----|-------|------|----------|
| IM | rapid | 30–90 min | N/A |
| IV | rapid | 15–30 min† | N/A |

* All parenterally administered aminoglycosides.
† Post–distribution peak occurs 30 min after the end of a 30-min infusion and 15 min after the end of a 1-hr infusion.

## NURSING IMPLICATIONS

### ASSESSMENT

■ **General Info:** Assess patient for infection (vital signs, wound appearance, sputum, urine, stool, WBC) at beginning of and throughout therapy.

❑ Obtain specimens for culture and sensitivity before initiating therapy. First dose may be given before receiving results.

❑ Evaluate eighth cranial nerve function by audiometry before and throughout therapy. Hearing loss is usually in the high-frequency range. Prompt recognition and intervention are essential in preventing permanent damage. Also monitor for vestibular dysfunction (vertigo, ataxia, nausea, vomiting). Eighth cranial nerve dysfunction is associated with persistently elevated peak aminoglycoside levels. Aminoglycosides should be discontinued if tinnitus or subjective hearing loss occurs.

❑ Monitor intake and output and daily weight to assess hydration status and renal function.

❑ Assess patient for signs of superinfection (fever, upper respiratory infection, vaginal itching or discharge, increasing malaise, diarrhea). Report to physician or other health care professional.

■ **Hepatic Encephalopathy:** Monitor neurologic status. Before administering oral medication, assess patient's ability to swallow.

■ *Lab Test Considerations:* Monitor renal function by urinalysis, specific gravity, BUN, creatinine, and CCr before and throughout therapy.

❑ May cause increased BUN, AST, ALT, serum alkaline phosphatase, bilirubin, creatinine, and LDH concentrations.

❑ May cause decreased serum calcium, magnesium, potassium, and sodium concentrations.

■ *Toxicity and Overdose:* Blood levels should be monitored periodically during therapy. Timing of blood levels is important in interpreting results. Draw blood for peak levels 1 hr after IM injection and 30 min after a 30-min IV infusion is completed. Trough levels should be drawn just before next dose. Peak level for **amikacin** and **kanamycin** should not exceed 35 mcg/ml; trough level should not exceed 5 mcg/ml. Peak level for **gentamicin** and **tobramycin** should not exceed 10 mcg/ml; trough level should not exceed 2 mcg/ml. Peak level for **netilmicin** should not exceed 16 mcg/ml; trough level should not exceed 2 mcg/ml. Peak level for **streptomycin** should not exceed 25 mcg/ml.

### POTENTIAL NURSING DIAGNOSES

■ Infection, risk for (Indications).

■ Sensory perception, disturbed (auditory) (Side Effects).

### IMPLEMENTATION

■ **General:** Do not confuse Amikin (amikacin) with Amicar (aminocaproic acid). Do not confuse Zagam (sparfloxacin) with Zyban (buproprion).

❑ Keep patient well hydrated (1500–2000 ml/day) during therapy.

■ **Preoperative Bowel Prep:** Neomycin is usually used in conjunction with erythromycin, a low-residue diet, and a cathartic or enema.

■ **PO:** May be administered without regard to meals.

■ **IM:** IM administration should be deep into a well-developed muscle. Alternate injection sites.

❑ **Amikacin**

■ **Intermittent Infusion:** Dilute 500 mg of amikacin in 100–200 ml of D5W, D10W, 0.9% NaCl, D5/0.9% NaCl, D5/0.45% NaCl, D5/0.25% NaCl, or LR. Solution may be pale yellow without decreased potency. Stable for 24 hr at room temperature.

■ *Rate:* Infuse over 30–60 min (over 1–2 hr for infants).

■ **Syringe Incompatibility:** ◆ heparin.

■ **Y-Site Compatibility:** ◆ acyclovir ◆ amifostine ◆ amiodarone ◆ aztreonam ◆ cisatracurium ◆ cyclophosphamide ◆ dexamethasone sodium phosphate ◆ diltiazem ◆ docetaxel ◆ enalaprilat ◆ esmolol ◆ etoposide ◆ filgrastim ◆ fluconazole ◆ fludarabine ◆ foscarnet ◆ furosemide ◆ gemcitabine ◆ granisetron ◆ idarubicin ◆ labetalol ◆ lorazepam ◆ magnesium sulfate ◆ melphalan ◆ midazolam ◆ morphine ◆ ondansetron ◆ paclitaxel ◆ perphenazine ◆ remifentanil ◆ sargramostim ◆ teniposide ◆ thiotepa ◆ vinorelbine ◆ warfarin ◆ zidovudine.

■ **Y-Site Incompatibility:** ◆ allopurinol sodium ◆ amophotericin B cholesteryl sulfate ◆ hetastarch ◆ propofol ◆ If aminoglycosides and penicillins or cephalosporins must be administered concurrently, administer in separate sites, at least 1 hr apart.

■ **Additive Incompatibility:** Manufacturer does not recommend admixing.

❑ **Gentamicin**

■ **Intermittent Infusion:** Dilute each dose in 50–200 ml of D5W, 0.9% NaCl, or LR to provide a concentration not to exceed 1 mg/ml. Also available in commercially mixed piggyback injections. Do not use solutions that are discolored or that contain a precipitate.

■ *Rate:* Infuse slowly over 30 min–2 hr. For pediatric patients, the volume of diluent may be reduced but should be sufficient to permit infusion over 30 min–2 hr.

■ **Syringe Incompatibility:** ◆ ampicillin ◆ cefamandole ◆ heparin.

■ **Y-Site Compatibility:** ◆ acyclovir ◆ alatrofloxacin ◆ amifostine ◆ amiodarone ◆ atracurium ◆ aztreonam ◆ ciprofloxacin ◆ cisatracurium ◆ cyclophosphamide ◆ cytarabine ◆ diltiazem ◆ docetaxel ◆ doxorubicin liposome ◆

enalaprilat ◆ esmolol ◆ etoposide ◆ famotidine ◆ fluconazole ◆ fludarabine ◆ foscarnet ◆ gatifloxacin ◆ gemcitabine ◆ granisetron ◆ hydromorphone ◆ insulin ◆ labetalol ◆ levofloxacin ◆ linezolid ◆ lorazepam ◆ magnesium sulfate ◆ melphalan ◆ meperidine ◆ meropenem ◆ midazolam ◆ morphine ◆ multivitamins ◆ ondansetron ◆ paclitaxel ◆ pancuronium ◆ perphenazine ◆ remifentanil ◆ sargramostim ◆ tacrolimus ◆ teniposide ◆ theophylline ◆ thiotepa ◆ tolazoline ◆ vecuronium ◆ vinorelbine ◆ vitamin B complex with C ◆ zidovudine.

■ **Y-Site Incompatibility:** ◆ allopurinol ◆ amphotericin B cholesteryl sulfate ◆ furosemide ◆ heparin ◆ hetastarch ◆ idarubicin ◆ indomethacin ◆ propofol ◆ warfarin.

■ **Additive Compatibility:** ◆ atracurium ◆ aztreonam ◆ bleomycin ◆ cimetidine ◆ ciprofloxacin ◆ metronidazole ◆ ofloxacin ◆ ranitidine.

■ **Additive Incompatibility:** ◆ amphotericin B ◆ heparin.

❑ **Kanamycin**

■ **Intermittent Infusion:** Dilute each 500 mg in 100–200 ml or each 1 g in 200–400 ml of D5W, D10W, D5/0.9% NaCl, 0.9% NaCl, or LR. Dilute in a proportionally smaller volume for pediatric patients. Darkening of solution does not alter potency.

■ *Rate:* Infuse slowly over 30–60 min.

■ **Syringe Incompatibility:** ◆ heparin.

■ **Y-Site Compatibility:** ◆ cyclophosphamide ◆ furosemide ◆ hydromorphone ◆ magnesium sulfate ◆ meperidine ◆ morphine ◆ perphenazine ◆ potassium chloride ◆ vitamin B complex with C.

■ **Additive Incompatibility:** Manufacturer does not recommend admixing with other antibacterial agents.

❑ **Netilmicin**

■ **Intermittent Infusion:** Dilute each dose in 50–200 ml of D5/LR, D5/0.9% NaCl, D5W, D10W, Ringer's or LR, 0.9% NaCl, 3% NaCl, or 5% NaCl. Dilute in a proportionally smaller volume for pediatric doses. Solution clear and colorless to pale yellow. Stable 72 hours at room temperature.

■ *Rate:* Infuse slowly over 30 min–2 hr.

■ **Syringe Incompatibility:** ◆ heparin.

■ **Y-Site Compatibility:** ◆ amifostine ◆ aminophylline ◆ aztreonam ◆ calcium gluconate ◆ cisatracurium ◆ docetaxel ◆ doxorubicin liposome ◆ etoposide ◆ filgrastim ◆ fludarabine ◆ gemcitabine ◆ granisetron ◆ melphalan ◆ remifentanil ◆ sargramostim ◆ teniposide ◆ thiotepa ◆ vinorelbine.

■ **Y-Site Incompatibility:** ◆ amphotericin B cholesteryl sulfate complex ◆ furosemide ◆ heparin ◆ propofol.

■ **Additive Compatibility:** ◆ aminocaproic acid ◆ atropine ◆ clindamycin ◆ dexamethasone sodium phosphate ◆ edetate calcium disodium ◆ fibrinolysin and deoxyribonuclease ◆ hydrocortisone sodium succinate ◆ metronidazole ◆ multivitamins ◆ potassium chloride ◆ vitamin B complex ◆ vitamin B complex with C.

❑ **Tobramycin**

■ **Intermittent Infusion:** Dilute each dose of tobramycin in 50–100 ml of D5W, D10W, D5/0.9% NaCl, 0.9%NaCl, Ringer's or LR to provide a concentration not >1 mg/ml. Pediatric doses may be diluted in proportionately smaller amounts. Stable for 24 hr at room temperature, 96 hr if refrigerated. Also available in commercially mixed piggyback injections.

■ *Rate:* Infuse slowly over 30–60 min in both adult and pediatric patients.

■ **Syringe Incompatibility:** ◆ clindamycin ◆ heparin.

■ **Y-Site Compatibility:** ◆ acyclovir ◆ amifostine ◆ amiodarone ◆ aztreonam ◆ ciprofloxacin ◆ cisatracurium ◆ cyclophosphamide ◆ diltiazem ◆ docetaxel ◆ doxorubicin liposome ◆ enalaprilat ◆ esmolol ◆ etoposide ◆ filgrastim ◆ fluconazole ◆ fludarabine ◆ foscarnet ◆ furosemide ◆ gemcitabine ◆ granisetron ◆ hydromorphone ◆ insulin ◆ labetalol ◆ magnesium sulfate ◆ melphalan ◆ meperidine ◆ midazolam ◆ morphine ◆ perphenazine ◆ remifentanil ◆ tacrolimus ◆ teniposide ◆ theophylline ◆ thiotepa ◆ tolazoline ◆ vinorelbine ◆ zidovudine.

■ **Y-Site Incompatibility:** ◆ allopurinol ◆ amphotericin B cholesteryl sulfate ◆ heparin ◆ hetastarch ◆ indomethacin ◆ propofol ◆ sargramostim.

■ **Additive Incompatibility:** Manufacturer recommends administering separately; do not admix.

■ **Topical:** Cleanse skin before application. Wear gloves during application.

## PATIENT/FAMILY TEACHING

■ **General Info:** Instruct patient to report signs of hypersensitivity, tinnitus, vertigo, hearing loss, rash, dizziness, or difficulty urinating.

❑ Advise patient of the importance of drinking plenty of liquids.

❑ Teach patients with a history of rheumatic heart disease or valve replacement the importance of using antimicrobial prophylaxis before invasive medical or dental procedures.

■ **PO:** Instruct patient to take as directed for full course of therapy. Missed doses should be taken as soon as possible if not almost time for next dose; do not double doses.

❑ Caution patient that medication may cause nausea, vomiting, or diarrhea.

■ **Topical:** Instruct patient to wash affected skin gently and pat dry. Apply a thin film of ointment. Apply occlusive dressing only if ordered by health care professional. Patient should assess skin and inform health care professional if skin irritation develops or infection worsens.

■ **Inhaln:** Instruct patient to take inhalation twice daily as close to 12 hr apart as possible; not <6 hr apart. Administer over 10–15 min period using a hand-held PARI LC PLUS reusable nebulizer with a *DeVilbiss Pulmo-Aide* compressor. Do not mix with dornase alpha in nebulizer. Instruct patient on multiple therapies to take others first and use tobramycin last. Tobramycin-induced bronchospasm may be reduced if tobramycin is administered after bronchodilators. Instruct patient to sit or stand upright during inhalation and breathe normally through mouthpiece of nebulizer. Nose clips may help patient breath through mouth.

## EVALUATION

**Clinical response to therapy can be evaluated by:** ■ Resolution of the signs and symptoms of infection. If no response is seen within 3–5 days, new cultures should be taken ■ Prevention of infection in intestinal surgery ■ Improved neurologic status in hepatic encephalopathy ■ Endocarditis prophylaxis.

## aminophylline, See BRONCHODILATORS (XANTHINES).

**High Alert**

# amiodarone
(am-ee-**oh**-da-rone)
Cordarone, Pacerone

*CLASSIFICATION(S):*
*Therapeutic: antiarrhythmics (class III)*

**Pregnancy Category D**

## INDICATIONS

■ Life-threatening ventricular arrhythmias unresponsive to less toxic agents. **Unlabeled uses:** ■ **PO:** Management of supraventricular tachyarrhythmias ■ **IV:** As part of the Advanced Cardiac Life Support (ACLS) and Pediatric Advanced Life Support (PALS) guidelines for the management of ventricular fibrillation/pulseless ventricular tachycardia after cardiopulmonary resuscitation and defibrillation have failed; also for other life-threatening tachyarrhythmias.

## ACTION

■ Prolongs action potential and refractory period ■ Inhibits adrenergic stimulation ■ Slows the sinus rate, increases PR and QT intervals, and decreases peripheral vascular resistance (vasodilation). **Therapeutic Effects:** ■ Suppression of arrhythmias.

## PHARMACOKINETICS

**Absorption:** IV administration results in complete bioavailability. Slowly and variably absorbed from the GI tract (35–65%).

**Distribution:** Distributed to and accumulates slowly in body tissues. Reaches high levels in fat, muscle, liver, lungs, and spleen. Crosses the placenta and enters breast milk.

**Protein Binding:** 96% bound to plasma proteins.

**Metabolism and Excretion:** Metabolized by the liver, excreted into bile. Minimal renal excretion. One metabolite has antiarrhythmic activity.

**Half-life:** 13–107 days.

## CONTRAINDICATIONS AND PRECAUTIONS

**Contraindicated in:** ■ Severe sinus node dysfunction ■ 2nd- and 3rd-degree AV block ■ Bradycardia (has caused syncope unless a pacemaker is in place) ■ Products containing benzyl alcohol should not be used in neonates ■ Pregnancy and lactation.

**Use Cautiously in:** ■ History of CHF ■ Thyroid disorders ■ Severe pulmonary or liver disease.

## ADVERSE REACTIONS AND SIDE EFFECTS*

■ **CNS:** dizziness, fatigue, malaise, headache, insomnia ■ **EENT:** corneal microdeposits, abnormal sense of smell, dry eyes, optic neuritis, optic neuropathy, photophobia ■ **Resp:** ADULT RESPIRATORY DISTRESS SYNDROME (ARDS), PULMONARY FIBROSIS ■ **CV:** CHF, WORSENING OF ARRHYTHMIAS, bradycardia, hypotension ■ **GI:** LIVER FUNCTION ABNORMALITIES, anorexia, constipation, nausea, vomiting, abdominal pain, abnormal sense of taste ■ **GU:** decreased libido, epididymitis ■ **Derm:** TOXIC EPIDERMAL NECROLYSIS, photosensitivity, blue discoloration ■ **Endo:** hypothyroidism, hyperthyroidism ■ **Neuro:** ataxia, involuntary movement, paresthesia, peripheral neuropathy, poor coordination, tremor.

## INTERACTIONS

**Drug-Drug:** ■ ↑ blood levels and may lead to toxicity from **digoxin** ( ↓ dose of digoxin by 50%) ■ ↑ blood levels and may lead to toxicity from other **class I antiarrhythmics (quinidine, procainamide, mexiletine, lidocaine,** or **flecainide**— ↓ doses of other drugs by 30–50%) ■ ↑ blood levels of **cyclosporine, dextromethorphan, methotrexate, phenytoin,** and **theophylline** ■ **Phenytoin** decreases amiodarone blood levels ■ Increases the activity of **warfarin** (decrease dose of warfarin by 33–50%) ■ Increased risk of bradyarrhythmias, sinus arrest, or AV heart block with **beta blockers** or **calcium channel blockers** ■ **Cholestyramine** may ↓ amiodarone blood levels ■ **Cimetidine** and **ritonavir** ↑ amiodarone blood levels ■ Risk of myocardial depression is ↑ by **volatile anesthetics.**

## ROUTE AND DOSAGE

### □ Ventricular Arrhythmias

■ **PO (Adults):** 800–1600 mg/day in 1–2 doses for 1–3 wk, then 600–800 mg/day in 1–2 doses for 1 mo, then 400 mg/day maintenance dose.

■ **PO (Children):** 10 mg/kg/day (800 mg/1.72 m²/day) for 10 days or until response or adverse reaction occurs, then 5 mg/kg/day (400 mg/1.72 m²/day) for several weeks, then decreased to 2.5 mg/kg/day (200 mg/1.72 m²/day) or lowest effective maintenance dose.

■ **IV (Adults):** 150 mg over 10 min, followed by 360 mg over the next 6 hr and then 540 mg over the next 18 hr. Continue infusion at 0.5 mg/min until oral therapy is initiated. If arrhythmia recurs, a small loading infusion of 150 mg over 10 min should be given; in addition, the rate of the maintenance infusion may be increased. *Conversion to initial oral therapy*—If duration of IV infusion was <1 wk, oral dose should be 800–1600 mg/day; if IV infusion was 1–3 wk, oral dose should be 600–800 mg/day; if IV infusion was >3 wk, oral dose should be 400 mg/day. *ACLS guidelines for pulseless VFib/VTach*—300 mg IV push, may repeat once after 3–5 min with 150 mg IV push (maximum cumulative dose 2.2 g/24 hr; unlabeled).

■ **IV: Intraosseous: (Children and infants):** *PALS guidelines for pulseless VFib/VTach* 5 mg/kg as a bolus; *perfusion tachycardia*—5 mg/kg loading dose over 20–60 min (maximum of 15 mg/kg/day; unlabeled)

### □ Supraventricular Tachycardia

■ **PO (Adults):** 600–800 mg/day for 1 wk or until desired response occurs or side effects develop, then decrease to 400 mg/day for 3 wk, then maintenance dose of 200–400 mg/day.

■ **PO (Children):** 10 mg/kg/day (800 mg/1.72 m²/day) for 10 days or until response or side effects occur, then 5 mg/kg/day (400 mg/1.72 m²/day) for several weeks, then decreased to 2.5 mg/kg/day (200 mg/1.72 m²/day) or lowest effective maintenance dose.

## AVAILABILITY (generic available)

■ *Tablets:* 200 mg$^{Rx}$, 400 mg$^{Rx}$ ■ Cost: 200 mg $194.87/60 ■ *Injection:* 50 mg/ml in 3-ml ampules$^{Rx}$ ■ Cost: $988.75/10 ampules.

TIME/ACTION PROFILE (suppression of ventricular arrhythmias)

|  | ONSET | PEAK | DURATION |
|---|---|---|---|
| PO | 2–3 days (up to 2–3 mos) | 3–7 hr | wks–mos |
| IV | 2 hr | 3–7 hr | unknown |

## NURSING IMPLICATIONS

### ASSESSMENT

■ **General Info:** ECG should be monitored continuously during IV therapy or initiation of oral therapy. Monitor heart rate and rhythm throughout therapy; PR prolongation, slight QRS widening, T-wave amplitude reduction with T-wave widening and bifurcation, and U waves may occur. QT prolongation may be associated with worsening of arrhythmias and should be monitored closely during IV therapy. Report bradycardia or increase in arrhythmias promptly; patients receiving IV therapy may require slowing rate, discontinuing infusion, or inserting a temporary pacemaker.

□ Assess for signs of pulmonary toxicity (rales/crackles, decreased breath sounds, pleuritic friction rub, fatigue, dyspnea, cough, pleuritic pain, fever). Chest x-ray and pulmonary function tests are recommended before therapy. Monitor chest x-ray every 3–6 mo during therapy to detect diffuse interstitial changes or alveolar infiltrates. Bronchoscopy or gallium radionuclide scan may also be used for diagnosis. Usually reversible after withdrawal, but fatalities have occurred.

■ **IV:** Assess patient for signs and symptoms of ARDS throughout therapy. Report dyspnea, tachypnea, or rales/crackles promptly. Bilateral, diffuse pulmonary infiltrates are seen on chest x-ray.

□ Monitor blood pressure frequently. Hypotension usually occurs during first several hours of therapy and is related to rate of infusion. If hypotension occurs, slow rate.

■ **PO:** Ophthalmic exams should be performed before and regularly during therapy and whenever visual changes (photophobia, halos around lights, decreased acuity) occur. May cause permanent loss of vision.

❏ Assess patient for signs of thyroid dysfunction, especially during initial therapy. Lethargy; weight gain; edema of the hands, feet, and periorbital region; and cool, pale skin suggest hypothyroidism and may require decrease in dose or discontinuation of therapy and thyroid supplementation. Tachycardia; weight loss; nervousness; sensitivity to heat; insomnia; and warm, flushed, moist skin suggest hyperthyroidism and may require discontinuation of therapy and treatment with antithyroid agents.

▪ **Lab Test Considerations:** Monitor liver and thyroid functions before and periodically throughout therapy. Drug effects persist long after discontinuation. Thyroid function abnormalities are common, but clinical thyroid dysfunction is uncommon.

❏ Monitor AST, ALT, and alkaline phosphatase at regular intervals during therapy, especially in patients receiving high maintenance dose. If liver function studies are 3 times normal or double in patients with elevated baseline levels or if hepatomegaly occurs, dose should be reduced.

❏ May cause asymptomatic elevations in ANA titer concentrations.

## POTENTIAL NURSING DIAGNOSES

▪ Cardiac output, decreased (Indications).
▪ Gas exchange, impaired (Side Effects).

## IMPLEMENTATION

❏ **High Alert:** Intravenous vasoactive medications are inherently dangerous; fatalities have occurred from medication errors involving amiodarone. Before administering, have second practitioner check original order, dosage calculations and infusion pump settings. Patients should be hospitalized and monitored closely during IV therapy and initiation of oral therapy. IV therapy should be administered only by physicians experienced in treating life-threatening arrhythmias. Do not confuse amiodarone with amrinone, now called inamrinone

▪ **General:** Hypokalemia and hypomagnesemia may decrease effectiveness or cause additional arrhythmias; correct before therapy.

❏ Assist patient during ambulation to prevent falls. Neurotoxicity (ataxia, proximal muscle weakness, tingling or numbness in fingers or toes, uncontrolled movements, tremors) is common during initial therapy, but may occur within 1 wk to several months of initiation of therapy and may persist for more than 1 yr after withdrawal. Dose reduction is recommended.

❏ Monitor closely when converting from IV to oral therapy, especially in geriatric patients.

▪ **PO:** May be administered with meals and in divided doses if GI intolerance occurs or if daily dose exceeds 1000 mg.

▪ **IV:** Administer via volumetric pump; drop size may be reduced, causing altered dosing with drop counter infusion sets.

❏ Infusions longer than 1 hr should not exceed 2 mg/ml unless administered through a central venous catheter.

❏ Administer through an in-line filter.

❏ Infusions exceeding 2 hr must be administered in glass or polyolefin bottles to prevent adsorption. However, polyvinyl chloride (PVC) tubing must be used during administration because concentrations and infusion rate recommendations have been based on PVC tubing.

▪ **Direct IV:** For cardiac arrest may administer 300 mg IV push. May repeat with 150 mg in 3–5 min.

▪ **Intermittent Infusion:** Recommended starting dose of about 1000 mg over 24 hr is administered during loading and maintenance infusions.

▪ **Initial loading dose:**

❏ Add 3 ml (150 mg) of amiodarone to 100 ml D5W for a concentration of 1.5 mg/ml.

▪ **Rate:** Administer rapidly over 10 min.

▪ **Loading Infusion:**

❏ Add 18 ml (900 mg) of amiodarone to 500 ml of D5W for a concentration of 1.8 mg/ml.

▪ **Rate:** Administer slowly, 360 mg over next 6 hr at a rate of 1 mg/min.

▪ **Maintenance Infusion:**

❏ Administer remainder of loading infusion.

▪ **Rate:** Administer 540 mg over the remaining 18 hr at a rate of 0.5 mg/min.

■ **Continuous Infusion:** After initial 24 hr, infusion may continue using a concentration of 1–6 mg/ml. Administer concentrations of >2 mg/ml via central venous catheter.

■ *Rate:* Administer at maintenance infusion rate of 0.5 mg/min (720 mg/24 hr). May be increased to achieve effective arrhythmia suppression but should not exceed 30 mg/min.

■ **Supplemental Infusions:** If breakthrough episodes of ventricular fibrillation or hemodynamically unstable ventricular tachycardia occur, dilute 150 mg of amiodarone in 100 ml of D5W.

■ *Rate:* Administer over 10 min to minimize hypotension.

■ **Y-Site Compatibility:** ◆ amikacin ◆ bretylium ◆ clindamycin ◆ dobutamine ◆ dopamine ◆ doxycycline ◆ erythromycin lactobionate ◆ esmolol ◆ gentamicin ◆ insulin ◆ isoproterenol ◆ labetalol ◆ lidocaine ◆ metronidazole ◆ midazolam ◆ morphine ◆ nitroglycerin ◆ norepinephrine ◆ penicillin G potassium ◆ phentolamine ◆ phenylephrine ◆ potassium chloride ◆ procainamide ◆ tobramycin ◆ vancomycin.

■ **Y-Site Incompatibility:** ◆ aminophylline ◆ heparin ◆ mezlocillin ◆ sodium bicarbonate.

■ **Additive Incompatibility:** ◆ aminophylline ◆ heparin ◆ mezlocillin ◆ sodium bicarbonate.

## PATIENT/FAMILY TEACHING

❑ Instruct patient to take amiodarone exactly as directed. If a dose is missed, do not take at all. Consult health care professional if more than two doses are missed.

❑ Inform patient that side effects may not appear until several days, weeks, or years after initiation of therapy and may persist for several months after withdrawal.

❑ Teach patients to monitor pulse daily and report abnormalities.

❑ Advise patients that photosensitivity reactions may occur through window glass, thin clothing, and sunscreens. Protective clothing and sunblock are recommended during and for 4 months after therapy. If photosensitivity occurs, dosage reduction may be useful.

❑ Inform patients that bluish discoloration of the face, neck, and arms is a possible side effect of this drug after prolonged use. This is usually reversible and will fade over several months. Notify health care professional if this occurs.

❑ Instruct male patients to notify health care professional if signs of epididymitis (pain and swelling in scrotum) occur. May require reduction in dose.

❑ Instruct patient to notify health care professional of medication regimen before treatment or surgery.

❑ Emphasize the importance of follow-up exams, including chest x-ray and pulmonary function tests every 3–6 mo and ophthalmic exams after 6 mo of therapy, and then annually.

## EVALUATION

**Effectiveness of therapy can be demonstrated by:** ■ Cessation of life-threatening ventricular arrhythmias. Adverse effects may take up to 4 months to resolve.

# amitriptyline
(a-mee-**trip**-ti-leen)
{Apo-Amitriptyline}, Elavil, Endep, {Levate}, {Novotriptyn}

*CLASSIFICATION(S):*
*Therapeutic: antidepressants*
*Pharmacologic: tricyclic antidepressants*

**Pregnancy Category D**

## INDICATIONS

■ Treatment of depression, often in conjunction with psychotherapy. **Unlabeled uses:** ■ Chronic pain syndromes.

## ACTION

■ Potentiates the effect of serotonin and norepinephrine in the CNS ■ Has significant anticholinergic properties. **Therapeutic Effects:** ■ Antidepressant action.

## PHARMACOKINETICS

**Absorption:** Well absorbed from the GI tract.
**Distribution:** Widely distributed.
**Protein Binding:** 95% bound to plasma proteins.
**Metabolism and Excretion:** Extensively metabolized by the liver. Some metabolites have antidepressant activity. Undergoes enterohepatic recir-

culation and secretion into gastric juices. Probably crosses the placenta and enters breast milk. **Half-life:** 10–50 hr.

## CONTRAINDICATIONS AND PRECAUTIONS

**Contraindicated in:** ■ Narrow-angle glaucoma ■ Pregnancy and lactation.

**Use Cautiously in:** ■ Geriatric patients (increased risk of adverse reactions) ■ Patients with pre-existing cardiovascular disease ■ Prostatic hypertrophy (increased risk of urinary retention) ■ History of seizures (threshold may be lowered).

## ADVERSE REACTIONS AND SIDE EFFECTS*

■ **CNS:** lethargy, sedation ■ **EENT:** blurred vision, dry eyes, dry mouth ■ **CV:** ARRHYTHMIAS , hypotension, ECG changes ■ **GI:** constipation, hepatitis, paralytic ileus ■ **GU:** urinary retention ■ **Derm:** photosensitivity ■ **Endo:** changes in blood glucose, gynecomastia ■ **Hemat:** blood dyscrasias ■ **Misc:** increased appetite, weight gain.

## INTERACTIONS

**Drug-Drug:** ■ Amitriptyline is metabolized in the liver by the cytochrome P450 2D6 enzyme, and its action may be affected by drugs that compete for metabolism by this enzyme, including other **antidepressants, phenothiazines, carbamazepine, class 1C antiarrhythmics** including **propafenone,** and **flecainide;** when these drugs are used concurrently with amitriptyline, dosage reduction of one or the other or both may be necessary. Concurrent use of other drugs that inhibit the activity of the enzyme, including **cimetidine, quinidine, amiodarone,** and **ritonavir,** may result in increased effects of amitriptyline ■ May cause hypotension, tachycardia, and potentially fatal reactions when used with **MAO inhibitors** (avoid concurrent use—discontinue 2 wk before starting amitriptyline) ■ Concurrent use with **SSRI antidepressants** may result in increased toxicity and should be avoided (**fluoxetine** should be stopped 5 wk before starting amitriptyline) ■ May prevent the therapeutic response to **guanethidine** ■ Concurrent use with **clonidine** may result in hypertensive crisis and should be avoided ■ Concurrent use with **levodopa** may

result in delayed or decreased absorption of levodopa or hypertension ■ Blood levels and effects may be decreased by **rifamycins (rifampin, rifapentine,** and **rifabutin)** ■ Concurrent use with **moxifloxaxin** or **sparfloxacin** increases the risk of adverse cardiovascular reactions ■ Additive CNS depression with other **CNS depressants** including **alcohol, antihistamines, clonidine, opioids,** and **sedative/ hypnotics** ■ **Barbiturates** may alter blood levels and effects ■ **Adrenergic** and **anticholinergic**side effects may be additive with other agents having **anticholinergic** properties ■ **Phenothiazines** or **oral contraceptives** increase levels and may cause toxicity ■ **Nicotine** may increase metabolism and alter effects.

**Drug-Natural Products:** ■ St. John's wort may decrease serum concentrations and efficacy ■ Concomitant use of **kava, valerian, skullcap, chamomile,** or **hops** can increase CNS depression ■ Increased anticholinergic effects with **angel's trumpet, jimson weed,** and **scopolia.**

## ROUTE AND DOSAGE

■ **PO (Adults):** 75 mg/day in divided doses; may be increased up to 150 mg/day or 50– 100 mg at bedtime, may increase by 25–50 mg up to 150 mg (in hospitalized patients, may initiate with 100 mg/day, increasing total daily dose up to 300 mg).

■ **PO (Geriatric Patients and Adolescents):** 10 mg tid and 20 mg at bedtime *or* 25 mg at bedtime initially, slowly increased to 100 mg/ day as a single bedtime dose or divided doses.

■ **IM (Adults):** 20–30 mg 4 times daily.

## AVAILABILITY (generic available)

■ *Tablets:* 10 mg$^{Rx}$, 25 mg$^{Rx}$, 50 mg$^{Rx}$, 75 mg$^{Rx}$, 100 mg$^{Rx}$, 150 mg$^{Rx}$ ■ Cost: 10 mg $17.90/100, 25 mg $35.75/100, 75 mg $85.25/ 100, 100 mg $108.00/100, 150 mg $108.86/ 100 ■ *Syrup:* 10 mg/5 ml$^{Rx}$ ■ *Injection:* 10 mg/ml$^{Rx}$.

TIME/ACTION PROFILE (antidepressant effect)

| | ONSET | PEAK | DURATION |
|---|---|---|---|
| PO | 2–3 wk (up to 30 days) | 2–6 wk | days–wks |
| IM | 2–3 wk | 2–6 wk | days–wks |

{ } = Available in Canada only.
*CAPITALS indicates life-threatening; underlines indicate most frequent.

# NURSING IMPLICATIONS

## ASSESSMENT

■ **General Info:** Monitor blood pressure and pulse before and during initial therapy. Notify physician or other health care professional of decreases in blood pressure (10–20 mmHg) or sudden increase in pulse rate. Patients taking high doses or with a history of cardiovascular disease should have ECG monitored before and periodically throughout therapy.

❑ Geriatric patients started on amitriptyline may be at an increased risk for falls; start with low dose and monitor closely.

■ **Depression:** Monitor mental status and affect. Assess for suicidal tendencies, especially during early therapy. Restrict amount of drug available to patient.

■ **Pain:** Assess intensity, quality, and location of pain periodically during therapy. May require several weeks for effects to be seen.

■ *Lab Test Considerations:* Assess leukocyte and differential blood counts, liver function, and serum glucose before and periodically during therapy. May cause an elevated serum bilirubin and alkaline phosphatase. May cause bone marrow depression. Serum glucose may be increased or decreased.

## POTENTIAL NURSING DIAGNOSES

■ Coping, ineffective (Indications).

■ Injury, risk for (Side Effects).

## IMPLEMENTATION

■ **General:** Do not confuse Elavil (amitriptyline) with Oruvail (ketoprofen).

❑ Dose increases should be made at bedtime because of sedation. Dose titration is a slow process; may take weeks to months. May give entire dose at bedtime. Sedative effect may be apparent before antidepressant effect is noted.

■ **PO:** Administer medication with or immediately after a meal to minimize gastric upset. Tablet may be crushed and given with food or fluids.

■ **IM:** For short-term IM administration only. Do not administer IV.

## PATIENT/FAMILY TEACHING

❑ Instruct patient to take medication exactly as directed. If a dose is missed, take as soon as possible unless almost time for next dose; if regimen is a single dose at bedtime, do not take in the morning because of side effects. Advise patient that drug effects may not be noticed for at least 2 wk. Abrupt discontinuation may cause nausea, vomiting, diarrhea, headache, trouble sleeping with vivid dreams, and irritability.

❑ May cause drowsiness and blurred vision. Caution patient to avoid driving and other activities requiring alertness until response to drug is known.

❑ Orthostatic hypotension, sedation, and confusion are common during early therapy, especially in geriatric patients. Protect patient from falls and advise patient to make position changes slowly.

❑ Advise patient to avoid alcohol or other CNS depressant drugs during and for 3–7 days after therapy has been discontinued.

❑ Instruct patient to notify health care professional if urinary retention occurs or if dry mouth or constipation persists. Sugarless candy or gum may diminish dry mouth, and an increase in fluid intake or bulk may prevent constipation. If symptoms persist, dose reduction or discontinuation may be necessary. Consult health care professional if dry mouth persists for more than 2 wk.

❑ Caution patient to use sunscreen and protective clothing to prevent photosensitivity reactions.

❑ Inform patient of need to monitor dietary intake. Increase in appetite may lead to undesired weight gain.

❑ Advise patient to notify health care professional if pregnancy is planned or suspected or if breastfeeding.

❑ Advise patient to notify health care professional of medication regimen before treatment or surgery. Medication should be discontinued as long as possible before surgery.

❑ Therapy for depression is usually prolonged and should be continued for at least 3 months to prevent relapse. Emphasize the importance of follow-up exams to monitor effectiveness and side effects.

## EVALUATION

**Effectiveness of therapy can be demonstrated by:** ■ Increased sense of well-being ❑ Renewed interest in surroundings ❑ Increased appetite ❑ Improved energy level ❑ Improved sleep ■ Decrease in chronic pain symptoms ■

Full therapeutic effects may be seen 2–6 wk after initiating therapy.

# amlodipine
(am-**loe**-di-peen)
Norvasc

## CLASSIFICATION(S):
**Therapeutic:** antihypertensives
**Pharmacologic:** calcium channel blockers

## Pregnancy Category C

## INDICATIONS
■ Alone or with other agents in the management of hypertension, angina pectoris, and vasospastic (Prinzmetal's) angina.

## ACTION
■ Inhibits the transport of calcium into myocardial and vascular smooth muscle cells, resulting in inhibition of excitation-contraction coupling and subsequent contraction. **Therapeutic Effects:** ■ Systemic vasodilation resulting in decreased blood pressure ■ Coronary vasodilation resulting in decreased frequency and severity of attacks of angina.

## PHARMACOKINETICS
**Absorption:** Well absorbed after oral administration (64–90%).
**Distribution:** Probably crosses the placenta.
**Protein Binding:** 95–98%.
**Metabolism and Excretion:** Mostly metabolized by the liver.
**Half-life:** 30–50 hr (increased in geriatric patients and patients with hepatic impairment)

## CONTRAINDICATIONS AND PRECAUTIONS
**Contraindicated in:** ■ Hypersensitivity ■ Blood pressure <90 mmHg.
**Use Cautiously in:** ■ Severe hepatic impairment (dosage reduction recommended) ■ Geriatric patients (dosage reduction recommended; increased risk of hypotension) ■ Aortic stenosis ■ History of CHF ■ Pregnancy, lactation, or children (safety not established).

## ADVERSE REACTIONS AND SIDE EFFECTS*
■ **CNS:** <u>headache</u>, dizziness, fatigue ■ **CV:** <u>peripheral edema</u>, angina, bradycardia, hypotension, palpitations ■ **GI:** gingival hyperplasia, nausea ■ **Derm:** flushing.

## INTERACTIONS
**Drug-Drug:** ■ Additive hypotension may occur when used concurrently with **fentanyl,** other **antihypertensives, nitrates,** acute ingestion of **alcohol,** or **quinidine** ■ Antihypertensive effects may be decreased by concurrent use of **nonsteroidal anti-inflammatory agents** ■ May increase the risk of neurotoxicity with **lithium.**
**Drug-Food:** ■ Blood levels and effects are increased by concurrent ingestion of **grapefruit juice.**

## ROUTE AND DOSAGE
■ **PO (Adults):** 5–10 mg once daily; *antihypertensive in fragile or small patients or patients already receiving other antihypertensives*—initiate at 2.5 mg/day, increase as required/tolerated (up to 10 mg/day) as an antihypertensive therapy with 2.5 mg/day in patients with hepatic insufficiency.
■ **PO (Geriatric Patients):** *Antihypertensive*—Initiate therapy at 2.5 mg/day, increase as required/tolerated (up to 10 mg/day); *antianginal*—initiate therapy at 5 mg/day, increase as required/tolerated (up to 10 mg/day).
❑ **Hepatic Impairment**
■ **PO (Adults):** *Antihypertensive*—Initiate therapy at 2.5 mg/day, increase as required/tolerated (up to 10 mg/day); *antianginal*—initiate therapy at 5 mg/day, increase as required/tolerated (up to 10 mg/day).

## AVAILABILITY
■ *Tablets:* 2.5 mg^Rx, 5 mg^Rx, 10 mg^Rx ■Cost: 2.5 mg $122.86/90, 5 mg $122.86/90, 10 mg $195.70/90 ■ benazepril (Lotrel)^Rx. See Appendix B.

TIME/ACTION PROFILE (cardiovascular effects)

|  | ONSET | PEAK | DURATION |
|---|---|---|---|
| PO | unknown | 6–9 | 24 hr |

{ } = Available in Canada only.
*CAPITALS indicates life-threatening; <u>underlines</u> indicate most frequent.

## NURSING IMPLICATIONS

### ASSESSMENT

- **General Info:** Monitor blood pressure and pulse before therapy, during dose titration, and periodically during therapy. Monitor ECG periodically during prolonged therapy.
- ❑ Monitor intake and output ratios and daily weight. Assess for signs of CHF (peripheral edema, rales/crackles, dyspnea, weight gain, jugular venous distention).
- **Angina:** Assess location, duration, intensity, and precipitating factors of patient's anginal pain.
- *Lab Test Considerations:* Total serum calcium concentrations are not affected by calcium channel blockers.

### POTENTIAL NURSING DIAGNOSES

- Tissue perfusion, ineffective (Indications).
- Pain, acute (Indications).

### IMPLEMENTATION

- **PO:** May be administered without regard to meals.

### PATIENT/FAMILY TEACHING

- **General Info:** Advise patient to take medication exactly as directed, even if feeling well. If a dose is missed, take as soon as possible unless almost time for next dose; do not double doses. May need to be discontinued gradually.
- ❑ Instruct patient on correct technique for monitoring pulse. Instruct patient to contact health care professional if heart rate is <50 bpm.
- ❑ Caution patient to change positions slowly to minimize orthostatic hypotension.
- ❑ May cause drowsiness or dizziness. Advise patient to avoid driving or other activities requiring alertness until response to the medication is known.
- ❑ Instruct patient on importance of maintaining good dental hygiene and seeing dentist frequently for teeth cleaning to prevent tenderness, bleeding, and gingival hyperplasia (gum enlargement).
- ❑ Instruct patient to avoid concurrent use of alcohol or OTC medications, especially cold preparations, without consulting health care professional.
- ❑ Advise patient to notify health care professional if irregular heartbeats, dyspnea, swelling of hands and feet, pronounced dizziness, nausea, constipation, or hypotension occurs or if headache is severe or persistent.
- ❑ Caution patient to wear protective clothing and use sunscreen to prevent photosensitivity reactions.
- ❑ Advise patient to inform health care professional of medication regimen before treatment or surgery.
- **Angina:** Instruct patient on concurrent nitrate or beta-blocker therapy to continue taking both medications as directed and to use SL nitroglycerin as needed for anginal attacks.
- ❑ Advise patient to contact health care professional if chest pain does not improve or worsens after therapy, if it occurs with diaphoresis, if shortness of breath occurs, or if severe, persistent headache occurs.
- ❑ Caution patient to discuss exercise restrictions with health care professional before exertion.
- **Hypertension:** Encourage patient to comply with other interventions for hypertension (weight reduction, low-sodium diet, smoking cessation, moderation of alcohol consumption, regular exercise, and stress management). Medication controls but does not cure hypertension.
- ❑ Instruct patient and family in proper technique for monitoring blood pressure. Advise patient to take blood pressure weekly and to report significant changes to health care professional.

### EVALUATION

**Effectiveness of therapy can be demonstrated by:** ■ Decrease in blood pressure ■ Decrease in frequency and severity of anginal attacks ❑ Decrease in need for nitrate therapy ❑ Increase in activity tolerance and sense of well-being.

## amoxicillin

(a-mox-i-**sil**-in)

Amoxil, {Apo-Amoxi}, DisperMox, {Novamoxin}, {Nu-Amoxi}, Trimox, Wymox

### *CLASSIFICATION(S):*

*Therapeutic: anti-infectives, antiulcer agents*

**Pharmacologic:** *aminopenicillins*

**Pregnancy Category B**

## INDICATIONS

■ Treatment of: ❑ Skin and skin structure infections ❑ Otitis media ❑ Sinusitis ❑ Respiratory infections ❑ Genitourinary infections ❑ Septicemia ■ Endocarditis prophylaxis ■ Management of ulcer disease due to *Helicobacter pylori.* **Unlabeled uses:** ■ Lyme disease.

## ACTION

■ Binds to bacterial cell wall, causing cell death. **Therapeutic Effects:** ■ Bactericidal action; spectrum is broader than penicillins. **Spectrum:** ■ Active against: ❑ Streptococci ❑ Pneumococci ❑ Enterococci ❑ *Haemophilus influenzae* ❑ *Escherichia coli* ❑ *Proteus mirabilis* ❑ *Neisseria meningitidis* ❑ *Shigella* ❑ *Chlamydia trachomatis* ❑ *Salmonella* ❑ *Borrelia burgdorferi* ❑ *H. pylori.*

## PHARMACOKINETICS

**Absorption:** Well absorbed from duodenum (75–90%). More resistant to acid inactivation than other penicillins.

**Distribution:** Diffuses readily into most body tissues and fluids. CSF penetration increased when meninges are inflamed. Crosses placenta; enters breast milk in small amounts.

**Metabolism and Excretion:** 70% excreted unchanged in the urine; 30% metabolized by the liver.

**Half-life:** 1–1.3 hr.

## CONTRAINDICATIONS AND PRECAUTIONS

**Contraindicated in:** ■ Hypersensitivity to penicillins ■ Tablets for oral suspension (Disper-Mox) contain aspartame; avoid in patients with phenylketonuria.

**Use Cautiously in:** ■ Severe renal insufficiency ( ↓ dose if CCr <30 ml/min) ■ Infectious mononucleosis ( ↑ risk of rash) ■ Has been used safely during pregnancy and lactation

## ADVERSE REACTIONS AND SIDE EFFECTS*

■ **CNS:** SEIZURES (high doses) ■ **GI:** PSEUDOMEMBRANOUS COLITIS, diarrhea, nausea, vomiting ■

**Derm:** rashes, urticaria ■ **Hemat:** blood dyscrasias ■ **Misc:** allergic reactions including ANAPHYLAXIS, SERUM SICKNESS, superinfection.

## INTERACTIONS

**Drug-Drug:** ■ **Probenecid** ↓ renal excretion and ↑ blood levels of amoxicillin—therapy may be combined for this purpose ■ May ↑ effect of **warfarin** ■ May ↓ effectiveness of **oral contraceptives**.

## ROUTE AND DOSAGE

❑ **Most Infections**

■ **PO (Adults and Children >20 kg):** 250–500 mg q 8 hr *or* 500–875 mg q 12 hr.

■ **PO (Children >3 mo):** 20–40 mg/kg/day in divided doses q 8 hr *or* 25–45 mg/kg/day individual doses q 12 hr.

■ **PO (Infants ≤3 mo):** up to 30 mg/kg/day in divided doses q 12 hr.

❑ *H. Pylori*

■ **PO (Adults):** *Triple therapy*—1000 mg amoxicillin twice daily with lansoprazole 30 mg twice daily and clarithromycin 500 mg twice daily for 14 days *or* 1000 mg amoxicillin twice daily with omeprazole 20 mg twice daily and clarithromycin 500 mg twice daily for 14 days *or* amoxicillin 1000 mg twice daily with esomeprazole 40 mg daily and clarithromycin 500 mg twice daily for 10 days. *Dual therapy*—1000 mg amoxicillin three times daily with lansoprazole 30 mg three times daily for 14 days.

❑ **Endocarditis Prophylaxis**

■ **PO (Adults):** 2 g 1 hr prior to procedure.

■ **PO (Children):** 50 mg/kg 1 hr prior to procedure.

❑ **Gonorrhea**

■ **PO (Adults and Children ≥40 kg):** single 3-g dose.

■ **PO (Children >2 yr and <40 kg):** 50 mg/kg with probenecid 25 mg/kg.

❑ **Renal Impairment**

■ **PO (Adults CCr 10–30 ml/min):** 250–500 mg q 12 hr.

❑ **Renal Impairment**

■ **PO (Adults CCr <10 ml/min):** 250–500 mg q 24 hr.

{ } = Available in Canada only.
*CAPITALS indicates life-threatening; underlines indicate most frequent.

## AVAILABILITY (generic available)

■ *Chewable tablets (cherry, banana, peppermint flavors):* 125 mg$^{Rx}$, 200 mg$^{Rx}$, 250 mg$^{Rx}$, 400 mg$^{Rx}$ ■ Cost: 125 mg $9.24/20, 200 mg $12.33/20, 400 mg $13.76/100 ■ *Tablets:* 500 mg$^{Rx}$, 875 mg$^{Rx}$ ■ Cost: 500 mg $10.40/20, 875 mg $21.22/20 ■ *Capsules:* 250 mg$^{Rx}$, 500 mg$^{Rx}$ ■ Cost: 250 mg $4.41/30, 500 mg $4.88/20 ■ *Suspension pediatric drops (bubblegum flavor):* 50 mg/ml$^{Rx}$ ■ Cost: 50 mg/ml $1.80/15 ml ■ *Tablets for oral suspension (strawberry):* 200 mg$^{Rx}$, 400 mg$^{Rx}$ ■ *Suspension (strawberry [125 mg/5 ml] and bubblegum [200 mg/5 ml, 250 mg/5 ml, 400 mg/5 ml] flavors):* 125 mg/5 ml$^{Rx}$, 200 mg/5 ml$^{Rx}$, 250 mg/5 ml$^{Rx}$, 400 mg/5 ml$^{Rx}$ ■ Cost: 125 mg/5ml $4.76/100 ml, 200 mg/5 ml $9.23/100 ml, 250 mg/5 ml $8.74/100 ml, 400 mg/5 ml $11.24/100 ml ■ clarithromycin and lansoprazole in a compliance package (Prevpac); with omeprazole and clarithromycin in a compliance package (Losec 1-2-3-A). See Appendix B.

TIME/ACTION PROFILE (blood levels)

| | ONSET | PEAK | DURATION |
|---|---|---|---|
| PO | 30 min | 1–2 hr | 8–12 hr |

## NURSING IMPLICATIONS

### ASSESSMENT

❑ Assess patient for infection (vital signs; appearance of wound, sputum, urine, and stool; WBC) at beginning of and throughout therapy.

❑ Obtain a history before initiating therapy to determine previous use of and reactions to penicillins or cephalosporins. Persons with a negative history of penicillin sensitivity may still have an allergic response.

❑ Observe for signs and symptoms of anaphylaxis (rash, pruritus, laryngeal edema, wheezing). Notify the physician or other health care professional immediately if these occur.

❑ Obtain specimens for culture and sensitivity prior to therapy. First dose may be given before receiving results.

❑ Monitor bowel function. Diarrhea, abdominal cramping, fever, and bloody stools should be reported to health care professional promptly as a sign of pseudomembra-nous colitis. May begin up to several weeks following cessation of therapy.

■ *Lab Test Considerations:* May cause increased serum alkaline phosphatase, LDH, AST, and ALT concentrations.

❑ May cause false-positive direct Coombs' test result.

## POTENTIAL NURSING DIAGNOSES

■ Infection, risk for (Indications, Side Effects).

■ Noncompliance (Patient/Family Teaching).

## IMPLEMENTATION

■ **PO:** Administer around the clock. May be given without regard to meals or with meals to decrease GI side effects. Capsule contents may be emptied and swallowed with liquids. Chewable tablets should be crushed or chewed before swallowing with liquids.

❑ Shake oral suspension before administering. Suspension may be given straight or mixed in formula, milk, fruit juice, water, or ginger ale. Administer immediately after mixing. Discard refrigerated reconstituted suspension after 10 days.

❑ Mix each *tablet for oral suspension (DisperMox)* in 2 teaspoons of water. Patient should drink entire mixture, rinse container with a small amount of water and drink to make sure entire dose is taken. Do not chew or swallow tablet. Tablets will not dissolve in mouth. Use only water to dissolve tablets, other liquids are not recommended. Store tablets at room temperature.

## PATIENT/FAMILY TEACHING

❑ Instruct patients to take medication around the clock and to finish the drug completely as directed, even if feeling better. Advise patients that sharing of this medication may be dangerous.

❑ Review use and preparation of *tablets for oral suspension (DisperMox)*.

❑ Instruct female patients taking oral contraceptives to use an alternate or additional nonhormonal method of contraception during therapy with amoxicillin and until next menstrual period.

❑ Advise patient to report the signs of superinfection (furry overgrowth on the tongue, vaginal itching or discharge, loose or foul-smelling stools) and allergy.

❑ Instruct patient to notify health care professional immediately if diarrhea, abdominal cramping, fever, or bloody stools occur and not to treat with antidiarrheals without consulting health care professionals.

❑ Instruct the patient to notify health care professional if symptoms do not improve.

❑ Teach patients with a history of rheumatic heart disease or valve replacement the importance of using antimicrobial prophylaxis before invasive medical or dental procedures.

### EVALUATION

**Clinical response to therapy can be evaluated by:** ■ Resolution of the signs and symptoms of infection. Length of time for complete resolution depends on the organism and site of infection ■ Endocarditis prophylaxis ■ Eradication of *H. pylori* with resolution of ulcer symptoms.

---

# amoxicillin/clavulanate
(a-mox-i-**sill**-in/klav-yoo-**lan**-ate)
Augmentin, Augmentin ES, Augmentin XR, {Clavulin}

### CLASSIFICATION(S):
*Therapeutic: anti-infectives*
*Pharmacologic: aminopenicillins/ beta lactamase inhibitors*

### Pregnancy Category B

### INDICATIONS

■ Treatment of a variety of infections including: ❑ Skin and skin structure infections ❑ Otitis media ❑ Sinusitis ❑ Respiratory tract infections ❑ Genitourinary tract infections ❑ Meningitis ❑ Septicemia.

### ACTION

■ Binds to bacterial cell wall, causing cell death; spectrum of amoxicillin is broader than penicillin. Clavulanate resists action of beta-lactamase, an enzyme produced by bacteria that is capable of inactivating some penicillins. **Therapeutic Effects:** ■ Bactericidal action against susceptible bacteria. **Spectrum:** ■ Active against: ❑ Streptococci ❑ Pneumococci ❑ Enterococci ❑ *Haemophilus influenzae* ❑ *Escherichia coli* ❑

*Proteus mirabilis* ❑ *Neisseria meningitidis* ❑ *Klebsiella pneumoniae* ❑ *Shigella* ❑ *Salmonella* ❑ *Moraxella catarrhalis.*

### PHARMACOKINETICS

**Absorption:** Well absorbed from the duodenum (75–90%). More resistant to acid inactivation than other penicillins.

**Distribution:** Diffuses readily into most body tissues and fluids. Does not readily enter brain/ CSF; CSF penetration is increased in the presence of inflamed meninges. Crosses the placenta and enters breast milk in small amounts.

**Metabolism and Excretion:** 70% excreted unchanged in the urine; 30% metabolized by the liver.

**Half-life:** 1–1.3 hr.

### CONTRAINDICATIONS AND PRECAUTIONS

**Contraindicated in:** ■ Hypersensitivity to penicillins ■ Hypersensitivity to clavulanate ■ Suspension and chewable tablets contain aspartame and should be avoided in phenylketonurics.

**Use Cautiously in:** ■ Severe renal insufficiency (dosage reduction necessary) ■ Infectious mononucleosis (increased incidence of rash) ■ Hepatic impairment (dose cautiously, monitor liver function).

### ADVERSE REACTIONS AND SIDE EFFECTS*

■ **CNS:** SEIZURES (high doses) ■ **GI:** PSEUDOMEMBRANOUS COLITIS, diarrhea, hepatic dysfunction, nausea, vomiting ■ **Derm:** rashes, urticaria ■ **Hemat:** blood dyscrasias ■ **Misc:** allergic reactions including ANAPHYLAXIS and SERUM SICKNESS, superinfection.

### INTERACTIONS

**Drug-Drug:** ■ **Probenecid** decreases renal excretion and increases blood levels of amoxicillin—therapy may be combined for this purpose ■ May potentiate the effect of **warfarin** ■ Concurrent **allopurinol** therapy increases risk of rash ■ May decrease the effectiveness of **hormonal contraceptives.**

---

{ } = Available in Canada only.
*CAPITALS indicates life-threatening; underlines indicate most frequent.

### ROUTE AND DOSAGE

❏ **Most Infections**

■ **PO (Adults and Children >40 kg): Tablets:** 1–500 mg tablet q 12 hr or 1–250 mg tablet q 8 hr. **Suspension:** 500 mg q 12 hr as 125 mg/5 ml or 250 mg/5 ml suspension.

❏ **Serious Infections and Respiratory Tract Infections**

■ **PO (Adults and Children >40 kg):** 1–875 mg tablet every 12 hr *or* 1–500 mg tablet q 8 hr; *acute bacterial sinusitis*—2000 mg q 12 hr for 10 days as extended release (XR) product; *community-acquired pneumonia*—2000 mg every 12 hr for 7–10 days as extended release (XR) product.

❏ **Recurrent/persistent acute otitis media due to** *S. pneumonia, H. influenzae,* **or** *M. catarrhalis* **in day-care children <2 yrs or in daycare**

■ **PO (Children <2 yr or in daycare):** 90 mg/kg/day in divided doses q 12 hr for 10 days (as ES formulation only).

❏ **Renal Impairment**

■ **PO (Adults):** *CCr 10–30 ml/min*—250–500 mg q 12 hr (do not use 875 mg tablet); *CCr <10 ml/min*—250–500 mg q 24 hr.

❏ **Otitis Media, Sinusitis, Lower Respiratory Tract Infections, Serious Infections**

■ **PO (Children ≥3 mo):** *200 mg/5 ml or 400 mg/5 ml suspension*—22.5 mg/kg q 12 hr; *125 mg/5 ml or 250 mg/5 ml suspension*—13.3 mg/kg q 8 hr.

❏ **Less Serious Infections**

■ **PO (Children ≥3 mo):** *200 mg/5 ml or 400 mg/5 ml suspension*—12.5 mg/kg q 12 hr *or* 6.6 mg/kg q 8 hr (as 125 mg/5 ml or 250 mg/5 ml suspension).

■ **PO (Children <3 mo):** 15 mg/kg q 12 hr (125 mg/ml suspension recommended).

### AVAILABILITY (generic available)

■ *Tablets:* 250 mg amoxicillin with 125 mg clavulanic acid[Rx], 500 mg amoxicillin with 125 mg clavulanate[Rx], 875 mg amoxicillin with 125 mg clavulanate[Rx] ■ Cost: 250 mg $281.12/100, 500 mg $80.74/20, 875 mg $107.77/20 ■ *Chewable tablets (125 mg and 250 mg are lemon-lime flavor; 200 mg and 400 mg are cherry-banana flavor):* 125 mg amoxicillin with 31.25 mg clavulanate[Rx], 200 mg amoxicillin with 28.5 mg clavulanate[Rx], 250 mg amoxicillin with 62.5 mg clavulanate[Rx], 400 mg amoxicillin with 57 mg clavulanate[Rx] ■ Cost: 125 mg $39.88/30, 200 mg $38.58/20, 250 mg $76.06/30, 400 mg $73.52/20 ■ *Extended-release tablets:* 1000 mg amoxicillin with 62.5 mg clavulanate ■ *Suspension (125 mg/5 ml and 250 mg/5 ml are orange flavor; 200 mg/5 ml, 400 mg/5 ml and 600 mg/5 mlare orange-raspberry flavor):* 125 mg amoxicillin with 31.25 mg clavulanic acid/5 ml[Rx], 200 mg amoxicillin with 28.5 mg clavulanic acid/5 ml[Rx], 250 mg amoxicillin with 62.5 mg clavulanate/5 ml[Rx], 400 mg amoxicillin with 57 mg clavulanic acid/5 ml[Rx], 600 mg amoxicillin with 42.9 mg clavulanate/5 ml(ES formulation) ■ Cost: 125 mg $27.11/100 ml, 200 mg $38.58/100 ml, 250 mg $ 51.77/100 ml, 400 mg $70.69/100 ml.

TIME/ACTION PROFILE (peak blood levels)

|    | ONSET | PEAK | DURATION |
|----|-------|------|----------|
| PO | 30 min | 1–2 hr | 8—12 hrhr |

### NURSING IMPLICATIONS

#### ASSESSMENT

❏ Assess patient for infection (vital signs; appearance of wound, sputum, urine, and stool; WBC) at beginning of and throughout therapy.

❏ Obtain a history before initiating therapy to determine previous use of and reactions to penicillins or cephalosporins. Persons with a negative history of penicillin sensitivity may still have an allergic response.

❏ Observe for signs and symptoms of anaphylaxis (rash, pruritus, laryngeal edema, wheezing). Notify the physician or other health care professional immediately if these occur.

❏ Obtain specimens for culture and sensitivity prior to therapy. First dose may be given before receiving results.

❏ Monitor bowel function. Diarrhea, abdominal cramping, fever, and bloody stools should be reported to health care professional promptly as a sign of pseudomembranous colitis. May begin up to several weeks following cessation of therapy.

■ *Lab Test Considerations:* May cause increased serum alkaline phosphatase, LDH, AST, and ALT concentrations. Elderly men and patients receiving prolonged treatment are at increased risk for hepatic dysfunction.

❑ May cause false-positive direct Coombs' test result.

## POTENTIAL NURSING DIAGNOSES

■ Infection, risk for (Indications, Side Effects).

■ Noncompliance (Patient/Family Teaching).

## IMPLEMENTATION

■ **PO:** Administer around the clock. May be given without regard to meals. May be given with meals to decrease GI side effects. Capsule contents may be emptied and swallowed with liquids. Chewable tablets should be crushed or chewed before swallowing with liquids. Shake oral suspension before administering. Refrigerated reconstituted suspension should be discarded after 10 days.

❑ Two 250-mg tablets are not bioequivalent to one 500-mg tablet; 250-mg tablets and 250-mg chewable tablets are also not interchangeable. Two 500–mg tablets are not interchangeable with one 1000–mg XR tablet; amounts of clavulanic acid and durations of action are different. Augmentin ES 600 (600 mg/5 ml) does not contain the same amount of clavulanic acid as any of the other Augmentin suspensions. Suspensions are not interchangeable.

❑ *Children:* Do not administer 250-mg chewable tablets to children <40 kg due to clavulanate content. Children <3 months should receive the 125-mg/5 ml oral solution.

## PATIENT/FAMILY TEACHING

❑ Instruct patients to take medication around the clock and to finish the drug completely as directed, even if feeling better. Advise patients that sharing of this medication may be dangerous.

❑ Instruct female patients taking oral contraceptives to use an alternate or additional method of contraception during therapy and until next menstrual period.

❑ Advise patient to report the signs of superinfection (furry overgrowth on the tongue, vaginal itching or discharge, loose or foul-smelling stools) and allergy.

❑ Instruct patient to notify health care professional immediately if diarrhea, abdominal cramping, fever, or bloody stools occur and not to treat with antidiarrheals without consulting health care professionals.

❑ Instruct the patient to notify health care professional if symptoms do not improve or if nausea or diarrhea persists when drug is administered with food.

## EVALUATION

**Clinical response to therapy can be evaluated by:** ■ Resolution of the signs and symptoms of infection. Length of time for complete resolution depends on the organism and site of infection.

# amphetamine mixtures
(am-**fet**-a-meen)
Amphetamine Salt, Adderall, Adderall XR

## CLASSIFICATION(S):
***Therapeutic:*** *central nervous system stimulants*

**Schedule II**

**Pregnancy Category C**

## INDICATIONS

■ Narcolepsy ■ ADHD.

## ACTION

■ Causes release of norepinephrine from nerve endings. Pharmacologic effects are: ■ CNS and respiratory stimulation ■ Vasoconstriction ■ Mydriasis (pupillary dilation). **Therapeutic Effects:** ■ Increased motor activity, mental alertness, and decreased fatigue in narcoleptic patients ■ Increased attention span in ADHD.

## PHARMACOKINETICS

**Absorption:** Well absorbed after oral administration.

**Distribution:** Widely distributed in body tissues, with high concentrations in the brain and CSF. Crosses placenta and enters breast milk.

**Metabolism and Excretion:** Some metabolism by the liver. Urinary excretion is pH-dependent. Alkaline urine promotes reabsorption and prolongs action.

**Half-life:** 10–30 hr (depends on urine pH).

## CONTRAINDICATIONS AND PRECAUTIONS

**Contraindicated in:** ■ Pregnancy or lactation ■ Hyperexcitable states including hyperthyroidism ■ Psychotic personalities ■ Suicidal or homicidal tendencies ■ Chemical dependence ■ Glaucoma.

**Use Cautiously in:** ■ Cardiovascular disease ■ Hypertension ■ Diabetes mellitus ■ Geriatric or debilitated patients.

## ADVERSE REACTIONS AND SIDE EFFECTS*

■ **CNS:** hyperactivity, insomnia, irritability, restlessness, tremor, dizziness, headache, cardiomyopathy (increased with prolonged use, high doses) ■ **CV:** palpitations, tachycardia, hypertension, hypotension ■ **GI:** anorexia, constipation, cramps, diarrhea, dry mouth, metallic taste, nausea, vomiting ■ **GU:** impotence, increased libido ■ **Derm:** urticaria ■ **Endo:** growth inhibition (with long term use in children) ■ **Misc:** psychological dependence.

## INTERACTIONS

**Drug-Drug:** ■ Use with **MAO inhibitors** or **meperidine** can result in hypertensive crisis ■ ↑ adrenergic effects with other **adrenergics** or **thyroid preparations** ■ **Drugs that alkalinize urine (sodium bicarbonate, acetazolamide)** ↓ excretion, ↑ effects ■ **Drugs that acidify urine (ammonium chloride, large doses of ascorbic acid)** ↓ effects ■ ↑ risk of hypertension and bradycardia with **beta blockers** ■ ↑ risk of arrhythmias with **digoxin** ■ **Tricyclic antidepressants** may ↑ effect of amphetamine but may ↑ risk of arrhythmias, hypertension, or hyperpyrexia.

**Drug-Food:** ■ **Foods that alkalinize the urine** (e.g., cranberry juice) can ↑ effect of amphetamine.

## ROUTE AND DOSAGE

Dose is expressed in total amphetamine content (amphetamine + dextroamphetamine).

❑ **Narcolepsy**

■ **PO (Adults and Children ≥ 12 yr):** 5–60 mg/day in divided doses; start with 10 mg/ day, increase by 10 mg/day at weekly intervals. Sustained-release capsules can be given once daily, tablets every 4–6 hr.

■ **PO (Children 6–12 yr):** 5 mg once daily; may increase by 5 mg/day at weekly intervals to a maximum of 60 mg/day.

❑ **ADHD**

■ **PO (Children ≥6 yr):** 5 mg/day 1–2 times daily; increase by 5 mg at weekly intervals. Sustained-release capsules can be given once daily, tablets every 4–6 hr. If starting therapy with extended release capsules, start with 10 mg once daily and increase by 10 mg/day at weekly intervals (up to 40 mg/day).

■ **PO (Children 3–5 yr):** 2.5 mg/day; increase by 2.5 mg at weekly intervals.

## AVAILABILITY (generic available)

Amount is expressed in total amphetamine content (amphetamine + dextroamphetamine).

■ *Tablets:* 5 mg$^{Rx}$, 7.5 mg$^{Rx}$, 10 mg$^{Rx}$, 12.5 mg$^{Rx}$, 15 mg$^{Rx}$, 20 mg$^{Rx}$, 30 mg$^{Rx}$ ■ *Extended-release capsules:* 10 mg$^{Rx}$, 20 mg$^{Rx}$, 30 mg$^{Rx}$.

TIME/ACTION PROFILE (CNS stimulation)

| | ONSET | PEAK | DURATION |
|---|---|---|---|
| PO | 1–2 hr | unknown | 4–10 hr |

## NURSING IMPLICATIONS

### ASSESSMENT

■ **General Info:** Monitor blood pressure, pulse, and respiration before and periodically during therapy.

❑ May produce a false sense of euphoria and well-being. Provide frequent rest periods and observe patient for rebound depression after the effects of the medication have worn off.

❑ Has high dependence and abuse potential. Tolerance to medication occurs rapidly; do not increase dose.

■ **ADHD:** Monitor weight biweekly and inform physician of significant loss. Monitor height periodically in children; inform physician of growth inhibition.

❑ Assess attention span, impulse control, motor and vocal tics, and interactions with others in children with ADHDs.

■ **Narcolepsy:** Observe and document frequency of narcoleptic episodes.

■ *Lab Test Considerations:*

❑ May interfere with urinary steroid determinations.

□ May cause ↑ plasma corticosteroid concentrations; greatest in evening.

## POTENTIAL NURSING DIAGNOSES

■ Thought processes, disturbed (Side Effects).

## IMPLEMENTATION

■ **PO:** Use the lowest effective dose.

□ May be taken without regard to food.

□ Extended-release capsules may be swallowed whole or opened and sprinkled on applesauce; swallow contents without chewing. Applesauce should be swallowed immediately; do not store. Do not divide contents of capsule; entire contents of capsule should be taken.

■ **ADHD:** When symptoms are controlled, dose reduction or interruption of therapy may be possible during summer months or may be given on each of the 5 school days, with medication-free weekends and holidays.

## PATIENT/FAMILY TEACHING

□ Instruct patient to take medication at least 6 hr before bedtime to avoid sleep disturbances. Missed doses should be taken as soon as remembered up to 6 hr before bedtime. Do not double doses. Instruct patient not to alter dose without consulting physician. Abrupt cessation of high doses may cause extreme fatigue and mental depression.

□ Inform patient that the effects of drug-induced dry mouth can be minimized by rinsing frequently with water or chewing sugarless gum or candies.

□ Advise patient to limit caffeine intake.

□ May impair judgment. Advise patient to use caution when driving or during other activities requiring alertness.

□ Inform patient that periodic holidays from the drug may be used to assess progress and decrease dependence.

□ Advise patient to notify physician if nervousness, restlessness, insomnia, dizziness, anorexia, or dry mouth becomes severe.

## EVALUATION

**Effectiveness of therapy can be demonstrated by:** ■ Improved attention span. Therapy should be interrupted and need reassessed

periodically ■ Decrease in narcoleptic symptoms.

# amphotericin B deoxycholate

(am-foe-**ter**-i-sin)

Fungizone

# amphotericin B cholesteryl sulfate

Amphotec

# amphotericin B lipid complex

Abelcet

# amphotericin B liposome

AmBisome

**CLASSIFICATION(S):**
**Therapeutic:** antifungals

**Pregnancy Category B**

## INDICATIONS

■ **IV:** Treatment of active, progressive, potentially fatal fungal infections ■ **Amphotericin B liposome:** Management of suspected fungal infections in febrile neutropenic patients □ Treatment of visceral leishmaniasis □ Treatment of crytococcal meningitis in HIV patients ■ **PO:** Treatment of oral candidiasis ■ **Topical:** Treatment of superficial fungal infections.

## ACTION

■ Binds to fungal cell membrane, allowing leakage of cellular contents ■ Toxicity (especially acute infusion reactions and nephrotoxicity) is less with lipid formulations. **Therapeutic Effects:** ■ Fungistatic action. **Spectrum:** ■ Active against: □ Aspergillosis □ Blastomycosis ■ *Candida* □ Coccidioidomycosis □ Cryptococcosis □ Histoplasmosis □ Leishmaniasis □ Mucormycosis.

## PHARMACOKINETICS

**Absorption:** Not absorbed orally. Topical and oral preparations are not significantly absorbed.

**Distribution:** After administration, distributed to body tissues and fluids. Poor penetration into CSF. *Cholesteryl*—taken up by liver, spleen, and bone marrow, then slowly released.

**Metabolism and Excretion:** Elimination is very prolonged. Detectable in urine up to 7 wk after discontinuation.

**Half-life:** Biphasic—initial phase, 24–48 hr; terminal phase, 15 days. *Cholesteryl*—28 hr. *Liposomal*—174 hr.

## CONTRAINDICATIONS AND PRECAUTIONS

**Contraindicated in:** ▪ Hypersensitivity ▪ Lactation.

**Use Cautiously in:** ▪ Renal impairment or electrolyte abnormalities ▪ Patients receiving concurrent leukocyte transfusions (increased risk of pulmonary toxicity with lipid complex formulation only) ▪ Pregnancy (has been used safely).

## ADVERSE REACTIONS AND SIDE EFFECTS*

▪ **CNS:** headache, dizziness, tremor ▪ **Resp:** dyspnea, hypoxia, wheezing ▪ **CV:** hypotension, arrhythmias ▪ **GI:** diarrhea, nausea, vomiting, abdominal pain, enlarged abdomen ▪ **GU:** nephrotoxicity, hematuria ▪ **F and E:** hypokalemia, hypocalcemia (cholesteryl only), hypomagnesemia ▪ **Hemat:** anemia, dyscrasias ▪ **Local:** phlebitis ▪ **MS:** arthralgia, myalgia ▪ **Neuro:** peripheral neuropathy ▪ **Misc:** HYPERSENSITIVITY REACTIONS, chills, fever, acute infusion reactions.

## INTERACTIONS

**Drug-Drug:** ▪ Increased risk of renal toxicity, bronchospasm, and hypotension with **antineoplastics** ▪ Concurrent use with **corticosteroids** or **corticotropin** increases the risk of hypokalemia and cardiac dysfunction ▪ Concurrent use with **zidovudine** may increase the risk of myelotoxicity and nephrotoxicity ▪ **Cyclosporine** increases the risk of nephrotoxicity ▪ Combined use with **flucytosine** increases antifungal activity but may increase the risk of toxicity from flucytosine ▪ Combined use with **azole antifungals** may induce resistance ▪ Increased risk of nephrotoxicity with other **nephrotoxic agents** ▪ **Thiazide diuretics, corticosteroids** may potentiate hypokalemia ▪ Hypokalemia from amphotericin increases the risk of **digoxin** toxicity ▪ Hypokalemia may

enhance the curariform effects of **neuromuscular blocking agents.**

## ROUTE AND DOSAGE

Specific dosage and duration of therapy depend on nature of infection being treated.

❑ **Amphotericin Deoxycholate (Fungizone)**

▪ **IV (Adults):** Give test dose of 1 mg, then initial dose of 0.25 mg/kg; increase daily doses slowly to 0.5–0.7 mg/kg (some infections may require 1.5 mg/kg/day; alternate-day dosing may be used).

▪ **IV (Children):** 0.25 mg/kg infused initially; increase by 0.25 mg/kg every other day to maximum of 1 mg/kg/day.

▪ **Topical (Adults and Children):** Apply 2–4 times daily.

▪ **PO (Adults and Children):** 1 ml 4 times daily.

❑ **Amphotericin B Cholesteryl Sulfate (Amphotec)**

▪ **IV (Adults and Children):** 3–4 mg/kg/day.

❑ **Amphotericin B Lipid Complex (Abelcet)**

▪ **IV (Adults and Children):** 5 mg/kg/day.

❑ **Amphotericin B Liposome (AmBisome)**

▪ **IV (Adults and Children):** *Suspected fungal infections*—3 mg/kg q 24 hr; *documented fungal infections*—3–5 mg/kg q 24 hr; *visceral leishmaniasis (immunocompetent patients)*—3 mg/kg q 24 hr on days 1–5, then 3 mg/kg on days 14 and 21; *visceral leishmaniasis (immunosuppressed patients)*—4 mg/kg q 24 hr on days 1–5, then 4 mg/kg on days 10, 17, 24, 31, and 38; *cryptococcal meningitis in HIV patients*—6 mg/kg/day

## AVAILABILITY

❑ **Amphotericin Deoxycholate**

▪ *Injection:* 50-mg vial[Rx] ▪ *Cream, lotion, ointment:* 3%[Rx] ▪ *Oral suspension:* 100 mg/ml in 24-ml bottles[Rx].

❑ **Amphotericin B Cholesteryl Sulfate**

▪ *Powder for injection:* 50 mg in 20-ml vial[Rx], 100 mg in 50-ml vial[Rx].

□ **Amphotericin B Lipid Complex**

■ *Suspension for injection:* 100 mg/20-ml vial<sup>Rx</sup>.

□ **Amphotericin B Liposome**

■ *Powder for injection:* 50–mg vial<sup>Rx</sup> ■ Cost: $188.40/vial.

TIME/ACTION PROFILE (blood levels)

|    | ONSET | PEAK | DURATION |
|----|-------|------|----------|
| IV | rapid | end of infu-<br>sion | 24 hr |

## NURSING IMPLICATIONS

### ASSESSMENT

□ Monitor patient closely during test dose and the first 1–2 hr of each dose for fever, chills, headache, anorexia, nausea, or vomiting. Premedicating with antipyretics, corticosteroids, antihistamines, meperidine, and antiemetics and maintaining sodium balance may decrease these reactions. Febrile reaction usually subsides within 4 hr after the infusion is completed.

□ Assess injection site frequently for thrombophlebitis or leakage. Drug is very irritating to tissues. Adding heparin to IV solution may decrease the likelihood of thrombophlebitis.

□ Monitor vital signs every 15–30 min during test dose and every 30 min for 2–4 hr after administration. Meperidine and dantrolene have been used to prevent and treat rigors. Assess respiratory status (lung sounds, dyspnea) daily. Notify physician of changes. If respiratory distress occurs, discontinue infusion immediately; anaphylaxis may occur. Equipment for cardiopulmonary resuscitation should be readily available.

□ Monitor intake and output and weigh daily. Adequate hydration (2000–3000 ml/day) may minimize nephrotoxicity.

■ *Lab Test Considerations:* Monitor CBC and platelet counts weekly, BUN and serum creatinine every other day while increasing dose and then twice weekly, and potassium and magnesium levels biweekly. Life-threatening hypokalemia may occur after each dose. If BUN exceeds 40 mg/100 ml or serum creatinine exceeds 3 mg/100 ml, dosage should be decreased or discontinued until renal function improves. May cause decreased hemoglobin, hematocrit, and magnesium levels.

### POTENTIAL NURSING DIAGNOSES

■ Infection, risk for (Indications).

### IMPLEMENTATION

■ **General:** Do not confuse amphotericin B cholesteryl sulfate (Amphotec) with amphotericin deoxycholate (Fungizone), amphotericin B lipid complex (Abelcet), or amphotericin B liposome (AmBisome); they are not interchangeable.

□ This drug should be administered IV only to hospitalized patients or those under close supervision. Diagnosis should be confirmed before administration.

□ **Amphotericin B Deoxycholate**

■ **IV:** Reconstitute 50-mg vial with 10 ml of sterile water for injection without bacteriostatic agent. Concentration equals 5 mg/ml. Shake until clear. Further dilute each 1 mg with at least 10 ml of D5W (pH >4.2) for a concentration of 100 mcg (0.1 mg)/ml. Do not use other diluents. Avoid use of precipitated solution. Use 20-gauge needle; change for each step of dilution. Wear gloves while handling.

□ Store in dark area. Reconstituted solution is stable for 24 hr at room temperature and for 1 wk if refrigerated.

■ **Test Dose:** Administer 1 mg in 20 ml of D5W over 10–30 min to determine patient tolerance. If medication is withheld for 7 days, restart at lowest dose level. In severe, life-threatening infections, test dose may be omitted.

■ **Intermittent Infusion:** Administer preferably through central line. If peripheral site is used, change site with each dose to prevent phlebitis. If an in-line filter is used, the mean pore diameter should be no less than 1 micron. Short-term exposure to light (8 hr) does not alter potency.

■ *Rate:* Administer slowly via infusion pump over 2–6 hr.

■ **Syringe Compatibility:** ◆ heparin.

- **Y-Site Compatibility:** ◆ aldesleukin ◆ diltiazem ◆ tacrolimus ◆ teniposide ◆ thiotepa ◆ zidovudine.
- **Y-Site Incompatibility:** ◆ allopurinol sodium ◆ amifostine ◆ aztreonam ◆ cefepime ◆ docetaxel ◆ doxorubicin liposome ◆ enalaprilat ◆ etoposide ◆ filgrastim ◆ fluconazole ◆ fludarabine ◆ foscarnet ◆ gemcitabine ◆ granisetron ◆ melphalan ◆ meropenem ◆ ondansetron ◆ paclitaxel ◆ piperacillin/tazobactam ◆ propofol ◆ vinorelbine.
- **Additive Compatibility:** ◆ heparin ◆ hydrocortisone ◆ sodium bicarbonate.
- **Additive Incompatibility:** ◆ calcium chloride ◆ calcium gluconate ◆ cimetidine ◆ diphenhydramine ◆ potassium chloride ◆ ranitidine.
- **Solution Incompatibility:** ◆ LR injection ◆ saline solutions.

□ **Amphotericin B Cholesteryl Sulfate**

- **IV:** Reconstitute 50-mg vial with 10 ml and 100-mg vial with 20 ml of sterile water for injection. Concentration equals 5 mg/ml. Shake gently until solids have dissolved. Solution may be opalescent. Further dilute with D5W for a concentration of 0.6 mg/ml. Do not use other diluents. Avoid use of precipitated solution. Use 20-gauge needle; change for each step of dilution. Wear gloves while handling.
- □ Refrigerate after reconstitution and further dilution; use within 24 hr.
- **Test Dose:** Administer 10 ml of the final preparation (containing 1.6–8.3 mg) over 15–30 min to determine patient tolerance. Observe patient closely for next 30 min. If medication is withheld for 7 days, restart at lowest dose level. In severe, life-threatening infections, test dose may be omitted.
- *Rate:* Administer at a rate of 1 mg/kg/hr via infusion pump. If patient tolerates infusion without adverse reactions, infusion time may be shortened to a minimum of 2 hr. If reactions occur or patient cannot tolerate volume, infusion time may be extended. Rapid infusions may cause hypotension, hypokalemia, arrhythmias, and shock.
- **Y-Site Compatibility:** ◆ acyclovir ◆ aminophylline ◆ ceftizoxime ◆ clindamycin ◆ fentanyl ◆ furosemide ◆ ganciclovir ◆ granisetron ◆ hydrocortisone ◆ ifosfamide ◆ lorazepam ◆ mannitol ◆ methotrexate ◆ methylprednisolone ◆ nitroglycerin ◆ trimethoprim/sulfamethoxazole ◆ vinblastine ◆ vincristine ◆ zidovudine.

- **Y-Site Incompatibility:** ◆ alfentanil ◆ amikacin ◆ ampicillin ◆ ampicillin/sulbactam ◆ atenolol ◆ aztreonam ◆ bretylium ◆ buprenorphine ◆ butorphanol ◆ calcium chloride ◆ calcium gluconate ◆ carboplatin ◆ cefazolin ◆ cefepime ◆ cefoperazone ◆ ceftazidime ◆ ceftriaxone ◆ chlorpromazine ◆ cimetidine ◆ cisatracurium ◆ cisplatin ◆ cyclophosphamide ◆ cyclosporine ◆ cytarabine ◆ diazepam ◆ digoxin ◆ diphenhydramine ◆ dobutamine ◆ dopamine ◆ doxorubicin ◆ doxorubicin liposome ◆ droperidol ◆ enalaprilat ◆ esmolol ◆ famotidine ◆ fluconazole ◆ fluorouracil ◆ gatifloxacin ◆ gentamicin ◆ haloperidol ◆ heparin ◆ hydromorphone ◆ imipenem/cilastatin ◆ labetalol ◆ leucovorin ◆ lidocaine ◆ magnesium sulfate ◆ meperidine ◆ mesna ◆ metoclopramide ◆ metoprolol ◆ metronidazole ◆ midazolam ◆ mitoxantrone ◆ morphine ◆ nalbuphine ◆ netilmicin ◆ naloxone ◆ ofloxacin ◆ ondansetron ◆ paclitaxel ◆ pentobarbital ◆ phenobarbital ◆ phenytoin ◆ piperacillin ◆ piperacillin/tazobactam ◆ potassium chloride ◆ prochlorperazine ◆ promethazine ◆ propranolol ◆ ranitidine ◆ remifentanil ◆ sodium bicarbonate ◆ ticarcillin ◆ ticarcillin-clavulanate ◆ tobramycin ◆ vancomycin ◆ vecuronium ◆ verapamil ◆ vinorelbine.
- **Additive Compatibility:** ◆ heparin.
- **Additive Incompatibility:** ◆ electrolytes.
- **Solution Incompatibility:** ◆ saline solutions.

□ **Amphotericin B Lipid Complex**

- **IV:** Prepare immediately before use. Shake vial gently until yellow sediment at bottom has dissolved. Withdraw dose from required number of vials with 18-gauge needle. Replace needle from syringe filled with amphotericin B lipid complex with 5-micron filter needle. Each filter needle may be used to filter the contents of no more than 4 vials. Insert filter needle of syringe into IV bag of D5W and empty contents of syringe into bag for a concentration of 1 mg/ml (2 mg/ml in pediatric patients or patients who cannot tolerate large volumes of fluid). Do not use admixtures containing foreign matter. Vials are for single use only; discard unused material.

- Refrigerate after dilution. May be stored in refrigerator for up to 48 hr and an additional 6 hr at room temperature.
- **Intermittent Infusion:** Do not use an in-line filter.
- **Rate:** Administer at a rate of 2.5 mg/kg/hr via infusion pump. If infusion exceeds 2 hr, mix contents by shaking infusion bag every 2 hr.
- **Y-Site Incompatibility:** Flush IV line with D5W before infusion or use a separate line.
- **Additive Incompatibility:** ♦ electrolytes.
- **Solution Incompatibility:** ♦ saline solutions.
- **Topical:** While wearing gloves, apply topical preparations liberally and rub in well. Shake lotion before applying. Do not use occlusive dressings. Discontinue if lesions worsen or signs of hypersensitivity develop.

## Amphotericin B Liposome

- **Intermittent Infusion:** To reconstitute, add 12 ml of sterile water without bacteriostatic agent to 50-ml vial for a concentration of 4 mg/ml. Immediately shake vial vigorously for at least 30 seconds until all particulate matter is completely dispersed. Withdraw appropriate volume for dilution. Using 5-micron filter, dilute in D5W for a concentration of 1–2 mg/ml. Lower concentrations may be used for infants and small children to provide sufficient volume for infusion. Reconstituted solution is stable for 24 hr if refrigerated. Diluted solution should be used within 6 hr of dilution.
- **Rate:** Administer over 2 hr. May be increased to 1 hr in patients who tolerate infusion well. If discomfort occurs during infusion, duration of infusion may be increased. May be administered through an in-line filter with pore diameter of at least 1 micron.
- **Y-Site Incompatibility:** If administered through an existing line, flush line with D5W before infusion or use separate lines.
- **Solution Incompatibility:** Do not dilute or admix with saline solutions, other medications, or solutions containing a bacteriostatic agent.

## PATIENT/FAMILY TEACHING

- **General Info:** Explain need for long duration of IV or topical therapy.
- **PO:** Instruct patient to swish medication around in mouth as long as possible before swallowing.
- **IV:** Inform patient of potential side effects and discomfort at IV site. Advise patient to notify health care professional if side effects occur.
- **Home Care Issue:** Instruct family or caregiver on dilution, rate, and administration of drug and proper care of IV equipment.
- **Topical:** Advise patient that topical preparations may stain clothing. Cream or lotion may be removed with soap and warm water; ointment may be removed with cleaning fluid.

## EVALUATION

**Effectiveness of therapy can be demonstrated by:** ■ Resolution of signs and symptoms of infection. Several weeks to months of therapy may be required to prevent relapse.

# ampicillin
(am-pi-**sil**-in)
{Ampicin}, {Apo-Ampi}, Marcillin, {Nu-Ampi}, {Novo-Ampicillin}, Omnipen, Penbritin, Principen, Polycillin, Totacillin

## CLASSIFICATION(S):
**Therapeutic:** anti-infectives
**Pharmacologic:** aminopenicillins

## Pregnancy Category B

## INDICATIONS

■ Treatment of the following infections: ❑ Skin and skin structure infections, soft-tissue infections ❑ Otitis media ❑ Sinusitis ❑ Respiratory infections ❑ Genitourinary infections ❑ Meningitis ❑ Septicemia ■ Endocarditis prophylaxis. **Unlabeled uses:** ■ Prevention of infection in certain high-risk patients undergoing cesarean section.

## ACTION

■ Binds to bacterial cell wall, resulting in cell death. **Therapeutic Effects:** ■ Bactericidal action; spectrum is broader than penicillin. **Spectrum:** ■ Active against: ❏ Streptococci ❏ Pneumococci ❏ Enterococci ❏ *Haemophilus influenzae* ❏ *Escherichia coli* ❏ *Proteus mirabilis* ❏ *Neisseria meningitidis* ❏ *N. gonorrhoeae* ❏ *Shigella* ❏ *Salmonella.*

## PHARMACOKINETICS

**Absorption:** Moderately absorbed from the duodenum (30–50%).

**Distribution:** Diffuses readily into body tissues and fluids. CSF penetration is increased in the presence of inflamed meninges. Crosses the placenta; enters breast milk in small amounts.

**Metabolism and Excretion:** Variably metabolized by the liver (12–50%). Renal excretion is variable (25–60% after oral dosing; 50–85% after IM administration).

**Half-life:** 1–1.5 hr (increased in renal impairment).

## CONTRAINDICATIONS AND PRECAUTIONS

**Contraindicated in:** ■ Hypersensitivity to penicillins.

**Use Cautiously in:** ■ Severe renal insufficiency (dosage reduction required if CCr <10 ml/min) ■ Infectious mononucleosis (increased incidence of rash) ■ Has been used during pregnancy and lactation.

## ADVERSE REACTIONS AND SIDE EFFECTS*

■ **CNS:** SEIZURES (high doses) ■ **GI:** PSEUDOMEMBRANOUS COLITIS, diarrhea, nausea, vomiting ■ **Derm:** rashes, urticaria ■ **Hemat:** blood dyscrasias ■ **Misc:** allergic reactions including ANAPHYLAXIS and SERUM SICKNESS, superinfection.

## INTERACTIONS

**Drug-Drug:** ■ **Probenecid** decreases renal excretion and increases blood levels of ampicillin—therapy may be combined for this purpose ■ Large doses may increase the risk of bleeding with **warfarin** ■ Incidence of rash increases with concurrent **allopurinol** therapy ■ May decrease the effectiveness of oral **hormonal contraceptives.**

## ROUTE AND DOSAGE

❏ **Respiratory and Soft-Tissue Infections**
■ **PO (Adults and Children ≥20 kg):** 250 mg q 6 hr.
■ **PO (Children <20 kg):** 50 mg/kg/day in divided doses q 6–8 hr.
■ **IM, IV (Adults and Children ≥40 kg):** 250–500 mg q 6 hr.
■ **IM, IV (Children <40 kg):** 25–50 mg/kg/day in divided doses q 6–8 hr.

❏ **Bacterial Meningitis Caused by *H. influenzae, Staphylococcus pneumoniae,* or *N. meningitidis* or Septicemia**
■ **IM, IV (Adults and Children):** 150–200 mg/kg/day in divided doses q 3–4 hr.

❏ **GI/GU Infections Other Than *N. gonorrhoeae***
■ **PO (Adults and Children >20 kg):** 500 mg q 6 hr (larger doses for more serious/chronic infections).
■ **PO (Children ≤20 kg):** 100 mg/kg/day in divided doses q 6 hr.

❏ **N. gonorrhoeae**
■ **PO (Adults):** 3.0 g with 1 g probenecid.
■ **IM, IV (Adults and Children ≥40 kg):** 500 mg q 6 hr.
■ **IM, IV (Children <40 kg):** 50 mg/kg/day in divided doses q 6–8 hr.

❏ **Urethritis Caused by *N. gonorrhoeae* in Men**
■ **IM, IV (Adults and Children ≥40 kg):** 500 mg, repeated 8–12 hr later; additional doses may be necessary for more complicated infections (prostatitis, epididymitis).

❏ **Prevention of Bacterial Endocarditus**
■ **IM, IV (Adults):** 2 g 30 min before procedure (gentamicin may be added for high-risk patients); additional 1 g may be given 6 hr later for high-risk patients.
■ **IM, IV (Children):** 50 mg/kg 30 min before procedure (gentamicin may be added for high-risk patients); additional 25 mg/kg may be given 6 hr later for high-risk patients.

❏ **Renal Impairment**
■ **(Adults and Children):** CCr ≤10 ml/min— Increase dosing interval to q 12–16 hr.

## AVAILABILITY

■ *Capsules:* 250 mg^Rx, 500 mg^Rx ■ *Suspension (wild cherry flavor):* 125 mg/5 ml^Rx,

250 mg/5 ml^{Rx}, 500 mg/5 ml^{Rx} ■ *Injection:* 125 mg^{Rx}, 250 mg^{Rx}, 1-, 2-, and 10-g vials^{Rx}.

TIME/ACTION PROFILE (blood levels)

| | ONSET | PEAK | DURATION |
|---|---|---|---|
| PO | rapid | 1.5–2 hr | 4–6 hr |
| IM | rapid | 1 hr | 4–6 hr |
| IV | rapid | end of infusion | 4–6 hr |

## NURSING IMPLICATIONS

### ASSESSMENT

❑ Assess patient for infection (vital signs, wound appearance, sputum, urine, stool, and WBC) at beginning of and throughout therapy.

❑ Obtain a history before initiating therapy to determine previous use and reactions to penicillins or cephalosporins. Persons with a negative history of penicillin sensitivity may still have an allergic response.

❑ Obtain specimens for culture and sensitivity before therapy. First dose may be given before receiving results.

❑ Observe patient for signs and symptoms of anaphylaxis (rash, pruritus, laryngeal edema, wheezing). Discontinue the drug and notify the physician or other health care professional immediately if these occur. Keep epinephrine, an antihistamine, and resuscitation equipment close by in the event of an anaphylactic reaction.

❑ Assess skin for "ampicillin rash," a nonallergic, dull red, macular or maculopapular, mildly pruritic rash.

■ *Lab Test Considerations:* May cause increased AST and ALT.

❑ May cause transient decreases in estradiol, total conjugated estriol, estriol-glucuronide, or conjugated estrone in pregnant women.

❑ May cause a false-positive direct Coombs' test result.

### POTENTIAL NURSING DIAGNOSES

■ Infection, risk for (Indications, Side Effects).

■ Noncompliance (Patient/Family Teaching).

## IMPLEMENTATION

■ **General:** Do not confuse with omnipen with imipenem.

❑ Reserve IM or IV route for moderately severe or severe infections or patients unable to take oral medication. Change to PO as soon as possible.

■ **PO:** Administer around the clock on an empty stomach at least 1 hr before or 2 hr after meals with a full glass of water. Capsules may be opened and mixed with water. Reconstituted oral suspensions retain potency for 7 days at room temperature and 14 days if refrigerated. Combination with probenecid should be used immediately after reconstitution.

■ **IM:** Reconstitute for IM or IV use by adding sterile water for injection 0.9–1.2 ml to the 125-mg vial, 0.9–1.9 ml to the 250-mg vial, 1.2–1.8 ml to the 500-mg vial, 2.4–7.4 ml to the 1-g vial, and 6.8 ml to the 2-g vial.

■ **Direct IV:** Add 5 ml of sterile or bacteriostatic water for injection to each 125-, 250-, or 500-mg vial or at least 7.4–10 ml of diluent to each 1- or 2-g vial.

■ *Rate:* Doses of 125–500 mg may be given over 3–5 min within 1 hr of reconstitution. Rapid administration may cause seizures.

■ **Intermittent Infusion:** Dilute in 50 ml or more of 0.9% NaCl, D5W, D5/0.45% NaCl, or LR solution for a concentration of no more than 30 mg/ml; administer within 4 hr (more stable in NaCl).

■ *Rate:* Administer doses over 10–15 min.

■ **Syringe Compatibility:** ♦ chloramphenicol ♦ heparin ♦ procaine.

■ **Syringe Incompatibility:** ♦ erythromycin lactobionate ♦ gentamicin ♦ kanamycin ♦ metoclopramide.

■ **Y-Site Compatibility:** ♦ acyclovir ♦ amifostine ♦ aztreonam ♦ clarithromycin ♦ cyclophosphamide ♦ docetaxel ♦ doxorubicin hydrochloride liposome ♦ enalaprilat ♦ esmolol ♦ etoposide ♦ famotidine ♦ filgrastim ♦ fludarabine ♦ foscarnet ♦ gatifloxacin ♦ gemcitabine ♦ granisetron ♦ heparin ♦ insulin, regular ♦ labetalol ♦ levofloxacin ♦ linezolid ♦ magnesium sulfate ♦ melphalan ♦ meperidine ♦ morphine ♦ multivitamins ♦ ofloxacin ♦ perphenazine ♦ phytonadione ♦ potassium chlo-

---

ride ◆ propofol ◆ remifentanil ◆ tacrolimus ◆ teniposide ◆ theophylline ◆ thiotepa ◆ tolazoline ◆ vitamin B complex with C.

■ **Y-Site Incompatibility:** ◆ amphotericin B cholesteryl sulfate ◆ epinephrine ◆ fluconazole ◆ hydralazine ◆ midazolam ◆ ondansetron ◆ sargramostim ◆ verapamil ◆ vinorelbine. If aminoglycosides and penicillins must be administered concurrently, administer in separate sites at least 1 hr apart.

■ **Additive Incompatibility:** ◆ amikacin ◆ gentamicin ◆ kanamycin ◆ tobramycin.

### PATIENT/FAMILY TEACHING

❑ Instruct patient to take medication around the clock and to finish the drug completely as directed, even if feeling better. Advise patients that sharing of this medication can be dangerous.

❑ Advise patient to report the signs of superinfection (furry overgrowth on the tongue, vaginal itching or discharge, loose or foul-smelling stools) and allergy.

❑ Advise patients taking oral contraceptives to use an alternate or additional nonhormonal method of contraception while taking ampicillin and until next menstrual period.

❑ Caution patient to notify health care professional if fever and diarrhea occur, especially if stool contains blood, pus, or mucus. Advise patient not to treat diarrhea without consulting health care professional. May occur up to several weeks after discontinuation of medication.

❑ Instruct the patient to notify health care professional if symptoms do not improve.

❑ Patients with a history of rheumatic heart disease or valve replacement need to be taught the importance of using antimicrobial prophylaxis before invasive medical or dental procedures.

### EVALUATION

**Clinical response to therapy can be evaluated by:** ■ Resolution of the signs and symptoms of infection. Length of time for complete resolution depends on the organism and site of infection ■ Endocarditis prophylaxis.

---

## ampicillin/sulbactam

(am-pi-**sil**-in/sul-**bak**-tam)
Unasyn

---

**CLASSIFICATION(S):**
**Therapeutic:** *anti-infectives*
**Pharmacologic:** *aminopenicillins/ beta lactamase inhibitors*

### Pregnancy Category B

### INDICATIONS

■ Treatment of the following infections: ❑ Skin and skin structure infections, soft-tissue infections ❑ Otitis media ❑ Sinusitis ❑ Respiratory infections ❑ Genitourinary infections ❑ Meningitis ❑ Septicemia.

### ACTION

■ Binds to bacterial cell wall, resulting in cell death; spectrum is broader than that of penicillin. Addition of sulbactam increases resistance to beta-lactamases, enzymes produced by bacteria that may inactivate ampicillin. **Therapeutic Effects:** ■ Bactericidal action. **Spectrum:** ■ Active against: ❑ Streptococci ❑ Pneumococci ❑ Enterococci ❑ *Haemophilus influenzae* ❑ *Escherichia coli* ❑ *Proteus mirabilis* ❑ *Neisseria meningitidis* ❑ *N. gonorrhoeae* ❑ *Shigella* ❑ *Salmonella* ❑ *Bacteroides fragilis* ❑ *Moraxella catarrhalis* ■ Use should be reserved for infections caused by beta-lactamase–producing strains.

### PHARMACOKINETICS

**Absorption:** Well absorbed from IM sites.
**Distribution:** Ampicillin diffuses readily into body tissues and fluids. CSF penetration is increased when meninges are inflamed. Crosses the placenta; enters breast milk in small amounts.
**Metabolism and Excretion:** Ampicillin is variably metabolized by the liver (12–50%). Renal excretion is also variable. Sulbactam is eliminated unchanged in urine.
**Half-life:** *Ampicillin*—1–1.5 hr; *sulbactam*—1–1.4 hr.

### CONTRAINDICATIONS AND PRECAUTIONS

**Contraindicated in:** ■ Hypersensitivity to penicillins or sulbactam.

**Use Cautiously in:** ■ Severe renal insufficiency (dosage reduction required if CCr <30 ml/min) ■ Infectious mononucleosis (increased incidence of rash) ■ Has been used during pregnancy and lactation (ampicillin).

## ADVERSE REACTIONS AND SIDE EFFECTS*

■ **CNS:** SEIZURES (high doses) ■ **GI:** PSEUDOMEM-BRANOUS COLITIS, diarrhea, nausea, vomiting ■ **Derm:** rashes, urticaria ■ **Hemat:** blood dyscrasias ■ **Local:** pain at IM site, pain at IV site ■ **Misc:** allergic reactions including ANAPHYLAXIS and SERUM SICKNESS, superinfection.

## INTERACTIONS

**Drug-Drug:** ■ **Probenecid** decreases renal excretion and increases blood levels of ampicillin—therapy may be combined for this purpose ■ May potentiate the effect of **warfarin** ■ Concurrent **allopurinol** therapy (increased incidence of rash) ■ May decrease the effectiveness of **hormonal contraceptives**.

## ROUTE AND DOSAGE

■ **IM, IV (Adults and Children ≥40 kg):** 1.5–3 g (1 g ampicillin plus 0.5 g sulbactam–2 g ampicillin plus 1 g sulbactam) q 6 hr (not to exceed 4 g sulbactam/day).

■ **IV (Children ≥1 yr):** 75 mg (50 mg ampicillin/25 mg sulbactam)/kg q 6 hr.

❑ **Renal Impairment**

■ **IM, IV (Adults ≥40 kg):** *CCr 15–29 ml/ min*—1.5–3 g (1 g ampicillin plus 0.5 g sulbactam–2 g ampicillin plus 1 g sulbactam) q 12 hr; *CCr 5–14*—1.5–3 g (1 g ampicillin plus 0.5 g sulbactam–2 g ampicillin plus 1 g sulbactam) q 24 hr.

## AVAILABILITY

■ *Injection:* 1 g ampicillin with 500 mg sulbactam$^{Rx}$, 2 g ampicillin with 1 g sulbactam$^{Rx}$.

TIME/ACTION PROFILE (blood levels)

| | ONSET | PEAK | DURATION |
|---|---|---|---|
| IM | rapid | 1 hr | 6–8 hr |
| IV | immediate | end of infusion | 6–8 hr |

## NURSING IMPLICATIONS

### ASSESSMENT

❑ Assess patient for infection (vital signs, wound appearance, sputum, urine, stool, and WBCs) at beginning and throughout therapy.

❑ Obtain a history before initiating therapy to determine previous use of and reactions to penicillins or cephalosporins. Persons with a negative history of penicillin sensitivity may still have an allergic response.

❑ Obtain specimens for culture and sensitivity before therapy. First dose may be given before receiving results.

❑ Observe patient for signs and symptoms of anaphylaxis (rash, pruritus, laryngeal edema, wheezing). Discontinue the drug and notify the physician or other health care professional immediately if these occur. Keep epinephrine, an antihistamine, and resuscitation equipment close by in the event of an anaphylactic reaction.

■ *Lab Test Considerations:* May cause increased AST, ALT, LDH, bilirubin, alkaline phosphatase, BUN, and creatinine.

❑ May cause decreased hemoglobin, hematocrit, RBC, WBC, neutrophils, and lymphocytes.

❑ May cause transient decreases in estradiol, total conjugated estriol, estriol-glucuronide, or conjugated estrone in pregnant women.

❑ May cause a false-positive Coombs' test result.

## POTENTIAL NURSING DIAGNOSES

■ Infection, risk for (Indications, Side Effects).

## IMPLEMENTATION

■ **IM:** Reconstitute for IM use by adding 3.2 ml of sterile water or 0.5% or 2% lidocaine HCl to the 1.5-g vial or 6.4 ml to the 3-g vial. Administer within 1 hr of preparation, deep IM into well-developed muscle.

■ **IV:** For IV use, add 3.2 ml of sterile water for injection to each 1.5-g vial and 6.4 ml to each 3-g vial for a concentration of 250 mg ampicillin/ml and 125 mg sulbactam/ml. Foaming should dissipate upon standing. Administer only clear solutions.

■ **Direct IV:** May be administered over 10–15 min (1–2 g) within 1 hr of reconstitution. More rapid administration may cause seizures.

■ **Intermittent Infusion:** Dilute immediately for infusion in 50–100 ml or more of 0.9% NaCl, D5W, D5/0.45% NaCl, or LR solution.

{ } = Available in Canada only.
*CAPITALS indicates life-threatening; underlines indicate most frequent.

Stability of solution varies from 2–8 hr at room temperature or 3–72 hr if refrigerated, depending on concentration and diluent.

■ *Rate:* Administer over 15–30 min.

■ **Y-Site Compatibility:** ◆ amifostine ◆ aztreonam ◆ cefepime ◆ docetaxel ◆ enalaprilat ◆ etoposide ◆ famotidine ◆ filgrastim ◆ fluconazole ◆ fludarabine ◆ gatifloxacin ◆ gemcitabine ◆ granisetron ◆ heparin ◆ insulin ◆ linezolid ◆ meperidine ◆ morphine ◆ paclitaxel ◆ remifentanil ◆ tacrolimus ◆ teniposide ◆ theophylline ◆ thiotepa.

■ **Y-Site Incompatibility:** ◆ amphotericin B cholesteryl sulfate complex ◆ ciprofloxacin ◆ idarubicin ◆ ondansetron ◆ sargramostim. If aminoglycosides and penicillins must be given concurrently, administer in separate sites at least 1 hr apart.

■ **Additive Compatibility:** aztreonam.

## PATIENT/FAMILY TEACHING

❏ Advise patient to report signs of superinfection (furry overgrowth on the tongue, vaginal itching or discharge, loose or foul-smelling stools) and allergy.

❏ Advise patients taking oral contraceptives to use an alternative or additional nonhormonal method of contraception while taking ampicillin/sulbactam and until next menstrual period.

❏ Caution patient to notify health care professional if fever and diarrhea occur, especially if stool contains blood, pus, or mucus. Advise patient not to treat diarrhea without consulting health care professional. May occur up to several weeks after discontinuation of medication.

❏ Instruct the patient to notify health care professional if symptoms do not improve.

## EVALUATION

**Clinical response to therapy can be evaluated by:** ■ Resolution of signs and symptoms of infection. Length of time for complete resolution depends on the organism and site of infection.

---

# amprenavir

(am-**pren**-a-veer)

Agenerase

---

**CLASSIFICATION(S):**
**Therapeutic:** *antiretrovirals*
**Pharmacologic:** *protease inhibitors*

## Pregnancy Category C

## INDICATIONS

■ Management of HIV infection in combination with other antiretrovirals.

## ACTION

■ Inhibits the action of HIV protease and prevents the cleavage of viral polyproteins. **Therapeutic Effects:** ■ Increased CD4 cell counts and decreased viral load with subsequent slowed progression of HIV and its sequelae.

## PHARMACOKINETICS

**Absorption:** Rapidly absorbed after oral administration; absorption from liquid formulation is 14%; less than from capsules.

**Distribution:** 90%; bound to plasma proteins.

**Metabolism and Excretion:** Mostly metabolized by the liver; <3% excreted unchanged by the kidneys.

**Half-life:** 7.1–10.6 hr.

## CONTRAINDICATIONS AND PRECAUTIONS

**Contraindicated in:** ■ Hypersensitivity ■ Concurrent use of bepredil, dihydroergotamine, ergotamine, midazolam, and triazolam (may cause serious, potentially fatal toxicity) ■ Concurrent use of rifampinor supplemental vitamin E ■ If amprenavir is used concurrently with ritonavir, flecainide and propafenone are contraindicated ■ Oral solution contains significant amounts of propylene glycol and is contraindicated in pregnancy, children <4 yrs, hepatic/renal impairment, concurrent disulfiram or metronidazole.

**Use Cautiously in:** ■ Hypersensitivity to sulfonamides ■ Hepatic impairment (dosage reduction required) ■ Hemophilia (may increase bleeding) ■ Diabetes mellitus (may worsen hyperglycemia) ■ Pregnancy or lactation (safety not established; breastfeeding not recommended in HIV-infected patients).

**Exercise Extreme Caution in:** ■ Concurrent use of amiodarone, parenteral lidocaine, tricyclic antidepressants, or quinidine (may produce potentially life-threatening drug interactions).

## ADVERSE REACTIONS AND SIDE EFFECTS*

■ **CNS:** depression/mood disorder ■ **GI:** diarrhea, nausea, taste disorders, vomiting ■ **Derm:** rash ■ **Endo:** hyperglycemia ■ **Metab:** hyperlipidemia, redistribution/accumulation of body fat.

## INTERACTIONS

**Drug-Drug:** ■ Increases blood levels and the risk of toxicity from **midazolam, triazolam,** ergot derivatives and pimozide; concurrent use is contraindicated; may also increase blood levels and effects of other benzodiazepines ■ Increases blood levels and the risk of toxicity from **amiodarone, lidocaine (parenteral), quinidine, tricyclic antidepressants,** and **warfarin**; careful monitoring is required ■ If ritonavir is used concurrently, additional use of **flecainide or propafenone** is contraindicated (increased risk of arrhythmias) ■ Significantly increases blood levels of **rifabutin**; decrease dose by 50% if used concurrently ■ May increase blood levels and toxicity of **HMG CoA reductase inhibitors, erythromycin, dapsone, itraconazole, ketoconazole alprazolam, diazepam, flurazepam, calcium channel blockers, clozapine, carbamazepime, cyclosporine** and **tacrolimus** and **loratadine** ■ Concurrent use with **sildenafil** increases the risk of priapism, hypotension, and visual changes ■ **Rifampin** significantly decreases blood levels and efficacy of amprenavir; concurrent use is contraindicated ■ **Phenobarbital, phenytoin, carbamazepine, dexamethasone efavirenz, delavirdine nevirapine** and **hormonal contraceptives** decrease amprenavir levels and may decrease antiretroviral activity ■ **Cimetidine, indinavir, lopinavir, ritonavir,** and **nelfinavir** may increase amprenavir levels (when used conconcurrently with **ritonavir**, amprenavir dosage should be decreased) ■ **Saquinavir** may decrease levels ■ **Antacids** and **didanosine** (due to buffer content) may decrease absorption (separate administration by 1 hr) ■ **Methadone** decreasese amprenavir levels and amprenavir decreases **methadone** levels; dosage adjustments may be necessary.

**Drug-Natural Products:** ■ Use with **St. John's wort** may cause decreased drug levels and effectiveness.

**Drug-Food:** ■ Ingestion of a **high-fat meal** may decrease absorption.

## ROUTE AND DOSAGE

■ **PO (Adults >13 yr >50 kg):** 1200 mg (eight 150-mg capsules) twice daily with other antiretrovirals.

■ **PO (Children 4–13 yr or Adolescents 13–16 yr ≤50 kg):** *Capsules*—20 mg/kg twice daily or 15 mg/kg 3 times daily with other antiretrovirals (not to exceed 2400 mg/day). *Oral solution*—22.5 mg/kg (1.5 ml/kg) twice daily or 17 mg/kg (1.1 ml/kg) three times daily (not to exceed 2800 mg/day).

❑ **Hepatic Impairment**
■ **PO (Adults):** *Child-Pugh score 5–8*—450 mg twice daily with other antiretrovirals; *Child-Pugh score 9–12*—300 mg twice daily with other antiretrovirals.

## AVAILABILITY

Both capsules and oral solution contain amounts of vitamin E that exceed the Reference Daily Intake (RDI).

■ *Capsules:* 50 mg^Rx, 150 mg^Rx ■ *Oral solution (grape–bubblegum–peppermint flavor):* 15 mg/ml^Rx.

TIME/ACTION PROFILE (blood levels)

| | ONSET | PEAK | DURATION |
|---|---|---|---|
| PO | rapid | 1–2 hr | 8–12 hr |

## NURSING IMPLICATIONS

### ASSESSMENT

❑ Assess patient for change in severity of HIV symptoms and for symptoms of opportunistic infections throughout therapy.
❑ Assess patient for allergy to sulfonamides. May exhibit cross-sensitivity.
❑ Assess patient for skin reactions throughout therapy. Reactions may be severe and life threatening. Discontinue therapy if severe reactions or moderate rashes with systemic symptoms occur.

■ *Lab Test Considerations:* Monitor viral load and CD4 cell count regularly during therapy. May cause increased serum glucose, cholesterol, and triglyceride levels.

## POTENTIAL NURSING DIAGNOSES

■ Infection, risk for (Indications).
■ Noncompliance (Patient/Family Teaching).

## IMPLEMENTATION

■ **General:** Administer antacids or didanosine at least 1 hr before or after amprenavir.
■ **PO:** May be administered with or without food. Avoid high-fat meals, which may decrease absorption. Capsules and oral solution may be stored at room temperature; do not refrigerate or freeze.
❑ Oral solution and capsules are not interchangeable on a mg-per-mg basis.

## PATIENT/FAMILY TEACHING

❑ Emphasize the importance of taking amprenavir exactly as directed. It must always be used in combination with other antiretroviral drugs. Do not take more than prescribed amount and do not stop taking without consulting health care professional. If a dose is missed, take as soon as remembered within 4 hr, then return to regular schedule. If more than 4 hr from scheduled dose, omit dose and take next scheduled dose; do not double doses.
❑ Instruct patient that amprenavir should not be shared with others.
❑ Inform patient that amprenavir does not cure AIDS or prevent associated or opportunistic infections. Amprenavir does not reduce the risk of transmission of HIV to others through sexual contact or blood contamination. Caution patient to use a condom and to avoid sharing needles or donating blood to prevent spreading the AIDS virus to others. Advise patient that the long-term effects of amprenavir are unknown at this time.
❑ Emphasize the importance of providing health care professional with accurate current drug history and notifying health care professional before taking any prescription or OTC medications because of potentially serious drug interactions. Vitamin E supplements should be avoided during amprenavir therapy.
❑ Some hormonal contraceptives decrease amprenavir levels and effectiveness; advise pa-

tient to use a nonhormonal form of contraception during therapy.
❑ Instruct patient to notify health care professional if nausea, vomiting, diarrhea, or rash occurs.
❑ Emphasize the importance of regular follow-up exams and blood counts to determine progress and monitor for side effects.

## EVALUATION

**Effectiveness of therapy can be demonstrated by:** ■ Delayed progression of AIDS and decreased opportunistic infections in patients with HIV ■ Decrease in viral load and increase in CD4 cell counts.

## anakinra

(a-na-**kin**-ra)
Kineret

### CLASSIFICATION(S):

*Therapeutic:* antirheumatics *(DMARD)*
*Pharmacologic:* interleukin antagonists

**Pregnancy Category B**

## INDICATIONS

■ Reduction of the signs and symptoms of moderately to severely active rheumatoid arthritis in patients who have failed other DMARDs (may be used in combination with other DMARDs other than tumor necrosis factor [TNF] blocking agents).

## ACTION

■ Blocks the destructive effects of interleukin-1 on cartilage and bone resorption by inhibiting its binding at specific tissue receptor sites. **Therapeutic Effects:** ■ Slowed progression of rheumatoid arthritis.

## PHARMACOKINETICS

**Absorption:** Well absorbed (95%) following subcut administration.

**Distribution:** Unknown.

**Metabolism and Excretion:** Unknown.

**Half-life:** 4–6 hr.

## CONTRAINDICATIONS AND PRECAUTIONS

**Contraindicated in:** ■ Hypersensitivity ■ Hypersensitivity to other *Escherichia coli*–derived products ■ Active infections.

**Use Cautiously in:** ■ Other chronic debilitating illness ■ Underlying immunosuppression ■ Renal impairment ■ Geriatric patients ■ Pregnancy, lactation, or children <18 yr(safety not established).

**Exercise Extreme Caution in:** ■ Concurrent use of TNF blocking agents such as etanercept (higher risk of serious infections).

## ADVERSE REACTIONS AND SIDE EFFECTS*

■ **CNS:** headache ■ **GI:** diarrhea, nausea ■ **Hemat:** neutropenia ■ **Local:** injection site reactions ■ **Misc:** INFECTIONS, hypersensitivity reactions (rare).

## INTERACTIONS

**Drug-Drug:** ■ ↑ risk of serious infection with **TNF blocking agents,** such as **etanercept** ■ May ↓ antibody response to and increase the risk of adverse reactions from **vaccines**; avoid concurrent administration of **live vaccines.**

## ROUTE AND DOSAGE

■ **Subcut (Adults ≥18 yr):** 100 mg/day.

## AVAILABILITY

■ *Solution for injection:* 100 mg/ml in 1-ml prefilled glass syringes^Rx.

TIME/ACTION PROFILE (clinical response)

|        | ONSET         | PEAK    | DURATION |
|--------|---------------|---------|----------|
| Subcut | within 12 wk  | unknown | unknown  |

# NURSING IMPLICATIONS

## ASSESSMENT

❏ Assess patient's range of motion and degree of swelling and pain in affected joints before and periodically during therapy.

❏ Assess for signs and symptoms of infection (fever, elevated WBC) prior to and periodically during therapy. Anakinra should not be instituted in patients with active infections

and should be discontinued if patient develops a serious infection.

❏ Observe patient for hypersensitivity reactions (urticaria, dyspnea, hypotension). Discontinue anakinra if severe reaction occurs. Medications (antihistamines, acetaminophen, corticosteroids, epinephrine) and equipment should be readily available in the event of a severe reaction.

■ *Lab Test Considerations:* Monitor neutrophil count prior to and during therapy, then monthly for 3 mo and quarterly thereafter for up to 1 yr.

## POTENTIAL NURSING DIAGNOSES

■ Mobility, impaired physical (Indications).

■ Pain, acute (Indications).

## IMPLEMENTATION

■ **General:** Administration of higher than recommended doses did not result in higher responses.

■ **Subcut:** Administer 1 dose/day. Do not administer solutions that are discolored or contain particulate matter. Provided in single–use 1–ml prefilled glass syringes.

## PATIENT/FAMILY TEACHING

❏ Inform patient of the signs and symptoms of hypersensitivity reactions and other adverse reactions. Advise patient of appropriate actions if reactions occur.

❏ Advise patients not to receive live vaccines during therapy with anakinra without consulting health care professional.

■ **Home Care Issues:** Instruct patient and family on preparation and correct technique for administration of injection and care and disposal of equipment. Caution patients and caregivers not to reuse needles, syringes, or drug product.

## EVALUATION

**Effectiveness of therapy can be demonstrated by:** ■ Reduction of signs and symptoms and slowed progression of moderate to severe active rheumatoid arthritis.

{ } = Available in Canada only.
*CAPITALS indicates life-threatening; underlines indicate most frequent.

## anastrazole

(a-**nass**-stra-zole)

Arimidex

**CLASSIFICATION(S):**
**Therapeutic:** antineoplastics
**Pharmacologic:** aromatase inhibitors

**Pregnancy Category D**

## INDICATIONS

■ Treatment of postmenopausal patients with hormone receptor-positive or unknown, locally advanced, or metastatic breast cancer ■ Treatment of advanced breast cancer in postmenopausal patients with disease progression despite tamoxifen therapy.

## ACTION

■ Inhibits the enzyme aromatase, which is partially responsible for conversion of precursors to estrogen. **Therapeutic Effects:** ■ Lowers levels of circulating estrogen, which may halt progression of estrogen-sensitive breast cancer.

## PHARMACOKINETICS

**Absorption:** 83–85% absorbed following oral administration.

**Distribution:** Unknown.

**Metabolism and Excretion:** 85% metabolized by the liver; 11% excreted renally.

**Half-life:** 50 hr.

## CONTRAINDICATIONS AND PRECAUTIONS

**Contraindicated in:** ■ Pregnancy.

**Use Cautiously in:** ■ Women with childbearing potential ■ Lactation or children (safety not established).

## ADVERSE REACTIONS AND SIDE EFFECTS*

■ **CNS:** headache, weakness, dizziness ■ **EENT:** pharyngitis ■ **Resp:** dyspnea, increased cough ■ **CV:** peripheral edema ■ **GI:** nausea, abdominal pain, anorexia, constipation, diarrhea, dry mouth, vomiting ■ **GU:** pelvic pain, vaginal bleeding, vaginal dryness ■ **Derm:** rash, sweating ■ **Metab:** weight gain ■ **MS:** back pain, bone pain ■ **Neuro:** paresthesia ■ **Misc:** hot flashes, pain.

## INTERACTIONS

**Drug-Drug:** ■ None significant.

## ROUTE AND DOSAGE

■ **PO (Adults):** 1 mg daily.

## AVAILABILITY

■ **Tablets:** 1 mg[Rx].

TIME/ACTION PROFILE (lowering of serum estradiol)

| | ONSET | PEAK | DURATION |
|---|---|---|---|
| PO | within 24 hr | 14 days | 6 days† |

†Following cessation of therapy.

# NURSING IMPLICATIONS

## ASSESSMENT

❑ Assess patient for pain and other side effects periodically throughout therapy.

■ **Lab Test Considerations:** May cause ↑ GTT, AST, ALT, alkaline phosphatase, total cholesterol, and LDL cholesterol levels.

## POTENTIAL NURSING DIAGNOSES

■ Pain, acute (Side Effects).

## IMPLEMENTATION

■ **General:** Take medication consistently with regard to food.

## PATIENT/FAMILY TEACHING

❑ Instruct patient to take medication as directed.

❑ Inform patient of potential for adverse reactions and advise her to notify health care professional if side effects are problematic.

❑ Advise patient that vaginal bleeding may occur during first few weeks after changing over from other hormonal therapy. Continued bleeding should be evaluated.

❑ Teach patient to report increase in pain so treatment can be initiated.

## EVALUATION

**Effectiveness of therapy can be demonstrated by:** ■ Slowing of disease progression in women with advanced breast cancer.

# ANGIOTENSIN II RECEPTOR ANTAGONISTS

**candesartan**
(can-de-**sar**-tan)
Atacand

**eprosartan**
(ep-roe-**sar**-tan)
Teveten

**irbesartan**
(ir-be-**sar**-tan)
Avapro

**losartan**
(loe-**sar**-tan)
Cozaar

**olmesartan**
(ole-me-**sar**-tan)
Benicar

**telmisartan**
(tel-mi-**sar**-tan)
Micardis

**valsartan**
(val-**sar**-tan)
Diovan

*CLASSIFICATION(S):*
*Therapeutic: antihypertensives*
*Pharmacologic: angiotensin II receptor antagonists*

**Pregnancy Category C (first trimester), D (second and third trimesters)**

## INDICATIONS

■ Management of hypertension ■ Treatment of type 2 diabetic nephropathy in patients with type 2 diabetes and hypertension (irbesartan and losartan only) ■ Management of CHF in patients who cannot tolerate ACE inhibitors (valsartan only) ■ Reduced risk of stroke in patients with CHF and left ventricular hypertrophy (losartan only).

## ACTION

■ Blocks vasoconstrictor and aldosterone-producing effects of angiotensin II at receptor sites, including vascular smooth muscle and the adrenal glands. **Therapeutic Effects:** ■ Lowering of blood pressure ■ Slowed progression of diabetic nephropathy (irbesartan, losartan) ■ Decreased hospitalizations in patients with CHF ■ Decreased risk of stroke.

## PHARMACOKINETICS

**Absorption:** *Candesartan*—Candesartan cilexetil is converted to candesartan in the GI tract where 15% is absorbed; *eprosartan*—13% absorbed; *irbesartan*—60–80% absorbed; *losartan*—well absorbed; with extensive first-pass hepatic metabolism, resulting in 33% bioavailability; *olmesartan*—26% absorbed; *telmisartan*—42–58% absorbed following oral administration (bioavailability ↑ hepatic impairment); *valsartan*—25% absorbed following oral administration.

**Distribution:** Unknown; *candesartan*—minimal penetration of the blood-brain barrier.

**Protein Binding:** *eprosartan*—98%; *olmesartan*—99%.

**Metabolism and Excretion:** *Candesartan*—Excreted mostly unchanged in urine and feces (via bile); minor metabolism by the liver; *eprosartan*—90% eliminated unchanged in feces via biliary elimination, 7% excreted in urine; *irbesartan*—some hepatic metabolism, some biliary excretion, some elimination as unchanged drug in urine; *losartan*—extensive first-pass hepatic metabolism; 14% is converted to an active metabolite. 4% of losartan is excreted unchanged by the kidneys; 6% of active metabolite is excreted unchanged by the kidneys, some biliary elimination; *olmesartan*—30–50% excreted unchanged in urine, remainder eliminated in feces via bile; *telmisartan*—excreted mostly unchanged in feces via biliary excretion, 11% metabolized by the liver; *valsartan*—20% metabolized by the liver; mostly excreted in feces via bile.

**Half-life:** *Candesartan*—9 hr; eprosartan—5–9 hr; *irbesartan*—11–15 hr; *losartan*—2 hr (6–9 hr for metabolite); *olmesartan*—13 hr; *telmisartan*—24 hr; *valsartan*—6 hr.

## CONTRAINDICATIONS AND PRECAUTIONS

**Contraindicated in:** ■ Hypersensitivity ■ Pregnancy or lactation.

**Use Cautiously in:** ■ CHF (may result in azotemia, oliguria, acute renal failure and/or death) ■ Volume- or salt-depleted patients or patients receiving high doses of diuretics (correct deficits before initiating therapy or initiate at lower doses) ■ Black patients (monotherapy may not be effective) ■ Impaired renal function due to primary renal disease or CHF (may worsen renal function) ■ Obstructive biliary disorders or hepatic impairment (lower initial doses of losartan, temisartan, or valsartan recommended) ■ Patients with childbearing potential ■ Children <18 yr (safety not established).

## ADVERSE REACTIONS AND SIDE EFFECTS*

■ **CNS:** dizziness, fatigue, headache ■ **CV:** hypotension ■ **GI:** diarrhea, drug-induced hepatitis ■ **GU:** RENAL FAILURE ■ **F and E:** hyperkalemia.

## INTERACTIONS

**Drug-Drug:** ■ **NSAIDs** may ↓ antihypertensive effects ■ ↑ antihypertensive effects with other **antihypertensives** and **diuretics**. Risk of hypotension ↑ by concurrent **diuretics** (use lower initial doses) and **nitrates** ■ Telmisartan ↑ serum **digoxin** levels ■ Concurrent use of **potassium-sparing diuretics** or **potassium supplements** may ↑ risk of hyperkalemia ■ Candesartan may ↑ serum **lithium** levels; monitoring is required.

## ROUTE AND DOSAGE

### ❏ Candesartan

■ **PO (Adults):** *As monotherapy*—16 mg once daily. *Patients receiving diuretics or who are volume depleted*—initiate therapy at a lower dose (range 2–32 mg/day as a single dose or divided into two daily doses).

### ❏ Renal Impairment

■ **PO (Adults):** Initiate therapy at a lower dose.

### ❏ Eprosartan

■ **PO (Adults):** 600 mg once daily, may also be given in divided doses twice daily (usual range 400–800 mg/day)

### ❏ Irbesartan

■ **PO (Adults):** *Hypertension*—150 mg once daily; may be increased to 300 mg once daily. *Patients receiving diuretics, who are volume depleted, or who are being hemodialyzed*—initiate with 75 mg/day. *Type 2 diabetic nephropathy*—300 mg once daily.

### ❏ Losartan

■ **PO (Adults):** *Hypertension*—50 mg/day initially (range 25–100 mg/day as a single daily dose or 2 divided doses). *Patients receiving diuretics or who are volume depleted*—25 mg/day initially; may be increased as tolerated. *Type 2 diabetic nephropathy*—50 mg once daily, may increase to 100 mg/daily depending on blood pressure response.

### ❏ Hepatic Impairment

■ **PO (Adults):** 25 mg/day initially; may be increased as tolerated.

### ❏ Olmesartan

■ **PO (Adults):** 20 mg/day (patients who are volume-depleted should be started on lower doses).

### ❏ Valsartan

■ **PO (Adults):** *Hypertension* 80 mg/day as a single dose initially in patients who are not receiving diuretics or other antihypertensives; may be increased to 160–320 mg/day; *CHF*—40 mg twice daily initially, may be titrated to 160 mg twice daily; concurrent ACE inhibitor and beta-blocker therapy not recommended; consider reduction of diuretics.

## AVAILABILITY

### ❏ Candesartan

■ *Tablets:* 4 mg^Rx, 8 mg^Rx, 16 mg^Rx, 32 mg^Rx ■ Cost: 4 mg $40.26/30, 8 mg $40.26/30, 16 mg $40.26/30, 32 mg $54.46/30 ■ hydrochlorothiazide (Atacand HCT; see Appendix B).

### ❏ Eprosartan

■ *Tablets:* 400 mg^Rx, 600 mg^Rx.

### ❏ Irbesartan

■ *Tablets:* 75 mg^Rx, 150 mg^Rx, 300 mg^Rx ■ Cost: 75 mg $41.05/30, 150 mg $43.21/30, 300 mg $51.95/30 ■ hydrochlorothiazide (Avalide^Rx; see Appendix B).

### ❏ Losartan

■ *Tablets:* 25 mg^Rx, 50 mg^Rx, 100 mg^Rx ■ Cost: 25 mg $128.73/90, 50 mg $42.90/30, 100 mg

$58.44/30 ■ hydrochlorothiazide (Hyzaar<sup>Rx</sup>; see Appendix B).

❏ **Olmesartan**

■ *Tablets:* 5 mg<sup>Rx</sup>, 20 mg<sup>Rx</sup>, 40 mg<sup>Rx</sup>.

❏ **Telmisartan**

■ *Tablets:* 40 mg<sup>Rx</sup>, 80 mg<sup>Rx</sup>.

❏ **Valsartan**

■ *Capsules:* 80 mg<sup>Rx</sup>, 160 mg<sup>Rx</sup> ■ Cost: 80 mg $139.75/100, 160 mg $151.70/100 ■ *Tablets:* 80 mg<sup>Rx</sup>, 160 mg<sup>Rx</sup>, 320 mg<sup>Rx</sup> ■ hydrochlorothiazide (Diovan HCT<sup>Rx</sup>; See Appendix B).

TIME/ACTION PROFILE (antihypertensive effect†)

| | ONSET | PEAK | DURATION |
|---|---|---|---|
| Candesartan | 2–4 hr | 6–8 hr | 24 hr |
| Eprosartan | 1–2 hr | unk | 12–24 hr |
| Irbesartan | within 2 hr | 3–14 hr | 24 hr |
| Losartan | unknown | 6 hr | 24 hr |
| Olmesartan | within 1 | 2 wk | 24 hr |
| Telmisartan | within 3 hr | unknown | 24 hr |
| Valsartan | within 2 hr | 4–6 hr | 24 hr |

†Maximum response may take 2–3 wk of treatment.

# NURSING IMPLICATIONS

## ASSESSMENT

❏ Assess blood pressure (lying down, sitting, standing) and pulse periodically during therapy.

❏ Monitor frequency of prescription refills to determine adherence.

❏ Assess patient for signs of angioedema (dyspnea, facial swelling). May rarely cause angioedema; more common in patients who have had angioedema with ACE inhibitors.

■ **CHF:** Monitor intake and output ratios and daily weight. Assess for peripheral edema and auscultate lungs for rales/crackles during therapy.

■ *Lab Test Considerations:* Monitor serum creatinine and urinary protein in patients treated for diabetic nephropathy. May rarely cause ↑ in BUN and serum creatinine.

❏ May cause ↑ serum bilirubin.

❏ May occasionally cause hyperkalemia.

❏ *Losartan* may cause transient ↑ of ALT and AST, hemoglobin, and hematocrit and ↓ uric acid concentrations.

## POTENTIAL NURSING DIAGNOSES

■ Injury, risk for (Adverse Reactions).

■ Noncompliance (Patient/Family Teaching).

## IMPLEMENTATION

■ **General:** Do not confuse Diovan (valsartan) with Zyban (buproprion). Do not confuse valsartan with losartan.

❏ Correct volume depletion, if possible, prior to initiation of therapy.

■ **PO:** May be administered without regard to meals.

## PATIENT/FAMILY TEACHING

❏ Emphasize the importance of continuing to take as directed, even if feeling well. Take missed doses as soon as remembered if not almost time for next dose; do not double doses. Medication controls but does not cure hypertension. Instruct patient to take medication at the same time each day. Gradual reduction of dose prior to discontinuation is suggested.

❏ Encourage patient to comply with additional interventions for hypertension (weight reduction, low-sodium diet, discontinuation of smoking, moderation of alcohol consumption, regular exercise, stress management).

❏ Instruct patient and family on proper technique for monitoring blood pressure. Advise them to check blood pressure at least weekly and to report significant changes.

❏ Caution patient to avoid sudden changes in position to decrease orthostatic hypotension. Use of alcohol, standing for long periods, exercising, and hot weather may increase orthostatic hypotension.

❏ Advise women of childbearing age to use contraception and notify health care professional if pregnancy is suspected or planned.

❏ May cause dizziness. Caution patient to avoid driving or other activities requiring alertness until response to medication is known.

❏ Advise patient to consult health care professional before taking any OTC or herbal cough, cold, or allergy remedies or other medications.

❏ Instruct patient to notify health care professional of medication regimen prior to treatment or surgery.

❏ Emphasize the importance of follow-up exams to evaluate effectiveness of medication.

## EVALUATION

**Effectiveness of therapy can be demonstrated by:** ■ Decrease in blood pressure without appearance of excessive side effects ■ Slowed progression of diabetic nephropathy ■ Decreased hospitalizations in patients with CHF ■ Reduced risk of stroke

---

# ANGIOTENSIN-CONVERTING ENZYME (ACE) INHIBITORS

**benazepril**
(ben-**aye**-ze-pril)
Lotensin

**captopril**
(**kap**-toe-pril)
Capoten

**enalapril/enalaprilat**
(e-**nal**-a-pril/e-**nal**-a-pril-at)
Vasotec, Vasotec IV

**fosinopril**
(foe-**sin**-oh-pril)
Monopril

**lisinopril**
(lyse-**in**-oh-pril)
Prinivil, Zestril

**moexipril**
(moe-**eks**-i-pril)
Univasc

**perindopril**
(pe-**rin**-do-pril)
Aceon

**quinapril**
(**kwin**-a-pril)
Accupril

**ramipril**
(ra-**mi**-pril)
Altace

**trandolapril**
(tran-**doe**-la-pril)
Mavik

*CLASSIFICATION(S):*
*Therapeutic: antihypertensives*
*Pharmacologic: ACE inhibitors*

**Pregnancy Category C (first trimester), D (second and third trimesters)**

## INDICATIONS

■ Alone or with other agents in the management of hypertension ■ **Captopril, enalapril, fosinopril, lisinopril, perindopril, quinapril, ramipril, trandolapril:** Management of CHF ■ **Captopril, lisinopril, ramipril, trandolapril:** Reduction of risk of death or development of CHF following MI ■ Slowed progression of left ventricular dysfunction into overt heart failure (selected agents) ■ **Ramipril:** Reduction of the risk of MI, stroke, and death from cardiovascular disease in patients at risk (>55 years old with a history of cardiovascular disease, stroke, peripheral vascular disease, or diabetes with another risk factor such as hypercholesterolemia or cigarette smoking) ■ **Captopril:** Decreased progression of diabetic nephropathy. **Unlabeled uses:** ■ **Lisinopril:** Prevention of migraine headaches.

## ACTION

■ ACE inhibitors block the conversion of angiotensin I to the vasoconstrictor angiotensin II. ACE also inactivates the vasodilator bradykinin and other vasodilatory prostaglandins. ACE inhibitors also increase plasma renin levels and reduce aldosterone levels. Net result is systemic vasodilation. **Therapeutic Effects:** ■ Lowering of blood pressure in hypertensive patients ■ Decreased afterload in patients with CHF ■ Decreased development of overt heart failure ■ Increased survival after MI (selected agents only) ■ Decreased progression of diabetic nephropathy (captopril only).

## PHARMACOKINETICS

**Absorption:** *Benazepril*—At least 37% absorbed following oral administration. *Captopril*—At least 75% following oral administration (decreased to 30–55% by food). *Enalapril*—60% absorbed following oral administration. *Enalaprilat*—IV administration results in complete bioavailability. *Fosinopril*—36% absorbed following oral administration. *Lisinopril*—25% absorbed following oral administration (much variability). *Moexipril*—Converted to moexiprilat (the active form) following oral administration; absorption is variable (decreased by food), resulting in 13% bioavailability as moexiprilat. *Perindopril*—75% absorbed following oral administration, rapidly converted to perindoprilat, the active metabolite (bioavailability for perindoprilat 35%). *Quinapril*—60% absorbed following oral administration (high-fat meal may decrease absorption). *Ramipril*—50–60% absorbed following oral administration. *Trandolapril*—Converted to trandolaprilat (the active form) following oral administration; bioavailability 10%, 70% for trandolaprilat.

**Distribution:** All ACE inhibitors cross the placenta. *Benazepril, benazeprilat, captopril, enalapril, enalaprilat,* and *fosinoprilat*—Enter breast milk in small amounts. *Lisinopril*—Minimal penetration of CNS. *Ramipril*—Probably does not enter breast milk. *Trandolapril*—Enters breast milk.

**Protein Binding:** *Benazepril*—96.7% (*benazeprilat*—95.3%), *fosinopril*—89–99.8%, *quinapril*—97%.

**Metabolism and Excretion:** *Benazepril*—Converted by the liver to benazeprilat, the active metabolite. 20% excreted by kidneys; 10–11% nonrenal (biliary elimination). *Captopril*—50% metabolized by the liver to inactive compounds, 50% excreted unchanged by the kidneys. *Enalapril, enalaprilat*—Enalapril is converted by the liver to enalaprilat, the active metabolite; 60% eliminated by the kidneys (20% as enalapril and 60% as enalaprilat; 33% eliminated in feces (6% as enalapril and 27% as enalaprilat). *Fosinopril*—Converted by the liver and GI mucosa to fosinoprilat, the active metabolite—50% eliminated by the kidneys; 50% fecal elimination. *Lisinopril*—100% eliminated by the kidneys. *Moexipril*—7% excreted in urine, 53% in feces. *Perindopril*—Converted by the liver to perindoprilat, the active metabolite. Perindoprilat and its metabolites are mostly eliminated by renal clearance. *Quinapril*—Converted by the liver, GI mucosa, and tissue to quinaprilat, the active metabolite: 61% eliminated by the kidneys; 37% fecal elimination. *Ramipril*—Metabolized by the liver to ramiprilat, the active metabolite; 60% eliminated by the kidneys; 40% fecal elimination. *Trandolapril*—Converted by liver to trandolaprilat; 33% excreted in urine as trandolaprilat, 66% in feces.

**Half-life:** *Benazeprilat*—10–11 hr. *Captopril*—<2 hr (increased in renal impairment). *Enalapril* and *enalaprilat*—11 hr (increased in renal impairment). *Fosinoprilat*—11.5 hr. *Lisinopril*—12 hr (increased in renal impairment). *Moexiprilat*—12 hr. *Perindoprilat*—10 hr, followed by a longer elimination half-life of 30–120 hr reflecting slow dissociation from tissue-binding sites and plasma. *Quinaprilat*—2 hr. *Ramiprilat*—13–17 hr (increased in renal impairment). *Trandolaprilat*—10 hr.

## CONTRAINDICATIONS AND PRECAUTIONS

**Contraindicated in:** ■ Hypersensitivity ■ Cross-sensitivity among ACE inhibitors may occur ■ Pregnancy ■ Angioedema (hereditary or idiopathic).

**Use Cautiously in:** ■ Renal impairment, hepatic impairment, hypovolemia, hyponatremia, elderly patients, concurrent diuretic therapy (initial dosage reduction recommended for most agents) ■ Black patients with hypertension (monotherapy less effective, may require additional therapy) ■ Aortic stenosis/hypertrophic cardiomyopathy ■ Cerebrovascular or cardiac insufficiency ■ Surgery/anesthesia (hypotension may be exaggerated) ■ Lactation or children (safety not established for most agents).

**Exercise Extreme Caution in:** ■ Family history of angioedema.

## ADVERSE REACTIONS AND SIDE EFFECTS*

■ **CNS:** dizziness, fatigue, headache, insomnia, weakness ■ **Resp:** <u>cough</u>, eosinophilic pneumonitis ■ **CV:** <u>hypotension</u>, angina pectoris, tachycardia ■ **GI:** <u>taste disturbances</u>, anorexia, diarrhea, nausea ■ **GU:** proteinuria, impotence, renal failure ■ **Derm:** rashes ■ **F and E:** hyperkalemia ■ **Hemat:** AGRANULOCYTOSIS , NEUTROPENIA (captopril only) ■ **Misc:** ANGIOEDEMA , fever.

## INTERACTIONS

**Drug-Drug:** ■ Excessive hypotension may occur with concurrent use of **diuretics** other **antihypertensives, nitrates, phenothiazines,** acute ingestion of **alcohol,** and during **surgery** or **general anesthesia** ■ Hyperkalemia may result from concurrent use of **potassium supplements, potassium-sparing diuretics, indomethacin, salt substitutes,** or **cyclosporine** ■ Antihypertensive response may be ↓ by **NSAIDs** ■ Absorption may be decreased by **antacids** ■ ↑ levels and may ↑ risk of **lithium** or **digoxin** toxicity ■ **Probenecid** ↓ elimination and ↑ levels of captopril ■ Risk of hypersensitivity reactions ↑ with **allopurinol** ■ **Capsaicin** may ↑ incidence of cough ■ **Rifampin** may ↓ effectiveness of enalapril ■ **Tetracycline** absorption is ↓ by quinapril (because of magnesium in tablets).

**Drug-Food:** ■ **Food** ↓ conversion of perindopril to perindoprilat.

## ROUTE AND DOSAGE

### ❑ Benazepril

■ **PO (Adults):** 5–10 mg once daily, increased gradually to maintenance dose of 20–40 mg/day as single dose or 2 divided doses (begin with 5 mg/day in patients receiving diuretics).

### ❑ Renal Impairment

■ **PO (Adults):** *CCr <30 ml/min*—Initiate therapy with 5 mg/day dose.

### ❑ Captopril

■ **PO (Adults):** *Hypertension*—12.5–25 mg 2–3 times daily, may be increased at 1–2 wk intervals up to 150 mg 3 times daily (usual dose 50 mg 3 times daily; begin with 6.25–12.5 mg 2–3 times daily in patients receiving diuretics). *CHF*—12.5 mg 2–3 times daily, may be increased up to 50–100 mg 3 times daily (range 12.5–450 mg/day). *Post-MI*—6.25-mg test dose, followed by 12.5 mg 3 times daily, may be increased up to 50 mg 3 times daily. *Diabetic nephropathy*—25 mg 3 times daily.

### ❑ Renal Impairment

■ **PO (Adults):** Initiate therapy at 6.25–12.5 mg 2–3 times daily.

### ❑ Enalapril/Enalaprilat

■ **PO (Adults):** *Hypertension*—5 mg/day, increased as required by response (usual range 10–40 mg/day in 1–2 divided doses; initiate therapy at 2.5 mg/day in patients receiving diuretics). *CHF*—2.5 mg 1–2 times daily, then 5 mg/day, increased as required by response (usual range 5–20 mg/day in 2 divided doses). *Asymptomatic left ventricular dysfunction*—2.5 mg twice daily, titrated upward to a target dose of 10 mg twice daily.

■ **IV (Adults):** 0.625–1.25 mg (0.625 mg if receiving diuretics) q 6 hr.

### ❑ Renal Impairment

■ **PO (Adults):** *CCr <30 ml/min*—Initiate therapy at 2.5 mg daily.

### ❑ Fosinopril

■ **PO (Adults):** *Hypertension*—10 mg once daily, may be increased as required (range 20–40 mg once daily), maximum 80 mg/day. *CHF*—10 mg once daily (5 mg in patients who have been vigorously diuresed), may be increased over several weeks up to 40 mg/day (usual range 20–40 mg/day).

### ❑ Lisinopril

■ **PO (Adults):** *Hypertension*—10 mg once daily, can be increased up to 20–40 mg/day (initiate therapy at 5 mg/day in patients receiving diuretics). *CHF*—2.5–5 mg once daily, can be increased up to 40 mg/day. *Improved survival after MI*—5 mg once daily for 2 days, then 10 mg daily for 6 wk.

### ❑ Renal Impairment

■ **PO (Adults):** *CCr >10 ml/min-<30 ml/min*—>5 mg/day initially; *CCr<10ml/min*—2.5 mg/day initially; may be titrated upward to 40 mg/day, based on response.

### ❑ Moexipril

■ **PO (Adults):** 7.5 mg once daily, may be increased as needed (usual range is 7.5–30 mg/day in 1–2 divided doses; begin with 3.75 mg in patients receiving diuretics).

### ❑ Renal Impairment

■ **PO (Adults):** *CCr <40 ml/min*—Initiate therapy at 3.75 mg once daily, may be titrated upward carefully to 15 mg/day.

### ❑ Perindopril

■ **PO (Adults):** 4 mg once daily, may be titrated upward to 16 mg/day as a single dose or

2 divided doses (begin with 2–4 mg/day in patients receiving diuretics).

■ **PO (Geriatric Patients):** *Hypertension*—4 mg once daily, may be titrated upward to 8 mg/day as a single dose or 2 divided doses; *CHF*—4 mg once daily.

❑ **Renal Impairment**

■ **PO (Adults):** *CCr >30 ml/min*—2 mg/day initially, may be titrated upward to 8 mg/day;—*CCr <30 ml/min*—safety not established.

❑ **Quinapril**

■ **PO (Adults):** *Hypertension*—10–20 mg once daily initially, may be titrated no more often than every 2 wk up to 80 mg/day in single or divided daily doses (initiate therapy at 10 mg/day in patients receiving diuretics). *CHF*—5 mg twice daily initially, may be titrated up to 40 mg/day.

❑ **Renal Impairment**

■ **PO (Adults):** *CCr >60 ml/min*—Initiate therapy at 10 mg/day; *CCr 30–60 ml/min*—Initiate therapy at 5 mg/day; *CCr <30 ml/min*—Initiate therapy at 2.5 mg/day.

❑ **Ramipril**

■ **PO (Adults):** *Hypertension*—2.5 mg once daily, may be increased slowly as needed up to 20 mg/day in 1–2 divided doses (initiate therapy at 1.25 mg/day in patients receiving diuretics). *CHF following MI*—1.25–2.5 mg twice daily initially, may be increased up to 5 mg twice daily.

❑ **Renal Impairment**

■ **PO (Adults):** *CCr <40 ml/min*—Initiate therapy at 1.25 mg once daily, may be slowly titrated up to 5 mg/day.

❑ **Trandolapril**

■ **PO (Adults):** *Hypertension in nonblack patients*—1 mg once daily; *hypertension in black patients*—2 mg once daily. May be increased weekly up to 4 mg once daily; twice daily dosing may be necessary in some patients (begin with 0.5 mg/day in patients receiving diuretics). *Heart failure post-MI or left ventricular dysfunction post-MI*—Initiate therapy at 1 mg once daily, titrate up to 4 mg once daily if possible.

❑ **Renal Impairment**

■ **PO (Adults):** *CCr <30 ml/min*—Initiate therapy at 0.5 mg once daily, may be slowly titrated upward.

❑ **Hepatic Impairment**

■ **PO (Adults):** Initiate therapy at 0.5 mg once daily, may be slowly titrated upward.

## AVAILABILITY

❑ **Benazepril**

■ *Tablets:* 5 mg^Rx, 10 mg^Rx, 20 mg^Rx, 40 mg^Rx
■ Cost: 5 mg $84.16/90, 10 mg $84.16/90, 20 mg $84.16/90, 40 mg $84.16/90 ■ amlodipine (Lotrel^Rx) and hydrochlorothiazide (Lotensin HCT^Rx). See Appendix B.

❑ **Captopril**

■ *Tablets:* 12.5 mg^Rx, 25 mg^Rx, 50 mg^Rx, 100 mg^Rx ■ Cost: *Capoten*—12.5 mg $97.10/100, 25 mg $104.98/100, 50 mg $180.01/100, 100 mg 239.72/100; *generic*—12.5 mg $62.70/100, 25 mg $68.75/100, 50 mg $118.22/100, 100 mg $129.95/100 ■ hydrochlorothiazide (Capozide^Rx). See Appendix B.

❑ **Enalapril**

■ *Tablets:* 2.5 mg^Rx, 5 mg^Rx, 10 mg^Rx, 20 mg^Rx ■ Cost: 2.5 mg $93.68/100, 5 mg $119.01/100, 10 mg $124.95/100, 20 mg $177.79/100 ■ diltiazem (Teczem^Rx), felodipine (Lexxel^Rx), hydrochlorothiazide (Vaseretic^Rx). See Appendix B.

❑ **Enalaprilat**

■ *Injection:* 1.25 mg/ml^Rx.

❑ **Fosinopril**

■ *Tablets:* 10 mg^Rx, 20 mg^Rx ■ Cost: 10 mg $99.24/90, 20 mg $99.24/90.

❑ **Lisinopril**

■ *Tablets:* 2.5 mg^Rx, 5 mg^Rx, 10 mg^Rx, 20 mg^Rx, 40 mg^Rx ■ Cost: *Prinivil*—2.5 mg $68.53/100, 5 mg $102.76/100, 10 mg $106.10/100, 20 mg $113.59/100, 40 mg $166.12/100; *Zestril*—2.5 mg $65.33/100, 5 mg $97.96/100, 10 mg $101.15/100, 20 mg $108.29/100, 40 mg $158.35/100 ■ hydrochlorothiazide (Prinzide^Rx, Zestoretic^Rx). See Appendix B.

◻ **Moexipril**

■ *Tablets:* 7.5 mg$^{Rx}$, 15 mg$^{Rx}$ ■ Cost: 7.5 mg $74.01/100, 15 mg $74.01/100 ■ hydrochlorothiazide (Uniretic$^{Rx}$).

◻ **Perindopril**

■ *Tablets:* 2 mg$^{Rx}$, 4 mg$^{Rx}$, 8 mg$^{Rx}$.

◻ **Quinapril**

■ *Tablets:* 5 mg$^{Rx}$, 10 mg$^{Rx}$, 20 mg$^{Rx}$, 40 mg$^{Rx}$ ■ Cost: 5 mg $101.30/90, 10 mg $101.30/90, 20 mg $101.30/90, 40 mg $101.30/90.

◻ **Ramipril**

■ *Capsules:* 1.25 mg$^{Rx}$, 2.5 mg$^{Rx}$, c, 5 mg$^{Rx}$, 10 mg$^{Rx}$ ■ Cost: 1.25 mg $89.38/100, 2.5 mg $108.11/100, 5 mg $118.03/100, 10 mg $141.96/100.

◻ **Trandolapril**

■ *Tablets:* 1 mg$^{Rx}$, 2 mg$^{Rx}$, 4 mg$^{Rx}$ ■ Cost: 1 mg $88.01/100, 2 mg $88.01/100, 4 mg $88.01/100 ■ verapamil (Tarka$^{Rx}$). See Appendix B.

TIME/ACTION PROFILE (effect on blood pressure—single dose†)

| | ONSET | PEAK | DURATION |
|---|---|---|---|
| Benazepril | within 1 hr | 2–4 hr | 24 hr |
| Captopril | 15–60 min | 60–90 min | 6–12 hr |
| Enalapril PO | 1 hr | 4–6 hr | 24 hr |
| Enalapril IV | 15 min | 1–4 hr | 6 hr |
| Fosinopril | within 1 hr | 2–6 hr | 24 hr |
| Lisinopril | 1 hr | 6 hr | 24 hr |
| Moexipril | within 1 hr | | up to 24 hr |
| Perindoprilat | unknown | 3–7 hr | 12–24 hr |
| Quinapril | within 1 hr | 2–4 hr | up to 24 hr |
| Ramipril | within 1–2 hr | 4–6.5 hr | 24 hr |
| Trandolapril | within 1 hr | 4–10 hr | up to 24 hr |

†Full effects may not be noted for several weeks.

# NURSING IMPLICATIONS

## ASSESSMENT

■ **Hypertension:** Monitor blood pressure and pulse frequently during initial dose adjustment and periodically during therapy. Notify health care professional of significant changes.

◻ Monitor frequency of prescription refills to determine adherence.

■ **CHF:** Monitor weight and assess patient routinely for resolution of fluid overload (peripheral edema, rales/crackles, dyspnea, weight gain, jugular venous distention).

■ *Lab Test Considerations:* Monitor BUN, creatinine, and electrolyte levels periodically. Serum potassium may be ↑ and BUN and creatinine transiently ↑, whereas sodium levels may be ↓. If ↑ BUN or serum creatinine concentrations occur, dose reduction or withdrawal may be required.

◻ Monitor CBC periodically during therapy. May rarely cause slight ↓ in hemoglobin and hematocrit.

◻ May cause ↑ AST, ALT, alkaline phosphatase, serum bilirubin, uric acid, and glucose.

◻ Assess urine protein prior to and periodically during therapy for up to 1 yr in patients with renal impairment or those receiving >150 mg/day of captopril. If excessive or ↑ proteinuria occurs, re-evaluate ACE inhibitor therapy.

◻ May cause positive ANA titer.

◻ *Captopril:* May cause false-positive test results for urine acetone.

◻ Monitor WBC with differential prior to initiation of therapy, monthly for the first 3–6 mo, and periodically thereafter for up to 1 yr in patients at risk for neutropenia (patients with renal impairment, collagen-vascular disease, or those receiving high doses) or at first sign of infection. Discontinue therapy if neutrophil count is <1000/mm$^3$.

## POTENTIAL NURSING DIAGNOSES

■ Cardiac output, decreased (Indications, Side Effects).

■ Noncompliance (Patient/Family Teaching).

## IMPLEMENTATION

■ **General:** Do not confuse Lotensin (benazepril) with Loniten (minoxidil) or Lovastatin. Do not confuse enalapril with Eldepryl (seligiline). Do not confuse Monopril (fosinopril) with Accupril (quinapril), minoxidil, or Monoket (isosorbide mononitrate). Do not confuse Prinivil (lisinopril) with Plendil (felodipine) or Prilosec (omeprazole). Do not confuse Accupril (quinapril) with Accutane (isotretinoin). Do not confuse Altace (ramipril) with Artane (trihexyphenidyl).

■ **PO:** Precipitous drop in blood pressure during first 1–3 hr following first dose may require volume expansion with normal saline but is not normally considered an indication for stopping therapy. Discontinuing diuretic therapy or increasing salt intake 1 week prior to initiation may decrease risk of hypotension. Monitor closely for at least 1 hr after blood pressure has stabilized. Resume diuretics if blood pressure is not controlled.

□ **Captopril**

□ Administer 1 hr before or 2 hr after meals. May be crushed if patient has difficulty swallowing. Tablets may have a sulfurous odor.

□ An oral solution may be prepared by crushing a 25-mg tablet and dissolving it in 25–100 ml of water. Shake for at least 5 min and administer within 30 min.

□ **Enalaprilat**

■ **Direct IV:** May be administered undiluted.

■ **Rate:** Administer over at least 5 min.

■ **Intermittent Infusion:** Dilute in up to 50 ml of D5W, 0.9% NaCl, D5/0.9% NaCl, or D5/LR. Diluted solution is stable for 24 hr.

■ **Rate:** Administer as a slow infusion.

■ **Y-Site Compatibility:** ◆ allopurinol ◆ amifostine ◆ amikacin ◆ aminophylline ◆ ampicillin ◆ ampicillin/sulbactam ◆ aztreonam ◆ butorphanol ◆ calcium gluconate ◆ cefazolin ◆ cefoperazone ◆ ceftazidime ◆ ceftizoxime ◆ chloramphenicol ◆ cimetidine ◆ cisatracurium ◆ cladribine ◆ clindamycin ◆ dextran 40 ◆ dobutamine ◆ docetaxel ◆ dopamine ◆ doxorubicin liposome ◆ erythromycin lactobionate ◆ esmolol ◆ etoposide phosphate ◆ famotidine ◆ fentanyl ◆ filgrastim ◆ ganciclovir ◆ gemcitabine ◆ gentamicin ◆ granisetron ◆ heparin ◆ hetastarch ◆ hydrocortisone sodium succinate ◆ labetalol ◆ lidocaine ◆ magnesium sulfate ◆ melphalan ◆ meropenem ◆ methylprednisolone sodium succinate ◆ metronidazole ◆ morphine ◆ nafcillin ◆ nitroprusside ◆ penicillin G potassium ◆ phenobarbital ◆ piperacillin ◆ piperacillin/tazobactam ◆ potassium chloride ◆ potassium phosphate ◆ propofol ◆ ranitidine ◆ remifentanil ◆ sodium acetate ◆ teniposide ◆ thiotepa ◆ tobramycin ◆ trimethoprim/sulfamethoxazole ◆ vancomycin ◆ vinorelbine.

■ **Y-Site Incompatibility:** ◆ amphotericin B ◆ amphotericin B cholesteryl sulfate ◆ cefepime ◆ phenytoin.

■ **Additive Compatibility:** ◆ dobutamine ◆ dopamine ◆ heparin ◆ meropenem ◆ nitroglycerin ◆ nitroprusside ◆ potassium chloride.

□ **Moexipril**

■ **PO:** Administer moexipril on an empty stomach, 1 hr prior to a meal.

□ **Ramipril**

■ **PO:** Capsules may be opened and sprinkled on applesauce, added to apple juice, or dissolved in 4 oz water for patients with difficulty swallowing. Effectiveness is same as capsule. Prepared mixtures can be stored for up to 24 hrs at room temperature or up to 48 hrs if refrigerated.

## PATIENT/FAMILY TEACHING

■ **General Info:** Instruct patient to take medication as directed at the same time each day, even if feeling well. Take missed doses as soon as possible but not if almost time for next dose. Do not double doses. Warn patient not to discontinue ACE inhibitor therapy unless directed by health care professional.

□ Caution patient to avoid salt substitutes or foods containing high levels of potassium or sodium unless directed by healthcare professional (see Appendix Q).

□ Caution patient to change positions slowly to minimize hypotension, particularly after initial dose. Patients should also be advised that exercising in hot weather may increase hypotensive effects.

□ Advise patient to consult health care professional before taking any OTC medications, especially cold remedies.

□ May cause dizziness. Caution patient to avoid driving and other activities requiring alertness until response to medication is known.

□ Advise patient to inform health care professional of medication regimen prior to treatment or surgery.

□ Advise patient that medication may cause impairment of taste that generally resolves within 8–12 wk, even with continued therapy.

□ Instruct patient to notify health care professional if rash; mouth sores; sore throat; fever; swelling of hands or feet; irregular heart beat; chest pain; dry cough; hoarseness; swelling of face, eyes, lips, or tongue; difficulty swallowing or breathing occur; or if taste impairment or skin rash persists. Persistent dry cough may occur and may not subside until medication is discontinued.

Consult health care professional if cough becomes bothersome. Also notify health care professional if nausea, vomiting, or diarrhea occurs and continues.

❑ Emphasize the importance of follow-up examinations to monitor progress.

■ **Hypertension:** Encourage patient to comply with additional interventions for hypertension (weight reduction, discontinuation of smoking, moderation of alcohol consumption, regular exercise, and stress management). Medication controls but does not cure hypertension.

❑ Instruct patient and family on correct technique for monitoring blood pressure. Advise them to check blood pressure at least weekly and to report significant changes to health care professional.

**EVALUATION**

**Effectiveness of therapy can be demonstrated by:** ■ Decrease in blood pressure without appearance of side effects ■ Decrease in signs and symptoms of CHF ■ Reduction of risk of death or development of CHF following MI ■ Decrease in progression of diabetic nephropathy (captopril).

**anistreplase, See THROMBOLYTIC AGENTS.**

# ANTIFUNGALS (TOPICAL)

**butenafine**

(byoo-**ten**-a-feen)

Lotrimin Ultra, Mentax

**ciclopirox**

(sye-kloe-**peer**-ox)

Loprox, Penlac

**clotrimazole**

(kloe-**trye**-ma-zole)

{Canesten}, {Clotrimaderm}, Fungoid, Lotrimin, Mycelex, Mycelex OTC, {Myclo}, {Neo-Zol}

**econazole**

(ee-**kon**-a-zole)

Spectazole

**haloprogin**

(hal-oh-**proe**-jin)

Halotex

**ketoconazole**

(kee-toe-**kon**-a-zole)

Nizoral

**miconazole**

(mye-**kon**-a-zole)

Breezee Mist Antifungal, Lotrimin AF, Maximum Strength Desenex Antifungal, Micatin, Monistat-Derm, Zeasorb-AF

**naftifine**

(**naff**-ti-feen)

Naftin

**nystatin**

(nye-**stat**-in)

Mycostatin, {Nadostine}, Nilstat, {Nyaderm}, Nystex, Pedi-Dri

**oxiconazole**

(ox-i-**kon**-a-zole)

Oxistat

**sulconazole**

(sul-**kon**-a-zole)

Exelderm

**terbinafine**

(ter-**bin**-a-feen)

Lamisil AT

**tolnaftate**

(tol-**naff**-tate)

Aftate, Dr. Scholl's Athlete's Foot Cream, Dr. Scholl's Maximum Strength Tritan, {Pitrez}, Quinsana Plus, Tinactin, Ting

**CLASSIFICATION(S):**

**Therapeutic:** antifungals (topical)

**Pregnancy Category A (nystatin), B (butenafine, ciclopirox, clotrimazole, haloprogin, naftifine,**

**nystatin, oxiconazole, terbinafine), C (econazole, ketoconazole, sulconazole), UK (miconazole, tolnaftate)**

## INDICATIONS

■ Treatment of a variety of cutaneous fungal infections, including cutaneous candidiasis, tinea pedis (athlete's foot), tinea cruris (jock itch), tinea corporis (ringworm), and tinea versicolor.

## ACTION

■ Butenafine, nystatin, clotrimazole, econazole, ketoconazole, miconazole, and oxiconazole affect the synthesis of the fungal cell wall, allowing leakage of cellular contents. **Therapeutic Effects:** ■ Fungistatic or fungicidal action depending on agent and concentration, with resultant decrease in symptoms of fungal infection.

## PHARMACOKINETICS

**Absorption:** Most agents are minimally, if at all, absorbed through intact skin.

**Distribution:** Distribution following topical administration not known. Action is primarily local.

**Metabolism and Excretion:** Metabolism and excretion not known following local application.

**Half-life:** *Ciclopirox*—1.7 hr; *miconazole*—24.1 hr (terminal).

## CONTRAINDICATIONS AND PRECAUTIONS

**Contraindicated in:** ■ Hypersensitivity to active ingredients, additives, preservatives, or bases ■ Some products contain alcohol or bisulfites and should be avoided in patients with known intolerance.

**Use Cautiously in:** ■ Nail and scalp infections (may require additional systemic therapy) ■ Pregnancy or lactation (safety not established).

## ADVERSE REACTIONS AND SIDE EFFECTS*

■ **Local:** burning, itching, local hypersensitivity reactions, redness, stinging.

## INTERACTIONS

**Drug-Drug:** ■ If sufficient ketoconazole is absorbed through skin, it may ↓ the metabolism of a number of other drugs, ↑ risk of toxicity (see ketoconazole, systemic monograph).

## ROUTE AND DOSAGE

❑ **Butenafine**

■ **Topical (Adults):** Apply once daily for 4 wk.

❑ **Ciclopirox**

■ **Topical (Adults):** *Cream/lotion*—Apply cream or lotion twice daily for up to 4 wk; *Topical solution (nail lacquer)*—Apply to nails at bedtime or 8 hr prior to washing for up to 48 wk ; *Shampoo*—5–10 ml applied to scalp, lather and leave on for 3 min, rinse; repeat twice weekly for 4 wk (at least 3 days between applications).

❑ **Clotrimazole**

■ **Topical (Adults):** Apply cream, solution, or lotion twice daily for 1–4 wk.

❑ **Econazole**

■ **Topical (Adults):** Apply cream once daily for tinea pedis, tinea cruris, or tinea versicolor. Apply twice daily for cutaneous candidiasis. Use for 2–4 wk.

❑ **Haloprogin**

■ **Topical (Adults):** Apply daily for 2–4 wk.

❑ **Ketoconazole**

■ **Topical (Adults):** Apply cream once daily for cutaneous candidiasis or twice daily for seborrheic dermatitis. For dandruff, use shampoo twice weekly (wait 3 days between treatments) for 4 wk, then intermittently.

❑ **Miconazole**

■ **Topical (Adults):** Apply cream, powder, or spray twice daily (once daily for tinea versicolor) for up to 1 mo.

❑ **Naftifine**

■ **Topical (Adults):** Apply cream once daily or gel twice daily.

❑ **Nystatin**

■ **Topical (Adults and Children):** Apply cream, ointment, or powder 2–3 times daily until healing is complete.

❏ **Oxiconazole**

■ **Topical (Adults and Children):** Apply cream or lotion 1–2 times daily for 2 wk–1 mo.

❏ **Sulconazole**

■ **Topical (Adults):** Apply 1–2 times daily (twice daily for tinea pedis).

❏ **Terbinafine**

■ **Topical (Adults):** Apply twice daily for tinea pedis or 1–2 times daily for tinea cruris or tinea corporis for 1–4 wk.

❏ **Tolnaftate**

■ **Topical (Adults):** Apply twice daily for 2–3 wk.

## AVAILABILITY

❏ **Butenafine**

■ *Cream:* 1%$^{Rx,\ OTC}$.

❏ **Ciclopirox**

■ *Cream:* 1%$^{Rx}$ ■ *Lotion:* 1%$^{Rx}$ ■ *Ointment:* 3%$^{OTC}$ ■ *Nail lacquer:* 8% solution (contains alcohol) in 3.3 ml bottles$^{Rx}$ ■ *Shampoo:* 1% solution in 120 ml bottles$^{Rx}$.

❏ **Clotrimazole**

■ *Cream:* {1%$^{Rx,\ OTC}$} ■ *Solution:* 1%$^{Rx,\ OTC}$ ■ *Lotion:* 1%$^{Rx,\ OTC}$ ■ betamethasone (Lotrisone)$^{Rx}$. See Appendix B.

❏ **Econazole**

■ *Cream:* 1%$^{Rx}$.

❏ **Haloprogin**

■ *Cream:* 1%$^{Rx}$ ■ *Solution:* 1%$^{Rx}$.

❏ **Ketoconazole**

■ *Cream:* 2%$^{Rx}$ ■ *Shampoo:* 2%$^{Rx,\ OTC}$.

❏ **Miconazole**

■ *Cream:* {2%$^{Rx,\ OTC}$} ■ *Lotion:* 2%$^{Rx}$ ■ *Powder:* 2%$^{OTC}$ ■ *Aerosol powder:* 2%$^{OTC}$ ■ *Spray:* 2%$^{OTC}$ ■ *Solution:* 2%(in alcohol)$^{OTC}$.

❏ **Naftifine**

■ *Cream:* {1%$^{Rx,\ OTC}$} ■ *Gel:* 1%$^{Rx,\ OTC}$.

❏ **Nystatin**

■ *Cream:* {100,000 units/gRx, OTC} ■ *Ointment:* {100,000 units/gRx, OTC} ■ *Powder:* {100,000 units/gRx, OTC} ■ triamcinolone (Mycogen II, Mycolog II, Myci-Triacet II, Mytrex)$^{Rx}$. See Appendix B.

❏ **Oxiconazole**

■ *Cream:* 1%$^{Rx}$ ■ *Lotion:* 1%$^{Rx}$.

❏ **Sulconazole**

■ *Cream:* 1%$^{Rx}$ ■ *Solution:* 1%$^{Rx}$.

❏ **Terbinafine**

■ *Spray:* 1%$^{OTC}$ ■ Cost: $58.40/30 ml.

❏ **Tolnaftate**

■ *Cream:* 1%$^{OTC}$ ■ *Solution:* 1%$^{OTC}$ ■ *Gel:* 1%$^{OTC}$ ■ *Powder:* 1%$^{OTC}$ ■ *Spray powder:* 1%$^{OTC}$ ■ *Spray liquid:* 1%$^{OTC}$.

TIME/ACTION PROFILE (resolution of symptoms/lesions)

| | ONSET | PEAK | DURATION |
|---|---|---|---|
| Butenafine | unknown | up to 4 wk | unknown |
| Ciclopirox | within 1st wk | unknown | 12 hr |
| Clotrimazole | within 1st wk | unknown | 12 hr |
| Miconazole | 2–3 days | 2 wk | 12–24 hr |

# NURSING IMPLICATIONS

## ASSESSMENT

❏ Inspect involved areas of skin and mucous membranes before and frequently during therapy. Increased skin irritation may indicate need to discontinue medication.

## POTENTIAL NURSING DIAGNOSES

■ Skin integrity, risk for impaired (Indications).

■ Infection, risk for (Indications).

## IMPLEMENTATION

■ **General:** Do not confuse Lotrim (clotrimazole) with Lotrisone (betamethasone/clotrimazole).

❏ Consult physician or other health care professional for proper cleansing technique before applying medication.

❏ Choice of vehicle is based on use. Ointments, creams, and liquids are used as primary therapy. Lotion is usually preferred in intertriginous areas; if cream is used, apply sparingly to avoid maceration. Powders are usually used as adjunctive therapy but may be used as primary therapy for mild conditions.

■ **Topical:** Apply small amount to cover affected area completely. Avoid the use of occlusive wrappings or dressings unless directed by physician or other health care professional.

- **Nail lacquer:** Avoid contact with skin other than skin immediately surrounding treated nail. Avoid contact with eyes or mucous membranes. Removal of unattached, infected nail, as frequently as monthly, by health care professional is needed with use of this medication. Up to 48 wk of daily application and professional removal may be required to achieve clear or almost clear nail. Six months of treatment may be required before results are noticed.
- **Ciclopirox or Ketoconazole shampoo:** Moisten hair and scalp thoroughly with water. Apply sufficient shampoo to produce enough lather to wash scalp and hair and gently massage it over the entire scalp area for approximately 1 min. Rinse hair thoroughly with warm water. Repeat process, leaving shampoo on hair for an additional 3 min. After the second shampoo, rinse and dry hair with towel or warm air flow. Shampoo twice a week for 4 wk with at least 3 days between each shampooing and then intermittently as needed to maintain control.
- **Triacetin:** For spray products, shake well. Dry affected areas before spraying. Spray onto affected nails, holding actuator down 1–2 seconds.

### PATIENT/FAMILY TEACHING

- ☐ Instruct patient to apply medication as directed for full course of therapy, even if feeling better. Emphasize the importance of avoiding the eyes.
- ☐ Caution patient that some products may stain fabric, skin, or hair. Check label information. Fabrics stained from cream or lotion can usually be cleaned by handwashing with soap and warm water; stains from ointments can usually be removed with standard cleaning fluids.
- ☐ Patients with athlete's foot should be taught to wear well-fitting, ventilated shoes and to change shoes and socks at least once a day.
- ☐ Advise patient to report increased skin irritation or lack of response to therapy to health care professional.
- **Nail lacquer:** File away loose nail and trim nails every 7 days after solution is removed with alcohol. Do not use nail polish on treated nails. Inform health care professional if

area of application shows signs of increased irritation (redness, itching, burning, blistering, swelling, oozing).

### EVALUATION

**Effectiveness of therapy can be demonstrated by:** ■ Decrease in skin irritation and resolution of infection. Early relief of symptoms may be seen in 2–3 days. For *Candida,* tinea cruris, and tinea corporis, 2 wk are needed, and for tinea pedis, therapeutic response may take 3–4 wk. Recurrent fungal infections may be a sign of systemic illness.

# ANTIFUNGALS (VAGINAL)

**butoconazole**

(byoo-toe-**kon**-a-zole)

Femstat-3, Gynezole-1, Mycelex-3

**clotrimazole**

(kloe-**trye**-ma-zole)

{Canesten}, {Clotrimaderm}, Fem-Care, Femizole, Gyne-Lotrimin, Mycelex, {Myclo-Gyne}, Trivagizole-3

**miconazole**

(mye-**kon**-a-zole)

Miconazole, Monistat, M-Zole 3

**nystatin**

(nye-**stat**-in)

Mycostatin, Nilstat

**terconazole**

(ter-**kon**-a-zole)

Terazol

**tioconazole**

(tye-oh-**kon**-a-zole)

{Gyne-Trosyd}, Vagistat

*CLASSIFICATION(S):*
*Therapeutic: antifungals (vaginal)*

**Pregnancy Category A (nystatin), B (clotrimazole, miconazole, nys-**

tatin), C (butoconazole, terconazole), UK (tioconazole)

## INDICATIONS

■ Treatment of vulvovaginal candidiasis.

## ACTION

■ Damages fungal cell membrane, allowing leakage of cellular contents. Not active against bacteria. **Therapeutic Effects:** ■ Inhibited growth and death of susceptible *Candida*, with decrease in accompanying symptoms of vulvovaginitis (vaginal burning, itching, discharge).

## PHARMACOKINETICS

**Absorption:** *Nystatin, miconazole,* and *tioconazole* are minimally absorbed; 5.5% of *butoconazole* is absorbed, 3–10% of *clotrimazole,* 5–15% of *terconazole* following intravaginal administration.

**Distribution:** Unknown. Action is primarily local.

**Metabolism and Excretion:** Small amounts of *clotrimazole* absorbed, rapidly metabolized.

**Half-life:** *Miconazole*—20–25 hr (following parenteral administration).

## CONTRAINDICATIONS AND PRECAUTIONS

**Contraindicated in:** ■ Hypersensitivity to active ingredients, additives, or preservatives ■ Butoconazole is contraindicated in the first trimester of pregnancy ■ Lactation (except terconazole).

**Use Cautiously in:** ■ Patients with recurrent vulvovaginal yeast infections ■ Lactation (safe use not established for terconazole).

## ADVERSE REACTIONS AND SIDE EFFECTS*

■ **CNS:** *terconazole*—headache ■ **Local:** irritation, sensitization, vulvovaginal burning ■ **Misc:** hypersensitivity reactions; *terconazole*—body pain.

## INTERACTIONS

**Drug-Drug:** ■ Concurrent use of vaginal miconazole with **warfarin** ↑ risk of bleeding/ bruising (appropriate monitoring recommended).

## ROUTE AND DOSAGE

❏ **Butoconazole**

■ **Vag (Adults and Adolescents):** *Vaginal cream*—1 applicatorful (5 g) at bedtime for 3 days *or* one applicatorful single dose (Gynezole●1).

❏ **Clotrimazole**

■ **Vag (Adults and Adolescents):** *Vaginal tablets*—100 mg at bedtime for 7 nights (preferred regimen for pregnancy) *or* 200 mg at bedtime for 3 nights *or* 500 mg (one 500-mg vaginal tablet) as a single bedtime dose. *Vaginal cream*—1 applicatorful (5 g) at bedtime for 3–7 days.

❏ **Miconazole**

■ **Vag (Adults and Adolescents):** *Vaginal suppositories*—one 200-mg or one 400-mg suppository at bedtime for 3 days *or* one 100-mg suppository at bedtime for 7 days. *Vaginal cream*—1 applicatorful at bedtime for 7 days. Combination packages contain both suppositories and cream; cream used for symptomatic management of itching. *Tampons (available in California only)*— One tampon (100 mg) inserted nightly for 7 days, retained overnight and removed the following morning.

❏ **Nystatin**

■ **Vag (Adults and Adolescents):** *Vaginal tablets*—100,000 units (1 tablet) daily for 2 wk.

❏ **Terconazole**

■ **Vag (Adults and Adolescents):** *Vaginal cream*—1 applicatorful (5 g) of 0.4% cream at bedtime for 7 days or 1 applicatorful (5 g) of 0.8% cream at bedtime for 3 days. *Vaginal suppositories*—1 suppository (80 mg) at bedtime for 3 days.

❏ **Tioconazole**

■ **Vag (Adults and Adolescents):** *Vaginal ointment*—1 applicatorful (4.6 g) at bedtime as a single dose.

## AVAILABILITY

❏ **Butoconazole**

■ *Vaginal cream:* 2%[OTC].

❏ **Clotrimazole**

■ *Vaginal tablets:* 100 mg[OTC], {200 mg[Rx]}, 500 mg[Rx], [OTC] ■ *Vaginal cream:* 1%[OTC], {2%[OTC]}.

❏ **Miconazole**

■ *Vaginal cream:* 2%$^{OTC}$ ■ *Vaginal suppositories:* 100 mg$^{OTC}$, 200 mg$^{Rx}$, $^{OTC}$, {400 mg$^{OTC}$} ■ *Tampons (available in California only):* 100 mg ■ combination package of 3 200-mg suppositories and 9-g tube of 2% cream$^{OTC}$.

❏ **Nystatin**

■ *Vaginal tablets:* 100,000 units$^{Rx}$.

❏ **Terconazole**

■ *Vaginal cream:* 0.4%$^{Rx}$, 0.8%$^{Rx}$ ■ Cost: 0.4% $33.82/45 g, 0.8% $33.82/20 g ■ *Vaginal suppositories:* 80 mg$^{Rx}$ ■Cost: $37.27/3 suppositories.

❏ **Tioconazole**

■ *Vaginal ointment:* 6.5%$^{OTC}$.

TIME/ACTION PROFILE

| | ONSET | PEAK | DURATION |
|---|---|---|---|
| All agents | rapid | unknown | 24 hr |

## NURSING IMPLICATIONS

### ASSESSMENT

❏ Inspect involved areas of skin and mucous membranes before and frequently during therapy. Increased skin irritation may indicate need to discontinue medication.

### POTENTIAL NURSING DIAGNOSES

■ Infection, risk for (Indications).
■ Skin integrity, risk for impaired (Indications).

### IMPLEMENTATION

■ **General:** Consult physician or other health care professional for proper cleansing technique before applying medication. Sitz baths and vaginal douches may be ordered concurrently with this therapy.
■ **Vag:** Applicators are supplied for vaginal administration.

### PATIENT/FAMILY TEACHING

❏ Instruct patient to apply medication as directed for full course of therapy, even if feeling better. Therapy should be continued during menstrual period.

❏ Instruct patient on proper use of vaginal applicator. Medication should be inserted high into the vagina at bedtime. Instruct patient to remain recumbent for at least 30 min after insertion. Advise use of sanitary napkins to prevent staining of clothing or bedding.

❏ Advise patient to consult health care professional regarding douching and intercourse during therapy. Vaginal medication may cause minor skin irritation in sexual partner. Advise patient to refrain from sexual contact during therapy or have male partner wear a condom. Some products may weaken latex contraceptive devices.

❏ Advise patient to report to health care professional increased skin irritation or lack of response to therapy. A second course may be necessary if symptoms persist.

## EVALUATION

**Clinical response to therapy can be evaluated by:** ■ Decrease in skin irritation and vaginal discomfort. Therapeutic response is usually seen after 1 wk. Diagnosis should be reconfirmed with smears or cultures before a second course of therapy to rule out other pathogens associated with vulvovaginitis. Recurrent vaginal infections may be a sign of systemic illness.

## aprepitant
(a-**prep**-i-tant)
Emend

### CLASSIFICATION(S):
*Therapeutic:* antiemetics
*Pharmacologic:* neurokinin antagonists

### Pregnancy Category B

## INDICATIONS

■ Prevention of acute and delayed nausea and vomiting caused by initial/repeat treatment with highly emetogenic chemotherapy (with other antiemetics).

## ACTION

■ Acts as a selective antagonist at substance P/neurokinin 1 (NK$_1$) receptors in the brain. **Therapeutic Effects:** ■ Decreased nausea and vomiting associated with chemotherapy ■ Augments the antiemetic effects of dexamethasone and 5–HT$_3$ antagonists (ondansetron).

## PHARMACOKINETICS

**Absorption:** 60–65% absorbed following oral administration.
**Distribution:** Crosses the blood brain barrier; remainder of distribution unknown.
**Metabolism and Excretion:** Mostly metabolized by the liver (CYP3A4 enzyme system); not renally excreted.
**Half-life:** 9–13 hr.

## CONTRAINDICATIONS AND PRECAUTIONS

**Contraindicated in:** ■ Lactation ■ Hypersensitivity ■ Concurrent use with pimozide (risk of life-threatening adverse cardiovascular reactions).
**Use Cautiously in:** ■ Concurrent use with any agents metabolized by CYP3A4 (see Drug-Drug Interactions) ■ Pregnancy (use only if clearly needed) ■ Children (safety not established).

## ADVERSE REACTIONS AND SIDE EFFECTS*

■ **CV:** dizziness, fatigue, weakness ■ **GI:** diarrhea ■ **Misc:** hiccups.

## INTERACTIONS

**Drug-Drug:** ■ Aprepitant inhibits, induces and is metabolized by the CYP3A4 enzyme system; it also induces the CYP2C9 system. Concurrent use with other medications that are metabolized by CYP3A4 may result in increased toxicity from these agents including **docetaxel, paclitaxel, etoposide, irinotecan, ifosfamide, imatinib, vinorelbine, vinblastine, vincristine, midazolam, triazolam,** and **alprazolam**; concurrent use should be undertaken with caution ■ Concurrent use with **drugs that significantly inhibit the CYP3A4 enzyme system** including (**ketoconazole, itraconazole, nefazodone, clarithromycin, ritonavir, nelfinavir,** and **diltiazem**) may ↑ blood levels and effects of aprepitant ■ Concurrent use with **drugs that induce the CYP3A4 enzyme system** including **rifampin, carbamazepine,** and **phenytoin** may ↓ blood levels and effects of aprepitant ■ ↑ blood levels and effects of **dexamethasone,** (regimen reflects a 50% dose reduction); a similar effect occurs with **methylprednisolone** ( ↓ IV dose by 25%, ↓ PO dose by 50% when used concurrently) ■ May ↓ the effects of **warfarin** (careful monitoring for 2 wk recommended), **oral contraceptives** (use alternate method), **tolbutamide** and **phenytoin.**

## ROUTE AND DOSAGE

■ **PO (Adults):** 125 mg 1 hr prior to chemotherapy, then 80 mg once daily for 2 days (with dexamethasone 12 mg PO 30 min prior to chemotherapy, then 8 mg once daily for 3 days and ondansetron 32 mg IV 30 min prior to chemotherapy).

## AVAILABILITY

■ *Capsules:* 80 mg$^{Rx}$, 125 mg$^{Rx}$.

TIME/ACTION PROFILE (antiemetic effect)

|    | ONSET | PEAK | DURATION |
|----|-------|------|----------|
| PO | 1 hr  | 4 hr* | 24 hr   |

*Blood level.

# NURSING IMPLICATIONS

## ASSESSMENT

❑ Assess nausea, vomiting, appetite, bowel sounds, and abdominal pain prior to and following administration.
❑ Monitor hydration, nutritional status, and intake and output. Patients with severe nausea and vomiting may require IV fluids in addition to antiemetics.
■ *Lab Test Considerations:* Monitor clotting status closely during the 2 wk period, especially at 7–10 days, following aprepitant therapy in patients on chronic warfarin therapy.
❑ May cause mild, transient ↑ in AST and ALT.

## POTENTIAL NURSING DIAGNOSES

■ Fluid volume, risk for deficit (Indications).
■ Nutrition, imbalanced: less than body requirements (Indications).

## IMPLEMENTATION

■ **General:** Aprepitant is given as part of a regimen that includes a corticosteroid and a 5–HT$_3$ antagonist (see Route & Dosage).

■ **PO:** Administer daily for 3 days. *Day 1—*administer 125 mg 1 hr prior to chemotherapy. *Days 2 and 3*—administer 80 mg once in the morning. May be administered without regard to food.

## PATIENT/FAMILY TEACHING

◻ Instruct patient to take aprepitant exactly as directed. Direct patient to read the patient package insert before starting therapy and to reread it each time the prescription is renewed.

◻ Advise patient to notify health care professional prior to taking any other prescription, OTC, or herbal products.

◻ Caution patient that aprepitant may decrease the effectiveness of oral contraceptives. Advise patient to use alternate nonhormal methods of contraception.

◻ Advise patient and family to use general measures to decrease nausea (begin with sips of liquids and small, nongreasy meals; provide oral hygiene; remove noxious stimuli from environment).

## EVALUATION

**Effectiveness of therapy can be demonstrated by:** ■ Decreased nausea and vomiting associated with chemotherapy.

# argatroban
(ar-**gat**-tro-ban)
Argatroban

*CLASSIFICATION(S):*
*Therapeutic:* anticoagulants
*Pharmacologic:* thrombin inhibitors

**Pregnancy Category B**

## INDICATIONS

■ Prophylaxis or treatment of thrombosis in patients with heparin-induced thrombocytopenia ■ As an anticoagulant in patients with or at risk for heparin-induced thrombocytopenia who are undergoing percutaneous coronary intervention (PCI).

## ACTION

■ Inhibits thrombin by binding to its receptor sites. Inhibition of thrombin prevents activation of factors V, VIII and XII; the conversion of fibrinogen to fibrin; platelet adhesion and aggregation. **Therapeutic Effects:** ■ Decreased thrombus formation and extension with decreased sequelae of thrombosis (emboli, postphlebitic syndromes).

## PHARMACOKINETICS

**Absorption:** IV administration results in complete bioavailability.
**Distribution:** Unknown.
**Metabolism and Excretion:** Mostly metabolized by the liver; excreted primarily in feces via biliary excretion. 16% excreted unchanged in urine, 14% excreted unchanged in feces.
**Half-life:** 39–51 min (increased in hepatic impairment).

## CONTRAINDICATIONS AND PRECAUTIONS

**Contraindicated in:** ■ Major bleeding ■ Hypersensitivity ■ Lactation.
**Use Cautiously in:** ■ Hepatic impairment (decreased initial infusion rate recommended) ■ Children <18 yr (safety not established) ■ Pregnancy (use only if clearly needed).

## ADVERSE REACTIONS AND SIDE EFFECTS*

■ **CV:** hypotens ■ **GI:** diarrhea, nausea, vomiting ■ **Hemat:** BLEEDING ■ **Misc:** allergic reactions including ANAPHYLAXIS, fever.

## INTERACTIONS

**Drug-Drug:** ■ Risk of bleeding may be increased by concurrent use of **antiplatelet agents, thrombolytic agents,** or **other anticoagulants.**
**Drug-Natural Products:** ■ Increased bleeding risk with **anise, arnica, chamomile, clove, feverfew, garlic, ginger, ginkgo, Panax ginseng,** and others.

## ROUTE AND DOSAGE

■ **IV (Adults):** 2 mcg/kg/min as a continuous infusion; adjust infusion rate on the basis of activated partial thromboplastin time (aPTT). *Patients undergoing PCI—350 mcg/kg* bolus followed by infusion at 25 mcg/kg/min, activated clotting time (ACT) should be assessed 5–10 min later. If ACT is 300–450 sec, procedure may be started. If ACT <300 sec, give additional bolus of 150 mcg/kg and increase infusion rate to 30 mg/kg/min. If ACT is >450 sec infusion rate should be decreased to 15 mcg/kg/min and ACT rechecked after 5–10 min. If thrombotic complications occur or ACT drops to <300 sec, an additional bolus of 150 mcg/kg may be given and the infusion rate increased to 40 mcg followed by ACT monitoring. If anticoagulation is required after surgery, lower infusion rates should be used.

◻ **Hepatic Impairment**

■ **IV (Adults):** 0.5 mcg/kg/min as a continuous infusion; adjust infusion rate on the basis of aPTT.

## AVAILABILITY

■ *Solution for injection (must be diluted 100-fold):* 250 mg/2.5 ml vial[Rx].

TIME/ACTION PROFILE (anticoagulant effect)

|      | ONSET     | PEAK    | DURATION |
|------|-----------|---------|----------|
| IV   | immediate | 1–3 hr  | 2–4 hr   |

## NURSING IMPLICATIONS

### ASSESSMENT

◻ Monitor vital signs periodically throughout therapy. Unexplained decreases in blood pressure may indicate hemorrhage. Assess patient for bleeding. Arterial and venous punctures, IM injections, and use of urinary catheters, nasotracheal intubation, and nasogastric tubes should be minimized. Noncompressible sites for IV access should be avoided. Monitor for blood in urine, lower back pain, pain or burning on urination. If bleeding cannot be controlled with pressure, decrease dose or discontinue argatroban immediately.

◻ Monitor for signs of anaphylaxis (rash, coughing, dyspnea) throughout therapy.

■ *Lab Test Considerations:* Monitor aPTT prior to initiation of continuous infusion, 2 hours after initiation of therapy, and periodically during therapy to confirm aPTT is within desired therapeutic range.

◻ For patients undergoing PCI, monitor ACT as described in Route and Dose section.

◻ Assess hemoglobin, hematocrit, and platelet count prior to, and periodically during, argatroban therapy. May cause decreased hemoglobin and hematocrit. Unexplained decreased in hematocrit may indicate hemorrhage.

◻ Use of argatroban concurrently with muliptle doses of warfarin will result in more prolonged prothrombin time and international normalized ratio (INR) (although there is not an increase in vitamin K-dependent factor $X_a$ activity) than when warfarin is used alone. Monitor INR daily during concomitant therapy. Repeat INR 4–6 hr after argatroban is discontinued. If the repeat value is below the desired therapeutic value for warfarin alone, restart argatroban therapy and continue until the desired therapeutic range for warfarin alone is reached. To obtain the INR for warfarin alone when the dose of argatroban is >2 mcg/kg/min the argatroban dose should be temporarily reduced to 2 mcg/kg/min; the INR for combined therapy may then be obtained 4–6 hr after argatroban dose was redeuced.

■ *Toxicity and Overdose:* There is no specific antidote for argatroban. If overdose occurs, discontinue argatroban. Anticoagulation parameters usually return to baseline within 2–4 hrs after discontinuation.

## POTENTIAL NURSING DIAGNOSES

■ Tissue perfusion, ineffective (Indications).

## IMPLEMENTATION

■ **General:** All parenteral anticoagulants should be discontinued before argatroban therapy is initiated. Oral anticoagulation may be initiated with maintenance dose of warfarin; do not administer loading dose. Discontinue argatroban therapy when INR for combined therapy is >4.

◻ Solution is slightly viscous, clear, and colorless to pale yellow. Do not administer solutions that are cloudy or contain particulate matter. Discard unused portion.

■ **Direct IV:** For patients undergoing PCI, initial bolus of 350 mcg/kg is administered followed by a continuous infusion of 25 mcg/kg/min.

■ *Rate:* Administer bolus over 3–5 min. See Route & Dose section for administration details.

■ **Continuous Infusion:** Dilute each 2.5 ml vial of argatroban in 250 ml of 0.9% NaCl, D5W, or lactated Ringer's solution for a concentration of 1 mg/ml. Mix by repeated inversion for 1 minute. Solution may show a slight haziness that disappears upon mixing. Solution is stable for 48 hours if refrigerated and protected from light.

■ **Rate:** Rate is based on patient weight. Administer at a rate of 2 mcg/kg/min. Dosage adjustment is made once steady state is reached (1–3 hours) until steady state aPTT is 1.5–3 times the initial baseline value (not to exceed 100 seconds).

■ **Y-Site Incompatibility:** Do not mix with other medications.

**PATIENT/FAMILY TEACHING**

❏ Inform patient of the purpose of argatroban.

❏ Instruct patient to notify health care professional immediately if any bleeding is noted.

**EVALUATION**

**Effectiveness of therapy can be demonstrated by:** ■ Decreased thrombus formation and extension ❏ Decreased sequelae of thrombosis (emboli, post-phlebitic syndromes).

## aripiprazole
(a-ri-**pip**-ra-zole)
Abilify

***CLASSIFICATION(S):***
***Therapeutic:*** *antipsychotics*
***Pharmacologic:*** *dihydrocarbostyril*

**Pregnancy Category C**

**INDICATIONS**

■ Treatment of schizophrenia.

**ACTION**

■ Psychotropic activity may be due to agonist activity at dopamine $D_2$ and serotonin 5–$HT_{1A}$ receptors and antagonist activity at the 5–$HT_{2A}$ receptor ■ Also has alpha$_1$ adrenergic blocking activity. **Therapeutic Effects:** ■ Decreased manifestations of schizophrenia.

**PHARMACOKINETICS**

**Absorption:** Well absorbed (87%) following oral administration.

**Distribution:** Extensive extravascular distribution.

**Protein Binding:** *aripiprazole and dehydroaripiprazole*—>99%.

**Metabolism and Excretion:** Mostly metabolized by the liver (CYP3A4 and CYP2D6 enzymes); one metabolite (dehydro-aripiprazole) has antipsychotic activity. 18% excreted unchanged in feces; <1% excreted unchanged in urine. A small percentage of patients are poor metabolizers and may need smaller doses.

**Half-life:** *Aripiprazole*—75 hr; *dehydro-aripiprazole*—94 hr.

**CONTRAINDICATIONS AND PRECAUTIONS**

**Contraindicated in:** ■ Hypersensitivity ■ Lactation.

**Use Cautiously in:** ■ Known cardiovascular or cerebrovascular disease ■ Conditions which cause hypotension (dehydration, treatment with antihypertensives or diuretics) ■ Concurrent ketoconazole or other potential CYP3A4 inhibitors (reduce aripiprazole dose by 50%) ■ Concurrent quinidine, fluoxetine, paroxetine or other potential CYP2D6 inhibitors ■ Concurrent carbamazepine or other potential CYP3A4 inducers ■ Pregnancy (use only if benefit outweighs risk to fetus) ■ Children and adolescents (safety not established).

**ADVERSE REACTIONS AND SIDE EFFECTS\***

■ **CNS:** confusion, depression, drowsiness, extrapyramidal reactions, hostility, lightheadedness, manic reactions, nervousness, ecchymosis, suicidal thought, tardive dyskinesia ■ **Resp:** dyspnea ■ **CV:** bradycardia, chest pain, edema, hypertension, orthostatic hypotension, tachycardia ■ **EENT:** conjunctivitis, ear pain ■ **GI:** anorexia, ↑ salivation, nausea, vomiting ■ **GU:** urinary incontinence ■ **Hemat:** anemia ■ **Derm:** dry skin, skin ulcer, sweating ■ **Metab:** weight loss ■ **MS:** muscle cramps, neck pain ■ **Neuro:** abnormal gait ■ **Misc:** NEUROLEPTIC MALIGNANT SYNDROME , ↓ heat regulation.

{ } = Available in Canada only.
*CAPITALS indicates life-threatening; underlines indicate most frequent.

## INTERACTIONS

**Drug-Drug:** ■ **Ketoconazole** or **other potential CYP3A4 inhibitors** decrease metabolism and increase effects (reduce aripiprazole dose by 50%) ■ **Quinidine, fluoxetine, paroxetine** or **other potential CYP2D6 inhibitors** decrease metabolism and increase effects (reduce aripiprazole dose by at least 50%) ■ Concurrent **carbamazepine** or **other potential CYP3A4 inducers** (double aripiprazole dose; then decrease to 10–15 mg/day when interfering drug is withdrawn).

## ROUTE AND DOSAGE

■ **PO (Adults):** *Starting and target dose*—10 or 15 mg/day as a single dose, doses up to 30 mg/day have been used; increments in dosing should not be made before 2 wk at a given dose.

## AVAILABILITY

■ *Tablets:* 10 mg$^{Rx}$, 15 mg$^{Rx}$, 20 mg$^{Rx}$, 30 mg$^{Rx}$.

TIME/ACTION PROFILE (antipsychotic effect)

|    | ONSET | PEAK | DURATION |
|----|-------|------|----------|
| PO | unknown | 2 wk | unknown |

# NURSING IMPLICATIONS

## ASSESSMENT

❑ Assess patient's mental status (orientation, mood, behavior) before and periodically during therapy.
❑ Monitor blood pressure (sitting, standing, lying), pulse, and respiratory rate before and periodically during therapy.
❑ Observe patient carefully when administering medication to ensure that medication is actually taken and not hoarded.
❑ Monitor patient for onset of akathisia (restlessness or desire to keep moving) and extrapyramidal side effects (*parkinsonian*—difficulty speaking or swallowing, loss of balance control, pill rolling, mask-like face, shuffling gait, rigidity, tremors; and *dystonic*—muscle spasms, twisting motions, twitching, inability to move eyes, weakness of arms or legs) periodically during therapy.
❑ Monitor for tardive dyskinesia (uncontrolled rhythmic movement of mouth, face, and extremities; lip smacking or puckering; puffing of cheeks; uncontrolled chewing; rapid or worm-like movements of tongue). Notify physician or other health care professional immediately if these symptoms occur, as these side effects may be irreversible.
❑ Monitor for development of neuroleptic malignant syndrome (fever, muscle rigidity, altered mental status, respiratory distress, tachycardia, seizures, diaphoresis, hypertension or hypotension, pallor, tiredness, loss of bladder control). Notify physician or other health care professional immediately if these symptoms occur.

■ *Lab Test Considerations:* May cause ↑ creatinine phosphokinase.

## POTENTIAL NURSING DIAGNOSES

■ Thought processes, disturbed (Indications).
■ Noncompliance (Patient/Family Teaching).

## IMPLEMENTATION

■ **PO:** Administer once daily without regard to meals.

## PATIENT/FAMILY TEACHING

❑ Advise patient to take medication exactly as directed and not to skip doses or double up on missed doses. If a dose is missed, it should be taken as soon as remembered unless almost time for the next dose.
❑ Inform patient of possibility of extrapyramidal symptoms and tardive dyskinesia. Instruct patient to report these symptoms immediately.
❑ Advise patient to make position changes slowly to minimize orthostatic hypotension.
❑ Medication may cause drowsiness and lightheadedness. Caution patient to avoid driving or other activities requiring alertness until response to medication is known.
❑ Caution patient to avoid taking alcohol or other CNS depressants concurrently with this medication.
❑ Advise patient that extremes in temperature should be avoided, because this drug impairs body temperature regulation.
❑ Advise patient to notify health care professional of medication regimen prior to treatment or surgery.
❑ Emphasize the importance of routine follow-up exams and continued participation in psychotherapy as indicated.

## EVALUATION

**Effectiveness of therapy can be demonstrated by:** ▪ Decrease in excitable, paranoic, or withdrawn behavior.

High Alert

## asparaginase
(a-**spare**-a-ji-nase)
Elspar, {Kidrolase}

**CLASSIFICATION(S):**
*Therapeutic: antineoplastics*
*Pharmacologic: enzymes*

## Pregnancy Category C

## INDICATIONS

▪ Part of combination chemotherapy in the treatment of acute lymphocytic leukemia (ALL).

## ACTION

▪ Catalyst in the conversion of asparagine (an amino acid) to aspartic acid and ammonia ▪ Depletes asparagine in leukemic cells. **Therapeutic Effects:** ▪ Death of leukemic cells.

## PHARMACOKINETICS

**Absorption:** Is absorbed from IM sites.
**Distribution:** Remains in the intravascular space. Poor penetration into the CSF.
**Metabolism and Excretion:** Slowly sequestered in the reticuloendothelial system.
**Half-life:** IV: 8–30 hr; IM: 39–49 hr.

## CONTRAINDICATIONS AND PRECAUTIONS

**Contraindicated in:** ▪ Previous hypersensitivity ▪ Pregnancy or lactation.
**Use Cautiously in:** ▪ History of hypersensitivity reactions ▪ Severe liver disease ▪ Renal or pancreatic disease ▪ CNS depression ▪ Clotting abnormalities ▪ Chronic debilitating illnesses ▪ Patients with childbearing potential.

## ADVERSE REACTIONS AND SIDE EFFECTS*

▪ **CNS:** SEIZURES, agitation, coma, confusion, depression, dizziness, fatigue, hallucinations, headache, irritability, somnolence ▪ **GI:** <u>nausea</u>, <u>vomiting</u>, anorexia, cramps, hepatotoxicity, pancreatitis, weight loss ▪ **Derm:** rashes, urticaria ▪ **Endo:** hyperglycemia ▪ **Hemat:** coagulation abnormalities, transient bone marrow depression ▪ **Metab:** hyperammonemia, hyperuricemia ▪ **Misc:** hypersensitivity reactions including ANAPHYLAXIS.

## INTERACTIONS

**Drug-Drug:** ▪ May negate the antineoplastic activity of **methotrexate** ▪ May enhance the hepatotoxicity of other **hepatotoxic drugs** ▪ Concurrent IV use with or immediately preceding **vincristine** and **prednisone** may result in increased neurotoxicity and hyperglycemia ▪ May alter the response to **live vaccines** (decreased antibody response, increased risk of adverse reactions).

## ROUTE AND DOSAGE

Various other regimens may be used.

❑ **Multiple-Agent Induction Regimen (in Combination with Vincristine and Prednisone)**
▪ **IV (Children):** 1000 IU/kg/day for 10 successive days beginning on day 22 of regimen.
▪ **IM (Children):** 6000 IU/m² on days 4, 7, 10, 13, 16, 19, 22, 25, 28.

❑ **Single-Agent Therapy for Acute Lymphocytic Leukemia**
▪ **IV (Adults and Children):** 200 IU/kg daily for 28 days.

❑ **Desensitization Regimen**
▪ **IV (Adults and Children):** Administer 1 IU, then double dose every 10 min until total dose for that day has been given or reaction occurs.

❑ **Test Dose.**
▪ **Intradermal (Adults and Children):** 2 IU.

## AVAILABILITY

▪*Injection:* 10,000-IU vial (with mannitol)^Rx.

TIME/ACTION PROFILE (depletion of asparagine)

| | ONSET | PEAK† | DURATION |
|---|---|---|---|
| IM | immediate | 14–24 hr | 23–33 days |
| IV | immediate | unknown | 23–33 days |

†Plasma levels of asparaginase.

---

{ } = Available in Canada only.
*CAPITALS indicates life-threatening; <u>underlines</u> indicate most frequent.

## NURSING IMPLICATIONS

### ASSESSMENT

❑ Monitor vital signs before and frequently during therapy. Inform physician if fever or chills occur.

❑ Monitor intake and output. Notify physician of significant discrepancies. Encourage patient to drink 2000–3000 ml/day to promote excretion of uric acid. Allopurinol and alkalinization of the urine may be used to prevent urate stone formation.

❑ Monitor for hypersensitivity reaction (urticaria, diaphoresis, facial swelling, joint pain, hypotension, bronchospasm). Epinephrine and resuscitation equipment should be readily available. Reaction may occur up to 2 hr after administration. If patient requires continued therapy, pegaspargase is an alternative.

❑ Assess nausea, vomiting, and appetite. Weigh weekly. An antiemetic may be given before administration.

❑ Monitor affect and neurologic status. Notify physician if depression, drowsiness, or hallucinations occur. Symptoms usually resolve 2–3 days after drug is discontinued.

■ *Lab Test Considerations:* Monitor CBC before and periodically throughout therapy. May alter coagulation studies. Platelets, PT, PTT, and thrombin time may be increased. May cause elevated BUN.

❑ Hepatotoxicity may be manifested by increased AST, ALT, alkaline phosphatase, bilirubin, or cholesterol. Liver function test results usually return to normal after therapy. May cause pancreatitis; monitor frequently for elevated amylase or glucose.

❑ Monitor blood glucose during therapy. May cause hyperglycemia treatable with fluids and insulin. May be fatal.

❑ May cause elevated serum and urine uric acid concentrations.

❑ May interfere with thyroid function tests.

### POTENTIAL NURSING DIAGNOSES

■ Injury, risk for (Side Effects).

■ Infection, risk for (Side Effects).

### IMPLEMENTATION

❑ *High Alert:* Fatalities have occurred with chemotherapeutic agents. Before administering, clarify all ambiguous orders; double check single, daily, and course-of-therapy dose limits; have second practitioner independently double check original order and dose calculations. Do not confuse asparaginase with pegaspargase.

■ **General:** Solution should be prepared in a biologic cabinet. Wear gloves, gown, and mask while handling medication. Discard equipment in specially designated containers (see Appendix M).

❑ If coagulopathy develops, apply pressure to venipuncture sites; avoid IM injections.

■ **Test Dose:** Intradermal test dose must be performed before initial dose; doses must be separated by more than 1 wk. Reconstitute vial with 5 ml of sterile water for injection or 0.9% NaCl for injection (without preservatives). Add 0.1 ml of this 2000-IU/ml solution to 9.9 ml additional diluent to yield a 20-IU/ml solution. Inject 0.1 ml (2 IU) intradermally. Observe site for 1 hr for formation of wheal. Wheal is indicative of a positive reaction.

■ **Desensitization Therapy:** Begin by administering 1 IU intravenously. Double dose every 10 min if hypersensitivity does not occur until full daily dose is administered.

■ **IM:** Prepare for IM dose by adding 2 ml of 0.9% NaCl for injection (without preservatives) to the 10,000-IU vial. Shake vial gently. Administer no more than 2 ml per injection site.

■ **Direct IV:** Prepare IV dose by diluting 10,000-IU vial with 5 ml of sterile water for injection or 0.9% NaCl (without preservatives). If gelatinous fibers are present, administration through a 5-micron filter will not alter potency. Administration through a 0.2-micron filter may cause loss of potency. Solution should be clear after reconstitution. Discard if cloudy. Stable for 8 hr if refrigerated.

■ *Rate:* Administer through Y-site of rapidly flowing IV of D5W or 0.9% NaCl over at least 30 min. Maintain IV infusion for 2 hr after dose.

■ **Y-Site Compatibility:** ◆ methotrexate ◆ sodium bicarbonate.

■ **Additive Incompatibility:** Information unavailable. Do not admix with other drugs.

### PATIENT/FAMILY TEACHING

❑ Instruct patient to notify health care professional if abdominal pain, severe nausea and vomiting, jaundice, fever, chills, sore throat, bleeding or bruising, excess thirst or urination, or mouth sores occur. Caution patient to avoid crowds and persons with known infections. Instruct patient to use soft toothbrush and electric razor, and to be especially careful to avoid falls. Patients should also be cautioned not to drink alcoholic beverages or take medication containing aspirin or NSAIDs because these may precipitate gastric bleeding.

❑ Advise patient of the need for contraception because of teratogenic effects of asparaginase.

❑ Instruct patient not to receive any vaccinations without advice of health care professional. Advise parents that this may alter immunization schedule.

❑ Emphasize need for periodic lab tests to monitor for side effects.

### EVALUATION

**Effectiveness of therapy can be demonstrated by:** ▪ Improvement of hematologic status in patients with leukemia.

---

## aspirin, See SALICYLATES.

---

## atenolol

(a-**ten**-oh-lole)

{Apo-Atenolol}, {Novo-Atenolol}, Tenormin

### CLASSIFICATION(S):

***Therapeutic:*** *antianginals, antihypertensives*

***Pharmacologic:*** *beta blockers*

### Pregnancy Category D

### INDICATIONS

▪ Management of hypertension ▪ Management of angina pectoris ▪ Prevention of MI.

### ACTION

▪ Blocks stimulation of beta$_1$(myocardial)-adrenergic receptors. Does not usually affect beta$_2$(pulmonary, vascular, uterine)-receptor sites. **Therapeutic Effects:** ▪ Decreased blood pressure and heart rate ▪ Decreased frequency of attacks of angina pectoris ▪ Prevention of MI.

### PHARMACOKINETICS

**Absorption:** 50–60% absorbed after oral administration.

**Distribution:** Minimal penetration of CNS. Crosses the placenta and enters breast milk.

**Metabolism and Excretion:** 40–50% excreted unchanged by the kidneys; remainder excreted in feces as unabsorbed drug.

**Half-life:** 6–9 hr.

### CONTRAINDICATIONS AND PRECAUTIONS

**Contraindicated in:** ▪ Uncompensated CHF ▪ Pulmonary edema ▪ Cardiogenic shock ▪ Bradycardia or heart block.

**Use Cautiously in:** ▪ Renal impairment (dosage reduction recommended if CCr ≤35 ml/min) ▪ Hepatic impairment ▪ Geriatric patients (increased sensitivity to beta blockers; initial dosage reduction recommended) ▪ Pulmonary disease (including asthma; beta selectivity may be lost at higher doses) ▪ Diabetes mellitus (may mask signs of hypoglycemia) ▪ Thyrotoxicosis (may mask symptoms) ▪ Patients with a history of severe allergic reactions (intensity of reactions may be increased) ▪ Pregnancy, lactation, or children (safety not established; all agents cross the placenta and may cause fetal/neonatal bradycardia, hypotension, hypoglycemia, or respiratory depression).

### ADVERSE REACTIONS AND SIDE EFFECTS*

▪ **CNS:** <u>fatigue</u>, <u>weakness</u>, anxiety, depression, dizziness, drowsiness, insomnia, memory loss, mental status changes, nervousness, nightmares ▪ **EENT:** blurred vision, stuffy nose ▪ **Resp:** bronchospasm, wheezing ▪ **CV:** BRADYCARDIA, CHF, PULMONARY EDEMA, hypotension, peripheral vasoconstriction ▪ **GI:** constipation, diarrhea, liver function abnormalities, nausea, vomiting ▪ **GU:** <u>impotence</u>, decreased libido, urinary frequency ▪ **Derm:** rashes ▪ **Endo:** hyperglycemia, hypoglycemia ▪ **MS:** arthralgia, back pain, joint pain ▪ **Misc:** drug-induced lupus syndrome.

---

{ } = Available in Canada only.
*CAPITALS indicates life-threatening; <u>underlines</u> indicate most frequent.

## INTERACTIONS

**Drug-Drug:** ■ **General anesthesia, IV phenytoin** and **verapamil** may cause additive myocardial depression ■ Additive bradycardia may occur with **digoxin** ■ Additive hypotension may occur with other **antihypertensives,** acute ingestion of **alcohol,** or **nitrates** ■ Concurrent use with **amphetamine, cocaine, ephedrine, epinephrine, norepinephrine, phenylephrine,** or **pseudoephedrine** may result in unopposed alpha-adrenergic stimulation (excessive hypertension, bradycardia) ■ Concurrent **thyroid** administration may decrease effectiveness ■ May alter the effectiveness of **insulins** or **oral hypoglycemic agents** (dosage adjustments may be necessary) ■ May decrease the effectiveness of **theophylline** ■ May decrease the beneficial beta$_1$-cardiovascular effects of **dopamine** or **dobutamine** ■ Use cautiously within 14 days of **MAO inhibitor** therapy (may result in hypertension).

## ROUTE AND DOSAGE

■ **PO (Adults):** *Antianginal*—50 mg once daily; may be increased after 1 wk to 100 mg/day (up to 200 mg/day). *Antihypertensive*—25–50 mg once daily; may be increased after 2 wk to 50–100 mg once daily. *MI*—50 mg (given 10 min after last IV dose), then 50 mg 12 hr later, then 100 mg/day as a single dose or in 2 divided doses for 6–9 days or until hospital discharge.

❑ **Renal Impairment**

■ **PO (Adults):** *CCr 15–35 ml/min*—dosage should not exceed 50 mg/day; *CCr <15 ml/min*—dosage should not exceed 50 mg every other day.

■ **IV (Adults):** *MI*—5 mg, followed by another 5 mg after 10 min; after 10 more min follow with oral dosing.

## AVAILABILITY (generic available)

■ *Tablets:* 25 mg$^{Rx}$, 50 mg$^{Rx}$, 100 mg$^{Rx}$ ■ Cost: 25 mg $15.79/60, 50 mg $10.50/60, 100 mg $81.20/60 ■ *Injection:* 500 mcg (0.5 mg)/ml$^{Rx}$ ■ chlorthalidone (Tenoretic)$^{Rx}$. See Appendix B.

TIME/ACTION PROFILE (cardiovascular effects)

|    | ONSET | PEAK | DURATION |
|----|-------|------|----------|
| PO | 1 hr | 2–4 hr | 24 hr |
| IV | rapid | 5 min | unknown |

## NURSING IMPLICATIONS

### ASSESSMENT

❑ Monitor blood pressure, ECG, and pulse frequently during dosage adjustment period and periodically throughout therapy.

❑ Monitor intake and output ratios and daily weights. Assess routinely for CHF (dyspnea, rales/crackles, weight gain, peripheral edema, jugular venous distention).

❑ Monitor frequency of prescription refills to determine adherence.

■ **Angina:** Assess frequency and characteristics of angina periodically throughout therapy.

■ *Lab Test Considerations:* May cause increased BUN, serum lipoprotein, potassium, triglyceride, and uric acid levels.

❑ May cause increased ANA titers.

❑ May cause increase in blood glucose levels.

■ *Toxicity and Overdose:* Monitor patients receiving beta blockers for signs of overdose (bradycardia, severe dizziness or fainting, severe drowsiness, dyspnea, bluish fingernails or palms, seizures). Notify physician immediately if these signs occur.

### POTENTIAL NURSING DIAGNOSES

■ Cardiac output, decreased (Side Effects).
■ Noncompliance (Patient/Family Teaching).

### IMPLEMENTATION

■ **PO:** Take apical pulse before administering drug. If <50 bpm or if arrhythmia occurs, withhold medication and notify physician or other health care professional.

■ **Direct IV:** IV therapy for acute MI should be initiated as soon as possible after patient arrives at the hospital.

❑ May be diluted in D5W, 0.9% NaCl, or D5/0.9% NaCl. Stable for 48 hr.

■ *Rate:* Administer 5 mg over 5 min, followed by another 5 mg 10 min later.

■ **Y-Site Compatibility:** ◆ meperidine ◆ meropenem ◆ morphine.

■ **Y-Site Incompatibility:** ◆ amphotericin B cholesteryl sulfate.

### PATIENT/FAMILY TEACHING

■ **General Info:** Instruct patient to take atenolol as directed at the same time each day, even if feeling well; do not skip or double up on missed doses. If a dose is missed, it should be taken as soon as possible up to 8 hr before next dose. Abrupt withdrawal may cause life-threatening arrhythmias, hypertension, or myocardial ischemia.

❑ Advise patient to make sure enough medication is available for weekends, holidays, and vacations. A written prescription may be kept in wallet in case of emergency.

❑ Teach patient and family how to check pulse and blood pressure. Instruct them to check pulse daily and blood pressure biweekly and to report significant changes.

❑ May cause drowsiness or dizziness. Caution patients to avoid driving or other activities that require alertness until response to the drug is known.

❑ Advise patients to change positions slowly to minimize orthostatic hypotension.

❑ Caution patient that atenolol may increase sensitivity to cold.

❑ Instruct patient to consult health care professional before taking any OTC medications, especially cold preparations, concurrently with this medication.

❑ Patients with diabetes should closely monitor blood glucose, especially if weakness, malaise, irritability, or fatigue occurs. Medication does not block sweating as a sign of hypoglycemia.

❑ Advise patient to notify health care professional if slow pulse, difficulty breathing, wheezing, cold hands and feet, dizziness, light-headedness, confusion, depression, rash, fever, sore throat, unusual bleeding, or bruising occurs.

❑ Instruct patient to inform health care professional of medication regimen before treatment or surgery.

❑ Advise patient to carry identification describing disease process and medication regimen at all times.

■ **Hypertension:** Reinforce the need to continue additional therapies for hypertension (weight loss, sodium restriction, stress reduction, regular exercise, moderation of alcohol consumption, and smoking cessation). Medication controls but does not cure hypertension.

## EVALUATION
**Effectiveness of therapy can be demonstrated by:** ■ Decrease in blood pressure ■ Reduction in frequency of angina ❑ Increase in activity tolerance ■ Prevention of MI.

# atomoxetine
(a-to-**mox**-e-teen)
Strattera

## CLASSIFICATION(S):
*Therapeutic:* agents for attention deficit disorder
*Pharmacologic:* selective nonepinephrine reuptake inhibitors

### Pregnancy Category C

## INDICATIONS
■ Treatment of Attention-Deficit/Hyperactivity Disorder (ADHD).

## ACTION
■ Selectively inhibits the presynaptic transporter of norepinephrine. **Therapeutic Effects:** ■ Increased attention span.

## PHARMACOKINETICS
**Absorption:** Well absorbed following oral administration.
**Distribution:** Unknown.
**Protein Binding:** 98%.
**Metabolism and Excretion:** Mostly metabolized by the liver (CYP2D6 enzyme pathway). A small percentage of the population are poor metabolizers and will have higher blood levels with increased effects).
**Half-life:** 5 hr.

## CONTRAINDICATIONS AND PRECAUTIONS
**Contraindicated in:** ■ Concurrent or within 2 wk therapy with MAO inhibitors ■ Narrow angle glaucoma.
**Use Cautiously in:** ■ Hypertension, tachycardia, cardiovascular or cerebrovascular disease ■ Concurrent albuterol or vasopressors (increases risk of adverse cardiovascular reactions) ■ Pregnancy (use only if benefits out-

weigh risks to fetus) ■ Lactation or children <6 yr (safety not established).

## ADVERSE REACTIONS AND SIDE EFFECTS*

■ **CNS:** dizziness, fatigue, mood swings; *Adults*—insomnia ■ **CV:** hypertension, orthostatic hypotension, tachycardia ■ **GI:** dyspepsia, nausea, vomiting; *Adults*—dry mouth, constipation ■ **Derm:** rash, urticaria ■ **GU:** *Adults*—dysmenorrhea, ejaculatory problems, ↓ libido, impotence, urinary hesitation, urinary retention ■ **Metab:** decreased appetite, weight/growth loss ■ **Misc:** allergic reactions including ANGIONEUROTIC EDEMA

## INTERACTIONS

**Drug-Drug:** ■ Concurrent use with **MAO inhibitors** may result in serious, potentially fatal reactions (do not use within 2 wk of each other) ■ Increased risk of cardiovascular effects with **albuterol** or **vasopressors** (use cautiously) ■ **Drugs which inhibit the CYP2D6 enzyme pathway (quinidine, fluoxetine, paroxetine)** will increase blood levels and effects, dosage ↓ recommended.

## ROUTE AND DOSAGE

■ **PO (Children and adolescents <70 kg):** 0.5 mg/kg/day initially, may be increased every 3 days to a daily target dose of 1.2 mg/kg, given as a single dose in the morning or evenly divided doses in the morning and late afternoon/early evening (not to exceed 1.4 mg/kg/day or 100 mg/day whichever is less). *If taking concurrent CYP2D6 inhibitor (quinidine, fluoxetine, paroxetine)*—0.5 mg/kg/day initially, may increase if needed to 1.2 mg/kg/day after 4 wk.

■ **PO (Adults, adolescents and children >70 kg):** 40 mg/day initially, may be increased every 3 days to a daily target dose of 80 mg/day given as a single dose in the morning or evenly divided doses in the morning and late afternoon/early evening; may be further increased after 2–4 wk up to 100 mg/day. *If taking concurrent CYP2D6 inhibitor (quinidine, fluoxetine, paroxetine)*—40 mg/day initially, may increase if needed to 80 mg/day after 4 wk.

❑ **Hepatic Impairment**

■ **PO (Adults and Children):** *Moderate hepatic impairment (Child-Pugh Class B)*—decrease initial and target dose by 50%; *Severe hepatic impairment (Child-Pugh Class C)*—decrease initial and target dose to 25% of normal.

## AVAILABILITY

■ *Capsules:* 10 mg$^{Rx}$, 18 mg$^{Rx}$, 25 mg$^{Rx}$, 20 mg$^{Rx}$, 60 mg$^{Rx}$.

### TIME/ACTION PROFILE

|    | ONSET | PEAK | DURATION |
|----|-------|------|----------|
| PO | unknown | 1–2 hr | 12–24 hr |

# NURSING IMPLICATIONS

## ASSESSMENT

❑ Assess attention span, impulse control, and interactions with others.

❑ Monitor blood pressure and pulse periodically during therapy.

❑ Monitor growth, body height and weight in children.

## POTENTIAL NURSING DIAGNOSES

■ Thought processes, disturbed (Indications).

■ Social interaction, impaired (Indications).

## IMPLEMENTATION

■ **PO:** Administer without regard to food.

## PATIENT/FAMILY TEACHING

❑ Instruct patient to take medication exactly as directed. Missed doses should be taken as soon as possible, but should not more than the total daily amount in any 24-hr period.

❑ Caution patient to consult health care professional prior to taking other prescription, OTC, dietary supplements, or herbal products.

❑ May cause dizziness. Caution patient to avoid driving or other activities requiring alertness until response to medication is known.

❑ Advise female patients to notify health care professional if pregnancy is planned or suspected or if they are breastfeeding.

❑ Advise parents to notify school nurse of medication regimen.

## EVALUATION

Effectiveness of therapy can be demonstrated by: ■ Improved attention span and social interactions in ADHD.

## atorvastatin, See HMG-CoA REDUCTASE INHIBITORS.

## atropine†

(at-ro-peen)

Atro-Pen

### CLASSIFICATION(S):

**Therapeutic:** *antiarrhythmics*
**Pharmacologic:** *anticholinergics, antimuscarinics*

### Pregnancy Category C

†See Appendix C for ophthalmic use.

### INDICATIONS

■ **IM:** Given preoperatively to decrease oral and respiratory secretions ■ **IV:** Treatment of sinus bradycardia and heart block ■ **PO:** Adjunctive therapy in the management of peptic ulcer and irritable bowel syndrome ■ **IV:** Reversal of adverse muscarinic effects of anticholinesterase agents (neostigmine, physostigmine, or pyridostigmine) ■ **IM, IV:** Treatment of anticholinesterase (organophosphate pesticide) poisoning.

### ACTION

■ Inhibits the action of acetylcholine at postganglionic sites located in: ■ Smooth muscle ■ Secretory glands ■ CNS (antimuscarinic activity) ■ Low doses decrease: ■ Sweating ■ Salivation ■ Respiratory secretions ■ Intermediate doses result in: ■ Mydriasis (pupillary dilation) ■ Cycloplegia (loss of visual accommodation) ■ Increased heart rate ■ GI and GU tract motility are decreased at larger doses. **Therapeutic Effects:** ■ Increased heart rate ■ Decreased GI and respiratory secretions ■ Reversal of muscarinic effects ■ May have a spasmolytic action on the biliary and genitourinary tracts.

### PHARMACOKINETICS

**Absorption:** Well absorbed following oral, subcut, or IM administration.

**Distribution:** Readily crosses the blood-brain barrier. Crosses the placenta and enters breast milk.

**Metabolism and Excretion:** Mostly metabolized by the liver; 30–50% excreted unchanged by the kidneys.

**Half-life:** 13–38 hr.

### CONTRAINDICATIONS AND PRECAUTIONS

**Contraindicated in:** ■ Hypersensitivity ■ Narrow-angle glaucoma ■ Acute hemorrhage ■ Tachycardia secondary to cardiac insufficiency or thyrotoxicosis.

**Use Cautiously in:** ■ Elderly and the very young (increased susceptibility to adverse reactions) ■ Intra-abdominal infections ■ Prostatic hypertrophy ■ Chronic renal, hepatic, pulmonary, or cardiac disease ■ Pregnancy and lactation (safety not established; IV administration may produce fetal tachycardia).

### ADVERSE REACTIONS AND SIDE EFFECTS*

■ **CNS:** drowsiness, confusion ■ **EENT:** blurred vision, cycloplegia, dry eyes, mydriasis ■ **CV:** tachycardia, palpitations ■ **GI:** dry mouth, constipation ■ **GU:** urinary hesitancy, retention ■ **Misc:** decreased sweating.

### INTERACTIONS

**Drug-Drug:** ■ ↑ anticholinergic effects with other **anticholinergics,** including **antihistamines, tricyclic antidepressants, quinidine,** and **disopyramide** ■ Anticholinergics may alter the absorption of other **orally administered drugs** by slowing motility of the GI tract ■ **Antacids** ↓ absorption of anticholinergics ■ May ↑ GI mucosal lesions in patients taking oral **potassium chloride** tablets.

### ROUTE AND DOSAGE

❑ **Preanesthesia (To Decrease Salivation/Secretions)**

■ **PO (Adults):** 2 mg.

■ **IM, IV, Subcut (Adults and Children >20 kg):** 0.4 mg (range 0.2–1 mg) 30–60 min preop.

■ **IM, Subcut (Children ≥20 kg):** 0.4 mg (range 0.2–1 mg) 30–60 min preop.

■ **IM, Subcut (Children 12–16 kg):** 0.3 mg 30–60 min preop.

■ **IM, Subcut (Children 7–9 kg):** 0.2 mg 30–60 min preop.

- **IM, Subcut (Children 3 kg):** 0.1 mg 30–60 min preop.

□ **Bradycardia**

- **IV (Adults):** 0.5–1.0 mg; may repeat as needed q 5 min (q 3–5 min in Advanced Cardiac Life Support guidelines) or 0.4–1 mg q 1–2 hr to a total of 3 mg or 0.04 mg/kg (total vagolytic dose).
- **IV (Children):** 0.01–0.03 mg/kg (range is 0.1–0.5 mg in children or up to 1 mg in adolescents); may repeat q 5 min up to a total dose of 1 mg in children (2 mg in adolescents).
- **Endotracheal: (Children):** use 2–10 times the IV dose.

□ **Reversal of Adverse Muscarinic Effects of Anticholinesterases**

- **IV (Adults):** 0.6–1.2 mg for each 0.5–2.5 mg of neostigmine methylsulfate or 10–20 mg of pyridostigmine bromide concurrently with anticholinesterase.

□ **Organophosphate Poisoning**

- **IM, IV (Adults):** 1–2 mg initially, then 2 mg q 5–60 min as needed. *Severe cases*—2–6 mg initially and repeated every 5–60 min as needed. May be followed by oral therapy. Pralidoxime may be given concurrently.
- **IM, IV (Children):** 0.05 mg/kg q 10–30 min as needed. Pralidoxime may be given concurrently.

□ **Anticholinergic Effects**

- **PO (Adults):** 400 mcg (0.4 mg)–600 mcg (0.6 mg) q 4–6 hr.
- **PO (Children):** 0.01 mg/kg (not to exceed 0.4 mg or 0.3 mg/m²/dose) q 4–6 hr.

**AVAILABILITY (generic available)**

- *Tablets:* 0.4 mg$^{Rx}$ ■ phenobarbital oral solution (Antrocol)$^{Rx}$. See Appendix B.
- *Injection:* 0.05 mg/ml$^{Rx}$, 0.1 mg/ml$^{Rx}$, 0.3 mg/ml$^{Rx}$, 0.4 mg/ml$^{Rx}$, 0.5 mg/ml$^{Rx}$, 0.8 mg/ml$^{Rx}$, 1 mg/ml$^{Rx}$, 2 mg/0.7 ml Auto-injector$^{Rx}$ ■ meperidine$^{Rx}$, neostigmine$^{Rx}$.

TIME/ACTION PROFILE (inhibition of salivation)

|  | ONSET | PEAK | DURATION |
|---|---|---|---|
| PO | 30 min | 30–60 min | 4–6 hr |
| IM, subcut | rapid | 15–50 min | 4–6 hr |
| IV | immediate | 2–4 min | 4–6 hr |

# NURSING IMPLICATIONS

## ASSESSMENT

□ Assess vital signs and ECG tracings frequently during IV drug therapy. Report any significant changes in heart rate or blood pressure, or increased ventricular ectopy or angina to physician promptly.

□ Monitor intake and output ratios in elderly or surgical patients because atropine may cause urinary retention.

□ Assess patients routinely for abdominal distention and auscultate for bowel sounds. If constipation becomes a problem, increasing fluids and adding bulk to the diet may help alleviate constipation.

- *Toxicity and Overdose:* If overdose occurs, physostigmine is the antidote.

## POTENTIAL NURSING DIAGNOSES

- Cardiac output, decreased (Indications).
- Oral mucous membrane, impaired (Side Effects).
- Constipation (Side Effects).

## IMPLEMENTATION

- **PO:** Oral doses of atropine are usually given 30 min before meals.
- **IM:** Intense flushing of the face and trunk may occur 15–20 min following IM administration. In children, this response is called "atropine flush" and is not harmful.
- **Direct IV:** Give IV undiluted or dilute in 10 ml of sterile water.
- *Rate:* Administer at a rate of 0.6 mg over 1 min. Do not add to IV solution. Inject through Y-tubing or 3-way stopcock. When given IV in doses less than 0.4 mg or over more than 1 min, atropine may cause paradoxical bradycardia, which usually resolves in approximately 2 min.
- **Syringe Compatibility:** ◆ butorphanol ◆ chlorpromazine ◆ cimetidine ◆ dimenhydrinate ◆ diphenhydramine ◆ droperidol ◆ fentanyl ◆ glycopyrrolate ◆ heparin ◆ hydromorphone ◆ hydroxyzine ◆ meperidine ◆ metoclopramide ◆ midazolam ◆ milrinone ◆ morphine ◆ nalbuphine ◆ ondansetron ◆ pentazocine ◆ perphenazine ◆ prochlorperazine ◆ promethazine ◆ ranitidine ◆ scopolamine ◆ sufentanil.
- **Y-Site Compatibility:** ◆ etomidate ◆ famotidine ◆ fenatanyl ◆ heparin ◆ hydrocortisone sodium succinate ◆ hydromorphone ◆ inam-

rinone ◆ meropenem ◆ methadone ◆ morphine ◆ nafcillin ◆ potassium chloride ◆ propofol ◆ sufentanil ◆ vitamin B complex with C. ■ **Y-Site Incompatibility:** ◆ thiopental.

### PATIENT/FAMILY TEACHING

❑ Instruct patient to take as directed. Take missed doses as soon as remembered unless almost time for next dose. Do not double doses.

❑ May cause drowsiness. Caution patients to avoid driving or other activities requiring alertness until response to medication is known.

❑ Instruct patient that oral rinses, sugarless gum or candy, and frequent oral hygiene may help relieve dry mouth.

❑ Caution patients that atropine impairs heat regulation. Strenuous activity in a hot environment may cause heat stroke.

❑ Instruct patient to consult health care professional before taking any OTC medications concurrently with atropine.

❑ Inform male patients with benign prostatic hypertrophy that atropine may cause urinary hesitancy and retention. Changes in urinary stream should be reported to health care professional.

### EVALUATION

**Effectiveness of therapy can be demonstrated by:** ■ Increase in heart rate ■ Dryness of mouth ■ Reversal of muscarinic effects.

---

## azathioprine

(ay-za-**thye**-oh-preen)
Azasan, Imuran

### CLASSIFICATION(S):

**Therapeutic:** immunosuppressants
**Pharmacologic:** purine antagonists

### Pregnancy Category D

### INDICATIONS

■ Prevention of renal transplant rejection (with corticosteroids, local radiation, or other cytotoxic agents) ■ Treatment of severe, active, erosive rheumatoid arthritis unresponsive to more conventional therapy. **Unlabeled uses:** ■ Management of Crohn's disease.

### ACTION

■ Antagonizes purine metabolism with subsequent inhibition of DNA and RNA synthesis. **Therapeutic Effects:** ■ Suppression of cell-mediated immunity and altered antibody formation.

### PHARMACOKINETICS

**Absorption:** Readily absorbed after oral administration.

**Distribution:** Crosses the placenta. Enters breast milk in low concentrations.

**Metabolism and Excretion:** Metabolized to mercaptopurine, which is further metabolized. Minimal renal excretion of unchanged drug.

**Half-life:** 3 hr.

### CONTRAINDICATIONS AND PRECAUTIONS

**Contraindicated in:** ■ Hypersensitivity ■ Concurrent use of mycophenolate ■ Pregnancy or lactation.

**Use Cautiously in:** ■ Infections ■ Malignancies ■ Decreased bone marrow reserve ■ Previous or concurrent radiation therapy ■ Other chronic debilitating illnesses ■ Severe renal impairment/oliguria (increased sensitivity) ■ Patients with childbearing potential.

### ADVERSE REACTIONS AND SIDE EFFECTS*

■ **EENT:** retinopathy ■ **Resp:** pulmonary edema ■ **GI:** <u>anorexia</u>, <u>hepatotoxicity</u>, <u>nausea</u>, <u>vomiting</u>, diarrhea, mucositis, pancreatitis ■ **Derm:** alopecia, rash ■ **Hemat:** <u>anemia</u>, <u>leukopenia</u>, <u>pancytopenia</u>, <u>thrombocytopenia</u> ■ **MS:** arthralgia ■ **Misc:** SERUM SICKNESS, <u>chills</u>, <u>fever</u>, Raynaud's phenomenon, retinopathy.

### INTERACTIONS

**Drug-Drug:** ■ Additive myelosuppression with **antineoplastics, cyclosporine,** and **myelosuppressive agents** ■ **Allopurinol** inhibits the metabolism of azathioprine, increasing toxicity. Dosage of azathioprine should be decreased by 25–33% with concurrent allopurinol ■ May decrease antibody response to live-

**virus vaccines** and increase the risk of adverse reactions.

**Drug-Natural Products:** ■ Concommitant use with **echinacea** and **melatonin** may interfere with immunosuppression.

## ROUTE AND DOSAGE

### ❑ Renal Allograft Rejection Prevention

■ **PO, IV (Adults and Children):** 3–5 mg/kg/day initially; maintenance dose 1–3 mg/kg/day.

### ❑ Rheumatoid Arthritis

■ **PO (Adults and Children):** 1 mg/kg/day for 6–8 wk, increase by 0.5 mg/kg/day q 4 wk until response or up to 2.5 mg/kg/day, then decrease by 0.5 mg/kg/day q 4–8 wk to minimal effective dose.

## AVAILABILITY (generic available)

■ *Tablets:* 50 mg$^{Rx}$, 75 mg$^{Rx}$, 100 mg$^{Rx}$ ■ *Injection:* 100-mg vial$^{Rx}$.

TIME/ACTION PROFILE

| | ONSET | PEAK | DURATION |
|---|---|---|---|
| PO (anti-inflammatory) | 6–8 wk | 12 wk | unknown |
| IV (immunosuppression) | days–wks | unknown | days–wks |

## NURSING IMPLICATIONS

### ASSESSMENT

■ **General Info:** Assess for infection (vital signs, sputum, urine, stool, WBC) during therapy.

❑ Monitor intake and output and daily weight. Decreased urine output may lead to toxicity with this medication.

■ **Rheumatoid Arthritis:** Assess range of motion; degree of swelling, pain, and strength in affected joints; and ability to perform activities of daily living before and periodically during therapy.

■ *Lab Test Considerations:* Monitor renal, hepatic, and hematologic functions before beginning therapy, weekly during the 1st mo, bimonthly for the next 2–3 mo, and monthly thereafter.

❑ Leukocyte count of <3000 or platelet count of <100,000/mm$^3$ may necessitate a reduction in dosage or temporary discontinuation.

❑ A ↓ in hemoglobin may indicate bone marrow suppression.

❑ Hepatotoxicity may be manifested by ↑ alkaline phosphatase, bilirubin, AST, ALT, and amylase concentrations. Usually occurs within 6 mo of transplant, rarely with rheumatoid arthritis, and is reversible on discontinuation of azathioprine.

❑ May ↓ serum and urine uric acid and plasma albumin.

## POTENTIAL NURSING DIAGNOSES

■ Infection, risk for (Indications).

## IMPLEMENTATION

■ **General:** Do not confuse Imuran (azathioprine) with IMDUR (isosorbide mononitrate).

❑ Protect transplant patients from staff members and visitors who may carry infection. Maintain protective isolation as indicated.

■ **PO:** May be administered with or after meals or in divided doses to minimize nausea.

■ **IV:** Reconstitute 100 mg with 10 ml of sterile water for injection. Swirl vial gently until completely dissolved. Reconstituted solution may be administered up to 24 hr after preparation.

❑ Solution should be prepared in a biologic cabinet. Wear gloves, gown, and mask while handling medication. Discard equipment in specially designated containers (see Appendix M).

■ **Intermittent Infusion:** Solution may be further diluted in 50 ml of 0.9% NaCl, 0.45% NaCl, or D5W. Do not admix.

■ *Rate:* Usually infused over 30–60 min; may range from 5 min–8 hr.

## PATIENT/FAMILY TEACHING

■ **General Info:** Instruct patient to take azathioprine exactly as directed. If a dose is missed on a once-daily regimen, omit dose; if on several-times-a-day dosing, take as soon as possible or double next dose. Consult health care professional if more than 1 dose is missed or if vomiting occurs shortly after dose is taken. Do not discontinue without consulting health care professional.

❑ Advise patient to report unusual tiredness or weakness; cough or hoarseness; fever or chills; lower back or side pain; painful or difficult urination; severe diarrhea; black, tarry stools; blood in urine; or transplant rejection to health care professional immediately.

◻ Reinforce the need for lifelong therapy to prevent transplant rejection.

◻ Instruct the patient to consult health care professional before taking any OTC medications or natural/herbal products, or receiving any vaccinations while taking this medication.

◻ Advise patient to avoid contact with persons with contagious diseases and persons who have recently taken oral poliovirus vaccine.

◻ This drug may have teratogenic properties. Advise patient to use contraception during and for at least 4 mo after therapy is completed.

◻ Emphasize the importance of follow-up exams and lab tests.

■ **Rheumatoid Arthritis:** Concurrent therapy with salicylates, NSAIDs, or corticosteroids may be necessary. Patient should continue physical therapy and adequate rest. Explain that joint damage will not be reversed; goal is to slow or stop disease process.

### EVALUATION

**Effectiveness of therapy can be demonstrated by:** ■ Prevention of transplant rejection ■ Decreased stiffness, pain, and swelling in affected joints in 6–8 wk in rheumatoid arthritis. Therapy is discontinued if no improvement in 12 wk.

---

## azithromycin
(aye-**zith**-row-my-sin)
Zithromax

### CLASSIFICATION(S):
**Therapeutic:** agents for atypical mycobacterium, anti-infectives
**Pharmacologic:** macrolides

### Pregnancy Category B

### INDICATIONS

■ Treatment of the following infections due to susceptible organisms: ◻ Upper respiratory tract infections, including streptococcal pharyngitis, acute bacterial exacerbations of chronic bronchitis and tonsillitis ◻ Lower respiratory tract infections, including bronchitis and pneumonia ◻ Acute otitis media ◻ Skin and skin structure infections ◻ Nongonococcal urethritis, cervicitis, gonorrhea, and chancroid ■ Prevention of disseminated *Mycobacterium avium* complex (MAC) infection in patients with advanced HIV infection. **Unlabeled uses:** ■ Prevention of bacterial endocarditis.

### ACTION

■ Inhibits protein synthesis at the level of the 50S bacterial ribosome. **Therapeutic Effects:** ■ Bacteriostatic action against susceptible bacteria. **Spectrum:** ■ Active against the following gram-positive aerobic bacteria: ◻ *Staphylococcus aureus* ◻ *Streptococcus pneumoniae* ◻ *Streptococcus pyogenes* (group A strep) ■ Active against these gram-negative aerobic bacteria: ◻ *Haemophilus influenzae* ◻ *Moraxella catarrhalis* ◻ *Neisseria gonorrhoeae* ■ Also active against: ◻ *Mycoplasma* ◻ *Legionella* ◻ *Chlamydia pneumoniae* ◻ *Ureaplasma urealyticum* ◻ *Borrelia burgdorferi* ◻ *M. avium* ■ Not active against methicillin-resistant *S. aureus*.

### PHARMACOKINETICS

**Absorption:** Rapidly absorbed (40%) after oral administration. IV administration results in complete bioavailability.

**Distribution:** Widely distributed to body tissues and fluids. Intracellular and tissue levels exceed those in serum; low CSF levels.

**Metabolism and Excretion:** Mostly excreted unchanged in bile; 4.5% excreted unchanged in urine.

**Half-life:** 11–14 hr after single dose; 2–4 days after several doses.

### CONTRAINDICATIONS AND PRECAUTIONS

**Contraindicated in:** ■ Hypersensitivity to azithromycin, erythromycin, or other macrolide anti-infectives.

**Use Cautiously in:** ■ Severe liver impairment (dosage adjustment may be required) ■ Severe renal impairment (CCr <10 ml/min) ■ Pregnancy, lactation, and children <6 mo (safety not established).

---

{ } = Available in Canada only.
*CAPITALS indicates life-threatening; underlines indicate most frequent.

## ADVERSE REACTIONS AND SIDE EFFECTS*

■ **CNS:** dizziness, drowsiness, fatigue, headache ■ **CV:** chest pain, palpitations ■ **GI:** PSEUDOMEMBRANOUS COLITIS, abdominal pain, diarrhea, nausea, cholestatic jaundice, dyspepsia, flatulence, melena ■ **GU:** nephritis, vaginitis ■ **Derm:** photosensitivity, rashes ■ **Endo:** hyperglycemia ■ **F and E:** hyperkalemia ■ **Misc:** ANGIOEDEMA,

## INTERACTIONS

**Drug-Drug:** ■ **Aluminum-** and **magnesium-containing antacids** decrease peak serum levels ■ **Nelfinavir** increases serum levels (monitor carefully). Similar anti-infectives have been known to increase serum levels and effects of **digoxin, theophylline, ergotamine, dihydroergotamine, triazolam, carbamazepine, cyclosporine,** and **phenytoin**; careful monitoring of concurrent use is recommended.

## ROUTE AND DOSAGE

❑ **Most Respiratory and Skin Infections**

■ **PO (Adults):** 500 mg on 1st day, then 250 mg/day for 4 more days (total dose of 1.5 g).

■ **PO (Children 2–15 yr):** 10 mg/kg (not >500 mg/dose) on 1st day, then 5 mg/kg (not >250 mg/dose) for 4 more days. *Pharyngitis/tonsilitis*—12 mg/kg once daily for 5 days.

❑ **Otitis media**

■ **PO (Children >6 mo):** 30 mg/kg single dose *or* 10 mg/kg/day as a single dose for 3 days *or* 10 mg/kg as a single dose on 1st day, then 5 mg/kg as a single dose daily for 4 more days.

❑ **Acute bacterial exacerbations of chronic bronchitis**

■ **PO (Adults):** 500 mg on 1st day, then 250 mg/day for 4 more days (total dose of 1.5 g) *or* 500 mg daily for 3 days.

❑ **Community-Acquired Pneumonia**

■ **IV, PO (Adults):** *More severe*—500 mg IV q 24 hr for at least 2 doses, then 500 mg PO q 24 hr for a total of 7–10 days; *less severe*—500 mg PO, then 250 mg/day PO for 4 more days.

■ **PO (Children >6 mo):** 10 mg/kg on 1st day, then 5 mg/kg for 4 more days.

❑ **Pelvic Inflammatory Disease**

■ **IV, PO (Adults):** 500 mg IV q 24 hr for 1–2 days, then 250 mg PO q 24 hr for a total of 7 days.

❑ **Endocarditis Prophylaxis**

■ **PO (Adults):** 500 mg 1 hr before procedure.

■ **PO (Children):** 15 mg/kg 1 hr before procedure.

❑ **Nongonococcal Urethritis, Cervicitis, Chancroid, Chlamydia**

■ **PO (Adults):** Single 1-g dose.

❑ **Gonorrhea**

■ **PO (Adults):** Single 2-g dose.

❑ **Prevention of Disseminated MAC Infection**

■ **PO (Adults):** 1.2 g once weekly (alone or with rifabutin).

## AVAILABILITY

■ *Capsules:* 250 mg$^{Rx}$ ■ *Tablets:* 250 mg$^{Rx}$, 500 mg$^{Rx}$, 600 mg$^{Rx}$ ■ *Powder for oral suspension (cherry, creme de vanilla, and banana flavor):* 1 g/pkt$^{Rx}$ ■ *Oral suspension (cherry, creme de vanilla and banana flavor):* 100 mg/5 ml in 15-ml bottles$^{Rx}$, 200 mg/5 ml in 15- and 22.5-ml bottles$^{Rx}$ ■ *Powder for injection:* 500 mg in 10-ml vials$^{Rx}$ ■ Cost: 500 mg $129.28/6 tabs.

TIME/ACTION PROFILE (serum)

| | ONSET | PEAK | DURATION |
|---|---|---|---|
| PO | rapid | 2.5–3.2 hr | 24 hr |
| IV | rapid | end of infusion | 24 hr |

# NURSING IMPLICATIONS

## ASSESSMENT

❑ Assess patient for infection (vital signs; appearance of wound, sputum, urine, and stool; WBC) at beginning of and throughout therapy.

❑ Obtain specimens for culture and sensitivity before initiating therapy. First dose may be given before receiving results.

❑ Observe for signs and symptoms of anaphylaxis (rash, pruritus, laryngeal edema, wheezing). Notify the physician or other health care professional immediately if these occur.

- **Lab Test Considerations:** May cause increased serum bilirubin, AST, ALT, LDH, and alkaline phosphatase concentrations.
- ❏ May cause elevated creatine phosphokinase, potassium, prothrombin time, BUN, serum creatinine, and blood glucose concentrations.
- ❏ May occasionally cause decreased WBC and platelet count.

## POTENTIAL NURSING DIAGNOSES

- Infection, risk for (Indications, Side Effects).
- Noncompliance (Patient/Family Teaching).

## IMPLEMENTATION

- **General:** Do not confuse azithromycin with erythromycin.
- **PO:** Administer 1 hr before or 2 hr after meals.
- ❏ For administration of single 1-g packet, thoroughly mix entire contents of packet with 2 oz (60 ml) of water. Drink entire contents immediately; add an additional 2 oz of water, mix and drink to assure complete consumption of dose. Do not use the single packet to administer doses other than 1000 mg of azithromycin. 1-g packet is not for pediatric use.
- **Intermittent Infusion:** Reconstitute by adding 4.8 ml of sterile water for injection to the 500-mg vial and shake until dissolved, for a concentration of 100 mg/ml. Because azithromycin is supplied under vacuum, standard 5-ml syringe should be used to ensure the exact amount of 4.8 ml of sterile water is dispensed. Do not administer solution containing particulate matter. Dilute further by transferring 5 ml of the 100 mg/ml solution to 250 ml or 500 ml of 0.9% NaCl, 0.45% NaCl, D5W, LR, D5/0.45% NaCl, or D5/LR for a concentration of 2 mg/ml or 1 mg/ml, respectively. Solution is stable for 24 hr at room temperature or for 7 days if refrigerated.
- **Rate:** Administer the 1 mg/ml solution over 3 hr or the 2 mg/ml solution over 1 hr. Do not administer as a bolus.

## PATIENT/FAMILY TEACHING

- ❏ Instruct patients to take medication as directed and to finish the drug completely, even if they are feeling better. Missed doses should be taken as soon as possible unless almost time for next dose; do not double doses. Advise patients that sharing of this medication may be dangerous.
- ❏ Instruct patient not to take azithromycin with food or antacids.
- ❏ May cause drowsiness and dizziness. Caution patient to avoid driving or other activities requiring alertness until response to medication is known.
- ❏ Advise patient to use sunscreen and protective clothing to prevent photosensitivity reactions.
- ❏ Advise patient to report the signs of superinfection (black, furry overgrowth on the tongue; vaginal itching or discharge; loose or foul-smelling stools).
- ❏ Instruct patient to notify health care professional if fever and diarrhea develop, especially if stool contains blood, pus, or mucus. Advise patient not to treat diarrhea without advice of health care professional.
- ❏ Advise patient to notify health care professional if pregnancy is planned or suspected.
- ❏ Advise patients being treated for nongonococcal urethritis or cervicitis that sexual partners should also be treated.
- ❏ Instruct patient to notify health care professional if symptoms do not improve.

## EVALUATION

**Clinical response to therapy can be evaluated by:** ■ Resolution of the signs and symptoms of infection. Length of time for complete resolution depends on the organism and site of infection.

# baclofen

(**bak**-loe-fen)
Lioresal

## CLASSIFICATION(S):

**Therapeutic:** antispasticity agents,
skeletal muscle relaxants (centrally
acting)

**Pregnancy Category C**

## INDICATIONS

■ **PO:** Treatment of reversible spasticity due to
multiple sclerosis or spinal cord lesions ■ **IT:**
Treatment of severe spasticity originating in the
spinal cord. **Unlabeled uses:** ■ Management of
pain in trigeminal neuralgia.

## ACTION

■ Inhibits reflexes at the spinal level. **Therapeutic Effects:** ■ Decreased muscle spasticity;
bowel and bladder function may also be improved.

## PHARMACOKINETICS

**Absorption:** Well absorbed after oral administration.
**Distribution:** Widely distributed; crosses the
placenta.
**Metabolism and Excretion:** 70–80% eliminated unchanged by the kidneys.
**Half-life:** 2.5–4 hr.

## CONTRAINDICATIONS AND PRECAUTIONS

**Contraindicated in:** ■ Hypersensitivity.
**Use Cautiously in:** ■ Patients in whom spasticity maintains posture and balance ■ Patients
with epilepsy (may ↓ seizure threshold) ■ Geriatric patients ( ↑ risk of CNS side effects) ■
Renal impairment ( ↓ dose may be required)
■ Pregnancy, lactation, and children (safety not
established).

## ADVERSE REACTIONS AND SIDE EFFECTS*

■ **CNS:** SEIZURES (IT), <u>dizziness</u>, <u>drowsiness</u>, <u>fa-
tigue</u>, <u>weakness</u>, confusion, depression, headache, insomnia ■ **EENT:** nasal congestion, tinnitus ■ **CV:** edema, hypotension ■ **GI:** <u>nausea</u>,
constipation ■ **GU:** frequency ■ **Derm:** pruritus,
rash ■ **Metab:** hyperglycemia, weight gain ■
**Neuro:** ataxia ■ **Misc:** hypersensitivity reactions, sweating.

## INTERACTIONS

**Drug-Drug:** ■ ↑ CNS depression with other
**CNS depressants** including **alcohol, antihistamines, opioid analgesics,** and **sedative/
hypnotics** ■ Use with **MAO inhibitors** may
lead to ↑ CNS depression or hypotension.
**Drug-Natural Products:** ■ Concomitant use of
**kava, valerian, chamomile,** or **hops** can ↑
CNS depression.

## ROUTE AND DOSAGE

■ **PO (Adults):** 5 mg 3 times daily. May increase q 3 days by 5 mg/dose up to 80 mg/
day (some patients may have a better response to 4 divided doses).
■ **IT (Adults):** 100–800 mcg/day infusion;
dose is determined by response during
screening phase.
■ **IT (Children):** 25–1200 mcg/day infusion
(average 275 mcg/day); dose is determined
by response during screening phase.

## AVAILABILITY (generic available)

■ **Tablets:** 10 mg$^{Rx}$, 20 mg$^{Rx}$ ■ Cost: 10 mg
$8.98/100, 20 mg $16.88/100 ■ **Intrathecal
injection:** 10 mg/20 ml (500 mcg/ml)$^{Rx}$, 10
mg/5 ml (2000 mcg/ml)$^{Rx}$.

TIME/ACTION PROFILE (effects on spasticity)

|    | ONSET | PEAK | DURATION |
|----|-------|------|----------|
| PO | hrs–wks | unknown | unknown |
| IT | 0.5–1 hr | 4 hr | 4–8 hr |

## NURSING IMPLICATIONS

### ASSESSMENT

■ **General Info:** Assess muscle spasticity before and periodically during therapy.
❑ Observe patient for drowsiness, dizziness, or
ataxia. May be alleviated by a change in dose.
■ **IT:** Monitor patient closely during test dose
and titration. Resuscitative equipment should
be immediately available for life-threatening
or intolerable side effects.

■ *Lab Test Considerations:* May cause ↑ in serum glucose, alkaline phosphatase, AST, and ALT levels.

## POTENTIAL NURSING DIAGNOSES

■ Mobility, impaired wheelchair (Indications).

■ Injury, risk for (Adverse Reactions).

## IMPLEMENTATION

■ **PO:** Administer with milk or food to minimize gastric irritation.

■ **IT:** For *screening phase,* dilute for a concentration of 50 mcg/ml with sterile preservative-free NaCl for injection. Test dose should be administered over at least 1 min. Observe patient for a significant decrease in muscle tone or frequency or severity of spasm. If response is inadequate, 2 additional test doses, each 24 hr apart, 75 mcg/1.5 ml and 100 mcg/2 ml respectively, may be administered. Patients with an inadequate response should not receive chronic IT therapy.

❑ Dose titration for implantable IT pumps is based on patient response. If no substantive response after dose increase, check pump function and catheter patency.

## PATIENT/FAMILY TEACHING

❑ Instruct patient to take baclofen as directed. Take a missed dose within 1 hr; do not double doses. Caution patient to avoid abrupt withdrawal of this medication because it may precipitate an acute withdrawal reaction (hallucinations, increased spasticity, seizures, mental changes, restlessness). Baclofen should be discontinued gradually over 2 wk or more.

❑ May cause dizziness and drowsiness. Advise patient to avoid driving or other activities requiring alertness until response to drug is known.

❑ Instruct patient to change positions slowly to minimize orthostatic hypotension.

❑ Advise patient to avoid concurrent use of alcohol or other CNS depressants while taking this medication.

❑ Instruct patient to notify health care professional if frequent urge to urinate or painful urination, constipation, nausea, headache, insomnia, tinnitus, depression, or confusion persists. Advise patient to report signs and symptoms of hypersensitivity (rash, itching) promptly.

■ **IT:** Caution patient and caregiver not to discontinue IT therapy abruptly. May result in fever, mental status changes, exaggerated rebound spasticity, and muscle rigidity. Advise patient not to miss scheduled refill appointments and to notify health care professional promptly if signs of withdrawal occur.

## EVALUATION

**Effectiveness of therapy can be demonstrated by:** ■ Decrease in muscle spasticity and associated musculoskeletal pain with an increased ability to perform activities of daily living ■ Decreased pain in patients with trigeminal neuralgia. May take weeks to obtain optimal effect.

# balsalazide
## (ba-**sal**-a-zide)
Colazal

*CLASSIFICATION(S):*
***Therapeutic:*** *gastrointestinal anti-inflammatories*

**Pregnancy Category B**

## INDICATIONS

■ Treatment of mild to moderately active ulcerative colitis.

## ACTION

■ Drug is metabolized in the colon to mesalamine (5-aminosalicylic acid), which is a local anti-inflammatory. **Therapeutic Effects:** ■ Reduction in the symptoms of ulcerative colitis.

## PHARMACOKINETICS

**Absorption:** Absorption is low and variable; drug is delivered intact to the colon.

**Distribution:** Mostly delivered intact to the colon; remainder of distribution unknown.

**Protein Binding:** ≥99%

**Metabolism and Excretion:** Following delivery to the colon, bacteria break balsalazide down into mesalamine (5-aminosalicylic acid) and an inactive metabolite; mostly excreted in feces.

**Half-life:** *Mesalamine*—12 hr (range 2–15 hr).

## CONTRAINDICATIONS AND PRECAUTIONS

**Contraindicated in:** ■ Hypersensitivity to salicylates or other metabolites.

**Use Cautiously in:** ■ Pyloric stenosis (may have prolonged gastric retention of capsules) ■ Pregnancy (use only if clearly needed) ■ Lactation and children (safety not established).

## ADVERSE REACTIONS AND SIDE EFFECTS*

■ **GI:** abdominal pain, diarrhea.

## INTERACTIONS

**Drug-Drug:** ■ None known.

## ROUTE AND DOSAGE

■ **PO (Adults):** 2.25 g three times daily (three 750 mg capsules three times daily) for 8–12 wks.

## AVAILABILITY

■ *Capsules:* 750 mg$^{Rx}$.

TIME/ACTION PROFILE (decreased symptoms)

|  | ONSET | PEAK | DURATION |
|----|-------|------|----------|
| PO | unknown | up to 8 wk | unknown |

## NURSING IMPLICATIONS

### ASSESSMENT

❑ Assess abdominal pain and frequency, quantity, and consistency of stools at the beginning of and throughout therapy.

❑ Assess patient for allergy to salicylates.

■ *Lab Test Considerations:* May cause elevated AST, ALT, serum alkaline phosphatase, gamma glutamyl transpepsidase (GGT), LDH, and bilirubin.

### POTENTIAL NURSING DIAGNOSES

■ Pain, acute (Indications).

■ Diarrhea (Indications).

### IMPLEMENTATION

■ **PO:** Administer 3 capsules three times a day for 8–12 wks.

## PATIENT/FAMILY TEACHING

❑ Instruct patient on the correct method of administration. Advise patient to take medication as directed, even if feeling better. If a dose is missed, it should be taken as soon as remembered unless almost time for next dose.

❑ Advise patient to notify health care professional if skin rash, difficulty breathing, or hives occur.

❑ Instruct patient to notify health care professional if symptoms do not improve after 1–2 mo of therapy.

## EVALUATION

**Clinical response to therapy can be evaluated by:** ■ Decrease in diarrhea and abdominal pain in patients with ulcerative colitis.

---

# basiliximab

(ba-sil-**ix**-i-mab)
Simulect

### CLASSIFICATION(S):

***Therapeutic:*** immunosuppressants
***Pharmacologic:*** monoclonal antibodies

### Pregnancy Category B

---

## INDICATIONS

■ Prevention of acute organ rejection in patients undergoing renal transplantation; used with corticosteroids and cyclosporine.

## ACTION

■ Binds to and blocks specific interleukin-2 (IL-2) receptor sites on activated T lymphocytes. **Therapeutic Effects:** ■ Prevention of acute organ rejection following renal transplantation.

## PHARMACOKINETICS

**Absorption:** IV administration results in complete bioavailability.

**Distribution:** Unknown.

**Metabolism and Excretion:** Unknown.

**Half-life:** 7.2 days.

## CONTRAINDICATIONS AND PRECAUTIONS

**Contraindicated in:** ■ Hypersensitivity ■ Pregnancy or lactation.
**Use Cautiously in:** ■ Women with childbearing potential ■ Geriatric patients.

## ADVERSE REACTIONS AND SIDE EFFECTS*

Noted for patients receiving corticosteroids and cyclosporine in addition to basiliximab. ■ **CNS:** dizziness, headache, insomnia, weakness ■ **EENT:** abnormal vision, cataracts ■ **Resp:** coughing ■ **CV:** HEART FAILURE, edema, hypertension, angina, arrhythmias, hypotension ■ **GI:** abdominal pain, constipation, diarrhea, dyspepsia, moniliasis, nausea, vomiting, GI bleeding, gingival hyperplasia, stomatitis ■ **Derm:** acne, wound complications, hypertrichosis, pruritus ■ **Endo:** hyperglycemia, hypoglycemia ■ **F and E:** acidosis, hypercholesterolemia, hyperkalemia, hyperuricemia, hypocalcemia, hypokalemia, hypophosphatemia ■ **Hemat:** bleeding, coagulation abnormalities ■ **MS:** back pain, leg pain ■ **Neuro:** tremor, neuropathy, paresthesia ■ **Misc:** hypersensitivity reactions including ANAPHYLAXIS, infection, weight gain, chills.

## INTERACTIONS

**Drug-Drug:** ■ Immunosuppression may be ↑ with other **immunosuppressants**.
**Drug-Natural Products:** ■ Concommitant use with **echinacea** and **melatonin** may interfere with immunosuppression.

## ROUTE AND DOSAGE

■ **IV (Adults and Children ≥35 kg):** 20 mg given 2 hr before transplantation; repeated 4 days after transplantation. Second dose should be withheld if complications or graft loss occurs.
■ **IV (Children <35 kg):** 10 mg given 2 hr before transplantation; repeated 4 days after transplantation. Second dose should be withheld if complications or graft loss occurs.

## AVAILABILITY

■ *Powder for reconstitution:* 20 mg/vial^Rx, 10 mg/vial^Rx.

TIME/ACTION PROFILE (effect on immune function)

| | ONSET | PEAK | DURATION |
|---|---|---|---|
| IV | 2 hr | unknown | 36 days |

## NURSING IMPLICATIONS

### ASSESSMENT

❑ Monitor for signs of anaphylactic or hypersensitivity reactions (hypotension, tachycardia, cardiac failure, dyspnea, wheezing, bronchospasm, pulmonary edema, respiratory failure, urticaria, rash, pruritus, sneezing) at each dose. Onset of symptoms is usually within 24 hr. Resuscitation equipment and medications for treatment of severe hypersensitivity should be readily available. If a severe hypersensitivity reaction occurs, basiliximab therapy should be permanently discontinued. Patients who have previously received basiliximab should only receive subsequent therapy with extreme caution.
❑ Monitor for infection (fever, chills, rash, sore throat, purulent discharge, dysuria). Notify physician immediately if these symptoms occur; may necessitate discontinuation of therapy.
■ *Lab Test Considerations:* May cause ↑ or ↓ hemoglobin, hematocrit, serum glucose, potassium, and calcium concentrations.
❑ May cause ↑ serum cholesterol levels.
❑ May cause ↑ BUN, serum creatinine, and uric acid concentrations.
❑ May cause ↓ serum magnesium, phosphate, and platelet levels.

### POTENTIAL NURSING DIAGNOSES

■ Infection, risk for (Side Effects).

### IMPLEMENTATION

■ **General:** Basiliximab is usually administered concurrently with cyclosporine and corticosteroids.
❑ Reconstitute with 2.5 ml or 5 ml of sterile water for injection for the 10 mg or 20 mg vial, respectively. Shake gently to dissolve powder.
■ **Direct IV:** May be administered undiluted. Bolus administration may be associated with nausea, vomiting, and local reactions (pain).
■ **Intermittent Infusion:** Dilute further with 25 ml or 50 ml of 0.9% NaCl or D5W for the 10 mg or 20 mg vial, respectively. Gently invert bag to mix; do not shake, to avoid foaming. Solution is clear to opalescent and colorless; do not administer solutions that are discolored or contain particulate matter. Discard unused portion. Administer within 4

hr or may be refrigerated for up to 24 hr. Discard after 24 hr.

- **Rate:** Administer over 20–30 min via peripheral or central line.
- **Compatibility:** Do not admix; do not administer in IV line containing other medications.

## PATIENT/FAMILY TEACHING

◘ Explain purpose of medication to patient. Explain that patient will need to resume lifelong therapy with other immunosuppressive drugs after completion of basiliximab course.

◘ May cause dizziness. Caution patient to avoid driving or other activities requiring alertness until response is known.

◘ Instruct patient to continue to avoid crowds and persons with known infections, because basiliximab also suppresses the immune system.

## EVALUATION

**Effectiveness of therapy can be demonstrated by:** ■ Prevention of acute organ rejection in patients receiving renal transplantation.

# beclomethasone, See CORTICOSTEROIDS (INHALATION), CORTICOSTEROIDS (NASAL).

# benazepril, See ANGIOTENSIN-CONVERTING ENZYME (ACE) INHIBITORS.

# benzathine penicillin G, See PENICILLINS.

# benzonatate

(ben-**zoe**-na-tate)

Tessalon

## CLASSIFICATION(S):

**Therapeutic:** allergy, cold, and cough remedies, antitussives (local anesthetic)

## Pregnancy Category C

## INDICATIONS

■ Relief of nonproductive cough due to minor throat or bronchial irritation from inhaled irritants or colds.

## ACTION

■ Anesthetizes cough or stretch receptors in vagal nerve afferent fibers found in lungs, pleura, and respiratory passages. May also decrease transmission of the cough reflex centrally. **Therapeutic Effects:** ■ Decrease in cough.

## PHARMACOKINETICS

**Absorption:** Unknown.
**Distribution:** Unknown.
**Metabolism and Excretion:** Unknown.
**Half-life:** Unknown.

## CONTRAINDICATIONS AND PRECAUTIONS

**Contraindicated in:** ■ Hypersensitivity to benzonatate. Cross-sensitivity with other ester-type local anesthetics (tetracaine, procaine, and others) may occur.
**Use Cautiously in:** ■ Pregnancy, lactation, or children <10 yr (safety not established).

## ADVERSE REACTIONS AND SIDE EFFECTS*

■ **CNS:** headache, mild dizziness, sedation ■ **EENT:** burning sensation in eyes, nasal congestion ■ **GI:** constipation, GI upset, nausea ■ **Derm:** pruritus, skin eruptions ■ **Misc:** chest numbness, chilly sensation, hypersensitivity reactions.

## INTERACTIONS

**Drug-Drug:** ■ Additive CNS depression may occur with **antihistamines, alcohol, opioids,** and **sedative/hypnotics.**

## ROUTE AND DOSAGE

■ **PO (Adults and Children ≥10 yr):** 100 mg 3 times daily (up to 600 mg/day).

## AVAILABILITY (generic available)

■ **Capsules:** 100 mg[Rx] ■ Cost: 100 mg $36.38/100.

TIME/ACTION PROFILE (antitussive effect)

| | ONSET | PEAK | DURATION |
|---|---|---|---|
| PO | 15–20 min | unknown | 3–8 hr |

## NURSING IMPLICATIONS

### ASSESSMENT

❑ Assess frequency and nature of cough, lung sounds, and amount and type of sputum produced. Unless contraindicated, maintain fluid intake of 1500–2000 ml to decrease viscosity of bronchial secretions.

### POTENTIAL NURSING DIAGNOSES

■ Airway clearance, ineffective (Indications).

### IMPLEMENTATION

■ **General:** Capsules should be swallowed whole. Do not chew, because release of benzonatate from capsules may cause local anesthetic effect and choking.

### PATIENT/FAMILY TEACHING

❑ Instruct patient to take exactly as directed. If a dose is missed, take as soon as possible unless almost time for next dose. Do not double doses.

❑ Caution patient not to chew capsules.

❑ Instruct patient to cough effectively: Sit upright and take several deep breaths before attempting to cough.

❑ Advise patient to minimize cough by avoiding irritants, such as cigarette smoke, fumes, and dust. Humidification of environmental air, frequent sips of water, and sugarless hard candy may also decrease the frequency of dry, irritating cough.

❑ Caution patient to avoid taking alcohol or other CNS depressants concurrently with this medication.

❑ May occasionally cause dizziness or drowsiness. Caution patient to avoid driving or other activities requiring alertness until response to the medication is known.

❑ Advise patient that any cough lasting more than 1 wk or accompanied by fever, chest pain, persistent headache, or skin rash warrants medical attention.

❑ Advise patient to notify health care professional if symptoms of overdose (seizures, restlessness, trembling) occur.

## EVALUATION

**Effectiveness of therapy can be demonstrated by:** ■ Decrease in frequency and intensity of cough without eliminating patient's cough reflex.

## benztropine

(benz-troe-peen)
{Apo-Benztropine}, Cogentin

### CLASSIFICATION(S):
**Therapeutic:** antiparkinson agents
**Pharmacologic:** anticholinergics

### Pregnancy Category C

### INDICATIONS

■ Adjunctive treatment of all forms of Parkinson's disease, including drug-induced extrapyramidal effects and acute dystonic reactions.

### ACTION

■ Blocks cholinergic activity in the CNS, which is partially responsible for the symptoms of Parkinson's disease ■ Restores the natural balance of neurotransmitters in the CNS. **Therapeutic Effects:** ■ Reduction of rigidity and tremors.

### PHARMACOKINETICS

**Absorption:** Well absorbed following PO and IM administration.
**Distribution:** Unknown.
**Metabolism and Excretion:** Unknown.
**Half-life:** Unknown.

### CONTRAINDICATIONS AND PRECAUTIONS

**Contraindicated in:** ■ Hypersensitivity ■ Children <3 yr ■ Narrow-angle glaucoma ■ Tardive dyskinesia.
**Use Cautiously in:** ■ Geriatric patients (increased risk of adverse reactions) ■ Prostatic hypertension ■ Seizure disorders ■ Cardiac arrhythmias ■ Pregnancy and lactation (safety not established).

### ADVERSE REACTIONS AND SIDE EFFECTS*

■ **CNS:** confusion, depression, dizziness, hallucinations, headache, sedation, weakness ■ **EENT:** blurred vision, dry eyes, mydriasis ■ **CV:**

arrhythmias, hypotension, palpitations, tachycardia ■ **GI:** <u>constipation</u>, <u>dry mouth</u>, ileus, nausea ■ **GU:** hesitancy, urinary retention ■ **Misc:** decreased sweating.

### INTERACTIONS

**Drug-Drug:** ■ Additive anticholinergic effects with **drugs sharing anticholinergic properties,** such as **antihistamines, phenothiazines, quinidine, disopyramide,** and **tricyclic antidepressants** ■ Counteracts the cholinergic effects of **bethanechol** ■ **Antacids** and **antidiarrheals** may decrease absorption.

**Drug-Natural Products:** ■ Increased anticholinergic effect with **angel's trumpet, jimson weed,** and **scopolia.**

### ROUTE AND DOSAGE

❑ **Parkinsonism**

■ **PO (Adults):** 1–2 mg/day in 1–2 divided doses (range 0.5–6 mg/day).

❑ **Acute Dystonic Reactions**

■ **IM, IV (Adults):** 1–2 mg, then 1–2 mg PO twice daily.

❑ **Drug-Induced Extrapyramidal Reactions**

■ **PO, IM, IV (Adults):** 1–4 mg given once or twice daily (1–2 mg 2–3 times daily may also be used PO).

### AVAILABILITY (generic available)

■ *Tablets:* 0.5 mg$^{Rx}$, 1 mg$^{Rx}$, 2 mg$^{Rx}$ ■ Cost: 0.5 mg $3.92/30, 1 mg $5.24/30, 2 mg $5.36/30 ■ *Injection:* 1 mg/ml$^{Rx}$.

TIME/ACTION PROFILE (antidyskinetic activity)

|        | ONSET      | PEAK        | DURATION |
|--------|------------|-------------|----------|
| PO     | 1–2 hr     | several days | 24 hr   |
| IM, IV | within min | unknown     | 24 hr    |

## NURSING IMPLICATIONS

### ASSESSMENT

■ **General Info:** Assess parkinsonian and extrapyramidal symptoms (restlessness or desire to keep moving, rigidity, tremors, pill rolling, mask-like face, shuffling gait, muscle spasms, twisting motions, difficulty speaking or swallowing, loss of balance control) before and throughout therapy.

❑ Assess bowel function daily. Monitor for constipation, abdominal pain, distention, or absence of bowel sounds.

❑ Monitor intake and output ratios and assess patient for urinary retention (dysuria, distended abdomen, infrequent voiding of small amounts, overflow incontinence).

❑ Patients with mental illness are at risk of developing exaggerated symptoms of their disorder during early therapy with benztropine. Withhold drug and notify physician or other health care professional if significant behavioral changes occur.

■ **IM/IV:** Monitor pulse and blood pressure closely and maintain bedrest for 1 hr after administration. Advise patients to change positions slowly to minimize orthostatic hypotension.

### POTENTIAL NURSING DIAGNOSES

■ Mobility, impaired physical (Indications).

■ Injury, risk for (Indications).

### IMPLEMENTATION

■ **PO:** Administer with food or immediately after meals to minimize gastric irritation. May be crushed and administered with food if patient has difficulty swallowing.

■ **IM:** Parenteral route is used only for dystonic reactions.

■ **Direct IV:** IV route is rarely used because onset is same as with IM route.

■ *Rate:* Administer at a rate of 1 mg over 1 min.

■ **Syringe Compatibility:** ◆ metoclopramide.

■ **Y-Site Compatibility:** ◆ fluconazole ◆ tacrolimus.

### PATIENT/FAMILY TEACHING

❑ Encourage patient to take benztropine as directed. Missed doses should be taken as soon as possible, up to 2 hr before the next dose. Taper gradually when discontinuing or a withdrawal reaction may occur (anxiety, tachycardia, insomnia, return of parkinsonian or extrapyramidal symptoms).

❑ May cause drowsiness or dizziness. Advise patient to avoid driving or other activities that require alertness until response to the drug is known.

❑ Instruct patient that frequent rinsing of mouth, good oral hygiene, and sugarless gum or candy may decrease dry mouth. Patient should notify health care professional if dryness persists (saliva substitutes may be used). Also, notify the dentist if dryness interferes with use of dentures.

❑ Caution patient to change positions slowly to minimize orthostatic hypotension.

❑ Instruct patient to notify health care professional if difficulty with urination, constipation, abdominal discomfort, rapid or pounding heartbeat, confusion, eye pain, or rash occurs.

❑ Advise patient to confer with health care professional before taking OTC medications, especially cold remedies, or drinking alcoholic beverages.

❑ Caution patient that this medication decreases perspiration. Overheating may occur during hot weather. Patient should notify health care professional if unable to remain indoors in an air-conditioned environment during hot weather.

❑ Advise patient to avoid taking antacids or antidiarrheals within 1–2 hr of this medication.

❑ Emphasize the importance of routine follow-up exams.

## EVALUATION

**Effectiveness of therapy can be demonstrated by:** ▪ Decrease in tremors and rigidity and an improvement in gait and balance. Therapeutic effects are usually seen 2–3 days after the initiation of therapy.

## betamethasone, See CORTICOSTEROIDS (SYSTEMIC), CORTICOSTEROIDS (TOPICAL/ LOCAL).

## betaxolol†

(be-**tax**-oh-lol)

Kerlone

*CLASSIFICATION(S):*
*Therapeutic: antihypertensives*

*Pharmacologic: beta blockers*

**Pregnancy Category C**

†See Appendix C for ophthalmic use.

## INDICATIONS

▪ Management of hypertension.

## ACTION

▪ Blocks stimulation of beta$_1$ (myocardial) adrenergic receptors. Does not usually affect beta$_2$ (pulmonary, vascular, uterine) receptor sites. **Therapeutic Effects:** ▪ Decreased blood pressure and heart rate.

## PHARMACOKINETICS

**Absorption:** Well absorbed after oral administration.

**Distribution:** Widely distributed.

**Metabolism and Excretion:** Mostly metabolized by the liver, 20% excreted unchanged by the kidneys.

**Half-life:** 15–20 hr.

## CONTRAINDICATIONS AND PRECAUTIONS

**Contraindicated in:** ▪ Uncompensated CHF ▪ Pulmonary edema ▪ Cardiogenic shock ▪ Bradycardia or heart block.

**Use Cautiously in:** ▪ Renal or hepatic impairment ▪ Geriatric patients (increased sensitivity to beta blockers; initial dosage reduction recommended) ▪ Pulmonary disease (including asthma; beta$_1$ selectivity may be lost at higher doses); avoid use if possible ▪ Diabetes mellitus ▪ Thyrotoxicosis ▪ Patients with a history of severe allergic reactions (intensity of reactions may be increased) ▪ Pregnancy, lactation, or children (safety not established; all agents cross the placenta and may cause fetal/neonatal bradycardia, hypotension, hypoglycemia, or respiratory depression).

## ADVERSE REACTIONS AND SIDE EFFECTS*

▪ **CNS:** fatigue, weakness, anxiety, depression, dizziness, drowsiness, insomnia, memory loss, mental status changes, nightmares ▪ **EENT:** blurred vision, stuffy nose ▪ **Resp:** bronchospasm, wheezing ▪ **CV:** BRADYCARDIA, CHF, PULMONARY EDEMA, hypotension, peripheral vasoconstriction ▪ **GI:** constipation, diarrhea, liver function abnormalities, nausea, vomiting ▪ **GU:** impotence, decreased libido, urinary frequency ▪

**Derm:** rashes ■ **Endo:** hyperglycemia, hypoglycemia ■ **MS:** arthralgia, back pain, joint pain ■ **Misc:** drug-induced lupus syndrome.

## INTERACTIONS

**Drug-Drug:** ■ **General anesthetics, IV phenytoin,** and **verapamil** may cause additive myocardial depression ■ Additive bradycardia may occur with **digoxin** ■ Additive hypotension may occur with other **antihypertensives,** acute ingestion of **alcohol,** or **nitrates** ■ Concurrent use with **amphetamine, cocaine, ephedrine, epinephrine, norepinephrine, phenylephrine,** or **pseudoephedrine** may result in unopposed alpha-adrenergic stimulation (excessive hypertension, bradycardia) ■ Concurrent **thyroid preparation** administration may decrease effectiveness ■ May alter the effectiveness of **insulins** or **oral hypoglycemic agents** (dosage adjustments may be necessary) ■ May decrease the effectiveness of **theophylline** ■ May decrease the beneficial beta₁-cardiovascular effects of **dopamine** or **dobutamine** ■ Use cautiously within 14 days of **MAO inhibitor** therapy (may result in hypertension).

## ROUTE AND DOSAGE

■ **PO (Adults):** 10 mg once daily, may be increased to 20 mg after 7 days; start with 5 mg in geriatric patients.

❑ **Renal Impairment**
■ **PO (Adults):** start with 5 mg once daily.

## AVAILABILITY

■ *Tablets:* 10 mg^Rx, 20 mg^Rx ■ Cost: 10 mg $82.63/100, 20 mg $123.95/100.

TIME/ACTION PROFILE (antihypertensive effect)

| | ONSET | PEAK | DURATION |
|---|---|---|---|
| PO | 3–4 hr | 3–4 hr | 24 hr |

## NURSING IMPLICATIONS

### ASSESSMENT

❑ Monitor blood pressure, ECG, and pulse frequently during dose adjustment and periodically during therapy.

❑ Monitor intake and output ratios and daily weights. Assess routinely for signs and symptoms of congestive heart failure (dyspnea, rales/crackles, weight gain, peripheral edema, jugular venous distention).

■ **Angina:** Assess frequency and characteristics of angina periodically during therapy.

■ *Lab Test Considerations:* May cause increased BUN, serum lipoprotein, potassium, triglyceride, and uric acid levels.

❑ May cause increased ANA titers.

❑ May cause increase in blood glucose levels.

■ *Toxicity and Overdose:* Monitor patients receiving beta blockers for signs of overdose (bradycardia, severe dizziness or fainting, severe drowsiness, dyspnea, bluish fingernails or palms, seizures). Notify physician or health care professional immediately if these signs occur.

❑ Glucagon has been used to treat bradycardia and hypotension.

### POTENTIAL NURSING DIAGNOSES

■ Cardiac output, decreased (Side Effects).

■ Noncompliance (Patient/Family Teaching).

### IMPLEMENTATION

■ **PO:** Take apical pulse before administering. If <50 bpm or if arrhythmia occurs, withhold medication and notify physician or other health care professional.

❑ May be administered without regard to food.

### PATIENT/FAMILY TEACHING

■ **General Info:** Instruct patient to take medication exactly as directed, at the same time each day, even if feeling well; do not skip or double up on missed doses. Take missed doses as soon as possible up to 4 hr before next dose. Abrupt withdrawal may precipitate life-threatening arrhythmias, hypertension, or myocardial ischemia.

❑ Advise patient to make sure enough medication is available for weekends, holidays, and vacations. A written prescription may be kept in wallet in case of emergency.

❑ Teach patient and family how to check pulse and blood pressure. Instruct them to check pulse daily and blood pressure biweekly and to report significant changes.

❏ May cause drowsiness or dizziness. Caution patients to avoid driving or other activities that require alertness until response to the drug is known.

❏ Advise patients to change positions slowly to minimize orthostatic hypotension.

❏ Caution patient that this medication may increase sensitivity to cold.

❏ Instruct patient to consult health care professional before taking any OTC medications, especially cold preparations, concurrently with this medication.

❏ Patients with diabetes should closely monitor blood glucose, especially if weakness, malaise, irritability, or fatigue occurs. Betaxolol may mask some signs of hypoglycemia, but sweating and dizziness may occur.

❏ Advise patient to notify health care professional if slow pulse, difficulty breathing, wheezing, cold hands and feet, dizziness, confusion, depression, rash, fever, sore throat, unusual bleeding, or bruising occurs.

❏ Instruct patient to inform health care professional of medication regimen before treatment or surgery.

❏ Advise patient to carry identification describing disease process and medication regimen at all times.

■ **Hypertension:** Reinforce the need to continue additional therapies for hypertension (weight loss, sodium restriction, stress reduction, regular exercise, moderation of alcohol consumption, and smoking cessation). Medication controls but does not cure hypertension.

## EVALUATION

**Effectiveness of therapy can be demonstrated by:** ■ Decrease in blood pressure without appearance of detrimental side effects.

---

# bethanechol
(be-**than**-e-kole)
Duvoid, Urabeth, Urecholine

### CLASSIFICATION(S):
**Therapeutic:** urinary tract stimulants
**Pharmacologic:** cholinergics

**Pregnancy Category C**

## INDICATIONS
■ Postpartum and postoperative nonobstructive urinary retention or urinary retention caused by neurogenic bladder.

## ACTION
■ Stimulates cholinergic receptors. Effects include: ■ Contraction of the urinary bladder ■ Decreased bladder capacity ■ Increased frequency of ureteral peristaltic waves ■ Increased tone and peristalsis in the GI tract ■ Increased pressure in the lower esophageal sphincter ■ Increased gastric secretions. **Therapeutic Effects:** ■ Bladder emptying.

## PHARMACOKINETICS
**Absorption:** Poorly absorbed after oral administration, requiring larger doses by mouth than subcutaneously.

**Distribution:** Does not cross the blood-brain barrier.

**Metabolism and Excretion:** Unknown.

**Half-life:** Unknown.

## CONTRAINDICATIONS AND PRECAUTIONS
**Contraindicated in:** ■ Hypersensitivity ■ Mechanical obstruction of the GI or GU tract.

**Use Cautiously in:** ■ History of asthma ■ Ulcer disease ■ Cardiovascular disease ■ Epilepsy ■ Hyperthyroidism ■ Sensitivity to cholinergic agents or effects ■ Children, pregnancy, and lactation (safety not established).

## ADVERSE REACTIONS AND SIDE EFFECTS*
■ **CNS:** headache, malaise ■ **EENT:** lacrimation, miosis ■ **Resp:** bronchospasm ■ **CV:** HEART BLOCK, SYNCOPE/CARDIAC ARREST, bradycardia, hypotension ■ **GI:** abdominal discomfort, diarrhea, nausea, salivation, vomiting ■ **GU:** urgency ■ **Misc:** flushing, sweating, hypothermia.

## INTERACTIONS
**Drug-Drug:** ■ **Quinidine** and **procainamide** may antagonize cholinergic effects ■ Additive cholinergic effects with **cholinesterase inhibitors** ■ Use with **ganglionic blocking agents** may result in severe hypotension ■ Do not use with **depolarizing neuromuscular blocking agents** ■ Effectiveness will be decreased by **anticholinergics**.

**Drug-Natural Products:** ■ Cholinergic effects may be antagonized by **angel's trumpet, jimson weed**, or **scopolia**.

## ROUTE AND DOSAGE

■ **PO (Adults):** 25–50 mg 3 times daily. Dose may be determined by administering 5–10 mg q 1–2 hr until response is obtained or total of 50 mg administered *or* by starting with 10 mg, giving 25 mg 6 hr later, then, if needed, 50 mg 6 hr later.
■ **PO (Children):** 0.2 mg/kg 3 times daily or 0.15 mg/kg 4 times daily.
■ **Subcut (Adults):** 5 mg 3–4 times daily. Dose may be determined by administering 2.5 mg q 15–30 min until response is obtained or total of 4 doses administered.
■ **Subcut (Children):** 0.06 mg/kg 3 times daily or 0.05 mg/kg 4 times daily.

## AVAILABILITY (generic available)

■ *Tablets:* 5 mg$^{Rx}$, 10 mg$^{Rx}$, 25 mg$^{Rx}$, 50 mg$^{Rx}$
■ Cost: 5 mg $2.75/100, 10 mg $2.95/100, 25 mg $3.95/100, 50 mg $7.25/100 ■ *Injection:* 5 mg/ml$^{Rx}$.

TIME/ACTION PROFILE (response on bladder muscle)

|        | ONSET      | PEAK      | DURATION |
| ------ | ---------- | --------- | -------- |
| PO     | 30–90 min  | 1 hr      | 6 hr     |
| Subcut | 5–15 min   | 15–30 min | 2 hr     |

## NURSING IMPLICATIONS

### ASSESSMENT

❑ Monitor blood pressure, pulse, and respirations before administering and for at least 1 hr after subcut administration.
❑ Monitor intake and output ratios. Palpate abdomen for bladder distention. Notify physician or other health care professional if drug fails to relieve condition for which it was prescribed. Catheterization may be ordered to assess postvoid residual.
■ *Lab Test Considerations:* May cause an increase in serum AST, amylase, and lipase concentrations.
■ *Toxicity and Overdose:* Observe patient for drug toxicity (sweating, flushing, abdominal cramps, nausea, salivation). If overdosage occurs, treatment includes atropine sulfate (specific antidote).

## POTENTIAL NURSING DIAGNOSES

■ Urinary elimination, impaired (Indications).

## IMPLEMENTATION

■ **General:** A test dose is usually employed before maintenance to determine minimum effective dose.
❑ Oral and subcut doses are *not* interchangeable.
■ **PO:** Administer medication on an empty stomach, 1 hr before or 2 hr after meals, to prevent nausea and vomiting.
■ **Subcut:** Parenteral solution is intended only for subcutadministration. Do not give IM or IV. Inadvertent IM or IV administration may cause cholinergic overstimulation (circulatory collapse, drop in blood pressure, abdominal cramps, bloody diarrhea, shock, and cardiac arrest).
❑ Do not use if solution is discolored or contains a precipitate.

## PATIENT/FAMILY TEACHING

❑ Instruct patient to take medication exactly as directed. Missed doses should be taken as soon as possible within 2 hr; otherwise, return to regular dosing schedule. Do not double doses.
❑ Caution patient to change positions slowly to minimize orthostatic hypotension.
❑ Advise patient to report abdominal discomfort, salivation, sweating, or flushing to health care professional.

## EVALUATION

**Effectiveness of therapy can be demonstrated by:** ■ Increase in bladder function and tone.

## bicalutamide

(bye-ka-**loot**-a-mide)
Casodex

*CLASSIFICATION(S):*
*Therapeutic:* antineoplastics

---

{ } = Available in Canada only.
*CAPITALS indicates life-threatening; underlines indicate most frequent.

*Pharmacologic: antiandrogens*

**Pregnancy Category X**

## INDICATIONS

■ Treatment of metastatic prostate carcinoma in conjunction with luteinizing hormone–releasing hormone (LHRH) analogues (goserelin, leuprolide).

## ACTION

■ Antagonizes the effects of androgen at the cellular level. **Therapeutic Effects:** ■ Decreased spread of prostate carcinoma.

## PHARMACOKINETICS

**Absorption:** Well absorbed after oral administration.

**Distribution:** Unknown.

**Protein Binding:** 96%.

**Metabolism and Excretion:** Mostly metabolized by the liver.

**Half-life:** 5.8 days.

## CONTRAINDICATIONS AND PRECAUTIONS

**Contraindicated in:** ■ Hypersensitivity ■ Pregnancy.

**Use Cautiously in:** ■ Moderate to severe liver impairment ■ Patients with childbearing potential ■ Lactation and children (safety not established).

## ADVERSE REACTIONS AND SIDE EFFECTS*

■ **CNS:** weakness, dizziness, headache, insomnia ■ **Resp:** dyspnea ■ **CV:** chest pain, hypertension, peripheral edema ■ **GI:** constipation, diarrhea, nausea, abdominal pain, increased liver enzymes, vomiting ■ **GU:** hematuria, impotence, incontinence, nocturia, urinary tract infections ■ **Derm:** alopecia, rashes, sweating ■ **Endo:** breast pain, gynecomastia ■ **Hemat:** anemia ■ **Metab:** hyperglycemia, weight loss ■ **MS:** back pain, pelvic pain, bone pain ■ **Neuro:** paresthesia ■ **Misc:** generalized pain, hot flashes, flu-like syndrome, infection.

## INTERACTIONS

**Drug-Drug:** ■ May increase the effect of **warfarin**.

## ROUTE AND DOSAGE

■ **PO (Adults):** 50 mg once daily (must be given concurrently with LHRH analogue or following surgical castration).

## AVAILABILITY

■ *Tablets:* 50 mg$^{Rx}$.

TIME/ACTION PROFILE (blood levels)

| | ONSET | PEAK | DURATION |
|---|---|---|---|
| PO | unknown | 31.3 hr | unknown |

# NURSING IMPLICATIONS

## ASSESSMENT

❑ Assess patient for adverse GI effects. Diarrhea is the most common cause of discontinuation of therapy.

■ *Lab Test Considerations:* Monitor serum prostate-specific antigen (PSA) periodically to determine response to therapy. If levels rise, assess patient for disease progression. May require periodic LHRH analogue administration without bicalutamide.

❑ Monitor liver function tests before and periodically during therapy. May cause elevated serum alkaline phosphatase, AST, ALT, and bilirubin concentrations. If transaminases increase >2 times normal, bicalutamide should be discontinued; levels usually return to normal after discontinuation.

❑ May cause increased BUN and serum creatinine, and decreased hemoglobin and WBCs.

## POTENTIAL NURSING DIAGNOSES

■ Diarrhea (Adverse Reactions).

## IMPLEMENTATION

■ **General:** Start treatment with bicalutamide at the same time as LHRH analogue.

■ **PO:** May be administered in the morning or evening, without regard to food.

## PATIENT/FAMILY TEACHING

❑ Instruct patient to take bicalutamide exactly as directed at the same time each day. Do not discontinue without consulting health care professional.

❑ Advise patient not to take other medications without consulting health care professional.

❑ Instruct patient to report severe or persistent diarrhea.

❏ Discuss with patient the possibility of hair loss. Explore methods of coping.

❏ Emphasize the importance of regular follow-up exams and blood tests to determine progress; monitor for side effects.

## EVALUATION

**Effectiveness of therapy can be demonstrated by:** ■ Decreased spread of prostate carcinoma.

## biperiden
(by-**per**-i-den)
Akineton

### CLASSIFICATION(S):
**Therapeutic:** antiparkinson agents
**Pharmacologic:** anticholinergics

### Pregnancy Category C

## INDICATIONS

■ Adjunctive treatment of all forms of Parkinson's disease, including drug-induced extrapyramidal effects and acute dystonic reactions.

## ACTION

■ Blocks cholinergic activity in the CNS, which is partially responsible for the symptoms of Parkinson's disease ■ Restores the natural balance of neurotransmitters in the CNS. **Therapeutic Effects:** ■ Reduction of rigidity and tremors.

## PHARMACOKINETICS

**Absorption:** Well absorbed after oral or IM administration.
**Distribution:** Unknown.
**Metabolism and Excretion:** Unknown.
**Half-life:** Unknown.

## CONTRAINDICATIONS AND PRECAUTIONS

**Contraindicated in:** ■ Hypersensitivity ■ Narrow-angle glaucoma ■ Bowel obstruction ■ Megacolon ■ Tardive dyskinesia.
**Use Cautiously in:** ■ Geriatric patients (increased risk of adverse reactions; lower doses may be necessary) ■ Prostatic enlargement ■

Seizure disorders ■ Cardiac arrhythmias ■ Pregnancy and lactation (safety not established).

## ADVERSE REACTIONS AND SIDE EFFECTS*

■ **CNS:** confusion, depression, dizziness, hallucinations, headache, sedation, weakness ■ **EENT:** blurred vision, dry eyes, mydriasis ■ **CV:** arrhythmias, hypotension, palpitations, tachycardia ■ **GI:** constipation, dry mouth, ileus, nausea ■ **GU:** hesitancy, urinary retention ■ **Misc:** decreased sweating.

## INTERACTIONS

**Drug-Drug:** ■ Additive anticholinergic effects with **drugs sharing anticholinergic properties,** such as **antihistamines, phenothiazines, quinidine, disopyramide,** and **tricyclic antidepressants** ■ Counteracts the cholinergic effects of **bethanechol** ■ **Antacids** or **antidiarrheals** may decrease absorption.
**Drug-Natural Products:** ■ Increased anticholinergic effects with **angel's trumpet** and **jimson weed** and **scopolia.**

## ROUTE AND DOSAGE

❏ **Parkinsonism**
■ **PO (Adults):** 2 mg 3–4 times daily initially (not to exceed 16 mg/day).
❏ **Extrapyramidal Reactions**
■ **PO (Adults):** 2 mg 1–3 times daily.
■ **IM, IV (Adults):** 2 mg, may repeat q 30 min (not to exceed 8 mg or 4 doses/24 hr).
■ **IM (Children):** 40 mcg (0.04 mg)/kg or 1.2 mg/m$^2$, may repeat q 30 min (not to exceed 4 doses/24 hr).

## AVAILABILITY

■ **Tablets:** 2 mg$^{Rx}$ ■ Cost: $29.76/100 ■ **Injection:** 5 mg/ml$^{Rx}$.

TIME/ACTION PROFILE (relief of symptoms)

| | ONSET | PEAK | DURATION |
|---|---|---|---|
| PO | unknown | unknown | unknown |
| IM | 10–30 min | unknown | unknown |
| IV | unknown | unknown | 1–8 hr |

{ } = Available in Canada only.
*CAPITALS indicates life-threatening; underlines indicate most frequent.

## NURSING IMPLICATIONS

### ASSESSMENT

- Assess parkinsonian and extrapyramidal symptoms (restlessness or desire to keep moving, rigidity, tremors, pill rolling, mask-like face, shuffling gait, muscle spasms, twisting motions, difficulty speaking or swallowing, loss of balance control) before and throughout therapy.
- Assess bowel function daily. Monitor for constipation, abdominal pain, distention, or the absence of bowel sounds.
- Monitor intake and output ratios and assess patient for urinary retention (dysuria, distended abdomen, infrequent voiding of small amounts, overflow incontinence).
- After parenteral administration, monitor pulse and blood pressure closely and maintain bed- rest for 1 hr. Advise patients to change positions slowly to minimize orthostatic hypotension.
- Patients with mental illness are at risk of developing exaggerated symptoms of their disorder during early therapy with this medication. Withhold drug and notify physician or other health care professional if significant behavioral changes occur.

### POTENTIAL NURSING DIAGNOSES

- Mobility, impaired physical (Indications).

### IMPLEMENTATION

- **PO:** Administer with food or immediately after meals to minimize gastric irritation.
- **Direct IV:** Administer each dose over at least 1 min to minimize hypotension and mild bradycardia.

### PATIENT/FAMILY TEACHING

- Advise patient to take medication exactly as directed. Missed doses should be taken as soon as possible up to 2 hr before the next dose. Drug should be tapered gradually when discontinuing or a withdrawal reaction may occur (anxiety, tachycardia, insomnia, return of parkinsonian or extrapyramidal symptoms).
- May cause drowsiness, dizziness, or blurred vision. Advise patient to avoid driving or other activities that require alertness until response to the drug is known.
- Caution patient to change positions slowly to minimize orthostatic hypotension.
- Advise patient that frequent mouth rinses, good oral hygiene, and sugarless gum or candy may decrease dry mouth. Patient should notify health care professional if dry mouth persists (saliva substitutes may be used). Also notify the dentist if dry mouth interferes with use of dentures.
- Instruct patient to notify health care professional if difficulty with urination, constipation, abdominal discomfort, rapid or pounding heartbeat, confusion, eye pain, or rash occurs.
- Advise patient to confer with health care professional before taking OTC medications, especially cold remedies, or drinking alcoholic beverages.
- Caution patient that this medication decreases perspiration. Overheating may occur during hot weather. Patients should notify health care professional if they cannot remain indoors in an air-conditioned environment during hot weather.
- Advise patient to avoid antacids or antidiarrheals within 1–2 hr of this medication.
- Emphasize the importance of routine follow-up exams.

### EVALUATION

**Effectiveness of therapy can be demonstrated by:** ▪ Decrease in tremors and rigidity and an improvement in gait and balance in Parkinson's disease ▪ Resolution of drug-induced extrapyramidal reactions.

---

## bisacodyl
(bis-a-**koe**-dill)
Bisac-Evac, {Bisaco-Lax}, {Bisacolax}, Caroid, Carter's Little Pills, Dacodyl, Deficol, Dulcagen, Dulcolax, Feen-a-Mint, Fleet Laxative, {Laxit}, Modane, Reliable Gentle Laxative, Theralax, Women's Gentle Laxative

### CLASSIFICATION(S):
**Therapeutic:** laxatives
**Pharmacologic:** stimulant laxatives

**Pregnancy Category UK**

## INDICATIONS

■ Treatment of constipation ■ Evacuation of the bowel before radiologic studies or surgery ■ Part of a bowel regimen in spinal cord injury patients.

## ACTION

■ Stimulates peristalsis ■ Alters fluid and electrolyte transport, producing fluid accumulation in the colon. **Therapeutic Effects:** ■ Evacuation of the colon.

## PHARMACOKINETICS

**Absorption:** Variable absorption follows oral administration; rectal absorption is minimal; action is local in the colon.

**Distribution:** Small amounts of metabolites excreted in breast milk.

**Metabolism and Excretion:** Small amounts absorbed are metabolized by the liver.

**Half-life:** Unknown.

## CONTRAINDICATIONS AND PRECAUTIONS

**Contraindicated in:** ■ Hypersensitivity ■ Abdominal pain ■ Obstruction ■ Nausea or vomiting (especially with fever or other signs of an acute abdomen).

**Use Cautiously in:** ■ Severe cardiovascular disease ■ Anal or rectal fissures ■ Excess or prolonged use (may result in dependence) ■ Products containing tannic acid (Clysodrast) should not be used as multiple enemas (increased risk of hepatotoxicity) ■ May be used during pregnancy and lactation.

## ADVERSE REACTIONS AND SIDE EFFECTS*

■ **GI:** <u>abdominal cramps</u>, nausea, diarrhea, rectal burning ■ **F and E:** hypokalemia (with chronic use) ■ **MS:** muscle weakness (with chronic use) ■ **Misc:** protein-losing enteropathy, tetany (with chronic use).

## INTERACTIONS

**Drug-Drug:** ■ **Antacids, histamine H$_2$-receptor agonists,** and **gastric acid–pump inhibitors** may remove enteric coating of tablets resulting in gastric irritation/dyspepsia ■ May decrease the absorption of other **orally ad-**ministered drugs because of increased motility and decreased transit time.

**Drug-Food:** ■ **Milk** may remove enteric coating of tablets, resulting in gastric irritation/dyspepsia.

## ROUTE AND DOSAGE

■ **PO (Adults and Children ≥12 yr):** 5–15 mg (up to 30 mg/day) as a single dose.
■ **PO (Children 3–11 yr):** 5–10 mg (0.3 mg/kg) as a single dose.
■ **Rect (Adults and Children ≥12 yr):** 10 mg single dose.
■ **Rect (Children 2–11 yr):** 5–10 mg single dose.
■ **Rect (Children <2 yr):** 5 mg single dose.

## AVAILABILITY (generic available)

■ *Enteric-coated tablets:* 5 mg$^{OTC}$ ■ *Enteric coated and delayed release:* 5 mg$^{OTC}$ ■ *Suppositories:* 5 mg$^{OTC}$, 10 mg$^{OTC}$ ■ *Rectal suspension:* 10 mg/30 ml$^{OTC}$ ■ tannic acid (Clysodrast$^{OTC}$), docusate (Dulcodos$^{OTC}$), hydroxypropyl methylcellulose (Fleet Bisacodyl Prep$^{OTC}$). Also in Bowel Preparation kits with Magnesium citrate (Evac-Q-Kwik$^{OTC}$, EZ-EM Prep Kit$^{OTC}$, LiquiPrep Bowel Evacuant$^{OTC}$, Tridate Bowel Cleansing Kit$^{OTC}$), Phosphate/biphosphate (Fleet Prep Kit. No. 1$^{OTC}$, Fleet Prep Kit No.2$^{OTC}$, Fleet Prep Kit No.3$^{OTC}$), sennosides (X-Prep Bowel Evacuant Kit #1$^{OTC}$), sennosides, magnesium citrate. magnesium sulfate (X-Prep Bowel Evacuant Kit #2$^{OTC}$). See Appendix B.

TIME/ACTION PROFILE (evacuation of bowel)

|        | ONSET      | PEAK    | DURATION |
|--------|------------|---------|----------|
| PO     | 6–12 hr    | unknown | unknown  |
| Rectal | 15–60 min  | unknown | unknown  |

# NURSING IMPLICATIONS

## ASSESSMENT

■ **General Info:** Assess patient for abdominal distention, presence of bowel sounds, and usual pattern of bowel function.
❑ Assess color, consistency, and amount of stool produced.

---

{ } = Available in Canada only.
*CAPITALS indicates life-threatening; <u>underlines</u> indicate most frequent.

## POTENTIAL NURSING DIAGNOSES

- Constipation (Indications).

## IMPLEMENTATION

- **General:** May be administered at bedtime for morning results.
- **PO:** Taking on an empty stomach will produce more rapid results.
  - Do not crush or chew enteric-coated tablets. Take with a full glass of water or juice.
  - Do not administer oral doses within 1 hr of milk or antacids; this may lead to premature dissolution of tablet and gastric or duodenal irritation.
- **Rect:** Suppository or enema can be given at the time a bowel movement is desired. Lubricate suppositories with water or water-soluble lubricant before insertion. Encourage patient to retain the suppository or enema 15–30 min before expelling.

## PATIENT/FAMILY TEACHING

- Advise patients, other than those with spinal cord injuries, that laxatives should be used only for short-term therapy. Prolonged therapy may cause electrolyte imbalance and dependence.
- Advise patient to increase fluid intake to at least 1500–2000 ml/day during therapy to prevent dehydration.
- Encourage patients to use other forms of bowel regulation (increasing bulk in the diet, increasing fluid intake, or increasing mobility). Normal bowel habits may vary from 3 times/day to 3 times/wk.
- Instruct patients with cardiac disease to avoid straining during bowel movements (Valsalva maneuver).
- Advise patient that bisacodyl should not be used when constipation is accompanied by abdominal pain, fever, nausea, or vomiting.

## EVALUATION

**Effectiveness of therapy can be demonstrated by:** ■ The patient's having a soft, formed bowel movement when used for constipation ■ Evacuation of colon before surgery or radiologic studies, or for patients with spinal cord injury.

---

## bismuth subsalicylate
**(biz**-muth sub-sa-**lis**-i-late)

Bismatrol, Bismed, Kaopectate, Pepto-Bismol, Pink Bismuth, {PMS-Bismuth Subsalicylate}

### CLASSIFICATION(S):
**Therapeutic:** *antidiarrheals, antiulcer agents*
**Pharmacologic:** *adsorbents*

### Pregnancy Category C

## INDICATIONS

■ Mild to moderate diarrhea ■ Nausea, abdominal cramping, heartburn, and indigestion that may accompany diarrheal illnesses ■ Treatment of ulcer disease associated with *Helicobacter pylori* (with anti-infectives). **Unlabeled uses:** ■ Treatment/ prevention of traveler's (enterotoxigenic *Escherichia coli*) diarrhea ■ Chronic infantile diarrhea.

## ACTION

■ Promotes intestinal adsorption of fluids and electrolytes ■ Decreases synthesis of intestinal prostaglandins. **Therapeutic Effects:** ■ Relief of diarrhea ■ Erradication of *h. pylori* with decreased recurrence of ulcer disease (with other agents).

## PHARMACOKINETICS

**Absorption:** Bismuth is not absorbed; salicylate split from parent compound is >90% absorbed from the small intestine. Salicylate is highly bound to albumin.

**Distribution:** Salicylate crosses the placenta and enters breast milk.

**Metabolism and Excretion:** Bismuth is excreted unchanged in the feces. Salicylate undergoes extensive hepatic metabolism.

**Half-life:** Salicylate—2–3 hr for low doses; 15–30 hr with larger doses.

## CONTRAINDICATIONS AND PRECAUTIONS

**Contraindicated in:** ■ Geriatric patients who may have fecal impaction ■ Children or teenagers during or after recovery from chickenpox or flu-like illness (contains salicylate) ■ Aspirin hypersensitivity; cross-sensitivity with NSAIDs or oil of wintergreen may occur.

**Use Cautiously in:** ■ Infants, geriatric or debilitated patients (impaction may occur) ■ Patients undergoing radiologic examination of the GI tract (bismuth is radiopaque) ■ Diabetes mellitus ■ Gout ■ Pregnancy or lactation (safety not established; avoid chronic use of large doses).

## ADVERSE REACTIONS AND SIDE EFFECTS*

■ **GI:** constipation, gray-black stools, impaction (infants, debilitated patients).

## INTERACTIONS

**Drug-Drug:** ■ If taken with **aspirin**, may ↑ the risk of salicylate toxicity ■ May ↓ absorption of **tetracycline** or **enoxacin** ■ May ↓ effectiveness of **probenecid** (large doses).

## ROUTE AND DOSAGE

■ **PO (Adults):** *Antidiarrheal*—2 tablets or 30 ml (15 ml of extra/maximum strength) q 30 min *or* 2 tablets q 60 min as needed (not to exceed 4.2 g/24 hr). *Antiulcer*—524 mg 4 times daily (as 2 tablets, 30 ml of regular strenth suspension or 15 ml of extra/maximum strength).

■ **PO (Children 9–12 yr):** 1 tablet or 15 ml (7.5 ml of extra/maximum strength) q 30–60 min (not to exceed 2.1 g/24 hr).

■ **PO (Children 6–9 yr):** 10 ml (5 ml of extra/maximum strength) q 30–60 min (not to exceed 1.4 g/24 hr).

■ **PO (Children 3–6 yr):** 5 ml (2.5 ml of extra/maximum strength) q 30–60 min (not to exceed 704 mg/24 hr).

## AVAILABILITY (generic available)

■ *Tablets:* 262 mg$^{OTC}$ ■ *Chewable tablets (cherry and other flavors):* 262 mg (contain calcium carbonate)$^{OTC}$, {300 mg$^{OTC}$} ■ *Liquid (cherry, carameland other flavors):* 262 mg/15 ml$^{OTC}$, {264 mg/15 ml$^{OTC}$}, 525 mg/15 ml$^{OTC}$ ■ *In combination with:* kaolin/pectin (Kaodene Non-Narcotic)$^{OTC}$, in a convenience package with metronidazole and tetracycline (Helidac). See Appendix B.

TIME/ACTION PROFILE (relief of diarrhea and other GI symptoms)

| | ONSET | PEAK | DURATION |
|---|---|---|---|
| PO | within 24 hr | unknown | unknown |

# NURSING IMPLICATIONS

## ASSESSMENT

■ **Diarrhea:** Assess the frequency and consistency of stools, presence of nausea and indigestion, and bowel sounds before and during therapy.

❑ Assess fluid and electrolyte balance and skin turgor for dehydration if diarrhea is prolonged.

■ **Ulcers:** Assess patient for epigastric or abdominal pain and frank or occult blood in the stool, emesis, or gastric aspirate.

■ *Lab Test Considerations:* Chronic high doses may cause falsely increased uric acid levels with colorimetric assay.

❑ May interfere with radiologic examination of the GI tract.

❑ May cause abnormal results with alkaline phosphatase, AST, and ALT tests.

❑ May cause ↓ potassium levels and serum T$_3$ and T$_4$ concentrations.

❑ Large doses of salicylates may also cause prolonged prothrombin time (PT).

❑ For additional lab test considerations related to salicylate content, see salicylates monograph.

## POTENTIAL NURSING DIAGNOSES

■ Diarrhea (Indications).
■ Constipation (Side Effects).

## IMPLEMENTATION

■ **PO:** Shake liquid before using. Chewable tablets may be chewed or allowed to dissolve before swallowing.

## PATIENT/FAMILY TEACHING

■ **General Info:** Instruct patient to take medication exactly as directed.

❑ Inform patient that medication may temporarily cause stools and tongue to appear gray-black.

❑ Instruct patient that this medication contains aspirin. Advise patient taking concurrent aspirin products to discontinue bismuth subsalicylate if tinnitus, ringing in the ears occurs.

■ **Diarrhea:** Instruct patient to notify health care professional if diarrhea persists for

---

{ } = Available in Canada only.
*CAPITALS indicates life-threatening; underlines indicate most frequent.

more than 2 days or if accompanied by a high fever.

❑ U.S. Centers for Disease Control and Prevention warn against giving salicylates to children or adolescents with varicella (chickenpox) or influenza-like or viral illnesses because of a possible association with Reye's syndrome.

■ **Ulcers:** Advise patient to consult health care professional before taking other OTC ulcer remedies concurrently with bismuth subsalicylate.

## EVALUATION

**Effectiveness of therapy can be demonstrated by:** ■ Decrease in diarrhea ■ Decrease in symptoms of indigestion ■ Prevention of traveler's diarrhea ■ Treatment of ulcers.

## bisoprolol

(bis-**oh**-proe-lol)
Monocor, Zebeta

**CLASSIFICATION(S):**
**Therapeutic:** antihypertensives
**Pharmacologic:** beta blockers

**Pregnancy Category C**

## INDICATIONS

■ Management of hypertension.

## ACTION

■ Blocks stimulation of $beta_1$(myocardial)-adrenergic receptors. Does not usually affect $beta_2$(pulmonary, vascular, uterine)-receptor sites. **Therapeutic Effects:** ■ Decreased blood pressure and heart rate.

## PHARMACOKINETICS

**Absorption:** Well absorbed after oral administration, but 20% undergoes first-pass hepatic metabolism.

**Distribution:** Unknown.

**Metabolism and Excretion:** 50% excreted unchanged by the kidneys; remainder renally excreted as metabolites; 2% excreted in feces.

**Half-life:** 9–12 hr.

## CONTRAINDICATIONS AND PRECAUTIONS

**Contraindicated in:** ■ Uncompensated CHF ■ Pulmonary edema ■ Cardiogenic shock ■ Bradycardia or heart block.

**Use Cautiously in:** ■ Renal impairment (dosage reduction recommended) ■ Hepatic impairment (dosage reduction recommended) ■ Geriatric patients (increased sensitivity to beta blockers; initial dosage reduction recommended) ■ Pulmonary disease (including asthma; $beta_1$ selectivity may be lost at higher doses); avoid use if possible ■ Diabetes mellitus (may mask signs of hypoglycemia) ■ Thyrotoxicosis (may mask symptoms) ■ Patients with a history of severe allergic reactions (intensity of reactions may be increased) ■ Pregnancy, lactation, or children (safety not established; all agents cross the placenta and may cause fetal/neonatal bradycardia, hypotension, hypoglycemia, or respiratory depression).

## ADVERSE REACTIONS AND SIDE EFFECTS*

■ **CNS:** <u>fatigue</u>, <u>weakness</u>, anxiety, depression, dizziness, drowsiness, insomnia, memory loss, mental status changes, nervousness, nightmares ■ **EENT:** blurred vision, stuffy nose ■ **Resp:** bronchospasm, wheezing ■ **CV:** BRADYCARDIA, CHF, PULMONARY EDEMA, hypotension, peripheral vasoconstriction ■ **GI:** constipation, diarrhea, liver function abnormalities, nausea, vomiting ■ **GU:** impotence, decreased libido, urinary frequency ■ **Derm:** rashes ■ **Endo:** hyperglycemia, hypoglycemia ■ **MS:** arthralgia, back pain, joint pain ■ **Misc:** drug-induced lupus syndrome.

## INTERACTIONS

**Drug-Drug:** ■ **General anesthetics, IV phenytoin,** and **verapamil** may cause additive myocardial depression ■ Additive bradycardia may occur with **digoxin** ■ Additive hypotension may occur with other **antihypertensives,** acute ingestion of **alcohol,** or **nitrates** ■ Concurrent use with **amphetamine, cocaine, ephedrine, epinephrine, norepinephrine, phenylephrine,** or **pseudoephedrine** may result in unopposed alpha-adrenergic stimulation (excessive hypertension, bradycardia) ■ Concurrent thyroid preparation administration may decrease effectiveness ■ May alter the effectiveness of **insulins** or **oral hypoglycemic agents** (dosage adjustments may be necessary) ■ May decrease the effectiveness of **theophyl-**

**line ■** May decrease the beneficial beta$_1$-cardiovascular effects of **dopamine** or **dobutamine** ■ Use cautiously within 14 days of **MAO inhibitor** therapy (may result in hypertension).

## ROUTE AND DOSAGE

■ **PO (Adults):** 5 mg once daily, may be increased to 10 mg once daily (range 2.5–20 mg/day).

❑ **Renal/Hepatic Impairment**

■ **PO (Adults):** *CCr <40 ml/min*—Initiate therapy with 2.5 mg/day, titrate cautiously.

## AVAILABILITY (generic available)

■ *Tablets:* 5 mg$^{Rx}$, 10 mg$^{Rx}$ ■ Cost: 5-mg and 10-mg tablets $35.75/30 tablets ■ hydrochlorothiazide (Ziac)$^{Rx}$. See Appendix B.

TIME/ACTION PROFILE (antihypertensive effect)

| | ONSET | PEAK | DURATION |
|---|---|---|---|
| PO | unknown | 1–4 hr | 24 hr |

# NURSING IMPLICATIONS

## ASSESSMENT

❑ Monitor blood pressure, ECG, and pulse frequently during dosage adjustment period and periodically throughout therapy.

❑ Monitor intake and output ratios and daily weights. Assess routinely for signs and symptoms of CHF (dyspnea, rales/crackles, weight gain, peripheral edema, jugular venous distention).

❑ Monitor frequency of prescription refills to determine adherence.

■ *Lab Test Considerations:* May cause increased BUN, serum lipoprotein, potassium, triglyceride, and uric acid levels.

❑ May cause increased ANA titers.

❑ May cause increase in blood glucose levels.

## POTENTIAL NURSING DIAGNOSES

■ Cardiac output, decreased (Side Effects).
■ Noncompliance (Patient/Family Teaching).

## IMPLEMENTATION

■ **PO:** Take apical pulse before administering. If <50 bpm or if arrhythmia occurs, withhold medication and notify physician or other health care professional.

❑ May be administered without regard to meals.

## PATIENT/FAMILY TEACHING

■ **General Info:** Instruct patient to take medication exactly as directed, at the same time each day, even if feeling well; do not skip or double up on missed doses. If a dose is missed, it should be taken as soon as possible up to 4 hr before next dose. Abrupt withdrawal may precipitate life-threatening arrhythmias, hypertension, or myocardial ischemia.

❑ Teach patient and family how to check pulse and blood pressure. Instruct them to check pulse daily and blood pressure biweekly and to report significant changes to health care professional.

❑ May cause drowsiness. Caution patients to avoid driving or other activities that require alertness until response to the drug is known.

❑ Advise patients to change positions slowly to minimize orthostatic hypotension.

❑ Caution patient that this medication may increase sensitivity to cold.

❑ Instruct patient to consult health care professional before taking any OTC medications, especially cold preparations, concurrently with this medication. Patients on antihypertensive therapy should also avoid excessive amounts of coffee, tea, and cola.

❑ Diabetics should closely monitor blood glucose, especially if weakness, malaise, irritability, or fatigue occurs. Medication does not block dizziness or sweating as signs of hypoglycemia.

❑ Advise patient to notify health care professional if slow pulse, difficulty breathing, wheezing, cold hands and feet, dizziness, light-headedness, confusion, depression, rash, fever, sore throat, unusual bleeding, or bruising occurs.

❑ Instruct patient to inform health care professional of medication regimen before treatment or surgery.

{ } = Available in Canada only.
*CAPITALS indicates life-threatening; underlines indicate most frequent.

❑ Advise patient to carry identification describing disease process and medication regimen at all times.

■ **Hypertension:** Reinforce the need to continue additional therapies for hypertension (weight loss, sodium restriction, stress reduction, regular exercise, moderation of alcohol consumption, and smoking cessation). Medication controls but does not cure hypertension.

## EVALUATION
**Effectiveness of therapy can be demonstrated by:** ■ Decrease in blood pressure.

---

# bivalirudin
(bi-val-i-**roo**-din)
Angiomax

## CLASSIFICATION(S):
**Therapeutic:** *anticoagulants*
**Pharmacologic:** *thrombin inhibitors*

### Pregnancy Category B

---

## INDICATIONS
■ Used in conjunction with aspirin to reduce the risk of acute ischemic complications in patients with unstable angina who are undergoing percutaneous transluminal angioplasty (PCTA).

## ACTION
■ Specifically and reversible inhibits thrombin by binding to its receptor sites. Inhibition of thrombin prevents activation of factors V, VIII and XII; the conversion of fibrinogen to fibrin; platelet adhesion and aggregation. **Therapeutic Effects:** ■ Decreased acute ischemic complications in patients with unstable angina (death, MI, or the urgent need for revascularization procedures).

## PHARMACOKINETICS
**Absorption:** IV administration results in complete bioavailability.
**Distribution:** Unknown.
**Metabolism and Excretion:** Cleared from plasma by a combination of renal mechanisms and proteolytic breakdown.
**Half-life:** 25 min (increased in renal impairment).

## CONTRAINDICATIONS AND PRECAUTIONS
**Contraindicated in:** ■ Active major bleeding ■ Hypersensitivity.

**Use Cautiously in:** ■ Any disease state associated with an increased risk of bleeding ■ Heparin-induced thrombocytopenia or heparin-induced thrombocytopenia-thrombosis syndrome ■ Patients with unstable angina not undergoing PCTA ■ Patients with other acute coronary syndromes ■ Concurrent use with other platelet aggregation inhibitors (safety not established) ■ Renal impairment (infusion rate reduction recommended if GFR <60 ml/min) ■ Lactation or children (safety not established) ■ Pregnancy (use only if clearly needed).

## ADVERSE REACTIONS AND SIDE EFFECTS*
■ **CNS:** headache, anxiety, insomnia, nervousness ■ **CV:** hypotension, bradycardia, hypertension ■ **GI:** nausea, abdominal pain, dyspepsia, vomiting ■ **Hemat:** BLEEDING ■ **Local:** injection site pain ■ **MS:** back pain ■ **Misc:** pain, fever, pelvic pain.

## INTERACTIONS
**Drug-Drug:** ■ Risk of bleeding may be increased by concurrent use of **abciximab, heparin, low-molecular-weight heparins/ heparinoids, ticlopidine, thrombolytic agents,** or any other **drugs that inhibit coagulation.**

## ROUTE AND DOSAGE
■ **IV (Adults):** 1 mg/kg as a bolus injection, followed by a 4-hr infusion at a rate of 2.5 mg/kg/hr. This may be followed by an additional infusion of 0.2 mg/kg/hr for up to 20 hr. Therapy should be initiated prior to PCTA and given in conjunction with aspirin.
❑ **Renal Impairment**
■ **IV (Adults):** *GFR 30–59 ml/min*—Reduce infusion dose by 20%; *GFR 10–29 ml/ min*—Reduce infusion dose by 60%; *Dialysis-dependent patients (off dialysis)*—Reduce infusion dose by 90%. Activated clotting time (ACT) should be monitored in all patients with renal impairment.

## AVAILABILITY
■ ***Powder for injection (requires reconstitution):*** 250 mg/vial[Rx].

TIME/ACTION PROFILE (anticoagulant effect)

| | ONSET | PEAK | DURATION |
|---|---|---|---|
| IV | immediate | Unk | 1–2 hr |

## NURSING IMPLICATIONS

### ASSESSMENT

❑ Assess patient for bleeding. Most common is oozing from the arterial access site for cardiac catheterization. Arterial and venous punctures, IM injections, and use of urinary catheters, nasotracheal intubation, and nasogastric tubes should be minimized. Noncompressible sites for IV access should be avoided. If bleeding cannot be controlled with pressure, discontinue bivalirudin immediately.

❑ Monitor vital signs. May cause bradycardia, hypertension, or hypotension. An unexplained decrease in blood pressure may indicate hemorrhage.

■ *Lab Test Considerations:* Assess hemoglobin, hematocrit, and platelet count prior to bivalirudin therapy and periodically during therapy. May cause decreased hemoglobin and hematocrit. An unexplained decrease in hematocrit may indicate hemorrhage.

❑ Monitor ACT periodically in patients with renal dysfunction.

### POTENTIAL NURSING DIAGNOSES

■ Tissue perfusion, ineffective (Indications).

### IMPLEMENTATION

■ **General:** Administer IV just prior to PTCA, in conjunction with aspirin 300 mg to 325 mg/day. Do not administer IM.

❑ Do not administer solutions that are discolored or contain particulate matter. Discard unused portion. Solution should be clear to slightly opalescent, colorless to slightly yellow.

■ **Direct IV:** Dilute by adding 5 ml of sterile water for injection to each 250 mg of bivalirudin and swirl until all material is dissolved. Dilute further with 50 ml of of D5W or 0.9% NaCl for a concentration of 5 mg/ml. Solution is stable for 24 hr if refrigerated.

■ *Rate:* Administer as a bolus injection.

■ **Intermittent Infusion:** Dilute by adding 5 ml of sterile water for injection to each 250 mg of bivalirudin and swirl until all material is dissolved. Dilute each vial further in 500 ml of of D5W or 0.9% NaCl for a concentration of 0.5 mg/ml. Diluted solution is stable for 24 hr at room temperature.

■ *Rate:* Initial direct IV dose is followed by a 4-hr infusion at a rate of 2.5 mg/kg/hr. After 4-hr infusion, if needed, an additional infusion may be administered at a rate of 0.2 mg/kg/hr for up to 20 hrs.

■ **Y-Site Incompatibility:** Administer through a separate line without mixing with other medications.

### PATIENT/FAMILY TEACHING

❑ Inform patient of the purpose of bivalirudin.

❑ Instruct patient to notify health care professional immediately if any bleeding is noted.

### EVALUATION

**Effectiveness of therapy can be demonstrated by:** ■ Decreased acute ischemic complications in patients with unstable angina (death, MI or the urgent need for revascularization procedures).

---

| High Alert |
|---|

## bleomycin

(blee-oh-**mye**-sin)
Blenoxane

### CLASSIFICATION(S):

***Therapeutic:*** *antineoplastics*
***Pharmacologic:*** *antitumor antibiotics*

**Pregnancy Category D**

### INDICATIONS

■ Treatment of: ❑ Lymphomas ❑ Squamous cell carcinoma ❑ Testicular embryonal cell carcinoma ❑ Choriocarcinoma ❑ Teratocarcinoma ■ Intrapleural administration to prevent the reaccumulation of malignant effusions.

## ACTION

■ Inhibits DNA and RNA synthesis. **Therapeutic Effects:** ■ Death of rapidly replicating cells, particularly malignant ones.

## PHARMACOKINETICS

**Absorption:** Well absorbed from IM and subcut sites. Absorption follows intrapleural and intraperitoneal administration.

**Distribution:** Widely distributed, concentrates in skin, lungs, peritoneum, kidneys, and lymphatics.

**Metabolism and Excretion:** 60–70% excreted unchanged by the kidneys.

**Half-life:** 2 hr (increased in renal impairment).

## CONTRAINDICATIONS AND PRECAUTIONS

**Contraindicated in:** ■ Hypersensitivity ■ Pregnancy or lactation.

**Use Cautiously in:** ■ Renal impairment (dosage reduction required if <35 ml/min) ■ Pulmonary impairment ■ Nonmalignant chronic debilitating illness ■ Geriatric patients (increased risk of pulmonary toxicity, age-related decrease in renal function) ■ Patients with childbearing potential.

## ADVERSE REACTIONS AND SIDE EFFECTS*

■ **CNS:** aggressive behavior, disorientation, weakness ■ **Resp:** PULMONARY FIBROSIS, pneumonitis ■ **CV:** hypotension, peripheral vasoconstriction ■ **GI:** anorexia, nausea, stomatitis, vomiting ■ **Derm:** hyperpigmentation, mucocutaneous toxicity, alopecia, erythema, rashes, urticaria, vesiculation ■ **Hemat:** anemia, leukopenia, thrombocytopenia ■ **Local:** pain at tumor site, phlebitis at IV site ■ **Metab:** weight loss ■ **Misc:** ANAPHYLACTOID REACTIONS, chills, fever.

## INTERACTIONS

**Drug-Drug:** ■ Hematologic toxicity ↑ with concurrent use of **radiation therapy** and other **antineoplastics** ■ Concurrent use with **cisplatin** ↓ elimination of bleomycin and may ↑ toxicity ■ ↑ risk of pulmonary toxicity with other **antineoplastics** or thoracic **radiation therapy** ■ **General anesthesia** ↑ the risk of pulmonary toxicity ■ ↑ risk of Raynaud's syndrome when used with **vinblastine**.

## ROUTE AND DOSAGE

Lymphoma patients should receive initial test doses of 2 units or less for the first 2 doses.

■ **IV, IM, Subcut (Adults and Children):** 0.25–0.5 unit/kg (10–20 units/m²) weekly or twice weekly initially. If favorable response, lower maintenance doses given (1 unit/day or 5 units/wk IM or IV). May also be given as continuous IV infusion at 0.25 unit/kg or 15 units/m²/day for 4–5 days.

■ **Intrapleural: (Adults):** 15–20 units instilled for 4 hr, then removed.

## AVAILABILITY

■ *Injection:* 15 units/vial^Rx, 30 units vial/^Rx ■ Cost: 15-unit vial $304.60, 30-unit vial $609.20.

TIME/ACTION PROFILE (tumor response)

| | ONSET | PEAK | DURATION |
| --- | --- | --- | --- |
| IV, IM, Subcut | 2–3 wk | unknown | unknown |

# NURSING IMPLICATIONS

## ASSESSMENT

❑ Monitor vital signs before and frequently during therapy.

❑ Assess for fever and chills. May occur 3–6 hr after administration and last 4–12 hr.

❑ Monitor for anaphylactic (fever, chills, hypotension, wheezing) and idiosyncratic (confusion, hypotension, fever, chills, wheezing) reactions. Keep resuscitation equipment and medications on hand. Lymphoma patients are at particular risk for idiosyncratic reactions that may occur immediately or several hours after therapy, usually after the first or second dose.

❑ Assess respiratory status for dyspnea and rales/crackles. Monitor chest x-ray before and periodically during therapy. Pulmonary toxicity occurs primarily in geriatric patients (age 70 or older) who have received 400 or more units or at lower doses in patients who received other antineoplastics or thoracic radiation. May occur 4–10 wk after therapy. Discontinue and do not resume bleomycin if pulmonary toxicity occurs.

❑ Assess nausea, vomiting, and appetite. Weigh weekly. Modify diet as tolerated. Antiemetics may be given before administration.

- **Lab Test Considerations:** Monitor CBC before and periodically during therapy. May cause thrombocytopenia and leukopenia (nadir occurs in 12 days and usually returns to pretreatment levels by day 17).
- Monitor baseline and periodic renal and hepatic function.

## POTENTIAL NURSING DIAGNOSES

- Injury, risk for (Side Effects).
- Body image, disturbed (Side Effects).

## IMPLEMENTATION

- **High Alert:** Fatalities have occurred with chemotherapeutic agents. Before administering, clarify all ambiguous orders; double check single, daily, and course-of-therapy dose limits; have second practitioner independently double check original order and dose calculations.
- **General:** Solution should be prepared in a biologic cabinet. Wear gloves, gown, and mask while handling medication. Discard equipment in specially designated containers.
- Lymphoma patients should receive a 1- or 2-unit test dose 2–4 hrs before initiation of therapy. Monitor closely for anaphylactic reaction. May not detect reactors.
- Premedication with acetaminophen, corticosteroids, and diphenhydramine may reduce drug fever and risk of anaphylaxis.
- Reconstituted solution is stable for 24 hr at room temperature and for 14 days if refrigerated.
- **IM, Subcut:** Reconstitute vial with 1–5 ml of sterile water for injection, 0.9% NaCl, or bacteriostatic water for injection. Do not reconstitute with diluents containing benzyl alcohol when used for neonates.
- **Direct IV:** Prepare IV doses by diluting 15-unit vial with at least 5 ml of 0.9% NaCl.
- **Rate:** Administer slowly over 10 min.
- **Syringe Compatibility:** ◆ cisplatin ◆ cyclophosphamide ◆ doxorubicin ◆ droperidol ◆ fluorouracil ◆ furosemide ◆ heparin ◆ leucovorin calcium ◆ methotrexate ◆ metoclopramide ◆ mitomycin ◆ vinblastine ◆ vincristine.
- **Y-Site Compatibility:** ◆ allopurinol ◆ amifostine ◆ aztreonam ◆ cefepime ◆ cisplatin ◆ cyclophosphamide ◆ doxorubicin ◆ doxorubi-

cin liposome ◆ droperidol ◆ etoposide phosphate ◆ filgrastim ◆ fludarabine ◆ fluorouracil ◆ gemcitabine ◆ granisetron ◆ heparin ◆ leucovorin calcium ◆ melphalan ◆ methotrexate ◆ metoclopramide ◆ mitomycin ◆ ondansetron ◆ paclitaxel ◆ piperacillin/tazobactam ◆ sargramostim ◆ teniposide ◆ thiotepa ◆ vinblastine ◆ vincristine ◆ vinorelbine.

- **Intrapleural:** Dissolve 60 units in 50–100 ml of 0.9% NaCl.
- May be administered through thoracotomy tube by physician. Position patient as directed.

## PATIENT/FAMILY TEACHING

- Instruct patient to notify health care professional if fever, chills, wheezing, faintness, diaphoresis, shortness of breath, prolonged nausea and vomiting, or mouth sores occur.
- Encourage patient not to smoke because this may worsen pulmonary toxicity.
- Explain to the patient that skin toxicity may manifest itself as skin sensitivity, hyperpigmentation (especially at skin folds and points of skin irritation), and skin rashes and thickening.
- Instruct patient to inspect oral mucosa for erythema and ulceration. If ulceration occurs, advise patient to use sponge brush and rinse mouth with water after eating and drinking. Opioid analgesics may be required if pain interferes with eating.
- Discuss with patient the possibility of hair loss. Explore coping strategies.
- Advise patient of the need for contraception.
- Instruct patient not to receive any vaccinations without advice of health care professional.
- Emphasize need for periodic lab tests to monitor for side effects.

## EVALUATION

**Effectiveness of therapy can be demonstrated by:** ■ Decrease in tumor size without evidence of hypersensitivity or pulmonary toxicity.

---

{ } = Available in Canada only.
*CAPITALS indicates life-threatening; <u>underlines</u> indicate most frequent.

# BRONCHODILATORS (XANTHINES)

## aminophylline
(am-in-**off**-i-lin)
Phyllocontin, Truphylline

## theophylline
(thee-**off**-i-lin)
Accurbron, {Apo-Theo LA}, Asmalix, Bronkodyl, Elixomin, Elixophyllin, Lanophyllin, Quibron-T, Respbid, Sustaire, Theobid, Theochron, Theoclear, Theospan, Theostat, Theo-Time, Theo-24, Theovent, Theo-X, T-Phyl, Uniphyl

### CLASSIFICATION(S):
**Therapeutic:** bronchodilators
**Pharmacologic:** xanthines

### Pregnancy Category C

## INDICATIONS

■ Long-term control of reversible airway obstruction caused by asthma or COPD. **Unlabeled uses:** ■ Respiratory and myocardial stimulant in apnea of infancy.

## ACTION

■ Inhibit phosphodiesterase, producing increased tissue concentrations of cyclic adenosine monophosphate (cAMP). Increased levels of cAMP result in: ■ Bronchodilation ■ CNS stimulation ■ Positive inotropic and chronotropic effects ■ Diuresis ■ Gastric acid secretion. Aminophylline is a salt of theophylline and releases free theophylline after administration. **Therapeutic Effects:** ■ Bronchodilation.

## PHARMACOKINETICS

**Absorption:** Aminophylline and oxtriphylline release theophylline after administration. *Aminophylline*—well absorbed from oral dosage forms; absorption from extended-release dosage forms is slow but complete. *Theophylline*—well absorbed from PO dosage forms; absorption from extended-release dosage forms is slow but complete.

**Distribution:** *Aminophylline*—widely distributed as theophylline; crosses the placenta; breast milk concentrations are 70% of plasma levels; not distributed into adipose tissue. *Theophylline*—widely distributed; crosses the placenta; breast milk concentrations are 70% of plasma levels; does not distribute into adipose tissue.

**Metabolism and Excretion:** *Aminophylline,* and *theophylline*—aminophylline and oxtriphylline are converted to theophylline; theophylline is metabolized by the liver (90%) to caffeine, which may accumulate in neonates; metabolites are renally excreted; 10% excreted unchanged by the kidneys.

**Half-life:** *Theophylline*—3–13 hr (increased in patients >60 yr, neonates, patients with CHF or liver disease; decreased in cigarette smokers and children).

## CONTRAINDICATIONS AND PRECAUTIONS

**Contraindicated in:** ■ Uncontrolled arrhythmias ■ Hyperthyroidism.

**Use Cautiously in:** ■ Geriatric patients (>60 yr), CHF, or liver disease (dosage reduction required) ■ Obese patients (dose should be based on lean body weight) ■ Has been used safely in pregnancy.

## ADVERSE REACTIONS AND SIDE EFFECTS*

■ **CNS:** SEIZURES, anxiety, headache, insomnia ■ **CV:** ARRHYTHMIAS, tachycardia, angina, palpitations ■ **GI:** nausea, vomiting, anorexia, cramps ■ **Neuro:** tremor.

## INTERACTIONS

**Drug-Drug:** ■ Additive CV and CNS side effects with **adrenergics (sympathomimetic)** ■ May decrease the therapeutic effect of **lithium** ■ **Nicotine** (cigarettes, gum, transdermal patches), **adrenergics, barbiturates, phenytoin, ketoconazole,** and **rifampin** may increase metabolism and may decrease effectiveness ■ **Erythromycin, beta blockers, clarithromycin, cimetidine, influenza vaccine, hormonal contraceptives, corticosteroids, disulfiram, fluvoxamine, interferons, mexiletine, thiabendazole,** some **fluoroquinolones,** and large doses of **allopurinol** decrease metabolism and may lead to toxicity ■ Increased risk of arrhythmias with **halothane** ■ **Isoniazid, carbamazepine,** and **loop diuretics** may increase or decrease theophylline levels.

**Drug-Natural Products:** ▪ Caffeine-containing herbs (**cola nut, guarana, mate, tea, coffee**) may increase **xanthine** serum levels and risk on CNS and CV side effects ▪ Decreased **xanthine** serum levels and effectiveness with **St. John's wort.**

**Drug-Food:** ▪ Excessive regular intake of **charcoal-broiled foods** may decrease effectiveness ▪ Excessive intake of **xanthine-containing foods** may increase the risk of CV and CNS side effects.

## ROUTE AND DOSAGE

Dose should be determined by theophylline serum level monitoring. Loading dose should be decreased or eliminated if theophylline preparation has been used in preceding 24 hr. Aminophylline is 79–86% theophylline. Extended-release (controlled-release, sustained-release) products may be given q 8–24 hr. Doses are expressed in theophylline.

▫ **Aminophylline/Theophylline**

▪ **PO (Adults):** *Loading dose*—6 mg/kg, then 3 mg/kg q 6 hr for 2 doses, then 3 mg/kg q 8 hr maintenance dose (up to 13 mg/kg or 900 mg/day).

▪ **PO (Adults with CHF):** *Loading dose*—6 mg/kg, then 2 mg/kg q 8 hr for 2 doses, then 1–2 mg/kg q 12 hr maintenance dose.

▪ **PO (Geriatric Patients and Patients with Cor Pulmonale):** 6 mg/kg loading dose, then 2 mg/kg q 6 hr for 2 doses, then 2 mg/kg q 8 hr maintenance dose.

▪ **PO (Children 9–16 yr or Young Adult Smokers):** *Loading dose*—6 mg/kg, then 3 mg/kg q 4 hr for 3 doses, then 3 mg/kg q 6 hr maintenance dose (up to 20 mg/kg/day in children 9–12 yr or 18 mg/kg/day in children 12–16 yr).

▪ **PO (Children 6 mo–9 yr):** *Loading dose*—4 mg/kg q 4 hr for 3 doses, then 4 mg/kg q 6 hr maintenance dose (up to 24 mg/kg/day).

▪ **PO, IV (Neonates—up to 40 wk Premature Postconception Age):** 1 mg/kg q 12 hr.

▪ **PO, IV (Neonates at Birth or 40 wk Postconception):** *Up to 4 wk postnatal age*—1–2 mg/kg q 12 hr; *4–8 wk postnatal age*—1–2 mg/kg q 8 hr; *over 8 wk postnatal age*—1–3 mg/kg q 6 hr.

▪ **IV (Adults):** *Loading dose*—4.7 mg/kg, then 0.55 mg/kg/hr for 12 hr, then 0.36 mg/kg/hr maintenance infusion rate.

▪ **IV (Adults with CHF):** *Loading dose*—4.7 mg/kg, then 0.39 mg/kg/hr for 12 hr, then 0.08–0.16 mg/kg/hr maintenance infusion rate.

▪ **IV (Geriatric Patients and Patients with Cor Pulmonale):** *Loading dose*—4.7 mg/kg, then 0.47 mg/kg/hr for 12 hr, then 0.24 mg/kg/hr maintenance infusion rate.

▪ **IV (Children 9–16 yr or Young Adult Smokers):** 4.7 mg/kg, then 0.79 mg/kg/hr for 12 hr, then 0.63 mg/kg/hr maintenance infusion rate.

▪ **IV (Children 6 mo–9 yr):** 4.7 mg/kg, then 0.95 mg/kg/hr for 12 hr, then 0.79 mg/kg/hr maintenance infusion rate.

▫ **Hepatic Impairment**

▪ **PO (Adults):** *Loading dose*—6 mg/kg, then 2 mg/kg q 8 hr for 2 doses, then 1–2 mg/kg q 12 hr maintenance dose.

▪ **IV (Adults):** *Loading dose*—4.7 mg/kg, then 0.39 mg/kg/hr for 12 hr, then 0.08–0.16 mg/kg/hr maintenance infusion rate.

## AVAILABILITY

▫ **Aminophylline**

▪ *Tablets:* 100 mg^Rx, 200 mg^Rx ▪ *Enteric-coated tablets:* 100 mg^Rx, 200 mg^Rx ▪ *Extended-release tablets:* 225 mg^Rx, {350 mg^Rx} ▪ *Oral solution:* 105 mg/5 ml^Rx ▪ *Suppositories:* 250 mg^Rx, 500 mg^Rx ▪ *Injection:* 250 mg/10 ml^Rx ▪ *Tablets:* 100 mg^Rx, 200 mg^Rx.

▫ **Theophylline**

▪ *Immediate-release tablets:* 100 mg^Rx, 125 mg^Rx, 200 mg^Rx, 250 mg^Rx, 300 mg^Rx ▪ *Timed-release tablets (8–12 hr):* 100 mg^Rx, 200 mg^Rx, 250 mg^Rx, 300 mg^Rx, 500 mg^Rx ▪ *Timed-release tablets (8–24 hr):* 100 mg^Rx, 200 mg^Rx, 300 mg^Rx, 450 mg^Rx ▪ *Timed-release tablets (12–24 hr):* 100 mg^Rx, 200 mg^Rx, 300 mg^Rx ▪ *Timed-release tablets (24 hr):* 400 mg^Rx, 600 mg^Rx ▪ *Immediate-release capsules:* 100 mg^Rx, 200 mg^Rx ▪ *Timed-release capsules (8–12 hr):* 50

$mg^{Rx}$, 60 $mg^{Rx}$, 65 $mg^{Rx}$, 75 $mg^{Rx}$, 100 $mg^{Rx}$, 125 $mg^{Rx}$, 130 $mg^{Rx}$, 200 $mg^{Rx}$, 250 $mg^{Rx}$, 260 $mg^{Rx}$ ■ *Timed-release capsules (12 hr):* 50 $mg^{Rx}$, 125 $mg^{Rx}$, 130 $mg^{Rx}$, 250 $mg^{Rx}$, 260 $mg^{Rx}$ ■ *Timed-release capsules (24 hr):* 100 $mg^{Rx}$, 200 $mg^{Rx}$, 300 $mg^{Rx}$ ■Cost: 100 mg $3.63/30, 200 mg $7.72/30, 300 mg $13.75/30 ■*Syrup (cherry):* 80 mg/15 $mg^{Rx}$, 150 mg/15 $ml^{Rx}$ ■ *Elixir (orange/raspberry, mixed fruit, and other flavors):* 80 mg/15 $ml^{Rx}$ ■ *Solution (tangerine and other flavors):* 80 mg/15 $ml^{Rx}$, 150 mg/15 $ml^{Rx}$ ■ *Injection (with dextrose):* 0.4 $mg/ml^{Rx}$, 0.8 $mg/ml^{Rx}$, 1.6 $mg/ml^{Rx}$, 2 $mg/ml^{Rx}$, 3.2 $mg/ml^{Rx}$, 4 $mg/ml^{Rx}$.

TIME/ACTION PROFILE (bronchodilation)

|  | ONSET† | PEAK | DURATION |
|---|---|---|---|
| Aminophylline PO | 15–60 min | 1–2 hr | 6–8 hr |
| Aminophylline PO–ER | unknown | 4–7 hr | 8–12 hr |
| Aminophylline IV | rapid | end of infusion | 6–8 hr |
| Theophylline PO | rapid | 1–2 hr | 6 hr |
| Theophylline PO–ER | delayed | 4–8 hr | 8–24 hr |
| Theophylline IV | rapid | end of infusion | 6–8 hr |

†Provided that a loading dose has been given and steady-state blood levels exist.

## NURSING IMPLICATIONS

### ASSESSMENT

- **General Info:** Assess blood pressure, pulse, respiratory status (rate, lung sounds, use of accessory muscles) before and throughout therapy. Ensure that oxygen therapy is correctly instituted during acute asthma attacks.
- ❑ Monitor intake and output ratios for an increase in diuresis or fluid overload.
- ❑ Patients with a history of cardiovascular problems should be monitored for chest pain and ECG changes (PACs, supraventricular tachycardia, PVCs, ventricular tachycardia). Resuscitative equipment should be readily available.
- ❑ Monitor pulmonary function tests before and periodically during therapy to determine therapeutic efficacy in patients with chronic bronchitis or emphysema.
- **Lab Test Considerations:** Monitor ABGs, acid-base, and fluid and electrolyte balance

in patients receiving parenteral therapy or whenever required by patient's condition.

- **Toxicity and Overdose:** Monitor drug levels routinely, especially in patients requiring high doses or during prolonged intensive therapy. Serum sample should be obtained at time of peak absorption. Peak levels should be evaluated 15–30 min after IV loading dose, 1–2 hr after rapid-acting forms, and 4–12 hr after extended-release forms. Therapeutic plasma levels range from 5–15 mcg/ml. Drug levels in excess of 20 mcg/ml are associated with toxicity. Caffeine ingestion may falsely elevate drug concentration levels.
- ❑ Observe patient for symptoms of drug toxicity (anorexia, nausea, vomiting, stomach cramps, diarrhea, confusion, headache, restlessness, flushing, increased urination, insomnia, tachycardia, arrhythmias, seizures). Notify physician or other health care professional immediately if these occur. Tachycardia, ventricular arrhythmias, or seizures may be the first sign of toxicity.

## POTENTIAL NURSING DIAGNOSES

- Airway clearance, ineffective (Indications).
- Activity intolerance (Indications).

## IMPLEMENTATION

- **General:** Administer around the clock to maintain therapeutic plasma levels. Once-a-day doses should be administered in the morning.
- ❑ Do not refrigerate elixirs, solutions, or syrups; crystals may form. Crystals should dissolve when liquid is warmed to room temperature.
- ❑ Wait at least 4–6 hr after stopping IV therapy to begin immediate-release oral dosage; for extended-release oral dosage form, give first oral dose at time of IV discontinuation.
- **PO:** Administer oral preparations with food or a full glass of water to minimize GI irritation. Food slows but does not reduce the extent of absorption. May be administered 1 hr before or 2 hr after meals for more rapid absorption. Use calibrated measuring device to ensure accurate dose of liquid preparations. Swallow tablets whole; do not crush, break, or chew enteric-coated or extended-release tablets (extended-release tablets may be broken if scored).
- ❑ Patients receiving once-daily doses of ≥13 mg/kg or ≥900 mg (whichever is less)

should avoid eating a high-fat-content morning meal or should take medication at least 1 hr before eating. Patients unable to comply with this regimen should be placed on alternative therapy.

- **IM:** Do not use if precipitate is present. May be caused by exposure to cold.

❑ Inject slowly; avoid IV administration.

❑ **Aminophylline**

- **IV:** May be diluted in D5W, D10W, D20W, 0.9% NaCl, 0.45% NaCl, D5/0.9% NaCl, D5/0.45% NaCl, D5/0.25% NaCl, or LR. Mixture is stable for 24 hr if refrigerated.

❑ Do not administer discolored or precipitated solution. Flush main IV line before administration.

❑ If extravasation occurs, local injection of 1% procaine and application of heat may relieve pain and promote vasodilation.

- **Loading Dose:** Administer over 20–30 min.

- *Rate:* Do not exceed 20–25 mg/min. Administer via infusion pump to ensure accurate dosage. Rapid administration may cause chest pain, dizziness, hypotension, tachypnea, flushing, arrhythmias, or a reaction to the solution or administration technique (chills; fever; redness, pain, or swelling at injection site).

- **Continuous Infusion:** Usually given as a loading dose in a small volume followed by continuous infusion in larger volume.

- *Rate:* See Route and Dosage section for rates.

- **Syringe Compatibility:** ◆ heparin ◆ metoclopramide.

- **Syringe Incompatibility:** ◆ doxapram.

- **Y-Site Compatibility:** ◆ allopurinol ◆ amifostine ◆ amphotericin B cholesteryl sulfate complex ◆ ceftazidime ◆ cimetidine ◆ cladribine ◆ docetaxel ◆ doxorubicin liposome ◆ enalaprilat ◆ esmolol ◆ etoposide ◆ famotidine ◆ filgrastim ◆ fluconazole ◆ fludarabine ◆ foscarnet ◆ gemcitabine ◆ granisetron ◆ inamrinone ◆ labetalol ◆ melphalan ◆ meropenem ◆ morphine ◆ netilmicin ◆ paclitaxel ◆ pancuronium ◆ piperacillin/tazobactam ◆ potassium chloride ◆ propofol ◆ ranitidine ◆ remifentanil ◆ sargramostim ◆ tacrolimus ◆ teniposide ◆ thiotepa ◆ tolazoline ◆ vecuronium ◆ vitamin B complex with vitamin C.

- **Y-Site Incompatibility:** ◆ amiodarone ◆ ciprofloxacin ◆ dobutamine ◆ hydralazine ◆ ondansetron ◆ vinorelbine ◆ warfarin

- **Additive Incompatibility:** Admixing is not recommended because of dose titration and incompatibilities.

❑ **Theophylline**

- **Continuous Infusion:** IV theophylline and 5% dextrose are packed in a moisture-barrier overwrap. Remove immediately before administration and squeeze bag to check for leaks. Discard if solution is not clear.

- **Loading Dose:** Administer over 20–30 min. If patient has had another form of theophylline before loading dose, serum theophylline level should be obtained and loading dose proportionally reduced.

- *Rate:* Do not exceed 20–25 mg/min. Rapid administration may cause chest pain, dizziness, hypotension, tachypnea, flushing, arrhythmias, or a reaction to the solution or administration technique (chills; fever; redness, pain, or swelling at injection site). Infusion rate may be increased after 12 hr. Administer via infusion pump to ensure accurate dosage. Monitor ECG continuously; tachyarrhythmias may occur.

- **Y-Site Compatibility:** ◆ acyclovir ◆ ampicillin ◆ ampicillin/sulbactam ◆ aztreonam ◆ cefazolin ◆ cefotetan ◆ ceftazidime ◆ ceftriaxone ◆ cimetidine ◆ cisatracurium ◆ clindamycin ◆ diltiazem ◆ dobutamine ◆ dopamine ◆ doxycycline ◆ erythromycin lactobionate ◆ famotidine ◆ fluconazole ◆ gentamicin ◆ haloperidol ◆ heparin ◆ hydrocortisone sodium succinate ◆ lidocaine ◆ methyldopate ◆ methylprednisolone sodium succinate ◆ metronidazole ◆ midazolam ◆ milrinone ◆ nafcillin ◆ nitroglycerin ◆ nitroprusside ◆ penicillin G potassium ◆ piperacillin ◆ potassium chloride ◆ ranitidine ◆ remifentanil ◆ ticarcillin ◆ ticarcillin/clavulanate ◆ tobramycin ◆ vancomycin.

- **Y-Site Incompatibility:** ◆ hetastarch ◆ phenytoin.

- **Additive Incompatibility:** Admixing is not recommended because of dose titration and incompatibilities.

---

{ } = Available in Canada only.
*CAPITALS indicates life-threatening; <u>underlines</u> indicate most frequent.

## PATIENT/FAMILY TEACHING

□ Emphasize the importance of taking only the prescribed dose at the prescribed time intervals. Missed doses should be taken as soon as possible or omitted if close to next dose.

□ Encourage the patient to drink adequate liquids (2000 ml/day minimum) to decrease the viscosity of the airway secretions.

□ Advise patient to avoid OTC cough, cold, or breathing preparations without consulting health care professional. These medications may increase side effects and cause arrhythmias.

□ Encourage patients not to smoke. A change in smoking habits may necessitate a change in dosage.

□ Advise patient to minimize intake of xanthine-containing foods or beverages (colas, coffee, chocolate) and not to eat charcoal-broiled foods daily.

□ Instruct patient not to change brands without consulting health care professional.

□ Advise patient to contact health care professional promptly if the usual dose of medication fails to produce the desired results, symptoms worsen after treatment, or toxic effects occur.

□ Emphasize the importance of having serum levels routinely tested every 6–12 mo.

## EVALUATION

**Effectiveness of therapy can be demonstrated by:** ■ Increased ease in breathing □ Clearing of lung fields on auscultation ■ Respiratory and myocardial stimulation in apnea of infancy.

---

**budesonide, See
CORTICOSTEROIDS (INHALATION),
CORTICOSTEROIDS (NASAL),
CORTICOSTEROIDS (SYSTEMIC).**

---

## bumetanide

(byoo-**met**-a-nide)

Bumex

**CLASSIFICATION(S):**

**Therapeutic:** diuretics
**Pharmacologic:** loop diuretics

**Pregnancy Category C**

## INDICATIONS

■ Edema: □ Due to congestive heart failure □ Hepatic or renal disease.

## ACTION

■ Inhibits the reabsorption of sodium and chloride from the loop of Henle and distal renal tubule ■ Increases renal excretion of water, sodium, chloride, magnesium, hydrogen, and calcium ■ May have renal and peripheral vasodilatory effects ■ Effectiveness persists in impaired renal function. **Therapeutic Effects:** ■ Diuresis and subsequent mobilization of excess fluid (edema, pleural effusions).

## PHARMACOKINETICS

**Absorption:** Well absorbed after oral or IM administration.

**Distribution:** Unknown.

**Protein Binding:** 94–96%.

**Metabolism and Excretion:** Partially metabolized by liver; 50% eliminated unchanged by kidneys and 20% excreted in feces.

**Half-life:** 60–90 min (6–15 hr in neonates).

## CONTRAINDICATIONS AND PRECAUTIONS

**Contraindicated in:** ■ Hypersensitivity ■ Cross-sensitivity with thiazides and sulfonamides may occur ■ Pre-existing uncorrected electrolyte imbalance, hepatic coma, or anuria.

**Use Cautiously in:** ■ Severe liver disease (may precipitate hepatic coma; concurrent use with potassium-sparing diuretics may be necessary) ■ Electrolyte depletion ■ Geriatric patients (difficulty assessing hearing status; increased risk of hypotension) ■ Diabetes mellitus ■ Increasing azotemia ■ Pregnancy, lactation, or children <18 yr (safety not established; bumetanide is a potent displacer of bilirubin and should be used cautiously in critically ill or jaundiced neonates because of risk of kernicterus).

## ADVERSE REACTIONS AND SIDE EFFECTS*

■ **CNS:** dizziness, encephalopathy, headache, insomnia, nervousness ■ **EENT:** hearing loss, tinnitus ■ **CV:** hypotension ■ **GI:** constipation, diarrhea, dry mouth, dyspepsia, nausea, vomiting ■ **GU:** excessive urination ■ **Derm:** photosensitivity, rashes ■ **Endo:** hyperglycemia ■ **F and E:** dehydration, hypochloremia, hypokalemia, hypomagnesemia, hyponatremia, hypovolemia, metabolic alkalosis ■ **Metab:** hyperglycemia, hyperuricemia ▪ **MS:** arthralgia, muscle cramps, myalgia ▪ **Misc:** increased BUN.

## INTERACTIONS

**Drug-Drug:** ▪ ↑ hypotension with **antihypertensives, nitrates,** or acute ingestion of **alcohol** ▪ ↑ risk of hypokalemia with other **diuretics, piperacillin, amphotericin B, stimulant laxatives,** and **corticosteroids** ▪ Hypokalemia may ↑ risk of **digoxin** toxicity ▪ ↓ **lithium** excretion, may cause toxicity ▪ ↑ risk of ototoxicity with **aminoglycosides** ▪ May ↑ the effectiveness of **warfarin, thrombolytic agents,** or **anticoagulants.**

## ROUTE AND DOSAGE

▪ **PO (Adults):** 0.5–2 mg/day as a single dose. Up to 2 additional doses may be given during the day q 4–5 hr (up to 10 mg/day).May also be given on alternate days or q 2–3 days.

▪ **IM, IV (Adults):** 0.5–1 mg/deg, may repeat q 2–3 hr as needed (up to 10 mg/day).

## AVAILABILITY (generic available)

▪ **Tablets:** 0.5 mg$^{Rx}$, 1 mg$^{Rx}$, 2 mg$^{Rx}$ ▪ Cost: *Bumex*—0.5 mg $39.82/100, 1 mg $55.91/100, 2 mg $94.51/100; *generic*—0.5 mg $17.43–30.20/100, 1 mg $40.33–55.91/100, 2 mg $68.17–73.18/100 ▪ **Injection:** 0.25 mg/ml$^{Rx}$ ▪ Cost: $16.20/2 ml, $27.00/4 ml, $76.80/10 ml.

TIME/ACTION PROFILE (diuretic effect)

| | ONSET | PEAK | DURATION |
|---|---|---|---|
| PO | 30–60 min | 1–2 hr | 3–6 hr |
| IM | 40 min | 1–2 hr | 4–6 hr |
| IV | within min | 15–45 min | 3–6 hr |

## NURSING IMPLICATIONS

### ASSESSMENT

❑ Assess fluid status during therapy. Monitor daily weight, intake and output ratios, amount and location of edema, lung sounds, skin turgor, and mucous membranes. Notify physician or other health care professional if thirst, dry mouth, lethargy, weakness, hypotension, or oliguria occurs.

❑ Monitor blood pressure and pulse before and during administration. Monitor frequen-

cy of prescription refills to determine compliance in patients treated for hypertension.

❑ Assess patients receiving digoxin for anorexia, nausea, vomiting, muscle cramps, paresthesia, and confusion ( ↑ risk of dioxin toxicity due to potassium-depleting effect of diuretic). Potassium supplements or potassium-sparing diuretics may be used concurrently to prevent hypokalemia.

❑ Assess patient for tinnitus and hearing loss. Audiometry is recommended for patients receiving prolonged high-dose IV therapy. Hearing loss is most common after rapid or high-dose IV administration in patients with decreased renal function or those taking other ototoxic drugs.

❑ Assess for allergy to sulfonamides.

▪ **Lab Test Considerations:** Monitor electrolytes, renal and hepatic function, serum glucose, and uric acid levels before and periodically during therapy. May cause ↓ serum potassium, calcium, and magnesium concentrations. May also cause ↑ BUN, serum glucose, creatinine, and uric acid levels.

❑ May cause an ↑ in urinary phosphate concentrations.

## POTENTIAL NURSING DIAGNOSES

▪ Fluid volume, excess (Indications).

▪ Fluid volume, risk for deficit (Side Effects).

## IMPLEMENTATION

▪ **General:** Do not confuse Bumex (bumetanide) with Buprenex (buprenorphine).

❑ Administer medication in the morning to prevent disruption of sleep cycle.

❑ IV is preferred over IM for parenteral administration.

▪ **PO:** Administer orally with food or milk to minimize gastric irritation.

▪ **Direct IV:** Administer undiluted.

▪ **Rate:** Administer slowly over 2 min.

▪ **Intermittent Infusion:** Dilute in D5W, 0.9% NaCl, or lactated Ringer's solution. Use reconstituted solution within 24 hr.

▪ **Rate:** May be administered over 12 hr for patients with renal impairment.

▪ **Y-Site Compatibility:** ◆ allopurinol sodium ◆ amifostine ◆ aztreonam ◆ cefepime ◆ cisatracurium ◆ cladribine ◆ diltiazem ◆ docetaxel

◆ etoposide ◆ filgrastim ◆ gemcitabine ◆ granisetron ◆ lorazepam ◆ melphalan ◆ meperidine ◆ milrinone ◆ morphine ◆ piperacillin/ tazobactam ◆ propofol ◆ remifentanil ◆ teniposide ◆ thiotepa ◆ vinorelbine.

■ **Y-Site Incompatibility:** ◆ midazolam.

## PATIENT/FAMILY TEACHING

■ **General Info:** Instruct patient to take bumetanide as directed. Take missed doses as soon as possible; do not double doses.

❑ Caution patient to make position changes slowly to minimize orthostatic hypotension. Caution patient that the use of alcohol, exercise during hot weather, or standing for long periods during therapy may enhance orthostatic hypotension.

❑ Instruct patient to consult health care professional regarding a diet high in potassium (see Appendix Q).

❑ Advise patient to consult health care professional before taking OTC medication concurrently with this therapy.

❑ Instruct patient to notify health care professional of medication regimen before treatment or surgery.

❑ Caution patient to use sunscreen and protective clothing to prevent photosensitivity reactions.

❑ Advise patient to contact health care professional immediately if muscle weakness, cramps, nausea, dizziness, numbness, or tingling of extremities occurs.

❑ Emphasize the importance of routine follow-up examinations.

■ **Hypertension:** Advise patients on antihypertensive regimen to continue taking medication even if feeling better. Bumetanide controls but does not cure hypertension.

❑ Reinforce the need to continue additional therapies for hypertension (weight loss, exercise, restricted sodium intake, stress reduction, regular exercise, moderation of alcohol consumption, cessation of smoking).

## EVALUATION

**Effectiveness of therapy can be demonstrated by:** ■ Decrease in edema ❑ Decrease in abdominal girth ❑ Increase in urinary output ■ Decrease in blood pressure ■ Decrease in serum calcium when used to manage hypercalcemia.

---

**bupivacaine, See EPIDURAL LOCAL ANESTHETICS.**

---

**High Alert**

## buprenorphine

(byoo-pre-**nor**-feen)

Buprenex, Subutex

### CLASSIFICATION(S):

**Therapeutic:** *opioid analgesics*

**Pharmacologic:** *opioid agonists/ antagonists*

**Schedule III**

**Pregnancy Category C**

### INDICATIONS

■ **IM, IV:** Management of moderate to severe acute pain ■ **SL:** Treatment of opioid dependence; suppresses withdrawal symptoms in opioid detoxification.

### ACTION

■ Binds to opiate receptors in the CNS ■ Alters the perception of and response to painful stimuli while producing generalized CNS depression ■ Has partial antagonist properties that may result in opioid withdrawal in physically dependent patients when used as an analgesic **Therapeutic Effects:** ■ **IM, IV:** Decreased severity of pain ■ **SL:** Suppression of withdrawal symptoms during detoxification and maintenance from heroin or other opioids. Produces a relatively mild withdrawal compared to other agents.

### PHARMACOKINETICS

**Absorption:** Well absorbed after IM and SL use; IV administration results in complete bioavailability.

**Distribution:** Crosses the placenta; enters breast milk. CNS concentration is 15–25% of plasma.

**Protein Binding:** 96%

**Metabolism and Excretion:** Mostly metabolized by the liver mostly via the CYP 3A4 enzyme system; one metabolite is active.

**Half-life:** 2–3 hr (parenteral).

## CONTRAINDICATIONS AND PRECAUTIONS

**Contraindicated in:** ■ Hypersensitivity ■ Lactation (enters breast milk).

**Use Cautiously in:** ■ Increased intracranial pressure ■ Severe renal, hepatic, or pulmonary disease ■ Hypothyroidism ■ Adrenal insufficiency ■ Alcoholism ■ Geriatric or debilitated patients (dosage reduction required) ■ Undiagnosed abdominal pain ■ Prostatic hypertrophy ■ Pregnancy, labor, or children <13 yr (safety not established; neonatal withdrawal may occur in infants born to patients receiving SL buprenorphine during pregnancy).

## ADVERSE REACTIONS AND SIDE EFFECTS*

■ **CNS:** confusion, dysphoria, hallucinations, sedation, dizziness, euphoria, floating feeling, headache, unusual dreams ■ **EENT:** blurred vision, diplopia, miosis (high doses) ■ **Resp:** respiratory depression ■ **CV:** hypertension, hypotension, palpitations ■ **GI:** nausea, constipation, dry mouth, ileus, vomiting ■ **GU:** urinary retention ■ **Derm:** sweating, clammy feeling ■ **Misc:** physical dependence, psychological dependence, tolerance.

## INTERACTIONS

**Drug-Drug:** ■ Use with extreme caution in patients receiving **MAO inhibitors** ( ↑ CNS and respiratory depression and hypotension— ↓ buprenorphine dose by 50%; may need to ↓ **MAO inhibitor** dose) ■ ↑ CNS depression with **alcohol, antihistamines, antidepressants,** and **sedative/hypnotics** ■ May ↓ effectiveness of other **opioid analgesics** ■ Inhibitors of the CYP 3A4 enzyme system including **azole antifungals (itraconazole, ketoconazole), erythromycin protease inhibitor antiretrovirals (ritonavir, indinavir, saquinavir)** ↑ blood levels and effects; dose reduction may be necessary during concurrent use ■ Inducers of the CYP 3A4 enzyme system including **carbamazepine rifampin** or **phenytoin** ↓ blood levels and effects; dose modification may be necessary during concurrent use ■ Concurrent abuse of IV buprenorphine and **benzodiazepines** may result in coma and death.

**Drug-Natural Products:** ■ Concomitant use of **kava, valerian, chamomile,** or **hops** can ↑ CNS depression.

## ROUTE AND DOSAGE

### ❏ Analgesia

■ **IM, IV (Adults):** 0.3 mg q 4–6 hr as needed. May repeat initial dose after 30 min (up to 0.3 mg q 4 hr or 0.6 mg q 6 hr); 0.6-mg doses should be given only IM.

■ **IM, IV (Children 2–12 yr):** 2–6 mcg (0.002–0.006 mg)/kg q 4–6 hr.

### ❏ Treatment of opioid dependence

■ **SL (Adults):** 12–16 mg/day as a single dose.

## AVAILABILITY

■ *Sublingual tablets:* 2 mg^Rx, 8 mg^Rx ■ naloxone (Suboxone). See Appendix B.

■ *Injection:* 300 mcg (0.3 mg)/ml^Rx.

TIME/ACTION PROFILE (analgesia)

|    | ONSET  | PEAK             | DURATION |
|----|--------|------------------|----------|
| IM | 15 min | 60 min           | 6 hr†    |
| IV | rapid  | less than 60 min | 6 hr†    |

†4–5 hr in children.

## NURSING IMPLICATIONS

### ASSESSMENT

■ **Pain:** Assess type, location, and intensity of pain before and 1 hr after IM and 5 min (peak) after IV administration. When titrating opioid doses, increases of 25–50% should be administered until there is either a 50% reduction in the patient's pain rating on a numerical or visual analog scale or the patient reports satisfactory pain relief. A repeat dose can be safely administered at the time of the peak if previous dose is ineffective and side effects are minimal. Single doses of 600 mcg (0.6 mg) should be administered IM. Patients requiring doses higher than 600 mcg (0.6 mg) should be converted to an opioid agonist. Buprenorphine is not recommended for prolonged use or as first-line therapy for acute or cancer pain.

{ } = Available in Canada only.
* CAPITALS indicates life-threatening; underlines indicate most frequent.

- An equianalgesic chart (see Appendix O) should be used when changing routes or when changing from one opioid to another.
- Assess level of consciousness, blood pressure, pulse, and respirations before and periodically during administration. If respiratory rate is <10/min, assess level of sedation. Dose may need to be decreased by 25–50%. Buprenorphine 0.3–0.4 mg has approximately equal analgesic and respiratory depressant effects to morphine 10 mg.
- Assess previous analgesic history. Antagonistic properties may induce withdrawal symptoms (vomiting, restlessness, abdominal cramps, increased blood pressure and temperature) in patients who are physically dependent on opioid agonists. Symptoms may occur up to 15 days after discontinuation and persist for 1–2 wk.
- Buprenorphine has a lower potential for dependence than other opioids; however, prolonged use may lead to physical and psychological dependence and tolerance. This should not prevent patient from receiving adequate analgesia. Most patients receiving buprenorphine for pain do not develop psychological dependence. If tolerance develops, changing to an opioid agonist may be required to relieve pain.
- **Opioid Dependence:** Assess patient for signs and symptoms of opioid withdrawal before and during therapy.
- *Lab Test Considerations:* May cause elevated serum amylase and lipase levels.
- Monitor liver function tests prior to and periodically during therapy for opioid dependence.
- *Toxicity and Overdose:* If an opioid antagonist is required to reverse respiratory depression or coma, naloxone (Narcan) is the antidote. Dilute the 0.4-mg ampule of naloxone in 10 ml of 0.9% NaCl and administer 0.5 ml (0.02 mg) by direct IV push every 2 min. For children and patients weighing <40 kg, dilute 0.1 mg of naloxone in 10 ml of 0.9% NaCl for a concentration of 10 mcg/ml and administer 0.5 mcg/kg every 1–2 min. Titrate dose to avoid withdrawal, seizures, and severe pain. Naloxone may not completely reverse respiratory depressant effects of buprenorphine; may require mechanical ventilation, oxygen, IV fluids, and vasopressors.

## POTENTIAL NURSING DIAGNOSES

- Pain, acute (Indications).
- Injury, risk for (Side Effects).
- Coping, ineffective (Indications).

## IMPLEMENTATION

- *High Alert:* Accidental overdosage of opioid analgesics has resulted in fatalities. Before administering, clarify all ambiguous orders; have second practitioner independently check original order, dose calculations, route of administration, and infusion pump programming. Do not confuse Buprenex (buprenorphine) with Bumex (bumetanide).
- **Pain:** Explain therapeutic value of medication before administration to enhance the analgesic effect.
- Regularly administered doses may be more effective than prn administration. Analgesic is more effective if given before pain becomes severe.
- Coadministration with nonopioid analgesics has additive effects and may permit lower opioid doses.
- **IM:** Administer IM injections deep into well-developed muscle. Rotate sites of injections.
- **Direct IV:** May give IV undiluted.
- *High Alert:* Administer slowly. Rapid administration may cause respiratory depression, hypotension, and cardiac arrest.
- **Syringe Compatibility:** ◆ midazolam ◆ heparin.
- **Y-Site Compatibility:** ◆ allopurinol ◆ amifostine ◆ aztreonam ◆ cefipime ◆ cisatracurium ◆ cladribine ◆ docetaxel ◆ etoposide ◆ filgrastim ◆ gatifloxacin ◆ granisetron ◆ linezolid ◆ melphalan ◆ piperacillin/tazobactam ◆ propofol ◆ remifentanil ◆ teniposide ◆ thiotepa ◆ vinorelbine.
- **Y-Site Incompatibility:** ◆ amphotericin B cholesteryl sulfate ◆ doxorubicin liposome.
- **Solution Compatibility:** ◆ 0.9% NaCl ◆ D5W ◆ D5/0.9% NaCl ◆ lactated Ringer's injection ◆ Ringer's injection.
- **Opioid Dependence:** Must be prescribed by health care professional with special training. Induction is usually started with buprenorphine (Subutex) over 3–4 days. Initial dose should be administered at least 4 hr after last opioid dose and preferably when early signs of opioid whitdrawal appear. Once patient is on a stable dose, maintenance therapy with buprenorphine/naloxone

(Suboxone) is preferred for continued, unsupervised treatment.

■ **SL:** Administer sublingually. Usually takes 2–10 min for tablets to dissolve. If more than one tablet is prescribed, place multiple tablets under the tongue or 2 at a time until all tablets are dissolved. Do not chew or swallow; decreases amount of medication absorbed.

## PATIENT/FAMILY TEACHING

■ **General Info:** Medication may cause drowsiness or dizziness. Advise patient to call for assistance when ambulating and to avoid driving or other activities requiring alertness until response to medication is known.

❑ Advise patient to avoid concurrent use of alcohol or other CNS depressants.

❑ Advise patient to notify health care professional before taking other Rx or OTC medication or herbal products.

■ **Pain:** Instruct patient on how and when to ask for pain medication.

❑ Encourage patients on bedrest to turn, cough, and deep-breathe every 2 hr to prevent atelectasis.

❑ Instruct patient to change positions slowly to minimize orthostatic hypotension.

❑ Advise patient that good oral hygiene, frequent mouth rinses, and sugarless gum or candy may decrease dry mouth.

■ **Opioid Dependence:** Instruct patient in the correct use of medication; directions for use must be followed exactly. Medication must be used regularly, not occasionally. Missed doses should be taken as soon as remembered; if almost time for next dose, skip missed dose and return to regular dosing schedule. Do not take 2 doses at once unless directed by health care professional. Do not discontinue use without consulting health care professional; abrupt discontinuation may cause withdrawal symptoms. If medication is discontinued, flush unused tablets down the toilet.

❑ Caution patient that buprenorphine may be a target for people who abuse drugs; store medications in a safe place to protect them from theft. Selling or giving this medication to others is against the law.

❑ Caution patient that injection of Suboxone can lead to bad withdrawal symptoms.

❑ Advise patient if admitted to the emergency room to inform treating physician and emergency room staff of physical dependence on opioids and of treatment regimen.

❑ Advise patient to notify health care professional promptly if faintness, dizziness, confusion, slowed breathing, skin or whites of eyes turn yellow, urine turns dark, light colored stools, decreased appetite, nausea, or abdominal pain occur.

## EVALUATION

**Effectiveness of therapy can be demonstrated by:** ■ Decrease in severity of pain without a significant alteration in level of consciousness or respiratory status ■ Suppression of withdrawal symptoms during detoxification and maintenance from heroin or other opioids.

# bupropion

(byoo-**proe**-pee-on)

Wellbutrin, Wellbutrin SR, Zyban

### CLASSIFICATION(S):

**Therapeutic:** antidepressants, smoking deterrents

### Pregnancy Category B

## INDICATIONS

■ Treatment of depression (with psychotherapy) ■ Smoking cessation (Zyban only). **Unlabeled uses:** ■ Treatment of ADHD in adults (SR only) ■ To increase sexual desire in women.

## ACTION

■ Decreases neuronal reuptake of dopamine in the CNS ■ Diminished neuronal uptake of serotonin and norepinephrine (less than tricyclic antidepressants). **Therapeutic Effects:** ■ Diminished depression ■ Decreased craving for cigarettes.

## PHARMACOKINETICS

**Absorption:** Although well absorbed, rapidly and extensively metabolized by the liver.
**Distribution:** Unknown.

**Metabolism and Excretion:** Extensively metabolized by the liver. Some conversion to active metabolites.

**Half-life:** 14 hr (active metabolites may have longer half-lives).

## CONTRAINDICATIONS AND PRECAUTIONS

**Contraindicated in:** ■ Hypersensitivity ■ History of seizures, bulimia, and anorexia nervosa ■ Concurrent MAO inhibitor or ritonavir therapy.

**Use Cautiously in:** ■ History of cranial trauma ■ Renal or hepatic impairment (dosage reduction recommended) ■ Recent history of MI ■ Geriatric patients (increased risk of drug accumulation; increased sensitivity to effects) ■ Unstable cardiovascular status ■ Pregnancy, lactation, or children (safety not established).

## ADVERSE REACTIONS AND SIDE EFFECTS*

■ **CNS:** SEIZURES, agitation, headache, insomnia, mania, psychoses ■ **GI:** dry mouth, nausea, vomiting, change in appetite, weight gain, weight loss ■ **Derm:** photosensitivity ■ **Endo:** hyperglycemia, hypoglycemia, syndrome of inappropriate ADH secretion ■ **Neuro:** tremor.

## INTERACTIONS

**Drug-Drug:** ■ ↑ risk of adverse reactions when used with **amantadine, levodopa** or **MAO inhibitors** (concurrent use of MAO inhibitors is contraindicated) ■ ↑ risk of seizures with **phenothiazines, antidepressants, theophylline, corticosteroids, OTC stimulants/anorectics,** or cessation of **alcohol** or **benzodiazepines** (avoid or minimize alcohol use) ■ Blood levels ↑ by **ritonavir** (avoid concurrent use) ■ **Carbamazepine** may decrease ↓ blood levels and effectiveness ■ Concurrent use with **nicotine** replacement may cause hypertension ■ ↑ risk of bleeding with **warfarin** ■ Bupropion and one of its metabolites inhibit the CYP 2D6 enzyme system and may ↑ levels and risk of toxicity from **antidepressants** (SSRIs and tricyclic), some **beta blockers, antiarrhythmics,** and **antipsychotics**.

## ROUTE AND DOSAGE

❑ **Depression**

■ **PO (Adults):** *Immediate-release*—100 mg twice daily initially; after 3 days may increase to 100 mg 3 times daily; after at least 4 wk of therapy, may increase up to 450 mg/day in divided doses (not to exceed 150 mg/dose; wait at least 6 hr between doses at the 300 mg/day dose or at least 4 hr between doses at the 450 mg/day dose). *Sustained-release*—150 mg once daily in the morning; after 3 days, may increase to 150 mg twice daily with at least 8 hr between doses; after at least 4 wk of therapy, may increase to a maximum daily dose 400 mg given as 200 mg twice daily.

❑ **Smoking cessation**

■ **PO (Adults):** *Zyban*—150 mg once daily for 3 days, then 150 mg twice daily for 7–12 wk (doses should be at least 8 hr apart).

## AVAILABILITY (generic available)

■ *Tablets:* 75 mg^Rx, 100 mg^Rx ■ Cost: 75 mg $84.10/100, 100 mg $112.19/100 ■ *Sustained-release tablets:* 100 mg^Rx, 150 mg^Rx, 200 mg^Rx ■ Cost: 100 mg $94.27/60, 150 mg $101.94/60.

TIME/ACTION PROFILE (antidepressant effect)

|  | ONSET | PEAK | DURATION |
| --- | --- | --- | --- |
| PO | 1–3 wk | unknown | unknown |

# NURSING IMPLICATIONS

## ASSESSMENT

❑ Monitor mood changes. Inform physician or other health care professional if patient demonstrates significant increase in anxiety, nervousness, or insomnia.

❑ Assess for suicidal tendencies, especially during early therapy. Restrict amount of drug available to patient.

■ *Lab Test Considerations:* Monitor hepatic and renal function closely in patients with kidney or liver impairment to prevent elevated serum and tissue bupropion concentrations.

## POTENTIAL NURSING DIAGNOSES

■ Coping, ineffective (Indications).

## IMPLEMENTATION

■ **General:** Do not confuse bupropion with buspirone. Do not confuse Zyban (bupropion) with Zagam (Sparfloxacin).

❏ Administer doses in equally spaced time increments throughout day to minimize the risk of seizures.

❏ May be initially administered concurrently with sedatives to minimize agitation. This is not usually required after the 1st wk of therapy.

❏ Insomnia may be decreased by avoiding bedtime doses.

❏ May be administered with food to lessen GI irritation.

❏ Nicotine patches, gum, inhalers, and spray may be used concurrently with bupropion.

■ **PO:** Sustained-release tablets should be swallowed whole; do not break, crush, or chew.

## PATIENT/FAMILY TEACHING

❏ Instruct patient to take bupropion exactly as directed. If a dose taken for depression is missed, take as soon as possible and space day's remaining doses evenly at not less than 4-hr intervals. Missed doses for smoking cessation should be omitted. Do not double doses or take more than prescribed. May require 4 wk or longer for full effects. Do not discontinue without consulting health care professional. May require gradual reduction before discontinuation.

❏ Bupropion may impair judgment or motor and cognitive skills. Caution patient to avoid driving and other activities requiring alertness until response to medication is known.

❏ Advise patient to avoid alcohol during therapy and to consult with health care professional before taking other medications with bupropion.

❏ Inform patient that frequent mouth rinses, good oral hygiene, and sugarless gum or candy may minimize dry mouth. If dry mouth persists for more than 2 wk, consult health care professional regarding use of saliva substitute.

❏ Advise patient to notify health care professional if rash or other troublesome side effects occur.

❏ Advise patient to use sunscreen and protective clothing to prevent photosensitivity reactions.

❏ Instruct female patients to inform health care professional if pregnancy is planned or suspected.

❏ Advise patient to notify health care professional of medication regimen before treatment or surgery.

❏ Emphasize the importance of follow-up exams to monitor progress. Encourage patient participation in psychotherapy.

■ **Smoking Cessation:** Smoking should be stopped during the 2nd week of therapy to allow for the onset of buprorion and to maximize the chances of quitting.

## EVALUATION

**Effectiveness of therapy can be demonstrated by:** ■ Increased sense of well-being ❏ Renewed interest in surroundings. Acute episodes of depression may require several months of treatment ■ Cessation of smoking.

# buspirone
(byoo-**spye**-rone)
BuSpar

***CLASSIFICATION(S):***
***Therapeutic:*** *antianxiety agents*

**Pregnancy Category B**

## INDICATIONS

■ Management of anxiety.

## ACTION

■ Binds to serotonin and dopamine receptors in the brain ■ Increases norepinephrine metabolism in the brain. **Therapeutic Effects:** ■ Relief of anxiety.

## PHARMACOKINETICS

**Absorption:** Rapidly absorbed.

**Distribution:** Unknown.

**Protein Binding:** 95% bound to plasma proteins.

**Metabolism and Excretion:** Extensively metabolized by the liver (CYP 3A4 enzyme system); 20–40% excreted in feces.

**Half-life:** 2–3 hr.

## CONTRAINDICATIONS AND PRECAUTIONS

**Contraindicated in:** ■ Hypersensitivity ■ Severe hepatic or renal impairment ■ Concurrent use of MAO inhibitors ■ Ingestion of large amounts of grapefruit juice.

**Use Cautiously in:** ■ Patients receiving other antianxiety agents (other agents should be slowly withdrawn to prevent withdrawal or rebound phenomenon) ■ Patients receiving other psychotropics ■ Pregnancy, lactation, and children (safety not established).

## ADVERSE REACTIONS AND SIDE EFFECTS*

■ **CNS:** <u>dizziness</u>, <u>drowsiness</u>, <u>excitement</u>, <u>fatigue</u>, <u>headache</u>, <u>insomnia</u>, <u>nervousness</u>, <u>weakness</u>, personality changes ■ **EENT:** <u>blurred vision</u>, <u>nasal congestion</u>, <u>sore throat</u>, <u>tinnitus</u>, altered taste or smell, conjunctivitis ■ **Resp:** chest congestion, hyperventilation, shortness of breath ■ **CV:** <u>chest pain</u>, <u>palpitations</u>, <u>tachycardia</u>, hypertension, hypotension, syncope ■ **GI:** <u>nausea</u>, abdominal pain, constipation, diarrhea, dry mouth, vomiting ■ **GU:** changes in libido, dysuria, urinary frequency, urinary hesitancy ■ **Derm:** <u>rashes</u>, alopecia, blisters, dry skin, easy bruising, edema, flushing, pruritus ■ **Endo:** irregular menses ■ **MS:** <u>myalgia</u> ■ **Neuro:** <u>incoordination</u>, <u>numbness</u>, <u>paresthesia</u>, tremor ■ **Misc:** <u>clamminess</u>, <u>sweating</u>, fever.

## INTERACTIONS

**Drug-Drug:** ■ Use with **MAO inhibitors** may result in hypertension and is not recommended ■ **Erythromycin, nefazodone, ketoconazole, itraconazole, ritonavir,** and other **inhibitors of CYP 3A4** ↑ blood levels and effects of buspirone; dose reduction is recommended (decrease to 2.5 mg twice daily with erythromycin, decrease to 2.5 mg once daily with nefazodone) ■ **Rifampin, dexamethasone, phenytoin, phenobarbital, carbamazepine,** and other **inducers of CYP 3A4** ↓ blood levels and effects of buspirone; dose adjustment may be necessary ■ Avoid concurrent use with **alcohol.**

**Drug-Natural Products:** ■ Concomitant use of **kava, valerian** or **chamomile** can ↑ CNS depression.

**Drug-Food:** ■ **Grapefruit juice** ↑ serum levels and effect; ingestion of large amounts of grapefruit juice is not recommended.

## ROUTE AND DOSAGE

■ **PO (Adults):** 5 mg 3 times daily; increase by 5 mg/day q 2–3 days as needed (not to exceed 60 mg/day). Usual dose is 20–30 mg/day.

## AVAILABILITY (generic available)

■ *Tablets:* 5 mg$^{Rx}$, 10 mg$^{Rx}$, 15 mg$^{Rx}$ ■ Cost: 5 mg $90.71/100, 10 mg $158.19/100, 15 mg $141.82/60.

TIME/ACTION PROFILE (relief of anxiety)

| | ONSET | PEAK | DURATION |
|---|---|---|---|
| PO | 7–10 days | 3–4 wk | unknown |

# NURSING IMPLICATIONS

## ASSESSMENT

❑ Assess degree and manifestations of anxiety before and periodically during therapy.

❑ Buspirone does not appear to cause physical or psychological dependence or tolerance. However, patients with a history of drug abuse should be assessed for tolerance or dependence. Restrict amount of drug available to these patients.

## POTENTIAL NURSING DIAGNOSES

■ Anxiety (Indications).

■ Injury, risk for (Side Effects).

## IMPLEMENTATION

■ **General:** Do not confuse buspirone with bupropion.

❑ Patients changing from other antianxiety agents should receive gradually decreasing doses. Buspirone will not prevent withdrawal symptoms.

■ **PO:** May be administered with food to minimize gastric irritation. Food slows but does not alter extent of absorption.

## PATIENT/FAMILY TEACHING

❑ Instruct patient to take buspirone exactly as directed. Take missed doses as soon as possible if not just before next dose; do not double doses. Do not take more than amount prescribed.

❑ May cause dizziness or drowsiness. Caution patient to avoid driving or other activities requiring alertness until response to the medication is known.

□ Advise patient to avoid concurrent use of alcohol or other CNS depressants.

□ Advise patient to consult health care professional before taking OTC medications or herbal products with this drug.

□ Instruct patient to notify health care professional if any chronic abnormal movements occur (dystonia, motor restlessness, involuntary movements of facial or cervical muscles) or if pregnancy is suspected.

□ Emphasize the importance of follow-up exams to determine effectiveness of medication.

## EVALUATION

**Effectiveness of therapy can be demonstrated by:** ■ Increase in sense of well-being □ Decrease in subjective feelings of anxiety. Some improvement may be seen in 7–10 days. Optimal results take 3–4 wk of therapy. Buspirone is usually used for short-term therapy (3–4 wk). If prescribed for long-term therapy, efficacy should be periodically assessed.

### High Alert

## busulfan
(byoo-**sul**-fan)
Busulfex, Myleran

*CLASSIFICATION(S):*
*Therapeutic: antineoplastics*
*Pharmacologic: alkylating agents*

**Pregnancy Category D**

## INDICATIONS

■ **PO:** Treatment of chronic myelogenous leukemia (CML) and bone marrow disorders ■ **IV:** With cyclophosphamide as a conditioning regimen before allogenic hematopoietic progenitor cell transplantation for CML.

## ACTION

■ Disrupts nucleic acid function and protein synthesis (cell-cycle phase–nonspecific). **Therapeutic Effects:** ■ Death of rapidly growing cells, especially malignant ones.

## PHARMACOKINETICS

**Absorption:** Rapidly absorbed from the GI tract.
**Distribution:** Unknown.
**Metabolism and Excretion:** Extensively metabolized by the liver.
**Half-life:** 2.5 hr.

## CONTRAINDICATIONS AND PRECAUTIONS

**Contraindicated in:** ■ Hypersensitivity ■ Failure to respond to previous courses ■ Pregnancy or lactation.

**Use Cautiously in:** ■ Active infections ■ Decreased bone marrow reserve ■ Obese patients (base dose on ideal body weight) ■ Other chronic debilitating diseases ■ Patients with childbearing potential.

## ADVERSE REACTIONS AND SIDE EFFECTS*

Incidence and severity of adverse reactions and side effects are increased with IV use. ■ **CNS:** *IV*—SEIZURES, CEREBRAL HEMORRHAGE/COMA, anxiety, confusion, depression, dizziness, headache, encephalopathy, mental status changes, weakness ■ **EENT:** *PO*—cataracts; *IV*—epistaxis, pharyngitis, ear disorders ■ **CV:** hepatic veno-oclusive disease ( ↑ allogenic transplantation) ■ **Resp:** *PO*—PULMONARY FIBROSIS.; *IV*—alveolar hemorrhage, asthma, atelectasis, cough, hemoptysis, hypoxia, pleural effusion, pneumonia, rhinitis, sinusitis ■ **CV:** *PO*—CARDIAC TAMPONADE (WITH HIGH-DOSE CYCLOPHOSPHAMIDE); *IV*—chest pain, hypotension, tachycardia, thrombosis, arrhythmias, atrial fibrillation, cardiomegaly, ECG changes, edema, heart block, hypertension, left-sided heart failure, pericardial effusion , ventricular extrasystoles ■ **GI:** *PO*—drug-induced hepatitis, nausea, vomiting.; *IV*—abdominal enlargement, anorexia, constipation, diarrhea, dry mouth, hematemesis, nausea, rectal discomfort, vomiting, abdominal pain, dyspepsia, hepatomegaly, pancreatitis, stomatitis ■ **GU:** oliguria, dysuria, hematuria ■ **Derm:** *PO*—itching, rashes, acne, alopecia, erythema nodosum, exfoliative dermatitis, hyperpigmentation ■ **Endo:** *PO*—sterility, gynecomastia ■ **F and E:** hypokalemia, hypomagnesemia, hypophosphatemia ■ **Hemat:** BONE MARROW DEPRESSION ■ **Local:** inflammation/pain at injection site ■ **Metab:** *PO and IV*—hyperuricemia.; *IV*—hyperglycemia ■ **MS:** arthralgia, myalgia, back pain ■ **Misc:** allergic reactions, chills, fever, infection.

### INTERACTIONS

**Drug-Drug:** ■ Concurrent or previous (within 72 hr) use of **acetaminophen** may ↓ elimination and ↑ toxicity ■ Concurrent use with high-dose **cyclophosphamide** in patients with thalassemia may result in cardiac tamponade ■ Concurrent use with **itraconazole** or **phenytoin** ↓ blood levels effectiveness ■ Long-term continuous therapy with **thioguanine** may ↑ risk of hepatic toxicity ■ ↑ bone marrow suppression with other **antineoplastics** or **radiation therapy** ■ May ↓ the antibody response to and ↑ risk of adverse reactions from **live-virus vaccines.**

### ROUTE AND DOSAGE

Many other regimens are used. See current protocols for up-to-date dosage.
- **PO (Adults):** *Induction*—1.8 mg/m²/day or 60 mcg (0.06 mg)/kg/day until WBCs <15,000/mm³. Usual dose is 4–8 mg/day (range 1–12 mg/day). *Maintenance*—1–3 mg/day.
- **PO (Children):** 0.06–0.12 mg/kg/day or 1.8–4.6 mg/m²/day initially. Titrate dose to maintain WBC of approximately 20,000/mm³.
- **IV (Adults):** 0.8 mg/kg q 6 hr (dose based on ideal body weight or actual weight, whichever is less; in obese patients, dosage should be based on adjusted ideal body weight) for 4 days (total of 16 doses); given in combination with cyclophosphamide.

### AVAILABILITY

■*Tablets:* 2 mg^Rx ■ *Solution for injection:* 6 mg/ml in 10 ml ampules (60 mg) Rx.

TIME/ACTION PROFILE (effects on blood counts)

|        | ONSET   | PEAK    | DURATION     |
|--------|---------|---------|--------------|
| PO     | 1–2 wk  | weeks   | up to 1 mo†  |
| IV     | unknown | unknown | 13 days‡     |

†Complete recovery may take up to 20 mo.
‡After administration of last dose.

## NURSING IMPLICATIONS

### ASSESSMENT

□ *High Alert:* Monitor for bone marrow depression. Assess for bleeding (bleeding gums, bruising, petechiae, guaiac stools, urine, emesis) and avoid IM injections and taking rectal temperatures. Apply pressure to venipuncture sites for at least 10 min. Assess for signs of infection (fever, chills, sore throat, cough, hoarseness, lower back or side pain, difficult or painful urination) during neutropenia. Anemia may occur. Monitor for increased fatigue, dyspnea, and orthostatic hypotension. Notify physician if these symptoms occur.

■ **General Info:** Monitor intake and output ratios and daily weights. Report significant changes in totals.

□ Monitor for symptoms of gout (increased uric acid, joint pain, lower back or side pain, swelling of feet or lower legs). Encourage patient to drink at least 2 L of fluid each day. Allopurinol may be given to decrease uric acid levels. Alkalinization of urine may be ordered to increase excretion of uric acid.

□ Assess for pulmonary fibrosis (fever, cough, shortness of breath) periodically during and after therapy. Discontinue therapy at the first sign of pulmonary fibrosis. Usually occurs 8 mo–10 yr (average 4 yr) after initiation of therapy.

■ **IV:** Premedicate patient with phenytoin before IV administration to minimize the risk of seizures.

□ Antiemetics should be administered before IV administration and on a fixed schedule throughout IV administration.

■ *Lab Test Considerations:* Monitor CBC with differential and platelet count before and weekly during therapy. The nadir of leukopenia occurs within 10–15 days and the nadir of WBC at 11–30 days. Recovery usually occurs within 12–20 wk. Notify physician if WBC is <15,000/mm³ or if a precipitous drop occurs. Institute thrombocytopenia precautions if platelet count is <150,000/mm³. Bone marrow depression may be severe and progressive, with recovery taking 1 mo–2 yr after discontinuation of therapy.

□ Monitor serum ALT, bilirubin, alkaline phosphatase, and uric acid before and periodically during therapy. May cause ↑ uric acid levels.

□ May cause false-positive cytology results of breast, bladder, cervix, and lung tissues.

## POTENTIAL NURSING DIAGNOSES

■ Body image, disturbed (Side Effects).

■ Injury, risk for (Side Effects).

■ Infection, risk for (Side Effects).

## IMPLEMENTATION

❑ *High Alert:* Fatalities have occurred with chemotherapeutic agents. Before administering, clarify all ambiguous orders; double check single, daily, and course-of-therapy dose limits; have second practitioner independently double check original order, calculations and infusion pump settings.

■ **PO:** Administer at the same time each day. Administer on an empty stomach to decrease nausea and vomiting.

■ **IV:** Solution for IV administration should be prepared in a biologic cabinet. Wear gloves, gown, and mask while handling IV medication. Discard IV equipment in specially designated containers.

■ **Intermittent Infusion:** Dilute with 10 times the volume of busulfan using 0.9% NaCl or D5W for a final concentration of ≥0.5 mg/ml. When drawing busulfan from vial, use needle with 5-micron nylon filter provided, remove calculated volume from vial, remove needle and filter, replace needle and inject busulfan into diluent. Do not use polycarbonate syringes with busulfan. Only use filters provided with busulfan. Always add busulfan to diluent, not diluent to busulfan. Solution diluted with 0.9% NaCl or D5W is stable for 8 hr at room temperature and solution diluted with 0.9% NaCl is stable for 12 hr if refrigerated. Administration must be completed during this time.

■ *Rate:* Administer via central venous catheter over 2 hr every 6 hr for 4 days for a total of 16 doses. Use infusion pump to administer entire dose over 2 hr.

■ **Y-Site Incompatibility:** Do not administer with other solutions. Flush catheter with 0.9% NaCl or D5W before and after administration.

## PATIENT/FAMILY TEACHING

❑ Instruct patient to take medication exactly as directed, at the same time each day, even if nausea and vomiting are a problem. Consult health care professional if vomiting occurs shortly after dose is taken. If a dose is missed, do not take at all; do not double doses.

❑ Advise patient to notify health care professional if fever; sore throat; signs of infection; lower back or side pain; difficult or painful urination; sores in the mouth or on the lips; chills; dyspnea; persistent cough; bleeding gums; bruising; petechiae; or blood in urine, stool, or emesis occurs. Instruct patient to use soft toothbrush and electric razor. Caution patient not to drink alcoholic beverages or take products containing aspirin or NSAIDs.

❑ Caution patient to avoid crowds and persons with known infections. Health care professional should be informed immediately if symptoms of infection occur.

❑ Discuss with patient the possibility of hair loss. Explore methods of coping.

❑ Review with patient the need for contraception during therapy. Women need to use contraception even if amenorrhea occurs.

❑ Instruct patient not to receive any vaccinations without advice of health care professional.

❑ Advise patient to notify health care professional if unusual bleeding; bruising; or flank, stomach, or joint pain occurs. Advise patients on long-term therapy to notify health care professional immediately if cough, shortness of breath, and fever occur or if darkening of skin, diarrhea, dizziness, fatigue, anorexia, confusion, or nausea and vomiting become pronounced.

❑ Inform patient of increased risk of a second malignancy with busulfan.

## EVALUATION

**Effectiveness of therapy can be demonstrated by:** ■ Decrease in leukocyte count to within normal limits ❑ Decreased night sweats ❑ Increase in appetite ❑ Increased sense of well-being. Therapy is resumed when leukocyte count reaches 50,000/mm³.

## BUTALBITAL COMPOUND
(byoo-**tal**-bi-tal)

**butalbital, acetaminophen†**

Axocet, Bucet, Bupap, Butex Forte, Dolgic, Marten-Tab, Phrenilin, Phrenilin Forte, Repap CF, Sedapap, Tencon, Triaprin

**butalbital, acetaminophen, caffeine†**

Endolor, Esgic, Esgic-Plus, Fioricet, Margesic, Medigesic, Repan, Triad

**butalbital, aspirin, caffeine‡**

Fiorinal, Fiortal, {Tecnal}

### CLASSIFICATION(S):

*Therapeutic: nonopioid analgesics (combination with barbiturate)*
*Pharmacologic: barbiturates*

**Schedule III (products with aspirin only)**

**Pregnancy Category D**

†For information on acetaminophen component in formulation, see acetaminophen monograph.

‡For information on aspirin component in formulation, see salicylates monograph.

### INDICATIONS

■ Management of mild to moderate pain.

### ACTION

■ Contain an analgesic (aspirin or acetaminophen) for relief of pain, a barbiturate (butalbital) for its sedative effect, and some contain caffeine, which may be of benefit in vascular headaches. **Therapeutic Effects:** ■ Decreased severity of pain with some sedation.

### PHARMACOKINETICS

**Absorption:** Well absorbed.
**Distribution:** Widely distributed; cross the placenta and enter breast milk.
**Metabolism and Excretion:** Mostly metabolized by the liver.
**Half-life:** 35 hr.

### CONTRAINDICATIONS AND PRECAUTIONS

**Contraindicated in:** ■ Hypersensitivity to individual components ■ Cross-sensitivity may occur ■ Comatose patients or those with pre-existing CNS depression ■ Uncontrolled severe pain ■ Aspirin should be avoided in patients with bleeding disorders or thrombocytopenia ■ Acetaminophen should be avoided in patients with severe hepatic or renal disease ■ Caffeine should be avoided in patients with severe cardiovascular disease ■ Pregnancy or lactation ■ Porphyria.

**Use Cautiously in:** ■ History of suicide attempt or drug addiction ■ Chronic alcohol use/abuse (for aspirin and acetaminophen content) ■ Geriatric patients (dosage reduction required) ■ Use should be short-term only ■ Children (safety not established).

### ADVERSE REACTIONS AND SIDE EFFECTS*

■ **CNS:** *caffeine*—drowsiness, hangover, delirium, depression, excitation, headache (with chronic use), insomnia, irritability, lethargy, nervousness, vertigo ■ **Resp:** respiratory depression ■ **CV:** *caffeine*—palpitations, tachycardia ■ **GI:** *caffeine*—constipation, diarrhea, epigastric distress, heartburn, nausea, vomiting ■ **Derm:** dermatitis, rash ■ **Misc:** hypersensitivity reactions including ANGIOEDEMA and SERUM SICKNESS, physical dependence, psychological dependence, tolerance.

### INTERACTIONS

**Drug-Drug:** ■ Additive CNS depression with other **CNS depressants,** including **alcohol, antihistamines, antidepressants, opioid analgesics,** and **sedative/hypnotics** ■ May increase the liver metabolism and decrease the effectiveness of other drugs including **hormonal contraceptives, chloramphenicol, acebutolol, propranolol, metoprolol, timolol, doxycycline, corticosteroids, tricyclic antidepressants, phenothiazines, phenylbutazone,** and **quinidine** ■ **MAO inhibitors, primidone,** and **valproic acid** may prevent metabolism and increase the effectiveness of butalbital ■ May enhance the hematologic toxicity of **cyclophosphamide.**

**Drug-Natural Products:** ■ **St. John's wort** may decrease barbiturate effect ■ Concurrent use of **kava, valerian, skullcap, chamomile,** or **hops** can increase CNS depression.

### ROUTE AND DOSAGE

■ **PO (Adults):** 1–2 capsules or tablets (50–100 mg butalbital) every 4 hr as needed for pain (not to exceed 4 g acetaminophen or aspirin/24 hr).

## AVAILABILITY (generic available)

■ *Tablets and capsules:* ■ Cost: $6.62/30 ■ aspirin, acetaminophen, caffeine, and codeine Rx. See Appendix B.

TIME/ACTION PROFILE

|    | ONSET | PEAK | DURATION |
|----|-------|------|----------|
| PO | 15–30 min | 1–2 hr | 2–6 hr |

## NURSING IMPLICATIONS

### ASSESSMENT

❏ Assess type, location, and intensity of pain before and 60 min following administration.

❏ Prolonged use may lead to physical and psychological dependence and tolerance. This should not prevent patient from receiving adequate analgesia. Most patients who receive butalbital compound for pain do not develop psychological dependence.

❏ Assess frequency of use. Frequent, chronic use may lead to daily headaches in headache-prone individuals because of physical dependence on caffeine and other components. Chronic headaches from overmedication are difficult to treat and may require hospitalization for treatment and prophylaxis.

### POTENTIAL NURSING DIAGNOSES

■ Pain, acute (Indications).

■ Injury, risk for (Side Effects).

### IMPLEMENTATION

■ **General:** Do not confuse Fiorinal with Fioricet.

❏ Explain therapeutic value of medication before administration to enhance the analgesic effect.

❏ Regularly administered doses may be more effective than prn administration. Analgesic is more effective if given before pain becomes severe.

❏ Medication should be discontinued gradually after long-term use to prevent withdrawal symptoms.

■ **PO:** Oral doses should be administered with food, milk, or a full glass of water to minimize GI irritation.

### PATIENT/FAMILY TEACHING

❏ Instruct patient to take medication exactly as directed. Do not increase dose because of the habit-forming potential of butalbital. If medication appears less effective after a few weeks, consult health care professional. Doses of acetaminophen or aspirin should not exceed the maximum recommended daily dose. Chronic excessive use of >4 g/day (2 g in chronic alcoholism) may lead to hepatotoxicity, renal or cardiac damage.

❏ Advise patients with vascular headaches to take medication at first sign of headache. Lying down in a quiet, dark room may also be helpful. Medications taken for prophylaxis should be continued.

❏ May cause drowsiness or dizziness. Advise patient to avoid driving and other activities requiring alertness until response to medication is known.

❏ Caution patient to avoid concurrent use of alcohol or other CNS depressants.

❏ Advise patient to use an additional nonhormonal method of contraception while taking butalbital compound.

### EVALUATION

**Effectiveness of therapy can be demonstrated by:** ■ Decrease in severity of pain without a significant alteration in level of consciousness.

---

## butenafine, See ANTIFUNGALS (TOPICAL).

---

## butoconazole, See ANTIFUNGALS (VAGINAL).

---

High Alert

## butorphanol

(byoo-**tor**-fa-nole)

Stadol, Stadol NS

---

**CLASSIFICATION(S):**
*Therapeutic:* opioid analgesics
*Pharmacologic:* opioid agonists/
antagonists

**Schedule IV**

**Pregnancy Category C**

## INDICATIONS

■ Management of moderate to severe pain ■ Analgesia during labor ■ Sedation before surgery ■ Supplement in balanced anesthesia.

## ACTION

■ Binds to opiate receptors in the CNS ■ Alters the perception of and response to painful stimuli while producing generalized CNS depression ■ Has partial antagonist properties that may result in opioid withdrawal in physically dependent patients. **Therapeutic Effects:** ■ Decreased severity of pain.

## PHARMACOKINETICS

**Absorption:** Well absorbed from IM sites and nasal mucosa.

**Distribution:** Crosses the placenta and enters breast milk.

**Metabolism and Excretion:** Mostly metabolized by the liver; 11–14% excreted in the feces. Minimal renal excretion.

**Half-life:** 3–4 hr.

## CONTRAINDICATIONS AND PRECAUTIONS

**Contraindicated in:** ■ Hypersensitivity ■ Patients physically dependent on opioids (may precipitate withdrawal).

**Use Cautiously in:** ■ Head trauma ■ Increased intracranial pressure ■ Severe renal, hepatic, or pulmonary disease (increase interval to q 6–8 hr initially in hepatic/renal impairment) ■ Hypothyroidism ■ Adrenal insufficiency ■ Alcoholism ■ Geriatric or debilitated patients (in geriatric patients, decrease usual dose by 50%; give at twice the usual interval initially) ■ Undiagnosed abdominal pain ■ Prostatic hypertrophy ■ Pregnancy, lactation, or children <18 yr (safety not established but has been used during labor—may cause respiratory depression in the newborn).

## ADVERSE REACTIONS AND SIDE EFFECTS*

■ **CNS:** confusion, dysphoria, hallucinations, sedation, euphoria, floating feeling, headache, unusual dreams ■ **EENT:** blurred vision, diplopia, miosis (high doses) ■ **Resp:** respiratory depression ■ **CV:** hypertension, hypotension, palpitations ■ **GI:** nausea, constipation, dry mouth, ileus, vomiting ■ **GU:** urinary retention ■ **Derm:** sweating, clammy feeling ■ **Misc:** physical dependence, psychological dependence, tolerance.

## INTERACTIONS

**Drug-Drug:** ■ Use with extreme caution in patients receiving **MAO inhibitors** (may produce severe, potentially fatal reactions—reduce initial dose of butorphanol to 25% of usual dose) ■ Additive CNS depression with **alcohol, antidepressants, antihistamines,** and **sedative/hypnotics** ■ May precipitate withdrawal in patients who are physically dependent on **opioids** and have not been detoxified ■ May decrease effects of concurrently administered **opioids**.

**Drug-Natural Products:** ■ Concomitant use of **kava, valerian, skullcap, chamomile,** or **hops** can increase CNS depression.

## ROUTE AND DOSAGE

■ **IM (Adults):** 2 mg q 3–4 hr as needed (range 1–4 mg).
■ **IV (Adults):** 1 mg q 3–4 hr as needed (range 0.5–2 mg).
■ **IM, IV (Geriatric Patients):** 1 mg q 4–6 hr, increased as necessary.
■ **Intranasal (Adults):** 1 mg (1 spray in 1 nostril) initially. An additional dose may be given 60–90 min later. This sequence may be repeated in 3–4 hr. If pain is severe, an initial dose of 2 mg (1 spray in each nostril) may be given. May be repeated in 3–4 hr.
■ **Intranasal (Geriatric Patients):** 1 mg (1 spray in 1 nostril) initially. An additional dose may be given 90–120 min later. This sequence may be repeated in 3–4 hr.

## AVAILABILITY (generic available)

■ *Injection:* 1 mg/ml^Rx, 2 mg/ml^Rx ■ *Intranasal solution:* 10 mg/ml, in 2.5-ml metered-dose spray pump (14–15 doses; 1 mg/spray)^Rx.

TIME/ACTION PROFILE (analgesia)

| | ONSET | PEAK | DURATION |
|---|---|---|---|
| IM | within 15 min | 30–60 min | 3–4 hr |
| IV | within mins | 4–5 min | 2–4 hr |
| Intranasal | within 15 min | 1–2 hr | 4–5 hr |

## NURSING IMPLICATIONS

### ASSESSMENT

❑ Assess type, location, and intensity of pain before and 30–60 min after IM, 5 min after IV, and 60–90 min after intranasal administration. When titrating opioid doses, increases of 25–50% should be administered until there is either a 50% reduction in the patient's pain rating on a numerical or visual analog scale or the patient reports satisfactory pain relief. A repeat dose can be safely administered at the time of the peak if previous dose is ineffective and side effects are minimal. Patients requiring doses higher than 4 mg should be converted to an opioid agonist. Butorphanol is not recommended for prolonged use or as first-line therapy for acute or cancer pain.

❑ An equianalgesic chart (see Appendix O) should be used when changing routes or when changing from one opioid to another.

❑ Assess blood pressure, pulse, and respirations before and periodically during administration. If respiratory rate is <10/min, assess level of sedation. Dosage may need to be decreased by 25–50%. Respiratory depression does not increase in severity, only in duration, with increased dosage.

❑ Assess previous analgesic history. Antagonistic properties may induce withdrawal symptoms (vomiting, restlessness, abdominal cramps, increased blood pressure and temperature) in patients who are physically dependent on opioid agonists.

❑ Butorphanol has a lower potential for dependence than other opioids; however, prolonged use may lead to physical and psychological dependence and tolerance. This should not prevent the patient from receiving adequate analgesia. Most patients receiving butorphanol for pain do not develop psychological dependence. If tolerance develops, changing to an opioid agonist may be required to relieve pain.

■ **Lab Test Considerations:** May cause elevated serum amylase and lipase levels.

■ **Toxicity and Overdose:** If an opioid antagonist is required to reverse respiratory depression or coma, naloxone (Narcan) is the antidote. Dilute the 0.4-mg ampule of naloxone in 10 ml of 0.9% NaCl and administer 0.5 ml (0.02 mg) by direct IV push every 2 min. For children and patients weighing <40 kg, dilute 0.1 mg of naloxone in 10 ml of 0.9% NaCl for a concentration of 10 mcg/ml and administer 0.5 mcg/kg every 1–2 min. Titrate dose to avoid withdrawal, seizures, and severe pain.

### POTENTIAL NURSING DIAGNOSES

■ Pain, acute (Indications).

■ Injury, risk for (Side Effects).

■ Sensory perception, disturbed (visual, auditory) (Side Effects).

### IMPLEMENTATION

❑ **High Alert:** Accidental overdosage of opioid analgesics has resulted in fatalities. Before administering, clarify all ambiguous orders; have second practitioner independently check original order, dose calculations, route of administration, and infusion pump programming. Do not confuse Stadol with Haldol.

■ **General:** Explain therapeutic value of medication before administration to enhance the analgesic effect.

❑ Regularly administered doses may be more effective than prn administration. Analgesic is more effective if given before pain becomes severe.

❑ Coadministration with nonopioid analgesics may have additive analgesic effects and permit lower opioid doses.

■ **IM:** Administer IM injections deep into well-developed muscle. Rotate sites of injections.

■ **Direct IV:** May give IV undiluted.

■ **Rate:** Administer over 3–5 min.

❑ **High Alert:** Rapid administration may cause respiratory depression, hypotension, and cardiac arrest.

■ **Syringe Compatibility:** ◆ atropine ◆ chlorpromazine ◆ cimetidine ◆ diphenhydramine ◆ droperidol ◆ fentanyl ◆ hydroxyzine ◆ meperidine ◆ methotrimeprazine ◆ metoclopramide ◆ midazolam ◆ morphine ◆ pentazocine ◆ perphenazine ◆ prochlorperazine ◆ promethazine ◆ scopolamine ◆ thiethylperazine.

■ **Syringe Incompatibility:** ◆ dimenhydrinate ◆ pentobarbital.

■ **Y-Site Compatibility:** ◆ allopurinol sodium ◆ amifostine ◆ aztreonam ◆ cefepime ◆ cladribine ◆ enalaprilat ◆ esmolol ◆ filgrastim ◆ fludarabine ◆ gatifloxacin ◆ granisetron ◆ labetalol ◆ linezolid ◆ melphalan ◆ paclitaxel ◆ piperacillin/tazobactam ◆ propofol ◆ sargramostim ◆ teniposide ◆ thiotepa ◆ vinorelbine. **Intranasal:** Administer 1 spray in 1 nostril.

## PATIENT/FAMILY TEACHING

❑ Instruct patient on how and when to ask for pain medication.

❑ Medication may cause drowsiness or dizziness. Advise patient to call for assistance when ambulating and to avoid driving or other activities requiring alertness until response to the medication is known.

❑ Encourage patients on bedrest to turn, cough, and deep-breathe every 2 hr to prevent atelectasis.

❑ Instruct patient to change positions slowly to minimize orthostatic hypotension.

❑ Caution patient to avoid concurrent use of alcohol or other CNS depressants with this medication.

❑ Advise patient that good oral hygiene, frequent mouth rinses, and sugarless gum or candy may decrease dry mouth.

■ **Intranasal:** Instruct patient on proper use of nasal spray. See package insert for detailed instructions. Instruct patient to replace protective clip and clear cover after use and to store the unit in the childresistant container. Caution patient that medication should not be used by anyone other than the person for whom it was prescribed. Excess medication should be disposed of as soon as it is no longer needed. To dispose of, unscrew cap, rinse bottle and pump with water, and dispose of in waste can.

❑ If 2-mg dose is prescribed, administer additional spray in other nostril. May cause dizziness and dysphoria. Patient should remain recumbent after administration of 2-mg dose until response to medication is known.

## EVALUATION

**Effectiveness of therapy can be demonstrated by:** ■ Decrease in severity of pain without a significant alteration in level of consciousness or respiratory status.

# cabergoline

(ka-**ber**-goe-leen)
Dostinex

*CLASSIFICATION(S):*
***Therapeutic:*** *antihyperprolactinemics*
***Pharmacologic:*** *dopamine antagonists*

Pregnancy Category C

## INDICATIONS

■ Treatment of hyperprolactinemia (idiopathic or pituitary in origin).

## ACTION

■ Inhibits secretion of prolactin by acting as a dopamine agonist. **Therapeutic Effects:** ■ Decreased secretion of prolactin.

## PHARMACOKINETICS

**Absorption:** Well absorbed but undergoes extensive first-pass hepatic metabolism.
**Distribution:** Widely distributed; concentrates in pituitary.
**Metabolism and Excretion:** Extensively metabolized by the liver; <4% excreted unchanged in urine.
**Half-life:** 63–69 hr.

## CONTRAINDICATIONS AND PRECAUTIONS

**Contraindicated in:** ■ Hypersensitivity to cabergoline or ergot alkaloids ■ Uncontrolled hypertension ■ Pregnancy or lactation.
**Use Cautiously in:** ■ Hepatic impairment ■ Children (safety not established).

## ADVERSE REACTIONS AND SIDE EFFECTS*

■ **CNS:** <u>dizziness</u>, <u>headache</u>, depression, drowsiness, fatigue, nervousness, vertigo, weakness ■ **EENT:** abnormal vision ■ **CV:** postural hypotension ■ **GI:** <u>constipation</u>, <u>nausea</u>, abdominal pain, dyspepsia, vomiting ■ **GU:** dysmenorrhea ■ **Endo:** breast pain ■ **Metab:** hot flashes ■ **Neuro:** paresthesia.

## INTERACTIONS

**Drug-Drug:** ■ Increased risk of hypotension with **antihypertensives** ■ Effectiveness may be decreased by **phenothiazines, butyrophenones (haloperidol), thioxanthenes,** or **metoclopramide** (avoid concurrent use).

## ROUTE AND DOSAGE

■ **PO (Adults):** 0.25 mg twice weekly; may be increased at 4-wk intervals up to 1 mg twice weekly.

## AVAILABILITY

■ ***Tablets:*** 0.5 mg$^{Rx}$ ■ Cost: $240.79/8 tablets.

TIME/ACTION PROFILE (effect on serum prolactin levels)

| | ONSET | PEAK | DURATION |
|---|---|---|---|
| PO | unknown | 4 wk | unknown |

# NURSING IMPLICATIONS

## ASSESSMENT

❑ Monitor blood pressure before and frequently during initial therapy. Initial doses >1 mg may cause orthostatic hypotension. Use with caution when administering concurrently with other medications that lower blood pressure. Supervise ambulation and transfer during initial dosing to prevent injury from hypotension.
■ *Lab Test Considerations:* Serum prolactin concentrations should be measured monthly until normalized (<20 mcg/liter in women and <15 mcg/liter in men).

## POTENTIAL NURSING DIAGNOSES

■ Injury, risk for (Side Effects).

## IMPLEMENTATION

■ **PO:** May be taken without regard to food.

## PATIENT/FAMILY TEACHING

❑ Instruct patient to take medication exactly as directed. If a dose is missed, take as soon as possible within 1 or 2 days. If not remembered until time of next dose, double dose. If nausea occurs, discuss with health care professional.

❑ May cause drowsiness and dizziness. Caution patient to avoid driving and other activities requiring alertness until response to medication is known.

❑ Advise patient to change positions slowly to minimize orthostatic hypotension.

❑ Caution patient to avoid concurrent use of alcohol during the course of therapy.

❑ Advise women to consult with health care professional regarding a nonhormonal method of birth control. Women should contact health care professional promptly if pregnancy is planned or suspected.

❑ Instruct patients taking cabergoline for pituitary tumors to inform health care professional immediately if signs of tumor enlargement (blurred vision, sudden headache, severe nausea, and vomiting) occur.

❑ Emphasize the importance of regular follow-up exams to determine effectiveness and monitor side effects.

### EVALUATION

**Effectiveness of therapy can be demonstrated by:** ■ Decrease in galactorrhea in patients with hyperprolactinemia ❑ After a normal serum prolactin level has been maintained for more than 6 mo, cabergoline may be discontinued. Serum prolactin levels should be monitored periodically to determine necessity of reinstituting cabergoline.

**calcifediol, See VITAMIN D COMPOUNDS.**

# calcitonin (salmon)
(kal-si-**toe**-nin)

Calcimar, Miacalcin, Osteocalcin, Salmonine

**CLASSIFICATION(S):**
**Therapeutic:** hypocalcemics
**Pharmacologic:** hormones

**Pregnancy Category C**

### INDICATIONS

■ **IM, Subcut:** Treatment of Paget's disease of bone ■ Adjunctive therapy for hypercalcemia ■ **IM, Subcut, Intranasal:** Management of postmenopausal osteoporosis.

### ACTION

■ Decreases serum calcium by a direct effect on bone, kidney, and GI tract ■ Promotes renal excretion of calcium. **Therapeutic Effects:** ■ Decreased rate of bone turnover ■ Lowering of serum calcium.

### PHARMACOKINETICS

**Absorption:** Completely absorbed from IM and subcut sites. Rapidly absorbed from nasal mucosa; absorption is 3% compared with parenteral administration.
**Distribution:** Unknown.
**Metabolism and Excretion:** Rapidly metabolized in kidneys, blood, and tissues.
**Half-life:** 70–90 min.

### CONTRAINDICATIONS AND PRECAUTIONS

**Contraindicated in:** ■ Hypersensitivity to salmon protein or gelatin diluent ■ Pregnancy or lactation (use not recommended).
**Use Cautiously in:** ■ Children (safety not established).

### ADVERSE REACTIONS AND SIDE EFFECTS*

■ **CNS:** headaches ■ **EENT:** *nasal only*—epistaxis, nasal irritation, rhinitis ■ **GI:** *IM, subcut*—nausea, vomiting, altered taste, diarrhea ■ **GU:** *IM, subcut*—urinary frequency ■ **Derm:** rashes ■ **Local:** injection site reactions ■ **MS:** *nasal*—arthralgia, back pain ■ **Misc:** allergic reactions including ANAPHYLAXIS, facial flushing, swelling, tingling, and tenderness in the hands.

### INTERACTIONS

**Drug-Drug:** ■ Previous bisphosphanate therapy, including **alendronate, risedronate, etidronate,** or **pamidronate** may decrease response to calcitonin.

### ROUTE AND DOSAGE

❑ **Postmenopausal osteoporosis**
■ **IM, Subcut (Adults):** 100 IU/day.
■ **Intranasal (Adults):** 200 IU/day.
❑ **Paget's disease**
■ **IM, Subcut (Adults):** 100 IU/day initially, after titration, maintenance dose is usually 50 IU/day or every other day.
❑ **Hypercalcemia**
■ **IM, Subcut (Adults):** 4 IU/kg q 12 hr; may be increased after 1–2 days to 8 IU/kg q 12

hr, and if necessaraftersalmon 2 more days may be increased to 8 IU q 6 hr.

## AVAILABILITY

■ *Injection:* 200 IU/ml in 2-ml vials^Rx ■ Cost: $34.00-53.40/vial ■ *Nasal spray:* 200 IU/actuation in 2-ml bottles^Rx ■ Cost: $56.72/bottle.

TIME/ACTION PROFILE

| | ONSET | PEAK | DURATION |
|---|---|---|---|
| IM, subcut† | Unknown | 2 hr | 6–8 hr |
| Intranasal‡ | rapid | 31–39 min | Unknown |

†Effects on serum calcium; effects on serum alkaline phophatase and urinary hydroxyproline in Paget's disease may require 6–24 months of continuous treatment.
‡Serum levels of administered calcitonin.

## NURSING IMPLICATIONS

### ASSESSMENT

❑ Observe patient for signs of hypersensitivity (skin rash, fever, hives, anaphylaxis, serum sickness). Keep epinephrine, antihistamines, and oxygen nearby in the event of a reaction.

❑ Assess patient for signs of hypocalcemic tetany (nervousness, irritability, paresthesia, muscle twitching, tetanic spasms, seizures) during the first several doses of calcitonin. Parenteral calcium, such as calcium gluconate, should be available in case of this event.

■ *Lab Test Considerations:* Serum calcium and alkaline phosphatase should be monitored periodically throughout therapy. These levels should normalize within a few months of initiation of therapy.

❑ Urine hydroxyproline (24 hr) may be monitored periodically in patients with Paget's disease.

### POTENTIAL NURSING DIAGNOSES

■ Pain, acute (Indications).
■ Injury, risk for (Indications, Side Effects).

### IMPLEMENTATION

■ **General:** Assess for sensitivity to calcitonin-salmon by administering an intradermal test dose on the inner aspect of the forearm prior to initiating therapy. Test dose is prepared in a dilution of 10 IU/ml by withdraw-ing 0.05 ml in a tuberculin syringe and filling to 1 ml with 0.9% NaCl for injection. Mix well and discard 0.9 ml. Administer 0.1 ml and observe site for 15 min. More than mild erythema or wheal constitutes positive response.

❑ Store solution in refrigerator.

■ **IM, Subcut:** Inspect injection site for the appearance of redness, swelling, or pain. Rotate injection sites. Subcut is the preferred route. Use IM route if dose exceeds 2 ml in volume. Use multiple sites to minimize inflammatory reaction.

❑ Do not administer solutions that are discolored or contain particulate matter.

## PATIENT/FAMILY TEACHING

■ **General Info:** Advise patient to take medication exactly as directed. If dose is missed and medication is scheduled for twice a day, take only if possible within 2 hr of correct time. If scheduled for daily dose, take only if remembered that day. If scheduled for every other day, take when remembered and restart alternate day schedule. If taking 1 dose 3 times weekly (Mon, Wed, Fri), take missed dose the next day and set each injection back 1 day; resume regular schedule the following week. Do not double doses.

❑ Instruct patient in the proper method of self-injection.

❑ Advise patient to report signs of hypercalcemic relapse (deep bone or flank pain, renal calculi, anorexia, nausea, vomiting, thirst, lethargy) or allergic response promptly.

❑ Reassure patient that flushing and warmth following injection are transient and usually last about 1 hr.

❑ Explain that nausea following injection tends to decrease even with continued therapy.

❑ Instruct patient to follow low-calcium diet if recommended by health care professional (see Appendix Q). Women with postmenopausal osteoporosis should adhere to a diet high in calcium and vitamin D.

■ **Osteoporosis:** Advise patients receiving calcitonin for the treatment of osteoporosis that exercise has been found to arrest and reverse bone loss. The patient should discuss any exercise limitations with health care professional before beginning program.

■ **Intranasal:** Instruct patient on correct use of nasal spray. Before first use, activate pump by holding upright and depressing white side arms down toward bottle 6 times until a fine spray is emitted. Following activation, place nozzle firmly in nostril with head in an upright position and depress the pump toward the bottle.

❏ Advise patient to notify health care professional if significant nasal irritation occurs.

## EVALUATION

**Effectiveness of therapy can be demonstrated by:** ■ Lowered serum calcium levels ■ Decreased bone pain ■ Slowed progression of postmenopausal osteoporosis. Significant increases in bone marrow density may be seen as early as a month after initiation of therapy.

---

**calcitriol, See VITAMIN D COMPOUNDS.**

---

High Alert

## CALCIUM SALTS

**calcium acetate (25% Ca or 12.6 mEq/g)**

(**kal**-see-um **ass**-e-tate)
Calphron, PhosLo

**calcium carbonate (40% Ca or 20 mEq/g)**

(**kal**-see-um **kar**-bo-nate)
Alka-Mints, Amitone, {Apo-Cal}, BioCal, Calcarb, Calci-Chew, Calciday, Calcilac, Calci-Mix, {Calcite}, {Calglycine}, Cal-Plus, {Calsan}, Caltrate, Chooz, Dicarbosil, Equilet, Gencalc, Liqui-Cal, Liquid Cal-600, Maalox Antacid Caplets, Mallamint, {Mylanta Lozenges}, Nephro-Calci, {Nu-Cal}, Os-Cal, Oysco, Oyst-Cal, Oystercal, Rolaids Calcium Rich, Surpass, Surpass Extra Strength, Titralac, Tums, Tums E-X

**calcium chloride (27% Ca or 13.6 mEq/g)**

(**kal**-see-um **kloh**-ride)

**calcium citrate (21% Ca or 12 mEq/g)**

(**kal**-see-um **si**-trate)
Cal-Citrate 250, Citrical, Citrical Liquitab

**calcium gluceptate (8.2% Ca or 4.1 mEq/g)**

(**kal**-see-um **gloo**-sep-tate)

**calcium gluconate (9% Ca or 4.5 mEq/g)**

(**kal**-see-um **gloo**-koh-nate)
Kalcinate

**calcium lactate (13% Ca or 6.5 mEq/g)**

(**kal**-see-um **lak**-tate)
Cal-Lac

**tricalcium phosphate (39% Ca or 19.5 mEq/g)**

Posture

*CLASSIFICATION(S):*
*Therapeutic: mineral and electrolyte replacements/supplements*

**Pregnancy Category C (calcium acetate, calcium chloride, calcium gluceptate, calcium gluconate injections), UK (calcium carbonate, calcium citrate, calcium lactate, tricalcium phosphate)**

## INDICATIONS

■ **PO, IV:** Treatment and prevention of hypocalcemia ■ **PO:** Adjunct in the prevention of postmenopausal osteoporosis ■ **IV:** Emergency treatment of hyperkalemia and hypermagnesemia and adjunct in cardiac arrest (calcium chloride, calcium gluconate). ■ **Calcium carbonate:** May be used as an antacid ■ **Calcium acetate:** Control of hyperphosphatemia in endstage renal disease.

## ACTION

■ Essential for nervous, muscular, and skeletal systems ■ Maintain cell membrane and capillary permeability ■ Act as an activator in the transmission of nerve impulses and contraction of cardiac, skeletal, and smooth muscle ■ Essential for bone formation and blood coagulation. **Therapeutic Effects:** ■ Replacement of calcium in deficiency states. Control of hyperphosphatemia in end-stage renal disease without promoting aluminum absorption (calcium acetate).

## PHARMACOKINETICS

**Absorption:** Absorption from the GI tract requires vitamin D. IV administration results in complete bioavailability.
**Distribution:** Readily enters extracellular fluid. Crosses the placenta and enters breast milk.
**Metabolism and Excretion:** Excreted mostly in the feces; 20% eliminated by the kidneys.
**Half-life:** Unknown.

## CONTRAINDICATIONS AND PRECAUTIONS

**Contraindicated in:** ■ Hypercalcemia ■ Renal calculi ■ Ventricular fibrillation.
**Use Cautiously in:** ■ Patients receiving digitalis glycosides ■ Severe respiratory insufficiency ■ Renal disease ■ Cardiac disease.

## ADVERSE REACTIONS AND SIDE EFFECTS*

■ **CNS:** syncope (IV only), tingling ■ **CV:** CARDIAC ARREST (IV only), arrhythmias, bradycardia ■ **GI:** constipation, nausea, vomiting ■ **GU:** calculi, hypercalciuria ■ **Local:** phlebitis (IV ONLY).

## INTERACTIONS

**Drug-Drug:** ■ Hypercalcemia increases the risk of **digoxin** toxicity ■ Chronic use with **antacids** in renal insufficiency may lead to milk-alkali syndrome ■ Ingestion by mouth decreases the absorption of orally administered **tetracyclines, fluoroquinolones, phenytoin,** and **iron salts** ■ Excessive amounts may decrease the effects of **calcium channel blockers** ■ Decreases absorption of **etidronate** and **risedronate** (do not take within 2 hr of calcium supplements) ■ May decrease the

effectiveness of **atenolol** ■ Concurrent use with **diuretics (thiazide)** may result in hypercalcemia ■ May decrease the ability of **sodium polystyrene sulfonate** to decrease serum potassium.
**Drug-Food:** ■ **Cereals, spinach,** or **rhubarb** may decrease the absorption of calcium supplements ■ Calcium acetate should not be given concurrently with other calcium supplements.

## ROUTE AND DOSAGE

Doses are expressed in mg, g, or mEq of calcium.
■ **PO (Adults):** *Prevention of hypocalcemia, treatment of depletion, osteoporosis*—1–2 g/day. *Antacid*—0.5–1.5 g as needed (calcium carbonate only). *Hyperphosphatemia in end-stage renal disease (calcium acetate only)*—Amount necessary to control serum phosphate and calcium.
■ **PO (Children):** *Supplementation*—45–65 mg/kg/day.
■ **PO (Infants):** *Neonatal hypocalcemia*—50–150 mg/kg (not to exceed 1 g).
■ **IV (Adults):** *Emergency treatment of hypocalcemia, cardiac standstill*—7–14 mEq. *Hypocalcemic tetany*—4.5–16 mEq; repeat until symptoms are controlled. *Hyperkalemia with cardiac toxicity*—2.25–14 mEq; may repeat in 1–2 min. *Hypermagnesemia*—7 mEq.
■ **IV (Children):** *Emergency treatment of hypocalcemia*—1–7 mEq. *Hypocalcemic tetany*—0.5–0.7 mEq/kg 3–4 times daily.
■ **IV (Infants):** *Emergency treatment of hypocalcemia*—<1 mEq. *Hypocalcemic tetany*—2.4 mEq/kg/day in divided doses.

## AVAILABILITY (generic available)

❑ **Calcium Acetate**
■ *Tablets:* 250 mg (65 mg Ca)$^{OTC}$, 667 mg (169 mg Ca)$^{OTC}$, 668 mg (169 mg Ca)$^{OTC}$, 1 g (250 mg Ca)$^{OTC}$ ■ *Capsules:* 500 mg (125 mg Ca)$^{OTC}$.

❑ **Calcium Carbonate**
■ *Tablets:* 500 mg (200 mg Ca)$^{OTC}$, 600 mg (240 mg Ca)$^{OTC}$, 650 mg (260 mg Ca)$^{OTC}$, 667 mg (266.8 mg Ca)$^{OTC}$, 1 g (400 mg Ca)$^{OTC}$, 1.25 g (500 mg Ca)$^{OTC}$, 1.5 g (600 mg Ca)$^{OTC}$ ■ *Chewable tablets:* 350 mg (300 mg Ca)$^{OTC}$,

{ } = Available in Canada only.
*CAPITALS indicates life-threatening; underlines indicate most frequent.

420 mg (168 mg Ca)$^{OTC}$, 450 mg $^{OTC}$, 500 mg (200 mg Ca)$^{OTC}$, 750 mg (300 mg Ca)$^{OTC}$, 1 g (400 mg Ca)$^{OTC}$, 1.25 g (500 mg Ca)$^{OTC}$ ▪ *Gum tablets:* 300 mg $^{OTC}$, 450 mg $^{OTC}$, 500 mg (200 mg Ca)$^{OTC}$ ▪ *Capsules:* 1.25 g (500 mg Ca)$^{OTC}$ ▪ *Lozenges:* 600 mg (240 mg Ca)$^{OTC}$ ▪ *Oral suspension:* 1.25 g (500 mg Ca)/5 ml$^{OTC}$ ▪ *Powder:* 6.5 g (2400 mg Ca)/packet$^{OTC}$.

❑ **Calcium Chloride**
▪ *Injection:* 10% (1.36 mEq/ml)$^{Rx}$.

❑ **Calcium Citrate**
▪ *Tablets:* 250 mg$^{OTC}$.

❑ **Calcium Gluceptate**
▪ *Injection:* 22% (0.9 mEq/ml)$^{Rx}$.

❑ **Calcium Gluconate**
▪ *Tablets:* 500 mg (45 mg Ca)$^{OTC}$, 650 mg (58.5 mg Ca)$^{OTC}$, 975 mg (87.75 mg Ca)$^{OTC}$, 1 g (90 mg Ca)$^{OTC}$ ▪ *Injection:* 10% (0.45 mEq/ml)$^{Rx}$.

❑ **Calcium Lactate**
▪ *Tablets:* 325 mg (42.45 mg Ca)$^{OTC}$, 500 mg$^{OTC}$, 650 mg (84.5 mg Ca)$^{OTC}$.

TIME/ACTION PROFILE (effects on serum calcium)

| | ONSET | PEAK | DURATION |
|---|---|---|---|
| PO | unknown | unknown | unknown |
| IV | immediate | immediate | 0.5–2 hr |

# NURSING IMPLICATIONS

## ASSESSMENT

▪ **Calcium Supplement/Replacement:** Observe patient closely for symptoms of hypocalcemia (paresthesia, muscle twitching, laryngospasm, colic, cardiac arrhythmias, Chvostek's or Trousseau's sign). Notify physician or other health care professional if these occur. Protect symptomatic patients by elevating and padding siderails and keeping bed in low position.

❑ Monitor blood pressure, pulse, and ECG frequently throughout parenteral therapy. May cause vasodilation with resulting hypotension, bradycardia, arrhythmias, and cardiac arrest. Transient increases in blood pressure may occur during IV administration, especially in geriatric patients or in patients with hypertension.

❑ Assess IV site for patency. Extravasation may cause cellulitis, necrosis, and sloughing.

❑ Monitor patient on digitalis glycosides for signs of toxicity.

▪ **Antacid:** When used as an antacid, assess for heartburn, indigestion, and abdominal pain. Inspect abdomen; auscultate bowel sounds.

▪ *Lab Test Considerations:* Monitor serum calcium or ionized calcium, chloride, sodium, potassium, magnesium, albumin, and parathyroid hormone (PTH) concentrations before and periodically throughout therapy for treatment of hypocalcemia.

❑ May cause decreased serum phosphate concentrations with excessive and prolonged use. When used to treat hyperphosphatemia in renal failure patients, monitor phosphate levels.

▪ *Toxicity and Overdose:* Assess patient for nausea, vomiting, anorexia, thirst, severe constipation, paralytic ileus, and bradycardia. Contact physician or other health care professional immediately if these signs of hypercalcemia occur.

## POTENTIAL NURSING DIAGNOSES

▪ Nutrition, imbalanced: less than body requirements (Indications).
▪ Injury, risk for, related to osteoporosis or electrolyte imbalance (Indications).

## IMPLEMENTATION

❑ *High Alert:* Errors with IV calcium gluceptate, gluconate, and chloride have occurred secondary to confusion over which salt is ordered. Clarify incomplete orders. Confusion has occurred with milligram doses of calcium chloride, calcium gluconate, and calcium gluceptate, which are not equal. Chloride and gluconate forms are routinely available on most hospital crash carts; physician should specify form of calcium desired. Doses should be expressed in mEq.

▪ **General:** Do not confuse Os-Cal (calcium carbonate) with Asacol (mesalamine).

❑ In arrest situations, the use of calcium chloride is now limited to patients with hyperkalemia, hypocalcemia, and calcium channel blocker toxicity.

▪ **PO:** Administer calcium carbonate or phosphate 1–1.5 hr after meals and at bedtime. Chewable tablets should be well chewed before swallowing. Dissolve effervescent tablets in glass of water. Follow oral doses with a full glass of water, except when using calcium carbonate as a phosphate binder in renal dialysis. Administer with meals for patients with hyperphosphatemia.

- **IM:** IM administration of calcium gluconate and calcium gluceptate may be tolerated in an emergency if IV administration is not feasible. For child, administer only in thigh. For adult, administer only in gluteal region. Do not administer calcium chloride IM.

- **IV:** IV solution should be warmed to body temperature and given through a small-bore needle in a large vein to minimize phlebitis. Do not administer through a scalp vein. May cause cutaneous burning sensation, peripheral vasodilation, and drop in blood pressure. Patient should remain recumbent for 30–60 min after IV administration.

- ❑ **High Alert:** Administer slowly. High concentrations may cause cardiac arrest.

- ❑ If infiltration occurs, discontinue IV. May be treated with application of heat, elevation, and local infiltration of normal saline, 1% procaine HCl, or hyaluronidase.

- ❑ Rapid administration may cause tingling, sensation of warmth, and a metallic taste. Halt infusion if these symptoms occur, and resume infusion at a slower rate when they subside.

- ❑ Do not administer solutions that are not clear or that contain a precipitate.

## ❑ Calcium Chloride

- **Direct IV:** May be administered undiluted by IV push.

- **Intermittent/Continuous Infusion:** May be diluted with D5W, D10W, 0.9% NaCl, D5/0.25% NaCl, D5/0.45% NaCl, D5/0.9% NaCl, or D5/LR.

- **Rate:** Maximum rate for adults is 0.7–1.4 mEq/min (0.5–1 ml of 10% solution); for children, 0.5 ml/min.

- **Syringe Compatibility:** ◆ milrinone.

- **Y-Site Compatibility:** ◆ dobutamine ◆ epinephrine ◆ esmolol ◆ gatifloxacin ◆ inamrinone ◆ morphine ◆ paclitaxel.

- **Y-Site Incompatibility:** ◆ amphotericin B cholesteryl sulfate ◆ propofol ◆ sodium bicarbonate.

## ❑ Calcium Gluceptate

- **Direct IV:** May be administered undiluted.

- **Rate:** Administer at a rate not to exceed 2 ml (1.8 mEq)/min for adults, 0.5 ml (0.45 mEq)/min for children. In exchange transfusion for neonates, 0.5 ml (0.45 mEq) is given after each 100 ml of citrated blood.

- **Intermittent Infusion:** May be further diluted in D5W, D10W, 0.9% NaCl, 0.45% NaCl, D5/LR, or LR. Solution should be clear; do not use if crystals are present.

- **Rate:** Do not exceed 200 mg/min.

## ❑ Calcium Gluconate

- **Direct IV:** Administer slowly by direct IV push.

- **Rate:** Maximum administration rate for adults is 1.5–2 ml/min.

- **Continuous Infusion:** May be further diluted in 1000 ml of D5W, D10W, D20W, D5/0.9% NaCl, 0.9% NaCl, D5/LR, or LR.

- **Rate:** Administer at a rate not to exceed 200 mg/min over 12–24 hr.

- **Syringe Incompatibility:** ◆ metoclopramide.

- **Y-Site Compatibility:** ◆ aldesleukin ◆ allopurinol ◆ amifostine ◆ aztreonam ◆ cefazolin ◆ cefepime ◆ ciprofloxacin ◆ cisatracurium ◆ cladribine ◆ dobutamine ◆ docetaxel ◆ doxorubicin liposome ◆ enalaprilat ◆ epinephrine ◆ etoposide ◆ famotidine ◆ filgrastim ◆ gatifloxacin ◆ gemcitabine ◆ granisetron ◆ labetalol ◆ linezolid ◆ melphalan ◆ midazolam ◆ milrinone ◆ netilmicin ◆ piperacillin/tazobactam ◆ potassium chloride ◆ prochlorperazine edisylate ◆ propofol ◆ remifentanil ◆ sargramostim ◆ tacrolimus ◆ teniposide ◆ thiotepa ◆ tolazoline ◆ vinorelbine ◆ vitamin B complex with C.

- **Y-Site Incompatibility:** ◆ amphotericin B cholesteryl sulfate ◆ fluconazole ◆ indomethacin.

## PATIENT/FAMILY TEACHING

- **General Info:** Instruct patient not to take enteric-coated tablets within 1 hr of calcium carbonate; this will result in premature dissolution of the tablets.

- ❑ Do not administer concurrently with foods containing large amounts of oxalic acid (spinach, rhubarb), phytic acid (brans, cereals), or phosphorus (milk or dairy products). Administration with milk products may lead to milk-alkali syndrome (nausea, vomiting, confusion, headache). Do not take within 1–2 hr of other medications if possible.

❑ Instruct patients on a regular schedule to take missed doses as soon as possible, then go back to regular schedule.

❑ Advise patient that calcium carbonate may cause constipation. Review methods of preventing constipation (increasing bulk in diet, increasing fluid intake, increasing mobility) and using laxatives. Severe constipation may indicate toxicity.

❑ Advise patient to avoid excessive use of tobacco or beverages containing alcohol or caffeine.

■ **Calcium Supplement:** Encourage patients to maintain a diet adequate in vitamin D (see Appendix Q).

■ **Osteoporosis:** Advise patients that exercise has been found to arrest and reverse bone loss. Patient should discuss any exercise limitations with health care professional before beginning program.

### EVALUATION

**Effectiveness of therapy can be demonstrated by:** ■ Increase in serum calcium levels ■ Decrease in the signs and symptoms of hypocalcemia ■ Resolution of indigestion ■ Control of hyperphosphatemia in patients with renal failure (calcium acetate only).

## candesartan, See ANGIOTENSIN II RECEPTOR ANTAGONISTS.

## capsaicin

(kap-**say**-sin)

{Axsam}, Capsin, Capzasin-P, Dolorac, No Pain-HP, Pain Doctor, Pain-X, R-Gel, Rid•a•Pain•HP, Zostrix, Zostrix-HP

### CLASSIFICATION(S):

***Therapeutic:*** *nonopioid analgesics (topical)*

**Pregnancy Category UK**

### INDICATIONS

■ Temporary management of pain due to rheumatoid arthritis and osteoarthritis ■ Treatment of pain associated with postherpetic neuralgia or diabetic neuropathy. **Unlabeled uses:** ■ Treatment of postmastectomy pain syndrome ■ Treatment of reflex sympathetic dystrophy syndrome.

### ACTION

■ May deplete and prevent the reaccumulation of a chemical (substance P) responsible for transmitting painful impulses from peripheral sites to the CNS. **Therapeutic Effects:** ■ Relief of discomfort associated with painful peripheral syndromes.

### PHARMACOKINETICS

**Absorption:** Unknown.
**Distribution:** Unknown.
**Metabolism and Excretion:** Unknown.
**Half-life:** Unknown.

### CONTRAINDICATIONS AND PRECAUTIONS

**Contraindicated in:** ■ Hypersensitivity to capsaicin or hot peppers ■ Not for use near eyes or on open or broken skin.
**Use Cautiously in:** ■ Pregnancy, lactation, or children <2 yr (safety not established).

### ADVERSE REACTIONS AND SIDE EFFECTS*

■ **Resp:** cough ■ **Derm:** transient burning.

### INTERACTIONS

**Drug-Drug:** ■ None significant.

### ROUTE AND DOSAGE

■ **Topical (Adults and Children ≥2 yr):** Apply to affected areas 3–4 times daily.

### AVAILABILITY

■ ***Cream:*** 0.025%ᴼᵀᶜ, 0.075%ᴼᵀᶜ ■Cost: 0.025% $11.94/60g, 0.075% $7.98/30g ■ ***Gel:*** 0.05%ᴼᵀᶜ ■Cost: 0.05% $9.84/20 g ■ ***Lotion:*** 0.025%ᴼᵀᶜ ■Cost: 0.025% $11.94/60, 0.075% $7.98/30 ■ ***Roll-on:*** 0.075%ᴼᵀᶜ ■Cost: 0.075% $7.98/30 g ■ methyl salicylate (Ziksᴼᵀᶜ). See Appendix B.

TIME/ACTION PROFILE

| | ONSET | PEAK | DURATION |
|---|---|---|---|
| top | 1–2 wk | 2–4 wk† | unknown |

†May take up to 6 wk for head and neck neuralgias.

## NURSING IMPLICATIONS

### ASSESSMENT

❑ Assess pain intensity and location before and periodically throughout therapy.

### POTENTIAL NURSING DIAGNOSES

■ Pain, chronic (Indications).

■ Noncompliance (Patient/Family Teaching).

### IMPLEMENTATION

■ **Topical:** Apply to affected area not more than 3–4 times daily. Avoid getting medication into eyes or on broken or irritated skin. Do not bandage tightly.

❑ Topical lidocaine may be applied during the first 1–2 wk of treatment to reduce initial discomfort.

### PATIENT/FAMILY TEACHING

❑ Instruct patient on the correct method for application of capsaicin. Rub cream into affected area well so that little or no cream is left on the surface. Gloves should be worn during application or hands should be washed immediately after application. If application is to hands for arthritis, do not wash hands for at least 30 min after application.

❑ Advise patient to apply missed doses as soon as possible unless almost time for next dose. Pain relief lasts only as long as capsaicin is used regularly.

❑ Advise patient that transient burning may occur with application, especially if applied fewer than 3–4 times daily. Burning usually disappears after the first few days but may continue for 2–4 wk or longer. Burning is increased by heat, sweating, bathing in warm water, humidity, and clothing. Burning usually decreases in frequency and intensity the longer capsaicin is used. Decreasing number of daily doses will not lessen burning but may decrease amount of pain relief and may prolong period of burning.

❑ Caution patient to flush area with water if capsaicin gets into eyes and to wash with warm, but not hot, soapy water if capsaicin gets on other sensitive areas of the body.

❑ Instruct patient with herpes zoster (shingles) not to apply capsaicin cream until lesions have healed completely.

❑ Advise patient to discontinue use and notify health care professional if pain persists longer than 1 month, worsens, or if signs of infection are present.

### EVALUATION

**Effectiveness of therapy can be demonstrated by:** ■ Decrease in discomfort associated with: ❑ Postherpetic neuropathy ❑ Diabetic neuropathy ❑ Rheumatoid arthritis ❑ Osteoarthritis. Pain relief usually begins within 1–2 wk with arthritis, 2–4 wk with neuralgias, and 4–6 wk with neuralgias of the head and neck.

## captopril, See ANGIOTENSIN-CONVERTING ENZYME (ACE) INHIBITORS.

## carbamazepine

(kar-ba-**maz**-e-peen)

{Apo-Carbamazepine}, Atretol, Carbatrol, Epitol, {Novo-Carbamaz}, Tegretol, {Tegretol CR}, Tegretol-XR, Teril

### CLASSIFICATION(S):
***Therapeutic:*** *anticonvulsants*

### Pregnancy Category C

### INDICATIONS

■ Prophylaxis of tonic-clonic, mixed, and complex-partial seizures ■ Management of pain in trigeminal neuralgia. **Unlabeled uses:** ■ Other forms of neurogenic pain ■ Prophylaxis and treatment of bipolar disorder.

### ACTION

■ Decreases synaptic transmission in the CNS by affecting sodium channels in neurons. **Therapeutic Effects:** ■ Prevention of seizures ■ Relief of pain in trigeminal neuralgia.

## PHARMACOKINETICS

**Absorption:** Absorption is slow but complete. Suspension produces earlier, higher peak and lower trough levels.

**Distribution:** Widely distributed. Crosses the blood-brain barrier. Crosses the placenta rapidly and enters breast milk in high concentrations.

**Metabolism and Excretion:** Extensively metabolized by the liver; epoxide metabolite has anticonvulsant and antineuralgic activity.

**Half-life:** *Carbamazapine*—single dose— 25–65 hr, chronic dosing—8–29 hr; *epoxide*—5–8 hr.

## CONTRAINDICATIONS AND PRECAUTIONS

**Contraindicated in:** ■ Hypersensitivity ■ Bone marrow depression ■ Pregnancy (use only if potential benefits outweigh risks to the fetus; additional vitamin K during last weeks of pregnancy has been recommended) ■ Lactation.

**Use Cautiously in:** ■ Cardiac disease ■ Hepatic disease ■ Older men with prostatic hypertrophy ■ Increased intraocular pressure.

## ADVERSE REACTIONS AND SIDE EFFECTS*

■ **CNS:** <u>ataxia</u>, <u>drowsiness</u>, fatigue, psychosis, vertigo ■ **EENT:** blurred vision, corneal opacities ■ **Resp:** pneumonitis ■ **CV:** CHF, hypertension, hypotension, syncope ■ **GI:** hepatitis ■ **GU:** hesitancy, urinary retention ■ **Derm:** photosensitivity, rashes, urticaria ■ **Endo:** syndrome of inappropriate antidiuretic hormone (SIADH) ■ **Hemat:** AGRANULOCYTOSIS, APLASTIC ANEMIA, THROMBOCYTOPENIA, eosinophilia, leukopenia ■ **Misc:** chills, fever, lymphadenopathy.

## INTERACTIONS

**Drug-Drug:** ■ ↓ levels/may ↓ effectiveness of **corticosteroids, doxycycline, felbamate, quinidine, warfarin, estrogen-containing contraceptives, barbiturates, cyclosporine, benzodiazepines, theophylline, lamotrigine, valproic acid, bupropion,** and **haloperidol** ■ **Danazol** ↑ blood levels (avoid concurrent use if possible) ■ Concurrent use (within 2 wk) of **MAO inhibitors** may result in hyperpyrexia, hypertension, seizures, and death ■ **Verapamil, diltiazem, propoxyphene, erythromycin, clarithromycin, SSRIs, antidepressants,** or **cimetidine** ↑ levels; may cause toxicity ■ May ↑ risk of hepatotoxicity from **isoniazid** ■ **Felbamate** ↓

carbamazepine levels but ↑ levels of active metabolite ■ May ↓ effectiveness and ↑ risk of toxicity from **acetaminophen** ■ May ↑ risk of CNS toxicity from **lithium** ■ May ↓ duration of action of **nondepolarizing neuromuscular blocking agents.**

**Drug-Food:** ■ **Grapefruit juice** ↑ serum levels and effect.

## ROUTE AND DOSAGE

■ **PO (Adults):** *Anticonvulsant*—200 mg twice daily (tablets) or 100 mg 4 times daily (suspension); increase by 200 mg/day q 7 days until therapeutic levels are achieved (range is 600–1200 mg/day in divided doses q 6–8 hr; not to exceed 1 g/day in 12–15-yr-olds. Extended-release products are given twice daily (XR, CR). *Antineuralgic*—100 mg twice daily or 50 mg 4 times daily (suspension); increase by up to 200 mg/day until pain is relieved, then maintenance dose of 200–1200 mg/day in divided doses (usual range, 400–800 mg/day).

■ **PO (Children 6–12 yr):** 100 mg twice daily (tablets) or 50 mg 4 times daily (suspension) increased by 100 mg weekly until therapeutic levels are obtained (usual range 400–800 mg/day; not to exceed 1 g/day). Extended-release products (XR, CR) are given twice.

■ **PO (Children <6 yr):** 10–20 mg/kg/day in 2–3 divided doses; may be increased by 100 mg/day at weekly intervals. Usual maintenance dose is 250–350 mg/day (not to exceed 400 mg/day).

## AVAILABILITY (generic available)

■ *Tablets:* 200 mg$^{Rx}$ ■ Cost: 200 mg $51.24/ 100 ■ *Chewable tablets:* 100 mg$^{Rx}$, {200 mg$^{Rx}$} ■ *Extended-release capsules:* 200 mg$^{Rx}$, 300 mg$^{Rx}$ ■ *Extended-release tablets:* 100 mg$^{Rx}$, 200 mg$^{Rx}$, 400 mg$^{Rx}$ ■ *Oral suspension (citrus/vanilla flavor):* 100 mg/5 ml$^{Rx}$.

TIME/ACTION PROFILE (anticonvulsant activity)

| | ONSET | PEAK | DURATION |
|---|---|---|---|
| PO | up to one month† | 4–5 hr‡ | 6–12 hr |
| PO-ER | up to one month† | 2–3–12 hr‡ | 12 hr |

†Onset of antineuralgic activity is 8–72 hr.
‡Listed for tablets; peak level occurs 1.5 hr after a chronic dose of suspension.

# NURSING IMPLICATIONS

## ASSESSMENT

- **Seizures:** Assess frequency, location, duration, and characteristics of seizure activity.
- **Trigeminal Neuralgia:** Assess for facial pain (location, intensity, duration). Ask patient to identify stimuli that may precipitate facial pain (hot or cold foods, bedclothes, touching face).
- *Lab Test Considerations:* Monitor CBC, including platelet count, reticulocyte count, and serum iron, weekly during the first 2 mo and yearly thereafter for evidence of potentially fatal blood cell abnormalities. Medication should be discontinued if bone marrow depression occurs.
- ❑ Liver function tests, urinalysis, and BUN should be routinely performed. May cause ↑ AST, ALT, serum alkaline phosphatase, bilirubin, BUN, urine protein, and urine glucose levels.
- ❑ Monitor serum ionized calcium levels every 6 mo or if seizure frequency increases. Thyroid function tests and ionized serum calcium concentrations may be ↓; hypocalcemia decreases seizure threshold.
- ❑ Monitor ECG and serum electrolytes before and periodically during therapy. May cause hyponatremia.
- ❑ May occasionally cause ↑ serum cholesterol, high-density lipoprotein, and triglyceride concentrations.
- ❑ May cause false-negative pregnancy test results with tests that determine human chorionic gonadotropin.
- *Toxicity and Overdose:* Serum blood levels should be routinely monitored during therapy. Therapeutic levels range from 6–12 mcg/ml.

## POTENTIAL NURSING DIAGNOSES

- Injury, risk for (Indications, Side Effects).
- Pain, chronic (Indications).

## IMPLEMENTATION

- **General:** Implement seizure precautions as indicated.
- **PO:** Administer medication with food to minimize gastric irritation. Tablets may be crushed if patient has difficulty swallowing. Do not crush or chew extended-release tablets. Extended-release capsules may be opened and the contents sprinkled on applesauce or other similar foods.
- ❑ Do not administer suspension simultaneously with other liquid medications or diluents; mixture produces an orange rubbery mass.

## PATIENT/FAMILY TEACHING

- **General Info:** Instruct patient to take carbamazepine around the clock, exactly as directed. If a dose is missed, take as soon as possible but not just before next dose; do not double doses. Notify health care professional if more than one dose is missed. Medication should be gradually discontinued to prevent seizures.
- ❑ May cause dizziness or drowsiness. Advise patients to avoid driving or other activities requiring alertness until response to medication is known.
- ❑ Instruct patients that fever, sore throat, mouth ulcers, easy bruising, petechiae, unusual bleeding, abdominal pain, chills, rash, pale stools, dark urine, or jaundice should be reported to health care professional immediately.
- ❑ Inform patient that coating of *Tegretol XR* is not absorbed, but is excreted in feces and may be visible in stool.
- ❑ Advise patient not to take alcohol or other CNS depressants concurrently with this medication.
- ❑ Caution patients to use sunscreen and protective clothing to prevent photosensitivity reactions.
- ❑ Inform patient that frequent mouth rinses, good oral hygiene, and sugarless gum or candy may help reduce dry mouth. Saliva substitute may be used. Consult dentist if dry mouth persists >2 wk.
- ❑ Advise female patients to use a nonhormonal form of contraception while taking carbamazepine.
- ❑ Instruct patient to notify health care professional of medication regimen before treatment or surgery.

{ } = Available in Canada only.
*CAPITALS indicates life-threatening; underlines indicate most frequent.

❏ Emphasize the importance of follow-up lab tests and eye exams to monitor for side effects.

■ **Seizures:** Advise patients to carry identification describing disease and medication regimen at all times.

## EVALUATION

**Effectiveness of therapy can be demonstrated by:** ■ Absence or reduction of seizure activity ■ Decrease in trigeminal neuralgia pain. Patients with trigeminal neuralgia who are pain-free should be re-evaluated every 3 mo to determine minimum effective dose.

---

**High Alert**

# carboplatin

(kar-boe-**pla**-tin)
Paraplatin, {Paraplatin-AQ}

*CLASSIFICATION(S):*
*Therapeutic:* antineoplastics
*Pharmacologic:* alkylating agents

**Pregnancy Category D**

---

## INDICATIONS

■ Advanced ovarian carcinoma (with other agents) ■ Palliative treatment of ovarian carcinoma unresponsive to other modalities.

## ACTION

■ Inhibits DNA synthesis by producing cross-linking of parent DNA strands (cell-cycle phase–nonspecific). **Therapeutic Effects:** ■ Death of rapidly replicating cells, particularly malignant ones.

## PHARMACOKINETICS

**Absorption:** IV administration results in complete bioavailability.

**Distribution:** Unknown.

**Protein Binding:** Platinum is irreversibly bound to plasma proteins.

**Metabolism and Excretion:** Excreted mostly by the kidneys.

**Half-life:** *Carboplatin*—2.6–5.9 hr (increased in renal impairment); *platinum*—5 days.

## CONTRAINDICATIONS AND PRECAUTIONS

**Contraindicated in:** ■ Hypersensitivity to carboplatin, cisplatin, or mannitol ■ Pregnancy or lactation.

**Use Cautiously in:** ■ Hearing loss ■ Electrolyte abnormalities ■ Renal impairment (dosage reduction recommended if creatinine <60 ml/min) ■ Active infections ■ Diminished bone marrow reserve (dosage reduction recommended) ■ Other chronic debilitating illnesses ■ Patients with childbearing potential.

## ADVERSE REACTIONS AND SIDE EFFECTS*

■ **CNS:** weakness ■ **EENT:** ototoxicity ■ **GI:** abdominal pain, nausea, vomiting, constipation, diarrhea, hepatitis, stomatitis ■ **GU:** gonadal suppression, nephrotoxicity ■ **Derm:** alopecia, rash ■ **F and E:** hypocalcemia, hypokalemia, hypomagnesemia, hyponatremia ■ **Hemat:** ANEMIA, LEUKOPENIA, THROMBOCYTOPENIA ■ **Metab:** hyperuricemia ■ **Neuro:** peripheral neuropathy ■ **Misc:** hypersensitivity reactions including ANAPHYLACTIC-LIKE REACTIONS.

## INTERACTIONS

**Drug-Drug:** ■ ↑ nephrotoxicity and ototoxicity with other **nephrotoxic** and **ototoxic drugs (aminoglycosides, loop diuretics)** ■ ↑ bone marrow depression with other **bone marrow–depressing drugs** or **radiation therapy** ■ May ↓ antibody response to **live-virus vaccines** and ↑ risk of adverse reactions.

## ROUTE AND DOSAGE

Other dosing formulas are used.

■ **IV (Adults):** *Initial treatment*—300 mg/m² with cyclophosphamide at 4-wk intervals. *Treatment of refractory tumors*—360 mg/m² as a single dose; may be repeated at 4-wk intervals, depending on response.

❏ **Renal Impairment**

■ **IV (Adults):** *CCr 41–59 ml/min*—initial dose 250 mg/m²; *CCr 16–40 ml/min*—initial dose 200 mg/m².

## AVAILABILITY

■ *Lyophilized powder for injection:* 50-mg vials^Rx, 150-mg vials^Rx, 450-mg vials^Rx ■ Cost: 50 mg $130.11/vial, 150 mg $390.30/vial, 450 mg $1170.93/vial ■ *Aqueous solution for injection:* 50/5ml vial<sup>Rx</sup>, 150 mg/15 ml vial<sup>Rx</sup>, 450 mg/45 ml/vial<sup>Rx</sup>.

TIME/ACTION PROFILE (effects on blood counts)

| | ONSET | PEAK | DURATION |
|---|---|---|---|
| IV | unknown | 21 days | 28 days |

## NURSING IMPLICATIONS

### ASSESSMENT

☐ Assess for nausea and vomiting; often occur 6–12 hr after therapy (1–4 hr for aqueous solution) and may persist for 24 hr. Prophylactic antiemetics may be used. Adjust diet as tolerated to maintain fluid and electrolyte balance and ensure adequate nutritional intake. May require discontinuation of therapy.

☐ Assess patients receiving *Paraplatin-AQ* for neurotoxicity (paresthesias in a stocking—glove distribution, areflexia, loss of proprioception and vibratory sensations). Discontinue therapy when symptoms are first observed. May progress further even after stopping therapy. May be irreversible.

☐ Monitor for bone marrow depression. Assess for bleeding (bleeding gums, bruising, petechiae, guaiac stools, urine, and emesis) and avoid IM injections and rectal temperatures if platelet count is low. Apply pressure to venipuncture sites for 10 min. Assess for signs of infection during neutropenia. Anemia may occur and may be cumulative; transfusions are frequently required. Monitor for increased fatigue, dyspnea, and orthostatic hypotension.

☐ Monitor for signs of anaphylaxis (rash, urticaria, pruritus, facial swelling, wheezing, tachycardia, hypotension). Discontinue medication immediately and notify physician if these occur. Epinephrine and resuscitation equipment should be readily available.

☐ Audiometry is recommended before initiation of therapy and subsequent doses. Ototoxicity manifests as tinitus and unilateral or bilateral hearing loss in high frequencies and becomes more frequent and severe with repeated doses. Ototoxicity is more pronounced in children.

■ *Lab Test Considerations:* Monitor CBC, differential, and clotting studies before and weekly during therapy. For *Paraplatin:* The nadirs of thrombocytopenia and leukopenia occur after 21 days and recover by 30 days after a dose. Nadir of granulocyte counts usually occurs after 21–28 days and recovers by day 35. Withhold subsequent doses until neutrophil count is >2000/mm³ and platelet count is >100,000/mm³. For *Paraplatin-AQ:* The nadirs of thrombocytopenia and leukopenia occur between days 18 and 23 and recover by day 39. Anemia also occurs with the same frequency and timing as thrombocytopenia and leukopenia.

☐ Monitor renal function and serum electrolytes before initiation of therapy and before each course of carboplatin. Nephrotoxicity with *Paraplatin-AQ* is cumulative and is potentiated by aminoglycoside antibiotics. Monitor serum creatinine, BUN, creatinine clearance, and magnesium, sodium, potassium, and calcium levels prior to initiating therapy and before each subsequent dose. May cause ↑ BUN and serum creatinine concentrations and ↓ CCr. May cause ↓ serum potassium, calcium, magnesium, and sodium concentrations. Renal function must return to normal before each dose of *Paraplatin-AQ* is given.

☐ Monitor hepatic function before and periodically during therapy. May cause ↑ serum bilirubin, alkaline phosphatase, and AST concentrations.

☐ *Paraplatin-AQ* may cause hyperuricemia, usually occurring 3–5 days after therapy. Allopurinol may be used to ↓ uric acid levels.

☐ *Paraplatin-AQ* may cause ↑ serum amylase levels.

### POTENTIAL NURSING DIAGNOSES

■ Infection, risk for (Adverse Reactions).
■ Injury, risk for (Side Effects).

### IMPLEMENTATION

☐ *High Alert:* Fatalities have occurred with chemotherapeutic agents. Before administering, clarify all ambiguous orders; double check single, daily, and course-of-therapy dose limits; have second practitioner independently double check original order, calculations and infusion pump settings. Do not

{ } = Available in Canada only.
*CAPITALS indicates life-threatening; <u>underlines</u> indicate most frequent.

confuse carboplatin with cisplatin. Do not confuse Paraplatin (carboplatin) with Platinol (cisplatin). Carboplatin should be administered in a monitored setting under the supervision of a physician experienced in cancer chemotherapy.

■ **General:** Solution should be prepared in a biologic cabinet. Wear gloves, gown, and mask while handling medication. Discard equipment in specially designated containers.

❑ Do not use aluminum needles or equipment during preparation or administration; aluminum reacts with the drug.

❑ **Paraplatin**

■ **Intermittent Infusion:** Reconstitute to a concentration of 10 mg/ml with sterile water for injection, D5W, or 0.9% NaCl for injection. May be further diluted in D5W or 0.9% NaCl to a concentration of 0.5 mg/ml. Stable for 8 hr at room temperature.

❑ May also be administered over 24 hr or by dividing total dose into 5 consecutive pulse doses; may decrease nausea and vomiting but does not decrease nephrotoxicity or ototoxicity.

■ *Rate:* Administer over 15–60 min.

■ **Y-Site Compatibility:** ◆ allopurinol ◆ amifostine ◆ aztreonam ◆ cefepime ◆ cladribine ◆ doxorubicin liposome ◆ etoposide phosphate ◆ filgrastim ◆ fludarabine ◆ gatifloxacin ◆ gemcitabine ◆ granisetron ◆ linezolid ◆ melphalan ◆ ondansetron ◆ paclitaxel ◆ piperacillin/tazobactam ◆ propofol ◆ sargramostim ◆ teniposide ◆ thiotepa ◆ topotecan ◆ vinorelbine.

❑ **Paraplatin-AQ**

■ **General:** Hydrate patient with 1–2 liters of fluid infused over 8–12 hr prior to therapy.

■ **Intermittent Infusion:** Adequate hydration and urinary output must be maintained for 24 hr following infusion.

■ **Intermittent Infusion:** Dilute Paraplatin-AQ with 2 liters of D5/0.45% NaCl containing 37.5 g of mannitol. Do not dilute with D5W. If diluted solution is not to be used within 6 hrs, protect solution from light. Do not refrigerate.

### PATIENT/FAMILY TEACHING

❑ Instruct patient to notify health care professional promptly if fever; chills; sore throat; signs of infection; lower back or side pain; difficult or painful urination; bleeding gums; bruising; pinpoint red spots on skin; blood in stools, urine, or emesis; increased fatigue, dyspnea, or orthostatic hypotension occurs.

❑ Caution patient to avoid crowds and persons with known infections. Instruct patient to use soft toothbrush and electric razor and to avoid falls. Caution patients not to drink alcoholic beverages or take medication containing aspirin or NSAIDs because they may precipitate gastric bleeding.

❑ Instruct patient to promptly report any numbness or tingling in extremities or face, decreased coordination, difficulty with hearing or ringing in the ears, unusual swelling, or weight gain to health care professional.

❑ Instruct patient not to receive any vaccinations without advice of health care professional and to avoid contact with persons who have received oral polio vaccine within the past several months.

❑ Advise patient of the need for contraception (if patient is not infertile as a result of surgical or radiation therapy).

❑ Instruct patient to inspect oral mucosa for erythema and ulceration. If ulceration occurs, advise patient to notify health care professional, rinse mouth with water after eating, and use sponge brush. Mouth pain may require treatment with opioids.

❑ Discuss with patient the possibility of hair loss. Explore methods of coping.

❑ Emphasize the need for periodic lab tests to monitor for side effects.

### EVALUATION

**Effectiveness of therapy can be demonstrated by:** ■ Decrease in size or spread of ovarian carcinoma.

---

## carisoprodol

(kar-i-**sop**-roe-dole)
Soma, Vanadom

### CLASSIFICATION(S):

***Therapeutic:*** *skeletal muscle relaxants (centrally acting)*

**Pregnancy Category UK**

## INDICATIONS

■ Adjunct to rest and physical therapy in the treatment of muscle spasm associated with acute painful musculoskeletal conditions.

## ACTION

■ Skeletal muscle relaxation, probably due to CNS depression. **Therapeutic Effects:** ■ Skeletal muscle relaxation.

## PHARMACOKINETICS

**Absorption:** Well absorbed after oral administration.

**Distribution:** Crosses the placenta; high concentrations in breast milk.

**Metabolism and Excretion:** Mostly metabolized by the liver.

**Half-life:** 8 hr.

## CONTRAINDICATIONS AND PRECAUTIONS

**Contraindicated in:** ■ Hypersensitivity to carisoprodol or to meprobamate ■ Porphyria or suspected porphyria.

**Use Cautiously in:** ■ Severe liver or kidney disease ■ Pregnancy, lactation, or children <12 yr (safety not established).

## ADVERSE REACTIONS AND SIDE EFFECTS*

■ **CNS:** <u>dizziness</u>, <u>drowsiness</u>, agitation, ataxia, depression, headache, insomnia, irritability, syncope ■ **Resp:** asthma attacks ■ **CV:** hypotension, tachycardia ■ **GI:** epigastric distress, hiccups, nausea, vomiting ■ **Derm:** flushing, rashes ■ **Hemat:** eosinophilia, leukopenia ■ **Misc:** ANA-PHYLACTIC SHOCK, fever, psychological dependence, severe idiosyncratic reaction.

## INTERACTIONS

**Drug-Drug:** ■ Additive CNS depression with other **CNS depressants** including **alcohol, antihistamines, opioid analgesics,** and **sedative/hypnotics.**

**Drug-Natural Products:** ■ Concomitant use of **kava, valerian, skullcap, chamomile,** or **hops** can increase CNS depression.

## ROUTE AND DOSAGE

■ **PO (Adults):** 350 mg 4 times daily.

■ **PO (Children 5–12 yr):** 6.25 mg/kg 4 times daily.

## AVAILABILITY (generic available)

■ *Tablets:* 350 mg^Rx ■ Cost: *Soma*—$265.32/100; *generic*—$22.32/100 ■ aspirin (Soma compound) and codeine^Rx. See Appendix B.

TIME/ACTION PROFILE (skeletal muscle relaxation)

| | ONSET | PEAK | DURATION |
|---|---|---|---|
| PO | 30 min | unknown | 4–6 hr |

# NURSING IMPLICATIONS

## ASSESSMENT

❑ Assess patient for pain, muscle stiffness, and range of motion before and periodically throughout therapy.

❑ Observe patient for idiosyncratic symptoms that may appear within minutes or hours of administration during the first dose. Symptoms include extreme weakness, quadriplegia, dizziness, ataxia, dysarthria, visual disturbances, agitation, euphoria, confusion, and disorientation. Usually subsides over several hours.

## POTENTIAL NURSING DIAGNOSES

■ Pain, acute (Indications).

■ Mobility, impaired bed (Indications).

■ Injury, risk for (Side Effects).

## IMPLEMENTATION

■ **General:** Do not confuse Soma with Soma Compound.

❑ Provide safety measures as indicated. Supervise ambulation and transfer of patients.

■ **PO:** Administer with food to minimize GI irritation. Give dose at bedtime.

## PATIENT/FAMILY TEACHING

❑ Instruct patient to take medication exactly as directed. Missed doses should be taken within 1 hr; if not, omit and return to regular dosing schedule. Do not double doses.

❑ Encourage patient to comply with additional therapies prescribed for muscle spasm (rest, physical therapy, heat, etc.).

{ } = Available in Canada only.
*CAPITALS indicates life-threatening; <u>underlines</u> indicate most frequent.

❑ May cause dizziness or drowsiness. Advise patient to avoid driving or other activities requiring alertness until response to drug is known.

❑ Instruct patient to change positions slowly to minimize orthostatic hypotension.

❑ Advise patient to avoid concurrent use of alcohol and other CNS depressants while taking this medication.

❑ Instruct patient to notify health care professional if signs of allergy (rash, hives, swelling of tongue or lips, dyspnea) or idiosyncratic reaction occur.

## EVALUATION

**Effectiveness of therapy can be demonstrated by:** ■ Decreased musculoskeletal pain and muscle spasticity ❑ Increased range of motion.

---

**High Alert**

# carmustine

(kar-**mus**-teen)

BCNU, BiCNU, Gliadel

*CLASSIFICATION(S):*
*Therapeutic: antineoplastics*
*Pharmacologic: alkylating agents*

**Pregnancy Category D**

---

## INDICATIONS

■ Alone or with other treatments (surgery, radiation) in the management of: ❑ Brain tumors ❑ Multiple myeloma ❑ Hodgkin's disease ❑ Other lymphomas.

## ACTION

■ Inhibits DNA and RNA synthesis (cell-cycle phase–nonspecific). **Therapeutic Effects:** ■ Death of rapidly replicating cells, especially malignant ones.

## PHARMACOKINETICS

**Absorption:** Following IV administration, absorption is complete. Following implantation, action is primarily local.

**Distribution:** Highly lipid soluble; readily penetrates CSF. Enters breast milk.

**Metabolism and Excretion:** Rapidly metabolized. Some metabolites have antineoplastic activity.

**Half-life:** *Biologic*—15–30 min; *chemical*—5 min.

## CONTRAINDICATIONS AND PRECAUTIONS

**Contraindicated in:** ■ Hypersensitivity ■ Pregnancy or lactation.

**Use Cautiously in:** ■ Infections ■ Depressed bone marrow reserve ■ Geriatric patients (consider age related decrease in body mass, renal/hepatic/cardiovascular function, concurrent medications and chronic illnesses) ■ Impaired pulmonary, hepatic, or renal function ■ Other chronic debilitating illnesses ■ Patients with childbearing potential.

## ADVERSE REACTIONS AND SIDE EFFECTS*

■ **Resp:** PULMONARY FIBROSIS, pulmonary infiltrates ■ **GI:** hepatotoxicity, nausea, vomiting, anorexia, diarrhea, esophagitis ■ **GU:** renal failure ■ **Derm:** alopecia ■ **Hemat:** LEUKOPENIA, THROMBOCYTOPENIA, anemia ■ **Local:** pain at IV site.

## INTERACTIONS

**Drug-Drug:** ■ ↑ bone marrow depression with other **antineoplastics** or **radiation therapy** ■ **Smoking** ↑ risk of pulmonary toxicity ■ May ↓ antibody response to **live-virus vaccines** and ↑ risk of adverse reactions ■ Myelosuppression may be ↑ by **cimetidine**.

## ROUTE AND DOSAGE

■ **IV (Adults and Children):** 150–200 mg/m$^2$ single dose every 6–8 wk *or* 75–100 mg/m$^2$/day for 2 days q 6 wk *or* 40 mg/m$^2$/day for 5 days q 6 wk.

■ **Intracavitary: (Adults):** Up to 61.6 mg (8 implants) placed in cavity created during surgical resection of brain tumor.

## AVAILABILITY

■ *Injection:* 100-mg vial$^{Rx}$ ■ Cost: $133.96/vial ■ *Intracavitary wafer:* 7.7 mg in packages of 8$^{Rx}$ ■ Cost: $12,700/8 wafers.

TIME/ACTION PROFILE (effect on platelet counts)

|  | ONSET | PEAK | DURATION |
|---|---|---|---|
| IV | days | 4–5 wk | 6 wk |

# NURSING IMPLICATIONS

## ASSESSMENT

❑ Monitor vital signs before and frequently during therapy.

❑ Monitor for bone marrow depression. Assess for bleeding (bleeding gums, bruising, petechiae, guaiac stools, urine, and emesis) and avoid IM injections and taking rectal temperatures if platelet count is low. Apply pressure to venipuncture sites for 10 min. Assess for signs of infection during neutropenia. Anemia may occur; monitor for increased fatigue, dyspnea, and orthostatic hypotension.

❑ Assess respiratory status for dyspnea or cough. Pulmonary toxicity usually occurs after high cumulative doses or several courses of therapy but may also occur following 1–2 courses of low doses. Symptoms may be rapid or gradual in onset; damage may be reversible or irreversible. Delayed pulmonary fibrosis may occur years after therapy. Notify physician promptly if symptoms occur.

❑ Monitor IV site closely. Carmustine is an irritant. Instruct patient to notify nurse immediately if discomfort occurs at IV site. Discontinue IV immediately if infiltration occurs. Ice may be applied to site. May cause hyperpigmentation of skin along vein.

❑ Monitor intake and output, appetite, and nutritional intake. Assess for nausea and vomiting, which occur within 2 hr of administration and persist for 4–6 hr. Administration of an antiemetic before and during therapy and adjusting diet as tolerated may help maintain fluid and electrolyte balance and nutritional status.

■ *Lab Test Considerations:* Monitor CBC with differential and platelet count before and throughout therapy. The nadir of thrombocytopenia occurs in 4–5 wk; the nadir of leukopenia in 5–6 wk. Recovery usually occurs in 6–7 wk but may take 10–12 wk after prolonged therapy. Withhold dose and notify physician if platelet count is <100,000/mm³ or leukocyte count is <4000/mm³. Anemia is usually mild.

❑ Monitor serum bilirubin, AST, ALT, and LDH before and periodically during therapy. May cause mild, reversible ↑ in AST, alkaline phosphatase, and bilirubin.

❑ Monitor BUN, serum creatinine, and uric acid before and periodically during therapy. Notify physician if BUN is elevated.

## POTENTIAL NURSING DIAGNOSES

■ Injury, risk for (Side Effects).

■ Body image, disturbed (Side Effects).

## IMPLEMENTATION

❑ *High Alert:* Fatalities have occurred with chemotherapeutic agents. Before administering, clarify all ambiguous orders; double check single, daily, and course-of-therapy dose limits; have second practitioner independently double check original order, calculations and infusion pump settings.

■ **General:** Solution should be prepared in a biologic cabinet. Wear gloves, gown, and mask while handling medication. Discard equipment in designated containers. Contact with skin may cause transient hyperpigmentation.

■ **Intermittent Infusion:** Dilute contents of each 100-mg vial with 3 ml of absolute ethyl alcohol provided as a diluent. Dilute this solution with 27 ml of sterile water for injection for a concentration of 3.3 mg/ml. Further dilute with 500 ml of D5W or 0.9% NaCl in a glass container.

❑ Solution is clear and colorless. Do not use vials that contain an oily film, which indicates decomposition. Reconstituted solution is stable for 24 hr when refrigerated and protected from light. Solution contains no preservatives; do not use as a multidose vial.

❑ IV lines may be flushed with 5–10 ml of 0.9% NaCl before and after carmustine infusion to minimize irritation at the injection site.

■ *Rate:* Administer dose over 1–2 hr. Rapid infusion rate may cause local pain, burning at site, and flushing. Facial flushing occurs within 2 hr and may persist for 4 hr.

■ **Y-Site Compatibility:** ◆ amifostine ◆ aztreonam ◆ cefepime ◆ etoposide ◆ filgrastim ◆ fludarabine ◆ gemcitabine ◆ granisetron ◆ melphalan ◆ ondansetron ◆ piperacillin/tazobactam ◆ sargramostim ◆ teniposide ◆ thiotepa ◆ vinorelbine.

■ **Additive Incompatibility:** ◆ allopurinol ◆ sodium bicarbonate.

## PATIENT/FAMILY TEACHING

❏ Instruct patient to notify health care professional if fever; chills; sore throat; signs of infection; lower back or side pain; difficult or painful urination; bleeding gums; bruising; petechiae; or blood in urine, stool, or emesis occurs. Caution patient to avoid crowds and persons with known infections. Instruct patient to use soft toothbrush and electric razor. Patients should be cautioned not to drink alcoholic beverages or to take products containing aspirin or NSAIDs.

❏ Instruct patient to notify health care professional if shortness of breath or increased cough occurs. Encourage patient not to smoke, because smokers are at greater risk for pulmonary toxicity.

❏ Instruct patient to inspect oral mucosa for redness and ulceration. If mouth sores occur, advise patient to use sponge brush and rinse mouth with water after eating and drinking. Stomatitis may require treatment with opioid analgesics.

❏ Discuss with patient the possibility of hair loss. Explore coping strategies.

❏ Advise patient of the need for contraception.

❏ Instruct patient not to receive any vaccinations without advice of health care professional.

❏ Emphasize need for periodic lab tests to monitor for side effects.

## EVALUATION

**Effectiveness of therapy can be demonstrated by:** ■ Decrease in size and spread of tumor ❏ Improvement in hematologic parameters in nonsolid cancers.

---

## carteolol

(**kar**-tee-oh-lole)
Cartrol

### CLASSIFICATION(S):

**Therapeutic:** antianginals, antihypertensives
**Pharmacologic:** beta blockers

### Pregnancy Category C

See Appendix C for ophthalmic use.

---

## INDICATIONS

■ Management of hypertension. **Unlabeled uses:** ■ Management of angina pectoris.

## ACTION

■ Blocks stimulation of beta$_1$(myocardial)- and beta$_2$(pulmonary, vascular, and uterine)-adrenergic receptor sites ■ Also has intrinsic sympathomimetic activity (ISA), which may reduce bradycardia. **Therapeutic Effects:** ■ Decreased heart rate and blood pressure.

## PHARMACOKINETICS

**Absorption:** 85% absorbed following oral administration.
**Distribution:** Unknown.
**Metabolism and Excretion:** Some metabolism by the liver, with conversion to at least one active compound (8-hydroxycarteolol); 50–70% excreted unchanged by the kidneys.
**Half-life:** 6–8 hr (8–12 hr for 8-hydroxycarteolol; both are increased in renal impairment).

## CONTRAINDICATIONS AND PRECAUTIONS

**Contraindicated in:** ■ Uncompensated CHF ■ Pulmonary edema ■ Cardiogenic shock ■ Bradycardia or heart block.
**Use Cautiously in:** ■ Renal impairment (increased dosing interval recommended) ■ Hepatic impairment ■ Geriatric patients (increased sensitivity to beta blockers; initial dosage reduction recommended) ■ Pulmonary disease (including asthma); avoid use if possible ■ Diabetes mellitus (may mask signs of hypoglycemia) ■ Thyrotoxicosis (may mask symptoms) ■ Patients with a history of severe allergic reactions (intensity of reactions may be increased) ■ Pregnancy, lactation, or children (safety not established; all agents cross the placenta and may cause fetal/neonatal bradycardia, hypotension, hypoglycemia, or respiratory depression).

## ADVERSE REACTIONS AND SIDE EFFECTS*

■ **CNS:** fatigue, weakness, anxiety, depression, dizziness, drowsiness, insomnia, memory loss, mental status changes, nightmares ■ **EENT:** blurred vision, dry eyes, nasal stuffiness ■ **Resp:** bronchospasm, wheezing ■ **CV:** BRADYCARDIA, CHF, PULMONARY EDEMA, orthostatic hypotension, peripheral vasoconstriction ■ **GI:** constipation, diarrhea, nausea ■ **GU:** impotence, decreased libido ■ **Derm:** itching, rashes ■ **Endo:** hyperglycemia, hypoglycemia ■ **MS:** arthralgia, back pain, muscle cramps ■ **Neuro:** paresthesia ■ **Misc:** drug-induced lupus syndrome.

## INTERACTIONS

**Drug-Drug:** ■ **General anesthetics, IV phenytoin,** and **verapamil** may cause additive myocardial depression ■ Additive bradycardia may occur with **digoxin** ■ Additive hypotension may occur with other **antihypertensives,** acute ingestion of **alcohol,** or **nitrates** ■ Concurrent use with **amphetamine, cocaine, ephedrine, epinephrine, norepinephrine, phenylephrine,** or **pseudoephedrine** may result in unopposed alpha-adrenergic stimulation (excessive hypertension, bradycardia) ■ Concurrent administration of **thyroid preparations** may decrease effectiveness ■ May alter the effectiveness of **insulins** or **oral hypoglycemic agents** (dosage adjustments may be necessary) ■ May decrease the effectiveness of **adrenergics** and **theophylline** ■ May decrease the beneficial beta-cardiovascular effects of **dopamine** or **dobutamine** ■ Use cautiously within 14 days of **MAO inhibitor** therapy (may result in hypertension) ■ Concurrent use with **clonidine** increases hypotension and bradycardia ■ May exaggerate withdrawal phenomenon from **clonidine** ■ Concurrent **NSAIDs** may decrease antihypertensive action.

## ROUTE AND DOSAGE

■ **PO (Adults):** 2.5 mg once daily, may be increased up to 10 mg/day.

❑ **Renal Impairment**

■ **PO (Adults):** *CCr 20-60 ml/min*—increase dosing interval to q 48 hr; *CCr <20ml/min*—increase dosing interval to q 72 hr.

## AVAILABILITY

■ *Tablets:* 2.5 mg^{Rx}, 5 mg^{Rx} ■ Cost: 2.5 mg $114.84/100, 5 mg $114.84/100.

TIME/ACTION PROFILE (cardiovascular effects)

| | ONSET | PEAK | DURATION |
|---|---|---|---|
| PO | unknown | 1–3 hr | ≥24 hr |

## NURSING IMPLICATIONS

### ASSESSMENT

■ **General Info:** Monitor blood pressure and pulse frequently during dosage adjustment period and periodically throughout therapy. Assess for orthostatic hypotension when assisting patient up from supine position.

❑ Monitor intake and output ratios and daily weight. Assess patient routinely for evidence of fluid overload (peripheral edema, dyspnea, rales/crackles, fatigue, weight gain, jugular venous distention).

■ **Hypertension:** Check frequency of refills to determine adherence.

■ **Angina:** Assess frequency and characteristics of angina periodically during therapy.

■ *Lab Test Considerations:* May cause increased BUN, serum lipoprotein, potassium, triglyceride, and uric acid levels.

❑ May cause increased ANA titers.

❑ May cause increase in blood glucose levels.

■ *Toxicity and Overdose:* Monitor patients receiving beta blockers for signs of overdose (bradycardia, severe dizziness or fainting, severe drowsiness, dyspnea, bluish fingernails or palms, seizures). Notify physician or other health care professional immediately if these signs occur.

### POTENTIAL NURSING DIAGNOSES

■ Cardiac output, decreased (Side Effects).
■ Noncompliance (Patient/Family Teaching).

### IMPLEMENTATION

■ **General:** Do not confuse carteolol with carvedilol.

❑ Discontinuation of concurrent clonidine should be gradual, with beta blocker discontinued first; then, after several days, discontinue clonidine.

■ **PO:** Take apical pulse before administering. If <50 bpm or if arrhythmia occurs, withhold medication and notify physician or other health care professional.

❑ Administer without regard to food.

### PATIENT/FAMILY TEACHING

■ **General Info:** Instruct patient to take medication exactly as directed, at the same time each day, even if feeling well; do not skip or double up on missed doses. If a dose is missed, it should be taken as soon as possible up to 4 hr before next dose. Abrupt withdrawal may precipitate life-threatening arrhythmias, hypertension, or myocardial ischemia.

▢ Advise patient to make sure enough medication is available for weekends, holidays, and vacations. A written prescription may be kept in wallet in case of emergency.

▢ Teach patient and family how to check pulse and blood pressure. Instruct them to check pulse daily and blood pressure biweekly. Advise patient to hold dose and contact health care professional if pulse is <50 bpm or blood pressure changes significantly.

▢ May cause drowsiness or dizziness. Caution patients to avoid driving or other activities that require alertness until response to the drug is known.

▢ Advise patient to change positions slowly to minimize orthostatic hypotension, especially during initiation of therapy or when dose is increased.

▢ Caution patient that this medication may increase sensitivity to cold.

▢ Instruct patient to consult health care professional before taking any OTC medications, especially cold preparations, concurrently with this medication.

▢ Diabetics should closely monitor blood glucose, especially if weakness, malaise, irritability, or fatigue occurs. Medication may mask some signs of hypoglycemia, but dizziness and sweating may still occur.

▢ Advise patient to notify health care professional if slow pulse, difficulty breathing, wheezing, cold hands and feet, dizziness, confusion, depression, rash, fever, sore throat, unusual bleeding, or bruising occurs.

▢ Instruct patient to inform health care professional of medication regimen before treatment or surgery.

▢ Advise patient to carry identification describing disease process and medication regimen at all times.

■ **Hypertension:** Reinforce the need to continue additional therapies for hypertension (weight loss, sodium restriction, stress reduction, regular exercise, moderation of alcohol consumption, and smoking cessation).

Medication controls but does not cure hypertension.

■ **Angina:** Caution patient to avoid overexertion with decrease in chest pain.

## EVALUATION

**Effectiveness of therapy can be demonstrated by:** ■ Decrease in blood pressure without appearance of detrimental side effects ■ Reduction in frequency of anginal attacks ▢ Increase in activity tolerance.

## carvedilol
(kar-**ve**-dil-ole)
Coreg

**CLASSIFICATION(S):**
**Therapeutic:** antihypertensives
**Pharmacologic:** beta blockers

**Pregnancy Category C**

## INDICATIONS

■ Hypertension ■ CHF (ischemic or cardiomyopathic) with digoxin, diuretics, and ACE inhibitors ■ Left ventricular dysfunction after myocardial infarction.

## ACTION

■ Blocks stimulation of beta$_1$ (myocardial) and beta (pulmonary, vascular, and uterine)-adrenergic receptor sites ■ Also has alpha$_1$ blocking activity, which may result in orthostatic hypotension. **Therapeutic Effects:** ■ Decreased heart rate and blood pressure ■ Improved cardiac output, slowing of the progression of CHF and decreased risk of death.

## PHARMACOKINETICS

**Absorption:** Well absorbed but rapidly undergoes extensive first-pass hepatic metabolism, resulting in 25–35% bioavailability. Food slows absorption.

**Distribution:** Unknown.

**Protein Binding:** 98%.

**Metabolism and Excretion:** Extensively metabolized, excreted in feces via bile, <2% excreted unchanged in urine.

**Half-life:** 7–10 hr.

## CONTRAINDICATIONS AND PRECAUTIONS

**Contraindicated in:** ■ Pulmonary edema ■ Cardiogenic shock ■ Bradycardia, heart block or sick sinus syndrome (unless a pacemaker is in place) ■ Uncompensated CHF requiring IV inotropic agents (wean before starting carvedilol) ■ Severe hepatic impairment ■ Asthma or other bronchospastic disorders.

**Use Cautiously in:** ■ CHF (condition may deteriorate during initial therapy) ■ Renal impairment ■ Hepatic impairment ■ Geriatric patients (increased sensitivity to beta blockers; initial dosage reduction recommended) ■ Diabetes mellitus (may mask signs of hypoglycemia) ■ Thyrotoxicosis (may mask symptoms) ■ Peripheral vascular disease ■ History of severe allergic reactions (intensity of reactions may be increased) ■ Pregnancy, lactation, or children (safety not established; all agents cross the placenta and may cause fetal/neonatal bradycardia, hypotension, hypoglycemia, or respiratory depression).

## ADVERSE REACTIONS AND SIDE EFFECTS*

■ **CNS:** dizziness, fatigue, weakness, anxiety, depression, drowsiness, insomnia, memory loss, mental status changes, nervousness, nightmares ■ **EENT:** blurred vision, dry eyes, nasal stuffiness ■ **Resp:** bronchospasm, wheezing ■ **CV:** BRADYCARDIA, CHF, PULMONARY EDEMA ■ **GI:** diarrhea, constipation, nausea ■ **GU:** impotence, decreased libido ■ **Derm:** itching, rashes ■ **Endo:** hyperglycemia, hypoglycemia ■ **MS:** arthralgia, back pain, muscle cramps ■ **Neuro:** paresthesia ■ **Misc:** drug-induced lupus syndrome.

## INTERACTIONS

**Drug-Drug:** ■ **General anesthetics, IV phenytoin, diltiazem,** and **verapamil** may cause ↑ myocardial depression ■ ↑ risk of bradycardia with **digoxin** ■ ↑ hypotension may occur with other **antihypertensives,** acute ingestion of **alcohol,** or **nitrates** ■ Concurrent use with **clonidine** ↑ hypotension and bradycardia ■ May ↑ withdrawal phenomenon from **clonidine** (discontinue carvedilol first) ■ Concurrent administration of **thyroid preparations** may ↓ effectiveness ■ May alter the effectiveness of **insulins** or **oral hypoglycemic**

agents (dose adjustments may be necessary) ■ May ↓ effectiveness of **theophylline** ■ May ↓ beneficial beta₁-cardiovascular effects of **dopamine** or **dobutamine** ■ Use cautiously within 14 days of **MAO inhibitor** therapy (may result in hypotension/bradycardia) ■ **Cimetidine** may ↑ toxicity from carvedilol ■ Concurrent **NSAIDs** may ↓ antihypertensive action ■ Effectiveness may be ↓ by **rifampin** ■ May ↑ serum **digoxin** levels ■ May ↑ blood levels of **cyclosporine** (monitor blood levels).

## ROUTE AND DOSAGE

■ **PO (Adults):** *Hypertension*—6.25 mg twice daily, may be increased q 7–14 days up to 25 mg twice daily; *CHF*—3.125 mg twice daily for 2 wk; may be increased to 6.25 mg twice daily. Dose may be doubled q 2 wk as tolerated (not to exceed 25 mg twice daily in patients <85 kg or 50 mg twice daily in patients >85 kg; *Left ventricular dysfunction after MI*—6.25 mg twice daily, increase after 3–10 days to 12.5 twice daily then to target dose of 25 mg twice daily; some patients may require lower initial doses and slower titration.

## AVAILABILITY

■ *Tablets:* 3.125 mg^Rx, 6.25 mg^Rx, 12.5 mg^Rx, 25 mg^Rx ■ Cost: all strengths $165.35/100.

TIME/ACTION PROFILE (cardiovascular effects)

|    | ONSET | PEAK | DURATION |
|----|-------|------|----------|
| PO | within 1 hr | 1–2 hr | 12 hr |

# NURSING IMPLICATIONS

## ASSESSMENT

■ **General Info:** Monitor blood pressure and pulse frequently during dose adjustment period and periodically during therapy. Assess for orthostatic hypotension when assisting patient up from supine position.

❏ Monitor intake and output ratios and daily weight. Assess patient routinely for evidence of fluid overload (peripheral edema, dyspnea, rales/crackles, fatigue, weight gain, jugular venous distention). Patients may experience worsening of symptoms during initiation of therapy for CHF.

■ **Hypertension:** Check frequency of refills to determine adherence.

■ *Lab Test Considerations:* May cause ↑ BUN, serum lipoprotein, potassium, triglyceride, and uric acid levels.

❏ May cause ↑ ANA titers.

❏ May cause ↑ in blood glucose levels.

■ *Toxicity and Overdose:* Monitor patients receiving beta blockers for signs of overdose (bradycardia, severe dizziness or fainting, severe drowsiness, dyspnea, bluish fingernails or palms, seizures). Notify physician or other health care professional immediately if these signs occur.

## POTENTIAL NURSING DIAGNOSES

■ Cardiac output, decreased (Side Effects).

■ Noncompliance (Patient/Family Teaching).

## IMPLEMENTATION

■ **General:** Do not confuse carvedilol with captopril or carteolol.

❏ Discontinuation of concurrent clonidine should be gradual, with carvedilol discontinued first over 1-2 week with limitation of physical activity; then, after several days, discontinue clonidine.

■ **PO:** Take apical pulse before administering. If <50 bpm or if arrhythmia occurs, withhold medication and notify physician or other health care professional.

❏ Administer with food to minimize orthostatic hypotension.

## PATIENT/FAMILY TEACHING

■ **General Info:** Instruct patient to take medication as directed, at the same time each day, even if feeling well. Do not skip or double up on missed doses. Take missed doses as soon as possible up to 4 hr before next dose. Abrupt withdrawal may precipitate life-threatening arrhythmias, hypertension, or myocardial ischemia.

❏ Advise patient to make sure enough medication is available for weekends, holidays, and vacations. A written prescription may be kept in wallet in case of emergency.

❏ Teach patient and family how to check pulse and blood pressure. Instruct them to check pulse daily and blood pressure biweekly. Advise patient to hold dose and contact health care professional if pulse is <50 bpm or blood pressure changes significantly.

❏ May cause drowsiness or dizziness. Caution patients to avoid driving or other activities that require alertness until response to the drug is known.

❏ Advise patient to change positions slowly to minimize orthostatic hypotension, especially during initiation of therapy or when dose is increased.

❏ Caution patient that this medication may increase sensitivity to cold.

❏ Instruct patient to consult health care professional before taking any OTC medications or herbal products, especially cold preparations, concurrently with this medication.

❏ Patients with diabetes should closely monitor blood glucose, especially if weakness, malaise, irritability, or fatigue occurs. Medication may mask some signs of hypoglycemia, but dizziness and sweating may still occur.

❏ Advise patient to notify health care professional if slow pulse, difficulty breathing, wheezing, cold hands and feet, dizziness, confusion, depression, rash, fever, sore throat, unusual bleeding, or bruising occurs.

❏ Instruct patient to inform health care professional of medication regimen before treatment or surgery.

❏ Advise patient to carry identification describing disease process and medication regimen at all times.

■ **Hypertension:** Reinforce the need to continue additional therapies for hypertension (weight loss, sodium restriction, stress reduction, regular exercise, moderation of alcohol consumption, and smoking cessation). Medication controls but does not cure hypertension.

## EVALUATION

**Effectiveness of therapy can be demonstrated by:** ■ Decrease in blood pressure without appearance of detrimental side effects ■ Decrease in severity of CHF.

## caspofungin

(kas-po-**fun**-gin)

Cancidas

## CLASSIFICATION(S):

*Therapeutic:* antifungals (systemic)

## INDICATIONS

■ Treatment of invasive aspergillosis in patients who are refractory to, or intolerant of, other therapies ■ Candidemia and associated serious infections (intra-abdominal abscesses, peritonitis, pleural space infections) ■ Esophageal candidiasis.

## ACTION

■ Inhibits the synthesis of β (1, 3)-D-glucan, a necessary component of the fungal cell wall. **Therapeutic Effects:** ■ Death of susceptible fungi.

## PHARMACOKINETICS

**Absorption:** IV administration results in complete bioavailability.
**Distribution:** Widely distributed to tissues.
**Protein Binding:** 97%.
**Metabolism and Excretion:** Slowly and extensively metabolized; <1.5% excreted unchanged in urine.
**Half-life:** Polyphasic: β *phase*—9–11 hr; ξ *phase*—40–50 hr.

## CONTRAINDICATIONS AND PRECAUTIONS

**Contraindicated in:** ■ Hypersensitivity ■ Concurrent use with cyclosporine.
**Use Cautiously in:** ■ Moderate hepatic impairment (decreased maintenance dose recommended) ■ Children <18 yr (safety not established).

## ADVERSE REACTIONS AND SIDE EFFECTS*

■ **CNS:** headache ■ **GI:** diarrhea, nausea, vomiting ■ **Derm:** flushing ■ **Local:** venous irritation at injection site ■ **Misc:** allergic reactions including ANAPHYLAXIS, fever.

## INTERACTIONS

**Drug-Drug:** ■ Concurrent use with **cyclosporine** is not recommended due to ↑ risk of hepatic toxicity ■ May ↓ blood levels and effects of **tacrolimus** ■ Blood levels and effectiveness may be decreased by **rifampin**; main-

tenance dose should be increased to 70 mg (in patients with normal liver function) ■ Blood levels and effectiveness may be also be ↓ by **efavirenz, nelfinavir, nevirapine, phenytoin, dexamethasone** or **carbamazepine** an increase in the maintenance dose to 70 mg should be considered in patients who are not clinically responding.

## ROUTE AND DOSAGE

■ **IV (Adults):** 70 mg initially followed by 50 mg daily, duration determined by clinical situation and response; *Esophageal candidiasis*—50 mg daily, duration determined by clinical situation and response.

❑ **Moderate Hepatic Impairment (Child-Pugh Score 5–6)**

■ **IV (Adults):** 70 mg initially followed by 35 mg daily, duration determined by clinical situation and response.

## AVAILABILITY

■ *Powder for injection:* 50 mg^Rx, 70 mg^Rx.

TIME/ACTION PROFILE

|  | ONSET | PEAK | DURATION |
|---|---|---|---|
| IV | unknown | end of infusion | 24 hr |

## NURSING IMPLICATIONS

### ASSESSMENT

❑ Assess patient for signs and symptoms of aspergillosis prior to and periodically during therapy.
❑ Monitor patient for signs of anaphylaxis (rash, dyspnea, stridor) during therapy.
■ *Lab Test Considerations:* May cause ↑ serum alkaline phosphatase, AST, ALT, eosinophils, and urine protein and RBCs. May also cause ↓ serum potassium, hemoglobin, hematocrit, and WBCs.

### POTENTIAL NURSING DIAGNOSES

■ Infection, risk for (Indications).

### IMPLEMENTATION

■ **Intermittent Infusion:** When diluting caspofungin, white cake should dissolve completely. Mix gently until a clear soluton is obtained. Do not use a solution that is cloudy, discolored, or contains precipitates. Solution must be used within 24 hr if refrigerated.

☐ To prepare for 70-mg or 50-mg administration, allow refrigerated vial to reach room temperature. Aseptically add 10.5 ml of 0.9% NaCl, sterile water or bacteriostatic water to the 70-mg or 50-mg vial. Solution may be stored for up to 1 hr at room temperature. Transfer 10 ml of 70-mg or 50-mg solution to an IV bag containing 250 ml of 0.9% NaCl, 0.45% NaCl, 0.225% NaCl, or LR for a concentration of 0.28 mg/ml or 0.20 mg/ml respectively. Dilute solution is stable for 24 hr at room temperature or 48 hr if refrigerated.

☐ If only 50-mg dose is available, to prepare 70-mg dose transfer a total of 14 ml from two 50-mg vials to the 250 ml of 0.9% NaCl, 0.45% NaCl, 0.225% NaCl, or LR.

☐ If reduced volume is medically necessary, 50-mg dose can be prepared by adding 10 ml of reconstituted solution to 100 ml of 0.9% NaCl, 0.45% NaCl, 0.225% NaCl, or LR for a concentration of 0.47 mg/ml.

☐ To prepare 35-mg dose for patients with hepatic insufficiency reconstitute one 50-mg vial. Transfer 7 ml for 250 ml or, if medically necessary, 100 ml of 0.9% NaCl, 0.45% NaCl, 0.225% NaCl, or LR for a concentration of 0.14 mg/ml or 0.34 mg/ml respectively.

■ *Rate:* Administer via slow IV infusion over approximately 1 hr.

■ **Y-Site Incompatibility:** Do not use diluents containing dextrose. Do not mix or infuse caspofungin with other medications.

**PATIENT/FAMILY TEACHING**

☐ Explain the purpose of caspofungin to patient and family.

**EVALUATION**

**Clinical response to therapy can be evaluated by:** ■ Decrease in signs and symptoms of aspergillosis. Duration of therapy is determined based on severity of underlying disease, recovery from immunosuppression, and clinical response.

**cefaclor, See CEPHALOSPORINS—SECOND GENERATION.**

**cefadroxil, See CEPHALOSPORINS—FIRST GENERATION.**

**cefazolin, See CEPHALOSPORINS—FIRST GENERATION.**

**cefdinir, See CEPHALOSPORINS—THIRD GENERATION.**

**cefditoren, See CEPHALOSPORINS—THIRD GENERATION.**

**cefepime, See CEPHALOSPORINS—THIRD GENERATION.**

**cefmetazole, See CEPHALOSPORINS—SECOND GENERATION.**

**cefonicid, See CEPHALOSPORINS—SECOND GENERATION.**

**cefoperazone, See CEPHALOSPORINS—THIRD GENERATION.**

**cefotaxime, See CEPHALOSPORINS—THIRD GENERATION.**

**cefotetan, See CEPHALOSPORINS—SECOND GENERATION.**

cefoxitin, See
**CEPHALOSPORINS—SECOND
GENERATION.**

cefpodoxime, See
**CEPHALOSPORINS—THIRD
GENERATION.**

cefprozil, See
**CEPHALOSPORINS—SECOND
GENERATION.**

ceftazidime, See
**CEPHALOSPORINS—THIRD
GENERATION.**

ceftibuten, See
**CEPHALOSPORINS—THIRD
GENERATION.**

ceftizoxime, See
**CEPHALOSPORINS—THIRD
GENERATION.**

ceftriaxone, See
**CEPHALOSPORINS—THIRD
GENERATION.**

cefuroxime, See
**CEPHALOSPORINS—SECOND
GENERATION.**

## celecoxib

(sel-e-**kox**-ib)
Celebrex

*CLASSIFICATION(S):*
*Therapeutic: antirheumatics,
nonsteroidal anti-inflammatory
agents*
*Pharmacologic: COX-2 inhibitors*

**Pregnancy Category C**

### INDICATIONS

■ Relief of signs and symptoms of osteoarthritis
■ Relief of signs and symptoms of rheumatoid arthritis in adults ■ Reduction of the number of adenomatous colorectal polyps in familial adenomatous polyposis (FAP), as an adjunct to usual care (endoscopic surveillance, surgery).

### ACTION

■ Inhibits the enzyme COX-2. This enzyme is required for the synthesis of prostaglandins ■ Has analgesic, anti-inflammatory, and antipyretic properties. **Therapeutic Effects:** ■ Decreased pain and inflammation caused by arthritis ■ Decreased number of colorectal polyps.

### PHARMACOKINETICS

**Absorption:** Bioavailability unknown.
**Distribution:** 97% bound to plasma proteins; extensive tissue distribution.
**Metabolism and Excretion:** Mostly metabolized by the liver; <3% excreted unchanged in urine and feces.
**Half-life:** 11 hr.

### CONTRAINDICATIONS AND PRECAUTIONS

**Contraindicated in:** ■ Hypersensitivity ■ Cross-sensitivity may exist with other NSAIDs, including aspirin ■ History of allergic-type reactions to sulfonamides ■ History of asthma, urticaria, or allergic-type reactions to aspirin or other NSAIDs, including the aspirin triad (asthma, nasal polyps, and severe hypersensitivity reactions to aspirin) ■ Advanced renal disease ■ Should not be used in late pregnancy (may cause premature closure of the ductus arteriosus).

**Use Cautiously in:** ■ Concurrent therapy with corticosteroids or anticoagulants, long duration of NSAID therapy, history of smoking, alcoholism, geriatric patients, or poor general health

{ } = Available in Canada only.
*CAPITALS indicates life-threatening; <u>underlines</u> indicate most frequent.

status (increased risk of GI bleeding) ▪ Pre-existing renal disease, heart failure, liver dysfunction, concurrent diuretic or ACE inhibitor therapy (increased risk of renal impairment) ▪ Hypertension or fluid retention ▪ Renal insufficiency (may precipitate acute renal failure) ▪ Serious dehydration (correct deficits before administering) ▪ Pre-existing asthma ▪ Pregnancy or children <18 yr (safety not established, use not recommended during late pregnancy).

**Exercise Extreme Caution in:** ▪ History of ulcer disease or GI bleeding.

## ADVERSE REACTIONS AND SIDE EFFECTS*

▪ **CNS:** dizziness, headache, insomnia ▪ **GI:** GI BLEEDING, abdominal pain, diarrhea, dyspepsia, flatulence, nausea ▪ **Derm:** rash.

## INTERACTIONS

**Drug-Drug:** ▪ Significant interactions may occur when celecoxib is coadministered with other drugs that inhibit the CYP450 2C9 enzyme system ▪ May decrease the effectiveness of **ACE inhibitors, thiazide diuretics,** and **furosemide** ▪ Although celecoxib may be used with **aspirin,** the combination may increase the risk of GI bleeding ▪ **Fluconazole** increases celecoxib blood levels (dosage reduction recommended) ▪ May increase the risk of bleeding with **warfarin** ▪ May increase serum **lithium** levels ▪ Does not inhibit the cardioprotective effect of low-dose **aspirin.**

## ROUTE AND DOSAGE

▪ **PO (Adults):** *Osteoarthritis*—200 mg/day as a single dose *or* 100 mg twice daily. *Rheumatoid arthritis*—100–200 mg twice daily. *Familial adenomatous polyosis*—400 mg twice daily.

## AVAILABILITY

▪ *Capsules:* 100 mg^Rx, 200 mg^Rx ▪ Cost: *100-mg capsules*—$148.72/100; *200-mg capsules*—$251.68/100.

TIME/ACTION PROFILE (pain reduction)

| | ONSET | PEAK | DURATION |
|---|---|---|---|
| PO | 24–48 hr | unknown | 12–24 hr† |

†After discontinuation.

## NURSING IMPLICATIONS

### ASSESSMENT

❑ Assess patient's range of motion, degree of swelling, and pain in affected joints before and periodically throughout therapy.

❑ Assess patient for allergy to sulfonamides, aspirin, or NSAIDs. Patients with these allergies should not receive celecoxib.

▪ *Lab Test Considerations:* May cause elevated AST and ALT levels.

❑ May cause hypophosphatemia and elevated BUN.

### POTENTIAL NURSING DIAGNOSES

▪ Mobility, impaired physical (Indications).

▪ Pain, acute (Indications).

### IMPLEMENTATION

▪ **General:** Do not confuse with Celexa (citalopram) or Cerebyx (fosphenytoin).

▪ **PO:** May be administered without regard to meals.

### PATIENT/FAMILY TEACHING

❑ Instruct patient to take celecoxib exactly as directed. Do not take more than prescribed dose. Increasing doses does not appear to increase effectiveness.

❑ Advise patient to notify health care professional promptly if signs or symptoms of GI toxicity (abdominal pain, black stools), skin rash, unexplained weight gain, or edema occurs. Patients should discontinue celecoxib and notify health care professional if signs and symptoms of hepatotoxicity (nausea, fatigue, lethargy, pruritus, jaundice, upper right quadrant tenderness, flu-like symptoms) occur.

❑ Advise patient to notify health care professional if pregnancy is planned or suspected.

❑ Advise patients with FAP to continue routine surveillance procedures.

### EVALUATION

**Effectiveness of therapy can be demonstrated by:** ▪ Reduction in joint pain in patients with osteoarthritis ▪ Reduction in joint tenderness, pain, and joint swelling in patients with rheumatoid arthritis ▪ Decreased number of colonic polyps in patients with FAP.

# cephalexin, See CEPHALOSPORINS—FIRST GENERATION.

## CEPHALOSPORINS—FIRST GENERATION

**cefadroxil**
(sef-a-**drox**-ill)
Duricef

**cefazolin**
(sef-**a**-zoe-lin)
Ancef

**cephalexin**
(sef-a-**lex**-in)
{Apo-Cephalex}, Biocef, Keflex, Keftab, {Novo-Lexin}, {Nu-Cephalex}

**cephapirin**
(sef-a-**pye**-rin)
Cefadyl

**cephradine**
(**sef**-re-deen)
Velosef

### CLASSIFICATION(S):
*Therapeutic:* anti-infectives
*Pharmacologic:* first-generation cephalosporins

### Pregnancy Category B

## INDICATIONS

■ Treatment of: ❑ Skin and skin structure infections (including burn wounds) ❑ Pneumonia ❑ Otitis media ❑ Urinary tract infections ❑ Bone and joint infections ❑ Septicemia (including endocarditis) caused by susceptible organisms ■ **Cefazolin, cephapirin, cephradine:** Perioperative prophylaxis ■ Not suitable for the treatment of meningitis.

## ACTION

■ Bind to bacterial cell wall membrane, causing cell death. **Therapeutic Effects:** ■ Bactericidal action against susceptible bacteria. **Spectrum:** ■ Active against many gram-positive cocci including: ❑ *Streptococcus pneumoniae* ❑ Group A beta-hemolytic streptococci ❑ Penicillinase-producing staphylococci ■ Not active against: ❑ Methicillin-resistant staphylococci ❑ *Bacteroides fragilis* ❑ *Enterococcus* ■ Limited activity against some gram-negative rods including: ❑ *Klebsiella pneumoniae* ❑ *Proteus mirabilis* ❑ *Escherichia coli.*

## PHARMACOKINETICS

**Absorption:** *Cefadroxil, cephalexin,* and *cephradine* are well absorbed following oral administration. *Cefazolin, cephapirin,* and *cephradine* are well absorbed following IM administration.

**Distribution:** Widely distributed. All cross the placenta and enter breast milk in low concentrations. Minimal CSF penetration.

**Metabolism and Excretion:** Excreted almost entirely unchanged by the kidneys.

**Half-life:** *Cefadroxil*—78–96 min; *cefazolin*—90–120 min; *cephalexin*—50–80 min; *cephalothin*—30–50 min; *cephapirin*—24–36 min; *cephradine*—48–80 min (all are increased in renal impairment).

## CONTRAINDICATIONS AND PRECAUTIONS

**Contraindicated in:** ■ Hypersensitivity to cephalosporins ■ Serious hypersensitivity to penicillins.

**Use Cautiously in:** ■ Renal impairment (dosage reduction and/or increased dosing interval recommended for: *cefadroxil* if CCr ≤50 ml/min, *cephradine* and *cephapirin* if CCr ≤20 ml/min, *cephalothin* if CCr ≤50 ml/min, *cefazolin* if CCr <55 ml/min) ■ History of GI disease, especially colitis ■ Geriatric patients (consider age-related decrease in body mass, renal/hepatic/cardiac function, concurrent medications and chronic disease states) ■ Pregnancy or lactation (half-life is shorter and blood levels lower during pregnancy; have been used safely).

## ADVERSE REACTIONS AND SIDE EFFECTS*

■ **CNS:** SEIZURES (high doses) ■ **GI:** PSEUDOMEM-BRANOUS COLITIS, diarrhea, nausea, vomiting, cramps ■ **GU:** interstitial nephritis (*cefadroxil* only) ■ **Derm:** rashes, urticaria ■ **Hemat:** blood dyscrasias, hemolytic anemia ■ **Local:** pain at IM site, phlebitis AT IV SITE ■ **Misc:** allergic reactions including ANAPHYLAXIS and SERUM SICKNESS, superinfection.

## INTERACTIONS

**Drug-Drug:** ■ **Probenecid** ↓ excretion and ↑ blood levels of renally excreted cephalosporins ■ Concurrent use of **loop diuretics** may ↑ risk of renal toxicity.

## ROUTE AND DOSAGE

### ❑ Cefadroxil

■ **PO (Adults):** *Group A beta-hemolytic streptococcal pharyngitis*—500 mg q 12 hr or 1 g q 24 hr for 10 days. *Skin and soft-tissue infections*—500 mg q 12 hr or 1 g q 24 hr. *Urinary tract infections*—500 mg–1 g q 12 hr or 1–2 g q 24 hr.

■ **PO (Children):** *Group A beta-hemolytic streptococcal pharyngitis*—15 mg/kg q 12 hr or 30 mg/kg q 24 hr for 10 days. *Skin and soft-tissue infections*—15 mg/kg q 12 hr or 30 mg/kg q 24 hr. *Urinary tract infections*—500 mg or 15 mg/kg q 12 hr.

### ❑ Renal Impairment

■ **PO (Adults):** *CCr 25–50 ml/min*—500 mg q 12 hr; *CCr 10–25 ml/min*—500 mg q 24 hr; *CCr 0–10 ml/min*—500 mg q 36 hr.

### ❑ Cefazolin

■ **IM, IV (Adults):** *Most infections*—250 mg–1.5 g q 6–8 hr. *Perioperative prophylaxis*—1 g within 60 min of incision, then q 8 hr for up to 24 hr.

■ **IM, IV (Children and Infants >1 mo):** 6.25–25 mg/kg q 6 hr or 8.3–33.3 mg/kg q 8 hr.

### ❑ Renal Impairment

■ **IM, IV (Adults):** *CCr 35–54 ml/min*—full dose q 8 hr or less frequently; *CCr 11–34 ml/min*—¹/₂ full dose q 12 hr; *CCr ≤10 ml/min*—¹/₂ full dose q 18–24 hr.

### ❑ Cephalexin

■ **PO (Adults):** *Most infections*—250–500 mg q 6 hr. *Cystitis, skin and soft-tissue infections, streptococcal pharyngitis*—500 mg q 12 hr.

■ **PO (Children):** *Most infections*—6.25–25 mg/kg q 6 hr. *Skin and soft-tissue infections, streptococcal pharyngitis*—12.5–50 mg/kg q 12 hr.

### ❑ Cephapirin

■ **IM, IV (Adults):** *Most infections*—0.5–1 g q 4–6 hr.

■ **IM, IV (Children >3 mo):** *Most infections*—10–20 mg/kg q 6 hr.

### ❑ Cephradine

■ **PO (Adults):** *Most infections*—250–500 mg q 6 hr *or* 500–1000 mg q 12 hr.

■ **PO (Children >9 mo):** *Most infections*—6.25–25 mg/kg q 6 hr.

### ❑ Renal Impairment

■ **PO (Adults):** *CCr 5–20 ml/min*—250 mg q 6 hr; *CCr <5 ml/min*—250 mg q 12 hr.

## AVAILABILITY

### ❑ Cefadroxil

■ *Capsules:* 500 mg[Rx] ■ *Tablets:* 1 g[Rx] ■ *Oral suspension (orange-pineapple flavor):* 125 mg/5 ml[Rx], 250 mg/5 ml[Rx], 500 mg/5 ml[Rx].

### ❑ Cefazolin

■ *Powder for injection:* 250 mg[Rx], 500 mg[Rx], 1 g[Rx], 5 g[Rx], 10 g[Rx], 20 g[Rx] ■ *Premixed containers:* 500 mg/50 ml D5W[Rx], 1 g/50 ml D5W[Rx].

### ❑ Cephalexin

■ *Capsules:* 250 mg[Rx], 500 mg[Rx] ■ Cost: *Keflex*—250-mg capsules $164.70/100; generic—250-mg capsules $15.00/100, 500-mg capsules $21.45/100 ■ *Tablets:* 250 mg[Rx], 500 mg[Rx] ■ Cost: *Keftab*—500-mg tablets $68.77/20; generic—250-mg $57.25/100 ■ *Oral suspension:* 100 mg/ml[Rx], 125 mg/5 ml[Rx], 250 mg/5 ml[Rx] ■ Cost: generic—125 mg/5ml $13.37/100 ml, 250 mg/5 ml $25.42/100 ml.

### ❑ Cephapirin

■ *Powder for injection:* 500 mg[Rx], 1 g[Rx], 2 g[Rx], 4 g[Rx], 20 g[Rx].

### ❑ Cephradine

■ *Capsules:* 250 mg[Rx], 500 mg[Rx] ■ *Oral suspension (fruit flavored):* 125 mg/5 ml[Rx], 250 mg/5 ml[Rx].

TIME/ACTION PROFILE (blood levels)

| | ONSET | PEAK | DURATION |
|---|---|---|---|
| Cefadroxil PO | rapid | 1.5–2 hr | 12–24 hr |
| Cefazolin IM | rapid | 1–2 hr | 6–12 hr |
| Cefazolin IV | rapid | end of infusion | 6–12 hr |
| Cephalexin PO | rapid | 1 hr | 6–12 hr |
| Cephapirin IM | rapid | 0.5 hr | 4–6 hr |
| Cephapirin IV | rapid | end of infusion | 4–6 hr |
| Cephradine PO | rapid | 1–2 hr | 6–12 hr |

## NURSING IMPLICATIONS

### ASSESSMENT

❑ Assess patient for infection (vital signs; appearance of wound, sputum, urine, and stool; WBC) at beginning and during therapy.

❑ Before initiating therapy, obtain a history to determine previous use of and reactions to penicillins or cephalosporins. Persons with a negative history of penicillin sensitivity may still have an allergic response.

❑ Obtain specimens for culture and sensitivity before initiating therapy. First dose may be given before receiving results.

❑ Observe patient for signs and symptoms of anaphylaxis (rash, pruritus, laryngeal edema, wheezing). Discontinue drug and notify physician or other health care professional immediately if these problems occur. Keep epinephrine, an antihistamine, and resuscitation equipment close by in case of an anaphylactic reaction.

■ *Lab Test Considerations:* May cause positive results for Coombs' test in patients receiving high doses or in neonates whose mothers were given cephalosporins before delivery.

❑ May cause ↑ serum AST, ALT, alkaline phosphatase, bilirubin, LDH, BUN, creatinine.

❑ May rarely cause leukopenia, neutropenia, agranulocytosis, thrombocytopenia, eosinophilia, lymphocytosis, and thrombocytosis.

## POTENTIAL NURSING DIAGNOSES

■ Infection, risk for (Indications, Side Effects).
■ Diarrhea (Adverse Reactions).

## IMPLEMENTATION

■ **PO:** Administer around the clock. May be administered on full or empty stomach. Administration with food may minimize GI irritation. Shake oral suspension well before administering. Refrigerate oral suspensions.

■ **IM:** Reconstitute IM doses with sterile or bacteriostatic water for injection or 0.9% NaCl for injection. May be diluted with lidocaine to minimize injection discomfort.

❑ Inject deep into a well-developed muscle mass; massage well.

■ **IV:** Monitor site frequently for thrombophlebitis (pain, redness, swelling). Change sites every 48–72 hr to prevent phlebitis.

❑ Do not use solutions that are cloudy or contain a precipitate.

❑ If aminoglycosides are administered concurrently, administer in separate sites, if possible, at least 1 hr apart. If second site is unavailable, flush line between medications.

■ **Direct IV:** Dilute in at least 1 g/10 ml of sterile water for injection. Do not use preparations containing benzyl alcohol for neonates.

■ *Rate:* Administer slowly over 3–5 min.

❑ **Cefazolin**

■ **Intermittent Infusion:** Reconstituted 500-mg or 1-g solution may be diluted in 50–100 ml of 0.9% NaCl, D5W, D10W, D5/0.25% NaCl, D5/0.45% NaCl, D5/09% NaCl, D5/LR. Solution is stable for 24 hr at room temperature and 96 hr if refrigerated.

■ *Rate:* Administer over 30–60 min.

■ **Syringe Compatibility:** ◆ heparin ◆ vitamin B complex.

■ **Syringe Incompatibility:** ◆ lidocaine.

■ **Y-Site Compatibility:** ◆ acyclovir ◆ allopurinol ◆ amifostine ◆ atracurium ◆ aztreonam ◆ calcium gluconate ◆ cyclophosphamide ◆ diltiazem ◆ docetaxel ◆ doxorubicin liposome ◆ enalaprilat ◆ esmolol ◆ etoposide ◆ famotidine ◆ filgrastim ◆ fluconazole ◆ fludarabine ◆ foscarnet ◆ gatifloxacin ◆ gemcitabine ◆ granisetron ◆ heparin ◆ insulin ◆ labetalol ◆ lidocaine ◆ linezolid ◆ magnesium sulfate ◆ melphalan ◆ meperidine ◆ midazolam ◆ morphine ◆ multivitamins ◆ ondansetron ◆ pancuronium ◆ perphenazine ◆ propofol ◆ ranitidine ◆ remifentanil ◆ sargramostim ◆ tacrolimus ◆ teniposide ◆ theophylline ◆ thiotepa ◆ vecuronium ◆ vitamin B complex with C ◆ warfarin.

■ **Y-Site Incompatibility:** ◆ amphotericin B cholesteryl sulfate ◆ idarubicin ◆ pentamidine ◆ vinorelbine.

❑ **Cephapirin**

■ **Intermittent Infusion:** Reconstituted solutions may be further diluted in 50–100 ml of 0.9% NaCl, D5W, D10W, D20W, D5/0.25% NaCl, D5/0.45% NaCl, D5/0.9% NaCl, or D5/LR. Stable for 24 hr at room temperature and 10 days if refrigerated.

■ *Rate:* Administer over at least 15–20 min.

■ **Continuous Infusion:** Solution may also be diluted in 500–1000 ml for continuous infusion.

■ **Y-Site Compatibility:** ◆ acyclovir ◆ cyclophosphamide ◆ famotidine ◆ heparin ◆ hydrocortisone sodium succinate ◆ hydromorphone ◆ magnesium sulfate ◆ meperidine ◆ morphine ◆ multivitamins ◆ perphenazine ◆ potassium chloride ◆ vitamin B complex with C ◆ warfarin.

**PATIENT/FAMILY TEACHING**

❑ Instruct patient to take medication around the clock at evenly spaced times and to finish the medication completely as directed, even if feeling better. Missed doses should be taken as soon as possible unless almost time for next dose; do not double doses. Instruct patient to use calibrated measuring device with liquid preparations. Advise patient that sharing this medication may be dangerous.

❑ Advise patient to report signs of superinfection (furry overgrowth on the tongue, vaginal itching or discharge, loose or foul-smelling stools) and allergy.

❑ Instruct patient to notify health care professional if fever and diarrhea develop, especially if diarrhea contains blood, mucus, or pus. Advise patient not to treat diarrhea without consulting health care professional.

**EVALUATION**

**Clinical response to therapy can be evaluated by:** ■ Resolution of signs and symptoms of infection. Length of time for complete resolution depends on the organism and site of infection ■ Decreased incidence of infection when used for prophylaxis.

# CEPHALOSPORINS— SECOND GENERATION

**cefaclor**

(**sef**-a-klor)

Ceclor, Ceclor CD

**cefmetazole**

(sef-**met**-a-zole)

Zefazone

**cefonicid**

(se-**fon**-i-sid)

Monocid

**cefotetan**

(sef-oh-**tee**-tan)

Cefotan

**cefoxitin**

(se-**fox**-i-tin)

Mefoxin

**cefprozil**

(sef-**proe**-zil)

Cefzil

**cefuroxime**

(se-fyoor-**ox**-eem)

Ceftin, Zinacef

**loracarbef**

(lore-a-**kar**-beff)

Lorabid

*CLASSIFICATION(S):*

***Therapeutic:*** *anti-infectives*

***Pharmacologic:*** *second-generation cephalosporins*

**Pregnancy Category B**

**INDICATIONS**

■ Treatment of: ❑ Respiratory tract infections ❑ Skin and skin structure infections ❑ Bone and joint infections (not cefmetazole, cefprozil, or loracarbef) □ Urinary tract and gynecologic infection (not cefprozil) □ Septicemia (not cefmetazole, cefprozil, or loracarbef) ■ **Cefotetan:** Intra-abdominal, gynecologic, and biliary tract infections ■ **Cefuroxime:** Meningitis ■ **Cefaclor, cefprozil, cefuroxime:** Otitis media ■ **Cefmetazole, cefonicid, ceforanide, cefotetan, cefoxitin, cefuroxime:** Perioperative prophylaxis.

## ACTION

■ Bind to bacterial cell wall membrane, causing cell death. **Therapeutic Effects:** ■ Bactericidal action. **Spectrum:** ■ Similar to that of first-generation cephalosporins but have ↑ activity against several other gram-negative pathogens including: □ *Haemophilus influenzae* □ *Escherichia coli* □ *Klebsiella pneumoniae* □ *Neisseria gonorrhoeae* (including penicillinase-producing strains) □ *Proteus* □ *Moraxella catarrhalis* ■ Cefotetan, and cefoxitin have activity against *Bacteroides fragilis* ■ Not active against methicillin-resistant staphylococci or enterococci.

## PHARMACOKINETICS

**Absorption:** Well absorbed following IM administration. *Cefaclor, cefprozil, cefuroxime,* and *loracarbef*—well absorbed following oral administration.

**Distribution:** Widely distributed. Penetration into CSF is poor, but adequate for cefuroxime to be used in treating meningitis. All cross the placenta and enter breast milk in low concentrations.

**Metabolism and Excretion:** Excreted primarily unchanged by the kidneys.

**Half-life:** *Cefaclor*—35–54 min; *cefmetazole*—72 min; *cefonicid*—270 min; *cefotetan*—3–4.6 hr; *cefoxitin*—40–60 min; *cefmetazole*—72 min; *cefprozil*—90 min; *cefuroxime*—80 min; *loracarbef*—1 hr (all are increased in renal impairment).

## CONTRAINDICATIONS AND PRECAUTIONS

**Contraindicated in:** ■ Hypersensitivity to cephalosporins ■ Serious hypersensitivity to penicillins.

**Use Cautiously in:** ■ Renal impairment ( ↓ dose/ ↑ dosing interval recommended for: *cefmetazole* if CCr ≤90 ml/min, *cefonicid* if CCr <80 ml/min, *cefotetan* if CCr ≤30 ml/min, *cefoxitin* if CCr ≤50 ml/min, *cefprozil* if CCr <30 ml/min, *cefuroxime* if CCr ≤20 ml/min, *loracarbef* if CCr <50 ml/min) ■ Geriatric, debilitated, or emaciated patients (may need supplemental vitamin K to prevent bleeding) ■ History of GI disease, especially colitis ■ Some oral dosage forms may contain aspartame and should be avoided in patients with phenylketonuria ■ Geriatric patients (consider age-related decrease in body mass, renal/hepatic/cardiac function, concurrent medications and chronic disease states) ■ Pregnancy and lactation (have been used safely).

## ADVERSE REACTIONS AND SIDE EFFECTS*

■ **CNS:** SEIZURES (high doses) ■ **GI:** PSEUDOMEMBRANOUS COLITIS , diarrheajaundice (ceftazidime), nausea, vomiting, cramps ■ **Derm:** rashes, urticaria ■ **Hemat:** bleeding (increased with cefmetazole, cefotetan), blood dyscrasias, hemolytic anemia ■ **Local:** pain at IM site, phlebitis AT IV SITE ■ **Misc:** allergic reactions including ANAPHYLAXIS and SERUM SICKNESS , superinfection.

## INTERACTIONS

**Drug-Drug:** ■ **Probenecid** ↓ excretion and increases blood levels ■ If **alcohol** is ingested within 48–72 hr of cefmetazole, or cefotetan, a disulfiram-like reaction may occur ■ Cefmetazole, and cefotetan may potentiate the effects of **anticoagulants** and ↑ risk of bleeding with **antiplatelet agents, thrombolytic agents, NSAIDs, plicamycin,** or **valproic acid**.

**Drug-Natural Products:** ■ Risk of bleeding with **cefmetazole** and **cefotetan** may be increased by **anise, arnica, chamomile, clove, fenugreek, feverfew, garlic, ginger, gingo, Panax ginseng, licorice, passionflower, turmeric, willow** and others.

## ROUTE AND DOSAGE

□ **Cefaclor**

■ **PO (Adults):** 250–500 mg q 8 hr or 375–500 mg q 12 hr as extended-release tablets.

---

- **PO (Children >1 mo):** 6.7–13.4 mg/kg q 8 hr or 10–20 mg/kg q 12 hr (up to 60 mg/kg/day or 1.5 g/day have been used).

## Cefmetazole

- **IV (Adults):** *Most infections*—2 g q 6–12 hr.

## Renal Impairment

- **IV (Adults):** *CCr 50–90 ml/min*—1–2 g 12 hr; *CCr 30–49 ml/min*—1–2 g 16 hr; *CCr 10–29 ml/min*—1–2 g 24 hr; *CCr <10 ml/min*—1–2 g 48 hr (after hemodialysis).

## Cefonicid

- **IM, IV (Adults):** *Most infections*—0.5–1 g q 24 hr. *Severe/life-threatening infections*—2 g q 24 hr.

## Renal Impairment

- **IM, IV (Adults):** *CCr 60–79 ml/min*—10–25 mg/kg q 24 hr; *CCr 40–59 ml/min*—8–20 mg/kg q 24 hr; *CCr 20–39 ml/min*—4–15 mg/kg q 24 hr; *CCr 10–19 ml/min*—4–15 mg/kg q 48 hr; *CCr 5–9 ml/min*—4–15 mg/kg q 3–5 days; *CCr <5 ml/min*—3–4 mg/kg q 3–5 days.

## Cefotetan

- **IM, IV (Adults):** *Most infections*—1–2 g q 12 hr. *Severe/life-threatening infections*—2–3 g q 12 hr. *Urinary tract infections*—500 mg–1 g q 12 hr *or* 1–2 g q 24 hr.

## Renal Impairment

- **IM, IV (Adults):** *CCr 10–30 ml/min*—Usual adult dose q 24 hr *or* ½ usual adult dose 12 hr; *<CCr 10 ml/min*—Usual adult dose q 48 hr *or* ¼ usual adult dose q 12 hr.

## Cefoxitin

- **IM, IV (Adults):** *Most infections*—1 g q 6–8 hr. *Severe infections*—1 g q 4 hr *or* 2 g q 6–8 hr. *Life-threatening infections*—2 g q 4 hr *or* 3 g q 6 hr. *Perioperative prophylaxis*—1–2 g within 60 min of incision, then q 6 hr for up to 24 hr.
- **IM, IV (Children and Infants >3 mo):** *Most infections*—13.3–26.7 mg/kg q 4 hr *or* 20–40 mg/kg q 6 hr.

## Renal Impairment

- **IM, IV (Adults):** *CCr 30–50 ml/min*—1–2 g q 8–12 hr; *CCr 10–29 ml/min*—1–2 g q 12–24 hr; *CCr 5–9 ml/min*—0.5–1 g q 12–24 hr; *CCr <5 ml/min*—0.5–1 g q 24–48 hr.

## Cefprozil

- **PO (Adults):** *Most infections*—250–500 mg q 12 hr *or* 500 mg q 24 hr.
- **PO (Children 6 mo–12 yr):** *Otitis media*—15 mg/kg q 12 hr.
- **PO (Children 2–12 yr):** *Pharyngitis/tonsillitis*—7.5 mg/kg q 12 hr.

## Renal Impairment

- **PO (Adults):** *CCr 0<130 ml/min*—½ of usual dose q 12 *or* 24 hr.

## Cefuroxime

- **PO (Adults and Children >12 yr):** *Most infections*—250–500 mg q 12 hr. *Urinary tract infections*—125–250 mg q 12 hr.
- **PO (Children <12 yr):** *Most infections*—125 mg q 12 hr as tablets. *Otitis media*—250 mg q 12 hr as tablets.
- **PO (Children 3 mo–12 yr):** *Otitis media, impetigo*—15 mg/kg q 12 hr as oral suspension. *Pharyngitis/tonsillitis*—10 mg/kg q 12 hr as oral suspension. *Acute bacterial maxillary sinusitis*—250 mg twice daily for 10 days in patients who can swallow tablets *or* 15 mg/kg twice daily for 10 days as oral suspension (up to 1000 mg/day).
- **IM, IV (Adults):** *Most infections*—750 mg–1.5 g q 8 hr. *Bacterial meningitis*—up to 3 g q 8 hr.
- **IM, IV (Children and Infants >3 mo):** *Most infections*—16.7–33.3 mg/kg q 8 hr *or* 15–50 mg/kg q 12 hr. *Bone infections*—50 mg/kg q 8 hr. *Bacterial meningitis*—50–60 mg/kg q 6 hr *or* 66.7–80 mg/kg q 8 hr.
- **IM, IV (Neonates):** *Most infections*—10–33.3 mg/kg q 8 hr *or* 15–50 mg/kg q 12 hr. *Bacterial meningitis*—33.3 mg/kg q 8 hr *or* 50 mg/kg q 12 hr.
- **PO (Children 6 mo–12 yr):** *Pharyngitis/skin and soft-tissue infections*—7.5 mg q 12 hr. *Otitis media*—15 mg/kg q 12 hr.

## Renal Impairment

- **IM, IV (Adults):** *CCr 10–20 ml/min*—750 mg q 12 hr; *CCr <10 ml/min*—750 mg q 24 hr.

## Loracarbef

- **PO (Adults):** *Most infections*—200–400 mg q 12 hr. *Cystitis*—200 mg q 24 hr.

## Renal Impairment

- **PO (Adults):** *CCr 10–49 ml/min*—half the usual dose every 12 hours *or* the usual dose q 24 hr. *<CCr 10 ml/min*—the usual adult dose given q 3–5 days.

## AVAILABILITY

❑ **Cefaclor**

■ *Capsules:* 250 mg$^{Rx}$, 500 mg$^{Rx}$ ■ *Extended-release tablets (CD):* 375 mg$^{Rx}$, 500 mg$^{Rx}$ ■ *Oral suspension (strawberry):* 125 mg/5 ml$^{Rx}$, 187 mg/5 ml$^{Rx}$, 250 mg/5 ml$^{Rx}$, 375 mg/5 ml$^{Rx}$.

❑ **Cefmetazole**

■ *Powder for injection:* 1 g$^{Rx}$, 2 g$^{Rx}$.

❑ **Cefonicid**

■*Powder for injection:* 500 mg$^{Rx}$, 1 g$^{Rx}$, 10 g$^{Rx}$.

❑ **Cefotetan**

■*Powder for injection:* 1 g$^{Rx}$, 2 g$^{Rx}$, 10 g$^{Rx}$.

❑ **Cefoxitin**

■*Powder for injection:* 1 g$^{Rx}$, 2 g$^{Rx}$, 10 g$^{Rx}$ ■*Premixed containers:* 1 g/50 ml D5W$^{Rx}$, 2 g/50 ml D5W$^{Rx}$.

❑ **Cefprozil**

■*Tablets:* 250 mg$^{Rx}$, 500 mg$^{Rx}$ ■Cost: 250 mg $355.37/100, 500 mg $723.88/60 ■ *Oral suspension (bubblegum flavor):* 125 mg/5 ml$^{Rx}$, 250 mg/5 ml$^{Rx}$.

❑ **Cefuroxime**

■ *Tablets:* 125 mg$^{Rx}$, 250 mg$^{Rx}$, 500 mg$^{Rx}$ ■ Cost: 250 mg $88.20/20, 500 mg $482.16/60 ■ *Oral suspension (tutti-frutti flavor):* 125 mg/5 ml$^{Rx}$ ■Cost: 125 mg/5 ml $36.08/100 ml ■ *Powder for injection:* 750 mg$^{Rx}$, 1.5 g$^{Rx}$, 7.5 g$^{Rx}$ ■*Premixed containers:* 750 mg/50 ml$^{Rx}$, 1.5 g/50 ml$^{Rx}$.

❑ **Loracarbef**

■ *Capsules:* 200 mg$^{Rx}$ ■ *Oral suspension (strawberry-bubblegum flavor):* 100 mg/5 ml$^{Rx}$.

### TIME/ACTION PROFILE

| | ONSET | PEAK | DURATION |
|---|---|---|---|
| Cefaclor PO | rapid | 30–60 min | 6–12 hr |
| Cefaclor PO-CD | unknown | unknown | 12 hr |

| | | | |
|---|---|---|---|
| Cefmetazole IV | rapid | end of infusion | 6–12 hr |
| Cefonicid IM | rapid | 60 min | 12–24 hr |
| Cefotetan IM | rapid | 1–3 hr | 12 hr |
| Cefotetan IV | rapid | end of infusion | 12 hr |
| Cefoxitin IM | rapid | 30 min | 4–8 hr |
| Cefoxitin IV | rapid | end of infusion | 4–8 hr |
| Cefprozil PO | unknown | 1–2 hr | 12–24 hr |
| Cefuroxime PO | unknown | 2 hr | 8–12 hr |
| Cefuroxime IM | rapid | end of infusion | 6–12 hr |
| Cefuroxime IV | rapid | end of infusion | 6–12 hr |
| Loracarbef PO | rapid | 0.5–1.2 hr | 12 hr |

## NURSING IMPLICATIONS

### ASSESSMENT

❑ Assess patient for infection (vital signs; appearance of wound, sputum, urine, and stool; WBC) at beginning and during therapy.

❑ Before initiating therapy, obtain a history to determine previous use of and reactions to penicillins or cephalosporins. Persons with a negative history of penicillin sensitivity may still have an allergic response.

❑ Obtain specimens for culture and sensitivity before initiating therapy. First dose may be given before receiving results.

❑ Observe patient for signs and symptoms of anaphylaxis (rash, pruritus, laryngeal edema, wheezing). Discontinue medication and notify physician or other health care professional immediately if these symptoms occur. Keep epinephrine, an antihistamine, and resuscitation equipment close by in the event of an anaphylactic reaction.

❑ Assess patient for renal dysfunction and adjust dose accordingly. Monitor for dose-related adverse CNS events (including seizures, myoclonus, encephalopathy) and nephrotoxicity.

■ *Lab Test Considerations:* May cause positive results for Coombs' test in patients receiving high doses or in neonates whose mothers were given cephalosporins before delivery.

❑ Monitor prothrombin time and assess patient for bleeding (guaiac stools; check for hema-

{ } = Available in Canada only.
* CAPITALS indicates life-threatening; underlines indicate most frequent.

turia, bleeding gums, ecchymosis) daily in high-risk patients or those receiving *cefmetazole*, or *cefotetan;* may cause hypoprothrombinemia.

❑ *Cefuroxime* may also cause false-negative blood glucose results with ferricyanide tests. Use glucose enzymatic or hexokinase tests to determine blood glucose.

❑ May cause ↑ serum AST, ALT, alkaline phosphatase, bilirubin, LDH, BUN, and creatinine.

❑ *Cefotetan, cephalothin,* and *cefoxitin* may cause falsely elevated test results for serum and urine creatinine; do not obtain serum samples within 2 hr of administration.

❑ May rarely cause leukopenia, neutropenia, agranulocytosis, thrombocytopenia, eosinophilia, lymphocytosis, and thrombocytosis.

**POTENTIAL NURSING DIAGNOSES**

■ Infection, risk for (Indications, Side Effects).

■ Diarrhea (Adverse Reactions).

■ Noncompliance (Patient/Family Teaching).

**IMPLEMENTATION**

■ **PO:** Administer around the clock. May be administered on full or empty stomach. Administration with food may minimize GI irritation. Shake oral suspension well before administering.

❑ Administer cefaclor extended-release tablets with food; do not crush, break, or chew.

❑ *Cefuroxime* tablets should be swallowed whole, not crushed; crushed tablets have a strong, persistent bitter taste. Tablets may be taken without regard to meals. Suspension must be taken with food. Shake well each time before using. Tablets and suspension are not interchangeable.

■ **IM:** Reconstitute IM doses with sterile or bacteriostatic water for injection or 0.9% NaCl for injection. May be diluted with lidocaine to minimize injection discomfort.

❑ Inject deep into a well-developed muscle mass; massage well.

❑ When administering 2-g dose of *cefonicid*, divide in half and inject into two large muscle mass sites.

■ **IV:** Change sites every 48–72 hr to prevent phlebitis. Monitor site frequently for thrombophlebitis (pain, redness, swelling).

❑ If aminoglycosides are administered concurrently, administer in separate sites if possi-

ble, at least 1 hr apart. If second site is unavailable, flush line between medications.

■ **Direct IV:** Dilute in at least 1 g/10 ml. Do not use preparations containing benzyl alcohol for neonates.

■ *Rate:* Administer slowly over 3–5 min.

❑ **Cefmetazole**

■ **Intermittent Infusion:** Reconstituted solution may be further diluted in 50–100 ml of 0.9% NaCl, D5W, or LR for a concentration of 1–20 mg/ml. Solution is stable for 24 hr at room temperature and 7 days if refrigerated.

■ *Rate:* Administer over 10–60 min.

■ **Y-Site Compatibility:** ◆ codeine ◆ cyclosporine ◆ diazepam ◆ digoxin ◆ dopamine ◆ esmolol ◆ furosemide ◆ hydrocortisone sodium succinate ◆ hydromorphone ◆ levothyroxine ◆ lorazepam ◆ magnesium sulfate ◆ meperidine ◆ midazolam ◆ morphine ◆ nalbuphine ◆ nitroglycerine ◆ ondansetron ◆ potassium chloride ◆ ranitidine ◆ Ringer's lactate ◆ sodium bicarbonate ◆ 0.9% NaCl.

■ **Y-Site Incompatibility:** ◆ diphenhydramine ◆ dobutamine ◆ droperidol ◆ erythromycin lactobionate ◆ haloperidol ◆ prochlorperazine ◆ promethazine.

❑ **Cefonicid**

■ **Intermittent Infusion:** Reconstituted solution may be further diluted in 50–100 ml of D5W, D10W, D5/LR, Ringer's or LR, D5/0.25% NaCl, D5/0.45% NaCl, D5/0.9% NaCl, or 0.9% NaCl. Solution may be colorless to light amber. Stable for 24 hr at room temperature and 72 hr if refrigerated.

■ *Rate:* Administer over 20–30 min.

■ **Y-Site Compatibility:** ◆ acyclovir ◆ amifostine ◆ aztreonam ◆ granisetron ◆ propofol ◆ teniposide ◆ thiotepa.

■ **Y-Site Incompatibility:** ◆ filgrastim ◆ sargramostim.

❑ **Cefotetan**

■ **Intermittent Infusion:** Reconstituted solution may be further diluted in 50–100 ml of D5W or 0.9% NaCl. Solution may be colorless or yellow. Solution is stable for 24 hr at room temperature or 96 hr if refrigerated.

■ *Rate:* Administer over 20–30 min.

■ **Y-Site Compatibility:** ◆ allopurinol ◆ amifostine ◆ aztreonam ◆ diltiazem ◆ docetaxel ◆ etoposide ◆ famotidine ◆ filgrastim ◆ fluconazole ◆ fludarabine ◆ gatifloxacin ◆ gemcitabine ◆ granisetron ◆ heparin ◆ insulin ◆ linezolid ◆ melphalan ◆ meperidine ◆ morphine ◆ paclitaxel ◆ propofol ◆ remifentanil ◆ sargramostim ◆ tacrolimus ◆ teniposide ◆ theophylline ◆ thiotepa.

■ **Y-Site Incompatibility:** ◆ promethazine ◆ vinorelbine.

❑ **Cefoxitin**

■ **Intermittent Infusion:** Reconstituted solution may be further diluted in 50–100 ml of D5W, D10W, 0.9% NaCl, D5/0.45% NaCl, D5/0.25% NaCl, D5/0.9% NaCl, D5/LR, Ringer's or LR. Stable for 24 hr at room temperature and 1 wk if refrigerated. Darkening of powder does not alter potency.

■ **Rate:** Administer over 15–30 min.

■ **Continuous Infusion:** May be diluted in 500–1000 ml for continuous infusion.

■ **Syringe Compatibility:** ◆ heparin.

■ **Y-Site Compatibility:** ◆ acyclovir ◆ amifostine ◆ amphotericin B cholesteryl sulfate ◆ aztreonam ◆ cyclophosphamide ◆ diltiazem ◆ docetaxel ◆ doxorubicin liposome ◆ etoposide ◆ famotidine ◆ fluconazole ◆ foscarnet ◆ gemcitabine ◆ granisetron ◆ hydromorphone ◆ linezolid ◆ magnesium sulfate ◆ meperidine ◆ morphine ◆ ondansetrol ◆ perphenazine ◆ propofol ◆ ranitidine ◆ remifentanil ◆ teniposide ◆ thiotepa.

■ **Y-Site Incompatibility:** Manufacturer recommends stopping other medications during infusion. ◆ filgrastim ◆ gatifloxacin ◆ pentamidine.

❑ **Cefuroxime**

■ **Intermittent Infusion:** Solution may be further diluted in 100 ml of 0.9% NaCl, D5W, D10W, D5/0.45% NaCl, or D5/0.9% NaCl. Stable for 24 hr at room temperature and 1 wk if refrigerated.

■ **Rate:** Administer over 15–60 min.

■ **Continuous Infusion:** May also be diluted in 500–1000 ml for continuous infusion.

■ **Y-Site Compatibility:** ◆ acyclovir ◆ allopurinol ◆ amifostine ◆ atracurium ◆ aztreonam ◆ cyclophosphamide ◆ diltiazem ◆ docetaxel ◆ etoposide ◆ famotidine ◆ fludarabine ◆ foscarnet ◆ gemcitabine ◆ granisetron ◆ hydromorphone ◆ linezolid ◆ melphalan ◆ meperidine ◆ morphine ◆ ondansetron ◆ pancuronium ◆

perphenazine ◆ propofol ◆ remifentanil ◆ sargramostim ◆ tacrolimus ◆ teniposide ◆ thiotepa ◆ vecuronium.

■ **Y-Site Incompatibility:** Manufacturer recommends temporarily discontinuing primary solution when administering cefuroxime via Y-site. ◆ filgrastim ◆ fluconazole ◆ midazolam ◆ vinorelbine.

## PATIENT/FAMILY TEACHING

❑ Instruct patient to take medication around the clock at evenly spaced times and to finish the medication completely, even if feeling better. Missed doses should be taken as soon as possible unless almost time for next dose; do not double doses. Advise patient that sharing of this medication may be dangerous.

❑ Advise patient to report signs of superinfection (furry overgrowth on the tongue, vaginal itching or discharge, loose or foul-smelling stools) and allergy.

❑ Caution patients that concurrent use of alcohol with *cefmetazole,* or *cefotetan* may cause a disulfiram-like reaction (abdominal cramps, nausea, vomiting, headache, hypotension, palpitations, dyspnea, tachycardia, sweating, flushing). Alcohol and alcohol-containing medications should be avoided during and for several days after therapy.

❑ Instruct patient to notify health care professional if fever and diarrhea develop, especially if stool contains blood, pus, or mucus. Advise patient not to treat diarrhea without consulting health care professional.

## EVALUATION

**Clinical response to therapy can be evaluated by:** ■ Resolution of signs and symptoms of infection. Length of time for complete resolution depends on the organism and site of infection ■ Decreased incidence of infection when used for prophylaxis.

# CEPHALOSPORINS—THIRD GENERATION

**cefdinir**

(**sef**-di-nir)

Omnicef

**cefditoren**

(sef-tye-**dor**-en)

Spectracef

**cefepime**

(**seff**-e-peem)

Maxipime

**cefoperazone**

(sef-oh-**per**-a-zone)

Cefobid

**cefotaxime**

(sef-oh-**taks**-eem)

Claforan

**cefpodoxime**

(sef-poe-**dox**-eem)

Vantin

**ceftazidime**

(sef-**tay**-zi-deem)

Ceptaz, Fortaz, Tazicef, Tazidime

**ceftibuten**

(sef-tye-**byoo**-ten)

Cedax

**ceftizoxime**

(sef-ti-**zox**-eem)

Cefizox

**ceftriaxone**

(sef-try-**ax**-one)

Rocephin

*CLASSIFICATION(S):*

*Therapeutic: anti-infectives*

*Pharmacologic: third-generation cephalosporins*

**Pregnancy Category B**

## INDICATIONS

■ Treatment of: ❑ Skin and skin structure infections ❑ Bone and joint infections ❑ Urinary and gynecologic infections including gonorrhea (ceftriaxone) or respiratory tract infections ❑ Intra-abdominal infections ❑ Septicemia ❑ Otitis media (cefdinir) ■ **Cefotaxime, ceftazidime, ceftizoxime, ceftriaxone:** Meningitis ■ **Ceftriaxone:** Perioperative prophylaxis ■ **Cefepime:** Empiric treatment of febrile neutropenic patients ■ **Ceftriaxone:** Single-dose treatment of acute bacterial otitis media ■ **Cefotaxime, ceftriaxone:** Lyme disease ■ **Cefdinir, cefditoren:** Acute exacerbations of chronic bronchitis.

## ACTION

■ Bind to the bacterial cell wall membrane, causing cell death. **Therapeutic Effects:** ■ Bactericidal action against susceptible bacteria. **Spectrum:** ■ Similar to that of second-generation cephalosporins, but activity against staphylococci is less, whereas activity against gram-negative pathogens is greater, even for organisms resistant to first- and second-generation agents ■ Notable is increased action against ❑ *Enterobacter* ❑ *Haemophilus influenzae* ❑ *Escherichia coli* ❑ *Klebsiella pneumoniae* ❑ *Neisseria* ❑ *Proteus* ❑ *Providencia* ❑ *Serratia* ❑ *Moraxella catarrhalis* ❑ *Borrelia burgdorferi* ■ Some agents have enhanced activity against: ❑ *Pseudomonas aeruginosa* (ceftazidime, cefoperazone) ■ All except ceftibuten, and cefpodoxime have some activity against anaerobes, including *Bacteroides fragilis.*

## PHARMACOKINETICS

**Absorption:** Well absorbed after IM administration. *Ceftibuten* and *cefpodoxime* are well absorbed after oral administration; *cefdinir* 16–25% absorbed after oral administration. Cefditoren is a prodrug and is broken down prior to absorption (14% absorbed).

**Distribution:** Widely distributed. Cross the placenta; enter breast milk in low concentrations. CSF penetration better than with first- and second-generation agents.

**Protein Binding:** *Cefoperazone* and *ceftriaxone* ≥90%.

**Metabolism and Excretion:** *Cefdinir, cefepime, ceftazidime, cefpodoxime, cefditoren,* and *ceftizoxime*—>85% excreted in urine. *Cefoperazone*—excreted in the bile. *Ceftibuten, ceftriaxone,* and *cefotaxime*—partly metabolized and partly excreted in the urine.

**Half-life:** *Cefdinir*—102 min; *cefditoren*—100 min; *cefepime*—120 min; *cefoperazone*—102–156 min; *cefotaxime*—60 min; *cefpodoxime*—120–180 min; *ceftazi-*

*dime*—114–120 min; *ceftibuten*—120–144 min; *ceftizoxime*—84–114 min; *ceftriaxone*—348–522 min (all except *cefoperazone* and *ceftriaxone* are increased in renal impairment).

## CONTRAINDICATIONS AND PRECAUTIONS

**Contraindicated in:** ■ Hypersensitivity to cephalosporins ■ Serious hypersensitivity to penicillins ■ Hypersensitivity to L -arginine (Ceptaz formulation only) ■ Carnitine deficiency or inborn errors of metabolism (cefditoren only).

**Use Cautiously in:** ■ Renal impairment (decreased dosing/increased dosing interval recommended for: *Cefdinir* if CCr <30 ml/min, *cefepime* if CCr ≤60 ml/min, *cefotaxime* if CCr <20 ml/min, *cefpodoxime* if CCr <30 ml/min, *ceftazidime* if CCr ≤50 ml/min, *ceftibuten* and *cefditoren* if CCr <50 ml/min, *ceftizoxime* if CCr ≤80 ml/min) ■ Severe hepatic/biliary impairment (dosage reduction/increased dosing interval recommended for *cefoperazone*) ■ Combined severe hepatic and renal impairment (dosage reduction/increased dosing interval recommended for *cefoperazone* and *ceftriaxone*) ■ Diabetes (*ceftibuten* and *cefdinir* suspension contain sucrose) ■ History of GI disease, especially colitis ■ Geriatric patients (consider age-related decrease in body mass, renal/hepatic/cardiac function, concurrent medications and chronic disease states) ■ Pregnancy and lactation (have been used safely).

## ADVERSE REACTIONS AND SIDE EFFECTS*

■ **CNS:** SEIZURES (high doses) ■ **GI:** PSEUDOMEMBRANOUS COLITIS , diarrhea, nausea, vomiting, cramps, janudice (ceftazidime), pseudolithiasis (ceftriaxone) ■ **Derm:** rashes, urticaria ■ **Hemat:** bleeding (increased with cefoperazone), blood dyscrasias, hemolytic anemia ■ **Local:** pain at IM site, phlebitis AT IV SITE ■ **Misc:** allergic reactions including ANAPHYLAXIS and SERUM SICKNESS , superinfection.

## INTERACTIONS

**Drug-Drug:** ■ **Probenecid** decreases excretion and increases serum levels (cefotaxime, cefpodoxime, ceftizoxime) ■ Ingestion of **alcohol** within 48–72 hr of cefoperazone may re-

sult in a disulfiram-like reaction ■ Cefoperazone may potentiate the effects of **anticoagulants** and increase the risk of bleeding with **antiplatelet agents, thrombolytic agents, plicamycin,** or **valproic acid** ■ Concurrent use of large doses of cephalosporins and **NSAIDs** may increase the risk of bleeding ■ Concurrent use of **loop diuretics** or **nephrotoxic agents** including **aminoglycosides** may increase the risk of nephrotoxicity ■ **Antacids** decrease absorption of cefdinir and cefpodoxime after antacid) ■ **Iron supplements** decrease absorption of cefdinir ■ **Antacids** and **H₂-receptor antagonists** decrease absorption of cefditoren (avoid concurrent use).

**Drug-Natural Products:** ■ Risk of bleeding with **cefoperazone** may be increased by **anise, arnica, chamomile, clove, fenugreek, feverfew, garlic, ginger, ginkgo, Panax ginseng, licorice, papain, passion flower, turmeric, willow, and others.**

## ROUTE AND DOSAGE

❑ **Cefdinir**

■ **PO (Adults ≥13 yr):** 300 mg q 12 hr *or* 600 mg q 24 hr (use q 12 hr dosing only for community-acquired pneumonia or skin and skin structure infections).

■ **PO (Children 6 mo–12 yr):** 7 mg/kg q 12 hr *or* 14 mg/kg q 24 hr.

❑ **Renal Impairment**

■ **PO (Adults):** *CCr <30 ml/min*—300 mg q 24 hr.

❑ **Cefditoren**

■ **PO (Adults):** 200–400 mg twice daily.

❑ **Renal Impairment**

■ **PO (Adults):** *CCr 30–50 ml/min*—dose should not exceed 200 mg twice daily; *CCr <30 ml/min*—dose should not exceed 200 mg once daily.

❑ **Cefepime**

■ **IM (Adults):** 0.5–1 g q 12 hr.

■ **IV (Adults):** 0.5–2 g q 12 hr.

■ **IM, IV (Children up to 40 kg):** 50 mg/kg q 12 hr (50 mg/kg q 8 hr in febrile neutropenic patients); in children >40 kg use adult dosing.

❑ **Renal Impairment**

- **IM, IV (Adults):** *CCr 30–60 ml/min—* 0.5–1 g q 12 hr *or* 2 g q 12–24 hr; *CCr 11–29 ml/min—*0.5–2 g q 24 hr; *CCr <11 ml/min—*250 mg–1 g q 24 hr.

□ **Cefoperazone**

- **IM, IV (Adults):** *Mild to moderate infections—*1–2 g q 12 hr. *Severe infections—* 2–4 g q 8 hr *or* 3–6 g q 12 hr.

**Hepatic/Renal Impairment**

- **IM, IV (Adults):** *Impaired hepatic function/biliary obstruction—*daily dose should not exceed 4 g; *combined hepatic and renal impairment—*daily dose should not exceed 1–2 g.

□ **Cefotaxime**

- **IM, IV (Adults):** *Most infections—*1 g q 12 hr. *Moderate or severe infections—*1–2 g q 6–8 hr. *Life-threatening infections—*2 g q 4 hr.

- **IM, IV (Children >1 mo):** 8.3–30 mg/kg q 4 hr *or* 12.5–45 mg/kg q 6 hr.

- **IV (Neonates 1–4 wk):** 50 mg/kg q 8 hr.

- **IV (Neonates ≤1 wk):** 50 mg/kg q 12 hr.

□ **Renal Impairment**

- **(Adults):** *CCr <20 ml/min—*decrease dose by 50%.

□ **Cefpodoxime**

- **PO (Adults):** *Most infections—*200 mg q 12 hr. *Skin and soft-tissue infections—* 400 mg q 12 hr. *Urinary tract infections/pharyngitis—*100 mg q 12 hr. *Gonorrhea—*200 mg single dose.

- **PO (Children 6 mo–12 yr):** *Pharyngitis/tonsillitis/otitis media—*5 mg/kg q 12 hr; may be given as 10 mg/kg once daily for otitis media (not to exceed 200 mg/day for pharyngitis/tonsillitis or 400 mg/day for otitis media).

□ **Renal Impairment**

- **PO (Adults):** *CCr <30 ml/min—*Increase dosing interval to q 24 hr.

□ **Ceftazidime**

- **IM, IV (Adults):** *Most infections—*500 mg–2 g q 8–12 hr. *Pneumonia and skin structure infections—*0.5–1 g q 8–12 hr. *Bone and joint infections—*2 g q 12 hr. *Severe and life-threatening infections—*2 g q 8 hr. *Complicated urinary tract infections—*500 mg q 8–12 hr. *Uncomplicated urinary tract infections—*250 mg q 12 hr.

- **IM, IV (Children 1 mo–12 yr):** 30–50 mg/kg q 8 hr.

- **IV (Neonates ≤4 wk):** 30 mg/kg q 12 hr.

□ **Renal Impairment**

- **IM, IV (Adults):** *CCr 31–50 ml/min—*1 g q 12 hr; *CCr 16–30 ml/min—*1 g q 24 hr; *CCr 6–15 ml/min—*500 mg q 24 hr; *CCr <5 ml/min—*500 mg q 48 hr.

□ **Ceftibuten**

- **PO (Adults and Children ≥12 yr):** 400 mg q 24 hr for 10 days.

- **PO (Children 6 mo–12 yr):** 9 mg/kg/day for 10 days (up to 400 mg/day).

□ **Renal Impairment**

- **PO (Adults):** *CCr 30–49 ml/min—*200 mg q 24 hr as capsules *or* 4.5 mg/kg q 24 hr as suspension; *CCr 5–29 ml/min—*100 mg q 24 hr as capsules *or* 2.25 mg/kg q 24 hr as suspension.

□ **Ceftizoxime**

- **IM, IV (Adults):** *Severe infections—*1–2 g q 8–12 hr. *Life-threatening infections—* 3–4 g q 8 hr. *Mild/moderate infections—*1 g q 8–12 hr. *Uncomplicated urinary tract infections—*500 mg q 12 hr.

- **IM, IV (Children >6 mo):** 50 mg/kg q 6–8 hr (not to exceed 200 mg/kg/day).

□ **Renal Impairment**

- **IM, IV (Adults):** *CCr 50–79 ml/min—*500 mg–1.5 g q 8 hr; *CCr 5–49 ml/min—*250 mg–1 g q 12 hr; *CCr 0–4 ml/min—*500 mg–1 g q 48 hr *or* 250–500 mg q 24 hr.

□ **Ceftriaxone**

- **IM, IV (Adults):** *Most infections—*0.5–1 g q 12 hr *or* 1–2 g q 24 hr. *Gonorrhea—*250 mg IM. *Meningitis—*2 g q 12 hr.

- **IM, IV (Children):** *Most infections—*25–37.5 mg/kg q 12 hr. *Meningitis—*100 mg/kg q 24 hr *or* 50 mg/kg q 12 hr. *Skin/soft-tissue infections—*50–75 mg/kg q 24 hr. *Acute otitis media—*50 mg/kg IM single dose.

**AVAILABILITY**

□ **Cefdinir**

- ***Oral suspension (strawberry):*** 125 mg/5 ml in 60- and 100-ml bottles[Rx] ■ Cost: $42.39/60 ml; $67.10/100 ml ■ ***Capsules:*** 300 mg[Rx] ■ Cost: $128.44/30 capsules

□ **Cefditoren**

- ***Tablets:*** 200 mg[Rx].

❑ **Cefepime**

■ *Powder for injection:* 500-mg, 1-g, 2-g vials$^{Rx}$, 1-g, 2-g piggyback bottles$^{Rx}$.

❑ **Cefoperazone**

■ *Powder for injection:* 1 g$^{Rx}$, 2 g$^{Rx}$ ■ *Premixed containers:* 1 g/50 ml$^{Rx}$, 2 g/50 ml$^{Rx}$.

❑ **Cefotaxime**

■ *Powder for injection:* 1 g$^{Rx}$, 2 g$^{Rx}$, 10 g$^{Rx}$ ■ *Premixed containers:* 1 g/50 ml$^{Rx}$, 2 g/50 ml$^{Rx}$.

❑ **Cefpodoxime**

■ *Tablets:* 100 mg$^{Rx}$, 200 mg$^{Rx}$ ■ *Oral suspension (lemon creme):* 50 mg/5 ml$^{Rx}$, 100 mg/5 ml$^{Rx}$.

❑ **Ceftazidime**

■ *Powder for injection:* 500 mg$^{Rx}$, 1 g$^{Rx}$, 2 g$^{Rx}$, 6 g$^{Rx}$, 10 g$^{Rx}$ ■ *Premixed containers:* 1 g/50 ml$^{Rx}$, 2 g/50 ml$^{Rx}$.

❑ **Ceftibuten**

■ *Capsules:* 400 mg$^{Rx}$ ■ *Oral suspension (cherry):* 90 mg/5 ml$^{Rx}$, 180 mg/5 ml$^{Rx}$.

❑ **Ceftizoxime**

■ *Powder for injection:* 500 mg$^{Rx}$, 1 g$^{Rx}$, 2 g$^{Rx}$, 10 g$^{Rx}$ ■ *Premixed containers:* 1 g/50 ml$^{Rx}$, 2 g/50 ml$^{Rx}$.

❑ **Ceftriaxone**

■ *Powder for injection:* 250 mg$^{Rx}$, 500 mg$^{Rx}$, 1 g$^{Rx}$, 2 g$^{Rx}$, 10 g$^{Rx}$ ■ *Premixed containers:* 1 g/50 ml$^{Rx}$, 2 g/50 ml$^{Rx}$.

TIME/ACTION PROFILE

| | ONSET | PEAK | DURATION |
|---|---|---|---|
| Cefdinir PO | rapid | 2–4 hr | 12–24 hr |
| Cefditoren PO | rapid | 0.5–3 hr | 12 hr |
| Cefepime IM | rapid | 1–2 hr | 12 hr |
| Cefepime IV | rapid | end of infusion | 12 hr |
| Cefoperazone IM | rapid | 1–2 hr | 12 hr |
| Cefoperazone IV | rapid | end of infusion | 12 hr |
| Cefotaxime IM | rapid | 0.5 hr | 4–12 hr |
| Cefotaxime IV | rapid | end of infusion | 4–12 hr |
| Cefpodoxime PO | unknown | 2–3 hr | 12 hr |
| Ceftazidime IM | rapid | 1 hr | 6–12 hr |
| Ceftazidime IV | rapid | end of infusion | 6–12 hr |
| Ceftibuten PO | rapid | 3 hr | 24 hr |
| Ceftizoxime IM | rapid | 0.5–1.5 hr | 6–12 hr |
| Ceftizoxime IV | rapid | end of infusion | 6–12 hr |
| Ceftriaxone IM | rapid | 1–2 hr | 12–24 hr |
| Ceftriaxone IV | rapid | end of infusion | 12–24 hr |

# NURSING IMPLICATIONS

## ASSESSMENT

❑ Assess patient for infection (vital signs; appearance of wound, sputum, urine, and stool; WBC) at beginning of and throughout therapy.

❑ Before initiating therapy, obtain a history to determine previous use of and reactions to penicillins or cephalosporins. Persons with a negative history of penicillin sensitivity may still have an allergic response.

❑ Obtain specimens for culture and sensitivity before initiating therapy. First dose may be given before receiving results.

❑ Observe patient for signs and symptoms of anaphylaxis (rash, pruritus, laryngeal edema, wheezing). Discontinue the drug and notify the physician or other health care professional immediately if these symptoms occur. Keep epinephrine, an antihistamine, and resuscitation equipment close by in the event of an anaphylactic reaction.

■ *Lab Test Considerations:* May cause positive results for Coombs' test in patients receiving high doses or in neonates whose mothers were given cephalosporins before delivery.

❑ Monitor prothrombin time and assess patient for bleeding (guaiac stools; check for hematuria, bleeding gums, ecchymosis) daily in patients receiving *cefoperazone* or *cefditoren*, as this agent may cause hypoprothrombinemia.

❑ May cause ↑ serum AST, ALT, alkaline phosphatase, bilirubin, LDH, BUN, and creatinine.

❑ May rarely cause leukopenia, neutropenia, agranulocytosis, thrombocytopenia, eosinophilia, lymphocytosis, and thrombocytosis.

| | | | |
|---|---|---|---|
| Ceftazidime IV | rapid | end of infusion | 6–12 hr |
| Ceftibuten PO | rapid | 3 hr | 24 hr |
| Ceftizoxime IM | rapid | 0.5–1.5 hr | 6–12 hr |
| Ceftizoxime IV | rapid | end of infusion | 6–12 hr |
| Ceftriaxone IM | rapid | 1–2 hr | 12–24 hr |
| Ceftriaxone IV | rapid | end of infusion | 12–24 hr |

## POTENTIAL NURSING DIAGNOSES

■ Infection, risk for (Indications, Side Effects).

■ Diarrhea (Adverse Reactions).

## IMPLEMENTATION

■ **General:** Cefditoren is not recommended for prolonged use since other piralate-containing compounds have caused clinical manifestations of carnitine deficiency when used over a period of months.

■ **PO:** Administer around the clock. May be administered on full or empty stomach. Administration with food may minimize GI irritation. Shake oral suspension well before administering. *Cefditoren* should be administered with meals to enhance absorption.

❑ Do not administer cefdinir or cefpodoxime within 2 hr before or after an antacid or cefdinir within 2 hr before or after iron supplements; may decrease absorption. Do not administer cefditoren concomitantly with antacids or other drugs taken to reduce stomach acid.

■ **IM:** Reconstitute IM doses with sterile or bacteriostatic water for injection or 0.9% NaCl for injection. May be diluted with lidocaine to minimize injection discomfort.

❑ Inject deep into a well-developed muscle mass; massage well.

■ **IV:** Monitor injection site frequently for phlebitis (pain, redness, swelling). Change sites every 48–72 hr to prevent phlebitis.

❑ If aminoglycosides are administered concurrently, administer in separate sites, if possible, at least 1 hr apart. If second site is unavailable, flush lines between medications.

■ **Direct IV:** Dilute in at least 1 g/10 ml. Avoid direct IV administration of *cefoperazone* and *ceftriaxone*. Do not use preparations containing benzyl alcohol for neonates.

■ *Rate:* Administer slowly over 3–5 min.

❑ **Cefepime**

■ **Intermittent Infusion:** Dilute in 50–100 ml for a concentration of 1–40 mg/ml with D5W, 0.9% NaCl, D10W, M/6 sodium lactate injection, D5/0.9% NaCl, D5/LR, D5/Normosol-R, or D5/Normosol-M injection.

❑ Solution is stable for 24 hr at room temperature and 7 days if refrigerated.

■ *Rate:* Administer over 30 min.

■ **Y-Site Compatibility:** ◆ ampicillin-sulbactam ◆ aztreonam ◆ bleomycin ◆ bumetanide ◆ buprenorphine ◆ butorphanol ◆ calcium gluconate ◆ carboplatin ◆ carmustine ◆ cyclophosphamide ◆ cytarabine ◆ dactinomycin ◆ dexamethasone sodium phosphate ◆ docetaxel ◆ doxorubicin liposome ◆ fluconazole ◆ fludarabine ◆ fluorouracil ◆ furosemide ◆ granisetron ◆ hydrocortisone sodium phosphate ◆ hydrocortisone sodium succinate ◆ hydromorphone ◆ imipenem-cilastatin ◆ leucovorin ◆ lorazepam ◆ melphalan ◆ mesna ◆ methotrexate ◆ methylprednisolone sodium succinate ◆ metronidazole ◆ paclitaxel ◆ piperacillin-tazobactam ◆ propofol ◆ ranitidine ◆ sargramostim ◆ sodium bicarbonate ◆ thiotepa ◆ ticarcillin-clavulanate ◆ trimethoprim-sulfamethoxazole ◆ zidovudine.

■ **Y-Site Incompatibility:** ◆ acyclovir ◆ amphotericin B ◆ amphotericin B cholesteryl sulfate ◆ chlordiazepoxide ◆ chlorpromazine ◆ cimetidine ◆ ciprofloxacin ◆ cisplatin ◆ dacarbazine ◆ daunorubicin ◆ diazepam ◆ diphenhydramine ◆ dobutamine ◆ dopamine ◆ doxorubicin ◆ droperidol ◆ enalaprilat ◆ etoposide ◆ famotidine ◆ filgrastim ◆ floxuridine ◆ ganciclovir ◆ haloperidol ◆ idarubicin ◆ ifosfamide ◆ magnesium sulfate ◆ mannitol ◆ mechlorethamine ◆ meperidine ◆ metoclopramide ◆ mitomycin ◆ mitoxantrone ◆ morphine ◆ nalbuphine ◆ ofloxacin ◆ ondansetron ◆ plicamycin ◆ prochlorperazine ◆ promethazine ◆ streptozocin ◆ vancomycin ◆ vinblastine ◆ vincristine.

❑ **Cefoperazone**

■ **Intermittent Infusion:** Reconstitute each gram with at least 2.8 ml of sterile or bacteriostatic water for injection or 0.9% NaCl. Shake vigorously and allow to stand for visualization and clarity. Solution may be colorless to straw colored. Each gram in solution should be further diluted in 20–40 ml of 0.9% NaCl, D5W, D10W, D5/0.25% NaCl, D5/0.9% NaCl, D5/LR, or LR. Solution is stable for 24 hr at room temperature and 5 days if refrigerated.

■ *Rate:* Administer over 15–30 min.

■ **Continuous Infusion:** For continuous infusion, concentration should be 2–25 mg/ml.

■ **Syringe Compatibility:** ◆ heparin.

■ **Y-Site Compatibility:** ◆ acyclovir ◆ allopurinol ◆ aztreonam ◆ cyclophosphamide ◆ docetaxel ◆ enalaprilat ◆ esmolol ◆ etoposide ◆ famotidine ◆ fludarabine ◆ foscarnet ◆ granisetron ◆ hydromorphone ◆ linezolid ◆ magnesium sulfate ◆ melphalan ◆ morphine ◆ propofol ◆ ranitidine ◆ teniposide ◆ thiotepa.

■ **Y-Site Incompatibility:** ◆ amifostine ◆ amphotericin B cholesteryl sulfate ◆ cisatracurium ◆ doxorubicin liposome ◆ filgrastim ◆ gatifloxacin ◆ gemcitabine ◆ labetalol ◆ meperidine ◆ ondansetron ◆ pentamidine ◆ perphenazine ◆ promethazine ◆ sargramostim ◆ vinorelbine.

❏ **Cefotaxime**

■ **Intermittent Infusion:** Reconstituted solution may be further diluted in 50–100 ml of D5W, D10W, LR, D5/0.25% NaCl, D5/0.45% NaCl, D5/0.9% NaCl, or 0.9% NaCl. Solution may appear light yellow to amber. Solution is stable for 24 hr at room temperature and 5 days if refrigerated.

■ *Rate:* Administer over 20–30 min.

■ **Syringe Compatibility:** ◆ heparin ◆ ofloxacin.

■ **Y-Site Compatibility:** ◆ acyclovir ◆ amifostine ◆ aztreonam ◆ cyclophosphamide ◆ diltiazem ◆ docetaxel ◆ etoposide ◆ famotidine ◆ fludarabine ◆ granisetron ◆ hydromorphone ◆ levofloxacin ◆ lorazepam ◆ magnesium sulfate ◆ melphalan ◆ meperidine ◆ midazolam ◆ morphine ◆ ondansetron ◆ perphenazine ◆ propofol ◆ remifentanil ◆ sargramostim ◆ teniposide ◆ thiotepa ◆ tolazoline ◆ vinorelbine.

■ **Y-Site Incompatibility:** ◆ allopurinol ◆ filgrastim ◆ fluconazole ◆ gemcitabine ◆ pentamidine.

❏ **Ceftazidime**

■ **Intermittent Infusion:** Reconstituted solution may be further diluted in at least 1 g/10 ml of 0.9% NaCl, D5W, D10W, D5/0.25% NaCl, D5/0.45% NaCl, D5/0.9% NaCl, or LR. Dilution causes $CO_2$ to form inside vial, resulting in positive pressure; vial may require venting after dissolution to preserve sterility of vial. Not required with L -arginine formulation (Ceptaz). Solution may appear yellow to amber; darkening does not alter potency. Solution is stable for 18 hr at room temperature and 7 days if refrigerated.

■ *Rate:* Administer over 15–30 min.

■ **Syringe Compatibility:** ◆ hydromorphone.

■ **Y-Site Compatibility:** ◆ acyclovir ◆ allopurinol ◆ amifostine ◆ aminophylline ◆ aztreonam

◆ ciprofloxacin ◆ diltiazem ◆ docetaxel ◆ enalaprilat ◆ etoposide ◆ esmolol ◆ famotidine ◆ filgrastim ◆ fludarabine ◆ foscarnet ◆ gatifloxacin ◆ gemcitabine ◆ granisetron ◆ heparin ◆ hydromorphone ◆ labetalol ◆ linezolid ◆ melphalan ◆ meperidine ◆ morphine ◆ ondansetron ◆ paclitaxel ◆ propofol ◆ ranitidine ◆ remifentanil ◆ tacrolimus ◆ teniposide ◆ theophylline ◆ thiotepa ◆ vinorelbine ◆ zidovudine.

■ **Y-Site Incompatibility:** ◆ alatrofloxacin ◆ amphotericin B cholesteryl sulfate ◆ doxorubicin liposome ◆ fluconazole ◆ idarubicin ◆ midazolam ◆ pentamidine ◆ warfarin.

❏ **Ceftizoxime**

■ **Intermittent Infusion:** Reconstituted solution may be further diluted in 50–100 ml of D5W, D10W, 0.9% NaCl, D5/0.25% NaCl, D5/0.45% NaCl, D5/0.9% NaCl, or LR. Solution is stable for 8 hr at room temperature and 48 hr if refrigerated.

■ *Rate:* Administer over 15–30 min.

■ **Y-Site Compatibility:** ◆ acyclovir ◆ allopurinol ◆ amifostine ◆ amphotericin B cholesteryl sulfate ◆ aztreonam ◆ docetaxel ◆ doxorubicin liposome ◆ enalaprilat ◆ esmolol ◆ etoposide ◆ famotidine ◆ fludarabine ◆ foscarnet ◆ gatifloxacin ◆ gemcitabine ◆ granisetron ◆ hydromorphone ◆ labetalol ◆ linezolid ◆ melphalan ◆ meperidine ◆ morphine ◆ ondansetron ◆ propofol ◆ ranitidine ◆ remifentanil ◆ sargramostim ◆ teniposide ◆ thiotepa ◆ vinorelbine.

■ **Y-Site Incompatibility:** ◆ filgrastim.

❏ **Ceftriaxone**

■ **Intermittent Infusion:** Reconstitute each 250-mg vial with 2.4 ml, each 500-mg vial with 4.8 ml, each 1-g vial with 9.6 ml, and each 2-g vial with 19.2 ml of sterile water for injection, 0.9% NaCl, or D5W for a concentration of 100 mg/ml. Solution may be further diluted in 50–100 ml of 0.9% NaCl, D5W, D10W, D5/0.45% NaCl, or LR. Solution may appear light yellow to amber. Solution is stable for 3 days at room temperature.

■ *Rate:* Administer over 15–30 min in adults and 10–30 min in newborns or children.

■ **Y-Site Compatibility:** ◆ acyclovir ◆ allopurinol ◆ amifostine ◆ aztreonam ◆ cisatracurium ◆ diltiazem ◆ docetaxel ◆ doxorubicin liposome ◆ etoposide ◆ famotidine ◆ fludarabine

◆ foscarnet ◆ gatifloxacin ◆ gemcitabine ◆ granisetron ◆ heparin ◆ linezolid ◆ melphalan ◆ meperidine ◆ methotrexate ◆ morphine ◆ paclitaxel ◆ propofol ◆ remifentanil ◆ sargramostim ◆ sodium bicarbonate ◆ tacrolimus ◆ teniposide ◆ theophylline ◆ thiotepa ◆ warfarin ◆ zidovudine.

■ **Y-Site Incompatibility:** ◆ alatrofloxacin ◆ amphotericin B cholesteryl sulfate ◆ filgrastim ◆ fluconazole ◆ labetalol ◆ pentamidine ◆ vinorelbine.

## PATIENT/FAMILY TEACHING

❑ Instruct patient to take medication at evenly spaced times and to finish the medication completely, even if feeling better. Missed doses should be taken as soon as possible unless almost time for next dose; do not double doses. Advise patient that sharing of this medication may be dangerous.

❑ Advise patient to report signs of superinfection (furry overgrowth on the tongue, vaginal itching or discharge, loose or foul-smelling stools) and allergy.

❑ Caution patients that concurrent use of alcohol with *cefoperazone* may cause a disulfiram-like reaction (abdominal cramps, nausea, vomiting, headache, hypotension, palpitations, dyspnea, tachycardia, sweating, flushing). Alcohol and alcohol-containing medications should be avoided during and for several days after therapy.

❑ Instruct patient to notify health care professional if fever and diarrhea develop, especially if stool contains blood, pus, or mucus. Advise patient not to treat diarrhea without consulting health care professional.

## EVALUATION

**Clinical response to therapy can be evaluated by:** ■ Resolution of the signs and symptoms of infection. Length of time for complete resolution depends on the organism and site of infection ■ Decreased incidence of infection when used for prophylaxis.

---

**cephapirin, See**
**CEPHALOSPORINS—FIRST**
**GENERATION.**

---

**cephradine, See**
**CEPHALOSPORINS—FIRST**
**GENERATION.**

---

## cetirizine

(se-ti-ra-zeen)
Zyrtec

### CLASSIFICATION(S):

**Therapeutic:** *allergy, cold, and cough remedies, antihistamines*
**Pharmacologic:** *piperazines (peripherally selective)*

**Pregnancy Category B**

## INDICATIONS

■ Relief of allergic symptoms caused by histamine release including: ❑ Seasonal and perennial allergic rhinitis ❑ Chronic urticaria.

## ACTION

■ Antagonizes the effects of histamine at $H_1$-receptor sites; does not bind to or inactivate histamine ■ Anticholinergic effects are minimal and sedation is dose–related. **Therapeutic Effects:** ■ Decreased symptoms of histamine excess (sneezing, rhinorrhea, ocular tearing and redness, pruritus).

## PHARMACOKINETICS

**Absorption:** Well absorbed following oral administration.
**Distribution:** Unknown.
**Metabolism and Excretion:** Excreted primarily unchanged by the kidneys.
**Half-life:** 8 hr (decreased in children, increased in renal impairment).

## CONTRAINDICATIONS AND PRECAUTIONS

**Contraindicated in:** ■ Hypersensitivity ■ Acute attacks of asthma ■ Not recommended for use during lactation.
**Use Cautiously in:** ■ Patients with hepatic or renal impairment (dosage reduction recommended if CCr ≤31 ml/min or hepatic function is impaired) ■ Geriatric patients (start with lower doses) ■ Pregnancy or children <2 yr (safety not established).

## ADVERSE REACTIONS AND SIDE EFFECTS*

■ **CNS:** dizziness, drowsiness, fatigue ■ **EENT:** pharyngitis ■ **GI:** dry mouth.

## INTERACTIONS

**Drug-Drug:** ■ Additive CNS depression may occur with **alcohol, opioid analgesics,** or **sedative/hypnotics.**

## ROUTE AND DOSAGE

■ **PO (Adults and children >6 yr):** 5–10 mg once daily.

■ **PO (Children 2–5 yr):** 2.5 mg once daily initially, may be increased to 5 mg once daily or 2.5 mg every 12 hr.

■ **PO (Children 6 mo –2 yr):** 2.5 mg once daily; may be increased to 2.5 mg every 12 hr children 12–23 mo.

❏ **Renal/Hepatic Impairment**

■ **PO (Adults):** *CCr ≤31 ml/min, hepatic impairment or hemodialysis*—5 mg once daily.

■ **PO (Children 6–11 yr):** start therapy at <5 mg/day.

## AVAILABILITY

■ **Tablets:** 5 mg$^{Rx}$, 10 mg$^{Rx}$ ■ Cost: $203.83/ 100 tablets (5 and 10 mg) ■ **Syrup (banana-grape):** 5 mg/5 ml$^{Rx}$ ■ Cost: $29.79/120 ml ■ pseudoephedrine (Zyrtec-D 12 Hour)$^{Rx}$ (See Appendix B).

TIME/ACTION PROFILE (antihistaminic effects)

| | ONSET | PEAK | DURATION |
|---|---|---|---|
| PO | 30 min | 4–8 hr | 24 hr |

# NURSING IMPLICATIONS

## ASSESSMENT

❏ Assess allergy symptoms (rhinitis, conjunctivitis, hives) before and periodically during therapy.

❏ Assess lung sounds and character of bronchial secretions. Maintain fluid intake of 1500–2000 ml/day to decrease viscosity of secretions.

■ *Lab Test Considerations:* May cause false-negative result in allergy skin testing.

## POTENTIAL NURSING DIAGNOSES

■ Airway clearance, ineffective (Indications).

■ Injury, risk for (Adverse Reactions).

## IMPLEMENTATION

■ **General:** Do not confuse Zyrtec (cetirizine) with Zantac (ranitidine) or Zyprexa (olanzapine).

■ **PO:** Administer once daily without regard to food.

## PATIENT/FAMILY TEACHING

❏ Instruct patient to take medication as directed.

❏ May cause dizziness and drowsiness. Caution patient to avoid driving or other activities requiring alertness until response to medication is known.

❏ Advise patient to avoid taking alcohol or other CNS depressants concurrently with this drug.

❏ Advise patient that good oral hygiene, frequent rinsing of mouth with water, and sugarless gum or candy may minimize dry mouth. Patient should notify dentist if dry mouth persists >2 wk.

❏ Instruct patient to contact health care professional if dizziness occurs or if symptoms persist.

## EVALUATION

**Effectiveness of therapy can be demonstrated by:** ■ Decrease in allergic symptoms.

| High Alert |
|---|

# chloral hydrate

(**klor**-al **hye**-drate)

Aquachloral, {Novo-Chlorhydrate}, {PMS-Chloral Hydrate}

## CLASSIFICATION(S):

*Therapeutic:* sedative/hypnotics

**Schedule IV**

**Pregnancy Category C**

{ } = Available in Canada only.
*CAPITALS indicates life-threatening; underlines indicate most frequent.

## INDICATIONS

■ Short-term sedative and hypnotic (effectiveness decreases after 2 wk of use) ■ Sedation or reduction of anxiety preoperatively (anesthetic adjunct).

## ACTION

■ Converted to trichloroethanol, which is the active drug. Has generalized CNS depressant properties. **Therapeutic Effects:** ■ Sedation or induction of sleep.

## PHARMACOKINETICS

**Absorption:** Well absorbed following oral or rectal administration.

**Distribution:** Widely distributed. Crosses the placenta and enters breast milk in low concentrations.

**Metabolism and Excretion:** Converted by liver to trichloroethanol, which is active. Trichloroethanol is, in turn, metabolized by the liver and kidneys to inactive compounds.

**Half-life:** *Trichloroethanol*—8–10 hr.

## CONTRAINDICATIONS AND PRECAUTIONS

**Contraindicated in:** ■ Hypersensitivity ■ Coma or pre-existing CNS depression ■ Uncontrolled severe pain ■ Pregnancy and lactation ■ Esophagitis, gastritis, or ulcer disease ■ Proctitis (rectal use) ■ Tartrazine hypersensitivity (some rectal products).

**Use Cautiously in:** ■ Hepatic dysfunction ■ Severe renal impairment ■ History of suicide attempt or substance abuse ■ Geriatric patients (dosage reduction recommended).

## ADVERSE REACTIONS AND SIDE EFFECTS*

■ **CNS:** excess sedation, disorientation, dizziness, hangover, headache, incoordination, irritability, paradoxical excitation (children) ■ **Resp:** respiratory depression ■ **GI:** diarrhea, nausea, vomiting, flatulence ■ **Derm:** rashes ■ **Misc:** tolerance, physical dependence, psychological dependence.

## INTERACTIONS

**Drug-Drug:** ■ Additive CNS depression with other **CNS depressants,** including **alcohol, antihistamines, antidepressants, sedative/ hypnotics,** and **opioid analgesics** ■ May potentiate **warfarin** ■ When given within 24 hr of IV **furosemide,** may cause diaphoresis,

changes in blood pressure, and flushing ■ May increase metabolism and decrease effects of **phenytoin**.

**Drug-Natural Products:** ■ Concomitant use of **kava, valerian, skullcap, chamomile,** or **hops** can increase CNS depression.

## ROUTE AND DOSAGE

■ **PO (Adults):** *Hypnotic*—500–1000 mg 15–30 min before bedtime. *Preoperative sedation*—500 mg–1 g 30 min before surgery. *Daytime sedation*—250 mg 3 times daily. Single dose/daily dose should not >2 g.

■ **PO (Geriatric Patients):** *Hypnotic*—250 mg 15–30 min before bedtime.

■ **Rect (Adults):** *Sedation*—325 mg 3 times daily. *Hypnotic*—500–1000 mg. Single dose/daily dose should not >2 g.

■ **PO, Rect (Children):** *Pre-electroencephalogram sedation*—20–25 mg/kg. *Sedation prior to dental/medical procedures*—50–75 mg/kg (not to exceed 1 g/single dose; unlabeled); single dose should not >1 g). *Hypnotic*—50 mg/kg.

## AVAILABILITY (generic available)

■ *Capsules:* 250 mg^Rx, 500 mg^Rx, 650 mg^Rx ■ *Syrup:* 250 mg/5 ml^Rx, 500 mg/5 ml^Rx ■ *Suppositories:* 325 mg^Rx, 500 mg^Rx.

TIME/ACTION PROFILE (sedation)

| | ONSET | PEAK | DURATION |
|---|---|---|---|
| PO | 30 min | 1 hr | 4–8 hr |
| Rectal | 0.5–1 hr | unknown | 4–8 hr |

# NURSING IMPLICATIONS

## ASSESSMENT

❑ Assess mental status, sleep patterns, and potential for abuse prior to administering this medication. Prolonged use may lead to physical and psychological dependence. Limit amount of drug available to the patient.

❑ Assess level of consciousness at time of peak effect. Notify physician or other health care professional if desired sedation does not occur or if paradoxical reaction occurs.

■ *Lab Test Considerations:* Interferes with tests for urinary 17-hydroxycorticosteroids and urinary catecholamines.

## POTENTIAL NURSING DIAGNOSES

- Sleep pattern disturbed (Indications).
- Anxiety (Indications).
- Injury, risk for (Side Effects).

## IMPLEMENTATION

- **High Alert:** Chloral hydrate overdosage has resulted in fatalities in children. Only accept orders written in milligrams, not volume (teaspoons) or concentration. Chloral hydrate should be administered to children only by trained staff in the health care setting. When administered to children for sedation before outpatient procedures, administer at the facility where procedure is to be performed. Continue monitoring until level of consciousness is safe for discharge.

- **General:** Before administering, reduce external stimuli and provide comfort measures to increase effectiveness of medication.

- Protect patient from injury. Place bed-side rails up. Assist with ambulation. Remove cigarettes from patients receiving hypnotic dose.

- **PO:** Capsules should be swallowed whole with a full glass of water or juice to minimize gastric irritation; do not chew. Dilute syrup in a half glass of water or juice.

- **Rect:** If suppository is too soft for insertion, chill in refrigerator for 30 min or run under cold water before removing foil wrapper.

## PATIENT/FAMILY TEACHING

- Instruct patient to take chloral hydrate exactly as directed. Missed doses should be omitted; do not double doses. If used for 2 wk or longer, abrupt withdrawal may result in CNS excitement, tremor, anxiety, hallucinations, and delirium.

- Chloral hydrate causes drowsiness and dizziness. Caution patient to avoid driving or other activities requiring alertness until response to medication is known.

- Caution patient that concurrent alcohol use may create an additive effect that results in tachycardia, vasodilation, flushing, headache, hypotension, and pronounced CNS depression. Alcohol and other CNS depressants should be avoided while taking chloral hydrate.

- Advise patient to discontinue use and notify health care professional if skin rash, dizziness, irritability, impaired thought processes, headache, or motor incoordination occurs.

## EVALUATION

**Effectiveness of therapy can be demonstrated by:** ■ Sedation ■ Improvement in sleep pattern.

# chlordiazepoxide

(klor-dye-az-e-**pox**-ide)

{Apo-Chlordiazepoxide}, Libritabs, Librium, {Novopoxide}

## CLASSIFICATION(S):

**Therapeutic:** antianxiety agents, sedative/hypnotics

**Pharmacologic:** benzodiazepines

**Schedule IV**

**Pregnancy Category D**

## INDICATIONS

■ Adjunct management of anxiety ■ Treatment of alcohol withdrawal.

## ACTION

■ Acts at many levels of the CNS to produce anxiolytic effect ■ Depresses the CNS, probably by potentiating GABA, an inhibitory neurotransmitter. **Therapeutic Effects:** ■ Sedation ■ Relief of anxiety.

## PHARMACOKINETICS

**Absorption:** Well absorbed from the GI tract. IM absorption may be slow and unpredictable.

**Distribution:** Widely distributed. Crosses the blood-brain barrier. Crosses the placenta; enters breast milk.

**Metabolism and Excretion:** Highly metabolized by the liver. Some products of metabolism are active as CNS depressants.

**Half-life:** 5–30 hr.

## CONTRAINDICATIONS AND PRECAUTIONS

**Contraindicated in:** ■ Hypersensitivity ■ Some products contain tartrazine and should be avoided in patients with known intolerance ■ Cross-sensitivity with other benzodiazepines may occur ■ Comatose patients or those with pre-existing CNS depression ■ Uncontrolled severe pain ■ Narrow-angle glaucoma ■ Porphyria ■ Pregnancy and lactation ■ Children ≤6 yr.

**Use Cautiously in:** ■ Hepatic dysfunction ■ Severe renal impairment ■ History of suicide attempt or substance abuse ■ Geriatric or debilitated patients (initial dosage reduction required).

## ADVERSE REACTIONS AND SIDE EFFECTS*

■ **CNS:** <u>dizziness</u>, <u>drowsiness</u>, hangover, headache, mental depression, paradoxical excitation ■ **EENT:** blurred vision ■ **GI:** constipation, diarrhea, nausea, vomiting ■ **Derm:** rashes ■ **Local:** <u>pain at IM site</u> ■ **Misc:** physical dependence, psychological dependence, tolerance.

## INTERACTIONS

**Drug-Drug:** ■ **Alcohol, antidepressants, antihistamines,** and **opioid analgesics**—concurrent use results in additive CNS depression ■ **Cimetidine, oral contraceptives, disulfiram, fluoxetine, isoniazid, ketoconazole, metoprolol, propoxyphene, propranolol,** or **valproic acid** may enhance effects ■ May decrease efficacy of **levodopa** ■ **Rifampin** or **barbiturates** may decrease effectiveness of chlordiazepoxide ■ Sedative effects may be decreased by **theophylline.**

**Drug-Natural Products:** ■ Concomitant use of **kava, valerian, skullcap, chamomile,** or **hops** can increase CNS depression.

## ROUTE AND DOSAGE

■ **PO (Adults):** *Alcohol withdrawal*—50–100 mg, repeated until agitation is controlled (up to 400 mg/day). *Anxiety*—5–25 mg 3–4 times daily.

■ **PO (Geriatric Patients or Debilitated Patients):** *Anxiety*—5 mg 2–4 times daily initially, increased as needed.

■ **PO (Children >6 yr):** *Anxiety*—5 mg 2–4 times daily, up to 10 mg 2–3 times daily.

■ **IM, IV (Adults):** *Alcohol withdrawal*—50–100 mg initially; may be repeated in 2–4 hr. *Anxiety*—50–100 mg initially, then 25–50 mg 3–4 times daily as required (25–50 mg initially in geriatric patients). *Preoperative sedation*—50–100 mg 1 hr preop.

■ **IM, IV (Geriatric Patients or Debilitated Patients):** *Anxiety/sedation*—25–50 mg/dose.

■ **IM, IV (Children >12 yr):** *Anxiety/sedation*—25–50 mg/dose.

## AVAILABILITY (generic available)

■ *Capsules:* 5 mg<sup>Rx</sup>, 10 mg<sup>Rx</sup>, 25 mg<sup>Rx</sup> ■ Cost: **Librium:** *5 mg*—$57.75/100; *10 mg*—$83.95/100; *25 mg*—$143.96/100; **generic:** *5 mg*—$9.88/100; *10 mg*—$21.00/100; *25 mg*—$22.66/100 ■ *Tablets:* 5 mg<sup>Rx</sup>, 10 mg<sup>Rx</sup>, 25 mg<sup>Rx</sup> ■ *Injection:* 100-mg ampule<sup>Rx</sup> ■ amitriptyline (Limbitrol DS)<sup>Rx</sup>, clidinium (Librax)<sup>Rx</sup>. See Appendix B.

TIME/ACTION PROFILE (sedation)

|    | ONSET | PEAK | DURATION |
|----|-------|------|----------|
| PO | 1–2 hr | 0.5–4 hr | up to 24 hr |
| IM | 15–30 min | unknown | unknown |
| IV | 1–5 min | unknown | 0.25–1 hr |

# NURSING IMPLICATIONS

## ASSESSMENT

■ **General Info:** Assess patient for anxiety and level of sedation (ataxia, dizziness, slurred speech) periodically throughout therapy.

❑ Monitor blood pressure, heart rate, and respiratory rate frequently when administering parenterally. Report significant changes immediately.

❑ Prolonged high-dose therapy may lead to psychological or physical dependence. Restrict the amount of drug available to patient.

■ **Alcohol Withdrawal:** Assess patient for tremors, agitation, delirium, and hallucinations. Protect patient from injury.

■ *Lab Test Considerations:* Patients on prolonged therapy should have CBC and liver function tests evaluated periodically. May cause an increase in serum bilirubin, AST, and ALT.

❑ May alter results of urine 17-ketosteroids and 17-ketogenic steroids. May cause decreased response on metyrapone tests and decreased thyroidal uptake of $^{123}$I and $^{131}$I.

## POTENTIAL NURSING DIAGNOSES

■ Anxiety (Indications).

■ Injury, risk for (Side Effects).

**IMPLEMENTATION**

■ **General:** Do not confuse Librium with Librax.

❑ IV administration is usually the preferred route for parenteral administration because of the slow, erratic absorption after IM administration.

❑ After parenteral administration, have patient remain recumbent and observe for 3–8 hr or longer, depending on patient's response.

❑ Equipment to maintain a patent airway should be immediately available when chlordiazepoxide is administered intravenously.

❑ Use parenteral solution immediately after reconstitution and discard any unused portion.

■ **PO:** Administer after meals or with milk to minimize GI irritation. Tablets may be crushed and taken with food or fluids if patient has difficulty swallowing.

■ **IM:** Reconstitute only with 2 ml of diluent provided by manufacturer. Do not use solution if opalescent or hazy. Agitate gently to minimize bubbling. Administer slowly, deep into a well-developed muscle mass to minimize pain at injection site. Solution reconstituted with IM diluent should not be given IV.

■ **Direct IV:** Reconstitute 100 mg in 5 ml of 0.9% NaCl or sterile water for injection. Do not use IM diluent.

■ *Rate:* Administer prescribed dose slowly over at least 1 min. Rapid administration may cause apnea, hypotension, bradycardia, or cardiac arrest.

■ **Y-Site Compatibility:** ◆ heparin ◆ hydrocortisone sodium succinate ◆ potassium chloride ◆ vitamin B complex with C.

**PATIENT/FAMILY TEACHING**

❑ Instruct patient to take chlordiazepoxide exactly as directed. If medication is less effective after a few weeks, check with health care professional; do not increase dose. Medication should be tapered at the completion of long-term therapy. Sudden cessation of medication may lead to withdrawal (insomnia, irritability, nervousness, tremors).

❑ May cause drowsiness or dizziness. Caution patient to avoid driving or other activities requiring alertness until response to medication is known.

❑ Advise patient to avoid the use of alcohol and other CNS depressants concurrently with this medication.

❑ Instruct patient to consult health care professional before taking OTC medications.

❑ Instruct patient to notify health care professional if pregnancy is planned or suspected.

**EVALUATION**

**Effectiveness of therapy can be demonstrated by:** ■ Decreased sense of anxiety ❑ Increased ability to cope ■ Decreased tremulousness and more rational ideation when used for alcohol withdrawal.

## chlorothiazide, See DIURETICS (THIAZIDE).

## chlorpheniramine

(klor-fen-**ir**-a-meen)

Aller-Chlor, Allergy, Chlo-Amine, Chlorate, Chlor-Trimeton, Chlor-Trimeton Allergy 4 Hour, Chlor-Trimeton Allergy 8 Hour, Chlor-Trimeton Allergy 12 Hour, {Chlor-Tripolon}, {Novo-Pheniram}, Pedia-Care Allergy Formula, Phenetron, Telechlor, Teldrin

### CLASSIFICATION(S):

*Therapeutic: allergy, cold, and cough remedies, antihistamines*

**Pregnancy Category B**

**INDICATIONS**

■ Relief of allergic symptoms caused by histamine release, including: ❑ Nasal allergies ❑ Allergic dermatoses ■ Management of severe allergic or hypersensitivity reactions, including anaphylaxis and transfusion reactions.

**ACTION**

■ Antagonizes the effects of histamine at $H_2$-receptor sites; does not bind to or inactivate histamine. **Therapeutic Effects:** ■ Decreased symptoms of histamine excess (sneezing, rhinorrhea, nasal and ocular pruritus, ocular tearing and redness).

## PHARMACOKINETICS

**Absorption:** Well absorbed following oral and parenteral administration.

**Distribution:** Widely distributed. Minimal amounts excreted in breast milk. Crosses the blood-brain barrier.

**Metabolism and Excretion:** Extensively metabolized by the liver.

**Half-life:** 12–15 hr.

## CONTRAINDICATIONS AND PRECAUTIONS

**Contraindicated in:** ■ Hypersensitivity ■ Acute attacks of asthma ■ Lactation (avoid use) ■ Known alcohol intolerance (some liquid forms).

**Use Cautiously in:** ■ Narrow-angle glaucoma ■ Liver disease ■ Geriatric patients (more susceptible to adverse reactions) ■ Pregnancy (safety not established).

## ADVERSE REACTIONS AND SIDE EFFECTS*

■ **CNS:** drowsiness, dizziness, excitation (in children) ■ **EENT:** blurred vision ■ **CV:** hypertension, arrhythmias, hypotension, palpitations ■ **GI:** dry mouth, constipation, obstruction ■ **GU:** retention, urinary hesitancy.

## INTERACTIONS

**Drug-Drug:** ■ Additive CNS depression with other **CNS depressants,** including **alcohol, opioid analgesics,** and **sedative/hypnotics** ■ **MAO inhibitors** intensify and prolong anticholinergic effects of antihistamines ■ Additive anticholinergic effects with other **drugs possessing anticholinergic properties,** including **antidepressants, atropine, haloperidol, phenothiazines, quinidine,** and **disopyramide.**

## ROUTE AND DOSAGE

■ **PO (Adults):** 4 mg q 4–6 hr *or* 8–12 mg of extended-release formulation q 8–12 hr (not to exceed 24 mg/day).

■ **PO (Geriatric Patients):** 4 mg twice daily *or* 8 mg of extended-release formulation at bedtime.

■ **PO (Children 6–12 yr):** 2 mg 3–4 times daily (not to exceed 12 mg/day).

■ **Subcut, IM, IV (Adults):** 5–40-mg single dose (not to exceed 40 mg/day).

■ **Subcut (Children):** 87.5 mcg (0.0875 mg)/kg or 2.5 mg/m$^2$ q 6 hr as needed.

## AVAILABILITY (generic available)

■ *Tablets:* 4 mg$^{Rx, OTC}$, 8 mg$^{Rx, OTC}$, 12 mg$^{Rx, OTC}$ ■ Cost: 4 mg $1.82/30, 8 mg $3.99/30, 12 mg $5.49/30 ■ *Chewable tablets (orange flavor):* 2 mg$^{Rx, OTC}$ ■ *Timed-release tablets:* 8 mg$^{Rx, OTC}$, 12 mg$^{Rx, OTC}$ ■ *Timed-release capsules:* 8 mg$^{Rx, OTC}$, 12 mg$^{Rx, OTC}$ ■ *Syrup:* 1 mg/5 mlRx, OTC, 2 mg/5 mlRx, OTC, {2.5 mg/5 mlRx, OTC} ■ *Injection:* 10 mg/ml$^{Rx}$, 100 mg/ml$^{Rx}$ ■ decongestantsRx, OTC. See Appendix B.

TIME/ACTION PROFILE (antihistaminic effects)

| | ONSET | PEAK | DURATION |
|---|---|---|---|
| PO | 15–30 min | 6 hr | 4–12 hr |
| PO–ER | unknown | unknown | 8–24 hr |
| Subcut | unknown | unknown | 4–12 hr |
| IM | unknown | unknown | 4–12 hr |
| IV | rapid | unknown | 4–12 hr |

# NURSING IMPLICATIONS

## ASSESSMENT

❑ Assess allergy symptoms (rhinitis, conjunctivitis, hives) prior to and periodically throughout therapy.

❑ Monitor pulse and blood pressure before initiating and throughout IV therapy.

❑ Assess lung sounds and character of bronchial secretions. Maintain fluid intake of 1500–2000 ml/day to decrease viscosity of secretions.

■ *Lab Test Considerations:* May cause false-negative reactions on allergy skin tests; discontinue 4 days prior to testing.

## POTENTIAL NURSING DIAGNOSES

■ Airway clearance, ineffective (Indications).

■ Injury, risk for (Adverse Reactions).

## IMPLEMENTATION

■ **PO:** Administer oral doses with food or milk to decrease GI irritation. Extended-release tablets and capsules should be swallowed whole; do not crush, break, or chew. Chewable tablets should not be swallowed whole; chew well before swallowing.

■ **Subcut, IM:** The 100-mg/ml solution is recommended for IM or subcut routes only. The

10-mg/ml solution may be used for IM, subcut, or IV.

- **Direct IV:** May be given undiluted. Use only the 10 mg/ml strength for IV administration.
- *Rate:* Administer each 10-mg dose over at least 1 min.

## PATIENT/FAMILY TEACHING

- ❏ Instruct patient to take chlorpheniramine exactly as directed.
- ❏ May cause drowsiness. Caution patient to avoid driving or other activities requiring alertness until response to drug is known.
- ❏ Caution patient to avoid using alcohol or other CNS depressants concurrently with this drug.
- ❏ Advise patient that good oral hygiene, frequent rinsing of mouth with water, and sugarless gum or candy may help relieve dryness of mouth.
- ❏ Instruct patient to contact health care professional if symptoms persist.

## EVALUATION

**Effectiveness of therapy can be demonstrated by:** ■ Decrease in allergic symptoms.

## chlorthalidone, See DIURETICS (THIAZIDE).

---

# chlorzoxazone
(klor-**zox**-a-zohn)
EZE-DS, Paraflex, Parafon Forte DSC, Relaxazone, Remular, Remular-S, Strifon Forte DSC

## CLASSIFICATION(S):
*Therapeutic: skeletal muscle relaxants (centrally acting)*

### Pregnancy Category UK

## INDICATIONS

- ■ Adjunct to rest and physical therapy in the treatment of muscle spasm associated with acute painful musculoskeletal conditions.

## ACTION

- ■ Skeletal muscle relaxation, probably due to CNS depression. **Therapeutic Effects:** ■ Skeletal muscle relaxation with decreased discomfort.

## PHARMACOKINETICS

**Absorption:** Readily absorbed after oral administration.

**Distribution:** Unknown.

**Metabolism and Excretion:** Mostly metabolized by the liver; <1% excreted unchanged in urine.

**Half-life:** 1.1 hr.

## CONTRAINDICATIONS AND PRECAUTIONS

**Contraindicated in:** ■ Hypersensitivity ■ Porphyria.

**Use Cautiously in:** ■ Underlying cardiovascular disease ■ Impaired renal or hepatic function ■ Pregnancy, lactation, or children (safety not established).

## ADVERSE REACTIONS AND SIDE EFFECTS*

- ■ **CNS:** <u>dizziness</u>, <u>drowsiness</u> ■ **GI:** GI BLEEDING, constipation, diarrhea, heartburn, nausea, vomiting ■ **Derm:** allergic dermatitis ■ **Hemat:** AGRANULOCYTOSIS, anemia ■ **Misc:** allergic reactions including ANGIOEDEMA.

## INTERACTIONS

**Drug-Drug:** ■ Increased risk of CNS depression with other **CNS depressants,** including **alcohol, antihistamines, antidepressants, sedative/hypnotics,** or **opioid analgesics.**
**Drug-Natural Products:** ■ Concomitant use of **kava, valerian, skullcap, chamomile,** or **hops** can increase CNS depression.

## ROUTE AND DOSAGE

- ■ **PO (Adults):** 250–750 mg 3–4 times daily.
- ■ **PO (Children):** 20 mg/kg or 600 mg/m²/day in 3–4 divided doses.

## AVAILABILITY (generic available)

- ■ *Tablets:* 250 mg$^{Rx}$, 500 mg$^{Rx}$ ■Cost: *250 mg generic*—$29.86/100; *500 mg Parafon Forte DSC*—$126.84/100; *generic*—$102.96/100.

---

TIME/ACTION PROFILE (skeletal muscle effects)

| | ONSET | PEAK | DURATION |
|---|---|---|---|
| PO | within 1 hr | 1–2 hr | 3–4 hr |

## NURSING IMPLICATIONS

### ASSESSMENT

❑ Assess patient for pain, muscle stiffness, and range of motion before and periodically throughout therapy.

### POTENTIAL NURSING DIAGNOSES

■ Pain, acute (Indications).
■ Mobility, impaired physical (Indications).
■ Injury, risk for (Side Effects).

### IMPLEMENTATION

■ **PO:** May be administered with meals to minimize gastric irritation. Tablets may be crushed and mixed with food or liquid for ease of administration.

### PATIENT/FAMILY TEACHING

❑ Instruct patient to take medication exactly as directed; do not take more than the prescribed amount. Missed doses should be taken within 1 hr of time ordered; otherwise, omit and return to normal dosage schedule. Do not double doses.
❑ Medication may cause drowsiness and dizziness. Caution patient to avoid driving or other activities requiring alertness until response to drug is known.
❑ Advise patient to avoid concurrent use of alcohol or other CNS depressants with this medication.
❑ If constipation becomes a problem, advise patient that increasing fluid intake and bulk in diet and stool softeners may alleviate this condition.

### EVALUATION

**Effectiveness of therapy can be demonstrated by:** ■ Relief of muscular spasm in acute skeletal muscle conditions.

---

## cholestyramine

(koe-less-**tear**-a-meen)

LoCHOLEST, LoCHOLEST Light, Prevalite, Questran, Questran Light

---

**CLASSIFICATION(S):**
**Therapeutic:** lipid-lowering agents
**Pharmacologic:** bile acid sequestrants

**Pregnancy Category C**

### INDICATIONS

■ Management of primary hypercholesterolemia ■ Pruritus associated with elevated levels of bile acids. **Unlabeled uses:** ■ Diarrhea associated with excess bile acids.

### ACTION

■ Bind bile acids in the GI tract, forming an insoluble complex. Result is increased clearance of cholesterol. **Therapeutic Effects:** ■ Decreased plasma cholesterol and low-density lipoproteins (LDLs) ■ Decreased pruritus.

### PHARMACOKINETICS

**Absorption:** Action takes place in the GI tract. No absorption occurs.
**Distribution:** No distribution.
**Metabolism and Excretion:** After binding bile acids, insoluble complex is eliminated in the feces.
**Half-life:** Unknown.

### CONTRAINDICATIONS AND PRECAUTIONS

**Contraindicated in:** ■ Hypersensitivity ■ Complete biliary obstruction ■ Some products contain aspartame and should be avoided in patients with phenylketonuria.
**Use Cautiously in:** ■ History of constipation.
**Exercise Extreme Caution in:** ■ Children (may cause intestinal obstruction; deaths have occurred).

### ADVERSE REACTIONS AND SIDE EFFECTS*

■ EENT: irritation of the tongue ■ **GI:** <u>abdominal discomfort</u>, <u>constipation</u>, <u>nausea</u>, fecal impaction, flatulence, hemorrhoids, perianal irritation, steatorrhea, vomiting ■ **Derm:** irritation, rashes ■ **F and E:** hyperchloremic acidosis ■ **Metab:** vitamin A, D, and K deficiency.

### INTERACTIONS

**Drug-Drug:** ■ May decrease absorption/effects of orally administered **acetaminophen, amiodarone, clindamycin, clofibrate, digoxin,**

diuretics, gemfibrozil, glipizide, corticosteroids, imipramine, mycophenolate, methotrexate, methyldopa, niacin, NSAIDs, penicillin, phenytoin, phosphates, propranolol, tetracyclines, tolbutamide, thyroid preparations, ursodiol, warfarin, and **fat-soluble vitamins (A, D, E, and K)** ▪ May decrease absorption of other **orally administered medications.**

## ROUTE AND DOSAGE

▪ **PO (Adults):** 4 g 1–2 times daily (initially, may be increased as needed/tolerated up to 24 g/day in 6 divided doses).
▪ **PO (Children):** 240 mg/kg/day in 2–3 divided doses (not >8 g/day).

## AVAILABILITY (generic available)

▪*Powder for suspension with aspartame (strawberry flavor [LoCHOLEST], unflavored [Prevalite, Questran Light]):* 4 g cholestyramine/packet or scoop$^{Rx}$ ▪Cost: *generic*—$70–$85/60 packets; *LoCHOLEST Light*—$97.55/60 packets; *Prevalite*—$82.02/60 packets; *Questran Light*—$90.34/60 packets ▪ *Powder for suspension (strawberry flavor [LoCHOLEST], unflavored [Questran, generic]):* 4 g cholestyramine/packet or scoop$^{Rx}$ ▪Cost: *generic*—$55–$85/60 packets; *LoCHOLEST*—$97.55/60 packets; *Questran*—$103.41/60 packets.

TIME/ACTION PROFILE (hypocholesterolemic effects)

| | ONSET | PEAK | DURATION |
|---|---|---|---|
| PO | 24–48 hr | 1–3 wk | 2–4 wk |

# NURSING IMPLICATIONS

## ASSESSMENT

▪ **Hypercholesterolemia:** Obtain a diet history, especially in regard to fat consumption.
▪ **Pruritus:** Assess severity of itching and skin integrity. Dose may be decreased when relief of pruritus occurs.
▪ **Diarrhea:** Assess frequency, amount, and consistency of stools.
▪ *Lab Test Considerations:* Serum cholesterol and triglyceride levels should be evaluated before initiating, frequently during first few months and periodically throughout therapy. Discontinue medication if paradoxical increase in cholesterol level occurs.

❑ May cause an increase in AST, ALT, phosphorus, chloride, and alkaline phosphatase and a decrease in serum calcium, sodium, and potassium levels.
❑ May also cause prolonged prothrombin times.

## POTENTIAL NURSING DIAGNOSES

▪ Constipation (Side Effects).
▪ Noncompliance (Patient/Family Teaching).

## IMPLEMENTATION

▪ **General:** Parenteral or water-miscible forms of fat-soluble vitamins (A, D, and K) and folic acid may be ordered for patients on chronic therapy.
▪ **PO:** Administer before meals.
❑ Scoops for powdered preparations may not be exchangable between products.
❑ Administer other medications 1 hr before or 4–6 hr after the administration of this medication.

## PATIENT/FAMILY TEACHING

❑ Instruct patient to take medication exactly as directed; do not skip doses or double up on missed doses.
❑ Instruct patient to take medication before meals. Mix cholestyramine with 4–6 oz water, milk, fruit juice, or other noncarbonated beverages. Shake vigorously. Slowly stir in a large glass. Rinse glass with small amount of additional beverage to ensure all medication is taken. May also mix with highly fluid soups, cereals, or pulpy fruits (applesauce, crushed pineapple). Allow powder to sit on fluid and hydrate for 1–2 min before mixing. Do not take dry. Variations in the color of cholestyramine do not alter stability.
❑ Advise patient that this medication should be used in conjunction with dietary restrictions (fat, cholesterol, carbohydrates, alcohol), exercise, and cessation of smoking.
❑ Explain that constipation may occur. Increase in fluids and bulk in diet, exercise, stool softeners, and laxatives may be required to minimize the constipating effects. Instruct patient to notify health care profes-

sional if constipation, nausea, flatulence, and heartburn persist or if stools become frothy and foul smelling.

◻ Advise patient to notify health care professional if unusual bleeding or bruising; petechiae; or black, tarry stools occur. Treatment with vitamin K may be necessary.

### EVALUATION

**Effectiveness of therapy can be demonstrated by:** ■ Decrease in serum low-density lipoprotein cholesterol levels. Therapy is usually discontinued if the clinical response remains poor after 3 mo of therapy ■ Decrease in severity of pruritus. Relief usually occurs 1–3 wk after therapy is initiated ■ Decrease in frequency and severity of diarrhea.

## choline and magnesium salicylates, See SALICYLATES.

## choline salicylate, See SALICYLATES.

## ciclopirox, See ANTIFUNGALS (TOPICAL).

## cidofovir

(sye-doe-**foe**-veer)
Vistide

*CLASSIFICATION(S):*
*Therapeutic:* antivirals

**Pregnancy Category C**

### INDICATIONS

■ Management of cytomegalovirus (CMV) retinitis in HIV-infected patients (with probenecid).

### ACTION

■ Suppresses replication of CMV by inhibiting viral DNA synthesis. **Therapeutic Effects:** ■ Slows progression of CMV retinitis; may not be curative.

### PHARMACOKINETICS

**Absorption:** IV administration results in complete bioavailability.

**Distribution:** Unknown.
**Metabolism and Excretion:** Excreted mostly unchanged by the kidneys.
**Half-life:** Unknown.

### CONTRAINDICATIONS AND PRECAUTIONS

**Contraindicated in:** ■ Hypersensitivity to cidofovir, probenecid, or sulfonamides ■ Serum Cr >1.5 mg/dl, CCr ≤55 ml/min, or urine protein ≥100 mg/dl (≥2+ proteinuria) ■ Concurrent use of foscarnet, amphotericin B, aminoglycoside anti-infectives, NSAIDs, or IV pentamidine.

**Use Cautiously in:** ■ Pregnancy or children (safety not established); breastfeeding is not recommended in HIV-positive patients.

**Exercise Extreme Caution in:** ■ Any condition or medication that increases the risk of dehydration.

### ADVERSE REACTIONS AND SIDE EFFECTS*

■ **CNS:** <u>headache</u>, <u>weakness</u> ■ **EENT:** decreased intraocular pressure, hearing loss, iritis, ocular hypotony, uveitis ■ **Resp:** <u>dyspnea</u>, pneumonia ■ **GI:** HEPATIC DYSFUNCTION, PANCREATITIS, <u>abdominal pain</u>, <u>nausea</u>, <u>vomiting</u>, anorexia, diarrhea ■ **GU:** RENAL FAILURE, <u>proteinuria</u> ■ **Derm:** alopecia, <u>rash</u> ■ **F and E:** decreased serum bicarbonate ■ **Hemat:** <u>neutropenia</u>, anemia ■ **Metab:** METABOLIC ACIDOSIS ■ **Misc:** <u>chills</u>, <u>fever</u>, <u>infection</u>.

### INTERACTIONS

**Drug-Drug:** ■ ↑ risk of nephrotoxicity with **aminoglycosides, amphotericin B, foscarnet,** and **pentamidine** and should be avoided; wait 7 days after giving other nephrotoxic agents ■ **Probenecid,** which is required concurrently, may interact with **acetaminophen, acyclovir, ACE inhibitors, barbiturates, benzodiazepines, bumetanide, methotrexate, famotidine, furosemide, NSAIDs, theophylline,** and **zidovudine.**

### ROUTE AND DOSAGE

■ **IV (Adults):** 5 mg/kg once weekly for 2 wk, followed by 5 mg/kg every 2 wk (must be given with probenecid).
◻ **Renal Impairment**
■ **IV (Adults):** *Increase in serum creatinine of 0.3–0.4 mg/dL*—decrease dose to 3 mg/kg; discontinue if serum creatinine increases ≥0.5 mg/dL over baseline.

## AVAILABILITY

■ *Solution for injection:* 75 mg/ml in 5-ml ampules[Rx].

### TIME/ACTION PROFILE

| | ONSET | PEAK | DURATION |
|---|---|---|---|
| IV | rapid | end of infusion | unknown |

## NURSING IMPLICATIONS

### ASSESSMENT

❑ Monitor vision for progression of CMV retinitis. Monitor ocular symptoms, intraocular pressure, and visual acuity periodically.

❑ Antiemetics and administration after a meal may minimize nausea and vomiting associated with probenecid. If allergic reactions occur in association with probenecid, pretreatment with antihistamines or acetaminophen should be considered.

❑ Monitor vital signs periodically. May cause fever, hypotension, and tachycardia. Monitor patients for early signs and symptoms of infection.

■ *Lab Test Considerations:* Renal function, measured by serum Cr and urine protein, must be monitored within 48 hr before each dose and throughout cidofovir therapy. In patients with proteinuria, administer IV hydration and repeat urine protein test. If renal function deteriorates, dose modification or temporary discontinuation should be considered.

❑ Monitor WBC before each dose. Granulocytopenia may occur.

❑ May cause hyperglycemia, hyperlipemia, hypocalcemia, hypokalemia, and elevated alkaline phosphatase, AST, and ALT.

### POTENTIAL NURSING DIAGNOSES

■ Infection, risk for (Indications).

### IMPLEMENTATION

Probenecid and saline prehydration must be given with cidofovir to minimize renal toxicity. *Probenecid* must be administered 2 g orally given 3 hr before, then 1 g given 2 hr and 8 hr after completion of cidofovir infusion. *Saline prehydration* with 1 L of 0.9% NaCl must be

given over 1–2 hr before cidofovir. A second liter over 1–3 hr is recommended concurrently with or after cidofovir.

❑ Patients receiving foscarnet, amphotericin B, aminoglycoside, NSAIDs, or IV pentamidine should wait at least 7 days after these agents to begin cidofovir.

■ **Intermittent Infusion:** Dilute in 100 ml of 0.9% NaCl. Solution is stable for 24 hr if refrigerated. Allow refrigerated solution to return to room temperature before administration.

■ *Rate:* Administer over 1 hr.

■ **Additive Incompatibility:** Information unavailable. Do not admix with other solutions or medications.

### PATIENT/FAMILY TEACHING

❑ Inform patient that cidofovir is not a cure for CMV retinitis and that retinitis may continue to progress during and after therapy.

❑ Inform patient that concurrent antiretroviral therapy may be continued. However, zidovudine therapy should be temporarily discontinued or decreased by 50% on the days of cidofovir therapy because of the effects of probenicid on zidovudine.

❑ Advise patient of the possibility of renal toxicity from cidofovir. Emphasize the importance of routine lab tests to monitor renal function.

❑ Inform patient that cidofovir may have teratogenic effects. Women should use contraception during and for 1 mo after therapy. Men should use barrier contraception during and for 3 mo after therapy.

❑ Discuss with patient the possibility of hair loss. Explore coping strategies.

❑ Advise patients to have routine ophthalmologic exams after cidofovir therapy.

### EVALUATION

**Effectiveness of therapy can be demonstrated by:** ■ Decrease in symptoms and arrest of progression of CMV retinitis in HIV-infected patients.

## cilostazol
(sil-**os**-tah-zol)
Pletal

**CLASSIFICATION(S):**
**Therapeutic:** *antiplatelet agents*
**Pharmacologic:** *platelet aggregation inhibitors*
**Pregnancy Category C**

## INDICATIONS

■ Reduction of the symptoms of intermittent claudication as measured by increased walking distance.

## ACTION

■ Inhibits the enzyme cyclic adenosine monophosphate (cAMP) phosphodiesterase III (PDE III), which results in increased cAMP in platelets and blood vessels, producing inhibition of platelet aggregation and vasodilation. **Therapeutic Effects:** ■ Reduced symptoms of intermittent claudication with improved walking distance.

## PHARMACOKINETICS

**Absorption:** Slowly absorbed after oral administration.
**Distribution:** Unknown.
**Protein Binding:** 95–98% bound to plasma proteins; one active metabolite is 97.4% bound, the other is 66% bound.
**Metabolism and Excretion:** Extensively metabolized by the liver, two metabolites have platelet aggregation inhibitory activity; metabolites are mostly excreted by the kidneys.
**Half-life:** *Cilostazol and its active metabolites—11–13* hr.

## CONTRAINDICATIONS AND PRECAUTIONS

**Contraindicated in:** ■ Hypersensitivity ■ CHF ■ Lactation.
**Use Cautiously in:** ■ Pregnancy or children (safety not established).

## ADVERSE REACTIONS AND SIDE EFFECTS*

■ **CNS:** <u>headache</u>, dizziness ■ **CV:** palpitations, tachycardia ■ **GI:** diarrhea.

## INTERACTIONS

**Drug-Drug:** ■ Concurrent administration of **ketoconazole, itraconazole, erythromycin, diltiazem, fluconazole, miconazole, fluvoxamine, fluoxetine, nefazodone, sertra-** line, or **omeprazole** decreases metabolism and increases levels and activity of cilostazol (use lower doses) ■ Concurrent use with **aspirin** has additive effects on platelet function.
**Drug-Food:** ■ **Grapefruit juice** inhibits metabolism and increases effects; concurrent use should be avoided.

## ROUTE AND DOSAGE

■ **PO (Adults):** 100 mg twice daily (50 mg twice daily if receiving inhibitors of cilostazol metabolism).

## AVAILABILITY

■ *Tablets:* 50 mg^Rx, 100 mg^Rx ■ Cost: 50 mg and 100 mg, $98.40/60.

TIME/ACTION PROFILE (symptom reduction)

|    | ONSET   | PEAK         | DURATION |
|----|---------|--------------|----------|
| PO | 2–4 wk  | up to 12 wk  | unknown  |

# NURSING IMPLICATIONS

## ASSESSMENT

❑ Assess patient for intermittent claudication before and throughout therapy.
■ *Lab Test Considerations:* May occasionally cause anemia, hyperlipemia, hyperuricemia, and albuminuria. May prolong bleeding time.

## POTENTIAL NURSING DIAGNOSES

■ Activity intolerance (Indications).

## IMPLEMENTATION

■ **PO:** Administer on an empty stomach, 1 hr before or 2 hr after meals.
❑ Do not administer with grapefruit juice. May increase cilostazol levels.

## PATIENT/FAMILY TEACHING

❑ Instruct patient to take cilostazol on an empty stomach, exactly as directed.
❑ May cause dizziness. Caution patient to avoid driving or other activities requiring alertness until response to medication is known.
❑ Advise patient to avoid smoking; nicotine constricts blood vessels.

## EVALUATION

Clinical response to therapy can be evaluated by: ■ Relief from cramping in calf muscles, buttocks, thighs, and feet during exercise

◻ Improvement in walking endurance. Therapeutic effects may be seen in 2–4 wk.

## cimetidine, See HISTAMINE H₂ ANTAGONISTS.

## ciprofloxacin, See FLUOROQUINOLONES.

**High Alert**

## cisplatin
(sis-**pla**-tin)
{Platinol}, Platinol-AQ

*CLASSIFICATION(S):*
*Therapeutic: antineoplastics*
*Pharmacologic: alkylating agents*

**Pregnancy Category D**

### INDICATIONS

■ Metastatic testicular and ovarian carcinoma ■ Advanced bladder cancer ■ Head and neck cancer ■ Cervical cancer ■ Lung cancer ■ Other tumors.

### ACTION

■ Inhibits DNA synthesis by producing cross-linking of parent DNA strands (cell-cycle phase–nonspecific). **Therapeutic Effects:** ■ Death of rapidly replicating cells, particularly malignant ones.

### PHARMACOKINETICS

**Absorption:** IV administration results in complete bioavailability.
**Distribution:** Widely distributed; accumulates for months; enters breast milk.
**Metabolism and Excretion:** Excreted mainly by the kidneys.
**Half-life:** 30–100 hr.

### CONTRAINDICATIONS AND PRECAUTIONS

**Contraindicated in:** ■ Hypersensitivity ■ Pregnancy or lactation.

**Use Cautiously in:** ■ Hearing loss ■ Renal impairment (dosage ↓ recommended) ■ CHF ■ Electrolyte abnormalities ■ Active infections ■ Bone marrow depression ■ Geriatric patients ( ↑ risk of nephrotoxicity, peripheral neuropathy) ■ Chronic debilitating illnesses ■ Patients with childbearing potential.

### ADVERSE REACTIONS AND SIDE EFFECTS*

■ **CNS:** SEIZURES, malaise, weakness ■ **EENT:** ototoxicity, tinnitus ■ **GI:** severe nausea, vomiting, diarrhea, hepatotoxicity ■ **GU:** nephrotoxicity, sterility ■ **Derm:** alopecia ■ **F and E:** hypocalcemia, hypokalemia, hypomagnesemia ■ **Hemat:** LEUKOPENIA, THROMBOCYTOPENIA, anemia ■ **Local:** phlebitis at IV site ■ **Metab:** hyperuricemia ■ **Neuro:** peripheral neuropathy ■ **Misc:** anaphylactoid reactions.

### INTERACTIONS

**Drug-Drug:** ■ ↑ nephrotoxicity and ototoxicity with other **nephrotoxic** and **ototoxic drugs (aminoglycosides, loop diuretics)** ■ ↑ risk of hypokalemia and hypomagnesemia with **loop diuretics** and **amphotericin B** ■ May ↓ **phenytoin** levels ■ ↑ bone marrow depression with other **antineoplastics** or **radiation therapy** ■ May ↓ antibody response to **live-virus vaccines** and ↑ adverse reactions.

### ROUTE AND DOSAGE

Other regimens are used.

■ **IV (Adults):** *Metastatic testicular tumors*—20 mg/m² daily for 5 days repeated q 3–4 wk. *Metastatic ovarian cancer*—75–100 mg/m², repeat q 4 wk in combination cyclophosphamide *or* 100 mg/m² q 3 wk if used as a single agent. *Advanced bladder cancer*—50–70 mg/m² q 3–4 wk as a single agent.

### AVAILABILITY (generic available)

■ *Powder for injection:* 10-mg, 50-mg vials^Rx ■ *Injection:* 1 mg/ml in 50- and 100-mg vials^Rx ■ Cost: 50 ml $249.48/vial, 100 ml $499.91/vial.

{ } = Available in Canada only.
*CAPITALS indicates life-threatening; underlines indicate most frequent.

TIME/ACTION PROFILE (effects on blood counts)

| | ONSET | PEAK | DURATION |
|---|---|---|---|
| IV | unknown | 18–23 days | 39 days |

# NURSING IMPLICATIONS

## ASSESSMENT

❏ Monitor vital signs frequently during administration. Report significant changes.

❏ Monitor intake and output and specific gravity frequently during therapy. Report discrepancies immediately. To reduce the risk of nephrotoxicity, maintain a urinary output of at least 100 ml/hr for 4 hr before initiating and for at least 24 hr after administration.

❏ Encourage patient to drink 2000–3000 ml/day to promote excretion of uric acid. Allopurinol and alkalinization of the urine may be used to help prevent uric acid nephropathy.

❏ Assess patency of IV site frequently during therapy. Cisplatin may cause severe irritation and necrosis of tissue if extravasation occurs. If a large amount of highly concentrated cisplatin solution extravasates, mix 4 ml of 10% sodium thiosulfate with 6 ml of sterile water or 1.6 ml of 25% sodium thiosulfate with 8.4 ml of sterile water and inject 1–4 ml (1 ml for each ml extravasated) through existing line or cannula. Inject subcut if needle has been removed. Sodium thiosulfate inactivates cisplatin.

❏ Severe and protracted nausea and vomiting usually occur 1–4 hr after a dose; vomiting may last for 24 hr. Administer parenteral antiemetic agents 30–45 min before therapy and routinely around the clock for the next 24 hr. Monitor amount of emesis and notify health care professional if emesis exceeds guidelines to prevent dehydration. Nausea and anorexia may persist for up to 1 wk.

❏ Monitor for bone marrow depression. Assess for bleeding (bleeding gums, bruising, petechiae, stools, urine, and emesis) and avoid IM injections and taking rectal temperatures if platelet count is low. Apply pressure to venipuncture sites for 10 min. Assess for signs of infection during neutropenia. Anemia may occur. Monitor for increased fatigue, dyspnea, and orthostatic hypotension.

❏ Monitor for signs of anaphylaxis (facial edema, wheezing, dizziness, fainting, tachycardia, hypotension). Discontinue medication immediately and report symptoms. Epinephrine and resuscitation equipment should be readily available.

❏ Medication may cause ototoxicity and neurotoxicity. Assess patient frequently for dizziness, tinnitus, hearing loss, loss of coordination, loss of taste, or numbness and tingling of extremities; may be irreversible. Notify health care professional promptly if these occur. Audiometry should be performed before initiation of therapy and before subsequent doses. Hearing loss is more frequent with children and usually occurs first with high frequencies and may be unilateral or bilateral.

❏ Monitor for inadvertent cisplatin overdose. Doses >100 mg/m$^2$/cycle once every 3–4 wk are rarely used. Differentiate daily doses from total dose/cycle. Symptoms of high cumulative doses include muscle cramps (localized, painful involuntary skeletal muscle contractions of sudden onset and short duration) and are usually associated with advanced stages of peripheral neuropathy.

■ *Lab Test Considerations:* Monitor CBC with differential and platelet count before and routinely throughout therapy. The nadir of leukopenia, thrombocytopenia, and anemia occurs within 18–23 days and recovery 39 days after a dose. Withhold further doses until WBC is >4000/mm$^3$ and platelet count is >100,000/mm$^3$.

❏ Monitor BUN, serum creatinine, and CCr before initiation of therapy and before each course of cisplatin to detect nephrotoxicity. May cause ↑ BUN and creatinine and ↓ calcium, magnesium, phosphate, sodium, and potassium levels that usually occur the 2nd wk after a dose. Do not administer additional doses until BUN is <25 mg/100 ml and serum creatinine is <1.5 mg/100 ml. May cause ↑ uric acid level, which usually peaks 3–5 days after a dose.

❏ May cause transiently ↑ serum bilirubin and AST concentrations.

❏ May cause positive Coombs' test result.

## POTENTIAL NURSING DIAGNOSES

■ Infection, risk for (Adverse Reactions).

■ Injury, risk for (Side Effects).

# IMPLEMENTATION

- **High Alert:** Fatalities have occurred with chemotherapeutic agents. Before administering, clarify all ambiguous orders; double check single, daily, and course-of-therapy dose limits; have second practitioner independently double check original order, calculations and infusion pump settings. Do not confuse with carboplatin. To prevent confusion, orders should include generic and brand names. Administer under the supervision of a physician experienced in the use of cancer chemotherapeutic agents.
- **General:** Solution should be prepared in a biologic cabinet. Wear gloves, gown, and mask while handling medication. If powder or solution comes in contact with skin or mucosa, wash thoroughly with soap and water. Discard equipment in specially designated containers (see Appendix M).
- Hydrate patient with at least 1–2 L of IV fluid 8–12 hr before initiating therapy with cisplatin. Amifostine may be administered to minimize nephrotoxicity.
- Do not use aluminum needles or equipment during preparation or administration. Aluminum reacts with this drug, forms a black or brown precipitate, and renders the drug ineffective.
- Unopened vials of powder and constituted solution must not be refrigerated.
- **Intermittent Infusion:** Reconstitute 10-mg vials with 10 ml of sterile water for injection and 50-mg vial with 50 ml. Stable for 20 hr if reconstituted with sterile water, for 72 hr with bacteriostatic water. Do not refrigerate, because crystals will form. Solution should be clear and colorless; discard if turbid or if it contains precipitates.
- Dilution in 2 L of 5% dextrose in 0.3% or 0.45% NaCl containing 37.5 g of mannitol is recommended.
- **Rate:** Infuse over 6–8 hr.
- **Continuous Infusion:** Has been administered as continuous infusion over 24 hr to 5 days with resultant decrease in nausea and vomiting.
- **High Alert:** Clarify dose to ensure cumulative dosage is not confused with daily dose; errors may be fatal.

- **Syringe Compatibility:** ◆ bleomycin ◆ cyclophosphamide ◆ doxapram ◆ doxorubicin ◆ droperidol ◆ fluorouracil ◆ furosemide ◆ heparin ◆ leucovorin calcium ◆ methotrexate ◆ metoclopramide ◆ mitomycin ◆ vinblastine ◆ vincristine.
- **Y-Site Compatibility:** ◆ allopurinol ◆ aztreonam ◆ bleomycin ◆ chlorpromazine ◆ cimetidine ◆ cladribine ◆ cyclophosphamide ◆ dexamethasone ◆ diphenhydramine ◆ doxorubicin ◆ doxorubicin liposome ◆ droperidol ◆ etoposide ◆ famotidine ◆ filgrastim ◆ fludarabine ◆ fluorouracil ◆ furosemide ◆ gatifloxacin ◆ ganciclovir ◆ gemcitabine ◆ granisetron ◆ granisetron ◆ heparin ◆ hydromorphone ◆ leucovorin calcium ◆ linezolid ◆ lorazepam ◆ melphalan ◆ methotrexate ◆ methylprednisolone ◆ metoclopramide ◆ mitomycin ◆ morphine ◆ ondansetron ◆ paclitaxel ◆ prochlorperazine edisylate ◆ promethazine ◆ propofol ◆ ranitidine ◆ sargramostim ◆ teniposide ◆ topotecan ◆ vinblastine ◆ vincristine ◆ vinorelbine.
- **Y-Site Incompatibility:** ◆ amifostine ◆ amphotericin B cholesteryl sulfate ◆ cefepime ◆ piperacillin/tazobactam ◆ thiotepa.
- **Additive Compatibility:** ◆ etoposide ◆ floxuridine ◆ ifosfamide ◆ leucovorin calcium ◆ magnesium sulfate ◆ mannitol ◆ ondansetron ◆ 0.9% NaCl ◆ D5/0.9% NaCl.
- **Additive Incompatibility:** ◆ fluorouracil ◆ mesna ◆ sodium bicarbonate ◆ thiotepa.

## PATIENT/FAMILY TEACHING

- Instruct patient to report pain at injection site immediately.
- Instruct patient to notify health care professional promptly if fever; chills; cough; hoarseness; sore throat; signs of infection; lower back or side pain; painful or difficult urination; bleeding gums; bruising; petechiae; blood in stools, urine, or emesis; increased fatigue; dyspnea; or orthostatic hypotension occurs. Caution patient to avoid crowds and persons with known infections. Instruct patient to use soft toothbrush and electric razor and to avoid falls. Caution patient not to drink alcoholic beverages or take medication containing aspirin or NSAIDs; may precipitate gastric bleeding.

---

{ } = Available in Canada only.
*CAPITALS indicates life-threatening; <u>underlines</u> indicate most frequent.

❏ Instruct patient to report promptly any numbness or tingling in extremities or face, difficulty with hearing or tinnitus, unusual swelling, or joint pain. .

❏ Instruct patient not to receive any vaccinations without advice of health care professional.

❏ Advise patient of the need for contraception, although cisplatin may cause infertility.

❏ Emphasize the need for periodic lab tests to monitor for side effects.

## EVALUATION

**Effectiveness of therapy can be demonstrated by:** ■ Decrease in size or spread of malignancies. Therapy should not be administered more frequently than every 3–4 wk, and only if lab values are within acceptable parameters and patient is not exhibiting signs of ototoxicity or other serious adverse effects.

---

# citalopram

(si-**tal**-oh-pram)

Celexa

**CLASSIFICATION(S):**
**Therapeutic:** antidepressants
**Pharmacologic:** selective serotonin reuptake inhibitors (SSRIs)

**Pregnancy Category C**

## INDICATIONS

■ Treatment of depression, often in conjunction with psychotherapy.

## ACTION

■ Selectively inhibits the reuptake of serotonin in the CNS. **Therapeutic Effects:** ■ Antidepressant action.

## PHARMACOKINETICS

**Absorption:** 80% absorbed after oral administration.

**Distribution:** Enters breast milk.

**Metabolism and Excretion:** Mostly metabolized by the liver (10% by CYP 3A4 and 2C19 enzymes); excreted unchanged in urine.

**Half-life:** 35 hr.

## CONTRAINDICATIONS AND PRECAUTIONS

**Contraindicated in:** ■ Hypersensitivity ■ Concurrent MAO inhibitor therapy.

**Use Cautiously in:** ■ History of mania ■ History of seizure disorder ■ Illnesses or conditions that are likely to result in altered metabolism or hemodynamic responses ■ Hepatic impairment or geriatric patients (lower doses recommended) ■ Severe renal impairment ■ Pregnancy, lactation, or children (safety not established).

## ADVERSE REACTIONS AND SIDE EFFECTS*

■ **CNS:** apathy, confusion, drowsiness, insomnia, weakness, agitation, amnesia, anxiety, decreased libido, dizziness, fatigue, impaired concentration, increased depression, migraine headache, suicide attempt ■ **EENT:** abnormal accommodation ■ **Resp:** cough ■ **CV:** postural hypotension, tachycardia ■ **GI:** abdominal pain, anorexia, diarrhea, dry mouth, dyspepsia, flatulence, increased saliva, nausea, altered taste, increased appetite, vomiting ■ **GU:** amenorrhea, dysmenorrhea, ejaculatory delay, impotence, polyuria ■ **Derm:** increased sweating, photosensitivity, pruritus, rash ■ **Metab:** decreased weight, increased weight ■**MS:** arthralgia, myalgia ■ **Neuro:** tremor, paresthesia ■ **Misc:** fever yawning.

## INTERACTIONS

**Drug-Drug:** ■ May cause serious, potentially fatal reactions when used with **MAO inhibitors** ; allow at least 14 days between citalopram and **MAO inhibitors** ■ Use cautiously with other **centrally acting drugs** (including **alcohol, antihistamines, opioid analgesics,** and **sedative/hypnotics**; concurrent use with **alcohol** is not recommended) ■ **Cimetidine** increases blood levels of citalopram ■ Serotonergic effects may be potentiated by **lithium** (concurrent use should be carefully monitored) ■**Ketoconazole, itraconazole, erythromycin,** and **omeprazole** may increase blood levels ■ **Carbamazepine** may decrease blood levels ■ May increase blood levels of **metoprolol** ■ Concurrent use with **tricyclic antidepressants** should be undertaken with caution because of altered pharmacokinetics ■ Concurrent use with **5-HT₁ agonists** used for migraine headaches may increase the risk of adverse reactions (weakness, hyperreflexia, incoordination).

**Drug-Natural Products:** ■ Increased risk of serotinergic side effects including serotonin syndrome with **St. John's wort** and **SAMe.**

## ROUTE AND DOSAGE

■ **PO (Adults):** 20 mg once daily initially, may be increased by 20 mg/day at weekly intervals, up to 60 mg/day (usual dose is 40 mg/day).

■ **PO (Geriatric Patients):** 20 mg once daily initially, may be increased to 40 mg/day only in nonresponding patients.

❏ **Hepatic Impairment**

■ **PO (Adults):** 20 mg once daily initially, may be increased to 40 mg/day only in nonresponding patients.

## AVAILABILITY

■ *Tablets:* 10 mg$^{Rx}$, 20 mg$^{Rx}$, 40 mg$^{Rx}$ ■ Cost: 20 mg $216.06/100, 40 mg $225.46/100 ■ *Oral solution (peppermint flavor):* 10 mg/5 ml$^{Rx}$ ■ Cost: 10 mg/5 ml $207.29/100 ml.

TIME/ACTION PROFILE (antidepressant effect)

| | ONSET | PEAK | DURATION |
|---|---|---|---|
| PO | 1–4 wk | unknown | unknown |

## NURSING IMPLICATIONS

### ASSESSMENT

■ **General Info:** Monitor mood changes throughout therapy.

❏ Assess for suicidal tendencies, especially during early therapy. Restrict amount of drug available to patient.

### POTENTIAL NURSING DIAGNOSES

■ Coping, ineffective (Indications).

■ Injury, risk for (Side Effects).

### IMPLEMENTATION

■ **General:** Do not confuse with Celebrex (celexicob) or Cerebyx (fosphenytoin) or Zyprexa (olanzapine).

■ **PO:** Administer as a single dose in the morning or evening without regard to food.

## PATIENT/FAMILY TEACHING

❏ Instruct patient to take citalopram exactly as directed.

❏ May cause drowsiness, dizziness, impaired concentration, and blurred vision. Caution patient to avoid driving and other activities requiring alertness until response to the drug is known.

❏ Advise patient to avoid alcohol or other CNS depressant drugs during therapy and to consult health care professional before taking other medications with citalopram.

❏ Caution patient to change positions slowly to minimize dizziness.

❏ Advise patient to use sunscreen and wear protective clothing to prevent photosensitivity reactions.

❏ Inform patient that frequent mouth rinses, good oral hygiene, and sugarless gum or candy may minimize dry mouth. If dry mouth persists for more than 2 wk, consult health care professional regarding use of saliva substitute.

❏ Instruct female patients to inform health care professional if pregnancy is planned or suspected, or if they plan to breastfeed an infant.

❏ Caution patients that citalopram should not be used for at least 14 days after discontinuing MAO inhibitors, and at least 14 days should be allowed after stopping citalopram before starting an MAO inhibitor.

❏ Emphasize the importance of follow-up exams to monitor progress. Encourage patient participation in psychotherapy as directed.

### EVALUATION

**Effectiveness of therapy can be demonstrated by:** ■ Increased sense of well-being ❏ Renewed interest in surroundings. May require 1–4 wk of therapy to obtain antidepressant effects.

## clarithromycin
(kla-**rith**-roe-mye-sin)
Biaxin, Biaxin XL

## CLASSIFICATION(S):

**Therapeutic:** *agents for atypical mycobacterium, anti-infectives, antiulcer agents*

**Pharmacologic:** *macrolides*

### Pregnancy Category C

## INDICATIONS

■ Treatment of respiratory tract infections including streptococcal pharyngitis, sinusitis, bronchitis and pneumonia ■ Treatment (with ethambutol) and prevention of disseminated *Mycobacterium avium* complex (MAC) ■ Treatment of following pediatric infections: ❑ Otitis media ❑ Sinusitis ❑ Pharyngitis ❑ Skin/skin structure infections ■ Part of a combination regimen for ulcer disease due to *Helicobacter pylori* ■ Endocarditis prophylaxis.

## ACTION

■ Inhibits protein synthesis at the level of the 50S bacterial ribosome. **Therapeutic Effects:** ■ Bacteriostatic action. **Spectrum:** ■ Active against these gram-positive aerobic bacteria: ❑ *Staphylococcus aureus* ❑ *Streptococcus pneumoniae* ❑ *Streptococcus pyogenes* (group A strep) ■ Active against these gram-negative aerobic bacteria: ❑ *Haemophilus influenzae* ❑ *Moraxella catarrhalis* ■ Also active against: ❑ *Mycoplasma* ❑ *Legionella* ❑ *H. pylori* ❑ *M. avium.*

## PHARMACOKINETICS

**Absorption:** Rapidly absorbed (50%) after oral administration.

**Distribution:** Widely distributed; tissue levels may exceed those in serum.

**Metabolism and Excretion:** 10–15% converted by the liver to 14-hydroxyclarithromycin, which has anti-infective activity; 20–30% excreted unchanged in urine. Metabolized by and also inhibits the CYP3A enzyme system.

**Half-life:** *250-mg dose*—3–4 hr; *500-mg dose*—5–7 hr.

## CONTRAINDICATIONS AND PRECAUTIONS

**Contraindicated in:** ■ Hypersensitivity to clarithromycin, erythromycin, or other macrolide anti-infectives ■ Concurrent use of pimozide ■ Pregnancy and lactation (avoid use during pregnancy unless no alternatives are available).

**Use Cautiously in:** ■ Severe liver or renal impairment (dosage adjustment required if CCr <30 ml/min).

## ADVERSE REACTIONS AND SIDE EFFECTS*

■ **CNS:** headache ■ **CV:** VENTRICULAR ARRHYTHMIAS ■ **GI:** PSEUDOMEMBRANOUS COLITIS, abdominal pain/discomfort, abnormal taste, diarrhea, dyspepsia, nausea.

## INTERACTIONS

**Drug-Drug:** ■ Clarithromycin is an inhibitor of the CYP3A enzyme system. Concurrent use with other agents metabolized by this system can ↑ levels and risk of toxicity ■ May ↑ risk of arrhythmias with **pimozide** ; concurrent use is contraindicated ■ Similar effects may occur with antiarrhythmics; ECG should be monitored for QTc prolongation and serum levels monitored ■ May ↑ serum levels and the risk of toxicity from **carbamazepine**, some **benzodiazepines (midazolam, triazolam, alprazolam), cyclosporine, buspirone, disopyramide, ergot alkaloids, felodipine, omeprazole, tacrolimus, digoxin,** or **theophylline** ■ **Ritonavir** ↑ increases blood levels ( ↓ clarithromycin dose in patients with CC <60 ml/min) ■ ↑ levels of **HMG-CoA reductase inhibitors** and may ↑ risk of rhabdomyolysis ■ May ↑ effect of **warfarin** and **sildenafil** (dosage reduction may be warranted) ■ May ↑ or ↓ effects of **zidovudine** ■ Blood levels are ↑ by **delavirdine** and **fluconazole** ■ Blood levels may be ↓ by **rifampin** and **rifabutin.**

## ROUTE AND DOSAGE

■ **PO (Adults):** *Pharyngitis/tonsillitis*—250 mg q 12 hr for 10 days; *Acute maxillary sinusitis*—500 mg q 12 hr for 14 days or 1000 mg once daily for 14 days as XL tablets; *Acute exacerbation of chronic bronchitis*—250–500 mg q 12 hr for 7–14 days or 1000 mg once daily for 7 days as XL tablets; *Community-Acquired pneumonia*—250 q 12 hr for 7–14 days or 1000 mg once daily for 7 days as XL tablets; *skin/skin structure infections*—250 mg q 12 hr for 7–14 days; *H. pylori*—500 mg 2–3 times daily with a proton pump inhibitor (lansoprazole or omeprazole) or ranitadine with or without amoxicillin for 10–14 days; *Endocarditis prophylaxis*—500 mg 1 hr before procedure; *MAC prophylaxis/treatment*—500 mg twice daily, for active infection another anti-mycobacterial is required.

- **PO (Children):** *Most infections*—7.5 mg/ kg q 12 hr for 10 days (up to 500 mg/dose for MAC). *Endocarditis prophylaxis*—15 mg/kg 1 hr before procedure.

❑ **Renal Impairment**
- **PO (Adults):** *CCr <30 ml/min*—250 mg 1-2 times daily, a 500-mg initial dose may be used.
- **PO (Children):** *CCr <30 ml/min*—decrease dose by 50% or double dosing interval.

## AVAILABILITY

■ *Tablets:* 250 mg$^{Rx}$, 500 mg$^{Rx}$ ■ Cost: 250-mg tablets—$79.34/20; 500-mg tablets—$248.58/60 ■ *Extended-release tablets:* 500 mg$^{Rx}$ ■ *Oral suspension (fruit punch and vanilla flavors):* 125 mg/5 ml$^{Rx}$, 250 mg/5 ml$^{Rx}$ ■ Cost: 125 mg/5 ml 50-ml bottle—$20.31; 250 mg/5 ml 50-ml bottle—$38.68 ■ amoxicillin and lansoprozole as part of a compliance package (Prevpac$^{Rx}$, Losec 1-2-3-A$^{Rx}$); omeprazole and metronidazole as part of a compliance package (Losec 1-2-3 M$^{Rx}$); See Appendix B.

TIME/ACTION PROFILE (serum levels)

| | ONSET | PEAK | DURATION |
|---|---|---|---|
| PO | unknown | 2 hr | 12 hr |
| PO-XL | unknown | 4 hr | 24 hr |

## NURSING IMPLICATIONS

### ASSESSMENT

- **General Info:** Assess patient for infection (vital signs; appearance of wound, sputum, urine, and stool; WBC) at beginning of and during therapy.
- ❑ Obtain specimens for culture and sensitivity before initiating therapy. First dose may be given before receiving results.
- **Ulcers:** Assess patient for epigastric or abdominal pain and frank or occult blood in the stool, emesis, or gastric aspirate.
- *Lab Test Considerations:* May rarely cause ↑ serum AST, ALT, and alkaline phosphatase concentrations.
- ❑ May occasionally cause ↑ BUN.

## POTENTIAL NURSING DIAGNOSES
- Infection, risk for (Indications, Side Effects).
- Noncompliance (Patient/Family Teaching).

## IMPLEMENTATION
- **PO:** Administer around the clock, without regard to meals. Food slows but does not decrease the extent of absorption.
- ❑ Administer XL tablets with food; do not crush, break or chew.
- ❑ Shake suspension well before administration. Store suspension at room temperature; do not refrigerate.
- ❑ Do not administer within 4 hr of zidovudine.

## PATIENT/FAMILY TEACHING
- ❑ Instruct patient to take medication around the clock and to finish the drug completely as directed, even if feeling better. Take missed doses as soon as possible, unless almost time for next dose. Do not double doses. Advise patient that sharing of this medication may be dangerous.
- ❑ Advise patient to report the signs of superinfection (black, furry overgrowth on the tongue; vaginal itching or discharge; loose or foul-smelling stools).
- ❑ Instruct patient to notify health care professional if fever and diarrhea develop, especially if stool contains blood, pus, or mucus. Advise patient not to treat diarrhea without consulting health care professional.
- ❑ Caution patients taking zidovudine that clarithromycin and zidovudine must be taken at least 4 hr apart.
- ❑ Advise patient to notify health care professional if pregnancy is planned or suspected.
- ❑ Instruct the patient to notify health care professional if symptoms do not improve within a few days.

## EVALUATION
**Clinical response to therapy can be evaluated by:** ■ Resolution of the signs and symptoms of infection. Length of time for complete resolution depends on the organism and site of infection ■ Treatment of ulcers ■ Endocarditis prophylaxis.

## clindamycin

(klin-da-**mye**-sin)

Cleocin, Cleocin T, Clinda-Derm, Clindets, C/T/S, {Dalacin C}, {Dalacin T}

*CLASSIFICATION(S):*
*Therapeutic: anti-infectives*

**Pregnancy Category B**

### INDICATIONS

■ **PO, IM, IV:** Treatment of: ❑ Skin and skin structure infections ❑ Respiratory tract infections ❑ Septicemia ❑ Intra-abdominal infections ❑ Gynecologic infections ❑ Osteomyelitis ❑ Endocarditis prophylaxis ■ **Topical:** Severe acne ■ **Vag:** Bacterial vaginosis. **Unlabeled uses:** ■ **PO, IM, IV:** Treatment of *Pneumocystis carinii* pneumonia, CNS toxoplasmosis, and babesiosis.

### ACTION

■ Inhibits protein synthesis in susceptible bacteria at the level of the 50S ribosome. **Therapeutic Effects:** ■ Bactericidal or bacteriostatic, depending on susceptibility and concentration. **Spectrum:** ■ Active against most gram-positive aerobic cocci, including: ❑ Staphylococci ❑ *Streptococcus pneumoniae* ❑ Other streptococci, but not enterococci ■ Has good activity against those anaerobic bacteria that cause bacterial vaginosis, including *Bacteroides fragilis, Gardnerella vaginalis, Mobiluncus* spp, *Mycoplasma hominis*, and *Corynebacterium* ■ Also active against *P. carinii* and *Toxoplasma gondii*.

### PHARMACOKINETICS

**Absorption:** Well absorbed following PO/IM administration. Minimal absorption following topical/vaginal use.

**Distribution:** Widely distributed. Does not significantly cross blood-brain barrier. Crosses the placenta; enters breast milk.

**Protein Binding:** 90%.

**Metabolism and Excretion:** Mostly metabolized by the liver.

**Half-life:** 2–3 hr.

### CONTRAINDICATIONS AND PRECAUTIONS

**Contraindicated in:** ■ Hypersensitivity ■ Previous pseudomembranous colitis ■ Severe liver impairment ■ Diarrhea ■ Known alcohol intolerance (topical solution, suspension).

**Use Cautiously in:** ■ Pregnancy or lactation (safety not established for systemic and topical; vaginal approved for use in 3rd trimester of pregnancy).

### ADVERSE REACTIONS AND SIDE EFFECTS*

■ **CNS:** dizziness, headache, vertigo ■ **CV:** arrhythmias, hypotension ■ **GI:** PSEUDOMEMBRANOUS COLITIS, diarrhea, bitter taste (IV only), nausea, vomiting ■ **Derm:** rashes ■ **Local:** phlebitis at IV site.

### INTERACTIONS

**Drug-Drug:** ■ **Kaolin/pectin** may decrease GI absorption ■ May enhance the neuromuscular blocking action of other **neuromuscular blocking agents** ■ **Topical:** Concurrent use with **irritants, abrasives,** or **desquamating agents** may result in additive irritation.

### ROUTE AND DOSAGE

■ **PO (Adults):** *Most infections*—150–300 mg q 6 hr. *P. carinii pneumonia*—1200–1800 mg/day in divided doses with 15–30 mg primaquine/day (unlabeled). *CNS toxoplasmosis*—1200–2400 mg/day in divided doses with pyrimethamine 50–100 mg/day (unlabeled).

■ **PO (Children >1 mo):** 2–5 mg/kg q 6 hr *or* 2.7–6.7 mg/kg q 8 hr. (Children ≤10 mg should receive at least 37.5 mg q 8 hr.)

■ **IM, IV (Adults):** *Most infections*—300–600 mg q 6–8 hr *or* 900 mg q 8 hr (up to 4.8 g/day IV has been used; single IM doses of >600 mg are not recommended). *P. carinii pneumonia*—2400–2700 mg/day in divided doses with primaquine (unlabeled). *Toxoplasmosis*—1200–4800 mg/day in divided doses with pyrimethamine.

■ **IM, IV (Children >1 mo):** 3.75–10 mg/kg (87.5–112.5 mg/m²) q 6 hr *or* 5–13.3 mg/kg (116.7–150 mg/m²) q 8 hr (300 mg/day minimum; up to 7.5 mg/kg q 6 hr for bone infections).

■ **IM, IV (Infants <1 mo):** 3.75–5 mg/kg q 6 hr *or* 5–6.7 mg/kg q 8 hr.

- **Vag (Adults and Adolescents):** 1 applicatorful (5 g) hs for 3 or 7 days (7 days in pregnant patients) *or* 1 suppository (100 mg) at bedtime for 3 nights.
- **Topical (Adults and Adolescents):** *Solution*—1% solution/suspension applied twice daily (range 1–4 times daily). *Gel*—1% gel applied twice daily.

## AVAILABILITY (generic available)

- *Capsules:* 75 mg$^{Rx}$, 150 mg$^{Rx}$, 300 mg$^{Rx}$ ▪ Cost: 75 mg $114.90/100, 150 mg $119.12/100, 300 mg $439.15/100 ▪ *Oral suspension:* 75 mg/5 ml$^{Rx}$ ▪ *Injection:* 150 mg/ml$^{Rx}$
- *Topical:* 1% lotion, gel, solution, suspension, single-use applicators$^{Rx}$ ▪ benzoyl peroxide (BenzaClin; See Appendix B).
- *Vaginal cream:* 2% cream$^{Rx}$ ▪ *Vaginal suppositories (ovules):* 100 mg$^{Rx}$.

TIME/ACTION PROFILE (blood levels)

| | ONSET | PEAK | DURATION |
|---|---|---|---|
| PO | rapid | 45 min | 6–8 hr |
| IM | rapid | 1.3 hr | 6–8 hr |
| IV | rapid | end of infusion | 6–8 hr |

# NURSING IMPLICATIONS

## ASSESSMENT

- ❑ Assess patient for infection (vital signs; appearance of wound, sputum, urine, and stool; WBC) at beginning of and throughout therapy.
- ❑ Obtain specimens for culture and sensitivity prior to initiating therapy. First dose may be given before receiving results.
- ❑ Monitor bowel elimination. Diarrhea, abdominal cramping, fever, and bloody stools should be reported to health care professional promptly as a sign of pseudomembranous colitis. This may begin up to several weeks following the cessation of therapy.
- ❑ Assess patient for hypersensitivity (skin rash, urticaria).
- **Lab Test Considerations:** Monitor CBC; may cause transient decrease in leukocytes, eosinophils, and platelets.
- ❑ May cause elevated alkaline phosphatase, bilirubin, CPK, AST, and ALT concentrations.

## POTENTIAL NURSING DIAGNOSES

- Infection, risk for (Indications, Side Effects).
- Diarrhea (Side Effects).

## IMPLEMENTATION

- **PO:** Administer with a full glass of water. May be given with meals. Shake liquid preparations well. Do not refrigerate. Stable for 14 days at room temperature.
- **IM:** Do not administer >600 mg in a single IM injection.
- **Intermittent Infusion:** Do not administer as an undiluted IV bolus. Dilute each 300 or 600 mg for IV administration with at least 50 ml and 900 or 1200 mg with at least 100 ml of D5W, D10W, D5/0.45% NaCl, D5/0.9% NaCl, D5/Ringer's injection, 0.9% NaCl, or LR for injection. Stable for 24 hr at room temperature. Crystals may occur if refrigerated, but dissolve when warmed to room temperature. Do not administer solution with undissolved crystals.
- *Rate:* Administer each 300 mg over a minimum of 10 min. Do not give more than 1200 mg in a single 1-hr infusion.
- **Continuous Infusion:** May also be initially administered as a single rapid infusion, followed by continuous IV infusion.
- *Rate:* May also administer at an infusion rate of 10–20 mg/min for 30 min, followed by a continuous infusion rate of 0.75–1.25 mg/min.
- **Syringe Compatibility:** ◆ amikacin ◆ aztreonam ◆ gentamicin ◆ heparin.
- **Syringe Incompatibility:** ◆ tobramycin.
- **Y-Site Compatibility:** ◆ amifostine ◆ amiodarone ◆ aztreonam ◆ cefepime ◆ cisatracurium ◆ cyclophosphamide ◆ diltiazem ◆ docetaxel ◆ doxorubicin liposome ◆ enalaprilat ◆ esmolol ◆ etoposide ◆ fludarabine ◆ foscarnet ◆ gatifloxacin ◆ gemcitabine ◆ granisetron ◆ heparin ◆ hydromorphone ◆ labetalol ◆ levofloxacin ◆ linezolid ◆ magnesium sulfate ◆ melphalan ◆ meperidine ◆ midazolam ◆ morphine ◆ multivitamins ◆ ondansetron ◆ perphenazine ◆ piperacillin/tazobactam ◆ propofol ◆ remifentanil ◆ sargramostim ◆ tacrolimus ◆ teniposide ◆ theophylline ◆ thiotepa ◆ vinorelbine ◆ vitamin B complex with C ◆ zidovudine.

- **Y-Site Incompatibility:** ◆ allopurinol ◆ filgrastim ◆ fluconazole ◆ idarubicin.
- **Vag:** Applicators are supplied for vaginal administration. When treating bacterial vaginosis, concurrent treatment of male partner is not usually necessary.
- **Topical:** Contact with eyes, mucous membranes, and open cuts should be avoided during topical application. If accidental contact occurs, rinse with copious amounts of cool water.
- Wash affected areas with warm water and soap, rinse, and pat dry prior to application. Apply to entire affected area.

## PATIENT/FAMILY TEACHING

- **General Info:** Instruct patient to take medication around the clock at evenly spaced times and to finish the drug completely as directed, even if feeling better. If a dose is missed, take as soon as possible unless almost time for next dose. Do not double doses. Advise patient that sharing of this medication may be dangerous.
- Instruct patient to notify health care professional immediately if diarrhea, abdominal cramping, fever, or bloody stools occur and not to treat with antidiarrheals without consulting health care professional.
- Advise patient to report signs of superinfection (furry overgrowth on the tongue, vaginal or anal itching or discharge).
- Notify health care professional if no improvement within a few days.
- Patients with a history of rheumatic heart disease or valve replacement need to be taught the importance of antimicrobial prophylaxis before invasive medical or dental procedures.
- **IV:** Inform patient that bitter taste occurring with IV administration is not clinically significant.
- **Vag:** Instruct patient on proper use of vaginal applicator. Insert high into vagina at bedtime. Instruct patient to remain recumbent for at least 30 min following insertion. Advise patient to use sanitary napkin to prevent staining of clothing or bedding. Continue therapy during menstrual period.
- Advise patient to refrain from vaginal sexual intercourse during treatment.
- Caution patient that mineral oil in clindamycin cream may weaken latex or rubber contraceptive devices. Such products should not be used within 72 hr of vaginal cream.
- **Topical:** Caution patient applying topical clindamycin that solution is flammable (vehicle is isopropyl alcohol). Avoid application while smoking or near heat or flame.
- Advise patient to notify health care professional if excessive drying of skin occurs.
- Advise patient to wait 30 min after washing or shaving area before applying.

### EVALUATION

**Clinical response to therapy can be evaluated by:** ■ Resolution of the signs and symptoms of infection. Length of time for complete resolution depends on the organism and site of infection ■ Endocarditis prophylaxis ■ Improvement in acne vulgaris lesions. Improvement should be seen in 6 wk but may take 8–12 wk for maximum benefit.

## clobetasol, See CORTICOSTEROIDS (TOPICAL/LOCAL).

## clocortolone, See CORTICOSTEROIDS (TOPICAL/LOCAL).

## clonazepam

(kloe-**na**-ze-pam)
Klonopin, {Rivotril}, {Syn-Clonazepam}

### CLASSIFICATION(S):
**Therapeutic:** *anticonvulsants*
**Pharmacologic:** *benzodiazepines*

Schedule IV

Pregnancy Category C

### INDICATIONS

■ Prophylaxis of: ❑ Petit mal ❑ Petit mal variant ❑ Akinetic ❑ Myoclonic seizures ■ Management of panic disorder. **Unlabeled uses:** ■ Uncontrolled leg movements during sleep ■ Neuralgias ■ Sedation.

## ACTION

■ Anticonvulsant effects may be due to presynaptic inhibition ■ Produces sedative effects in the CNS, probably by stimulating inhibitory GABA receptors. **Therapeutic Effects:** ■ Prevention of seizures.

## PHARMACOKINETICS

**Absorption:** Well absorbed from the GI tract. **Distribution:** Probably crosses the blood-brain barrier and the placenta. **Metabolism and Excretion:** Mostly metabolized by the liver. **Half-life:** 18–50 hr.

## CONTRAINDICATIONS AND PRECAUTIONS

**Contraindicated in:** ■ Hypersensitivity to clonazepam or other benzodiazepines ■ Severe liver disease.

**Use Cautiously in:** ■ Narrow-angle glaucoma ■ Chronic respiratory disease ■ History of porphyria ■ Do not discontinue abruptly ■ Pregnancy, lactation, or children (safety not established; chronic use during pregnancy may result in withdrawal in the neonate).

## ADVERSE REACTIONS AND SIDE EFFECTS*

■ **CNS:** <u>behavioral changes</u>, <u>drowsiness</u> ■ **EENT:** abnormal eye movements, diplopia, nystagmus ■ **Resp:** increased secretions ■ **CV:** palpitations ■ **GI:** constipation, diarrhea, hepatitis ■ **GU:** dysuria, nocturia, urinary retention ■ **Hemat:** anemia, eosinophilia, leukopenia, thrombocytopenia ■ **Neuro:** <u>ataxia</u>, hypotonia ■ **Misc:** fever, physical dependence, psychological dependence, tolerance.

## INTERACTIONS

**Drug-Drug:** ■ **Alcohol, antidepressants, antihistamines,** other **benzodiazepines,** and **opioid analgesics**—concurrent use results in additive CNS depression ■ **Cimetidine, hormonal contraceptives, disulfiram, fluoxetine, isoniazid, ketoconazole, metoprolol, propoxyphene, propranolol,** or **valproic acid** may decrease the metabolism of clonazepam, enhancing its actions ■ May decrease efficacy of **levodopa** ■ **Rifampin** or **barbiturates** may increase the metabolism and decrease effectiveness of clonazepam ■ Sedative effects may be decreased by **theophylline** ■ May increase serum **phenytoin** levels ■ **Phenytoin** may decrease serum clonazepam levels.

**Drug-Natural Products:** ■ Concomitant use of **kava, valerian, skullcap, chamomile,** or **hops** can increase CNS depression.

## ROUTE AND DOSAGE

■ **PO (Adults):** 0.5 mg 3 times daily; may increase by 0.5–1 mg q 3rd day. Total daily maintenance dose not to exceed 20 mg. *Panic disorder*—0.125 mg twice daily; increase after 3 days toward target dose of 1 mg/day (some patients may require up to 4 mg/day).

■ **PO (Children <10 yr or 30 kg):** Initial daily dose 0.01–0.03 mg/kg/day (not to exceed 0.05 mg/kg/day) given in 2–3 equally divided doses; increase by no more than 0.25–0.5 mg q 3rd day until therapeutic blood levels are reached (not to exceed 0.2 mg/kg/day).

## AVAILABILITY (generic available)

■ *Tablets:* 0.5 mg^Rx, 1 mg^Rx, 2 mg^Rx ■ Cost: *Klonopin*—0.5 mg $73.99/100; 1 mg $84.40/100; 2 mg $116.96/100; *generic*—0.5 mg $71.37/100; 1 mg $77.80/100; 2 mg $112.82/100.

TIME/ACTION PROFILE (anticonvulsant activity)

| | ONSET | PEAK | DURATION |
|---|---|---|---|
| PO | 20–60 min | 1–2 hr | 6–12 hr |

# NURSING IMPLICATIONS

## ASSESSMENT

❑ Observe and record intensity, duration, and location of seizure activity.
❑ Assess degree and manifestations of anxiety and mental status prior to and periodically during therapy.
❑ Assess patient for drowsiness, unsteadiness, and clumsiness. These symptoms are dose related and most severe during initial therapy; may decrease in severity or disappear with continued or long-term therapy.
■ *Lab Test Considerations:* Patients on prolonged therapy should have CBC and liver

function test results evaluated periodically. May cause an increase in serum bilirubin, AST, and ALT.

❑ May cause decreased thyroidal uptake of sodium iodide, $^{123}$I, and $^{131}$I.

■ *Toxicity and Overdose:* Therapeutic serum concentrations are 20–80 mg/ml.

## POTENTIAL NURSING DIAGNOSES

■ Injury, risk for (Indications, Side Effects).

## IMPLEMENTATION

■ **General:** Do not confuse clonazepam with clonidine or clorazepate.

❑ Institute seizure precautions for patients on initial therapy or undergoing dose manipulations.

■ **PO:** Administer with food to minimize gastric irritation. Tablets may be crushed if patient has difficulty swallowing.

## PATIENT/FAMILY TEACHING

❑ Instruct patient to take medication exactly as directed. Missed doses should be taken within 1 hr or omitted; do not double doses. Abrupt withdrawal of clonazepam may cause status epilepticus, tremors, nausea, vomiting, and abdominal and muscle cramps.

❑ Medication may cause drowsiness or dizziness. Advise patient to avoid driving or other activities requiring alertness until response to drug is known.

❑ Caution patient to avoid taking alcohol or other CNS depressants concurrently with this medication.

❑ Advise patient to notify health care professional of medication regimen prior to treatment or surgery.

❑ Instruct patient and family to notify health care professional of unusual tiredness, bleeding, sore throat, fever, clay-colored stools, yellowing of skin, or behavioral changes.

❑ Patient on anticonvulsant therapy should carry identification at all times describing disease process and medication regimen.

❑ Emphasize the importance of follow-up exams to determine effectiveness of the medication.

## EVALUATION

**Effectiveness of therapy can be demonstrated by:** ■ Decrease or cessation of seizure activity without undue sedation. Dosage adjust-

ments may be required after several months of therapy ■ Decrease in frequency and severity of panic attacks ■ Relief of leg movements during sleep ■ Decrease in pain from neuralgia.

# clonidine
(**klon**-i-deen)
Catapres, Catapres-TTS, {Dixarit}, Duraclon

## CLASSIFICATION(S):
*Therapeutic:* antihypertensives
*Pharmacologic:* adrenergics (centrally acting)

## Pregnancy Category C

## INDICATIONS

■ **PO, Transdermal:** Management of mild to moderate hypertension ■ **Epidural:** Management of cancer pain unresponsive to opioids alone. **Unlabeled uses:** ■ Management of opioid withdrawal.

## ACTION

■ Stimulates alpha-adrenergic receptors in the CNS; which results in decreased sympathetic outflow inhibiting cardioacceleration and vasoconstriction centers ■ Prevents pain signal transmission to the CNS by stimulating alpha-adrenergic receptors in the spinal cord. **Therapeutic Effects:** ■ Decreased blood pressure ■ Decreased pain.

## PHARMACOKINETICS

**Absorption:** Well absorbed from the GI tract and skin. Enters systemic circulation following epidural use. Some absorption follows sublingual administration.

**Distribution:** Widely distributed; enters CNS. Crosses the placenta readily; enters breast milk in high concentrations.

**Metabolism and Excretion:** Mostly metabolized by the liver; 40–50% eliminated unchanged in urine.

**Half-life:** *Plasma*—12–22 hr; *CNS*—1.3 hr.

## CONTRAINDICATIONS AND PRECAUTIONS

**Contraindicated in:** ■ Hypersensitivity ■ *Epidural*—injection site infection, anticoagulant therapy, or bleeding problems.

Use Cautiously in: ■ Serious cardiac or cerebrovascular disease ■ Renal insufficiency ■ Geriatric patients (dosage reduction may be required) ■ Pregnancy or lactation (safety not established).

## ADVERSE REACTIONS AND SIDE EFFECTS*

■ **CNS:** drowsiness, depression, dizziness, nervousness, nightmares ■ **CV:** bradycardia, hypotension (increased with epidural), palpitations ■ **GI:** dry mouth, constipation, nausea, vomiting ■ **GU:** impotence ■ **Derm:** rash, sweating ■ **F and E:** sodium retention ■ **Metab:** weight gain ■ **Misc:** withdrawal phenomenon.

## INTERACTIONS

**Drug-Drug:** ■ Additive sedation with **CNS depressants,** including **alcohol, antihistamines, opioid analgesics,** and **sedative/ hypnotics** ■ Additive hypotension with other **antihypertensives** and **nitrates** ■ Additive bradycardia with **myocardial depressants,** including **beta blockers** ■ **MAO inhibitors, amphetamines, beta blockers, prazosin,** or **tricyclic antidepressants** may decrease antihypertensive effect ■ Withdrawal phenomenon may be increased by discontinuation of **beta blockers** ■ Epidural clonidine prolongs the effects of epidurally administered **local anesthetics** ■ May decrease effectiveness of **levodopa** ■ Increased risk of adverse cardiovascular reactions with **verapamil.**

## ROUTE AND DOSAGE

■ **PO (Adults):** *Hypertension (initial dose)*—100 mcg (0.1 mg) bid, increase by 100–200 mcg (0.1–0.2 mg)/day q 2–4 days. *Usual maintenance dose* is 200–600 mcg (0.2–0.6 mg)/day in 2–3 divided doses (up to 2.4 mg/day). *Urgent treatment*—200 mcg (0.2 mg) loading dose, then 100 mcg (0.1 mg) q hr until blood pressure is controlled or 800 mcg (0.8 mg) total has been administered; follow with maintenance dosing. *Opioid withdrawal*—300 mcg (0.3 mg)–1.2 mg/day, may be decreased by 50%/ day for 3 days, then discontinued or decreased by 100–200 mcg (0.1–0.2 mg)/day.

■ **PO (Geriatric Patients):** 100 mcg (0.1 mg) at bedtime initially, increased as needed.

■ **PO (Children):** 50–400 mcg (0.05–0.4 mg) twice daily.

■ **Transdermal (Adults):** *Hypertension*—Transdermal system delivering 100–300 mcg (0.1–0.3 mg)/24 hr applied every 7 days. Initiate with 100 mcg (0.1 mg)/24 hr system; dosage increments may be made q 1–2 wk when system is changed.

■ **Epidural: (Adults):** 30 mcg/hr initially; titrated according to need.

■ **Epidural: (Children):** 0.5 mcg/kg/hr initially; titrated according to need.

## AVAILABILITY (generic available)

■ *Tablets:* {25 mcg (0.025 mg)[Rx]}, 100 mcg (0.1 mg)[Rx], 200 mcg (0.2 mg)[Rx], 300 mcg (0.3 mg)[Rx] ■ Cost: *Catapres*—0.1 mg $72.11/100, 0.2 mg $110.32/100, 0.3 mg $138.43/100; *generic*—0.1 mg $18.58/100, 0.2 mg $31.10/ 100, 0.3 mg $34.85/100 ■ *Transdermal systems:* Catapres-TTS 1[Rx] contains 2.5 mg total clonidine content, releases 0.1 mg/24 hr; Catapres-TTS 2[Rx] contains 5 mg total clonidine content, releases 0.2 mg/24 hr; Catapres-TTS 3[Rx] contains 7.5 mg total clonidine content, releases 0.3 mg/24 hr ■ *Solution for epidural injection:* 100 mcg/ml in 10-ml vials[Rx], 500 mcg/ml in 10-ml vials[Rx] ■ chlorthalidone (Combipres)[Rx]. See Appendix B.

TIME/ACTION PROFILE (PO, TD = antihypertensive effect; epidural = analgesia)

| | ONSET | PEAK | DURATION |
|---|---|---|---|
| PO | 30–60 min | 2–4 hr | 8–12 hr |
| Transdermal | 2–3 days | unknown | 7 days† |
| Epidural | unknown | unknown | unknown |

†8 hr following removal of patch.

## NURSING IMPLICATIONS

### ASSESSMENT

■ **General Info:** Monitor intake and output ratios and daily weight, and assess for edema daily, especially at beginning of therapy.
❏ Monitor blood pressure and pulse frequently during initial dosage adjustment and periodi-

cally throughout therapy. Report significant changes.

■ **Pain:** Assess location, character, and intensity of pain prior to, frequently during first few days, and routinely throughout administration.

❏ Monitor for fever as potential sign of catheter infection.

■ **Opioid Withdrawal:** Monitor patient for signs and symptoms of opioid withdrawal (tachycardia, fever, runny nose, diarrhea, sweating, nausea, vomiting, irritability, stomach cramps, shivering, unusually large pupils, weakness, difficulty sleeping, gooseflesh).

■ *Lab Test Considerations:* May cause transient increase in blood glucose levels.

❏ May cause decreased urinary catecholamine and vanillylmandelic acid (VMA) concentrations; these may increase on abrupt withdrawal.

❏ May cause weakly positive Coombs' test result.

## POTENTIAL NURSING DIAGNOSES

■ Pain, acute (Indications).
■ Injury, risk for (Side Effects).

## IMPLEMENTATION

■ **General:** Do not confuse Catapres (clonidine) with Cataflam (diclofenac).

❏ Do not confuse clonidine with clonazepam (Klonopin).

❏ In the perioperative setting, continue clonidine up to 4 hr prior to surgery and resume as soon as possible thereafter. Do not interrupt *transdermal clonidine* during surgery. Monitor blood pressure carefully.

■ **PO:** Administer last dose of the day at bedtime.

■ **Transdermal:** Transdermal system should be applied once every 7 days. May be applied to any hairless site; avoid cuts or calluses. Absorption is greater when placed on chest or upper arm and decreased when placed on thigh. Rotate sites. Wash area with soap and water; dry thoroughly before application. Apply firm pressure over patch to ensure contact with skin, especially around edges. Remove old system and discard. System includes a protective adhesive overlay to be applied over medication patch to ensure adhesion, should medication patch loosen.

## PATIENT/FAMILY TEACHING

■ **General Info:** Instruct patient to take clonidine at the same time each day, even if feeling well. If a dose is missed, take as soon as remembered. If more than 1 oral dose in a row is missed or if transdermal system is late in being changed by 3 or more days, consult health care professional. All routes of clonidine should be gradually discontinued over 2–4 days to prevent rebound hypertension.

❏ Advise patient to make sure enough medication is available for weekends, holidays, and vacations. A written prescription may be kept in wallet in case of emergency.

❏ Clonidine may cause drowsiness, which usually diminishes with continued use. Advise patient to avoid driving or other activities requiring alertness until response to medication is known.

❏ Caution patient to avoid sudden changes in position to decrease orthostatic hypotension. Use of alcohol, standing for long periods, exercising, and hot weather may increase orthostatic hypotension.

❏ If dry mouth occurs, frequent mouth rinses, good oral hygiene, and sugarless gum or candy may decrease effect. If dry mouth continues for more than 2 wk, consult health care professional.

❏ Caution patient to avoid concurrent use of alcohol or other CNS depressants with this medication.

❏ Advise patient to consult health care professional before taking any OTC cough, cold, or allergy remedies.

❏ Advise patient to notify health care professional of medication regimen prior to treatment or surgery.

❏ Advise patient to notify health care professional if itching or redness of skin (with transdermal patch), mental depression, swelling of feet and lower legs, paleness or cold feeling in fingertips or toes, or vivid dreams or nightmares occur. May require discontinuation of therapy, especially with depression.

■ **Hypertension:** Encourage patient to comply with additional interventions for hypertension (weight reduction, low-sodium diet, discontinuation of smoking, moderation of alcohol consumption, regular exercise, and stress management). Medication helps control but does not cure hypertension.

▫ Instruct patient and family on proper technique for blood pressure monitoring. Advise them to check blood pressure at least weekly and report significant changes.

▪ **Transdermal:** Instruct patient on proper application of transdermal system. Do not cut or trim unit. Transdermal system can remain in place during bathing or swimming.

## EVALUATION

**Effectiveness of therapy can be demonstrated by:** ▪ Decrease in blood pressure ▪ Decrease in severity of pain ▪ Decrease in the signs and symptoms of opioid withdrawal.

---

## clopidogrel

(kloh-**pid**-oh-grel)

Plavix

**CLASSIFICATION(S):**

**Therapeutic:** antiplatelet agents
**Pharmacologic:** platelet aggregation inhibitors

**Pregnancy Category B**

---

## INDICATIONS

▪ Reduction of atherosclerotic events (MI, stroke, vascular death) in patients at risk for such events including recent MI, acute coronary syndrome (unstable angina/non–Q-wave MI), stroke, or peripheral vascular disease.

## ACTION

▪ Inhibits platelet aggregation by irreversibly inhibiting the binding of ATP to platelet receptors. **Therapeutic Effects:** ▪ Decreased occurrence of atherosclerotic events in patients at risk.

## PHARMACOKINETICS

**Absorption:** Well absorbed following oral administration; rapidly metabolized to an active antiplatelet compound. Parent drug has no antiplatelet activity.

**Distribution:** Unknown.

**Protein Binding:** Clopidogrel—98%; active metabolite—94%.

**Metabolism and Excretion:** Rapidly and extensively converted by the liver to its active metabolite, which is then eliminated 50% in urine and 45% in feces.

**Half-life:** 8 hr (active metabolite).

## CONTRAINDICATIONS AND PRECAUTIONS

**Contraindicated in:** ▪ Hypersensitivity ▪ Pathologic bleeding (peptic ulcer, intracranial hemorrhage) ▪ Lactation.

**Use Cautiously in:** ▪ Patients at risk for bleeding (trauma, surgery, or other pathologic conditions) ▪ History of GI bleeding/ulcer disease ▪ Severe hepatic impairment ▪ Pregnancy or children (safety not established; use in pregnancy only if clearly indicated).

## ADVERSE REACTIONS AND SIDE EFFECTS*

Incidence of adverse reactions similar to that of aspirin. ▪ **CNS:** depression, dizziness, fatigue, headache ▪ **EENT:** epistaxis ▪ **Resp:** cough, dyspnea ▪ **CV:** chest pain, edema, hypertension ▪ **GI:** GI BLEEDING, abdominal pain, diarrhea, dyspepsia, gastritis ▪ **Derm:** pruritus, purpura, rash ▪ **Hemat:** BLEEDING, NEUTROPENIA, THROMBOTIC THROMBOCYTPENIC PURPURA ▪ **Metab:** hypercholesterolemia ▪ **MS:** arthralgia, back pain ▪ **Misc:** fever, hypersensitivity reactions.

## INTERACTIONS

**Drug-Drug:** ▪ Concurrent **abciximab, eptifibatide, tirofiban, aspirin, NSAIDs, heparin, heparanoids, thrombolytic agents, ticlopidine,** or **warfarin** may ↑ risk of bleeding ▪ May ↓ metabolism and ↑ effects of **phenytoin, tolbutamide, tamoxifen, torsemide, fluvastatin,** and many **NSAIDs.**

**Drug-Natural Products:** ▪ ↑ bleeding risk with **anise, arnica, chamomile, clove, fenugreek, feverfew, garlic, ginger, ginkgo, Panax ginseng,** and others.

## ROUTE AND DOSAGE

▫ **Recent MI, stroke, or peripheral vascular disease**

▪ **PO (Adults):** 75 mg once daily.

---

❏ **Acute coronary syndrome**

■ **PO (Adults):** 300 mg initially, then 75 mg once daily; aspirin 75–325 mg once daily should be given concurrently.

## AVAILABILITY

■ *Tablets:* 75 mg^Rx ■ Cost: $342.22/90.

TIME/ACTION PROFILE (effects on platelet function)

|  | ONSET | PEAK | DURATION |
|---|---|---|---|
| PO | within 24 hr | 3–7 days | 5 days† |

†Following discontinuation.

## NURSING IMPLICATIONS

### ASSESSMENT

❏ Assess patient for symptoms of stroke, peripheral vascular disease, or MI periodically during therapy.

❏ Monitor patient for signs of thrombotic thrombocytic purpura (thrombocytopenia, microangiopathic hemolytic anemia, neurologic findings, renal dysfunction, fever). May rarely occur, even after short exposure (<2 wk). Requires prompt treatment.

■ *Lab Test Considerations:* Monitor bleeding time during therapy. Prolonged bleeding time, which is time- and dose-dependent, is expected.

❏ Monitor CBC with differential and platelet count periodically during therapy. Neutropenia and thrombocytopenia may rarely occur.

❏ May cause ↑ serum bilirubin, hepatic enzymes, total cholesterol, nonprotein nitrogen (NPN), and uric acid concentrations.

### POTENTIAL NURSING DIAGNOSES

■ Injury, risk for (Indications, Side Effects).

### IMPLEMENTATION

■ **General:** Discontinue clopidogrel 5–7 days before planned surgical procedures.

■ **PO:** Administer once daily without regard to food.

### PATIENT/FAMILY TEACHING

❏ Instruct patient to take medication exactly as directed. Missed doses should be taken as soon as possible unless almost time for next dose; do not double doses.

❏ Advise patient to notify health care professional promptly if fever, chills, sore throat, or unusual bleeding or bruising occurs.

❏ Advise patient to notify health care professional of medication regimen prior to treatment or surgery.

❏ Instruct patient to avoid taking OTC medications containing aspirin or NSAIDs without consulting health care professional.

### EVALUATION

**Effectiveness of therapy can be demonstrated by:** ■ Prevention of stroke, MI, and vascular death in patients at risk.

## clorazepate

(klor-**az**-e-pate)

{Apo-Clorazepate}, Gen-XENE, {Novo-Clopate}, Tranxene, Tranxene-SD

### CLASSIFICATION(S):

*Therapeutic: anticonvulsants, sedative/hypnotics*
*Pharmacologic: benzodiazepines*

**Schedule IV**

**Pregnancy Category UK**

## INDICATIONS

■ Treatment of anxiety ■ Management of alcohol withdrawal ■ Management of simple partial seizures.

## ACTION

■ Acts at many levels in the CNS to produce anxiolytic effect and CNS depression (by stimulating inhibitory GABA receptors) ■ Produces skeletal muscle relaxation (by inhibiting spinal polysynaptic afferent pathways) ■ Also has anticonvulsant effect (enhances presynaptic inhibition). **Therapeutic Effects:** ■ Relief of anxiety ■ Sedation ■ Prevention of seizures.

## PHARMACOKINETICS

**Absorption:** Well absorbed from the GI tract as desmethyldiazepam.

**Distribution:** Widely distributed. Crosses the placenta; enters breast milk.

**Metabolism and Excretion:** Metabolized by the liver; some conversion to active compounds.
**Half-life:** 48 hr.

## CONTRAINDICATIONS AND PRECAUTIONS

**Contraindicated in:** ▪ Hypersensitivity ▪ Cross-sensitivity with other benzodiazepines may occur ▪ Pre-existing CNS depression ▪ Severe uncontrolled pain ▪ Narrow-angle glaucoma ▪ Pregnancy or lactation.

**Use Cautiously in:** ▪ Pre-existing hepatic dysfunction ▪ Patients who may be suicidal or have been addicted to drugs in the past ▪ Geriatric or debilitated patients (dosage reduction required) ▪ Severe pulmonary disease.

## ADVERSE REACTIONS AND SIDE EFFECTS*

▪ **CNS:** <u>dizziness</u>, <u>drowsiness</u>, <u>lethargy</u>, hangover, headache, mental depression, paradoxical excitation ▪ **EENT:** blurred vision ▪ **Resp:** respiratory depression ▪ **GI:** constipation, diarrhea, nausea, vomiting ▪ **Derm:** rashes ▪ **Misc:** physical dependence, psychological dependence, tolerance.

## INTERACTIONS

**Drug-Drug:** ▪ **Alcohol, antidepressants, antihistamines,** and **opioid analgesics**—concurrent use results in ↑ CNS depression ▪ **Cimetidine, hormonal contraceptives, disulfiram, fluoxetine, isoniazid, ketoconazole, metoprolol, propoxyphene, propranolol,** or **valproic acid** may ↓ the metabolism of clorazepate, ↑ its actions ▪ May ↓ efficacy of **levodopa** ▪ **Rifampin** or **barbiturates** may ↓ the metabolism and ↓ effectiveness of clorazepate ▪ Sedative effects may be ↓ by **theophylline.**

**Drug-Natural Products:** ▪ Concomitant use of **kava, valerian,** or **chamomile** ↑ CNS depression.

## ROUTE AND DOSAGE

▪ **PO (Adults):** *Anxiety*—7.5–15 mg 2–4 times daily *or* 15 mg at bedtime initially. May also be given in a single dose of 11.25–22.5 mg at bedtime. *Alcohol withdrawal*—30 mg initially, then 15 mg 2–4 times daily on 1st day, then gradually decreased over subsequent days. *Anticonvulsant*—7.5 mg 3 times daily; can increase by no more than 7.5 mg/day at weekly intervals (daily dose not to exceed 90 mg).

▪ **PO (Geriatric Patients or Debilitated Patients):** *Anxiety*—3.75–15 mg/day, may be increased.

▪ **PO (Children 9–12 yr):** *Anticonvulsant*—7.5 mg twice daily initially, may increase by 7.5 mg/wk (not to exceed 60 mg/day).

## AVAILABILITY

▪ *Tablets:* 3.75 mg$^{Rx}$, 7.5 mg$^{Rx}$, 11.25 mg$^{Rx}$, 15 mg$^{Rx}$, 22.5 mg$^{Rx}$ ▪ *Capsules:* 3.75 mg$^{Rx}$, 7.5 mg$^{Rx}$, 15 mg$^{Rx}$.

TIME/ACTION PROFILE (sedation)

|    | ONSET | PEAK | DURATION |
|----|-------|------|----------|
| PO | 1–2 hr | 1–2 hr | up to 24 hr† |

†May last longer in geriatric patients.

## NURSING IMPLICATIONS

### ASSESSMENT

▪ **General Info:** Assess for drowsiness, unsteadiness, and clumsiness. Symptoms are dose related and most severe during initial therapy; may decrease in severity or disappear with continued or long-term therapy.

▫ Prolonged high-dose therapy may lead to psychological or physical dependence. Restrict amount of drug available to patient.

▪ **Anxiety:** Assess degree and manifestations of anxiety prior to and periodically during therapy.

▪ **Alcohol Withdrawal:** Assess patient experiencing alcohol withdrawal for tremors, agitation, delirium, and hallucinations. Protect from injury.

▪ **Seizures:** Observe and record intensity, duration, and location of seizure activity.

▪ *Lab Test Considerations:* Patients on prolonged therapy should have CBC and liver function tests evaluated periodically. May cause an ↑ in serum bilirubin, AST, and ALT.

□ May cause ↓ thyroidal uptake of sodium iodide $^{123}$I and $^{131}$I.

## POTENTIAL NURSING DIAGNOSES

■ Anxiety (Indications).

■ Injury, risk for (Indications, Side Effects).

## IMPLEMENTATION

■ **General:** Do not confuse clorazepate with clonazepam.

■ **PO:** If gastric irritation is a problem, may be administered with food or fluids. Capsule should be swallowed whole; do not open.

□ Avoid administration of antacids within 1 hr of medication, because absorption of clorazepate may be delayed.

## PATIENT/FAMILY TEACHING

■ **General Info:** Instruct patient to take medication as directed, not to skip or double up on missed doses. Abrupt withdrawal may cause status epilepticus, tremors, nausea, vomiting, and abdominal and muscle cramps.

□ May cause drowsiness or dizziness. Advise patient to avoid driving or other activities requiring alertness until response to drug is known.

□ Caution patient to avoid alcohol or other CNS depressants concurrently with this medication.

□ Instruct patient to contact health care professional immediately if pregnancy is suspected.

□ Advise patient to notify health care professional of medication regimen prior to treatment or surgery.

□ Instruct patient and family to notify health care professional of unusual tiredness, bleeding, sore throat, fever, clay-colored stools, yellowing of skin, or behavioral changes.

□ Emphasize the importance of follow-up exams to determine effectiveness of the medication.

■ **Seizures:** Patients on anticonvulsant therapy should carry identification describing disease process and medication regimen at all times.

## EVALUATION

**Effectiveness of therapy can be demonstrated by:** ■ Increase in sense of well-being ■ Decrease in subjective feelings of anxiety ■ Control of acute alcohol withdrawal ■ Decrease or cessation of seizure activity without undue sedation.

---

**clotrimazole, See ANTIFUNGALS (TOPICAL), ANTIFUNGALS (VAGINAL).**

---

**cloxacillin, See PENICILLINS, PENICILLINASE RESISTANT.**

---

## clozapine

(**kloe**-za-peen)

Clozaril

*CLASSIFICATION(S):*
*Therapeutic: antipsychotics*

**Pregnancy Category B**

## INDICATIONS

■ Schizoprenia unresponsive to or intolerant of standard therapy with other antipsychotics ■ To reduce recurrent suicidal behavior in schizophrenic patients.

## ACTION

■ Binds to dopamine receptors in the CNS ■ Also has anticholinergic and alpha-adrenergic blocking activity ■ Produces fewer extrapyramidal reactions and less tardive dyskinesia than standard antipsychotics but carries high risk of hematologic abnormalities. **Therapeutic Effects:** ■ Diminished schizophrenic behavior. Diminished suicidal behavior.

## PHARMACOKINETICS

**Absorption:** Well absorbed after oral administration.

**Distribution:** Rapid and extensive distribution; crosses blood-brain barrier and placenta.

**Protein Binding:** 95%.

**Metabolism and Excretion:** Mostly metabolized on first pass through the liver.

**Half-life:** 8–12 hr.

## CONTRAINDICATIONS AND PRECAUTIONS

**Contraindicated in:** ■ Hypersensitivity ■ Bone marrow depression ■ Lactation ■ Severe CNS depression/coma.

**Use Cautiously in:** ■ Prostatic enlargement ■ Narrow-angle glaucoma ■ Malnourished patients or patients with cardiovascular, hepatic, or renal disease (use lower initial dose, titrate more slowly) ■ Diabetes ■ Seizure disorder ■ Children <16 yr (safety not established).

## ADVERSE REACTIONS AND SIDE EFFECTS*

■ **CNS:** NEUROLEPTIC MALIGNANT SYNDROME, SEIZURES, dizziness, sedation ■ **EENT:** visual disturbances ■ **CV:** MYOCARDITIS, hypotension, tachycardia, ECG changes, hypertension ■ **GI:** constipation, abdominal discomfort, dry mouth, increased salivation, nausea, vomiting ■ **Derm:** rash, sweating ■ **Endo:** hyperglycemia ■ **Hemat:** AGRANULOCYTOSIS, LEUKOPENIA ■ **Neuro:** extrapyramidal reactions ■ **Misc:** fever, weight gain.

## INTERACTIONS

**Drug-Drug:** ■ ↑ anticholinergic effects with other **agents having anticholinergic properties,** including **antihistamines, quinidine, disopyramide,** and **antidepressants** ■ Concurrent use with **SSRI antidepressants** ↑ blood levels and risk of toxicity (especially **fluvoxamine**) ■ ↑ CNS depression with **alcohol, antidepressants, antihistamines, opioid analgesics,** or **sedative/hypnotics** ■ ↑ hypotension with **nitrates,** acute ingestion of **alcohol,** or **antihypertensives** ■ ↑ risk of bone marrow suppression with **antihypertensives** or **radiation therapy** ■ Use with **lithium** ↑ risk of adverse CNS reactions, including seizures.

**Drug-Natural Products:** ■ Caffeine-containing herbs (**cola nut, tea, coffee**) may increase serum levels and side effects ■ **St. John's wort** may decrease blood levels and efficacy.

## ROUTE AND DOSAGE

■ **PO (Adults):** 25 mg 1–2 times daily initially; increase by 25–50 mg/day over a period of 2 wk up to target dose of 300–450 mg/day. May increase by up to 100 mg/day once or twice further (not to exceed 900 mg/day). Treatment should be continued for at least 2 yr in patients with suicidal behavior.

## AVAILABILITY (generic available)

■ **Tablets:** 25 mg$^{Rx}$, 100 mg$^{Rx}$.

**TIME/ACTION PROFILE** (antipsychotic effect)

| | ONSET | PEAK | DURATION |
|---|---|---|---|
| PO | unknown | wks | 4–12 hr |

## NURSING IMPLICATIONS

### ASSESSMENT

❏ Monitor patient's mental status (delusions, hallucinations, and behavior) before and periodically throughout therapy.

❏ Monitor blood pressure (sitting, standing, lying) and pulse rate before and frequently during initial dosage titration.

❏ Observe patient carefully when administering medication to ensure that medication is actually taken and not hoarded.

❏ Monitor for signs of myocarditis (unexplained fatigue, dyspnea, tachypnea, fever, chest pain, palpitations, other signs and symptoms of heart failure, ECG changes, such as ST-T wave abnormalities, arrhythmia, or tachycardia during first month of therapy). If these occur, clozapine should be discontinued and not restarted.

❏ Monitor patient for onset of akathisia (restlessness or desire to keep moving) and extrapyramidal side effects (*parkinsonian—* difficulty speaking or swallowing, loss of balance control, pill-rolling motion, mask-like face, shuffling gait, rigidity, tremors and dystonic muscle spasms, twisting motions, twitching, inability to move eyes, weakness of arms or legs) every 2 mo during therapy and 8–12 wk after therapy has been discontinued. Notify physician or other health care professional if these symptoms occur; reduction in dose or discontinuation of medication may be necessary. Trihexyphenidyl or diphenhydramine may be used to control these symptoms.

❏ Although not yet reported for clozapine, monitor for possible tardive dyskinesia (uncontrolled rhythmic movement of mouth, face, and extremities, lip smacking or puckering, puffing of cheeks, uncontrolled chewing, rapid or worm-like movements of tongue). Report these symptoms immediately; may be irreversible.

- Monitor frequency and consistency of bowel movements. Increasing bulk and fluids in the diet may help to minimize constipation.
- Clozapine lowers the seizure threshold. Institute seizure precautions for patients with history of seizure disorder.
- Transient fevers may occur, especially during first 3 wk of therapy. Fever is usually self-limiting but may require discontinuation of medication. Also, monitor for development of neuroleptic malignant syndrome (fever, respiratory distress, tachycardia, seizures, diaphoresis, hypertension or hypotension, pallor, tiredness). Notify physician immediately if these symptoms occur.

- **Lab Test Considerations:** Monitor WBC and differential count before initiation of therapy and WBC weekly for the first 6 months, then biweekly throughout therapy and weekly for 4 wk after discontinuation of clozapine. Because of the risk of agranulocytosis, clozapine is available only in a 1-wk supply through the **Clozaril Patient Management System,** which combines WBC testing, patient monitoring, and controlled distribution through participating pharmacies. If WBC is <3000 mm³ or granulocyte count is <1500 mm³, withhold clozapine, increase frequency of WBC monitoring according to management system guidelines, and monitor patient for signs and symptoms of infection.

- **Toxicity and Overdose:** Overdose is treated with activated charcoal and supportive therapy. Monitor patient for several days because of risk of delayed effects.
- Avoid use of epinephrine and its derivatives when treating hypotension, and avoid quinidine and procainamide when treating arrhythmias.

## POTENTIAL NURSING DIAGNOSES

- Violence, risk for other-directed (Indications).
- Thought processes, disturbed (Indications).
- Injury, risk for (Side Effects).

## IMPLEMENTATION

- **PO:** Administer capsules with food or milk to decrease gastric irritation.

## PATIENT/FAMILY TEACHING

- Instruct patient to take medication exactly as directed. Patients on long-term therapy may need to discontinue gradually over 1–2 wk.
- Inform patient of possibility of extrapyramidal symptoms. Instruct patient to report these symptoms immediately.
- Advise patient to change positions slowly to minimize orthostatic hypotension.
- May cause seizures and drowsiness. Caution patient to avoid driving or other activities requiring alertness while taking clozapine.
- Caution patient to avoid concurrent use of alcohol, other CNS depressants, and OTC medications without consulting health care professional.
- Instruct patient to use frequent mouth rinses, good oral hygiene, and sugarless gum or candy to minimize dry mouth.
- Advise patient to notify health care professional of medication regimen before treatment or surgery.
- Instruct patient to notify health care professional promptly if unexplained fatigue, dyspnea, tachypnea, chest pain, palpitations, sore throat, fever, lethargy, weakness, malaise, or flu-like symptoms occur or if pregnancy is planned or suspected.
- Advise patient of need for continued medical follow-up for psychotherapy, eye exams, and laboratory tests.

## EVALUATION

**Effectiveness of therapy can be demonstrated by:** ■ Diminished schizophrenic behavior ■ Diminished suicidal behavior.

**High Alert**

# codeine
**(koe**-deen)
{Paveral}

## CLASSIFICATION(S):
**Therapeutic:** allergy, cold, and cough remedies, antitussives, opioid analgesics
**Pharmacologic:** opioid agonists

**Schedule I, II, IV, V (depends on content)**

**Pregnancy Category C**

# INDICATIONS

- Management of mild to moderate pain ■ Antitussive (in smaller doses). **Unlabeled uses:** ■ Management of diarrhea.

# ACTION

- Binds to opiate receptors in the CNS. Alters the perception of and response to painful stimuli while producing generalized CNS depression ■ Decreases cough reflex ■ Decreases GI motility. **Therapeutic Effects:** ■ Decreased severity of pain ■ Suppression of the cough reflex ■ Relief of diarrhea.

# PHARMACOKINETICS

**Absorption:** 50% absorbed from the GI tract. Completely absorbed from IM sites. Oral and parenteral doses are not equal.

**Distribution:** Widely distributed. Crosses the placenta; enters breast milk.

**Metabolism and Excretion:** Mostly metabolized by the liver; 10% converted to morphine, 5–15% excreted unchanged in urine.

**Half-life:** 2.5–4 hr.

# CONTRAINDICATIONS AND PRECAUTIONS

**Contraindicated in:** ■ Hypersensitivity.

**Use Cautiously in:** ■ Head trauma ■ Increased intracranial pressure ■ Severe renal, hepatic, or pulmonary disease ■ Hypothyroidism ■ Adrenal insufficiency ■ Alcoholism ■ Geriatric or debilitated patients (dosage reduction required; more susceptible to CNS depression, constipation) ■ Undiagnosed abdominal pain ■ Prostatic hypertrophy ■ Has been used during labor; respiratory depression may occur in the newborn ■ Pregnancy or lactation (avoid chronic use).

# ADVERSE REACTIONS AND SIDE EFFECTS*

- **CNS:** confusion, sedation, dysphoria, euphoria, floating feeling, hallucinations, headache, unusual dreams ■ **EENT:** blurred vision, diplopia, miosis ■ **Resp:** respiratory depression ■ **CV:** hypotension, bradycardia ■ **GI:** constipation, nausea, vomiting ■ **GU:** urinary retention ■ **Derm:** flushing, sweating ■ **Misc:** physical dependence, psychological dependence, tolerance.

# INTERACTIONS

**Drug-Drug:** ■ Use with extreme caution in patients receiving **MAO inhibitors** (reduce initial dosage to 25% of usual dose) ■ Additive CNS depression with **alcohol, antidepressants, antihistamines,** and **sedative/hypnotics** ■ Administration of **partial antagonists (buprenorphine, butorphanol, nalbuphine,** or **pentazocine)** may precipitate opioid withdrawal in physically dependent patients ■ **Nalbuphine** or **pentazocine** may decrease analgesia.

**Drug-Natural Products:** ■ Concomitant use of **kava, valerian, skullcap, chamomile,** or **hops** can increase CNS depression.

# ROUTE AND DOSAGE

- **PO (Adults):** *Analgesic*—15–60 mg q 3–6 hr as needed. *Antitussive*—10–20 mg q 4–6 hr as needed (not to exceed 120 mg/day). *Antidiarrheal*—30 mg up to 4 times daily.
- **PO (Children 6–12 yr):** *Analgesic*—0.5 mg/kg (15 mg/m²) q 4–6 hr (up to 4 times daily) as needed. *Antitussive*—5–10 mg q 4–6 hr as needed (not to exceed 60 mg/day). *Antidiarrheal*—0.5 mg/kg up to 4 times daily.
- **PO (Children 2–5 yr):** *Analgesic*—0.5 mg/kg (15 mg/m²) q 4–6 hr (up to 4 times daily) as needed. *Antitussive*—0.25 mg/kg up to 4 times daily. *Antidiarrheal*—0.5 mg/kg up to 4 times daily.
- **IM, IV, Subcut (Adults):** *Analgesic*—15–60 mg q 4–6 hr as needed.
- **IM, IV, Subcut (Infants and Children):** *Analgesic*—0.5 mg/kg (15 mg/m²) q 4–6 hr as needed.

# AVAILABILITY (generic available)

- **Tablets:** 15 mg$^{Rx}$, 30 mg$^{Rx}$, 60 mg$^{Rx}$ ■ Cost: 15 mg $37.41/100, 30 mg $40.27/100, 60 mg $73.77/100 ■ **Oral solution:** {10 mg/5 ml$^{Rx}$}, 15 mg/5 ml$^{Rx}$ ■ **Injection:** 30 mg/ml$^{Rx}$, 60 mg/ml$^{Rx}$ ■ antihistamines, decongestants, antipyretics, caffeine, butalbital, and nonopioid analgesics$^{Rx}$. See Appendix B.

TIME/ACTION PROFILE (analgesia)

| | ONSET | PEAK | DURATION |
|---|---|---|---|
| PO | 30–45 min | 60–120 min | 4 hr |
| IM | 10–30 min | 30–60 min | 4 hr |
| Subcut | 10–30 min | unknown | 4 hr |

{ } = Available in Canada only.
* CAPITALS indicates life-threatening; underlines indicate most frequent.

## NURSING IMPLICATIONS

### ASSESSMENT

■ **General Info:** Assess blood pressure, pulse, and respirations before and periodically during administration. If respiratory rate is <10/min, assess level of sedation. Physical stimulation may be sufficient to prevent significant hypoventilation. Dose may need to be decreased by 25–50%. Initial drowsiness will diminish with continued use.

❑ Assess bowel function routinely. Prevention of constipation should be instituted with increased intake of fluids, bulk, and laxatives to minimize constipating effects. Stimulant laxatives should be administered routinely if opioid use exceeds 2–3 days, unless contraindicated.

■ **Pain:** Assess type, location, and intensity of pain before and 1 hr (peak) after administration. When titrating opioid doses, increases of 25–50% should be administered until there is either a 50% reduction in the patient's pain rating on a numerical or visual analog scale or the patient reports satisfactory pain relief. A repeat dose can be safely administered at the time of the peak if previous dose is ineffective and side effects are minimal.

❑ An equianalgesic chart (see Appendix O) should be used when changing routes or when changing from one opioid to another.

❑ Prolonged use may lead to physical and psychological dependence and tolerance. This should not prevent patient from receiving adequate analgesia. Most patients who receive codeine for pain do not develop psychological dependence. If progressively higher doses are required, consider conversion to a stronger opioid.

■ **Cough:** Assess cough and lung sounds during antitussive use.

■ *Lab Test Considerations:* May cause increased plasma amylase and lipase concentrations.

■ *Toxicity and Overdose:* If an opioid antagonist is required to reverse respiratory depression or coma, naloxone (Narcan) is the antidote. Dilute the 0.4-mg ampule of naloxone in 10 ml of 0.9% NaCl and administer 0.5 ml (0.02 mg) by direct IV push every 2 min. For children and patients weighing <40 kg, dilute 0.1 mg of naloxone in 10 ml of 0.9% NaCl for a concentration of 10 mcg/ml and administer 0.5 mcg/kg every 2 min. Titrate dose to avoid withdrawal, seizures, and severe pain.

### POTENTIAL NURSING DIAGNOSES

■ Pain, acute (Indications).

■ Sensory perception, disturbed (visual, auditory) (Side Effects).

■ Injury, risk for (Side Effects).

### IMPLEMENTATION

❑ *High Alert:* Accidental overdosage of opioid analgesics has resulted in fatalities. Before administering, clarify all ambiguous orders; have second practitioner independently check dose calculations, route of administration, and infusion pump programming. Do not confuse codeine with Cardene (nicardipine) or Lodine (etodolac).

■ **General:** Explain therapeutic value of medication before administration to enhance the analgesic effect.

❑ Regularly administered doses may be more effective than prn administration. Analgesic is more effective if given before pain becomes severe.

❑ Coadministration with nonopioid analgesics may have additive analgesic effects and permit lower doses.

❑ Medications should be discontinued gradually after long-term use to prevent withdrawal symptoms.

❑ When combined with nonopioid analgesics (aspirin, acetaminophen) #2 = 15 mg, #3 = 30 mg, #4 = 60 mg codeine. Codeine as an individual drug is a Schedule II substance. In combination with other drugs, tablet form is Schedule III, liquid is Schedule IV, and elixir or cough suppressant is Schedule V (see Appendix N).

■ **PO:** Oral doses may be administered with food or milk to minimize GI irritation.

■ **IM, Subcut:** Do not administer solution that is more than slightly discolored or contains a precipitate.

■ **Direct IV:** Codeine is usually administered IM or subcut, but slow IV injection has been used.

■ **Syringe Compatibility:** ◆ glycopyrrolate ◆ hydroxyzine.

## PATIENT/FAMILY TEACHING

- ❑ Instruct patient on how and when to ask for pain medication.
- ❑ Codeine may cause drowsiness or dizziness. Advise patient to call for assistance when ambulating or smoking. Caution ambulatory patient to avoid driving or other activities requiring alertness until response to medication is known.
- ❑ Advise patient to change positions slowly to minimize orthostatic hypotension.
- ❑ Caution patient to avoid concurrent use of alcohol or other CNS depressants with this medication.
- ❑ Encourage patient to turn, cough, and breathe deeply every 2 hr to prevent atelectasis.
- ❑ Advise patient that good oral hygiene, frequent mouth rinses, and sugarless gum or candy may decrease dry mouth.

## EVALUATION

**Effectiveness of therapy can be demonstrated by:** ■ Decrease in severity of pain without a significant alteration in level of consciousness or respiratory status ■ Suppression of cough ■ Control of diarrhea.

---

**High Alert**

## colchicine
(**kol**-chi-seen)

*CLASSIFICATION(S):*
*Therapeutic:* antigout agents

**Pregnancy Category D**

---

## INDICATIONS

■ Acute attacks of gouty arthritis (larger doses) ■ Prevention of recurrences of gout (smaller doses). **Unlabeled uses:** ■ Treatment of hepatic cirrhosis and familial Mediterranean fever.

## ACTION

■ Interferes with the functions of WBCs in initiating and perpetuating the inflammatory response to monosodium urate crystals. **Therapeutic Effects:** ■ Decreased pain and inflammation in acute attacks of gout ■ Prevention of recurrent attacks of gout.

## PHARMACOKINETICS

**Absorption:** Absorbed from the GI tract, then re-enters GI tract from biliary secretions, when more absorption may occur.

**Distribution:** Concentrates in WBCs.

**Metabolism and Excretion:** Partially metabolized by the liver. Secreted in bile back into GI tract; eliminated in the feces. Small amount excreted in the urine.

**Half-life:** 20 min (plasma), 60 hr (WBCs).

## CONTRAINDICATIONS AND PRECAUTIONS

**Contraindicated in:** ■ Hypersensitivity ■ Pregnancy ■ Severe renal (CCr <10 ml/min) or GI disease.

**Use Cautiously in:** ■ Elderly or debilitated patients (toxicity may be cumulative) ■ Renal impairment (dosage reduction suggested if CCr <50 ml/min; total IV dose not >2 mg) ■ Lactation or children (safety not established).

## ADVERSE REACTIONS AND SIDE EFFECTS*

■ **GI:** <u>diarrhea</u>, <u>nausea</u>, <u>vomiting</u>, abdominal pain ■ **GU:** anuria, hematuria, renal damage ■ **Derm:** alopecia ■ **Hemat:** AGRANULOCYTOSIS, APLASTIC ANEMIA, leukopenia, thrombocytopenia ■ **Local:** phlebitis at IV site ■ **Neuro:** peripheral neuritis.

## INTERACTIONS

**Drug-Drug:** ■ Additive bone marrow depression may occur with **bone marrow depressants** or **radiation therapy** ■ Additive adverse GI effects with **NSAIDs** ■ May cause reversible malabsorption of **vitamin B$_{12}$.**

## ROUTE AND DOSAGE

■ **PO (Adults):** *Treatment of acute attacks*—0.5–1.2 mg, then 0.5–0.6 mg q 1–2 hr *or* 1–1.2 mg q 2 hr until relief, GI side effects, or a total cumulative dose of 8 mg is achieved. *Prophylaxis*—0.5–0.6 mg daily (may be used up to 3 times daily or as little as 1–4 times weekly). If surgery is planned, give 3 times daily for 3 days before and 3 days after procedure.

- **IV (Adults):** *Treatment of acute attack*—2 mg initially, then 0.5 mg q 6 hr *or* 1 mg q 6–12 hr, until relief or cumulative dose of 4 mg has been given. Other regimens may use lower doses. *Prophylaxis*—0.5–1 mg 1–2 times daily. Other regimens may use lower doses.

## AVAILABILITY (generic available)

- **Tablets:** 0.5 mg$^{Rx}$, 0.6 mg$^{Rx}$, {1 mg$^{Rx}$} ■ Cost: 0.5 mg $34.51/100, 0.6 mg $26.44/100, 1 mg $30.99/100 ■ *Injection:* 0.5 mg/ml in 2-ml ampules$^{Rx}$.

TIME/ACTION PROFILE (anti-inflammatory activity)

|  | ONSET | PEAK | DURATION |
|---|---|---|---|
| PO | 12 hr | 24–72 hr | unknown |
| IV | within 6–12 hr | unknown | unknown |

## NURSING IMPLICATIONS

### ASSESSMENT

- ❑ **High Alert:** Assess patient for toxicity (weakness, abdominal discomfort, nausea, vomiting, diarrhea, delerium, seizures, sense of suffocation, dilated pupils, difficulty swallowing, ascending paralysis, oliguria), withhold drug and report symptoms immediately.
- ❑ Assess involved joints for pain, mobility, and edema throughout therapy. During initiation of therapy, monitor for drug response every 1–2 hr.
- ❑ Monitor intake and output ratios. Fluids should be encouraged to promote a urinary output of at least 2000 ml/day.
- ■ **Lab Test Considerations:** In patients receiving prolonged therapy, monitor baseline and periodic CBC; report significant decrease in values. May cause decreased platelet count, leukopenia, aplastic anemia, and agranulocytosis.
- ❑ May cause an increase in AST and alkaline phosphatase.
- ❑ May cause false-positive results for urine hemoglobin.
- ❑ May interfere with results of urinary 17-hydroxycorticosteroid concentrations.
- ■ **Toxicity and Overdose:** Assess patient for toxicity (weakness, abdominal discomfort, nausea, vomiting, diarrhea). If these symptoms occur, discontinue medication and notify physician or other health care profes-

sional. Opioids may be needed to treat diarrhea.

## POTENTIAL NURSING DIAGNOSES

- ■ Pain, acute (Indications).
- ■ Walking, impaired (Indications).

## IMPLEMENTATION

- ❑ **High Alert:** Colchicine overdose can be fatal. Cumulative dose by any route should not exceed 4 mg. Limit IV doses to a maximum of 1-2 mg in patients who have recently received oral colchicine. Cumulative dose should not exceed 2 mg in geriatric and renal patients. After dosing limit has been reached, do not administer any additional colchicine by any route for 21 days. Do not administer oral and IV colchicine concurrently.
- ■ **General:** Intermittent therapy with 3 days between courses may be used to decrease risk of toxicity.
- ■ **PO:** Administer oral doses with food to minimize gastric irritation. Oral route is preferred.
- ■ **IV:** Avoid extravasation; may cause necrosis of skin and soft tissue.
- ■ **Direct IV:** May be administered undiluted. If a lower concentration is desired, may dilute to a volume of 10–20 ml with sterile water or 0.9% NaCl for injection. Do not administer solutions that are turbid.
- ■ **Rate:** Administer slowly over 2–10 min. Rapid administration may cause cardiac arrhythmias.
- ■ **Y-Site Incompatibility:** Do not dilute colchicine with or inject into IV tubing containing D5W, solutions containing a bacteriostatic agent, or any other solution that might change the pH of the colchicine solution because precipitation will occur.

## PATIENT/FAMILY TEACHING

- ❑ Review medication administration schedule. If dose is missed, take as soon as remembered unless almost time for next dose. Do not double doses.
- ❑ Instruct patients taking prophylactic doses not to increase to therapeutic doses during an acute attack to prevent toxicity. An NSAID or corticosteroid, preferably via intrasynovial injection, should be used to treat acute attacks.

◻ Advise patient to follow recommendations of health care professional regarding weight loss, diet, and alcohol consumption.

◻ Instruct patient to report nausea, vomiting, abdominal pain, diarrhea, unusual bleeding, bruising, sore throat, fatigue, malaise, or rash promptly. Medication should be withheld if gastric symptoms, indicative of toxicity, occur.

◻ Surgery may precipitate an acute attack of gout. Advise patient to confer with health care professional regarding dose 3 days before surgical or dental procedures.

## EVALUATION
**Effectiveness of therapy can be demonstrated by:** ▪ Decrease in pain and swelling in affected joints within 12 hr ◻ Relief of symptoms within 24–48 hr ▪ Prevention of acute gout attacks.

## coleseveIam
(koe-le-**sev**-e-lam)
Welchol,

### CLASSIFICATION(S):
**Therapeutic:** lipid-lowering agents
**Pharmacologic:** bile acid sequestrants

### Pregnancy Category B

## INDICATIONS
▪ Adjunctive therapy to diet and exercise for the reduction of LDL cholesterol in patients with primary hypercholesterolemia; may be used alone or in combination with hepatic hydroxymethylglutaryl coenzyme A (HMG-CoA) reductase inhibitor.

## ACTION
▪ Binds bile acids in the GI tract ▪ Result in increased clearance of cholesterol.**Therapeutic Effects:** ▪ Decreased cholesterol.

## PHARMACOKINETICS
**Absorption:** Not absorbed; action is primarily local in the GI tract.
**Distribution:** Unknown.

**Metabolism and Excretion:** Unknown.
**Half-life:** Unknown.

## CONTRAINDICATIONS AND PRECAUTIONS
**Contraindicated in:** ▪ Hypersensitivity ▪ Bowel obstruction
**Use Cautiously in:** ▪ Triglycerides >300 mg/dl ▪ Dysphagia, swallowing disorders, severe GI molitlity disorders, or major GI tract surgery ▪ Pregnancy, lactation, or children (safety not established).

## ADVERSE REACTIONS AND SIDE EFFECTS*
▪ **GI:** constipation, dyspepsia.

## INTERACTIONS
**Drug-Drug:** ▪ May decrease blood levels of sustained-release form of **verapamil**.

## ROUTE AND DOSAGE
▪ **PO (Adults):** 3 tablets twice daily or 6 tablets once daily; may be increased to 7 tablets daily.

## AVAILABILITY
▪ **Tablets:** 625 mg.

TIME/ACTION PROFILE (cholesterol-lowering effect)

| | ONSET | PEAK | DURATION |
|---|---|---|---|
| PO | 24–48 hr | 2 wk | unknown |

## NURSING IMPLICATIONS

### ASSESSMENT
◻ Obtain a diet history, especially in regard to fat consumption.
▪ **Lab Test Considerations:** Serum total cholesterol, LDL, and triglyceride levels should be evaluated before initiating, and periodically throughout, the therapy.

### POTENTIAL NURSING DIAGNOSES
▪ Constipation (Side Effects).
▪ Noncompliance (Patient/Family Teaching).

## IMPLEMENTATION

- **PO:** Administer once or twice daily with meals. Colesevelam should be taken with a liquid.

## PATIENT/FAMILY TEACHING

- ❑ Instruct patient to take medication exactly as directed; do not skip doses or double up on missed doses.
- ❑ Advise patient that this medication should be used in conjunction with diet restrictions (fat, cholesterol, carbohydrates, alcohol), exercise, and cessation of smoking.

## EVALUATION

**Effectiveness of therapy can be demonstrated by:** ■ Decrease in serum total choesterol, LDL cholesterol, and apolipoprotein levels.

# colestipol

(koe-**les**-ti-pole)

Colestid

***CLASSIFICATION(S):***

***Therapeutic:*** *lipid-lowering agents*
***Pharmacologic:*** *bile acid seques-trants*

**Pregnancy Category UK**

## INDICATIONS

■ Management of primary hypercholesterolemia ■ Pruritus associated with elevated levels of bile acids. **Unlabeled uses:** ■ Diarrhea associated with excess bile acids.

## ACTION

■ Bind bile acids in the GI tract, forming an insoluble complex. Result is increased clearance of cholesterol. **Therapeutic Effects:** ■ Decreased plasma cholesterol and LDL ■ Decreased pruritus.

## PHARMACOKINETICS

**Absorption:** Action takes place in the GI tract. No absorption occurs.

**Distribution:** No distribution.

**Metabolism and Excretion:** After binding bile acids, insoluble complex is eliminated in the feces.

**Half-life:** Unknown.

## CONTRAINDICATIONS AND PRECAUTIONS

**Contraindicated in:** ■ Hypersensitivity ■ Complete biliary obstruction ■ Some products contain aspartame and should be avoided in patients with phenylketonuria.

**Use Cautiously in:** ■ History of constipation.

**Exercise Extreme Caution in:** ■ Children (may cause intestinal obstruction; deaths have occurred).

## ADVERSE REACTIONS AND SIDE EFFECTS*

■ **EENT:** irritation of the tongue ■ **GI:** <u>abdominal discomfort</u>, <u>constipation</u>, <u>nausea</u>, fecal impaction, flatulence, hemorrhoids, perianal irritation, steatorrhea, vomiting ■ **Derm:** irritation, rashes ■ **F and E:** hyperchloremic acidosis ■ **Metab:** vitamin A, D, and K deficiency.

## INTERACTIONS

**Drug-Drug:** ■ May decrease absorption/effects of orally administered **acetaminophen, amiodarone, clindamycin, clofibrate, digoxin, diuretics, gemfibrozil, glipizide, corticosteroids, imipramine, mycophenolate, methotrexate, methyldopa, niacin, NSAIDs, penicillin, phenytoin, phosphates, propranolol, tetracyclines, tolbutamide, thyroid preparations, ursodiol, warfarin,** and **fat-soluble vitamins (A, D, E, and K)** ■ May decrease absorption of other **orally administered medications.**

## ROUTE AND DOSAGE

■ **PO (Adults):** *Granules*—5 g 1–2 times daily, may be increased q 1–2 mo up to 30 g/day in 1–2 doses. *Tablets*—2 g 1–2 times daily, may be increased q 1–2 mo up to 16 g/day in 1–2 doses.

## AVAILABILITY

■ *Granules for suspension (unflavored):* 5 g/packet or scoop<sup>Rx</sup> ■ Cost: $49.89/30 packets; $146.66/90 packets; $59.43/300-g cannister; $99.05/500-g cannister ■ *Flavored granules for suspension with aspartame (orange flavor):* 5 g/packet or scoop<sup>Rx</sup> ■ Cost: $99.61/60 packets or $63.59/450-g cannister ■ *Tablets:* 1 g<sup>Rx</sup> ■ Cost: $46.08/120 tablets.

TIME/ACTION PROFILE (hypocholesterolemic effects)

| | ONSET | PEAK | DURATION |
|---|---|---|---|
| PO | 24–48 hr | 1 mo | 1 mo |

## NURSING IMPLICATIONS

### ASSESSMENT

- **Hypercholesterolemia:** Obtain a diet history, especially in regard to fat consumption.
- **Pruritus:** Assess severity of itching and skin integrity. Dose may be decreased when relief of pruritus occurs.
- **Diarrhea:** Assess frequency, amount, and consistency of stools.
- **Lab Test Considerations:** Serum cholesterol and triglyceride levels should be evaluated before initiating, frequently during first few months and periodically throughout therapy. Discontinue medication if paradoxical increase in cholesterol level occurs.
- ❑ May cause an increase in AST, ALT, phosphorus, chloride, and alkaline phosphatase and a decrease in serum calcium, sodium, and potassium levels.
- ❑ May also cause prolonged PT.

### POTENTIAL NURSING DIAGNOSES

- Constipation (Side Effects).
- Noncompliance (Patient/Family Teaching).

### IMPLEMENTATION

- **General:** Parenteral or water-miscible forms of fat-soluble vitamins (A, D, K) and folic acid may be ordered for patients on chronic therapy.
- **PO:** Administer before meals.
- ❑ Scoops for powdered preparations may not be exchangable between products.
- ❑ Administer other medications 1 hr before or 4–6 hr after the administration of this medication.
- ❑ Colestipol tablets should be swallowed whole; do not crush, break, or chew.

### PATIENT/FAMILY TEACHING

- ❑ Instruct patient to take medication exactly as directed; do not skip doses or double up on missed doses.
- ❑ Instruct patient to take medication before meals. Colestipol can be mixed with water, juice, or carbonated beverages. Slowly stir in a large glass. Rinse glass with small amount of additional beverage to ensure all medication is taken. May also mix with highly fluid soups, cereals, or pulpy fruits (applesauce, crushed pineapple). Allow powder to sit on fluid and hydrate for 1–2 min before mixing. Do not take dry.
- ❑ Advise patient that this medication should be used in conjunction with diet restrictions (fat, cholesterol, carbohydrates, alcohol), exercise, and cessation of smoking.
- ❑ Explain that constipation may occur. Increase in fluids and bulk in diet, exercise, stool softeners, and laxatives may be required to minimize the constipating effects. Instruct patient to notify health care professional if constipation, nausea, flatulence, and heartburn persist or if stools become frothy and foul smelling.
- ❑ Advise patient to notify health care professional if unusual bleeding or bruising; petechiae; or black, tarry stools occur. Treatment with vitamin K may be necessary.

### EVALUATION

**Effectiveness of therapy can be demonstrated by:** ■ Decrease in serum LDL cholesterol levels. Therapy is usually discontinued if the clinical response remains poor after 3 mo of therapy ■ Decrease in severity of pruritus. Relief usually occurs 1–3 wk after therapy is initiated ■ Decrease in frequency and severity of diarrhea.

## CONTRACEPTIVES, HORMONAL
## MONOPHASIC ORAL
## CONTRACEPTIVES

**ethinyl estradiol/desogestrel**

**(eth**-in-il es-tra-**dye**-ole/dess-oh-**jes**-trel)

Desogen, Ortho-Cept

**ethinyl estradiol/drospirenone**

**(eth**-in-il es-tra-**dye**-ole/droe-**spy**-re-nown)

Yasmin

**ethinyl estradiol/ethynodiol**

(**eth**-in-il es-tra-**dye**-ole/e-thye-noe-**dye**-ole)
Demulen, Demulen 1/35

**ethinyl estradiol/levonorgestrel**

(**eth**-in-il es-tra-**dye**-ole/lee-voe-nor-**jes**-trel)
Alesse, Aviane-28, Levlen, Nordette

**ethinyl estradiol/norethindrone**

(**eth**-in-il es-tra-**dye**-ole/nor-eth-**in**-drone)
Brevicon, Genora 0.5/35, Genora 1/35, Junel 21 1/20, Junel 21 1.5/20, Loestrin 21 1.5/30, Loestrin 21 1/20, Microgestin, Modicon, N.E.E. 1/35, Nelova 0.5/35E, Nelova 1/35E, Norcept-E 1/35, Norethin 1/35E, Norinyl 1+ 35, Norlestrin 1/50, Norlestrin 2.5/50, Nortrel, Ortho-Novum 1/35, Ovcon 35, Ovcon 50

**ethinyl estradiol/norgestimate**

(**eth**-in-il es-tra-**dye**-ole/nor-**jest**-i-mate)
Ortho-Cyclen, Sprintec

**ethinyl estradiol/norgestrel**

(**eth**-in-il es-tra-**dye**-ole/nor-**jess**-trel)
Cryselle, Lo/Ovral, Ovral

**mestranol/norethindrone**

(**mes**-tre-nole/nor-eth-**in**-drone)
Genora 1/50, Nelova 1/50M, Norethin 1/50M, Norinyl 1+50, Ortho-Novum 1/50, Yasmin

# BIPHASIC ORAL CONTRACEPTIVES

**ethinyl estradiol/norethindrone**

(**eth**-in-il es-tra-**dye**-ole/nor-eth-**in**-drone)
Kariva, Mircette, Nelova 10/11, Ortho-Novum 10/11

# TRIPHASIC ORAL CONTRACEPTIVES

**ethinyl estradiol/desogestrel**

(**eth**-in-il es-tra-**dye**-ole/dess-oh-**jes**-trel)
Cyclessa

**ethinyl estradiol/norethindrone**

(**eth**-in-il es-tra-**dye**-ole/nor-eth-**in**-drone)
Necor 7/7/7, Nortrel 7/7/7, Ortho-Novum 7/7/7, Tri-Norinyl

**norgestimate/ethinyl estradiol**

(**eth**-in-il es-tra-**dye**-ole/nor-**jes**-ti-mate)
Ortho Tri-Cyclen, Ortho Tri-Cyclen Lo

**ethinyl estradiol/norgestrel**

(**eth**-in-il ess-tra-**dye**-ole/nor-**jes**-trel)
Enpresse, Portia, Tri-Levlen, Triphasil

# EXTENDED-CYCLE ORAL CONTRACEPTIVE

**ethinyl estradiol/levonergestrel**

(**eth**-in-il ess-tra-**dye**-ole/lee-voe-nor-**jess**-trel)

# PROGESTIN-ONLY ORAL CONTRACEPTIVES

**norethindrone**

(nor-eth-**in**-drone)
Errin, Ortho Micronor, Camila, Jolivette, Nor-Q D

**norgestrel**

(nor-**jes**-trel)
Ovrette

# PROGRESSIVE ESTROGEN ORAL CONTRACEPTIVES

**norethindrone/ethinyl acetate**

(nor-eth-**in**-drone/**eth**-in-il a-se-tate)
Estrostep, Estrostep Fe

# CONTRACEPTIVE IMPLANT

**levonorgestrel**

(**lee**-voe-nor-jes-trel)

Norplant, Mirena

# EMERGENCY CONTRACEPTIVE

**levonorgestrel/ethinyl estradiol**

(**lee**-voe-nor-jes-trel/**eth**-in-il ess-tra-**dye**-ole)

Preven

**levonorgestrel**

(**lee**-voe-nor-jes-trel)

Plan B

# INJECTABLE CONTRACEPTIVE

**estradiol cypionate/medroxyprogesterone acetate**

(ess-tra-**dye**-ole sip-**eye**-oh-nate/me-**drox**-ee-proe-jess-te-rone**a**-se-tate)

Lunelle

**medroxyprogesterone**

(me-**drox**-ee-proe-jess-te-rone)

Depo-Provera

# INTRAUTERINE CONTRACEPTIVE

**levonorgestrel**

(**lee**-voe-nor-jess-trel)

Mirena

# Vaginal Ring Contraceptive

**ethinyl estradiol/etonogestrel**

(**eth**-in-il ess-tra-**dye**-ole /e-toe-noe-**jess**-trel)

NuvaRing

# Transdermal Contraceptive

**ethinyl estradiol/norelgestromin**

(**eth**-in-il ess-tra-**dye**-ole /nor-el-**jess**-troe-min)

Ortho Evra

*CLASSIFICATION(S):*
*Therapeutic:* contraceptive hormones

**Pregnancy Category X**

## INDICATIONS

■ Prevention of pregnancy ■ Regulation of menstrual cycle ■ Emergency contraception (some products) ■ Management of acne in women >14 yr who desire contraception, have no health problems, and have failed topical treatment.

## ACTION

■ **Monophasic Oral Contraceptives:** Provide a fixed dosage of estrogen/progestin over a 21-day cycle. Ovulation is inhibited by suppression of follicle-stimulating hormone (FSH) and luteinizing hormone (LH). May alter cervical mucus and the endometrial environment, preventing penetration by sperm and implantation of the egg ■ **Biphasic Oral Contraceptives:** Ovulation is inhibited by suppression of FSH and LH. May alter cervical mucus and the endometrial environment, preventing penetration by sperm and implantation of the egg. In addition, smaller dose of progestin in phase 1 allows for proliferation of endometrium. Larger amount in phase 2 allows for adequate secretory development ■ **Triphasic Oral Contraceptives:** Ovulation is inhibited by suppression of FSH and LH. May alter cervical mucus and the endometrial environment, preventing penetration by sperm and implantation of the egg. Varying doses of estrogen/progestin may more closely mimic natural hormonal fluctuations ■ **Extended-cycle:** Provides continuous estrogen/progestin for 84 days, then off for 7 days, resulting in 4 menstrual periods/year ■ **Progressive Estrogen:** Contains constant amount of progestin with 3 progressive doses of estrogen ■ **Progestin-Only Contraceptives/Contraceptive Implant/Intrauterine Levonorgestrel:** Mechanism not clearly known. May alter cervical mucus and the endometrial environment, preventing penetration by sperm and implantation of the egg. Ovulation may also be suppressed ■ **Estradiol/Medroxyprogesterone and Medroxyprogesterone Injection:** Inhibits gonadotropin secretion, follicle maturation, and ovulation. Also produces endometrial thinning ■ **Emergency Contraceptive Pills (ECPs):** Inhibit ovulation/fertilization; may also alter tubal transport of sperm/egg and prevent implantation ■ **Vaginal Ring, Transdermal Patch:** inhibits ovulation, decreases sperm entry into uterus, and decreases likelihood of implantation ■ **Anti-acne effect:** Combination of estrogen/progestin may increase sex hormone binding globulin (SHBG) resulting is decreased unbound testosterone, which may be a cause of acne. **Therapeutic Effects:** ■ Prevention of pregnancy ■ Decreased severity of acne.

## PHARMACOKINETICS

**Absorption:** *Ethinyl estradiol*—raidly absorbed; *norethindrone*—65% absorbed; *Desogesrtrel and levonorgestrel*—100% aborbed. Others are well absorbed after oral administration. Slowly absorbed from implant or IM injection.Some absorption follows intrauterine implantation.

**Distribution:** Unknown.

**Protein Binding:** *Ethinyl estradiol*—97–98%.

**Metabolism and Excretion:** *Ethinyl estradiol and norethindrone*—undergo extensive first pass hepatic metabolism. *Mestranol*—is rapidly converted to ethinyl estradol. *Desogestrel*—is rapidly metabolized to 3-keto-desogestgrel, the active metabolite. Most agents are metabolized by the liver.

**Half-life:** *Ethinyl estradiol*—6–20 hr; *Levonorgestrel*—45 hr; *Norethindrone*—5–14 hr; *Desogestrel (metabolite)*—38hr ±20 hr; *Norgestimate (metabolite)*—12–20 hr; others—unknown.

## CONTRAINDICATIONS AND PRECAUTIONS

**Contraindicated in:** ■ Pregnancy ■ History of thromboembolic disorders, cardiovascular disease, cerebrovascular disease, liver tumors, or gallbladder disease ■ Hypersensitivity to parabens (injectable only) ■ Lactation (avoid use) ■ *Intrauterine levonorgestrel only*—Intrauterine anomoly, postpartum endometriosis, pelvic inflammatory disease, liver disease, genital actinomycosis, immunosuppression, IV drug abuse, untreated genitourinary infection, history of ec-

topic pregnancy ■ Some products contain tartrazine and should be avoided in patients with known hypersensitivity intolerance.

**Use Cautiously in:** ■ Surgical procedures (depending on procedure, may want to discontinue 2–4 wk before surgery) ■ History of cigarette smoking or age >30–35 yr (increased risk of cardiovascular or thromboembolic phenomenon) ■ Presence of other cardiovascular risk factors (obesity, hyperglycemia, elevated lipids, hypertension) ■ History of diabetes mellitus, bleeding disorders, concurrent anticoagulant therapy or headaches.

**Exercise Extreme Caution in:** ■ Products containing >50 mcg estrogen (increased risk of thromboembolic disorders and other vascular problems) ■ Prepubertal girls (safety not established).

## ADVERSE REACTIONS AND SIDE EFFECTS*

■ **CNS:** depression, migraine headache ■ **EENT:** contact lens intolerance, optic neuritis, retinal thrombosis ■ **CV:** CEREBRAL HEMORRHAGE, CEREBRAL THROMBOSIS, CORONARY THROMBOSIS, PULMONARY EMBOLISM, edema, hypertension, Raynaud's phenomenon, thromboembolic phenomena, thrombophlebitis ■ **GI:** abdominal cramps, bloating, cholestatic jaundice, gallbladder disease, liver tumors, nausea, vomiting ■ **GU:** amenorrhea, breakthrough bleeding, dysmenorrhea, spotting, *Intrauterine levonerogestrel only*—uterine imbedment/uterine rupture ■ **Derm:** melasma, rash ■ **Endo:** hyperglycemia ■ **Misc:** weight change.

## INTERACTIONS

**Drug-Drug:** ■ Oral contraceptive efficacy may be ↓ by **penicillins, ampicillin, chloramphenicol, dihydroergotamine, mineral oil, oral neomycin, sulfonamides, barbiturates, chronic alcohol use, carbamazepine,** (systemic) **corticosteroids, griseofulvin, phenylbutazone, phenytoin, topiramate, primidone, modafinil, rifampin,** some **protease inhibitor antiretrovirals** (including **ritonavir**), or **tetracyclines** ■ May ↑ effects/risk of toxicity from **tricyclic antidepressants,** some **benzodiazepines, beta blockers, caffeine, corticosteroids, cyclosporine,** and **theophylline** ■ ↑ risk of hepatic toxicity with **dantrolene** (estrogen only) ■ **Carbamazepine** or **phenytoin** may ↓ efficacy of contraceptive implants ■ **Smoking** ↑

risk of thromboembolic phenomena (estrogen only) ■ May interfere with the effectiveness of **bromocriptine** ■ May ↓ levels of **acetaminophen, temazepam, lorazepam, oxazepam, salicylic acid,** or **morphine** ■ *Yasmin product only*—concurrent use with **NSAIDs, potassium-sparing diuretics, potasssium supplements, ACE inhibitors, angiotensin II receptor antagonists,** or **heparin** may result in hyperkalemia.

**Drug-Natural Products:** ■ Concomitant use with **St. John's wort** may ↓ contraceptive efficacy and cause breakthrough bleeding and irregular menses ■ ↑ caffeine levels and side effects with caffeine-containing herbs (**cola nut, tea, coffee**).

## ROUTE AND DOSAGE

❏ **Monophasic Oral Contraceptives**

■ **PO (Adults):** On 21-day regimen, take first tablet on first Sunday after menses begin (take on Sunday if menses begin on Sunday) for 21 days, then skip 7 days and begin again. Regimen may also be started on first day of menses, continue for 21 days, then skip 7 days and begin again. Some regimens contain 7 placebo tablets, so that 1 tablet is taken every day for 28 days.

❏ **Biphasic Oral Contraceptives**

■ **PO (Adults):** Given in 2 phases. First phase is 10 days of smaller amount of progestin. Second phase is larger amount of progestin. Amount of estrogen remains constant for same length of time (total of 21 days), then skip 7 days and begin again. Some regimens contain 7 placebo tablets for 28-day regimen.

❏ **Triphasic Oral Contraceptives**

■ **PO (Adults):** Progestin amount varies throughout 21-day cycle. Estrogen component stays the same or may vary. Some regimens contain 7 placebo tablets for 28-day regimen.

❏ **Extended-cycle contraceptive**

■ **PO (Adults):** Start taking first active pill on first Sunday after menses start (if first day is Sunday, start then), continue for 84 days of active pill, followed by 7 days of placebo tablets, then resume 84/7 cycle again.

❏ **Progestin-Only Oral Contraceptives**

■ **PO (Adults):** Start on first day of menses. Taken daily and continuously.

❏ **Progressive Estrogen Oral Contraceptives**

■ **PO (Adults):** Estrogen amount increases q 7 days throughout 21-day cycle. Progestin component stays the same. Some regimens contain 7 placebo tablets for 28-day regimen.

❏ **Contraceptive Implant**

■ **Subdermal: (Adults):** 6 capsules implanted subdermally during first 7 days of menses or immediately after abortion; replaced q 5 yr.

❏ **Emergency Contraceptive**

■ **PO (Adults and Adolescents):** Given within 72 hr of unprotected intercourse and repeated 12 hr later. *Plan B*—1 tablet followed by 1 more tablet 12 hr later; *Preven*—2 tablets followed by 2 more tablets 12 hr later; *Ovral*—2 white tablets; *Lo/Ovral*—4 white tablets; *Levlen, Nordette*—4 light orange tablets; *Triphasil, Tri-Levlen*—4 yellow tablets.

❏ **Injectable Contraceptive**

**estradiol/medroxyprogesterone (Lunelle)**

■ **IM (Adults):** 0.5 ml (contains 5 mg estradiol cypionate/25 mg medroxyprogesterone acetate) within first 5 days of menses, within 5 days of a complete first trimester abortion or no earlier than 4 weeks postpartum if not breastfeeding. If breastfeeding, give 6 wk postpartum; repeat q 28–30 days.

**medroxyprogesterone (Depo-Provera)**

■ **IM (Adults):** 150 mg within first 5 days of menses or within 5 days postpartum, if not breastfeeding. If breastfeeding, give 6 wk postpartum; repeat q 3 mo.

❏ **Vaginal Ring Contraceptive**

■ **Vag (Adults):** One ring inserted on or prior to day 5 of menstrual cycle. Ring is left in place for 3 wk, then removed for 1 wk, then a new ring is inserted.

❏ **Transdermal Patch**

■ **Transdermal (Adults):** Patch is applied on day 1 of menstrual cycle (or convenient day in first week), changed weekly thereafter for

3 weeks. Week 4 is patch-free. Cycle is then repeated.

□ **Acne**

■ **PO (Adults):** Ortho Tri-Cyclen only, taken daily for 21 days, off for 7 days.

## AVAILABILITY

□ **Combination Estrogen/Progestin Oral Contraceptives**

■ *Oral contraceptive tablets:* Usually in monthly packs with enough (21) active tablets to complete a 28-day cycle. Some contain 7 inert tablets to complete the cycle with or without supplemental iron[Rx] ■ Cost: *Alesse-28*—$98.85/3 cycles; *Demulen 1/35*—$197.83/6 cycles; *Desogen*—$171.17/6 cycles; *Loestrin Fe 1/20*—$165.83/5 cycles; *Loestrin 1.5/30*—$165.43/5 cycles; *Lo-Ovral 28*—$204.23/6 cycles; *Nordette*—$31.93/1 cycle; *Ortho-Cept*—$196.66/6 cycles; *Ortho-Novum 1/35*—$196.66/6 cycles; *Ortho-Novum 7-7-7*—$196.66/6 cycles; *Ortho-Cyclen*—$196.66/6 cycles; *Ortho Tri-Cyclen*—$196.66/6 cycles; *Tri-Levlen*—$95.50/3 cycles.

□ **Extended-cycle contraceptive**

■ *Tablets:* 84 active tablets containing 0.03 mg ethinyl estradiol and 0.15 mg levonorgestrel and 7 inactive tablets.

□ **Levonorgestrel**

■ *Emergency contraceptives:* 4 tablets containing 0.25 mg levonorgestrel and 0.05 of ethinyl estradiol packaged with a pregnancy test (Preven)[Rx], 2 tablets containing 0.75 mg levonorgestrel (Plan B)[Rx] ■ Cost: *Preven*—$19.94/kit ■ *Implant:* Package of 6 implantable capsules containing 36 mg of levonorgestrel each[Rx] ■ Cost: $475.00/implant ■ *Intrauterine system:* contains 52 mg norgestrel, (releases 20 mcg/day)[Rx].

□ **Estradiol/Medroxyprogesterone**

■ *Injectable suspension:* estradiol 5 mg/25 mg medroxyprogesterone per 0.5 ml/ml[Rx].

□ **Medroxyprogesterone**

■ *Injectable:* 150 mg/ml[Rx].

□ **Vaginal Ring Contraceptive**

■ *Ring:* delivers 0.015 mg ethinyl estradiol and 0.120 mg etonogestrel/day.

□ **Transdermal Patch**

■ *Patch:* contains 0.75 mg ethinyl estradiol and 6 mg of norelgestromin; releases 20 mg ethinyl estradiol/150 mg norelgestromin per 24 hr.

TIME/ACTION PROFILE (prevention of pregnancy)

| | ONSET | PEAK | DURATION |
|---|---|---|---|
| PO | 1 mo | 1 mo | 1 mo† |
| Implant | 1 mo | 1 mo | 5 yr |
| Intrauterine system | 1 mo | 1 mo | 5 yr |
| IM | 1 mo | 1 mo | 3 mo |

†Only during month of taking contraceptive.

# NURSING IMPLICATIONS

## ASSESSMENT

■ **General Info:** Assess blood pressure before and periodically throughout therapy.

■ **Acne:** Assess skin lesion before and periodically during therapy.

■ *Lab Test Considerations:* Monitor hepatic function periodically during therapy.

□ *Estrogens only*—May cause ↑ serum glucose, sodium, triglyceride, VHDL, total cholesterol, prothrombin, and factors VII, VIII, IX, and X levels. May cause ↓ LDL and antithrombin III levels.

□ May cause false interpretations of thyroid function tests, false ↑ in norepinephrine platelet-induced aggregability, and false ↓ in metyrapone tests.

□ *Progestins only*—May cause ↑ LDL concentrations. May cause ↓ serum alkaline phosphatase and HDL concentrations.

## POTENTIAL NURSING DIAGNOSES

■ Noncompliance (Patient/Family Teaching).

## IMPLEMENTATION

■ **PO:** Oral doses may be administered with or immediately after food to reduce nausea.

□ For extended-cycle tablets, take active tablets (pink) for 84 days and followed by the placebo tablets (white) for 7 days.

■ **Levonorgestrel Implant:** 6-capsule implant is inserted subdermally in midportion of upper arm about 8–10 cm above the elbow crease. Health care professionals attempting insertion or removal should be instructed in the procedures before attempting them.

- **IM:** Shake vial vigorously just before use to ensure uniform suspension. Administer deep IM into gluteal or deltoid muscle. If period between injections is >14 wk, determine that patient is not pregnant before administering the drug.

## PATIENT/FAMILY TEACHING

❏ Instruct patient to take oral medication as directed at the same time each day. Pills should be taken in proper sequence and kept in the original container.

❏ *If single daily dose is missed:* Take as soon as remembered; if not until next day, take 2 tablets and continue on regular dosing schedule. *If 2 days in a row are missed:* Take 2 tablets a day for the next 2 days and continue on regular dosing schedule, using a second method of birth control for the remaining cycle. *If 3 days in a row are missed:* Discontinue medication and use another form of birth control until period begins or pregnancy is ruled out; then begin a new cycle of tablets. *For 28-day dosing schedule:* If schedule is followed for first 21 days and 1 dose is missed of the last 7 tablets, it is important to take the 1st tablet of next month's cycle on the regularly scheduled day.

❏ Advise patient taking *extended-cycle tablets* that withdrawal bleeding should occur during the 7 days following discontinuation of the pink (active) tablets. If withdrawal bleeding does not occur, notify health care professional.

❏ For initial use of extended cycle tablets, caution patient to use a nonhormonal method of contraception until she has taken the first 7 days of pink (active) tablets. Each 91–day cycle should start on the same day of the week. If started later than the proper day or 2 or more days are missed, a second nonhormonal method of contraception should be used until she has taken the pink tablet for 7 days. Transient spotting or bleeding may occur. If bleeding is persistent or prolonged, notify health care professional.

❏ Advise patient of the need to use another form of contraception for the first 3 wk when beginning to use oral contraceptives.

❏ Advise patient that a second method of birth control should also be used during each cycle in which any of the following are used: *Oral contraceptives*—ampicillin, corticosteroids, antiretroviral protease inhibitors, barbiturates, carbamazepine, chloramphenicol, dihydroergotamine, corticosteroids (systemic), griseofulvin, mineral oil, oral neomycin, penicillin V, phenylbutazone, primidone, rifampin, sulfonamides, tetracyclines, or valproic acid. *Levonorgestrel implant*—carbamazepine or phenytoin.

❏ Explain dosage schedule and maintenance routine. Discontinuing medication suddenly may cause withdrawal bleeding.

❏ If nausea becomes a problem, advise patient that eating solid food often provides relief.

❏ Advise patient to report signs and symptoms of fluid retention (swelling of ankles and feet, weight gain), thromboembolic disorders (pain, swelling, tenderness in extremities, headache, chest pain, blurred vision), mental depression, hepatic dysfunction (yellowed skin or eyes, pruritus, dark urine, light-colored stools), or abnormal vaginal bleeding.Women with a strong family history of breast cancer, fibrocystic breast disease, abnormal mammograms or cervical dysplasia should be monitored for breast cancer at least yearly.

❏ Instruct patient to stop taking medication and notify health care professional if pregnancy is suspected.

❏ Caution patient that cigarette smoking during estrogen therapy may increase risk of serious side effects, especially for women over age 35.

❏ Caution patients to use sunscreen and protective clothing to prevent increased pigmentation.

❏ Caution patient that oral contraceptives do not protect against HIV or other sexually transmitted diseases.

❏ Advise patient to notify health care professional of medication regimen before treatment or surgery.

❏ Emphasize the importance of routine follow-up physical exams including blood pressure; breast, abdomen, and pelvic examinations; and Papanicolaou smears every 6–12 mo.

■ **Transdermal:** Instruct patient on application of patch. First patch should be applied within 24 hrs of menstrual period. If applied after Day 1 of menstrual period, a nonhormonal method of contraception should be used for the next 7 days. Day of application becomes *Patch Change Day*. Patches are worn for 1 wk and changed on the same day of each wk for 3 wks. Week 4 is patch-free. Withdrawal bleeding is expected during this time.

❑ Apply patch to clean, dry, intact, healthy skin on buttock, abdomen, upper outer arm, or upper torso in a place where it won't be rubbed by tight clothing. Do not place on skin that is red, irritated or cut, and do not place on breasts. Do not apply make-up, creams, lotions, powders, or other topical products to area of patch application.

❑ To apply patch open foil pouch by tearing along edge using fingers. Peel pouch apart and open flat. Grasp a corner of the patch firmly and remove gently from foil pouch. Use fingernail to lift one corner of the patch and peel patch **and** the plastic liner off the foil liner. Do not remove clear liner as patch is removed. Peel away half of the clear liner without touching sticky surface. Apply the sticky surface and remove the rest of the liner. Press down firmly with palm of hand for 10 seconds; make sure the edges stick well.

❑ On *Patch Change Day* remove patch and apply new one immediately. Used patch still contains some active hormones; fold in half so it sticks to itself and throw away. Apply new patches to a new spot to prevent skin irritation; may be applied in same anatomic area.

❑ Following patch-free week, apply a new patch on *Patch Change Day*, the day after Day 28, no matter when the menstrual cycle begins

❑ If patch becomes partially or completely detached for less than 1 day, reapply patch or apply new patch. If patch is detached for more than 1 day, apply a new patch immediately and use a nonhormonal form of contraception for the next 7 days. Cycle will now start over with a new *Patch Change Day*. If patch is no longer sticky, apply a new patch; do not use tape or wraps to keep patch in place.

❑ If patch is not changed on *Patch Change Day* in the first week of the cycle, apply new patch immediately upon remembering and use a nonhormonal method of contraception for next 7 days. If patch change is missed in for 1 or 2 days during Week 2 or 3, apply new patch immediately and apply next patch on usual *Patch Change Day*. No backup contraception is needed. If patch change is missed for more than 2 days during Week 2 or 3, stop the cycle and start a new 4-wk contraceptive cycle by applying new patch immediately and using a nonhormonal method of contraception for the next 7 days. If patch is not removed on *Patch Change Day* in Week 4, remove as soon as remembered and start next cycle on usual *Patch Change Day*. No additional contraception is needed.

■ **NuvaRing:** *If a hormonal contraceptive was not used in the past month,* insert *NuvaRing* between Day 1 and 5 of the menstrual cycle (Day 1 = first day of menstrual period), even if bleeding has not finished. Use a nonhormonal method of birth control other than a diaphragm during the first 7 days of ring use. *If switching from a combination estrogen/progesterone oral contraceptive,* insert *NuvaRing* any time during first 7 days after last tablet and no later than the day a new pill cycle would have started. No extra birth control is needed. *If switching from a mini-pill,* start using *NuvaRing* on any day of the month; do not skip days between last pill and first day of *NuvaRing* use. *If switching from an implant,* start using *NuvaRing* on same day implant is removed. *If switching from an injectable contraceptive,* start using *NuvaRing* on the day when next injection is due. *If switching from a progestin-containing IUD,* start using *NuvaRing* on the same day as IUD is removed. A nonhormonal method of contraception, other than the diaphragm, should be used for the first 7 days of *NuvaRing* use when switching from the mini-pill, implant, injectable contraceptive, or IUD.

❑ *NuvaRing* comes in a reclosable foil pouch. Instruct patient to wash hands, then remove *NuvaRing* from pouch; keep pouch for ring disposal. Using the position of comfort (lying down, squatting, or standing with one leg up), hold *NuvaRing* between thumb and index finger and press opposite sides of the ring together. Gently push folded ring into vagina. Exact position is not important for function of *NuvaRing*. Most women do not feel *NuvaRing* once it is in place. If discomfort is felt, *NuvaRing* may not be inserted far enough into vagina; use finger to push further into vagina. *There is no danger of NuvaRing being pushed in too far or getting lost.* Once inserted, leave *NuvaRing* in place for 3 wks.

❏ Remove ring 3 wks after insertion on same day and time of insertion. Remove by hooking finger under forward rim or by holding ring between index and middle finger and pulling out. Place ring in foil pouch and dispose; do not throw in toilet. Menstrual period will usually start 2–3 days after ring is removed and may not have finished before next ring is inserted. To continue contraceptive protection, new ring must be inserted 1 wk after last one was removed, even if menstrual period has not stopped.

❏ If *NuvaRing* slips out of vagina and has been out less than 3 hrs, contraceptive protection is still in place. *NuvaRing* can be rinsed in cool to tepid water and should be reinserted as soon as possible. If ring is lost, insert a new ring and continue same schedule as lost ring. If *NuvaRing* has been out of vagina for more than 3 hrs, a nonhormonal method of contraception, other than a diaphragm, should be used for the next 7 days.

❏ *If NuvaRing has been left in for an extra wk or less (4 wks total or less)*, remove and insert a new ring after a 1 wk ring-free break. If *NuvaRing* has been left in place for more than 4 wks, woman should check to be sure she is not pregnant. A nonhormonal method of contraception, other than a diaphragm, must be used for the next 7 days.

## EVALUATION

**Effectiveness of therapy can be demonstrated by:** ■ Prevention of pregnancy ■ Regulation of the menstrual cycle ■ Decrease in acne.

# CORTICOSTEROIDS (INHALATION)

**beclomethasone**
(be-kloe-**meth**-a-sone)
{Beclodisk}, {Becloforte}, QVAR

**budesonide**
(byoo-**dess**-oh-nide)
Pulmicort

**flunisolide**
(floo-**niss**-oh-lide)
AeroBid, {Bronalide}

**fluticasone**
(floo-**ti**-ka-sone)
Flovent

**triamcinolone**
(trye-am-**sin**-oh-lone)
Azmacort, Azmacort HFA

*CLASSIFICATION(S):*
*Therapeutic: antiasthmatics, corticosteroids*
*Pharmacologic: corticosteroids (inhalation)*

**Pregnancy Category B (budesonide), C (all others)**

## INDICATIONS

■ Asthma (maintenance/prophylactic; long-term control) ■ May decrease the need for systemic corticosteroids and delay lung damage associated with asthma.

## ACTION

■ Potent, locally acting anti-inflammatory and immune modifier. **Therapeutic Effects:** ■ Decreased frequency and severity of asthma ■ Prevention of pulmonary damage from asthma.

## PHARMACOKINETICS

**Absorption:** *Beclomethasone—20%; budesonide—39%; flunisolide—40%; fluticasone—30%(aerosol), 13.5% (powder); triamcino-*

*lone*—25%. Action is primarily local after inhalation.

**Distribution:** 10–25% is deposited in airways if a spacer device is not used. With a spacer, more drug may reach the respiratory tract. All cross the placenta and enter breast milk in small amounts.

**Protein Binding:** *Budenoside*—85–90%; *fluticasone*—91%.

**Metabolism and Excretion:** *Beclomethasone*—after inhalation, beclomethasone dipropionate is converted to beclomethasone monopropionate, an active metabolite that adds to its potency, <10% excreted in feces and urine; *budenoside, flunisolide, fluticasone,* and *triamcinolone*—metabolized by the liver after absorption from lungs. *Budenoside*—60% excreted in urine, smaller amounts in feces; *flunisolide*—50% excreted in urine, 50% in feces; *fluticasone*—<5% excreted in urine and feces; *triamcinolone*—40% excreted in urine, 60% in feces.

**Half-life:** *Beclomethasone*—0.5 hr; *budesonide*—2–3 hr; *flunisolide*—1.8 hr; *fluticasone*—7.8 hr; *triamcinolone*—88 min.

## CONTRAINDICATIONS AND PRECAUTIONS

**Contraindicated in:** ■ Some products contain chlorofluorocarbon (CFC) propellants, alcohol, propylene, or polyethylene glycol and should be avoided in patients with known hypersensitivity or intolerance ■ Acute attack of asthma/status asthmaticus.

**Use Cautiously in:** ■ Active untreated infections ■ Patients with diabetes or glaucoma ■ Patients with underlying immunosuppression (due to disease or concurrent therapy) ■ Systemic corticosteroid therapy (should not be abruptly discontinued; additional corticosteroids needed in stress or trauma) ■ Pregnancy, lactation, or children <5 yr (safety not established; prolonged or high-dose therapy may lead to complications).

## ADVERSE REACTIONS AND SIDE EFFECTS*

■ **CNS:** *Budesonide, fluticasone*—headache; *Fluticasone*—agitation, depression, fatigue, insomnia, restlessness ■ **EENT:** dysphonia, hoarseness, oropharyngeal fungal infections, cataracts; *Fluticasone*—nasal stuffiness/sinusitis ■ **Resp:** bronchospasm, cough, wheezing ■ **GI:** dry mouth, esophageal candidiasis; *Bude-*

*sonide*—dyspepsia, gastroenteritis; *Fluticasone*—nausea ■ **Endo:** adrenal suppression (increased dose, long-term therapy only), decreased growth (children) ■ **MS:** *Budesonide*—back pain; *Fluticasone*—muscle soreness ■ **Misc:** CHURG-STRAUSS SYNDROME; *Budesonide*—flu-like syndrome.

## INTERACTIONS

**Drug-Drug:** ■ **Ketoconazole** ↓ metabolism and ↑ levels of budesonide and fluticasone.

## ROUTE AND DOSAGE

❏ **Beclomethasone**

■ **Inhaln (Adults and adolescents):** *Previously therapy of bronchodilators alone*—40 – 80 mcg twice daily; *previously therapy of inhaled corticosteroids*—40 – 160 mcg twice daily (up to 320 mcg twice daily).

■ **Inhaln (Children 5–11 yr):** 40 mcg twice daily (up to 80 mcg twice daily).

❏ **Budesonide**

■ **Inhaln (Adults [Pulmicort turbuhaler dose form]):** *Previous control with bronchodilators alone*—1–2 inhalations twice daily (200 mcg/inhalation); *previous control on other inhaled corticosteroids*—1–2 inhalations twice daily (up to 4 inhalations twice daily); *previous control on oral corticosteroids*—2–4 inhalations twice daily (up to 4 inhalations twice daily).

■ **Inhaln (Children ≥6 yr [Pulmicort Turbhaler dose form]):** *Previous control on bronchodilators alone*—1–2 inhalations twice daily (200 mcg/inhalation); *previous control on other inhaled corticosteroids*—1–2 inhalations twice daily; *previous control on oral corticosteroids*—Not to exceed 2 inhalations twice daily.

■ **Inhaln (Children 12 mos–8 yr [Pulmicort Respules dose form]):** —*Previous control on bronchodilators alone*—0.25 mg/day as a single dose or twice daily in divided doses; *previous control on other inhaled corticosteroids*—0.5 mg/day as a single dose or twice daily in divided doses; *previous control on oral corticosteroids*—1 mg/day as a single dose or twice daily in divided doses.

❏ **Flunisolide**

■ **Inhaln (Adults and Children >6 yr):** 2 inhalations twice daily (250 mcg/ inhalation;

not to exceed 8 inhalations/day in adults or 4 inhalations/day in children).

❑ **Fluticasone (Aerosol Inhaler)**

■ **Inhaln (Adults and Adolescents):** *Previous control on bronchodilators alone*—88 mcg twice daily initially, may be increased up to 440 mcg twice daily; *previous control on other inhaled corticosteroids*—88–220 mcg twice daily initially, up to 440 mcg twice daily; *previous control included systemic corticosteroids*—880 mcg twice daily.

❑ **Fluticasone (Dry Powder Inhaler)**

■ **Inhaln (Adults and Adolescents):** *Previous control on bronchodilators alone*—100 mcg twice daily initially, may be increased up to 500 mcg twice daily; *previous control on other inhaled corticosteroids*—100–250 mcg twice daily initially, up to 500 mcg twice daily; *previous control on systemic corticosteroids*—1000 mcg twice daily.

■ **Inhaln (Children 4–11 yr):** 50 mcg twice daily initially, may be increased up to 100 mcg twice daily.

❑ **Triamcinolone**

■ **Inhaln (Adults and Children >12 yr):** 2 inhalations 3–4 times daily *or* 4 inhalations twice daily (100 mcg/ inhalation; not to exceed 16 inhalations/day).

■ **Inhaln (Children 6–12 yr):** 1–2 inhalations 3–4 times daily *or* 2–4 inhalations twice daily (100 mcg/ inhalation; not to exceed 12 inhalations/day).

### AVAILABILITY

❑ **Beclomethasone**

■ *Inhalation aerosol:* 40 mcg/metered inhalation in 7.3-g canister (100 metered inhalations)$^{Rx}$, {50 mcg/metered inhalation in 16.8-g canister (200 metered inhalations)$^{Rx}$}, 80mcg/ metered inhalation in 7.3-g canister (100 metered inhalations) $^{Rx}$, {250 mcg/metered inhalation in 80- or 200-metered-inhalation canisters$^{Rx}$} ■ Cost: 40 mcg/metered inhalation $41.32/7.3–g canister; 80 mcg metered inhalation $52.04/7.3–g canister ■ *Inhalation capsules:* {100 mcg$^{Rx}$}, {200 mcg$^{Rx}$.}

❑ **Budesonide**

■ *Inhalation powder:* 200 mcg/metered inhalation in 200-metered-inhalation inhaler$^{Rx}$ ■ *Inhalation suspension (Respules):* 0.25 mg/2 ml$^{Rx}$, 0.5 mg/2 ml$^{Rx}$.

❑ **Flunisolide**

■ *Inhalation aerosol:* 250 mcg/metered inhalation in 7-g canisters (100 metered inhalations)$^{Rx}$.

❑ **Fluticasone**

■ *Inhalation aerosol:* 44 mcg/metered inhalation in 7.9-g (60 metered inhalations) and 13-g (120 metered inhalations) canisters$^{Rx}$, 110 mcg/metered inhalation in 13-g canisters (120 metered inhalations)$^{Rx}$, 220 mcg/metered inhalation in 13-g canisters (120 metered inhalations)$^{Rx}$ ■ Cost: 44 mcg $50.77/each ■ *Dry powder inhaler (Diskhaler):* 50 mcg$^{Rx}$, 100 mcg$^{Rx}$, 250 mcg$^{Rx}$ Rotadisk blister. ■ salmeterol (Advair Diskus)$^{Rx}$. See Appendix B.

❑ **Triamcinolone**

■ *Inhalation aerosol:* 100 mcg/metered inhalation in 20-g canister (240 metered inhalations)$^{Rx}$ ■ Cost: 100 mcg $68.58/each.

TIME/ACTION PROFILE (improvement in symptoms)

| | ONSET | PEAK | DURATION |
|---|---|---|---|
| Inhalation | within 24 hr‡ | 1–4 wk† | unknown |

†Improvement in pulmonary function; decreased airway responsiveness may take longer.
‡2-8 days for budenoside Respule.

## NURSING IMPLICATIONS

### ASSESSMENT

❑ Monitor respiratory status and lung sounds. Pulmonary function tests may be assessed periodically during and for several months after a transfer from systemic to inhalation corticosteroids.

❑ Assess patients changing from systemic corticosteroids to inhalation corticosteroids for signs of adrenal insufficiency (anorexia, nausea, weakness, fatigue, hypotension, hypoglycemia) during initial therapy and periods of stress. If these signs appear, notify physician

{ } = Available in Canada only.
*CAPITALS indicates life-threatening; underlines indicate most frequent.

or other health care professional immediately; condition may be life-threatening.

❑ Monitor for withdrawal symptoms (joint or muscular pain, lassitude, depression) during withdrawal from oral corticosteroids.

■ *Lab Test Considerations:* Periodic adrenal function tests may be ordered to assess degree of hypothalamic-pituitary-adrenal (HPA) axis suppression in chronic therapy. Children and patients using higher than recommended doses are at highest risk for HPA suppression.

❑ May cause ↑ serum and urine glucose concentrations if significant absorption occurs.

❑ Monitor growth rate in children; use lowest possible dose.

## POTENTIAL NURSING DIAGNOSES

■ Airway clearance, ineffective (Indications).
■ Infection, risk for (Side Effects).

## IMPLEMENTATION

■ **General:** After the desired clinical effect has been obtained, attempts should be made to decrease dose to lowest amount required to control symptoms. Gradually decrease dose every 2–4 wk as long as desired effect is maintained. If symptoms return, dose may briefly return to starting dose.

❑ When switching from other beclomethasone inhalers containing CFCs to *QVAR*, start at 1/2 the dose of the CFC inhaler, because of smaller particle size and increased delivery **Inhaln:** Allow at least 1 min between inhalations of aerosol medication.

## PATIENT/FAMILY TEACHING

■ **General Info:** Advise patient to take medication as directed. Take missed doses as soon as remembered unless almost time for next dose. Advise patient not to discontinue medication without consulting health care professional; gradual decrease is required.

❑ Advise patients using inhalation corticosteroids and bronchodilator to use bronchodilator first and to allow 5 min to elapse before administering the corticosteroid, unless otherwise directed by health care professional.

❑ Advise patient that inhalation corticosteroids should not be used to treat an acute asthma attack but should be continued even if other inhalation agents are used.

❑ Patients using inhalation corticosteroids to control asthma may require systemic corticosteroids for acute attacks. Advise patient to use regular peak flow monitoring to determine respiratory status.

❑ Caution patient to avoid smoking, known allergens, and other respiratory irritants. Patients who have not been immunized should also avoid exposure to chickenpox or measles.

❑ Advise patient to notify physician if sore throat or sore mouth occurs.

❑ Instruct patient whose systemic corticosteroids have been recently reduced or withdrawn to carry a warning card indicating the need for supplemental systemic corticosteroids in the event of stress or severe asthma attack unresponsive to bronchodilators.

❑ Inform patient that beclomethasone aerosol may have different taste and sensation than inhalers containing CFC propellant.

■ **Metered-Dose Inhaler:** Instruct patient in the proper use of the metered-dose inhaler. Most inhalers require priming before first use. There are 3 methods of using a metered-dose inhaler. Shake inhaler well. (1) Take a drink of water to moisten the throat; place the inhaler mouthpiece 2 finger-widths away from mouth; tilt head back slightly; while activating inhaler, take a slow, deep breath for 3–5 sec, hold the breath for 10 sec, and breathe out slowly. (2) Exhale, close lips firmly around mouthpiece, administer during 2nd half of inhalation, and hold breath for as long as possible to ensure deep instillation of medication. (3) Use a spacer. Consult health care professional to determine method desired before instruction. Allow 1–2 min between inhalations. Rinse mouth with water or mouthwash after each use to minimize fungal infections, dry mouth, and hoarseness. Wash inhalation assembly at least daily in warm running water (see Appendix F).

■ **Pulmicort Turbuhaler (budesonide):** Advise patient to follow instructions supplied. Before first-time use, prime unit by turning cover and lifting off; hold upright with mouthpiece up and twist brown grip fully to right, then to left; repeat. To administer dose, hold upright, twist brown grip fully to right, then to left, listening for click. Turn head away from inhaler and exhale (do not blow into inhaler). Do not shake. Place mouthpiece between lips and inhale forcefully. Repeat procedure if 2nd dose required. Replace cover; rinse mouth with water (do not swallow).

■ **Flovent Rotadisk:** Advise patient to follow instructions for the administration of the contents of each blister via breath-activated Diskhaler device.

## EVALUATION

**Effectiveness of therapy can be demonstrated by:** ■ Management of the symptoms of chronic asthma ■ Prevention of pulmonary damage that results from chronic asthma.

---

## CORTICOSTEROIDS (NASAL)

### beclomethasone
(be-kloe-**meth**-a-sone)
Beconase, Beconase AQ, Vancenase, Vancenase AQ 84 mcg

### budesonide
(byoo-**dess**-oh-nide)
Rhinocort, Rhinocort Aqua

### flunisolide
(floo-**niss**-oh-lide)
Nasalide, Nasarel, {Rhinalar}

### fluticasone
(floo-**ti**-ka-sone)
Flonase

### mometasone
(moe-**met**-a-sone)
Nasonex

### triamcinolone
(trye-am-**sin**-oh-lone)
Nasacort, Nasacort AQ, Tri-Nasal

*CLASSIFICATION(S):*

*Therapeutic: allergy, cold, and cough remedies, corticosteroids*
*Pharmacologic: corticosteroids (nasal)*

**Pregnancy Category C**

---

## INDICATIONS

■ Seasonal and perennial allergic rhinitis. allergic rhinitis and other chronic nasal inflammatory conditions, including nasal polyps.

## ACTION

■ Potent, locally acting anti-inflammatory and immune modifier. **Therapeutic Effects:** ■ Decrease in symptoms of allergic rhinitis.

## PHARMACOKINETICS

**Absorption:** *Beclomethasone*—absorption is rapid; *budesonide*—small amounts absorbed; *flunisolide*—50% absorbed; *fluticasone*—<2% absorbed; Action of all agents is primarily local following nasal use; systemic absorption is minimal at recommended doses; *mometasone*—negligible absorption.

**Distribution:** Small portions of corticosteroids administered nasally are swallowed. All agents cross the placenta and enter breast milk in small amounts.

**Metabolism and Excretion:** Following absorption from nasal mucosa, corticosteroids are rapidly and extensively metabolized by the liver.

**Half-life:** *Beclomethasone*—1.5 hr; *budesonide*—2 hr (plasma); *flunisolide*—1–2 hr; *fluticasone*—3 hr; *mometasone*—5.8 hr; *triamcinolone*—4 hr (due to prolonged absorption).

## CONTRAINDICATIONS AND PRECAUTIONS

**Contraindicated in:** ■ Some products contain fluorocarbon propellants, alcohol, propylene, or polyethylene glycol and should be avoided in patients with known hypersensitivity or intolerance.

**Use Cautiously in:** ■ Active untreated infections ■ Patients with diabetes or glaucoma ■ Patients with underlying immunosuppression (due to disease or concurrent therapy) ■ Systemic corticosteroid therapy (should not be abruptly discontinued when intranasal therapy is started) ■ Recent nasal trauma or surgery (wound healing may be impaired by nasal corticosteroids) ■ Pregnancy or lactation (safety not established; prolonged or high-dose therapy may lead to complications).

## ADVERSE REACTIONS AND SIDE EFFECTS*

■ **CNS:** dizziness, headache (increased with triamcinolone) ■ **EENT:** loss of sense of smell (flunisolide only), nasal burning, nasal irritation, sneezing attacks, throat itching (budesonide only), nasal bleeding ■ **GI:** abdominal pain, loss of sense of taste (flunisolide only), esophageal candidiasis ■ **Endo:** adrenal suppression (increased dose, long-term therapy only).

## INTERACTIONS

**Drug-Drug:** ■ None significant at recommended doses.

## ROUTE AND DOSAGE

❑ **Beclomethasone**

■ **Intranasal (Adults and Children >12 yr):** *Beconase, Vancenase*—1 metered spray in each nostril 2–4 times daily (42–50 mcg/spray); *Beconase AQ*—1–2 sprays in each nostril twice daily (42 mcg/spray); *Vancenase AQ 84 mcg*—1–2 sprays in each nostril once daily (84 mcg/spray); not to exceed 1 mg/day total.

■ **Intranasal (Children 6–12 yr):** *Beconase, Vancenase*—1 metered spray in each nostril 3 times daily (42–50 mcg/spray); *Beconase AQ*—1 metered spray in each nostril twice daily, may increase to 2 sprays in each nostril twice daily; (42 mcg/spray); *Vancenase AQ 84 mcg*—1–2 sprays in each nostril once daily (84 mcg/spray;)not to exceed 500 mcg/day.

■ **Intranasal (Adults and Children ≥6 yr):** *Vancenase AQ*—1 spray in each nostril(84 mcg/spray) once daily.

❑ **Budesonide**

■ **Intranasal (Adults and Children ≥6 yr):** *Rhinocort*—2 sprays in each nostril twice daily or 4 sprays in each nostril once daily; *Rhinocort Aqua*—1 spray in each nostril once daily; not to exceed 4 sprays in each nostril once daily in adults or 2 sprays in each nostril once daily in children 6–11 yr (32 mcg/spray);

❑ **Flunisolide**

■ **Intranasal (Adults and Children >14 yr):** 2 sprays in each nostril 2 times daily; dosage should be decreased to lowest effective amount and discontinued when possible (25 mcg/spray; not to exceed 16 metered sprays/day).

■ **Intranasal (Children 6–14 yr):** 1 spray in each nostril three time daily or 2 sprays in each nostril twice daily; dosage should be decreased to lowest effective amount and discontinued when possible (25 mcg/metered spray; not to exceed 8 metered sprays/day).

❑ **Fluticasone**

■ **Intranasal (Adults):** 2 sprays in each nostril once daily or 1 spray in each nostril twice daily after several days; decrease to 1 spray in each nostril once daily (50 mcg/metered spray; not to exceed 4 metered sprays/day).

■ **Intranasal (Children >4 yr and Adolescents):** 1 spray in each nostril once daily (50 mcg/metered spray); not to exceed 200 mcg/day total dose.

❑ **Mometasone**

■ **Intranasal (Adults and Children >12 yr):** 2 sprays in each nostril (50 mcg/spray) once daily.

■ **Intranasal (Children 2–11 yr):** 1 spray in each nostril (50 mcg/spray) once daily.

❑ **Triamcinolone**

■ **Intranasal (Adults):** *Nasacort, Nasacort AQ, Tri-Nasal*—2 sprays in each nostril once daily (50–55 mcg/metered spray; not to exceed 8 metered sprays/day); —

■ **Intranasal (Children 6–11 yr):** *Nasacort*—2 sprays in each nostril once daily; *Nasacort AQ*—One spray in each nostil once daily.

## AVAILABILITY

❑ **Beclomethasone**

■ *Nasal aerosol:* 42 mcg/metered spray in 25-g canister (200 metered sprays)[Rx], {50 mcg/metered spray in 16.8-g canister (200 metered sprays)[Rx] } ■ *Nasal solution:* 42 mcg/metered spray in 25-g bottles (200 metered sprays)[Rx], 50 mcg/metered spray in 25-g bottles (200 metered sprays)[Rx], 84 mcg/metered spray in 25-g bottles (200 metered sprays)[Rx] ■ Cost: 42 mcg $54.82/each.

❑ **Budesonide**

■ *Nasal aerosol:* 32 mcg/metered spray in 7-g canister (200 metered sprays)[Rx] ■ Cost: $43.31/each.

❏ **Flunisolide**

■ *Nasal solution:* 25 mcg/spray in 25-ml bottle (200 metered sprays)$^{Rx}$.

❏ **Fluticasone**

■ *Nasal spray:* 50 mcg/metered spray in 9-g bottle (120 metered sprays)$^{Rx}$ ■ Cost: $57.71/ 17 g.

❏ **Mometasone**

■ *Nasal spray:* 50 mcg/metered spray in 17-g bottle (120 sprays)$^{Rx}$ ■ Cost: $57.71/16 g.

❏ **Triamcinolone**

■ *Nasal spray:* 55 mcg/metered spray in 15-g canister (100 metered sprays)$^{Rx}$, 50 mcg/metered spray in 15–ml bottle (Tri-Nasal) ■ Cost: $38.34/15 g.

TIME/ACTION PROFILE (improvement in symptoms)

| | ONSET | PEAK | DURATION |
|---|---|---|---|
| Beclomethasone | 3 days | up to 3 wk | unknown |
| Budesonide | 104 hr | 3–7 days (up to 3 wk) | unknown |
| Flunisolide | few days | up to 3 wk | unknown |
| Fluticasone | few days | unknown | unknown |
| Mometasone | within 2 days | 1–2 wk | unknown |
| Triamcinolone | 12 hr-a few days | 2–3 wk | unknown |

## NURSING IMPLICATIONS

### ASSESSMENT

❏ Monitor degree of nasal stuffiness, amount and color of nasal discharge, and frequency of sneezing.

❏ Patients on long-term therapy should have periodic otolaryngologic examinations to monitor nasal mucosa and passages for infection or ulceration.

■ *Lab Test Considerations:* Periodic adrenal function tests may be ordered to assess degree of hypothalamic-pituitary-adrenal (HPA) axis suppression in chronic therapy. Children and patients using higher than recommended doses are at highest risk for HPA suppression.

## POTENTIAL NURSING DIAGNOSES

■ Airway clearance, ineffective (Indications).

■ Infection, risk for (Side Effects).

## IMPLEMENTATION

■ **General:** After the desired clinical effect has been obtained, attempts should be made to decrease dose to lowest amount. Gradually decrease dose every 2–4 wk as long as desired effect is maintained. If symptoms return, dose may briefly return to starting dose.

■ **Intranasal:** Patients also using a topical decongestant should be given a decongestant 5–15 min before corticosteroid nasal spray. If patient is unable to breathe freely through nasal passages, instruct patient to blow nose gently in advance of medication administration.

## PATIENT/FAMILY TEACHING

❏ Advise patient to take medication exactly as directed. If a dose is missed, take as soon as remembered unless almost time for next dose.

❏ Caution patient not to exceed maximal daily dose of 4 sprays/nostril.

❏ Instruct patient in correct technique for administering nasal spray (see Appendix F). Most nasal sprays include directions with pictures. Instruct patient to read patient informations sheet prior to use. Shake well before use. Warn patient that temporary nasal stinging may occur.

❏ Advise patient to store canister with valve downward. Canister should not be stored in cold areas or in high humidity and should be used within 3 mo (beclomethasone, flunisolide) or within 6 mo of opening aluminum pouch. Advise patient to save inhaler for beclomethasone or dexamethasone; refills may be available.

❏ Instruct patient to notify health care professional if symptoms do not improve within 1 mo or if nasal discharge becomes purulent.

## EVALUATION

**Effectiveness of therapy can be demonstrated by:** ■ Resolution of nasal stuffiness, discharge, and sneezing in seasonal or perennial rhinitis.

{ } = Available in Canada only.
*CAPITALS indicates life-threatening; underlines indicate most frequent.

## CORTICOSTEROIDS (SYSTEMIC)

### short-acting corticosteroids

**cortisone**

**(kor-**ti-sone)
{Cortone}, Cortone Acetate

**hydrocortisone**

**(hye-droe-kor-**ti-sone)
A-hydroCort, Cortef, Hydrocortone, Solu-Cortef

### intermediate-acting corticosteroids

**methylprednisolone**

**(meth-ill-pred-niss-**oh-lone)
A-Methapred, depMedalone, Depo-Medrol, Depoject, Depopred, Duralone, Medralone, Medrol, Solu-Medrol

**prednisolone**

**(pred-niss-**oh-lone)
Articulose, Cotolone, Delta-Cortef, Hydeltrasol, Key-Pred, Nor-Pred, OrapredPediapred, Predacort, Predate, Pred-Ject, Prednisol, Prelone

**prednisone**

**(pred-**ni-sone)
Cordrol, Deltasone, Liquid Pred, Meticorten, Orasone, Panasol-S, Pred-Pak, Prednicen-M, Prednicot, Sterapred

**triamcinolone**

**(trye-am-sin-**oh-lone)
Amcort, Aristocort, Aristospan, Atolone, Clinacort, Kenacort, Kenaject, Kenalog, Tac, Triam-A, Triam Forte, Triamolone, Triamonide, Tri-Kort, Trilog, Trilone, Tristoject

### long-acting corticosteroids

**betamethasone**

(bay-ta-**meth-**a-sone)
{Betnelan}, {Betnesol}, Celestone, Cel-U-Jec, {Selestoject}

**budesonide**

**(byoo-des-**oh-nide)
Entocort EC

**dexamethasone**

(dex-a-**meth-**a-sone)
Cortastat, Dalalone, Decadrol, Decadron, Decaject, Deronil, Dexacorten, Dexameth, Dexasone, Dexone, Hexadrol, Primethasone, Solurex

**CLASSIFICATION(S):**

*Therapeutic: antiasthmatics, corticosteroids*

*Pharmacologic: corticosteroids (systemic)*

**Pregnancy Category C (prednisolone), UK (all others)**

## INDICATIONS

■ **Cortisone, hydrocortisone:** Management of adrenocortical insufficiency; chronic use in other situations is limited because of mineralocorticoid activity ■ **Betamethasone, dexamethasone, prednisolone, prednisone, methylprednisolone, triamcinolone:** Used systemically and locally in a wide variety of chronic diseases including: ❑ Inflammatory ❑ Allergic ❑ Hematologic ❑ Neoplastic ❑ Autoimmune disorders ❑ With other immunosuppressants in the prevention of organ rejection in tranplatation surgery ■ Asthma ■ Some agents are suitable for alternate-day dosing in the management of chronic illness (methylprednisolone, prednisolone, prednisone, triamcinolone) ■ Replacement therapy in adrenal insufficiency (not dexamethasone) ■ **Dexamethasone:** Management of cerebral edema ❑ Diagnostic agent in adrenal disorders ■ **Budesonide:** Treatment of mild to moderate Crohn's disease. **Unlabeled uses:** ■ Short-term administration to high-risk mothers before delivery to prevent respiratory distress syndrome in the newborn (betamethasone, dexamethasone) ■ Adjunctive therapy of hypercalcemia ■ Management of acute spinal cord injury (methylprednisolone) ■ Adjunctive management of nausea and vomiting from chemotherapy.

## ACTION

■ In pharmacologic doses, all agents suppress inflammation and the normal immune response ■ All agents have numerous intense metabolic effects (see Adverse Reactions and Side Effects) ■ Suppress adrenal function at chronic doses of *betamethasone*—0.6 mg/day; *cortisone, hydrocortisone*—20 mg/day; *dexamethasone*—0.75 mg/day; *methylprednisolone*—4 mg/day; *prednisone/prednisolone*—5 mg/day; *triamcinolone*—4 mg/day ■ **Cortisone, hydrocortisone:** Replace endogenous cortisol in deficiency states ■ **Cortisone, hydrocortisone:** Also have potent mineralocorticoid (sodium-retaining) activity ■ **Prednisolone, prednisone:** Have minimal mineralocorticoid activity ■ **Betamethasone, dexamethasone, methylprednisolone, triamcinolone:** Have negligible mineralocorticoid activity ■ **Budesonide:** local anti-inflammatory activity in the lumen of the GI tract. **Therapeutic Effects:** ■ Suppression of inflammation and modification of the normal immune response ■ Replacement therapy in adrenal insufficiency ■ **Budesonide:** improvement in symptoms/sequelae of Crohn's disease.

## PHARMACOKINETICS

**Absorption:** Well absorbed after oral administration. Sodium phosphate and sodium succinate salts are rapidly absorbed after IM administration. Acetate, acetonide, diacetate, hexacetonide, and tebutate salts are slowly but completely absorbed after IM administration. Absorption from local sites (intra-articular, intralesional) is slow but complete. Budesonide is rapidly inactivated following absorption.

**Distribution:** All are widely distributed, cross the placenta, and probably enter breast milk.

**Metabolism and Excretion:** All are metabolized mostly by the liver. *Cortisone* is converted by the liver to hydrocortisone. *Prednisone* is converted by the liver to prednisolone, which is then metabolized by the liver.

**Half-life:** *Betamethasone*—3–5 hr (plasma), 36–54 hr (tissue); adrenal suppression lasts 3.25 days. *Budesonide*—2.0–3.6 hr. *Cortisone*—0.5 hr (plasma), 8–12 hr (tissue); adrenal suppression lasts 1.25–1.5 days. *Dexamethasone*—3–4.5 hr (plasma), 36–54 hr (tissue); adrenal suppression lasts 2.75 days. *Hydrocortisone*—1.5–2 hr (plasma), 8–12 hr (tissue); adrenal suppression lasts 1.25–1.5 days. *Methylprednisolone*—>3.5 hr (plasma), 18–36 hr (tissue); adrenal suppression lasts 1.25–1.5 days. *Prednisolone*—2.1–3.5 hr (plasma), 18–36 hr (tissue); adrenal suppression lasts 1.25–1.5 days. *Prednisone*—3.4–3.8 hr (plasma), 18–36 hr (tissue); adrenal suppression lasts 1.25–1.5 days. *Triamcinolone*—2–>5 hr (plasma), 18–36 hr (tissue); adrenal suppression lasts 2.25 days.

## CONTRAINDICATIONS AND PRECAUTIONS

**Contraindicated in:** ■ Active untreated infections (may be used in patients being treated for some forms of meningitis) ■ Lactation (avoid chronic use) ■ Known alcohol, bisulfite, or tartrazine hypersensitivity or intolerance (some products contain these and should be avoided in susceptible patients).

**Use Cautiously in:** ■ Chronic treatment (will lead to adrenal suppression; use lowest possible dose for shortest period of time) ■ Children (chronic use will result in decreased growth; use lowest possible dose for shortest period of time) ■ Stress (surgery, infections); supplemental doses may be needed ■ Potential infections may mask signs (fever, inflammation) ■ Pregnancy (safety not established).

## ADVERSE REACTIONS AND SIDE EFFECTS*

Adverse reactions/side effects are much more common with high-dose/long-term therapy. ■ **CNS:** depression, euphoria, headache, increased intracranial pressure (children only), personality changes, psychoses, restlessness ■ **EENT:** cataracts, increased intraocular pressure ■ **CV:** hypertension ■ **GI:** PEPTIC ULCERATION, anorexia, nausea, vomiting ■ **Derm:** acne, decreased wound healing, ecchymoses, fragility, hirsutism, petechiae ■ **Endo:** adrenal suppression, hyperglycemia ■ **F and E:** fluid retention (long-term high doses), hypokalemia, hypokalemic alkalosis ■ **Hemat:** THROMBOEMBOLISM, thrombophlebitis ■ **Metab:** weight gain, weight loss ■ **MS:** muscle wasting, osteoporosis, aseptic necrosis of joints, muscle pain ■ **Misc:** cushingoid appearance (moon face, buffalo hump), increased susceptibility to infection.

### INTERACTIONS

**Drug-Drug:** ■ ↑ risk of hypokalemia with **thiazide** and **loop diuretics, amphotericin B, piperacillin,** or **ticarcillin** ■ Hypokalemia may ↑ risk of **digoxin** toxicity ■ May increase requirement for **insulin** or **oral hypoglycemic agents** ■ **Phenytoin, phenobarbital,** and **rifampin** ↑ metabolism; may ↓ effectiveness ■ **Hormonal contraceptives** may ↓ metabolism ■ ↑ risk of adverse GI effects with **NSAIDs** (including aspirin) ■ At chronic doses that suppress adrenal function, may ↓ antibody response to and ↑ risk of adverse reactions from **live-virus vaccines** ■ May ↑ risk of tendon rupture from **fluoroquinolones** ■ Concurrent use may ↓ the response to **somatrem** or **somatropin** at doses of 12.5–18.8 mg/m²/day of oral cortisone ■ **Antacids** ↓ absorption of prednisone and dexamethasone ■ **Ketoconazole, itraconazole, ritonavir, indinavir, saquinavir,** and **erythromycin** ↑ blood levels and effects (dosage reduction budesonide and methylprednisolone may be necessary) ■ May decrease **salicylate** and **isoniazid** levels and effectiveness ■ May antagonize the effects of **anticholinesterases** in myastenia gravis.

**Drug-Food:** ■ **Grapefruit juice** ↑ serum levels and effects of methylprednisolone and budesonide (avoid concurrent use).

### ROUTE AND DOSAGE

□ **Betamethasone**

■ **PO (Adults):** 0.6 mg–7.2 mg/day as single daily dose or in divided doses.

■ **PO (Children):** *Adrenocortical insufficiency*—17.5 mcg/kg (500 mcg/m²)/day in 3 divided doses. *Other uses*—62.5–250 mcg/kg (1.875–7.5 mg/m²)/day in 3 divided doses.

■ **IM, IV (Adults):** Up to 9 mg of betamethasone sodium phosphate or 0.5–9 mg IM as betamethasone sodium phosphate/acetate suspension. *Prevention of respiratory distress syndrome in newborn*—12 mg IM daily for 2–3 days before delivery (unlabeled).

■ **IM (Children):** *Adrenocortical insufficiency*—17.5 mcg/kg (500 mcg/m²)/day in 3 divided doses every 3rd day or 5.8–8.75

mcg/kg (166–250 mcg/m²)/day as a single dose. *Other uses*—20.8–125 mcg/kg (0.625–3.75 mg/m²) of the base q 12–24 hr.

□ **Budesonide**

■ **PO (Adults):** 9 mg once daily for up to 8 wk; can be tapered to 6 mg/day for 2 wk prior to discontinuing. Course may be repeated.

□ **Cortisone**

■ **PO (Adults):** 25–300 mg/day as a single dose or in divided doses.

■ **PO (Children):** *Adrenocortical insufficiency*—0.7 mg/kg (20–25 mg/m²)/day in divided doses. *Other uses*—2.5–10 mg/kg (75–300 mg/m²)/day as a single dose or in divided doses.

■ **IM (Adults):** 20–300 mg/day.

■ **IM (Children):** *Adrenocortical insufficiency*—0.7 mg/kg (37.5 mg/m²) q 3 days or 0.23–0.35 mg/kg (12.5 mg/m²)/day. *Other uses*—0.83–5 mg/kg (25–150 mg/m²) q 12–24 hr.

□ **Dexamethasone (Adrenocortical Insufficiency/Anti-inflammatory/Most Other Uses)**

■ **PO (Adults):** 0.5–9 mg daily in single or divided doses.

■ **PO (Children):** *Adrenocortical insufficiency*—23.3 mcg/kg (670 mcg/m²/day) in 3 divided doses. *Other uses*—83.3–333.3 mcg/kg (2.5–10 mg/m²)/day in 3–4 divided doses. *Acute asthma*—0.6 mg/kg/day for 2 days.

■ **IV (Adults):** *Dexamethasone phosphate*—0.5–24 mg/day (up to 1 mg/kg as a single dose has been used).

■ **IM (Adults):** *Dexamethasone acetate*—8–16 mg q 1–3 wk.

□ **Dexamethasone (Cerebral Edema)**

■ **IM, IV (Adults):** *Dexamethasone phosphate*—10 mg initially IV, 4 mg q 6 hr, may be decreased to 2 mg q 8–12 hr, then change to PO.

■ **PO (Adults):** 2 mg q 8–12 hr.

□ **Dexamethasone (Suppression Test)**

■ **PO (Adults):** 1 mg at 11 PM or 0.5 mg q 6 hr for 48 hr.

◻ **Hydrocortisone**

▪ **PO (Adults):** 20–240 mg/day in 1–4 divided doses.

▪ **PO (Children):** *Adrenocortical insufficiency*—0.56 mg/kg (15–20 mg/m²)/day as a single dose or in divided doses. *Other uses*—2–8 mg/kg/day (60–240 mg/m²/day) as a single dose or in divided doses.

▪ **IM, IV (Adults):** *Hydrocortisone sodium succinate/sodium phosphate*—100–500 mg q 2–6 hr (range 100–8000 mg/day). Hydrocortisone sodium phosphate may also be given subcut.

▪ **IM, IV (Children):** *Adrenocortical insufficiency: hydrocortisone sodium succinate/ sodium phosphate*—0.186–0.28 mg/kg/day (10–12 mg/m²)/day in 3 divided doses. *Other uses: hydrocortisone sodium succinate/ sodium phosphate*—0.666–4 mg/kg (20–120 mg/m²) q 12–24 hr (phosphate or succinate). Hydrocortisone sodium phosphate may also be given subcut.

◻ **Methylprednisolone**

▪ **PO (Adults):** *Multiple sclerosis*—160 mg/day for 7 days, then 64 mg every other day for 1 mo. *Other uses*—4–48 mg/day as a single dose or in divided doses.

▪ **PO (Children):** *Adrenocortical insufficiency*—117 mcg/kg (3.33 mg/m²)/day in 3 divided doses. *Other uses*—0.417 mg/kg– 1.67 mg/kg (12.5–50 mg/m²)/day in 3–4 divided doses.

▪ **Rect (Adults):** 40 mg 3–7 times weekly for at least 2 wk.

▪ **Rect (Children):** 0.5–1 mg/kg (15–30 mg/ m²) daily or every other day for at least 1 wk.

▪ **IM, IV (Adults):** *Most uses: methylprednisolone sodium succinate*—10–40 mg, repeated as needed. *High-dose "pulse" therapy: methylprednisolone sodium succinate*—30 mg/kg IV q 4–6 hr up to 72 hr. *Multiple sclerosis: methylprednisolone sodium succinate*—160 mg/day for 7 days, then 64 mg every other day for 1 mo. *Adjunctive therapy of* Pneumocystis carinii *pneumonia in AIDS patients: methylprednisolone sodium succinate*—30 mg twice daily for 5 days, then 30 mg once daily for 5 days, 15 mg once daily for 10 days. *Acute spinal cord injury: methylprednisolone so-dium succinate*—30 mg/kg over 15 min initially, followed 45 min later with 5.4 mg/ kg/hr for 23 hr (unlabeled).

▪ **IM, IV (Children):** *Adrenocortical insufficiency: methylprednisolone sodium succinate*—117 mcg/kg (3.33 mg/m²)/day in 3 divided doses. *Acute spinal cord injury: methylprednisolone sodium succinate*—30 mg/kg over 15 min initially, then 45 min later initiate continuous infusion of 5.4 mg/ kg/hr for 23 hr (unlabeled). *Other uses: methylprednisolone sodium succinate*— 139–835 mcg/kg (4.16–25 mg/m²) q 12–24 hr.

▪ **IM (Adults):** *Methylprednisolone acetate*—40–120 mg daily, weekly, or every 2 wk.

◻ **Prednisolone**

▪ **PO (Adults):** *Most uses*—5–60 mg/day single dose or divided doses. *Multiple sclerosis*—200 mg/day for 7 days, then 80 mg every other day for 1 mo.

▪ **PO (Children):** *Adrenocortical insufficiency*—0.14 mg/kg (4 mg/m²)/day in 3 divided doses. *Other uses*—0.5–2 mg/kg (15–60 mg/m²)/day in 3–4 divided doses.

▪ **IM, IV (Adults):** *Prednisolone sodium phosphate*—4–60 mg/day.

▪ **IM (Children):** *Adrenocortical insufficiency: prednisolone sodium phosphate/ acetate*—0.14 mg/kg (4 mg/m²)/day in 3 divided doses q 3 days or 0.046–0.07 mg/kg (1.33–2 mg/m²) once daily. *Other uses*— 0.166–1 mg/kg (5–30 mg/m²) q 12–24 hr.

▪ **IM (Adults):** *Prednisolone acetate*—4–60 mg/day. *Prednisolone sodium acetate/ phosphate*—25–100 mg (total); may repeat q 3 days–4 wk.

◻ **Prednisone**

▪ **PO (Adults):** *Most uses*—5–60 mg/day single dose or divided doses. *Multiple sclerosis*—200 mg/day for 1 wk, then 80 mg every other day for 1 mo. *Adjunctive therapy of* Pneumocystis carinii *pneumonia in AIDS patients*—40 mg twice daily for 5 days, then 40 mg once daily for 5 days, then 20 mg once daily for 10 days.

▪ **PO (Children ≥10 yr):** *Nephrosis*—20 mg 4 times daily initially.

- **PO (Children 4–10 yr):** *Nephrosis*—15 mg 4 times daily initially.

- **PO (Children 18 mo–4 yr):** *Nephrosis*—7.5–10 mg 4 times daily initially.

### ❏ Triamcinolone

- **PO (Adults):** *Adrenocortical insufficiency*—4–12 mg/day as a single dose or in divided doses. *Other uses*—4–48 mg/day (up to 60 mg/day) as a single dose or in divided doses.

- **PO (Children):** *Adrenocortical insufficiency*—117 mcg/kg/day (3.3 mg/m²/day) as a single dose or in divided doses. *Other uses*—416 mcg–1.7 mg/kg /day (12.5–50 mg/m²/day) as a single dose or in divided doses. Some conditions may require up to 2 mg/kg/day.

- **IM (Adults):** *Triamcinolone acetonide*—40–80 mg q 4 wk. *Triamcinolone diacetate*—40 mg weekly.

- **IM (Children):** *Triamcinolone acetonide*—40 mg q 4 wk or 30–200 mcg/kg (1–6.25 mg/m²) q 1–7 days. *Triamcinolone diacetate*—40 mg weekly.

## AVAILABILITY

### ❏ Betamethasone

■ *Tablets:* {0.5 mg$^{Rx}$}, 0.6 mg$^{Rx}$ ■ *Syrup:* 0.6 mg/5 ml$^{Rx}$ ■ *Effervescent tablets:* {0.5 mg$^{Rx}$} ■ *Extended-release tablets:* {1 mg$^{Rx}$} ■ *Solution for injection (sodium phosphate):* 3 mg/ml$^{Rx}$ ■ *Suspension for injection (Phosphate/acetate):* 6 mg (total)/ml$^{Rx}$.

### ❏ Budesonide

■ *Capsules:* 3 mg.

### ❏ Cortisone

■ *Tablets:* 5 mg$^{Rx}$, 10 mg$^{Rx}$, 25 mg$^{Rx}$ ■ *Suspension for injection:* 50 mg/ml$^{Rx}$.

### ❏ Dexamethasone

■ *Tablets:* 0.25 mg$^{Rx}$, 0.5 mg$^{Rx}$, 0.75 mg$^{Rx}$, 1 mg$^{Rx}$, 1.5 mg$^{Rx}$, 2 mg$^{Rx}$, 4 mg$^{Rx}$, 6 mg$^{Rx}$ ■ *Elixir:* 0.5 mg/5 ml$^{Rx}$ ■ *Oral solution:* 0.5 mg/5 ml$^{Rx}$, 1 mg/ml$^{Rx}$ ■ *Solution for injection (sodium phosphate):* 4 mg/ml$^{Rx}$, 10 mg/ml$^{Rx}$, 20 mg/ml$^{Rx}$, 24 mg/ml$^{Rx}$ ■ *Suspension for injection (acetate):* 8 mg/ml$^{Rx}$, 16 mg/ml$^{Rx}$.

### ❏ Hydrocortisone

■ *Tablets:* 5 mg$^{Rx}$, 10 mg$^{Rx}$, 20 mg$^{Rx}$ ■ *Oral suspension:* 10 mg/5 ml$^{Rx}$ ■ *Suspension for injection (base):* 25 mg/ml$^{Rx}$, 50 mg/ml$^{Rx}$ ■ *Suspension for injection (acetate):* 25 mg/ml$^{Rx}$, 50 mg/ml$^{Rx}$ ■ *Solution for injection (sodium phosphate):* 50 mg/ml$^{Rx}$ ■ *Powder for injection (sodium succinate):* 100 mg$^{Rx}$, 250 mg$^{Rx}$, 500 mg$^{Rx}$, 1 g$^{Rx}$.

### ❏ Methylprednisolone

■ *Tablets:* 2 mg$^{Rx}$, 4 mg$^{Rx}$, 8 mg$^{Rx}$, 16 mg$^{Rx}$, 24 mg$^{Rx}$, 32 mg$^{Rx}$ ■ *Solution for injection:* 40 mg$^{Rx}$, 125 mg$^{Rx}$, 500 mg$^{Rx}$, 1 g$^{Rx}$, 2 g$^{Rx}$ ■ *Suspension for injection:* 20 mg/ml$^{Rx}$, 40 mg/ml$^{Rx}$, 80 mg/ml$^{Rx}$ ■ *Enema:* 40 mg$^{Rx}$.

### ❏ Prednisolone

■ *Tablets:* 4 mg$^{Rx}$, 5 mg$^{Rx}$, 8 mg$^{Rx}$, 16 mg$^{Rx}$, 24 mg$^{Rx}$, 32 mg$^{Rx}$ ■ *Syrup:* 15 mg/5 ml$^{Rx}$ ■ *Oral solution:* 3 mg/ml$^{Rx}$, 5 mg/ml$^{Rx}$ ■ *Solution for injection (sodium phosphate):* 20 mg/ml$^{Rx}$ ■ *Suspension for injection (acetate):* 25 mg/ml, 50 mg/ml$^{Rx}$ ■ *Suspension for injection (sodium phosphate/acetate):* 100 mg (total)/ml$^{Rx}$ ■ *Suspension for injection (tebutate):* 20 mg/ml$^{Rx}$.

### ❏ Prednisone

■ *Tablets:* 1 mg$^{Rx}$, 2.5 mg$^{Rx}$, 5 mg$^{Rx}$, 10 mg$^{Rx}$, 20 mg$^{Rx}$, 50 mg$^{Rx}$ ■Cost: 1 mg $6.63/100, 2.5 mg $7.01/100, 5 mg $8.32/100, 10 mg $8.46/100, 20 mg $7.18/30, 50 mg $2.18/8 ■ *Oral solution:* 5 mg/5 ml$^{Rx}$, 5 mg/1 ml$^{Rx}$ ■ *Syrup:* 5 mg/5 ml$^{Rx}$.

### ❏ Triamcinolone

■ *Tablets:* 1 mg$^{Rx}$, 2 mg$^{Rx}$, 4 mg$^{Rx}$, 8 mg$^{Rx}$, 16 mg$^{Rx}$ ■ *Oral syrup:* 2 mg/5 ml$^{Rx}$, 4 mg/5 ml$^{Rx}$ ■ *Suspension for injection (acetonide):* 3 mg/ml$^{Rx}$, 10 mg/ml$^{Rx}$, 40 mg/ml$^{Rx}$ ■ *Suspension for injection (diacetate):* 25 mg/ml$^{Rx}$, 40 mg/ml$^{Rx}$ ■ *Suspension for injection (hexacetonide):* 5 mg/ml$^{Rx}$, 20 mg/ml$^{Rx}$.

TIME/ACTION PROFILE (anti-inflammatory activity)

| | ONSET | PEAK | DURATION |
| --- | --- | --- | --- |
| Betamethasone PO | unknown | 1–2 hr | 3.25 days |
| Betamethasone sodium phosphate IM, IV | rapid | unknown | unknown |

| | | | |
|---|---|---|---|
| Betamethasone acetate/sodium phosphate IM | 1–3 hr | unknown | 1 wk |
| Budesonide PO | unknown | unknown | unknown |
| Cortisone PO | rapid | 2 hr | 1.25–1.5 days |
| Cortisone IM | slow | 20–48 hr | 1.25–1.5 days |
| Dexamethasone PO | unknown | 1–2 hr | 2.75 days |
| Dexamethasone IM, IV (phosphate) | rapid | unknown | 2.75 days |
| Dexamethasone IM (acetate) | unknown | 8 hr | 6 days |
| Hydrocortisone PO | unknown | 1–2 hr | 1.25–1.5 days |
| Hydrocortisone sodium succinate IM | rapid | 1 hr | variable |
| Hydrocortisone IV | rapid | unknown | unknown |
| Methylprednisolone PO | unknown | 1–2 hr | 1.25–1.5 days |
| Methylprednisolone IM (acetate) | 6–48 hr | 4–8 days | 1–4 wk |
| Methylprednisolone IM, IV (succinate) | rapid | unknown | unknown |
| Prednisolone PO | unknown | 1–2 hr | 1.25–1.5 days |
| Prednisolone IM, IV (phosphate) | rapid | 1 hr | unknown |
| Prednisolone IM (acetate) | slow | unknown | unknown |
| Prednisone PO | hr | unknown | 1.25–1.5 days |
| Triamcinolone PO | unknown | 1–2 hr | 2.25 days |
| Triamcinolone IM (acetonide) | 24–48 hr | unknown | 1–6 wk |
| Triamcinolone IM (diacetonide) | slow | unknown | 4 days–4 wk |

## NURSING IMPLICATIONS

### ASSESSMENT

- These drugs are indicated for many conditions. Assess involved systems before and periodically during therapy.
- Assess patient for signs of adrenal insufficiency (hypotension, weight loss, weakness, nausea, vomiting, anorexia, lethargy, confusion, restlessness) before and periodically during therapy.
- Monitor intake and output ratios and daily weights. Observe patient for peripheral edema, steady weight gain, rales/crackles, or dyspnea. Notify physician or other health care professional if these occur.

- Children should have periodic evaluations of growth.
- **Cerebral Edema:** Assess patient for changes in level of consciousness and headache during therapy.
- **Budesonide:** Assess signs of Crohn's disease (diarrhea, crampy abdominal pain, fever, bleeding from rectum) during therapy.
- *Lab Test Considerations:* Monitor serum electrolytes and glucose. May cause hyperglycemia, especially in persons with diabetes. May cause hypokalemia. Patients on prolonged courses of therapy should routinely have hematologic values, serum electrolytes, and serum and urine glucose evaluated. May ↓ WBCs. May cause hyperglycemia, especially in persons with diabetes. May ↓ serum potassium and calcium and ↑ serum sodium concentrations.
- Guaiac-test stools. Promptly report presence of guaiac-positive stools.
- May ↑ serum cholesterol and lipid values. May ↓ uptake of thyroid $^{123}$I or $^{131}$I.
- Suppress reactions to allergy skin tests.
- Periodic adrenal function tests may be ordered to assess degree of hypothalamic-pituitary-adrenal axis suppression in systemic and chronic topical therapy. **Dexamethasone Suppression Test:** To diagnose Cushing's syndrome: Obtain baseline cortisol level; administer dexamethasone at 11 PM and obtain cortisol levels at 8 AM the next day. Normal response is a ↓ cortisol level.
- Alternative method: Obtain baseline 24-hr urine for 17-hydroxycorticosteroid (OHCS) concentrations, then begin 48-hr administration of dexamethasone. Second 24-hr urine for 17-OHCS is obtained after 24 hr of dexamethasone.

## POTENTIAL NURSING DIAGNOSES

- Infection, risk for (Side Effects).
- Body image, disturbed (Side Effects).

### IMPLEMENTATION

- **General:** Do not confuse prednisone with methylprednisolone or primidone.
- If dose is ordered daily or every other day, administer in the morning to coincide with the body's normal secretion of cortisol. Peri-

{ } = Available in Canada only.
*CAPITALS indicates life-threatening; underlines indicate most frequent.

ods of stress, such as surgery, may require supplemental systemic corticosteroids. Patients with mild to moderate Crohn's disease may be switched from oral prednisolone without adrenal insufficiency by gradually decreasing prednisolone doses and adding budesonide.

■ **PO:** Administer with meals to minimize GI irritation.

❏ Tablets may be crushed and administered with food or fluids for patients with difficulty swallowing. Capsules should be swallowed whole; do not crush, break, or chew.

❏ Use calibrated measuring device to ensure accurate dosage of liquid forms.

❏ Avoid consumption of grapefruit juice during therapy with budesonide or methylprednisolone.

■ **IM, Subcut:** Shake suspension well before drawing up. IM doses should not be administered when rapid effect is desirable. Do not dilute with other solution or admix. Do not administer suspensions IV.

❏ **Betamethasone**

■ **Direct IV:** Only betamethasone sodium phosphate may be given IV. Administer undiluted.

■ *Rate:* Administer over at least 1 min.

■ **Intermittent Infusion:** May be administered as infusion in D5W, 0.9% NaCl, Ringer's solution, D5/Ringer's solution, or D5/LR.

■ **Y-Site Compatibility:** ◆ heparin ◆ potassium chloride ◆ vitamin B complex with C.

❏ **Dexamethasone**

■ **Direct IV:** May be given undiluted. Do not administer suspension IV.

■ *Rate:* Administer over 1 min.

■ **Intermittent Infusion:** May be added to D5W or 0.9% NaCl solution. Administer infusions at prescribed rate. Diluted solution should be used within 24 hr.

❏ **Dexamethasone Sodium Phosphate**

■ **Syringe Compatibility:** ◆ granisetron ◆ metoclopramide ◆ ranitidine ◆ sufentanil.

■ **Syringe Incompatibility:** ◆ doxapram ◆ glycopyrrolate.

■ **Y-Site Compatibility:** ◆ acyclovir ◆ allopurinol ◆ amifostine ◆ amikacin ◆ amphotericin B cholesteryl sulfate ◆ aztreonam ◆ cefepime ◆ cisatracurium ◆ cisplatin ◆ cladribine ◆ cyclo-

phosphamide ◆ cytarabine ◆ docetaxel ◆ doxorubicin ◆ doxorubicin liposome ◆ etoposide ◆ famotidine ◆ fentanyl ◆ filgrastim ◆ fluconazole ◆ fludarabine ◆ foscarnet ◆ gatifloxacin ◆ gemcitabine ◆ granisetron ◆ heparin ◆ hydromorphone ◆ levofloxacin ◆ linezolid ◆ lorazepam ◆ melphalan ◆ meperidine ◆ meropenem ◆ methadone ◆ morphine ◆ ondansetron ◆ paclitaxel ◆ piperacillin/tazobactam ◆ potassium ◆ propofol ◆ remifentanil ◆ sargramostim ◆ sodium bicarbonate ◆ sufentanil ◆ tacrolimus ◆ teniposide ◆ theophylline ◆ thiotepa ◆ vinorelbine ◆ vitamin B complex with C ◆ zidovudine.

■ **Y-Site Incompatibility:** ◆ ciprofloxacin ◆ idarubicin ◆ midazolam ◆ topotecan.

■ **Additive Compatibility:** ◆ aminophylline ◆ bleomycin ◆ cimetidine ◆ furosemide ◆ granisetron ◆ lidocaine ◆ meropenem ◆ mitomycin ◆ nafcillin ◆ netilmicin ◆ ranitidine

■ **Additive Incompatibility:** ◆ daunorubicin ◆ vancomycin.

❏ **Hydrocortisone**

■ **Direct IV:** Reconstitute with provided solution (i.e., Act-O-Vials) or 2 ml of bacteriostatic water or saline for injection.

■ *Rate:* Administer each 100 mg over at least 30 sec. Doses 500 mg and larger should be infused over at least 10 min.

■ **Intermittent/Continuous Infusion:** May be added to 50–1000 ml of D5W, 0.9% NaCl, or D5/0.9% NaCl. Administer infusions at prescribed rate. Diluted solutions should be used within 24 hr.

❏ **Hydrocortisone Sodium Phosphate**

■ **Syringe Compatibility:** ◆ metoclopramide.

■ **Y-Site Compatibility:** ◆ allopurinol ◆ amifostine ◆ aztreonam ◆ cefepime ◆ cladribine ◆ docetaxel ◆ etoposide ◆ famotidine ◆ filgrastim ◆ fluconazole ◆ fludarabine ◆ gemcitabine ◆ granisetron ◆ melphalan ◆ ondansetron ◆ paclitaxel ◆ piperacillin/tazobactam ◆ teniposide ◆ thiotepa ◆ vinorelbine.

■ **Y-Site Incompatibility:** ◆ sargramostim.

■ **Additive Compatibility:** ◆ amikacin ◆ amphotericin B ◆ bleomycin ◆ sodium bicarbonate.

❏ **Hydrocortisone Sodium Succinate**

■ **Syringe Compatibility:** ◆ metoclopramide ◆ thiopental.

■ **Y-Site Compatibility:** ◆ acyclovir ◆ allopurinol ◆ amifostine ◆ aminophylline ◆ amphotericin B cholesteryl sulfate ♦ ampicillin ♦ atracurium ♦ atropine ♦ aztreonam ♦ calcium gluconate ♦ cefepime ♦ cephalothin ♦ cephapirin ♦ chlordiazepoxide ♦ chlorpromazine ♦ cisatracurium ♦ cladribine ♦ cyanocobalamin ♦ cytarabine ♦ digoxin ♦ diphenhydramine ♦ docetaxel ♦ dopamine ♦ doxorubicin liposome ♦ droperidol ♦ edrophonium ♦ enalaprilat ♦ epinephrine ♦ esmolol ♦ conjugated estrogens ♦ ethacrynate ♦ etoposide ♦ famotidine ♦ fentanyl ♦ filgrastim ♦ fludarabine ♦ fluorouracil ♦ foscarnet ♦ furosemide ♦ gatifloxacin ♦ gemcitabine ♦ granisetron ♦ heparin ♦ hydralazine ♦ inamrinone ♦ insulin ♦ isoproterenol ♦ kanamycin ♦ lidocaine ♦ linezolid ♦ lorazepam ♦ magnesium ♦ melphalan ♦ meperidine ♦ methoxamine ♦ methylergonovine ♦ minocycline ♦ morphine ♦ neostigmine ♦ norepinephrine ♦ ondansetron ♦ oxacillin ♦ oxytocin ♦ paclitaxel ♦ pancuronium ♦ penicillin G potassium ♦ pentazocine ♦ phytonadione ♦ piperacillin/tazobactam ♦ procainamide ♦ prochlorperazine edisylate ♦ propofol ♦ propranolol ♦ pyridostigmine ♦ remifentanil ♦ scopolamine ♦ sodium bicarbonate ♦ succinylcholine ♦ tacrolimus ♦ teniposide ♦ theophylline ♦ thiotepa ♦ trimethobenzamide ♦ vecuronium ♦ vinorelbine.

■ **Y-Site Incompatibility:** ♦ ciprofloxacin ♦ diazepam ♦ idarubicin ♦ midazolam ♦ phenytoin ♦ sargramostim.

■ **Additive Compatibility:** ♦ amikacin ♦ aminophylline ♦ amphotericin ♦ daunorubicin ♦ diphenhydramine ♦ magnesium sulfate ♦ mitoxantrone ♦ potassium chloride ♦ vitamin B complex with C.

■ **Additive Incompatibility:** ♦ bleomycin

❏ **Methylprednisolone**

■ **Direct IV:** Reconstitute with provided solution (Act-O-Vials, Univials, ADD-Vantage vials) or 2 ml of bacteriostatic water (with benzyl alcohol) for injection.

■ **Rate:** May be administered direct IV push over 1 to several minutes.

■ **Intermittent/Continuous Infusion:** May be diluted further in D5W, 0.9% NaCl, or D5/0.9% NaCl and administered as intermittent or continuous infusion at the prescribed rate. Solution may form a haze upon dilution.

❏ **Methylprednisolone Sodium Succinate**

■ **Syringe Compatibility:** ♦ granisetron ♦ metoclopramide.

■ **Y-Site Compatibility:** ♦ acyclovir ♦ amifostine ♦ amphotericin B cholesteryl sulfate ♦ aztreonam ♦ cefepime ♦ cisplatin ♦ cladribine ♦ cyclophosphamide ♦ cytarabine ♦ dopamine ♦ doxorubicin ♦ doxorubicin liposome ♦ enalaprilat ♦ famotidine ♦ fludarabine ♦ gatifloxacin ♦ granisetron ♦ heparin ♦ inamrinone ♦ linezolid ♦ melphalan ♦ meperidine ♦ methotrexate ♦ metronidazole ♦ midazolam ♦ morphine ♦ piperacillin/tazobactam ♦ remifentanil ♦ sodium bicarbonate ♦ tacrolimus ♦ teniposide ♦ theophylline ♦ thiotepa ♦ topotecan.

■ **Y-Site Incompatibility:** ♦ allopurinol ♦ ciprofloxacin ♦ docetaxel ♦ etoposide ♦ filgrastim ♦ gemcitabine ♦ ondansetron ♦ paclitaxel ♦ propofol ♦ sargramostim ♦ vinorelbine

■ **Additive Compatibility:** ♦ cimetidine ♦ granisetron ♦ heparin ♦ ranitidine ♦ theophylline.

❏ **Prednisolone**

■ **Direct IV:** Do not use the acetate form of this drug for IV administration.

■ **Rate:** Prednisolone sodium phosphate IV may be administered direct IV push at a rate of no more than 10 mg/min.

■ **Intermittent Infusion:** May be added to 50–1000 ml of D5W or 0.9% NaCl. Stable for 24 hr.

■ **Rate:** Administer infusions at prescribed rate.

■ **Y-Site Compatibility:** ♦ heparin ♦ potassium chloride ♦ vitamin B complex with C.

■ **Additive Compatibility:** ♦ ascorbic acid ♦ cephalothin ♦ cytarabine ♦ erythromycin lactobionate ♦ fluorouracil ♦ heparin ♦ penicillin G potassium ♦ penicillin G sodium ♦ vitamin B complex with C.

■ **Additive Incompatibility:** ♦ calcium gluceptate ♦ methotrexate ♦ polymyxin B sulfate.

## PATIENT/FAMILY TEACHING

■ **General Info:** Instruct patient on correct technique of medication administration. Advise patient to take medication as directed. Take missed doses as soon as remembered unless almost time for next dose. Do not double doses. Stopping the medication suddenly may result in adrenal insufficiency (anorexia, nausea, weakness, fatigue, dyspnea, hypotension, hypoglycemia). If these signs appear, notify health care professional immediately. This can be life threatening.

❑ Corticosteroids cause immunosuppression and may mask symptoms of infection. Instruct patient to avoid people with known contagious illnesses and to report possible infections immediately.

❑ Caution patient to avoid vaccinations without first consulting health care professional.

❑ Review side effects with patient. Instruct patient to inform health care professional promptly if severe abdominal pain or tarry stools occur. Patient should also report unusual swelling, weight gain, tiredness, bone pain, bruising, nonhealing sores, visual disturbances, or behavior changes.

❑ Advise patient to notify health care professional of medication regimen before treatment or surgery.

❑ Discuss possible effects on body image. Explore coping mechanisms.

❑ Instruct patient to inform health care professional if symptoms of underlying disease return or worsen.

❑ Advise patient to carry identificationdescribing disease process and medication regimen in the event of emergency in which patient cannot relate medical history.

❑ Explain need for continued medical follow-up to assess effectiveness and possible side effects of medication. Periodic lab tests and eye exams may be needed.

■ **Long-term Therapy:** Encourage patient to eat a diet high in protein, calcium, and potassium, and low in sodium and carbohydrates (see Appendix Q). Alcohol should be avoided during therapy.

## EVALUATION

**Effectiveness of therapy can be demonstrated by:** ■ Decrease in presenting symptoms with minimal systemic side effects ■ Suppression of the inflammatory and immune responses in autoimmune disorders, allergic reactions, and neoplasms ■ Management of symptoms in adrenal insufficiency ■ Improvement of symptoms/sequelae of Crohn's disease (decreased frequency of liquid stools, decreased abdominal complaints, improved sense of well being).

# CORTICOSTEROIDS (TOPICAL/LOCAL)

**alclometasone**

(al-kloe-**met**-a-sone)

Aclovate

**amcinonide**

(am-**sin**-oh-nide)

Cyclocort

**betamethasone**

(bay-ta-**meth**-a-sone)

Alphatrex, Beben, {Betacort}, {Betaderm}, Betatrex, Beta-Val, {Betnovate}, {Celestoderm}, Dermabet, Diprolene, Diprosone, {Ectosone}, Luxiq, Maxivate, {Metaderm}, {Novobetamet}, Occlucort, {Prevex}, Teladar, {Topilene}, {Topisone}, Uticort, Valisone, Valnac

**clobetasol**

(kloe-**bay**-ta-sol)

{Dermovate}, Embeline E, Temovate

**clocortolone**

(kloe-**kor**-toe-lone)

Cloderm

**desonide**

(**des**-oh-nide)

DesOwen, Tridesilon

**desoximetasone**

(dess-ox-i-**met**-a-sone)

Topicort

**dexamethasone**

(dex-a-**meth**-a-sone)

Aeroseb-Dex, Decadron, Decaspray

**diflorasone**

(dye-**flor**-a-sone)

Florone, Maxiflor, Psorcon

**fluocinolone**

(floo-oh-**sin**-oh-lone)

Bio-Syn, Derma-Smoothe/FS, Fluocet, {Fluoderm}, {Fluolar}, Fluonid, {Fluonide}, Flurosyn, FS Shampoo, Synalar, {Synamol}, Synemol

**fluocinonide**
(floo-oh-**sin**-oh-nide)
Fluocin, Licon, {Lidemol}, Lidex, {Lyderm}, {Topsyn}

**flurandrenolide**
(flure-an-**dren**-oh-lide)
Cordran, {Drenison}

**fluticasone**
(floo-**tik**-a-sone)
Cutivate

**halcinonide**
(hal-**sin**-oh-nide)
Halog

**halobetasol**
(hal-oh-**bay**-ta-sol)
Ultravate

**hydrocortisone**
(hye-droe-**kor**-ti-sone)
Acticort, Aeroseb-HC, Ala-Cort, Ala-Scalp, Alphaderm, Anusol HC, Bactine, {Barriere-HC}, CaldeCORT Anti-Itch, Carmol HC, Cetacort, {Cortacet}, Cortaid, {Cortate}, Cort-Dome, {Cortef Feminine Itch}, Cortenema, Corticaine, {Corticreme}, Cortifair, Cortifoam, Cortizone, Dermacort, DermiCort, Dermtex HC, {Emo-Cort}, FoilleCort, Gynecort, Hemril-HC, Hi-Cor, Hycort, {Hyderm}, Hydro-Tex, Hytone, LactiCare-HC, Lanacort 9-1-1, Lemoderm, Locoid, {Novohydrocort}, Nutracort, Orabase-HCA, Pandel, Penecort, Pharma-Cort, Prevex HC, Proctocort, Rhulicort, Synacort, Texacort, {Unicort}, Westcort

**methylprednisolone**
(meth-il-pred-**nis**-oh-lone)
Medrol

**mometasone**
(moe-**met**-a-sone)
{Elocom}, Elocon

**prednicarbate**
(pred-ni-**kar**-bate)
Dermatop

**triamcinolone**
(trye-am-**sin**-oh-lone)
Aristocort, Delta-Tritex, Flutex, Kenalog, Kenonel, {Triaderm}, {Trianide}

**CLASSIFICATION(S):**
**Therapeutic:** *corticosteroids*
**Pharmacologic:** *corticosteroids (topical)*
**Pregnancy Category C**

### INDICATIONS

■ Management of various allergic/immunologic skin problems.

### ACTION

■ Topical/local corticosteroids have anti-inflammatory, antipruritic and vasoconstrictive properties. Application results in inhibition of macrophage/leukocyte migration due to decreased vascular dilation and permeability. If systemically absorbed for prolonged periods of time, topical/local corticosteroids may produce adrenal suppression. **Therapeutic Effects:** ■ Decreased edema, erythema and pruritus.

### PHARMACOKINETICS

**Absorption:** Prolonged use on large surface areas, application of large amounts, or use of occlusive dressings will produce systemic absorption and adrenal suppression. Absorption is increased in children/growing adolescents due to large body surface area to weight ratio.

**Distribution:** Remain primarily at site of action.

**Metabolism and Excretion:** Usually metabolized in skin; some have been modified to resist local metabolism and have a prolonged local effect.

**Half-life:** *Betamethasone*—3–5 hr (plasma), 36–54 hr (tissue); adrenal suppression lasts 3.25 days. *Dexamethasone*—3–4.5 hr (plasma), 36–54 hr (tissue); adrenal suppression lasts 2.75 days. *Hydrocortisone*—1.5–2 hr (plasma), 8–12 hr (tissue); adrenal suppression lasts 1.25–1.5 days. *Triamcinolone*—2– >5 hr (plasma), 18–36 hr (tissue); adrenal suppression lasts 2.25 days.

## CONTRAINDICATIONS AND PRECAUTIONS

**Contraindicated in:** ■ Hypersensitivity or known intolerance to corticosteroids or components of vehicles (ointment or cream base, preservative, alcohol) ■ Untreated bacterial or viral infections.

**Use Cautiously in:** ■ Hepatic dysfunction ■ Diabetes mellitus, cataracts, glaucoma, or tuberculosis (use of large amounts of high-potency agents may worsen condition) ■ Patients with pre-existing skin atrophy ■ Geriatric patients (infrequent, brief use recommended in patients with skin atrophy) ■ Pregnancy, lactation, or children/growing adolescents (chronic high-dose usage may result in adrenal suppression in mother, growth suppression in children; children may be more susceptible to adrenal and growth suppression). Low-potency agents, unfluorinated agents recommended in children; safety of augmented betamethasone dipropionate, clobetasol, desoximetasone, and halobetasol not established. Some agents are approved for pediatric use. Should not be used for the routine management of diaper dermatoses.

## ADVERSE REACTIONS AND SIDE EFFECTS*

■ **Derm:** allergic contact dermatitis, atrophy, burning, dryness, edema, folliculitis, hypersensitivity reactions, hypertrichosis, hypopigmentation, irritation, maceration, miliaria, perioral dermatitis, secondary infection, striae ■ **Misc:** adrenal suppression (increased dose, long-term therapy).

## INTERACTIONS

**Drug-Drug:** ■ None significant.

## ROUTE AND DOSAGE

■ **Topical (Adults and Children):** 1–4 times daily (depends on product, preparation, and condition being treated).

■ **Rect (Adults):** hydrocortisone: *Retention enema*—100 mg nightly for 21 days or until remission occurs; *aerosol foam*—90 mg 1– 2 times/day for 2–3 wk; then adjusted.

## AVAILABILITY

❑ **Alclometasone**
■ *Cream:* 0.05%^Rx ■ *Ointment:* 0.05%^Rx.

❑ **Amcinonide**
■ *Cream:* 0.1%^Rx ■ *Lotion:* 0.1%^Rx ■ *Ointment:* 0.1%^Rx.

❑ **Betamethasone**
■ *Cream:* 0.01%^Rx, 0.025%^Rx, 0.05%^Rx, 0.1%^Rx ■ *Gel:* 0.05%^Rx, 0.25%^Rx ■ *Lotion:* 0.025%^Rx, 0.05%^Rx, 0.1%^Rx ■ *Ointment:* 0.05%^Rx, 0.1%^Rx ■ *Aerosol:* 0.1%^Rx.

❑ **Clobetasol**
■ *Cream:* 0.05%^Rx ■ *Ointment:* 0.05%^Rx ■ *Foam:* 0.05%^Rx ■ *Scalp solution:* 0.05%^Rx.

❑ **Clocortolone**
■ *Cream:* 0.1%^Rx.

❑ **Desonide**
■ *Cream:* 0.05%^Rx ■ *Ointment:* 0.05%^Rx ■ *Lotion:* 0.05%^Rx.

❑ **Desoximetasone**
■ *Cream:* 0.05%^Rx, 0.25%^Rx ■ *Gel:* 0.05%^Rx ■ *Ointment:* 0.25%^Rx.

❑ **Dexamethasone**
■ *Cream:* 1%^Rx ■ *Aerosol:* 0.01%^Rx, 0.04%^Rx.

❑ **Diflorasone**
■ *Cream:* 0.05%^Rx ■ *Ointment:* 0.05%^Rx.

❑ **Fluocinolone**
■ *Cream:* 0.01%^Rx, 0.02%^Rx, 0.025%^Rx ■ *Ointment:* 0.025%^Rx ■ *Solution:* 0.01%^Rx ■ *Shampoo:* 0.01%^Rx ■ *Oil:* 0.01%^Rx.

❑ **Fluocinonide**
■ *Cream:* 0.05%^Rx ■ *Gel:* 0.05%^Rx ■ *Ointment:* 0.05%^Rx ■ *Solution:* 0.05%^Rx.

❑ **Flurandrenolide**
■ *Cream:* 0.025%^Rx, 0.05%^Rx ■ *Ointment:* 0.025%^Rx, 0.05%^Rx ■ *Lotion:* 0.05%^Rx ■ *Tape:* 4 mcg/m²^Rx.

❏ **Fluticasone**

■ *Cream:* $0.05\%^{Rx}$ ■ *Ointment:* $0.005\%^{Rx}$.

❏ **Halcinonide**

■ *Cream:* $0.025\%^{Rx}$, $0.1\%^{Rx}$ ■ *Ointment:* $0.1\%^{Rx}$ ■ *Solution:* $0.1\%^{Rx}$.

❏ **Halobetasol**

■ *Cream:* $0.05\%^{Rx}$ ■ *Ointment:* $0.05\%^{Rx}$.

❏ **Hydrocortisone**

■ *Cream:* $0.5\%^{Rx, OTC}$, $1\%^{Rx, OTC}$, $2.5\%^{Rx}$ ■ *Gel:* $0.5\%^{Rx, OTC}$, $1\%^{Rx, OTC}$ ■ *Ointment:* $0.5\%^{Rx, OTC}$, $1\%^{Rx, OTC}$ ■ *Lotion:* $0.25\%^{Rx}$, $0.5\%^{Rx, OTC}$, $1\%^{Rx, OTC}$, $2\%^{Rx}$, $2.5\%^{Rx}$ ■ *Solution:* $1\%^{Rx}$ ■ *Spray:* $0.5\%^{Rx, OTC}$, $1\%^{Rx, OTC}$ ■ *Enema:* 100 mg$^{Rx}$ ■ *Rectal aerosol:* 90 mg$^{Rx}$.

❏ **Methylprednisolone**

■ *Ointment:* $0.25\%^{Rx}$, $1\%^{Rx}$.

❏ **Mometasone**

■ *Cream:* $0.1\%^{Rx}$ ■Cost: 0.1% \$40.27/45 g ■ *Ointment:* $0.1\%^{Rx}$ ■Cost: 0.1% \$40.27/45 g ■ *Lotion:* $0.1\%^{Rx}$ ■Cost: 0.1% \$23.84/30ml.

❏ **Prednicarbate**

■ *Cream:* $0.1\%^{Rx}$.

❏ **Triamcinolone**

■ *Cream:* $0.025\%^{Rx}$, $0.1\%^{Rx}$, $0.5\%^{Rx}$ ■ *Ointment:* $0.025\%^{Rx}$, $0.1\%^{Rx}$, $0.5\%^{Rx}$ ■ *Lotion:* $0.025\%^{Rx}$, $0.1\%^{Rx}$ ■*Spray:* 2 sec/spray$^{Rx}$ ■acetic acid, antifungals, anti-infectives, antihistamines, urea, and benzoyl peroxide in various otic and topical preparations. See Appendix B.

TIME/ACTION PROFILE (response depends on condition being treated)

| | ONSET | PEAK | DURATION |
|---|---|---|---|
| Topical | min–hrs | hrs–days | hrs–days |

# NURSING IMPLICATIONS

## ASSESSMENT

❏ Assess affected skin before and daily during therapy. Note degree of inflammation and pruritus. Notify physician or other health care professional if symptoms of infection (increased pain, erythema, purulent exudate) develop.

■ *Lab Test Considerations:* Periodic adrenal function tests may be ordered to assess degree of hypothalamic-pituitary-adrenal (HPA) axis suppression in chronic topical therapy. Children and patients with dose applied to a large area, using an occlusive dressing, or using high-potency products are at highest risk for HPA suppression.

❏ May cause increased serum and urine glucose concentrations if significant absorption occurs.

## POTENTIAL NURSING DIAGNOSES

■ Skin integrity, risk for impaired (Indications).

■ Infection, risk for (Side Effects).

## IMPLEMENTATION

■ **General:** Choice of vehicle depends on site and type of lesion. Ointments are more occlusive and preferred for dry, scaly lesions. Creams should be used on oozing or intertriginous areas, where the occlusive action of ointments might cause folliculitis or maceration. Creams may be preferred for esthetic reasons even though they may dry skin more than ointments. Gels, aerosols, lotions, and solutions are useful in hairy areas.

■ **Topical:** Apply *ointments, creams,* or *gels* sparingly as a thin film to clean, slightly moist skin. Wear gloves. Apply occlusive dressing only if specified by physician or other health care professional.

❏ Apply *lotion, solution,* or *gel* to hair by parting hair and applying a small amount to affected area. Rub in gently. Protect area from washing, clothing, or rubbing until medication has dried. Hair may be washed as usual but not right after applying medication.

❏ Use *aerosols* by shaking well and spraying on affected area, holding container 3–6 in. away. Spray for about 2 seconds to cover an area the size of a hand. Do not inhale. If spraying near face, cover eyes.

## PATIENT/FAMILY TEACHING

❏ Instruct patient on correct technique of medication administration. Emphasize importance of avoiding the eyes. If a dose is missed, it should be applied as soon as re-

{ } = Available in Canada only.
*CAPITALS indicates life-threatening; underlines indicate most frequent.

membered unless almost time for the next dose.

❑ Caution patient to use only as directed. Avoid using cosmetics, bandages, dressings, or other skin products over the treated area unless directed by health care professional.

❑ Advise parents of pediatric patients not to apply tight-fitting diapers or plastic pants on a child treated in the diaper area; these garments work as an occlusive dressing and may cause more of the drug to be absorbed.

❑ Caution women that medication should not be used extensively, in large amounts, or for protracted periods if they are pregnant or planning to become pregnant.

❑ Advise patient to consult health care professional before using medicine for condition other than indicated.

❑ Instruct patient to inform health care professional if symptoms of underlying disease return or worsen or if symptoms of infection develop.

### EVALUATION
**Effectiveness of therapy can be demonstrated by:** ■ Resolution of skin inflammation, pruritus, or other dermatologic conditions.

## cortisone, See CORTICOSTEROIDS (SYSTEMIC).

## cromolyn, See MAST CELL STABILIZERS.

## cyanocobalamin, See VITAMIN B₁₂ PREPARATIONS.

## cyclobenzaprine
(sye-kloe-**ben**-za-preen)
Flexeril

*CLASSIFICATION(S):*
*Therapeutic: skeletal muscle relaxants (centrally acting)*

**Pregnancy Category B**

### INDICATIONS
■ Management of acute painful musculoskeletal conditions associated with muscle spasm. **Unlabeled uses:** ■ Management of fibromyalgia.

### ACTION
■ Reduces tonic somatic muscle activity at the level of the brainstem. Structurally similar to tricyclic antidepressants. **Therapeutic Effects:** ■ Reduction in muscle spasm and hyperactivity without loss of function.

### PHARMACOKINETICS
**Absorption:** Well absorbed from the GI tract.
**Distribution:** Unknown.
**Protein Binding:** 93%.
**Metabolism and Excretion:** Mostly metabolized by the liver.
**Half-life:** 1–3 days.

### CONTRAINDICATIONS AND PRECAUTIONS
**Contraindicated in:** ■ Hypersensitivity ■ Should not be used within 14 days of MAO inhibitor therapy ■ Immediate period after MI ■ Severe or symptomatic cardiovascular disease ■ Cardiac conduction disturbances ■ Hyperthyroidism.
**Use Cautiously in:** ■ Cardiovascular disease ■ Pregnancy, lactation, and children <15 yr (safety not established).

### ADVERSE REACTIONS AND SIDE EFFECTS*
■ **CNS:** dizziness, drowsiness, confusion, fatigue, headache, nervousness ■ **EENT:** dry mouth, blurred vision ■ **CV:** arrhythmias ■ **GI:** constipation, dyspepsia, nausea, unpleasant taste ■ **GU:** urinary retention.

### INTERACTIONS
**Drug-Drug:** ■ Additive CNS depression with other **CNS depressants,** including **alcohol, antihistamines, opioid analgesics,** and **sedative/hypnotics** ■ Additive anticholinergic effects with **drugs possessing anticholinergic properties,** including **antihistamines, antidepressants, atropine, disopyramide, haloperidol,** and **phenothiazines** ■ Avoid use within 14 days of **MAO inhibitors** (hyperpyretic crisis, seizures, and death may occur) ■ May blunt the response to **guanadrel** or **guanethidine.**

**Drug-Natural Products:** ■ Concomitant use of kava, valerian, skullcap, chamomile, or hops can increase CNS depression.

## ROUTE AND DOSAGE

■ **PO (Adults):** *Acute painful musculoskeletal conditions*—10 mg 3 times daily (range 20–40 mg/day in 2–4 divided doses; not to exceed 60 mg/day). *Fibromyalgia*—5–40 mg at bedtime (unlabeled).

## AVAILABILITY (generic available)

■ *Tablets:* 10 mg$^{Rx}$ ■ Cost: *Flexeril*—$36.83/30; *generic*—$25.89/30.

TIME/ACTION PROFILE (skeletal muscle relaxation)

| | ONSET | PEAK† | DURATION |
|---|---|---|---|
| PO | within 1 hr | 3–8 hr | 12–24 hr |

†Full effects may not occur for 1–2 wk.

## NURSING IMPLICATIONS

### ASSESSMENT

❑ Assess patient for pain, muscle stiffness, and range of motion before and periodically throughout therapy.

### POTENTIAL NURSING DIAGNOSES

■ Pain, acute (Indications).
■ Mobility, impaired physical (Indications).
■ Injury, risk for (Side Effects).

### IMPLEMENTATION

■ **General:** Do not confuse cyclobenzaprine with cyproheptadine.
■ **PO:** May be administered with meals to minimize gastric irritation.

### PATIENT/FAMILY TEACHING

❑ Instruct patient to take medication exactly as directed; do not take more than the prescribed amount. Missed doses should be taken within 1 hr of time ordered; otherwise, return to normal dosage schedule. Do not double doses.
❑ Medication may cause drowsiness, dizziness, and blurred vision. Caution patient to avoid driving or other activities requiring alertness until response to drug is known.

❑ Advise patient to avoid concurrent use of alcohol or other CNS depressants with this medication.
❑ If constipation becomes a problem, advise patient that increasing fluid intake and bulk in diet and stool softeners may alleviate this condition.
❑ Advise patient to notify health care professional if symptoms of urinary retention (distended abdomen, feeling of fullness, overflow incontinence, voiding small amounts) occur.
❑ Inform patient that good oral hygiene, frequent mouth rinses, and sugarless gum or candy may help relieve dry mouth.

### EVALUATION

**Effectiveness of therapy can be demonstrated by:** ■ Relief of muscular spasm in acute skeletal muscle conditions. Maximum effects may not be evident for 1–2 wk. Use is usually limited to 2–3 wk; however, has been effective for at least 12 wk in the management of fibromyalgia.

**High Alert**

## cyclophosphamide
(sye-kloe-**fos**-fa-mide)
Cytoxan, Neosar, {Procytox}

### CLASSIFICATION(S):
***Therapeutic:*** *antineoplastics, immunosuppressants*
***Pharmacologic:*** *alkylating agents*

**Pregnancy Category D**

### INDICATIONS

■ Alone or with other modalities in the management of: ❑ Hodgkin's disease ❑ Malignant lymphomas ❑ Multiple myeloma ❑ Leukemias ❑ Mycosis fungoides ❑ Neuroblastoma ❑ Ovarian carcinoma ❑ Breast carcinoma and a variety of other tumors ■ Minimal change nephrotic syndrome in children. **Unlabeled uses:** ■ Severe active rheumatoid arthritis or Wegener's granulomatosis.

{ } = Available in Canada only.
*CAPITALS indicates life-threatening; underlines indicate most frequent.

## ACTION

■ Interferes with DNA replication and RNA transcription, ultimately disrupting protein synthesis (cell-cycle phase–nonspecific). **Therapeutic Effects:** ■ Death of rapidly replicating cells, particularly malignant ones ■ Also has immunosuppressant action in smaller doses.

## PHARMACOKINETICS

**Absorption:** Inactive parent drug is well absorbed from the GI tract. Converted to active drug by the liver.

**Distribution:** Widely distributed. Limited penetration of the blood-brain barrier. Crosses the placenta; enters breast milk.

**Metabolism and Excretion:** Converted to active drug by the liver; 30% eliminated unchanged by the kidneys.

**Half-life:** 4–6.5 hr.

## CONTRAINDICATIONS AND PRECAUTIONS

**Contraindicated in:** ■ Hypersensitivity ■ Pregnancy or lactation.

**Use Cautiously in:** ■ Active infections ■ Bone marrow depression ■ Other chronic debilitating illnesses ■ Patients with childbearing potential.

## ADVERSE REACTIONS AND SIDE EFFECTS*

■ **Resp:** PULMONARY FIBROSIS ■ **CV:** MYOCARDIAL FIBROSIS, hypotension ■ **GI:** anorexia, nausea, vomiting ■ **GU:** HEMORRHAGIC CYSTITIS, hematuria ■ **Derm:** alopecia ■ **Endo:** gonadal suppression, syndrome of inappropriate antidiuretic hormone (SIADH) ■ **Hemat:** LEUKOPENIA, thrombocytopenia, anemia ■ **Metab:** hyperuricemia ■ **Misc:** secondary neoplasms.

## INTERACTIONS

**Drug-Drug:** ■ **Phenobarbital** or **rifampin** may increase the toxicity of cyclophosphamide ■ Concurrent **allopurinol** or **thiazide diuretics** may exaggerate bone marrow depression ■ May prolong neuromuscular blockade from **succinylcholine** ■ Cardiotoxicity may be additive with other **cardiotoxic agents (cytarabine, daunorubicin, doxorubicin)** ■ May decrease serum **digoxin** levels ■ Additive bone marrow depression with other **antineoplastics** or **radiation therapy** ■ May potentiate the effects of **warfarin** ■ May decrease antibody response to **live-virus vaccines** and increase

the risk of adverse reactions ■ Prolongs the effects of **cocaine.**

## ROUTE AND DOSAGE

Many regimens are used.

■ **PO (Adults):** 1–5 mg/kg/day.

■ **PO (Children):** *Induction*—2–8 mg/kg/day (60–250 mg/m²/day) in divided doses for 6 days or longer. *Maintenance*—2–5 mg/kg (50–150 mg/m²/day) twice weekly.

■ **IV (Adults):** 40–50 mg/kg in divided doses over 2–5 days *or* 10–15 mg/kg q 7–10 days *or* 3–5 mg/kg twice weekly *or* 1.5–3 mg/kg/day. Other regimens may use larger doses.

■ **IV (Children):** *Induction*—2–8 mg/kg/day (60–250 mg/m²/day) in divided doses for 6 days or longer. Total dose for 7 days may be given as a single weekly dose. *Maintenance*—10–15 mg/kg every 7–10 days or 30 mg/kg q 3–4 wk.

## AVAILABILITY (generic available)

■ *Tablets:* 25 mg^Rx, 50 mg^Rx ■ Cost: 25 mg $203.22/100, 50 mg $372.96/100 ■ *Injection:* 100 mg^Rx, 200 mg^Rx, 500 mg^Rx, {750 mg^Rx}, 1 g^Rx, 2 g^Rx ■ Cost: 100 mg $6.45, 200 mg $12.25, 500 mg $25.71, 1 g $51.43, 2 g $102.89.

TIME/ACTION PROFILE (effects on blood counts)

|        | ONSET  | PEAK       | DURATION |
|--------|--------|------------|----------|
| PO, IV | 7 days | 7–15 days  | 21 days  |

# NURSING IMPLICATIONS

## ASSESSMENT

❏ Monitor blood pressure, pulse, respiratory rate, and temperature frequently during administration. Report significant changes.

❏ Monitor urinary output frequently during therapy. To reduce the risk of hemorrhagic cystitis, fluid intake should be at least 3000 ml/day for adults and 1000–2000 ml/day for children. May be administered with mesna.

❏ Monitor for bone marrow depression. Assess for bleeding (bleeding gums, bruising, petechiae, guaiac stools, urine, and emesis) and avoid IM injections and taking rectal temperatures if platelet count is low. Apply pressure to venipuncture sites for 10 min. Assess for signs of infection during neutropenia. Anemia may occur. Monitor for increased fatigue, dyspnea, and orthostatic hypotension.

◻ Assess nausea, vomiting, and appetite. Weigh weekly. Antiemetics may be given 30 min before administration of medication to minimize GI effects. Anorexia and weight loss can be minimized by feeding frequent light meals.

◻ Encourage patient to drink 2000–3000 ml/ day to promote excretion of uric acid. Alkalinization of the urine may be used to help prevent uric acid nephropathy.

◻ Assess cardiac and respiratory status for dyspnea, rales/crackles, weight gain, edema. Pulmonary toxicity may occur after prolonged therapy. Cardiotoxicity may occur early in therapy and is characterized by symptoms of CHF.

■ **Lab Test Considerations:** Monitor CBC with differential and platelet count before and periodically during therapy. The nadir of leukopenia occurs in 7–12 days (recovery in 17–21 days). Leukocytes should be maintained at 2500–4000/mm³. May also cause thrombocytopenia (nadir 10–15 days), and rarely causes anemia.

◻ Monitor BUN, creatinine, and uric acid before and frequently during therapy to detect nephrotoxicity.

◻ Monitor ALT, AST, LDH, and serum bilirubin before and frequently during therapy to detect hepatotoxicity.

◻ Urinalysis should be evaluated before initiating therapy and frequently during therapy to detect hematuria or change in specific gravity indicative of SIADH.

◻ May suppress positive reactions to skin tests for *Candida*, mumps, *Trichophyton*, and tuberculin purified-protein derivative (PPD). May also produce false-positive results in Papanicolaou smears.

## POTENTIAL NURSING DIAGNOSES

■ Infection, risk for (Side Effects).
■ Body image, disturbed (Side Effects).

## IMPLEMENTATION

◻ **High Alert:** Fatalities have occurred with chemotherapeutic agents. Before administering, clarify all ambiguous orders; double check single, daily, and course-of-therapy dose limits; have second practitioner independently double check original order, calculations and infusion pump settings. Do not confuse cyclophosphamide with cyclosporine. Do not confuse Cytoxan (cyclophosphamide) with Cytozar (cytarabine) or Cytotec (misoprostol).

■ **PO:** Administer medication on an empty stomach. If severe gastric irritation develops, medication may be given with food.

◻ Oral solution can be formed by diluting powder for injection in aromatic elixir to a concentration of 1–5 mg of cyclophosphamide/ ml. Reconstituted preparations should be refrigerated and used within 2 wk.

■ **IV:** Solution for IV administration should be prepared in a biologic cabinet. Wear gloves, gown, and mask while handling IV medication. Discard IV equipment in specially designated containers.

◻ Prepare IV solution by diluting each 100 mg with 5 ml of sterile water or bacteriostatic water for injection containing parabens. Shake solution gently and allow to stand until clear. Use solution without bacteriostatic water within 6 hr. Solution prepared with bacteriostatic water is stable for 24 hr at room temperature, 6 days if refrigerated.

■ **Direct IV:** Administer reconstituted solution directly.

■ **Rate:** Administer at a rate of 100 mg over 1 min.

■ **Intermittent Infusion:** May be further diluted in up to 250 ml of D5W, 0.9% NaCl, D5/0.9% NaCl, 0.45% NaCl, LR, or dextrose/ Ringer's solution.

■ **Syringe Compatibility:** ◆ bleomycin ◆ cisplatin ◆ doxapram ◆ doxorubicin ◆ droperidol ◆ fluorouracil ◆ furosemide ◆ heparin ◆ leucovorin calcium ◆ methotrexate ◆ metoclopramide ◆ mitomycin ◆ vinblastine ◆ vincristine.

■ **Y-Site Compatibility:** ◆ allopurinol ◆ amifostine ◆ amikacin ◆ ampicillin ◆ aztreonam ◆ bleomycin ◆ cefamandole ◆ cefazolin ◆ cefepime ◆ cefoperazone ◆ cefotaxime ◆ cefoxitin ◆ cefuroxime ◆ chloramphenicol ◆ chlorpromazine ◆ cimetidine ◆ cisplatin ◆ cladribine ◆ clindamycin ◆ dexamethasone ◆ diphenhydramine ✦ doxorubicin ✦ doxorubicin liposome ✦ doxycycline ✦ droperidol ✦ erythromycin lactobionate ✦ etoposide phosphate ✦ famotidine ✦ filgrastim ✦ fludarabine ✦ fluorouracil ✦ furosemide ✦ ganciclovir ✦ gatifloxacin ✦ gemcitabine ✦ gentamicin ✦ granisetron ✦ heparin ✦ hydromorphone ✦ idarubicin ✦ kanamycin ✦ leucovorin calcium ✦ linezolid ✦ lorazepam ✦ melphalan ✦ methotrexate ✦ methylprednisolone ✦ metoclopramide ✦ metronidazole ✦ minocycline ✦ mitomycin ✦ morphine ✦ nafcillin ✦ ondansetron ✦ oxacillin ✦ paclitaxel ✦ penicillin G potassium ✦ piperacillin ✦ piperacillin/tazobactam ✦ prochlorperazine ✦ promethazine ✦ propofol ✦ ranitidine ✦ sargramostim ✦ sodium bicarbonate ✦ teniposide ✦ thiotepa ✦ ticarcillin ✦ ticarcillin/clavulanate ✦ tobramycin ✦ topotecan ✦ trimethoprim/sulfamethoxazole ✦ vancomycin ✦ vinblastine ✦ vincristine ✦ vinorelbine.

■ **Y-Site Incompatibility:** ✦ amphotericin B cholesteryl sulfate.

■ **Additive Compatibility:** ✦ fluorouracil ✦ methotrexate ✦ mitoxantrone ✦ ondansetron.

## PATIENT/FAMILY TEACHING

❑ Instruct patient to take dose in early morning. Emphasize need for adequate fluid intake for 72 hr after therapy. Patient should void frequently to decrease bladder irritation from metabolites excreted by the kidneys. Report hematuria immediately. If a dose is missed, health care professional should be contacted.

❑ Instruct patient to notify health care professional promptly if fever; sore throat; signs of infection; lower back or side pain; difficult or painful urination; sores in the mouth or on the lips; yellow discoloration of skin or eyes; bleeding gums; bruising; petechiae; blood in urine, stool, or emesis; unusual swelling; joint pain; shortness of breath; or confusion occurs. Caution patient to avoid crowds and persons with known infections. Instruct patient to use soft toothbrush and electric razor and to avoid falls. Patient should also be cautioned not to drink alcoholic beverages or to take products containing aspirin or NSAIDs; may precipitate GI hemorrhage.

❑ Advise patient that this medication may cause sterility and menstrual irregularities or cessation of menses. This drug is also teratogenic,

and contraceptive measures should continue for at least 4 mo after completion of therapy.

❑ Discuss with patient the possibility of hair loss. Explore methods of coping. May also cause darkening of skin and fingernails.

❑ Instruct patient not to receive any vaccinations without advice of health care professional.

## EVALUATION

**Effectiveness of therapy can be demonstrated by:** ■ Decrease in size or spread of malignant tumors ■ Improvement of hematologic status in patients with leukemia. Maintenance therapy is instituted if leukocyte count remains between 2500 and 4000/mm³ and if patient does not demonstrate serious side effects ■ Management of minimal change nephrotic syndrome in children.

---

## cyclosporine†

(**sye**-kloe-spor-een)
Neoral, Sandimmune, Gengraf

### CLASSIFICATION(S):

**Therapeutic:** *immunosuppressants, antirheumatics ((DMARD)*
**Pharmacologic:** *polypeptides (cyclic)*

### Pregnancy Category C

See Appendix C for ophthalmic use.

## INDICATIONS

■ **PO, IV:** Prevention and treatment of rejection in renal, cardiac, and hepatic transplantation (with corticosteroids) ■ **PO:** Treatment of severe active rheumatoid arthritis (Neoral only) ■ Treatment of severe recalcitrant psoriasis in adult nonimmunocompromised patients (Neoral only). **Unlabeled uses:** ■ Management of recalcitrant ulcerative colitis.

## ACTION

■ Inhibits normal immune responses (cellular and humoral) by inhibiting interleukin-2, a factor necessary for initiation of T-cell activity. **Therapeutic Effects:** ■ Prevention of rejection reactions ■ Slowed progression of rheumatoid arthritis or psoriasis.

## PHARMACOKINETICS

**Absorption:** Erratically absorbed (range 10–60%) after oral administration, with significant first-pass metabolism by the liver. Microemulsion (Neoral) has better bioavailability.
**Distribution:** Widely distributed, mainly into extracellular fluid and blood cells. Crosses the placenta; enters breast milk.
**Protein Binding:** 90%.
**Metabolism and Excretion:** Extensively metabolized by the liver; excreted in bile, small amounts excreted unchanged in urine.
**Half-life:** Children—7 hr; adults—19 hr.

## CONTRAINDICATIONS AND PRECAUTIONS

**Contraindicated in:** ■ Hypersensitivity to cyclosporine or polyoxyethylated castor oil (vehicle for IV form) ■ Should not be given to pregnant or lactating women unless benefits outweigh risks ■ Disulfiram therapy or known alcohol intolerance (IV and oral liquid dosage forms contain alcohol) ■ Psoriasis patients receiving immunosuppressants or radiation.
**Use Cautiously in:** ■ Severe hepatic impairment (dosage reduction recommended) ■ Renal impairment (frequent dosage changes may be necessary) ■ Active infection ■ Children (larger or more frequent doses may be required).

## ADVERSE REACTIONS AND SIDE EFFECTS*

■ **CNS:** SEIZURES, <u>tremor</u>, confusion, flushing, headache, psychiatric problems ■ **CV:** <u>hypertension</u> ■ **GI:** <u>diarrhea</u>, <u>hepatotoxicity</u>, <u>nausea</u>, <u>vomiting</u>, abdominal discomfort, anorexia ■ **GU:** <u>nephrotoxicity</u> ■ **Derm:** <u>hirsutism</u>, acne ■ **F and E:** hyperkalemia, hypomagnesemia ■ **Hemat:** anemia, leukopenia, thrombocytopenia ■ **Metab:** hyperlipidemia, hyperuricemia ■ **Neuro:** hyperesthesia, paresthesia ■ **Misc:** <u>gingival hyperplasia</u>, <u>hypersensitivity reactions</u>, <u>infections</u>.

## INTERACTIONS

**Drug-Drug:** ■ ↑ blood levels and/or risk of toxicity with **amphotericin B, aminoglycosides, amiodarone, anabolic steroids,** some **calcium channel blockers, cimetidine, colchicine, danazol, erythromycin, fluconazole, fluoroquinolones, ketoconazole, itraconazole, metoclopramide, methotrexate, miconazole, NSAIDs, melphalan,** or **hormonal contraceptives** ■ ↑ immunosuppression with other **immunosuppressants** (cyclophosphamide, azathioprine, corticosteroids) ■ **Quinupristin/dalfopristin** ↑ cyclosporine levels ■ **Barbiturates, phenytoin, rifampin, rifabutin carbamazepine,** or **sulfonamides** may ↓ effect of cyclosporine ■ ↑ risk of hyperkalemia with **potassium-sparing diuretics, potassium supplements,** or **ACE inhibitors** ■ ↑ serum levels/ risk of toxicity from **digoxin** ( ↓ digoxin dose by 50%) ■ Prolongs the action of **neuromuscular blocking agents** ■ ↑ risk of seizures with **imipenem/cilastatin** ■ May ↓ antibody response to **live-virus vaccines** and ↑ risk of adverse reactions ■ ↑ risk of rhabdomyolysis with **HMG-CoA reductase inhibitors** ■ Concurrent use with **tacrolimus** should be avoided ■ **Orlistat** ↓ absorption; avoid concurrent use.

**Drug-Natural Products:** ■ Concomitant use with, **echinacea,** and **melatonin** may interfere with immunosuppression ■ Use with **St. John's wort** may cause ↓ serum levels and organ rejection for transplant patients ■ Some **HIV protease inhibitos** may ↑ blood levels and the risk of toxicity.

**Drug-Food:** ■ Concurrent ingestion of **grapefruit or grapefruit juice** ↑ absorption and should be avoided ■ **Food** ↓ absorption of microemulsion products (Neoral).

## ROUTE AND DOSAGE

Doses are adjusted on the basis of serum level monitoring.

❑ **Prevention of Transplant Rejection**

■ **PO (Adults and Children):** 12–15 mg/kg/day (first dose before transplant) for 1–2 wk, taper by 5% weekly to maintenance dose of 5–10 mg/kg/day. Children may require larger or more frequent dosing because of faster clearance.

■ **IV (Adults and Children):** 2–6 mg/kg/day initially, change to PO as soon as possible. Children may require larger or more frequent dosing because of faster clearance.

---

{ } = Available in Canada only.
*CAPITALS indicates life-threatening; <u>underlines</u> indicate most frequent.

❏ **Rheumatoid Arthritis (Neoral only)**

■ **PO (Adults):** 2.5 mg/kg/day given in 2 divided doses; may increase by 0.5–0.75 mg/kg/day after 8 and 12 weeks, up to 4 mg/kg/day. Decrease dose by 25–50% if adverse reactions occur.

❏ **Severe Psoriasis (Neoral only)**

■ **PO (Adults):** 2.5 mg/kg/day given in 2 divided doses, for at least 4 wk; then may increase by 0.5 mg/kg/day q 2 wk, up to 4 mg/kg/day. Decrease dose by 25–50% if adverse reactions occur.

## AVAILABILITY (generic available)

■ *Microemulsion soft gelatin capsules (Neoral):* 25 mg[Rx], 100 mg[Rx] ■Cost: 25 mg $45.85/30, 100 mg, $183.21/30 caps ■ *Microemulsion oral solution (Neoral):* 100 mg/ml[Rx] ■Cost: $332.83/50 ml ■ *Soft gelatin capsules:* 25 mg[Rx], 100 mg[Rx] ■ *Oral solution:* 100 mg/ml[Rx] ■ *Injection:* 50 mg/ml in 5-ml ampules[Rx].

TIME/ACTION PROFILE (blood levels)

| | ONSET | PEAK | DURATION |
|---|---|---|---|
| PO | unknown† | 3.5 hr | unknown |
| IV | unknown | end of infusion | unknown |

†Onset of action in rheumatoid arthritis is 4–8 wk and may last 4 wk after discontinuation; for psoriasis, onset is 2–6 wk and lasts 6 wk following discontinuation.

## NURSING IMPLICATIONS

### ASSESSMENT

■ **General Info:** Monitor intake and output ratios, daily weight, and blood pressure during therapy. Report significant changes.

■ **Prevention of Transplant Rejection:** Assess for symptoms of organ rejection throughout therapy.

■ **IV:** Monitor patient for signs and symptoms of hypersensitivity (wheezing, dyspnea, flushing of face or neck) continuously during at least the first 30 min of each treatment and frequently thereafter. Oxygen, epinephrine, and equipment for treatment of anaphylaxis should be available with each IV dose.

■ **Arthritis:** Assess pain and limitation of movement prior to and during administration.

❏ Prior to initiating therapy, perform a physical exam including blood pressure on 2 occasions to determine baseline. Monitor blood pressure every 2 wk during initial 3 mo, then monthly if stable. If hypertension occurs, dose should be reduced.

■ **Psoriasis:** Assess skin lesions prior to and during therapy.

■ *Lab Test Considerations:* Serum creatinine, BUN, CBC, magnesium, potassium, uric acid, and lipids should be measured at baseline, every 2 wk during initial therapy, and then monthly if stable. Nephrotoxicity may occur; report significant increases.

❏ May cause hepatotoxicity; monitor for ↑ AST, ALT, alkaline phosphatase, amylase, and bilirubin.

❏ May cause ↑ serum potassium and uric acid levels and ↓ serum magnesium levels.

❏ Serum lipid levels may be ↑ .

■ *Toxicity and Overdose:* Serum cyclosporine levels should be evaluated periodically during therapy. Dose may be adjusted daily, in response to levels, during initiation of therapy. Guidelines for desired serum levels will vary among institutions.

## POTENTIAL NURSING DIAGNOSES

■ Infection, risk for (Side Effects).

■ Pain, acute (Indications).

## IMPLEMENTATION

■ **General:** Do not confuse cyclosporine with cyclophosphamide or cycloserine.

❏ Given with other immunosuppressive agents. Protect transplant patients from staff and visitors who may carry infection. Maintain protective isolation as indicated.

❏ Microemulsion products (Neoral) and other products (Sandimmune) are not interchangeable.

■ **PO:** Draw up oral solution in the pipette provided with the medication. Mix oral solution with milk, chocolate milk, or orange juice, preferably at room temperature. Stir well and drink at once. Use a glass container and rinse with more diluent to ensure that total dose is taken. Administer oral doses with meals. Wipe pipette dry; do not wash after use.

■ **Intermittent Infusion:** Dilute each 1 ml (50 mg) of IV concentrate immediately before use with 20–100 ml of D5W or 0.9% NaCl for injection. Solution is stable for 24 hr in D5W. In 0.9% NaCl, it is stable for 6 hr

in a polyvinylchloride container and 12 hr in a glass container at room temperature.
- **Rate:** Infuse slowly over 2–6 hr via infusion pump.
- **Continuous Infusion:** May be administered over 24 hr.
- **Y-Site Compatibility:** ✦ alatrofloxacin ✦ gatifloxacin ✦ linezolid ✦ propofol ✦ sargramostim.
- **Y-Site Incompatibility:** ✦ amphotericin B cholesteryl sulfate.
- **Additive Incompatibility:** ✦ magnesium sulfate.

## PATIENT/FAMILY TEACHING

- Instruct patient to take medication at the same time each day and with regard to food, as directed. Do not skip doses or double up on missed doses. Take missed doses as soon as remembered within 12 hr. Do not discontinue medication without advice of health care professional.
- Reinforce the need for lifelong therapy to prevent transplant rejection. Review symptoms of rejection for transplanted organ, and stress need to notify health care professional immediately if they occur.
- Instruct patient to avoid grapefruit and grapefruit juice to prevent interaction with cyclosporine.
- Advise patient of common side effects (nephrotoxicity, increased blood pressure, hand tremors, increased facial hair, gingival hyperplasia).
- Teach patient the correct method for monitoring blood pressure. Instruct patient to notify health care professional of significant changes in blood pressure or if hematuria, increased frequency, cloudy urine, decreased urine output, fever, sore throat, tiredness, or unusual bruising occurs.
- Instruct patient on proper oral hygiene. Meticulous oral hygiene and dental examinations for teeth cleaning and plaque control every 3 mo will help decrease gingival inflammation and hyperplasia.
- Instruct patient to consult health care professional before taking any OTC medications or receiving any vaccinations while taking this medication.

- Advise patient to notify health care professional if pregnancy is planned or suspected.
- Emphasize the importance of follow-up exams and lab tests.

## EVALUATION

**Effectiveness of therapy can be demonstrated by:** ■ Prevention of rejection of transplanted tissues ■ Decrease in severity of pain ❑ Increased ease of joint movement ■ Decrease in progression of psoriasis.

# cyproheptadine

(si-proe-**hep**-ta-deen)
Periactin, PMS-Cyproheptadine

## CLASSIFICATION(S):
**Therapeutic:** allergy, cold, and cough remedies, antihistamines

**Pregnancy Category B**

## INDICATIONS

■ Relief of allergic symptoms caused by histamine release including: ❑ Seasonal and perennial allergic rhinitis ❑ Chronic urticaria ❑ Cold urticaria. **Unlabeled uses:** ■ Stimulation of appetite.

## ACTION

■ Antagonizes the effects of histamine at H-receptor sites; does not bind to or inactivate histamine ■ Also blocks the effects of serotonin, which may result in increased appetite. **Therapeutic Effects:** ■ Decreased symptoms of histamine excess (sneezing, rhinorrhea, nasal and ocular pruritus, ocular tearing and redness) ■ Decreased cold urticaria.

## PHARMACOKINETICS

**Absorption:** Apparently well absorbed after oral dosing.

**Distribution:** Unknown.

**Metabolism and Excretion:** Mostly metabolized by the liver.

**Half-life:** Unknown.

## CONTRAINDICATIONS AND PRECAUTIONS

**Contraindicated in:** ■ Hypersensitivity ■ Acute attacks of asthma ■ Lactation ■ Known alcohol intolerance (syrup only).
**Use Cautiously in:** ■ Geriatric patients ■ Narrow-angle glaucoma ■ Liver disease ■ Pregnancy (safety not established).

## ADVERSE REACTIONS AND SIDE EFFECTS*

■ **CNS:** <u>drowsiness</u>, excitation (increased in children) ■ **EENT:** <u>blurred vision</u> ■ **CV:** arrhythmias, hypotension, palpitations ■ **GI:** <u>dry mouth</u>, constipation ■ **GU:** hesitancy, retention ■ **Derm:** photosensitivity, rashes ■ **Misc:** weight gain.

## INTERACTIONS

**Drug-Drug:** ■ Additive CNS depression with other **CNS depressants**, including **alcohol, opioid analgesics**, and **sedative/hypnotics** ■ **MAO inhibitors** may intensify and prolong the anticholinergic effects of **antihistamines.**

## ROUTE AND DOSAGE

■ **PO (Adults):** 4 mg q 8 hr (range 4–20 mg/day in 3 divided doses; up to 0.5 mg/kg/day).
■ **PO (Children 6–14 yr):** 2–4 mg q 8–12 hr (not to exceed 16 mg/day).
■ **PO (Children 2–6 yr):** 2 mg q 8–12 hr (not to exceed 12 mg/day).

## AVAILABILITY (generic available)

■ **Tablets:** 4 mg$^{Rx}$, {4 mg$^{OTC}$} ■ Cost: 4 mg$^{Rx}$ $4.79/30 ■ **Syrup:** 2 mg/5 ml$^{Rx}$, {2 mg/5 ml$^{OTC}$} ■ Cost: 2 mg/5 ml$^{Rx}$ $7.47/120 ml.

TIME/ACTION PROFILE (antihistaminic effects)

|    | ONSET | PEAK | DURATION |
|----|-------|------|----------|
| PO | 15–60 min | 1–2 hr | 8 hr |

# NURSING IMPLICATIONS

## ASSESSMENT

■ **Allergy:** Assess symptoms (rhinitis, conjunctivitis, hives) prior to and periodically throughout therapy.
❑ Assess lung sounds and respiratory function prior to and periodically throughout therapy. May cause thickening of bronchial secre-

tions. Maintain fluid intake of 1500–2000 ml/day to decrease viscosity of secretions.
■ **Appetite Stimulant:** Monitor food intake and weight routinely.
■ **Lab Test Considerations:** May cause false-negative reactions on allergy skin tests; discontinue 72 hr prior to testing.
❑ Increased serum amylase and prolactin concentrations may occur when cyproheptadine is administered with a thyrotropin-releasing hormone.

## POTENTIAL NURSING DIAGNOSES

■ Airway clearance, ineffective (Indications).
■ Injury, risk for (Side Effects).

## IMPLEMENTATION

■ **General:** Do not confuse cyproheptadine with cyclobenzaprine.
■ **PO:** Administer with food, water, or milk to minimize gastric irritation.

## PATIENT/FAMILY TEACHING

❑ Instruct patient to take cyproheptadine exactly as directed. Missed dose should be taken as soon as remembered. Do not double doses. Syrup should be accurately measured using calibrated medication cup or measuring device.
❑ Medication may cause drowsiness. Advise patient to avoid driving or other activities requiring alertness until response to the drug is known.
❑ Advise patient to use sunscreen and protective clothing to prevent a photosensitivity reaction.
❑ Caution patient to avoid concurrent use of alcohol and other CNS depressants.
❑ Advise patient that frequent mouth rinses, good oral hygiene, and sugarless gum or candy may decrease dry mouth. Patient should notify dentist if dry mouth persists for >2 wk.

## EVALUATION

**Effectiveness of therapy can be demonstrated by:** ■ Alleviation of allergic symptoms ❑ Alleviation of cold urticaria ■ Improvement of appetite.

| High Alert |

# cytarabine

(sye-**tare**-a-been)

Ara-C, cytosine arabinoside, {Cytosar}, Cytosar-U, DepoCyt

## CLASSIFICATION(S):

**Therapeutic:** *antineoplastics*
**Pharmacologic:** *antimetabolites*

## Pregnancy Category D

## INDICATIONS

■ **IV:** Used mainly in combination chemotherapeutic regimens for the treatment of leukemias and non-Hodgkin's lymphomas ■ **IT:** Treatment of lymphomatous meningitis.

## ACTION

■ Inhibits DNA synthesis by inhibiting DNA polymerase (cell-cycle S-phase–specific). **Therapeutic Effects:** ■ Death of rapidly replicating cells, particularly malignant ones.

## PHARMACOKINETICS

**Absorption:** Absorption occurs from subcut sites, but blood levels are lower than with IV administration; IT administration results in negligible systemic exposure.

**Distribution:** Widely distributed; IV- and subcut-administered cytarabine crosses the blood-brain barrier but not in sufficient quantities. Crosses the placenta.

**Metabolism and Excretion:** Metabolized mostly by the liver; <10% excreted unchanged by the kidneys. Metabolism to inactive drug in the CSF is negligible because the enzyme that metabolizes it is present in very low concentrations in the CSF.

**Half-life:** *IV, subcut*—1–3 hr; *IT*—100–236 hr.

## CONTRAINDICATIONS AND PRECAUTIONS

**Contraindicated in:** ■ Hypersensitivity ■ Pregnancy or lactation ■ Active meningeal infection (IT only).

**Use Cautiously in:** ■ Active infections ■ Decreased bone marrow reserve ■ Renal/hepatic disease ■ Other chronic debilitating illnesses ■ Patients with childbearing potential.

## ADVERSE REACTIONS AND SIDE EFFECTS*

■ **CNS:** CNS dysfunction (high dose), confusion, drowsiness, headache ■ **EENT:** corneal toxicity (high dose), hemorrhagic conjunctivitis (high dose) ■ **Resp:** PULMONARY EDEMA (high dose) ■ **CV:** edema ■ **GI:** nausea, vomiting, hepatitis, hepatotoxicity, severe GI ulceration (high dose), stomatitis ■ **GU:** urinary incontinence ■ **Derm:** alopecia, rash ■ **Endo:** sterility ■ **Hemat:** *(less with IT use)*—anemia, leukopenia, thrombocytopenia ■ **Metab:** hyperuricemia ■ **Neuro:** *Intrathecal only*—CHEMICAL ARACHNOIDITIS, abnormal gait ■ **Misc:** cytarabine syndrome, fever.

## INTERACTIONS

**Drug-Drug:** ■ Additive bone marrow depression with other **antineoplastics** or **radiation therapy** ■ Increased risk of cardiomyopathy when used in high-dose regimens with **cyclophosphamide** ■ May decrease antibody response to **live-virus vaccines** and increase the risk of adverse reactions ■ May decrease absorption of **digoxin** tablets ■ May decrease the efficacy of **gentamicin** when used to treat *Klebsiella pneumoniae* infections ■ Recent treatment with **asparaginase** may increase the risk of pancreatitis ■ Additive neurotoxicity with concurrently administered **IT antineoplastics** (IT only).

## ROUTE AND DOSAGE

Dosage regimens vary widely.

■ **IV (Adults):** *Induction dose*—200 mg/m²/day for 5 days q 2 wk as a single agent *or* 2–6 mg/kg/day (100–200 mg/m²/day) as a single daily dose *or* in 2–3 divided doses for 5–10 days or until remission occurs as part of combination chemotherapy. *Maintenance*—70–200 mg/m²/day for 2–5 days monthly. *Refractory leukemias/lymphomas*—3 g/m² q 12 hr for up to 12 doses.

■ **Subcut, IM (Adults):** *Maintenance*—1–1.5 mg/kg q 1–4 wk.

■ **IT (Adults):** *Depo Cyt Induction*—50 mg (intraventricular or lumbar puncture) every 14 days for 2 doses (weeks 1 and 3); *con-*

*solidation*—50 mg (intraventricular or lumbar puncture) every 14 days for 3 doses (weeks 5, 7 and 9), followed by one additional dose at week 13; *maintenance*—50 mg (intraventricular or lumbar puncture) every 28 days for 4 doses (weeks 17, 21, 25, and 29). If drug-related neurotoxicity occurs, dosage should be reduced to 25 mg or discontinued (dexamethasone 4 mg PO/IV twice daily for 5 days should be started concurrently with IT cytarabine).

## AVAILABILITY (generic available)

■ *Powder for injection:* 100 mg$^{Rx}$, 500 mg$^{Rx}$, 1 g$^{Rx}$, 2 g$^{Rx}$ ■ *Sustained-release liposome injection for IT use:* 50 ml/5-ml vial$^{Rx}$.

TIME/ACTION PROFILE (IV, subcut—effects on WBCs; IT—levels in CSF)

| | ONSET | PEAK | DURATION |
|---|---|---|---|
| Subcut, IV (1st phase) | 24 hr | 7–9 days | 12 days |
| Subcut, IV (2nd phase) | 15–24 days | 15–24 days | 25–34 days |
| IT | rapid | 5 hr | 14–28 days |

# NURSING IMPLICATIONS

## ASSESSMENT

■ **General Info:** Monitor for bone marrow depression. Assess for bleeding (bleeding gums, bruising, petechiae, guaiac stools, urine, and emesis) and avoid IM injections and taking rectal temperatures if platelet count is low. Apply pressure to venipuncture sites for 10 min. Assess for signs of infection during neutropenia. Anemia may occur. Monitor for increased fatigue, dyspnea, and orthostatic hypotension.

❑ Monitor intake and output ratios and daily weights. Report significant changes in totals.

❑ Monitor for symptoms of gout (increased uric acid, joint pain, edema). Encourage patient to drink at least 2 L of fluid each day. Allopurinol may decrease uric acid levels. Alkalinization of urine may increase excretion of uric acid.

❑ Assess nutritional status. Nausea and vomiting may occur within 1 hr of administration, especially if IV dose is administered rapidly, less severe if medication is infused slowly. Administering an antiemetic prior to and periodically throughout therapy and adjusting diet as tolerated may help maintain fluid and electrolyte balance and nutritional status.

❑ Monitor patient for development of *cytarabine* or *ara-C syndrome* (fever, myalgia, bone pain, chest pain, maculopapular rash, conjunctivitis, malaise), which usually occurs 6–12 hr following administration. Corticosteroids may be used for treatment or prevention. If patient responds to corticosteroids, continue cytarabine and corticosteroids.

❑ Assess patient for respiratory distress and pulmonary edema. Occurs with high doses rarely; may be fatal.

❑ Monitor patient for signs of anaphylaxis (rash, dyspnea, swelling). Epinephrine, corticosteroids, and resuscitation equipment should be readily available.

■ **IT:** Chemical arachnoiditis (nausea, vomiting, headache, fever, back pain, CSF pleocytosis and neck rigidity, neck pain, or meningism) is an expected side effect of IT cytarabine. Incidence and severity of symptoms may be decreased with coadministration of dexamethasone.

❑ Monitor patients receiving IT therapy continuously for the development of neurotoxicity (myelopathy, personality changes, dysarthria, ataxia, confusion, somnolence, coma). If neurotoxicity develops, decrease amount of subsequent doses and discontinue if neurotoxicity persists. Risk may be increased if cytarabine is administered intrathecally and IV within a few days.

■ *Lab Test Considerations:* Monitor CBC with differential and platelet count prior to and frequently throughout therapy. Leukocyte counts begin to drop within 24 hr of administration. The initial nadir occurs in 7–9 days. After a small rise in the count, the second, deeper nadir occurs 15–24 days after administration. Platelet counts begin to fall 5 days after a dose, with a nadir at 12–15 days. Leukocyte and thrombocyte counts usually begin to rise 10 days after the nadirs. Therapy is usually withdrawn if leukocyte count is <1000/mm$^3$ or platelet count is <50,000/mm$^3$. Bone marrow aspirations are recommended every 2 wk until remission occurs.

❑ Renal (BUN and creatinine) and hepatic function (AST, ALT, bilirubin, alkaline phosphatase, and LDH) should be monitored prior to and routinely throughout therapy.

❏ May cause increased uric acid concentrations.

## POTENTIAL NURSING DIAGNOSES

■ Infection, risk for (Adverse Reactions).

■ Injury, risk for (Side Effects).

## IMPLEMENTATION

❏ *High Alert:* Fatalities have occurred with chemotherapeutic agents. Before administering, clarify all ambiguous orders; double check single, daily, and course-of-therapy dose limits; have second practitioner independently double check original order, calculations and infusion pump settings. Do not confuse cytarabine with Cytoxan (cyclophosphamide). Do not confuse Cytosar (cytarabine) with Cytovene (ganciclovir) or Cytoxan. Do not confuse high-dose and regular therapy. Fatalities have occurred with high-dose therapy.

■ **General:** Solution should be prepared in a biologic cabinet. Wear gloves, gown, and mask while handling IV medication. Discard IV equipment in specially designated containers (see Appendix M).

❏ May be given subcut, direct IV, intermittent IV, continuous IV, or IT.

■ **IV, Subcut:** Reconstitute 100-mg vials with 5 ml of bacteriostatic water for injection with benzyl alcohol 0.9% for a concentration of 20 mg/ml. Reconstitute 500-mg vials with 10 ml for a concentration of 50 mg/ml, 1-g vials with 10 ml, and 2-g vials with 20 ml for a concentration of 100 mg/ml. Reconstituted solution is stable for 48 hr. Do not administer a cloudy or hazy solution.

■ **Direct IV:** Administer each 100 mg direct IV push over 1–3 min.

■ **Intermittent Infusion:** May be further diluted in 100 ml of 0.9% NaCl or D5W. May also be diluted in D10W, D5/0.9% NaCl, Ringer's solution, LR, or D5/LR.

■ *Rate:* Infuse over 30 min.

■ **Continuous Infusion:** Rate and concentration for IV infusion are ordered individually by physician.

■ **Syringe Compatibility:** ◆ metoclopramide.

■ **Y-Site Compatibility:** ◆ amifostine ◆ aztreonam ◆ cefepime ◆ chlorpromazine ◆ cimeti-dine ◆ cladribine ◆ diphenhydramine ◆ droperidol ◆ famotidine ◆ filgrastim ◆ fludarabine ◆ furosemide ◆ gatifloxacin ◆ granisetron ◆ heparin ◆ hydrocortisone ◆ hydromorphone ◆ idarubicin ◆ linezolid ◆ lorazepam ◆ melphalan ◆ methotrexate ◆ methylprednisolone ◆ metoclopramide ◆ morphine ◆ ondansetron ◆ paclitaxel ◆ piperacillin/tazobactam ◆ prochlorperazine ◆ promethazine ◆ propofol ◆ ranitidine ◆ sargramostim ◆ teniposide ◆ thiotepa ◆ vinorelbine.

■ **Y-Site Incompatibility:** ◆ ganciclovir.

■ **Additive Compatibility:** ◆ etoposide ◆ methotrexate ◆ mitoxantrone ◆ potassium chloride ◆ prednisolone sodium phosphate ◆ sodium bicarbonate ◆ vincristine.

■ **Additive Incompatibility:** ◆ fluorouracil ◆ heparin ◆ regular insulin ◆ nafcillin ◆ oxacillin ◆ penicillin G sodium.

■ **IT:** Patients receiving *liposomal cytarabine* should be started on dexamethasone 4 mg twice daily PO or IV for 5 days beginning on the day of liposomal cytarabine injection.

❏ Allow vial to warm to room temperature. Gently agitate or invert vial to resuspend particles immediately before withdrawal from vial. No further reconstitution or dilution is required with *liposomal cytarabine.* Reconstitute *conventional cytarabine* with preservative-free 0.9% NaCl or autologous spinal fluid. Use immediately to prevent bacterial contamination.

❏ Liposomal cytarabine must be used within 4 hr of withdrawal from the vial. Discard unused portions. Inject directly into CSF via intraventricular reservoir or by direct injection into lumbar sac. Do not use in-line filters.

❏ Instruct patient to lie flat for 1 hr following IT injection. Monitor for immediate toxic reactions.

## PATIENT/FAMILY TEACHING

❏ Caution patient to avoid crowds and persons with known infections. Report symptoms of infection (fever, chills, cough, hoarseness, sore throat, lower back or side pain, painful or difficult urination) immediately.

❏ Instruct patient to report unusual bleeding. Advise patient of thrombocytopenia precautions (use soft toothbrush and electric razor, avoid falls, do not drink alcoholic beverages or take medication containing aspirin or NSAIDs; may precipitate gastric bleeding).

❏ Instruct patient to inspect oral mucosa for redness and ulceration. If mouth sores occur, advise patient to use sponge brush and rinse mouth with water after eating and drinking. Stomatitis may require treatment with opioid analgesics.

❏ Advise patient that this medication may have teratogenic effects. Contraception should be used during therapy and for at least 4 mo after therapy is concluded.

❏ Instruct patient not to receive any vaccinations without advice of health care professional.

❏ Emphasize the need for periodic lab tests to monitor for side effects.

■ **IT:** Inform patient about the expected side effects (headache, nausea, vomiting, fever) and about early signs of neurotoxicity. Instruct patient to notify health care professional if these signs occur.

❏ Emphasize the importance of taking dexamethasone with lyposomal cytarabine.

## EVALUATION

**Effectiveness of therapy can be demonstrated by:** ■ Improvement of hematopoietic values in leukemias ■ Decrease in size and spread of the tumor in non-Hodgkin's lymphomas. Therapy is continued every 2 wk until patient is in complete remission or thrombocyte count or leukocyte count falls below acceptable levels ■ Treatment of lymphomatous meningitis.

# daclizumab

(da-**kliz**-yoo-mab)

Zenapax

*CLASSIFICATION(S):*

*Therapeutic: immunosuppressants*
*Pharmacologic: monoclonal antibodies*

**Pregnancy Category C**

## INDICATIONS

■ Prevention of acute organ rejection during renal transplantation (with cyclosporine and corticosteroids).

## ACTION

■ Binds specifically to interleukin-2 (IL-2) receptor sites on activated lymphocytes, acting as an IL-2 receptor antagonist. This prevents further activation of lymphocytes and allograft rejection. **Therapeutic Effects:** ■ Prevention of renal allograft rejection.

## PHARMACOKINETICS

**Absorption:** IV administration results in complete bioavailability.

**Distribution:** Crosses the placenta.

**Metabolism and Excretion:** Binds to lymphocytes.

**Half-life:** 20 days.

## CONTRAINDICATIONS AND PRECAUTIONS

**Contraindicated in:** ■ Hypersensitivity.

**Use Cautiously in:** ■ Geriatric patients ■ Pregnancy, lactation, or children (has been used in children; increased risk of hypertension and dehydration).

## ADVERSE REACTIONS AND SIDE EFFECTS*

■ **CNS:** dizziness, fatigue, headache, insomnia ■ **Resp:** PULMONARY EDEMA, coughing, dyspnea ■ **CV:** chest pain, edema, hypertension ( ↑ in children), hypotension, tachycardia ■ **GI:** abdominal discomfort, constipation, diarrhea ( ↑ in children), dyspepsia, epigastric pain, nausea, pyrosis, vomiting ( ↑ in children) ■ **GU:** dysu-

ria, oliguria, renal tubular necrosis ■ **Derm:** acne, impaired wound healing, pruritus ( ↑ in children) ■ **Hemat:** thrombosis ■ **MS:** arthralgia, back pain, musculoskeletal pain ■ **Neuro:** tremor ■ **Misc:** Allergic reactions including ANAPHYLAXIS, fever ( ↑ in children), post-operative pain ( ↑ in children), urinary and respiratory tract infection ( ↑ in children).

## INTERACTIONS

**Drug-Drug:** ■ None known.

**Drug-Natural Products:** ■ Concomitant use with **astragalus, echinacea,** and **melatonin** may interfere with immunosuppression.

## ROUTE AND DOSAGE

■ **IV (Adults and Children):** 1 mg/kg, with 1st dose given no more than 24 hr before transplantation, then q 2 wk for a total of 5 doses.

## AVAILABILITY

■ *Concentrate for injection (must be diluted):* 25 mg/5 ml in 5-ml vials[Rx].

TIME/ACTION PROFILE (saturation of IL-2 receptors)

| | ONSET | PEAK | DURATION |
|---|---|---|---|
| IV | rapid | after 5th dose | 120 days† |

†Post-transplantation.

# NURSING IMPLICATIONS

## ASSESSMENT

■ **General Info:** Assess for fluid overload (monitor weight and intake and output, assess for edema and rales/crackles). Notify physician if patient has experienced 3% or more weight gain in the previous week. Obtain chest x-ray within 24 hr before beginning therapy. Fluid-overloaded patients are at high risk of developing pulmonary edema. Monitor vital signs and breath sounds closely.

❑ Monitor for signs of anaphylactic or hypersensitivity reactions (hypotension, bronchospasms, wheezing, laryngeal edema, pulmonary edema, cyanosis, hypoxia, respiratory arrest, cardiac arrhythmia, cardiac arrest, peripheral edema, loss of consciousness, fever, rash, urticaria, diaphoresis, pruritus, and/or injection site reactions) at each dose. Resuscitation equipment should be readily available. If a severe hypersensitivity reaction occurs, therapy with daclizumab should be permanently discontinued.

❑ Monitor for infection (fever, chills, rash, sore throat, purulent discharge, dysuria). Notify physician immediately if these symptoms occur; may necessitate discontinuation of therapy.

## POTENTIAL NURSING DIAGNOSES

■ Infection, risk for (Side Effects).
■ Fluid volume, excess (Side Effects).

## IMPLEMENTATION

■ **General:** Daclizumab is usually administered concurrently with cyclosporine and corticosteroids.
❑ Daclizumab should be used only by physicians experienced in the management of organ transplantation.
■ **Intermittent Infusion:** Dilute daclizumab with 50 ml of 0.9% NaCl. Gently invert bag to mix; do not shake to avoid foaming. Solution is clear and colorless; do not administer solutions that are discolored or contain particulate matter. Discard unused portion. Administer within 4 hr or may be refrigerated for up to 24 hr. Discard after 24 hr.
■ *Rate:* Administer over 15 min via peripheral or central line.
■ **Compatibility:** Do not admix; do not administer in IV line containing other medications. If line must be used for other medications, flush with 0.9% NaCl before and after daclizumab.

## PATIENT/FAMILY TEACHING

❑ Explain that patient will need to resume lifelong therapy with other immunosuppressive drugs after completion of daclizumab course.
❑ May cause dizziness. Caution patient to avoid driving or other activities requiring alertness until response is known.
❑ Instruct patient to continue to avoid crowds and persons with known infections; this drug also suppresses the immune system.
❑ Instruct patient not to receive any vaccinations and to avoid contact with persons receiving oral polio vaccine without advice of health care professional.

## EVALUATION

**Effectiveness of therapy can be demonstrated by:** ■ Prevention of acute organ rejection.

## dalteparin, See HEPARINS (LOW MOLECULAR WEIGHT)/ HEPARINOIDS.

# dantrolene
(**dan**-troe-leen)
Dantrium

## CLASSIFICATION(S):
*Therapeutic: skeletal muscle relaxants (direct acting)*

**Pregnancy Category C**

## INDICATIONS

■ **PO:** Treatment of spasticity associated with: ❑ Spinal cord injury ❑ Stroke ❑ Cerebral palsy ❑ Multiple sclerosis ■ Prophylaxis of malignant hyperthermia ■ **IV:** Emergency treatment of malignant hyperthermia. **Unlabeled uses:** ■ Management of neuroleptic malignant syndrome.

## ACTION

■ Acts directly on skeletal muscle, causing relaxation by decreasing calcium release from sarcoplasmic reticulum in muscle cells ■ Prevents intense catabolic process associated with malignant hyperthermia. **Therapeutic Effects:** ■ Reduction of muscle spasticity ■ Prevention of malignant hyperthermia.

## PHARMACOKINETICS

**Absorption:** 35% absorbed after oral administration.
**Distribution:** Unknown.
**Metabolism and Excretion:** Almost entirely metabolized by the liver.
**Half-life:** 8.7 hr.

## CONTRAINDICATIONS AND PRECAUTIONS

**Contraindicated in:** ■ No contraindications to IV form in treatment of hyperthermia ■ Pregnancy and lactation ■ Situations in which spasticity is used to maintain posture or balance.

**Use Cautiously in:** ■ Cardiac, pulmonary, or previous liver disease ■ Women, patients >35 yr (increased risk of hepatotoxicity).

## ADVERSE REACTIONS AND SIDE EFFECTS*

■ **CNS:** <u>drowsiness</u>, <u>muscle weakness</u>, confusion, dizziness, headache, insomnia, malaise, nervousness ■ **EENT:** excessive lacrimation, visual disturbances ■ **Resp:** pleural effusions ■ **CV:** changes in BP, tachycardia ■ **GI:** HEPATOTOX-ICITY, <u>diarrhea</u>, anorexia, cramps, dysphagia, GI bleeding, vomiting ■ **GU:** crystalluria, dysuria, frequency, impotence, incontinence, nocturia ■ **Derm:** pruritus, sweating, urticaria ■ **Hemat:** eosinophilia ■ **Local:** irritation at IV site, phlebitis ■ **MS:** myalgia ■ **Misc:** chills, drooling, fever.

## INTERACTIONS

**Drug-Drug:** ■ Additive CNS depression with **CNS depressants,** including **alcohol, antihistamines, opioid analgesics, sedative/ hypnotics,** and parenteral **magnesium sulfate** ■ Increased risk of hepatotoxicity with other **hepatotoxic agents** or **estrogens** ■ Increased risk of arrhythmias with **verapamil**.

**Drug-Natural Products:** ■ Concomitant use of **kava, valerian, skullcap, chamomile,** or **hops** can increase CNS depression.

## ROUTE AND DOSAGE

■ **PO (Adults):** *Spasticity*—25 mg/day initially; increase by 25 mg/day q 4–7 days until desired response or total of 100 mg 4 times daily is reached. *Prevention of malignant hyperthermia*—4–8 mg/kg/day in 3–4 divided doses for 1–2 days before procedure, last dose 3–4 hr preop. *Post-hyperthermic crisis follow-up*—4–8 mg/kg/day in 3–4 divided doses for 1–3 days after IV treatment.

■ **PO (Children >5 yr):** *Spasticity*—0.5 mg/ kg twice daily; increase by 0.5 mg/kg/day q 4–7 days until desired response is obtained or dosage of 3 mg/kg 4 times daily is reached (not to exceed 400 mg/day). *Prevention of malignant hyperthermia*—4–8 mg/kg/day in 3–4 divided doses for 1–2 days before procedure, last dose 3–4 hr preop. *Post-hyperthermic crisis follow-up*—4–8

mg/kg/day in 3–4 divided doses for 1–3 days after IV treatment.

■ **IV (Adults and Children):** *Treatment of malignant hyperthermia*—at least 1 mg/kg (up to 3 mg/kg), continued until symptoms decrease or a cumulative dose of 10 mg/kg has been given. If symptoms reappear, dosage may be repeated. *Prevention of malignant hyperthermia*—2.5 mg/kg before anesthesia.

## AVAILABILITY

■ ***Capsules:*** 25 mg$^{Rx}$, 50 mg$^{Rx}$, 100 mg$^{Rx}$ ■ ***Powder for injection:*** 20 mg/vial$^{Rx}$.

TIME/ACTION PROFILE (effects on spasticity)

|     | ONSET | PEAK | DURATION |
|-----|-------|------|----------|
| PO  | 1 wk  | unknown | 6–12 hr |
| IV  | rapid | rapid | unknown |

# NURSING IMPLICATIONS

## ASSESSMENT

■ **General Info:** Assess bowel function periodically. Persistent diarrhea may warrant discontinuation of therapy.

■ **Muscle Spasticity:** Assess neuromuscular status and muscle spasticity before initiating therapy and periodically during its course to determine response to therapy.

■ **Malignant Hyperthermia:** Assess previous anesthesia history of all surgical patients. Also assess for family history of reactions to anesthesia (malignant hyperthermia or perioperative death).

❑ Monitor ECG, vital signs, electrolytes, and urine output continuously when administering IV for malignant hyperthermia.

❑ Monitor patient for difficulty swallowing and choking during meals on the day of administration.

■ *Lab Test Considerations:* Monitor liver function frequently during therapy. Liver function abnormalities (elevated AST, ALT, alkaline phosphatase, bilirubin, GGTP) may require discontinuation of therapy.

❑ Renal function and CBC should be evaluated before and periodically during therapy in patients receiving prolonged therapy.

## POTENTIAL NURSING DIAGNOSES

- Mobility, impaired physical (Indications).
- Pain, acute (Indications).
- Injury, risk for (Side Effects).

## IMPLEMENTATION

- **General:** Do not confuse Dantrium (dantrolene) with danazol.
- **PO:** If gastric irritation becomes a problem, may be administered with food. Oral suspensions may be made by opening capsules and adding them to fruit juices or other liquid. Drink immediately after mixing.
- Oral dose for spasticity should be divided into 4 doses/day.
- **Direct IV:** Reconstitute each 20 mg with 60 ml of sterile water for injection without a bacteriostatic agent for a concentration of 333 mcg/ml. Shake until solution is clear. Solution must be used within 6 hr. Protect diluted solution from direct light.
- **Rate:** Administer each single dose by rapid continuous IV push through Y-tubing or 3-way stopcock. Follow immediately with subsequent doses as indicated. Medication is very irritating to tissues; observe infusion site frequently to avoid extravasation.
- **Intermittent Infusion:** Prophylactic dose has been administered as an infusion.
- **Rate:** Administer over 1 hr before anesthesia.

## PATIENT/FAMILY TEACHING

- **General Info:** Advise patient not to take more medication than the amount prescribed to minimize risk of hepatotoxicity and other side effects. If a dose is missed, do not take unless remembered within 1 hr. Do not double doses.
- May cause dizziness, drowsiness, visual disturbances, and muscle weakness. Advise patient to avoid driving and other activities requiring alertness until response to drug is known. After IV dose for surgery, patients may experience decreased grip strength, leg weakness, light-headedness, and difficulty swallowing for up to 48 hr. Caution patients to avoid activities requiring alertness and to use caution when walking down stairs and eating during this period.
- Advise patient to avoid taking alcohol or other CNS depressants concurrently with this medication.
- Instruct patient to notify health care professional if rash; itching; yellow eyes or skin; dark urine; or clay-colored, bloody, or black, tarry stools occur or if nausea, weakness, malaise, fatigue, or diarrhea persists. May require discontinuation of therapy.
- Advise patient to wear sunscreen and protective clothing to prevent photosensitivity reactions.
- Emphasize the importance of follow-up exams to check progress in long-term therapy and blood tests to monitor for side effects.
- **Malignant Hyperthermia:** Patients with malignant hyperthemia should carry identification describing disease process at all times.

## EVALUATION

**Effectiveness of therapy can be demonstrated by:** ■ Relief of muscle spasm in musculoskeletal conditions. One wk or more may be required to see improvement; if there is no observed improvement in 45 days, the medication is usually discontinued ■ Prevention of or decrease in temperature and skeletal rigidity in malignant hyperthermia.

## darbepoetin

(dar-be-**poh**-e-tin)

Aranesp

**CLASSIFICATION(S):**
**Therapeutic:** antianemics
**Pharmacologic:** hormones (rDNA)

**Pregnancy Category C**

## INDICATIONS

■ Anemia associated with chronic renal failure ■ Chemotherapy-induced anemia in patients with non-myeloid malignancies.

## ACTION

■ Stimulates erythropoiesis (production of red blood cells) **Therapeutic Effects:** ■ Maintains and may elevate red blood cell counts, decreasing the need for transfusions.

## PHARMACOKINETICS

**Absorption:** 30–50% following subcut administration; IV administration results in complete bioavailability.

**Distribution:** Confined to the intravascular space
**Metabolism and Excretion:** Unknown.
**Half-life:** *subcut*—49 hr; *IV*—21 hr.

## CONTRAINDICATIONS AND PRECAUTIONS

**Contraindicated in:** ■ Hypersensitivity ■ Uncontrolled hypertension.

**Use Cautiously in:** ■ History of hypertension ■ Underlying hematologic diseases, including hemolytic anemia, sickle-cell anemia, thalassemia and porphyria (safety not established) ■ Pregnancy, lactation or children (safety not established).

## ADVERSE REACTIONS AND SIDE EFFECTS*

■ **CNS:** SEIZURES, dizziness, fatigue, headache, weakness ■ **Resp:** cough, dyspnea, bronchitis ■ **CV:** ARRHYTHMIAS, CHF, MI, STROKE, edema, hypertension, hypotension, chest pain, transient ischemic attack, thrombotic events ■ **GI:** abdominal pain, nausea, diarrhea, vomiting, constipation ■ **Derm:** pruritus ■ **Hemat:** pure red cell aplasia ■ **MS:** myalgia, arthralgia, back pain, limb pain ■ **Misc:** fever, allergic reactions, flu-like syndrome, sepsis.

## INTERACTIONS

**Drug-Drug:** ■ None reported.

## ROUTE AND DOSAGE

❑ **Anemia due to Chronic Renal Failure**

■ **IV, Subcut (Adults):** *Starting treatment with darbepoetin (no previous epoetin)*— 0.45 mcg/kg once weekly; adjust dose to attain target hemoglobin of 12 g/dl. Dosage adjustments should be made monthly in increments or decrements of 25% of current dose. Some patients may dosed every 2 weeks. *Conversion from epoetin to darbepoetin*—weekly epoetin dose <2500 units = 6.25 mcg/week darbepoetin, weekly epoetin dose 2500-4999 units = 12.5 mcg/week darbepoetin, weekly epoetin dose 5000-10,999 units = 25 mcg/week darbepoetin, weekly epoetin dose 11,000-17,999 units = 40 mcg/week darbepoetin, weekly epoetin dose 18,000-33,999 units = 60 mcg/week darbe-

poetin, weekly epoetin dose 34,000-89,999 units = 100 mcg/week darbepoetin, weekly epoetin dose >90,000 units = 200 mcg/week darbepoetin.

❑ **Anemia due to Chemotherapy**

■ **Subcut (Adults):** 2.25 mcg/kg initially. Adjust dose to attain target hemoglobin. If hemoglobin increases by <1.0 g/dL after 6 weeks of therapy, dose should be increased up to 4.5 mcg/kg. If hemoglobin increases by >1.0 g/dL in 2-weeks or if the hemoglobin >12 g/dL, decrease dose by approximately 25%. If the hemoglobin >13 g/dL, temporarily withhold until hemoglobin falls to 12 g/dL. Restart at a dose approximately 25% < the previous dose.

## AVAILABILITY

■ *Albumin solution for injection:* 25 mcg/ml 1-ml vial[Rx], 40 mcg/ml 1-ml vial[Rx], 60 mcg/ml 1-ml vial[Rx], 100 mcg/ml 1-ml vial[Rx], 150 mcg/ml 0.75-ml vial[Rx], 200 mcg/ml 1-ml vial[Rx], 300 mcg/ml 1-ml vial[Rx], 500 mcg/ml 1-ml vial[Rx] ■ Cost: 25 mcg $124.69/vial, 40 mcg $199.50/vial, 60 mcg $299.25/vial, 100 mcg $498.75/vial, 150 mcg $748.13/vial, 200 mcg $997.50/vial ■ *Pre-filled syringes:* 60 mcg/0.5 ml[Rx], 100 mcg/0.5 ml[Rx], 200 mcg/0.5 ml[Rx].

TIME/ACTION PROFILE (increase in RBCs)

| | ONSET | PEAK | DURATION |
|---|---|---|---|
| IV, subcut | 2–6 wks | unknown | unknown |

# NURSING IMPLICATIONS

## ASSESSMENT

❑ Monitor blood pressure before and during therapy. Inform physician or other health care professional if severe hypertension is present or if blood pressure begins to increase. Additional antihypertensive therapy may be required during initiation of therapy.
❑ Monitor response for symptoms of anemia (fatigue, dyspnea, pallor).
❑ Monitor dialysis shunts (thrill and bruit) and status of artificial kidney during hemodialysis. Heparin dose may need to be increased to prevent clotting. Patients with underlying

vascular disease should be monitored for impaired circulation.

- Monitor for allergic reactions (rash, utricaria). Discontinue darbepoetin if signs of anaphylaxis (dyspnea, laryngeal swelling) occur.
- **Lab Test Considerations:** May cause ↑ in WBCs and platelets. May ↓ bleeding times.
- Monitorserum ferritin, transferrin, and iron levels prior to and during therapy to assess need for concurrent iron therapy. Transferrin saturation should be at least 20% and ferritin should be at least 100 ng/ml.
- Monitor hemoglobin before and weekly during initial therapy, for 4 wk after a change in dose, and regularly after target range has been reached and maintenance dose is determined. Monitor other hematopoietic parameters (CBC with differential and platelet count) before and periodically duringtherapy. Hemoglobin increases of more than 1.0 g/dl in any 2-week period, increase the likelihood of cardiac arrest, neurologic events (seizures, stroke), hypertensive reactions, CHF, vascular thrombosis/ischemia/infarction, acute MI, and fluid overload/edema. Decrease dose by 25% and monitor hemoglobin weekly for 4 wk. If hemoglobin continues to increase, temporarily withhold until hemoglobin begins to decrease; then reinitiate at a dose 25% lower than previous dose.
- If increase in hemoglobin is less than 1 g/dl over 4 wks and iron stores are adequate, dose may be increased by 25% of previous dose.
- Monitor renal function studies and electrolytes closely; resulting increased sense of well-being may lead to decreased compliance with other therapies for renal failure.

## POTENTIAL NURSING DIAGNOSES

- Activity intolerance (Indications).

## IMPLEMENTATION

- **General:** Transfusions are still required for severe symptomatic anemia. Supplemental iron should be initiated with darbepoetin and continued during therapy. Correct deficiencies of folic acid or vitamin $B_{12}$ prior to therapy.
- Institute seizure precautions in patients who experience greater than a 1.0 g/dl increase in hemoglobin in a 2-wk period or exhibit any change in neurologic status.

- For conversion from epoetin alfa to darbepoetin, if epoetin was administered 2-3 times/wk administer darbepoetin once a week. If patient was receiving epoetin once/ wk, darbepoetin may be administered once every 2 wks. Route of administration should remain consistent.
- Dose adjustments should not be more frequent than once/month.
- Do not shake vial; inactivation of medication may occur. Do not administer vials containing solution that is discolored or contains particulate matter. Discard vial immediately after withdrawing dose. Do not pool unused portions.
- **Subcut:** This route is often used for patients not requiring dialysis.
- **Direct IV:** Administer undiluted.
- *Rate:* May be administered as direct injection or bolus into IV tubing or via venous line at end of dialysis session.
- **Y-Site Incompatibility:** Do not administer in conjunction with other drugs or solutions.

## PATIENT/FAMILY TEACHING

- **General Info:** Explain rationale for concurrent iron therapy (increased red blood cell production requires iron).
- Discuss possible return of menses and fertility in women of childbearing age. Patient should discuss contraceptive options with health care professional.
- Discuss ways of preventing self-injury in patients at risk for seizures. Driving and activities requiring continuous alertness should be avoided.
- Stress importance of compliance with dietary restrictions, medications, and dialysis. Foods high in iron and low in potassium include liver, pork, veal, beef, mustard and turnip greens, peas, eggs, broccoli, kale, blackberries, strawberries, apple juice, watermelon, oatmeal, and enriched bread. Darbepoetin will result in increased sense of well-being, but it does not cure underlying disease.
- **Home Care Issues:** Home dialysis patients determined to be able to safely and effectively administer darbepoetin should be taught proper dosage, administration technique, and disposal of equipment. *Information for Patients and Caregivers* should be provided to patient along with medication.

## EVALUATION

**Clinical response to therapy can be evaluated by:** ■ Increase in hemoglobin not to exceed 12 g/dl with improvement in symptoms of anemia in patients with chronic renal failure.

---

High Alert

# daunorubicin citrate liposome

(daw-noe-**roo**-bi-sin**sy**-trate**lye**-poe-sohm)

DaunoXome

*CLASSIFICATION(S):*
*Therapeutic: antineoplastics*
*Pharmacologic: anthracyclines*

**Pregnancy Category D**

---

## INDICATIONS

■ Management of advanced Kaposi's sarcoma in HIV-infected patients.

## ACTION

■ Forms a complex with DNA, which subsequently inhibits DNA and RNA synthesis (cell-cycle phase–nonspecific) ■ Encapsulation in a liposome increases uptake by tumor and decreases systemic toxicity. **Therapeutic Effects:** ■ Death of rapidly replicating cells, particularly malignant ones. Also has immunosuppressive properties.

## PHARMACOKINETICS

**Absorption:** Administered IV only, resulting in complete bioavailability. DaunoXome is released from the liposome after uptake by tumor.

**Distribution:** Widely distributed. Crosses the placenta.

**Metabolism and Excretion:** Extensively metabolized by the liver. Converted partially to a compound that also has antineoplastic activity (daunorubicinol); 40% eliminated by biliary excretion.

**Half-life:** *Daunorubicin citrate liposome*—55.4 hr. *Daunorubicinol*—26.7 hr.

## CONTRAINDICATIONS AND PRECAUTIONS

**Contraindicated in:** ■ Hypersensitivity to daunorubicin or any other components in the formulation ■ Pregnant or lactating women.

**Use Cautiously in:** ■ Active infections or decreased bone marrow reserve ■ Geriatric patients or patients with other chronic debilitating illnesses ■ May reactivate skin lesions produced by previous radiation therapy ■ Hepatic or renal impairment (dosage reduction recommended if serum creatinine >3 mg/dl or serum bilirubin >1.2 mg/dl) ■ Patients who have received previous anthracycline therapy or who have underlying cardiovascular disease (increased risk of cardiotoxicity) ■ Patients with childbearing potential ■ Children (safety not established for DaunoXome).

## ADVERSE REACTIONS AND SIDE EFFECTS*

■ **CNS:** fatigue, headache, depression, dizziness, insomnia, malaise ■ **EENT:** rhinitis, abnormal vision, sinusitis ■ **CV:** CARDIOTOXICITY, chest pain, edema ■ **GI:** abdominal pain, anorexia, constipation, diarrhea, nausea, stomatitis, tenesmus, vomiting ■ **GU:** red urine, gonadal suppression ■ **Derm:** alopecia, increased sweating, pruritus ■ **Hemat:** anemia, leukopenia, thrombocytopenia ■ **Local:** phlebitis at IV site ■ **Metab:** hyperuricemia ■ **MS:** back pain, arthralgia, myalgia ■ **Neuro:** neuropathy ■ **Misc:** *DaunoXome*—allergic reactions, chills, fever, back pain, flushing, chest tightness, influenza-like symptoms.

## INTERACTIONS

**Drug-Drug:** ■ Additive myelosuppression with other **antineoplastics** ■ May decrease antibody response to **live-virus vaccines** and increase risk of adverse reactions ■ **Cyclophosphamide** increases the risk of cardiotoxicity.

## ROUTE AND DOSAGE

Other dose regimens are used. In adults, cumulative dose should not exceed 550 mg/m² (450 mg/m² if previous chest radiation).

■ **IV (Adults):** 40 mg/m² q 2 wk.

▫ **Renal Impairment**
■ **IV (Adults):** *Serum creatinine >3 mg/dl*—reduce dose by 50%.

---

❏ **Hepatic Impairment**

■ **IV (Adults):** *Serum bilirubin 1.2–3 mg/ dl*—reduce dose by 25%; *serum bilirubin >3 mg/dl*—reduce dose by 50%.

**AVAILABILITY (generic available)**

■ *Liposomal dispersion for injection:* 2 mg/ml in 25-ml vial$^{Rx}$.

TIME/ACTION PROFILE (effects on blood counts)

| | ONSET | PEAK | DURATION |
|---|---|---|---|
| IV | unknown | unknown | unknown |

## NURSING IMPLICATIONS

### ASSESSMENT

❏ Monitor vital signs before and frequently during therapy.

❏ Assess patient for back pain, flushing, and chest tightness. Usually occurs during first 5 min of infusion and subsides with interruption of therapy. Symptoms do not usually recur when infusion is restarted at a slower rate.

❏ Monitor for bone marrow depression. Assess for bleeding (bleeding gums; bruising; petechiae; guaiac stools, urine, and emesis) and avoid IM injections and taking rectal temperatures if platelet count is low. Apply pressure to venipuncture sites for 10 min. Assess for signs of infection during neutropenia. Anemia may occur. Monitor for increased fatigue, dyspnea, and orthostatic hypotension.

❏ Assess IV site frequently for inflammation or infiltration. Instruct patient to notify nurse immediately if pain or irritation at injection site occurs. If extravasation occurs, infusion must be stopped and restarted in another vein to avoid damage to subcut tissue. Notify physician immediately.

❏ Monitor intake and output, appetite, and nutritional intake. Assess for nausea and vomiting, which, although mild, may persist for 24–48 hr. Administration of an antiemetic before and periodically during therapy and adjusting diet as tolerated may help maintain fluid and electrolyte balance and nutritional status. Encourage fluid intake of 2000–3000 ml/day. Allopurinol and alkalinization of the urine may be used to help prevent urate stone formation.

❏ Assess patient for evidence of cardiotoxicity, which manifests as CHF (peripheral edema, dyspnea, rales/crackles, weight gain, jugular venous distention) and usually occurs 1–6 mo after initiation of therapy. Chest x-ray, echocardiography, ECGs, and radionuclide angiography determination of ejection fraction may be ordered before and periodically throughout therapy. A 30% decrease in QRS voltage and decrease in systolic ejection fraction are early signs of cardiotoxicity. Patients who receive total cumulative doses >550/ mm$^2$, who have a history of cardiac disease, or who have received mediastinal radiation are at greater risk of developing cardiotoxicity. May be irreversible and fatal, but usually responds to early treatment.

■ *Lab Test Considerations:* Monitor uric acid levels.

❏ Monitor CBC and differential before each course of therapy. May cause severe bone marrow depression, especially granulocytopenia. Repeat blood counts before each dose and do not administer if absolute granulocyte count is <750 cells/mm$^3$.

❏ Monitor hepatic and renal function before each dose.

### POTENTIAL NURSING DIAGNOSES

■ Infection, risk for (Adverse Reactions).

■ Cardiac output, decreased (Side Effects).

### IMPLEMENTATION

❏ *High Alert:* Fatalities have occurred with chemotherapeutic agents. Before administering, clarify all ambiguous orders; double check single, daily, and course-of-therapy dose limits; have second practitioner independently double check original order, calculations and infusion pump settings. Do not confuse daunorubicin citrate liposome (DaunoXome) with daunorubicin hydrochloride (Cerubidine) or with doxorubicin (Adriamycin, Rubex) or doxorubicin hydorchloride liposome (Doxil). To prevent confusion, orders should include generic and brand name.

■ **General:** Solution should be prepared in a biologic cabinet. Wear gloves, gown, and mask while handling IV medication. Discard IV equipment in specially designated containers.

■ **Intermittent Infusion:** Dilute with D5W for a concentration of 1 mg/ml. Do not use an in-line filter for infusion. Reconstituted infusion may be stored for up to 6 hr in refrigerator.

■ *Rate:* Administer dose over 1 hr.

■ **Additive Incompatibility:** Information unavailable. Do not admix with other solutions or medications.

## PATIENT/FAMILY TEACHING

❏ Instruct patient to notify health care professional if fever; chills; sore throat; signs of infection; bleeding gums; bruising; petechiae; or blood in urine, stool, or emesis occurs. Caution patient to avoid crowds and persons with known infections. Instruct patient to use soft toothbrush and electric razor. Patient should be cautioned not to drink alcoholic beverages or take products containing aspirin or NSAIDs.

❏ Instruct patient to inspect oral mucosa for erythema and ulceration. If ulceration occurs, advise patient to use sponge brush and rinse mouth with water after eating and drinking. Stomatitis pain may require management with opioid analgesics. Period of highest risk is 3–7 days after administration of dose.

❏ Instruct patient to notify health care professional immediately if irregular heartbeat, shortness of breath, or swelling of lower extremities occurs.

❏ Discuss with patient possibility of hair loss. Explore methods of coping. Regrowth of hair usually begins within 5 wk after discontinuing therapy.

❏ Inform patient that medication may turn urine reddish color for 1–2 days after administration.

❏ Inform patient that this medication may cause irreversible gonadal suppression. Advise patient that this medication may have teratogenic effects. Contraception should be used during therapy and for at least 4 mo after therapy is concluded.

❏ Instruct patient not to receive any vaccinations without advice of health care professional.

❏ Emphasize the need for periodic lab tests to monitor for side effects.

## EVALUATION

**Effectiveness of therapy can be demonstrated by:** ■ Arrested progression of Kaposi's sarcoma in patients with HIV infection. Therapy is continued until there is evidence of progression (new visceral sites of involvement, progression of visceral disease, development of 10 or more new cutaneous lesions or 25% increase in the number of lesions at baseline, change in character of >25% of lesions from flat to raised, increase in surface area of lesions) or until complications of HIV disease preclude continuation of therapy.

**High Alert**

# daunorubicin hydrochloride
(daw-noe-**roo**-bi-sinhye-dro-**klor**-ide)
Cerubidine

*CLASSIFICATION(S):*
*Therapeutic: antineoplastics*
*Pharmacologic: anthracyclines*

**Pregnancy Category D**

## INDICATIONS

■ In combination with other antineoplastics in the treatment of leukemias.

## ACTION

■ Forms a complex with DNA, which subsequently inhibits DNA and RNA synthesis (cell-cycle phase-nonspecific). **Therapeutic Effects:** ■ Death of rapidly replicating cells, particularly malignant ones. Also has immunosuppressive properties.

## PHARMACOKINETICS

**Absorption:** Administered IV only, resulting in complete bioavailability.

**Distribution:** Widely distributed. Crosses the placenta.

**Metabolism and Excretion:** Extensively metabolized by the liver. Converted partially to a compound that also has antineoplastic activity (daunorubicinol); 40% eliminated by biliary excretion.

**Half-life:** *Daunorubicin*—18.5 hr. *Daunorubicinol*—26.7 hr.

## CONTRAINDICATIONS AND PRECAUTIONS

**Contraindicated in:** ■ Hypersensitivity to daunorubicin or any other components in the formulation ■ Symptomatic CHF/arrhythmias ■ Pregnant or lactating women.

**Use Cautiously in:** ■ Active infections or decreased bone marrow reserve ■ Geriatric patients or patients with other chronic debilitating illnesses (dosage reduction recommended for patients ≥60 yr) ■ May reactivate skin lesions produced by previous radiation therapy ■ Hepatic or renal impairment (dosage reduction recommended if serum creatinine >3 mg/dl or serum bilirubin >1.2 mg/dl) ■ Patients who have received previous anthracycline therapy or who have underlying cardiovascular disease (increased risk of cardiotoxicity) ■ Patients with childbearing potential.

## ADVERSE REACTIONS AND SIDE EFFECTS*

■ **EENT:** rhinitis, abnormal vision, sinusitis ■ **CV:** CARDIOTOXICITY, arrhythmias ■ **GI:** nausea, vomiting, esophagitis, hepatotoxicity, stomatitis ■ **GU:** red urine, gonadal suppression ■ **Derm:** alopecia ■ **Hemat:** anemia, leukopenia, thrombocytopenia ■ **Local:** phlebitis at IV site ■ **Metab:** hyperuricemia ■ **Misc:** chills, fever.

## INTERACTIONS

**Drug-Drug:** ■ Additive myelosuppression with other **antineoplastics** ■ May decrease antibody response to **live-virus vaccines** and increase risk of adverse reactions ■ **Cyclophosphamide** increases the risk of cardiotoxicity ■ Increased risk of hepatic toxicity with other **hepatotoxic agents**.

## ROUTE AND DOSAGE

Other dose regimens are used. In adults, cumulative dose should not exceed 550 mg/m² (450 mg/m² if previous chest radiation).

■ **IV (Adults <60 yr):** 45 mg/m²/day for 3 days in first course, then for 2 days of second course (as part of combination regimen).

■ **IV (Adults ≥60 yr):** 30 mg/m²/day for 3 days in first course, then for 2 days of sec-

ond course (as part of combination regimen).

■ **IV (Children >2 yr):** 25 mg/m² once weekly (as part of combination regimen). In children <2 yr or BSA <0.5 m², dosage should be determined on a mg/kg basis.

## AVAILABILITY (generic available)

■ *Powder for injection:* 20 mg/vial$^{Rx}$ ■ *Solution for injection:* 5 mg/ml in 4-ml vials (20 mg)$^{Rx}$.

TIME/ACTION PROFILE (effects on blood counts)

| | ONSET | PEAK | DURATION |
|---|---|---|---|
| IV | 7–10 days | 10–14 days | 21 days |

# NURSING IMPLICATIONS

## ASSESSMENT

❑ Monitor vital signs before and frequently during therapy.

❑ Monitor for bone marrow depression. Assess for bleeding (bleeding gums; bruising; petechiae; guaiac stools, urine, and emesis) and avoid IM injections and taking rectal temperatures if platelet count is low. Apply pressure to venipuncture sites for 10 min. Assess for signs of infection during neutropenia. Anemia may occur. Monitor for increased fatigue, dyspnea, and orthostatic hypotension.

❑ Assess IV site frequently for inflammation or infiltration. Instruct patient to notify nurse immediately if pain or irritation at injection site occurs. If extravasation occurs, infusion must be stopped and restarted in another vein to avoid damage to subcut tissue. Notify physician immediately. Daunorubicin is a vesicant. Standard treatments include local injections of steroids and application of ice compresses.

❑ Monitor intake and output, appetite, and nutritional intake. Assess for nausea and vomiting, which, although mild, may persist for 24–48 hr. Administration of an antiemetic before and periodically during therapy and adjusting diet as tolerated may help maintain fluid and electrolyte balance and nutritional status. Encourage fluid intake of 2000–3000 ml/day. Allopurinol and alkalinization of the urine may be used to help prevent urate stone formation.

◻ Assess patient for evidence of cardiotoxicity, which manifests as CHF (peripheral edema, dyspnea, rales/crackles, weight gain, jugular venous distention) and usually occurs 1–6 mo after initiation of therapy. Chest x-ray, echocardiography, ECGs, and radionuclide angiography determination of ejection fraction may be ordered before and periodically throughout therapy. A 30% decrease in QRS voltage and decrease in systolic ejection fraction are early signs of cardiotoxicity. Patients who receive total cumulative doses >550/mm², who have a history of cardiac disease, or who have received mediastinal radiation are at greater risk of developing cardiotoxicity. May be irreversible and fatal, but usually responds to early treatment.

■ *Lab Test Considerations:* Monitor uric acid levels.

◻ *Daunorubicin hydrochloride:* Monitor CBC and differential before and periodically throughout therapy. The leukocyte count nadir occurs 10–14 days after administration. Recovery usually occurs within 21 days after administration of daunorubicin.

◻ Monitor AST, ALT, LDH, and serum bilirubin. May cause transiently elevated serum alkaline phosphatase, bilirubin, and AST concentrations.

## POTENTIAL NURSING DIAGNOSES

■ Infection, risk for (Adverse Reactions).
■ Cardiac output, decreased (Side Effects).

## IMPLEMENTATION

◻ *High Alert:* Fatalities have occurred with chemotherapeutic agents. Before administering, clarify all ambiguous orders; double check single, daily, and course-of-therapy dose limits; have second practitioner independently double check original order, calculations and infusion pump settings. Do not confuse daunorubicin hydrochloride (Cerubidine) with daunorubicin citrate liposome (DaunoXome) or with doxorubicin (Adriamycin, Rubex) or doxorubicin hydrochloride liposome (Doxil). To prevent confusion, orders should include generic and brand name.

■ **General:** Solution should be prepared in a biologic cabinet. Wear gloves, gown, and mask while handling IV medication. Discard IV equipment in specially designated containers.

■ **IV:** Reconstitute each 20 mg with 4 ml of sterile water for injection for a concentration of 5 mg/ml. Shake gently to dissolve. Reconstituted medication is stable for 24 hr at room temperature, 48 hr if refrigerated. Protect from sunlight.

◻ Do not use aluminum needles when reconstituting or injecting daunorubicin, as aluminum darkens the solution.

■ **Direct IV:** Dilute further in 10–15 ml of 0.9% NaCl. Administer direct IV push through Y-site into free-flowing infusion of 0.9% NaCl or D5W.

■ *Rate:* Administer over at least 2–3 min. Rapid administration rate may cause facial flushing or erythema along the vein.

■ **Intermittent Infusion:** Has also been diluted in 50 or 100 ml of 0.9% NaCl.

■ *Rate:* Administer 50 ml over 10–15 min or 100 ml over 30–45 min.

■ **Y-Site Compatibility:** ♦ amifostine ♦ etoposide ♦ filgrastim ♦ gemcitabine ♦ granisetron ♦ melphalan ♦ methotrexate ♦ ondansetron ♦ sodium bicarbonate ♦ teniposide ♦ thiotepa ♦ vinorelbine.

■ **Y-Site Incompatibility:** ♦ allopurinol ♦ aztreonam ♦ cefepime ♦ fludarabine ♦ piperacillin/tazobactam.

■ **Additive Incompatibility:** Manufacturer does not recommend admixing daunorubicin hydrochloride.

## PATIENT/FAMILY TEACHING

◻ Instruct patient to notify health care professional if fever; chills; sore throat; signs of infection; bleeding gums; bruising; petechiae; or blood in urine, stool, or emesis occurs. Caution patient to avoid crowds and persons with known infections. Instruct patient to use soft toothbrush and electric razor. Patient should be cautioned not to drink alcoholic beverages or take products containing aspirin or NSAIDs.

◻ Instruct patient to inspect oral mucosa for erythema and ulceration. If ulceration occurs, advise patient to use sponge brush and rinse mouth with water after eating and drinking. Stomatitis pain may require management with opioid analgesics. Period of highest risk is 3–7 days after administration of dose.

□ Instruct patient to notify health care professional immediately if irregular heartbeat, shortness of breath, or swelling of lower extremities occurs.

□ Discuss with patient possibility of hair loss. Explore methods of coping. Regrowth of hair usually begins within 5 wk after discontinuing therapy.

□ Inform patient that medication may turn urine reddish color for 1–2 days after administration.

□ Inform patient that this medication may cause irreversible gonadal suppression. Advise patient that this medication may have teratogenic effects. Contraception should be used during therapy and for at least 4 mo after therapy is concluded.

□ Instruct patient not to receive any vaccinations without advice of health care professional.

□ Emphasize the need for periodic lab tests to monitor for side effects.

## EVALUATION

**Effectiveness of therapy can be demonstrated by:** ■ Improvement of hematologic status in patients with leukemia.

## delavirdine

(de-**la**-veer-deen)
Rescriptor

### CLASSIFICATION(S):
**Therapeutic:** antiretrovirals
**Pharmacologic:** non-nucleoside reverse transcriptase inhibitors

### Pregnancy Category C

## INDICATIONS

■ Treatment of HIV infection in combination with other antiretrovirals.

## ACTION

■ Binds to reverse transcriptase, inhibiting viral DNA synthesis. **Therapeutic Effects:** ■ Decreased viral load and increased CD4 cell count

■ Slowed progression of HIV infection and decreased severity of its sequelae.

## PHARMACOKINETICS

**Absorption:** 85% absorbed after oral administration, increased when tablet is dispersed in water.
**Distribution:** Unknown.
**Protein Binding:** 98%.
**Metabolism and Excretion:** Extensively metabolized by the liver; <5% excreted unchanged in urine.
**Half-life:** 5.8 hr.

## CONTRAINDICATIONS AND PRECAUTIONS

**Contraindicated in:** ■ Hypersensitivity ■ Concurrent use of astemizole, benzodiazepines and antiarrhythmics, dihydropyridine, calcium channel blockers (nifedipine), ergot alkaloids, amphetamines, and sildenafil (may result in excessive sedation, vasoconstriction, or arrhythmias).
**Use Cautiously in:** ■ Impaired hepatic function ■ Achlorhydria (requires acidic environment for absorption) ■ Pregnancy, lactation, or children (safety not established; HIV-infected patients should not breastfeed).

## ADVERSE REACTIONS AND SIDE EFFECTS*

■ **CNS:** fatigue, headache ■ **GI:** diarrhea, increased amylase, increased liver enzymes, nausea, vomiting ■ **Derm:** rash, pruritus ■ **Misc:** fat redistribution.

## INTERACTIONS

**Drug-Drug:** ■ Delavirdine inhibits the hepatic drug-metabolizing enzyme CYP P3A4 and ↑ blood levels of **sedative/hypnotics antiarrhythmics** , **calcium channel blockers** , **ergot alkaloids** , **sildenafil** , and **pimozide** ; this may result in potentially life-threatening adverse reactions (avoid concurrent use) ■ Concurrent administration of **clarithromycin** significantly ↑ levels of both agents ■ Concurrent administration with **didanosine** ↓ levels of both agents (separate doses by 1 hr) ■ **Fluoxetine** and **ketoconazole** ↑ delavirdine levels ■ **Antacids** ↓ absorption (do not use within 1 hr of each other) ■ **Histamine blockers** ↓ absorption (avoid chronic use) ■ Levels are ↓ by **rifabutin, rifampin, phenytoin, phenobarbital,** and **carbamazepine** (avoid concurrent use) ■ ↑ levels of **amprenavir, indinavir,** and **saquinavir** (dosage reductions may be necessary) ■ Concurrent use with **saquinavir** may ↑ risk of liver dysfunction. **Drug-Natural Products:** ■ Use with **St. John's wort** may ↓ levels and effectiveness, including development of drug resistance.

## ROUTE AND DOSAGE

■ **PO (Adults):** 400 mg 3 times daily.

## AVAILABILITY

■ *Tablets:* 100 mg$^{Rx}$, 200 mg$^{Rx}$.

TIME/ACTION PROFILE (blood levels)

|    | ONSET | PEAK | DURATION |
|----|-------|------|----------|
| PO | rapid | 1 hr | 8 hr |

## NURSING IMPLICATIONS

### ASSESSMENT

❑ Assess patient for change in severity of HIV symptoms and for symptoms of opportunistic infections throughout therapy.

■ *Lab Test Considerations:* Monitor viral load and CD4 cell counts regularly during therapy.

❑ May cause ↑ serum AST and ALT concentrations.

❑ May cause ↓ in neutrophil counts.

### POTENTIAL NURSING DIAGNOSES

■ Infection, risk for (Indications).

■ Noncompliance (Patient/Family Teaching).

### IMPLEMENTATION

■ **PO:** Administer without regard to food. Tablets should be taken whole or dispersed in water. To prepare dispersion, add 4 tablets to at least 3 oz water and allow to stand for a few minutes. Stir mixture until a uniform dispersion occurs. Dispersion should be consumed promptly, followed by rinsing the glass and swallowing rinse to consume entire dose.

❑ Do not administer within 1 hr of antacids or didanosine.

❑ Patients with achlorhydria should take delavirdine with an acidic beverage such as orange juice or cranberry juice.

### PATIENT/FAMILY TEACHING

❑ Emphasize the importance of taking delavirdine exactly as directed, at evenly spaced times throughout day. Do not take more than prescribed amount and do not stop taking without consulting health care professional. Take missed doses as soon as remembered; do not double doses.

❑ Instruct patient that delavirdine should not be shared with others.

❑ Advise patient to avoid taking other medications, prescription or OTC, without consulting health care professional.

❑ Inform patient that delavirdine does not cure AIDS or prevent associated or opportunistic infections. Delavirdine does not reduce the risk of transmission of HIV to others through sexual contact or blood contamination. Caution patient to use a condom and avoid sharing needles or donating blood to prevent spreading the AIDS virus to others. Advise patient that the long-term effects of delavirdine are unknown at this time.

❑ Emphasize the importance of regular follow-up exams and blood counts to determine progress and monitor for side effects.

### EVALUATION

**Effectiveness of therapy can be demonstrated by:** ■ Delayed progression of AIDS and decreased opportunistic infections in patients with HIV ■ Improved CD4 cell count and decrease in viral load.

## desipramine

(dess-**ip**-ra-meen)

Norpramin, {Pertofrane}

*CLASSIFICATION(S):*

*Therapeutic:* antidepressants

*Pharmacologic:* tricyclic antidepressants

**Pregnancy Category C**

## INDICATIONS

■ Treatment of depression, often in conjunction with psychotherapy. **Unlabeled uses:** ■ Chronic pain syndromes.

## ACTION

■ Potentiates the effect of serotonin and norepinephrine in the CNS ■ Has significant anticholinergic properties. **Therapeutic Effects:** ■ Antidepressant action (may develop only over several weeks).

## PHARMACOKINETICS

**Absorption:** Well absorbed from the GI tract.
**Distribution:** Widely distributed.
**Protein Binding:** 90–92%.
**Metabolism and Excretion:** Extensively metabolized by the liver. One metabolite is pharmacologically active (2-hydroxydesipramine). Undergoes enterohepatic recirculation and secretion into gastric juices. Small amounts enter breast milk.
**Half-life:** 12–27 hr.

## CONTRAINDICATIONS AND PRECAUTIONS

**Contraindicated in:** ■ Narrow-angle glaucoma ■ Pregnancy and lactation.
**Use Cautiously in:** ■ Geriatric patients ■ Patients with pre-existing cardiovascular disease ■ Prostatic hypertrophy (increased susceptibility to urinary retention) ■ History of seizures (threshold may be lowered).

## ADVERSE REACTIONS AND SIDE EFFECTS*

■ **CNS:** drowsiness, fatigue ■ **EENT:** blurred vision, dry eyes, dry mouth ■ **CV:** ARRHYTHMIAS, hypotension, ECG changes ■ **GI:** constipation, drug-induced hepatitis, paralytic ileus ■ **GU:** urinary retention ■ **Derm:** photosensitivity ■ **Endo:** changes in blood glucose, gynecomastia ■ **Hemat:** blood dyscrasias ■ **Misc:** increased appetite, weight gain.

## INTERACTIONS

**Drug-Drug:** ■ Desipramine is metabolized in the liver by the cytochrome P450 2D6 enzyme and its action may be affected by drugs which compete for metabolism by or alter the activity of this enzyme including **other antidepressants, phenothiazines, carbamazepine, class 1C antiarrhythmics (propafenone, flecainide, encainide)**; when used concurrently dosage reduction of one or the other or both may be necessary. Concurrent use of other drugs that inhibit the activity of the enzyme, including **cimetidine, quinidine, amiodarone,** and **ritonavir** may result in increased

effects ■ May cause hypotension, tachycardia, and potentially fatal reactions when used with **MAO inhibitors** (avoid concurrent use—discontinue 2 wk prior to) ■ Concurrent use with **SSRI antidepressants** may result in increased toxicity and should be avoided (fluoexetine should be stopped 5 wk before) ■ May prevent the therapeutic response to **guanethidine** ■ Concurrent use with **clonidine** may result in hypertensive crisis and should be avoided ■ **Phenytoin** may decrease levels and effectiveness; larger doses of desipramine may be required to treat depression ■ Concurrent use with **levodopa** may result in delayed/decreased absorption of levodopa or hypertension ■ Blood levels and effects may be decreased by **rifamycins, carbamazepine,** and **barbiturates** ■ Concurrent use with **moxifloxacin** or **sparfloxacin** increases the risk of adverse cardiovascular reactions ■ Additive CNS depression with other **CNS depressants** including **alcohol, antihistamines, clonidine, opioid analgesics,** and **sedative/hypnotics** ■ **Barbiturates** may alter blood levels and effects ■ **Adrenergic** and **anticholinergic** side effects may be additive with other **agents having these properties** ■ **Hormonal contraceptives** increase levels and may cause toxicity ■ **Cigarette smoking** may increase metabolism and alter effects.

**Drug-Natural Products:** ■ Concomitant use of **kava, valerian, skullcap, chamomile,** or **hops** can increase CNS depression ■ Increased anticholinergic effects with **angel's trumpet, jimson weed,** and **scopolia.**

## ROUTE AND DOSAGE

■ **PO (Adults):** 100–200 mg/day as a single dose or in divided doses (up to 300 mg/day).

■ **PO (Geriatric Patients):** 25–50 mg/day in divided doses (up to 150 mg/day).

■ **PO (Children >12 yr):** 25–50 mg/day in divided doses, increased as needed up to 100 mg/day.

■ **PO (Children 6–12 yr):** 10–30 mg/day (1–5 mg/kg/day) in divided doses.

## AVAILABILITY (generic available)

■ *Tablets:* 10 mg$^{Rx}$, 25 mg$^{Rx}$, 50 mg$^{Rx}$, 75 mg$^{Rx}$, 100 mg$^{Rx}$, 150 mg$^{Rx}$.

TIME/ACTION PROFILE (antidepressant effect)

| | ONSET | PEAK | DURATION |
|---|---|---|---|
| PO | 2–3 wk | 2–6 wk | days–wks |

# NURSING IMPLICATIONS

## ASSESSMENT

❑ Monitor mental status and affect. Assess for suicidal tendencies, especially during early therapy. Restrict amount of drug available to patient.

❑ Monitor blood pressure and pulse prior to and during initial therapy. Notify physician or other health care professional of decreases in blood pressure (10–20 mm Hg) or sudden increase in pulse rate. Patients taking high doses or with a history of cardiovascular disease should have ECG monitored prior to and periodically throughout therapy.

■ *Lab Test Considerations:* Assess leukocyte and differential blood counts, liver function, and serum glucose periodically. May cause an elevated serum bilirubin and alkaline phosphatase. May cause bone marrow depression. Serum glucose may be increased or decreased.

## POTENTIAL NURSING DIAGNOSES

■ Coping, ineffective (Indications).
■ Injury, risk for (Side Effects).

## IMPLEMENTATION

■ **General:** Do not confuse desipramine with clomipramine, imipramine, or nortriptyline.

❑ Dose increases should be made at bedtime because of sedation. Dose titration is a slow process; may take weeks to months. May give entire dose at bedtime.

■ **PO:** Administer medication with or immediately after a meal to minimize gastric upset. Tablet may be crushed and given with food or fluids.

## PATIENT/FAMILY TEACHING

❑ Instruct patient to take medication exactly as directed. If a dose is missed, take as soon as possible unless almost time for next dose; if regimen is a single dose at bedtime, do not take in the morning because of side effects. Advise patient that drug effects may not be noticed for at least 2 wk. Abrupt discontinuation may cause nausea; vomiting; diarrhea; headache; trouble sleeping, with vivid dreams; and irritability.

❑ May cause drowsiness and blurred vision. Caution patient to avoid driving and other activities requiring alertness until response to drug is known.

❑ Orthostatic hypotension, sedation, and confusion are common during early therapy, especially in the elderly. Protect patient from falls and advise patient to make position changes slowly.

❑ Advise patient to avoid alcohol or other CNS depressant drugs during and for 3–7 days after therapy has been discontinued.

❑ Instruct patient to notify health care professional if urinary retention occurs or if dry mouth or constipation persists. Sugarless candy or gum may diminish dry mouth, and an increase in fluids or bulk may prevent constipation. If symptoms persist, dose reduction or discontinuation may be necessary. Consult health care professional if dry mouth persists for more than 2 wk.

❑ Caution patient to use sunscreen and protective clothing to prevent photosensitivity reactions.

❑ Inform patient of need to monitor dietary intake. Increase in appetite may lead to undesired weight gain.

❑ Advise patient to notify health care professional of medication regimen prior to treatment or surgery.

❑ Therapy for depression is usually prolonged. Emphasize the importance of follow-up exams to monitor effectiveness and side effects.

## EVALUATION

**Effectiveness of therapy can be demonstrated by:** ■ Increased sense of well-being ❑ Renewed interest in surroundings ❑ Increased appetite ❑ Improved energy level ❑ Improved sleep ■ Decrease in chronic pain symptoms ■ Full therapeutic effects may be seen 2–6 wk after initiating therapy.

# desirudin

(des-i-**rude**-in)
Iprivask

**CLASSIFICATION(S):**
**Therapeutic:** anticoagulants
**Pharmacologic:** thrombin inhibitors

**Pregnancy Category C**

## INDICATIONS

■ Prevention of deep-vein thrombosis (DVT) after hip-replacement surgery.

## ACTION

■ Selectively inhibits free and clot-bound thrombin. Inhibition of thrombin prevents activation of factors V, VIII and XII; conversion of fibrinogen to fibrin; platelet adhesion and aggregation. **Therapeutic Effects:** ■ Decreased incidence of DVT and subsequent pulmonary embolism after hip-replacement surgery.

## PHARMACOKINETICS

**Absorption:** Completely absorbed following subcut administration.

**Distribution:** Binds specifically and directly to thrombin.

**Metabolism and Excretion:** 40–50% excreted unchanged by kidneys; some metabolism in kidneys and by pancreatic enzymes.

**Half-life:** 2 hr.

## CONTRAINDICATIONS AND PRECAUTIONS

**Contraindicated in:** ■ Hypersensitivity to natural or recombinant hirudins ■ Active bleeding ■ Coagulation disorders.

**Use Cautiously in:** ■ Renal impairment (dosage change recommended if CCr ≤60 ml/min) ■ Geriatric patients (due to age-related renal impairment) ■ Hepatic impairment ■ Pregnancy (use only if benefits to mother outweigh fetal risk) ■ Lactation, children (safety not established).

**Exercise Extreme Caution in:** ■ Spinal/epidural anesthesia (increased risk of spinal/epidural hematomas and their sequelae, especially when used with NSAIDs, platelet inhibitors or other anticoagulants).

## ADVERSE REACTIONS AND SIDE EFFECTS*

■ **GI:** nausea ■ **Hemat:** BLEEDING, anemia ■ **Local:** injection site reactions, wound secretion.

## INTERACTIONS

**Drug-Drug:** ■ **Dextran 40, systemic corticosteroids, thrombolytics,** and other **anticoagulants** ↑ risk of bleeding (discontinue if possible, if not monitor laboratory and clinical status closely) ■ Agents altering platelet function including **salicylates, NSAIDs, clopidogrel, ticlopidine, dipyridamole,** and **glycoprotein IIb/IIIa antagonists** also ↑ risk of bleeding.

## ROUTE AND DOSAGE

■ **Subcut (Adults):** 15 mg every 12 hr, start 5–15 min prior to surgery, but after regional block (if used), for up to 12 days.

❑ **Renal Impairment**
■ **Subcut (Adults):** *CCr 31–60 ml/min*—start with 5 mg every 12 hr; further doses determined by daily aPTT; *CCr <31 ml/min*—start with 1.7 mg every 12 hr; further doses determined by daily aPTT.

## AVAILABILITY

■ *Lyophilized powder for injection (requires reconstitution with specific diluent):* 15.75 mg/vial with 0.6 ml ampule of diluent (contains mannitol, delivers 15 mg dose).

TIME/ACTION PROFILE (effect on aPTT)

| | ONSET | PEAK | DURATION |
|---|---|---|---|
| Subcut | rapid | 1–3 hr | 12 hr |

# NURSING IMPLICATIONS

## ASSESSMENT

❑ Assess patient for signs of bleeding (bleeding gums, nosebleed, unusual bruising; black, tarry stools; hematuria; fall in hematocrit of blood pressure; guaiac-positive stools; bleeding from surgical site). Notify physician if these occur.

❑ Assess patient for evidence of thrombosis. Symptoms depend on area of involvement. Notify physician immediately; may require urgent treatment.

❑ Monitor patients with epidural catheters frequently for signs of neurological impairment (midline back pain, numbness or weakness in lower limbs, bowel and/or bladder dysfunction). Notify physician immediately if these occur.

❑ Observe injection sites for hematomas, ecchymosis, or inflammation.

■ *Lab Test Considerations:* Monitor activated partial thromboplastin time (aPTT) daily in patients with increased risk of bleeding and/or renal impairment. Monitor serum creatinine daily in patients with renal impairment. Peak aPTT should not exceed two times control. Reduce dose or discontinue desirudin until aPTT is <2 times control; resume at a lower dose.

❑ If a patient is switched from oral anticoagulants to desirudin or from desirudin to oral anticoagulants, measure anticoagulant activity closely.

❑ Thrombin time is not suitable for monitoring desirudin.

❑ Monitor CBC. If hematocrit ↓ unexpectedly, assess patient for potential bleeding sites.

## POTENTIAL NURSING DIAGNOSES

■ Tissue perfusion, ineffective (Indications).
■ Injury, risk for (Adverse Reactions).

## IMPLEMENTATION

■ **General:** Reconstitute each vial with 0.5 ml of diluent provided for a concentration of 15.75 mg of desirudin/0.5 ml. Shake vial gently until fully reconstituted to a clear colorless solution. Do not administer solutions that are discolored, cloudy, or contain a particulate matter. Reconstituted solution should be used immediately, but is stable for 24 hr at room temperature and protected from light. Discard unused solution.

■ **Subcut:** Withdraw all reconstituted solution into syringe with a 26 or 27-gauge, 1/2 inch length needle. Inject entire contents subcutaneously which will deliver 15 mg. Patient should be sitting or lying down during administration. Rotate sites between left and right anterolateral and left and right posterolateral thigh or abdominal wall. Inject entire length of needle while pinching skin between thumb and forefinger; continue to pinch skin throughout injection. Do not rub injection site following injection to prevent bruising.

■ **Syringe Incompatibility:** Do not mix with other diluents or medications.

## PATIENT/FAMILY TEACHING

❑ Advise patient to report symptoms of unusual bleeding or bruising to health care professional immediately.

❑ Instruct patient not to take aspirin, NSAIDs, or herbal products during therapy without consulting health care professional.

## EVALUATION

**Effectiveness of therapy can be demonstrated by:** ■ Decreased incidence of DVT and subsequent pulmonary embolism after hip-replacement surgery.

# desloratadine
(dess-lor-**a**-ta-deen)
Clarinex

## CLASSIFICATION(S):
*Therapeutic: allergy, cold, and cough remedies, antihistamines*

**Pregnancy Category C**

## INDICATIONS

■ Nasal and non-nasal symptoms of allergic rhinitis (seasonal and perennial) ■ Chronic idiopathic urticaria.

## ACTION

■ Blocks peripheral effects of histamine released during allergic reactions. **Therapeutic Effects:** ■ Decreased symptoms of allergic reactions (nasal stuffiness, red swollen eyes). Decreased pruritus, reduction in number and size of hives in chronic idiopathic urticaria.

## PHARMACOKINETICS

**Absorption:** Well absorbed; absorption for orally-disintegrating tablets and oral tablets is identical.

**Distribution:** Enters breast milk.

**Metabolism and Excretion:** Extensively metabolized to 3-hydroxydesloratadine, an active metabolite; small percentage of patients may be slow metabolizers.

**Half-life:** 27 hr.

## CONTRAINDICATIONS AND PRECAUTIONS

**Contraindicated in:** ■ Hypersensitivity ■ Lactation.

**Use Cautiously in:** ■ Patients with hepatic or renal impairment ( ↓ dose to 5 mg every other day) ■ Geriatric patients ( ↑ risk of adverse reactions) ■ Pregnancy or children <12 yr (safety not established).

## ADVERSE REACTIONS AND SIDE EFFECTS*

■ **CNS:** drowsiness (rare) ■ **EENT:** pharyngitis ■ **GI:** dry mouth ■ **Misc:** allergic reactions including ANAPHYLAXIS.

## INTERACTIONS

**Drug-Drug:** ■ The following interactions may occur, but are less likely to occur with desloratidine than with more sedating antihistamines ■ **MAO inhibitors** may intensify and prolong effects of antihistamines ■ ↑ CNS depression may occur with other **CNS depressants** including **alcohol, antidepressants, opioids,** and **sedative/hypnotics**.

## ROUTE AND DOSAGE

■ **PO (Adults and Children ≥12 yr):** 5 mg once daily.
❑ **Renal/Hepatic Impairment**
■ **PO (Adults and Children ≥12 yr):** 5 mg every other day.

## AVAILABILITY

■ ***Tablets:*** 5 mg<sup>Rx</sup> ■ ***Orally-disintegrating tablets (RediTabs):*** 5 mg<sup>Rx</sup>.

TIME/ACTION PROFILE (antihistaminic effects)

|     | ONSET | PEAK | DURATION |
| --- | --- | --- | --- |
| PO | unknown | 3 hr | 24 hr |

## NURSING IMPLICATIONS

### ASSESSMENT

❑ Assess allergy symptoms (rhinitis, conjunctivitis, hives) before and periodically during therapy.
❑ Assess lung sounds and character of bronchial secretions. Maintain fluid intake of 1500–2000 ml/day to decrease viscosity of secretions.
■ *Lab Test Considerations:* May cause false-negative result on allergy skin testing.

### POTENTIAL NURSING DIAGNOSES

■ Airway clearance, ineffective (Indications).
■ Injury, risk for (Adverse Reactions).

### IMPLEMENTATION

■ **PO:** May be administered without regard to meals. *For rapidly disintegrating tablets (Reditabs):* Place on tongue. Tablet disintegrates rapidly. May be taken with or without water. Administer immediately after opening the blister.

### PATIENT/FAMILY TEACHING

❑ Instruct patients to take desloratidine as directed. Do not increase dose or frequency; does not increase effectiveness and may increase side effects.
❑ May rarely cause drowsiness. Caution patient to avoid driving or other activities requiring alertness until response to medication is known.
❑ Advise patient to avoid taking alcohol or other CNS depressants concurrently with this drug.
❑ Advise patient that good oral hygiene, frequent rinsing of mouth with water, and sugarless gum or candy may minimize dry mouth. Patient should notify dentist if dry mouth persists >2 wk.

### EVALUATION

**Effectiveness of therapy can be demonstrated by:** ■ Decrease in allergic symptoms.

## desmopressin

(des-moe-**press**-in)
DDAVP, DDAVP Rhinal Tube, DDAVP Rhinyle Drops, Octostim, Stimate

### CLASSIFICATION(S):
***Therapeutic:*** hormones
***Pharmacologic:*** antidiuretic hormones

**Pregnancy Category B**

## INDICATIONS

■ **Intranasal:** Management of primary nocturnal enuresis unresponsive to other treatment modalities ■ **PO, Subcut, IV, Intranasal:** Treatment of diabetes insipidus caused by a deficiency of vasopressin ■ **Intranasal:** Controls bleeding in certain types of hemophilia and von Willebrand's disease.

## ACTION

■ An analogue of naturally occurring vasopressin (antidiuretic hormone). Primary action is enhanced reabsorption of water in the kidneys. **Therapeutic Effects:** ■ Prevention of nocturnal enuresis ■ Maintenance of appropriate body water content in diabetes insipidus ■ Control of bleeding in certain types of hemophilia or von Willebrand's disease.

## PHARMACOKINETICS

**Absorption:** 5% absorbed following oral administration; some 10–20% absorbed from nasal mucosa.

**Distribution:** Distribution not fully known. Enters breast milk.

**Metabolism and Excretion:** Unknown.

**Half-life:** 75 min.

## CONTRAINDICATIONS AND PRECAUTIONS

**Contraindicated in:** ■ Hypersensitivity ■ Hypersensitivity to chlorobutanol ■ Patients with type IIB or platelet-type (pseudo) von Willebrand's disease.

**Use Cautiously in:** ■ Angina pectoris ■ Hypertension ■ Pregnancy or lactation (safety not established).

## ADVERSE REACTIONS AND SIDE EFFECTS*

■ **CNS:** drowsiness, headache, listlessness ■ **EENT:** *intranasal*—nasal congestion, rhinitis ■ **Resp:** dyspnea ■ **CV:** hypertension, hypotension, tachycardia (large IV doses only) ■ **GI:** mild abdominal cramps, nausea ■ **GU:** vulval pain ■ **Derm:** flushing ■ **F and E:** water intoxication/hyponatremia ■ **Local:** phlebitis at IV site.

## INTERACTIONS

**Drug-Drug:** ■ **Chlorpropamide, clofibrate,** or **carbamazepine** may enhance the antidiuretic response to desmopressin ■ **Demeclocycline, lithium,** or **norepinephrine** may diminish the antidiuretic response to desmopressin ■ Large doses may enhance the effects of **vasopressors.**

## ROUTE AND DOSAGE

❑ **Primary Nocturnal Enuresis**
■ **Intranasal (Adults and Children ≥6 yr):** 20 mcg (10 mcg in each nostril) at bedtime (range 10–40 mcg).

❑ **Diabetes Insipidus**
■ **PO (Adults):** 0.05 mg twice daily; adjusted as needed (usual range 0.1–1.2 mg/day in 2–3 divided doses).
■ **PO (Children):** 0.05 mg daily initially; adjusted as needed.
■ **Intranasal (Adults):** *Using nasal tube delivery system or spray pump (0.1 mg/ml)*—0.1–0.4 ml/day as a single dose or 2–3 divided doses.
■ **Intranasal (Children 3 mo–12 yr):** *Using nasal tube delivery system or spray pump (0.1 mg/ml)*—0.05–0.3 ml/day as a single dose or 2 divided doses.
■ **Subcut, IV (Adults):** 2–4 mcg/day in 2 divided doses.

❑ **Antihemorrhagic**
■ **IV (Adults and Children >3 mo):** 0.3 mcg/kg repeated as needed.
■ **Intranasal (Adults and Children ≥50 kg):** 1 spray (150 mcg) in each nostril.
■ **Intranasal (Adults and Children <50 kg):** 1 spray in one nostril (150 mcg).

## AVAILABILITY

■ *Tablets:* 0.1 mg^Rx, 0.2 mg^Rx ■ *Nasal spray pump:* 10 mcg/spray—5-ml bottle (0.1 mg/ml) contains 50 doses (DDAVP)^Rx ■ *Rhinal tube delivery system-nasal solution:* 2.5-ml vials with applicator tubes (0.1 mg/ml)^Rx ■ *Nasal solution:* 1.5 mg/ml (150 mcg/dose) in 2.5-ml bottle (contains 25 doses)^Rx ■ *Injection:* 4 mcg/ml^Rx, 15 mcg/ml^Rx.

TIME/ACTION PROFILE (PO, intranasal = antidiuretic effect; IV = effect on factor VIII activity)

| | ONSET | PEAK | DURATION |
|---|---|---|---|
| PO | 1 hr | 4–7 hr | unknown |
| Intranasal | 1 hr | 1–5 hr | 8–20 hr |
| IV | within min | 15–30 min | 3 hr† |

†4–24 hr in mild hemophilia A.

# NURSING IMPLICATIONS

## ASSESSMENT

- **General Info:** Chronic intranasal use may cause tolerance or if administered more frequently than every 24–48 hr IV tachyphylaxis (short-term tolerance) may develop.
- **Nocturnal Enuresis:** Monitor frequency of enuresis throughout therapy.
- **Diabetes Insipidus:** Monitor urine and plasma osmolality and urine volume frequently. Assess patient for symptoms of dehydration (excessive thirst, dry skin and mucous membranes, tachycardia, poor skin turgor). Weigh patient daily and assess for edema.
- **Hemophilia:** Monitor plasma factor VIII coagulant, factor VIII antigen, and ristocetin cofactor. May also assess activated partial thromboplastin time (aPTT) for hemophilia A and skin bleeding time for von Willebrand's disease. Assess patient for signs of bleeding.
- ❑ Monitor blood pressure and pulse during IV infusion.
- ❑ Monitor intake and output and adjust fluid intake (especially in children and elderly) to avoid overhydration in patients receiving desmopressin for hemophilia.
- *Toxicity and Overdose:* Signs and symptoms of water intoxication include confusion, drowsiness, headache, weight gain, difficulty urinating, seizures, and coma.
- ❑ Treatment of overdose includes decreasing dosage and, if symptoms are severe, administration of furosemide.

## POTENTIAL NURSING DIAGNOSES

- Fluid volume, deficit (Indications).
- Fluid volume, excess (Adverse Reactions).

## IMPLEMENTATION

- **General:** IV desmopressin has 10 times the antidiuretic effect of intranasal desmopressin.
- **PO:** Begin oral doses 12 hr after last intranasal dose. Monitor response closely.
- **Diabetes Insipidus:** Parenteral dose for antidiuretic effect is administered direct IV or subcut.
- **Hemophilia:** Parenteral dose for control of bleeding is administered via IV infusion. If used preoperatively, administer 30 min prior to procedure.
- **Direct IV:** Administer each dose over 1 min for diabetes insipidus.
- **Intermittent Infusion:** Dilute each dose in 50 ml of 0.9% NaCl for adults and children >10 kg and in 10 ml in children weighing <10 kg.
- *Rate:* Infuse slowly over 15–30 min for hemophilia. **Intranasal:** If intranasal dose is used preoperatively, administer 2 hr before procedure.

## PATIENT/FAMILY TEACHING

- **General Info:** Advise patient to notify health care professional if bleeding is not controlled or if headache, dyspnea, heartburn, nausea, abdominal cramps, vulval pain, or severe nasal congestion or irritation occurs.
- ❑ Caution patient to avoid concurrent use of alcohol with this medication.
- **Diabetes Insipidus:** Instruct patient on intranasal administration. Medication is supplied with a flexible calibrated catheter (rhinyle). Draw solution into rhinyle. Insert one end of tube into nostril, blow on the other end to deposit solution deep into nasal cavity. An air-filled syringe may be attached to the plastic catheter for children, infants, or obtunded patients. Tube should be rinsed under water after each use.
- ❑ If nasal spray is used, prime pump prior to first use by pressing down 4 times. Caution patient that nasal spray should not be used beyond the labeled number of sprays; subsequent sprays may not deliver accurate dose. Do not attempt to transfer remaining solution to another bottle.
- ❑ If a dose is missed, instruct patient to take it as soon as remembered but not if it is almost time for the next dose. Do not double doses.

❑ Advise patient that rhinitis or upper respiratory infection may decrease effectiveness of this therapy. If increased urine output occurs, patient should contact health care professional for dosage adjustment.

❑ Patients with diabetes insipidus should carry identification at all times describing disease process and medication regimen.

### EVALUATION

**Effectiveness of therapy can be demonstrated by:** ■ Decreased frequency of nocturnal enuresis ■ Decrease in urine volume ❑ Relief of polydipsia ❑ Increased urine osmolality ■ Control of bleeding in hemophilia.

---

## desonide, See CORTICOSTEROIDS (TOPICAL/LOCAL).

---

## desoximetasone, See CORTICOSTEROIDS (TOPICAL/LOCAL).

---

## dexamethasone, See CORTICOSTEROIDS (SYSTEMIC), CORTICOSTEROIDS (TOPICAL/LOCAL).

---

## dexmedetomidine

(dex-me-de-**to**-mi-deen)

Precedex

***CLASSIFICATION(S):***
***Therapeutic:*** sedative/hypnotics

**Pregnancy Category C**

### INDICATIONS

■ Sedation of initially intubated and mechanically ventilated patients during treatment in an intensive care setting; should not be used for >24 hr.

### ACTION

■ Acts as a relatively selective alpha-adrenergic agonist with sedative properties. **Therapeutic Effects:** ■ Sedation.

### PHARMACOKINETICS

**Absorption:** IV administration results in complete bioavailability.

**Distribution:** Unknown.

**Protein Binding:** 94%.

**Metabolism and Excretion:** Mostly metabolized by the liver, some metabolism by P450 enzyme system. Metabolites are mostly excreted in urine.

**Half-life:** 2 hr.

### CONTRAINDICATIONS AND PRECAUTIONS

**Contraindicated in:** ■ Hypersensitivity.

**Use Cautiously in:** ■ Hepatic impairment (lower doses may be required) ■ Advanced heart block ■ Geriatric patients (increased risk of bradycardia and hypotension in patients ≥65 yr ■ Pregnancy, lactation or children (safety not established).

### ADVERSE REACTIONS AND SIDE EFFECTS*

■ **Resp:** hypoxia ■ **CV:** BRADYCARDIA, SINUS ARREST, hypotension, transient hypertension ■ **GI:** nausea, vomiting ■ **Hemat:** anemia ■ **Misc:** fever.

### INTERACTIONS

**Drug-Drug:** ■ Sedation is enhanced by **anesthetics,** other **sedative/hypnotics,** and **opioid analgesics.**

**Drug-Natural Products:** ■ Concomitant use of **kava, valerian, skullcap, chamomile,** or **hops** can increase CNS depression.

### ROUTE AND DOSAGE

■ **IV (Adults):** *Loading infusion*—1 mcg/kg over 10 min followed by *maintenance infusion* of 0.2–0.7 mcg/kg/hr for maximum of 24 hrs; rate is adjusted to achieve desired level of sedation.

### AVAILABILITY

■ *Injection:* 100 mcg/ml in 2-ml ampules and vials[Rx].

TIME/ACTION PROFILE (sedation)

|    | ONSET | PEAK | DURATION |
|----|-------|------|----------|
| IV | rapid | unknown | unknown |

## NURSING IMPLICATIONS

### ASSESSMENT

❑ Assess level of sedation throughout therapy. Dose is adjusted based on level of sedation.

❑ Monitor ECG and blood pressure continuously throughout therapy. May cause hypotension, bradycardia, and sinus arrest.

■ *Toxicity and Overdose:* Atropine IV may be used to modify the vagal tone.

### POTENTIAL NURSING DIAGNOSES

■ Anxiety (Indications).

### IMPLEMENTATION

■ **General:** Dexmedetomidine should be administered only in intensive care settings with continuous monitoring.

■ **Continuous Infusion:** To prepare infusion, withdraw 2 ml of dexmedetomidine and add to 48 ml of 0.9 NaCl for a total of 50 ml. Shake gently. Solution should be clear; do not administer solutions that are discolored or contain particulate matter. Ampules and vials are for single use only.

■ *Rate:* Administer *loading infusion* over 10 minutes, followed by *maintenance infusion* of 0.2–0.7 mcg/kg/hr. Adjust dose to achieve desired level of sedation. Administer via infusion pump to ensure accurate rate.

■ **Y-Site Compatibility:** ◆ 0.9% NaCl ◆ 20% mannitol ◆ atracurium ◆ atropine ◆ D5W ◆ etomidate ◆ fentanyl ◆ glycopyrrolate ◆ midazolam ◆ mivacurium ◆ morphine ◆ pancuronium ◆ phenylephrine ◆ plasma substitute ◆ succinylcholine ◆ thiopental ◆ vecuronium.

■ **Y-Site Incompatibility:** ◆ blood ◆ plasma ◆ serum.

### PATIENT/FAMILY TEACHING

❑ Explain to patient and family the purpose of the medication.

### EVALUATION

**Effectiveness of therapy can be demonstrated by:** ■ Sedation for up to 24 hr.

---

# dexmethylphenidate
(dex-meth-ill-**fen**-i-date)
Focalin

---

## INDICATIONS

■ Adjunctive treatment of ADHD.

## ACTION

■ Produces CNS and respiratory stimulation with weak sympathomimetic activity. **Therapeutic Effects:** ■ Increased attention span in ADHD.

## PHARMACOKINETICS

**Absorption:** Readily absorbed following oral administration.

**Distribution:** Unknown.

**Metabolism and Excretion:** Mostly metabolized by the liver; inactive metabolites are renally excreted.

**Half-life:** 2.2 hr.

## CONTRAINDICATIONS AND PRECAUTIONS

**Contraindicated in:** ■ Hypersensitivity ■ Hyperexcitable states (marked anxiety, agitation, or tension) ■ Hyperthyroidism ■ Psychotic personalities, suicidal or homicidal tendencies ■ Glaucoma ■ Motor tics, family history or diagnosis of Tourette's syndrome ■ Concurrent use of MAO inhibitors ■ Should not be used to treat depression or prevent/treat normal fatigue ■ Psychoses (may exacerbate symptoms).

**Use Cautiously in:** ■ History of cardiovascular disease ■ Hypertension ■ Diabetes mellitus ■ Geriatric/debilitated patients ■ Continual use (may result in psychological or physical dependence) ■ Seizure disorders (may lower seizure threshold) ■ Pregnancy, lactation, or children <6 yr (safety not established; use in pregnancy only if clearly needed).

## ADVERSE REACTIONS AND SIDE EFFECTS*

■ **CNS:** insomnia, nervousness ■ **EENT:** visual disturbances ■ **CV:** tachycardia ■ **GI:** <u>abdominal pain</u>, anorexia, nausea ■ **Metab:** growth suppression, weight loss (may occur with prolonged use) ■ **Neuro:** twitching ■ **Misc:** fever.

## INTERACTIONS

**Drug-Drug:** ■ Concurrent use with or use within 14 days following discontinuation of **MAO inhibitors** may result in hypertensive crisis and is contraindicated ■ May ↓ effects of **antihypertensives** ■ May ↑ effects of **vasopressors** ■ May cause serious adverse reactions with **clonidine** ■ May ↑ effects of **warfarin phenobarbital phenytoin** some **antidepressants**; dosage adjustments may be necessary.

## ROUTE AND DOSAGE

■ **PO (Children ≥6 yr):** *Patients not previously taking methylphenidate*—2.5 mg twice daily, may be increased weekly as needed up to 10 mg twice daily; *Patients currently taking methylphenidate*—starting dose is 1/2 of the methylphenidate dose, up to 10 mg twice daily.

## AVAILABILITY

■ *Tablets:* 2.5 mg^Rx, 5 mg^Rx, 10 mg^Rx.

TIME/ACTION PROFILE (improvement in symptoms)

|    | ONSET | PEAK | DURATION |
|----|-------|------|----------|
| PO | 7 days | 1 mo | unknown |

## NURSING IMPLICATIONS

### ASSESSMENT

❑ Assess child's attention span, impulse control, and interactions with others. Therapy may be interrupted at intervals to determine whether symptoms are sufficient to continue therapy.

❑ Monitor blood pressure, pulse, and respiration before administering and periodically during therapy.

❑ Monitor growth, both height and weight, in children on long-term therapy.

❑ Dexmethylphenidate has the potential for dependence and abuse. Prolonged use may result in tolerance.

■ *Lab Test Considerations:* Monitor CBC, differential, and platelet count periodically in patients receiving prolonged therapy.

## POTENTIAL NURSING DIAGNOSES

■ Thought processes, disturbed (Side Effects).

## IMPLEMENTATION

■ **PO:** Administer twice daily at least 4 hr apart without regard to meals.

## PATIENT/FAMILY TEACHING

❑ Instruct patient to take medication exactly as directed. If more than prescribed amount is taken notify health care professional immediately. If a dose is missed, take the remaining doses for that day at regularly spaced intervals; do not double doses. Take the last dose before 6 PM to minimize the risk of insomnia. Instruct patient not to alter dose without consulting health care professional. Abrupt cessation with high doses may cause extreme fatigue and mental depression.

❑ Inform patient that sharing this medication may be dangerous.

❑ Advise patient to check weight 2–3 times weekly and report weight loss to health care professional.

❑ Advise patient to consult with health care professional prior to taking other prescription, OTC, or herbal products concurrently with dexmethylphenidate.

❑ May rarely cause dizziness or drowsiness. Caution patient to avoid driving or activities requiring alertness until response to medication is known.

❑ Inform patient that health care professional may order periodic holidays from the drug to assess progress and to decrease dependence.

❑ Advise patient to notify health care professional if pregnancy is planned or suspected, or if breastfeeding.

❑ Caution patients to inform health care professional if they have ever abused or been dependent on alcohol or drugs, or if they are now abusing or dependent on alcohol or drugs.

❑ Emphasize the importance of routine follow-up exams to monitor progress.

❑ Advise parents to notify school nurse of medication regimen.

## EVALUATION

**Effectiveness of therapy can be demonstrated by:** ■ Improved attention span, decreased impulsiveness and hyperactivity in ADHD.

---

# dextroamphetamine

(dex-troe-am-**fet**-a-meen)
Dexedrine, Dextrostat

*CLASSIFICATION(S):*
*Therapeutic:* central nervous system stimulants
*Pharmacologic:* amphetamines

Schedule II

Pregnancy Category C

## INDICATIONS

■ Narcolepsy ■ Adjunct management of ADHD.

## ACTION

■ Produces CNS stimulation by releasing norepinephrine from nerve endings. Pharmacologic effects: ■ CNS and respiratory stimulation ■ Vasoconstriction ■ Mydriasis (pupillary dilation) ■ Contraction of the urinary bladder sphincter. **Therapeutic Effects:** ■ Increased motor activity and mental alertness and decreased fatigue in narcoleptic patients ■ Increased attention span in ADHD.

## PHARMACOKINETICS

**Absorption:** Well absorbed.

**Distribution:** Widely distributed; high concentrations in brain and CSF. Crosses the placenta; enters breast milk; potentially embryotoxic.

**Metabolism and Excretion:** Some metabolism by the liver. Urinary excretion is pH-dependent. Alkaline urine promotes reabsorption and prolongs action.

**Half-life:** 10–12 hr (6.8 hr in children).

## CONTRAINDICATIONS AND PRECAUTIONS

**Contraindicated in:** ■ Pregnancy or lactation ■ Hyperexcitable states, including hyperthyroidism ■ Psychotic personalities ■ Suicidal or homicidal tendencies ■ Glaucoma ■ Some products contain tartrazine and should be avoided in patients with known hypersensitivity.

**Use Cautiously in:** ■ Cardiovascular disease ■ Hypertension ■ Diabetes mellitus ■ History of substance abuse ■ Elderly/ debilitated patients ■ Continual use (may produce psychological dependence or physical addiction).

## ADVERSE REACTIONS AND SIDE EFFECTS*

■ **CNS:** hyperactivity, insomnia, restlessness, tremor, depression, dizziness, headache, irritability ■ **CV:** palpitations, tachycardia, arrhythmias, hypertension, hypotension ■ **GI:** anorexia, constipation, cramps, diarrhea, dry mouth, metallic taste, nausea, vomiting ■ **GU:** impotence, increased libido ■ **Derm:** urticaria ■ **Misc:** physical dependence, psychological dependence.

## INTERACTIONS

**Drug-Drug:** ■ ↑ adrenergic effects with other **adrenergics** ■ Use with **MAO inhibitors** can result in hypertensive crisis ■ Alkalinizing the urine (**sodium bicarbonate, acetazolamide**) prolongs effect ■ Acidification of urine (**ammonium chloride**, large doses of **ascorbic acid**) ↓ effect ■ **Phenothiazines** may decrease the effect of dextroamphetamine ■ May antagonize the response to **antihypertensives** ■ ↑ risk of cardiovascular side effects with **beta blockers** or **tricyclic antidepressants.**

**Drug-Natural Products:** ■ Use with caffeine-containing herbs (**guarana, tea, coffee**) ↑ stimulant effect.

## ROUTE AND DOSAGE

❑ **Attention-Deficit Hyperactivity Disorder**

■ **PO (Adults):** 5–60 mg/day in divided doses. Sustained-release capsules should not be used as initial therapy.

■ **PO (Children ≥6 yr):** 5 mg 1–2 times daily, increase by 5 mg at weekly intervals. Sustained-release capsules should not be used as initial therapy.

■ **PO (Children 3–5 yr):** 2.5 mg/day, increase by 2.5 mg at weekly intervals.

❑ **Narcolepsy**

■ **PO (Adults):** 5–60 mg/day single dose or in divided doses. Sustained-release capsules should not be used as initial therapy.

■ **PO (Children ≥12 yr):** 10 mg/day, increase by 10 mg/day at weekly intervals until response is obtained or adult dose is reached.

■ **PO (Children 6–12 yr):** 5 mg/day, increase by 5 mg/day at weekly intervals until response is obtained or adult dose is reached.

## AVAILABILITY (generic available)

■ *Tablets:* 5 mg$^{Rx}$ ■ Cost: 5 mg $35.23/100 ■ *Sustained-release capsules:* 5 mg$^{Rx}$, 10 mg$^{Rx}$, 15 mg$^{Rx}$.

### TIME/ACTION PROFILE (CNS stimulation)

|  | ONSET | PEAK | DURATION |
|---|---|---|---|
| PO | 1–2 hr | unknown | 2–10 hr |
| PO-ER | unknown | unknown | up to 24 hr |

# NURSING IMPLICATIONS

## ASSESSMENT

- ■ **General Info:** Monitor blood pressure, pulse, and respiration before administering and periodically during therapy.
- ■ **ADHD:** Monitor weight biweekly and inform physician of significant loss. Monitor height periodically in children; report growth inhibition.
- ❑ Assess attention span, impulse control, motor and vocal tics, and interactions with others.
- ■ **Narcolepsy:** Observe and document frequency of narcoleptic episodes.
- ❑ May produce a false sense of euphoria and well-being. Provide frequent rest periods and observe patient for rebound depression after the effects of the medication have worn off.
- ❑ Has high dependence and abuse potential. Tolerance to medication occurs rapidly; do not increase dose.
- ■ *Lab Test Considerations:* May interfere with urinary steroid determinations.
- ❑ May cause ↑ plasma corticosteroid concentrations; greatest in evening.

## POTENTIAL NURSING DIAGNOSES

- ■ Thought processes, disturbed (Side Effects).

## IMPLEMENTATION

- ■ **General:** Do not confuse Adderall (dextroamphetamine/amphetamine) with Inderal (propranolol).
- ❑ Therapy should utilize the lowest effective dose.
- ■ **PO:** Sustained-release capsules should be swallowed whole; do not break, crush, or chew.

- ■ **ADHD:** When symptoms are controlled, dose reduction or interruption of therapy may be possible during summer months or may be given on each of the 5 school days with medication-free weekends and holidays.

## PATIENT/FAMILY TEACHING

- ■ **General Info:** Instruct patient to take medication at least 6 hr before bedtime to avoid sleep disturbances. Take missed doses as soon as remembered up to 6 hr before bedtime. Do not double doses. Instruct patient not to alter dose without consulting health care professional. Abrupt cessation of high doses may cause extreme fatigue and mental depression.
- ❑ Inform patient that the effects of drug-induced dry mouth can be minimized by rinsing frequently with water or chewing sugarless gum or candies.
- ❑ Advise patient to avoid the intake of large amounts of caffeine.
- ❑ Medication may impair judgment. Advise patients to use caution when driving or during other activities requiring alertness.
- ❑ Advise patient to notify health care professional if nervousness, restlessness, insomnia, dizziness, anorexia, or dry mouth becomes severe.
- ❑ Inform patient that periodic holiday from the drug may be ordered to assess progress and decrease dependence.

## EVALUATION

**Effectiveness of therapy can be demonstrated by:** ■ Improved attention span. Therapy should be interrupted and need reassessed periodically ■ Decrease in narcoleptic symptoms.

## dextromethorphan

(dex-troe-meth-**or**-fan)

{Balminil DM}, Benylin Adult, Benylin Pediatric, {Broncho-Grippol-DM}, {Calmylin #1}, Children's Hold, Creo-Terpin, Delsym, DexAlone, {DM Syrup}, Drixoral Liquid Cough Caps, Hold, {Koffex},

Mediquell, {Neo-DM}, {Ornex•DM}, Pertussin Cough Suppressant, Pertussin CS, Pertussin ES, {Robidex}, Robitussin Cough Calmers, Robitussin Maximum Strength Cough Suppressant, Robitussin Pediatric, {Sedatuss}, Sucrets Cough Control Formula, Vicks Formula 44 Pediatric Formula

### CLASSIFICATION(S):

***Therapeutic:*** *allergy, cold, and cough remedies, antitussives*

### Pregnancy Category UK

## INDICATIONS

■ Symptomatic relief of coughs caused by minor viral upper respiratory tract infections or inhaled irritants ■ Most effective for chronic nonproductive cough ■ A common ingredient in nonprescription cough and cold preparations.

## ACTION

■ Suppresses the cough reflex by a direct effect on the cough center in the medulla. Related to opioids structurally but has no analgesic properties. **Therapeutic Effects:** ■ Relief of irritating nonproductive cough.

## PHARMACOKINETICS

**Absorption:** Rapidly absorbed from the GI tract. Extended-release product is slowly absorbed.

**Distribution:** Unknown. Probably crosses the placenta and enters breast milk.

**Metabolism and Excretion:** Metabolized to dextrorphan, an active metabolite. Dextromethorphan and dextrorphan are renally excreted.

**Half-life:** Unknown.

## CONTRAINDICATIONS AND PRECAUTIONS

**Contraindicated in:** ■ Hypersensitivity ■ Patients taking MAO inhibitors or SSRIs ■ Should not be used for chronic productive coughs ■ Some products contain alcohol and should be avoided in patients with known intolerance.

**Use Cautiously in:** ■ Cough that lasts more than 1 wk or is accompanied by fever, rash, or headache—health care professional should be consulted ■ Diabetes (some products contain sucrose) ■ Pregnancy (has been used safely) ■

Lactation or children <2 yr (safety not established).

## ADVERSE REACTIONS AND SIDE EFFECTS*

■ **CNS:** *high dose*—dizziness, sedation ■ **GI:** nausea.

## INTERACTIONS

**Drug-Drug:** ■ Use with **MAO inhibitors** may result in serotonin syndrome (nausea, confusion, changes in blood pressure); concurrent use should be avoided ■ Additive CNS depression with **antihistamines, alcohol, antidepressants, sedative/hypnotics,** or **opioid analgesics** ■ **Amiodarone, fluoxetine,** or **quinidine** may increase blood levels and adverse reactions from dextromethorphan.

## ROUTE AND DOSAGE

■ **PO (Adults and Children >12 yr):** 10–20 mg q 4 hr *or* 30 mg q 6–8 hr *or* 60 mg of extended-release preparation bid (not to exceed 120 mg/day).

■ **PO (Children 6–12 yr):** 5–10 mg q 4 hr *or* 15 mg q 6–8 hr *or* 30 mg of extended-release preparation q 12 hr (not to exceed 60 mg/day).

■ **PO (Children 2–6 yr):** 2.5–5 mg q 4 hr *or* 7.5 mg q 6–8 hr *or* 15 mg of extended-release preparation q 12 hr (not to exceed 30 mg/day).

## AVAILABILITY

■ ***Gelcaps:*** 30 mg$^{OTC}$ ■ ***Lozenges:*** 2.5 mg$^{OTC}$, 5 mg$^{OTC}$ ■ ***Liquid:*** 3.5 mg/5 ml$^{OTC}$, 7.5 mg/5 ml$^{OTC}$, 15 mg/5 ml$^{OTC}$ ■ ***Syrup:*** 15 mg/15 ml$^{OTC}$, 10 mg/5 ml$^{OTC}$ ■ Cost: 15 mg/15 ml $2.40/120 ml ■ ***Extended-release suspension:*** 30 mg/5 ml$^{OTC}$ ■ antihistamines, decongestants, and expectorants in cough and cold preparations$^{OTC}$. See Appendix B.

TIME/ACTION PROFILE (cough suppression)

| | ONSET | PEAK | DURATION |
|---|---|---|---|
| PO | 15–30 min | unknown | 3–6 hr† |
| PO-ER | unknown | unknown | 9–12 hr |

†Up to 8 hr for gelcaps.

## NURSING IMPLICATIONS

### ASSESSMENT

■ **General Info:** Assess frequency and nature of cough, lung sounds, and amount and type of sputum produced. Unless contraindicated, maintain fluid intake of 1500–2000 ml to decrease viscosity of bronchial secretions.

## POTENTIAL NURSING DIAGNOSES

■ Airway clearance, ineffective (Indications).

## IMPLEMENTATION

■ **General:** Do not confuse Benylin (dextromethorphan) with Benadryl (diphenhydramine).

❑ Dextromethorphan 15–30 mg is equivalent in cough suppression to codeine 8–15 mg.

■ **PO:** Do not give fluids immediately after administering to prevent dilution of vehicle. Shake oral suspension well before administration.

## PATIENT/FAMILY TEACHING

❑ Instruct patient to cough effectively: Sit upright and take several deep breaths before attempting to cough.

❑ Advise patient to minimize cough by avoiding irritants, such as cigarette smoke, fumes, and dust. Humidification of environmental air, frequent sips of water, and sugarless hard candy may also decrease the frequency of dry, irritating cough.

❑ Caution patient to avoid taking alcohol or other CNS depressants concurrently with this medication.

❑ May occasionally cause dizziness. Caution patient to avoid driving or other activities requiring alertness until response to the medication is known.

❑ Advise patient that any cough lasting over 1 wk or accompanied by fever, chest pain, persistent headache, or skin rash warrants medical attention.

## EVALUATION

**Effectiveness of therapy can be demonstrated by:** ■ Decrease in frequency and intensity of cough without eliminating patient's cough reflex.

## diazepam
(dye-**az**-e-pam)

{Apo-Diazepam}, Diastat, {Diazemuls}, Dizac, D-Val, {Novodipam}, {PMS-Diazepam}, Valium, {Vivol}

## CLASSIFICATION(S):

**Therapeutic:** antianxiety agents, anticonvulsants, sedative/hypnotics, skeletal muscle relaxants (centrally acting)
**Pharmacologic:** benzodiazepines

## Schedule IV

## Pregnancy Category D

## INDICATIONS

■ Adjunct in the management of: ❑ Anxiety ❑ Preoperative sedation ❑ Conscious sedation ■ Provides light anesthesia and anterograde amnesia ■ Treatment of status epilepticus/uncontrolled seizures ■ Skeletal muscle relaxant ■ Management of the symptoms of alcohol withdrawal.

## ACTION

■ Depresses the CNS, probably by potentiating GABA, an inhibitory neurotransmitter ■ Produces skeletal muscle relaxation by inhibiting spinal polysynaptic afferent pathways ■ Has anticonvulsant properties due to enhanced presynaptic inhibition. **Therapeutic Effects:** ■ Relief of anxiety ■ Sedation ■ Amnesia ■ Skeletal muscle relaxation ■ Decreased seizure activity.

## PHARMACOKINETICS

**Absorption:** Rapidly absorbed from the GI tract. Absorption from IM sites may be slow and unpredictable. Well absorbed (90%) from rectal mucosa.
**Distribution:** Widely distributed. Crosses the blood-brain barrier. Crosses the placenta; enters breast milk.
**Metabolism and Excretion:** Highly metabolized by the liver. Some products of metabolism are active as CNS depressants.
**Half-life:** 20–70 hr (up to 200 hr for metabolites).

## CONTRAINDICATIONS AND PRECAUTIONS

**Contraindicated in:** ■ Hypersensitivity ■ Cross-sensitivity with other benzodiazepines may occur ■ Comatose patients ■ Pre-existing CNS depression ■ Uncontrolled severe pain ■ Narrow-angle glaucoma ■ Pregnancy or lactation ■ Some products contain alcohol, propylene glycol, or tartrazine and should be avoided in patients with known hypersensitivity or intolerance.

**Use Cautiously in:** ■ Hepatic dysfunction ■ Severe renal impairment ■ History of suicide attempt or drug dependence ■ Geriatric or debilitated patients (dosage reduction required) ■ Children (dosage should not exceed 0.25 mg/kg).

## ADVERSE REACTIONS AND SIDE EFFECTS*

■ **CNS:** dizziness, drowsiness, lethargy, depression, hangover, headache, paradoxical excitation ■ **EENT:** blurred vision ■ **Resp:** respiratory depression ■ **CV:** hypotension (IV only) ■ **GI:** constipation, diarrhea, nausea, vomiting ■ **Derm:** rashes ■ **Local:** pain (IM), phlebitis (IV), venous thrombosis ■ **Misc:** physical dependence, psychological dependence, tolerance.

## INTERACTIONS

**Drug-Drug:** ■ **Alcohol, antidepressants, antihistamines,** and **opioid analgesics**—concurrent use results in additive CNS depression ■ **Cimetidine, hormonal contraceptives, disulfiram, fluoxetine, isoniazid, ketoconazole, metoprolol, propoxyphene, propranolol,** or **valproic acid** may decrease the metabolism of diazepam, enhancing its actions ■ May decrease the efficacy of **levodopa** ■ **Rifampin** or **barbiturates** may increase the metabolism and decrease effectiveness of diazepam ■ Sedative effects may be decreased by **theophylline**.

**Drug-Natural Products:** ■ Concomitant use of **kava, valerian, skullcap, chamomile,** or **hops** can increase CNS depression.

## ROUTE AND DOSAGE

❑ **Antianxiety/Anticonvulsant**
■ **PO (Adults):** 2–10 mg 2–4 times daily.
■ **PO (Children >6 mo):** 1–2.5 mg 3–4 times daily; may be increased.

❑ **Precardioversion**
■ **IV (Adults):** 5–15 mg 5–10 min precardioversion.

❑ **Pre-endoscopy**
■ **IV (Adults):** 2.5–20 mg.

■ **IM (Adults):** 5–10 mg 30 min pre-endoscopy.

❑ **Status Epilepticus/Acute Seizure Activity**
■ **IV (Adults):** 5–10 mg, may repeat q 10–15 min to a total of 30 mg, may repeat regimen again in 2–4 hr (IM route may be used if IV route unavailable); larger doses may be required.
■ **IM, IV (Children ≥5 yr):** 1 mg q 2–5 min to a total of 10 mg, repeat q 2–4 hr.
■ **IM, IV (Children 1 mo–5 yr):** 0.2–0.5 mg q 2–5 min to maximum of 5 mg.
■ **Rect (Adults):** 0.2 mg/kg; may repeat 4–12 hr later.
■ **Rect (Children 6–11 yr):** 0.3 mg/kg; may repeat 4–12 hr later.
■ **Rect (Children 2–5 yr):** 0.5 mg/kg; may repeat 4–12 hr later.

❑ **Skeletal Muscle Relaxation**
■ **PO (Adults):** 2–10 mg 3–4 times daily or 15–30 mg of extended-release form once daily.
■ **PO (Geriatric Patients or Debilitated Patients):** 2–2.5 mg 1–2 times daily initially.
■ **PO (Children):** 1–2.5 mg 3–4 times daily.
■ **IM, IV (Adults):** 5–10 mg; may repeat in 2–4 hr (larger doses may be required for tetanus).
■ **IM, IV (Geriatric Patients or Debilitated Patients):** 2–5 mg; may repeat in 2–4 hr (larger doses may be required for tetanus).
■ **IM, IV (Children ≥5 yr):** *Tetanus*—5–10 mg q 3–4 hr.
■ **IM, IV (Children >1 mo):** *Tetanus*—1–2 mg q 3–4 hr.

❑ **Alcohol Withdrawal**
■ **PO (Adults):** 10 mg 3–4 times in first 24 hr, decrease to 5 mg 3–4 times daily.
■ **IM, IV (Adults):** 10 mg initially, then 5–10 mg in 3–4 hr as needed; larger or more frequent doses have been used.

❑ **Psychoneurotic Reactions**
■ **IM, IV (Adults):** 2–10 mg, may be repeated in 3–4 hr.

## AVAILABILITY (generic available)

■ *Tablets:* 2 mg^Rx, 5 mg^Rx, 10 mg^Rx ■ Cost: *Valium*—2 mg $49.84/100, *generic*—$6.99/100; *Valium*—5 mg $77.83/100, *generic*—$10.84/100; *Valium*—10 mg $120.12/100, *generic*—$19.83/100 ■ *Oral solution:* 5 mg/ ml (Intensol)$^{Rx}$, 5 mg/5 ml$^{Rx}$ ■ *Injection:* 5 mg/ml (contains 10% alcohol and 40% propylene glycol)$^{Rx}$ ■ *Rectal gel delivery system:* 2.5 mg$^{Rx}$, 10 mg$^{Rx}$, 15 mg$^{Rx}$, 20 mg$^{Rx}$ ■ *Sterile emulsion for injection:* 5 mg/ml (contains egg phospholipids and soybean oil)$^{Rx}$.

TIME/ACTION PROFILE (sedation)

| | ONSET | PEAK | DURATION |
|---|---|---|---|
| PO | 30–60 min | 1–2 hr | up to 24 hr |
| IM | within 20 min | 0.5–1.5 hr | unknown |
| IV | 1–5 min | 15–30 min | 15–60 min† |
| Rectal | unknown | 1–2 hr | 4–12 hr |

†In status epilepticus, anticonvulsant duration is 15–20 min.

## NURSING IMPLICATIONS

### ASSESSMENT

- **General Info:** Monitor blood pressure, pulse, and respiratory rate prior to and periodically throughout therapy and frequently during IV therapy.
- Assess IV site frequently during administration; diazepam may cause phlebitis and venous thrombosis.
- Prolonged high-dose therapy may lead to psychological or physical dependence. Restrict amount of drug available to patient. Observe depressed patients closely for suicidal tendencies.
- **Anxiety:** Assess degree of anxiety and level of sedation (ataxia, dizziness, slurred speech) prior to and periodically throughout therapy.
- **Seizures:** Observe and record intensity, duration, and location of seizure activity. The initial dose of diazepam offers seizure control for 15–20 min after administration. Institute seizure precautions.
- **Muscle Spasms:** Assess muscle spasm, associated pain, and limitation of movement prior to and throughout therapy.
- **Alcohol Withdrawal:** Assess patient experiencing alcohol withdrawal for tremors, agitation, delirium, and hallucinations. Protect patient from injury.
- *Lab Test Considerations:* Hepatic and renal function and CBC should be evaluated

periodically throughout course of prolonged therapy.

## POTENTIAL NURSING DIAGNOSES

- Anxiety (Indications).
- Mobility, impaired physical (Indications).
- Injury, risk for (Side Effects).

## IMPLEMENTATION

- **General:** Do not confuse diazepam with lorazepam or ditropan.
- Patient should be kept on bedrest and observed for at least 3 hr following parenteral administration.
- If opioid analgesics are used concurrently with parenteral diazepam, decrease opioid dose by $\frac{1}{3}$ and titrate dose to effect.
- **PO:** Tablets may be crushed and taken with food or water if patient has difficulty swallowing. Swallow sustained-release capsules whole; do not crush, break, or chew.
- Mix Intensol preparation with liquid or semisolid food such as water, juices, soda, applesauce, or pudding. Administer entire amount immediately. Do not store.
- **IM:** IM injections are painful and erratically absorbed. If IM route is used, inject deeply into deltoid muscle for maximum absorption.
- **IV:** Resuscitation equipment should be available when diazepam is administered IV.
- **Direct IV:** For IV administration do not dilute or mix with any other drug. If direct IV push is not feasible, administer IV push into tubing as close to insertion site as possible. Continuous infusion is not recommended because of precipitation in IV fluids and absorption of diazepam into infusion bags and tubing. Injection may cause burning and venous irritation; avoid small veins.
- *Rate:* Administer slowly at a rate of 5 mg over at least 1 min. Infants and children should receive total dose over a minimum of 3–5 min. Rapid injection may cause apnea, hypotension, bradycardia, or cardiac arrest.
- **Syringe Compatibility:** ♦ cimetidine.
- **Syringe Incompatibility:** ♦ doxapram ♦ glycopyrrolate ♦ heparin ♦ hydromorphone ♦ nalbuphine ♦ sufentanil.
- **Y-Site Compatibility:** ♦ dobutamine ♦ nafcillin ♦ quinidine gluconate ♦ sufentanil.

- **Y-Site Incompatibility:** ◆ amphotericin B cholesteryl sulfate ◆ atracurium ◆ cefepime ◆ diltiazem ◆ fluconazole ◆ foscarnet ◆ gatifloxacin ◆ heparin ◆ hydromorphone ◆ linezolid ◆ meropenem ◆ pancuronium ◆ potassium chloride ◆ propofol ◆ vecuronium ◆ vitamin B complex with C.
- **Sterile emulsion for injection (Dizac):** For IV use only. Use strict aseptic technique. Do not dilute, ampule is for single use; discard unused portion. Do not use filters >5 microns; restricts flow and causes breakdown of emulsion. Administer within 6 hr of drawing up, flush line at end of administration and after 6 hr to remove residual.
- **Incompatibility:** ◆ glycopyrrolate ◆ morphine
- **Rect:** Do not repeat *Diastat* rectal dose more than 5 times/mo or 1 episode every 5 days. Round dose up to next available dose unit.
- ❑ Diazepam injection has been used for rectal administration. Instill via catheter or cannula fitted to the syringe or directly from a 1-ml syringe inserted 4–5 cm into the rectum. A dilution of diazepam injection with propylene glycol containing 1 mg/ml has also been used.
- ❑ Do not dilute with other solutions, IV fluids, or medications.

### PATIENT/FAMILY TEACHING

- **General Info:** Instruct patient to take medication exactly as directed and not to take more than prescribed or increase dose if less effective after a few weeks without checking with health care professional. Abrupt withdrawal of diazepam may cause insomnia, unusual irritability or nervousness, and seizures. Advise patient that sharing of this medication may be dangerous.
- ❑ Medication may cause drowsiness, clumsiness, or unsteadiness. Advise patient to avoid driving or other activities requiring alertness until response to medication is known.
- ❑ Caution patient to avoid taking alcohol or other CNS depressants concurrently with this medication.
- ❑ Advise patient to notify health care professional if pregnancy is suspected or planned.
- ❑ Emphasize the importance of follow-up examinations to determine effectiveness of the medication.

- **Seizures:** Patients on anticonvulsant therapy should carry identification describing disease process and medication regimen at all times.
- ❑ Carefully review patient/caregiver package insert for Diastat rectal gel with caregiver prior to administration.

### EVALUATION

**Effectiveness of therapy can be demonstrated by:** ■ Decrease in anxiety level. Full therapeutic antianxiety effects occur after 1–2 wk of therapy ■ Decreased recall of surgical or diagnostic procedures ■ Control of seizures ■ Decrease in muscle spasms ■ Decreased tremulousness and more rational ideation when used for alcohol withdrawal.

---

# DICLOFENAC†
(dye-**kloe**-fen-ak)

**diclofenac potassium**
Cataflam, {Voltaren Rapide}

**diclofenac sodium**
{Apo-Diclo}, {Novo-Difenac}, Nu-Diclo, Voltaren, {Voltaren-SR}

**dicofenac topical**
Solaraze

## CLASSIFICATION(S):
*Therapeutic: nonopioid analgesics, nonsteroidal anti-inflammatory agents*

**Pregnancy Category B (first trimester)**

†For ophthalmic use see Appendix C.

---

### INDICATIONS

■ **PO:** Management of inflammatory disorders including: ❑ Rheumatoid arthritis ❑ Osteoarthritis ❑ Ankylosing spondylitis ■ Relief of mild to moderate pain of dysmenorrhea ■ **Topical:** Treatment of actinic keratoses.

### ACTION

■ Inhibits prostaglandin synthesis. **Therapeutic Effects:** ■ Suppression of pain and inflammation.

## PHARMACOKINETICS

**Absorption:** Well absorbed after oral administration. Oral diclofenac sodium is a delayed-release dosage form. Diclofenac potassium is an immediate-release dosage form. 10% of topically applied diclofenac is systemically absorbed.

**Distribution:** Crosses the placenta; enters breast milk.

**Protein Binding:** >99%.

**Metabolism and Excretion:** ≥50% metabolized on first pass through the liver.

**Half-life:** 1.2–2 hr.

## CONTRAINDICATIONS AND PRECAUTIONS

**Contraindicated in:** ■ Hypersensitivity to diclofenac or other components of formulation ■ Cross-sensitivity may occur with other NSAIDs including aspirin ■ Active GI bleeding/ulcer disease.

**Use Cautiously in:** ■ Severe cardiovascular/renal/hepatic disease ■ History of porphyria ■ History of ulcer disease ■ Geriatric patients (dosage reduction recommended; more susceptible to adverse reactions) ■ Bleeding tendency or concurrent anticoagulant therapy ■ Pregnancy, lactation, and children (safety not established; not recommended for use during second half of pregnancy).

## ADVERSE REACTIONS AND SIDE EFFECTS*

For oral diclofenac unless noted. ■ **CNS:** dizziness, drowsiness, headache ■ **CV:** hypertension ■ **GI:** GI BLEEDING, abdominal pain, dyspepsia, heartburn, diarrhea, hepatotoxicity ■ **GU:** acute renal failure, dysuria, frequency, hematuria, nephritis, proteinuria ■ **Derm:** eczema, photosensitivity, rashes ■ **F and E:** edema ■ **Hemat:** prolonged bleeding time ■ **Local:** *Topical only*—contact dermatitis, dry skin, exfoliation, rash ■ **Misc:** allergic reactions including ANAPHYLAXIS.

## INTERACTIONS

Primarily noted for oral administration.

**Drug-Drug:** ■ Concurrent use with **aspirin** may decrease effectiveness ■ Additive adverse GI effects with **aspirin**, other **NSAIDs, colchi-** cine, **corticosteroids**, or **alcohol** ■ Chronic use with **acetaminophen** may increase the risk of adverse renal reactions ■ May decrease the effectiveness of **diuretics, antihypertensives, insulins,** or **hypoglycemic agents** ■ Increases serum **digoxin** levels (dosage adjustment may be necessary) ■ May increase levels and increase the risk of toxicity from **cyclosporine, lithium,** or **methotrexate** ■ **Probenecid** increases risk of toxicity from diclofenac ■ Increased risk of bleeding with some **cephalosporins, plicamycin, thrombolytic agents, antiplatelet agents,** or **anticoagulants** ■ Increased risk of adverse hematologic reactions with **antineoplastics** or **radiation therapy** ■ Concurrent use with **potassium-sparing diuretics** increases risk of hyperkalemia ■ Concurrent use with **gold compounds** may increase the risk of adverse renal reactions ■ Concurrent use of oral **NSAIDs** during topical diclofenac therapy should be minimized.

**Drug-Natural Products:** ■ Increased bleeding risk with **anise, arnica, chamomile, clove, dong quai, fenugreek, feverfew, garlic, ginger, ginkgo, Panax ginseng,** and others.

## ROUTE AND DOSAGE

### ❑ Diclofenac Potassium

■ **PO (Adults):** *Analgesic/antidysmenorrheal*—100 mg initially, then 50 mg 3 times daily as needed; *rheumatoid arthritis*—50 mg 3–4 times daily, after initial resopnse reduce to lowest dose that controls symptoms (usual maintenance dose 25 mg 3 times daily); *osteoarthritis*—50 mg 2–3 times daily, after initial response reduce to lowest dose that controls symptoms; *ankylosing spondylitis*—25 mg 4–5 times daily, after initial response reduce to lowest dose that controls symptoms.

### ❑ Diclofenac Sodium

■ **PO (Adults):** *Rheumatoid arthritis*—50 mg 3–4 times daily, after initial resopnse reduce to lowest dose that controls symptoms (usual maintenance dose 25 mg 3 times daily).

■ **Topical (Adults):** Apply to lesions twice daily for 60–90 days.

---

## AVAILABILITY (generic available)

- **Diclofenac potassium immediate-release tablets:** 50 mg$^{Rx}$, 75 mg$^{Rx}$ ■ Cost: *Cataflam*—50 mg$^{Rx}$ $183.82/100 ■ **Diclofenac sodium delayed-release (enteric-coated) tablets:** 25 mg$^{Rx}$, 50 mg$^{Rx}$, 75 mg$^{Rx}$ ■ Cost: *Voltaren*—25 mg$^{Rx}$ $68.82/100, 50 mg$^{Rx}$ $134.23/100, 75 mg$^{Rx}$ $154.44/100 ■**Diclofenac sodium extended-release tablets:** {75 mg$^{Rx}$}, {100 mg$^{Rx}$} ■ **Suppositories:** {50 mg$^{Rx}$}, {100 mg$^{Rx}$} ■ **Gel:** 3% in 25- and 50-g tubes$^{Rx}$ ■ 200 mcg misoprostol (Arthrotec)$^{Rx}$. See Appendix B.

### TIME/ACTION PROFILE

|  | ONSET | PEAK | DURATION |
|---|---|---|---|
| PO (inflammation) | few days–1 wk | 2 wk or more | unknown |
| PO (pain) | 30 min | unknown | up to 8 hr |
| Topical | Unk | 30 days* | unknown |

*Complete healing of lesions following cessation of therapy.

## NURSING IMPLICATIONS

### ASSESSMENT

- **General Info:** Patients who have asthma, aspirin-induced allergy, and nasal polyps are at increased risk for developing hypersensitivity reactions.
- **Pain:** Assess pain and limitation of movement; note type, location, and intensity before and 30–60 min after administration.
- **Arthritis:** Assess arthritic pain (note type, location, intensity) and limitation of movement before and periodically during therapy.
- **Lab Test Considerations:** Diclofenac has minimal effect on bleeding time and platelet aggregation.
- ❑ May cause decreased hemoglobin, hematocrit, leukocyte, and platelet counts.
- ❑ Monitor liver function tests within 8 wk of initiating diclofenac therapy and periodically during therapy. May cause elevated serum alkaline phosphatase, LDH, AST, and ALT concentrations.
- ❑ Monitor BUN, serum creatinine, and electrolytes periodically during therapy. May cause increased BUN, serum creatinine, and electrolyte concentrations and decreased urine electrolyte concentrations.
- ❑ May cause decreased serum and increased urine uric acid concentrations.

## POTENTIAL NURSING DIAGNOSES

- Pain, acute (Indications).
- Mobility, impaired physical (Indications).

## IMPLEMENTATION

- **General:** Do not confuse Cataflam (diclofenac) with Catapres (clonidine).
- ❑ Administration in higher than recommended doses does not provide increased effectiveness but may cause increased side effects.
- **PO:** Administer after meals, with food, or with an antacid containing aluminum or magnesium to minimize gastric irritation. May take first 1–2 doses on an empty stomach for more rapid onset. Do not crush or chew enteric-coated or sustained-release tablets.
- **Dysmenorrhea:** Administer as soon as possible after the onset of menses. Prophylactic treatment has not been shown to be effective.
- **Topical:** Gel should be applied to intact skin; do not use on open wounds.

## PATIENT/FAMILY TEACHING

- **PO:** Instruct patient to take diclofenac with a full glass of water and to remain in an upright position for 15–30 min after administration. If a dose is missed, take as soon as possible within 1–2 hr if taking once or twice a day or unless almost time for next dose if taking more than twice a day. Do not double doses.
- ❑ Caution patient to avoid concurrent use of alcohol, aspirin, acetaminophen, other NSAIDs, or other OTC medications without consulting health care professional.
- ❑ May cause drowsiness or dizziness. Caution patient to avoid driving or other activities requiring alertness until response to medication is known.
- ❑ Instruct patient to notify health care professional of medication regimen before treatment or surgery.
- ❑ Caution patient to wear sunscreen and protective clothing to prevent photosensitivity reactions.
- ❑ Advise patient to consult health care professional if rash, itching, visual disturbances, tinnitus, weight gain, edema, black stools, persistent headache, or influenza-like syndrome (chills, fever, muscle aches, pain) occurs.

■ **Topical:** Advise patient to minimize use of concurrent NSAIDs during topical therapy.

## EVALUATION

**Effectiveness of therapy can be demonstrated by:** ■ Decrease in severity of mild-to-moderate pain ❑ Increased ease of joint movement. Patients who do not respond to one NSAID may respond to another. May require 2 wk or more for maximum effects.

## dicloxacillin, See PENICILLINS, PENICILLINASE RESISTANT.

## dicyclomine

(dye-**sye**-kloe-meen)

Bentyl, {Bentylol}, {Formulex}, {Spasmoban}

**CLASSIFICATION(S):**
***Therapeutic:*** *antispasmodics*
***Pharmacologic:*** *anticholinergics*

**Pregnancy Category UK**

## INDICATIONS

■ Management of irritable bowel syndrome in patients who do not respond to usual interventions (sedation/change in diet).

## ACTION

■ May have a direct and local effect on GI smooth muscle, reducing motility and tonc. **Therapeutic Effects:** ■ Decreased GI motility.

## PHARMACOKINETICS

**Absorption:** Well absorbed after oral and IM administration.

**Distribution:** Unknown.

**Metabolism and Excretion:** 80% eliminated in urine, 10% in feces.

**Half-life:** 1.8 hr (initial phase), 9–10 hr (terminal phase).

## CONTRAINDICATIONS AND PRECAUTIONS

**Contraindicated in:** ■ Hypersensitivity ■ Obstruction of the GI or GU tract ■ Reflux esopha-

gitis ■ Severe ulcerative colitis (risk of paralytic ileus) ■ Unstable cardiovascular status ■ Glaucoma ■ Myasthenia gravis ■ Infants <6 mo ■ Lactation.

**Use Cautiously in:** ■ High environmental temperatures (risk of heat prostration) ■ Hepatic/renal impairment ■ Autonomic neuropathy ■ Cardiovascular disease ■ Prostatic hyperplasia ■ Geriatric patients (increased risk of adverse reactions) ■ Pregnancy (safety not established).

## ADVERSE REACTIONS AND SIDE EFFECTS*

■ **CNS:** confusion (increased in geriatric patients), drowsiness, light-headedness (IM only) ■ **EENT:** blurred vision, increased intraocular pressure ■ **CV:** palpitations, tachycardia ■ **GI:** PARALYTIC ILEUS, constipation, heartburn, decreased salivation, dry mouth, nausea, vomiting ■ **GU:** impotence, urinary hesitancy, urinary retention ■ **Derm:** decreased sweating ■ **Endo:** decreased lactation ■ **Local:** pain/redness at IM site ■ **Misc:** allergic reactions including ANAPHYLAXIS.

## INTERACTIONS

**Drug-Drug:** ■ Additive anticholinergic effects with other **anticholinergics,** including **antihistamines, quinidine,** and **disopyramide** ■ May alter the absorption of **other orally administered drugs** by slowing motility of the GI tract ■ **Antacids** or **adsorbent antidiarrheals** decrease the absorption of anticholinergics ■ May increase GI mucosal lesions in patients taking oral **potassium chloride** tablets ■ Increased risk of adverse cardiovascular reactions with **cyclopropane** anesthesia.

## ROUTE AND DOSAGE

■ **PO (Adults):** 10–20 mg 3–4 times daily (up to 160 mg/day).

■ **PO (Children ≥2 yr):** 10 mg 3–4 times daily, adjusted as tolerated.

■ **PO (Children 6 mo–2 yr):** 5–10 mg 3–4 times daily, adjusted as tolerated.

■ **IM (Adults):** 20 mg q 4–6 hr, adjusted as tolerated.

## AVAILABILITY

■ ***Tablets:*** {10 mg$^{Rx}$}, 20 mg$^{Rx}$ ■ Cost: *Bentyl*—20 mg $42.24/100; *generic*—10 mg

---

{ } = Available in Canada only.
*CAPITALS indicates life-threatening; underlines indicate most frequent.

$7.91/30, 20 mg $7.67/30 ▪ *Capsules:* 10 mg$^{Rx}$, 20 mg$^{Rx}$ ▪ Cost: *Bentyl*—10 mg $29.58/100; *generic*—$21–$25.48 ▪ *Syrup:* 10 mg/5 ml$^{Rx}$ ▪ Cost: *Bentyl*—$32.88/480 ml ▪ *Solution for injection:* 10 mg/ml$^{Rx}$.

TIME/ACTION PROFILE (antispasmodic effect)

| | ONSET | PEAK | DURATION |
|---|---|---|---|
| PO, IM | unknown | unknown | unknown |

## NURSING IMPLICATIONS

### ASSESSMENT

❑ Assess patient for symptoms of irritable bowel syndrome (abdominal cramping, alternating constipation and diarrhea, mucus in stools) before and periodically during therapy.
❑ Assess patient routinely for abdominal distention and auscultate for bowel sounds. If constipation becomes a problem, increasing fluids and adding bulk to the diet may help alleviate the constipating effects of the drug.
❑ Monitor intake and output ratios; may cause urinary retention.
▪ *Lab Test Considerations:* Antagonizes effects of pentagastrin and histamine during the gastric acid secretion test. Avoid administration for 24 hr preceding the test.
▪ *Toxicity and Overdose:* Severe anticholinergic symptoms may be reversed with physostigmine or neostigmine.

### POTENTIAL NURSING DIAGNOSES

▪ Pain, acute (Indications).
▪ Diarrhea (Indications).

### IMPLEMENTATION

▪ **PO:** Administer dicyclomine 30 min–1 hr before meals.
▪ **IM:** Monitor patient after administration; may cause light-headedness and irritation at injection site.

### PATIENT/FAMILY TEACHING

❑ Instruct patient to take dicyclomine exactly as directed and not to take more than the prescribed amount. Missed doses should be taken as soon as remembered if not just before next dose.
❑ Medication may cause drowsiness and blurred vision. Caution patient to avoid driv-

ing or other activities requiring alertness until response to the medication is known.
❑ Inform patient that frequent oral rinses, sugarless gum or candy, and good oral hygiene may help relieve dry mouth. Consult health care professional regarding use of saliva substitute if dry mouth persists for more than 2 wk.
❑ Advise patient receiving dicyclomine to make position changes slowly to minimize the effects of drug-induced orthostatic hypotension.
❑ Caution patient to avoid extremes of temperature. This medication decreases the ability to sweat and may increase the risk of heat stroke.
❑ Advise patient to consult health care professional before taking any OTC medications concurrently with this therapy.
❑ Advise patient to notify health care professional immediately if eye pain or increased sensitivity to light occurs. Emphasize the importance of routine eye exams throughout therapy.

### EVALUATION

**Effectiveness of therapy can be demonstrated by:** ▪ A decrease in the symptoms of irritable bowel syndrome.

## didanosine

(dye-**dan**-oh-seen)
ddI, dideoxyinosine, Videx, Videx EC

### CLASSIFICATION(S):
**Therapeutic:** *antiretrovirals*
**Pharmacologic:** *nucleoside reverse transcriptase inhibitors*

### Pregnancy Category B

### INDICATIONS

▪ HIV infection (with other antiretrovirals).

### ACTION

▪ Inhibits viral replication by interfering with viral RNA-directed DNA polymerase (reverse transcriptase). Converted intracellularly by the phosphorylation process to its active form. **Therapeutic Effects:** ▪ Increase in CD4 cell counts and decreased viral load, with decreased incidence of opportunistic infections and slowed progression in HIV-infected patients.

## PHARMACOKINETICS

**Absorption:** Rapidly degrades at gastric pH. Buffers in formulation neutralize gastric acid and allow for maximal absorption (33–37%). **Distribution:** CSF levels are 21% of plasma levels in adults.

**Metabolism and Excretion:** Metabolized as a purine; 55% eliminated by the kidneys (18% as unchanged drug; urinary excretion is less in children).
**Half-life:** 1.6 hr (0.8 hr in children).

## CONTRAINDICATIONS AND PRECAUTIONS

**Contraindicated in:** ■ Hypersensitivity ■ Phenylketonuria (tablets contain aspartame) ■ Lactation ■ Concurrent use of ribavirin or allopurinol.

**Use Cautiously in:** ■ History of gout ■ Patients on sodium-restricted diets (tablets contain 264.5 mg sodium) ■ Renal impairment (dosage modification required if CCr <60 ml/min; increased risk of pancreatitis) ■ History of seizures ■ Diabetes mellitus ■ Children (increased risk of pancreatitis).

## ADVERSE REACTIONS AND SIDE EFFECTS*

■ **CNS:** SEIZURES , headache, dizziness, insomnia, lethargy, pain, weakness ■ **EENT:** rhinitis, ear pain, epistaxis, optic neuritis, parotid gland enlargement, photophobia, retinal depigmentation, sialoadenitis ■ **Resp:** cough, asthma ■ **CV:** arrhythmias, edema, hypertension, vasodilation ■ **GI:** LIVER FAILURE , PANCREATITIS , anorexia, diarrhea, liver function abnormalities, nausea, vomiting, abdominal pain, constipation, dry mouth, dyspepsia, flatulence, hepatic steatosis, stomatitis ■ **GU:** urinary frequency ■ **Derm:** alopecia, ecchymoses, rash ■ **Endo:** hyperglycemia ■ **Hemat:** granulocytopenia, anemia, bleeding, leukopenia ■ **Metab:** LACTIC ACIDOSIS , hyperlipidemia, hyperuricemia, weight loss ■ **MS:** RHABDOMYOLYSIS , arthritis, myalgia ■ **Neuro:** peripheral neuropathy, poor coordination ■ **Misc:** chills, fever, anaphylactoid reactions.

## INTERACTIONS

**Drug-Drug:** ■ **Ribavirin** and **allopurinol** ↑ levels and risk of toxicity (concurrent use not recommended) ■ Concurrent use with **ganciclovir** ↑ levels (dosage adjustments may be necessary ■ **Methadone** ↓ levels of didanosine (dose adjustments may be necessary) ■ Buffers in didanosine ↑ absorption of **ketoconazole, itraconazole, dapsone, tetracyclines,** and **fluoroquinolones** (do not administer within 2 hr of didanosine) ■ ↑ risk of peripheral neuropathy **isoniazid, phenytoin, zalcitabine, stavudine, ethambutol,** and **chloramphenicol** (use cautiously) ■ ↑ risk of pancreatitis with other **alcohol, thiazide diuretics, IV pentamidine, tetracyclines** (use with extreme caution) ■ ↑ risk of bone marrow depression with other **drugs causing bone marrow depression** ■ Concurrent **stavudine** during pregnancy ↑ the risk of fetal lactic acidosis.

**Drug-Food:** ■ Administration **food** decreases absorption by 50%.

## ROUTE AND DOSAGE

When tablets are used, adults and children >1 yr should receive 2 tablets/dose to ensure adequate buffering. Children <1 yr may receive 1 tablet. Tablets and buffered powder are not interchangeable because of differences in bioavailabilty. Twice-daily dosing is preferred in children.

■ **PO (Adults ≥60 kg):** *Tablets*—200 mg bid; *Videx EC capsules*—400 mg once daily; *buffered powder packets*—250 mg bid.

■ **PO (Adults <60 kg):** *Tablets*—125 mg bid; *Videx EC Capsules*—250 mg once daily; *buffered powder packets*—167 mg q 12 hr.

■ **PO (Children):** *Tablets*—90–120 mg/m² q 12 hr; *buffered powder packets*—112.5–150 mg/m² q 12 hr.

■ **PO (Children with BSA 1.1–1.4 m²):** *Tablets*—100 mg q 12 hr; *reconstituted pediatric powder*—125 mg q 12 hr.

■ **PO (Children with BSA 0.8–1 m²):** *Tablets*—75 mg q 12 hr; *reconstituted pediatric powder*—94 mg q 12 hr.

- **PO (Children with BSA 0.5–0.7 m²):** *Tablets*—50 mg q 12 hr; *reconstituted pediatric powder*—62 mg q 12 hr.
- **PO (Children with BSA <0.4 m²):** *Tablets*—25 mg q 12 hr; *reconstituted pediatric powder*—31 mg q 12 hr.

❏ **Renal Impairment**

- **PO (Adults >60 kg):** *CCr 30–59 ml/min*—*Tablets*—100 mg q 12 hr; *Videx EC Capsules*—200 mg once daily; *buffered powder packets*—100 mg q 12 hr; *CCr 10–29 ml/min*—*Tablets*—150 mg q 24 hr; *Videx EC Capsules*—125 mg once daily; *buffered powder packets*—167 mg q 24 hr; *CCr <10 ml/min*—*Tablets*—100 mg q 24 hr; *Videx EC Capsules*—125 mg once daily; *buffered powder packets*—100 mg q 24 hr.
- **PO (Adults <60 kg):** *CCr 30–59 ml/min*—*Tablets*—75 mg q 12 hr; *Videx EC Capsules*—125 mg once daily; *buffered powder packets*—100 mg q 12 hr; *CCr 10–29 ml/min*—*Tablets*—100 mg q 24 hr; *Videx EC Capsules*—125 mg once daily; *buffered powder packets*—100 mg q 24 hr; *CCr <10 ml/min*—*Tablets*—75 mg q 24 hr; *buffered powder packets*—100 mg q 24 hr.

## AVAILABILITY

■ *Chewable/dispersible buffered tablets:* 25 mg^Rx, 50 mg^Rx, 100 mg^Rx, 150 mg^Rx ■ *Buffered powder packets for oral solution (sweetened):* 100 mg^Rx, 167 mg^Rx, 250 mg^Rx, 375 mg^Rx ■ *Delayed-release capsules (with enteric-coated beadlets):* 125 mg^Rx, 200 mg^Rx, 250 mg^Rx, 400 mg^Rx ■ *Pediatric powder for oral solution (requires reconstitution):* 10 mg/ml^Rx, 20 mg/ml^Rx.

TIME/ACTION PROFILE (retroviral plasma levels)

| | ONSET | PEAK | DURATION |
|---|---|---|---|
| PO | unknown | 0.25–1.5 hr | 12 hr |

# NURSING IMPLICATIONS

## ASSESSMENT

- ❏ Monitor patient for change in severity of HIV symptoms and for symptoms of opportunistic infection before and throughout therapy.
- ❏ Monitor patient for peripheral neuropathy (distal numbness, tingling, or pain in feet or hands) throughout therapy. Dose may need to be decreased.
- ❏ Monitor patient for symptoms of pancreatitis (abdominal pain, nausea, vomiting, increased amylase, lipase, or triglyceride concentrations). If amylase is elevated 1.5–2 times the normal limit and/or the patient has symptoms of pancreatitis, didanosine should be discontinued. Pancreatitis may be fatal.
- ■ *Lab Test Considerations:* Monitor viral load and CD4 count before and routinely during therapy to determine response.
- ❏ Monitor CBC, hepatic function, and uric acid concentrations throughout therapy. May cause leukopenia, granulocytopenia, thrombocytopenia, and anemia. May cause elevated AST, ALT, alkaline phosphatase, bilirubin, uric acid, amylase, lipase, and triglyceride concentrations. Lactic acidosis may occur with hepatic toxicity causing hepatic steatosis; may be fatal, especially in women.
- ❏ May cause hyperglycemia.
- ❏ Monitor serum potassium concentrations routinely. Diarrhea from buffer may cause a decrease in serum potassium concentrations.

## POTENTIAL NURSING DIAGNOSES

- ■ Infection, risk for (Indications, Side Effects).
- ■ Injury, risk for (Side Effects).

## IMPLEMENTATION

- ■ **General:** Commonly identified by abbreviation "ddI," but generic and brand names should be used when ordering to prevent errors.
- ❏ If diarrhea develops in patients taking buffered powder for oral solution, chewable/dispersible buffered tablets may cause less diarrhea.
- ❏ If solution or powder spills or leaks, a wet mop or damp sponge should be used for cleaning to avoid generation of dust. Clean surface with soap and water as needed.
- ■ **PO:** Administer every 12 hr on an empty stomach, 30 min before or 2 hr after meals. Do not administer ketoconazole, dapsone, tetracyclines, or fluoroquinolones within 2 hr (6 hr for ciprofloxacin) of didanosine.
- ❏ Tablets should be chewed thoroughly, manually crushed, or dispersed in at least 1 oz water before administration. To disperse, add 1 or 2 tablets to at least 1 oz water and stir until a uniform dispersion forms. Dispersion should be taken immediately.

□ Buffered powder for oral solution should be mixed in at least 4 oz water; do not mix with fruit juice or other acid-containing liquid. Stir 2–3 min until the powder dissolves completely. Solution should be taken immediately.

□ Solution for pediatric use is mixed by pharmacist and is stable for 30 days if refrigerated. Shake admixture immediately before administering.

## PATIENT/FAMILY TEACHING

□ Instruct patient on the importance of taking didanosine exactly as directed, even if feeling better. Caution patient not to share or trade this medication with others.

□ May cause dizziness. Caution patient to avoid driving or other activities requiring alertness until response to medication is known.

□ Inform patient that didanosine may cause hyperglycemia. Advise patient to notify health care professional if increased thirst or hunger; unexplained weight loss; increased urination; fatigue; or dry, itchy skin occurs.

□ Advise patient to consult health care professional before taking other medications concurrently with didanosine.

□ Caution patient to avoid crowds and persons with known infections.

□ Advise patient to notify health care professional immediately if numbness or tingling of the hands or feet, stomach pain, nausea, or vomiting occurs.

□ Caution patient to use a condom to prevent transmission of HIV and not to share needles with anyone.

□ Children should have dilated retinal exams every 3–6 mo or if there is a change in vision throughout therapy.

□ Emphasize the importance of regular exams to monitor for side effects.

## EVALUATION

**Effectiveness of therapy can be demonstrated by:** ■Decreased incidence of opportunistic infection and slowed progression of HIV infection.

# diflorasone, See CORTICOSTEROIDS (TOPICAL/LOCAL).

**High Alert**

# digoxin
(di-**jox**-in)
Digitek, Lanoxicaps, Lanoxin

## CLASSIFICATION(S):
*Therapeutic: antiarrhythmics, inotropics*
*Pharmacologic: digitalis glycosides*

**Pregnancy Category C**

## INDICATIONS
■ Treatment of CHF ■ Tachyarrhythmias □ Atrial fibrillation and atrial flutter (slows ventricular rate) □ Paroxysmal atrial tachycardia.

## ACTION
■ Increases the force of myocardial contraction ■ Prolongs refractory period of the AV node ■ Decreases conduction through the SA and AV nodes. **Therapeutic Effects:** ■ Increased cardiac output (positive inotropic effect) and slowing of the heart rate (negative chronotropic effect).

## PHARMACOKINETICS
**Absorption:** 60–85% absorbed after oral administration of tablets; 75–80% absorbed after administration of elixir. Absorption from liquid-filled capsules is 90–100%; 80% absorbed from IM sites, but this route is not recommended because of extreme pain and irritation.
**Distribution:** Widely distributed; crosses the placenta and enters breast milk.
**Metabolism and Excretion:** Excreted almost entirely unchanged by the kidneys.
**Half-life:** 36–48 hr (increased in renal impairment).

## CONTRAINDICATIONS AND PRECAUTIONS
**Contraindicated in:** ■ Hypersensitivity ■ Uncontrolled ventricular arrhythmias ■ AV block ■

Idiopathic hypertrophic subaortic stenosis ■ Constrictive pericarditis ■ Known alcohol intolerance (elixir only).

**Use Cautiously in:** ■ Electrolyte abnormalities (hypokalemia, hypercalcemia, and hypomagnesemia may predispose to toxicity) ■ Geriatric patients (very sensitive to toxic effects) ■ MI ■ Renal impairment (dosage reduction required) ■ Obese patients (dose should be based on ideal body weight) ■ Pregnancy and lactation (although safety has not been established, has been used during pregnancy without adverse effects on the fetus).

## ADVERSE REACTIONS AND SIDE EFFECTS*

■ **CNS:** fatigue, headache, weakness ■ **EENT:** blurred vision, yellow vision ■ **CV:** ARRHYTHMIAS, bradycardia, ECG changes ■ **GI:** anorexia, nausea, vomiting, diarrhea ■ **Endo:** gynecomastia ■ **Hemat:** thrombocytopenia.

## INTERACTIONS

**Drug-Drug:** ■ **Thiazide** and **loop diuretics, mezlocillin, piperacillin, ticarcillin, amphotericin B,** and **corticosteroids,** which cause hypokalemia, may increase the risk of toxicity ■ Excessive use of **laxatives** may also cause hypokalemia and increase the risk of digoxin toxicity ■ **Quinidine, quinine, cyclosporine, amiodarone, verapamil, diltiazem, propafenone,** and **diclofenac** increase serum levels and may lead to toxicity (serum level monitoring/dosage reduction recommended) ■ **Spironolactone** increases halflife (reduced dosage/increased dosing interval may be required) ■ Additive bradycardia may occur with **beta blockers** and other **antiarrhythmics (quinidine, disopyramide)** ■ Absorption is decreased by concurrent **antacids, kaolin/pectin, cholestyramine,** or **colestipol** ■ **Thyroid hormones** may decrease therapeutic effects.

**Drug-Natural Products:** ■ **Licorice** and stimulant natural products (**aloe**) may increase the risk of potassium depletion ■ **St. John's wort** may decrease digoxin levels and effect.

**Drug-Food:** ■ Concurrent ingestion of a **high-fiber meal** may decrease absorption.

## ROUTE AND DOSAGE

For rapid effect, a larger initial loading/digitalizing dose should be given in several divided doses over 12–24 hr. Maintenance doses are determined for digoxin by renal function. All dosing must be evaluated by individual response. In general, doses required for atrial arrhythmias are higher than those for inotropic effect. When determining dosage, consider that bioavailability of gelatin capsules (Lanoxicaps) is greater than that of tablets.

■ **IV (Adults):** *Digitalizing dose*—0.6–1 mg (10–15 mcg/kg) given as 50% of the dose initially and additional fractions given at 4–8-hr intervals.

■ **IV (Children >10 yr):** *Digitalizing dose*—8–12 mcg/kg given as 50% of the dose initially and additional fractions given at 4–8-hr intervals.

■ **IV (Children 5–10 yr):** *Digitalizing dose*—15–30 mcg/kg given as 50% of the dose initially and additional fractions given at 4–8-hr intervals.

■ **IV (Children 2–5 yr):** *Digitalizing dose*—25–35 mcg/kg given as 50% of the dose initially and additional fractions given at 4–8-hr intervals.

■ **IV (Children 1–24 mo):** *Digitalizing dose*—30–50 mcg/kg given as 50% of the dose initially and additional fractions given at 4–8-hr intervals.

■ **IV (Infants—full term):** 20–30 mcg/kg given as 50% of the dose initially and additional fractions given at 4–8-hr intervals.

■ **IV (Infants—premature):** *Digitalizing dose*—15–25 mcg/kg given as 50% of the dose initially and additional fractions given at 4–8-hr intervals.

■ **PO (Adults):** *Digitalizing dose*—0.75–1.25 mg (10–15 mg/kg) given as 50% of the dose initially and additional fractions given at 4–8-hr intervals. *Maintenance dose*—0.063–0.5 mg/day as tablets or 0.350–0.5 mg/day as gelatin capsules, depending on patient's lean body weight, renal function, and serum level.

■ **PO (Adults):** Maintenance dose = Loading dose × (daily loss/100); where percentage of daily loss = 14+ (CCr/5). CCr should be corrected to 70 kg body weight or 1.73 m².

■ **PO (Children >10 yr):** *Digitalizing dose*—10–15 mcg/kg given as 50% of the dose initially and additional fractions given at 6–8-hr intervals. *Maintenance dose*—25–35% of the loading dose given daily as a single dose.

- **PO (Children 5–10 yr):** *Digitalizing dose*—20–35 mcg/kg given as 50% of the dose initially and additional fractions given at 6–8-hr intervals . *Maintenance dose*—25–35% of the loading dose given daily in 2 divided doses.

- **PO (Children 2–5 yr):** *Digitalizing dose*—30–40 mcg/kg given as 50% of the dose initially and additional fractions given at 6–8-hr intervals. *Maintenance dose*—25–35% of the loading dose given daily in 2 divided doses.

- **PO (Children 1–24 mo):** *Digitalizing dose*—35–60 mcg/kg given as 50% of the dose initially and additional fractions given at 6–8-hr intervals. *Maintenance dose*—25–35% of the loading dose given daily in 2 divided doses.

- **PO (Infants—full term):** *Digitalizing dose*—25–35 mcg/kg given as 50% of the dose initially and additional fractions given at 6–8-hr intervals. *Maintenance dose*—25–35% of the loading dose given daily in 2 divided doses.

- **PO (Infants—premature):** *Digitalizing dose*—20–30 mcg/kg given as 50% of the dose initially and additional fractions given at 6–8-hr intervals. *Maintenance dose*—20–30% of the loading dose given daily in 2 divided doses.

### AVAILABILITY

■ *Tablets:* 0.125 mg$^{Rx}$, 0.25 mg$^{Rx}$, 0.5 mg$^{Rx}$ ■ Cost: *Lanoxin*—0.125 mg $21.32/100, 0.25 mg $21.32/100; *generic*—$8.79/100 ■ *Capsules:* 0.05 mg$^{Rx}$, 0.1 mg$^{Rx}$, 0.2 mg$^{Rx}$ ■ *Pediatric elixir (lime flavor):* 0.05 mg/ml$^{Rx}$ ■ *Injection:* 0.25 mg/ml$^{Rx}$ ■ *Pediatric injection:* 0.1 mg/ml$^{Rx}$.

TIME/ACTION PROFILE (antiarrhythmic or inotropic effects, provided that a loading dose has been given)

| | ONSET | PEAK | DURATION |
|---|---|---|---|
| Digoxin–PO | 30–120 min | 2–6 hr | 2–4 days† |
| Digoxin–IM | 30 min | 4–6 hr | 2–4 days† |
| Digoxin–IV | 5–30 min | 1–5 hr | 2–4 days† |

†Duration listed is that for normal renal function; in impaired renal function, duration will be longer.

## NURSING IMPLICATIONS

### ASSESSMENT

❑ Monitor apical pulse for 1 full min before administering. Withhold dose and notify physician if pulse rate is <60 bpm in an adult, <70 bpm in a child, or <90 bpm in an infant. Also notify physician or health care professional promptly of any significant changes in rate, rhythm, or quality of pulse.

❑ Monitor blood pressure periodically in patients receiving IV digoxin.

❑ Monitor ECG throughout IV administration and periodically during therapy. Notify physician or health care professional if bradycardia or new arrhythmias occur.

❑ Observe IV site for redness or infiltration; extravasation can lead to tissue irritation and sloughing.

❑ Monitor intake and output ratios and daily weights. Assess for peripheral edema, and auscultate lungs for rales/crackles throughout therapy.

❑ Before administering initial loading dose, determine whether patient has taken any digitalis preparations in the preceding 2–3 wk.

■ *Lab Test Considerations:* Serum electrolyte levels (especially potassium, magnesium, and calcium) and renal and hepatic functions should be evaluated periodically during therapy. Notify physician or other health care professional before giving dose if patient is hypokalemic. Hypokalemia, hypomagnesemia, or hypercalcemia may make the patient more susceptible to digitalis toxicity.

■ *Toxicity and Overdose:* Therapeutic serum digoxin levels range from 0.5–2 ng/ml. Serum levels may be drawn 4–10 hr after a dose is administered, although they are usually drawn immediately before the next dose.

❑ Observe patient for signs and symptoms of toxicity. In adults and older children, the first signs of toxicity usually include abdominal pain, anorexia, nausea, vomiting, visual disturbances, bradycardia, and other arrhythmias. In infants and small children, the first symptoms of overdose are usually cardiac arrhythmias. If these appear, withhold drug and notify physician or health care professional immediately.

▫ If signs of toxicity occur and are not severe, discontinuation of digitalis glycoside may be all that is required.

▫ If hypokalemia is present and renal function is adequate, potassium salts may be administered. Do not administer if hyperkalemia or heart block exists.

▫ Correction of arrhythmias resulting from digitalis toxicity may be attempted with lidocaine, procainamide, quinidine, propranolol, or phenytoin. Temporary ventricular pacing may be useful in advanced heart block.

▫ Treatment of life-threatening arrhythmias may include administration of digoxin immune Fab (Digibind), which binds to the digitalis glycoside molecule in the blood and is excreted by the kidneys.

## POTENTIAL NURSING DIAGNOSES

■ Cardiac output, decreased (Indications).

## IMPLEMENTATION

▫ **High Alert:** Digoxin has a narrow therapeutic range. Medication errors associated with digoxin include miscalculation of pediatric dosages and insufficient monitoring of digoxin levels in chronic or subacute use. Have second practitioner independently check original order and dose calculations. Monitor therapeutic drug levels.

■ **General:** For rapid digitalization, the initial dose is higher than the maintenance dose; 25–50% of the total digitalizing dose is given initially. The remainder of the dose will be administered in 25% increments at 4–8 hr intervals.

▫ When changing from parenteral to oral dosage forms, dosage adjustments may be necessary because of pharmacokinetic variations in percentage of digoxin absorbed: 100 mcg (0.1 mg) digoxin injection or 100 mcg (0.1 mg) liquid-filled capsule = 125 mcg (0.125 mg) tablet or 125 mcg (0.125 mg) of elixir.

■ **PO:** Oral preparations can be administered without regard to meals. Tablets can be crushed and administered with food or fluids if patient has difficulty swallowing. Use calibrated measuring device for liquid preparations. Do not alternate between dosage forms; bioavailability of capsules is not equal to that of tablets or elixir.

■ **IM:** Administer deep into gluteal muscle and massage well to reduce painful local reactions. Do not administer more than 2 ml of digoxin in each IM site. IM administration is not generally recommended.

■ **Direct IV:** IV doses may be given undiluted or each 1 ml may be diluted in 4 ml of sterile water, 0.9% NaCl, D5W, or LR for injection. Less diluent will cause precipitation. Use diluted solution immediately. Do not use solution that is discolored or contains precipitate.

■ *Rate:* Administer each dose through Y-site injection over a minimum of 5 min.

■ **Syringe Compatibility:** ◆ heparin ◆ milrinone.

■ **Y-Site Compatibility:** ◆ ciprofloxacin ◆ cisatracurium ◆ diltiazem ◆ famotidine ◆ gatifloxacin ◆ linezolid ◆ meperidine ◆ meropenem ◆ midazolam ◆ milrinone ◆ morphine ◆ potassium chloride ◆ remifentanil ◆ tacrolimus ◆ vitamin B complex with C.

■ **Y-Site Incompatibility:** ◆ amphotericin B cholesteryl sulfate ◆ fluconazole ◆ foscarnet. ◆ propofol.

■ **Additive Incompatibility:** Manufacturer recommends that digoxin not be admixed with other drugs.

## PATIENT/FAMILY TEACHING

▫ Instruct patient to take medication exactly as directed, at the same time each day. Missed doses should be taken within 12 hr of scheduled dose or not taken at all. Do not double doses. Consult health care professional if doses for 2 or more days are missed. Do not discontinue medication without consulting health care professional.

▫ Teach patient to take pulse and to contact health care professional before taking medication if pulse rate is <60 or >100.

▫ Review signs and symptoms of digitalis toxicity with patient and family. Advise patient to notify health care professional immediately if these or symptoms of CHF occur. Inform patient that these symptoms may be mistaken for those of colds or flu.

▫ Instruct patient to keep digoxin tablets in their original container and not to mix in pill boxes with other medications; they may look similar to and may be mistaken for other medications.

▫ Advise patient that sharing of this medication can be dangerous.

▫ Caution patient to avoid concurrent use of OTC and herbal medications without consulting health care professional. Advise patient to avoid taking antacids or antidiarrheals within 2 hr of digoxin.

◻ Advise patient to notify health care professional of this medication regimen before treatment.

◻ Patients taking digoxin should carry identification describing disease process and medication regimen at all times.

◻ *High Alert:* Emphasize the importance of routine follow-up exams to determine effectiveness and to monitor for toxicity.

### EVALUATION

**Effectiveness of therapy can be demonstrated by:** ■ Decrease in severity of CHF ■ Increase in cardiac output ■ Decrease in ventricular response in atrial tachyarrhythmias ■ Termination of paroxysmal atrial tachycardia.

---

## digoxin immune Fab

(di-**jox**-in im-**myoon**fab)

Digibind, DigiFab

### CLASSIFICATION(S):

***Therapeutic:*** *antidotes*
***Pharmacologic:*** *antibody fragments*

### Pregnancy Category C

### INDICATIONS

■ Serious life-threatening overdosage with digoxin.

### ACTION

■ An antibody produced in sheep that binds antigenically to unbound digoxin in serum. **Therapeutic Effects:** ■ Binding and subsequent removal of digoxin, preventing toxic effects in overdose.

### PHARMACOKINETICS

**Absorption:** Administered IV only, resulting in complete bioavailability.

**Distribution:** Widely distributed throughout extracellular space.

**Metabolism and Excretion:** Excreted by the kidneys as the bound complex (digoxin immune Fab plus digoxin).

**Half-life:** 14–20 hr.

### CONTRAINDICATIONS AND PRECAUTIONS

**Contraindicated in:** ■ No known contraindications.

**Use Cautiously in:** ■ Known hypersensitivity to sheep proteins or products ■ Children, pregnancy, or lactation (safety not established).

### ADVERSE REACTIONS AND SIDE EFFECTS*

■ **CV:** re-emergence of atrial fibrillation, re-emergence of CHF ■ **F and E:** HYPOKALEMIA.

### INTERACTIONS

**Drug-Drug:** ■ Prevents therapeutic response to **digoxin**.

### ROUTE AND DOSAGE

*Digibind*—38 mg of digoxin immune Fab will bind 0.5 mg of digoxin. Each vial contains 38 mg of digoxin immune Fab; *DigiFab*—40 mg of digoxin immune Fab will bind 0.5 mg of digoxin. Each vial contains 40 mg of digoxin immune Fab.

◻ **Known Amount of Digoxin Ingested (Administered)**

■ **IV (Adults and Children):** *For digitalis glycoside toxicity due to digoxin tablets, oral solution, or IM digoxin*—dose of digoxin ingested (mg) × 0.8/1000 × 38. *For digitalis glycoside toxicity due to digoxin capsules, IV digoxin*—dose of digoxin ingested (mg)/0.5 × 38.

◻ **Known Serum Digoxin Concentrations (SDCs)**

■ **IV (Adults and Children):** *Digibind*—Dose (mg)=SDC (nanograms/ml) × body weight (kg)/100 × 38; *DigiFab*—SDC (nanograms/ml) × body weight (kg)/100 × 40.

◻ **Unknown Amount Ingested/SDCs Unavailable**

■ **IV (Adults and Children):** *Digibind*—760 mg (20 vials); *DigiFab*—800 mg (20 vials).

---

{ } = Available in Canada only.
*CAPITALS indicates life-threatening; underlines indicate most frequent.

□ **Toxicity during chronic digoxin therapy**
■ **IV (Adults and Children):** *Digibind*—228 mg (6 vials); *DigiFab*—240 mg (6 vials).

## AVAILABILITY

■ *Powder for injection, lyophilized (Digibind):* 38 mg/vial[Rx] ■ *Powder for injection, lyophilized (DigiFab):* 40 mg/vial[Rx].

TIME/ACTION PROFILE (reversal of arrhythmias and hyperkalemia; reversal of inotropic effect may take several hr)

| | ONSET | PEAK | DURATION |
|---|---|---|---|
| IV | 30 min (variable) | unknown | 2–6 hr |

## NURSING IMPLICATIONS

### ASSESSMENT

□ Monitor ECG, pulse, blood pressure, and body temperature before and during treatment. Patients with atrial fibrillation may develop a rapid ventricular response as a result of decreased digoxin levels.

□ Assess patient for increase in signs of CHF (peripheral edema, dyspnea, rales/crackles, weight gain).

■ *Lab Test Considerations:* Monitor serum digoxin levels before administration.

□ Monitor serum potassium levels frequently during treatment. Before treatment, hyperkalemia usually coexists with toxicity. Levels may decrease rapidly; hypokalemia should be treated promptly.

□ Free serum digoxin levels fall rapidly after administration. Total serum concentrations rise suddenly after administration but are bound to the Fab molecule and are inactive. Total serum concentrations will decrease to undetectable levels within several days. Serum digoxin levels are not valid for 5–7 days after administration.

### POTENTIAL NURSING DIAGNOSES

■ Knowledge, deficient, related to medication regimen (Patient/Family Teaching).

### IMPLEMENTATION

■ **General:** Cardiopulmonary resuscitation equipment and medications should be available during administration.

□ Delay redigitalization for several days until the elimination of digoxin immune Fab from the body is complete.

■ **Intermittent Infusion:** Reconstitute each vial in 4 ml of sterile water for injection and mix gently. Solution will contain a concentration of 9.5 mg/ml (Digibind) or 10 mg/ml (DigiFab). May be further diluted with 0.9% NaCl for IV infusion. Reconstituted solution should be used immediately but is stable for 4 hr if refrigerated.

□ In infants and small children, monitor for fluid overload. For small doses, a reconstituted 38-mg vial can be diluted with 34 ml of 0.9% NaCl (Digibind) or 36 ml of 0.9% NaCl (DigiFab) for a concentration of 1 mg/ml. Administer with a tuberculin syringe.

■ *Rate:* Administer reconstituted solution by IV infusion through a 0.22-micron membrane filter over 15–30 min. If cardiac arrest is imminent, rapid direct IV injection may be used. Do not use rapid direct injection in other patients because of increased risk of adverse reactions.

■ **Incompatibility:** Information unavailable. Do not mix with other drugs or solutions.

### PATIENT/FAMILY TEACHING

□ Explain the procedure and purpose of the treatment to the patient.

□ Instruct patient notify health care provider immediately if signs of delayed allergic reaction (rash, pruritus, urticaria) occur after hospital discharge.

### EVALUATION

**Effectiveness of therapy can be demonstrated by:** ■ Resolution of signs and symptoms of digoxin toxicity □ Decreased digoxin or level without major side effects.

## dihydrotachysterol, See VITAMIN D COMPOUNDS.

# diltiazem

(dil-**tye**-a-zem)

{Apo-Diltiaz}, Cardizem, Cardizem LA, CartiaXT, Dilacor XR, Diltia XT, {Novo-Diltiazem}, Nu-Diltiaz, {Syn-Diltiazem}, Tiamate, Tiazac

*CLASSIFICATION(S):*
*Therapeutic: antianginals, antiarrhythmics (class IV), antihypertensives*
*Pharmacologic: calcium channel blockers*
**Pregnancy Category C**

## INDICATIONS

■ □ Hypertension □ Angina pectoris and vasospastic (Prinzmetal's) angina □ Supraventricular tachyarrhythmias and rapid ventricular rates in atrial flutter or fibrillation. **Unlabeled uses:** ■ Management of Raynaud's syndrome.

## ACTION

■ Inhibits transport of calcium into myocardial and vascular smooth muscle cells, resulting in inhibition of excitation-contraction coupling and subsequent contraction. **Therapeutic Effects:** ■ Systemic vasodilation resulting in decreased blood pressure ■ Coronary vasodilation resulting in decreased frequency and severity of attacks of angina ■ Suppression of arrhythmias.

## PHARMACOKINETICS

**Absorption:** Well absorbed, but rapidly metabolized after oral administration.
**Distribution:** Unknown.
**Protein Binding:** 70–80%.
**Metabolism and Excretion:** Mostly metabolized by the liver (CYP 3A4 enzyme system).
**Half-life:** 3.5–9 hr.

## CONTRAINDICATIONS AND PRECAUTIONS

**Contraindicated in:** ■ Hypersensitivity ■ Sick sinus syndrome ■ 2nd- or 3rd-degree AV block (unless an artificial pacemaker is in place) ■ Blood pressure <90 mmHg ■ Recent MI or pulmonary congestion ■ Concurrent use of rifampin.
**Use Cautiously in:** ■ Severe hepatic impairment ( ↓ dose recommended) ■ Geriatric patients ( ↓ dose/slower IV infusion rate recommended; ↑ risk of hypotension; consider age-related decrease in body mass, decreased hepatic/renal/cardiac function, concurrent drug therapy and other disease states) ■ Severe renal impairment ■ Serious ventricular arrhythmias or CHF ■ Pregnancy, lactation, or children (safety not established).

## ADVERSE REACTIONS AND SIDE EFFECTS*

■ **CNS:** abnormal dreams, anxiety, confusion, dizziness, drowsiness, headache, nervousness, psychiatric disturbances, weakness ■ **EENT:** blurred vision, disturbed equilibrium, epistaxis, tinnitus ■ **Resp:** cough, dyspnea ■ **CV:** ARRHYTHMIAS, CHF, peripheral edema, bradycardia, chest pain, hypotension, palpitations, syncope, tachycardia ■ **GI:** abnormal liver function studies, anorexia, constipation, diarrhea, dry mouth, dysgeusia, dyspepsia, nausea, vomiting ■ **GU:** dysuria, nocturia, polyuria, sexual dysfunction, urinary frequency ■ **Derm:** dermatitis, erythema multiforme, flushing, increased sweating, photosensitivity, pruritus/urticaria, rash ■ **Endo:** gynecomastia, hyperglycemia ■ **Hemat:** anemia, leukopenia, thrombocytopenia ■ **Metab:** weight gain ■ **MS:** joint stiffness, muscle cramps ■ **Neuro:** paresthesia, tremor ■ **Misc:** STEVENS-JOHNSON SYNDROME, gingival hyperplasia.

## INTERACTIONS

**Drug-Drug:** ■ ↑ hypotension may occur when used with **fentanyl**, other **antihypertensives, nitrates,** acute ingestion of **alcohol,** or **quinidine** ■ Antihypertensive effects may be ↓ by **NSAIDs** ■ Serum **digoxin** levels may be increased ■ Concurrent use with **beta blockers, digoxin, disopyramide,** or **phenytoin** may result in bradycardia, conduction defects, or CHF ■ **Phenobarbital** and **phenytoin** may ↑ metabolism and ↓ effectiveness ■ May ↓ metabolism of and ↑ risk of toxicity from **cyclosporine, quinidine,** or **carbamazepine** ■ **Cimetidine** and **ranitidine** ↑ blood levels and effects ■ May increase or decrease the effects of **lithium** or **theophylline.**
**Drug-Food:** ■ **Grapefruit juice** increases serum levels and effect.

## ROUTE AND DOSAGE

■ **PO (Adults):** 30–120 mg 3–4 times daily or 60–120 mg twice daily as SR capsules or 180–240 mg once daily as CD or XR capsules or LA tablets (up to 360 mg/day).

■ **IV (Adults):** 0.25 mg/kg; may repeat in 15 min with a dose of 0.35 mg/kg. May follow with continuous infusion at 10 mg/hr (range 5–15 mg/hr) for up to 24 hr.

## AVAILABILITY (generic available)

■ *Tablets:* 30 mg$^{Rx}$, 60 mg$^{Rx}$, 90 mg$^{Rx}$, 120 mg$^{Rx}$ ■ Cost: *generic*—30 mg $40.73/100; 60 mg $65.70/100; 90 mg $89.46/100; 120 mg $116.34/100 ■ *Extended (sustained)-release capsules:* 60 mg$^{Rx}$, 90 mg$^{Rx}$, 120 mg$^{Rx}$, 180 mg$^{Rx}$, 240 mg$^{Rx}$, 300 mg$^{Rx}$, 360 mg$^{Rx}$, 420 mg$^{Rx}$ ■ Cost: *Cardizem CD*—120 mg $119.81/90, 180 mg $144.58/90, 240 mg $205.10/90, 300 mg $265.82/90; *Dilacor XR*—120 mg $107.71/100, 180 mg $126.82/100, 240 mg $144.46/100; *Tiazac*—120 mg $95.86/90, 180 mg $115.58/90, 240 mg $164.15/90, 300 mg $212.66/90, 360 mg $216.77/90, 420 mg $227.19/90 ■ *Extended-release tablets (Cardizem LA):* 120 mg$^{Rx}$, 180 mg$^{Rx}$, 240 mg$^{Rx}$, 300 mg$^{Rx}$, 360 mg$^{Rx}$, 420 mg$^{Rx}$ ■ *Injection:* 5 mg/ml in 10-ml vials$^{Rx}$, 25 mg ready-to-use syringes (Lyo-Ject)$^{Rx}$ ■ enalapril (Teczem$^{Rx}$). See Appendix B.

TIME/ACTION PROFILE

|  | ONSET | PEAK | DURATION |
|---|---|---|---|
| PO | 30 min | 2–3 hr | 6–8 hr |
| PO–SR | unknown | unknown | 12 hr |
| PO–CD, XR, LA | unknown | 14 days† | up to 24 hr |
| IV | 2–5 min | 2–4 hr | unknown |

†Maximum antihypertensive effect with chronic therapy.

# NURSING IMPLICATIONS

## ASSESSMENT

■ **General Info:** Monitor blood pressure and pulse before therapy, during dose titration, and periodically during therapy. Monitor ECG periodically during prolonged therapy. May cause prolonged PR interval.

❏ Monitor intake and output ratios and daily weight. Assess for signs of CHF (peripheral edema, rales/crackles, dyspnea, weight gain, jugular venous distention).

❏ Monitor frequency of prescription refills to determine adherence.

❏ Patients receiving digoxin concurrently with calcium channel blockers should have routine serum digoxin levels checked and be monitored for signs and symptoms of digoxin toxicity.

■ **Angina:** Assess location, duration, intensity, and precipitating factors of patient's anginal pain.

■ **Arrhythmias:** Monitor ECG continuously during administration. Report bradycardia or prolonged hypotension promptly. Emergency equipment and medication should be available. Monitor blood pressure and pulse before and frequently during administration.

■ **Lab Test Considerations:** Total serum calcium concentrations are not affected by calcium channel blockers.

❏ Monitor serum potassium periodically. Hypokalemia ↑ the risk of arrhythmias and should be corrected.

❏ Monitor renal and hepatic functions periodically during long-term therapy. May cause ↑ in hepatic enzymes after several days of therapy, which return to normal on discontinuation of therapy.

## POTENTIAL NURSING DIAGNOSES

■ Pain, acute (Indications).

■ Cardiac output, decreased (Adverse Reactions).

## IMPLEMENTATION

■ **General:** Do not confuse Cardizem (diltiazem) with Cardene (nicardipine). Do not confuse Cardizem LA with Cardene SR. Do not confuse Tiazac (diltiazem) with Ziac (bisprolol/hydrochlorothiazide).

■ **PO:** May be administered without regard to meals. May be administered with meals if GI irritation becomes a problem.

❏ Do not open, crush, break, or chew sustained-release capsules or tablets. Empty tablets that appear in stool are not significant. Crush and mix diltiazem with food or fluids for patients having difficulty swallowing.

■ **Direct IV:** May be administered undiluted.

■ *Rate:* Administer each dose as a bolus over 2 min.

■ **Continuous Infusion:** Dilute 125 mg in 100 ml, 250 mg in 250 ml, or 250 mg in 500 ml of 0.9% NaCl, D5W, or D5/0.45% NaCl for concentrations of 1 mg/ml, 0.83 mg/ml, or 0.45 mg/ml, respectively. Solution is stable for 24 hr at room temperature or if refrigerated.

■ *Rate:* Initial infusion should be administered at a rate of 10 mg/hr. May increase in increments of 5 mg/hr, up to 15 mg/hr if further reduction in heart rate is required. Some patients may respond to a rate of 5 mg/hr. Infusion may be continued up to 24 hr.

■ **Y-Site Compatibility:** ♦ albumin ♦ amikacin ♦ amphotericin B ♦ aztreonam ♦ bretylium ♦ bumetanide ♦ cefazolin ♦ cefotaxime ♦ cefotetan ♦ cefoxitin ♦ ceftazidime ♦ ceftriaxone ♦ cefuroxime ♦ cimetidine ♦ ciprofloxacin ♦ clindamycin ♦ digoxin ♦ dobutamine ♦ dopamine ♦ doxycycline ♦ epinephrine ♦ erythromycin lactobionate ♦ esmolol ♦ fentanyl ♦ fluconazole ♦ gentamicin ♦ hydromorphone ♦ imipenem/cilastatin ♦ labetalol ♦ lidocaine ♦ lorazepam ♦ meperidine ♦ metoclopramide ♦ metronidazole ♦ midazolam ♦ milrinone ♦ morphine ♦ multivitamins ♦ nitroprusside ♦ nitroglycerin ♦ norepinephrine ♦ oxacillin ♦ penicillin G potassium ♦ pentamidine ♦ piperacillin ♦ potassium chloride ♦ potassium phosphate ♦ ranitidine ♦ theophylline ♦ ticarcillin ♦ ticarcillin/clavulanate ♦ tobramycin ♦ trimethoprim/sulfamethoxazole ♦ vancomycin. ♦ vecuronium.

■ **Y-Site Incompatibility:** ♦ diazepam ♦ furosemide ♦ phenytoin ♦ rifampin ♦ thiopental.

## PATIENT/FAMILY TEACHING

■ **General Info:** Advise patient to take medication exactly as directed at the same time each day, even if feeling well. Take missed doses as soon as possible unless almost time for next dose; do not double doses. May need to be discontinued gradually.

❏ Instruct patient on correct technique for monitoring pulse. Instruct patient to contact health care professional if heart rate is <50 bpm.

❏ Caution patient to change positions slowly to minimize orthostatic hypotension.

❏ May cause drowsiness or dizziness. Advise patient to avoid driving or other activities requiring alertness until response to the medication is known.

❏ Instruct patient on importance of maintaining good dental hygiene and seeing dentist frequently for teeth cleaning to prevent tenderness, bleeding, and gingival hyperplasia (gum enlargement).

❏ Instruct patient to avoid concurrent use of alcohol or OTC medications, especially cough and cold preparations, without consulting health care professional.

❏ Advise patient to notify health care professional if irregular heartbeats, dyspnea, swelling of hands and feet, pronounced dizziness, nausea, constipation, or hypotension occurs or if headache is severe or persistent.

❏ Caution patient to wear protective clothing and use sunscreen to prevent photosensitivity reactions.

■ **Angina:** Instruct patient on concurrent nitrate or beta-blocker therapy to continue taking both medications as directed and to use SL nitroglycerin as needed for anginal attacks.

❏ Advise patient to contact health care professional if chest pain does not improve, worsens after therapy, or occurs with diaphoresis; if shortness of breath occurs; or if severe, persistent headache occurs.

❏ Caution patient to discuss exercise restrictions with health care professional before exertion.

■ **Hypertension:** Encourage patient to comply with other interventions for hypertension (weight reduction, low-sodium diet, smoking cessation, moderation of alcohol consumption, regular exercise, and stress management). Medication controls but does not cure hypertension.

❏ Instruct patient and family in proper technique for monitoring blood pressure. Advise patient to take blood pressure weekly and to report significant changes to health care professional.

## EVALUATION

**Effectiveness of therapy can be demonstrated by:** ■ Decrease in blood pressure ■ Decrease in frequency and severity of anginal attacks ❏ Decrease in need for nitrate therapy ❏ Increase in activity tolerance and sense of wellbeing ■ Suppression and prevention of tachyarrhythmias.

---

**dimenhydrinate**
(dye-men-**hye**-dri-nate)

{Apo-Dimenhydrinate}, Calm X, Dimetabs, Dinate, Dramamine, Dramanate, {Gravol}, Hydrate, {PMS-Dimenhydrinate}, {Traveltabs}, Triptone Caplets

## CLASSIFICATION(S):

*Therapeutic: antiemetics, antihistamines*

**Pregnancy Category B**

## INDICATIONS

■ Nausea, vomiting, dizziness, and vertigo accompanying motion sickness.

## ACTION

■ Inhibits vestibular stimulation ■ Has significant CNS depressant, anticholinergic, antihistaminic, and antiemetic properties. **Therapeutic Effects:** ■ Decreased vestibular stimulation, which may prevent motion sickness.

## PHARMACOKINETICS

**Absorption:** Well absorbed after oral or IM administration.

**Distribution:** Probably crosses the placenta and enters breast milk.

**Metabolism and Excretion:** Metabolized by the liver.

**Half-life:** Unknown.

## CONTRAINDICATIONS AND PRECAUTIONS

**Contraindicated in:** ■ Hypersensitivity ■ Some products contain alcohol or tartrazine; in patients with known intolerance.

**Use Cautiously in:** ■ Narrow-angle glaucoma ■ Seizure disorders ■ Prostatic hypertrophy.

## ADVERSE REACTIONS AND SIDE EFFECTS*

■ **CNS:** drowsiness, dizziness, headache, paradoxical excitation (children) ■ **EENT:** blurred vision, tinnitus ■ **CV:** hypotension, palpitations ■ **GI:** anorexia, constipation, diarrhea, dry mouth ■ **GU:** dysuria, frequency ■ **Derm:** photosensitivity ■ **Local:** pain at IM site.

## INTERACTIONS

**Drug-Drug:** ■ ↑ CNS depression with other **antihistamines, alcohol, opioid analgesics,** and **sedative/hypnotics** ■ May mask signs or symptoms of ototoxicity in patients receiving **ototoxic drugs (aminoglycosides, ethacrynic acid)** ■ ↑ anticholinergic properties with **tricyclic antidepressants, quinidine,** or **disopyramide** ■ **MAO inhibitors** intensify and prolong the anticholinergic effects of antihistamines.

## ROUTE AND DOSAGE

■ **PO (Adults):** 50–100 mg q 4 hr (not to exceed 400 mg/day).
■ **PO (Children 6–12 yr):** 25–50 mg q 6–8 hr (not to exceed 300 mg/day).
■ **Rect (Adults):** 50–100 mg q 6–8 hr.
■ **Rect (Children 8–12 yr):** 25–50 mg q 8–12 hr.
■ **Rect (Children 6–8 yr):** 12.5–25 mg q 8–12 hr.
■ **IM, IV (Adults):** 50 mg q 4 hr as needed.
■ **IM, IV (Children):** 1.25 mg/kg (37.5 mg/m²) q 6 hr as needed (not to exceed 300 mg/day).

## AVAILABILITY (generic available)

■ *Tablets:* 50 mg^OTC ■ *Chewable tablets (orange flavor):* 50 mg^OTC ■ *Capsules:* {50 mg^OTC} ■ *Extended-release capsules:* {25 mg^OTC} ■ *Elixir (cherry flavor):* 12.5 mg/5 ml^OTC, {15 mg/5 ml^OTC} ■ *Liquid:* 12.5 mg/4 ml^OTC ■ *Suppositories:* {50 mg^OTC}, {100 mg^OTC} ■ *Injection:* 50 mg/ml^Rx ■ Cost: $4.00/10 ml.

TIME/ACTION PROFILE (anti–motion sickness, antiemetic activity)

|      | ONSET      | PEAK    | DURATION |
|------|------------|---------|----------|
| PO   | 15–60 min  | 1–2 hr  | 3–6 hr   |
| Rect | 30–45 min  | unknown | 6–12 hr  |
| IM   | 20–30 min  | 1–2 hr  | 3–6 hr   |
| IV   | rapid      | unknown | 3–6 hr   |

# NURSING IMPLICATIONS

## ASSESSMENT

❑ Assess nausea, vomiting, bowel sounds, and abdominal pain before and after administration of this drug. Dimenhydrinate may mask the signs of an acute abdomen.

❑ Monitor intake and output, including emesis. Assess for signs of dehydration (excessive thirst, dry skin and mucous membranes, tachycardia, increased urine specific gravity, poor skin turgor).

- **Lab Test Considerations:** Will cause false-negative allergy skin test results; discontinue 72 hr before testing.

## POTENTIAL NURSING DIAGNOSES

- Fluid volume, risk for deficit (Indications).
- Nutrition, imbalanced: less than body requirements (Indications).
- Injury, risk for (Side Effects).

## IMPLEMENTATION

- **General:** When used for prophylaxis of motion sickness, administer at least 30 min and preferably 1–2 hr before exposure to conditions that may precipitate motion sickness.
- **PO:** Use calibrated measuring device when administering liquid dose.
- **IM:** Administer into well-developed muscle; massage well.
- **Direct IV:** Dilute 50 mg in 10 ml of 0.9% NaCl for injection.
- **Rate:** Inject over 2 min.
- **Syringe Compatibility:** ◆ atropine ◆ codeine ◆ droperidol ◆ fentanyl ◆ heparin ◆ hydromorphone ◆ meperidine ◆ metoclopromide ◆ morphine ◆ pentazocine ◆ perphenazine ◆ ranitidine ◆ scopolamine.
- **Syringe Incompatibility:** ◆ butorphanol ◆ chlorpromazine ◆ glycopyrrolate ◆ hydroxyzine ◆ midazolam ◆ nalbuphine ◆ pentobarbital ◆ prochlorperazine ◆ promethazine ◆ thiopental.
- **Y-Site Compatibility:** ◆ acyclovir.
- **Y-Site Incompatibility:** ◆ aminophylline ◆ heparin ◆ hydrocortisone sodium succinate ◆ phenobarbital ◆ phenytoin ◆ prednisolone ◆ prochlorperazine ◆ promethazine.
- **Solution Compatibility:** D5W, 0.45% NaCl, 0.9% NaCl, Ringer's solution, lactated Ringer's solution, dextrose/saline combinations, or dextrose/Ringer's combinations.

## PATIENT/FAMILY TEACHING

- May cause drowsiness. Advise patient to avoid driving or other activities requiring alertness until response to the drug is known.
- Inform patient that this medication may cause dry mouth. Frequent oral rinses, good oral hygiene, and sugarless gum or candy may minimize this effect.
- Caution patient to avoid alcohol and other CNS depressants concurrently with this medication.
- Advise patient to use sunscreen and protective clothing to prevent photosensitivity reactions.

## EVALUATION

**Effectiveness of therapy can be demonstrated by:** ■ Prevention or decreased severity of nausea and vomiting, vertigo, or motion sickness.

## dinoprostone

(dye-noe-**prost**-one)

Cervidil Vaginal Insert, Prepidil Endocervical Gel, Prostin E Vaginal Suppository

### CLASSIFICATION(S):

**Therapeutic:** cervical ripening agents
**Pharmacologic:** oxytocics, prostaglandins

### Pregnancy Category C

## INDICATIONS

■ Endocervical Gel, Vaginal Insert ❑ Used to "ripen" the cervix in pregnancy at or near term when induction of labor is indicated ■ Vaginal Suppository ❑ Induction of midtrimester abortion ❑ Management of missed abortion up to 28 wk ❑ Management of nonmetastatic gestational trophoblastic disease (benign hydatidiform mole).

## ACTION

■ Produces contractions similar to those occurring during labor at term by stimulating the myometrium (oxytocic effect) ■ Initiates softening, effacement, and dilation of the cervix ("ripening") ■ Also stimulates GI smooth muscle. **Therapeutic Effects:** ■ Initiation of labor ■ Expulsion of fetus.

## PHARMACOKINETICS

**Absorption:** Rapidly absorbed.

**Distribution:** Unknown. Action is mostly local.

**Metabolism and Excretion:** Metabolized by enzymes in lung, kidneys, spleen, and liver tissue.

**Half-life:** Unknown.

## CONTRAINDICATIONS AND PRECAUTIONS

**Contraindicated in:** ■ Hypersensitivity to prostaglandins or additives in the gel or suppository ■ The gel/insert should be avoided in situations in which prolonged uterine contractions should be avoided, including: ❑ Previous cesarean section or uterine surgery ❑ Cephalopelvic disproportion ❑ Traumatic delivery or difficult labor ❑ Multiparity (≥6 term pregnancies) ❑ Hyperactive or hypertonic uterus ❑ Fetal distress (if delivery is not imminent) ❑ Unexplained vaginal bleeding ❑ Placenta previa ❑ Vasa previa ❑ Active herpes genitalis ❑ Obstetric emergency requiring surgical intervention ❑ Situations in which vaginal delivery is contraindicated ■ Presence of acute pelvic inflammatory disease or ruptured membranes ■ Concurrent oxytocic therapy (wait for 30 min after removing insert before using oxytocin).

**Use Cautiously in:** ■ Uterine scarring ■ Asthma ■ Hypotension ■ Cardiac disease ■ Adrenal disorders ■ Anemia ■ Jaundice ■ Diabetes mellitus ■ Epilepsy ■ Glaucoma ■ Pulmonary, renal, or hepatic disease ■ Multiparity (up to 5 previous term pregnancies).

## ADVERSE REACTIONS AND SIDE EFFECTS*

Endocervical Gel, Vaginal Insert ■ **GU:** uterine contractile abnormalities, warm feeling in vagina ■ **MS:** back pain ■ **Misc:** fever.

Suppository ■ **CNS:** <u>headache</u>, drowsiness, syncope ■ **Resp:** coughing, dyspnea, wheezing ■ **CV:** <u>hypotension</u>, hypertension ■ **GI:** <u>diarrhea</u>, <u>nausea</u>, <u>vomiting</u> ■ **GU:** UTERINE RUPTURE, urinary tract infection, uterine hyperstimulation, vaginal/uterine pain ■ **Misc:** allergic reactions including ANAPHYLAXIS, chills, fever.

## INTERACTIONS

**Drug-Drug:** ■ Augments the effects of other **oxytocics.**

## ROUTE AND DOSAGE

❑ **Cervical Ripening**

■ **Vag (Adults, Cervical):** *Endocervical gel*—0.5 mg; if response is unfavorable, may repeat in 6 hr (not to exceed 1.5 mg/24 hr). *Vaginal insert*—one 10-mg insert.

❑ **Abortifacient**

■ **Vag (Adults):** One 20-mg suppository, repeat q 3–5 hr (not to exceed 240 mg total or longer than 48 hr).

## AVAILABILITY

■*Endocervical gel (Prepidil):* 0.5 mg dinoprostone in 3 g of gel vehicle in a prefilled syringe with catheters^Rx ■ Cost: $796.93/5 syringes ■ *Vaginal insert (Cervidil):* 10 mg^Rx ■Cost: $183.46/each ■ *Vaginal suppository (Prostin E Vaginal):* 20 mg^Rx.

TIME/ACTION PROFILE

| | ONSET | PEAK | DURATION |
|---|---|---|---|
| Cervical ripening (gel) | rapid | 30–45 min | unknown |
| Cervical ripening (insert) | rapid | unknown | 12 hr |
| Abortion time (suppository) | 10 min | 12–24 hr | 2–3 hr |

# NURSING IMPLICATIONS

## ASSESSMENT

■ **Abortifacient:** Monitor frequency, duration, and force of contractions and uterine resting tone. Opioid analgesics may be administered for uterine pain.

❑ Monitor temperature, pulse, and blood pressure periodically throughout therapy. Dinoprostone-induced fever (elevation >1.1°C or 2°F) usually occurs within 15–45 min after insertion of suppository. This returns to normal 2–6 hr after discontinuation or removal of suppository from vagina.

❑ Auscultate breath sounds. Wheezing and sensation of chest tightness may indicate hypersensitivity reaction.

❑ Assess for nausea, vomiting, and diarrhea in patients receiving suppository. Vomiting and diarrhea occur frequently. Patient should be premedicated with antiemetic and antidiarrheal.

- Monitor amount and type of vaginal discharge. Notify physician or other health care professional immediately if symptoms of hemorrhage (increased bleeding, hypotension, pallor, tachycardia) occur.
- **Cervical Ripening:** Monitor uterine activity, fetal status, and dilation and effacement of cervix continuously throughout therapy. Assess for hypertonus, sustained uterine contractility, and fetal distress. Insert should be removed at the onset of active labor.

## POTENTIAL NURSING DIAGNOSES

- Knowledge, deficient, related to medication regimen (Patient/Family Teaching).

## IMPLEMENTATION

- **Abortifacient:** Warm the suppository to room temperature just before use.
- Wear gloves when handling unwrapped suppository to prevent absorption through skin.
- Patient should remain supine for 10 min after insertion of suppository; then she may be ambulatory.
- **Vaginal Insert:** Place vaginal insert transversely in the posterior vaginal fornix immediately after removing from foil package. Warming of insert and sterile conditions are not required. Use vaginal insert only with a retrieval system. Use minimal amount of water-soluble lubricant during insertion; avoid excess because it may hamper release of dinoprostone from insert. Patient should remain supine for 2 hr after insertion, then may ambulate.
- Vaginal insert delivers dinoprostone 0.3 mg/hr over 12 hr. Remove insert at the onset of active labor, before amniotomy, or after 12 hr.
- Oxytocin should not be used during or less than 30 min after removal of insert.
- **Endocervical Gel:** Determine degree of effacement before insertion of the endocervical catheter. Do not administer above the level of the internal os. Use a 20-mm endocervical catheter if no effacement is present and a 10-mm catheter if the cervix is 50% effaced.
- Use caution to prevent contact of dinoprostone gel with skin. Wash hands thoroughly with soap and water after administration.

- Bring gel to room temperature just before administration. Do not force warming with external sources (water bath, microwave). Remove peel-off seal from end of syringe; then remove the protective end cap and insert end cap into plunger stopper assembly in barrel of syringe. Aseptically remove catheter from package. Firmly attach catheter hub to syringe tip; click is evidence of attachment. Fill catheter with sterile gel by pushing plunger to expel air from catheter before administration to patient. Gel is stable for 24 mo if refrigerated.
- Patient should be in dorsal position with cervix visualized using a speculum. Introduce gel with catheter into cervical canal using sterile technique. Administer gel by gentle expulsion from syringe and then remove catheter. Do not attempt to administer small amount of gel remaining in syringe. Use syringe for only 1 patient; discard syringe, catheter, and unused package contents after using.
- Patient should remain supine for 15–30 min after administration to minimize leakage from cervical canal.
- Oxytocin may be administered 6–12 hr after desired response from dinoprostone gel. If no cervical/uterine response to initial dose of dinoprostone is obtained, repeat dose may be administered in 6 hr.

## PATIENT/FAMILY TEACHING

- **General Info:** Explain purpose of medication and vaginal exams.
- **Abortifacient:** Instruct patient to notify health care professional immediately if fever and chills, foul-smelling vaginal discharge, lower abdominal pain, or increased bleeding occurs.
- Provide emotional support throughout therapy.
- **Cervical Ripening:** Inform patient that she may experience a warm feeling in her vagina during administration.
- Advise patient to notify health care professional if contractions become prolonged.

## EVALUATION

**Effectiveness of therapy can be demonstrated by:** ■ Complete abortion. Continuous administration for more than 2 days is not usually recommended ■ Cervical ripening and induction of labor.

# diphenhydramine (oral, parenteral)

(dye-fen-**hye**-dra-meen)

{Allerdryl}, Allergy Medication, AlerMax, Banophen, Benadryl Dye-Free Allergy, Benadryl Allergy, Benadryl, Compoz, Compoz Nighttime Sleep Aid, Diphen AF, Diphen Cough, Diphenhist, Dormin, Genahist, 40 Winks, Hyrexin- 50, {Insomnal}, Maximum Strength Nytol, Maximum Strength Sleepinal, Midol PM, Miles Nervine, Nighttime Sleep Aid, Nytol, Scot-Tussin Allergy DM, Siladril, Silphen, Sleep-Eze 3, Sleepwell 2-night, Sominex, Snooze Fast, Sominex, Tusstat, Twilite, Unisom Nighttime Sleep-Aid

## CLASSIFICATION(S):

*Therapeutic: allergy, cold, and cough remedies, antihistamines, antitussives*

**Pregnancy Category B**

## INDICATIONS

■ Relief of allergic symptoms caused by histamine release including: ❑ Anaphylaxis ❑ Seasonal and perennial allergic rhinitis ❑ Allergic dermatoses ■ Parkinson's disease and dystonic reactions from medications ■ Mild nighttime sedation ■ Prevention of motion sickness ■ Antitussive (syrup only).

## ACTION

■ Antagonizes the effects of histamine at $H_1$-receptor sites; does not bind to or inactivate histamine ■ Significant CNS depressant and anticholinergic properties. **Therapeutic Effects:** ■ Decreased symptoms of histamine excess (sneezing, rhinorrhea, nasal and ocular pruritus, ocular tearing and redness, urticaria) ■ Relief of acute dystonic reactions ■ Prevention of motion sickness ■ Suppression of cough.

## PHARMACOKINETICS

**Absorption:** Well absorbed after oral or IM administration.

**Distribution:** Widely distributed. Crosses the placenta; enters breast milk.

**Metabolism and Excretion:** 95% metabolized by the liver.

**Half-life:** 2.4–7 hr.

## CONTRAINDICATIONS AND PRECAUTIONS

**Contraindicated in:** ■ Hypersensitivity ■ Acute attacks of asthma ■ Lactation ■ Known alcohol intolerance (some liquid products).

**Use Cautiously in:** ■ Geriatric patients (more susceptible to adverse drug reactions; dosage reduction recommended) ■ Severe liver disease ■ Narrow-angle glaucoma ■ Seizure disorders ■ Prostatic hypertrophy ■ Pregnancy (safety not established).

## ADVERSE REACTIONS AND SIDE EFFECTS*

■ **CNS:** <u>drowsiness</u>, dizziness, headache, paradoxical excitation (increased in children) ■ **EENT:** blurred vision, tinnitus ■ **CV:** hypotension, palpitations ■ **GI:** <u>anorexia</u>, <u>dry mouth</u>, constipation, diarrhea ■ **GU:** dysuria, frequency, urinary retention ■ **Derm:** photosensitivity ■ **Local:** pain at IM site.

## INTERACTIONS

**Drug-Drug:** ■ ↑ risk of CNS depression with other **antihistamines, alcohol, opioid analgesics,** and **sedative/hypnotics** ■ ↑ anticholinergic effects with **tricyclic antidepressants, quinidine,** or **disopyramide** ■ **MAO inhibitors** intensify and prolong the anticholinergic effects of antihistamines.

**Drug-Natural Products:** ■ Concomitant use of **kava, valerian,** or **chamomile,** can ↑ CNS depression.

## ROUTE AND DOSAGE

■ **PO (Adults):** *Antihistaminic/antiemetic/antivertiginic*—25–50 mg q 4–6 hr. *Antitussive*—25 mg q 4 hr as needed. *Antidyskinetic*—25 mg 3 times daily (up to 50 mg 4 times daily). *Sedative/hypnotic*—50 mg 20–30 min before bedtime.

■ **PO (Children 6–12 yr):** *Antihistaminic*—12.5–25 mg q 4–6 hr. *Antiemetic/antivertiginic*—1–1.5 mg/kg q 4–6 hr as needed

(not to exceed 300 mg/day). *Antitussive*—
12.5 mg q 4 hr (not to exceed 75 mg/day).
- **PO (Children 2–6 yr):** *Antihistaminic*—
6.25–12.5 mg q 4–6 hr. *Antiemetic/antiv-
ertiginic*—1–1.5 mg/kg q 4–6 hr as needed
(not to exceed 300 mg/day). *Antitussive*—
6.25 mg q 4 hr (not to exceed 25 mg/24
hr).
- **IM, IV (Adults):** 10–50 mg q 2–3 hr as
needed (may need up to 100-mg dose, not to
exceed 400 mg/day).
- **IM, IV (Children):** 1.25 mg/kg (37.5 mg/
m²) 4 times daily (not to exceed 300 mg/
day).

## AVAILABILITY (generic available)

- *Capsules:* 25 mg^Rx, ᴼᵀᶜ, 50 mg^Rx, ᴼᵀᶜ ■Cost:
25 mg $22.77/100, 50 mg $30.71/100 ■ *Tablets:* 25 mg^Rx, ᴼᵀᶜ, 50 mg^Rx, ᴼᵀᶜ ■ *Chewable
tablets (grape flavor):* 25 mg^Rx, ᴼᵀᶜ ■*Elixir
(cherry and other flavors):* 12.5 mg/5
mlRx, OTC ■ *Syrup (cherry and raspberry
flavor):* 12.5 mg/5 mlRx, OTC ■ *Injection:*
10 mg/ml^Rx, 50 mg/ml^Rx ■ analgesics, decongestants, and expectorants, in OTC pain, sleep,
cough, and cold preparations. See Appendix B.

TIME/ACTION PROFILE (antihistaminic effects)

| | ONSET | PEAK | DURATION |
|---|---|---|---|
| PO | 15–60 min | 1–4 hr | 4–8 hr |
| IM | 20–30 min | 1–4 hr | 4–8 hr |
| IV | rapid | unknown | 4–8 hr |

## NURSING IMPLICATIONS

### ASSESSMENT

- **General Info:** Diphenhydramine has multiple uses. Determine why the medication was
ordered and assess symptoms that apply to
the individual patient.
- **Prevention and Treatment of Anaphylaxis:** Assess for urticaria and for patency of
airway.
- **Allergic Rhinitis:** Assess degree of nasal
stuffiness, rhinorrhea, and sneezing.
- **Parkinsonism and Extrapyramidal Reactions:** Assess movement disorder before and
after administration.
- **Insomnia:** Assess sleep patterns.

- **Motion Sickness:** Assess nausea, vomiting,
bowel sounds, and abdominal pain.
- **Cough Suppressant:** Assess frequency and
nature of cough, lung sounds, and amount
and type of sputum produced. Unless contraindicated, maintain fluid intake of 1500–
2000 ml daily to decrease viscosity of bronchial secretions.
- **Pruritus:** Assess degree of itching, skin
rash, and inflammation.
- *Lab Test Considerations:* Diphenhydramine may decrease skin response to allergy
tests. Discontinue 4 days before skin testing.

### POTENTIAL NURSING DIAGNOSES

- Sleep pattern disturbed (Indications).
- Fluid volume, risk for deficit (Indications).
- Injury, risk for (Side Effects).

### IMPLEMENTATION

- **General:** Do not confuse Benadryl (diphenhydramine) with Benylin (dextromethorphan).
- ❏ When used for insomnia, administer 20 min
before bedtime and schedule activities to
minimize interruption of sleep.
- ❏ When used for prophylaxis of motion
sickness, administer at least 30 min and
preferably 1–2 hr before exposure to conditions that may precipitate motion sickness.
- **PO:** Administer with meals or milk to minimize GI irritation. Capsule may be emptied
and contents taken with water or food.
- **IM:** Administer into well-developed muscle.
Avoid subcut injections.
- **Direct IV:** May give undiluted. May be further diluted in 0.9% NaCl, 0.45% NaCl, D5W,
D10W, D5/0.9% NaCl, D5/0.45% NaCl, D5/
0.25% NaCl, Ringer's solution, LR, and dex-
trose/Ringer's combinations.
- *Rate:* Inject 25 mg over at least 1 min.
- **Syringe Compatibility:** ◆ atropine ◆ butorphanol ◆ chlorpromazine ◆ cimetidine ◆ dimenhydrinate ◆ droperidol ◆ fentanyl ◆ fluphenazine ◆ glycopyrrolate ◆ hydromorphone
◆ hydroxyzine ◆ meperidine ◆ metoclopramide ◆ midazolam ◆ morphine ◆ nalbuphine ◆
pentazocine ◆ perphenazine ◆ prochlorperazine ◆ promethazine ◆ ranitidine ◆ scopolamine ◆ sufentanil.

■ **Syringe Incompatibility:** ◆ haloperidol ◆ pentobarbital ◆ thiopental.

■ **Y-Site Compatibility:** ◆ acyclovir ◆ aldesleukin ◆ amifostine ◆ aztreonam ◆ ciprofloxacin ◆ cisatracurium ◆ cisplatin ◆ cladribine ◆ cyclophosphamide ◆ cytarabine ◆ docetaxel ◆ doxorubicin ◆ doxorubicin liposome ◆ etoposide phosphate ◆ famotidine ◆ fentanyl ◆ filgrastim ◆ fluconazole ◆ fludarabine ◆ gatifloxacin ◆ gemcitabine ◆ granisetron ◆ heparin ◆ hydrocortisone ◆ hydromorphone ◆ idarubicin ◆ linezolid ◆ melphalan ◆ meperidine ◆ meropenem ◆ methadone ◆ methotrexate ◆ morphine ◆ ondansetron ◆ paclitaxel ◆ piperacillin/tazobactam ◆ potassium chloride ◆ propofol ◆ remifentanil ◆ sargramostim ◆ sufentanil ◆ tacrolimus ◆ teniposide ◆ thiotepa ◆ vinorelbine ◆ vitamin B complex with C.

■ **Y-Site Incompatibility:** ◆ allopurinol ◆ amphotericin B cholesteryl sulfate ◆ cefepime ◆ foscarnet.

## PATIENT/FAMILY TEACHING

❑ Instruct patient to take medication as directed; do not exceed recommended amount. Caution patient not to use oral OTC diphenhydramine products with any other product containing diphenhydramine, including products used topically.

❑ May cause drowsiness. Advise patient to avoid driving or other activities requiring alertness until response to drug is known.

❑ Inform patient that this drug may cause dry mouth. Frequent oral rinses, good oral hygiene, and sugarless gum or candy may minimize this effect. Notify dentist if dry mouth persists for more than 2 wk.

❑ Advise patient to use sunscreen and protective clothing to prevent photosensitivity reactions.

❑ Caution patient to avoid use of alcohol and other CNS depressants concurrently with this medication.

❑ Advise patients taking diphenhydramine in OTC preparations to notify health care professional if symptoms worsen or persist for more than 7 days.

## EVALUATION

**Effectiveness of therapy can be demonstrated by:** ■ Prevention of or decreased urticaria in anaphylaxis or other allergic reactions ■ Decreased dyskinesia in parkinsonism and extrapyramidal reactions ■ Sedation when used as a sedative/hypnotic ■ Prevention of or decrease in nausea and vomiting caused by motion sickness ■ Decrease in frequency and intensity of cough without eliminating cough reflex.

## diphenoxylate/atropine
(dye-fen-**ox**-i-late/**a**-troe-peen)
Logen, Lomanate, Lomotil, Lonox
## difenoxin/atropine
(dye-fen-**ox**-in/**a**-troe-peen)
Motofen

**CLASSIFICATION(S):**
**Therapeutic:** antidiarrheals
**Pharmacologic:** anticholinergics

**Schedule V (diphenoxylate/atropine), IV difenoxin/atropine)**

**Pregnancy Category C**

## INDICATIONS

■ Adjunctive therapy in the treatment of diarrhea.

## ACTION

■ Inhibits excess GI motility ■ Structurally related to opioid analgesics but has no analgesic properties ■ Atropine added to discourage abuse. **Therapeutic Effects:** ■ Decreased GI motility with subsequent decrease in diarrhea.

## PHARMACOKINETICS

**Absorption:** Well absorbed from the GI tract.
**Distribution:** Enters breast milk.
**Metabolism and Excretion:** *Diphenoxylate*—mostly metabolized by the liver with some conversion to an active antidiarrheal compound (difenoxin). *Difenoxin*—metabolized by the liver. Minimal excretion in urine.
**Half-life:** *Diphenoxylate*—2.5 hr; *difenoxin*—4.5 hr.

## CONTRAINDICATIONS AND PRECAUTIONS

**Contraindicated in:** ■ Hypersensitivity ■ Severe liver disease ■ Infectious diarrhea (due to *Escherichia coli*, *Salmonella*, or *Shigella*) ■ Diarrhea associated with pseudomembranous colitis ■ Dehydrated patients ■ Narrow-angle glaucoma

■ Children <2 yr ■ Known alcohol intolerance (some liquid diphenoxylate/atropine products only).

**Use Cautiously in:** ■ Patients physically dependent on opioids ■ Inflammatory bowel disease ■ Geriatric patients (more sensitive to effects) ■ Children (more sensitive to effects, espcially Down's syndrome patients) ■ Prostatic hypertrophy ■ Pregnancy, lactation, or children <12 yr (safety not established for difenoxin/atropine in children <12 yr; dipehoxylate/atropine should not be used in children <2 yr).

## ADVERSE REACTIONS AND SIDE EFFECTS*

■ **CNS:** dizziness, confusion, drowsiness, headache, insomnia, nervousness ■ **EENT:** blurred vision, dry eyes ■ **CV:** tachycardia ■ **GI:** constipation, dry mouth, epigastric distress, ileus, nausea, vomiting ■ **GU:** urinary retention ■ **Derm:** flushing.

## INTERACTIONS

**Drug-Drug:** ■ Additive CNS depression with other **CNS depressants** including **alcohol, antihistamines, opioid analgesics,** and **sedative/hypnotics** ■ Additive anticholinergic properties with other **drugs having anticholinergic properties,** including **tricyclic antidepressants** and **disopyramide** ■ Use with **MAO inhibitors** may result in hypertensive crisis.

**Drug-Natural Products:** ■ Increased anticholinergic effects with **angel's trumpet, jimson wccd,** and **scopolia.**

## ROUTE AND DOSAGE

### ❑ Difenoxin/Atropine

Doses given are in terms of difenoxin—each tablet contains 1 mg difenoxin with 0.025 mg of atropine.

■ **PO (Adults):** 2 tablets initially, then 1 tablet after each loose stool or every 3–4 hr as needed (not to exceed 8 tablets/day).

### ❑ Diphenoxylate/Atropine

Adult doses given are in terms of diphenoxylate—each tablet contains 2.5 mg diphenoxylate with 0.025 mg of atropine; pediatric doses are given in mg of diphenoxylate and in ml of diphenoxylate/atropine liquid; each 5 ml of liq-

uid contains 2.5 mg diphenoxylate with 0.025 mg of atropine.

■ **PO (Adults):** 5 mg 3–4 times daily initially, then 5 mg once daily as needed (not to exceed 20 mg/day).

■ **PO (Children):** *use liquid only*—0.3–0.4 mg/kg/day in 4 divided doses.

## AVAILABILITY

### ❑ Difenoxin/Atropine

■ *Tablets:* 1 mg difenoxin/0.025 mg atropine$^{Rx}$.

### ❑ Diphenoxylate/Atropine

■ *Tablets:* 2.5 mg diphenoxylate/0.025 mg atropine$^{Rx}$ ■ Cost: 2.5 mg–0.025 mg $55.89/100 ■ *Liquid (cherry flavor):* 2.5 mg diphenoxylate/0.025 mg atropine per 5 ml$^{Rx}$ ■ Cost: 2.5 mg–0.025 mg/5 ml $16.51/60 ml.

TIME/ACTION PROFILE (antidiarrheal action)

| | ONSET | PEAK | DURATION |
|---|---|---|---|
| Difenoxin–PO | 45–60 min | 2 hr | 3–4 hr |
| Diphenoxy-late–PO | 45–60 min | 2 hr | 3–4 hr |

# NURSING IMPLICATIONS

## ASSESSMENT

❑ Assess the frequency and consistency of stools and bowel sounds prior to and throughout therapy.

❑ Assess patient's fluid and electrolyte balance and skin turgor for dehydration.

■ *Lab Test Considerations:* Liver function tests should be evaluated periodically during prolonged therapy.

❑ Diphenoxylate/atropine may cause increased serum amylase concentrations.

## POTENTIAL NURSING DIAGNOSES

■ Diarrhea (Indications).

■ Constipation (Side Effects).

## IMPLEMENTATION

■ **General:** Do not confuse Lomotil with Lamictal (lamontrigine) or Lamisil (terbinafine).

❑ Risk of dependence increases with high-dose, long-term use. Atropine has been added to discourage abuse.

---

{ } = Available in Canada only.
*CAPITALS indicates life-threatening; underlines indicate most frequent.

■ **PO:** Diphenoxylate/atropine tablets may be administered with food if GI irritation occurs. Tablets may be crushed and administered with patient's fluid of choice. Use calibrated measuring device for liquid preparations.

## PATIENT/FAMILY TEACHING

❑ Instruct patient to take medication exactly as directed. Do not take more than the prescribed amount because of the habit-forming potential and risk of overdose in children. If on a scheduled dosing regimen, missed doses should be taken as soon as possible unless almost time for next dose. Do not double doses.

❑ Medication may cause drowsiness. Advise patient to avoid driving or other activities requiring alertness until response to drug is known.

❑ Advise patient that frequent mouth rinses, good oral hygiene, and sugarless gum or candy may relieve dry mouth.

❑ Caution patient to avoid alcohol and other CNS depressants concurrently with this medication.

❑ Advise patient to inform health care professional of medication regimen prior to treatment or surgery.

❑ Instruct patient to notify health care professional if diarrhea persists or if fever, abdominal pain, or palpitations occur.

## EVALUATION

**Effectiveness of therapy can be demonstrated by:** ■ Decrease in diarrhea. Treatment of acute diarrhea should be continued for 24–36 hr before it is considered ineffective.

## dipyridamole

(dye-peer-**id**-a-mole)

{Apo-Dipyridamole}, Dipridacot, {Novodipiradol}, Persantine, Persantine IV

### CLASSIFICATION(S):

**Therapeutic:** antiplatelet agents, diagnostic agents (coronary vasodilators)

**Pharmacologic:** platelet adhesion inhibitors

## Pregnancy Category B

## INDICATIONS

■ **PO:** Prevention of thromboembolism in patients with prosthetic heart valves (with warfarin) ■ Maintains patency after surgical grafting procedures, including coronary artery bypass (with aspirin) ■ **IV:** Diagnostic agent in lieu of exercise during thallium myocardial perfusion imaging.

## ACTION

■ **PO:** Decreases platelet aggregation by inhibiting the enzyme phosphodiesterase ■ **IV:** Produces coronary vasodilation by inhibiting adenosine uptake. **Therapeutic Effects:** ■ **PO:** Inhibition of platelet aggregation and subsequent thromboembolic events ■ **IV:** In diagnostic thallium imaging, dipyridamole dilates normal coronary arteries, reducing flow to vessels that are narrowed and causing abnormal thallium distribution.

## PHARMACOKINETICS

**Absorption:** Moderately absorbed (30–60%) after oral administration.

**Distribution:** Widely distributed. Crosses the placenta; enters breast milk.

**Metabolism and Excretion:** Metabolized by the liver; excreted in the bile.

**Half-life:** 10 hr.

## CONTRAINDICATIONS AND PRECAUTIONS

**Contraindicated in:** ■ Hypersensitivity.

**Use Cautiously in:** ■ Hypotensive patients ■ Patients with platelet defects ■ Pregnancy (although safety not established, has been used without harm during pregnancy) ■ Lactation or children <12 yr (safety not established).

## ADVERSE REACTIONS AND SIDE EFFECTS*

■ **CNS:** dizziness, headache, syncope; *IV only*— transient cerebral ischemia, weakness ■ **Resp:** *IV only*—bronchospasm ■ **CV:** *IV only*—MI, hypotension, arrhythmias, flushing ■ **GI:** nausea, diarrhea, GI upset, vomiting ■ **Derm:** rash.

## INTERACTIONS

**Drug-Drug:** ■ Additive effects with **aspirin** on platelet aggregation ■ Risk of bleeding may be increased when used with **anticoagulants, thrombolytic agents, NSAIDs, cefamandole, cefoperazone, cefotetan, plicamycin, valproic acid,** or **sulfinpyrazone** ■ Increased risk of hypotension with **alcohol** ■ **Theophylline** may negate the effects of dipyridamole during diagnostic thallium imaging.

## ROUTE AND DOSAGE

- **PO (Adults):** 225–400 mg/day in 3–4 divided doses.
- **IV (Adults):** 570 mcg/kg; maximum dose 60 mg.

## AVAILABILITY (generic available)

■ *Tablets:* 25 mg$^{Rx}$, 50 mg$^{Rx}$, 75 mg$^{Rx}$, {100 mg$^{Rx}$} ■ Cost: *Persantine*—25 mg $40.28/100, 50 mg $64.91/100, 75 mg $86.82/100; *generic*—25 mg $2.52/100, 50 mg $4.13/100, 75 mg $5.93/100 ■ aspirin (Aggrenox$^{Rx}$). See Appendix B.

■ *Injection:* 10 mg/2 ml$^{Rx}$.

TIME/ACTION PROFILE (PO = antiplatelet activity, IV = coronary vasodilation)

| | ONSET | PEAK | DURATION |
|---|---|---|---|
| PO | unknown | unknown | unknown |
| IV | unknown | 6.5 min† | 30 min |

†From start of infusion.

## NURSING IMPLICATIONS

### ASSESSMENT

- **PO:** Monitor blood pressure and pulse before instituting therapy and regularly during period of dosage adjustment.
- **IV:** Monitor vital signs during and for 10–15 min after infusion. Obtain ECG in at least 1 lead. If severe chest pain or bronchospasm occurs, administer IV aminophylline 50–250 mg at a rate of 50–100 mg over 30–60 sec. If hypotension is severe, place patient in a supine position with head tilting down. If chest pain is unrelieved with aminophylline 250 mg, administer nitroglycerin SL. If chest pain is still unrelieved, treat as myocardial infarction.
- **Lab Test Considerations:** Bleeding time should be monitored periodically throughout therapy.

## POTENTIAL NURSING DIAGNOSES

- Cardiac output, decreased (Indications).
- Pain, acute (Indications).

## IMPLEMENTATION

- **PO:** Administer with a full glass of water at least 1 hr before or 2 hr after meals for faster absorption. If GI irritation occurs, may be administered with or immediately after meals. Tablets may be crushed and mixed with food if patient has difficulty swallowing. Pharmacist may make a suspension.
- **Intermittent Infusion:** Dilute in at least a 1:2 ratio of 0.45% NaCl, 0.9% NaCl, or D5W for a total volume of 20–50 ml. Undiluted dipyridamole may cause venous irritation.
- **Rate:** Infuse dose over 4 min.

## PATIENT/FAMILY TEACHING

- **PO:** Instruct patient to take medication at evenly spaced intervals as directed. If a dose is missed, take as soon as remembered unless the next scheduled dose is within 4 hr. Do not double doses. Benefit of medication may not be apparent to patient; encourage patient to continue taking medication as directed.
- Caution patient to change positions slowly to minimize orthostatic hypotension.
- Advise patient to avoid the use of alcohol, as it may potentiate the hypotensive effects. Tobacco products should also be avoided because nicotine causes vasoconstriction.
- Advise patient to consult health care professional before taking OTC medications concurrently with this medication. Aspirin should be taken only if directed and only in dose prescribed. Advise patient to discuss alternatives for pain relief or fever.
- Instruct patient to notify health care professional if unusual bleeding or bruising occurs. Concurrent use of aspirin or warfarin may increase risk of bleeding but is commonly used with specific indications.
- Advise patient to notify health care professional of medication regimen and whether using concurrent aspirin or warfarin therapy.
- **IV:** Instruct patient to notify health care professional immediately if dyspnea or chest pain occurs.

{ } = Available in Canada only.
*CAPITALS indicates life-threatening; underlines indicate most frequent.

## EVALUATION

**Effectiveness of therapy can be demonstrated by:** ■ Prevention of postoperative thromboembolic complications associated with prosthetic heart valves ■ Maintenance of patency after surgical graft procedures ■ Coronary vasodilation in thallium myocardial perfusion imaging.

# disopyramide
(dye-soe-**peer**-a-mide)
Norpace, Norpace CR, {Rythmodan}, {Rythmodan-LA}

### CLASSIFICATION(S):
**Therapeutic:** antiarrhythmics (class I)

### Pregnancy Category C

## INDICATIONS

■ Suppression/prevention of unifocal and multifocal PVCs, paired PVCs, and ventricular tachycardia. **Unlabeled uses:** ■ Treatment/prevention of supraventricular tachyarrhythmias.

## ACTION

■ Decreases myocardial excitability and conduction velocity ■ Has anticholinergic properties ■ Little effect on heart rate but has a direct negative inotropic effect. **Therapeutic Effects:** ■ Suppression of ventricular arrhythmias.

## PHARMACOKINETICS

**Absorption:** Well absorbed from the GI tract.
**Distribution:** Widely distributed; enters breast milk.
**Metabolism and Excretion:** Metabolized by the liver; 10% excreted unchanged in the feces, 50% excreted unchanged by the kidneys.
**Half-life:** 8–18 hr (increased in hepatic or renal impairment).

## CONTRAINDICATIONS AND PRECAUTIONS

**Contraindicated in:** ■ Hypersensitivity ■ Cardiogenic shock ■ 2nd-degree and 3rd-degree heart block ■ Sick sinus syndrome (without a pacemaker).
**Use Cautiously in:** ■ CHF or left ventricular dysfunction (dosage reduction recommended) ■ Hepatic or renal insufficiency (dosage reduction recommended if CCr ≤40 ml/min) ■ Prostatic enlargement ■ Myasthenia gravis ■ Glaucoma ■ Children, pregnancy, or lactation (safety not established).

## ADVERSE REACTIONS AND SIDE EFFECTS*

■ **CNS:** dizziness, fatigue, headache ■ **EENT:** blurred vision, dry eyes, dry throat ■ **CV:** CHF, arrhythmias, AV block, dyspnea, edema, hypotension ■ **GI:** constipation, dry mouth, abdominal pain, flatulence, nausea ■ **GU:** urinary hesitancy, urinary retention ■ **Endo:** hypoglycemia ■ **Misc:** impaired temperature regulation.

## INTERACTIONS

**Drug-Drug:** ■ May potentiate anticoagulant effect of **warfarin** ■ **Rifampin, phenobarbital,** and **phenytoin** may decrease blood levels and effectiveness ■ **Cimetidine** or **erythromycin** may decrease metabolism and increase blood levels ■ May have additive toxic cardiac effects when used with other **antiarrhythmics** (prolonged conduction and decreased cardiac output), especially **verapamil**—avoid using disopyramide for 48 hr before or 24 hr after ■ Anticholinergic side effects may be additive with other **drugs having anticholinergic properties,** including **antihistamines** and **tricyclic antidepressants** ■ Increased risk of arrhythmias with **pimozide.**

**Drug-Natural Products:** ■ Increased anticholinergic effects with **angel's trumpet, jimson weed,** and **scopolia.**

## ROUTE AND DOSAGE

- **PO (Adults >50 kg):** 150 mg q 6 hr (as immediate-release capsules) or 300 mg q 12 hr (as CR or LA dosage form; not to exceed 800 mg/day).
- **PO (Adults <50 kg or Patients with Poor Left Ventricular Function):** 100 mg q 6–8 hr (as immediate-release capsules) or 200 mg q 12 hr (as CR or LA dosage form).
- **PO (Children 12–18 yr):** 6–15 mg/kg daily, in divided doses q 6 hr.
- **PO (Children 4–12 yr):** 10–15 mg/kg daily in divided doses q 6 hr.
- **PO (Children 1–4 yr):** 10–20 mg/kg daily in divided doses q 6 hr.
- **PO (Children <1 yr):** 10–30 mg/kg daily in divided doses q 6 hr.
- ❑ **Renal Impairment**

■ **PO (Adults):** *CCr >40 ml/min or patients with hepatic impairment*—100 mg q 6 hr; *CCr 30–40 ml/min*—100 mg q 8 hr; *CCr 15–30 ml/min*—100 mg q 12 hr; *CCr <15 ml/min*—100 mg q 24 hr as immediate-release dosage form

## AVAILABILITY (generic available)

■ *Capsules:* 100 mg$^{Rx}$, 150 mg$^{Rx}$ ■ *Extended-release capsules:* 100 mg$^{Rx}$, 150 mg$^{Rx}$ ■ *Extended-release tablets:* {150 mg$^{Rx}$} ■ *Injection:* {10 mg/ml$^{Rx}$}.

TIME/ACTION PROFILE (antiarrhythmic effects)

|  | ONSET | PEAK | DURATION |
|---|---|---|---|
| PO | 0.5–3.5 hr | 2.5 hr | 1.5–8.5 hr |
| PO-CR | 0.5–3.5 hr | 4.9 hr | 12 hr |

# NURSING IMPLICATIONS

## ASSESSMENT

❑ Monitor blood pressure, pulse, and ECG before and routinely throughout therapy. Check pulse before administering medication; withhold and notify physician or other health care professional if <60 or >120 bpm or if changes in rhythm.

❑ Monitor intake and output ratios and daily weight; assess for edema and urinary retention daily.

❑ Assess patient for signs of congestive heart failure (peripheral edema, rales/crackles, dyspnea, weight gain, jugular venous distention). Notify physician or other health care professional if these occur.

■ *Lab Test Considerations:* Renal and hepatic functions and serum potassium levels should be evaluated periodically throughout therapy.

❑ May cause elevated serum BUN, cholesterol, and triglyceride levels.

❑ May cause decreased blood glucose concentrations.

## POTENTIAL NURSING DIAGNOSES

■ Cardiac output, decreased (Indications).

■ Oral mucous membrane, impaired (Side Effects).

## IMPLEMENTATION

■ **General:** When changing from quinidine sulfate or procainamide to disopyramide, regular maintenance dose of disopyramide may be given 6–12 hr after last dose of quinidine sulfate or 3–6 hr after last dose of procainamide.

❑ Extended-release form (CR or LA formulations) is indicated for maintenance therapy only. When changing from regular form to extended-release forms, give the first dose of extended-release form 6 hr after the last regular dose.

■ **PO:** Administer medication on an empty stomach, 1 hr before or 2 hr after meals. CR and LA forms must be swallowed whole; do not break open, crush, or chew.

❑ Pharmacist may prepare a suspension with 100 mg capsules and cherry syrup.

## PATIENT/FAMILY TEACHING

❑ Advise patient to take medication around the clock, exactly as directed. Do not discontinue medication without consulting health care professional. If a dose is missed, take as soon as remembered unless within 4 hr of next dose. Do not double doses.

❑ Medication may cause dizziness. Caution patients to avoid driving or other activities requiring alertness until response to medication is known.

❑ Instruct patient to change positions slowly to minimize orthostatic hypotension.

❑ Advise patient that frequent mouth rinses, good oral hygiene, and sugarless gum or candy may help relieve dry mouth.

❑ Caution patient to avoid extremes of temperature, because this medication may cause impairment of body temperature regulation. Patient should use sunscreen and protective clothing to prevent photosensitivity reactions.

❑ Advise patient to consult health care professional before taking OTC medications or alcohol concurrently with this medication.

❑ If constipation becomes a problem, advise patient that increasing bulk and fluids in the diet and exercising may minimize constipation.

{ } = Available in Canada only.
*CAPITALS indicates life-threatening; underlines indicate most frequent.

❑ Instruct patient to notify health care professional if dry mouth, difficult urination, constipation, or blurred vision persists.

## EVALUATION

**Effectiveness of therapy can be demonstrated by:** ■ Suppression of PVCs and ventricular tachycardia ■ Prevention of further arrhythmias.

# DIURETICS (POTASSIUM-SPARING)

## amiloride
(a-**mill**-oh-ride)
Midamor

## spironolactone
(speer-oh-no-**lak**-tone)
Aldactone, {Novospiroton}

## triamterene
(trye-**am**-ter-een)
Dyrenium

### CLASSIFICATION(S):
**Therapeutic:** diuretics
**Pharmacologic:** potassium-sparing diuretics

### Pregnancy Category B (amiloride, triamterene), UK (spironolactone)

## INDICATIONS

■ Counteract potassium loss caused by other diuretics ■ Used with other agents (thiazides) to treat edema or hypertension ■ Hyperaldosteronism (spironolactone only). **Unlabeled uses:** ■ **Spironolactone:** Management of CHF (low doses).

## ACTION

■ Cause loss of sodium bicarbonate and calcium while saving potassium and hydrogen ions. **Therapeutic Effects:** ■ Weak diuretic and antihypertensive response when compared with other diuretics ■ Conservation of potassium.

## PHARMACOKINETICS

**Absorption:** *Amiloride*—15–25% absorbed from the GI tract; *spironolactone*—>90% absorbed; *triamterene*—30–70% absorbed.

**Distribution:** *Amiloride* and *triamterene*—widely distributed; *spironolactone*—crosses the placenta; enters breast milk.

**Protein Binding:** *spironolactone* and *canrenone*—>90%.

**Metabolism and Excretion:** *Amiloride*—50% eliminated unchanged in urine, 40% excreted unabsorbed in the feces; *spironolactone*—converted by the liver to its active diuretic compound (canrenone); *triamterene*—partially metabolized by the liver, some excretion of unchanged drug.

**Half-life:** *Amiloride*—6–9 hr; *spironolactone*—13–24 hr (canrenone); *triamterene*—100–150 min.

## CONTRAINDICATIONS AND PRECAUTIONS

**Contraindicated in:** ■ Hypersensitivity ■ Hyperkalemia.

**Use Cautiously in:** ■ Hepatic dysfunction ■ Geriatric or debilitated patients or patients with diabetes mellitus (increased risk of hyperkalemia,presence of age-related renal dysfunction; dosage adjustments may be necessary)) ■ Renal insufficiency (BUN >30 mg/dl or CCr <30 ml/min) ■ History of gout or kidney stones (triamterene only) ■ Pregnancy, lactation, or children (safety not established).

## ADVERSE REACTIONS AND SIDE EFFECTS*

■ **CNS:** dizziness; *spironolactone only*—clumsiness, headache ■ **CV:** arrhythmias ■ **GI:** *amiloride*—constipation, GI irritation (increased with spironolactone) ■ **GU:** impotence, *triamterene*—bluish urine, nephrolithiasis ■ **Derm:** *triamterene*—photosensitivity ■ **Endo:** *spironolactone*—gynecomastia ■ **F and E:** <u>hyperkalemia</u>, hyponatremia ■ **Hemat:** *spironolactone and triamterene*—dyscrasias ■ **MS:** muscle cramps ■ **Misc:** allergic reactions.

## INTERACTIONS

**Drug-Drug:** ■ ↑ hypotension with acute ingestion of **alcohol**, other **antihypertensives**, or **nitrates** ■ Use with **ACE inhibitors, angiotensin II receptor antagonists, indomethacin, potassium supplements**, or **cyclosporine** ↑ risk of hyperkalemia ■ ↓ **lithium** excretion ■ Effectiveness may be ↓ by **NSAIDs** ■ Spironolactone may ↑ effects of **digoxin** ■ Triamterene ↓ effects of **folic acid** (leucovorin should be used) ■ Triamterene may ↑ risk of toxicity from **amantadine**.

## ROUTE AND DOSAGE

❑ **Amiloride**

■ **PO (Adults):** 5–10 mg/day (up to 20 mg).

❑ **Spironolactone**

■ **PO (Adults):** 25–400 mg/day as a single dose or 2–4 divided doses. *CHF*—12.5–25 mg/day (unlabeled use).

■ **PO (Children):** 1–3 mg/kg/day (30–90 mg/m²/day as a single dose or 2–4 divided doses (not to exceed 3 times initial dose).

❑ **Triamterene**

■ **PO (Adults):** 100 mg twice daily (not to exceed 300 mg/day; lower doses in combination products).

■ **PO (Children):** 2–4 mg/kg/day (120 mg/ m²/day) in divided doses given daily or every other day (not to exceed 6 mg/kg/day or 300 mg/day).

## AVAILABILITY

❑ **Amiloride**

■ *Tablets:* 5 mg^Rx ■ Cost: $57.65/100 ■ hydrochlorothiazide (Moduretic^Rx, {Moduret}^Rx). See Appendix B.

❑ **Spironolactone**

■ *Tablets:* 25 mg^Rx, 50 mg^Rx, 100 mg^Rx ■ Cost: *Aldactone*—25 mg $55.75/100, 50 mg $97.91/100, 100 mg $164.16/100; *generic*— 25 mg $8.94/100 ■ hydrochlorothiazide (Aldactazide^Rx, {Novo-Spirozine^Rx}, Spirazide^Rx). See Appendix B.

❑ **Triamterene**

■ *Capsules:* 50 mg^Rx, 100 mg^Rx ■ Cost: 50 mg $94.52/100, 100 mg $171.88/100 ■ *Tablets:* {50 mg^Rx}, {100 mg^Rx} ■ hydrochlorothiazide (Apo-Triazide^Rx, Dyazide^Rx, Maxzide^Rx, {Novo-Triamzide}^Rx). See Appendix B.

TIME/ACTION PROFILE (diuretic effect)

|  | ONSET | PEAK | DURATION |
|---|---|---|---|
| Amiloride | 2 hr† | 6–10 hr† | 24 hr† |
| Spironolactone | unknown | 2–3 days‡ | 2–3 days‡ |
| Triamterene | 2–4 hr† | 1–several days‡ | 7–9 hr† |

†Single dose.
‡Multiple doses.

## NURSING IMPLICATIONS

### ASSESSMENT

❑ Monitor intake and output ratios and daily weight during therapy.

❑ If medication is given as an adjunct to antihypertensive therapy, monitor blood pressure before administering.

❑ Monitor response of signs and symptoms of hypokalemia (weakness, fatigue, U wave on ECG, arrhythmias, polyuria, polydipsia). Assess patient frequently for development of hyperkalemia (fatigue, muscle weakness, paresthesia, confusion, dyspnea, cardiac arrhythmias). Patients who have diabetes mellitus or kidney disease and geriatric patients are at increased risk of developing these symptoms.

❑ Periodic ECGs are recommended in patients receiving prolonged therapy.

■ *Lab Test Considerations:* Serum potassium levels should be evaluated before and routinely during therapy. Withhold drug and notify physician or other health care professional if patient becomes hyperkalemic.

❑ Monitor BUN, serum creatinine, and electrolytes before and periodically during therapy. May cause ↑ serum magnesium, uric acid, BUN, creatinine, potassium, plasma renin activity, and urinary calcium excretion levels. May also cause ↓ sodium levels.

❑ Discontinue potassium-sparing diuretics 3 days before a glucose tolerance test because of risk of severe hyperkalemia.

❑ *Spironolactone* may cause false ↑ of plasma cortisol concentrations. Spironolactone should be withdrawn 4–7 days before test.

❑ Monitor platelet count and total and differential leukocyte count periodically during therapy in patients taking *triamterene*.

### POTENTIAL NURSING DIAGNOSES

■ Fluid volume, excess (Indications).

### IMPLEMENTATION

■ **PO:** Administer in AM to avoid interrupting sleep pattern.

❑ Administer with food or milk to minimize gastric irritation and to increase bioavailability.

---

{ } = Available in Canada only.
*CAPITALS indicates life-threatening; underlines indicate most frequent.

❏ *Triamterene* capsules may be opened and contents mixed with food or fluids for patients with difficulty swallowing.

### PATIENT/FAMILY TEACHING

■ **General Info:** Emphasize the importance of continuing to take this medication, even if feeling well. Instruct patient to take medication at the same time each day. Take missed doses as soon as remembered unless almost time for next dose. Do not double doses.

❏ Caution patient to avoid salt substitutes and foods that contain high levels of potassium or sodium unless prescribed by health care professional.

❏ May cause dizziness. Caution patient to avoid driving or other activities requiring alertness until response to medication is known.

❏ Advise patient to consult with health care professional before taking any OTC decongestants, cough or cold preparations, or appetite suppressants concurrently with this medication because of potential for increased blood pressure.

❏ Advise patients taking *triamterene* to use sunscreen and protective clothing to prevent photosensitivity reactions.

❏ Instruct patient to notify health care professional of medication regimen before treatment or surgery.

❏ Inform patient that *triamterene* may cause bluish-colored urine.

❏ Advise patient to notify health care professional if muscle weakness or cramps; fatigue; or severe nausea, vomiting, or diarrhea occurs.

❏ Emphasize the need for follow-up exams to monitor progress.

■ **Hypertension:** Reinforce need to continue additional therapies for hypertension (weight loss, restricted sodium intake, stress reduction, moderation of alcohol intake, regular exercise, and cessation of smoking). Medication helps control but does not cure hypertension.

❏ Teach patient and family the correct technique for checking blood pressure weekly.

### EVALUATION

**Effectiveness of therapy can be demonstrated by:** ■ Increase in diuresis and decrease in edema while maintaining serum potassium level in an acceptable range ■ Decrease in blood pressure ■ Prevention of hypokalemia in patients taking diuretics ■ Treatment of hyperaldosteronism.

---

# DIURETICS (THIAZIDE)

**chlorothiazide**
(klor-oh-**thye**-a-zide)
Diuril

**chlorthalidone (thiazide–like)**
(klor-**thal**-i-doan)
{Apo-Chlorthalidone}, Hygroton, Thalitone, {Uridon}

**hydrochlorothiazide**
(hye-droe-klor-oh-**thye**-a-zide)
{Apo-Hydro}, Esidrex, HCTZ, Hydro-chlor, Hydro-D, HydroDIURIL, Microzide, {Neo-Codema}, Novo-Hydrazide, Oretic, {Urozide}

*CLASSIFICATION(S):*
*Therapeutic: antihypertensives, diuretics*
*Pharmacologic: thiazide diuretics, thiazide-like diuretics*

**Pregnancy Category B**

### INDICATIONS

■ Management of mild to moderate hypertension ■ Treatment of edema associated with: ❏ CHF ❏ Renal dysfunction ❏ Cirrhosis ❏ Corticosteroid therapy ❏ Estrogen therapy.

### ACTION

■ Increases excretion of sodium and water by inhibiting sodium reabsorption in the distal tubule ■ Promotes excretion of chloride, potassium, magnesium, and bicarbonate ■ May produce arteriolar dilation. **Therapeutic Effects:** ■ Lowering of blood pressure in hypertensive patients and diuresis with mobilization of edema.

### PHARMACOKINETICS

**Absorption:** All are rapidly absorbed after oral administration.

**Distribution:** Distributed into extracellular space. All cross the placenta and enter breast milk.

**Metabolism and Excretion:** All are excreted mainly unchanged by the kidneys.

**Half-life:** *Chlorothiazide*—1–2 hr; *chlorthalidone*—35–50 hr; *hydrochlorothiazide*—6–15 hr.

## CONTRAINDICATIONS AND PRECAUTIONS

**Contraindicated in:** ■ Hypersensitivity ■ Cross-sensitivity with other thiazides or sulfonamides may exist ■ Some products contain tartrazine and should be avoided in patients with known intolerance ■ Anuria ■ Lactation.

**Use Cautiously in:** ■ Renal or severe hepatic impairment ■ Pregnancy (jaundice or thrombocytopenia may be seen in the newborn).

## ADVERSE REACTIONS AND SIDE EFFECTS*

■ **CNS:** dizziness, drowsiness, lethargy, weakness ■ **CV:** hypotension ■ **GI:** anorexia, cramping, hepatitis, nausea, vomiting ■ **Derm:** photosensitivity, rashes ■ **Endo:** hyperglycemia ■ **F and E:** hypokalemia, dehydration, hypercalcemia, hypochloremic alkalosis, hypomagnesemia, hyponatremia, hypophosphatemia, hypovolemia ■ **Hemat:** blood dyscrasias ■ **Metab:** hyperuricemia, elevated lipids ■ **MS:** muscle cramps ■ **Misc:** pancreatitis.

## INTERACTIONS

**Drug-Drug:** ■ Additive hypotension with other **antihypertensives,** acute ingestion of **alcohol,** or **nitrates** ■ Additive hypokalemia with **corticosteroids, amphotericin B, mezlocillin, piperacillin,** or **ticarcillin** ■ Decreases the excretion of **lithium** ■ **Cholestyramine** or **colestipol** decreases absorption ■ Hypokalemia increases risk of **digoxin** toxicity ■ **NSAIDs** may decrease effectiveness ■ **Allopurinol** may increase the risk of hypersensitivity reactions.

**Drug-Natural Products:** ■ **Licorice** and **stimulant laxative** herbs (**aloe, cascara sagrada, senna**) may increase risk of potassium depletion ■ Concomitant use with **ginkgo** may decrease antihypertensive effects.

## ROUTE AND DOSAGE

When used as a diuretic in adults, may be given every other day or 2–3 days/week.

❑ **Chlorothiazide**

■ **PO (Adults):** 250 mg–1 g/day as a single dose or in divided doses.
■ **PO (Children ≥6 mos):** 10–20 mg/kg/day as a single dose or in 2 divided doses.
■ **IV (Adults):** *Diuretic*—250 mg q 6–12 hr. *Antihypertensive*—500 mg–1 g/day as a single dose or 2 divided doses.

❑ **Chlorthalidone**

■ **PO (Adults):** 25–100 mg once daily.
■ **PO (Children):** 2 mg/kg (60 mg/m$^2$) daily for 3 days/wk.

❑ **Hydrochlorothiazide**

■ **PO (Adults):** *Hypertension*—12.5 mg/day initially (range 12.5–100 mg/day in 1–2 doses up to 200 mg/day; not to exceed 50 mg/day for hypertension).
■ **PO (Children >6 mo):** 1–2 mg/kg (30–60 mg/m$^2$/day) in 1–2 divided doses.
■ **PO (Children <6 mo):** Up to 3 mg/kg/day.

## AVAILABILITY

❑ **Chlorothiazide**

■ *Tablets:* 250 mg$^{Rx}$, 500 mg$^{Rx}$ ■ *Oral suspension:* 250 mg/5 m$^{Rx}$ ■ *Powder for injection:* 500 mg$^{Rx}$ ■ methyldopa, reserpine$^{Rx}$. See Appendix B.

❑ **Chlorthalidone**

■ *Tablets:* 25 mg$^{Rx}$, 50 mg$^{Rx}$, 100 mg$^{Rx}$ ■ atenolol, clonidine, reserpine$^{Rx}$. See Appendix B.

❑ **Hydrochlorothiazide**

■ *Tablets:* 25 mg$^{Rx}$, 50 mg$^{Rx}$, 100 mg$^{Rx}$ ■ Cost: *HydroDIURIL*—25 mg $16.82/100, 50 mg $24.83/100; *generic*—25 mg $3.43/100, 50 mg $4.23/100, 100 mg $6.97 ■ *Capsules:* 12.5 mg$^{Rx}$ ■ Cost: *Microzide*—$40.95/100 ■ *Oral solution:* 10 mg/ml$^{Rx}$, 100 mg/ml$^{Rx}$ ■ spironolactone, triamterene, bisoprolol, hydralazine, moexipril, reserpine, timolol$^{Rx}$. See Appendix B.

TIME/ACTION PROFILE (diuretic effect)

| | ONSET | PEAK | DURATION |
|---|---|---|---|
| Chlorothiazide | 2 hr | 4 hr | 6–12 hr |
| Chlorthalidone | 2 hr | 2 hr | 48–72 hr |

| | | | |
|---|---|---|---|
| Hydrochloro-thiazide† | 2 hr | 3–6 hr | 6–12 hr |

†Onset of antihypertensive effect is 3–4 days and does not become maximal for 7–14 days of dosing.

## NURSING IMPLICATIONS

### ASSESSMENT

- **General Info:** Monitor blood pressure, intake, output, and daily weight and assess feet, legs, and sacral area for edema daily.
- Assess patient, especially if taking digitalis glycosides, for anorexia, nausea, vomiting, muscle cramps, paresthesia, and confusion. Notify physician or other health care professional if these signs of electrolyte imbalance occur. Patients taking digoxin are at risk of digoxin toxicity because of the potassium-depleting effect of the diuretic.
- Assess patient for allergy to sulfonamides.
- **Hypertension:** Monitor blood pressure before and periodically throughout therapy.
- Monitor frequency of prescription refills to determine compliance.
- *Lab Test Considerations:* Monitor electrolytes (especially potassium), blood glucose, BUN, serum creatinine, and uric acid levels before and periodically throughout therapy.
- May cause increase in serum and urine glucose in diabetic patients.
- May cause an increase in serum bilirubin, calcium, creatinine, and uric acid, and a decrease in serum magnesium, potassium, sodium, and urinary calcium concentrations.
- May cause decreased serum protein-bound iodine (PBI) concentrations.
- May cause increased serum cholesterol, low-density lipoprotein, and triglyceride concentrations.

### POTENTIAL NURSING DIAGNOSES

- Fluid volume, excess (Indications).
- Fluid volume, risk for deficit (Side Effects).

### IMPLEMENTATION

- **General:** Administer in the morning to prevent disruption of sleep cycle.
- Intermittent dose schedule may be used for continued control of edema.
- **PO:** May give with food or milk to minimize GI irritation. Tablets may be crushed and mixed with fluid to facilitate swallowing.

- **Intermittent Infusion:** Reconstitute chlorothiazide with at least 18 ml of sterile water for injection for a concentration of 25 mg/ml. Shake to dissolve. Stable for 24 hr at room temperature. May be diluted further with D5W or 0.9% NaCl.

### PATIENT/FAMILY TEACHING

- **General Info:** Instruct patient to take this medication at the same time each day. If a dose is missed, take as soon as remembered but not just before next dose is due. Do not double doses.
- Instruct patient on use of calibrated dropper for measuring hydrochlorothiazide concentrated oral solution.
- Instruct patient to monitor weight biweekly and notify health care professional of significant changes.
- Caution patient to change positions slowly to minimize orthostatic hypotension. This may be potentiated by alcohol.
- Advise patient to use sunscreen and protective clothing to prevent photosensitivity reactions.
- Instruct patient to discuss dietary potassium requirements with health care professional (see Appendix Q).
- Instruct patient to notify health care professional of medication regimen before treatment or surgery.
- Advise patient to report muscle weakness, cramps, nausea, vomiting, diarrhea, or dizziness to health care professional.
- Emphasize the importance of routine follow-up exams.
- **Hypertension:** Advise patients to continue taking the medication even if feeling better. Medication controls but does not cure hypertension.
- Encourage patient to comply with additional interventions for hypertension (weight reduction, low-sodium diet, regular exercise, smoking cessation, moderation of alcohol consumption, and stress management).
- Instruct patient and family in correct technique for monitoring weekly blood pressure.
- Advise patient to consult health care professional before taking OTC medication, especially cough or cold preparations, concurrently with this therapy.

## EVALUATION

**Effectiveness of therapy can be demonstrated by:** ■ Decrease in blood pressure ■ Increase in urine output ◻ Decrease in edema.

High Alert

# dobutamine
(doe-**byoo**-ta-meen)
Dobutrex

*CLASSIFICATION(S):*
*Therapeutic: inotropics*
*Pharmacologic: adrenergics*

**Pregnancy Category B**

## INDICATIONS

■ Short-term (<48 hr) management of heart failure caused by depressed contractility from organic heart disease or surgical procedures.

## ACTION

■ Stimulates beta$_1$(myocardial)-adrenergic receptors with relatively minor effect on heart rate or peripheral blood vessels. **Therapeutic Effects:** ■ Increased cardiac output without significantly increased heart rate.

## PHARMACOKINETICS

**Absorption:** Administered by IV infusion only, resulting in complete bioavailability.
**Distribution:** Unknown.
**Metabolism and Excretion:** Metabolized by the liver and other tissues.
**Half-life:** 2 min.

## CONTRAINDICATIONS AND PRECAUTIONS

**Contraindicated in:** ■ Hypersensitivity to dobutamine or bisulfites ■ Idiopathic hypertrophic subaortic stenosis.

**Use Cautiously in:** ■ History of hypertension (increased risk of exaggerated pressor response) ■ MI ■ Atrial fibrillation (pretreatment with digitalis glycosides recommended) ■ History of ventricular atopic activity (may be exacerbated) ■ Hypovalemia (correct before administration) ■ Pregnancy or lactation (safety not established) ■ Children (has been used safely in children, although risk of tachycardia is increased).

## ADVERSE REACTIONS AND SIDE EFFECTS*

■ **CNS:** headache ■ **Resp:** shortness of breath ■ **CV:** <u>hypertension</u>, <u>increased heart rate</u>, <u>premature ventricular contractions</u>, angina pectoris, arrhythmias, hypotension, palpitations ■ **GI:** nausea, vomiting ■ **Local:** phlebitis ■ **Misc:** hypersensitivity reactions including skin rash, fever, bronchospasm or eosinophilia, nonanginal chest pain.

## INTERACTIONS

**Drug-Drug:** ■ Use with **nitroprusside** may have a synergistic effect on increasing cardiac output ■ **Beta blockers** may negate the effect of dobutamine ■ Increased risk of arrhythmias or hypertension with some **anesthetics (cyclopropane, halothane)**, **MAO inhibitors, oxytocics,** or **tricyclic antidepressants**.

## ROUTE AND DOSAGE

■ **IV (Adults and Children):** Start with low infusion rates (0.5–1 mcg/kg/min), titrated at intervals of a few minutes, guided by the patient's response (range 2–20 mcg/kg/min, up to 40 mcg/kg/min).

## AVAILABILITY

■ *Injection:* 12.5 mg/ml in 20-ml vial$^{Rx}$.

TIME/ACTION PROFILE (inotropic effects)

|     | ONSET    | PEAK   | DURATION    |
|-----|----------|--------|-------------|
| IV  | 1–2 min  | 10 min | brief (min) |

# NURSING IMPLICATIONS

## ASSESSMENT

◻ Monitor blood pressure, heart rate, ECG, pulmonary capillary wedge pressure (PCWP), cardiac output, CVP, and urinary output continuously during the administration. Report significant changes in vital signs or arrhythmias. Consult physician for parameters for pulse, blood pressure, or ECG changes for adjusting dosage or discontinuing medication.

{ } = Available in Canada only.
*CAPITALS indicates life-threatening; <u>underlines</u> indicate most frequent.

□ Palpate peripheral pulses and assess appearance of extremities routinely throughout dobutamine administration. Notify physician if quality of pulse deteriorates or if extremities become cold or mottled.

■ **Lab Test Considerations:** Monitor potassium concentrations during therapy; may cause hypokalemia.

□ Monitor electrolytes, BUN, creatinine, and prothrombin time weekly during prolonged therapy.

■ **Toxicity and Overdose:** If overdose occurs, reduction or discontinuation of therapy is the only treatment necessary because of the short duration of dobutamine.

## POTENTIAL NURSING DIAGNOSES

■ Cardiac output, decreased (Indications).
■ Tissue perfusion, ineffective (Indications).

## IMPLEMENTATION

□ **High Alert:** IV vasoactive medications are potentially dangerous. Have second practitioner independently check original order, dosage calculations and infusion pump settings. Do not confuse dobutamine with dopamine. If available as floor stock, store in separate areas.

■ **General:** Correct hypovolemia with volume expanders before initiating dobutamine therapy.

□ Administer into a large vein and assess administration site frequently. Extravasation may cause pain and inflammation.

■ **IV:** Reconstitute 250-mg vial with 10 ml of sterile water or D5W for injection. If not completely dissolved, add another 10 ml of diluent. Dilute in at least 50 ml of D5W, 0.9% NaCl, sodium lactate, 0.45% NaCl, D5/0.45% NaCl, D5/0.9% NaCl, D5/LR, or LR. Standard concentrations range from 250 mcg/ml to 1000 mcg/ml. Concentrations should not exceed 5 mg of dobutamine per ml. Slight pink color of solution does not alter potency. Solution is stable for 24 hr at room temperature.

■ **Continuous Infusion:** Administer via infusion pump. Rate of administration is titrated according to patient response (heart rate, presence of ectopic activity, blood pressure, urine output, CVP, PCWP, cardiac output). Dose should be titrated so heart rate does not increase by >10% of baseline.

■ **Y-Site Compatibility:** ◆ amifostine ◆ amiodarone ◆ atracurium ◆ aztreonam ◆ bretylium ◆ calcium chloride ◆ calcium gluconate ◆ ciprofloxacin ◆ cisatracurium ◆ cladribine ◆ diazepam ◆ diltiazem ◆ docetaxel ◆ dopamine ◆ doxorubicin liposome ◆ enalaprilat ◆ epinephrine ◆ etoposide ◆ famotidine ◆ fentanyl ◆ fluconazole ◆ gatifloxacin ◆ gemcitabine ◆ granisetron ◆ haloperidol ◆ hydromorphone ◆ inamrinone ◆ insulin ◆ labetalol ◆ levofloxacin ◆ lidocaine ◆ linezolid ◆ lorazepam ◆ magnesium sulfate ◆ meperidine ◆ milrinone ◆ morphine ◆ nitroglycerin ◆ nitroprusside ◆ norepinephrine ◆ pancuronium ◆ potassium chloride ◆ propofol ◆ ranitidine ◆ remifentanil ◆ streptokinase ◆ tacrolimus ◆ theophylline ◆ thiotepa ◆ tolazoline ◆ vecuronium ◆ verapamil ◆ zidovudine.

■ **Y-Site Incompatibility:** ◆ alatrofloxacin ◆ acyclovir ◆ alteplase ◆ aminophylline ◆ amphotericin B cholesteryl sulfate ◆ cefepime ◆ foscarnet ◆ indomethacin ◆ phytonadione ◆ piperacillin/tazobactam ◆ thiopental ◆ warfarin.

## PATIENT/FAMILY TEACHING

□ Explain to patient the rationale for instituting this medication and the need for frequent monitoring.

□ Advise patient to inform nurse immediately if chest pain; dyspnea; or numbness, tingling, or burning of extremities occurs.

□ Instruct patient to notify nurse immediately of pain or discomfort at the site of administration.

■ **Home Care Issues:** Instruct caregiver on proper care of IV equipment.

□ Instruct caregiver to report signs of worsening CHF (shortness of breath, orthopnea, decreased exercise tolerance), abdominal pain, and nausea or vomiting to health care professional promptly.

## EVALUATION

**Effectiveness of therapy can be demonstrated by:** ■ Increase in cardiac output □ Improved hemodynamic parameters □ Increased urine output.

**High Alert**

# docetaxel
(doe-se-**tax**-el)

Taxotere

**CLASSIFICATION(S):**
*Therapeutic:* antineoplastics
*Pharmacologic:* taxoids

**Pregnancy Category D**

## INDICATIONS
■ Locally advanced or metastatic breast cancer ■ Locally advanced or metastatic non–small-cell lung cancer.

## ACTION
■ Interferes with normal cellular microtubule function required for interphase and mitosis. **Therapeutic Effects:** ■ Death of rapidly replicating cells, particularly malignant ones.

## PHARMACOKINETICS
**Absorption:** IV administration results in complete bioavailability.
**Distribution:** Unknown.
**Metabolism and Excretion:** Extensively metabolized by the liver; metabolites undergo fecal elimination.
**Half-life:** 11.1 hr.

## CONTRAINDICATIONS AND PRECAUTIONS
**Contraindicated in:** ■ Hypersensitivity ■ Hypersensitivity to polysorbate 80 ■ Known alcohol intolerance ■ Neutrophil count <1500/mm³ ■ Liver impairment (serum bilirubin >upper limit of normal, ALT and/or AST >1.5 times upper limit of normal, with alkaline phosphatase >2.5 times upper limit of normal) ■ Pregnancy or lactation.
**Use Cautiously in:** ■ Patients with childbearing potential.

## ADVERSE REACTIONS AND SIDE EFFECTS*
■ **CNS:** <u>fatigue</u>, <u>weakness</u> ■ **Resp:** bronchospasm ■ **CV:** ASCITES, CARDIAC TAMPONADE, PERICARDIAL EFFUSION, PULMONARY EDEMA, <u>peripheral edema</u> ■ **GI:** <u>diarrhea</u>, <u>nausea</u>, <u>stomatitis</u>, <u>vomiting</u> ■ **Derm:** <u>alopecia</u>, <u>rashes</u>, dermatitis, desquamation, edema, erythema, nail disorders ■ **Hemat:** <u>anemia</u>, <u>thrombocytopenia</u>, leukopenia ■ **Local:** injection site reactions ■ **MS:** <u>myalgia</u>, arthral-

gia ■ **Neuro:** neurosensory deficits, peripheral neuropathy ■ **Misc:** hypersensitivity reactions, including ANAPHYLAXIS.

## INTERACTIONS
**Drug-Drug:** ■ ↑ bone marrow depression may occur with other **antineoplastics** or **radiation therapy** ■ **Cyclosporine, ketoconazole, erythromycin,** or **troleandomycin** may significantly alter the effects of docetaxel.

## ROUTE AND DOSAGE
■ **IV (Adults):** *Breast cancer*—60–100 mg/m² every 3 wk; *Non–small-cell lung cancer*—75 mg/m² every 3 wk.

## AVAILABILITY
■ *Injection concentrate:* 20 mg/0.5 ml polysorbate 80 with diluent (13% ethanol)$^{Rx}$, 80 mg/2 ml polysorbate 80 with diluent (13% ethanol)$^{Rx}$ ■ Cost: 20 mg/0.5 ml $329.18/0.5 ml, 80 mg $1316.70/2 ml.

TIME/ACTION PROFILE (effect on blood counts)

|    | ONSET | PEAK | DURATION |
|----|-------|------|----------|
| IV | rapid | 5–9 days | 7 days |

# NURSING IMPLICATIONS

## ASSESSMENT
❑ Monitor vital signs before and after administration.
❑ Assess infusion site for patency. Docetaxel is not a vesicant. If extravasation occurs, discontinue docetaxel immediately and aspirate the IV needle. Apply cold compresses to the site for 24 hr.
❑ Monitor for hypersensitivity reactions continuously during infusion. These are most common after the first and second doses of docetaxel. Reactions may consist of bronchospasm, hypotension, and/or erythema. Mild to moderate reactions may be treated symptomatically and infusion slowed or stopped until reaction subsides. Severe reactions require discontinuation of therapy and symptomatic treatment. Do not readminister docetaxel to patients with previous severe reactions. Severe edema may also occur. Weigh

patients before each treatment. Fluid accumulation may result in edema, ascites, and pleural or pericardial effusions. Pretreatment with corticosteroids (such as dexamethasone 8 mg PO twice daily for 5 days, starting 1 day before docetaxel) is recommended to minimize edema and hypersensitivity reactions. PO furosemide may be used to treat edema.

❑ Monitor for bone marrow depression. Assess for bleeding (bleeding gums, bruising, petechiae; guaiac stools, urine, and emesis) and avoid IM injections and taking rectal temperatures if platelet count is low. Apply pressure to venipuncture sites for 10 min. Assess for signs of infection during neutropenia. Anemia may occur. Monitor for increased fatigue, dyspnea, and orthostatic hypotension.

❑ Assess patient for rash. May occur on feet or hands but may also occur on arms, face, or thorax, usually with pruritus. Rash usually occurs within 1 wk after infusion and resolves before next infusion.

❑ Assess for development of neurosensory deficit (paresthesia, dysesthesia, pain, burning). May also cause weakness. Pyridoxine may be used to minimize symptoms. Severe symptoms may require dose reduction or discontinuation.

❑ Assess patient for arthralgia and myalgia, which are usually relieved by nonopioid analgesics but may be severe enough to require treatment with opioid analgesics.

▪ *Lab Test Considerations:* Monitor CBC and differential before each treatment. Frequently causes neutropenia (<2000 neutrophils/mm³); may require dose adjustment. If the neutrophil count is less than 1500/mm³, dose should be held. Neutropenia is reversible and not cumulative. The nadir is 8 days, with a duration of 7 days. May also cause thrombocytopenia and anemia.

❑ Monitor liver function studies (AST, ALT, alkaline phosphatase, bilirubin) before each cycle. Doses are usually held if levels are elevated.

## POTENTIAL NURSING DIAGNOSES

▪ Infection, risk for (Adverse Reactions).
▪ Injury, risk for (Adverse Reactions).

## IMPLEMENTATION

❑ *High Alert:* Fatalities have occurred with chemotherapeutic agents. Before administering, clarify all ambiguous orders; double

check single, daily, and course-of-therapy dose limits; have second practitioner independently double check original order, calculations and infusion pump settings. Do not confuse Taxotere (docetaxel) with Taxol (paclitaxel).

▪ **General:** Solution should be prepared in a biologic cabinet. Wear gloves, gown, and mask while handling medication. Discard IV equipment in specially designated containers.

▪ **Continuous Infusion:** Before dilution, allow vials to stand at room temperature for 5 min. Withdraw entire contents of diluent vial and transfer to vial of docetaxel. Rotate vial gently for 15 sec to mix. Do not shake. Solution should be clear but may contain foam at top. Allow to stand for a few minutes to allow foam to dissipate. All foam need not dissipate before continuing preparation. To prepare the solution for infusion, withdraw the required amount of 10 mg/ml solution into syringe and inject into 250 ml of 0.9% NaCl or D5W for a concentration of 0.3–0.9 mg/ml. Rotate infusion container to mix infusion thoroughly. Do not administer solutions that are cloudy or contain a precipitate. Solution does not require an in-line filter. Dilute solutions are stable for 8 hr if refrigerated or at room temperature.

▪ *Rate:* Administer over 1 hr.

▪ **Y-Site Compatibility:** ♦ acyclovir ♦ amifostine ♦ amikacin ♦ aminophylline ♦ ampicillin ♦ ampicillin/sulbactam ♦ aztreonam ♦ bumetanide ♦ buprenorphine ♦ butorphanol ♦ calcium gluconate ♦ cefazolin ♦ cefepime ♦ cefoperazone ♦ cefotaxime ♦ cefotetan ♦ cefoxitin ♦ ceftazidime ♦ ceftizoxime ♦ ceftriaxone ♦ cefuroxime ♦ chlorpromazine ♦ cimetidine ♦ ciprofloxacin ♦ clindamycin ♦ diphenhydramine ♦ dobutamine ♦ dopamine ♦ doxycycline ♦ droperidol ♦ enalaprilat ♦ famotidine ♦ fluconazole ♦ furosemide ♦ ganciclovir ♦ gemcitabine ♦ gentamicin ♦ granisetron ♦ haloperidol ♦ heparin ♦ hydrocortisone ♦ hydromorphone ♦ imipenem/cilastatin ♦ leucovorin ♦ lorazepam ♦ magnesium sulfate ♦ mannitol ♦ meperidine ♦ meropenem ♦ mesna ♦ metoclopramide ♦ metronidazole ♦ minocycline ♦ morphine ♦ netilmicin ♦ ofloxacin ♦ ondansetron ♦ piperacillin ♦ piperacillin/tazobactam ♦ potassium chloride ♦ prochlorperazine ♦ promethazine ♦ ranitidine ♦ sodium bicarbonate ♦ ticarcillin ♦ ticarcillin/clavulanate ♦

tobramycin ✦ trimethoprim/sulfamethoxazole ✦ vancomycin ✦ zidovudine.

■ **Y-Site Incompatibility:** ✦ amphotericin B ✦ doxorubicin liposome ✦ methylprednisolone ✦ nalbuphine.

■ **Additive Incompatibility:** Information unavailable. Do not admix with other drugs or solutions.

## PATIENT/FAMILY TEACHING

❑ Advise patient to notify health care professional if fever >101°F; chills; sore throat; signs of infection; bleeding gums; bruising; petechiae; or blood in urine, stool, or emesis occur. Caution patient to avoid crowds and persons with known infections. Instruct patient to use soft toothbrush and electric razor.

❑ Patient should be cautioned not to drink alcoholic beverages or take products containing aspirin or NSAIDs.

❑ Fatigue is a frequent side effect of docetaxel. Advise patient that frequent rest periods and pacing of activities may minimize fatigue.

❑ Instruct patient to notify health care professional if abdominal pain, yellow skin, weakness, paresthesia, gait disturbances, swelling of the feet, or joint or muscle aches occur.

❑ Instruct patient to inspect oral mucosa for redness and ulceration. If mouth sores occur, advise patient to use sponge brush and rinse mouth with water after eating and drinking.

❑ Discuss with patient the possibility of hair loss. Complete hair loss usually begins after 1 or 2 treatments and is reversible after discontinuation of therapy. Explore coping strategies.

❑ Instruct patient not to receive any vaccinations without advice of health care professional.

❑ Emphasize the need for periodic lab tests to monitor for side effects.

## EVALUATION

**Effectiveness of therapy can be demonstrated by:** ■ Decrease in size or spread of malignancy in women with advanced breast cancer ■ Decrease in size or spread of malig-

nancy in locally advanced or metastatic non–small-cell lung cancer.

# DOCUSATE
(**dok**-yoo-sate)

### docusate calcium
DC Softgels, Stool softener, Stool softener DC, Surfak

### docusate sodium
Colace, Correctol Stool Softener Soft Gels, Diocto, Docu, DOS Softgels, DOSS, DSS, ex-lax Stool Softener, Genasoft, Modane Soft, Silace, Stool Softener, Therevac SB

## CLASSIFICATION(S):
**Therapeutic:** laxatives
**Pharmacologic:** stool softeners

### Pregnancy Category C

## INDICATIONS

■ **PO:** Prevention of constipation (in patients who should avoid straining, such as after MI or rectal surgery) ■ **Rect:** Used as enema to soften fecal impaction.

## ACTION

■ Promotes incorporation of water into stool, resulting in softer fecal mass ■ May also promote electrolyte and water secretion into the colon. **Therapeutic Effects:** ■ Softening and passage of stool.

## PHARMACOKINETICS

**Absorption:** Small amounts may be absorbed from the small intestine after oral administration. Absorption from the rectum is not known.
**Distribution:** Unknown.
**Metabolism and Excretion:** Amounts absorbed after oral administration are eliminated in bile.
**Half-life:** Unknown.

## CONTRAINDICATIONS AND PRECAUTIONS

**Contraindicated in:** ■ Hypersensitivity ■ Abdominal pain, nausea, or vomiting, especially when associated with fever or other signs of an acute abdomen.

**Use Cautiously in:** ■ Excessive or prolonged use may lead to dependence ■ Should not be used if prompt results are desired ■ Has been used during pregnancy and lactation.

## ADVERSE REACTIONS AND SIDE EFFECTS*

■ **EENT:** throat irritation ■ **GI:** mild cramps ■ **Derm:** rashes.

## INTERACTIONS

**Drug-Drug:** ■ None significant.

## ROUTE AND DOSAGE

❑ **Docusate Calcium**

■ **PO (Adults):** 240 mg once daily.
■ **PO (Children ≥6 yr and Adults with Minimal Requirements):** 50–150 mg once daily.

❑ **Docusate Sodium**

■ **PO (Adults and Children >12 yr):** 50–500 mg once daily.
■ **PO (Children 6–12 yr):** 40–120 mg once daily.
■ **PO (Children 3–6 yr):** 20–60 mg once daily.
■ **PO (Children <3 yr):** 10–40 mg once daily.
■ **Rect (Adults):** 50–100 mg or 1 unit containing 283 mg docusate sodium, soft soap, and glycerin.

## AVAILABILITY (generic available)

❑ **Docusate Calcium**

■ *Capsules:* 50 mg^OTC, 240 mg^OTC.

❑ **Docusate Sodium**

■ *Tablets:* 100 mg^OTC ■ Cost: $4.25/100 ■ *Capsules:* 50 mg^OTC, 100 mg^OTC, 120 mg^OTC, 240 mg^OTC, 250 mg^OTC ■ *Syrup:* 20 mg/5 ml^OTC ■ *Liquid:* 150 mg/15 ml^OTC ■ *Solution:* 50 mg/5 ml^OTC ■ *Enema:* 283 mg/3.9-g capsule^OTC ■ stimulant laxatives^OTC. See Appendix B.

TIME/ACTION PROFILE (softening of stool)

| | ONSET | PEAK | DURATION |
|---|---|---|---|
| PO | 24–48 hr (up to 3–5 days) | unknown | unknown |
| Rectal | 2–15 min | unknown | unknown |

## NURSING IMPLICATIONS

### ASSESSMENT

❑ Assess patient for abdominal distention, presence of bowel sounds, and usual pattern of bowel function.
❑ Assess color, consistency, and amount of stool produced.

### POTENTIAL NURSING DIAGNOSES

■ Constipation (Indications).

### IMPLEMENTATION

■ **General:** This medication does not stimulate intestinal peristalsis.
■ **PO:** Administer with a full glass of water or juice. May be administered on an empty stomach for more rapid results.
❑ Oral solution may be diluted in milk or fruit juice to decrease bitter taste.
❑ Do not administer within 2 hr of other laxatives, especially mineral oil. May cause increased absorption.

### PATIENT/FAMILY TEACHING

❑ Advise patients that laxatives should be used only for short-term therapy. Long-term therapy may cause electrolyte imbalance and dependence.
❑ Encourage patients to use other forms of bowel regulation, such as increasing bulk in the diet, increasing fluid intake (6–8 full glasses/day), and increasing mobility. Normal bowel habits are variable and may vary from 3 times/day to 3 times/wk.
❑ Instruct patients with cardiac disease to avoid straining during bowel movements (Valsalva maneuver).
❑ Advise patient not to use laxatives when abdominal pain, nausea, vomiting, or fever is present.
❑ Advise patient not to take docusate within 2 hr of other laxatives.

### EVALUATION

**Effectiveness of therapy can be demonstrated by:** ■A soft, formed bowel movement, usually within 24–48 hr. Therapy may take 3–5 days for results. Rectal dosage forms produce results within 2–15 min.

# dofetilide

(doe-**fet**il-ide)

Tikosyn

**CLASSIFICATION(S):**

**Therapeutic:** *antiarrhythmics (class III)*

**Pregnancy Category C**

## INDICATIONS

■ Maintenance of normal sinus rhythm (delay in time to recurrence of atrial fibrillation/atrial flutter [AF/AFl]) in patients with AF/AFl of greater than 1-wk duration, and who have been converted to normal sinus rhythm ■ For the conversion of atrial fibrillation and atrial flutter to normal sinus rhythm.

## ACTION

■ Blocks cardiac ion channels responsible for transport of potassium ■ Increases monophasic action potential duration ■ Increases effective refractory period. **Therapeutic Effects:** ■ Prevention of recurrent AF/AFl ■ Conversion of AF/AFl to normal sinus rhythm

## PHARMACOKINETICS

**Absorption:** Well absorbed (>90%) following oral administration.

**Distribution:** Unknown.

**Metabolism and Excretion:** 80% excreted by kidneys via cationic renal secretion, mostly as unchanged drug; 20% excreted as inactive metabolites; some metabolism in the liver via cytochrome P450 system (CYP 3A4 isoenzyme)

**Half-life:** 10 hr.

## CONTRAINDICATIONS AND PRECAUTIONS

**Contraindicated in:** ■ Hypersensitivity ■ Congenital or acquired prolonged QT syndromes ■ Baseline QT interval or QTc of >440 msec (500 msec in patients with ventricular conduction abnormalities) ■ Creatinine clearance (CCr) <20 ml/min ■ Concurrent use of verapamil or agents which inhibit the renal cation transport system including cimetidine, ketoconazole, trimethoprim, megestrol or prochlorperazine ■ Lactation (use should be avoided).

**Use Cautiously in:** ■ Underlying electrolyte abnormalities (increased risk of serious arrhythmias; correct prior to administration) ■ CCr 20–60 ml/min (dosage reduction recommended) ■ Severe hepatic impairment ■ Pregnancy (use only when benefit to patient outweighs potential risk to fetus) ■ Children <18 yr (safety not established).

## ADVERSE REACTIONS AND SIDE EFFECTS*

■ **CNS:** <u>dizziness</u>, <u>headache</u> ■ **CV:** VENTRICULAR ARRHYTHMIAS, <u>chest pain</u>, QT interval prolongation..

## INTERACTIONS

**Drug-Drug:** ■ Concurrent use of renal cation transport inhibitors including **cimetidine, trimethoprim,** and **ketoconazole** increases blood levels and the risk of serious arrhythmias and is contraindicated ■ **Amiloride, metformin, megestrol, prochlorperazine,** and **triamterene** may have similar effects ■ Blood levels and risk of arrhythmias is also increased by **verapamil**; concurrent use is contraindicated and a 2-day washout period is recommended) ■ Inhibitors of the cytochrome P450 system (CY P450 3A4 isoenzyme) including **macrolide anti-infectives, azole antifungals, protease inhibitor antiretrovirials, SSRI antidepressants, amiodarone, cannabinoids, diltiazem, nefazodone, quinine,** and **zafirlukast** may also increase blood levels and the risk of arrhythmias and concurrent use should be undertaken with caution ■ Should not be used concurrently with other **class I or III antiarrhythmics** due to increased risk of arrhythmias ■ **Phenothiazines** and **tricyclic antidepressants** also prolong QT interval and should not be used concurrently with dofetilide ■ Hypokalemia or hypomagnesemia from **potassium-depleting diuretics** increases the risk of arrhythmias; correct abnormalities prior to administration ■ Concurrent use of **digoxin** may also increase the risk of arrhythmias.

**Drug-Food:** ■ **Grapefruit juice** may increase levels; avoid concurrent use.

## ROUTE AND DOSAGE

Dosing should be adjusted according to renal function and assessment of QT interval.

- **PO (Adults):** *Starting dose*—500 mcg twice daily; *maintenance dose*—250 mcg twice daily (not to exceed 500 mcg twice daily).

□ **Renal Impairment**

- **PO (Adults): CCr 40–60 ml/min:** *Starting dose*—250 mcg twice daily; *maintenace dose*—125 mcg twice daily; **CCr 20– 40 ml/min:** *Starting dose*—125 mcg twice daily; *maintenace dose*—125 mcg once daily.

## AVAILABILITY

- **Capsules:** 125 mcg, 250 mcg, 500 mcg.

TIME/ACTION PROFILE (blood levels)

|  | ONSET | PEAK | DURATION |
|---|---|---|---|
| PO | within hours | 2-3 hr† | 12-24 hr |

†Steady state levels are achieved after 2–3 days.

## NURSING IMPLICATIONS

### ASSESSMENT

□ Monitor ECG, pulse, and blood pressure continuously throughout initiation or therapy and for at least 3 days, then periodically throughout therapy. QTc should be evaluated prior to initiation of therapy and every 3 months throughout therapy. If QTc exceeds 440 msec (500 msec in patients with ventricular conduction abnormalities), dofetilide should be discontinued and patient should be carefully monitored until QTc returns to baseline.

□ Assess the patient's medication history including OTC, Rx, and natural/herbal products, with emphasis on those that interact with dofetilide (see Interactions).

- **Lab Test Considerations:** Creatinine clearance must be calculated for all patients prior to administration and every 3 months throughout therapy.

### POTENTIAL NURSING DIAGNOSES

- Cardiac output, decreased (Indications).

### IMPLEMENTATION

- **General:** Dolfetilide must be initiated or reinitiated in a setting that provides continuous ECG monitoring and has personnel trained in the management of serious ventricular arrhythmias. Due to the potential for life-threatening ventricular arrhythmias, do-

fetilide is usually used for patients with highly symptomatic AF/AFl.

□ Patients with AF should be anticoagulated according to usual protocol prior to electrical or pharmacological cardioversion.

□ Make sure patient has an adequate supply of dofetilide prior to discharge to prevent interruption of therapy.

□ Patients should not be discharged from the hospital within 12 hrs of electrical or pharmacological conversion to normal sinus rhythm.

- **PO:** Administer at the same time each day without regard to food.

### PATIENT/FAMILY TEACHING

□ Instruct patient to take medication exactly as directed, even if feeling well. If a dose is missed, do not double next dose. Take next dose at usual time.

□ Patient should read the patient package insert prior to initiation of therapy and reread it each time therapy is renewed. Emphasize the need for compliance with therapy, the potential for drug interactions, and the need for periodic monitoring to minimize the risk of serious arrhythmias.

□ Instruct patient or family member on how to take pulse. Advise patient to report changes in pulse rate or rhythm to health care professional.

□ May cause dizziness. Caution patient to avoid driving or other activities requiring alertness until response to medication is known.

□ Advise patient to inform health care professional of medication regimen prior to treatment or surgery.

□ Instruct patient not to take OTC medications with dofetilide without consulting health care professional.

□ Advise patient to consult health care professional immediately if they faint, become dizzy, or have fast heartbeats. If health care professional is unavailable instruct patient to go to nearest hospital emergency department, take remaining dofetilide capsules, and show them to the doctor or nurse. If symptoms associated with altered electrolyte balance such as excessive or prolonged diarrhea, sweating, or vmoiting or loss of appetite or thirst occur health care professional should also be notified immediately.

❑ Emphasize the importance of routine follow-up exams to monitor progress.

## EVALUATION

**Clinical response to therapy can be evaluated by:** ■ Prevention of recurrent AF/AFl ■ Conversion of AF/AFl to normal sinus rhythm ❑ If patients do not convert to normal sinus rhythm within 24 hr of initiation of therapy, electrical conversion should be considered.

# dolasetron
(dol-**a**-se-tron)
Anzemet

## CLASSIFICATION(S):
**Therapeutic:** antiemetics
**Pharmacologic:** 5 HT$_3$ antagonists

**Pregnancy Category B**

## INDICATIONS

■ Prevention of nausea and vomiting associated with emetogenic chemotherapy ■ Prevention and treatment of postoperative nausea/vomiting.

## ACTION

■ Blocks the effects of serotonin at receptor sites (selective antagonist) located in vagal nerve terminals and in the chemoreceptor trigger zone in the CNS. **Therapeutic Effects:** Decreased incidence and severity of nausea/vomiting associated with emetogenic chemotherapy or surgery.

## PHARMACOKINETICS

**Absorption:** Well absorbed but rapidly metabolized to hydrodolasetron, the active metabolite.
**Distribution:** Unknown.
**Metabolism and Excretion:** 61% of hydrodolasetron is excreted unchanged by the kidneys.
**Half-life:** *Hydrodolasetron*—8.1 hr (shorter in children).

## CONTRAINDICATIONS AND PRECAUTIONS

**Contraindicated in:** ■ Hypersensitivity.
**Use Cautiously in:** ■ Patients with risk factors for prolongation of cardiac conduction intervals (hypokalemia, hypomagnesemia, concurrent diuretic or antiarrhythmic therapy, congenital QT syndrome, cumulative high-dose anthracycline therapy) ■ Pregnancy or lactation (safety not established).

## ADVERSE REACTIONS AND SIDE EFFECTS*

■ **CNS:** <u>headache</u> (increased in cancer patients), dizziness, fatigue, syncope ■ **CV:** bradycardia, ECG changes, hypertension, hypotension, tachycardia ■ **GI:** diarrhea, dyspepsia ■ **GU:** oliguria ■ **Derm:** pruritus ■ **Misc:** chills, fever, pain.

## INTERACTIONS

**Drug-Drug:** ■ Concurrent **diuretic** or **antiarrhythmic** therapy or cumulative **high-dose anthracycline therapy** may increase the risk of conduction abnormalities ■ Blood levels and effects of hydrodolasteron are increased by **atenolol** and **cimetidine** ■ Blood levels and effects of hydrodolasteron are decreased by **rifampin**.

## ROUTE AND DOSAGE

❑ **Prevention of Chemotherapy-Induced Nausea/Vomiting**
■ **PO (Adults):** 100 mg given within 1 hr before chemotherapy.
■ **PO (Children 2–16 yr):** 1.8 mg/kg given within 1 hr before chemotherapy (not to exceed 100 mg).
■ **IV (Adults and Children ≥2 yr):** 1.8 mg/kg given 30 min before chemotherapy (usual dose in adults is 100 mg; not to exceed 100 mg in children).

❑ **Prevention/Treatment of Postoperative Nausea/Vomiting**
■ **PO (Adults):** 100 mg given within 2 hr before surgery.
■ **PO (Children 2–16 yr):** 1.2 mg/kg (up to 100 mg/dose) given within 2 hr before surgery.
■ **IV (Adults):** 12.5 mg given 15 min before cessation of anesthesia (prevention) or as soon as nausea or vomiting begins (treatment).
■ **IV (Children 2–16 yr):** 0.35 mg/kg (up to 12.5 mg) given 15 min before cessation of

anesthesia (prevention) or as soon as nausea or vomiting begins (treatment).

## AVAILABILITY

■ *Tablets:* 50 mg^Rx, 100 mg^Rx ■ Cost: 50 mg $155.88/5, 100 mg $343.20/5 ■ *Injection:* 12.5 mg/0.625 ml ampules^Rx, 20 mg/ml in 5-ml vials^Rx ■ Cost: 20 mg/ml $155.88/5 ml.

TIME/ACTION PROFILE (antiemetic effect)

|    | ONSET   | PEAK      | DURATION    |
|----|---------|-----------|-------------|
| PO | unknown | 1–2 hr    | up to 24 hr |
| IV | unknown | 15–30 min | up to 24 hr |

## NURSING IMPLICATIONS

### ASSESSMENT

❑ Assess patient for nausea, vomiting, abdominal distention, and bowel sounds before and after administration.

❑ Monitor vital signs after administration. IV administration may be followed by severe hypotension, bradycardia, and syncope.

### POTENTIAL NURSING DIAGNOSES

■ Nutrition, imbalanced: less than body requirements (Indications).

### IMPLEMENTATION

■ **PO:** Administer within 1 hr before chemotherapy or 2 hr before surgery.

❑ Injectable dolasetron may be mixed in apple or apple-grape juice for oral dosing for pediatric patients. May be stored at room temperature for 2 hr before use.

■ **IV:** Administer 30 min before chemotherapy, 15 min before cessation of anesthesia, or postoperatively if nausea and vomiting occur shortly after surgery.

■ **Direct IV:** May be administered undiluted.

■ *Rate:* Administer over at least 30 sec.

■ **Intermittent Infusion:** May be diluted in 50 ml of 0.9% NaCl, D5W, D5/0.45% NaCl, D5/LR, LR, or 10% mannitol solution. Solution is clear and colorless. Stable for 24 hr at room temperature or 48 hr if refrigerated after dilution.

■ *Rate:* Administer each dose as an IV infusion over up to 15 min.

■ **Y-Site Incompatibility:** Manufacturer recommends not admixing with other medications. Flush infusion line before and after administration.

## PATIENT/FAMILY TEACHING

❑ Advise patient to notify health care professional if nausea or vomiting occurs.

## EVALUATION

**Effectiveness of therapy can be demonstrated by:** ■ Prevention of nausea and vomiting associated with emetogenic cancer chemotherapy ■ Prevention and treatment of postoperative nausea and vomiting.

# donepezil

(doe-**nep**-i-zill)

Aricept

## CLASSIFICATION(S):

*Therapeutic: anti-Alzheimer's agents*

*Pharmacologic: cholinergics (cholinesterase inhibitors)*

**Pregnancy Category C**

## INDICATIONS

■ Treatment of mild to moderate dementia associated with Alzheimer's disease.

## ACTION

■ Improves cholinergic function by inhibiting acetylcholinesterase. **Therapeutic Effects:** ■ May temporarily lessen some of the dementia associated with Alzheimer's disease ■ Does not alter the course of the disease.

## PHARMACOKINETICS

**Absorption:** Well absorbed after oral administration.

**Distribution:** Unknown.

**Protein Binding:** 96%.

**Metabolism and Excretion:** Partially metabolized by the liver (CYP2D6 and CYP3A4 enyzmes) and partially excreted by kidneys (17% unchanged). Two metabolites are pharmacologically active.

**Half-life:** 70 hr.

## CONTRAINDICATIONS AND PRECAUTIONS

**Contraindicated in:** ■ Hypersensitivity to donepezil or piperidine derivatives.

**Use Cautiously in:** ■ Patients with underlying cardiac disease, especially sick sinus syndrome or supraventricular conduction defects ■ Patients with a history of ulcer disease or those currently taking NSAIDs ■ Patients with a history of seizures ■ Patients with a history of asthma or obstructive pulmonary disease ■ Pregnancy, lactation, or children (safety not established).

## ADVERSE REACTIONS AND SIDE EFFECTS*

■ **CNS:** headache, abnormal dreams, depression, dizziness, drowsiness, fatigue, insomnia, syncope ■ **CV:** atrial fibrillation, hypertension, hypotension, vasodilation ■ **GI:** diarrhea, nausea, anorexia, vomiting ■ **GU:** frequent urination ■ **Derm:** ecchymoses ■ **Metab:** hot flashes, weight loss ■ **MS:** arthritis, muscle cramps.

## INTERACTIONS

**Drug-Drug:** ■ Exaggerates muscle relaxation from **succinylcholine** ■ Interferes with the action of **anticholinergics** ■ Increases the cholinergic effects of **bethanechol** ■ May increase the risk of GI bleeding from **NSAIDs** ■ **Quinidine** and **ketoconazole** decrease the metabolism of donepezil ■ **Rifampin, carbamazepine, dexamethasone, phenobarbital,** and **phenytoin** induce the enzymes that metabolize donepezil and may decrease its effects.

**Drug-Natural Products:** ■ **Angel's trumpet, jimson weed,** and **scopolia** may antagonize cholinergic effects.

## ROUTE AND DOSAGE

■ **PO (Adults):** 5 mg once daily; after 4–6 wk may increase to 10 mg once daily (dose should not exceed 5 mg/day in frail, elderly females).

## AVAILABILITY

■ **Tablets:** 5 mg^Rx, 10 mg^Rx ■ Cost: 5 mg $131.31/30 tablets, 10 mg $131.31/30 tablets.

TIME/ACTION PROFILE (improvement in symptoms)

| | ONSET | PEAK | DURATION |
|---|---|---|---|
| PO | unknown | several wk | 6 wk† |

†Return to baseline after discontinuation.

## NURSING IMPLICATIONS

### ASSESSMENT

❑ Assess cognitive function (memory, attention, reasoning, language, ability to perform simple tasks) periodically throughout therapy.
❑ Monitor heart rate periodically during therapy. May cause bradycardia.

### POTENTIAL NURSING DIAGNOSES

■ Thought processes, disturbed (Indications).
■ Injury, risk for (Indications).

### IMPLEMENTATION

■ **PO:** Administer in the evening just before going to bed. May be taken without regard to food.

### PATIENT/FAMILY TEACHING

❑ Emphasize the importance of taking donepezil daily, as directed. Missed doses should be skipped and regular schedule returned to the following day. Do not take more than prescribed; higher doses do not increase effects but may increase side effects.
❑ Caution patient and caregiver that donepezil may cause dizziness.
❑ Advise patient and caregiver to notify health care professional if nausea, vomiting, diarrhea, or changes in color of stool occur or if new symptoms occur or previously noted symptoms increase in severity.
❑ Advise patient and caregiver to notify health care professional of medication regimen before treatment or surgery.
❑ Emphasize the importance of follow-up exams to monitor progress.

### EVALUATION

**Clinical response to therapy can be evaluated by:** ■ Improvement in cognitive function (memory, attention, reasoning, language, ability to perform simple tasks) in patients with Alzheimer's disease.

**High Alert**

## dopamine
(**dope**-a-meen)
Intropin, {Revimine}

{ } = Available in Canada only.
*CAPITALS indicates life-threatening; underlines indicate most frequent.

## CLASSIFICATION(S):
*Therapeutic: inotropics, vasopressors*
*Pharmacologic: adrenergics*
**Pregnancy Category C**

## INDICATIONS

■ Adjunct to standard measures to improve: ❑ Blood pressure ❑ Cardiac output ❑ Urine output in treatment of shock unresponsive to fluid replacement.

## ACTION

■ Small doses (0.5–3 mcg/kg/min) stimulate dopaminergic receptors, producing renal vasodilation ■ Larger doses (2–10 mcg/kg/min) stimulate dopaminergic and beta$_1$-adrenergic receptors, producing cardiac stimulation and renal vasodilation ■ Doses greater than 10 mcg/kg/min stimulate alpha-adrenergic receptors and may cause renal vasoconstriction. **Therapeutic Effects:** ■ Increased cardiac output, increased blood pressure, and improved renal blood flow.

## PHARMACOKINETICS

**Absorption:** Administered IV only, resulting in complete bioavailability.

**Distribution:** Widely distributed but does not cross the blood-brain barrier.

**Metabolism and Excretion:** Metabolized in liver, kidneys, and plasma.

**Half-life:** 2 min.

## CONTRAINDICATIONS AND PRECAUTIONS

**Contraindicated in:** ■ Tachyarrhythmias ■ Pheochromocytoma ■ Hypersensitivity to bisulfites (some products).

**Use Cautiously in:** ■ Hypovolemia ■ Myocardial infarction ■ Occlusive vascular diseases ■ Pregnancy, lactation, and children (safety not established).

## ADVERSE REACTIONS AND SIDE EFFECTS*

■ **CNS:** headache ■ **EENT:** mydriasis (high dose) ■ **Resp:** dyspnea ■ **CV:** <u>arrhythmias</u>, <u>hypotension</u>, angina, ECG change, palpitations, vasoconstriction ■ **GI:** nausea, vomiting ■ **Derm:** piloerection ■ **Local:** irritation at IV site.

## INTERACTIONS

**Drug-Drug:** ■ Use with **MAO inhibitors, ergot alkaloids** (ergotamine), **doxapram, guanethidine, guanadrel,** or some **antidepressants** results in severe hypertension ■ Use with IV **phenytoin** may cause hypotension and bradycardia ■ Use with **general anesthetics** may result in arrhythmias ■ **Beta blockers** may antagonize cardiac effects.

## ROUTE AND DOSAGE

■ **IV (Adults):** *Dopaminergic (renal vasodilation) effects—0.5–3 mcg/kg/min. Beta-adrenergic (cardiac stimulation) effects— 2–10 mcg/kg/min. Alpha-adrenergic (increased peripheral vascular resistance) effects—10 mcg/kg/min; infusion rate may be increased as needed.*

■ **IV (Children):** 5–20 mcg/kg/min, depending on desired response (0.5–3 mcg/kg/min has been used to improve renal blood flow).

## AVAILABILITY (generic available)

■ *Injection for dilution:* 40 mg/ml$^{Rx}$, 80 mg/ml$^{Rx}$, 160 mg/ml$^{Rx}$ ■ *Premixed injection:* 0.8 mg/ml, 1.6 mg/ml, and 3.2 mg/ml in 250- and 500-ml D5W$^{Rx}$.

TIME/ACTION PROFILE (hemodynamic effects)

|     | ONSET | PEAK | DURATION |
|-----|-------|------|----------|
| IV  | 1–2 min | up to 10 min | <10 min |

# NURSING IMPLICATIONS

## ASSESSMENT

❑ Monitor blood pressure, heart rate, pulse pressure, ECG, pulmonary capillary wedge pressure (PCWP), cardiac output, CVP, and urinary output continuously during administration. Report significant changes in vital signs or arrhythmias. Consult physician for parameters for pulse, blood pressure, or ECG changes for adjusting dosage or discontinuing medication.

❑ Monitor urine output frequently throughout administration. Report decreases in urine output promptly.

❑ Palpate peripheral pulses and assess appearance of extremities routinely throughout dopamine administration. Notify physician if quality of pulse deteriorates or if extremities become cold or mottled.

❑ If hypotension occurs, administration rate should be increased. If hypotension continues, more potent vasoconstrictors (norepinephrine) may be administered.

■ *Toxicity and Overdose:* If excessive hypertension occurs, rate of infusion should be decreased or temporarily discontinued until blood pressure is decreased. Although additional measures are usually not necessary because of short duration of dopamine, phentolamine may be administered if hypertension continues.

## POTENTIAL NURSING DIAGNOSES

■ Cardiac output, decreased (Indications).
■ Tissue perfusion, ineffective (Indications).

## IMPLEMENTATION

❑ *High Alert:* IV vasoactive medications are potentially dangerous. Have second practitioner independently check original order, dosage calculations and infusion pump settings. Do not confuse dopamine with dobutamine. If both are available as floor stock, store in separate areas.

■ **General:** Correct hypovolemia with volume expanders before initiating dopamine therapy.

❑ Extravasation may cause severe irritation, necrosis, and sloughing of tissue. Administer into a large vein and assess administration site frequently. If extravasation occurs, affected area should be infiltrated liberally with 10–15 ml of 0.9% NaCl containing 5–10 mg of phentolamine. Reduce proportionally for pediatric patients. Infiltration within 12 hr of extravasation produces immediate hyperemic changes.

■ **Continuous Infusion:** Dilute 200–400 mg in 250–500 ml of 0.9% NaCl, D5W, D5/LR, D5/0.45% NaCl, D5/0.9% NaCl, or LR for IV infusion. Concentrations commonly used are 800 mcg/ml or 0.8 mg/ml (200 mg/250 ml) when fluid expansion is not problematic and 1.6 mg/ml (400 mg/250 ml) or 3.2 mg/ml (800 mg/250 ml) when patient is on fluid restriction or a slower rate is desired. Dilute immediately before administration. Yellow or brown discoloration indicates decomposi-

tion. Discard solution that is cloudy, discolored, or contains a precipitate. Solution is stable for 24 hr.

■ *Rate:* Administer at a rate of 0.5–5 mcg/kg/min, and increase by 1–4 mcg/kg/min at 10- to 30-min intervals until desired dosage is obtained. Infusion must be administered via infusion pump to ensure precise amount delivered. Rate of administration is titrated according to patient response (blood pressure, heart rate, urine flow, peripheral perfusion, presence of ectopic activity, cardiac output); see infusion rate chart. Decrease rate gradually when discontinuing to prevent marked decreases in blood pressure.

■ **Y-Site Compatibility:** ◆ alatrofloxacin ◆ aldesleukin ◆ amifostine ◆ amiodarone ◆ amrinone ◆ atracurium ◆ aztreonam ◆ cefmetazole ◆ ciprofloxacin ◆ cladribine ◆ diltiazem ◆ dobutamine ◆ enalaprilat ◆ epinephrine ◆ esmolol ◆ famotidine ◆ fentanyl ◆ fluconazole ◆ foscarnet ◆ gatifloxacin ◆ granisetron ◆ haloperidol ◆ heparin ◆ hydrocortisone sodium succinate ◆ hydromorphone ◆ labetalol ◆ levofloxacin ◆ lidocaine ◆ linezolid ◆ lorazepam ◆ meperidine ◆ methylprednisolone ◆ metronidazole ◆ midazolam ◆ milrinone ◆ morphine ◆ nitroglycerin ◆ nitroprusside ◆ norepinephrine ◆ ondansetron ◆ pancuronium ◆ piperacillin/tazobactam ◆ potassium chloride ◆ propofol ◆ ranitidine ◆ sargramostim ◆ streptokinase ◆ tacrolimus ◆ theophylline ◆ thiotepa ◆ tirofiban ◆ tolazoline ◆ vecuronium ◆ verapamil ◆ vitamin B complex with C ◆ warfarin ◆ zidovudine.

■ **Y-Site Incompatibility:** ◆ acyclovir ◆ alteplase ◆ cefepime ◆ indomethacin ◆ insulin ◆ thiopental.

## PATIENT/FAMILY TEACHING

❑ Explain to patient the rationale for instituting this medication and the need for frequent monitoring.

❑ Advise patient to inform nurse immediately if chest pain; dyspnea; numbness, tingling, or burning of extremities occurs.

❑ Instruct patient to inform nurse immediately of pain or discomfort at the site of administration.

## EVALUATION

**Effectiveness of therapy can be demonstrated by:** ■ Increase in blood pressure ❑ Increase in peripheral circulation ❑ Increase in urine output.

---

# doxazosin

(dox-**ay**-zoe-sin)

Cardura

### CLASSIFICATION(S):

*Therapeutic:* antihypertensives
*Pharmacologic:* peripherally acting antiadrenergics

### Pregnancy Category C

## INDICATIONS

■ Hypertension (alone or with other agents) ■ Symptomatic benign prostatic hyperplasia (BPH).

## ACTION

■ Dilates both arteries and veins by blocking postsynaptic alpha₁-adrenergic receptors. **Therapeutic Effects:** ■ Lowering of blood pressure.

## PHARMACOKINETICS

**Absorption:** Well absorbed following oral administration.

**Distribution:** Probably enters breast milk; rest of distribution unknown.

**Protein Binding:** 98–99%.

**Metabolism and Excretion:** Extensively metabolized by the liver.

**Half-life:** 22 hr.

## CONTRAINDICATIONS AND PRECAUTIONS

**Contraindicated in:** ■ Hypersensitivity.

**Use Cautiously in:** ■ Hepatic dysfunction ■ Geriatric patients or patients with impaired renal function (increased risk of hypotension) ■ Pregnancy, lactation, or children (safety not established).

## ADVERSE REACTIONS AND SIDE EFFECTS*

■**CNS:** dizziness, headache, depression, drowsiness, fatigue, nervousness, weakness ■ **EENT:** abnormal vision, blurred vision, conjunctivitis, epistaxis ■ **Resp:** dyspnea ■ **CV:** first-dose orthostatic hypotension, arrhythmias, chest pain, edema, palpitations ■ **GI:** abdominal discomfort, constipation, diarrhea, dry mouth, flatulence, nausea, vomiting ■ **GU:** decreased libido, sexual dysfunction ■ **Derm:** flushing, rash, urticaria ■ **MS:** arthralgia, arthritis, gout, myalgia.

## INTERACTIONS

**Drug-Drug:** ■ ↑ risk of hypotension with acute ingestion of **alcohol, sildenafil vardenafil** other **antihypertensives,** or **nitrates** ■ May ↓ antihypertensive effect of **clonidine.**

## ROUTE AND DOSAGE

■ **PO (Adults):** *Hypertension*—1 mg once daily, may be gradually increased at 2-wk intervals to 2–16 mg/day; incidence of postural hypotension greatly increased at doses >4 mg/day. *BPH*—1 mg once daily, may be gradually increased to 8 mg/day.

## AVAILABILITY (generic available)

■ *Tablets:* 1 mg^Rx, 2 mg^Rx, 4 mg^Rx, 8 mg^Rx ■ Cost: 1 mg $109.18/100, 2 mg $109.18/100, 4 mg $114.60/100, 8 mg $120.34/100.

TIME/ACTION PROFILE (antihypertensive effect)

| | ONSET | PEAK | DURATION |
|---|---|---|---|
| PO | 1–2 hr | 2–6 hr | 24 hr |

# NURSING IMPLICATIONS

## ASSESSMENT

■ **General Info:** Monitor blood pressure and pulse 2–6 hr after first dose, with each increase in dose, and periodically during therapy. Report significant changes.

❑ Assess patient for first-dose orthostatic hypotension and syncope. Incidence may be dose related. Observe patient closely during this period and take precautions to prevent injury.

❑ Monitor intake and output ratios and daily weight, and assess for edema daily, especially at beginning of therapy. Report weight gain or edema.

■ **BPH:** Assess patient for symptoms of prostatic hyperplasia (urinary hesitancy, feeling of incomplete bladder emptying, interruption of urinary stream, impairment of size and force of urinary stream, terminal urinary dribbling, straining to start flow, dysuria, urgency) prior to and periodically during therapy.

## POTENTIAL NURSING DIAGNOSES

- Urinary elimination, impaired (Indications).
- Injury, risk for (Side Effects).

## IMPLEMENTATION

- **General:** Do not confuse Cardura (doxazosin) with Cardene (nicardipine) or Ridaura (auranofin).
- Administer daily dose at bedtime.
- **Hypertension:** May be administered concurrently with a diuretic or other antihypertensive.

## PATIENT/FAMILY TEACHING

- **General Info:** Emphasize the importance of continuing to take this medication, even if feeling well. Instruct patient to take medication at the same time each day. Take missed doses as soon as remembered unless almost time for next dose. Do not double doses.
- Doxazosin may cause drowsiness or dizziness. Advise patient to avoid driving or other activities requiring alertness until response to medication is known.
- Caution patient to change positions slowly to decrease orthostatic hypotension.
- Advise patient to consult health care professional before taking any cough, cold, or allergy remedies or herbal products.
- Emphasize the importance of follow-up visits to determine effectiveness of therapy.
- **Hypertension:** Instruct patient and family on proper technique for blood pressure monitoring. Advise them to check blood pressure at least weekly and report significant changes.
- Encourage patient to comply with additional interventions for hypertension (weight reduction, low-sodium diet, smoking cessation, moderation of alcohol consumption, regular exercise, and stress management).

## EVALUATION

**Effectiveness of therapy can be demonstrated by:** ■ Decrease in blood pressure without appearance of side effects ■ Decrease in urinary symptoms of BPH.

## doxepin

(**dox**-e-pin)
Sinequan, {Triadapin}, Zonalon

### CLASSIFICATION(S):

**Therapeutic:** antianxiety agents, antidepressants, antihistamines (topical)
**Pharmacologic:** tricyclic antidepressants

### Pregnancy Category UK

## INDICATIONS

■ **PO:** Management of various forms of endogenous depression (with psychotherapy) ■ Treatment of anxiety ■ **Topical:** Short-term control of pruritus associated with: ◻ Eczematous dermatitis ◻ Lichen simplex chronicus. **Unlabeled uses:** ■ **PO:** Management of chronic pain syndromes ◻ Management of pruritus.

## ACTION

■ **PO:** Prevents the reuptake of norepinephrine and serotonin by presynaptic neurons; resultant accumulation of neurotransmitters potentiates their activity ■ Also possesses significant anticholinergic properties ■ **Topical:** Antipruritic action due to antihistaminic properties. **Therapeutic Effects:** ■ **PO:** Relief of depression ■ Decreased anxiety ■ **Topical:** Decreased pruritus.

## PHARMACOKINETICS

**Absorption:** Well absorbed from the GI tract, although much is metabolized on first pass through the liver. Some systemic absorption follows topical application.

**Distribution:** Widely distributed. Enters breast milk; probably crosses the placenta.

**Metabolism and Excretion:** Metabolized by the liver. Some conversion to active antidepressant compound. May re-enter gastric juice via secretion from enterohepatic circulation, where more absorption may occur.

**Half-life:** 8–25 hr.

## CONTRAINDICATIONS AND PRECAUTIONS

**Contraindicated in:** ■ Hypersensitivity ■ Some products contain bisulfites and should be avoided in patients with known intolerance ■ Untreated narrow-angle glaucoma ■ Period immediately after myocardial infarction ■ Pregnancy or lactation.

**Use Cautiously in:** ■ Geriatric patients (initial dosage reduction recommended) ■ Pre-existing cardiovascular disease (increased risk of adverse reactions) ■ Prostatic enlargement (more susceptible to urinary retention) ■ Seizures.

## ADVERSE REACTIONS AND SIDE EFFECTS*

■ **CNS:** fatigue, sedation, agitation, confusion, hallucinations ■ **EENT:** blurred vision, increased intraocular pressure ■ **CV:** hypotension, arrhythmias, ECG abnormalities ■ **GI:** constipation, dry mouth, hepatitis, increased appetite, nausea, paralytic ileus ■ **GU:** urinary retention ■ **Derm:** photosensitivity, rashes ■ **Hemat:** blood dyscrasias ■ **Misc:** hypersensitivity reactions.

## INTERACTIONS

Apply to both topical and oral use.

**Drug-Drug:** ■ Doxepin is metabolized in the liver by the cytochrome P450 2D6 enzyme and its action may be affected by drugs that compete for metabolism by this enzyme including other **antidepressants, phenothiazines, carbamazepine, class 1C antiarrhythmics (propafenone, flecainide)**; when used concurrently, dosage reduction of one or the other or both may be necessary. Concurrent use of other drugs that inhibit the activity of the enzyme, including **cimetidine, quinidine, amiodarone,** and **ritonavir,** may result in increased effects of doxepin ■ May cause hypotension, tachycardia, and potentially fatal reactions when used with **MAO inhibitors** (avoid concurrent use—discontinue 2 wk prior to doxepin) ■ Concurrent use with **SSRI antidepressants** may result in increased toxicity and should be avoided (fluoxetine should be stopped 5 wk before) ■ May prevent the therapeutic response to **guanethidine** ■ Concurrent use with **clonidine** may result in hypertensive crisis and should be avoided ■ Concurrent use with **levodopa** may result in delayed/decreased absorption of levodopa or hypertension ■ Blood levels and effects may be decreased by **rifamycins** ■ Concurrent use with **sparfloxacin** increases the risk of adverse cardiovascular reactions ■ Additive CNS depression with other **CNS depressants** including **alcohol, antihistamines, clonidine, opioid analgesics,** and **sedative/hypnotics** ■ **Barbiturates** may alter blood levels and effects ■ **Adrenergic** and **anticholinergic** side effects may be additive with other **agents having these properties** ■ **Phenothiazines** or **oral contraceptives** increase levels and may cause toxicity ■ **Smoking** may increase metabolism and alter effects.

**Drug-Natural Products:** ■ Concomitant use of **kava, valerian, skullcap, chamomile,** or **hops** can increase CNS depression ■ Increased anticholinergic effects with **angel's trumpet, jimson weed,** and **scopolia.**

## ROUTE AND DOSAGE

■ **PO (Adults):** *Antidepressant/anti-anxiety*—25 mg 3 times daily, may be increased as needed (up to 150 mg/day in outpatients or 300 mg/day in inpatients; some patients may require only 25–50 mg/day). Once stabilized, entire daily dose may be given at bedtime. *Antipruritic*—10 mg at bedtime initially, may be increased up to 25 mg.

■ **PO (Geriatric Patients):** *Antidepressant*—25–50 mg/day initially, may be increased as needed.

■ **Topical (Adults):** Apply 4 times daily (wait 3–4 hr between applications) for up to 8 days.

## AVAILABILITY (generic available)

■ *Capsules:* 10 mg$^{Rx}$, 25 mg$^{Rx}$, 50 mg$^{Rx}$, 75 mg$^{Rx}$, 100 mg$^{Rx}$, 150 mg$^{Rx}$ ■ Cost: *Sinequan*—10 mg $39.42/100, 25 mg $55.83/100, 50 mg $77.10/100, 75 mg $121.83/100, 100 mg $133.21/100, 150 mg $272.80/100; *generic*—10 mg $15.83/100, 25 mg $19.43/100, 50 mg $33.20/100, 75 mg $40.24/100, 100 mg $45.82/100, 150 mg $62.10/100 ■ *Oral concentrate:* 10 mg/ml$^{Rx}$ ■ *Topical cream:* 5%$^{Rx}$.

TIME/ACTION PROFILE (antidepressant activity)

| | ONSET | PEAK | DURATION |
|---|---|---|---|
| PO | 2–3 wk | up to 6 wk | days–weeks |

# NURSING IMPLICATIONS

## ASSESSMENT

- **General Info:** Monitor blood pressure and pulse rate prior to and during initial therapy. Patients taking high doses or with a history of cardiovascular disease should have ECG monitored prior to and periodically throughout therapy.
- **Depression:** Assess mental status frequently. Confusion, agitation, and hallucinations may occur during initiation of therapy and may require dosage reduction. Monitor mood changes. Assess for suicidal tendencies, especially during early therapy. Restrict amount of drug available to patient.
- **Anxiety:** Assess degree and manifestations of anxiety prior to and throughout therapy.
- **Pain:** Assess the type, location, and severity of pain prior to and periodically throughout therapy.
- **Topical:** Assess pruritic area prior to and periodically throughout therapy.
- **Lab Test Considerations:** Monitor WBC and differential blood counts, hepatic function, and serum glucose periodically. May cause elevated serum bilirubin and alkaline phosphatase levels. May cause bone marrow depression. Serum glucose may be increased or decreased.

## POTENTIAL NURSING DIAGNOSES

- Coping, ineffective (Indications).
- Injury, risk for (Side Effects).

## IMPLEMENTATION

- **General:** Do not confuse doxepin with doxycycline.
- May be given as a single dose at bedtime to minimize sedation during the day. Dose increases should be made at bedtime because of sedation. Dose titration is a slow process; may take weeks to months.
- **PO:** Administer medication with or immediately following a meal to minimize gastric irritation. Capsules may be opened and mixed with foods or fluids if patient has difficulty swallowing.
- Oral concentrate must be diluted in at least 120 ml of water, milk, or fruit juice. Do not mix with carbonated beverages or grape juice. Use calibrated measuring device to ensure accurate amount.
- **Topical:** Apply thin film of doxepin cream only to affected areas, and rub in gently. Apply only to affected skin; not for ophthalmic, oral, or intravaginal use.

## PATIENT/FAMILY TEACHING

- **General Info:** Inform patient that systemic side effects may occur with oral or topical use.
- May cause drowsiness and blurred vision. Caution patient to avoid driving and other activities requiring alertness until response to the medication is known.
- Orthostatic hypotension, sedation, and confusion are common during early therapy, especially in geriatric patients. Protect patient from falls and advise patient to change positions slowly.
- Advise patient to avoid alcohol or other CNS depressant drugs during and for at least 3–7 days after therapy has been discontinued.
- Instruct patient to notify health care professional if urinary retention occurs or if dry mouth or constipation persists. Sugarless candy or gum may diminish dry mouth, and an increase in fluid intake or bulk may prevent constipation. If symptoms persist, dosage reduction or discontinuation may be necessary. Consult health care professional if dry mouth persists for more than 2 wk.
- Advise patient to notify health care professional of medication regimen prior to treatment or surgery.
- **PO:** Instruct patient to take medication exactly as directed. If a dose is missed, take as soon as possible unless almost time for next dose; if regimen is a single dose at bedtime, do not take in the morning because of side effects. Advise patient that drug effects may not be noticed for at least 2 wk. Abrupt discontinuation may cause nausea, vomiting, diarrhea, headache, trouble sleeping with vivid dreams, and irritability.
- Caution patient to use sunscreen and protective clothing to prevent photosensitivity reactions.

- Inform patient of need to monitor dietary intake. Increase in appetite is possible and may lead to undesired weight gain.
- Therapy for depression is usually prolonged. Emphasize the importance of follow-up exams to monitor effectiveness and side effects.
- **Topical:** Instruct patient to apply medication exactly as directed; do not use more medication than directed, apply to a larger area than directed, use more often than directed, or use longer than 8 days.
- Inform patient that topical preparation may cause burning, stinging, swelling, increased itching, or worsening of eczema. Notify health care professional if these symptoms become bothersome.
- Caution patient not to use occlusive dressings; may increase systemic absorption.
- Advise patient to notify health care professional if excessive drowsiness occurs with topical application. Number of applications per day, amount of cream applied, or area of application may be reduced. May require discontinuation of therapy.

## EVALUATION

**Effectiveness of therapy can be demonstrated by:** ■ Increased sense of well-being □ Renewed interest in surroundings □ Increased appetite □ Improved energy level □ Improved sleep ■ Decrease in anxiety ■ Decrease in chronic pain. Patients may require 2–6 wk of oral therapy before full therapeutic effects of medication are evident ■ Decrease in pruritus associated with eczema.

---

**doxercalciferol, See VITAMIN D COMPOUNDS.**

---

| High Alert |
| --- |

# doxorubicin hydrochloride

(dox-oh-**roo**-bi-sin hye-droe-**klor**-ide)

Adriamycin PFS, Adriamycin RDF, Rubex

### *CLASSIFICATION(S):*

***Therapeutic:*** *antineoplastics*
***Pharmacologic:*** *anthracyclines*

| Pregnancy Category D |
| --- |

## INDICATIONS

■ Alone or with other modalities in the treatment of various solid tumors including: □ Breast □ Ovarian □ Bladder □ Bronchogenic carcinoma □ Malignant lymphomas and leukemias.

## ACTION

■ Inhibits DNA and RNA synthesis by forming a complex with DNA; action is cell-cycle S-phase–specific ■ Also has immunosuppressive properties ■**Therapeutic Effects:** ■ Death of rapidly replicating cells, particularly malignant ones.

## PHARMACOKINETICS

**Absorption:** Administered IV only, resulting in complete bioavailability.

**Distribution:** Widely distributed; does not cross the blood-brain barrier; extensively bound to tissues.

**Metabolism and Excretion:** Mostly metabolized by the liver. Converted by liver to an active compound. Excreted predominantly in the bile, 50% as unchanged drug. Less than 5% eliminated unchanged in the urine.

**Half-life:** 16.7 hr.

## CONTRAINDICATIONS AND PRECAUTIONS

**Contraindicated in:** ■ Hypersensitivity ■ Pregnancy or lactation.

**Use Cautiously in:** ■ History of cardiac disease or high cumulative doses of anthracyclines ■ Depressed bone marrow reserve ■ Liver impairment (reduce dose if serum bilirubin >1.2 mg/dl) ■ Children, geriatric patients, mediastinal radiation, concurrent cyclophosphamide (risk of cardiotoxicity) ■ Patients with childbearing potential.

## ADVERSE REACTIONS AND SIDE EFFECTS*

■ **Resp:** recall pneumonitis ■ **CV:** CARDIOMYOPATHY, ECG changes ■ **GI:** diarrhea, esophagitis, nausea, stomatitis, vomiting ■ **GU:** red urine ■ **Derm:** alopecia, photosensitivity ■ **Endo:** sterility, prepubertal growth failure with temporary gonadal impairment (children only) ■ **Hemat:** anemia, leukopenia, thrombocytopenia ■ **Local:** phlebitis at IV site, tissue necrosis ■**Metab:** hyperuricemia ■ **Misc:** hypersensitivity reactions.

## INTERACTIONS

**Drug-Drug:** ■ ↑ bone marrow depression with other **antineoplastics** or **radiation therapy** ■ Pediatric patients who have received concurrent doxorubicin and **dactinomycin** have an ↑ risk of recall pneumonitis at variable times following local radiation therapy ■ May ↑ skin reactions at previous **radiation therapy** sites ■ If **paclitaxel** is administered first, clearance of doxorubicin is ↓ and the incidence and severity of neutropenia and stomatitis are ↑ (problem is diminished if doxorubicin is administered first) ■ Hematologic toxicity is ↑ and prolonged by concurrent use of **cyclosporine**; risk of coma and seizures is also ↑ ■ Incidence and severity of neutropenia and thrombocytopenia are ↑ by concurrent **progesterone** ■ **Phenobarbital** may ↑ clearance and decrease effects of doxorubicin ■ Doxorubicin may ↓ metabolism and ↑ effects of **phenytoin** ■ **Streptozocin** may ↑ the half-life of doxorubicin (dosage ↓ of doxorubicin recommended) ■ May ↑ risk of hemorrhagic cystitis from **cyclophosphamide** or hepatitis from **mercaptopurine** ■ Cardiac toxicity may be ↑ by **radiation therapy** or **cyclophosphamide** ■ May ↓ antibody response to **live-virus vaccines** and ↑ risk of adverse reactions.

## ROUTE AND DOSAGE

Other regimens are used.

■ **IV (Adults):** 60–75 mg/m² daily, repeat q 21 days; or 25–30 mg/m² daily for 2–3 days, repeat q 3–4 wk or 20 mg/m²/wk. Total cumulative dose should not exceed 550 mg/m² without monitoring of cardiac function or 400 mg/m² in patients with previous chest radiation or other cardiotoxic chemotherapy.

■ **IV (Children):** 30 mg/m²/day for 3 days every 4 wk.

◻ **Hepatic Impairment**

■ **IV (Adults):** Serum bilirubin 1.2–3 mg/dl—50% of usual dose; serum bilirubin 3.1–5 mg/dl—25% of usual dose.

## AVAILABILITY (generic available)

■ **Powder for injection:** 10-mg, 20-mg, 50-mg, 100-mg, 150-mg vials<sup>Rx</sup> ■ **Injection:** 2 mg/ml<sup>Rx</sup> ■ Cost: $56.34/5 ml, $112.66/10 ml, $281.68/25 ml, $1104.13/100 ml.

## TIME/ACTION PROFILE (effect on blood counts)

| | ONSET | PEAK | DURATION |
|---|---|---|---|
| IV | 10 days | 14 days | 21–24 days |

# NURSING IMPLICATIONS

## ASSESSMENT

■ **General Info:** Monitor blood pressure, pulse, respiratory rate, and temperature frequently during administration. Report significant changes.

◻ Monitor for bone marrow depression. Assess for bleeding (bleeding gums, bruising, petechiae, guaiac stools, urine, and emesis) and avoid IM injections and taking rectal temperatures if platelet count is low. Apply pressure to venipuncture sites for 10 min. Assess for signs of infection during neutropenia. Anemia may occur. Monitor for increased fatigue, dyspnea, and orthostatic hypotension.

◻ Monitor intake and output ratios, and report occurrence of significant discrepancies. Encourage fluid intake of 2000–3000 ml/day. Allopurinol and alkalinization of the urine may be used to decrease serum uric acid levels and to help prevent urate stone formation.

◻ Severe and protracted nausea and vomiting may occur as early as 1 hr after therapy and may last 24 hr. Administer parenteral antiemetics 30–45 min prior to therapy and routinely around the clock for the next 24 hr as indicated. Monitor amount of emesis and notify physician or other health care professional if emesis exceeds guidelines to prevent dehydration.

◻ Monitor for development of signs of cardiac toxicity, which may be either acute and transient (ST segment depression, flattened T wave, sinus tachycardia, and extrasystoles) or late onset (usually occurs 1–6 mo after initiation of therapy) and characterized by intractable CHF (peripheral edema, dyspnea, rales/crackles, weight gain). Chest x-ray, echocardiography, ECGs, and radionuclide angiography may be ordered prior to and periodically during therapy. Cardiotoxicity is more prevalent in children younger than 2 yr and geriatric patients. Dexrazoxane may be used to prevent cardiotoxicity in patients receiving cumulative doses of >300 mg/m$^2$.

❑ Assess injection site frequently for redness, irritation, or inflammation. Doxorubicin is a vesicant but may infiltrate painlessly even if blood returns on aspiration of infusion needle. Severe tissue damage may occur if doxorubicin extravasates. If extravasation occurs, stop infusion immediately, restart, and complete dose in another vein. Local infiltration of antidote is not recommended. Apply ice packs and elevate and rest extremity for 24–48 hr to reduce swelling, then resume normal activity as tolerated. If swelling, redness, and/or pain persists beyond 48 hr, immediate consultation for possible debridement is indicated.

❑ Assess oral mucosa frequently for development of stomatitis. Increased dosing interval and/or decreased dosing is recommended if lesions are painful or interfere with nutrition.

■ **Lab Test Considerations:** Monitor CBC and differential prior to and periodically during therapy. The WBC nadir occurs 10–14 days after administration, and recovery usually occurs by the 21st day. Thrombocytopenia and anemia may also occur. Increased dosing interval and/or decreased dose is recommended if ANC is <1000 cells/mm$^3$ and/or platelet count is <50,000 cells/mm$^3$.

❑ Monitor renal (BUN and creatinine) and hepatic (AST, ALT, LDH, and serum bilirubin) function prior to and periodically during therapy. Dose reduction is required for bilirubin >1.2 mg/dl or serum creatinine >3 mg/dl.

❑ May cause ↑ serum and urine uric acid concentrations.

## POTENTIAL NURSING DIAGNOSES

■ Infection, risk for (Adverse Reactions).
■ Cardiac output, decreased (Adverse Reactions).

## IMPLEMENTATION

❑ **High Alert:** Fatalities have occurred with incorrect administration of chemotherapeutic agents. Before administering, clarify all ambiguous orders; double check single, daily, and course-of-therapy dose limits; have second practitioner independently double check original order, calculations and infusion pump settings. Do not confuse doxoru-

bicin hydrochloride (Adriamycin, Rubex) with doxorubicin hydrochloride liposome (Doxil) or with daunorubicin hydrochloride (Cerubidine) or daunorubicin citrate liposome (DaunoXome) or with idarubicin. Do not confuse adriamycin with idamycin. Clarify orders that do not include generic and brand names.

■ **General:** Solution should be prepared in a biologic cabinet. Wear gloves, gown, and mask while handling medication. Discard IV equipment in specially designated containers (see Appendix M).

❑ Aluminum needles may be used to administer doxorubicin but should not be used during storage, because prolonged contact results in discoloration of solution and formation of a dark precipitate. Solution is red.

■ **Direct IV:** Dilute each 10 mg with 5 ml of 0.9% NaCl (nonbacteriostatic) for injection. Shake to dissolve completely. Do not add to IV solution. Reconstituted medication is stable for 24 hr at room temperature and 48 hr if refrigerated. Protect from sunlight.

■ **Rate:** Administer each dose over 3–5 minutes through Y-site of a free-flowing infusion of 0.9% NaCl or D5W. Facial flushing and erythema along involved vein frequently occur when administration is too rapid.

■ **Syringe Compatibility:** ◆ bleomycin ◆ cisplatin ◆ cyclophosphamide ◆ droperidol ◆ leucovorin calcium ◆ methotrexate ◆ metoclopramide ◆ mitomycin ◆ vincristine.

■ **Syringe Incompatibility:** ◆ furosemide ◆ heparin.

■ **Y-Site Compatibility:** ◆ amifostine ◆ aztreonam ◆ bleomycin ◆ chlorpromazine ◆ cimetidine ◆ cisplatin ◆ cladribine ◆ cyclophosphamide ◆ dexamethasone ◆ diphenhydramine ◆ droperidol ◆ etoposide phosphate ◆ famotidine ◆ filgrastim ◆ fludarabine ◆ fluorouracil ◆ gatifloxacin ◆ gemcitabine ◆ granisetron ◆ hydromorphone ◆ leucovorin calcium ◆ linezolid ◆ lorazepam ◆ lorazepam ◆ melphalan ◆ methotrexate ◆ methylprednisolone ◆ metoclopramide ◆ mitomycin ◆ morphine ◆ ondansetron ◆ paclitaxel ◆ prochlorperazine edisylate ◆ promethazine ◆ ranitidine ◆ sargramostim ◆ sodium bicarbonate ◆ teniposide ◆ thiotepa ◆ topotecan ◆ vinblastine ◆ vincristine ◆ vinorelbine.

■ **Y-Site Incompatibility:** ◆ allopurinol ◆ amphotericin B cholesteryl sulfate ◆ cefepime ◆

ganciclovir ◆ piperacillin/tazobactam. ◆ propofol

## PATIENT/FAMILY TEACHING

❑ Instruct patient to notify health care professional promptly if fever; sore throat; signs of infection; bleeding gums; bruising; petechiae; blood in stools, urine, or emesis; increased fatigue; dyspnea; or orthostatic hypotension occurs. Caution patient to avoid crowds and persons with known infections. Instruct patient to use soft toothbrush and electric razor and to avoid falls. Caution patient not to drink alcoholic beverages or take medication containing aspirin or NSAIDs, because these may precipitate gastric bleeding.

❑ Instruct patient to report pain at injection site immediately.

❑ Instruct patient to inspect oral mucosa for erythema and ulceration. If ulceration occurs, advise patient to use sponge brush, rinse mouth with water after eating and drinking, and confer with health care professional if mouth pain interferes with eating. Pain may require treatment with opioid analgesics. The risk of developing stomatitis is greatest 5–10 days after a dose; the usual duration is 3–7 days.

❑ Advise patient that this medication may have teratogenic effects. Contraception should be used during and for at least 4 mo after therapy is concluded. Inform patient before initiating therapy that this medication may cause irreversible gonadal suppression.

❑ Instruct patient to notify health care professional immediately if irregular heartbeat, shortness of breath, swelling of lower extremities, or skin irritation (swelling, pain, or redness of feet or hands) occurs.

❑ Discuss the possibility of hair loss with patient. Explore methods of coping. Regrowth usually occurs 2–3 mo after discontinuation of therapy.

❑ Instruct patient not to receive any vaccinations without advice of health care professional.

❑ Inform patient that medication may cause urine to appear red for 1–2 days.

❑ Instruct patient to notify health care professional if skin irritation occurs at site of previous radiation therapy.

❑ Advise family and/or caregivers to take precautions (i.e., latex gloves) in handling body fluids for at least 5 days posttreatment.

❑ Emphasize the need for periodic lab tests to monitor for side effects.

## EVALUATION

**Effectiveness of therapy can be demonstrated by:** ■ Decrease in size or spread of malignancies in solid tumors ■ Improvement of hematologic status in leukemias

### High Alert

# doxorubicin hydrochloride liposome

(dox-oh-**roo**-bi-sin hye-droe-**klor**-ide**lye**-poe-sohm)
Doxil

### CLASSIFICATION(S):
**Therapeutic:** antineoplastics
**Pharmacologic:** anthracyclines

### Pregnancy Category D

## INDICATIONS

■ AIDS-related Kaposi's sarcoma (KS) in patients cannot tolerate conventional therapy ■ Metastatic ovarian carcinoma when disease is refractory to both paclitaxel- and platinum-based chemotherapy regimens.

## ACTION

■ Inhibits DNA and RNA synthesis by forming a complex with DNA; action is cell-cycle S-phase–specific ■ Also has immunosuppressive properties ■ Encapsulation in a liposome increases uptake by tumors, prolongs action, and may decrease some toxicity. **Therapeutic Effects:** ■ Death of rapidly replicating cells, particularly malignant ones.

## PHARMACOKINETICS

**Absorption:** Administered IV only, resulting in complete bioavailability.

**Distribution:** Widely distributed; does not cross the blood-brain barrier; extensively bound to tissues ( ↑ concentrations delivered to KS lesions due to liposomal carrier)

**Metabolism and Excretion:** Mostly metabolized by the liver with conversion to an active compound. Excreted mostly in bile, 50% as unchanged drug. <5% eliminated unchanged in the urine.

**Half-life:** 55 hr.

## CONTRAINDICATIONS AND PRECAUTIONS

**Contraindicated in:** ■ Hypersensitivity ■ Pregnancy or lactation.

**Use Cautiously in:** ■ Pre-existing cardiac disease or ↑ cumulative doses of anthracyclines ■ Depressed bone marrow reserve ■ Liver impairment (dosage reduction required if serum bilirubin >1.2 mg/dl) ■ Children, geriatric patients, prior mediastinal radiation, concurrent cyclophosphamide (increased risk of cardiotoxicity) ■ Patients with childbearing potential.

## ADVERSE REACTIONS AND SIDE EFFECTS*

■ **CNS:** weakness ■ **CV:** CARDIOMYOPATHY ■ **GI:** nausea, diarrhea, increased alkaline phosphatase, moniliasis, stomatitis, vomiting ■ **Derm:** alopecia, palmar-plantar erythrodysesthesia ■ **Hemat:** anemia, leukopenia, thrombocytopenia ■ **Local:** injection site reactions ■ **Misc:** ANAPHYLACTOID ALLERGIC REACTIONS, acute infusion-related reactions, fever.

## INTERACTIONS

**Drug-Drug:** ■ ↑ bone marrow depression with other **antineoplastics** or **radiation therapy** ■ Pediatric patients who have received concurrent doxorubicin and **dactinomycin** have ↑ risk of recall pneumonitis following local radiation therapy ■ May ↑ skin reactions at previous **radiation therapy** sites ■ If **paclitaxel** is administered first, clearance of doxorubicin is ↓ and incidence and severity of neutropenia and stomatitis are ↑ (problem is less if doxorubicin is administered first) ■ Hematologic toxicity is ↑ by concurrent use of **cyclosporine**; risk of coma and seizures is also ↑ ■ Incidence and severity of neutropenia and thrombocytopenia are ↑ by concurrent **progesterone** ■ **Phenobarbital** may ↑ clearance and ↓ effects of doxorubicin ■ Doxorubicin may ↓ metabolism and ↑ effects of

**phenytoin** ■ **Streptozocin** may ↑ the half-life of doxorubicin (dosage reduction of doxorubicin recommended) ■ May ↑ risk of hemorrhagic cystitis from **cyclophosphamide** or hepatitis from **mercaptopurine** ■ Cardiac toxicity may be ↑ by **radiation therapy** or **cyclophosphamide** ■ May ↓ antibody response to **live-virus vaccines** and ↑ risk of adverse reactions.

## ROUTE AND DOSAGE

Other regimens are used.

■ **IV (Adults):** *AIDS-related KS*—20 mg/m² every 3 wk; *metastatic ovarian cancer*— 40—50 mg/m² every 4 wk.

## AVAILABILITY

■ *Liposomal dispersion for injection:* 20 mg/10 ml in 10-ml and 25 ml vials^Rx ■ Cost: 10 ml $796.50/vial, 25 ml $1991.25/vial.

TIME/ACTION PROFILE (effect on blood counts)

|    | ONSET | PEAK | DURATION |
|----|-------|------|----------|
| IV | 10 days | 14 days | 21–24 days |

# NURSING IMPLICATIONS

## ASSESSMENT

■ **General Info:** Monitor blood pressure, pulse, respiratory rate, and temperature frequently during administration. Report significant changes.

❑ Monitor for acute infusion-related reactions consisting of flushing, shortness of breath, facial swelling, headache, chills, chest pain, back pain, chest or throat tightness, fever, tachycardia, pruritus, rash, cyanosis, syncope, bronchospasm, asthma, apnea, which may be accompanied by hypotension. Reactions usually resolve over 1 day and are usually limited to first dose. Slowing infusion rate may minimize this reaction. Reaction is thought to be due to liposome.

❑ Observe patient for signs and symptoms of anaphylaxis (rash, pruritus, laryngeal edema, wheezing). Discontinue the drug and notify physician or other health care professional immediately if these problems occur. Keep epinephrine, an antihistamine, and resuscitation equipment close by in case of an anaphylactic reaction.

- Monitor for bone marrow depression. Assess for bleeding (bleeding gums, bruising, petechiae, guaiac stools, urine, and emesis) and avoid IM injections and taking rectal temperatures if platelet count is low. Apply pressure to venipuncture sites for 10 min. Assess for signs of infection during neutropenia. Anemia may occur. Monitor for increased fatigue, dyspnea, and orthostatic hypotension.

- Monitor intake and output ratios, and report occurrence of significant discrepancies. Encourage fluid intake of 2000–3000 ml/day. Allopurinol and alkalinization of the urine may be used to decrease serum uric acid levels and to help prevent urate stone formation.

- Severe and protracted nausea and vomiting may occur as early as 1 hr after therapy and may last 24 hr. Parenteral antiemetics should be administered 30–45 min prior to therapy and routinely around the clock for the next 24 hr as indicated. Monitor amount of emesis and notify physician or other health care professional if emesis exceeds guidelines to prevent dehydration.

- Monitor for development of signs of cardiac toxicity, which may be either acute and transient (ST segment depression, flattened T wave, sinus tachycardia, and extrasystoles) or late onset (usually occurs 1–6 mo after initiation of therapy) and characterized by intractable CHF (peripheral edema, dyspnea, rales/crackles, weight gain). Chest x-ray, echocardiography, ECGs, and radionuclide angiography may be ordered prior to and periodically during therapy. Cardiotoxicity is more prevalent in children younger than 2 yr and geriatric patients. Dexrazoxane may be used to prevent cardiotoxicity in patients receiving cumulative doses of >300 mg/m².

- Assess injection site frequently for redness, irritation, or inflammation. Doxorubicin is a vesicant but may infiltrate painlessly even if blood returns on aspiration of infusion needle. Severe tissue damage may occur if doxorubicin extravasates. If extravasation occurs, stop infusion immediately, restart, and complete dose in another vein. Local infiltration of antidote is not recommended. Apply ice packs and elevate and rest extremity for 24–48 hr to reduce swelling, then resume normal activity as tolerated. If swelling, redness, and/or pain persists beyond 48 hr, immediate consultation for possible debridement is indicated.

- Assess oral mucosa frequently for development of stomatitis. Increased dosing interval and/or decreased dosing is recommended if lesions are painful or interfere with nutrition.

- Monitor for skin toxicity with prolonged use; palmar-plantar erythrodysesthesia usually occurs after 6 wk of treatment and consists of swelling, pain, and erythema of the hands and feet. This may progress to desquamation but usually regresses after 2 wk. In severe cases, modification of future doses of doxorubicin hydrochloride liposome may be necessary.

- **Lab Test Considerations:** Monitor CBC and differential prior to and periodically during therapy. The WBC nadir occurs 10–14 days after administration, and recovery usually occurs by the 21st day. Thrombocytopenia and anemia may also occur. ↑ dosing interval and/or ↓ dose is recommended if ANC is <1000 cells/mm³ and/or platelet count is <50,000 cells/mm³.

- Monitor renal (BUN and creatinine) and hepatic (AST, ALT, LDH, and serum bilirubin) function prior to and periodically during therapy. Dose reduction is required for bilirubin >1.2 mg/dl or serum creatinine >3 mg/dl.

- May cause ↑ serum and urine uric acid concentrations.

## POTENTIAL NURSING DIAGNOSES

- Infection, risk for (Adverse Reactions).
- Cardiac output, decreased (Adverse Reactions).

## IMPLEMENTATION

- **High Alert:** Fatalities have occurred with incorrect administration of chemotherapeutic agents. Before administering, clarify all ambiguous orders; double check single, daily, and course-of-therapy dose limits; have second practitioner independently double check original order, calculations and infusion pump settings. Do not confuse doxorubicin hydrochloride liposome (Doxil) with doxorubicin hydrochloride (Adriamycin, Rubex) or with daunorubicin hydrochloride (Cerubidine) or daunorubicin citrate liposome (DaunoXome). Clarify orders that do not include generic and brand names.

■ **General:** Solution should be prepared in a biologic cabinet. Wear gloves, gown, and mask while handling medication. Discard IV equipment in specially designated containers.

❏ Aluminum needles may be used to administer doxorubicin but should not be used during storage, because prolonged contact results in discoloration of solution and formation of a dark precipitate. Solution is red.

■ **Intermittent Infusion:** Dilute the dose of doxorubicin hydrochloride liposome, up to 90 mg, in 250 ml of D5W. Do not dilute with other diluents or diluents containing a bacteriostatic agent. Solution is not clear, but a translucent red liposomal dispersion. Do not use in-line filters. Refrigerate diluted solutions and administer within 24 hr of dilution.

■ *Rate:* Initial rate of infusion should be 1 mg/min to minimize risk of infusion reactions. If no reactions occur, increase rate to complete administration within 1 hr. Do not administer as a bolus or undiluted solution. Rapid infusion may increase infusion-related reactions.

■ **Y-Site Compatibility:** ◆ acyclovir ◆ allopurinol ◆ aminophylline ◆ ampicillin ◆ aztreonam ◆ bleomycin ◆ butorphanol ◆ calcium gluconate ◆ carboplatin ◆ cefazolin ◆ cefepime ◆ cefoxitin ◆ ceftizoxime ◆ ceftriaxone ◆ chlorpromazine ◆ cimetidine ◆ ciprofloxacin ◆ cisplatin ◆ clindamycin ◆ cyclophosphamide ◆ cytarabine ◆ dacarbazine ◆ dexamethasone sodium phosphate ◆ diphenhydramine ◆ dobutamine ◆ dopamine ◆ droperidol ◆ enalaprilat ◆ etoposide ◆ famotidine ◆ fluconazole ◆ fluorouracil ◆ furosemide ◆ ganciclovir ◆ gentamicin ◆ granisetron ◆ haloperidol ◆ heparin ◆ hydrocortisone sodium succinate ◆ hydromorphone ◆ ifosfamide ◆ leucovorin ◆ lorazepam ◆ magnesium sulfate ◆ mesna ◆ methotrexate ◆ methylprednisolone sodium succinate ◆ metronidazole ◆ netilmicin ◆ ondansetron ◆ piperacillin ◆ potassium chloride ◆ prochlorperazine ◆ ranitidine ◆ ticarcillin ◆ ticarcillin/clavulanate ◆ tobramycin ◆ trimethoprim/sulfamethoxazole ◆ vancomycin ◆ vinblastine ◆ vincristine ◆ vinorelbine ◆ zidovudine.

■ **Y-Site Incompatibility:** ◆ amphotericin B ◆ amphotericin B cholesteryl sulfate complex ◆

buprenorphine ◆ cefoperazone ◆ ceftazidime ◆ docetaxel ◆ mannitol ◆ meperidine ◆ metoclopramide ◆ mitoxantrone ◆ morphine ◆ ofloxacin ◆ paclitaxel ◆ piperacillin/tazobactam ◆ promethazine ◆ sodium bicarbonate.

■ **Additive Incompatibility:** Do not admix with other solutions or medications.

## PATIENT/FAMILY TEACHING

❏ Instruct patient to notify health care professional promptly if fever; sore throat; signs of infection; bleeding gums; bruising; petechiae; blood in stools, urine, or emesis; increased fatigue; dyspnea; or orthostatic hypotension occurs. Caution patient to avoid crowds and persons with known infections. Instruct patient to use soft toothbrush and electric razor and to avoid falls. Caution patient not to drink alcoholic beverages or take medication containing aspirin or NSAIDs, because these may precipitate gastric bleeding.

❏ Instruct patient to report pain at injection site immediately.

❏ Instruct patient to inspect oral mucosa for erythema and ulceration. If ulceration occurs, advise patient to use sponge brush, rinse mouth with water after eating and drinking, and confer with health care professional if mouth pain interferes with eating. Pain may require treatment with opioid analgesics. The risk of developing stomatitis is greatest 5–10 days after a dose; the usual duration is 3–7 days.

❏ Advise patient that this medication may have teratogenic effects. Contraception should be used during and for at least 4 mo after therapy is concluded. Inform patient before initiating therapy that this medication may cause irreversible gonadal suppression.

❏ Instruct patient to notify health care professional immediately if irregular heartbeat, shortness of breath, swelling of lower extremities, or skin irritation (swelling, pain, or redness of feet or hands) occurs.

❏ Discuss the possibility of hair loss with patient. Explore methods of coping. Regrowth usually occurs 2–3 mo after discontinuation of therapy.

❏ Instruct patient not to receive any vaccinations without advice of health care professional.

❏ Inform patient that medication may cause urine to appear red for 1–2 days.

❑ Instruct patient to notify health care professional if skin irritation occurs at site of previous radiation therapy.

❑ Advise family and/or caregivers to take precautions (i.e., latex gloves) in handling body fluids for at least 5 days posttreatment.

❑ Emphasize the need for periodic lab tests to monitor for side effects.

## EVALUATION

**Effectiveness of therapy can be demonstrated by:** ■ Decrease in size or spread of malignancies in solid tumors ■ Arrested progression of KS in patients with HIV infection.

## doxycycline, See TETRACYCLINES.

## droperidol

(droe-**per**-i-dole)

Inapsine

*CLASSIFICATION(S):*
*Therapeutic: sedative/hypnotics*
*Pharmacologic: butyrophenones*

**Pregnancy Category C**

## INDICATIONS

■ Used to produce tranquilization and as an adjunct to general and regional anesthesia. **Unlabeled uses:** ■ Useful in decreasing postoperative or postprocedure nausea and vomiting.

## ACTION

■ Similar to haloperidol—alters the action of dopamine in the CNS. **Therapeutic Effects:** ■ Tranquilization ■ Suppression of nausea and vomiting in selected situations.

## PHARMACOKINETICS

**Absorption:** Well absorbed following IM administration.

**Distribution:** Appears to cross the blood-brain barrier and placenta.

**Metabolism and Excretion:** Mainly metabolized by the liver. Only 10% excreted unchanged by the kidneys.

**Half-life:** 2.2 hr.

## CONTRAINDICATIONS AND PRECAUTIONS

**Contraindicated in:** ■ Hypersensitivity ■ Known intolerance ■ Narrow-angle glaucoma ■ Bone marrow depression ■ CNS depression ■ Severe liver or cardiac disease ■ Known or suspected QT prolongation.

**Use Cautiously in:** ■ Geriatric, debilitated, or severely ill patients (smaller doses should be used) ■ Diabetic patients ■ Respiratory insufficiency ■ Prostatic hypertrophy ■ CNS tumors ■ Intestinal obstruction ■ Seizures (may lower seizure threshold) ■ Severe liver disease ■ Pregnancy, lactation, and children <2 yr (although safety not established, droperidol has been used during cesarean section without respiratory depression in the newborn) ■ Age >65 yr, concurrent benzodiazepines, volatile anesthetics, IV opioids (may increase risk of serious arrhythmias); use lower initial doses.

**Exercise Extreme Caution in:** ■ Patients with risk factors for prolonged QT syndrome (CHF, bradycardia, diuretic use, cardiac hypertrophy, hypokalemia, hypomagnesema or other drugs known to prolong QT interval.

## ADVERSE REACTIONS AND SIDE EFFECTS*

■ **CNS:** SEIZURES, extrapyramidal reactions, abnormal EEG, anxiety, confusion, dizziness, excessive sedation, hallucinations, hyperactivity, mental depression, nightmares, restlessness, tardive dyskinesia ■ **CV:** ARRHYTHMIAS (including torsades de pointes), QT prolongation ■ **EENT:** blurred vision, dry eyes ■ **Resp:** bronchospasm, laryngospasm ■ **CV:** hypotension, tachycardia ■ **GI:** constipation, dry mouth ■ **Misc:** chills, facial sweating, shivering.

## INTERACTIONS

**Drug-Drug:** ■ Additive hypotension with **antihypertensives** or **nitrates** ■ Additive CNS depression with other **CNS depressants,** including **alcohol, antihistamines, antidepressants, opioid analgesics,** and other **sedatives** ■ Concurrent use of **drugs known to prolong QT interval** (increased risk of potentially life-threatening arrhythmias).

**Drug-Natural Products:** ■ Concomitant use of **kava, valerian, skullcap, chamomile,** or **hops** can increase CNS depression.

{ } = Available in Canada only.
*CAPITALS indicates life-threatening; underlines indicate most frequent.

## ROUTE AND DOSAGE

❏ **Premedication/Use Without Premedication in Diagnostic Procedures**

■ **IV, IM (Adults):** 2.5–initially, 30–60 min prior to induction of anesthesia; additional doses of 1.25 mg IV may be needed, but should be undertaken with caution.

■ **IM, IV (Children 2–12 yr):** 0.1 mg/kg maximum initial dose.

❏ **Adjunct to General Anesthesia**

■ **IV (Adults):** 2.5 mg additional doses of 1.25 mg IV may be needed, but should be undertaken with caution.

■ **IM, IV (Children 2–12 yr):** 0.1 mg/kg maximum initial dose.

❏ **Adjunct in Regional Anesthesia**

■ **IM, IV (Adults):** 2.5 mg.

❏ **Antiemetic**

■ **IV (Adults):** 0.5–1.25 mg q 4 hr as needed (unlabeled).

## AVAILABILITY (generic available)

■ *Injection:* 2.5 mg/ml[Rx].

TIME/ACTION PROFILE (sedation)

| | ONSET | PEAK | DURATION* |
|---|---|---|---|
| IM, IV | 3–10 min | 30 min | 2–4 hr |

*Listed as duration of tranquilization; alterations in consciousness may last up to 12 hr.

## NURSING IMPLICATIONS

### ASSESSMENT

■ **General Info:** Monitor blood pressure and heart rate frequently throughout course of therapy. Report significant changes immediately. Hypotension may be treated with parenteral fluids if hypovolemia is a causal factor. Vasopressors (norepinephrine, phenylephrine) may be needed. Avoid use of epinephrine, because droperidol reverses its pressor effects and may cause paradoxical hypotension.

❏ Assess 12–lead ECG in all patients prior to administration to determine if prolonged QT interval is present. Do not administer to patients with a prolonged QT interval. Monitor ECG prior to, during, and for 2–3 hr after treatment to monitor for arrhythmias.

❏ Assess patient for level of sedation following administration.

❏ Observe patient for extrapyramidal symptoms (dystonia, oculogyric crisis, extended neck, flexed arms, tremor, restlessness, hyperactivity, anxiety) throughout therapy. Notify physician or other health care professional should these occur. An anticholinergic antiparkinsonian agent may be used to treat these symptoms.

■ **Nausea and Vomiting:** Assess nausea, vomiting, hydration status, bowel sounds, and abdominal pain prior to and following administration.

## POTENTIAL NURSING DIAGNOSES

■ Injury, risk for (Side Effects).

## IMPLEMENTATION

■ **Direct IV:** Administer undiluted.

■ *Rate:* Administer each dose slowly over at least 1 min.

■ **Intermittent Infusion:** May be added to 250 ml of D5W, 0.9% NaCl, or LR.

■ *Rate:* Administer by slow IV infusion. Titrate according to patient response.

■ **Syringe Compatibility:** ◆ atropine ◆ bleomycin ◆ butorphanol ◆ chlorpromazine ◆ cimetidine ◆ cisplatin ◆ cyclophosphamide ◆ dimenhydrinate ◆ diphenhydramine ◆ doxorubicin ◆ fentanyl ◆ glycopyrrolate ◆ hydroxyzine ◆ meperidine ◆ metoclopramide ◆ midazolam ◆ mitomycin ◆ morphine ◆ nalbuphine ◆ pentazocine ◆ perphenazine ◆ prochlorperazine ◆ promethazine ◆ scopolamine ◆ vinblastine ◆ vincristine.

■ **Syringe Incompatibility:** ◆ fluorouracil ◆ furosemide ◆ heparin ◆ leucovorin calcium ◆ methotrexate ◆ pentobarbital.

■ **Y-Site Compatibility:** ◆ amifostine ◆ aztreonam ◆ bleomycin ◆ buprenorphine ◆ cisatracurium ◆ cisplatin ◆ cyclophosphamide ◆ cytarabine ◆ doxorubicin ◆ doxorubicin liposome ◆ filgrastim ◆ fluconazole ◆ fludarabine ◆ granisetron ◆ hydrocortisone sodium succinate ◆ idarubicin ◆ melphalan ◆ meperidine ◆ metoclopramide ◆ mitomycin ◆ ondansetron ◆ paclitaxel ◆ potassium chloride ◆ propofol ◆ sargramostim ◆ teniposide ◆ thiotepa ◆ vinblastine ◆ vincristine ◆ vinorelbine ◆ vitamin B complex with C.

■ **Y-Site Incompatibility:** ◆ allopurinol sodium ◆ amphotericin B cholesteryl sulfate complex ◆ cefepime ◆ cefmetazole ◆ fluorouracil ◆ foscarnet ◆ furosemide ◆ leucovorin calcium ◆ nafcillin ◆ piperacillin/tazobactam.

■ **Additive Incompatibility:** ◆ barbiturates.

## PATIENT/FAMILY TEACHING

❑ Caution patient to change positions slowly to minimize orthostatic hypotension.

❑ Medication causes drowsiness. Advise patient to call for assistance during ambulation and transfer.

## EVALUATION

**Effectiveness of therapy can be demonstrated by:** ■ General quiescence and reduced motor activity ■ Decreased nausea and vomiting.

# drotrecogin

(dro-tre-**coe**-gin)
Xigris

### CLASSIFICATION(S):

**Therapeutic:** anti-infectives
**Pharmacologic:** activated protein C, human

## Pregnancy Category C

## INDICATIONS

■ To reduce mortality in adult patients with sepsis.

## ACTION

■ Probably acts by suppressing widespread inflammation associated with sepsis. **Therapeutic Effects:** ■ Decrease mortality due to sepsis.

## PHARMACOKINETICS

**Absorption:** IV administration results in complete bioavailability.
**Distribution:** Unknown.
**Metabolism and Excretion:** Unknown.
**Half-life:** Unknown.

## CONTRAINDICATIONS AND PRECAUTIONS

**Contraindicated in:** ■ Hypersensitivity ■ Patients with a high risk of bleeding, including those with ❑ active internal bleeding ❑ recent (within 3 months) stroke ❑ recent (within 2 months) intracranial or intraspinal injury or severe head trauma ❑ any trauma associated with an increased risk of life-threatening bleeding ❑ presence of an epidural catheter ❑ intracranial neoplasm/mass lesion/cerebral herniation ■ Patients not expected to survive due to pre-existing medical condition(s) ■ HIV-positive patients with CD-4 cell counts ≤50/mm³ ■ Chronic dialysis patients ■ Patients who have undergone bone marrow, lung, liver, pancreas or small bowel transplantation ■ Lactation.

**Use Cautiously in:** ■ Concurrent therapeutic heparin therapy (≥15 units/kg/hr), recent (within 3 days) thrombolytic therapy, recent (within 7 days) oral anticoagulants or glycoprotein IIb/IIIa inhibitors, recent (within 7 days) aspirin therapy >650 mg/day or other platelet inhibitors ■ Platelet count <30,000 x 10⁶/L ■ Prothrombin time - INR >3.0 ■ Recent (within 6 wk) GI bleeding ■ Recent (within 3 mos) ischemic stroke ■ Intracranial arteriovenous malformation or aneurysm ■ Known bleeding diathesis ■ Chronic severe hepatic disease ■ Any other serious bleeding risk ■ Surgical procedures (discontinue 2 hr before; resume 12 hr after if hemostasis is achieved) ■ Pregnancy (use only if clearly needed) ■ Children (safety not established).

## ADVERSE REACTIONS AND SIDE EFFECTS*

■ **Hemat:** BLEEDING.

## INTERACTIONS

**Drug-Drug:** ■ Risk of serious bleeding may be increased by **antiplatelet agents, anticoagulants, thrombolytic agents,** or **other agents that may affect coagulation.**

**Drug-Natural Products:** ■ Risk of bleeding may be increased by **anise, arnica, chamomile, clove, dong quai, feverfew, garlic, ginger, gingko, Panax ginseng** and others.

## ROUTE AND DOSAGE

■ **IV (Adults):** 24 mcg/kg/hr for 96 hr.

## AVAILABILITY

■ *Powder for intravenous infusion (requires reconstitution):* 5-mg vial^Rx, 20-mg vial^Rx.

TIME/ACTION PROFILE (activity)

| | ONSET | PEAK | DURATION |
|---|---|---|---|
| IV | unknown | end of infu-sion | unknown |

## NURSING IMPLICATIONS

### ASSESSMENT

❑ Assess patient for signs of bleeding and hemorrhage (bleeding gums; nosebleed; unusual bruising; tarry, black stools; hematuria; fall in hematocrit or blood pressure; guaiac-positive stools, urine, or nasogastric aspirate) throughout therapy. If clinically important bleeding occurs, stop drotrecogin infusion immediately. Assess other agents used that may affect coagulation. Once hemostasis is achieved, reinstitution of drotrecogin may be reconsidered.

❑ Assess patient for infection (vital signs; appearance of wound, sputum, urine, and stool; WBC) at beginning of and throughout therapy.

■ **Lab Test Considerations:** Most patients with severe sepsis have coagulopathy prolonging activated partial thromboplastin time (aPTT) and prothrombin time (PT). Drotrecogin may also affect aPTT, but has minimal effect on PT. Use PT to monitor coagulation status of patients receiving drotrecogin.

### POTENTIAL NURSING DIAGNOSES

■ Tissue perfusion, ineffective, impaired (Indications).

### IMPLEMENTATION

■ **General:** Drotrecogin should be discontinued 2 hr prior to invasive surgical procedures or procedures with a risk of bleeding. Once hemostasis is achieved, drotrecogin may be started 12 hr after the procedure.

■ **Intermittent Infusion:** Calculate dose and number of 5-mg or 20-mg vials needed (vials contain excess to facilitate delivery. Reconstitute 5-mg vials with 2.5 ml and 20-mg vials with 10 ml sterile water for injection for a concentration of 2 mg/ml. Add sterile water slowly to vial; avoid inverting or shaking. Gently swirl until powder is completely dissolved. Reconstituted solution must be diluted further with 0.9% NaCl for a concentration of 100–200 mcg/ml if using an infusion pump or a concentration of 100–1000 mcg/

ml if using a syringe pump. Withdraw amount of reconstituted solution needed from vial and add to infusion bag of 0.9% NaCl; direct stream to side of the bag to avoid agitating solution. Gently invert bag to mix. Reconstituted solution must be used within 3 hr and IV administration must be completed within 12 hr of preparation of IV solution. Do not administer if discolored or contains particulate matter.

■ **Rate:** Administer at a rate of 24 mcg/kg/hr for 96 hr.

■ **Y-Site Incompatibility:** Administer via a dedicated IV line or a dedicated lumen of a multilumen central venous catheter.

■ **Solution Compatibility:** May be administered only with 0.9% NaCl, LR, dextrose or dextrose and saline mixtures.

### PATIENT/FAMILY TEACHING

❑ Explain purpose of medication to patient.

### EVALUATION

**Effectiveness of therapy can be demonstrated by:** ■ Reduction of mortality in adult patients with severe sepsis.

## dutasteride
(doo-**tas**-te-ride)
Duagen

### CLASSIFICATION(S):
**Therapeutic:** benign prostatic hyperplasia (BPH) agents
**Pharmacologic:** androgen inhibitors

### Pregnancy Category X

## INDICATIONS

■ Management of the symptoms of benign prostatic hyperplasia (BPH) in men with an enlarged prostate gland.

## ACTION

■ Inhibits the enzyme 5-alpha-reductase, which is responsible for converting testosterone to its potent metabolite 5-alpha-dihydrotestosterone in the prostate gland and other tissues. 5-Alpha-dihydrotestosterone is partly responsible for prostatic hyperplasia. **Therapeutic Effects:** ■

Reduced prostate size with associated decrease in urinary symptoms.

## PHARMACOKINETICS

**Absorption:** Well absorbed (60%) following oral administration; also absorbed through skin.

**Distribution:** 11.5% of serum concentration partitions into semen.

**Protein Binding:** 99% bound to albumin; 96.6% bound to alpha-1 glycoprotein.

**Metabolism and Excretion:** Mostly metabolized by the liver via the CYP 3A4 metabolic pathway; metabolites are excreted in feces.

**Half-life:** 5 wk.

## CONTRAINDICATIONS AND PRECAUTIONS

**Contraindicated in:** ■ Hypersensitivity ■ Cross-sensitivity with other 5-alpha-reductase inhibitors may occur ■ Women ■ Children.

**Use Cautiously in:** ■ Hepatic impairment.

## ADVERSE REACTIONS AND SIDE EFFECTS*

■ **GU:** decreased libido, ejaculation disorders, impotence ■ **Endo:** gynecomastia.

## INTERACTIONS

**Drug-Drug:** ■ Blood levels and effects may be increased by **ritonavir, ketoconazole, verapamil, diltiazem, cimetidine, ciprofloxacin,** or other **CYP 3A4 enzyme inhibitors**.

## ROUTE AND DOSAGE

■ **PO (Adults):** 0.5 mg once daily.

## AVAILABILITY

■ *Soft gelatin capsules:* 0.5 mg$^{Rx}$.

TIME/ACTION PROFILE (reduction in dihydrotestosterone levels†)

| | ONSET | PEAK | DURATION |
|---|---|---|---|
| PO | unknown | 1-2 wk | unknown |

†Symptoms may only improve over 3–12 mo.

## NURSING IMPLICATIONS

### ASSESSMENT

❏ Assess patient for symptoms of prostatic hypertrophy (urinary hesitancy, feeling of incomplete bladder emptying, interruption of urinary stream, impairment of size and force of urinary stream, terminal urinary dribbling, straining to start flow, dysuria, urgency) before and periodically throughout therapy.

❏ Digital rectal examinations should be performed before and periodically throughout therapy for BPH.

■ *Lab Test Considerations:* Serum prostate-specific antigen (PSA) concentrations, which are used to screen for prostate cancer, decrease by about 20% within the 1st mo of therapy and stabilize at about 50% of the pretreatment level within 6 mo. New baseline PSA concentrations should be established at 3 and 6 mo of therapy and evaluated periodically throughout therapy.

### POTENTIAL NURSING DIAGNOSES

■ Urinary elimination, impaired (Indications).

### IMPLEMENTATION

■ **PO:** Administer once daily with or without meals. Do not crush, break, or chew capsule.

### PATIENT/FAMILY TEACHING

❏ Instruct patient to take dutasteride at the same time each day as directed, even if symptoms improve or are unchanged. If a dose is missed, take as soon as remembered later in the day or omit dose. Do not make up by taking double doses the next day.

❏ Caution patient that sharing of dutasteride may be dangerous.

❏ Inform patient that the volume of ejaculate may be decreased during therapy but that this will not interfere with normal sexual function.

❏ Caution patient that dutasteride poses a potential risk to a male fetus. Women who are pregnant or may become pregnant should avoid exposure to semen of a partner taking

{ } = Available in Canada only.
*CAPITALS indicates life-threatening; underlines indicate most frequent.

dutasteride and should not handle dutasteride because of the potential for absorption.

❑ Advise patient to avoid donating blood for at least 6 mo after last dose of dutasteride to prevent a pregnant female from receiving dutasteride through a blood transfusion.

❑ Emphasize the importance of periodic follow-up exams to determine whether a clinical response has occurred.

## EVALUATION

**Clinical response to therapy can be evaluated by:** ■ Decrease in urinary symptoms of BPH.

## econazole, See ANTIFUNGALS (TOPICAL).

## efavirenz

(e-**fav**-i-renz)
Sustiva

### CLASSIFICATION(S):
**Therapeutic:** antiretrovirals
**Pharmacologic:** non-nucleoside reverse transcriptase inhibitors

### Pregnancy Category C

### INDICATIONS
■ HIV infection (incombination with one or more other antiretroviral agents).

### ACTION
■ Inhibits HIV reverse transcriptase, which results in disruption of DNA synthesis. **Therapeutic Effects:** ■ Slowed progression of HIV infection and decreased occurrence of sequelae ■ Increases CD4 cell counts and decreases viral load.

### PHARMACOKINETICS
**Absorption:** 50% absorbed when ingested following a high-fat meal.
**Distribution:** 99.5–99.75% bound to plasma proteins; enters CSF.
**Metabolism and Excretion:** Mostly metabolized by the liver.
**Half-life:** *Following single dose*—52–76 hr. *Following multiple doses*—40–55 hr.

### CONTRAINDICATIONS AND PRECAUTIONS
**Contraindicated in:** ■ Hypersensitivity ■ Concurrent midazolam, triazolam, or ergot derivatives.
**Use Cautiously in:** ■ History of mental illness or substance abuse ■ History of hepatic impairment (including hepatitis B or C infection or concurrent therapy with hepatotoxic agents) ■ Children (increased incidence of rash) ■ Pregnancy or lactation (use in pregnancy only if other options have been exhausted; breastfeeding not recommended in HIV-infected patients).

### ADVERSE REACTIONS AND SIDE EFFECTS*
■ **CNS:** abnormal dreams, depression, dizziness, drowsiness, fatigue, headache, impaired concentration, insomnia, nervousness ■ **GI:** nausea, abdominal pain, anorexia, diarrhea, dyspepsia, flatulence ■ **GU:** hematuria, renal calculi ■ **Derm:** RASH, increased sweating, pruritus ■ **Neuro:** hypoesthesia.

### INTERACTIONS
**Drug-Drug:** ■ ↑ levels of **midazolam, triazolam,** or **ergot alkaloids** when used concurrently; may result in potentially serious adverse reactions including arrhythmias, CNS, and respiratory depression ■ Induces (stimulates) the hepatic cytochrome P450 3A4 enzyme system and would be expected to influence the effects of other drugs that are metabolized by this system; efavirenz itself is also metabolized by this system ■ ↑ risk of CNS depression with other **CNS depressants,** including **alcohol, antidepressants, antihistamines,** and **opioid analgesics** ■ Concurrent use with **ritonavir** ↑ levels of both agents and the likelihood of adverse reactions, especially hepatotoxicity ■ May alter the effectiveness of **hormonal contraceptives** ■ Reduces **indinavir** blood levels (indinavir dosage increase recommended) ■ ↓ **saquinavir** blood levels (avoid using saquinavir as the only protease inhibitor with efavirenz) ■ May alter the effects of **warfarin.**
**Drug-Natural Products:** ■ Use with **St. John's wort** may cause ↓ levels and effectiveness, including development of drug resistance.
**Drug-Food:** ■ Ingestion following a high-fat meal increases absorption by 50%.

### ROUTE AND DOSAGE
■ **PO (Adults and Children >40 kg):** 600 mg once daily.
■ **PO (Children 32.5–40 kg):** 400 mg once daily.
■ **PO (Children 25–32.5 kg):** 350 mg once daily.
■ **PO (Children 20–25 kg):** 300 mg once daily.

{ } = Available in Canada only.
* CAPITALS indicate life-threatening; underlines indicate most frequent.

- **PO (Children 15–20 kg):** 250 mg once daily.
- **PO (Children 10–15 kg):** 200 mg once daily.

## AVAILABILITY

- **Capsules:** 50 mg$^{Rx}$, 100 mg$^{Rx}$, 200 mg$^{Rx}$ ▪ Cost: 50 mg $36.00/30, 100 mg $71.94/30, 200 mg $431.95/30 ▪ **Tablets:** 600 mg$^{Rx}$ ▪ Cost: 600 mg $431.85/30.

TIME/ACTION PROFILE (blood levels)

|    | ONSET | PEAK | DURATION |
|----|-------|------|----------|
| PO | rapid | 3–5 hr | 24 hr |

# NURSING IMPLICATIONS

## ASSESSMENT

- Assess for change in severity of HIV symptoms and for symptoms of opportunistic infections during therapy.
- Assess patient for rash, especially during 1st mo of therapy. Onset is usually within 2 wk and resolves with continued therapy within 1 mo. May range from mild maculopapular with erythema and pruritus to exfoliative dermatitis and Stevens-Johnson syndrome. Occurs more often and may be more severe in children. If rash is severe or accompanied by blistering, desquamation, mucosal involvement, or fever, therapy must be discontinued immediately. Efavirenz may be reinstated concurrently with antihistamines or corticosteroids in patients discontinuing due to rash.
- Assess patient for CNS and psychiatric symptoms (dizziness, impaired concentration, somnolence, abnormal dreams, insomnia) throughout therapy. Symptoms usually begin during 1st or 2nd day of therapy and resolve after 2–4 wk. Administration at bedtime may minimize symptoms. Concurrent use with alcohol or psychoactive agents may cause additive CNS symptoms.
- **Lab Test Considerations:** Monitor viral load and CD4 cell count regularly during therapy.
- Monitor liver function tests in patients with a history of hepatitis B or C. May cause ↑ serum AST, ALT, and GGT concentrations. If moderate to severe liver function test abnormalities occur, efavirenz doses should be held until levels return to normal. Discontin-

ue if liver function abnormalities recur when therapy is resumed.
- May cause ↑ in total cholesterol and serum triglyceride levels.
- May cause false-positive urine cannabinoid results.

## POTENTIAL NURSING DIAGNOSES

- Infection, risk for (Indications).
- Noncompliance (Patient/Family Teaching).

## IMPLEMENTATION

- **PO:** May be administered with or without food. Avoid taking with a high-fat meal.

## PATIENT/FAMILY TEACHING

- Emphasize the importance of taking efavirenz as directed. It must always be used in combination with other antiretroviral drugs. Do not take more than prescribed amount and do not stop taking without consulting health care professional. Take missed doses as soon as remembered; do not double doses.
- Instruct patient that efavirenz should not be shared with others.
- May cause dizziness, impaired concentration, or drowsiness. Caution patient to avoid driving or other activities requiring alertness until response to medication is known.
- Advise patient to avoid taking other medications, prescription or OTC, or herabl productswithout consulting health care professional.
- Inform patient that efavirenz does not cure AIDS or prevent associated or opportunistic infections. Efavirenz does not reduce the risk of transmission of HIV to others through sexual contact or blood contamination. Caution patient to use a condom and to avoid sharing needles or donating blood to prevent spreading the AIDS virus to others. Advise patient that the long-term effects of efavirenz are unknown at this time.
- Advise patients taking oral contraceptives to use a nonhormonal method of birth control during efavirenz therapy and to notify health care professional if they become pregnant while taking efavirenz.
- Instruct patient to notify health care professional immediately if rash occurs.
- Emphasize the importance of regular follow-up exams and blood counts to determine progress and monitor for side effects.

## EVALUATION

**Effectiveness of therapy can be demonstrated by:** ■ Delayed progression of AIDS and decreased opportunistic infections in patients with HIV ■ Decrease in viral load and increase in CD4 cell counts.

# eletriptan
(e-le-**trip**-tan)
Relpax

### CLASSIFICATION(S):
**Therapeutic:** vascular headache suppressants
**Pharmacologic:** 5 HT₁ agonists

**Pregnancy Category C**

## INDICATIONS

■ Acute treatment of migraine headache.

## ACTION

■ Acts as an agonist at specific 5-hydroxy-tryptamine receptor sites in intracranial blood vessels and sensory trigeminal nerves. **Therapeutic Effects:** ■ Cranial vessel vasoconstriction with resultant decrease in migraine headache.

## PHARMACOKINETICS

**Absorption:** 50% absorbed after oral administration.
**Distribution:** Enters breast milk.
**Metabolism and Excretion:** Mostly metabolized by the liver via the CYP 3A4 enzyme system.
**Half-life:** 4 hr.

## CONTRAINDICATIONS AND PRECAUTIONS

**Contraindicated in:** ■ Hypersensitivity ■ Hemiplegic or basilar migraine ■ Ischemic cardiovascular, cerebrovascular, or peripheral vascular syndromes (including ischemic bowel disease) ■ History of significant cardiovascular disease ■ Uncontrolled hypertension ■ Severe hepatic impairment ■ Should not be used within 24 hr of other 5-HT₁ agonists or ergot-type compounds (dihydroergotamine) ■ Should not be used within 72 hr of potent CYP3A4 inhibitors in-

cluding ketoconazole, itraconazole, nefazodone, clarithromycin, ritonavir, and nelfinavir.
**Use Cautiously in:** ■ Geriatric patients ■ Pregnancy, lactation, or children <18 yr (safety not established; use during pregnancy only if potential benefits justify potential risk to fetus).
**Exercise Extreme Caution in:** ■ Cardiovascular risk factors (hypertension, hypercholesterolemia, cigarette smoking, obesity, diabetes, strong family history, menopausal women or men >40 yr); use only if cardiovascular status has been evaluated and determined to be safe and 1st dose is administered under supervision.

## ADVERSE REACTIONS AND SIDE EFFECTS*

■ **CNS:** dizziness, drowsiness, weakness ■ **CV:** chest tightness/pressure ■ **GI:** abdominal pain, dry mouth, dysphagia, nausea ■ **Neuro:** paresthesia.

## INTERACTIONS

**Drug-Drug:** ■ Blood levels and risk of adverse reactions are increased by potent **CYP3A4 inhibitors** (including **ketoconazole, itraconazole, nefazodone, clarithromycin, ritonavir,** and **nelfinavir**); use within 72 hr is contraindicated ■ Concurrent use (within 24 hr of each other) with ergot-containing drugs (**dihydroergotamine**) may result in prolonged vasospastic reactions and should be avoided.

## ROUTE AND DOSAGE

■ **PO (Adults):** 20 or 40 mg; may be repeated in 2 hr if initial response is inadequate (not to exceed 80 mg/24 hr or treatment of 3 headaches/mo).

## AVAILABILITY

■ **Tablets:** 20 mg^Rx, 40 mg^Rx.

TIME/ACTION PROFILE (decreased migraine pain)

| | ONSET | PEAK | DURATION |
|---|---|---|---|
| PO | within 2 hr | 2 hr | up to 24 hr |

## NURSING IMPLICATIONS

### ASSESSMENT

❑ Assess pain location, intensity, character, duration and associated symptoms (photopho-

nia, phonophobia, nausea, vomiting) during migraine attack.

**POTENTIAL NURSING DIAGNOSES**

▪ Pain, acute (Indications).

**IMPLEMENTATION**

▪ **PO:** Administer at the first sign of a headache. If after the initial dose, headache improves but then returns, dose may be repeated at least 2 hr after initial dose. If initial dose is ineffective, second dose is unlikely to be effective.

**PATIENT/FAMILY TEACHING**

❑ Instruct patient that eletriptan should only be used during a migraine attack. Eletriptan is used for treatment of a migraine attack, not for prevention.

❑ Instruct patient to take eletriptan at the first sign of a migraine, but may be administered at any time during attack. Allow at least 2 hr between doses and do not use more than 80 mg/day or 3 attacks/mo.

❑ Caution patient not to take eletriptan within 24 hr of other vascular headache suppressants.

❑ Advise patient that lying down in a darkened room after eletriptan administration may further help relieve headache.

❑ Advise patient to notify health care professional if she plans or suspects pregnancy, or if breastfeeding.

❑ Advise patient to notify health care professional before next dose of eletriptan if pain or tightness in the chest occurs. If chest pain is severe or does not subside, notify health care professional immediately. If feelings of tingling, heat, flushing, heaviness, pressure, drowsiness, dizziness, tiredness, or sickness develop, discuss with health care provider at next visit.

❑ May cause drowsiness or dizziness. Caution patient to avoid driving or other activities requiring alertness until response to medication is known.

❑ Advise patient to avoid alcohol, which aggravates headaches, during therapy.

**EVALUATION**

**Effectiveness of therapy can be demonstrated by:** ▪ Relief of migraine attack.

**enalapril/enalaprilat, See ANGIOTENSIN-CONVERTING ENZYME (ACE) INHIBITORS.**

**enoxacin, See FLUOROQUINOLONES.**

**enoxaparin, See HEPARINS (LOW MOLECULAR WEIGHT)/ HEPARINOIDS.**

**entacapone**
(en-**tak**-a-pone)
Comtan

**CLASSIFICATION(S):**
**Therapeutic:** antiparkinson agents
**Pharmacologic:** catechol-O-methyltransferase inhibitors

**Pregnancy Category C**

**INDICATIONS**

▪ With levodopa/carbidopa to treat idiopathic Parkinson's disease when signs and symptoms of end-of-dose "wearing-off" (so-called fluctuating patients) occur.

**ACTION**

▪ Acts as a selective and reversible inhibitor of the enzyme catechol-O-methyltransferase (COMT) ▪ Inhibition of this enzyme prevents the breakdown of levodopa, increasing availability to the CNS. **Therapeutic Effects:** ▪ Prolongs duration of response to levodopa with end-of-dose motor fluctuations ▪ Decreased signs and symptoms of Parkinson's disease.

**PHARMACOKINETICS**

**Absorption:** 35% absorbed following oral administration; absorption is rapid.
**Distribution:** Unknown.
**Protein Binding:** 98%.
**Metabolism and Excretion:** Minimal amounts excreted unchanged; highly metabolized followed by biliary excretion.
**Half-life:** *Initial phase*—0.4–0.7 hr; *second phase*—2.4 hr.

## CONTRAINDICATIONS AND PRECAUTIONS

**Contraindicated in:** ■ Hypersensitivity ■ Concurrent nonselective MAO inhibitor therapy
**Use Cautiously in:** ■ Hepatic impairment ■ Concurrent use of drugs that are metabolized by COMT ■ Pregnancy, lactation, or children (safety not established)

## ADVERSE REACTIONS AND SIDE EFFECTS*

■ **CNS:** NEUROLEPTIC MALIGNANT SYNDROME, dizziness, hallucinations, syncope ■ **Resp:** pulmonary infiltrates, pleural effusion, pleural thickening ■ **CV:** hypotension ■ **GI:** abdominal pain, diarrhea, nausea (during initiation), retroperitoneal fibrosis ■ **GU:** brownish-orange discoloration of urine ■ **MS:** RHABDOMYOLYSIS ■ **Neuro:** dyskinesia.

## INTERACTIONS

**Drug-Drug:** ■ Concurrent use with selective **MAO inhibitors** is not recommended; both agents inhibit the metabolic pathways of catecholamines ■ Concurrent use of drugs that are metabolized by COMT such as **isoproterenol, epinephrine, norepinephrine, dopamine, dobutamine, methyldopa,** and **bitolterol** may ↑ risk of tachycardia, increased blood pressure, and arrhythmias ■ **Probenecid, cholestyramine, erythromycin, rifampin, ampicillin,** and **chloramphenicol** may interfere with biliary elimination of entacapone; concurrent use should be undertaken with caution.

## ROUTE AND DOSAGE

■ **PO (Adults):** 200 mg with each dose of levodopa/carbidopa up to a maximum of 8 times daily.

## AVAILABILITY

■ *Tablets:* 200 mg^Rx. ■ levodopa/carbidopa (Stalevo), see Appendix B.

TIME/ACTION PROFILE (inhibition of COMT)

|    | ONSET | PEAK | DURATION |
|----|-------|------|----------|
| PO | unknown | unknown | up to 8 hr |

## NURSING IMPLICATIONS

### ASSESSMENT

■ **General Info:** Assess parkinsonian and extrapyramidal symptoms (restlessness or desire to keep moving, rigidity, tremors, pill rolling, mask-like face, shuffling gait, muscle spasms, twisting motions, difficulty speaking or swallowing, loss of balance control) prior to and during therapy. Dyskinesia may increase with therapy.
❏ Monitor patient for development of diarrhea. Usually occurs within 4 to 12 wk of start of therapy, but may occur as early as the first week and as late as months after initiation of therapy.
❏ Monitor patient for signs similar to neuroleptic malignant syndrome (elevated temperature, muscular rigidity, altered consciousness, elevated CPK). Symptoms have been associated with rapid dose reduction or withdrawal of other dopaminergic drugs. Withdrawal should be gradual.

### POTENTIAL NURSING DIAGNOSES

■ Mobility, impaired physical (Indications).
■ Injury, risk for (Indications).

### IMPLEMENTATION

■ **PO:** Always administer entacapone with levodopa/carbidopa. Entacapone has no antiparkinsonism effects of its own.

### PATIENT/FAMILY TEACHING

❏ Encourage patient to take entacapone as directed. Missed doses should be taken as soon as possible, up to 2 hr before the next dose. Taper gradually when discontinuing or a withdrawal reaction may occur.
❏ May cause dizziness or hallucinations. Advise patient to avoid driving or other activities that require alertness until response to the drug is known.
❏ Inform patient that nausea may occur, especially at initiation of therapy. Therapy may cause change in urine color to brownish orange.
❏ Caution patient to change positions slowly to minimize orthostatic hypotension.
❏ Instruct patient to notify health care professional if pregnancy is planned or suspected.

---

{ } = Available in Canada only.
*CAPITALS indicates life-threatening; <u>underlines</u> indicate most frequent.

❑ Emphasize the importance of routine follow-up exams.

## EVALUATION

**Effectiveness of therapy can be demonstrated by:** ■ Decreased signs and symptoms of Parkinson's disease.

---

# EPIDURAL LOCAL ANESTHETICS

**bupivacaine**

(byoo-**pi**-vi-kane)

Marcaine, Sensorcaine

**levobupivacaine**

(**lee**-voe-byoo-**pi**-vi-kane)

Chirocaine

**ropivacaine**

(**roe**-pi-vi-kane)

Naropin

*CLASSIFICATION(S):*

*Therapeutic: epidural local anesthetics, anesthetics—topical/local*

**Pregnancy Category C (bupivacaine, ropivacaine), B (levobupivacaine)**

---

## INDICATIONS

■ May be combined with epidural opioids or clonidine in the management of severe acute or chronic pain. Low doses of epidural anesthetics act synergistically with opioids, allowing for use of lower doses of opioids and fewer systemic opioid side effects (constipation, nausea, respiratory depression, hypotension) ❑ Compared with other local anesthetics, these agents are better able to block nerve fibers that carry pain, with minimal effect on sensory and motor fibers.

## ACTION

■ Local anesthetics inhibit initiation and conduction of sensory nerve impulses by altering the influx of sodium and efflux of potassium in neurons, slowing or stopping pain transmission. Epidural administration allows action to take place at the level of the spinal nerve roots immediately adjacent to the site of administra-tion. The catheter is placed as close as possible to the dermatomes (skin surface areas innervated by a single spinal nerve or group of spinal nerves) that, when blocked, will produce the most effective spread of analgesia for the site of injury. **Therapeutic Effects:** ■ Decreased pain; low doses have minimal effect on sensory or motor function; higher doses may produce complete motor blockade. Catheter placement allows localization of effect.

## PHARMACOKINETICS

**Absorption:** Systemic absorption follows epidural administration, but amount absorbed depends on dose.

**Distribution:** Agents are lipid soluble, which selectively keeps them in the epidural space and limits systemic absorption. If systemic absorption occurs, these agents are widely distributed and cross the placenta.

**Metabolism and Excretion:** Small amounts that may reach systemic circulation are mostly metabolized by the liver. Because only small amounts are cleared by the kidneys, renal function has minimal impact.

**Half-life:** *Bupivacaine*—5 hr (after epidural use); *levobupivacaine*—1.3 hr (after IV administration); *ropivacaine*—3 hr (after epidural use).

## CONTRAINDICATIONS AND PRECAUTIONS

**Contraindicated in:** ■ Hypersensitivity; cross-sensitivity with other amide local anesthetics may occur (etidocaine, lidocaine, mepivacaine, prilocaine) ■ Bupivacaine contains bisulfites and should be avoided in patients with known intolerance.

**Use Cautiously in:** ■ Concurrent use of other local anesthetics ■ Liver disease ■ Concurrent use of anticoagulants (including low-dose heparin and low-molecular-weight heparins/heparinoids) increases the risk of spinal/epidural hematomas ■ Children (safety not established).

## ADVERSE REACTIONS AND SIDE EFFECTS*

Noted primarily for use in pain management. ■ **CNS:** SEIZURES, headache, irritability, slow speech, twitching ■ **EENT:** tinnitus ■ **CV:** CARDIO-VASCULAR COLLAPSE, arrhythmias, bradycardia, hypotension ■ **GI:** metallic taste ■ **GU:** urinary retention ■ **Derm:** pruritus ■ **F and E:** acidosis

■ **Neuro:** circumoral tingling/numbness ■ **Misc:** allergic reactions, fever.

## INTERACTIONS

**Drug-Drug:** ■ Additive toxicity may occur with concurrent use of other **amide local anesthetics** (including **lidocaine, mepivacaine,** and **prilocaine**).

## ROUTE AND DOSAGE

❏ **Bupivacaine**

■ **Epidural: (Adults):** Epidural analgesia: 0.0625–0.125% solution (0.625–1.25 mg/ml). *Partial to moderate motor block—* 25–50 mg as a 0.25% solution q 3 hr; *moderate to complete motor block*—50–100 mg as a 0.5% solution q 3 hr; *complete motor block*—75–150 mg as a 0.75% solution q 3 hr.

❏ **Levobupivacaine**

■ **Epidural: (Adults):** *Epidural for surgery*—50–150 mg as a 0.5–0.75% solution. *Epidural for cesarean section*—100–150 mg as a 0.5% solution. *Labor anesthesia (epidural bolus)*—25–50 mg as a 0.25% solution. *Postoperative pain management (epidural infusion)*—5–25 mg/hr as a 0.25% solution.

❏ **Ropivacaine**

■ **Epidural: (Adults):** *Major Nerve block*— 7.5 mg/ml for up to 72 hr; *Postoperative pain*—0.2% solution (2 mg/ml). *Lumbar epidural continuous infusion*—12–20 mg/ hr (6–10 ml/hr). *Thoracic epidural continuous infusion*—8–16 mg/hr (4–8 ml/hr).

## AVAILABILITY

❏ **Bupivacaine**

■ *Solution for injection (with and without preservatives):* 0.25%$^{Rx}$, 0.5%$^{Rx}$, 0.75%$^{Rx}$ ■ epinephrine$^{Rx}$.

❏ **Levobupivacaine**

■ *Solution for injection:* 2.5 mg/ml in 10- and 30-ml vials$^{Rx}$, 5 mg/ml in 10- and 30-ml vials$^{Rx}$, 7.5 mg/ml in 10- and 30-ml vials$^{Rx}$.

❏ **Ropivacaine (Preservative-Free)**

■ *Solution for injection:* 0.2%$^{Rx}$, 0.5%$^{Rx}$, 0.75%$^{Rx}$, 1%$^{Rx}$.

TIME/ACTION PROFILE (analgesia)

| | ONSET | PEAK | DURATION |
|---|---|---|---|
| Epidural | 10–30 min | unknown | 2-8 hr† |

†Duration of anesthetic block.

## NURSING IMPLICATIONS

### ASSESSMENT

■ **Systemic Toxicity:** Assess for systemic toxicity (circumoral tingling and numbness, ringing in ears, metallic taste, slow speech, irritability, twitching, seizures, cardiac dysrhythmias) each shift. Report to anesthesiologist. Treatment includes removal of local anesthetic from analgesic solution.

■ **Orthostatic Hypotension:** Assess heart rate and blood pressure, including orthostatic blood pressure prior to ambulation, regularly until dose is stabilized and it is clear that hypotension is not a problem. Mild hypotension is common because of the effect of local anesthetic block of nerve fibers on the sympathetic nervous system, causing vasodilation. Significant hypotension and bradycardia may occur, especially when rising from a prone position or following large dose increases or boluses. Treatment of unresolved hypotension may include hydration, decreasing the epidural infusion rate, and/or removal of local anesthetic from analgesic solution.

■ **Unwanted Motor and Sensory Deficit:** The goal of adding low-dose local anesthetics to epidural opioids for pain management is to provide analgesia, not to produce anesthesia. Patients should be able to ambulate if their condition allows, and epidural analgesic should not hamper this important recovery activity. However, many factors, including location of the epidural catheter, local anesthetic dose, and variability in patient response, can result in patients experiencing unwanted motor and sensory deficits. Pain is the first sensation lost, followed by temperature, touch, proprioception, and skeletal muscle tone.

❏ Assess for sensory deficit every shift. Ask patient to point to numb and tingling skin areas (numbness and tingling at the incision site is common and usually normal).

{ } = Available in Canada only.
*CAPITALS indicates life-threatening; underlines indicate most frequent.

❑ Assess patient for motor deficit. Ask patient to bend the knees and lift the buttocks off the mattress. Most are able to do this without difficulty. Determine patient's ability to bear weight. Provide assistance when ambulating as needed. Notify anesthesiologist of unwanted motor and sensory deficits.

❑ Unwanted motor and sensory deficits often can be corrected with simple treatment. For example, a change in position may relieve temporary sensory loss in an extremity. Minor extremity muscle weakness is often treated by decreasing the epidural infusion rate and keeping the patient in bed until the weakness resolves. Sometimes removing the local anesthetic from the analgesic solution is necessary, such as when signs of local anesthetic toxicity are detected or when simple treatment of motor and sensory deficits has been unsuccessful.

## POTENTIAL NURSING DIAGNOSES

■ Pain, acute, acute (Indications).
■ Mobility, impaired physical.

## IMPLEMENTATION

See Route and Dosage section.

## PATIENT/FAMILY TEACHING

❑ Instruct patient to notify nurse if signs or symptoms of systemic toxicity occur.

❑ Advise patient to request assistance during ambulation until orthostatic hypotension and motor deficits are ruled out.

## EVALUATION

**Effectiveness of therapy can be demonstrated by:** ■ Decrease in postoperative pain without unwanted sensory or motor deficits.

| High Alert |
| --- |

## epinephrine
(e-pi-**nef**-rin)
Adrenalin, Ana-Guard, AsthmaHaler Mist, AsthmaNefrin (racepineph-rine), EpiPen, microNefrin, Neph-ron, Primatene, Sus-Phrine, S-2

### CLASSIFICATION(S):
**Therapeutic:** *antiasthmatics, bronchodilators, vasopressors*
**Pharmacologic:** *adrenergics*

## Pregnancy Category C
See Appendix C for ophthalmic use.

## INDICATIONS

■ **Subcut, IV, Inhaln:** Management of reversible airway disease due to asthma or COPD ■ **Subcut, IV:** Management of severe allergic reactions ■ **IV, Intracardiac, Intratracheal, Intraosseous (part of advanced cardiac life support [ACLS] and pediatric advanced life support [PALS] guidelines):** Management of cardiac arrest (unlabeled) ■ **Local/Spinal:** Adjunct in the localization/prolongation of anesthesia.

## ACTION

■ Results in the accumulation of cyclic adenosine monophosphate (cAMP) at beta-adrenergic receptors ■ Affects both $beta_1$(cardiac)-adrenergic receptors and $beta_2$(pulmonary)-adrenergic receptor sites ■ Produces bronchodilation ■ Also has alpha-adrenergic agonist properties, which result in vasoconstriction ■ Inhibits the release of mediators of immediate hypersensitivity reactions from mast cells. **Therapeutic Effects:** ■ Bronchodilation ■ Maintenance of heart rate and blood pressure ■ Localization/prolongation of local/spinal anesthetic.

## PHARMACOKINETICS

**Absorption:** Well absorbed following subcut administration; some absorption may occur following repeated inhalation of large doses.
**Distribution:** Does not cross the blood-brain barrier; crosses the placenta and enters breast milk.
**Metabolism and Excretion:** Action is rapidly terminated by metabolism and uptake by nerve endings.
**Half-life:** Unknown.

## CONTRAINDICATIONS AND PRECAUTIONS

**Contraindicated in:** ■ Hypersensitivity to adrenergic amines ■ Some products may contain bisulfites or fluorocarbons (in some inhalers) and should be avoided in patients with known hypersensitivity or intolerance.
**Use Cautiously in:** ■ Cardiac disease ■ Hypertension ■ Hyperthyroidism ■ Diabetes ■ Glaucoma (except for ophthalmic use) ■ Elderly patients (more susceptible to adverse reactions; may require dosage reduction) ■ Pregnancy

(near term), lactation, and children <2 yr (safety not established) ■ Excessive use may lead to tolerance and paradoxical bronchospasm (inhaler).

## ADVERSE REACTIONS AND SIDE EFFECTS*

■ **CNS:** <u>nervousness</u>, <u>restlessness</u>, <u>tremor</u>, headache, insomnia ■ **Resp:** paradoxical bronchospasm (excessive use of inhalers) ■ **CV:** <u>angina</u>, <u>arrhythmias</u>, <u>hypertension</u>, <u>tachycardia</u> ■ **GI:** nausea, vomiting ■ **Endo:** hyperglycemia.

## INTERACTIONS

**Drug-Drug:** ■ Concurrent use with other **adrenergic agents** will have additive adrenergic side effects ■ Use with **MAO inhibitors** may lead to hypertensive crisis ■ **Beta blockers:** may negate therapeutic effect.

**Drug-Natural Products:** ■ Use with caffeine-containing herbs (**cola nut, guarana, mate, tea, coffee**) increases stimulant effect.

## ROUTE AND DOSAGE

■ **Subcut, IM (Adults):** *Anaphylactic reactions/asthma*—0.1–0.5 mg (single dose not to exceed 1 mg); may repeat q 10–15 min for anaphylactic shock or q 20 min–4 hr for asthma. *Epinephrine suspension*—0.5 mg subcut initially; may repeat 0.5–1.5 mg q 6 hr.

■ **Subcut (Children):** *Anaphylactic reactions/asthma*—0.01 mg/kg or 0.3 mg/m$^2$ (not to exceed 0.5 mg/dose) q 15 min for 2 doses, then q 4 hr. *Epinephrine suspension*—0.025 mg/kg (0.625 mg/m$^2$) subcut; may be repeated q 6 hr (not to exceed 0.75 mg in children ≤30 kg).

■ **IV (Adults):** *Severe anaphylaxis*—0.1–0.25 mg q 5–15 min; may be followed by 1–4 mcg/min continuous infusion. *Cardiopulmonary resuscitation (ACLS guidelines)*—1 mg q 3–5 min; *Bradycardia (ACLS guidelines)*—2–10 mcg/min).

■ **IV (Children):** *Severe anaphylaxis*—0.1 mg (less in younger children); may be followed by 0.1 mcg/kg/min continuous infusion (may be increased up to 1.5 mcg/kg/min). *Symptomatic bradycardia/pulseless arrest (PALS guidelines)*—0.01 mg/kg, may be repeated q 3–5 min higher doses (up to

0.1–0.2 mg/kg) may be considered; may also be given by the intraosseous route. May also be given by the endotracheal route in doses 2–10 times the IV dose diluted to a volume of 3–5 ml with normal saline followed by several positive pressure ventilations.

■ **Inhaln (Adults and Children ≥4 yr):** *Metered-dose inhaler*—1 inhalation (160–250 mcg), may be repeated after 1–2 min; additional doses may be repeated q 3 hr. *Inhalation solution*—1 inhalation of 1% solution; may be repeated after 1–2 min; additional doses may be given q 3 hr. *Racepinephrine*—Via hand nebulizer, 2–3 inhalations of 2.25% solution; may repeat in 5 min with 2–3 more inhalations, up to 4–6 times daily.

■ **Intracardiac (Adults):** 0.3–0.5 mg.

■ **Endotracheal: (Adults):** *Cardiopulmonary resuscitation (ACLS guidelines)*—2.0–2.5 mg.

■ **Topical (Adults and Children ≥6 yr):** *Nasal decongestant*—Apply 1% solution as drops, spray, or with a swab.

■ **Intraspinal: (Adults and Children):** 0.2–0.4 ml of 1:1000 solution.

■ **With Local Anesthetics: (Adults and Children):** Use 1:200,000 solution with local anesthetic.

## AVAILABILITY (generic available)

■*Inhalation aerosol:* 0.125% (≥300 inhalations/15 ml)$^{OTC}$, 0.5% (≥300 inhalations/15 ml)$^{OTC}$, 300 mcg/spray (≥300 inhalations/15 ml)$^{OTC}$ ■*Inhalation solution:* 1%$^{OTC}$ ■*Injection:* 10 mcg/ml$^{Rx}$, 100 mcg /ml$^{Rx}$, 500 mcg/ml$^{Rx}$, 1 mg/ml$^{Rx}$ ■ *Suspension for injection:* 5 mg/ml$^{Rx}$ ■*Autoinjector:* 0.15 mg$^{Rx}$, 0.3 mg$^{Rx}$ ■ *Topical solution:* 0.1%$^{Rx}$.

TIME/ACTION PROFILE (bronchodilation)

| | ONSET | PEAK | DURATION |
|---|---|---|---|
| Inhaln | 3–5 min | unknown | 1–3 hr |
| Subcut | 6–12 min | 20 min | <1–4 hr |
| IM | 6–12 min | unknown | <1–4 hr |
| IV | rapid | 20 min | 20–30 min |

{ } = Available in Canada only.
*CAPITALS indicates life-threatening; <u>underlines</u> indicate most frequent.

## NURSING IMPLICATIONS

### ASSESSMENT

■ **Bronchodilator:** Assess lung sounds, respiratory pattern, pulse, and blood pressure before administration and during peak of medication. Note amount, color, and character of sputum produced, and notify physician or other health care professional of abnormal findings.

❑ Monitor pulmonary function tests before initiating therapy and periodically throughout course to determine effectiveness of medication.

❑ Observe for paradoxical bronchospasm (wheezing). If condition occurs, withhold medication and notify physician or other health care professional immediately.

❑ Observe patient for drug tolerance and rebound bronchospasm. Patients requiring more than 3 inhalation treatments in 24 hr should be under close supervision. If minimal or no relief is seen after 3–5 inhalation treatments within 6–12 hr, further treatment with aerosol alone is not recommended.

❑ Assess for hypersensitivity reaction (rash; urticaria; swelling of the face, lips, or eyelids). If condition occurs, withhold medication and notify physician or other health care professional immediately.

■ **Vasopressor:** Monitor blood pressure, pulse, ECG, and respiratory rate frequently during IV administration. Continuous ECG monitoring, hemodynamic parameters, and urine output should be monitored continuously during IV administration.

❑ Monitor for chest pain, arrhythmias, heart rate >110 bpm, and hypertension. Consult physician for parameters of pulse, blood pressure, and ECG changes for adjusting dosage or discontinuing medication.

■ **Shock:** Assess volume status. Hypovolemia should be corrected prior to administering epinephrine IV.

■ **Nasal Decongestant:** Assess patient for nasal and sinus congestion prior to and periodically during therapy.

■ *Lab Test Considerations:* May cause transient decrease in serum potassium concentrations with nebulization or at higher than recommended doses.

❑ May cause an increase in blood glucose and serum lactic acid concentrations.

■ *Toxicity and Overdose:*

❑ Symptoms of overdose include persistent agitation, chest pain or discomfort, decreased blood pressure, dizziness, hyperglycemia, hypokalemia, seizures, tachyarrhythmias, persistent trembling, and vomiting.

❑ Treatment includes discontinuing adrenergic bronchodilator and other beta-adrenergic agonists and symptomatic, supportive therapy. Cardioselective beta blockers are used cautiously, because they may induce bronchospasm.

### POTENTIAL NURSING DIAGNOSES

■ Airway clearance, ineffective (Indications).
■ Tissue perfusion, ineffective (Indications).

### IMPLEMENTATION

❑ *High Alert:* Patient harm or fatalities have occurred from medication errors with epinephrine. Epinephrine is available in various concentrations, strengths, and percentages and is used for different purposes. Packaging labels may be easily confused or the products incorrectly diluted. Dilutions should be prepared by a pharmacist. IV doses should be expressed in milligrams not ampoules, concentration or volume. Prior to administration, have second practitioner independently check original order, dosage calculations, concentration, route of administration, and infusion pump settings.

■ **General Info:** Medication should be administered promptly at the onset of bronchospasm.

❑ Use a tuberculin syringe with a 26-gauge $\frac{1}{2}$-in. needle for subcut injection to ensure that correct amount of medication is administered. Suspension is for subcut use only.

❑ Tolerance may develop with prolonged or excessive use. Effectiveness may be restored by discontinuing for a few days and then readministering.

❑ Do not use solutions that are pinkish or brownish or that contain a precipitate.

❑ For anaphylactic shock, volume replacement should be administered concurrently with epinephrine. Antihistamines and corticosteroids may be used in conjunction with epinephrine.

■ **IM, Subcut:** Medication can cause irritation of tissue. Rotate injection sites to prevent tissue necrosis. Massage injection sites well after administration to enhance absorption and to decrease local vasoconstriction. Avoid IM administration in gluteal muscle. Shake suspension well before administering; inject promptly to prevent settling.

- **IV:** Dilute 1 mg (1 ml) of 1:1000 solution in at least 10 ml of 0.9% NaCl for injection to prepare a 1:10,000 solution. Discard any solution not used within 24 hr of preparation.

- **Direct IV:** Administer each 1 mg (10 ml) of 1:10,000 solution over at least 1 min; more rapid administration may be used during cardiac resuscitation. Follow each dose with 20 ml IV flush.

- **Intermittent Infusion:** In severe anaphylactic shock, 0.1–0.25-mg dose may be repeated every 5–15 min.

- **Rate:** Administer over 5–10 min.

- **Continuous Infusion:** *For cardiac arrest*—add 30 mg epinephrine (30 ml of 1:1000 solution) to 250 ml of D5W or 0.9% NaCl. *For profound bradycardia or hypotension*—add 1 mg or 1:1000 solution to 500 ml 0.9% NaCl. Administer through Y-site via infusion pump to ensure accurate dosage.

- **Rate:** *For cardiac arrest*—administer at a rate of 100 ml/hr. Titrate to response. *For profound bradycardia or hypotension*—administer at a rate of 1–5 ml/min for a 2–10 mcg/min infusion.

- **Syringe Compatibility:** ♦ doxapram ♦ heparin ♦ milrinone.

- **Y-Site Compatibility:** ♦ atracurium ♦ calcium chloride ♦ calcium gluconate ♦ cisatracurium ♦ diltiazem ♦ dobutamine ♦ dopamine ♦ famotidine ♦ fentanyl ♦ furosemide ♦ heparin ♦ hydrocortisone sodium succinate ♦ hydromorphone ♦ inamrinone ♦ labetalol ♦ levofloxacin ♦ lorazepam ♦ midazolam ♦ milrinone ♦ morphine ♦ nitroglycerin ♦ norepinephrine ♦ pancuronium ♦ phytonadione ♦ potassium chloride ♦ propofol ♦ ranitidine ♦ remifentanil ♦ vecuronium ♦ vitamin B complex with C ♦ warfarin.

- **Y-Site Incompatibility:** ♦ ampicillin ♦ thiopental.

- **Additive Compatibility:** ♦ cimetidine ♦ ranitidine.

- **Additive Incompatibility:** ♦ aminophylline ♦ sodium bicarbonate. **Inhaln:** When using epinephrine inhalation solution, 10 drops of 1% base solution should be placed in the reservoir of the nebulizer.

- ❏ The 2.25% inhalation solution of racepinephrine must be diluted for use in the combination nebulizer/respirator.

- ❏ Allow 1–2 min to elapse between inhalations of epinephrine inhalation solution, epinephrine inhalation aerosol, or epinephrine bitartrate inhalation aerosol to make certain the second inhalation is necessary.

- ❏ When epinephrine is used concurrently with corticosteroid or ipratropium inhalations, administer bronchodilator first and other medications 5 min apart to prevent toxicity from inhaled fluorocarbon propellants.

- **Endotracheal:** Epinephrine can be injected directly into the bronchial tree via the endotracheal tube if the patient has been intubated. Perform 5 rapid insufflations; forcefully administer 10 ml containing 2.0–2.5 mg epinephrine (1 mg/ml) directly into tube; follow with 5 quick insufflations.

## PATIENT/FAMILY TEACHING

- **General Info:** Instruct patient to take medication exactly as directed. If on a scheduled dosing regimen, take a missed dose as soon as possible; space remaining doses at regular intervals. Do not double doses. Caution patient not to exceed recommended dose; may cause adverse effects, paradoxical bronchospasm, or loss of effectiveness of medication.

- ❏ Instruct patient to contact health care professional immediately if shortness of breath is not relieved by medication or is accompanied by diaphoresis, dizziness, palpitations, or chest pain.

- ❏ Advise patient to consult health care professional before taking any OTC medications or alcoholic beverages concurrently with this therapy. Caution patient also to avoid smoking and other respiratory irritants.

- **Inhaln:** Review correct administration technique (aerosolization, IPPB, metered-dose inhaler) with patient. See Appendix F for administration with metered-dose inhaler. Wait 1–5 min before administering next dose. Mouthpiece should be washed after each use.

❏ Do not spray inhaler near eyes.

❏ Instruct patient to save inhaler; refill canisters may be available.

❏ Advise patients to use bronchodilator first if using other inhalation medications, and allow 5 min to elapse before administering other inhalant medications, unless otherwise directed.

❏ Advise patient to rinse mouth with water after each inhalation dose to minimize dry mouth.

❏ Advise patient to maintain adequate fluid intake (2000–3000 ml/day) to help liquefy tenacious secretions.

❏ Advise patient to consult health care professional if respiratory symptoms are not relieved or worsen after treatment or if chest pain, headache, severe dizziness, palpitations, nervousness, or weakness occurs.

❏ Instruct patient to notify health care professional if contents of one canister are used up in less than 2 wk.

■ **Autoinjector:** Instruct patients using autoinjector for anaphylactic reactions to remove gray safety cap, placing black tip on thigh at right angle to leg. Press hard into thigh until auto-injector functions, hold in place several seconds, remove, and discard properly. Massage injected area for 10 sec.

## EVALUATION

**Effectiveness of therapy can be demonstrated by:** ■ Prevention or relief of bronchospasm ❏ Increase in ease of breathing ❏ Prevention of bronchospasm or reduction of frequency of acute asthma attacks in patients with chronic asthma ❏ Prevention of exercise-induced asthma ■ Reversal of signs and symptoms of anaphylaxis ■ Increase in cardiac rate and output, when used in cardiac resuscitation ■ Increase in blood pressure, when used as a vasopressor ■ Localization of local anesthetic ■ Decrease in sinus and nasal congestion.

High Alert

# epirubicin

(ep-i-**roo**-bi-sin)

Ellence

## CLASSIFICATION(S):

**Therapeutic:** antineoplastics
**Pharmacologic:** anthracyclines

## Pregnancy Category D

## INDICATIONS

■ A component of adjuvant therapy for evidence of axillary tumor involvement following resection of primary breast cancer.

## ACTION

■ Inhibits DNA and RNA synthesis by forming a complex with DNA. **Therapeutic Effects:** ■ Death of rapidly replicating cells, particularly malignant ones.

## PHARMACOKINETICS

**Absorption:** IV administration results in complete bioavailability.

**Distribution:** Rapidly and widely distributed; concentrates in RBCs.

**Metabolism and Excretion:** Extensively and rapidly metabolized by the liver and other tissues.

**Half-life:** 35 hr.

## CONTRAINDICATIONS AND PRECAUTIONS

**Contraindicated in:** ■ Hypersensitivity to epirubicin, other anthracyclines, or related compounds ■ Baseline neutrophil count <1500 cells/mm³ ■ Severe myocardial insufficiency or recent MI ■ Previous anthracyclines up to the maximum cumulative dose ■ Severe hepatic dysfunction ■ Pregnancy or lactation ■ Concurrent cimetidine therapy.

**Use Cautiously in:** ■ Severe renal impairment (serum creatinine >5 mg/dl); lower doses should be considered ■ Hepatic impairment (dosage reduction recommended for bilirubin >1.2 mg/dl or AST >2–4 times upper limit of normal) ■ Female patients ≥70 yr (increased risk of toxicity) ■ Depressed bone marrow reserve ■ Patients with childbearing potential ■ Pediatric patients (safety not established; increased risk of acute cardiotoxicity and chronic CHF).

## ADVERSE REACTIONS AND SIDE EFFECTS*

■ **CNS:** lethargy ■ **CV:** CARDIOTOXICITY (dose-related) ■ **GI:** nausea, vomiting, anorexia, diarrhea, mucositis ■ **Derm:** alopecia, flushing, itching, photosensitivity, radiation-recall reaction, rash, skin/nail hyperpigmentation ■ **Endo:** gonadal suppression ■ **Hemat:** LEUKOPENIA, anemia, thrombocytopenia ■ **Local:** injection site reactions, phlebitis at IV site, tissue necrosis ■ **Metab:** hot flashes, hyperuricemia ■ **Misc:** ANAPHYLAXIS, INFECTION.

## INTERACTIONS

**Drug-Drug:** ■ **Cimetidine** increases blood levels and the risk of serious toxicity; concurrent use should be avoided ■ Additive hematologic and gastrointestinal toxicity with other **antineoplastics** or **radiation therapy** ■ May decrease the antibody response to **live-virus vaccines** and increase the risk of adverse reactions.

## ROUTE AND DOSAGE

■ **IV (Adults):** 100–120 mg/m² repeated in 3–4 wk cycles (total dose may be given on day 1 or split and given in equally divided doses on day 1 and day 8 of each cycle (combination regimens may employ concurrent 5-fluorouracil and cyclophosphamide).

❑ **Hepatic Impairment**

■ **IV (Adults):** *Bilirubin 1.2—3 mg/dl or AST 2–4 times upper limit of normal*—use 50% of recommended starting dose; *bilirubin >3 mg/dl or AST >4 times upper limit of normal*—use 25% of recommended starting dose.

## AVAILABILITY

■ *Solution for injection (red):* 50-mg/25-ml single-use vial^Rx, 200-mg/100-ml single-use vial^Rx.

TIME/ACTION PROFILE (effect on WBCs)

| | ONSET | PEAK | DURATION |
|---|---|---|---|
| IV | unknown | 10–14 days | 21 days |

## NURSING IMPLICATIONS

### ASSESSMENT

■ **General Info:** Monitor for bone marrow depression. Assess for bleeding (bleeding gums, bruising, petechiae, guaiac stools, urine, and emesis) and avoid IM injections and taking rectal temperatures if platelet count is low. Apply pressure to venipuncture sites for 10 min. Assess for signs of infection during neutropenia. Anemia may occur.

Monitor for increased fatigue, dyspnea, and orthostatic hypotension.

❑ Severe nausea and vomiting may occur. Parenteral antiemetic agents should be administered 30–45 min prior to therapy and routinely around the clock for the next 24 hr as indicated. Monitor amount of emesis and notify physician or other health care professional if emesis exceeds guidelines to prevent dehydration.

❑ Cardiac function, measured by ECG and a multigated radionuclide angiography (MUGA) scan or an ECHO, should be measured prior to therapy. Repeated evaluations of left ventricular ejection fraction should be performed during therapy. Monitor for development of signs of cardiac toxicity, which may occur early (ST-T wave changes, sinus tachycardia, and extrasystoles) or late (may occur months to years after termination of therapy). Delayed cardiac toxicity is characterized by cardiomyopathy, tachycardia, peripheral edema, dyspnea, rales/crackles, weight gain, hepatomegaly, ascites, pleural effusion. Toxicity is usually dependent on cumulative dose.

❑ Assess injection site frequently for redness, irritation, or inflammation. Burning or stinging during infusion may indicate infiltration and infusion should be discontinued and restarted in another vein. Epirubicin is a vesicant but may infiltrate painlessly even if blood returns on aspiration of infusion needle. Severe tissue damage may occur if epirubicin extravasates. If extravasation occurs, stop infusion immediately, restart, and complete dose in another vein.

❑ Assess oral mucosa frequently for development of stomatitis (pain, burning, erythema, ulcerations, bleeding, infection). Increased dosing interval and/or decreased dosing is recommended if lesions are painful or interfere with nutrition.

■ *Lab Test Considerations:* Monitor CBC and differential before and during each cycle of therapy. Epirubicin should not be administered to patients with a baseline neutrophil count <1500 cells/mm³. The WBC nadir occurs 10–14 days after administration, and recovery usually occurs by the 21st day. Severe thrombocytopenia and anemia may also occur.

❑ Monitor renal (BUN and creatinine) and hepatic (AST, ALT, LDH, and serum bilirubin) function prior to and periodically throughout therapy. Dose reduction is required for bilirubin >1.2 mg/dl, AST 2–4 times the upper limit of normal, or serum creatinine >5 mg/dl.

## POTENTIAL NURSING DIAGNOSES

■ Infection, risk for (Adverse Reactions).
■ Cardiac output, decreased (Adverse Reactions).

## IMPLEMENTATION

❑ *High Alert:* Fatalities have occurred with incorrect administration of chemotherapeutic agents. Before administering, clarify all ambiguous orders; double check single, daily, and course-of-therapy dose limits; have second practitioner independently double check original order, calculations and infusion pump settings. Epirubicin should be administered only under the supervision of a physician experienced in the use of cancer chemotherapeutic agents.

■ **General:** Solution should be prepared in a biologic cabinet. Wear gloves, gown, and mask while handling medication. Discard IV equipment in specially designated containers.

❑ Prophylactic anti-infective therapy with trimethoprim/sulfamethoxazole or a fluoroquinolone and antiemetic therapy should be administered prior to administration of epirubicin.

❑ Do not administer subcut or IM.

■ **Intermittent Infusion:** Administer undiluted. Use epirubicin within 24 hr of penetration of rubber stopper. Discard unused solution.

■ *Rate:* Administer each dose over 3–5 min through Y-site of a free-flowing infusion of 0.9% NaCl or D5W. Do not administer via direct IV push. Facial flushing and erythema along involved vein frequently occur when administration is too rapid. Venous sclerosis may result from injection into a small vein or repeated injections into the same vein. Avoid veins over joints or in extremities with compromised venous or lymphatic drainage.

■ **Syringe Incompatibility:** Do not mix in syringe with other drugs or with alkaline solutions ◆ fluorouracil ◆ heparin.

## PATIENT/FAMILY TEACHING

❑ Instruct patient to notify health care professional promptly if fever; sore throat; signs of infection; bleeding gums; bruising; petechiae; blood in stools, urine, or emesis; increased fatigue; dyspnea; or orthostatic hypotension occurs. Caution patient to avoid crowds and persons with known infections. Instruct patient to use soft toothbrush and electric razor and to avoid falls. Patient should be cautioned not to drink alcoholic beverages or take medication containing aspirin or NSAIDs, because these may precipitate gastric bleeding.

❑ Instruct patient to report pain at injection site immediately.

❑ Instruct patient to inspect oral mucosa for erythema and ulceration. If ulceration occurs, advise patient to use sponge brush, rinse mouth with water after eating and drinking, and confer with health care professional if mouth pain interferes with eating. Pain may require treatment with opioid analgesics. Patients usually recover by the third week of therapy.

❑ Advise patient that this medication may have teratogenic effects. Contraception should be used during and for at least 4 mo after therapy is concluded. Inform patient before initiating therapy that this medication may cause irreversible gonadal suppression.

❑ Instruct patient to avoid taking cimetidine, OTC or Rx, during therapy, and to consult health care professional prior to taking other OTC medications.

❑ Instruct patient to notify health care professional immediately if vomiting, dehydration, fever, evidence of infection, symptoms of CHF, or pain at injection site occurs. Patients should be informed of the risk of irreversible cardiac damage and treatment-related leukemia.

❑ Discuss the possibility of hair loss with patient. Explore methods of coping. Regrowth usually occurs 2–3 mo after discontinuation of therapy.

❑ Instruct patient not to receive any vaccinations without advice of health care professional.

❑ Inform patient that medication may cause urine to appear red for 1–2 days.

❑ Instruct patient to notify health care professional if skin irritation occurs at site of previous radiation therapy. May cause hyperpigmentation of the skin and nails. Advise patient to use sunscreen and protective clothing to prevent photosensitivity reactions.

❑ Emphasize the need for periodic lab tests to monitor for side effects.

## EVALUATION

**Effectiveness of therapy can be demonstrated by:** ■ Decrease in size or spread of malignancies in patients with axillary node tumor involvement following resection of primary breast cancer.

# eplerenone

(e-**ple**-re-none)

Inspra

### CLASSIFICATION(S):

**Therapeutic:** antihypertensives
**Pharmacologic:** aldosterone antagonists

### Pregnancy Category B

## INDICATIONS

■ Hypertension (alone, or with other agents).

## ACTION

■ Blocks the effects of aldosterone by attaching to mineralocorticoid receptors. **Therapeutic Effects:** ■ Lowering of blood pressure.

## PHARMACOKINETICS

**Absorption:** Well absorbed following oral administration.
**Distribution:** Unknown.
**Metabolism and Excretion:** Mostly metabolized by the liver (CYP3A4 enzyme system); <5% excreted unchanged by the kidneys.
**Half-life:** 4–6 hr.

## CONTRAINDICATIONS AND PRECAUTIONS

**Contraindicated in:** ■ Serum potassium >5.5 mEq/L ■ Type 2 diabetes with microalbuminuria (increased risk of hyperkalemia) ■ Serum creatinine >2.0 mg/dL in males or >1.8 mg/dL in females ■ CCr <50 ml/min ■ Concurrent use of

potassium-sparing diuretics ■ Concurrent use of strong inhibitors of the CYP3A4 enzyme system (ketoconazole, itraconazole) ■ Lactation.

**Use Cautiously in:** ■ Severe hepatic impairment ■ Concurrent use of ACE inhibitors or angiotensin II receptor antagonists (increased risk of hyperkalemia) ■ Pregnancy (use only if clearly needed) ■ Children (safety not established).

## ADVERSE REACTIONS AND SIDE EFFECTS*

■ **CNS:** dizziness, fatigue ■ **GI:** abnormal liver function tests, abdominal pain, diarrhea ■ **GU:** albuminuria ■ **Endo:** abnormal vaginal bleeding, gynecomastia ■ **F and E:** HYPERKALEMIA ■ **Metab:** hypercholesterolemia, hypertriglyceridemia ■ **Misc:** flu-like symptoms.

## INTERACTIONS

**Drug-Drug:** ■ Concurrent use of strong inhibitors of the CYP3A4 enzyme system (**ketoconazole, itraconazole**) significantly ↑ effects of eplerenone and should be avoided. Concurrent use of weak inhibitors of the CYP3A4 enzyme system (**erythromycin, saquinavir, fluconazole, verapamil**) may ↑ effects of eplerenone; initial dose of eplerenone should be ↓ by 50% ■ **NSAIDs** may ↓ antihypertensive effects ■ Concurrent use of **ACE inhibitors** or **Angiotensin II receptor blockers** may ↑ risk of hyperkalemia.

## ROUTE AND DOSAGE

■ **PO (Adults):** 50 mg once daily initially; may be increased to 50 mg twice daily; *patients receiving concurrent weak CYP3A4 inhibitors (erythromycin, saquinavir, verapamil, fluconazole)*—25 mg once daily initially.

## AVAILABILITY

■ *Tablets:* 25 mg[Rx], 50 mg[Rx], 100 mg[Rx].

TIME/ACTION PROFILE (antihypertensive effect)

|    | ONSET   | PEAK | DURATION |
|----|---------|------|----------|
| PO | Unknown | 4 wk | Unknown  |

# NURSING IMPLICATIONS

## ASSESSMENT

❏ Monitor blood pressure periodically during therapy.

❏ Monitor prescription refills to determine adherence.

■ *Lab Test Considerations:* May cause hyperkalemia. Monitor serum potassium levels every 2 wk for the first 1–2 mo, then monthly thereafter.

❏ May cause ↓ serum sodium and ↑ serum triglyceride, cholesterol, ALT, GGT, creatinine, and uric acid levels.

## POTENTIAL NURSING DIAGNOSES

■ Cardiac output, decreased (Indications).

■ Noncompliance (Patient/Family Teaching).

## IMPLEMENTATION

■ **PO:** Administer once daily. May be increased to twice daily if response is inadequate.

## PATIENT/FAMILY TEACHING

❏ Instruct patient to take medication as directed at the same time each day, even if feeling well.

❏ Encourage patient to comply with additional interventions for hypertension (weight reduction, discontinuation of smoking, moderation of alochol consumption, regular exercise, stress management). Medication controls, but does not cure, hypertension.

❏ Instruct patient and family on correct technique for monitoring blood pressure. Advise them to monitor blood pressure at least weekly, and notify health care professional of significant changes.

❏ Inform patient not to use potassium supplements, salt substitutes containing potassium, or other Rx or OTC medications without consulting health care professional.

❏ May cause dizziness. Caution patient to avoid driving or other activities requiring alertness until response to medication is known.

❏ Advise patient to inform health care professional of treatment regimen prior to treatment or surgery.

## EVALUATION

**Effectiveness of therapy can be demonstrated by:** ■ Decrease in blood pressure without appearance of side effects.

# epoetin
(e-**poe**-e-tin)

Epogen, EPO, {Eprex}, erythropoietin, Procrit

### CLASSIFICATION(S):
**Therapeutic:** antianemics
**Pharmacologic:** hormones

### Pregnancy Category C

## INDICATIONS

■ Treatment of anemia associated with chronic renal failure ■ Management of anemia secondary to zidovudine (AZT) therapy in HIV-infected patients ■ Management of anemia from chemotherapy in patients with nonmyeloid malignancies ■ Reduction of need for transfusions after surgery.

## ACTION

■ Stimulates erythropoiesis (production of red blood cells). **Therapeutic Effects:** ■ Maintains and may elevate RBCs, decreasing the need for transfusions.

## PHARMACOKINETICS

**Absorption:** Well absorbed after subcut administration.
**Distribution:** Unknown.
**Metabolism and Excretion:** Unknown.
**Half-life:** 4–13 hr.

## CONTRAINDICATIONS AND PRECAUTIONS

**Contraindicated in:** ■ Hypersensitivity to albumin or mammalian cell-derived products ■ Uncontrolled hypertension ■ Patients with erythropoietin levels >200 mU/ml.
**Use Cautiously in:** ■ History of seizures ■ History of porphyria ■ Pregnancy or lactation.

## ADVERSE REACTIONS AND SIDE EFFECTS*

■ **CNS:** SEIZURES, headache ■ **CV:** hypertension, thrombotic events (hemodialysis patients) ■ **Derm:** transient rashes ■ **Endo:** restored fertility, resumption of menses.

## INTERACTIONS

**Drug-Drug:** ■ May increase the requirement for **heparin** anticoagulation during hemodialysis.

## ROUTE AND DOSAGE

❏ **Anemia of Chronic Renal Failure**

■ **Subcut, IV (Adults):** 50–100 units/kg 3 times weekly initially, then adjust dosage based on hematocrit.

■ **Subcut, IV (Children):** 50 units/kg 3 times weekly initially, then adjust dosage based on hematocrit.

❏ **Anemia Secondary to AZT Therapy**

■ **Subcut, IV (Adults):** 100 units/kg 3 times weekly for 8 wk; if inadequate response, may increase by 50–100 units/kg every 4–8 wk, up to 300 units/kg 3 times weekly.

❏ **Anemia from Chemotherapy**

■ **Subcut (Adults):** 150 units/kg 3 times weekly; may increase after 8 wk up to 300 units/kg 3 times weekly.

❏ **Surgery**

■ **Subcut (Adults):** 300 units/kg/day for 10 days before surgery, day of surgery, and 4 days after *or* 600 units/kg 21, 14, and 7 days before surgery and on day of surgery.

## AVAILABILITY

■ *Injection:* 2000 units/ml$^{Rx}$, 3000 units/ml$^{Rx}$, 4000 units/ml$^{Rx}$, 10,000 units/ml$^{Rx}$, 20,000 units/ml$^{Rx}$.

TIME/ACTION PROFILE (increase in RBCs)

| | ONSET† | PEAK | DURATION |
|---|---|---|---|
| IV, subcut | 7–10 days | within 2 mos | 2 wk‡ |

†Increase in reticulocytes.
‡After discontinuation.

## NURSING IMPLICATIONS

### ASSESSMENT

❏ Monitor blood pressure before and throughout therapy. Inform physician or other health care professional if severe hypertension is present or if blood pressure begins to increase. Additional antihypertensive therapy may be required during initiation of therapy.

❏ Monitor response for symptoms of anemia (fatigue, dyspnea, pallor).

❏ Monitor dialysis shunts (thrill and bruit) and status of artificial kidney during hemodialysis. Heparin dose may need to be increased to prevent clotting. Patients with underlying vascular disease should be monitored for impaired circulation.

■ **Lab Test Considerations:** May cause increase in WBCs and platelets. May decrease bleeding times.

❏ Serum ferritin, transferrin, and iron levels should also be monitored to assess need for concurrent iron therapy. Transferrin saturation should be at least 20% and ferritin should be at least 100 ng/ml.

■ **Anemia of Chronic Renal Failure:** Hematocrit should be monitored before and twice weekly during initial therapy, for 2–6 wk after a change in dose, and regularly after target range (30–36%) has been reached and maintenance dose is determined. Other hematopoietic parameters (CBC with differential and platelet count) should also be monitored before and periodically throughout therapy. If hematocrit increases more than 4 points in a 2-wk period, the likelihood of hypertensive reaction and seizures increases. Dose should be decreased and hematocrit monitored twice weekly for 2–6 wk. Dosage adjustment may be needed. If hematocrit is increasing and approaching 36%, dose is reduced to maintain suggested target hematocrit range. If increase in hematocrit continues and exceeds 36%, dose should be withheld until hematocrit begins to decrease; epoetin is then reinitiated at a lower dose. If hematocrit increase of 5–6 points is not achieved after an 8-wk period and iron stores are adequate, dose may be incrementally increased at 4–6-wk intervals until desired response is attained.

❏ Monitor renal function studies and electrolytes closely; resulting increased sense of well-being may lead to decreased compliance with other therapies for renal failure. Increases in BUN, creatinine, uric acid, phosphorus, and potassium may occur.

■ **Anemia Secondary to Zidovudine Therapy:** Before initiating therapy, determine serum erythropoietin level before transfusion. Patients receiving zidovudine with endogenous serum erythropoietin levels >500 mU/ml may not respond to therapy. Monitor hematocrit weekly during dosage adjustment. If response does not reduce transfusion requirements or increase hematocrit effectively after 8 wk of therapy, dose may be increased by 50–100 units/kg 3 times weekly. Evaluate response and adjust dose by 50–100 units/ kg every 4–8 wk thereafter. If a satisfactory response is not obtained with a dose of 300 units/kg 3 times weekly, it is unlikely that a higher dose will produce a response. Once the desired response is attained, maintenance dose is titrated based on variations of zidovudine dose and intercurrent infections. If hematocrit exceeds 40%, discontinue dose until hematocrit drops to 36%, then decrease dose by 25%.

■ **Anemia from Chemotherapy:** Monitor hematocrit weekly until stable. Patients with lower baseline serum erythropoietin levels may respond more rapidly; not recommended if levels >200 mU/ml. If response is not adequate after 8 wk of therapy, dose may be increased up to 300 units/kg 3 times weekly. If no response is obtained to this dose, it is unlikely that higher doses will produce a response. If hematocrit exceeds 40%, hold dose until it falls to 36%, then decrease dose by 25%. If initial dose response is >4 percentage points in any 2-wk period, reduce dose.

■ **Surgery:** Determine that hematocrit is >10 to ≤13 g/dl before therapy.

## POTENTIAL NURSING DIAGNOSES

■ Activity intolerance (Indications).
■ Noncompliance (Patient/Family Teaching).

## IMPLEMENTATION

■ **General:** Transfusions are still required for severe symptomatic anemia. Supplemental iron should be initiated with epoetin and continued throughout therapy.

❑ Institute seizure precautions in patients who experience greater than a 4-point increase in hematocrit in a 2-wk period or exhibit any change in neurologic status. Risk of seizures is greatest during the first 90 days of therapy.

❑ Do not shake vial; inactivation of medication may occur. Discard vial immediately after withdrawing dose from single-use 1-ml vial. Refrigerate multidose 2-ml vial; stable for 21 days after initial entry.

■ **Subcut:** This route is often used for patients not requiring dialysis.

❑ May be admixed in syringe immediately before administration with 0.9% NaCl with ben-

zyl alcohol 0.9% in a 1:1 ratio to prevent injection site discomfort.

■ **Direct IV:** Administer undiluted.

■ *Rate:* May be administered as direct injection or bolus into IV tubing or via venous line at end of dialysis session.

## PATIENT/FAMILY TEACHING

■ **General Info:** Explain rationale for concurrent iron therapy (increased red blood cell production requires iron).

❑ Discuss possible return of menses and fertility in women of childbearing age. Patient should discuss contraceptive options with health care professional.

❑ Discuss ways of preventing self-injury in patients at risk for seizures. Driving and activities requiring continuous alertness should be avoided.

■ **Anemia of Chronic Renal Failure:** Stress importance of compliance with dietary restrictions, medications, and dialysis. Foods high in iron and low in potassium include liver, pork, veal, beef, mustard and turnip greens, peas, eggs, broccoli, kale, blackberries, strawberries, apple juice, watermelon, oatmeal, and enriched bread. Epoetin will result in increased sense of well-being, but it does not cure underlying disease.

■ **Home Care Issues:** Home dialysis patients determined to be able to safely and effectively administer epoetin should be taught proper dosage, administration technique, and disposal of equipment. *Information for Home Dialysis Patients* should be provided to patient along with medication.

## EVALUATION

**Clinical response to therapy can be evaluated by:** ■ Increase in hematocrit to 30–36% with improvement in symptoms of anemia in patients with chronic renal failure ■ Increase in hematocrit in anemia secondary to zidovudine therapy ■ Increase in hematocrit in patients with anemia resulting from chemotherapy ■ Reduction of need for transfusions after surgery.

**eprosartan, See ANGIOTENSIN II RECEPTOR ANTAGONISTS.**

| High Alert |
| --- |

# eptifibatide
(ep-ti-**fib**-a-tide)
Integrilin

## CLASSIFICATION(S):
***Therapeutic:*** *antiplatelet agents*
***Pharmacologic:*** *glycoprotein IIb/IIIa inhibitors*

**Pregnancy Category B**

## INDICATIONS

■ Treatment of acute coronary syndrome (unstable angina/non–Q-wave MI), including patients who will be managed medically and those who will undergo percutaneous coronary intervention (PCI) that may consist of percutaneous transluminal angioplasty (PCTA) or atherectomy ■ Treatment of patients undergoing PCI ■ Usually used concurrently with aspirin and heparin.

## ACTION

■ Decreases platelet aggregation by reversibly antagonizing the binding of fibrinogen to the glycoprotein IIb/IIIa binding site on platelet surfaces. **Therapeutic Effects:** ■ Inhibition of platelet aggregation resulting in decreased incidence of new MI, death, or refractory ischemia, reducing the need for repeat urgent cardiac intervention.

## PHARMACOKINETICS

**Absorption:** IV administration results in complete bioavailability.
**Distribution:** Unknown.
**Metabolism and Excretion:** 50% excreted by the kidneys.
**Half-life:** 2.5 hr.

## CONTRAINDICATIONS AND PRECAUTIONS

**Contraindicated in:** ■ Hypersensitivity ■ Active internal bleeding or history of bleeding within previous 30 days ■ Severe uncontrolled hypertension (systolic BP >200 mmHg and/or diastolic BP >110 mmHg) ■ Major surgical procedure within 6 wk ■ History of hemorrhagic stroke or other stroke within 30 days ■ Concurrent use of other glycoprotein IIb/IIIa receptor antagonists ■ Platelet count <100,000/mm³ ■ Severe renal insufficiency (serum creatinine ≥4 mg/dl) or dependency on renal dialysis.

**Use Cautiously in:** ■ Geriatric patients (increased risk of bleeding) ■ Renal insufficiency (decrease initial dose and infusion rate if infusion serum creatinine ≥2 mg/dl but <4 mg/dl) ■ Pregnancy, lactation, or children (safety not established; use in pregnancy only if clearly needed).

## ADVERSE REACTIONS AND SIDE EFFECTS*

Noted for patients receiving heparin and aspirin in addition to eptifibatide. ■ **CV:** hypotension ■ **Hemat:** BLEEDING (including GI and intracranial bleeding, hematuria, and hematomas).

## INTERACTIONS

**Drug-Drug:** ■ Increased risk of bleeding with other drugs that affect hemostasis (**heparins, warfarin, NSAIDs, thrombolytic agents, abciximab, dipyridamole, ticlopidine, clopidogrel,** some **cephalosporins, plicamycin, valproates**).
**Drug-Natural Products:** ■ Increased bleeding risk with **arnica, chamomile, clove, dong quai, feverfew, garlic, ginger, ginkgo,** and **Panax ginseng.**

## ROUTE AND DOSAGE

❑ **Acute Coronary Syndrome**

■ **IV (Adults ≤121 kg):** 180 mcg/kg as a loading dose, followed by 2 mcg/kg/min (maximum 15 mg/hr) until hospital discharge or surgical intervention (up to 72 hr). Infusion rate may be decreased to 0.5 mcg/kg/min during PCI and continued for 20–24 hr following.

■ **IV (Adults >121 kg):** maximum of 22.6 mg as a bolus, followed by 15 mg/hr as a maximum infusion rate.

❑ **Percutaneous Coronary Intervention without Acute Coronary Syndrome**

■ **IV (Adults):** 135 mcg/kg as a loading dose, immediately before PCI, followed by 0.5 mcg/kg/min as a continuous infusion for 20–

24 hr. Infusion should be discontinued prior to coronary artery bypass graft surgery.

◻ **Renal Impairment**
■ **IV (Adults):** *SrCr >2 mg/dl and <4 mg/dl*—use 135 mcg/kg loading dose and 0.5 mcg/kg/min infusion.

## AVAILABILITY
■ *Solution for injection:* 20 mg/10 ml in 10-ml vials^Rx, 75 mg/100 ml in 100-ml vials^Rx.

TIME/ACTION PROFILE (effects on platelet function)

|     | ONSET | PEAK | DURATION |
|-----|-------|------|----------|
| IV  | immediate | following bolus | brief† |

†Inhibition is reversible following cessation of infusion.

## NURSING IMPLICATIONS

### ASSESSMENT
◻ Assess patient for bleeding. Most common sites are arterial access site for cardiac catheterization or GI or GU tract. Arterial and venous punctures, IM injections, and use of urinary catheters, nasotracheal intubation, and NG tubes should be minimized. Noncompressible sites for IV access should be avoided. If bleeding cannot be controlled with pressure, discontinue eptifibatide and heparin immediately.
■ *Lab Test Considerations:* Prior to eptifibatide therapy, assess hemoglobin or hematocrit, platelet count, serum creatinine, and PT/aPTT. Activated clotting time (ACT) should also be measured in patients undergoing PCI.
◻ Maintain the aPTT between 50 and 70 sec unless PCI is to be performed. Maintain ACT between 300 and 350 sec during PCI.
◻ Arterial sheath should not be removed unless aPTT <45 sec.
◻ If platelet count decreases to <100,000 and is confirmed, eptifibatide and heparin should be discontinued and condition monitored and treated.

### POTENTIAL NURSING DIAGNOSES
■ Tissue perfusion, ineffective (Indications).

### IMPLEMENTATION
◻ *High Alert:* Accidental overdosage of anti-platelet medications has resulted in patient harmor death from internal hemorrhage or intracranial bleeding. Have second practitioner independently check original order, dosage calculations, and infusion pump settings.
■ **General:** Most patients receive heparin and aspirin concurrently with eptifibatide.
◻ After PCI, femoral artery sheath may be removed during eptifibatide treatment only after heparin has been discontinued and its effects mostly reversed.
◻ Do not administer solutions that are discolored or contain particulate matter. Discard unused portion.
■ **Direct IV,** *High Alert:* Withdraw appropriate loading dose from bolus vial (20 mg/10ml vial) into a syringe. Administer undiluted.
■ *Rate:* Administer via IV push over 1–2 min.
■ **Intermittent Infusion:** Administer undiluted directly from the 100-ml vial via an infusion pump. Spike the 100-ml vial in the center of the stopper top with a vented infusion set.
■ *Rate:* Rate is based on patient weight. See Route and Dosage section.
■ **Y-Site Compatibility:** ◆ 0.9% NaCl ◆ D5/0.9% NaCl ◆ up to 60 meq KCl ◆ alteplase ◆ atropine ◆ dobutamine ◆ heparin ◆ lidocaine ◆ meperidine ◆ metoprolol ◆ midazolam ◆ morphine ◆ nitroglycerin ◆ verapamil.
■ **Y-Site Incompatibility:** ◆ furosemide.

### PATIENT/FAMILY TEACHING
◻ Inform patient of the purpose of eptifibatide.
◻ Instruct patient to notify health care professional immediately if any bleeding is noted.

### EVALUATION
**Effectiveness of therapy can be demonstrated by:** ■Inhibition of platelet aggregation, resulting in decreased incidence of new MI, death, or refractory ischemia with the need for repeat urgent cardiac intervention.

---

**ergocalciferol, See VITAMIN D COMPOUNDS.**

---

**ergonovine**
(er-goe-**noe**-veen)

ergometrine, Ergotrate

*CLASSIFICATION(S):*
*Therapeutic: none assigned*
*Pharmacologic: oxytocics*
**Pregnancy Category UK**

## INDICATIONS

■ Prevention and treatment of postpartum or postabortion hemorrhage caused by uterine atony or involution. **Unlabeled uses:** ■ As a diagnostic agent to provoke coronary artery spasm.

## ACTION

■ Directly stimulates uterine and vascular smooth muscle. **Therapeutic Effects:** ■ Uterine contraction.

## PHARMACOKINETICS

**Absorption:** Well absorbed after oral or IM administration.
**Distribution:** Unknown.
**Metabolism and Excretion:** Unknown. Probably metabolized by the liver.
**Half-life:** Unknown.

## CONTRAINDICATIONS AND PRECAUTIONS

**Contraindicated in:** ■ Hypersensitivity ■ Avoid chronic use ■ Should not be used to induce labor.
**Use Cautiously in:** ■ Hypertensive or eclamptic patients (increased susceptibility to hypertensive and arrhythmogenic side effects) ■ Severe hepatic or renal disease ■ Sepsis ■ Third stage of labor.

## ADVERSE REACTIONS AND SIDE EFFECTS*

■ **CNS:** dizziness, headache ■ **EENT:** tinnitus ■ **Resp:** dyspnea ■ **CV:** arrhythmias, chest pain, hypertension, palpitations ■ **GI:** nausea, vomiting ■ **Derm:** sweating ■ **Misc:** allergic reactions.

## INTERACTIONS

**Drug-Drug:** ■ Excessive vasoconstriction may result when used with other **vasopressors,** such as **dopamine** or **nicotine** ■ May increase

the risk of adverse reactions with **bromocriptine.**

## ROUTE AND DOSAGE

❑ **Oxytocic**
■ **PO, SL (Adults):** 0.2–0.4 mg q 6–12 hr (usual course is 48 hr).
■ **IM, IV (Adults):** 200 mcg (0.2 mg) q 2–4 hr for up to 5 doses.

❑ **Provocative Agent for Coronary Artery Spasm**
■ **IV (Adults):** 50 mcg (0.05 mg) q 5 min until chest pain occurs or a total dose of 400 mcg (0.4 mg) has been given (unlabeled).

## AVAILABILITY

■*Tablets:* 0.2 mg^Rx ■*Injection:* 0.2 mg/ml^Rx, {0.25 mg/ml^Rx}.

TIME/ACTION PROFILE (uterine contractions)

| | ONSET | PEAK | DURATION |
|---|---|---|---|
| PO | 5–15 min | unknown | ≥3 hr |
| IM | 2–5 min | unknown | ≥3 hr |
| IV | immediate | unknown | 45 min |

# NURSING IMPLICATIONS

## ASSESSMENT

❑ Monitor blood pressure, pulse, and respirations every 15–30 min until transfer to the postpartum unit, then every 1–2 hr. Report hypertension, chest pain, arrhythmias, headache, or change in neurologic status.
❑ Monitor amount and type of vaginal discharge. Report symptoms of hemorrhage (increased bleeding, hypotension, pallor, tachycardia) immediately.
❑ Palpate uterine fundus; note position and consistency. Notify physician or other health care professional if fundus fails to contract in response to ergonovine. Assess patient for severe cramping; dose may be decreased.
❑ Assess for signs of ergotism (cold, numb fingers and toes; nausea; vomiting; diarrhea; headache; muscle pain; weakness).
❑ If patient fails to respond to ergonovine, check serum calcium level. Correction of hypocalcemia may restore responsiveness.

- **Lab Test Considerations:** May cause decreased serum prolactin level, which inhibits synthesis of breast milk.
- **Toxicity and Overdose:** Toxicity, initially manifested as ergotism, may cause seizures and gangrene. Seizures are treated with anticonvulsants. Vasodilators and heparin may be ordered to improve circulation to extremities.

## POTENTIAL NURSING DIAGNOSES

- Tissue perfusion, ineffective (Indications).
- Injury, risk for (Side Effects).

## IMPLEMENTATION

- **General:** Do not administer solution that is discolored or contains a precipitate.
- **PO:** Administration is usually limited to 48 hr postpartum, by which time the danger of hemorrhage from uterine atony has passed.
- ❑ Tablets may be administered SL.
- **IM:** The preferred route is IM. Firm uterine contractions are produced within a few minutes. Dose may need to be repeated every 2–4 hr for full therapeutic effect.
- **Direct IV:** The IV route is reserved for severe uterine bleeding. Dilute with 5 ml of 0.9% NaCl.
- **Rate:** Administer slow IV push over at least 1 min through Y-site injection of an IV of D5W or 0.9% NaCl.

## PATIENT/FAMILY TEACHING

- ❑ Review symptoms of toxicity with patient. Instruct the patient to report occurrence of these immediately.
- ❑ Inform patient that uterine cramping demonstrates effectiveness of therapy.
- ❑ Explain need for pad count to determine degree of bleeding. Instruct patient to report immediately an increase in degree of bleeding or passage of clots.
- ❑ Instruct patient to report breastfeeding difficulties.
- ❑ Caution patient not to smoke while receiving ergonovine; nicotine is also a vasoconstrictor.

## EVALUATION

**Effectiveness of therapy can be demonstrated by:** ■ Uterine contraction and cramping in the prevention or cessation of uterine hemorrhage after delivery or abortion ■ Vaso-constriction of the coronary arteries when used as a diagnostic agent.

# ergotamine

(er-**got**-a-meen)

{Ergomar}, Ergostat, {Gynergen}

## dihydroergotamine

(dye-hye-droe-er-**got**-a-meen)

D.H.E. 45, {Dihydroergotamine-Sandoz}, Migranal

## CLASSIFICATION(S):

**Therapeutic:** vascular headache suppressants

**Pharmacologic:** alpha-adrenergic blockers

### Pregnancy Category X

## INDICATIONS

- Vascular headaches including: ❑ Migraine ❑ Cluster headaches.

## ACTION

- In therapeutic doses, produces vasoconstriction of dilated blood vessels by stimulating alpha-adrenergic and serotonergic (5-HT) receptors ■ Larger doses may produce alpha-adrenergic blockade and vasodilation. **Therapeutic Effects:** ■ Constriction of dilated carotid artery bed with resolution of vascular headache.

## PHARMACOKINETICS

**Absorption:** *Ergotamine*—Unpredictably absorbed (60%) from the GI tract (may be enhanced by caffeine). Sublingual absorption is very poor. *Dihydroergotamine*—rapidly absorbed after IM and subcut administration, 32% absorbed from nasal mucosa.

**Distribution:** Ergotamine crosses the blood-brain barrier and enters breast milk.

**Protein Binding:** *Dihydroergotamine*—90%; *ergotamine*—93–98%.

**Metabolism and Excretion:** Both ergotamine and dihydroergotamine are 90% metabolized by the liver (CYP 3A4 enzyme system). Some metabolites are active.

**Half-life:** *Ergotamine* (2 phases)—2.7 hr first phase; 21 hr second phase. *Dihydroergotamine* (2 phases)—2.3 min–1.45 hr first phase; 10–32 hr second phase.

## CONTRAINDICATIONS AND PRECAUTIONS

**Contraindicated in:** ■ Serious infections ■ Peripheral vascular disease ■ Cardiovascular disease ■ Uncontrolled hypertension ■ Severe renal or liver disease ■ Malnutrition ■ Known alcohol intolerance (dihydroergotamine injection only) ■ Pregnancy ■ Lactation ■ Concurrent use of protease inhibitors and macrolide anti-infectives.

**Use Cautiously in:** ■ Illnesses associated with peripheral vascular pathology such as diabetes mellitus ■ Children <6 yr (safety not established).

## ADVERSE REACTIONS AND SIDE EFFECTS*

■ **CNS:** dizziness ■ **EENT:** rhinitis (nasal) ■ **CV:** MI, angina pectoris, arterial spasm, intermittent claudication, sinus bradycardia, sinus tachycardia ■ **GI:** abdominal pain, nausea, vomiting, altered taste (nasal), diarrhea, polydipsia ■ **MS:** extremity stiffness, muscle pain, stiff neck, stiff shoulders ■ **Neuro:** leg weakness, numbness or tingling in fingers or toes ■ **Misc:** fatigue.

## INTERACTIONS

**Drug-Drug:** ■ Concurrent use of potent inhibitors of the CYP 3A4 enzyme system, including protease inhibitors (**ritonavir, nelfinavir,** and **indinavir**) some macrolide anti-infectives (**erythromycin, clarithromycin**) and some azole antifungals **ketoconazole, itraconazole**) may result in vasospasm, cerebral or peripheral ischemia and is contraindicated ■ Concurrent use with **beta blockers, hormonal contraceptives, vasoconstrictors,** or **nicotine** (heavy smoking) may ↑ risk of peripheral vasoconstriction ■ Dihydroergotamine antagonizes the antianginal effects of **nitrates** ■ Concurrent use with **vasoconstrictors** may have ↑ effects (avoid concurrent use) ■ Concurrent use with **almotriptan, frovatriptan, naratriptan, rizatriptan, sumatriptan,** and **zolmitriptan** may result in prolonged vasoconstriction (allow 24 hr between use).

## ROUTE AND DOSAGE

❑ **Ergotamine**

■ **PO, SL (Adults):** 1–2 mg initially, then 1–2 mg q 30 min until attack subsides or a total

of 6 mg has been given. Should not be used more than twice weekly, with at least 5 days between courses; 1–2 mg PO at bedtime daily for 10–14 days have been used to terminate series of cluster headaches.

❑ **Dihydroergotamine**

■ **IM, Subcut (Adults):** 1 mg; may repeat in 1 hr to a total of 3 mg (not to exceed 3 mg/day or 6 mg/wk).
■ **IM, Subcut (Children ≥6 yr):** 0.5 mg; may be repeated in 1 hr.
■ **IV (Adults):** 0.5 mg; may repeat in 1 hr (not to exceed 2 mg/day or 6 mg/wk). For chronic intractable headache, 0.5–1 mg q 8 hr may be given until relief is obtained (not to exceed 6 mg/wk).
■ **IV (Children ≥6 yr):** 0.25 mg; may be repeated in 1 hr.
■ **IV (Children and Adolescents 12–16 yr):** *Severe, acute migraine*—0.25–0.5 mg; 1–2 more doses may be given q 20 min.
■ **IV (Children 9–12 yr):** *Severe, acute migraine*—0.2 mg; 1–2 more doses may be given q 20 min.
■ **IV (Children 6–9 yr):** *Severe, acute migraine*—0.1–0.15 mg; 1–2 more doses may be given q 20 min.
■ **Intranasal (Adults):** 1 spray (0.5 mg) in each nostril, repeat after 15 min (2 mg total dose); not to exceed 3 mg/24 hr or 4 mg/wk.

## AVAILABILITY

❑ **Ergotamine**

■ *Sublingual tablets:* 2 mg^Rx ■ *Tablets:* 1 mg^Rx.

❑ **Dihydroergotamine**

■ *Injection:* 1 mg/ml (contains alcohol)^Rx ■ *Nasal spray:* 4 mg/1 ml in 1-ml ampules with nasal spray applicator^Rx ■ Cost: $81.67/4 ml ■ *Ergotamine*—caffeine, barbiturates, and belladonna alkaloids in preparations for vascular headaches^Rx. See Appendix B.

TIME/ACTION PROFILE (relief of headache)

| | ONSET | PEAK | DURA-TION |
|---|---|---|---|
| PO | 1–2 hr (variable) | 1–5 hr | unknown |
| Nasal | within 30 min | unknown | unknown |

{ } = Available in Canada only.
*CAPITALS indicates life-threatening; underlines indicate most frequent.

| | | | |
|---|---|---|---|
| SL | unknown | unknown | unknown |
| IM, sub-cut | 15–30 min | 15 min–2 hr | 8 hr |
| IV | <5 min | 15 min–2 hr | 8 hr |

# NURSING IMPLICATIONS

## ASSESSMENT

- ❑ Assess frequency, location, duration, and characteristics (pain, nausea, vomiting, visual disturbances) of chronic headaches. During acute attack, assess type, location, and intensity of pain before and 60 min after administration.
- ❑ Monitor blood pressure and peripheral pulses periodically during therapy. Report significant hypertension.
- ❑ Assess for signs of ergotism (cold, numb fingers and toes; nausea; vomiting; headache; muscle pain; weakness).
- ❑ Assess for nausea and vomiting. Ergotamine stimulates the chemoreceptor trigger zone. For adults, metoclopramide 10 mg IV may be administered 3–5 min before administration of dihydroergotamine IV. In children, metoclopramide or a phenothiazine antiemetic may be given orally as prophylaxis 1 hr before administration of dihydroergotamine IV. Oral administration may decrease risk of extrapyramidal and other side effects encountered with IV administration.
- ■ *Toxicity and Overdose:* Toxicity is manifested by severe ergotism (chest pain, abdominal pain, persistent paresthesia in the extremities) and gangrene. Vasodilators, dextran, or heparin may be ordered to improve circulation.

## POTENTIAL NURSING DIAGNOSES

- ■ Pain, acute (Indications).
- ■ Injury, risk for (Side Effects).

## IMPLEMENTATION

- ■ **General:** Administer as soon as patient reports prodromal symptoms or headache. **SL:** Allow tablet to dissolve under tongue. Do not allow patient to eat, drink, or smoke while tablet is dissolving.
- ■ **Direct IV:** Dihydroergotamine may be administered undiluted.
- ■ *Rate:* Administer over 1 min.

## PATIENT/FAMILY TEACHING

- ■ **General Info:** Instruct patient to take ergotamine at the first sign of an impending head-

ache and not to exceed the maximum dose prescribed.
- ❑ Encourage patient to rest in a quiet, dark room after taking ergotamine.
- ❑ Review symptoms of toxicity. Instruct patient to report these promptly.
- ❑ Caution patient not to smoke and to avoid exposure to cold; these vasoconstrictors may further impair peripheral circulation.
- ❑ May cause dizziness. Caution patient to avoid driving and other activities requiring alertness until response to the drug is known.
- ❑ Advise patient to avoid alcohol, which may precipitate vascular headaches.
- ❑ Instruct female patients to inform health care professional if they plan or suspect pregnancy. Ergotamine should not be taken during pregnancy.
- ■ **Subcut, IM:** Inject at the first sign of a headache and repeat at 1-hr intervals up to 3 doses. Once minimal effective dose is determined, adjust dose for subsequent attacks.
- ■ **Intranasal:** Instruct patient in proper use of nasal spray. Prime nasal sprayer 4 times before dose. Administer 1 spray to each nostril followed in 15 min by an additional spray in each nostril for a total of 4 sprays. Do not tilt head or sniff after spray. Do not use more than amount instructed. Discard ampule within 8 hr of opening. Do not refrigerate. Assembly may be used for 4 treatments; then discard.
- ❑ Advise patient not to use these medications to prevent a headache if there are no symptoms or if headache is different from typical migraine.
- ❑ Instruct patient to notify health care professional if numbness or tingling in fingers or toes; pain, tightness, or discomfort in chest; muscle pain or cramps in arms or legs; weakness in legs; temporary speeding or slowing of heart rate; or swelling or itching occurs.

## EVALUATION

**Effectiveness of therapy can be demonstrated by:** ■ Relief of pain from vascular headaches.

# ertapenem
(er-ta-**pen**-em)
Invanz

## CLASSIFICATION(S):
**Therapeutic:** *anti-infectives*
**Pharmacologic:** *carbapenems*

### Pregnancy Category B

## INDICATIONS

■ Moderate to severe: ❑ complicated intra-abdominal infections ❑ complicated skin and skin structure infections ❑ community acquired pneumonia ❑ complicated urinary tract infections (including pyelonephritis) ❑ acute pelvic infections including postpartum endomyometritis, septic abortion, and post surgical gynecologic infections.

## ACTION

■ **Therapeutic Effects:** ■ Bactericidal action against susceptible bacteria. **Spectrum:** ■ Active against the following aerobic gram-positive organisms *Staphylococcus aureus* (methicillin-susceptible strains only), *Streptococcus agalactiae, S. pneumoniae* (penicillin-susceptible strains only), and *S. pyogenes* ■ Also active against the following gram-negative aerobic organisms *Escherichia coli, Haemophilus influenzae* (beta-lactamase negative strains), *Klebsiella pneumonia,* and *Moraxella catarrhalis.* ■ Addition anaerobic spectrum includes *Bacteroides fragilis, B. distasonis, B. ovatus, B. thetaiotamicron, B. uniformis, Clostridium clostrioforme, Eubacterium lentum, Peptostreptococcus, Porphyromonas asaccharolytica,* and *Prevotella bivia.*

## PHARMACOKINETICS

**Absorption:** 90% after IM administration; IV administration results in complete bioavailability.

**Distribution:** Enters breast milk.

**Metabolism and Excretion:** Mostly excreted by the kidneys.

**Half-life:** 1.8 hr (increased in renal impairment).

## CONTRAINDICATIONS AND PRECAUTIONS

**Contraindicated in:** ■ Hypersensitivity ■ Cross-sensitivity may occur with penicillins, cephalosporins and other carbapenems ■ Hypersensitivity to lidocaine (may be used as a diluent for IM administration).

**Use Cautiously in:** ■ History of multiple hypersensitivity reactions ■ Seizure disorders ■ Geriatric patients ( ↑ sensitivity and age-related ↓ in renal function) ■ Renal impairment ■ Pregnancy, lactation or children <18 yr (safety not established, use during lactation only when benefits outweigh risks, use in pregnancy only if clearly needed).

## ADVERSE REACTIONS AND SIDE EFFECTS*

■ **CNS:** SEIZURES, headache ■ **GI:** PSEUDOMEMBRANOUS COLITIS, diarrhea, nausea, vomiting ■ **GU:** vaginitis ■ **Local:** phlebitis at IV site, pain at IM site ■ **Misc:** hypersensitivity reaction including ANAPHYLAXIS.

## INTERACTIONS

**Drug-Drug:** ■ **Probenecid** decreases excretion and increases blood levels.

## ROUTE AND DOSAGE

■ **IV, IM (Adults):** 1 g once daily.
❑ **Renal Impairment**
■ **IM, IV (Adults):** *CCr ≤30 ml/min/1.73m²*—500 mg once daily.

## AVAILABILITY

■ *powder for IV infusion (requires reconstitution):* 1 g/vial<sup>Rx</sup>.

TIME/ACTION PROFILE (blood levels)

| | ONSET | PEAK | DURATION |
|---|---|---|---|
| IM | rapid | 2 hr | 24 hr |
| IV | rapid | end of infusion | 24 hr |

# NURSING IMPLICATIONS

## ASSESSMENT

❑ Assess patient for infection (vital signs; appearance of wound, sputum, urine, and stool; WBC) at beginning of and during therapy.

❑ Obtain a history before initiating therapy to determine previous use of and reactions to penicillins, cephalosporins or carbapenems.

Persons with a negative history of penicillin sensitivity may still have an allergic response.
◻ Obtain specimens for culture and sensitivity before initiating therapy. First dose may be given before receiving results.
◻ Observe patient for signs and symptoms of anaphylaxis (rash, pruritus, laryngeal edema, wheezing). Discontinue the drug and notify the physician immediately if these occur. Have epinephrine, an antihistamine, and resuscitative equipment close by in the event of an anaphylactic reaction.
■ *Lab Test Considerations:* May cause ↑ AST, ALT, serum alkaline phosphatase levels.
◻ May cause ↑ platelet and eosinophil counts.

## POTENTIAL NURSING DIAGNOSES

■ Infection, risk for (Indications, Side Effects).

## IMPLEMENTATION

■ **IM:** Reconstitute 1-g vial with 3.2 ml of 1% lidocaine without epinephrine. Shake well to form solution. Immediately withdraw contents and inject deep into large muscle mass. Use reconstituted solution within 1 hr.
■ **Intermittent Infusion:** Reconstitute 1-g vial with 10 ml of sterile or bacteriostatic water for injection or 0.9% NaCl and shake well. Transfer the resulting solution to 50 ml of 0.9% NaCl. Administer within 6 hr of reconstitution.
■ *Rate:* Administer over 30 min. Do not administer direct IV.
■ **Y-Site Incompatibility:** Do not infuse with other medications.

## PATIENT/FAMILY TEACHING

◻ Advise patient to report the signs of superinfection (black, furry overgrowth on the tongue; vaginal itching or discharge; loose or foul-smelling stools) and allergy. Consult health care professional before treating with antidiarrheals.
◻ Caution patient to notify health care professional if fever and diarrhea occur, especially if stool contains blood, pus, or mucus. Advise patient not to treat diarrhea without consulting health care professional. May occur up to several weeks after discontinuation of medication.

## EVALUATION

**Clinical response to therapy can be evaluated by:** ■ Resolution of the signs and symptoms of infection. Length of time for complete resolution depends on the organism and site of infection.

# ERYTHROMYCIN†
## (eh-rith-roe-**mye**-sin)

**erythromycin base**
{Apo-Erythro-EC}, E-Base, E-Mycin, {Erybid}, Eryc, Ery-Tab, {Erythromid}, {Novo-rythro}, PCE

**erythromycin estolate**
Ilosone, {Novo-rythro}

**erythromycin ethylsuccinate**
{Apo-Erythro-ES}, E.E.S., EryPed

**erythromycin gluceptate**

**erythromycin lactobionate**
Erythrocin

**erythromycin stearate**
Erythrocin, {Novo-rythro}

**erythromycin (topical)**
Akne-Mycin, Del-Mycin, A/T/S, E/Gel, Emgel, Erycette, Erygel, Ery-Max, Erysol, ETS, {Sans-Acne}, Staticin, Theramycin Z, T-Stat

*CLASSIFICATION(S):*
*Therapeutic: anti-infectives*
*Pharmacologic: macrolides*

**Pregnancy Category B**

†See Appendix C for ophthalmic use.

## INDICATIONS

■ **IV, PO:** Infections caused by susceptible organisms including: ◻ Upper and lower respiratory tract infections ◻ Otitis media (with sulfonamides) ◻ Skin and skin structure infections ◻ Pertussis ◻ Diphtheria ◻ Erythrasma ◻ Intestinal amebiasis ◻ Pelvic inflammatory disease ◻ Nongonococcal urethritis ◻ Syphilis ◻ Legionnaires' disease ◻ Rheumatic fever ■ Useful when penicillin is the most appropriate drug but cannot be used because of hypersensitivity, including: ◻ Streptococcal infections ◻ Treatment of syphilis or gonorrhea ■ **Topical:** Treatment of acne.

## ACTION

■ Suppresses protein synthesis at the level of the 50S bacterial ribosome. **Therapeutic Effects:** ■ Bacteriostatic action against susceptible bacteria. **Spectrum:** ■ Active against many gram-positive cocci, including: ❑ Streptococci ❑ Staphylococci ■ Gram-positive bacilli, including: ❑ *Clostridium* ❑ *Corynebacterium* ■ Several gram-negative pathogens, notably: ❑ *Neisseria* ❑ *Legionella pneumophila* ■ *Mycoplasma* and *Chlamydia* are also usually susceptible.

## PHARMACOKINETICS

**Absorption:** Well absorbed from the duodenum after oral administration. Absorption of enteric-coated products is delayed. Minimal absorption may follow topical or ophthalmic use.

**Distribution:** Widely distributed. Minimal CNS penetration. Crosses placenta; enters breast milk.

**Protein Binding:** 70–80%; 96% for estolate.

**Metabolism and Excretion:** Partially metabolized by the liver, excreted mainly unchanged in the bile; small amounts excreted unchanged in the urine.

**Half-life:** 1.4–2 hr.

## CONTRAINDICATIONS AND PRECAUTIONS

**Contraindicated in:** ■ Hypersensitivity ■ Hepatic dysfunction (estolate salt) ■ Concurrent pimozide or sparfloxacin ■ Known alcohol intolerance (most topicals) ■ Tartrazine sensitivity (some products contain tartrazine—FDC yellow dye #5) ■ Pregnancy (estolate salt) ■ Products containing benzyl alcohol should be avoided in neonates.

**Use Cautiously in:** ■ Liver/renal disease ■ Geriatric patients ( ↑ risk of ototoxicity if parenteral dose >4 g/day, ↑ risk of QTc prolongation) ■ Salts other than the estolate may be used in pregnancy to treat chlamydial infections or syphilis.

## ADVERSE REACTIONS AND SIDE EFFECTS*

■ **CNS:** seizures (rare) ■ **EENT:** ototoxicity ■ **CV:** QT C PROLONGATION (may result in Torsades de Pointes), VENTRICULAR ARRHYTHMIAS, ■ **GI:** nausea, vomiting, abdominal pain, cramping, diarrhea, drug-induced hepatitis, infantile hypertrophic pyloric stenosis, drug-induced pancreatitis (rare) ■ **Derm:** rashes ■ **Local:** phlebitis at IV site ■ **Misc:** allergic reactions, superinfection.

## INTERACTIONS

**Drug-Drug:** ■ Concurrent use with **pimozide** or **sparfloxacin** ↑ risk of serious arrhythmias (concurrent use contraindicated) ■ ↑ blood levels and effects of **silfenafil** (use lower sildenafil dose) ■ Concurrent **rifabutin** or **rifampin** may ↓ effect of erythromycin and ↑ risk of adverse GI reactions ■ ↑ levels and risk of toxicity from **alfentanil, alprazolam, buspirone, clozapine, bromocriptine, theophylline, carbamazepine, cyclosporine, cylostazol diazepam, disopyramide, ergot alkaloids, felodipine, warfarin, methylprednisolone, midazolam, quinidine, rifabutin, tacrolimus, triazolam,** or **vinblastine** ■ Concurrent **HMG-CoA reductase inhibitors** ↑ risk of myopathy/rhabdomyolysis ■ May ↑ serum **digoxin** levels in a few patients ■ **Theophylline** may ↓ blood levels ■ Beneficial effects may be ↓ by **clindamycin** or **lincomycin**.

## ROUTE AND DOSAGE

250 mg of erythromycin base, estolate, or stearate = 400 mg of erythromycin ethylsuccinate.

❑ **Most Infections**

■ **PO (Adults):** *Base, estolate, stearate*—250 mg q 6 hr, *or* 333 mg q 8 hr, *or* 500 mg q 12 hr. *Ethylsuccinate*—400 mg q 6 hr *or* 800 mg q 12 hr.

■ **PO (Children):** 7.5–12.5 mg/kg q 6 hr *or* 12.5–25 mg/kg q 12 hr (up to 100 mg/kg/day).

■ **IV (Adults):** *Gluceptate and lactobionate only*—250–500 mg (up to 1 g) q 6 hr.

■ **IV (Children):** *Gluceptate and lactobionate only*—3.75–5 mg/kg q 6 hr.

❑ **Acne**

■ **Topical (Adults and Children >12 yr):** 2% ointment, gel, or solution bid.

## AVAILABILITY (generic available)

❑ **Erythromycin Base**

■ *Enteric-coated tablets:* 250 mg^Rx, 333 mg^Rx ■ *Tablets with polymer-coated particles:* 333 mg^Rx, 500 mg^Rx ■ *Film-coated*

---

{ } = Available in Canada only.
*CAPITALS indicates life-threatening; underlines indicate most frequent.

*tablets:* 500 mg$^{Rx}$ ■ *Delayed-release capsules:* 250 mg$^{Rx}$.

❑ **Erythromycin Estolate**
■ *Tablets:* 500 mg$^{Rx}$ ■ *Capsules:* 250 mg$^{Rx}$ ■ *Oral suspension (orange flavor):* 125 mg/5 ml$^{Rx}$ ■ *Oral suspension (cherry flavor):* 250 mg/5 ml$^{Rx}$.

❑ **Erythromycin Ethylsuccinate**
■ *Chewable tablets (fruit flavor):* 200 mg$^{Rx}$ ■ *Tablets:* 400 mg$^{Rx}$ ■ *Oral suspension (fruit flavor, cherry):* 200 mg/5 ml$^{Rx}$ ■ *Oral suspension (orange, banana flavors):* 400 mg/5 ml$^{Rx}$ ■ *Drops (fruit flavor):* 100 mg/2.5 ml$^{Rx}$.

❑ **Erythromycin Glucepate**
■ *Powder for injection:* 500 mg$^{Rx}$, 1 g$^{Rx}$.

❑ **Erythromycin Lactobionate**
■ *Powder for injection:* 500 mg$^{Rx}$, 1 g$^{Rx}$.

❑ **Erythromycin Stearate**
■ *Film-coated tablets:* 250 mg$^{Rx}$.

❑ **Topical Preparations**
■ *Topical ointment:* 2%$^{Rx}$ ■ *Topical gel:* 2%$^{Rx}$ ■ *Topical solution:* 2%$^{Rx}$ ■ Cost: *Benzamycin*—$58.94/23.3 g, $102.53/46.6 g ■ sulfisoxazole (Eryzole, Pediazole)$^{Rx}$ and benzoyl peroxide (Benzamycin)$^{Rx}$. See Appendix B.

TIME/ACTION PROFILE (blood levels)

|  | ONSET | PEAK | DURATION |
|---|---|---|---|
| PO | 1 hr | 1–4 hr | 6–12 hr |
| IV | rapid | end of infusion | 6–12 hr |

## NURSING IMPLICATIONS

### ASSESSMENT

❑ Assess patient for infection (vital signs; appearance of wound, sputum, urine, and stool; WBC) at beginning of and during therapy.
❑ Obtain specimens for culture and sensitivity before initiating therapy. First dose may be given before receiving results.
■ *Lab Test Considerations:* Liver function tests should be performed periodically on patients receiving high-dose, long-term therapy.
❑ May cause ↑ serum bilirubin, AST, ALT, and alkaline phosphatase concentrations.

❑ May cause false ↑ of urinary catecholamines.

## POTENTIAL NURSING DIAGNOSES

■ Infection, risk for (Indications, Side Effects).
■ Noncompliance (Patient/Family Teaching).

## IMPLEMENTATION

■ **General:** Do not confuse erythromycin with azithromycin. Do not confuse Erythrocin (erythromycin) with Ethmozine (morizocine).
■ **PO:** Administer around the clock. *Erythromycin film-coated tablets (base and stearate)* are absorbed better on an empty stomach, at least 1 hr before or 2 hr after meals; may be taken with food if GI irritation occurs. *Enteric-coated erythromycin (base and estolate)* may be taken without regard to meals. *Erythromycin ethylsuccinate* is best absorbed when taken with meals. Take each dose with a full glass of water.
❑ Use calibrated measuring device for liquid preparations. Shake well before using.
❑ Chewable tablets should be crushed or chewed and not swallowed whole.
❑ Do not crush or chew delayed-release capsules or tablets; swallow whole. *Erythromycin base delayed-release capsules* may be opened and sprinkled on applesauce, jelly, or ice cream immediately before ingestion. Entire contents of the capsule should be taken.
■ **IV:** Add 10 ml of sterile water for injection without preservatives to 250- or 500-mg vials and 20 ml to 1-g vial. Solution is stable for 7 days after reconstitution if refrigerated.
■ **Intermittent Infusion:** Dilute further in 100–250 ml of 0.9% NaCl or D5W.
■ *Rate:* Administer slowly over 20–60 min to avoid phlebitis. Assess for pain along vein; slow rate if pain occurs; apply ice and notify physician or other health care professional if unable to relieve pain.
■ **Continuous Infusion:** May also be administered as an infusion in a dilution of 1 g/liter of 0.9% NaCl, D5W, or LR over 4 hr.

❑ **Erythromycin Glucepate**
■ **Syringe Incompatibility:** ◆ heparin.
■ **Additive Compatibility:** ◆ calcium gluconate ◆ heparin ◆ hydrocortisone sodium succinate ◆ potassium chloride ◆ sodium bicarbonate.

- **Additive Incompatibility:** ◆ pentobarbital ◆ secobarbital.

◻ **Erythromycin Lactobionate**

- **Syringe Incompatibility:** ◆ heparin.

- **Y-Site Compatibility:** ◆ acyclovir ◆ amiodarone ◆ cyclophosphamide ◆ diltiazem ◆ enalaprilat ◆ esmolol ◆ famotidine ◆ foscarnet ◆ heparin ◆ hydromorphone ◆ idarubicin ◆ labetalol ◆ lorazepam ◆ magnesium sulfate ◆ meperidine ◆ midazolam ◆ morphine ◆ multivitamins ◆ perphenazine ◆ tacrolimus ◆ theophylline ◆ vitamin B complex with C ◆ zidovudine.

- **Y-Site Incompatibility:** ◆ fluconazole.

- **Additive Compatibility:** ◆ cimetidine ◆ hydrocortisone sodium succinate ◆ pentobarbital ◆ potassium chloride ◆ ranitidine ◆ sodium bicarbonate.

- **Additive Incompatibility:** ◆ heparin ◆ metoclopramide ◆ vitamin B complex with C.

- **Topical:** Cleanse area before application. Wear gloves during application.

### PATIENT/FAMILY TEACHING

◻ Instruct patient to take medication around the clock and to finish the drug completely as directed, even if feeling better. Missed doses should be taken as soon as remembered, with remaining doses evenly spaced throughout day. Advise patient that sharing of this medication may be dangerous.

◻ May cause nausea, vomiting, diarrhea, or stomach cramps; notify health care professional if these effects persist or if severe abdominal pain, yellow discoloration of the skin or eyes, darkened urine, pale stools, or unusual tiredness develops. May cause infantile hypertrophic pyloric stenosis in infants; notify health care professional if vomiting and irritability occur.

◻ Advise patient to report signs of superinfection (black, furry overgrowth on the tongue; vaginal itching or discharge; loose or foul-smelling stools).

◻ Instruct patient to notify health care professional if symptoms do not improve.

### EVALUATION

**Clinical response to therapy can be evaluated by:** ■ Resolution of the signs and symptoms of infection. Length of time for complete resolution depends on the organism and site of infection ■ Improvement of acne lesions.

## escitalopram
(ess-sit-**al**-o-pram)
Lexapro

### CLASSIFICATION(S):
**Therapeutic:** antidepressants
**Pharmacologic:** selective serotonin reuptake inhibitors (SSRIs)

### Pregnancy Category C

### INDICATIONS
■ Treatment of depression, often in conjunction with psychotherapy.

### ACTION
■ Selectively inhibits the reuptake of serotonin in the CNS. **Therapeutic Effects:** ■ Antidepressant action.

### PHARMACOKINETICS
**Absorption:** 80% absorbed following oral administration.

**Distribution:** Enters breast milk.

**Metabolism and Excretion:** Mostly metabolized by the liver (primarily CYP3A4 and CYP2C19 isoenzymes); 7% excreted unchanged by kidneys.

**Half-life:** Increased in geriatric patients and patients with hepatic impairment.

### CONTRAINDICATIONS AND PRECAUTIONS
**Contraindicated in:** ■ Hypersensitivity ■ Concurrent MAO inhibitors ■ Concurrent use of citalopram.

**Use Cautiously in:** ■ History of mania (may activate mania/hypomania) ■ History of seizures ■ Patients at risk for suicide ■ Hepatic impairment (dosage reduction recommended) ■ Severe renal impairment ■ Pregnancy or children (safety not established) ■ Lactation (may cause adverse effects in infant; risk/benefit should be considered).

## ADVERSE REACTIONS AND SIDE EFFECTS*

■ **CNS:** insomnia, dizziness, drowsiness, fatigue ■ **GI:** diarrhea, nausea, abdominal pain, constipation, dry mouth, indigestion ■ **GU:** anorgasmia, decreased libido, ejaculatory delay, impotence ■ **Derm:** increased sweating ■ **Endo:** syndrome on inappropriate secretion of antidiuretic hormone (SIADH) ■ **F and E:** hyponatremia ■ **Metab:** increased appetite.

## INTERACTIONS

**Drug-Drug:** ■ May cause serious, potentially fatal reactions when used with **MAO inhibitors**; allow at least 14 days between escitalopram and **MAO inhibitors** ■ Use cautiously with other **centrally acting drugs** (including **alcohol, antihistamines, opioid analgesics,** and **sedative/hypnotics**; concurrent use with **alcohol** is not recommended) ■ Concurrent use with **sumatriptan** or other **5–HT₃ agonist vascular headache suppressants** may result in weakness, hyperreflexia, and incoordination ■ **Cimetidine** increases blood levels of escitalopram ■ Serotonergic effects may be potentiated by **lithium** (concurrent use should be carefully monitored) ■ **Carbamazepine** may decrease blood levels ■ May increase blood levels of **metoprolol** ■ Concurrent use with **tricyclic antidepressants** should be undertaken with caution because of altered pharmacokinetics.
**Drug-Natural Products:** ■ Increased risk of serotonin syndrome with **St. John's wort** and **SAMe.**

## ROUTE AND DOSAGE

■ **PO (Adults):** 10 mg once daily, may be increased to 20 mg once daily after one week.
❏ **Hepatic Impairment**
■ **PO (Adults):** 10 mg once daily.
■ **PO (Geriatric Patients):** 10 mg once daily.

## AVAILABILITY

■ ***Tablets:*** 5 mg^Rx, 10 mg^Rx, 20 mg^Rx ■ ***Oral solution (peppermint):*** 10 mg/5 ml in 240–ml bottles^Rx.

TIME/ACTION PROFILE (antidepressant effect)

| | ONSET | PEAK | DURATION |
|---|---|---|---|
| PO | within 1–4 wk | Unknown | Unknown |

## NURSING IMPLICATIONS

### ASSESSMENT

❏ Monitor mood changes during therapy.
❏ Assess for suicidal tendencies, especially during early therapy. Restrict amount of drug available to patient.

### POTENTIAL NURSING DIAGNOSES

■ Coping, ineffective (Indications).
■ Injury, risk for (Side Effects).

### IMPLEMENTATION

■ **General:** Do not administer escitalopram and citalopram concomitantly.
■ **PO:** Administer as a single dose in the morning or evening without regard to meals.

### PATIENT/FAMILY TEACHING

❏ Instruct patient to take escitalopram exactly as directed.
❏ May cause dizziness. Caution patient to avoid driving or other activities requiring alertness until response to medication is known.
❏ Advise patient to avoid alcohol and other CNS-depressant drugs during therapy and to consult a health care professional before taking other Rx or OTC medications or herbal products.
❏ Instruct female patients to notify health care professional if pregnancy is planned or suspected or if they plan to breastfeed an infant.
❏ Caution patients that escitalopram should not be used for at least 14 days after discontinuing MAO inhibitors, and at least 14 days should be allowed after stopping escitalopram before starting an MAO inhibitor.

### EVALUATION

**Effectiveness of therapy can be demonstrated by:** ■ Increased sense of well-being ❏ Renewed interest in surroundings. May require 1–4 wk of therapy to obtain antidepressant effects.

High Alert

## esmolol

**(es**-moe-lole)
Brevibloc

## INDICATIONS

■ Management of sinus tachycardia and supraventricular arrhythmias.

## ACTION

■ Blocks stimulation of beta$_1$(myocardial)-adrenergic receptors. Does not usually affect beta$_2$(pulmonary, vascular, or uterine)-receptor sites. **Therapeutic Effects:** ■ Decreased heart rate ■ Decreased AV conduction.

## PHARMACOKINETICS

**Absorption:** IV administration results in complete bioavailability.
**Distribution:** Rapidly and widely distributed.
**Metabolism and Excretion:** Metabolized by enzymes in RBCs and liver.
**Half-life:** 9 min.

## CONTRAINDICATIONS AND PRECAUTIONS

**Contraindicated in:** ■ Uncompensated CHF ■ Pulmonary edema ■ Cardiogenic shock ■ Bradycardia or heart block ■ Known alcohol intolerance.

**Use Cautiously in:** ■ Geriatric patients (increased sensitivity to the effects of beta blockers) ■ Thyrotoxicosis (may mask symptoms) ■ Diabetes mellitus (may mask symptoms of hypoglycemia) ■ Patients with a history of severe allergic reactions (intensity of reactions may be increased) ■ Pregnancy, lactation, or children (safety not established; neonatal bradycardia, hypotension, hypoglycemia, and respiratory depression may occur rarely).

## ADVERSE REACTIONS AND SIDE EFFECTS*

■ **CNS:** fatigue, agitation, confusion, dizziness, drowsiness, weakness ■ **CV:** hypotension, peripheral ischemia ■ **GI:** nausea, vomiting ■ **Derm:** sweating ■ **Local:** injection site reactions.

## INTERACTIONS

**Drug-Drug:** ■ **General anesthesia,** IV **phenytoin,** and **verapamil** may cause additive myocardial depression ■ Additive bradycardia may occur with **digoxins** ■ Additive hypotension may occur with other **antihypertensives,** acute ingestion of **alcohol,** or **nitrates** ■ Concurrent use with **amphetamine, cocaine, ephedrine, epinephrine, norepinephrine, phenylephrine,** or **pseudoephedrine** may result in unopposed alpha-adrenergic stimulation (excessive hypertension, bradycardia) ■ Concurrent **thyroid** administration may decrease effectiveness ■ May alter the effectiveness of **insulins** or **oral hypoglycemic agents** (dosage adjustments may be necessary) ■ May decrease the effectiveness of **theophylline** ■ May decrease the beneficial beta cardiovascular effects of **dopamine** or **dobutamine** ■ Use cautiously within 14 days of **MAO inhibitor** therapy (may result in hypertension).

## ROUTE AND DOSAGE

■ **IV (Adults):** *Antiarrhythmic*—500-mcg/kg loading dose over 1 min initially, followed by 50-mcg/kg/min infusion for 4 min; if no response within 5 min, give 2nd loading dose of 500 mcg/kg over 1 min, then increase infusion to 100 mcg/kg/min for 4 min. If no response, repeat loading dose of 500 mcg/kg over 1 min and increase infusion rate by 50-mcg/kg/min increments (not to exceed 200 mcg/kg/min for 48 hr). As therapeutic end point is achieved, eliminate loading doses and decrease dosage increments to 25 mg/kg/min. *Intraoperative antihypertensive/antiarrhythmic*—250–500-mcg/kg loading dose over 1 min initially, followed by 50-mcg/kg/min infusion for 4 min; if no response within 5 min, give 2nd loading dose of 250–500 mcg/kg over 1 min, then increase infusion to 100 mcg/kg/min for 4 min. If no response, repeat loading dose of 250–500 mcg/kg over 1 min and increase infusion rate by 50-mcg/kg/min increments (not to exceed 200 mcg/kg/min for 48 hr).

■ **IV (Children):** *Antiarrhythmic*—50 mcg/kg/min, may be increased q 10 min up to 300 mcg/kg/min.

## AVAILABILITY

■ *Solution for injection (prediluted for use as loading dose):* 10 mg/ml in 10-ml vials^Rx ■ *Solution for injection (must be diluted before use):* 250 mg/ml in 10-ml vials^Rx.

TIME/ACTION PROFILE (antiarrhythmic effect)

|  | ONSET | PEAK | DURATION |
|---|---|---|---|
| IV | within minutes | unknown | 1–20 min |

## NURSING IMPLICATIONS

### ASSESSMENT

❑ Monitor blood pressure, ECG, and pulse frequently during dosage adjustment period and periodically throughout therapy. The risk of hypotension is greatest within the first 30 min of initiating esmolol infusion.

❑ Monitor intake and output ratios and daily weights. Assess routinely for signs and symptoms of CHF (dyspnea, rales/crackles, weight gain, peripheral edema, jugular venous distention).

❑ Assess infusion site frequently throughout therapy. Concentrations >10 mg/ml may cause redness, swelling, skin discoloration, and burning at the injection site. Do not use butterfly needles for administration. If venous irritation occurs, stop the infusion and resume at another site.

■ *Toxicity and Overdose:* Monitor patients receiving esmolol for signs of overdose (bradycardia, severe dizziness or fainting, severe drowsiness, dyspnea, bluish fingernails or palms, seizures). Notify physician immediately if these signs occur.

❑ IV glucagon and symptomatic care are used in the treatment of esmolol overdose. Because of the short action of esmolol, discontinuation of therapy may relieve acute toxicity.

### POTENTIAL NURSING DIAGNOSES

■ Cardiac output, decreased (Side Effects).

### IMPLEMENTATION

❑ *High Alert:* IV vasoactive medications are inherently dangerous. Esmolol is available in different concentrations; fatalities have occured when loading dose vial is confused with concentrated solution for injection, which contains 2,500 mg in 10 ml (250 mg/ml) and must be diluted. Before administering, have second practitioner independently check original order, dosage calculations, and infusion pump settings. Do not confuse Brevibloc (esmolol) with Brevital (methohexital). If both are available as floor stock, store in separate areas.

■ **General:** To convert to other antiarrhythmics following esmolol administration, administer the 1st dose of the antiarrhythmic agent and decrease the esmolol dose by 50% after 30 min. If an adequate response is maintained for 1 hr following the 2nd dose of the antiarrhythmic agent, discontinue esmolol.

■ **Direct IV:** The 10-mg/ml strength may be administered undiluted.

■ **Intermittent Infusion:** To dilute for infusion, remove 20 ml from a 500-ml bag of D5W, D5/LR, D5/0.45% NaCl, D5/0.9% NaCl, 0.45% NaCl, 0.9% NaCl, or LR. Add 5 g of esmolol to the bottle for a concentration of 10 mg/ml. Solution is clear, colorless to light yellow; stable for 24 hr at room temperature.

■ *Rate:* The loading dose of esmolol is administered over 1 min, followed by a maintenance dose via IV infusion over 4 min. If the response is not adequate, procedure is repeated every 5 min with an increase in the maintenance dose. Titration of dose is based on desired heart rate or undesired decrease in blood pressure. The maintenance dose should not exceed 200 mcg/kg/min and can be administered for up to 48 hr. Esmolol infusions should not be abruptly discontinued; eliminate loading doses and decrease dosage by 25 mcg/kg/min.

■ **Y-Site Compatibility:** ◆ amikacin ◆ aminophylline ◆ amiodarone ◆ ampicillin ◆ atracurium ◆ butorphanol ◆ calcium chloride ◆ cefazolin ◆ cefmetazole ◆ cefoperazone ◆ ceftazidime ◆ ceftizoxime ◆ chloramphenicol ◆ cimetidine ◆ clindamycin ◆ diltiazem ◆ dopamine ◆ enalaprilat ◆ erythromycin lactobionate ◆ famotidine ◆ fentanyl ◆ gatifloxacin ◆ gentamicin ◆ heparin ◆ hydrocortisone sodium succinate ◆ insulin ◆ labetalol ◆ linezolid ◆ magnesium sulfate ◆ methyldopate ◆ metronidazole ◆ midazolam ◆ morphine ◆ nafcillin ◆ nitroprusside ◆ norepinephrine ◆ pancuronium ◆ penicillin G potassium ◆ phenytoin ◆ piperacillin ◆ polymyxin B ◆ potassium chloride ◆ potassium phosphate ◆ propofol ◆ ranitidine ◆ sodium acetate ◆ streptomycin ◆ tacrolimus

♦ tobramycin ♦ trimethoprim/sulfamethoxazole ♦ vancomycin ♦ vecuronium.

■ **Y-Site Incompatibility:** ♦ furosemide ♦ warfarin.

## PATIENT/FAMILY TEACHING

❑ May cause drowsiness. Caution patients receiving esmolol to call for assistance during ambulation or transfer.

❑ Advise patients to change positions slowly to minimize orthostatic hypotension.

❑ Patients with diabetes should closely monitor blood glucose, especially if weakness, malaise, irritability, or fatigue occurs. Medication does not block dizziness or sweating as signs of hypoglycemia.

## EVALUATION

**Effectiveness of therapy can be demonstrated by:** ■ Control of arrhythmias without appearance of detrimental side effects.

## esomeprazole
(es-o-**mep**-ra-zole)
Nexium

### CLASSIFICATION(S):
**Therapeutic:** antiulcer agents
**Pharmacologic:** proton-pump inhibitors

### Pregnancy Category B

## INDICATIONS

■ GERD including: ❑ erosive esophagitis ■ With amoxicillin and clarithromycin to eradicate *Helicobacter pylori* in duodenal ulcer disease or history of duodenal ulcer disease.

## ACTION

■ Binds to an enzyme on gastric parietal cells in the presence of acidic gastric pH, preventing the final transport of hydrogen ions into the gastric lumen. **Therapeutic Effects:** ■ Diminished accumulation of acid in the gastric lumen with lessened gastroesophageal reflux ■ Healing of duodenal ulcers.

## PHARMACOKINETICS

**Absorption:** 90% absorbed following oral administration; food decreases absorption.

**Distribution:** Unknown.

**Protein Binding:** 97%.

**Metabolism and Excretion:** Extensively metabolized by the liver (cytochrome P450 [CY P450] system, primarily CY P2 C19 isoenzyme); <1% excreted unchanged in urine.

**Half-life:** 1.0–1.5 hr.

## CONTRAINDICATIONS AND PRECAUTIONS

**Contraindicated in:** ■ Hypersensitivity ■ Lactation (not recommended).

**Use Cautiously in:** ■ Severe hepatic impairment (daily dose should not exceed 20 mg) ■ Pregnancy (use only if clearly needed) ■ Children <18 yr (safety not established).

## ADVERSE REACTIONS AND SIDE EFFECTS*

■ **CNS:** headache ■ **GI:** abdominal pain, constipation, diarrhea, dry mouth, flatulence, nausea.

## INTERACTIONS

**Drug-Drug:** ■ May ↓ absorption and effects of drugs where gastric pH is a determinant of bioavailability, including **digoxin, ketoconazole,** and **iron salts** ■ May ↑ risk of bleeding with **warfarin** (monitor INR and PT).

## ROUTE AND DOSAGE

❑ **Gastroesophageal Reflux Disease**

■ **PO (Adults):** *Healing of erosive esophagitis*—20 mg or 40 mg once daily for 4–8 wks; *maintenance of healing of erosive esophagitis*—20 mg once daily; *symptomatic GERD*—20 mg once daily for 4 wks (additional 4 wks may be considered for nonresponders).

❑ ***H. pylori* Eradication to Reduce the Risk of Duodenal Ulcer Recurrence (Triple Therapy)**

■ **PO (Adults):** 40 mg once daily for 10 days with amoxicillin 1000 mg twice daily for 10 days and clarithromycin 500 mg twice daily for 10 days.

❑ **Severe Hepatic Impairment**
■ **PO (Adults):** Daily dose should not exceed 20 mg.

## AVAILABILITY

■ **Delayed-release capsules:** 20 mg<sup>Rx</sup>, 40 mg<sup>Rx</sup> ■ Cost: 20 mg $124.33/30, 40 mg $124.33/30.

TIME/ACTION PROFILE (blood levels*)

| | ONSET | PEAK | DURATION |
|---|---|---|---|
| PO | rapid | 1.6 hr | 24 hr |

*Resolution of symptoms takes 5–8 days.

## NURSING IMPLICATIONS

### ASSESSMENT

❑ Assess patient routinely for epigastric or abdominal pain and frank or occult blood in the stool, emesis, or gastric aspirate.
■ **Lab Test Considerations:** May cause ↑ serum creatinine, uric acid, total bilirubin, alkaline phosphatase, AST, and ALT.
❑ May alter hemoglobin, WBC, platelets, serum sodium, potassium, and thyroxine levels.

### POTENTIAL NURSING DIAGNOSES

■ Pain, acute (Indications).

### IMPLEMENTATION

■ **General:** Antacids may be used while taking esomeprazole.
■ **PO:** Administer at least 1 hr before meals. Capsules should be swallowed whole.
❑ For patients with difficulty swallowing, place 1 tbsp of applesauce in an empty bowl. Open capsule and carefully empty the pellets inside onto applesauce. Mix pellets with applesauce and swallow immediately. Applesauce should not be hot and should be soft enough to swallow without chewing. Do not store applesauce mixture for future use. Tap water, orange juice, apple juice, and yogurt have also been used. Do not crush or chew pellets.

### PATIENT/FAMILY TEACHING

❑ Instruct patient to take medication as directed for the full course of therapy, even if feeling better. Take missed doses as soon as remembered but not if almost time for next dose. Do not double doses.

❑ Advise patient to avoid alcohol, products containing aspirin or NSAIDs, and foods that may cause an increase in GI irritation.
❑ Advise patient to report onset of black, tarry stools; diarrhea; abdominal pain; or persistent headache to health care professional promptly.

### EVALUATION

**Clinical response to therapy can be evaluated by:** ■ Decrease in abdominal pain or prevention of gastric irritation and bleeding. Healing of duodenal ulcers can be seen on x-ray examination or endoscopy ■ Decrease in symptoms of GERD. Sustained resolution of symptoms usually occurs in 5–8 days. Therapy is continued for 4–8 wk after initial episode.

## ESTRADIOL

(es-tra-**dye**-ole)
Estrace, Gynodiol

### estradiol cypionate
depGynogen, Depo-Estradiol, Depogen, Dura-Estrin, E-Cypionate, Estragyn LA 5, Estro-Cyp, Estrofem, Estroject-LA, Estro-L.A.

### estradiol valerate
Clinagen LA, Delestrogen, Dioval, Duragen, Estra-L, Estro-Span, {Femogex}, Gynogen L.A., Menaval, Valergen

### estradiol transdermal system
Alora, Climara, Esclim, Estraderm, FemPatch, Vivelle

### estradiol vaginal tablet
Vagifem

### estradiol vaginal ring
Femring, Estring

**CLASSIFICATION(S):**
**Therapeutic:** hormones
**Pharmacologic:** estrogens

**Pregnancy Category X**

### INDICATIONS
■ **PO, IM, Transdermal:** Replacement of estrogen (HRT) to diminish moderate to severe

vasomotor symptoms of menopause and of various estrogen deficiency states including: ❏ Female hypogonadism ❏ Ovariectomy ❏ Primary ovarian failure ■ Treatment and prevention of postmenopausal osteoporosis (not vaginal dosage forms) ■ **PO:** Inoperable metastatic postmenopausal breast or prostate carcinoma ■ **Vag:** Management of atrophic vaginitis that may occur with menopause (low dose), bothersome systemic symptoms of menopause (higher dose) ■ Concurrent use of progestin is recommended during cyclical therapy to decrease the risk of endometrial carcinoma in patients with an intact uterus.

## ACTION

■ Estrogens promote growth and development of female sex organs and the maintenance of secondary sex characteristics in women ■ Metabolic effects include reduced blood cholesterol, protein synthesis, and sodium and water retention. **Therapeutic Effects:** ■ Restoration of hormonal balance in various deficiency states, including menopause ■ Treatment of hormone-sensitive tumors.

## PHARMACOKINETICS

**Absorption:** Well absorbed after oral administration. Readily absorbed through skin and mucous membranes.

**Distribution:** Widely distributed. Crosses the placenta and enters breast milk.

**Metabolism and Excretion:** Mostly metabolized by the liver and other tissues. Enterohepatic recirculation occurs, and more absorption may occur from the GI tract.

**Half-life:** Unknown.

## CONTRAINDICATIONS AND PRECAUTIONS

**Contraindicated in:** ■ Thromboembolic disease ■ Undiagnosed vaginal bleeding ■ Pregnancy (may result in harm to the fetus) ■ Lactation.

**Use Cautiously in:** ■ Underlying cardiovascular disease ■ Severe hepatic or renal disease ■ May increase the risk of endometrial carcinoma ■ History of porphyria.

## ADVERSE REACTIONS AND SIDE EFFECTS*

■ **CNS:** headache, dizziness, lethargy ■ **EENT:** intolerance to contact lenses, worsening of myopia or astigmatism ■ **CV:** MI, THROMBOEMBOLISM, edema, hypertension ■ **GI:** nausea, weight changes, anorexia, increased appetite, jaundice, vomiting ■ **GU:** *women*—amenorrhea, dysmenorrhea, breakthrough bleeding, cervical erosions, loss of libido, vaginal candidiasis;; *men*—impotence, testicular atrophy ■ **Derm:** oily skin, acne, pigmentation, urticaria ■ **Endo:** gynecomastia (men), hyperglycemia ■ **F and E:** hypercalcemia, sodium and water retention ■ **MS:** leg cramps ■ **Misc:** breast tenderness.

## INTERACTIONS

**Drug-Drug:** ■ May alter requirement for **warfarin, oral hypoglycemic agents,** or **insulins** ■ **Barbiturates** or **rifampin** may ↓ effectiveness ■ **Smoking** ↑ risk of adverse CV reactions.

## ROUTE AND DOSAGE

Estrogens should be used in the lowest doses for the shortest period of time consistent with desired therapeutic outcome.

❏ **Symptoms of Menopause, Atrophic Vaginitis, Female Hypogonadism, Ovarian Failure/Osteoporosis**

■ **PO (Adults):** 0.5–2 mg daily or in a cycle.

■ **IM (Adults):** 1–5 mg monthly (estradiol cypionate) *or* 10–20 mg (estradiol valerate) monthly.

■ **Transdermal (Adults):** *Alora, Estraderm*—50- or 100-mcg/24-hr transdermal patch applied twice weekly. *Climara*—50–100-mcg/24-hr patch applied weekly. *FemPatch*—25-mcg/24-hr patch applied q 7 days. *Vivelle*—37.5–100-mcg transdermal patch applied twice weekly. Progestin may be administered for 10–14 days of each month.

■ **Vag (Adults):** *Cream*—2–4 g (0.2–0.4 mg estradiol) daily for 1–2 wk, then decrease to 1–2 g/day for 1–2 wk; then maintenance dose of 1 g 1–3 times weekly for 3 wk, then off for 1 wk; then repeat cycle once vaginal mucosa has been restored; *Vaginal ring (Estring)*—2-mg (releases 7.5 mcg estradiol/24 hr)q 3 mo; *Vaginal ring (Femr-*

{ } = Available in Canada only.
*CAPITALS indicates life-threatening; underlines indicate most frequent.

*ing)*—12.4 mg (releases 50 mcg estradiol/ 24 hr)q 3 mo or 24.8 mg (releases 100 mcg estradiol/24 hr)q 3 mo (*Femring* requires concurrent progesterone) *Vaginal tablet*— 25-mcg once daily for 2 wk, then twice weekly.

❑ **Postmenopausal Breast Carcinoma**

■ **PO (Adults):** 10 mg 3 times daily.

❑ **Prostate Carcinoma**

■ **PO (Adults):** 1–2 mg 3 times daily.

■ **IM (Adults):** 30 mg q 1–2 wk (estradiol valerate).

## AVAILABILITY

■ *Tablet:* 0.5 mg$^{Rx}$, 1 mg$^{Rx}$, 2 mg$^{Rx}$ ■ Cost: 1 mg $57.22/100, 2 mg $83.56/100 ■ *Injection (valerate in oil):* 10 mg/ml$^{Rx}$, 20 mg/ml$^{Rx}$, 40 mg/ml$^{Rx}$ ■ *Injection (cypionate in oil):* 5 mg/ml$^{Rx}$ ■ *Transdermal system:* 25 mcg/ 24-hr release rate$^{Rx}$, 37.5 mcg /24-hr release rate$^{Rx}$, 50 mcg/24-hr release rate$^{Rx}$, 75 mcg/24-hr release rate$^{Rx}$, 100 mcg/24-hr release rate$^{Rx}$ ■ Cost: 100 mcg $29.99/8 patches ■ *Vaginal cream:* 100 mcg/g$^{Rx}$ ■ *Vaginal ring (Estring):* 2 mg (releases 7.5 mcg/day over 90 days)$^{Rx}$ ■ *Vaginal ring (Femring):* 12.4 mg (releases 50 mcg/day over 90 days)$^{Rx}$, 24.8 mg (releases 100 mcg/day over 90 days)$^{Rx}$ ■ *Vaginal tablet:* 25 mcg$^{Rx}$.

TIME/ACTION PROFILE (estrogenic effects)

| | ONSET | PEAK | DURATION |
|---|---|---|---|
| PO | unknown | unknown | unknown |
| IM | unknown | unknown | unknown |
| TD | unknown | unknown | 3–4 days (Estraderm), 7 days (Climara) |
| Vaginal ring | unknown | unknown | 90 days |
| Vaginal tablet | unknown | unknown | 3–4 days |

# NURSING IMPLICATIONS

## ASSESSMENT

❑ Assess blood pressure before and periodically during therapy.

❑ Monitor intake and output ratios and weekly weight. Report significant discrepancies or steady weight gain.

■ **Menopause:** Assess frequency and severity of vasomotor symptoms.

■ *Lab Test Considerations:* May cause ↑ HDL, phospholipids, and triglycerides and ↓ serum LDL and total cholesterol concentrations.

❑ May cause ↑ serum glucose, sodium, cortisol, prolactin, prothrombin, and factor VII, VIII, IX, and X levels. May ↓ serum folate, pyridoxine, antithrombin III, and urine pregnanediol concentrations.

❑ Monitor hepatic function before and periodically during therapy.

❑ May cause false interpretations of thyroid function tests, false ↑ in norepinephrine platelet-induced aggregability, and false ↓ in metyrapone tests.

❑ May cause hypercalcemia in patients with metastatic bone lesions.

## POTENTIAL NURSING DIAGNOSES

■ Sexual dysfunction (Indications).

## IMPLEMENTATION

■ **General:** Do not confuse Estraderm (estradiol) with Testaderm (testosterone).

■ **PO:** Administer with or immediately after food to reduce nausea.

■ **Vag:** Manufacturer provides applicator with cream. Dose is marked on the applicator. Wash applicator with mild soap and warm water after each use. **Transdermal:** When switching from PO form, begin transdermal therapy 1 wk after the last dose or when symptoms reappear.

■ **IM:** Injection has oil base. Roll syringe to ensure even dispersion. Administer deep IM. Avoid IV administration.

## PATIENT/FAMILY TEACHING

■ **General Info:** Instruct patient to take medication as directed. Take missed doses as soon as remembered as long as it is not just before next dose. Do not double doses.

❑ Explain dose schedule and maintenance routine. Discontinuing medication suddenly may cause withdrawal bleeding.

❑ If nausea becomes a problem, advise patient that eating solid food often provides relief.

❑ Advise patient to report signs and symptoms of fluid retention (swelling of ankles and feet, weight gain), thromboembolic disorders (pain, swelling, tenderness in extremities, headache, chest pain, blurred vision), mental depression, or hepatic dysfunction (yellowed skin or eyes, pruritus, dark urine, light-colored stools) to health care professional.

❑ Instruct patient to stop taking medication and notify health care professional if pregnancy is suspected.

❑ Advise patient to notify health care professional of medication regimen before treatment or surgery.

❑ Caution patient that cigarette smoking during estrogen therapy may cause increased risk of serious side effects, especially for women over age 35.

❑ Caution patient to use sunscreen and protective clothing to prevent increased pigmentation.

❑ Advise patient treated for osteoporosis that exercise has been found to arrest and reverse bone loss. The patient should discuss any exercise limitations with health care professional before beginning program.

❑ Inform patient that estrogens should not be used to decrease risk of cardiovascular disease. Estrogens may increase risk of cardiovascular disease and breast cancer.

❑ Emphasize the importance of routine follow-up physical exams, including blood pressure; breast, abdomen, and pelvic examinations; Papanicolaou smears every 6–12 mo; and mammogram every 12 mo or as directed. Health care professional will evaluate possibility of discontinuing medication every 3–6 mo. If on continuous (not cyclical) therapy or without concurrent progestins, endometrial biopsy may be recommended, if uterus is intact.

■ **Vag:** Instruct patient in the correct use of applicator. Patient should remain recumbent for at least 30 min after administration. May use sanitary napkin to protect clothing, but do not use tampon. If a dose is missed, do not use the missed dose, but return to regular dosing schedule.

❑ Instruct patient to use applicator provided with vaginal tablet. Insert as high up in the vagina as comfortable, without using force.

■ **Vaginal Ring:** Instruct patient to press ring into an oval and insert into the upper third of the vaginal vault. Exact position is not critical. Once ring is inserted, patient should not feel anything. If discomfort is felt, ring is probably not in far enough; gently push farther into vagina. Leave in place continuously for 90 days. Ring does not interfere with sexual intercourse. If straining at defecation makes ring move to lower vagina, push up with finger. If expelled totally, rinse ring with lukewarm water and reinsert. To remove, hook a finger through the ring and pull it out.

■ **Transdermal:** Instruct patient to wash and dry hands first. Apply disc to intact skin on hairless portion of abdomen (do not apply to breasts or waistline). Press disc for 10 sec to ensure contact with skin (especially around edges). Avoid areas where clothing may rub disc loose. Change site with each administration to prevent skin irritation. Do not reuse site for 1 wk. disc may be reapplied if it falls off.

## EVALUATION

**Effectiveness of therapy can be demonstrated by:** ■ Resolution of menopausal vasomotor symptoms ■ Decreased vaginal and vulvar itching, inflammation, or dryness associated with menopause ■ Normalization of estrogen levels in patients with ovariectomy or hypogonadism ■ Control of the spread of advanced metastatic breast or prostate cancer ■ Prevention of osteoporosis.

# estradiol cypionate/ medroxyprogesterone acetate, See CONTRACEPTIVES, HORMONAL.

# estrogens, conjugated
**(ess-troe-jenz)**
Cenestin, {C.E.S.}, {Congest}, Premarin

**estrogens, conjugated (synthetic, A)**
Cenestin

*CLASSIFICATION(S):*
*Therapeutic:* hormones
*Pharmacologic:* estrogens

**Pregnancy Category X**

## INDICATIONS

■ **PO:** Part of HRT in the of moderate to severe vasomotor symptoms of menopause ■ Estrogen deficiency states, including: ❏ Female hypogonadism ❏ Ovariectomy ❏ Primary ovarian failure ■ Postmenopausal osteoporosis ■ Advanced inoperable metastatic breast and prostatic carcinoma ■ **IM, IV:** Uterine bleeding resulting from hormonal imbalance ■ **Vag:** Management of atrophic vaginitis ■ Concurrent use of progestin is recommended during cyclical therapy to decrease the risk of endometrial carcinoma in patients with an intact uterus.

## ACTION

■ Estrogens promote the growth and development of female sex organs and the maintenance of secondary sex characteristics in women ■ Metabolic effects include reduced blood cholesterol, protein synthesis, and sodium and water retention. **Therapeutic Effects:** ■ Restoration of hormonal balance in various deficiency states and treatment of hormone-sensitive tumors.

## PHARMACOKINETICS

**Absorption:** Well absorbed after oral administration. Readily absorbed through skin and mucous membranes.

**Distribution:** Widely distributed. Crosses placenta and enters breast milk.

**Metabolism and Excretion:** Mostly metabolized by liver and other tissues. Enterohepatic recirculation occurs, with more absorption from GI tract.

**Half-life:** Unknown.

## CONTRAINDICATIONS AND PRECAUTIONS

**Contraindicated in:** ■ Thromboembolic disease ■ Undiagnosed vaginal bleeding ■ Pregnancy (may result in harm to the fetus) ■ Lactation.

**Use Cautiously in:** ■ Underlying cardiovascular disease ■ Severe hepatic or renal disease ■ May increase the risk of endometrial carcinoma.

## ADVERSE REACTIONS AND SIDE EFFECTS*

(systemic use) ■ **CNS:** <u>headache</u>, dizziness, lethargy, mental depression ■ **EENT:** <u>intolerance to contact lenses</u>, worsening of myopia or astigmatism ■ **CV:** MI, THROMBOEMBOLISM, <u>edema</u>, <u>hypertension</u> ■ **GI:** <u>nausea</u>, <u>weight changes</u>, an-

orexia, increased appetite, jaundice, vomiting ■ **GU:** *women*—<u>amenorrhea</u>, <u>breakthrough bleeding</u>, <u>dysmenorrhea</u>, cervical erosion, loss of libido, vaginal candidiasis; *men*— impotence, <u>testicular atrophy</u> ■ **Derm:** <u>acne</u>, <u>oily skin</u>, pigmentation, urticaria ■ **Endo:** <u>gynecomastia</u> (men), hyperglycemia ■ **F and E:** hypercalcemia, sodium and water retention ■ **MS:** leg cramps ■ **Misc:** <u>breast tenderness</u>.

## INTERACTIONS

**Drug-Drug:** ■ May alter requirement for **warfarin, oral hypoglycemic agents,** or **insulins** ■ **Barbiturates** or **rifampin** may ↓ effectiveness ■ **Smoking** ↑ risk of adverse cardiovascular reactions.

**Drug-Natural Products:** ■ **St. John's wort** may ↓ levels and effect.

## ROUTE AND DOSAGE

❏ **Ovariectomy, Primary Ovarian Failure**

■ **PO (Adults):** 1.25 mg daily or in a cycle.

❏ **Osteoporosis/Menopausal Symptoms**

■ **PO (Adults):** 0.3–1.25 mg daily or in a cycle.

❏ **Hypogonadism**

■ **PO (Adults):** 2.5–7.5 mg daily or in a cycle.

❏ **Inoperable Breast Carcinoma—Men and Postmenopausal Women**

■ **PO (Adults):** 10 mg tid.

❏ **Inoperable Prostate Carcinoma**

■ **PO (Adults):** 1.25–2.5 mg tid.

❏ **Uterine Bleeding**

■ **IM, IV (Adults):** 25 mg, may repeat in 6–12 hr if necessary.

❏ **Atrophic Vaginitis**

■ **Vag (Adults):** 1.25–2.5 mg (2–4 g cream) daily for 3 wk, off for 1 wk, then repeat.

## AVAILABILITY (generic available)

■ *Tablets:* 0.3 mg^Rx, 0.45 mg^Rx, 0.625 mg^Rx, 0.9 mg^Rx, 1.25 mg^Rx, 2.5 mg^Rx ■ Cost: *Premarin*—0.625 mg $75.54/100 ■ *Powder for injection:* 25 mg/vial^Rx ■ *Vaginal cream:* 0.625 mg/g^Rx ■ Cost: $57.64/42.5 gm tube ■ medroxyprogesterone in compliance package (Prempro^Rx and Premphase^Rx). See Appendix B.

TIME/ACTION PROFILE (estrogenic effects†)

| | ONSET | PEAK | DURATION |
|---|---|---|---|
| PO | rapid | unknown | 24 hr |
| IM | delayed | unknown | 6–12 hr |
| IV | rapid | unknown | 6–12 hr |

†Tumor response may take several weeks.

## NURSING IMPLICATIONS

### ASSESSMENT

- **General Info:** Assess blood pressure before and periodically during therapy.
- Monitor intake and output ratios and weekly weight. Report significant discrepancies or steady weight gain.
- **Menopause:** Assess frequency and severity of vasomotor symptoms.
- *Lab Test Considerations:* May cause ↑ HDL, phospholipids, and triglycerides, and ↓ serum LDL and total cholesterol concentrations.
- May cause ↑ serum glucose, sodium, cortisol, prolactin, prothrombin, and factor VII, VIII, IX, and X levels. May ↓ serum folate, pyridoxine, antithrombin III, and urine pregnanediol concentrations.
- Monitor hepatic function before and periodically during therapy.
- May cause false interpretations of thyroid function tests, false increases in norepinephrine platelet-induced aggregability, and false ↓ in metyrapone tests.
- May cause hypercalcemia in patients with metastatic bone lesions.

### POTENTIAL NURSING DIAGNOSES

- Sexual dysfunction (Indications).

### IMPLEMENTATION

- **General:** Estrogens should be used in the lowest doses for the shortest period of time consistent with desired therapeutic outcome.
- **PO:** Administer with or immediately after food to reduce nausea.
- **Vag:** Manufacturer provides applicator with cream. Dose is marked on the applicator. Wash applicator with mild soap and warm water after each use.

- **IM:** To reconstitute, withdraw at least 5 ml of air from dry container and then slowly introduce the sterile diluent against the container side. Gently agitate container to dissolve; do not shake vigorously. Solution is stable for 60 days if refrigerated. Do not use if precipitate is present or if solution is darkened.
- IV is preferred parenteral route because of rapid response.
- **Direct IV:** Reconstitute as for IM. Inject into distal port tubing of free-flowing IV of 0.9% NaCl, D5W, or lactated Ringer's solution.
- *Rate:* Administer slowly (no faster than 5 mg/min) to prevent flushing.
- **Y-Site Compatibility:** ◆ heparin ◆ potassium chloride ◆ vitamin B complex with C.
- **Additive Incompatibility:** ◆ ascorbic acid or acidic solutions.

### PATIENT/FAMILY TEACHING

- **General Info:** Instruct patient to take oral medication as directed. Take missed doses as soon as remembered, but not just before next dose. Do not double doses.
- Explain dosage schedule and maintenance routine. Discontinuing medication suddenly may cause withdrawal bleeding. Bleeding is anticipated during the week when conjugated estrogens are withheld.
- If nausea becomes a problem, advise patient that eating solid food often provides relief.
- Advise patient to report signs and symptoms of fluid retention (swelling of ankles and feet, weight gain), thromboembolic disorders (pain, swelling, tenderness in extremities; headache; chest pain; blurred vision), depression, hepatic dysfunction (yellowed skin or eyes, pruritus, dark urine, light-colored stools), or abnormal vaginal bleeding to health care professional.
- Instruct patient to stop taking medication and notify health care professional if pregnancy is suspected.
- Caution patient that cigarette smoking during estrogen therapy may increase risk of serious side effects, especially for women over age 35.
- Caution patient to use sunscreen and protective clothing to prevent increased pigmentation.

❑ Advise patient to notify health care professional of medication regimen before treatment or surgery.

❑ Advise patient treated for osteoporosis that exercise has been found to arrest and reverse bone loss. The patient should discuss any exercise limitations with health care professional before beginning program.

❑ Emphasize the importance of routine follow-up physical exams, including blood pressure; breast, abdomen, and pelvic examinations; Papanicolaou smears every 6–12 mo; and mammogram every 12 mo or as directed. Health care professional will evaluate possibility of discontinuing medication every 3–6 mo. If on continuous (not cyclical) therapy or without concurrent progestins, endometrial biopsy may be recommended if uterus is intact.

❑ Inform patient that estrogens should not be used to decrease risk of cardiovascular disease. Estrogens may increase risk of cardiovascular disease and breast cancer.

■ **Vag:** Instruct patient in the correct use of applicator. Patient should remain recumbent for at least 30 min after administration. May use sanitary napkin to protect clothing, but do not use tampon. If a dose is missed, do not use the missed dose, but return to regular dosing schedule.

## EVALUATION

**Effectiveness of therapy can be demonstrated by:** ■ Resolution of menopausal vasomotor symptoms ❑ Decreased vaginal and vulvar itching, inflammation, or dryness associated with menopause ■ Normalization of estrogen levels in patients with ovariectomy or hypogonadism ■ Control of the spread of advanced metastatic breast or prostate cancer ■ Prevention of osteoporosis.

## estropipate

(ess-troe-**pi**-pate)
Ogen, Ortho-Est, piperazine estrone sulfate

### CLASSIFICATION(S):
**Therapeutic:** hormones
**Pharmacologic:** estrogens

**Pregnancy Category X**

## INDICATIONS

■ **PO:** As part of HRT in the treatment of vasomotor symptoms of menopause ■ Treatment of various estrogen deficiency states, including: ❑ Female hypogonadism ❑ Ovariectomy ❑ Primary ovarian failure ■ Adjunctive therapy of postmenopausal osteoporosis ■ **Vag:** Management of atrophic vaginitis ■ Concurrent use of progestin is recommended during cyclical therapy to decrease the risk of endometrial carcinoma in patients with an intact uterus.

## ACTION

■ Estrogens promote the growth and development of female sex organs and the maintenance of secondary sex characteristics in women ■ Metabolic effects include reduced blood cholesterol, protein synthesis, and sodium and water retention. **Therapeutic Effects:** ■ Restoration of hormonal balance in various deficiency states.

## PHARMACOKINETICS

**Absorption:** Well absorbed after oral administration. Readily absorbed through skin and mucous membranes.

**Distribution:** Widely distributed. Crosses the placenta and enters breast milk.

**Metabolism and Excretion:** Mostly metabolized by the liver and other tissues. Enterohepatic recirculation occurs, and more absorption may occur from the GI tract.

**Half-life:** Unknown.

## CONTRAINDICATIONS AND PRECAUTIONS

**Contraindicated in:** ■ Thromboembolic disease ■ Undiagnosed vaginal bleeding ■ Pregnancy (may result in harm to the fetus) ■ Lactation.
**Use Cautiously in:** ■ Underlying cardiovascular disease ■ Severe hepatic or renal disease ■ May increase the risk of endometrial carcinoma.

## ADVERSE REACTIONS AND SIDE EFFECTS*

(systemic use) ■ **CNS:** <u>headache</u>, dizziness, lethargy, mental depression ■ **EENT:** <u>intolerance to contact lenses</u>, worsening of myopia or astigmatism ■ **CV:** MI, THROMBOEMBOLISM, <u>edema</u>, hypertension ■ **GI:** <u>nausea</u>, <u>weight changes</u>, anorexia, increased appetite, jaundice, vomiting ■ **GU:** women—<u>amenorrhea</u>, <u>breakthrough bleeding</u>, <u>dysmenorrhea</u>, cervical erosion, loss of libido, vaginal candidiasis; *men*—impotence, testicular atrophy ■ **Derm:** acne, oily skin, pigmentation, urticaria ■ **Endo:** gynecomastia (men), hyperglycemia ■ **F and E:** hypercalcemia, sodium and water retention ■ **MS:** leg cramps ■ **Misc:** breast tenderness.

## INTERACTIONS

**Drug-Drug:** ■ May alter requirement for **warfarin, oral hypoglycemic agents,** or **insulins** ■ **Barbiturates** or **rifampin** may decrease effectiveness ■ **Smoking** increases the risk of adverse cardiovascular reactions.

## ROUTE AND DOSAGE

❑ **Vasomotor Symptoms of Menopause/ Atrophic Vaginitis/Osteoporosis**

■ **PO (Adults):** 0.75–6 mg daily or in a cycle.

■ **Vag (Adults):** 3–6 mg (2–4 g of 0.15% cream) daily for 3 wk, then off for 1 wk, then repeat cycle.

❑ **Female Hypogonadism/Ovarian Failure**

■ **PO (Adults):** 1.5–9 mg daily or in a cycle.

## AVAILABILITY (generic available)

■ *Tablets:* 0.75 mg$^{Rx}$, 1.5 mg$^{Rx}$, 3 mg$^{Rx}$, 6 mg estropipate$^{Rx}$ ■ Cost: 0.75 mg $41.28/100, 1.5 mg $57.67/100, 3 mg$100.39/100, 6 mg $129.83/100 ■ *Vaginal cream:* 1.5 mg/g$^{Rx}$.

TIME/ACTION PROFILE (estrogenic effects)

| | ONSET | PEAK | DURATION |
|---|---|---|---|
| PO | unknown | unknown | 24 hr |

## NURSING IMPLICATIONS

### ASSESSMENT

■ **General Info:** Assess blood pressure before and periodically throughout therapy.

❑ Monitor intake and output ratios and weekly weight. Report significant discrepancies or steady weight gain.

■ **Menopause:** Assess frequency and severity of vasomotor symptoms.

■ *Lab Test Considerations:* May cause increased HDL, phospholipids, and triglycerides, and decreased serum LDL and total cholesterol concentrations.

❑ May cause increased serum glucose, sodium, cortisol, prolactin, prothrombin, and factor VII, VIII, IX, and X levels. May decrease serum folate, pyridoxine, antithrombin III, and urine pregnanediol concentrations.

❑ Monitor hepatic function before and periodically throughout therapy.

❑ May cause false interpretations of thyroid function tests, false increases in norepinephrine platelet-induced aggregability, and false decreases in metyrapone tests.

## POTENTIAL NURSING DIAGNOSES

■ Sexual dysfunction (Indications).

## IMPLEMENTATION

■ **PO:** Administer PO doses with or immediately after food to reduce nausea.

■ **Vag:** Manufacturer provides applicator with cream. Dose is marked on the applicator. Wash applicator with mild soap and warm water after each use.

## PATIENT/FAMILY TEACHING

■ **General Info:** Instruct patient to take oral medication as directed. If a dose is missed, take as soon as remembered as long as it is not just before next dose. Do not double doses.

❑ Explain medication schedule to women on 21-day cycle followed by 7 days of not taking medication. Encourage patient to take medication at the same time each day.

❑ If nausea becomes a problem, advise patient that eating solid food often provides relief.

❑ Advise patient to report signs and symptoms of fluid retention (swelling of ankles and feet, weight gain), thromboembolic disorders (pain, swelling, or tenderness in extremities; headache; chest pain; blurred vision), mental depression, hepatic dysfunction (yellowed skin or eyes, pruritus, dark urine, light-colored stools), or abnormal vaginal bleeding to health care professional.

❑ Instruct patient to stop taking medication and notify health care professional if pregnancy is suspected.

❑ Caution patient that cigarette smoking during estrogen therapy may increase risk of serious side effects, especially for women over age 35.

❑ Caution patient to use sunscreen and protective clothing to prevent increased pigmentation.

❑ Advise patient to notify health care professional of medication regimen before treatment or surgery.

❑ Advise patient treated for osteoporosis that exercise has been found to arrest and reverse bone loss. The patient should discuss any exercise limitations with health care professional before beginning program.

❑ Emphasize the importance of routine follow-up physical exams, including blood pressure; breast, abdomen, and pelvic examinations; Papanicolaou smears every 6–12 mo; and mammogram every 12 mo or as directed. Health care professional will evaluate possibility of discontinuing medication every 3–6 mo. If on continuous (not cyclical) therapy or without concurrent progestins, endometrial biopsy may be recommended, if uterus is intact.

■ **Vag:** Instruct patient in the correct use of applicator. Patient should remain recumbent for at least 30 min after administration. May use sanitary napkin to protect clothing, but do not use tampon. If a dose is missed, do not use the missed dose, but return to regular dosing schedule.

## EVALUATION

**Effectiveness of therapy can be demonstrated by:** ■ Resolution of menopausal vasomotor symptoms ❑ Decreased vaginal and vulvar itching, inflammation, or dryness associated with menopause ■ Normalization of estrogen levels in patients with ovariectomy or hypogonadism ■ Prevention of osteoporosis.

---

## etanercept

(e-**tan**-er-sept)

Enbrel

### CLASSIFICATION(S):

***Therapeutic:*** *antirheumatics (DMARDs)*
***Pharmacologic:*** *anti-TNF agents*

**Pregnancy Category B**

---

## INDICATIONS

■ To decrease progression and reduce signs and symptoms of moderately to severely active rheumatoid arthritis in patients with inadequate response to other disease-modifying agents. May be used with methotrexate.

## ACTION

■ Binds to tumor necrosis factor (TNF), making it inactive. TNF is a mediator of inflammatory response. **Therapeutic Effects:** ■ Decreased inflammation and slowed progression of rheumatoid arthritis.

## PHARMACOKINETICS

**Absorption:** 60% absorbed after subcut administration.

**Distribution:** Unknown.

**Metabolism and Excretion:** Unknown.

**Half-life:** 115 hr (range 98–300 hr).

## CONTRAINDICATIONS AND PRECAUTIONS

**Contraindicated in:** ■ Hypersensitivity ■ Sepsis ■ Lactation ■ Untreated infections.

**Use Cautiously in:** ■ Pre-existing or recent demyelinating disorders (multiple sclerosis, myelitis, optic neuritis) ■ History of tuberculosis (increased risk of reactivation) ■ Underlying chronic diseases which may predispose to infections (advanced or poorly-controlled diabetes mellitus) ■ Latex allergy (needle cover of diluent syringe contains latex) ■ Children with significant exposure to varicella virus (temporarily discontinue etanercept; consider varicella zoster immune globulin) ■ Pregnancy (use only if needed).

## ADVERSE REACTIONS AND SIDE EFFECTS*

■ **CNS:** <u>headache</u>, dizziness, weakness. ■ **EENT:** <u>rhinitis</u>, pharyngitis, sinusitis. ■ **Resp:** <u>upper respiratory tract infection</u>, cough, respiratory disorder. ■ **GI:** abdominal pain, dyspepsia. ■ **Derm:** rash. ■ **Hemat:** pancytopenia. ■ **Local:** <u>injection site reactions</u>. ■ **Misc:** INFECTIONS.

## INTERACTIONS

**Drug-Drug:** ■ May decrease the antibody response to **live-virus vaccine** and increase the risk of adverse reactions (do not administer concurrently).

## ROUTE AND DOSAGE

- **Subcut (Adults):** 25 mg twice weekly.
- **Subcut (Children 4–17 yr):** 0.4 mg/kg (not to exceed 25 mg/dose) twice weekly for 3 mo.

## AVAILABILITY

- *Powder for injection:* 25 mg/vial[Rx].

TIME/ACTION PROFILE (symptom reduction)

| | ONSET | PEAK | DURATION |
|---|---|---|---|
| Subcut | 2–4 wk | unknown | unknown |

## NURSING IMPLICATIONS

### ASSESSMENT

- ❏ Assess patient's range of motion, degree of swelling, and pain in affected joints before and periodically throughout therapy.
- ❏ Assess patient for injection site reaction (erythema, pain, itching, swelling). Reactions are usually mild to moderate and last 3–5 days after injection.
- ❏ Monitor patients who develop a new infection while taking etanercept closely. Discontinue therapy in patients who develop a serious infection or sepsis. Do not initiate therapy in patients with active infections.

### POTENTIAL NURSING DIAGNOSES

- Mobility, impaired physical (Indications).
- Pain, acute (Indications).

### IMPLEMENTATION

- **General:** Needle cover of diluent syringe contains latex and should not be handled by people with latex allergies.
- **Subcut:** Reconstitute with 1 ml of the bacteriostatic sterile water supplied by manufacturer. Inject diluent slowly into vial to avoid foaming. Some foaming will occur. Swirl gently for dissolution; do not shake or vigorously agitate to prevent excess foaming. Solution should be clear and colorless; do not administer solution that is discolored or contains particulate matter. Withdraw solution into syringe. Some foam may remain in vial. Amount in syringe should approximate 1 ml. Do not filter reconstituted solution during preparation or administration. Administer as soon as possible after reconstitution; stable up to 6 hr if refrigerated.

- ❏ May be injected into abdomen, thigh, or upper arm. Rotate sites. Do not administer within 1 inch of an old site or into area that is tender, red, hard, or bruised.
- **Syringe Incompatibility:** Do not mix with other solutions or dilute with other diluents.

### PATIENT/FAMILY TEACHING

- ❏ Instruct patient on self-administration technique, storage, and disposal of equipment. First injection should be administered under the supervision of health care professional. Provide patient with a puncture-proof container for used equipment.
- ❏ Advise patient not to receive live vaccines during therapy. Parents should be advised that children should complete immunizations to date before initiation of etanercept. Patients with significant exposure to varicella virus (chickenpox) should temporarily discontinue therapy and varicella immune globulin should be considered.
- ❏ Advise patient that methotrexate, analgesics, NSAIDs, corticosteroids, and salicylates may be continued during therapy.
- ❏ Instruct patient to notify health care professional if upper respiratory or other infections occur. Therapy may need to be discontinued if serious infection occurs.

### EVALUATION

**Effectiveness of therapy can be demonstrated by:** ▪ Reduction in symptoms of rheumatoid arthritis. Symptoms may return within 1 mo of discontinuation of therapy.

---

**ethinyl estradiol/desogestrel, See CONTRACEPTIVES, HORMONAL.**

---

**ethinyl estradiol/drospirenone, See CONTRACEPTIVES, HORMONAL.**

---

**ethinyl estradiol/ethynodiol, See CONTRACEPTIVES, HORMONAL.**

---

{ } = Available in Canada only.
*CAPITALS indicates life-threatening; underlines indicate most frequent.

**ethinyl estradiol/etonogestrel, See CONTRACEPTIVES, HORMONAL.**

**ethinyl estradiol/levonorgestrel, See CONTRACEPTIVES, HORMONAL.**

**ethinyl estradiol/norelgestromin, See CONTRACEPTIVES, HORMONAL.**

**ethinyl estradiol/norethindrone, See CONTRACEPTIVES, HORMONAL.**

**ethinyl estradiol/norgestimate, See CONTRACEPTIVES, HORMONAL.**

**ethinyl estradiol/norgestrel, See CONTRACEPTIVES, HORMONAL.**

## etidronate
(eh-tih-**droe**-nate)
Didronel

*CLASSIFICATION(S):*
*Therapeutic: bone resorption in-hibitors, hypocalcemics*
*Pharmacologic: biphosphonates*

**Pregnancy Category B (oral), C (intravenous)**

### INDICATIONS

■ Treatment of Paget's disease of bone ■ Treatment and prophylaxis of heterotopic calcification associated with total hip replacement or spinal cord injury ■ Used with other agents (saline diuresis) in the management of hypercalcemia associated with malignancies.

### ACTION

■ Blocks the growth of calcium hydroxyapatite crystals by binding to calcium phosphate.

**Therapeutic Effects:** ■ Decreased bone resorption and turnover.

### PHARMACOKINETICS

**Absorption:** Absorption is generally poor (1–6%) after oral administration.

**Distribution:** Half of the absorbed dose is bound to hydroxyapatite crystals in areas of increased osteogenesis.

**Metabolism and Excretion:** Unabsorbed drug is eliminated in the feces; 50% of the absorbed dose is excreted unchanged by the kidneys.

**Half-life:** 5–7 hr.

### CONTRAINDICATIONS AND PRECAUTIONS

**Contraindicated in:** ■ Hypersensitivity ■ Severe renal impairment (serum creatinine >5 mg/dl) ■ Hypercalcemia due to hyperparathyroidism.

**Use Cautiously in:** ■ Long bone fractures ■ CHF ■ Hypocalcemia ■ Hypovitaminosis D ■ Moderate renal impairment (dosage reduction recommended if serum creatinine 2.5–4.9 mg/dl) ■ Pregnancy, lactation, or children (safety not established).

### ADVERSE REACTIONS AND SIDE EFFECTS*

■ **GI:** diarrhea, nausea; *IV*—loss of taste, metallic taste ■ **GU:** nephrotoxicity ■ **Derm:** rash ■ **MS:** bone pain, bone tenderness, microfractures.

### INTERACTIONS

**Drug-Drug:** ■ **Antacids, mineral supplements,** or **buffers** (as in didanosine) containing **calcium, aluminum, iron,** or **magnesium** may decrease the absorption of etidronate ■ Hypocalcemic effect may be additive with **calcitonin.**

**Drug-Food:** ■ Foods containing large amounts of **calcium, aluminum, iron,** or **magnesium** may decrease the absorption of etidronate.

### ROUTE AND DOSAGE

❑ **Paget's Disease**

■ **PO (Adults):** 5–10 mg/kg/day single dose for up to 6 mo *or* 11–20 mg/kg/day for not more than 3 mo.

□ **Heterotopic Ossification (Hip Replacement)**

■ **PO (Adults):** 20 mg/kg/day for 1 mo before and 3 mo after surgery.

□ **Heterotopic Ossification (Spinal Cord Injury)**

■ **PO (Adults):** 20 mg/kg/day for 2 wk, then decreased to 10 mg/kg/day for 10 wk.

□ **Hypercalcemia**

■ **PO (Adults):** 20 mg/kg/day for 30–90 days.

■ **IV (Adults):** 7.5 mg/kg/day for 3 days; has also been given as a single dose of 25–30 mg/kg over 24 hr. May be followed by oral therapy.

## AVAILABILITY

■ *Tablets:* 200 mg^{Rx}, 400 mg^{Rx} ■ Cost: 200 mg $148.43/60, 400 mg $296.80/60 ■ *Injection:* 50 mg/ml in 6-ml ampules^{Rx}.

TIME/ACTION PROFILE

| | ONSET | PEAK | DURATION |
|---|---|---|---|
| PO (Paget's disease) | 1 mo† | unknown | 1 yr |
| PO (heterotopic calcification) | unknown | unknown | several months |
| IV‡ (hypercalcemia) | 24 hr | 3 days | 11 days |

†As measured by decreased urinary hydroxyproline.
‡As measured by decreased urinary calcium excretion.

## NURSING IMPLICATIONS

### ASSESSMENT

■ **General Info:** Assess patient for bone pain, weakness, or loss of function before and throughout therapy. Bone pain may persist or increase in patients with Paget's disease; it usually subsides days to months after therapy is discontinued. Confer with physician or other health care professional regarding analgesic to control pain.

■ **Heterotopic Ossification:** Monitor for inflammation and pain at the site and loss of function if ossification occurs near a joint.

■ **Hypercalcemia:** Monitor symptoms of hypercalcemia (nausea, vomiting, anorexia, weakness, constipation, thirst, and cardiac arrhythmias).

□ Observe patient carefully for evidence of hypocalcemia (paresthesia, muscle twitching, laryngospasm, colic, cardiac arrhythmias, and Chvostek's or Trousseau's sign). Protect symptomatic patients by elevating and padding side rails; keep bed in low position. Risk of hypocalcemia is greatest after 3 days of continuous IV therapy.

■ *Lab Test Considerations:* Etidronate interferes with bone uptake of technetium 99 in diagnostic scans.

□ *Paget's disease:* Decreased urinary excretions of hydroxyproline and serum alkaline phosphatase are often the first clinical signs of effectiveness. These values are monitored every 3 mo. Treatment is restarted when levels return to 75% of pretreatment values. Serum phosphate levels are also monitored before and 4 wk after beginning therapy. Dosage may be reduced if serum phosphate is elevated without corresponding decrease in urinary excretion of hydroxyproline or serum alkaline phosphatase.

□ *Hypercalcemia:* Monitor serum calcium and albumin levels to determine effectiveness of therapy.

□ Monitor BUN and creatine before and periodically throughout course of therapy. Stable or reversible increases in BUN and creatinine may occur in patients with hypercalcemia.

## POTENTIAL NURSING DIAGNOSES

■ Pain, acute (Indications, Side Effects).

■ Injury, risk for (Indications).

## IMPLEMENTATION

■ **General:** Do not confuse etidronate with etomidate.

■ **Hypercalcemia:** Used as adjunctive treatment after IV hydration and loop diuretics have restored urine output.

□ Oral doses may be started on the day after the last IV infusion.

■ **PO:** Administer on empty stomach, because food decreases absorption.

■ **Intermittent Infusion:** Dilute in at least 250 ml of 0.9% NaCl or D5W. Solution is

stable for 48 hr. Oral etidronate may be started on the day after last infusion.
■ *Rate:* Infuse doses of 7.5 mg/kg/day over at least 2 hr.
■ **Continuous Infusion:** May also dilute 25–30 mg/kg single dose in 1000 ml of 0.9% NaCl.
■ *Rate:* Administer over 24 hr.

## PATIENT/FAMILY TEACHING

❑ Advise patient to take as directed. If dose is missed, take as soon as remembered unless almost time for next dose. Do not double up on doses. Dose should not be taken within 2 hr of eating (especially products high in calcium) or taking vitamins or antacids, because absorption will be impaired.
❑ Instruct patient to notify health care professional if diarrhea occurs. Health care professional may divide the dose throughout the day to control diarrhea.
❑ Encourage patients to comply with diet recommendations. Diet should contain adequate amounts of calcium and vitamin D (see Appendix Q).
❑ Advise patient to notify health care professional if pain appears or worsens during therapy.
❑ Explain to patient receiving IV dose that metallic taste is not uncommon and usually disappears in a few hours.
❑ Advise patient to report signs of hypercalcemic relapse (bone pain, anorexia, nausea, vomiting, thirst, lethargy) to health care professional promptly.
❑ Emphasize need for keeping follow-up appointments to monitor progress, even after medication is discontinued, to detect relapse.

## EVALUATION

**Effectiveness of therapy can be demonstrated by:** ■ Lowered serum calcium levels ■ Decreased bone pain and fractures in Paget's disease ■ Prevention or treatment of heterotopic ossification. Normal serum calcium levels are usually attained in 2–8 days in hypercalcemia associated with bony metastasis. Therapy may be repeated once after 1 wk.

## etodolac

(ee-**toe**-doe-lak)
Lodine, Lodine XL

**CLASSIFICATION(S):**
*Therapeutic:* antirheumatics, nonopioid analgesics
*Pharmacologic:* pyranocarboxylic acid

**Pregnancy Category C**

## INDICATIONS

■ Osteoarthritis ■ Rheumatoid arthritis ■ Mild to moderate pain (not XL tablets).

## ACTION

■ Inhibits prostaglandin synthesis ■ Also has uricosuric action. **Therapeutic Effects:** ■ Suppression of inflammation ■ Decreased severity of pain.

## PHARMACOKINETICS

**Absorption:** Well absorbed after oral administration.
**Distribution:** Widely distributed,
**Protein Binding:** >99%.
**Metabolism and Excretion:** Mostly metabolized by the liver; <1% excreted unchanged in urine.
**Half-life:** 6–7 hr (single dose); 7.3 hr (chronic dosing).

## CONTRAINDICATIONS AND PRECAUTIONS

**Contraindicated in:** ■ Hypersensitivity ■ Active GI bleeding or ulcer disease ■ Cross-sensitivity may exist with other NSAIDs, including aspirin.
**Use Cautiously in:** ■ Severe cardiovascular, renal, or hepatic disease ■ History of ulcer disease ■ Pregnancy (not recommended for use during second half of pregnancy) ■ Lactation or children (safety not established).

## ADVERSE REACTIONS AND SIDE EFFECTS*

■ **CNS:** depression, dizziness, drowsiness, insomnia, malaise, nervousness, syncope, weakness ■ **EENT:** blurred vision, photophobia, tinnitus ■ **Resp:** asthma ■ **CV:** CHF, edema, hypertension, palpitations ■ **GI:** GI BLEEDING, dyspepsia, abdominal pain, constipation, diarrhea, drug-induced hepatitis, dry mouth, flatulence, gastritis, nausea, stomatitis, thirst, vomiting ■ **GU:** dysuria, renal failure, urinary frequency ■ **Derm:** ecchymoses, flushing, hyperpigmentation, pruritus, rashes, sweating ■ **Hemat:** anemia, prolonged bleeding time, thrombocytopenia ■ **Misc:** allergic reactions including ANAPHYLAXIS, ANGIOEDEMA, STEVENS-JOHNSON SYNDROME, chills, fever.

## INTERACTIONS

**Drug-Drug:** ■ Concurrent use with **aspirin** may decrease effectiveness ■ Additive adverse GI effects with **aspirin,** other **NSAIDs, potassium supplements, corticosteroids, antiplatelet agents,** or **alcohol** ■ Chronic use with **acetaminophen** may increase the risk of adverse renal reactions ■ May decrease the effectiveness of **diuretic** or **antihypertensive** therapy ■ May increase serum **lithium** levels and increase the risk of toxicity ■ Increases the risk of toxicity from **methotrexate** ■ Increased risk of bleeding with **cefamandole, cefotetan, cefoperazone, valproic acid, plicamycin, thrombolytic agents, antiplatelet agents,** or **anticoagulants** ■ Increased risk of adverse hematologic reactions with **antineoplastics** or **radiation therapy** ■ May increase the risk of nephrotoxicity from **cyclosporine.**

**Drug-Natural Products:** ■ Increased risk of bleeding with **arnica, chamomile, clove, dong quai, fever few, garlic, ginko,** and **Panax ginseng.**

## ROUTE AND DOSAGE

■ **PO (Adults):** *Analgesia*—200–400 mg q 6–8 hr (not to exceed 1200 mg/day). *Osteoarthritis/rheumatoid arthritis*—300 mg 2–3 times daily, 400 mg twice daily, or 500 mg twice daily; may also be given as 400–1200 mg once daily as XL tablets.

## AVAILABILITY (generic available)

■ *Capsules:* 200 mg<sup>Rx</sup>, 300 mg<sup>Rx</sup> ■ Cost: 200 mg $106.13/100, 300 mg $120.22/100 ■ *Tablets:* 400 mg<sup>Rx</sup>, 500 mg<sup>Rx</sup> ■ *Extended-release tablets (XL):* 400 mg<sup>Rx</sup>, 600 mg<sup>Rx</sup>.

TIME/ACTION PROFILE (analgesic effect)

| | ONSET | PEAK | DURATION |
|---|---|---|---|
| PO (analgesic) | 0.5 hr | 1–2 hr | 4–12 hr |
| PO (anti-inflammatory) | days–wks | unknown | 6–12 hr† |

†Up to 24 hr as XL (extended-release) tablet.

## NURSING IMPLICATIONS

### ASSESSMENT

■ **General Info:** Patients who have asthma, aspirin-induced allergy, and nasal polyps are at increased risk for developing hypersensitivity reactions. Monitor for rhinitis, asthma, and urticaria.

■ **Osteoarthritis/Rheumatoid Arthritis:** Assess pain and range of movement before and 1–2 hr after administration.

■ **Pain:** Assess location, duration, and intensity of the pain before and 60 min after administration.

■ *Lab Test Considerations:* May cause decreased hemoglobin, hematocrit, leukocyte, and platelet counts.

❑ Monitor liver function tests within 8 wk of initiating etodolac therapy and periodically during therapy. May cause elevated serum alkaline phosphatase, LDH, AST, and ALT concentrations.

❑ Monitor BUN, serum creatinine, and electrolytes periodically during therapy. May cause increased BUN, serum creatinine, and electrolyte concentrations and decreased urine electrolyte concentrations.

❑ May cause decreased serum and increased urine uric acid concentrations.

### POTENTIAL NURSING DIAGNOSES

■ Pain, acute (Indications).

■ Mobility, impaired physical (Indications).

### IMPLEMENTATION

■ **General:** Do not confuse Lodine (etodolac) with codeine or iodine.

❑ Administration in higher-than-recommended doses does not provide increased effectiveness but may cause increased side effects.

■ **PO:** For rapid initial effect, administer 30 min before or 2 hr after meals. May be administered with food, milk, or antacids containing aluminum or magnesium to decrease GI irritation.

❑ Do not crush, break, or chew extended-release tablets.

## PATIENT/FAMILY TEACHING

❏ Advise patients to take etodolac with a full glass of water and to remain in an upright position for 15–30 min after administration.

❏ Instruct patient to take medication exactly as directed. If a dose is missed, take as soon as possible within 1–2 hr if taking twice/day, or unless almost time for next dose if taking more than twice/day. Do not double doses.

❏ Etodolac may occasionally cause drowsiness or dizziness. Advise patient to avoid driving or other activities requiring alertness until response to the medication is known.

❏ Caution patient to avoid the concurrent use of alcohol, aspirin, acetaminophen, NSAIDs, or other OTC medications without consultation with health care professional.

❏ Advise patient to inform health care professional of medication regimen before treatment or surgery.

❏ Advise patient to consult health care professional if rash, itching, visual disturbances, tinnitus, weight gain, edema, black stools, persistent headache, or influenza-like syndrome (chills, fever, muscle aches, pain) occurs.

## EVALUATION

**Effectiveness of therapy can be demonstrated by:** ■ Decreased severity of pain ■ Improved joint mobility. Patients who do not respond to one NSAID may respond to another. May require 2 wk or more for maximum anti-inflammatory effects.

**High Alert**

# ETOPOSIDES

(e-**toe**-poe-sides)

**etoposide**
VePesid, VP-16

**etoposide phosphate**
Etopophos

*CLASSIFICATION(S):*
*Therapeutic: antineoplastics*
*Pharmacologic: podophyllotoxin derivatives*

**Pregnancy Category D**

## INDICATIONS

■ Refractory testicular neoplasms ■ Small cell lung carcinoma ■ Used alone and with other modalities (other antineoplastics, radiation therapy, surgery): ❏ neoplasms **Unlabeled uses:** ■ Lymphomas and some leukemias.

## ACTION

■ Damages DNA before mitosis (cycle-dependent and phase-specific). **Therapeutic Effects:** ■ Death of rapidly replicating cells, particularly malignant ones.

## PHARMACOKINETICS

**Absorption:** Variably absorbed after oral administration. After IV administration, etoposide phosphate is rapidly converted to etoposide.

**Distribution:** Rapidly distributed, does not appear to enter the CSF but probably crosses placenta; enters breast milk.

**Protein Binding:** 97%.

**Metabolism and Excretion:** Some metabolism by the liver with biliary excretion, 44% excreted in feces; 45% excreted unchanged by the kidneys.

**Half-life:** 7 hr (range 3–12 hr).

## CONTRAINDICATIONS AND PRECAUTIONS

**Contraindicated in:** ■ Hypersensitivity ■ Pregnancy ■ Lactation ■ Known intolerance to benzyl alcohol, ethyl alcohol, polyethylene glycol (IV etoposide only), or dextran (IV etoposide phosphate only).

**Use Cautiously in:** ■ Patients with childbearing potential ■ Active infections ■ Decreased bone marrow reserve ■ Renal/hepatic impairment (dosage modification may be necessary) ■ Other chronic debilitating illnesses.

## ADVERSE REACTIONS AND SIDE EFFECTS*

■ **CNS:** drowsiness, fatigue, headache, vertigo ■ **Resp:** PULMONARY EDEMA, bronchospasm ■ **CV:** CHF, MI, hypotension (IV) ■ **GI:** nausea, vomiting ■ **Derm:** alopecia ■ **Endo:** sterility ■ **Hemat:** leukopenia, thrombocytopenia ■ **Local:** phlebitis at IV site ■ **MS:** muscle cramps ■ **Neuro:** peripheral neuropathy ■ **Misc:** allergic reactions including ANAPHYLAXIS, fever.

## INTERACTIONS

**Drug-Drug:** ■ ↑ bone marrow depression with other **antineoplastics** or **radiation**

therapy ■ May alter immune response to **live-virus vaccines** and ↑ risk of adverse reactions.

## ROUTE AND DOSAGE

Other regimens are used.

### ◻ Testicular Neoplasms

■ **IV (Adults):** 50–100 mg/m² daily for 5 days; repeat every 3–4 wk up to 100 mg/m² on days 1, 3, and 5 every 3–4 wk.

### ◻ Small-Cell Carcinoma of the Lung

■ **PO (Adults):** 70 mg/m² (rounded to the nearest 50 mg)/day for 4 days, repeated every 3–4 wk up to 100 mg/m² (rounded to the nearest 50 mg)/day for 5 days every 3–4 wk.

■ **IV (Adults):** 35 mg/m² daily for 4 days up to 50 mg/m² daily for 5 days every 3–4 wk.

## AVAILABILITY

### ◻ Etoposide

■ *Capsules:* 50 mg^Rx ■ *Injection:* 20 mg/ml^Rx ■ Cost: $136.49/5 ml, $665.38/25 ml, $1296.64/50 ml.

### ◻ Etoposide Phosphate

■ *Powder for injection:* 100 mg/vial (with dextran)^Rx ■ Cost: $124.14/vial.

TIME/ACTION PROFILE (noted as effects on blood counts)

| | ONSET | PEAK | DURATION |
|----|----------|-----------|----------|
| PO | 7–14 days | 9–16 days | 20 days |
| IV | 7–14 days | 9–16 days | 20 days |

# NURSING IMPLICATIONS

## ASSESSMENT

◻ Monitor blood pressure before and every 15 min during infusion. If hypotension occurs, stop infusion and notify physician or other health care professional. After stabilizing blood pressure with IV fluids and supportive measures, infusion may be resumed at slower rate.

◻ Monitor for hypersensitivity reaction (fever, chills, pruritus, urticaria, bronchospasm, tachycardia, hypotension). If these occur, stop infusion and notify physician. Keep epinephrine, an antihistamine, corticosteroids, volume expanders, and resuscitative equipment close by in the event of an anaphylactic reaction.

◻ Assess for signs of infection (fever, chills, cough, hoarseness, lower back or side pain, sore throat, difficult or painful urination). Notify physician if these symptoms occur.

◻ Assess for bleeding (bleeding gums, bruising, petechiae, guaiac test stools, urine, and emesis). Avoid IM injections and taking rectal temperatures. Apply pressure to venipuncture sites for 10 min.

◻ Monitor intake and output, appetite, and nutritional intake. Etoposide causes nausea and vomiting in 30% of patients. Prophylactic antiemetics may decrease frequency and duration of nausea and vomiting.

◻ Adjust diet as tolerated to help maintain fluid and electrolyte balance and nutritional status.

■ *Lab Test Considerations:* Monitor CBC and differential before and periodically during therapy. The nadir of leukopenia occurs in 7–14 days. Notify physician if leukocyte count is <1000/mm³. The nadir of thrombocytopenia occurs in 9–16 days. Notify physician if the platelet count is <75,000/mm³. Recovery of leukopenia and thrombocytopenia occurs in 20 days.

◻ Monitor liver function studies (AST, ALT, LDH, bilirubin) and renal function studies (BUN, creatinine) before and periodically during therapy to detect hepatotoxicity and nephrotoxicity.

◻ May cause ↑ uric acid. Monitor levels periodically during therapy.

## POTENTIAL NURSING DIAGNOSES

■ Injury, risk for (Side Effects).
■ Infection, risk for (Side Effects).

## IMPLEMENTATION

◻ *High Alert:* Fatalities have occurred with incorrect administration of chemotherapeutic agents. Before administering, clarify all ambiguous orders; double check single, daily, and course-of-therapy dose limits; have second practitioner independently double check original order, calculations and infusion pump settings. Do not confuse VePesid (etoposide) with Versed (midazolam). Do not confuse etoposide (VePesid) with etoposide phosphate (Etopophos).

■ **General:** Solution should be prepared in a biologic cabinet. Wear gloves, gown, and mask while handling medication. Discard equipment in designated containers.

❏ Avoid contact with skin. Use Luer-Lok tubing to prevent accidental leakage. If contact with skin occurs, immediately wash skin with soap and water.

■ **PO:** Capsules should be refrigerated.

❏ **Etoposide (VePesid)**

■ **Intermittent Infusion:** Dilute 5-ml vial with 250–500 ml of D5W or 0.9% NaCl for a concentration of 200–400 mcg/ml. The 200-mcg/ml solution is stable for 96 hr. The 400-mcg/ml solution is stable for 48 hr. Concentrations >400 mcg/ml are not recommended, because crystallization is likely. Discard solution if crystals are present.

■ *Rate:* Infuse slowly over 30–60 min. Temporary hypotension may occur with infusion rates shorter than 30 min.

■ **Y-Site Compatibility:** ◆ allopurinol ◆ amifostine ◆ aztreonam ◆ cladribine ◆ doxorubicin liposome ◆ fludarabine ◆ gemcitabine ◆ granisetron ◆ melphalan ◆ methotrexate ◆ mitoxandrone ◆ ondansetron ◆ paclitaxel ◆ piperacillin/tazobactam ◆ sargramostim ◆ sodium bicarbonate ◆ teniposide ◆ thiotepa ◆ topotecan ◆ vinorelbine.

■ **Y-Site Incompatibility:** ◆ cefepime ◆ filgrastim ◆ idarubicin.

■ **Additive Compatibility:** ◆ carboplatin ◆ cisplatin ◆ cytarabine ◆ floxuridine ◆ fluorouracil ◆ ifosfamide ◆ ondansetron.

❏ **Etoposide phosphate (Etopophos)**

■ **Intermittent Infusion:** Reconstitute each vial with 5 or 10 ml of sterile water, D5W, or 0.9% NaCl for a concentration of 20 or 10 mg/ml, respectively.

❏ May be administered undiluted or diluted to a concentration as low as 0.1 mg/ml with D5W or 0.9% NaCl.

❏ Reconstituted solutions are stable for 24 hr at room temperature or if refrigerated.

■ *Rate:* Administer over at least 5–10 min.

■ **Y-Site Compatibility:** ◆ acyclovir ◆ amikacin ◆ aminophylline ◆ ampcillin ◆ ampicillin/sulbactam ◆ aztreonam ◆ bleomycin ◆ bumetanide ◆ buprenorphine ◆ butorphanol ◆ calcium gluconate ◆ carboplatin ◆ carmustine ◆

cefazolin ◆ cefoperazone ◆ cefotaxime ◆ cefotetan ◆ cefoxitin ◆ ceftazidime ◆ ceftizoxime ◆ ceftriaxone ◆ cefuroxime ◆ cimetidine ◆ ciprofloxacin ◆ cisplatin ◆ clindamycin ◆ cyclophosphamide ◆ cytarabine ◆ dacarbazine ◆ dactinomycin ◆ daunorubicin ◆ diphenhydramine ◆ dobutamine ◆ dopamine ◆ doxorubicin ◆ doxycycline ◆ droperidol ◆ enalaprilat ◆ famotidine ◆ floxuridine ◆ fluconazole ◆ fludarabine ◆ fluorouracil ◆ furosemide ◆ ganciclovir ◆ gatifloxacin ◆ gemcitabine ◆ gentamicin ◆ granisetron ◆ haloperidol ◆ heparin ◆ hydrocortisone ◆ hydromorphone ◆ idarubicin ◆ ifosfamide ◆ leucovorin calcium ◆ linezolid ◆ lorazepam ◆ magnesium sulfate ◆ mannitol ◆ meperidine ◆ mesna ◆ methotrexate ◆ metoclopramide ◆ metronidazole ◆ minocycline ◆ mitoxantrone ◆ morphine ◆ nalbuphine ◆ netilmicin ◆ ofloxacin ◆ ondansetron ◆ paclitaxel ◆ piperacillin ◆ piperacillin/tazobactam ◆ plicamycin ◆ potassium chloride ◆ promethazine ◆ ranitidine ◆ sodium bicarbonate ◆ streptozocin ◆ teniposide ◆ thiotepa ◆ ticarcillin ◆ ticarcillin/clavulanate ◆ tobramycin ◆ trimethoprim/sulfamethoxazole ◆ vancomycin ◆ vinblastine ◆ vincristine ◆ zidovudine

■ **Y-Site Incompatibility:** ◆ amphotericin B ◆ cefepime ◆ chlorpromazine ◆ imipenem/cilastatin ◆ methylprednisolone ◆ mitomycin ◆ prochlorperazine

## PATIENT/FAMILY TEACHING

❏ Instruct patient to take etoposide exactly as directed, even if nausea or vomiting occurs. If vomiting occurs shortly after dose is taken, consult physician. If a dose is missed, do not take at all.

❏ Advise patient to notify health care professional if fever; chills; sore throat or other signs of infection; bleeding gums; bruising; petechiae; or blood in urine, stool, or emesis occurs. Caution patient to avoid crowds and persons with known infections. Instruct patient to use soft toothbrush and electric razor. Caution patient not to drink alcoholic beverages or take products containing aspirin or NSAIDs.

❏ Instruct patient to notify health care professional if rapid heartbeat, difficulty breathing, abdominal pain, yellow skin, weakness, paresthesia, or gait disturbances occur.

❏ Instruct patient to inspect oral mucosa for redness and ulceration. If mouth sores oc-

cur, advise patient to use sponge brush and rinse mouth with water after eating and drinking. Viscous lidocaine swishes may be used if pain interferes with eating. Stomatitis pain may require treatment with opioid analgesics.
- ❑ Discuss with patient the possibility of hair loss. Explore coping strategies.
- ❑ Advise patient to use contraception.
- ❑ Instruct patient not to receive any vaccinations without advice of physician.
- ❑ Emphasize the need for periodic lab tests to monitor for side effects.

## EVALUATION

**Effectiveness of therapy can be demonstrated by:** ■ Decrease in size or spread of malignancies in solid tumors ■ Improvement of hematologic status in leukemias.

---

# ezetimibe
(e-**zet**-i-mibe)
Zetia

### CLASSIFICATION(S):
**Therapeutic:** lipid-lowering agents
**Pharmacologic:** cholesterol absorption inhibitors

### Pregnancy Category C

## INDICATIONS

■ Alone or with other agents (HMG-CoA reductase inhibitors) in the management of dyslipidemias including primary hypercholesterolemia, homozygous familial hypercholesterolemia and homozygous sitosterolemia.

## ACTION

■ Inhibits absorption of cholesterol in the small intestine. **Therapeutic Effects:** ■ Lowering of cholesterol, a known risk factor for atherosclerosis.

## PHARMACOKINETICS

**Absorption:** Following absoption, rapidly converted to ezetimibe-glucaronide, which is active. Bioavailability is variable.
**Distribution:** Unknown.

**Metabolism and Excretion:** Undergoes enterhepatic recycling, mostly eliminated in feces, minimal renal excretion.
**Half-life:** 22 hr.

## CONTRAINDICATIONS AND PRECAUTIONS

**Contraindicated in:** ■ Hypersensitivity ■ Acute liver disease or unexplained laboratory evidence of liver disease (when used with HMG-CoA reductase inhibitor) ■ Moderate or severe hepatic insufficiency ■ Concurrent use of fibrates.
**Use Cautiously in:** ■ Lactation (use only if benefit to mother outweighs possible risks to infant) ■ Pregnancy or children <10 yr (safety not established).

## ADVERSE REACTIONS AND SIDE EFFECTS*

■ **GI:** increased hepatic transaminases (with HMG-CoA reductase inhibitors).

## INTERACTIONS

**Drug-Drug:** ■ Effects may be ↓ by **cholestyramine** or other **bile acid sequestrants** ■ Concurrent use of **fibrates** may ↑ blood levels of ezetimibe and also ↑ the risk of cholelithiasis ■ **Cyclosporine** may ↑ ezetimibe levels.

## ROUTE AND DOSAGE

■ **PO (Adults):** 10 mg once daily.

## AVAILABILITY

■ *Tablets:* 10 mg.

TIME/ACTION PROFILE

| | ONSET | PEAK | DURATION |
|---|---|---|---|
| PO | unknown | unknown | unknown |

# NURSING IMPLICATIONS

## ASSESSMENT

- ❑ Obtain a diet history, especially with regard to fat consumption.
- ■ *Lab Test Considerations:* Serum cholesterol and triglyceride levels should be evaluated before initiating, after 2–4 wk of therapy, and periodically thereafter.

❑ May cause elevated liver transaminases when administered with HMG-CoA reductase inhibitors. Monitor liver enzymes prior to initiation and throughout therapy according to recommendations of HMG-CoA reductase inhibitor. Elevations are usually asymptomatic and return to baseline with continued therapy.

## POTENTIAL NURSING DIAGNOSES

■ Noncompliance, related to diet and medication regimen (Patient/Family Teaching).

## IMPLEMENTATION

■ **PO:** Administer without regard to meals. May be taken at the same time as HMG-CoA reductase inhibitors.

## PATIENT/FAMILY TEACHING

❑ Instruct patient to take medication exactly as directed, at the same time each day, even if feeling well. Take missed doses as soon as remembered, but do not take more than 1 dose/day. Medication helps control but does not cure elevated serum cholesterol levels.

❑ Advise patient that this medication should be used in conjunction with diet restrictions (fat, cholesterol, carbohydrates, alcohol), exercise, and cessation of smoking. Ezetimibe does not assist with weight loss.

❑ Instruct female patients to notify health care professional promptly if pregnancy is planned or suspected or if breast feeding. If regimen includes HMG-CoA reductase inhibitors, they are contraindicated in pregnancy.

❑ Instruct patient to notify health care professional if unexplained muscle pain, tenderness, or weakness occur.

❑ Advise patient to avoid taking OTC medications or natural/herbal products without consulting health care professional.

❑ Advise patient to notify health care professional of medication regimen prior to treatment or surgery.

❑ Emphasize the importance of follow-up exams to determine effectiveness and to monitor for side effects.

## EVALUATION

**Effectiveness of therapy can be demonstrated by:** ■ Decrease in serum LDL and total cholesterol levels ❑ Increase in HDL cholesterol levels.

# famciclovir

(fam-**sye**-kloe-veer)

Famvir

*CLASSIFICATION(S):*
*Therapeutic: antivirals*

## Pregnancy Category B

## INDICATIONS

■ Acute herpes zoster infections (shingles) ■ Treatment/suppression of recurrent herpes genitalis in immunocompetent patients ■ Treatment of recurrent mucocutaneous herpes simplex virus (HSV) infection in HIV-infected patients.

## ACTION

■ Inhibits viral DNA synthesis in herpes-infected cells only. **Therapeutic Effects:** ■ Decreased duration of herpes zoster infection with decreased duration of viral shedding ■ Decreased lesion formation and improved healing in recurrent HSV infection.

## PHARMACOKINETICS

**Absorption:** Following absorption, famciclovir is rapidly converted in the intestinal wall to penciclovir, the active compound.

**Distribution:** Unknown.

**Metabolism and Excretion:** Penciclovir is mostly excreted by the kidneys.

**Half-life:** *Penciclovir*—2.1–3 hr (increased in renal impairment).

## CONTRAINDICATIONS AND PRECAUTIONS

**Contraindicated in:** ■ Hypersensitivity.

**Use Cautiously in:** ■ Patients with impaired renal function (increased dosage interval/decreased dose recommended if CCr <40–60 ml/min) ■ Geriatric patients (because of age-related decrease in renal function) ■ Pregnancy, lactation, or children <18 yr (safety not established).

## ADVERSE REACTIONS AND SIDE EFFECTS*

■ **CNS:** <u>headache</u>, dizziness, fatigue ■ **GI:** diarrhea, nausea, vomiting.

## INTERACTIONS

**Drug-Drug:** ■ **Probenecid** increases plasma concentration of penciclovir.

## ROUTE AND DOSAGE

❑ **Herpes Zoster**

■ **PO (Adults):** 500 mg q 8 hr for 7 days.

❑ **Renal Impairment**

■ **PO (Adults):** *CCr 40–59 ml/min*—500 mg q 12 hr; *CCr 20–39ml/min*—500 mg q 24 hr; *CCr <20 ml/min*—250 mg q 24 hr.

❑ **Recurrent Herpes Simplex Infections**

■ **PO (Adults):** 125 mg q 12 hr for 5 days.

❑ **Renal Impairment**

■ **PO (Adults):** *CCr <39 ml/min*—125 mg q 24 hr for 5 days.

❑ **Suppression of Recurrent Herpes Simplex Infections**

■ **PO (Adults):** 250 mg q 12 hr for up to 1 yr.

❑ **Renal Impairment**

■ **PO (Adults):** *CCr 20–39 ml/min*—125 mg q 12 hr for 5 days; *CCr <20 ml/min*—125 mg q 24 hr for 5 days.

❑ **Herpes Simplex in HIV-Infected Patients**

■ **PO (Adults):** 500 mg q 12 hr for 7 days.

❑ **Renal Impairment**

■ **PO (Adults):** *CCr 20–39 ml/min*—500 mg q 24 hr for 7 days; *CCr <20 ml/min*—250 mg q 24 hr for 7 days.

## AVAILABILITY

■ *Tablets:* 125 mg$^{Rx}$, 250 mg$^{Rx}$, 500 mg$^{Rx}$ ■ Cost: 125 mg $101.40/30, 250 mg $110.25/30, 500 mg $221.30/30.

TIME/ACTION PROFILE (penciclovir blood levels)

|  | ONSET | PEAK | DURATION |
|---|---|---|---|
| PO | rapid | 0.9 hr | 8–12 hr |

# NURSING IMPLICATIONS

## ASSESSMENT

❑ Assess lesions prior to and daily during therapy.

❑ Assess patient for postherpetic neuralgia periodically during and following therapy.

## POTENTIAL NURSING DIAGNOSES

■ Skin integrity, risk for impaired (Indications).

■ Infection, risk for (Indications, Patient/Family Teaching).

## IMPLEMENTATION

■ **General:** Famciclovir therapy should be started as soon as herpes zoster is diagnosed, at least within 72 hr, preferably within 48 hr.

■ **PO:** Famciclovir may be administered without regard to meals.

## PATIENT/FAMILY TEACHING

❑ Instruct patient to take famciclovir exactly as directed for the full course of therapy. If a dose is missed, take as soon as remembered if not just before next dose.

❑ Inform patient that famciclovir does not prevent the spread of infection to others. Until all lesions have crusted, precautions should be taken around others who have not had chickenpox or varicella vaccine or people who are immunosuppressed.

❑ Advise patient that condoms should be used during sexual contact and that no sexual contact should be made while lesions are present.

❑ Instruct women with genital herpes to have yearly Papanicolaou smears because these women may be more likely to develop cervical cancer.

## EVALUATION

**Effectiveness of therapy can be demonstrated by:** ■ Decrease in time to full crusting, loss of vesicles, loss of ulcers, and loss of crusts in patients with acute herpes zoster (shingles) ■ Crusting over and healing of lesions in genital herpes and in recurrent mucocutaneous HSV infection in HIV-infected patients ■ Prevention of recurrence of herpes genitalis.

## famotidine, See HISTAMINE H₂ ANTAGONISTS.

## felodipine
(fe-**loe**-di-peen)
Plendil, {Renedil}

### CLASSIFICATION(S):
**Therapeutic:** antianginals, antihypertensives
**Pharmacologic:** calcium channel blockers

### Pregnancy Category C

## INDICATIONS

■ Management of hypertension, angina pectoris, and vasospastic (Prinzmetal's) angina.

## ACTION

■ Inhibits the transport of calcium into myocardial and vascular smooth muscle cells, resulting in inhibition of excitation-contraction coupling and subsequent contraction. **Therapeutic Effects:** ■ Systemic vasodilation resulting in decreased blood pressure ■ Coronary vasodilation resulting in decreased frequency and severity of attacks of angina.

## PHARMACOKINETICS

**Absorption:** Well absorbed after oral administration, but extensively metabolized, resulting in decreased bioavailability.

**Distribution:** Unknown.

**Protein Binding:** >99%.

**Metabolism and Excretion:** Mostly metabolized; minimal amounts excreted unchanged by kidneys.

**Half-life:** 11–16 hr.

## CONTRAINDICATIONS AND PRECAUTIONS

**Contraindicated in:** ■ Hypersensitivity (cross-sensitivity may occur) ■ Sick sinus syndrome ■ 2nd- or 3rd-degree AV block (unless an artificial pacemaker is in place) ■ Blood pressure <90 mmHg.

**Use Cautiously in:** ■ Severe hepatic impairment (dosage reduction recommended) ■ Geriatric patients (dosage reduction recommended; increased risk of hypotension) ■ Severe renal impairment ■ History of serious ventricular arrhythmias or CHF ■ Pregnancy, lactation, or children (safety not established).

## ADVERSE REACTIONS AND SIDE EFFECTS*

■ **CNS:** <u>headache</u>, abnormal dreams, anxiety, confusion, dizziness, drowsiness, nervousness, psychiatric disturbances, weakness ■ **EENT:** blurred vision, disturbed equilibrium, epistaxis, tinnitus ■ **Resp:** cough, dyspnea ■ **CV:** ARRHYTH-MIAS, CHF, <u>peripheral edema</u>, bradycardia, chest pain, hypotension, palpitations, syncope, tachycardia ■ **GI:** abnormal liver function studies, anorexia, constipation, diarrhea, dry mouth, dysgeusia, dyspepsia, nausea, vomiting ■ **GU:** dysuria, nocturia, polyuria, sexual dysfunction, urinary frequency ■ **Derm:** dermatitis, erythema multiforme, flushing, increased sweating, photosensitivity, pruritus/urticaria, rash ■ **Endo:** gynecomastia, hyperglycemia ■ **Hemat:** anemia, leukopenia, thrombocytopenia ■ **Metab:** weight gain ■ **MS:** joint stiffness, muscle cramps ■ **Neuro:** paresthesia, tremor ■ **Misc:** STEVENS-JOHNSON SYNDROME, gingival hyperplasia.

## INTERACTIONS

**Drug-Drug:** ■ Additive hypotension may occur when used concurrently with **fentanyl**, other **antihypertensives, nitrates,** acute ingestion of **alcohol,** or **quinidine** ■ Antihypertensive effects may be decreased by concurrent use of **NSAIDs** ■ Concurrent use with **beta blockers, digoxin, disopyramide,** or **phenytoin** may result in bradycardia, conduction defects, or CHF ■ **Ketoconazole, itraconazole, propranolol** and **erythromycin** decrease metabolism, increase blood levels and the risk of toxicity (dosage reduction may be necessary).

**Drug-Food:** ■ **Grapefruit juice** increases blood levels and effects (avoid concurrent use).

## ROUTE AND DOSAGE

■ **PO (Adults):** 5 mg/day (2.5 mg/day in geriatric patients); may increase q 2 wk (range 5–10 mg/day; not to exceed 10 mg/day).

## AVAILABILITY

■ *Extended-release tablets:* 2.5 mg^Rx, 5 mg^Rx, 10 mg^Rx ■ Cost: 2.5 mg $29.81/30, 5 mg $29.81/30, 10 mg $53.54/30 ■ with enalapril (Lexxel and Lexxel2)^Rx. See Appendix B.

TIME/ACTION PROFILE (antihypertensive effect)

| | ONSET | PEAK | DURATION |
|---|---|---|---|
| PO | 1 hr | 2–4 hr | up to 24 hr |

# NURSING IMPLICATIONS

## ASSESSMENT

■ **General Info:** Monitor blood pressure and pulse before therapy, during dosage titration, and periodically throughout therapy. Monitor ECG periodically during prolonged therapy.

❑ Monitor intake and output ratios and daily weight. Assess for signs of CHF (peripheral edema, rales/crackles, dyspnea, weight gain, jugular venous distention).

■ **Angina:** Assess location, duration, intensity, and precipitating factors of patient's anginal pain.

■ **Hypertension:** Check frequency of refills to monitor adherence.

■ *Lab Test Considerations:* Total serum calcium concentrations are not affected by calcium channel blockers.

❑ Monitor serum potassium periodically. Hypokalemia increases the risk of arrhythmias and should be corrected.

❑ Monitor renal and hepatic functions periodically during long-term therapy. May cause increase in hepatic enzymes after several days of therapy, which return to normal upon discontinuation of therapy.

## POTENTIAL NURSING DIAGNOSES

■ Tissue perfusion, ineffective (Indications).
■ Pain, acute (Indications).

## IMPLEMENTATION

■ **General:** Do not confuse Plendil (felodipine) with pindolol.

■ **PO:** May be administered without regard to meals. May be administered with meals if GI irritation becomes a problem.

❑ Do not crush, break, or chew sustained-release tablets. Empty tablets that appear in stool are not significant.

## PATIENT/FAMILY TEACHING

■ **General Info:** Advise patient to take medication exactly as directed, even if feeling well. If a dose is missed, take as soon as possible unless almost time for next dose; do not double doses. May need to be discontinued gradually.

❑ Instruct patient on correct technique for monitoring pulse. Instruct patient to contact health care professional if heart rate is <50 bpm.

❑ Caution patient to change positions slowly to minimize orthostatic hypotension.

❑ May cause drowsiness or dizziness. Advise patient to avoid driving or other activities requiring alertness until response to the medication is known.

❑ Instruct patient on importance of maintaining good dental hygiene and seeing dentist frequently for teeth cleaning to prevent tenderness, bleeding, and gingival hyperplasia (gum enlargement).

❑ Instruct patient to avoid concurrent use of alcohol or OTC medications, especially cold preparations, without consulting health care professional.

❑ Advise patient to notify health care professional if irregular heartbeat, dyspnea, swelling of hands and feet, pronounced dizziness, nausea, constipation, or hypotension occurs or if headache is severe or persistent.

❑ Caution patient to wear protective clothing and to use sunscreen to prevent photosensitivity reactions.

❑ Advise patient to inform health care professional of medication regimen before treatment or surgery.

■ **Angina:** Instruct patient on concurrent nitrate or beta-blocker therapy to continue taking both medications as directed and to use SL nitroglycerin as needed for anginal attacks.

❑ Advise patient to contact health care professional if chest pain does not improve or worsens after therapy, occurs with diaphoresis or shortness of breath, or if severe, persistent headache occurs.

❑ Caution patient to discuss exercise restrictions with health care professional before exertion.

■ **Hypertension:** Encourage patient to comply with other interventions for hypertension (weight reduction, low-sodium diet, smoking cessation, moderation of alcohol consumption, regular exercise, and stress management). Medication controls but does not cure hypertension.

❑ Instruct patient and family in proper technique for monitoring blood pressure. Advise patient to take blood pressure weekly and to report significant changes.

## EVALUATION

**Effectiveness of therapy can be demonstrated by:** ■ Decrease in blood pressure ■ Decrease in frequency and severity of anginal attacks ❑ Decrease in need for nitrate therapy ❑ Increase in activity tolerance and sense of well-being.

## fenofibrate

(fen-o-**fi**-brate)
Lofibra, Tricor

### CLASSIFICATION(S):

**Therapeutic:** lipid-lowering agents
**Pharmacologic:** fibric acid derivatives

### Pregnancy Category C

## INDICATIONS

■ With dietary therapy to decrease LDL cholesterol, total cholesterol, triglycerides, and apoliporotein B in adult patients with hypercholesterolemia or mixed dyslipidemia ■ With dietary management in the treatment of hypertriglyceridemia (types IV and V hyperlipidemia) in patients who are at risk for pancreatitis and do not respond to nondrug therapy.

## ACTION

■ Fenofibric acid primarily inhibits triglyceride synthesis. **Therapeutic Effects:** ■ Lowering of triglycerides with subsequent decreased risk of pancreatitis.

## PHARMACOKINETICS

**Absorption:** Well absorbed (60%) after oral administration; absorption is increased by food.
**Distribution:** Unknown.
**Protein Binding:** 99%.
**Metabolism and Excretion:** Rapidly converted to fenofibric acid, which is the active metabolite; fenofibric acid is metabolized by the liver.

Fenofibric acid and its metabolites are primarily excreted in urine (60%).
**Half-life:** 20 hr.

## CONTRAINDICATIONS AND PRECAUTIONS

**Contraindicated in:** ■ Hypersensitivity ■ Hepatic impairment (including primary biliary cirrhosis) ■ Pre-existing gallbladder disease ■ Severe renal impairment ■ Concurrent use of HMG-CoA reductase inhibitors ■ Lactation.

**Use Cautiously in:** ■ Concurrent warfarin therapy ■ Pregnancy or children (use in pregnancy only if benefits outweigh risks to the fetus; safety not established).

## ADVERSE REACTIONS AND SIDE EFFECTS*

■ **CNS:** fatigue/weakness, headache ■ **CV:** arrhythmias ■ **GI:** cholelithiasis, pancreatitis ■ **Derm:** rash, urticaria ■ **MS:** rhabdomyolysis ■ **Misc:** hypersensitivity reactions.

## INTERACTIONS

**Drug-Drug:** ■ ↑ anticoagulant effects of **warfarin** ■ Concurrent use with **HMG-CoA reductase inhibitors** ↑ risk of rhabdomyolysis (combined use should be avoided) ■ Absorption is ↓ by **bile acid sequestrants** (fenofibrate should be given 1 hr before or 4–6 hr after) ■ ↑ risk of nephrotoxicity with **cyclosporine**.

## ROUTE AND DOSAGE

■ **PO (Adults):** *Hypercholesterolemia*—160 mg/day initially; *Hypertriglyceridemia*—54—160 mg/day initially, may be increased q 4–8 wk up to 160 mg/day as needed; *Geriatric patients*—54 mg/day initially.
◻ **Renal Impairment**
■ **PO (Adults):** *CCr <50 ml/min*—54 mg/day initially.

## AVAILABILITY

■ *Tablets:* 54 mg^Rx, 160 mg^Rx.

TIME/ACTION PROFILE (lowering of triglycerides)

| | ONSET | PEAK | DURATION |
|---|---|---|---|
| PO | unknown | 2 wk | unknown |

## NURSING IMPLICATIONS

### ASSESSMENT

◻ Obtain a diet history, especially with regard to fat consumption. Every attempt should be made to obtain normal serum triglyceride levels with diet, exercise, and weight loss in obese patients before fenofibrate therapy is instituted.
◻ Assess patient for cholelithiasis. If symptoms occur, gallbladder studies are indicated. Therapy should be discontinued if gallstones are found.
■ *Lab Test Considerations:* Monitor serum lipids before therapy to determine consistent elevations, then monitor periodically during therapy.
◻ Monitor serum AST and ALT periodically during therapy. May cause ↑ levels. Therapy should be discontinued if levels rise >3 times the normal limit.
◻ If patient develops muscle tenderness during therapy, CPK levels should be monitored. If CPK levels are markedly ↑ or myopathy occurs, therapy should be discontinued.
◻ May cause mild to moderate ↓ in hemoglobin, hematocrit, and WBCs. Monitor periodically during first 12 mo of therapy. Levels usually stabilize during long-term therapy.
◻ Patients taking anticoagulants concurrently should have prothrombin levels monitored frequently until levels stabilize.

### POTENTIAL NURSING DIAGNOSES

■ Noncompliance (Patient/Family Teaching).

### IMPLEMENTATION

■ **General:** Patients should be placed on a triglyceride-lowering diet before therapy and remain on this diet throughout therapy.
◻ Dose may be increased after repeated serum triglyceride levels every 4–8 wk.
■ **PO:** Administer with meals.

### PATIENT/FAMILY TEACHING

◻ Instruct patient to take medication as directed, not to skip doses or double up on missed doses. Medication helps control but does not cure elevated serum triglyceride levels.
◻ Advise patient that this medication should be used in conjunction with diet restrictions

---

{ } = Available in Canada only.
*CAPITALS indicate life-threatening; underlines indicate most frequent.

(fat, cholesterol, carbohydrates, alcohol), exercise, and cessation of smoking.

❑ Instruct patient to notify health care professional if unexplained muscle pain, tenderness, or weakness occurs, especially if accompanied by fever or malaise.

❑ Instruct female patients to notify health care professional promptly if pregnancy is planned or suspected.

❑ Advise patient to notify health care professional of medication regimen before treatment or surgery.

❑ Emphasize the importance of follow-up exams to determine effectiveness and to monitor for side effects.

## EVALUATION

**Effectiveness of therapy can be demonstrated by:** ■ Decrease in serum triglycerides to normal levels. Therapy should be discontinued in patients who do not have an adequate response in 2 mo of therapy.

## fenoldopam
(fen-**ole**-doe-pam)
Corlopam

*CLASSIFICATION(S):*
*Therapeutic: antihypertensives*
*Pharmacologic: vasodilators*

**Pregnancy Category B**

## INDICATIONS

■ Short-term (<48 hr), in-hospital management of hypertensive emergencies, including malignant hypertension with end-organ deterioration.

## ACTION

■ Acts as an agonist at dopamine $d_1$-like receptors ■ Also binds to alpha-adrenergic receptors ■ Acts as a vasodilator. **Therapeutic Effects:** ■ Rapid lowering of blood pressure.

## PHARMACOKINETICS

**Absorption:** IV administration results in complete bioavailability.
**Distribution:** Unknown.
**Metabolism and Excretion:** Mostly metabolized by the liver; 90% of metabolites are excreted in urine, 10% in feces.
**Half-life:** 5–10 min.

## CONTRAINDICATIONS AND PRECAUTIONS

**Contraindicated in:** ■ Hypersensitivity to fenoldopam or sulfites ■ Concurrent beta blocker therapy (will prevent reflex tachycardia).

**Use Cautiously in:** ■ Glaucoma or intraocular hypertension ■ Pregnancy, lactation, or children (safety not established).

## ADVERSE REACTIONS AND SIDE EFFECTS*

■ **CNS:** headache, nervousness/anxiety, dizziness ■ **CV:** hypotension, tachycardia, ECG changes, peripheral edema ■ **GI:** nausea, abdominal pain, constipation, diarrhea, vomiting ■ **Derm:** flushing, sweating ■ **F and E:** hypokalemia ■ **Local:** injection site reactions ■ **MS:** back pain.

## INTERACTIONS

**Drug-Drug:** ■ Concurrent use with **beta blockers** may result in excessive hypotension (concurrent use should be avoided).

## ROUTE AND DOSAGE

■ **IV (Adults):** 0.01–1.6 mcg/kg/min.

## AVAILABILITY

■ *Concentrate for injection:* 10 mg/ml in 5-ml single-use ampules (with sodium meta-bisulfite)$^{Rx}$.

TIME/ACTION PROFILE (effect on blood pressure)

|    | ONSET | PEAK | DURATION |
|----|-------|------|----------|
| IV | rapid | 15 min | 1–4 hr |

# NURSING IMPLICATIONS

## ASSESSMENT

❑ Monitor blood pressure, heart rate, and ECG frequently throughout therapy; continuous monitoring is preferred. Consult physician for parameters.

■ *Lab Test Considerations:* Monitor serum potassium concentrations every 6 hr during therapy. May cause hypokalemia. Treat with oral or IV potassium supplementation.

## POTENTIAL NURSING DIAGNOSES

■ Tissue perfusion, ineffective (Indications).

## IMPLEMENTATION

- **General:** Administer via continuous infusion; do not use bolus doses. Avoid hypotension and rapid decreases in blood pressure. Initial dose titration should occur no more frequently than every 15 min and less frequently as desired blood pressure is reached. Increments of 0.05 to 0.1 mcg/kg/min are recommended for titration. Lower initial doses (0.03 to 0.1 mcg/kg/min) titrated slowly have been associated with less reflex tachycardia than higher initial doses.
- ❑ Infusion can be abruptly discontinued or gradually tapered before discontinuation. Oral therapy with other antihypertensives can begin anytime after the blood pressure is stable. Do not administer beta blockers concurrently with fenoldopam.
- **Continuous Infusion:** Dilute 4 ml (40 mg of drug) with 1000 ml, 2 ml (20 mg of drug) with 500 ml, or 1 ml (10 mg of drug) with 250 ml of 0.9% NaCl or D5W for a concentration of 40 mcg/ml. Solution is stable for 24 hrs. Discard unused solution.
- ❑ Avoid extravasation.
- ***Rate:*** Rate is based on body weight and desired speed and extent of effect. Administer via infusion pump to ensure accurate dosage rate.
- **Additive Incompatibility:** Information unavailable. Do not admix with other medications.

### PATIENT/FAMILY TEACHING

- ❑ Explain purpose of medication to patient.
- ❑ Advise patient to report headache or pain at the injection site.

### EVALUATION

**Effectiveness of therapy can be demonstrated by:** ■ Decrease in blood pressure without the appearance of side effects.

### High Alert

## fentanyl (oral transmucosal)

**(fen**-ta-nil)

Actiq

### CLASSIFICATION(S):

***Therapeutic:*** *opioid analgesics*
***Pharmacologic:*** *opioid agonists*

### Schedule II

### Pregnancy Category C

### INDICATIONS

■ Management of breakthrough cancer pain in patients with malignancies who are already receiving and are tolerant to opioid therapy for their underlying cancer pain.

### ACTION

■ Binds to opiate receptors in the CNS, altering response to and perception of pain. **Therapeutic Effects:** ■ Decreased pain.

### PHARMACOKINETICS

**Absorption:** Initial rapid absorption (25%) from buccal mucosa is followed by more prolonged absorption (25%) from GI tract (combined bioavailability 50%).

**Distribution:** Highly lipid soluble; rapidly distributes to brain, heart, lungs, kidneys, and spleen, followed by slower distribution to muscle and fat.

**Metabolism and Excretion:** Mostly metabolized by liver and intestinal mucosa; <7% excreted unchanged in urine.

**Half-life:** 7 hr.

### CONTRAINDICATIONS AND PRECAUTIONS

**Contraindicated in:** ■ Hypersensitivity ■ Management of acute or postoperative pain ■ Opioid-naive (nontolerant) patients ■ Lactation.

**Use Cautiously in:** ■ Bradyarrhythmias ■ Concurrent use of CNS active drugs ■ Chronic pulmonary disease or predisposition to hypoventilation ■ Hepatic or renal impairment ■ Pregnancy or children <16 yr (safety not established).

**Exercise Extreme Caution in:** ■ Increased intracranial pressure or altered consciousness.

### ADVERSE REACTIONS AND SIDE EFFECTS*

Includes effects seen with concurrent use of longer-acting opioids. ■ **CNS:** <u>dizziness</u>, <u>drowsi-</u>

ness, abnormal thinking, confusion, hallucinations, headache, insomnia, nervousness,
weakness ■ **EENT:** abnormal vision ■ **Resp:** RES-
PIRATORY DEPRESSION, dyspnea ■ **CV:** hypotension ■
**GI:** nausea, constipation, dry mouth, vomiting ■
**Derm:** pruritus, rash, sweating ■ **Neuro:** abnormal gait.

## INTERACTIONS

**Drug-Drug:** ■ Should not be used within 14
days of **MAO inhibitors** because of possible
severe and unpredictable reactions ■ Concurrent use of other **CNS depressants,** including
**sedative/hypnotics, antidepressants,** other
**opioid analgesics, skeletal muscle relax-
ants, sedating antihistamines,** or **alcohol**
may produce ↑ ↑ sedation, hypoventilation,
and hypotension ■ Some **hepatic enzyme inhibitors,** including **erythromycin, ketoconazole,** and some **protease inhibitor antiretroviral agents** will ↓ metabolism and effects, which may lead to profound sedation,
hypoventilation, and hypotension ■ Administration of **partial-antagonist opioid analgesics**
or **opioid antagonists** will precipitate withdrawal in physically dependent patients ■ **Buprenorphine, nalbuphine,** or **pentazocine**
may decrease analgesia.

## ROUTE AND DOSAGE

■ **Transmucosal: (Adults):** *Dose titration—*
One 200 mcg *Actiq* unit dissolved in mouth
(see Implementation section) over 15 min;
additional unit may be used 15 min after first
unit is completed. If more than one unit is
required per episode (as evaluated over several episodes), dose may be increased as
required to control pain. Optimal usage/titra-
tion should result in using no more than 4
units/day.

## AVAILABILITY

■ *Lozenge on a stick (berry flavor):* 200
mcg[Rx], 400 mcg[Rx], 600 mcg[Rx], 800 mcg[Rx],
1200 mcg[Rx], 1600 mcg[Rx] ■ Cost: 200 mcg
$178.25/24, 400 mcg $230.00/24, 600 mcg
$281.25/24, 800 mcg $332.50/24, 1200 mcg
$433.75/24, 1600 mcg $536.25/24.

TIME/ACTION PROFILE (analgesia)

| | ONSET | PEAK | DURATION |
|---|---|---|---|
| Oral/tran-smucosal | rapid | 15–30 min | several hrs |

## NURSING IMPLICATIONS

### ASSESSMENT

❏ Monitor type, location, and intensity of pain
before and 15 min after administration of
transmucosal fentanyl.

❏ Assess blood pressure, pulse, and respirations before and periodically during administration. If respiratory rate is <10 min, assess
level of sedation. Physical stimulation may be
sufficient to prevent hypoventilation. Subsequent doses may need to be decreased by
25–50%. Patients tolerant to opioid analgesics are usually tolerant to the respiratory
depressant effects also.

■ *Toxicity and Overdose:* If an opioid antagonist is required to reverse respiratory
depression or coma, naloxone (Narcan) is
the antidote. Dilute the 0.4-mg ampule of
naloxone in 10 ml of 0.9% NaCl and administer 0.5 ml (0.02 mg) by direct IV push
every 2 min. For patients weighing <40 kg,
dilute 0.1 mg of naloxone in 10 ml of 0.9%
NaCl for a concentration of 10 mcg/ml and
administer 0.5 mcg every 2 min. Use extreme
caution when titrating dose in patients physically dependent on opioid analgesics to avoid
withdrawal, seizures, and severe pain.

### POTENTIAL NURSING DIAGNOSES

■ Pain, acute (Indications).
■ Injury, risk for (Adverse Reactions).

### IMPLEMENTATION

❏ *High Alert:* Accidental overdosage of opioid
analgesicshas resulted in fatalities. Before administering, clarify all ambiguous orders;
have second practitioner independently
check original order and dose calculations.

■ **General:** Patients considered opioid-tolerant
are those who are taking ≥60 mg of oral
morphine/day, 50 mcg transdermal fentanyl/
hr, or an equianalgesic dose of another
opioid for ≥1 wk.

❏ *High Alert:* Supplied in individually sealed
child-resistant foil pouches. Dose may be
lethal to a child; keep out of reach of children.

■ **Transmucosal:** Open the foil package immediately before use. Instruct patient to
place unit in the mouth between the cheek
and lower gum, moving it from one side to
the other using the handle. Patient should
suck, not chew, the lozenge. If it is chewed

and swallowed, lower peak concentrations and lower bioavailability may occur. Instruct patient to consume lozenge over 15-min period; longer or shorter periods may be less efficacious. If signs of excessive opioid effects occur, remove from patient's mouth immediately and decrease future doses.

❏ Initial dose for breakthrough pain should be 200 mcg. Six 200-mcg units should be prescribed and should be used before increasing to a higher dose. If one unit is ineffective, a second unit may be started 15 min after the completion of the first unit. Do not use more than 2 units during a single episode of breakthrough pain during titration phase. With each new dose during titration, 6 units should be prescribed, allowing treatment of several episodes of breakthrough pain. Adequate dose is determined based on effective analgesia with acceptable side effects. Side effects during titration period are usually greater than after effective dose is determined.

❏ Once an effective dose is determined, instruct patient to limit dose to 4 units/day. If >4 units/day are required, consider increasing the dose of the long-acting opioid.

❏ Discontinue with a gradual decrease in dose to prevent signs and symptoms of abrupt withdrawal.

❏ To dispose of remaining unit, remove drug matrix from handle by grasping with tissue paper and separating with a twisting motion. Flush remaining drug matrix down toilet. Drug remaining on handle may be removed by placing under running warm water until dissolved. Dispose of drug-free handle according to institutional protocol. *High Alert:* Partially consumed units are no longer protected by child-resistant pouch; dose may still be fatal. A temporary child-resistant storage bottle is provided for partially consumed units that cannot be disposed of properly.

### PATIENT/FAMILY TEACHING

❏ Instruct patient in proper use, storage, and disposal of unit. Advise patient to notify health care professional if excessive opioid effects occur or if >4 units/day are required to control pain.

❏ Caution patient to make position changes slowly to minimize orthostatic hypotension.

❏ Medication causes dizziness and drowsiness. Advise patient to call for assistance during ambulation and transfer, and to avoid driving or other activities requiring alertness until response to medication is known.

❏ Instruct patient to avoid concurrent use of alcohol or other CNS depressants.

❏ Inform patient that this drug contains sugar and may cause dry mouth. Advise patient to maintain good oral hygiene regualr dental exams.

### EVALUATION

**Effectiveness of therapy can be demonstrated by:** ■ Decrease in severity of pain during episodes of breakthrough pain in patients receiving long-acting opioids.

---

**High Alert**

# fentanyl (parenteral)
**(fen**-ta-nil)
Sublimaze

*CLASSIFICATION(S):*
*Therapeutic: opioid analgesics*
*Pharmacologic: opioid agonists*

**Schedule II**

**Pregnancy Category C**

---

### INDICATIONS

■ Analgesic supplement to general anesthesia; usually with other agents (ultra–short-acting barbiturates, neuromuscular blocking agents, and inhalation anesthetics) to produce balanced anesthesia ■ Induction/maintenance of anesthesia (with oxygen or oxygen/nitrous oxide and a neuromuscular blocking agents) ■ Neuroleptanalgesia/neuroleptanesthesia (with or without nitrous oxide) ■ Supplement to regional/local anesthesia ■ Preoperative and postoperative analgesia. **Unlabeled uses:** ■ Continuous IV infusion as part of PCA.

## ACTION

■ Binds to opiate receptors in the CNS, altering the response to and perception of pain ■ Produces CNS depression. **Therapeutic Effects:** ■ Supplement in anesthesia ■ Decreased pain.

## PHARMACOKINETICS

**Absorption:** Well absorbed after IM administration.

**Distribution:** Unknown.

**Metabolism and Excretion:** Mostly metabolized by the liver, 10–25% excreted unchanged by the kidneys.

**Half-life:** 0.5–3.6 hr (increased after cardiopulmonary bypass and in geriatric patients)

## CONTRAINDICATIONS AND PRECAUTIONS

**Contraindicated in:** ■ Hypersensitivity; crosssensitivity among agents may occur ■ Known intolerance.

**Use Cautiously in:** ■ Geriatric, debilitated, or critically ill patients ■ Diabetes ■ Severe pulmonary or hepatic disease ■ CNS tumors ■ Increased intracranial pressure ■ Head trauma ■ Adrenal insufficiency ■ Undiagnosed abdominal pain ■ Hypothyroidism ■ Alcoholism ■ Cardiac disease (arrhythmias) ■ Pregnancy, lactation, and children <2 yr (safety not established).

## ADVERSE REACTIONS AND SIDE EFFECTS*

■ **CNS:** confusion, paradoxical excitation/delirium, postoperative depression, postoperative drowsiness ■ **EENT:** blurred/double vision ■ **Resp:** APNEA, LARYNGOSPASM, allergic bronchospasm, respiratory depression ■ **CV:** arrhythmias, bradycardia, circulatory depression, hypotension ■ **GI:** biliary spasm, nausea/vomiting ■ **Derm:** facial itching ■ **MS:** skeletal and thoracic muscle rigidity.

## INTERACTIONS

**Drug-Drug:** ■ Avoid use in patients who have received **MAO inhibitors** within the previous 14 days (may produce unpredictable, potentially fatal reactions) ■ Additive CNS and respiratory depression with other **CNS depressants,** including **alcohol, antihistamines, antidepressants,** other **sedative/hypnotics,** and other **opioid analgesics** ■ Increased risk of hypotension with **benzodiazepines** ■ **Nalbuphine, buprenorphine,** or **pentazocine** may decrease analgesia.

## ROUTE AND DOSAGE

❏ **Preoperative Use**

■ **IM (Adults):** 50–100 mcg (0.05–0.1 mg) or 0.7–1.4 mcg/kg 30–60 min before surgery.

❏ **Adjunct to General Anesthesia**

■ **IV (Adults):** *Low dose–minor surgery*—2 mcg (0.002 mg)/kg. *Moderate dose–major surgery*—2–20 mcg (0.002–0.02 mg)/kg. *High dose–major surgery*—20–50 mcg (0.02–0.05 mg)/kg.

❏ **Adjunct to Regional Anesthesia**

■ **IM, IV (Adults):** 50–100 mcg (0.05–0.1 mg).

❏ **Postoperative Use (Recovery Room)**

■ **IM (Adults):** 50–100 mcg; may repeat in 1–2 hr.

❏ **General Anesthesia**

■ **IV (Adults):** 50–100 mcg (0.05–0.1 mg)/kg (up to 150 mcg/kg).

■ **IV (Children 2–12 yr):** 2–3 mcg/kg.

## AVAILABILITY (generic available)

■*Injection:* 0.05 mg/ml^Rx ■ droperidol (Innovar)^Rx. See Appendix B.

## TIME/ACTION PROFILE (analgesia*)

|  | ONSET | PEAK | DURATION |
|---|---|---|---|
| IM | 7–15 min | 20–30 min | 1–2 hr |
| IV | 1–2 min | 3–5 min | 0.5–1 hr |

*Respiratory depression may last longer than analgesia.

# NURSING IMPLICATIONS

## ASSESSMENT

■ **General Info:** Monitor respiratory rate and blood pressure frequently throughout therapy. Report significant changes immediately. The respiratory depressant effects of fentanyl may last longer than the analgesic effects. Initial doses of other opioids should be reduced by 25–33% of the usually recommended dose. Monitor closely.

■ **IV, IM:** Assess type, location, and intensity of pain before and 30 min after IM administration or 3–5 min after IV administration when fentanyl is used to treat pain.

■ *Lab Test Considerations:* May cause elevated serum amylase and lipase concentrations.

■ *Toxicity and Overdose:* Symptoms of toxicity include respiratory depression, hypotension, arrhythmias, bradycardia, and asystole. Atropine may be used to treat bradycardia. If respiratory depression persists after surgery, prolonged mechanical ventilation may be required. If an opioid antagonist is required to reverse respiratory depression or coma, naloxone (Narcan) is the antidote. Dilute the 0.4-mg ampule of naloxone in 10 ml of 0.9% NaCl and administer 0.5 ml (0.02 mg) by direct IV push every 2 min. For children and patients weighing <40 kg, dilute 0.1 mg of naloxone in 10 ml of 0.9% NaCl for a concentration of 10 mcg/ml and administer 0.5 mcg/kg every 2 min. Titrate dose to avoid withdrawal, seizures, and severe pain. Administration of naloxone in these circumstances, especially in cardiac patients, has resulted in hypertension and tachycardia, occasionally causing left ventricular failure and pulmonary edema.

## POTENTIAL NURSING DIAGNOSES

■ Pain, acute (Indications).

■ Breathing pattern, ineffective (Adverse Reactions).

■ Injury, risk for (Side Effects).

## IMPLEMENTATION

❑ *High Alert:* Accidental overdosage of opioid analgesics has resulted in fatalities. Before administering, clarify all ambiguous orders; have second practitioner independently check original order, dose calculations, route of administration, and infusion pump programming. Do not confuse fentanyl with sufentanil.

■ **General:** Benzodiazepines may be administered before or after administration of fentanyl to reduce the induction dose requirements, decrease the time to loss of consciousness, and produce amnesia. This combination may also increase the risk of hypotension.

❑ *High Alert:* Opioid antagonists, oxygen, and resuscitative equipment should be readily available during the administration of fentanyl. Fentanyl derivatives should be administered IV only in monitored anesthesia care settings (operating room, emergency department, ICU) with immediate access to life-support equipment and should be administered only by personnel trained in resuscitation and emergency airway management.

■ **Direct IV:** Administer undiluted.

■ *Rate:* Injections should be administered slowly over 1–3 min. Slow IV administration may reduce the incidence and severity of muscle rigidity, bradycardia, or hypotension. Neuromuscular blocking agents may be administered concurrently to decrease muscle rigidity.

■ **Intermittent Infusion:** May be diluted in D5W or 0.9% NaCl.

■ **Syringe Compatibility:** ◆ atracurium ◆ atropine ◆ butorphanol ◆ chlorpromazine ◆ cimetidine ◆ dimenhydrinate ◆ diphenhydramine ◆ droperidol ◆ heparin ◆ hydromorphone ◆ hydroxyzine ◆ meperidine ◆ metoclopramide ◆ midazolam ◆ morphine ◆ pentazocine ◆ perphenazine ◆ prochlorperazine edisylate ◆ promethazine ◆ ranitidine ◆ scopolamine.

■ **Syringe Incompatibility:** ◆ pentobarbital.

■ **Y-Site Compatibility:** ◆ alatrofloxacin ◆ atracurium ◆ diltiazem ◆ dobutamine ◆ dopamine ◆ enalaprilat ◆ epinephrine ◆ esmolol ◆ etomidate ◆ furosemide ◆ gatifloxacin ◆ heparin ◆ hydrocortisone sodium succinate ◆ hydromorphone ◆ labetalol ◆ levofloxacin ◆ linezolid ◆ lorazepam ◆ midazolam ◆ milrinone ◆ morphine ◆ nafcillin ◆ nitroglycerin ◆ norepinephrine ◆ pancuronium ◆ potassium chloride ◆ propofol ◆ ranitidine ◆ sargramostim ◆ thiopental ◆ vecuronium ◆ vitamin B complex with C.

■ **Additive Compatibility:** ◆ bupivacaine.

■ **Additive Incompatibility:** ◆ methohexital ◆ pentobarbital ◆ thiopental.

## PATIENT/FAMILY TEACHING

❑ Discuss the use of anesthetic agents and the sensations to expect with the patient before surgery.

❑ Explain pain assessment scale to patient.

❑ Caution patient to change positions slowly to minimize orthostatic hypotension.

❑ Medication causes dizziness and drowsiness. Advise patient to call for assistance during ambulation and transfer and to avoid driving or other activities requiring alertness for 24 hr after administration during outpatient surgery.

❑ Instruct patient to avoid alcohol or other CNS depressants for 24 hr after administration for outpatient surgery.

### EVALUATION

**Effectiveness of therapy can be demonstrated by:** ■ General quiescence ❑ Reduced motor activity ■ Pronounced analgesia.

---

**High Alert**

# fentanyl (transdermal)
**(fen**-ta-nil)
Duragesic

*CLASSIFICATION(S):*
*Therapeutic: opioid analgesics, anesthetic adjuncts*
*Pharmacologic: opioid agonists*

**Schedule II**

**Pregnancy Category C**

---

### INDICATIONS

■ Management of chronic pain in patients requiring opioid analgesic therapy ■ Transdermal fentanyl is not recommended for the control of postoperative, mild, or intermittent pain.

### ACTION

■ Binds to opiate receptors in the CNS, altering the response to and perception of pain. **Therapeutic Effects:** ■ Decrease in severity of chronic pain.

### PHARMACOKINETICS

**Absorption:** Well absorbed (92% of dose) through skin surface under transdermal patch, creating a depot in the upper skin layers. Release from transdermal system into systemic circulation increases gradually to a constant rate, providing continuous delivery for 72 hr.

**Distribution:** Crosses the placenta; enters breast milk.

**Metabolism and Excretion:** Mostly metabolized by the liver; 10–25% excreted unchanged by the kidneys.

**Half-life:** 17 hr after removal of a single application patch, increases to 21 hr after removal

of multiple patches (because of continued release from deposition of drug in skin layers).

### CONTRAINDICATIONS AND PRECAUTIONS

**Contraindicated in:** ■ Hypersensitivity to fentanyl or adhesives ■ Known intolerance ■ Acute pain (onset not rapid enough) ■ Alcohol intolerance (small amounts of alcohol released into skin).

**Use Cautiously in:** ■ Patients >60 yr, cachectic or debilitated patients (dosage reduction suggested because of altered drug disposition) ■ Diabetes ■ Patients with severe pulmonary or hepatic disease ■ CNS tumors ■ Increased intracranial pressure ■ Head trauma ■ Adrenal insufficiency ■ Undiagnosed abdominal pain ■ Hypothyroidism ■ Alcoholism ■ Cardiac disease (particularly bradyarrhythmias) ■ Fever (increases release of fentanyl from delivery system) ■ Titration period (additional analgesics may be required) ■ Pregnancy, lactation, and children <2 yr (safety not established).

### ADVERSE REACTIONS AND SIDE EFFECTS*

■ **CNS:** confusion, sedation, weakness, dizziness, restlessness ■ **Resp:** APNEA, bronchoconstriction, laryngospasm, respiratory depression ■ **CV:** bradycardia ■ **GI:** anorexia, constipation, dry mouth, nausea, vomiting ■ **Derm:** sweating, erythema ■ **Local:** application site reactions ■ **MS:** skeletal and thoracic muscle rigidity ■ **Misc:** physical dependence, psychological dependence.

### INTERACTIONS

**Drug-Drug:** ■ Avoid use in patients who have received **MAO inhibitors** within the previous 14 days (may produce unpredictable, potentially fatal reactions) ■ Additive CNS and respiratory depression with other **CNS depressants,** including **alcohol, antihistamines, antidepressants, sedative/hypnotics,** and other **opioids.**

**Drug-Natural Products:** ■ Concomitant use of **kava, valerian, skullcap, chamomile,** or **hops** can increase CNS depression.

### ROUTE AND DOSAGE

■ **Transdermal (Adults):** 25 mcg/hr is the initial dose; patients who have not been receiving opioids should receive not more that 25 mcg/hr. To calculate the dosage of transdermal fentanyl required in patients who are already receiving opioid analgesics, assess the 24-hr requirement of currently used opioid. Using the equianalgesic table in Appendix O, convert this to an equivalent amount of morphine/24 hr. Conversion to fentanyl transdermal may be accomplished by using the fentanyl conversion table ( Appendix O). During dosage titration, additional short-acting opioids should be available for any breakthrough pain that may occur. Morphine 10 mg IM or 60 mg PO q 4 hr (60 mg/24 hr IM or 360 mg/24 hr PO) is considered to be approximately equivalent to transdermal fentanyl 100 mcg/hr. Transdermal patch lasts 72 hr in most patients. Some patients require a new patch every 48 hr.

■ **Transdermal (Adults >60 yr, Debilitated, or Cachectic Patients):** Initial 'dose should be 25 mcg/hr unless previous opioid use was >135 mg morphine PO/day (or other opioid equivalent).

## AVAILABILITY

■ *Transdermal systems:* 25 mcg/hr[Rx], 50 mcg/hr[Rx], 75 mcg/hr[Rx], 100 mcg/hr[Rx] ■ Cost: 25 mcg/hr $64.07/5 systems, 50 mcg/hr $106.82/5 systems, 75 mcg/hr $169.52/5 systems, 100 mcg/hr $213.23/5 systems.

TIME/ACTION PROFILE (decreased pain)

| | ONSET | PEAK | DURATION |
|---|---|---|---|
| Transdermal | 6 hr† | 12–24 hr | 72 hr‡ |

†Achievement of blood levels associated with analgesia. Maximal response and dose titration may take up to 6 days.
‡While patch is worn.

## NURSING IMPLICATIONS

### ASSESSMENT

❏ Assess type, location, and intensity of pain before and 24 hr after application and periodically throughout therapy. Pain should be monitored frequently during initiation of therapy and dosage changes to assess need for supplementary analgesics for breakthrough pain.

❏ Assess blood pressure, pulse, and respirations before and periodically during adminis-

tration. If respiratory rate is <10/min, assess level of sedation. Physical stimulation may be sufficient to prevent significant hypoventilation. Dose may need to be decreased by 25–50%. Initial drowsiness will diminish with continued use.

❏ Prolonged use may lead to physical and psychological dependence and tolerance. This should not prevent patient from receiving adequate analgesia. Most patients who receive opioid analgesics for pain do not develop psychological dependence.

❏ Progressively higher doses may be required to relieve pain with long-term therapy. It may take up to 6 days after increasing doses to reach equilibrium, so patients should wear higher dose through 2 applications before increasing dose again.

❏ Assess bowel function routinely. Prevention of constipation should be instituted with increased intake of fluids and bulk, and laxatives to minimize constipating effects. Stimulant laxatives should be administered routinely if opioid use exceeds 2–3 days, unless contraindicated.

■ *Lab Test Considerations:* May increase plasma amylase and lipase levels.

■ *Toxicity and Overdose:* If an opioid antagonist is required to reverse respiratory depression or coma, naloxone (Narcan) is the antidote. Dilute the 0.4-mg ampule of naloxone in 10 ml of 0.9% NaCl and administer 0.5 ml (0.02 mg) by direct IV push every 2 min. For patients weighing <40 kg, dilute 0.1 mg of naloxone in 10 ml of 0.9% NaCl for a concentration of 10 mcg/ml and administer 0.5 mcg/kg every 2 min. Titrate dose to avoid withdrawal, seizures, and severe pain. Monitor patient closely; dose may need to be repeated or may need to be administered as an infusion because of long duration of action despite removal of patch.

## POTENTIAL NURSING DIAGNOSES

■ Pain, acute (Indications).
■ Injury, risk for (Side Effects).

## IMPLEMENTATION

❏ *High Alert:* Accidental overdosage of opioid narcotics has resulted in fatalities. Before administering, clarify all ambiguous orders;

have second practitioner independently check original order and dose calculations.

■ **General:** Supplemental doses of short-acting opioid analgesics should be used to manage pain until relief is obtained with the transdermal system. Patients may continue to require supplemental opioids for breakthrough pain. If >100 mcg/hr is required, use multiple transdermal systems.

❑ Dosage is titrated based on the patient's report of pain until adequate analgesia (50% reduction in patient's pain rating on numerical or visual analogue scale or patient reports satisfactory relief) is attained. Dose is determined by calculating the previous 24-hr analgesic requirement and converting to the equianalgesic morphine dose using Appendix O. The conversion ratio from morphine to transdermal fentanyl is conservative; 50% of patients may require a dose increase after initial application. Increase after 3 days based on required daily doses of supplemental analgesics. Increases should be based on ratio of 90 mg/24 hr of oral morphine to 25 mcg/hr increase in transdermal fentanyl dose.

❑ Coadministration with nonopioid analgesics may have additive analgesic effects and permit lower opioid doses.

❑ To convert to another opioid analgesic, remove transdermal fentanyl system and begin treatment with half the equianalgesic dose of the new analgesic in 12–18 hr.

❑ Medication should be discontinued gradually after long-term use to prevent withdrawal symptoms. **Transdermal:** Apply system to flat, nonirritated, and nonirradiated site such as chest, back, flank, or upper arm. If skin preparation is necessary, use clear water and clip, do not shave, hair. Allow skin to dry completely before application. Apply immediately after removing from package. Do not alter the system (i.e., cut) in any way before application. Remove liner from adhesive layer and press firmly in place with palm of hand for 30 sec, especially around the edges, to make sure contact is complete. For continued use, remove used system and fold so that adhesive edges are together. Flush system down toilet immediately on removal. Apply new system to a different site. Discard unused systems by removing from pouch and flushing down toilet.

## PATIENT/FAMILY TEACHING

❑ Instruct patient in how and when to ask for pain medication.

❑ Instruct patient in correct method for application and disposal of transdermal system. May be worn while bathing, showering, or swimming.

❑ Medication may cause drowsiness or dizziness. Caution patient to call for assistance when ambulating or smoking and to avoid driving or other activities requiring alertness until response to medication is known.

❑ Advise patient to change positions slowly to minimize dizziness.

❑ Caution patient to avoid concurrent use of alcohol or other CNS depressants with this medication.

❑ Advise patient that fever, electric blankets, heating pads, saunas, hot tubs, and heated water beds increase the release of fentanyl from the patch.

❑ Advise patient that good oral hygiene, frequent mouth rinses, and sugarless gum or candy may decrease dry mouth.

## EVALUATION

**Effectiveness of therapy can be demonstrated by:** ■ Decrease in severity of pain without a significant alteration in level of consciousness, respiratory status, or blood pressure.

## fexofenadine
(fex-oh-**fen**-a-deen)
Allegra

**CLASSIFICATION(S):**
**Therapeutic:** *allergy, cold, and cough remedies, antihistamines*

**Pregnancy Category C**

## INDICATIONS

■ Relief of symptoms of seasonal allergic rhinitis ■ Management of chronic idiopathic urticaria.

## ACTION

■ Antagonizes the effects of histamine at peripheral histamine–1 ($H_1$) receptors, including pruritus and urticaria ■ Also has a drying effect on the nasal mucosa. **Therapeutic Effects:** ■

Decreased sneezing, rhinorrhea, itchy eyes, nose, and throat associated with seasonal allergies ■ Decreased urticaria.

## PHARMACOKINETICS

**Absorption:** Rapidly absorbed after oral administration.

**Distribution:** Unknown.

**Metabolism and Excretion:** 80% excreted in urine, 11% excreted in feces.

**Half-life:** 14.4 hr (increased in renal impairment).

## CONTRAINDICATIONS AND PRECAUTIONS

**Contraindicated in:** ■ Hypersensitivity.

**Use Cautiously in:** ■ Impaired renal function (increased dosing interval recommended) ■ Pregnancy, lactation, or children <12 yr (safety not established).

## ADVERSE REACTIONS AND SIDE EFFECTS*

■ **CNS:** drowsiness, fatigue ■ **GI:** dyspepsia ■ **Endo:** dysmenorrhea.

## INTERACTIONS

**Drug-Drug:** ■ **Magnesium and aluminum-containing antacids** decrease absorption and may decrease effectiveness.

**Drug-Food:** ■ **Apple, orange,** and **grapefruit juice** decrease absorption any may decrease effectiveness.

## ROUTE AND DOSAGE

■ **PO (Adults and Children ≥12 yr):** 60 mg twice daily, or 180 mg once daily.

■ **PO (Children 6–11 yr):** 30 mg twice daily.

❑ **Renal Impairment**

■ **PO (Adults):** 60 mg once daily as a starting dose.

■ **PO (Children 6–11 yr):** 30 mg once daily as a starting dose.

## AVAILABILITY

■ *Tablets:* 30 mg^Rx, 60 mg^Rx, 180 mg^Rx ■ *Capsules:* 60 mg^Rx ■ Cost: $99.42/100 ■ pseudoephedrine (Allegra-D^Rx). See Appendix B.

**TIME/ACTION PROFILE** (antihistaminic effect)

| | ONSET | PEAK | DURATION |
|---|---|---|---|
| PO | within 1 hr | 2–3 hr | 12–24 hr |

# NURSING IMPLICATIONS

## ASSESSMENT

❑ Assess allergy symptoms (rhinitis, conjunctivitis, hives) before and periodically throughout therapy.

❑ Assess lung sounds and character of bronchial secretions. Maintain fluid intake of 1500–2000 ml/day to decrease viscosity of secretions.

■ *Lab Test Considerations:* Will cause false-negative reactions on allergy skin tests; discontinue 3 days before testing.

## POTENTIAL NURSING DIAGNOSES

■ Airway clearance, ineffective (Indications).

■ Injury, risk for (Adverse Reactions).

## IMPLEMENTATION

■ **PO:** Administer with food or milk to decrease GI irritation. Capsules and tablets should be taken with water or milk, not juice.

## PATIENT/FAMILY TEACHING

❑ Instruct patient to take medication as directed. If a dose is missed, take as soon as remembered unless almost time for next dose.

❑ Inform patient that drug may cause drowsiness, although it is less likely to occur than with other antihistamines. Avoid driving or other activities requiring alertness until response to drug is known.

❑ Instruct patient to contact health care professional if symptoms persist.

## EVALUATION

**Effectiveness of therapy can be demonstrated by:** ■ Decrease in allergic symptoms ■ Decrease in urticaria.

# filgrastim

(fil-**gra**-stim)
Neupogen, G-CSF, granulocyte colony stimulating factor

### CLASSIFICATION(S):
**Therapeutic:** colony-stimulating factors

## Pregnancy Category C

## INDICATIONS

■ Prevention of febrile neutropenia and associated infection in patients who have received bone marrow–depressing antineoplastics for the treatment of nonmyeloid malignancies ■ Reduction of time for neutrophil recovery and duration of fever in patients undergoing induction and consolidation chemotherapy for acute myelogenous leukemia ■ Reduction of time to neutrophil recovery and sequelae of neutropenia in patients with nonmyeloid malignancies undergoing myeloablative chemotherapy followed by bone marrow transplantation ■ Mobilization of hematopoietic progenitor cells into peripheral blood for collection by leukapheresis ■ Management of severe chronic neutropenia. **Unlabeled uses:** ■ Neutropenia associated with HIV infection.

## ACTION

■ A glycoprotein, filgrastim binds to and stimulates immature neutrophils to divide and differentiate. Also activates mature neutrophils. **Therapeutic Effects:** ■ Decreased incidence of infection in patients who are neutropenic from chemotherapy or other causes ■ Improved harvest of progenitor cells for bone marrow transplantation.

## PHARMACOKINETICS

**Absorption:** Well absorbed after subcut administration.
**Distribution:** Unknown.
**Metabolism and Excretion:** Unknown.
**Half-life:** 3.5 hr.

## CONTRAINDICATIONS AND PRECAUTIONS

**Contraindicated in:** ■ Hypersensitivity to filgrastim or *Escherichia coli*–derived proteins. **Use Cautiously in:** ■ Malignancy with myeloid characteristics ■ Pre-existing cardiac disease ■ Pregnancy, lactation, or children (safety not established).

## ADVERSE REACTIONS AND SIDE EFFECTS*

■ **Hemat:** excessive leukocytosis ■ **Local:** pain, redness at subcut site ■ **MS:** medullary bone pain.

## INTERACTIONS

**Drug-Drug:** ■ Simultaneous use with **antineoplastics** may have adverse effects on rapidly proliferating neutrophils—avoid use for 24 hr before and 24 hr after chemotherapy ■ **Lithium** may potentiate the release of neutrophils; concurrent use should be undertaken cautiously.

## ROUTE AND DOSAGE

❑ **After Myelosuppressive Chemotherapy**
■ **IV, Subcut (Adults):** 5 mcg/kg/day as a single injection daily for up to 2 wk. Dosage may be increased by 5 mcg/kg during each cycle of chemotherapy, depending on blood counts.

❑ **After Bone Marrow Transplantation**
■ **IV, Subcut (Adults):** 10 mcg/kg/day as a 4- or 24-hr IV infusion or as a continuous subcut infusion; initiate at least 24 hr after chemotherapy and at least 24 hr after bone marrow transplantation. Subsequent dosage is adjusted according to blood counts.

❑ **Peripheral Blood Progenitor Cell Collection and Therapy**
■ **Subcut (Adults):** 10 mcg/kg/day as a bolus or continuous infusion for at least 4 days before first leukapheresis and continued until last leukapheresis; dosage modification suggested if WBC >100,000 cells/mm³.

❑ **Severe Chronic Neutropenia**
■ **Subcut (Adults):** *Congenital neutropenia*—6 mcg/kg twice daily. *Idiopathic/cyclical neutropenia*—5 mcg/kg daily (decrease if ANC remains >10,000/mm³).

## AVAILABILITY

■ *Injection:* 300 mcg/ml in 1- and 1.6-ml vials^Rx.

## TIME/ACTION PROFILE

| | ONSET | PEAK | DURATION |
|---|---|---|---|
| IV, subcut | unknown | unknown | 4 days† |

†Return of neutrophil count to baseline.

# NURSING IMPLICATIONS

## ASSESSMENT

❑ Monitor heart rate, blood pressure, and respiratory status before and periodically during therapy.

❑ Assess bone pain throughout therapy. Pain is usually mild to moderate and controllable with nonopioid analgesics, but may require treatment with opioid analgesics, especially in patients receiving high-dose IV therapy.

■ *Lab Test Considerations: After chemotherapy*, obtain a CBC with differential, including examination for the presence of blast cells, and platelet count before chemotherapy and twice weekly during therapy to avoid leukocytosis. Monitor ANC. A transient rise is seen 1–2 days after initiation of therapy, but therapy should not be discontinued until ANC >10,000/mm$^3$.

❑ *After bone marrow transplant*, the daily dose is titrated by the neutrophil response. When the ANC is >1000/mm$^3$ for 3 consecutive days, the dose should be reduced by 5 mcg/kg/day. If the ANC remains >1000/mm$^3$ for 3 or more consecutive days, filgrastim is discontinued. If the ANC decreases to <1000/mm$^3$, filgrastim should be resumed at 5 mcg/kg/day.

❑ *For chronic severe neutropenia*, monitor CBC with differential and platelet count twice weekly during initial 4 wk of therapy and during 2 wk after any dose adjustment.

❑ May cause decreased platelet count and transient increases in uric acid, LDH, and alkaline phosphatase concentrations.

## POTENTIAL NURSING DIAGNOSES

■ Infection, risk for (Indications).

■ Pain, acute (Side Effects).

## IMPLEMENTATION

■ **General:** Administer no earlier than 24 hr after cytotoxic chemotherapy, at least 24 hr after bone marrow infusion, and not during the 24 hr before administration of chemotherapy.

❑ Refrigerate; do not freeze. Do not shake. May warm to room temperature for up to 6 hr before injection. Discard if left at room temperature for >6 hr. Vial is for 1-time use only.

■ **Subcut:** If dose requires >1 ml of solution, may be divided into 2 injection sites.

❑ May also be administered as a continuous subcut infusion over 24 hr after bone marrow transplantation.

■ **Continuous Infusion:** Dilute in D5W to produce a concentration of >15 mcg of filgrastim/ml. If the final concentration is 2–15 mcg/ml, human albumin in a concentration of 2 mg/ml must be added to D5W before filgrastim to prevent adsorption of the components of the drug delivery system. Refrigerate; do not freeze. Do not shake. May warm to room temperature for up to 6 hr before injection. Vial is for 1-time use only.

■ *Rate: After chemotherapy* dose is administered via infusion over 15–30 min.

❑ *After chemotherapy* dose may also be administered as a continuous infusion.

❑ *After bone marrow transplant*, dose should be administered as an infusion over 4 or 24 hr.

■ **Y-Site Compatibility:** ◆ acyclovir ◆ allopurinol ◆ amikacin ◆ aminophylline ◆ ampicillin ◆ ampicillin/sulbactam ◆ aztreonam ◆ bleomycin ◆ bumetanide ◆ buprenorphine ◆ butorphanol ◆ calcium gluconate ◆ carboplatin ◆ carmustine ◆ cefazolin ◆ cefotetan ◆ ceftazidime ◆ chlorpromazine ◆ cimetidine ◆ cisplatin ◆ cyclophosphamide ◆ cytarabine ◆ dacarbazine ◆ daunorubicin ◆ diphenhydramine ◆ doxorubicin ◆ doxycycline ◆ droperidol ◆ enalaprilat ◆ famotidine ◆ floxuridine ◆ fluconazole ◆ fludarabine ◆ ganciclovir ◆ haloperidol ◆ hydrocortisone ◆ hydromorphone ◆ idarubicin ◆ ifosfamide ◆ leucovorin calcium ◆ lorazepam ◆ mechlorethamine ◆ melphalan ◆ meperidine ◆ mesna ◆ methotrexate ◆ metoclopramide ◆ miconazole ◆ minocycline ◆ mitoxantrone ◆ morphine ◆ nalbuphine ◆ netilmicin ◆ ondansetron ◆ plicamycin ◆ potassium chloride ◆ promethazine ◆ ranitidine ◆ sodium bicarbonate ◆ streptozocin ◆ ticarcillin ◆ ticarcillin/clavulanate ◆ tobramycin ◆ trimethoprim/sulfamethoxazole ◆ vancomycin ◆ vinblastine ◆ vincristine ◆ vinorelbine ◆ zidovudine.

---

{ } = Available in Canada only.

\* CAPITALS indicates life-threatening; <u>underlines</u> indicate most frequent.

■ **Y-Site Incompatibility:** ◆ amphotericin B ◆ cefepime ◆ cefonicid ◆ cefoperazone ◆ cefotaxime ◆ cefoxitin ◆ ceftizoxime ◆ ceftriaxone ◆ cefuroxime ◆ clindamycin ◆ dactinomycin ◆ etoposide ◆ fluorouracil ◆ furosemide ◆ heparin ◆ mannitol ◆ methylprednisolone sodium succinate ◆ metronidazole ◆ mezlocillin ◆ mitomycin ◆ piperacillin ◆ prochlorperazine ◆ thiotepa.

### PATIENT/FAMILY TEACHING

■ **Home Care Issues:** Instruct patient on correct technique and proper disposal for home administration. Caution patient not to reuse needle, vial, or syringe. Provide patient with a puncture-proof container for needle and syringe disposal.

### EVALUATION

**Effectiveness of therapy can be demonstrated by:** ■ Decreased incidence of infection in patients who receive bone marrow–depressing antineoplastics ■ Reduction of duration and sequelae of neutropenia after bone marrow transplantation ■ Reduction of the incidence and duration of sequelae of neutropenia in patients with severe chronic neutropenia ■ Improved harvest of progenitor cells for bone marrow transplantation.

---

## finasteride
(fi-**nas**-teer-ide)
Propecia, Proscar

### CLASSIFICATION(S):
**Therapeutic:** hair regrowth stimulants
**Pharmacologic:** androgen inhibitors

### Pregnancy Category X

---

### INDICATIONS

■ Benign prostatic hyperplasia (BPH) ■ Androgenetic alopecia (male pattern baldness) in men only.

### ACTION

■ Inhibits the enzyme 5-alpha-reductase, which is responsible for converting testosterone to its potent metabolite 5-alpha-dihydrotestosterone in prostate, liver, and skin; 5-alpha-dihydrotestosterone is partially responsible for prostatic hyperplasia and hair loss. **Therapeutic Effects:** ■ Reduced prostate size with associated decrease in urinary symptoms ■ Decreases hair loss; promotes hair regrowth.

## PHARMACOKINETICS

**Absorption:** Well absorbed after oral administration (63%).

**Distribution:** Enters prostatic tissue and crosses the blood-brain barrier. Remainder of distribution not known.

**Protein Binding:** 90%.

**Metabolism and Excretion:** Mostly metabolized; 39% excreted in urine as metabolites; 57% excreted in feces.

**Half-life:** 6 hr (range 6–15 hr; slightly increased in patients >70 yr).

## CONTRAINDICATIONS AND PRECAUTIONS

**Contraindicated in:** ■ Hypersensitivity ■ Women.

**Use Cautiously in:** ■ Patients with hepatic impairment or obstructive uropathy.

## ADVERSE REACTIONS AND SIDE EFFECTS*

■ **GU:** decreased libido, decreased volume of ejaculate, impotence.

## INTERACTIONS

**Drug-Drug:** ■ None noted.

## ROUTE AND DOSAGE

■ **PO (Adults):** *BPH*—5 mg once daily (Proscar); *androgenetic alopecia*—1 mg/day (Propecia).

## AVAILABILITY

■ *Tablets:* 1 mg^Rx (Propecia), 5 mg^Rx (Proscar) ■Cost: *Propecia*—1 mg $49.35/30; *Proscar*—5 mg $266.25/100.

TIME/ACTION PROFILE (reduction in dihydrotestosterone levels†)

| | ONSET | PEAK | DURATION |
|---|---|---|---|
| PO | rapid | 8 hr | 2 wk |

†Clinical effects as noted by urinary tract symptoms and hair regrowth may not be evident for several months and remain for 4 mo after discontinuation.

## NURSING IMPLICATIONS

### ASSESSMENT

❏ Assess for symptoms of prostatic hypertrophy (urinary hesitancy, feeling of incomplete bladder emptying, interruption of urinary stream, impairment of size and force of urinary stream, terminal urinary dribbling, straining to start flow, dysuria, urgency) before and periodically during therapy.

❏ Digital rectal examinations should be performed before and periodically during therapy for BPH.

■ *Lab Test Considerations:* Serum prostate-specific antigen (PSA) concentrations, which are used to screen for prostate cancer, may be evaluated before and periodically during therapy. Finasteride may cause a ↓ in serum PSA levels.

### POTENTIAL NURSING DIAGNOSES

■ Urinary elimination, impaired (Indications).

### IMPLEMENTATION

■ **PO:** Administer once daily with or without meals.

### PATIENT/FAMILY TEACHING

❏ Instruct patient to take finasteride as directed, even if symptoms improve or are unchanged. At least 6–12 mo of therapy may be necessary to determine whether or not an individual will respond to finasteride.

❏ Inform patient that the volume of ejaculate may be decreased during therapy but that this will not interfere with normal sexual function. Sexual dysfunction side effects will diminish over time.

❏ Caution patient that finasteride poses a potential risk to a male fetus. Women who are pregnant or may become pregnant should avoid exposure to semen of a partner taking finasteride and should not handle crushed finasteride because of the potential for absorption.

❏ Emphasize the importance of periodic follow-up exams to determine whether a clinical response has occurred.

### EVALUATION

**Clinical response to therapy can be evaluated by:** ■ Decrease in urinary symptoms of benign prostatic hyperplasia ■ Hair regrowth in androgenetic alopecia. Evidence of hair growth usually requires 3 mo or longer. Continued use is recommended to sustain benefit. Withdrawal leads to reversal of effect within 12 mo.

## fluconazole

(floo-**kon**-a-zole)

Diflucan

**CLASSIFICATION(S):**

**Therapeutic:** antifungals (systemic)

**Pregnancy Category C**

### INDICATIONS

■ **PO, IV:** Fungal infections caused by susceptible organisms, including: ❏ Oropharyngeal or esophageal candidiasis ❏ Serious systemic candidal infections ❏ Urinary tract infections ❏ Peritonitis ❏ Cryptococcal meningitis ■ Prevention of candidiasis in patients who have undergone bone marrow transplantation ■ **PO:** Single-dose oral treatment of vaginal candidiasis.

### ACTION

■ Inhibits synthesis of fungal sterols, a necessary component of the cell membrane. **Therapeutic Effects:** ■ Fungistatic action against susceptible organisms ■ May be fungicidal in higher concentrations. **Spectrum:** ■ *Cryptococcus neoformans* ■ *Candida* spp.

### PHARMACOKINETICS

**Absorption:** Well absorbed after oral administration.

**Distribution:** Widely distributed, good penetration into CSF, eye, and peritoneum.

**Metabolism and Excretion:** >80% excreted unchanged by the kidneys; <10% metabolized by the liver.

**Half-life:** 30 hr (increased in renal impairment).

---

{ } = Available in Canada only.
*CAPITALS indicates life-threatening; underlines indicate most frequent.

## CONTRAINDICATIONS AND PRECAUTIONS

**Contraindicated in:** ▪ Hypersensitivity to fluconazole or other azole antifungals ▪ Concurrent use with pimozide.

**Use Cautiously in:** ▪ Renal impairment (dosage reduction required if CCr <50 ml/min) ▪ Underlying liver disease ▪ Pregnancy, lactation, or children (safety not established).

## ADVERSE REACTIONS AND SIDE EFFECTS*

Incidence of adverse reactions is increased in HIV patients. ▪ **CNS:** headache ▪ **GI:** HEPATOTOXICITY, abdominal discomfort, diarrhea, nausea, vomiting ▪ **Derm:** exfoliative skin disorders including STEVENS-JOHNSON SYNDROME.

## INTERACTIONS

**Drug-Drug:** ▪ ↑ activity of **warfarin** ▪ **Rifampin, rifabutin,** and **isoniazid** ↓ levels ▪ Fluconazole at doses >200 mg/day may inhibit the CYP3A4 enzyme system and effect the activity of drugs metabolized by this system ▪ ↑ hypoglycemic effects of **tolbutamide, glyburide,** or **glipizide** ▪ ↑ levels and risk of toxicity from **cyclosporine, rifabutin, tacrolimus, theophylline, zidovudine, alfentanil,** and **phenytoin.** ▪ ↑ levels and effects of **benzodiazepines, zolpidem, bispirone, nisoldipine, tricyclic antidepressants,** and **losartan.**

## ROUTE AND DOSAGE

❑ **Oropharyngeal Candidiasis**
▪ **PO, IV (Adults):** 200 mg initially, then 100 mg daily for at least 2 wk.
▪ **PO, IV (Children >6 mos):** 3 mg/kg/day for at least 2 wk.

❑ **Esophageal Candidiasis**
▪ **PO, IV (Adults):** 200 mg initially, then 100 mg once daily for at least 3 wk or 2 wk after symptomatic improvement (up to 400 mg/day).
▪ **PO, IV (Children >6 mos):** 3 mg/kg/day for at least 3 wk or 2 wk after symptomatic improvement.

❑ **Vaginal Candidiasis**
▪ **PO (Adults):** 150-mg single dose.

❑ **Other Candidiasis**
▪ **PO, IV (Adults):** 50–400 mg/day.

❑ **Cryptococcal Meningitis**
▪ **PO, IV (Adults):** *Treatment*—400 mg once daily until favorable clinical response, then 200–400 mg once daily for at least 10–12 wk after clearing of CSF; change to oral therapy as soon as possible. *Suppressive therapy*—200 mg once daily.
▪ **PO, IV (Children >6 mos):** 6—12 mg/kg/day for at least 10—12 wk after clearing of CSF; change to oral therapy as soon as possible. *Suppressive therapy*—6 mg/kg/day.

❑ **Prevention of Candidiasis after Bone Marrow Transplant**
▪ **PO, IV (Adults):** 400 mg once daily; begin several days before procedure if severe neutropenia is expected, and continue for 7 days after ANC >1000 /mm$^3$.

❑ **Renal Impairment**
▪ **PO, IV (Adults):** *CCr 11–50 ml/min*—50% of the usual dose.

## AVAILABILITY (generic available)

▪ *Tablets:* 50 mg$^{Rx}$, 100 mg$^{Rx}$, 150 mg$^{Rx}$, 200 mg$^{Rx}$ ▪ Cost: 50 mg $/30, 100 mg $231.34/30, 150 mg $154.59/12, 200 mg $397.30/30 ▪ *Oral suspension (orange flavor):* 50 mg/5 ml in 35-ml bottle$^{Rx}$, 200 mg/5 ml in 35-ml bottle$^{Rx}$ ▪ *Injection:* 2 mg/ml in 100- or 200-ml bottles/containers$^{Rx}$.

TIME/ACTION PROFILE (blood levels)

| | ONSET | PEAK | DURATION |
|---|---|---|---|
| PO | unknown | 1–2 hr | 24 hr |
| IV | rapid | end of infu-sion | 24 hr |

# NURSING IMPLICATIONS

## ASSESSMENT

❑ Assess infected area and monitor CSF cultures before and periodically during therapy.
❑ Specimens for culture should be taken before instituting therapy. Therapy may be started before results are obtained.
▪ *Lab Test Considerations:* Monitor BUN and serum creatinine before and periodically during therapy; patients with renal dysfunction will require dose adjustment.
❑ Monitor liver function tests before and periodically during therapy. May cause ↑ AST, ALT, serum alkaline phosphate, and bilirubin concentrations.

## POTENTIAL NURSING DIAGNOSES
- Infection, risk for (Indications).

## IMPLEMENTATION
- **General:** Do not confuse Diflucan (fluconazole) with Diprivan (propofol).
- **PO:** Shake oral suspension well before administration.
- **Intermittent Infusion:** Open overwrap immediately before infusion. Inner bag may have slight opacity that will diminish gradually. Do not administer solution that is cloudy or has a precipitate. Check for leaks by squeezing inner bag. If leaks are found, discard container as unsterile.
- Do not set tubing as part of a series of connections as this may cause air embolism.
- **Rate:** Infuse at a maximum rate of 200 mg/hr.
- **Y-Site Compatibility:** ◆ acyclovir ◆ aldesleukin ◆ allopurinol ◆ amifostine ◆ amikacin ◆ aminophylline ◆ ampicillin/sulbactam ◆ aztreonam ◆ benztropine ◆ cefazolin ◆ cefepime ◆ cefotetan ◆ cefoxitin ◆ chlorpromazine ◆ cimetidine ◆ cisatracurium ◆ dexamethasone sodium phosphate ◆ diltiazem ◆ diphenhydramine ◆ dobutamine ◆ docetaxel ◆ dopamine ◆ doxorubicin liposome ◆ droperidol ◆ etoposide ◆ famotidine ◆ filgrastim ◆ fludarabine ◆ foscarnet ◆ ganciclovir ◆ gatifloxacin ◆ gemcitabine ◆ gentamicin ◆ granisetron ◆ heparin ◆ hydrocortisone ◆ immune globulin ◆ leucovorin ◆ linezolid ◆ lorazepam ◆ melphalan ◆ meperidine ◆ meropenem ◆ metoclopramide ◆ metronidazole ◆ midazolam ◆ morphine ◆ nafcillin ◆ nitroglycerin ◆ ondansetron ◆ oxacillin ◆ paclitaxel ◆ pancuronium ◆ penicillin G potassium ◆ phenytoin ◆ piperacillin/tazobactam ◆ prochlorperazine ◆ promethazine ◆ propofol ◆ ranitidine ◆ remifentanil ◆ sargramostim ◆ tacrolimus ◆ teniposide ◆ theophylline ◆ thiotepa ◆ ticarcillin/clavulanate ◆ tobramycin ◆ vancomycin ◆ vecuronium ◆ vinorelbine ◆ zidovudine.
- **Y-Site Incompatibility:** ◆ amphotericin B ◆ amphotericin B cholesteryl sulfate complex ◆ ampicillin ◆ calcium gluconate ◆ cefotaxime ◆ ceftazidime ◆ ceftriaxone ◆ cefuroxime ◆ chloramphenicol ◆ clindamycin ◆ diazepam ◆ digoxin ◆ erythromycin lactobionate ◆ furosemide ◆ haloperidol ◆ hydroxyzine ◆ imipenem/cilastatin ◆ pentamidine ◆ piperacillin ◆ ticarcillin ◆ trimethoprim/sulfamethoxazole.
- **Additive Incompatibility:** Manufacturer does not recommend admixing.

## PATIENT/FAMILY TEACHING
- Instruct patient to take medication as directed, even if feeling better. Doses should be taken at the same time each day. Take missed doses as soon as remembered, but not if almost time for next dose. Do not double doses.
- Instruct patient to notify health care professional if abdominal pain, fever, or diarrhea becomes pronounced, if signs and symptoms of liver dysfunction (unusual fatigue, anorexia, nausea, vomiting, jaundice, dark urine, or pale stools) occur, or if no improvement is seen within a few days of therapy.

## EVALUATION
**Effectiveness of therapy can be demonstrated by:** ■ Resolution of clinical and laboratory indications of fungal infections. Full course of therapy may require weeks or months of treatment after resolution of symptoms ■ Prevention of candidiasis in patients who have undergone bone marrow transplantation ■ Decrease in skin irritation and vaginal discomfort in patients with vaginal candidiasis. Diagnosis should be reconfirmed with smears or cultures before a second course of therapy to rule out other pathogens associated with vulvovaginitis. Recurrent vaginal infections may be a sign of systemic illness.

## fludrocortisone
(floo-droe-**kor**-ti-sone)
Florinef

**CLASSIFICATION(S):**
**Therapeutic:** hormones
**Pharmacologic:** corticosteroids (mineralocorticoid)

**Pregnancy Category C**

## INDICATIONS

■ Sodium loss and hypotension associated with adrenocortical insufficiency (given with hydrocortisone or cortisone) ■ Management of sodium loss due to congenital adrenogenital syndrome (congenital adrenal hyperplasia). **Unlabeled uses:** ■ Idiopathic orthostatic hypotension (with increased sodium intake) ■ Type IV renal tubular acidosis.

## ACTION

■ Causes sodium reabsorption, hydrogen and potassium excretion, and water retention by its effects on the distal renal tubule. **Therapeutic Effects:** ■ Maintenance of sodium balance and blood pressure in patients with adrenocortical insufficiency.

## PHARMACOKINETICS

**Absorption:** Well absorbed following oral administration.
**Distribution:** Widely distributed; probably enters breast milk.
**Protein Binding:** High.
**Metabolism and Excretion:** Mostly metabolized by the liver.
**Half-life:** 3.5 hr.

## CONTRAINDICATIONS AND PRECAUTIONS

**Contraindicated in:** ■ Hypersensitivity.
**Use Cautiously in:** ■ CHF ■ Addison's disease (patients may have exaggerated response) ■ Pregnancy, lactation, or children (safety not established).

## ADVERSE REACTIONS AND SIDE EFFECTS*

■ **CNS:** dizziness, headache ■ **CV:** CHF, arrhythmias, edema, hypertension ■ **GI:** anorexia, nausea ■ **Endo:** adrenal suppression, weight gain ■ **F and E:** hypokalemia, hypokalemic alkalosis ■ **MS:** arthralgia, muscular weakness, tendon contractures ■ **Neuro:** ascending paralysis ■ **Misc:** hypersensitivity reactions.

## INTERACTIONS

**Drug-Drug:** ■ Use with **thiazide or loop diuretics, mezlocillin, piperacillin,** or **amphotericin B** may result in ↑ risk of hypokalemia ■ Hypokalemia may ↑ risk of **digoxin** toxicity ■ May produce prolonged neuromuscular blockade following the use of **nondepolarizing neuromuscular blocking agents** ■

**Phenobarbital** or **rifampin** may ↑ metabolism and ↓ effectiveness of fludrocortisone.
**Drug-Food:** ■ Large amounts of **salt** or **sodium-containing foods** may cause excessive sodium retention and potassium loss.

## ROUTE AND DOSAGE

■ **PO (Adults):** *Adrenocortical insufficiency*—100 mcg/day (range 100 mcg 3 times weekly—200 mcg daily). Doses as small as 50 mcg daily may be required by some patients. Use with 10–37.5 mg cortisone daily or 10–30 mg hydrocortisone daily. *Adrenogenital syndrome*—100–200 mcg/day. *Idiopathic hypotension*—50–200 mcg/day (unlabeled).
■ **PO (Children):** 50–100 mcg/day.

## AVAILABILITY (generic available)

■ *Tablets:* 100 mcg (0.1 mg)[Rx].

TIME/ACTION PROFILE (mineralocorticoid activity)

| | ONSET | PEAK | DURATION |
|---|---|---|---|
| PO | unknown | unknown | 1–2 days |

# NURSING IMPLICATIONS

## ASSESSMENT

❑ Monitor blood pressure periodically during therapy. Report significant changes. Hypotension may indicate insufficient dose.

❑ Monitor for fluid retention (weigh daily, assess for edema, and auscultate lungs for rales/crackles).

❑ Monitor patients with Addison's disease closely and stop treatment if a significant increase in weight or blood pressure, edema, or cardiac enlargement occurs. Patients with Addison's disease are more sensitive to the action of fludrocortisone and may have an exaggerated response.

■ *Lab Test Considerations:* Monitor serum electrolytes periodically during therapy. Fludrocortisone causes ↓ serum potassium levels.

## POTENTIAL NURSING DIAGNOSES

■ Fluid volume, deficit (Indications).
■ Fluid volume, excess (Side Effects).

## IMPLEMENTATION

■ **PO:** Tablets are scored and may be broken if dose adjustment is necessary.

## PATIENT/FAMILY TEACHING

❏ Instruct patient to take medication as directed. Take missed doses as soon as remembered but not just before next dose is due. Explain that lifelong therapy may be necessary and that abrupt discontinuation may lead to addisonian crisis. Patient should keep an adequate supply available at all times.

❏ Advise patient to follow dietary modification prescribed by health care professional. Instruct patient to follow a diet high in potassium (see Appendix Q). Amount of sodium allowed in diet varies with pathophysiology.

❏ Instruct patient to inform health care professional if weight gain or edema, muscle weakness, cramps, nausea, anorexia, or dizziness occurs.

❏ Advise patient to carry identification at all times describing disease process and medication regimen.

## EVALUATION

**Effectiveness of therapy can be demonstrated by:** ■ Normalization of fluid and electrolyte balance without the development of hypokalemia or hypertension.

---

## flumazenil

(flu-**maz**-e-nil)

{Anexate}, Romazicon

### CLASSIFICATION(S):

**Therapeutic:** antidotes
**Pharmacologic:** benzodiazepines

### Pregnancy Category C

---

## INDICATIONS

■ Completely or partially reverses the effects of benzodiazepines used as general anesthetics, or during diagnostic or therapeutic procedures ■ Management of intentional or accidental overdose of benzodiazepines.

## ACTION

■ Flumazenil is a benzodiazepine derivative that antagonizes the CNS depressant effects of benzodiazepine compounds. It has no effect on CNS depression from other causes, including opioids, alcohol, barbiturates, or general anesthetics. **Therapeutic Effects:** ■ Reversal of benzodiazepine effects.

## PHARMACOKINETICS

**Absorption:** IV administration results in complete bioavailability.

**Distribution:** Unknown.

**Metabolism and Excretion:** Metabolism of flumazenil occurs primarily in the liver.

**Half-life:** 41–79 min.

## CONTRAINDICATIONS AND PRECAUTIONS

**Contraindicated in:** ■ Hypersensitivity to flumazenil or benzodiazepines ■ Patients receiving benzodiazepines for life-threatening medical problems, including status epilepticus or increased intracranial pressure, should not be given flumazenil ■ Serious cyclic antidepressant overdosage.

**Use Cautiously in:** ■ Mixed CNS depressant overdosage (effects of other agents may emerge when benzodiazepine effect is removed) ■ History of seizures (seizures are more likely to occur in patients who are experiencing sedative/hypnotic withdrawal, who have recently received repeated doses of benzodiazepines, or who have a previous history of seizure activity) ■ Head injury (may increase intracranial pressure and risk of seizures) ■ Pregnancy, lactation, or children <2 yr (safety not established).

## ADVERSE REACTIONS AND SIDE EFFECTS*

■ **CNS:** SEIZURES, <u>dizziness</u>, agitation, confusion, drowsiness, emotional lability, fatigue, headache, sleep disorders ■ **EENT:** abnormal hearing, abnormal vision, blurred vision ■ **CV:** arrhythmias, chest pain, hypertension ■ **GI:** <u>nausea</u>, <u>vomiting</u>, hiccups ■ **Derm:** flushing, sweating ■ **Local:** pain/injection-site reactions, phlebitis ■ **Neuro:** paresthesia ■ **Misc:** rigors, shivering.

---

{ } = Available in Canada only.
*CAPITALS indicates life-threatening; <u>underlines</u> indicate most frequent.

## INTERACTIONS

**Drug-Drug:** ■ None significant.

## ROUTE AND DOSAGE

❑ **Reversal of Conscious Sedation or General Anesthesia**

■ **IV (Adults):** 0.2 mg. Additional doses may be given at 1-min intervals until desired results are obtained, up to a total dose of 1 mg. If resedation occurs, regimen may be repeated at 20-min intervals, not to exceed 3 mg/ hr.

■ **IV (Children):** 0.01 mg/kg (up to 0.2 mg); if the desired level of consciousness is not obtained after waiting an additional 45 sec, further injections of 0.01 mg/kg (up to 0.2 mg) can be administered and repeated at 60-sec intervals when necessary (up to a maximum of 4 additional times) to a maximum total dose of 0.05 mg/kg or 1 mg, whichever is lower. The dose should be individualized based on the patient's response.

❑ **Suspected Benzodiazepine Overdose**

■ **IV (Adults):** 0.2 mg. Additional 0.3 mg may be given 30 sec later. Further doses of 0.5 mg may be given at 1-min intervals, if necessary, to a total dose of 3 mg. Usual dose required is 1–3 mg. If resedation occurs, additional doses of 0.5 mg/min for 2 min may be given at 20-min intervals (given no more than 1 mg at a time, not to exceed 3 mg per hour).

■ **IV (Children):** Unlabeled: 100 mcg (0.1 mg)/kg up to a cumulative dose of 1 mg.

## AVAILABILITY

■ *Injection:* 0.1 mg/ml in 5- and 10-ml vials^Rx
■ Cost: $471.02/5-ml vial, $749.33/10-ml vial.

TIME/ACTION PROFILE (reversal of benzodiazepine effects)

| | ONSET | PEAK | DURATION |
|---|---|---|---|
| IV | 1–2 min | 6–10 min | 1–2 hr† |

†Depends on dose/concentration of benzodiazepine and dose of flumazenil.

## NURSING IMPLICATIONS

### ASSESSMENT

■ **General Info:** Assess level of consciousness and respiratory status before and throughout therapy. Observe patient for at least 2 hr after administration for the appearance of resedation. Hypoventilation may occur.

■ **Overdose:** Attempt to determine time of ingestion and amount and type of benzodiazepine taken. Knowledge of agent ingested allows an estimate of duration of CNS depression.

## POTENTIAL NURSING DIAGNOSES

■ Injury, risk for (Indications).
■ Poisoning, risk for (Indications).

## IMPLEMENTATION

■ **General:** Ensure that patient has a patent airway before administration of flumazenil.

❑ Observe IV site frequently for redness or irritation. Administer through a free-flowing IV infusion into a large vein to minimize pain at the injection site.

❑ Optimal emergence should be undertaken slowly to decrease undesirable effects including confusion, agitation, emotional lability, and perceptual distortion.

❑ Institute seizure precautions. Seizures are more likely to occur in patients who are experiencing sedative/hypnotic withdrawal, patients who have recently received repeated doses of benzodiazepines, or those who have a previous history of seizure activity. Seizures may be treated with benzodiazepines, barbiturates, or phenytoin. Larger than normal doses of benzodiazepines may be required.

■ **Suspected Benzodiazepine Overdose:** If no effects are seen after administration of flumazenil, consider other causes of decreased level of consciousness (alcohol, barbiturates, opioid analgesics).

■ **Direct IV:** May be administered undiluted or diluted in syringe with D5W, 0.9% NaCl, or LR. Diluted solution should be discarded after 24 hr.

■ *Rate:* Administer each dose over 15–30 sec into free-flowing IV in a large vein.

## PATIENT/FAMILY TEACHING

❑ Flumazenil does not consistently reverse the amnestic effects of benzodiazepines. Provide patient and family with written instructions for postprocedure care. Inform family that patient may appear alert at the time of discharge but the sedative effects of the benzodiazepine may recur. Instruct patient to avoid driving or other activities requiring alertness for at least 24 hr after discharge.

❑ Instruct patient not to take any alcohol or nonprescription drugs for at least 18–24 hr after discharge.

❑ Resumption of usual activities should occur only when no residual effects of the benzodiazepine remain.

### EVALUATION

**Clinical response to therapy can be evaluated by:** ■ Improved level of consciousness ❑ Decrease in respiratory depression caused by benzodiazepines.

---

**flunisolide, See CORTICOSTEROIDS (INHALATION), CORTICOSTEROIDS (NASAL).**

---

**fluocinolone, See CORTICOSTEROIDS (TOPICAL/ LOCAL), CORTICOSTEROIDS (TOPICAL/LOCAL).**

---

## FLUOROQUINOLONES
(floor-oh-**kwin**-oh-lones)

**alatrofloxacin**
(a-la-troe-**flox**-a-sin)
Trovan (IV)

**ciprofloxacin†**
(sip-roe-**flox**-a-sin)
Cipro, Cipro XR

**enoxacin**
(ee-**nox**-a-sin)
Penetrex

**gatifloxacin**
(ga-ti-**flox**-a-sin)
Tequin

**gemifloxacin**
(gem-i-**flox**-a-sin)
Factive

**levofloxacin**
(le-voe-**flox**-a-sin)
Levaquin

**lomefloxacin**
(loe-me-**flox**-a-sin)
Maxaquin

**moxifloxacin†**
(mox-i-**flox**-a-sin)
Avelox

**norfloxacin†**
(nor-**flox**-a-sin)
Noroxin

**ofloxacin†**
(oh-**flox**-a-sin)
Floxin

**sparfloxacin**
(spar-**flox**-a-sin)
Zagam

**trovafloxacin**
(troe-va-**flox**-a-sin)
Trovan (oral)

***CLASSIFICATION(S):***
***Therapeutic:*** *anti-infectives*

**Pregnancy Category C**

†See Appendix C for ophthalmic use.

### INDICATIONS

■ **PO, IV:** Treatment of: ❑ Urinary tract and gynecologic infections ❑ Gonorrhea (some agents) ❑ Prostatitis (ciprofloxacin, levofloxacin, ofloxacin) ❑ Respiratory tract infections including sinusitis (not enoxacin or norfloxacin) ❑ Skin and skin structure infections (alatrofloxacin, gatifloxacin, levofloxacin, trovafloxacin, moxifloxacin, ciprofloxacin, ofloxacin) ❑ Bone and joint infections (ciprofloxacin) ❑ Infectious diarrhea (ciprofloxacin) ❑ Intraabdominal infections (ciprofloxacin with metronidazole, alatrofloxacin, trovafloxacin) ■

---

{ } = Available in Canada only.
*CAPITALS indicates life-threatening; underlines indicate most frequent.

Perioperative prophylaxis before transurethral procedures (lomefloxacin) or colorectal procedures (alatrofloxacin, trovafloxacin) ■ Hospital-acquired pneumonia or complicated intra-abdominal infection (alatrofloxacin, trovafloxacin) ■ Febrile neutropenia (ciprofloxacin) ■ Post-exposure treatment of inhalational anthrax (ciprofloxacin).

## ACTION

■ Inhibit bacterial DNA synthesis by inhibiting DNA gyrase. **Therapeutic Effects:** ■ Death of susceptible bacteria. **Spectrum:** ■ Broad activity includes many gram-positive pathogens: ❑ Staphylococci including methicillin-resistant *Staphylococcus aureus* and *Staphylococcus epidermidis* ❑ *Streptococcus pneumoniae* ❑ *Bacillus anthracis* ■ Gram-negative spectrum notable for activity against: ❑ *Escherichia coli* ❑ *Klebsiella* spp ❑ *Enterobacter* ❑ *Salmonella* ❑ *Shigella* ❑ *Proteus vulgaris* ❑ *Providencia stuartii* ❑ *Providencia rettgeri* ❑ *Morganella morganii* ❑ *Pseudomonas aeruginosa* ❑ *Serratia* ❑ *Haemophilus* spp ❑ *Acinetobacter* ❑ *Neisseria gonorrhoeae* and *Neisseria meningitidis* ❑ *Moraxella catarrhalis* ❑ *Yersinia* ❑ *Vibrio* ❑ *Brucella* ❑ *Campylobacter* ❑ *Aeromonas* spp ■ Active against the following anaerobic pathogens: ❑ *Bacteroides fragilis* and *Bacteroides intermedius* (alatrofloxacin, sparfloxacin, trovafloxacin) ❑ and *Clostridium welchii* ❑ *Gardnerella vaginalis* ❑ *Peptococcus niger* ❑ *Peptostreptococcus* spp ■ Additional spectrum includes: ❑ *Chlamydia pneumoniae* and *Chlamydia trachomatis* ❑ *Legionella pneumoniae* ❑ *Mycobacterium tuberculosis* ❑ *Mycoplasma pneumoniae* ❑ *Urea urealyticum.*

## PHARMACOKINETICS

**Absorption:** Well absorbed after oral administration (*ciprofloxacin*—70%; *enoxacin, moxifloxacin*—90%; *gatifloxacin*—96%; *gemifloxacin*—71%; *levofloxacin*—99%; *lomefloxacin*—95–98%; *norfloxacin*—30–40%; *ofloxacin*—89%; *sparfloxacin*—92%; *trovafloxacin*—88%; after IV administration alatrofloxacin is rapidly converted to trovafloxacin).

**Distribution:** Widely distributed. High tissue and urinary levels are achieved. All agents appear to cross the placenta. *Ciprofloxacin, ofloxacin,* and *sparfloxacin* enter breast milk.

**Metabolism and Excretion:** *Ciprofloxacin*—15% metabolized by the liver, 40–50% excreted unchanged by the kidneys;

*enoxacin*—>40% excreted unchanged by the kidneys, 20% metabolized by the liver, <10% excreted unchanged in urine; *gatifloxacin*—70% excreted unchanged in urine; *gemifloxacin*—Minimal metabolism, 61% excreted unchanged in feces, 36% excreted unchanged in urine; *levofloxacin*—87% excreted unchanged in urine, small amounts metabolized; *lomefloxacin*—65% excreted unchanged by the kidneys, 10% excreted unchanged in feces; *moxifloxacin*—mostly metabolized by the liver, 20% excreted unchanged in urine, 25% excreted unchanged in feces; *norfloxacin*—10% metabolized by the liver, 30% excreted unchanged by the kidneys, 30% excreted unchanged in feces; *ofloxacin*—70–80% excreted unchanged by the kidneys; *sparfloxacin*—partially metabolized by the liver, 10% excreted unchanged in urine; *trovafloxacin*—partially metabolized by the liver, 50% excreted unchanged in urine.

**Half-life:** *Ciprofloxacin*—4 hr; *enoxacin*—3–6 hr; *gatifloxacin*—7.1–7.8 hr; *gemifloxacin*—7 hr (range 4–12 hr); *levofloxacin*—6–8 hr; *lomefloxacin*—8 hr; *moxifloxacin*—12 hr; *norfloxacin*—6.5 hr; *ofloxacin*—5–7 hr (all are increased in renal impairment); *sparfloxacin*—20 hr; *trovafloxacin*—11 hr.

## CONTRAINDICATIONS AND PRECAUTIONS

**Contraindicated in:** ■ Hypersensitivity. Cross-sensitivity among agents may occur (including cinoxacin and nalidixic acid) ■ Pregnancy or Children <18 yr (except for post-exposure inhalational or cutaneous anthrax) ■ **Sparfloxacin:** ❑ History of photosensitivity to other agents; unavoidable exposure to sun; bright, natural light; or UV rays ❑ *Gatifloxacin, gemifloxacin, moxifloxacin, sparfloxacin*—concurrent use of amiodarone, disopyramide, erythromycin, pentamidine, phenothiazines, pimozide, procainamide, quinidine, sotalol, or tricyclic antidepressants ❑ Known QT prolongation or concurrent use of agents causing prolongation.

**Use Cautiously in:** ■ Underlying CNS pathology ■ Renal impairment (dosage reduction if CCr ≤50 ml/min for ciprofloxacin, levofloxacin, ofloxacin, sparfloxacin; ≤30 ml/min for enoxacin, norfloxacin, moxifloxacin; <40 ml/min for gatifloxacin, gemifloxacin or lomefloxacin) ■ Cirrhosis (dose reduction for alatrofloxacin/trovafloxacin recommended) ■ Geriatric patients, dialysis patients (increased risk of adverse reactions) ■ Lactation (safety not established except for post-exposure inhalational or cutaneous anthrax).

## ADVERSE REACTIONS AND SIDE EFFECTS*

■ **CNS:** SEIZURES, dizziness, drowsiness, headache, insomnia, acute psychoses, agitation, confusion, hallucinations, increased intracranial pressure, light-headedness, tremors ■ **CV:** *moxifloxacin, sparfloxacin*—ARRHYTHMIAS, QT prolongation, vasodilation ■ **GI:** HEPATOTOXICITY (ALATROFLOXACIN AND TROVAFLOXACIN ONLY), PSEUDOMEMBRANOUS COLITIS, abdominal pain, diarrhea, nausea, altered taste ■ **GU:** interstitial cystitis, vaginitis ■ **Derm:** photosensitivity (increased with lomefloxacin), phototoxicity (sparfloxacin), rash ■ **Endo:** hyperglycemia, hypoglycemia ■ **Local:** phlebitis at IV site ■ **MS:** tendinitis, tendon rupture ■ **Misc:** hypersensitivity reactions including ANAPHYLAXIS, STEVENS-JOHNSON SYNDROME, lymphadenopathy.

## INTERACTIONS

**Drug-Drug:** ■ ↑ risk of serious adverse cardiovascular reactions with concurrent use of gatifloxacin, gemifloxacin, moxifloxacin or sparfloxacin and **amiodarone, bepridil, disopyramide, erythromycin, pentamidine, phenothiazines, pimozide, procainamide, quinidine, sotalol, tricyclic antidepressants** ■ Intravenous **morphine** significantly ↓ the absorption of trovafloxacin ■ ↑ serum **theophylline** levels and may lead to toxicity ■ Administration with **antacids, iron salts, bismuth subsalicylate, sucralfate,** and **zinc salts** decreases absorption of fluoroquinolones ■ May alter the effects of **warfarin** ■ Serum levels of fluoroquinolones may be decreased by **antineoplastics** ■ **Cimetidine** may interfere with elimination of fluoroquinolones ■ Beneficial effects of ciprofloxacin may be antagonized by **nitrofurantoin** ■ **Probenecid** ↓ renal elimination of fluoroquinolones ■ **Digoxin** levels may be ↑ by concurrent enoxacin ■ Fluoroquinolones may ↑ risk of nephrotoxicity from **cyclosporine** ■ Concurrent use of ciprofloxacin with **foscarnet** may ↑ risk of seizures ■ Concurrent therapy with **corticosteroids** may ↑ the risk of tendon rupture ■ Gatifloxacin may exaggerate hypoglycemia when used with **oral hypoglycemic agents.**

**Drug-Natural Products:** ■ **Fennel** ↓ the absorption of ciprofloxacin.

**Drug-Food:** ■ Absorption is impaired by **concurrent tube feeding** (because of metal cations) ■ Ciprofloxacin should not be taken with **milk** or **yogurt** alone, but may be taken with other dietary calcium ■ Absorption of norfloxacin is decreased by **food** and/or **dairy products** (take 1 hr before or 2 hr after).

## ROUTE AND DOSAGE

❏ **Alatrofloxacin**

■ **IV (Adults):** *Serious infections*—300 mg q 24 hr. *Other infections*—200 mg q 24 hr. *Perioperative prophylaxis*—200 mg 30 min–4 hr before surgery.

❏ **Ciprofloxacin**

■ **PO (Adults):** *Most infections*—500–750 mg q 12 hr. *Urinary tract infections*—250–500 mg q 12 hr; *or* 1000 mg q 24 hr for 10–14 days as extended-release tablets. *Uncomplicated urinary tract infections*—100 mg q 12 hr for 3 days *or* 500 mg q 24 hr for 3 days as extended-release tablets. *Gonorrhea*—250-mg single dose. *Inhalational anthrax (post exposure) or cutaneous anthrax*—500 mg q 12 hr for 60 days.

■ **PO (Children):** *Inhalational anthrax (post exposure) or cutaneous anthrax*—15 mg/kg q 12 hr for 60 days (not to exceed 500 mg/dose).

■ **IV (Adults):** *Most infections*—400 mg q 12 hr. *Urinary tract infections*—200 mg q 12 hr. *Inhalational anthrax (post exposure)*—400 mg q 12 hr for 60 days.

■ **IV (Children):** *Inhalational anthrax (post exposure)*—10 mg/kg q 12 hr for 60 days (not to exceed 400 mg/dose).

❏ **Renal Impairment**

■ **PO (Adults):** *CCr 30–50 ml/min*—250–500 mg q 12 hr; *CCr 5–29 ml/min*—250–500 mg q 18 hr.

■ **IV (Adults):** *CCr 5–29 ml/min*—200–400 mg q 18–24 hr.

## ❑ Enoxacin

■ **PO (Adults):** *Complicated urinary tract infections*—400 mg q 12 hr. *Uncomplicated urinary tract infections*—200 mg q 12 hr. *Gonorrhea*—400-mg single dose.

## ❑ Renal Impairment

■ **PO (Adults):** *CCr* ≤*30 ml/min*—50% of the recommended dose q 12 hr.

## ❑ Gatifloxacin

■ **PO, IV (Adults):** *Acute bacterial exacerbation of chronic bronchitis, skin/skin structure infections, complicated urinary tract infections, acute pyelonephritis*—400 mg q 24 hr for 7–10 days. *Acute sinusitis*—400 mg q 24 hr for 10 days. *Community-acquired pneumonia*—400 mg q 24 hr for 7–14 days. *Uncomplicated urinary tract infections, cystitis*—400-mg single dose or 200 mg q 24 hr for 3 days. *Uncomplicated urethral gonorrhea in men or endocervical/rectal gonorrhea in women*—400-mg single dose.

## ❑ Renal Impairment

■ **PO, IV (Adults):** *CCr <40 ml/min*—400 mg initially, then 200 mg every 24 hr.

## ❑ Gemifloxacin

■ **PO (Adults):** *Acute bacterial exacerbation of chronic bronchitis*—320 mg once daily for 5 days; *Community-acquired-pneumonia (CAP)*—320 mg once daily for 7 days.

## ❑ Renal Impairment

■ **PO (Adults):** *CCr ≤ 40 ml/min*—AECB 160 mg once daily for 5 days; *CAP*—160 mg once daily for 7 days.

## ❑ Levofloxacin

■ **PO, IV (Adults):** 250–750 mg q 24 hr.

## ❑ Renal Impairment

■ **PO, IV (Adults):** *Most Infections:—CCr 20–49 ml/min*—500 mg initially then 250 mg q 24 hr; *CCr 10–19 ml/min*—500 mg initially then 250 mg q 48 hr. *Urinary tract infections:—CCr 10–19 ml/min*—250 mg q 48 hr.

## ❑ Lomefloxacin

■ **PO (Adults):** *Bronchitis/urinary tract infections*—400 mg once daily. *Perioperative prophylaxis (transurethral surgery)*—400 mg 2–6 hr before surgery.

## ❑ Renal Impairment

■ **PO (Adults):** *CCr ≤40 ml/min*—400 mg initially, then 200 mg once daily.

## ❑ Moxifloxacin

■ **PO, IV (Adults):** *Community-acquired pneumonia/bacterial sinusitis*—400 mg once daily for 10 days. *Acute bacterial exacerbation of chronic bronchitis*—400 mg once daily for 5 days. *Uncomplicated skin/skin structure infections*—400 mg/day for 7 days.

## ❑ Norfloxacin

■ **PO (Adults):** *Urinary tract infections*—400 mg q 12 hr. *Gonorrhea*—800-mg single dose.

## ❑ Renal Impairment

■ **PO (Adults):** *CCr ≤30 ml/min*—400 mg once daily.

## ❑ Ofloxacin

■ **PO, IV (Adults):** *Most infections*—400 mg q 12 hr. *Prostatitis/chlamydial infections*—300 mg q 12 hr. *Urinary tract infections*—200 mg q 12 hr. *Gonorrhea*—400-mg single dose.

## ❑ Renal Impairment

■ **PO, IV (Adults):** *CCr 20–50 ml/min*—100% of the usual dose q 24 hr; *CCr <20 ml/min*—50% of the usual dose q 24 hr.

## ❑ Sparfloxacin

■ **PO (Adults):** 400 mg initially, then 200 mg q 24 hr for 10 days.

## ❑ Renal Impairment

■ **PO (Adults):** *CCr <50 ml/min*—400 mg initially, then 200 mg q 48 hr.

## ❑ Trovafloxacin

■ **PO (Adults):** *Most infections*—100–200 mg q 24 hr. *Gonorrhea*—100-mg single dose. *Perioperative prophylaxis*—200 mg 30 min–4 hr before surgery.

## AVAILABILITY

## ❑ Alatrovafloxacin

■ *Concentrated solution for injection:* 200 mg/40 ml[Rx], 300 mg/60 ml[Rx].

## ❑ Ciprofloxacin

■ *Tablets:* 250 mg[Rx], 500 mg[Rx], 750 mg[Rx] ■ Cost: 500 mg $435.00/100 ■ *Extended-release tablets:* 500 mg[Rx] ■ *Oral suspension (strawberry flavor):* 250 mg/5 ml in 100-ml bottle[Rx], 500 mg/5 ml in 100-ml bottle[Rx] ■ *Injection:* 200 mg/20 ml[Rx], 400 mg/40 ml[Rx], 200 mg/100 ml premixed in D5W[Rx], 400 mg/200 ml premixed in D5W[Rx], 1200 mg/120 ml bulk package^Rx ∎ hydrocortisone Cipro HC Otic^Rx (see Appendix B).

❑ **Enoxacin**

∎ *Tablets:* 200 mg^Rx, 400 mg^Rx ∎Cost: 400 mg $70.22/20

❑ **Gatifloxacin**

∎ *Tablets:* 200 mg^Rx, 400 mg^Rx ∎Cost: 400 mg $411.16/50 ∎ *Injection:* 200 mg/20-ml vial^Rx, 400 mg/20-ml vial.

❑ **Levofloxacin**

∎ *Tablets:* 250 mg^Rx, 500 mg^Rx, 750 mg^Rx ∎ Cost: 500 mg $892.87/100 ∎ *Concentrated solution for injection:* 500 mg/20 ml^Rx ∎ *Premixed solution for injection:* 250 mg^Rx, 500 mg^Rx.

❑ **Lomefloxacin**

∎ *Tablets:* 400 mg^Rx ∎ Cost: 400 mg $138.68/ 20.

❑ **Moxifloxacin**

∎ *Tablets:* 400 mg^Rx ∎ *Injection, premixed:* 400 mg/250-ml bags^Rx.

❑ **Norfloxacin**

∎ *Tablets:* 400 mg^Rx ∎ Cost: 400 mg $81.05/ 20.

❑ **Ofloxacin**

∎ *Tablets:* 200 mg^Rx, 300 mg^Rx, 400 mg^Rx ∎ Cost: 400 mg $101.90/20 ∎*Injection:* 20 mg/ ml^Rx, 40 mg/ml^Rx ∎*Premixed injection:* 200 mg/50 ml^Rx, 400 mg/100 ml^Rx.

❑ **Sparfloxacin**

∎ *Tablets:* 200 mg^Rx.

❑ **Trovafloxacin**

∎*Tablets:* 100 mg^Rx, 200 mg^Rx ∎Cost: 100 mg $193.60/30.

TIME/ACTION PROFILE (blood levels)

| | ONSET | PEAK | DURATION |
|---|---|---|---|
| Alatrovafloxacin IV | rapid | end of infusion | 24 hr |
| Ciprofloxacin— PO | rapid | 1–2 hr | 12 hr |
| Ciprofloxacin— PO-ER | rapid | 1–4 hr | 24 hr |
| Ciprofloxacin— IV | rapid | end of infusion | 12 hr |
| Enoxacin—PO | rapid | 1–3 hr | 12 hr |
| Gatifloxacin—PO | rapid | 1–2 hr | 24 hr |
| Gatifloxacin—IV | rapid | end of infusion | 24 hr |
| Gemifloxacin— PO | rapid | 0.5—2 hr | 24 hr |
| Levofloxacin— PO | rapid | 1–2 hr | 24 hr |
| Levofloxacin—IV | rapid | end of infusion | 24 hr |
| Lomefloxacin— PO | rapid | unknown | 24 hr |
| Moxifloxacin— PO | within 1 hr | 1–3 hr | 24 hr |
| Moxifloxacin—IV | rapid | end of infusion | 24 hr |
| Norfloxacin—PO | rapid | 2–3 hr | 12 hr |
| Ofloxacin—PO | rapid | 1–2 hr | 12 hr |
| Ofloxacin—IV | rapid | end of infusion | 12 hr |
| Sparfloxacin— PO | rapid | 3–6 hr | 24 hr |
| Trovafloxacin— PO | rapid | 1 hr | 24 hr |

## NURSING IMPLICATIONS

### ASSESSMENT

❑ Assess patient for infection (vital signs; appearance of wound, sputum, urine, and stool; WBC; urinalysis; frequency and urgency of urination; cloudy or foul-smelling urine) prior to and during therapy.

❑ Obtain specimens for culture and sensitivity before initiating therapy. First dose may be given before receiving results. To prevent development of resistant bacteria, therapy should only be used to treat infections that are proven or strongly suspected to be caused by susceptible bacteria.

❑ Observe patient for signs and symptoms of anaphylaxis (rash, pruritus, laryngeal edema, wheezing). Discontinue drug and notify physician or other health care professional immediately if these problems occur. Keep epinephrine, an antihistamine, and resuscitation equipment close by in case of an anaphylactic reaction. Patients taking *gemifloxacin* who are at greater risk for rash are those receiving gemifloxacin for >7 days, <40 yrs of age, females, and postmenopausal females receiving hormone replacement therapy.

∎ *Lab Test Considerations:* Alatrovafloxacin and trovafloxacin may cause potentially fatal hepatitis. Monitor for ↑ serum AST,

{ } = Available in Canada only.
*CAPITALS indicates life-threatening; underlines indicate most frequent.

ALT, LDH, bilirubin, and alkaline phosphatase. Monitor liver function tests and pancreatic tests in patients who develop symptoms consistent with hepatitis and/or pancreatitis. Therapy should be discontinued.

❑ Other fluoroquinolones may cause ↑ serum AST, ALT, LDH, bilirubin, and alkaline phosphatase.

❑ May also cause ↓ WBC; ↑ or ↓ serum glucose; and glucosuria, hematuria, proteinuria, and albuminuria.

❑ Ciprofloxacin and norfloxacin may also cause crystalluria and ↑ BUN and serum creatinine concentrations.

❑ Moxifloxacin may cause hyperglycemia, hyperlipidemia, and altered prothrombin time. It may also cause ↑ WBC; ↑ serum calcium, chloride, albumin, and globulin; and ↓ glucose, hemoglobin, RBCs, neutrophils, eosinophils, and basophils.

❑ Monitor prothrombin time closely in patients receiving fluoroquinolones and warfarin; may enhance the anticoagulant effects of warfarin.

## POTENTIAL NURSING DIAGNOSES

■ Infection, risk for (Patient/Family Teaching).

## IMPLEMENTATION

■ **General:** Do confuse norfloxacin with Norflex (orphenadrine).

❑ Because of potentially fatal hepatic toxicity associated with the use of alatrofloxacin and trovafloxacin, their use should be strictly limited to one of several very specific infections that is serious and life or limb threatening; therapy must be initiated in an inpatient facility and must be judged to be a situation where benefit outweighs possible risks. Therapy should not be more than 14 days and should be immediately discontinued if any signs/symptoms of liver dysfunction occur.

❑ Intravenous morphine significantly reduces the absorption of *oral trovafloxacin*. IV morphine should be administered 2 hr after *oral trovafloxacin* is administered in a fasting state or 4 hr after food.

■ **PO:** Administer *norfloxacin, ofloxacin*, and *enoxacin* on an empty stomach 1 hr before or 2 hr after meals, with a full glass of water. *Moxifloxacin, gemifloxacin*, and *trovafloxacin* may be administered without regard to meals. Antacids containing magnesium or aluminum, iron, or zinc preparations should

not be taken within 4 hr before and 2 hr (8 hr for moxifloxacin) after administration.

❑ If gastric irritation occurs, ciprofloxacin and lomefloxacin may be administered with meals. Food slows and may slightly decrease absorption.

❑ Milk and yogurt decrease the absorption of ciprofloxacin. Do not administer concurrently.

❑ Ciprofloxacin 5% and 10% oral suspension should not be administered through a feeding tube due to unusual physical characteristics. Shake solution for 15 seconds prior to administration. Do not chew microcapsules in solution.

❑ *Gemifloxacin* and *ciprofloxacin extended-release tablets* should be swallowed whole; do not crush, break, or chew.

❑ **Alatrovafloxacin**

■ **Intermittent Infusion:** Dilute with D5W, 0.45% NaCl, D5/0.45% NaCl, D5/0.9% NaCl, or D5/LR for a concentration of 1–2 mg/ml. Discard unused portion.

■ *Rate:* Administer over 60 min.

■ **Y-Site Compatibility:** ◆ amikacin ◆ cyclosporine ◆ dopamine ◆ droperidol ◆ fentanyl ◆ gentamicin ◆ ketorolac ◆ lorazepam ◆ LR ◆ midazolam ◆ nitroglycerin ◆ ondansetron ◆ potassium chloride ◆ propofol ◆ sodium bicarbonate ◆ 0.45% NaCL ◆ tobramycin ◆ vancomycin.

■ **Y-Site Incompatibility:** Incompatible with 0.9% NaCl and LR over time. Temporarily discontinue other solutions when administering alatrofloxacin. Flush line before and after administration. Lines may be flushed with 0,9% NaCL; incompatibility only occurs with prolonged exposure. ◆ aztreonam ◆ ceftazidine ◆ ceftriaxone ◆ dobutamine ◆ famotidine ◆ furosemide ◆ heparin ◆ insulin ◆ magnesium sulfate ◆ midazolam ◆ morphine ◆ piperacillin/tazobactam ◆ ticarcillin/clavulanate.

■ **Additive Incompatibility:** Do not admix with other medications.

❑ **Ciprofloxacin**

■ **Intermittent Infusion:** Dilute to a concentration of 1–2 mg/ml with 0.9% NaCl or D5W. Stable for 14 days at refrigerated or room temperature.

■ *Rate:* Administer over 60 min into a large vein to minimize venous irritation.

■ **Y-Site Compatibility:** ◆ amifostine ◆ aztreonam ◆ calcium gluconate ◆ ceftazidime ◆ cisatracurium ◆ digoxin ◆ diltiazem ◆ diphenhydramine ◆ dobutamine ◆ docetaxel ◆ dopamine ◆ doxorubicin liposome ◆ etoposide ◆ gemcitabine ◆ gentamicin ◆ granisetron ◆ lidocaine ◆ linezolid ◆ lorazepam ◆ LR ◆ metoclopramide ◆ midazolam ◆ midodrine ◆ piperacillin ◆ potassium acetate ◆ potassium chloride ◆ promethazine ◆ ranitidine ◆ remifentanil ◆ 0.9% NaCL ◆ tacrolimus ◆ teniposide ◆ thiotepa ◆ tobramycin ◆ verapamil.

■ **Y-Site Incompatibility:** Manufacturer recommends temporarily discontinuing other solutions when administering ciprofloxacin. ◆ aminophylline ◆ amphotericin B ◆ ampicillin/sulbactam ◆ cefuroxime ◆ clindamycin ◆ floxacillin ◆ heparin ◆ sodium bicarbonate ◆ ticarcillin.

❑ **Gatifloxacin**

■ **Intermittent Infusion:** Dilute to a concentration of 2 mg/ml with D5W, 0.9% NaCl, D5LR, or D5/0.9% NaCl. Solution is stable for 14 days if refrigerated or at room temperature.

■ *Rate:* Administer over 60 min. Avoid rapid or bolus IV infusion.

■ **Y-Site Compatibility:** ◆ acyclovir ◆ alfentanil ◆ amikacin ◆ aminophylline ◆ ampicillin ◆ ampicillin/sulbactam ◆ aztreonam ◆ bretylium ◆ buprenorphine ◆ butorphanol ◆ calcium chloride ◆ calcium gluconate ◆ carboplatin ◆ cefazolin ◆ cefotetan ◆ ceftazidime ◆ ceftizoxime ◆ ceftriaxone ◆ chlorpromazine ◆ cimetidine ◆ cisatracurium ◆ cisplatin ◆ clindamycin ◆ cyclophosphamide ◆ cyclosporine ◆ cytarabine ◆ digoxin ◆ diphenhydramine ◆ dobutamine ◆ dopamine ◆ doxorubicin ◆ droperidol ◆ enalaprilat ◆ esmolol ◆ etoposide ◆ famotidine ◆ fentanyl ◆ fluconazole ◆ fluorouracil ◆ ganciclovir ◆ gemcitabine ◆ gentamicin ◆ granisetron ◆ haloperidol ◆ hydrocortisone sodium succinate ◆ hydromorphone ◆ ifosfamide ◆ imipenem/cilastatin ◆ labetalol ◆ leucovoran ◆ lidocaine ◆ lorazepam ◆ magnesium sulfate ◆ mannitol ◆ meperidine ◆ mesna ◆ methotrexate ◆ methylprednisolone ◆ metoclopramide ◆ metronidazole ◆ midazolam ◆ mitoxantrone ◆ morphine ◆ nalbuphine ◆ naloxone ◆ nitroglycerin ◆ ondansetron ◆ paclitaxel ◆ pentamidine ◆ pentobarbital ◆ phenobarbital ◆ potassium chloride ◆ prochlorperazine ◆ promethazine ◆ propranolol ◆ ranitidine ◆ remifentanil ◆ sodium bicarbonate ◆ sodium phosphates ◆ sufentanil ◆ theophylline ◆ ticarcillin ◆ ticarcillin/clavulanate ◆ tobramycin ◆ trimethoprim/sulfamethoxazole ◆ vecuronium ◆ verapamil ◆ vinblastine ◆ vincristine ◆ vinorelbine ◆ zidovudine.

■ **Y-Site Incompatibility:** Do not mix or administer with other medications. Temporarily discontinue other solutions when administering gatifloxacin. Flush IV line before and after administration. ◆ amphotericin B ◆ amphotericin B cholesteryl sulfate ◆ cefoperazone ◆ cefoxitin ◆ diazepam ◆ furosemide ◆ heparin ◆ phenytoin ◆ piperacillin ◆ piperacillin/tazobactam ◆ potassium phosphates ◆ vancomycin.

❑ **Levofloxacin**

■ **Intermittent Infusion:** Dilute to a concentration of 5 mg/ml with 0.9% NaCl, D5W, D5/0.9% NaCl, D5/0.45% NaCl, D5/LR, 5% sodium bicarbonate, D5, Plasmalyte 56, or sodium lactate. Also available in premixed bottles and flexible containers with D5W, which need no further dilution. Discard unused solution. Diluted solution is stable for 72 hr at room temperature and 14 days if refrigerated.

■ *Rate:* Administer by infusion over at least 60 min. Avoid rapid bolus injection.

■ **Y-Site Compatibility:** ◆ amikacin ◆ aminophylline ◆ ampicillin ◆ caffeine citrate ◆ cefotaxime ◆ cimetidine ◆ clindamycin ◆ dexamethasone ◆ dobutamine ◆ dopamine ◆ epinephrine ◆ fentanyl ◆ gentamicin ◆ isoproterenol ◆ lidocaine ◆ linezolid ◆ lorazepam ◆ metoclopramide ◆ morphine ◆ oxacillin ◆ pancuronium ◆ penicillin G ◆ phenobarbital ◆ phenylephrine ◆ sodium bicarbonate ◆ vancomycin.

■ **Y-Site Incompatibility:** ◆ acyclovir ◆ alprostadil ◆ furosemide ◆ heparin ◆ indomethacin ◆ nitroglycerin ◆ nitroprusside ◆ propofol.

■ **Additive Compatibility:** ◆ potassium chloride.

□ **Moxifloxacin**

■ **Intermittent Infusion:** Premix bags should not be further diluted. Use transfer set whose piercing pin does not require excessive force; insert with a gentle twisting motion until pin is firmly seated.

■ **Rate:** Administer over 60 min. Avoid rapid or bolus infusion.

■ **Solution Compatibility:** ◆ 0.9% NaCl ◆ D5W ◆ D10W ◆ LR

■ **Y-Site Incompatibility:** Temporarily discontinue administration of other solutions during moxifloxacin.

□ **Ofloxacin**

■ **Intermittent Infusion:** Dilute to a concentration of 4 mg/ml with 0.9% NaCl, D5W, D5/0.9% NaCl, D5/LR, 5% sodium bicarbonate, D5, Plasmalyte 56, or sodium lactate. Also available in premixed bottles and flexible containers with D5W that need no further dilution. Discard unused solution.

■ **Rate:** Administer by infusion only over at least 60 min.

■ **Y-Site Compatibility:** ◆ ampicillin ◆ cisatracurium ◆ docetaxel ◆ etoposide ◆ gemcitabine ◆ granisetron ◆ linezolid ◆ propofol ◆ remifentanil ◆ thiotepa.

■ **Y-Site Incompatibility:** ◆ amphotericin B cholesteryl sulfate ◆ cefepime ◆ doxorubicin liposome.

**PATIENT/FAMILY TEACHING**

□ Instruct patient to take medication as directed at evenly spaced times and to finish drug completely, even if feeling better. Missed doses should be taken as soon as possible, unless almost time for next dose. Do not double doses. Advise patient that sharing of this medication may be dangerous. Caution patients that fluoroquinolones should only be used to treat bacterial infections; they are not effective against viral infections, such as the common cold.

□ Advise patients to notify health care professional immediately if they are taking theophylline.

□ Encourage patient to maintain a fluid intake of at least 1500–2000 ml/day to prevent crystalluria.

□ Advise patient that antacids or medications containing iron or zinc will decrease absorption and should not be taken within 2 hr before *norfloxacin* or *ofloxacin*; 3 hr before *gemifloxacin*; 4 hr before *moxifloxacin* or *trovafloxacin*; 6 hr before *ciprofloxacin* or *lomefloxacin*; or 8 hr before *enoxacin* and 2 hr (*moxifloxacin*—8 hr) after taking this medication.

□ May cause dizziness and drowsiness. Caution patient to avoid driving or other activities requiring alertness until response to medication is known.

□ Advise patient to notify health care professional of any personal or family history of QTc prolongation or proarrhythmic conditions such as recent hypokalemia, significant bradycardia, or recent myocardial ischemia. Patients with this history should not receive fluoroquinolones.

□ Caution patient to use sunscreen and protective clothing to prevent phototoxicity reactions during and for 5 days after therapy. Notify health care professional if a sunburn-like reaction or skin eruption occurs.

□ Instruct patients being treated for gonorrhea that partners also must be treated.

□ Instruct patient to consult health care professional before taking any other Rx or OTC medications, or herbal products or supplements.

□ Advise patient to report signs of superinfection (furry overgrowth on the tongue, vaginal itching or discharge, loose or foul-smelling stools).

□ Instruct patient to notify health care professional if fever and diarrhea develop, especially if stool contains blood, pus, or mucus. Advise patient not to treat diarrhea without consulting health care professional.

□ Instruct patient to notify health care professional immediately if rash or tendon pain or inflammation occur. Therapy should be discontinued.

**EVALUATION**

**Clinical response to therapy can be evaluated by:** ■ Resolution of the signs and symptoms of infection. Time for complete resolution depends on organism and site of infection ■ Resolution of the signs and symptoms of urinary tract infection □ Negative urine culture ■ Post exposure treatment of inhalational anthrax or cutaneous anthrax.

## fluorouracil

(flure-oh-**yoor**-a-sill)

Adrucil, Efudex, Fluoroplex, 5-FU

*CLASSIFICATION(S):*
*Therapeutic: antineoplastics*
*Pharmacologic: antimetabolites*

**Pregnancy Category D**

### INDICATIONS

■ **IV:** Used alone and in combination with other modalities (surgery, radiation therapy, other antineoplastics) in the treatment of: ❑ Colon cancer ❑ Breast cancer ❑ Rectal cancer ❑ Gastric cancer ❑ Pancreatic carcinoma ■ **Topical:** Management of multiple actinic (solar) keratoses and superficial basal cell carcinomas.

### ACTION

■ Inhibits DNA and RNA synthesis by preventing thymidine production (cell-cycle S-phase–specific). **Therapeutic Effects:** ■ Death of rapidly replicating cells, particularly malignant ones.

### PHARMACOKINETICS

**Absorption:** Minimal absorption (5–10%) after topical application.

**Distribution:** Widely distributed; concentrates and persists in tumors.

**Metabolism and Excretion:** Converted to an active metabolite; undergoes hepatic metabolism with small amounts excreted unchanged in urine.

**Half-life:** 20 hr.

### CONTRAINDICATIONS AND PRECAUTIONS

**Contraindicated in:** ■ Hypersensitivity ■ Pregnancy or lactation.

**Use Cautiously in:** ■ Infections ■ Depressed bone marrow reserve ■ Other chronic debilitating illnesses ■ Obese patients, patients with edema or ascites (dose should be based on ideal body weight).

### ADVERSE REACTIONS AND SIDE EFFECTS*

More likely to occur with systemic use than with topical use. ■ **CNS:** acute cerebellar dysfunction ■ **GI:** diarrhea, nausea, stomatitis, vomiting ■ **Derm:** alopecia, maculopapular rash, local inflammatory reactions (topical only), melanosis of nails, nail loss, palmar-plantar erythrodysesthesia, phototoxicity ■ **Endo:** sterility ■ **Hemat:** anemia, leukopenia, thrombocytopenia ■ **Local:** thrombophlebitis ■ **Misc:** fever.

### INTERACTIONS

**Drug-Drug:** ■ Combination chemotherapy with **irinotecan** may produce unacceptable toxicity (dehydration, neutropenia, sepsis) ■ Additive bone marrow depression with other **bone marrow depressants,** including other **antineoplastics** and **radiation therapy** ■ May decrease antibody response to **live-virus vaccines** and increase risk of adverse reactions.

### ROUTE AND DOSAGE

Doses may vary greatly, depending on tumor, patient condition, and protocol used.

❑ **Advanced Colorectal Cancer**

■ **IV (Adults):** 370 mg/m² preceded by leucovorin *or* 425 mg/m² preceded by leucovorin daily for 5 days. May be repeated q 4–5 wk.

❑ **Other Tumors**

■ **IV (Adults):** *Initial dose*—12 mg/kg/day for 4 days, then 1 day of rest, then 6 mg/kg every other day for 4–5 doses *or* 7–12 mg/kg/day for 4 days followed by 3-day rest, then 7–10 mg/kg q 3–4 days for 3 doses. *Maintenance*—7–12 mg/kg q 7–10 days *or* 300–500 mg/m²/day for 4–5 days, repeated monthly (no single daily dose should exceed 800 mg). **Poor-Risk Patients:** 3–6 mg/kg/day on days 1–3, 3 mg/kg/day on days 5, 7, 9 (not to exceed 400 mg/dose). Doses of 370–425 mg/m²/day for 5 days have been used in combination with leucovorin.

❑ **Actinic (Solar) Keratoses/Superficial Basal Cell Carcinomas**

■ **Topical (Adults):** *Actinic/solar keratoses*—1% solution or cream 1–2 times daily to lesions on head, neck, or chest; 2–5%

solution or cream may be needed for hands. *Superficial basal cell carcinomas*—5% solution or cream twice daily for 3–6 wk (up to 12 wk).

## AVAILABILITY

■ *Injection:* 50 mg/ml in 10-ml ampules or 10-, 20-, and 100-ml vials$^{Rx}$ ■ Cost: $2.87/10 ml vial, $5.74/20 ml vial ■ *Cream:* 1%$^{Rx}$, 5%$^{Rx}$ ■ *Solution:* 1%$^{Rx}$, 2%$^{Rx}$, 5%$^{Rx}$.

TIME/ACTION PROFILE (IV = effects on blood counts, Top = dermatologic effects)

|  | ONSET | PEAK | DURATION |
|---|---|---|---|
| IV | 1–9 days | 9–21 days (nadir) | 30 days |
| Top | 2–3 days | 2–6 wk | 1–2 mo |

# NURSING IMPLICATIONS

## ASSESSMENT

■ **General Info:** Monitor vital signs before and frequently during therapy.

❑ Assess mucous membranes, number and consistency of stools, and frequency of vomiting. Assess for signs of infection (fever, chills, sore throat, cough, hoarseness, pain in lower back or side, difficult or painful urination). Assess for bleeding (bleeding gums; bruising; petechiae; and guaiac test stools, urine, and emesis). Avoid IM injections and taking rectal temperatures. Apply pressure to venipuncture sites for 10 min. Notify physician if symptoms of toxicity (stomatitis or esophagopharyngitis, uncontrollable vomiting, diarrhea, GI bleeding, myocardial ischemia, leukocyte count <3500/mm$^3$, platelet count <100,000/mm$^3$, or hemorrhage from any site) occur; drug will need to be discontinued. May be reinitiated at a lower dose when side effects have subsided.

❑ Assess IV site frequently for inflammation or infiltration. Patient should notify nurse if pain or irritation at injection site occurs. May cause thrombophlebitis. If extravasation occurs, infusion must be stopped and restarted in another vein to avoid damage to subcut tissue. Report immediately. Standard treatment includes application of ice compresses.

❑ Assess skin for palmar-plantar erythrodysesthesia (tingling of hands and feet followed by pain, erythema, and swelling) throughout therapy.

❑ Monitor intake and output, appetite, and nutritional intake. GI effects usually occur on 4th day of therapy. Adjusting diet as tolerated may help maintain fluid and electrolyte balance and nutritional status.

❑ Monitor patient for cerebellar dysfunction (weakness, ataxia, dizziness). This may persist after discontinuation of therapy.

■ **Topical:** Inspect involved skin before and throughout therapy.

■ *Lab Test Considerations:* May cause a decrease in plasma albumin.

❑ Hepatic (AST, ALT, LDH, and serum bilirubin), renal, and hematologic (hematocrit, hemoglobin, leukocyte, platelet count) functions should be monitored before and periodically throughout therapy. CBC should be monitored daily during IV therapy. Report WBC of <3500/mm$^3$ or platelets <100,000/mm$^3$ immediately; they are criteria for discontinuation. Nadir of leukopenia usually occurs in 9–14 days, with recovery by day 30. May also cause thrombocytopenia.

❑ May cause an increase in urine excretion of 5-hydroxyindoleacetic acid (5-HIAA).

## POTENTIAL NURSING DIAGNOSES

■ Infection, risk for (Side Effects).

■ Nutrition, imbalanced: less than body requirements (Side Effects).

## IMPLEMENTATION

❑ *High Alert:* Fatalities have occurred with incorrect administration of chemotherapeutic agents. Before administering, clarify all ambiguous orders; double check single, daily, and course-of-therapy dose limits; have second practitioner independently double check original order, calculations and infusion pump settings. The number 5 in 5-fluorouracil is part of the drug name and does not refer to the dosage.

■ **General:** Solution should be prepared in a biologic cabinet. Wear gloves, gown, and mask while handling IV medication. Discard IV equipment in specially designated containers.

■ **Direct IV:** May be administered undiluted.

■ *Rate:* Rapid IV push administration (over 1–2 min) is most effective, but there is a more rapid onset of toxicity.

■ **Intermittent Infusion:** May be diluted with D5W or 0.9% NaCl.

❑ Use plastic IV tubing and IV bags to maintain greater stability of medication. Solution is stable for 24 hr at room temperature; do not refrigerate. Solution is colorless to faint yellow. Discard highly discolored or cloudy solution. If crystals form, dissolve by warming solution to 140°F, shaking vigorously, and cooling to body temperature.

■ *Rate:* Onset of toxicity is greatly delayed by administering an infusion over 2–8 hr.

■ **Syringe Compatibility:** ◆ bleomycin ◆ cisplatin ◆ cyclophosphamide ◆ furosemide ◆ heparin ◆ leucovorin ◆ methotrexate ◆ metoclopramide ◆ mitomycin ◆ vinblastine ◆ vincristine.

■ **Syringe Incompatibility:** ◆ droperidol ◆ epirubicin.

■ **Y-Site Compatibility:** ◆ allopurinol ◆ amifostine ◆ aztreonam ◆ bleomycin ◆ cefepime ◆ cisplatin ◆ cyclophosphamide ◆ doxorubicin ◆ doxorubicin liposome ◆ etoposide ◆ fludarabine ◆ furosemide ◆ gatifloxacin ◆ gemcitabine ◆ granisetron ◆ heparin ◆ hydrocortisone ◆ leucovorin ◆ linezolid ◆ mannitol ◆ melphalan ◆ methotrexate ◆ metoclopramide ◆ mitomycin ◆ paclitaxel ◆ piperacillin/tazobactam ◆ potassium chloride ◆ propofol ◆ sargramostim ◆ teniposide ◆ thiotepa ◆ vinblastine ◆ vincristine ◆ vitamin B complex with C.

■ **Y-Site Incompatibility:** ◆ amphotericin B cholesteryl sulfate complex ◆ droperidol ◆ filgrastim ◆ topotecan ◆ vinorelbine.

■ **Additive Compatibility:** ◆ bleomycin ◆ cyclophosphamide ◆ D5/LR ◆ etoposide ◆ floxuridine ◆ ifosfamide ◆ methotrexate ◆ mitoxantrone ◆ vincristine.

■ **Additive Incompatibility:** ◆ carboplatin ◆ cisplatin ◆ cytarabine ◆ diazepam ◆ doxorubicin ◆ fentanyl ◆ leucovorin ◆ metoclopramide ◆ morphine.

■ **Topical:** Consult physician before administering topical preparations to determine which skin preparation regimen should be followed. Tight occlusive dressings are not advised because of irritation to surrounding healthy tissue. A loose gauze dressing for cosmetic purposes is usually preferred. Wear gloves when applying medication. Do not use metallic applicator.

## PATIENT/FAMILY TEACHING

■ **General Info:** Instruct patient to notify health care professional if fever; chills; sore throat; signs of infection; yellowing of skin or eyes; abdominal pain; joint or flank pain; swelling of feet or legs; bleeding gums; bruising; petechiae; or blood in urine, stool, or emesis occurs. Caution patient to avoid crowds and persons with known infections. Instruct patient to use soft toothbrush and electric razor. Patients should be cautioned not to drink alcoholic beverages or take products containing aspirin or NSAIDs.

❑ Advise patient to rinse mouth with clear water after eating and drinking and to avoid flossing to minimize stomatitis. Viscous lidocaine may be used if mouth pain interferes with eating. Stomatitis pain may require treatment with opioid analgesics.

❑ Discuss with patient the possibility of hair loss. Explore methods of coping.

❑ Review with patient the need for contraception during therapy.

❑ Caution patient to use sunscreen and protective clothing to prevent phototoxicity reactions.

❑ Instruct patient not to receive any vaccinations without advice of health care professional.

❑ Emphasize the importance of routine follow-up lab tests to monitor progress and to check for side effects.

■ **Topical:** Instruct patient in correct application of solution or cream. Emphasize importance of avoiding the eyes; caution should also be used when applying medication near mouth and nose. If patient uses clean finger to self-administer, emphasize importance of washing hands thoroughly after application. Explain that erythema, scaling, and blistering with pruritus and burning sensation are expected. Therapy is discontinued when erosion, ulceration, and necrosis occur in 2–6 wk (10–12 wk for basal cell carcinomas). Skin heals 4–8 wk later.

## EVALUATION

**Effectiveness of therapy can be demonstrated by:** ■ Tumor regression ■ Removal of solar keratoses or superficial basal cell skin cancers.

# fluoxetine
(floo-**ox**-uh-teen)
Prozac, Prozac Weekly, Sarafem

## CLASSIFICATION(S):
**Therapeutic:** *antidepressants*
**Pharmacologic:** *selective serotonin reuptake inhibitors (SSRIs)*

## Pregnancy Category B

## INDICATIONS

■ Various forms of depression, often in conjunction with psychotherapy (including depression in geriatric patients) ■ OCD ■ Bulimia nervosa ■ Panic disorder ■ **Sarafem:** Management of premenstrual dysphoric disorder (PMDD). **Unlabeled uses:** ■ Anorexia nervosa ❏ ADHD ❏ Diabetic neuropathy ❏ Fibromyalgia ❏ Obesity ❏ Raynaud's phenomenon.

## ACTION

■ Selectively inhibits the reuptake of serotonin in the CNS. **Therapeutic Effects:** ■ Antidepressant action ■ Decreased behaviors associated with ■ panic disorder ■ bulimia ■ Decreased mood alterations associated with PMDD.

## PHARMACOKINETICS

**Absorption:** Well absorbed after oral administration.
**Distribution:** Crosses the blood-brain barrier.
**Protein Binding:** 94.5%.
**Metabolism and Excretion:** Converted by the liver to norfluoxetine, another antidepressant compound; fluoxetine and norfluoxetine are mostly metabolized by the liver; 12% excreted by kidneys as unchanged fluoxetine, 7% as unchanged norfluoxetine.
**Half-life:** 1–3 days (norfluoxetine 5–7 days).

## CONTRAINDICATIONS AND PRECAUTIONS

**Contraindicated in:** ■ Hypersensitivity ■ Concurrent use or use within 14 days of discontinuing MAO inhibitors (fluoxetine should be discontinued 5 weeks before MAO therapy is initiated).

**Use Cautiously in:** ■ Severe hepatic or renal impairment (lower/less frequent dose may be necessary) ■ History of seizures ■ Debilitated patients ( ↑ risk of seizures) ■ Diabetes mellitus ■ Patients with concurrent chronic illness, or multiple drug therapy (dosage adjustments may be necessary) ■ Patients with impaired hepatic function (lower doses/increased dosing interval may be necessary) ■ Pregnancy or lactation (although safety not established, has been used without harm during pregnancy).

## ADVERSE REACTIONS AND SIDE EFFECTS*

■ CNS: SEIZURES, anxiety, drowsiness, headache, insomnia, nervousness, abnormal dreams, dizziness, fatigue, hypomania, mania, weakness ■ EENT: stuffy nose, visual disturbances ■ **Resp:** cough ■ CV: chest pain, palpitations ■ GI: diarrhea, abdominal pain, abnormal taste, anorexia, constipation, dry mouth, dyspepsia, nausea, vomiting, weight loss ■ GU: sexual dysfunction, urinary frequency ■ **Derm:** excessive sweating, pruritus, erythema nodosum, flushing, rashes ■ **Endo:** dysmenorrhea ■ **MS:** arthralgia, back pain, myalgia ■ **Neuro:** tremor ■ **Misc:** allergic reactions, fever, flu-like syndrome, hot flashes, sensitivity reaction.

## INTERACTIONS

**Drug-Drug:** ■ **Discontinue use of MAO inhibitors** for 14 days before fluoxetine therapy; combined therapy may result in confusion, agitation, seizures, hypertension, and hyperpyrexia (serotonin syndrome). Fluoxetine should be discontinued for at least 5 wk before MAO inhibitor therapy is initiated ■ Inhibits the activity of cytochrome P450 2D6 enzyme in the liver and increases the effects of drugs metabolized by this enzyme system ■ **Medications that inhibit the P450 enzyme system** (including **ritonavir, saquinavir,** and **efavirenz**) may increase the risk of developing the serotonin syndrome). For concurrent use with **ritonavir** decrease fluoxetine dose by 70%; if initiating fluoxetine, start with 10 mg/day dose ■ Decreases metabolism and increases effects of **alprazolam** (decrease alprazolam dose by 50%) ■ ↑ CNS depression with **alcohol, antihistamines,** other **antidepressants, opioid analgesics,** or **sedative/hypnotics** ■ ↑ risk of side effects and adverse reactions with other **antidepressants, tryptophan, risperidone,** or **phenothiazines** ■ May ↑ effectiveness/risk of toxicity from **carbamazepine, clozapine,**

digoxin, **haloperidol, phenytoin, lithium, or warfarin.** ■ May ↓ the effects of **buspirone** ■ **Cyproheptadine** may decrease or reverse effects of fluoxetine ■ May ↑ sensitivity to **adrenergics** and increase the risk of serotonin syndrome ■ May alter the activity of other **drugs that are highly bound to plasma proteins.**
**Drug-Natural Products:** ■ ↑ risk of serotonin syndrome with **St. John's wort** and **SAMe.**

## ROUTE AND DOSAGE

■ **PO (Adults):** *Depression, OCD*—20 mg/day in the morning. After several weeks, may increase by 20 mg/day at weekly intervals. Doses greater than 20 mg/day should be given in 2 divided doses, in the morning and at noon (not to exceed 80 mg/day). Patients who have been stabilized on the 20 mg/day dose may be switched over to delayed-release capsules (Prozac Weekly) at dose of 90 mg weekly, initiated 7 days after the last 20 mg dose. *Panic disorder*—10 mg/day initially, may increase after one week to 20 mg/day (usual dose is 20 mg, but may be increased as needed/tolerated up to 60 mg/day). *Bulimia nervosa*—60 mg/day (may need to titrate up to dosage over several days). *PMDD*—20 mg/day (not to exceed 80 mg/day) *or* 20 mg/day starting 14 days prior to expected onset on menses, continued through first full day of menstruation, repeated with each cycle.

■ **PO (Geriatric Patients):** *Depression*—10 mg/day in the morning initially, may be increased (not to exceed 60 mg/day).

■ **PO (Children 7–17 yr):** *adolescents and higher weight children*—10 mg/day may be increased after 2 wk to 20 mg/day; additional increases may be made after several more weeks (range 20–60 mg/day); *lower weight children*—10 mg/day initially, may be increased after several more weeks (range 20–30 mg/day).

## AVAILABILITY (generic available)

■ *Tablets:* 10 mgRx ■ *Capsules:* 10 mgRx, 20 mgRx, 40 mgRx ■ Cost: 10 mg $324.71/100, 20 mg $333.07/100, 40 mg $199.85/30; *generic*—10 mg 260.09/100, 20 mg 266.40/100 ■ *Delayed-release capsules (Prozac Week-*

*ly):* 90 mgRx ■ Cost: $84.94/4 tabs ■ *Oral solution (mint flavor):* 20 mg/5 mlRx ■ Cost: $147.91/120 ml; *generic*—$118.00/120 ml.

TIME/ACTION PROFILE (antidepressant effect)

| | ONSET | PEAK | DURATION |
|---|---|---|---|
| PO | 1–4 wk | unknown | 2 wk |

## NURSING IMPLICATIONS

### ASSESSMENT

■ **General Info:** Monitor mood changes. Inform physician or other health care professional if patient demonstrates significant increase in anxiety, nervousness, or insomnia.
□ Assess for suicidal tendencies, especially during early therapy. Restrict amount of drug available to patient.
□ Monitor appetite and nutritional intake. Weigh weekly. Notify physician or other health care professional of continued weight loss. Adjust diet as tolerated to support nutritional status.
□ Assess patient for sensitivity reaction (urticaria, fever, arthralgia, edema, carpal tunnel syndrome, rash, hives, lymphadenopathy, respiratory distress) and notify physician or other health care professional if present; symptoms usually resolve by stopping fluoxetine but may require administration of antihistamines or corticosteroids.
■ **OCD:** Assess patient for frequency of obsessive-compulsive behaviors. Note degree to which these thoughts and behaviors interfere with daily functioning.
■ **Bulimia Nervosa:** Assess frequency of binge eating and vomiting duringtherapy.
■ **PMDD:** Monitor patient's mood prior to and periodically during therapy.
■ *Lab Test Considerations:* Monitor CBC and differential periodically during therapy. Notify physician or other health care professional if leukopenia, anemia, thrombocytopenia, or increased bleeding time occurs.
□ Proteinuria and mild ↑ in AST may occur during sensitivity reactions.

□ May cause ↑ in serum alkaline phosphatase, ALT, BUN, creatine phosphokinase; hypouricemia, hypocalcemia, hypoglycemia or hyperglycemia, and hyponatremia.

## POTENTIAL NURSING DIAGNOSES

■ Coping, ineffective (Indications).

■ Injury, risk for (Side Effects).

## IMPLEMENTATION

■ **General:** Do not confuse Sarafem (fluoxetine) with Serophene (clomiphene).

■ **PO:** Administer as a single dose in the morning. Some patients may require increased amounts, in divided doses, with a 2nd dose at noon.

□ May be administered with food to minimize GI irritation.

## PATIENT/FAMILY TEACHING

□ Instruct patient to take fluoxetine exactly as directed. If a dose is missed, omit and return to regular schedule. Do not double doses or discontinue without consulting health care professional; discontinuation may cause anxiety, insomnia, nervousness.

□ May cause drowsiness, dizziness, impaired judgment, and blurred vision. Caution patient to avoid driving and other activities requiring alertness until response to the drug is known.

□ Advise patient to avoid alcohol or other CNS depressant drugs during therapy and to consult health care professional before taking other medications or natural/herbal products with fluoxetine.

□ Caution patient to change positions slowly to minimize dizziness.

□ Inform patient that frequent mouth rinses, good oral hygiene, and sugarless gum or candy may minimize dry mouth. If dry mouth persists for more than 2 wk, consult health care professional regarding use of saliva substitute.

□ Instruct female patients to inform health care professional if pregnancy is planned or suspected.

□ Caution patient to wear protective clothing and use sunscreen to prevent photosensitivity reactions.

□ Inform patient that medication may cause decreased libido.

□ Advise patient to notify health care professional if symptoms of sensitivity reaction occur or if headache, nausea, anorexia, anxiety, or insomnia persists.

□ Emphasize the importance of follow-up exams to monitor progress. Encourage patient participation in psychotherapy.

## EVALUATION

**Effectiveness of therapy can be demonstrated by:** ■ Increased sense of well-being □ Renewed interest in surroundings. May require 1–4 wk of therapy to obtain antidepressant effects ■ Decrease in obsessive-compulsive behaviors ■ Decrease in binge eating and vomiting in patients with bulimia nervosa ■ Decreased incidence frequency of panic attacks ■ Decreased mood alterations associated with PMDD.

# FLUPHENAZINE

(floo-**fen**-a-zeen)

**fluphenazine decanoate**
{Modecate}, {Modecate Concentrate}, Prolixin Decanoate

**fluphenazine enanthate**
{Moditen Enanthate}, Prolixin Enanthate

**fluphenazine hydrochloride**
{Apo-Fluphenazine}, {Moditen HCl}, {Moditen HCl-HP}, Permitil, Prolixin

## CLASSIFICATION(S):

**Therapeutic:** *antipsychotics*
**Pharmacologic:** *phenothiazines*

**Pregnancy Category C**

## INDICATIONS

■ Acute and chronic psychoses.

## ACTION

■ Alter the effects of dopamine in the CNS ■ Possess anticholinergic and alpha-adrenergic blocking activity. **Therapeutic Effects:** ■ Diminished signs and symptoms of psychoses.

## PHARMACOKINETICS

**Absorption:** Well absorbed after PO/IM administration. Decanoate and enanthate salts in sesame oil have delayed onset and prolonged

action because of delayed release from oil vehicle and subsequent delayed release from fatty tissues.
**Distribution:** Widely distributed. Cross the blood-brain barrier. Cross the placenta; enter breast milk.
**Protein Binding:** ≥90%.
**Metabolism and Excretion:** Highly metabolized by the liver; undergo enterohepatic recirculation.
**Half-life:** *Fluphenazine hydrochloride*—4.7–15.3 hr; *fluphenazine enanthate*—3.7 days; *fluphenazine decanoate*—6.8–9.6 days.

## CONTRAINDICATIONS AND PRECAUTIONS

**Contraindicated in:** ■ Hypersensitivity ■ Cross-sensitivity with other phenothiazines may exist ■ Narrow-angle glaucoma ■ Bone marrow depression ■ Severe liver or cardiovascular disease ■ Hypersensitivity to sesame oil (decanoate and enanthate salts) ■ Some products contain alcohol or tartrazine and should be avoided in patients with known intolerance ■ Concurrent pimozide.
**Use Cautiously in:** ■ Geriatric or debilitated patients (initial dosage reduction may be necessary) ■ Diabetes mellitus ■ Respiratory disease ■ Prostatic hypertrophy ■ CNS tumors ■ Epilepsy ■ Intestinal obstruction ■ Pregnancy or lactation (safety not established).

## ADVERSE REACTIONS AND SIDE EFFECTS*

■ **CNS:** <u>extrapyramidal reactions</u>, sedation, tardive dyskinesia ■ **EENT:** blurred vision, dry eyes, lens opacities ■ **CV:** hypotension, tachycardia ■ **GI:** anorexia, constipation, drug-induced hepatitis, dry mouth, ileus ■ **GU:** urinary retention ■ **Derm:** <u>photosensitivity</u>, pigment changes, rashes ■ **Endo:** galactorrhea ■ **Hemat:** AGRANULOCYTOSIS, leukopenia ■ **Misc:** allergic reactions, hyperthermia.

## INTERACTIONS

**Drug-Drug:** ■ **Pimozide** may have additive adverse cardiovascular effects (QT prolongation); concurrent use should be avoided ■ Additive hypotension with **antihypertensives** ■ Additive CNS depression with other **CNS depressants,** including **alcohol, antidepressants,** antihistamines, MAO inhibitors, opioids, sedative/hypnotics, or general anesthetics ■ **Phenobarbital** may increase metabolism and decrease effectiveness ■ Concurrent use with **lithium** may produce any of the following—decreased fluphenazine absorption, increased excretion of lithium, increased risk of extrapyramidal reactions, or masking of the early signs of lithium toxicity ■ Concurrent **meperidine** may produce excess sedation and hypotension ■ **Aluminum-containing antacids** or **adsorbent antidiarrheals, charcoal (kaolin)** may decrease oral absorption ■ Increased risk of agranulocytosis with **antithyroid drugs** ■ May decrease anti-Parkinson activity of **levodopa** and **bromocriptine** ■ Decrease vasopressor response to **epinephrine** and **norepinephrine** ■ Decrease antihypertensive effect of **guanethidine** ■ Concurrent use with **beta blockers** may result in inhibition of metabolism of one or both drugs, producing an increased response ■ Increased risk of anticholinergic effects with other **agents having anticholinergic properties,** including **antihistamines, tricyclic antidepressants, disopyramide,** or **quinidine** ■ May decrease the pharmacologic affects of **amphetamines**.

## ROUTE AND DOSAGE

❑ **Fluphenazine Decanoate**
■ **IM, Subcut (Adults):** 12.5–25 mg initially; may be repeated q 1–4 wk. Dosage may be slowly increased as needed (not to exceed 100 mg/dose).
■ **IM, Subcut (Children ≥12 yr):** 6.25–18.75 mg initially; may be repeated q 1–3 wk. Dosage may be slowly increased as needed to 25 mg.
■ **IM, Subcut (Children 5–12 yr):** 3.125–12.5 mg initially; may be repeated q 1–3 wk. Dosage may be slowly increased.

❑ **Fluphenazine Enanthate**
■ **IM, Subcut (Adults):** 25 mg q 1–3 wk. May be slowly increased as needed (not to exceed 100 mg/dose).

❑ **Fluphenazine Hydrochloride**
■ **PO (Adults):** *Initial dose*—2.5–10 mg/day in divided doses q 6–8 hr. *Maintenance dose*—1–5 mg/day.

- **PO (Children):** 0.25–0.75 mg 1–4 times daily.
- **PO, IM (Geriatric Patients or Debilitated Patients):** 1–2.5 mg/day initially.
- **IM (Adults):** 1.25–2.5 mg q 6–8 hr.

## AVAILABILITY (generic available)

■ *Fluphenazine decanoate injection:* 25 mg/ml$^{Rx}$, {100 mg/ml$^{Rx}$} ■ *Fluphenazine enanthate injection:* 25 mg/ml$^{Rx}$ ■ *Fluphenazine hydrochloride tablets:* 1 mg$^{Rx}$, 2.5 mg$^{Rx}$, 5 mg$^{Rx}$, 10 mg$^{Rx}$ ■ *Fluphenazine hydrochloride elixir (orange flavor):* 2.5 mg/5 ml$^{Rx}$ ■ *Fluphenazine hydrochloride concentrate:* 5 mg/ml$^{Rx}$ ■ *Fluphenazine hydrochloride injection:* 2.5 mg/ml$^{Rx}$, {10 mg/ml$^{Rx}$}.

TIME/ACTION PROFILE (antipsychotic activity)

| | ONSET | PEAK | DURATION |
|---|---|---|---|
| PO hydro-chloride | 1 hr | unknown | 6–8 hr |
| IM hydro-chloride | 1 hr | 1.5–2 hr | 6–8 hr |
| IM enanthate | 24–72 hr | unknown | 1–3 wk |
| IM deca-noate | 24–72 hr | unknown | ≥4 wk |

## NURSING IMPLICATIONS

### ASSESSMENT

❏ Assess patient's mental status (orientation, mood, behavior) before and periodically throughout therapy.
❏ Monitor blood pressure (sitting, standing, lying), ECG, pulse, and respiratory rate before and frequently during the period of dosage adjustment. May cause Q-wave and T-wave changes in ECG.
❏ Observe patient carefully when administering oral medication to ensure that medication is actually taken and not hoarded.
❏ Assess fluid intake and bowel function. Increased bulk and fluids in the diet help minimize constipation.
❏ Monitor patient for onset of akathisia (restlessness or desire to keep moving) and extrapyramidal side effects (*parkinsonian—*difficulty speaking or swallowing, loss of balance control, pill rolling, mask-like face, shuffling gait, rigidity, tremors; *dystonic—*muscle spasms, twisting motions, twitching, inability to move eyes, weakness of arms or

legs) every 2 mo during therapy and 8–12 wk after therapy has been discontinued. Reduction in dosage or discontinuation of medication may be necessary. Trihexyphenidyl or diphenhydramine may be used to control these symptoms.
❏ Monitor for tardive dyskinesia (uncontrolled rhythmic movement of mouth, face, and extremities; lip smacking or puckering; puffing of cheeks; uncontrolled chewing; rapid or worm-like movements of tongue). Report immediately; may be irreversible.
❏ Monitor for development of neuroleptic malignant syndrome (fever, respiratory distress, tachycardia, seizures, diaphoresis, hypertension or hypotension, pallor, tiredness, severe muscle stiffness, loss of bladder control). Report immediately.
- *Lab Test Considerations:* CBC, liver function tests, and ocular examinations should be evaluated periodically during therapy. May cause decreased hematocrit, hemoglobin, leukocytes, granulocytes, and platelets. May cause elevated bilirubin, AST, ALT, and alkaline phosphatase. Agranulocytosis may occur after 4–10 wk of therapy with recovery 1–2 wk after discontinuation. May recur if medication is restarted. Liver function abnormalities may require discontinuation of therapy.
❏ May cause false-positive or false-negative pregnancy tests and false-positive urine bilirubin test results.

### POTENTIAL NURSING DIAGNOSES

- Thought processes, disturbed (Indications).
- Noncompliance (Patient/Family Teaching).

### IMPLEMENTATION

- **General:** Slight yellow to amber color does not alter potency.
❏ To prevent contact dermatitis, avoid getting liquid preparations on hands and wash hands thoroughly if spillage occurs.
❏ Injectable forms must be drawn up with a dry syringe and dry 21-gauge needle to prevent clouding of the solution.
- **PO:** Dilute concentrate just before administration in 120–240 ml of water, milk, carbonated beverage, soup, or tomato or fruit juice. Do not mix with beverages containing caffeine (cola, coffee), tannics (tea), or pectinates (apple juice).
- **Subcut:** Fluphenazine decanoate and enanthate are dissolved in sesame oil for long

duration of action. They may be administered subcut or IM.

■ **IM:** IM dose is usually 30–50% of oral dose. Because fluphenazine hydrochloride has a shorter duration of action, it is used initially to determine the patient's response to the drug and to treat the acutely agitated patient.

❏ Administer deep IM, using a dry syringe and 21-gauge needle, into dorsal gluteal site. Instruct patient to remain recumbent for 30 min to prevent hypotension.

## PATIENT/FAMILY TEACHING

❏ Advise patient to take medication exactly as directed and not to skip doses or double up on missed doses. If a dose is missed, take within 1 hr or skip dose and return to regular schedule if taking more than 1 dose/day; take as soon as possible unless almost time for next dose if taking 1 dose/day. Abrupt withdrawal may lead to gastritis, nausea, vomiting, dizziness, headache, tachycardia, and insomnia.

❏ Inform patient of possibility of extrapyramidal symptoms and tardive dyskinesia. Caution patient to report these symptoms immediately to health care professional.

❏ Advise patient to change positions slowly to minimize orthostatic hypotension.

❏ Medication may cause drowsiness. Caution patient to avoid driving or other activities requiring alertness until response to medication is known.

❏ Caution patient to avoid taking alcohol or other CNS depressants concurrently with this medication.

❏ Advise patient to use sunscreen and protective clothing when exposed to the sun. Exposed surfaces may develop a blue-gray pigmentation, which may fade after discontinuation of the medication. Extremes of temperature should also be avoided because this drug impairs body temperature regulation.

❏ Advise patient that good oral hygiene, frequent rinsing of mouth with water, and sugarless gum or candy may help relieve dry mouth. Health care professional should be notified if dry mouth persists beyond 2 wk.

❏ Inform patient that this medication may turn urine pink to reddish-brown.

❏ Instruct patient to notify health care professional promptly if sore throat, fever, unusual bleeding or bruising, rash, weakness, tremors, visual disturbances, dark-colored urine, or clay-colored stools occur.

❏ Advise patient to notify health care professional of medication regimen before treatment or surgery.

❏ Emphasize the importance of routine follow-up exams, including ocular exams, with long-term therapy and continued participation in psychotherapy.

## EVALUATION

**Effectiveness of therapy can be demonstrated by:** ■ Decrease in excitable, paranoic, or withdrawn behavior.

# flurandrenolide, See CORTICOSTEROIDS (TOPICAL/LOCAL).

# flurazepam

(flur-**az**-e-pam)

{Apo-Flurazepam}, Dalmane, {Novo-flupam}, {Somnol}

*CLASSIFICATION(S):*
*Therapeutic: sedative/hypnotics*
*Pharmacologic: benzodiazepines*

Schedule IV

Pregnancy Category UK

## INDICATIONS

■ Short-term management of insomnia (<4 wk).

## ACTION

■ Depresses the CNS, probably by potentiating GABA, an inhibitory neurotransmitter. **Therapeutic Effects:** ■ Relief of insomnia.

## PHARMACOKINETICS

**Absorption:** Well absorbed after oral administration.

**Distribution:** Widely distributed; crosses blood-brain barrier. Probably crosses the placenta and enters breast milk. Accumulation of drug occurs with chronic dosing.

**Protein Binding:** 97% (one of the active metabolites).

**Metabolism and Excretion:** Metabolized by the liver; some metabolites have hypnotic activity.

**Half-life:** 2.3 hr (half-life of active metabolite may be 30–200 hr).

## CONTRAINDICATIONS AND PRECAUTIONS

**Contraindicated in:** ■ Hypersensitivity ■ Cross-sensitivity with other benzodiazepines may exist ■ Pre-existing CNS depression ■ Severe uncontrolled pain ■ Narrow-angle glaucoma ■ Pregnancy or lactation.

**Use Cautiously in:** ■ Hepatic dysfunction (dosage reduction may be necessary) ■ History of suicide attempt or drug dependence ■ Geriatric or debilitated patients (initial dosage reduction may be necessary) ■ Children <15 yr (safety not established).

## ADVERSE REACTIONS AND SIDE EFFECTS*

■ **CNS:** confusion, daytime drowsiness, decreased concentration, dizziness, headache, lethargy, mental depression, paradoxical excitation ■ **EENT:** blurred vision ■ **GI:** constipation, diarrhea, nausea, vomiting ■ **Derm:** rashes ■ **Neuro:** ataxia ■ **Misc:** physical dependence, psychological dependence, tolerance.

## INTERACTIONS

**Drug-Drug:** ■ Concurrent use with **alcohol, antidepressants, antihistamines,** and **opioids** may result in additive CNS depression ■ **Cimetidine, hormonal contraceptives, disulfiram, fluoxetine, isoniazid, ketoconazole, metoprolol, propoxyphene, propranolol,** or **valproic acid** may decrease the metabolism of flurazepam, enhancing its actions ■ May decrease efficacy of **levodopa** ■ **Rifampin** or **barbiturates** may increase the metabolism and decrease effectiveness of flurazepam ■ Sedative effects may be decreased by **theophylline**.

**Drug-Natural Products:** ■ Concomitant use of **kava, valerian, skullcap, chamomile,** or **hops** can increase CNS depression.

## ROUTE AND DOSAGE

■ **PO (Adults):** 15–30 mg at bedtime.
■ **PO (Geriatric Patients or Debilitated Patients):** 15 mg initially, may be increased.

## AVAILABILITY (generic available)

■ **Capsules:** 15 mgRx, 30 mgRx ■ Cost: *Dalmane*—15 mg $29.43/30, 30 mg $32.09/30; generic—15 mg $16.64/30, 30 mg $17.68/30 ■ **Tablets:** 15 mgRx, 30 mgRx.

TIME/ACTION PROFILE (hypnotic activity)

|    | ONSET | PEAK | DURATION |
|----|-------|------|----------|
| PO | 15–45 min | 0.5–1 hr | 7–8 hr |

# NURSING IMPLICATIONS

## ASSESSMENT

❑ Assess sleep patterns before and periodically throughout therapy.
❑ Prolonged therapy may lead to psychological or physical dependence. Restrict amount of drug available to patient, especially if patient is depressed or suicidal, or has a history of addiction.

## POTENTIAL NURSING DIAGNOSES

■ Sleep pattern disturbed (Indications).
■ Injury, risk for (Side Effects).

## IMPLEMENTATION

■ **General:** Do not confuse flurazepam with temazepam.
❑ Supervise ambulation and transfer of patients after administration. Remove cigarettes. Side rails should be raised and call bell within reach at all times.
■ **PO:** Capsules may be opened and mixed with food or fluids for patients having difficulty swallowing.

## PATIENT/FAMILY TEACHING

❑ Advise patient to take medication exactly as directed. Discuss the importance of preparing environment for sleep (dark room, quiet, avoidance of nicotine and caffeine).
❑ Medication may cause daytime drowsiness. Caution patient to avoid driving and other activities requiring alertness until response to medication is known.
❑ Caution patient to avoid taking alcohol or other CNS depressants concurrently with this medication.

❑ Instruct patient to contact health care professional immediately if pregnancy is planned or suspected.

## EVALUATION

**Effectiveness of therapy can be demonstrated by:** ▪ Improvement in sleep patterns. Maximum hypnotic properties are apparent 2–3 nights after initiating therapy and may last 1–2 nights after therapy is discontinued.

---

# flutamide
(**floo**-ta-mide)
Eulexin

## CLASSIFICATION(S):
**Therapeutic:** antineoplastics
**Pharmacologic:** antiandrogens

### Pregnancy Category D

---

## INDICATIONS

▪ Treatment of prostate carcinoma in conjunction with luteinizing hormone–releasing hormone (LHRH) analogues such as leuprolide.

## ACTION

▪ Antagonizes the effects of androgen (testosterone) at the cellular level. **Therapeutic Effects:** ▪ Decreased growth of prostate carcinoma, an androgen-sensitive tumor.

## PHARMACOKINETICS

**Absorption:** Well absorbed after oral administration.
**Distribution:** Unknown.
**Metabolism and Excretion:** Mostly metabolized by the liver. Some conversion to another antiandrogenic compound (2-hydroxyflutamide).
**Half-life:** Unknown.

## CONTRAINDICATIONS AND PRECAUTIONS

**Contraindicated in:** ▪ Hypersensitivity ▪ Severe hepatic impairment.
**Use Cautiously in:** ▪ Severe cardiovascular disease.

## ADVERSE REACTIONS AND SIDE EFFECTS*

Side effects primarily caused by LHRH antagonist. ▪ **CNS:** anxiety, confusion, drowsiness, mental depression, nervousness ▪ **CV:** edema, hypertension ▪ **GI:** HEPATOTOXICITY, diarrhea, nausea, vomiting ▪ **GU:** impotence, loss of libido ▪ **Derm:** photosensitivity, rash ▪ **Endo:** gynecomastia ▪ **Misc:** hot flashes.

## INTERACTIONS

**Drug-Drug:** ▪ Acts synergistically with **LHRH analogues (leuprolide).**

## ROUTE AND DOSAGE

▪ **PO (Adults):** 250 mg q 8 hr; given concurrently with leuprolide.

## AVAILABILITY

▪ *Capsules:* 125 mg$^{Rx}$, {250 mg$^{Rx}$}.

TIME/ACTION PROFILE

| | ONSET | PEAK | DURATION |
|---|---|---|---|
| PO | unknown | unknown | unknown |

## NURSING IMPLICATIONS

### ASSESSMENT

❑ Monitor for diarrhea, nausea, and vomiting. Adjust diet as tolerated. Notify physician if these symptoms become severe.

▪ *Lab Test Considerations:* May cause elevated AST, ALT, bilirubin, and serum creatinine values. Monitor ALT before therapy, monthly for the first 4 mo of therapy, and periodically thereafter. If ALT rises above 2 times the upper limit of normal, flutamide should be discontinued immediately. Liver function tests should also be obtained at the first sign of nausea, vomiting, abdominal pain, fatigue, anorexia, or hyperbilirubinemia.

❑ May cause increased plasma estradiol and testosterone concentrations.

### POTENTIAL NURSING DIAGNOSES

▪ Sexual dysfunction (Side Effects).

---

{ } = Available in Canada only.
*CAPITALS indicates life-threatening; underlines indicate most frequent.

## IMPLEMENTATION

■ **General:** Used in combination with LHRH agonist, such as leuprolide.

## PATIENT/FAMILY TEACHING

❑ Explain that flutamide must be taken in conjunction with leuprolide. Instruct patient to take flutamide exactly as directed. If a dose is missed, take as soon as possible unless almost time for next dose. Do not double doses.

❑ Warn patient that side effects such as hot flashes, loss of sex drive, impotence, and breast enlargement may be caused by the LHRH agonist. The primary side effect of flutamide alone is diarrhea, but the combination of drugs is necessary to achieve the therapeutic effect.

❑ Advise patient to notify health care professional immediately if dark urine, itching, loss of appetite, nausea, vomiting, pain in right side, or yellow eyes or skin occurs. Hepatotoxicity usually resolves when flutamide is discontinued, but it may be progressive and fatal; requires immediate medical attention.

## EVALUATION

**Effectiveness of therapy can be demonstrated by:** ■ Decrease in the spread of prostate cancer.

---

## fluticasone, See CORTICOSTEROIDS (INHALATION), CORTICOSTEROIDS (NASAL), CORTICOSTEROIDS (TOPICAL/ LOCAL).

---

## fluvastatin, See HMG-CoA REDUCTASE INHIBITORS.

---

## folic acid

(**foe**-lika-sid)

{Apo-Folic}, folate, Folvite, {Novofolacid}, vitamin B

### CLASSIFICATION(S):

**Therapeutic:** antianemics, vitamins
**Pharmacologic:** water soluble vitamins

## Pregnancy Category A

## INDICATIONS

■ Prevention and treatment of megaloblastic and macrocytic anemias ■ Given during pregnancy to promote normal fetal development.

## ACTION

■ Required for protein synthesis and red blood cell function. Stimulates the production of red blood cells, white blood cells, and platelets. Necessary for normal fetal development. **Therapeutic Effects:** ■ Restoration and maintenance of normal hematopoiesis.

## PHARMACOKINETICS

**Absorption:** Well absorbed from the GI tract and IM and subcut sites.

**Distribution:** Half of all stores are in the liver. Enters breast milk. Crosses the placenta.

**Protein Binding:** Extensive.

**Metabolism and Excretion:** Converted by the liver to its active metabolite, dihydrofolate reductase. Excess amounts are excreted unchanged by the kidneys.

**Half-life:** Unknown.

## CONTRAINDICATIONS AND PRECAUTIONS

**Contraindicated in:** ■ Uncorrected pernicious anemia (neurologic damage will progress despite correction of hematologic abnormalities) ■ Preparations containing benzyl alcohol should not be used in newborns.

**Use Cautiously in:** ■ Undiagnosed anemias.

## ADVERSE REACTIONS AND SIDE EFFECTS*

■ **Derm:** rashes ■ **Misc:** fever.

## INTERACTIONS

**Drug-Drug:** ■ **Pyrimethamine, methotrexate, trimethoprim,** and **triamterene** prevent the activation of folic acid (leucovorin should be used instead) ■ Absorption of folic acid is decreased by **sulfonamides** (including **sulfasalazine**), **anatacids,** and **cholestyramine** ■ Folic acid requirements are increased by **estrogens, phenytoin, phenobarbital, primidone, carbamazepine,** or **corticosteroids.**

## ROUTE AND DOSAGE

☐ **Therapeutic Dose**

■ **PO, IM, IV, Subcut (Adults and Children):** Up to 1 mg/day.

☐ **Maintenance Dose**

■ **PO, IM, IV, Subcut (Adults and Children >4 yr):** 0.4 mg/day.

■ **PO, IM, IV, Subcut (Adults, Pregnant or Lactating):** 0.8 mg/day.

■ **PO, IM, IV, Subcut (Children <4 yr):** Up to 0.3 mg/day.

■ **PO, IM, IV, Subcut (Infants):** 0.1 mg/day.

## AVAILABILITY (generic available)

■ *Tablets:* 0.1 mg$^{Rx}$, 0.4 mg$^{Rx}$, 0.8 mg$^{Rx}$, 1 mg$^{Rx}$, {5 mg$^{Rx}$} ■ Cost: 0.1 mg $2.08/100, 0.4 mg $2.15/100, 0.8 mg $2.48/100, 1 mg $4.17/100 ■ *Injection:* 5 mg/ml$^{Rx}$, 10 mg/ml$^{Rx}$ ■ other vitamins and minerals as multiple vitaminsRx, OTC.

TIME/ACTION PROFILE (increase in reticulocyte count)

|  | ONSET | PEAK | DURATION |
|---|---|---|---|
| PO, IM, subcut, IV | 3–5 days | 5–10 days | unknown |

## NURSING IMPLICATIONS

### ASSESSMENT

☐ Assess patient for signs of megaloblastic anemia (fatigue, weakness, dyspnea) before and periodically throughout therapy.

■ *Lab Test Considerations:* Monitor plasma folic acid levels, hemoglobin, hematocrit, and reticulocyte count before and periodically during therapy.

☐ May cause decrease in serum concentrations of vitamin B when given in high continuous doses.

### POTENTIAL NURSING DIAGNOSES

■ Nutrition, imbalanced: less than body requirements (Indications).

■ Activity intolerance (Indications).

### IMPLEMENTATION

■ **General:** Do not confuse folic acid with folinic acid (leucovorin calcium).

☐ Because of infrequency of solitary vitamin deficiencies, combinations are commonly administered (see Appendix B).

☐ May be given subcut, deep IM, or IV when PO route is not feasible.

■ **PO:** Antacids should be given at least 2 hr after folic acid; folic acid should be given 2 hr before or 4–6 hr after cholestyramine.

■ **IV:** Solution ranges from yellow to orange-yellow in color.

■ **Direct IV:** Administer at a rate of 5 mg over at least 1 min.

■ **Continuous Infusion:** May be added to hyperalimentation solution.

■ **Y-Site Compatibility:** ◆ famotidine.

■ **Additive Compatibility:** ◆ D20W.

■ **Additive Incompatibility:** ◆ D50W ◆ calcium gluconate.

### PATIENT/FAMILY TEACHING

☐ Encourage patient to comply with diet recommendations of health care professional. Explain that the best source of vitamins is a well-balanced diet with foods from the four basic food groups. A diet low in vitamin B and folate will be used to diagnose folic acid deficiency without concealing pernicious anemia.

☐ Foods high in folic acid include vegetables, fruits, and organ meats; heat destroys folic acid in foods.

☐ Patients self-medicating with vitamin supplements should be cautioned not to exceed RDA. The effectiveness of megadoses for treatment of various medical conditions is unproven and may cause side effects.

☐ Explain that folic acid may make urine more intensely yellow.

☐ Instruct patient to notify health care professional if rash occurs, which may indicate hypersensitivity.

☐ Emphasize the importance of follow-up exams to evaluate progress.

### EVALUATION

**Effectiveness of therapy can be demonstrated by:** ■ Reticulocytosis 2–5 days after beginning therapy ☐ Resolution of symptoms of megaloblastic anemia.

**fondaparinux, See HEPARINS (LOW MOLECULAR WEIGHT)/ HEPARINOIDS.**

---

## formoterol

(for-**mo**-te-role)

Foradil

**CLASSIFICATION(S):**
**Therapeutic:** bronchodilators
**Pharmacologic:** adrenergics

**Pregnancy Category C**

### INDICATIONS

■ Long-term maintenance treatment of asthma ■ Prevention of bronchospasm in reversible obstructive airways disease, including ■ Long-term management of bronchoconstriction associated with COPD including chronic bronchitis and emphysema ■ Acute prevention of exercise-induced bronchospasm, when used on an occasional, as needed, basis.

### ACTION

■ Produces accumulation of cyclic adenosine monophosphate (cAMP) at beta-adrenergic receptors, resulting in relaxation of airway smooth muscle ■ Relatively specific for beta$_2$ (pulmonary) receptors. **Therapeutic Effects:** ■ Bronchodilation.

### PHARMACOKINETICS

**Absorption:** Following inhalation, majority of inhaled drug is swallowed and absorbed.
**Distribution:** Unknown.
**Metabolism and Excretion:** Mostly metabolized by the liver; 10–18% excreted unchanged in urine.
**Half-life:** 10 hr.

### CONTRAINDICATIONS AND PRECAUTIONS

**Contraindicated in:** ■ Hypersensitivity ■ Acute attack of asthma (onset of action is delayed).
**Use Cautiously in:** ■ Cardiovascular disease (including angina and hypertension) ■ Diabetes ■ Glaucoma ■ Hyperthyroidism ■ Pheochromocytoma ■ Excessive use (may lead to tolerance and paradoxical bronchospasm) ■ Pregnancy, lactation, or children <5 yr (may inhibit contractions during labor; use only if potential benefits outweigh risks).

### ADVERSE REACTIONS AND SIDE EFFECTS*

■ **CNS:** dizziness, fatigue, headache, insomnia, malaise, nervousness ■ **Resp:** PARADOXICAL BRONCHOSPASM ■ **CV:** angina, arrhythmias, hypertension, hypotension, palpitations, tachycardia ■ **GI:** dry mouth, nausea ■ **F and E:** hypokalemia ■ **Metab:** hyperglycemia, metabolic acidosis ■ **MS:** muscle cramps ■ **Neuro:** tremor ■ **Misc:** allergic reactions including ANAPHYLAXIS.

### INTERACTIONS

**Drug-Drug:** ■ Concurrent use with **MAO inhibitors**, **tricyclic antidepressants** or other agents that may prolong the QTc interval may result in serious arrhythmias and should be undertaken with extreme caution. ■ ↑ risk of hypokalemia with **theophylline, corticosteroids, potassium-losing diuretics.** ■ **Beta blockers** may ↓ therapeutic effects of formoterol ■ ↑ adrenergic effects may occur with concurrent use of **adrenergics**.

### ROUTE AND DOSAGE

❏ **Maintenance Treatment of Asthma**
■ **Inhaln (Adults and Children ≥ 5 yr):** 1 capsule (12 mcg) every 12 hr using the Aerolizer Inhaler.

❏ **Prevention of Exercise-Induced Bronchospasm**
■ **Inhaln (Adults and Children ≥12 yr):** 1 capsule (12 mcg) at least 15 min before exercise on an occasional as-needed basis.

### AVAILABILITY

■ *Capsule for Aerolizer use:* 12 mcg[Rx].

TIME/ACTION PROFILE (bronchodilation)

| | ONSET | PEAK | DURATION |
|---|---|---|---|
| inhalation | 15 min | 1–3 hr | 12 hr |

## NURSING IMPLICATIONS

### ASSESSMENT

❏ Assess lung sounds, pulse, and blood pressure before administration and during peak of medication. Note amount, color, and character of sputum produced. Closely monitor patients on higher dose for adverse effects.

❑ Monitor pulmonary function tests before initiating and periodically therapy to determine effectiveness of medication.

❑ Observe for paradoxical bronchospasm (wheezing). If condition occurs, withhold medication and notify physician or other health care provider immediately.

❑ Monitor ECG periodically during therapy. May cause prolonged QTc interval.

❑ Monitor patient for signs of anaphylaxis (dyspnea, rash, laryngeal edema) throughout therapy.

■ **Lab Test Considerations:** May cause ↑ serum glucose and decreased serum potassium.

## POTENTIAL NURSING DIAGNOSES

■ Airway clearance, ineffective (Indications).

## IMPLEMENTATION

■ **General:** Place capsule in the well of the Aerolizer Inhaler with dry hands; do not expose to moisture. The capsule is pierced by pressing and releasing the buttons on the side of the device. Medication is dispersed into the air stream when patient inhales rapidly and deeply through mouthpiece. Capsules are only to be used with Aerolizer Inhaler and should not be taken orally. Store capsules in the blister and only remove immediately before use. Store inhaler in a level, horizontal position. Aerolizer Inhaler should never be washed and should be kept dry.

❑ Do not use a spacer with fomoterol. **Inhaln:** To use, pull off the Aerolizer cover. Hold the base of the inhaler firmly, and twist mouthpiece in the direction of the arrow to open. Push the buttons in to make sure four pins are visible in the capsule well on each side. Remove capsule from blister pack immediately before use. Separate one blistered capsule by tearing at perforations. With foil-side up, fold back along perforation and flatten. Starting at slit, tear off corner; separate and peel foil from paper backing and remove capsule. Place capsule in the capsule chamber in the base of the Aerolizer Inhaler. Never place a capsule directly into the mouthpiece. Twist the mouthpiece back to the closed position. With the mouthpiece upright, simultaneously press both buttons only once. A click should be heard as the capsule is being pierced. Release buttons; if buttons stick in depressed position grasp wings on buttons and retract before inhalation. With patient sitting or standing in a comfortable upright position, exhale fully. Do not exhale into the device. Tilt head back slightly and breathe in rapidly but steadily. A sweet taste will be experienced and a whirring noise heard. If no whirring is heard, the capsule may be stuck. Open inhaler and loosen capsule allowing it to spin freely. Do not repeatedly press buttons to loosen capsule. Hold breath for as long as comfortably possible after removing inhaler from mouth. Open inhaler to see if any powder is still in capsule. If powder is found, repeat inhalation steps. After use, open, remove and discard empty capsule.

## PATIENT/FAMILY TEACHING

❑ Instruct patient to take fomoterol as directed. Do not discontinue therapy without discussing with health care professional, even if feeling better. If on a scheduled dosing regimen, take a missed dose as soon as remembered, spacing remaining doses at regular intervals. Do not double doses. Use a rapid-acting bronchodilator if symptoms occur before next dose is due. Caution patient not to use more than 2 times a day or less than 12 hr apart; may cause adverse effects, paradoxical bronchospasm, or loss of effectiveness of medication.

❑ Instruct patient on correct technique for use of Aerolizer Inhaler. Advise patient always to use new Aerolizer Inhaler that comes with each refill. Take sticker with "use by" date written by pharmacist from the outside of the box and place it on the Aerolizer Inhaler cover. If the date is blank, count 4 months from the date of purchase and write date on sticker. Use new inhaler and blister pack following the "use by" date.

❑ Inform patient that in rare cases capsule might break into small pieces. These pieces should be retained by the screen in the inhaler, however in rare instances tiny pieces may reach mouth or throat after inhalation. Shattering of capsule is less likely to happen if storage conditions are strictly followed, capsules removed from blister immediately before use, and capsules are only pierced once.

❑ Advise patient to have a rapid-acting bronchodilator available for use at all times for symptomatic relief of acute asthma attacks.

❑ Instruct patient to contact health care professional immediately if shortness of breath is not relieved by medication or nausea, vomiting, shakiness, headache, fast or irregular heartbeat, or sleeplessness occur.

❑ Instruct patient to notify health care professional if there is no response to the usual dose of fomoterol. Asthma and treatment regimen should be re-evaluated and corticosteroids should be considered. Need for increased use to treat symptoms indicates decrease in asthma control and need to reevaluate therapy.

❑ Advise patient to consult health care professional before taking any OTC medications, herbal/alternative products or alcohol concurrently with this therapy. Caution patient also to avoid smoking and other respiratory irritants.

❑ Advise patient to notify health care professional if pregnancy is planned or suspected, or if nursing.

## EVALUATION

**Effectiveness of therapy can be demonstrated by:** ■ Prevention bronchospasm.

## foscarnet

(foss-**kar**-net)

Foscavir

*CLASSIFICATION(S):*
*Therapeutic:* antivirals

**Pregnancy Category C**

## INDICATIONS

■ Treatment of cytomegalovirus (CMV) retinitis in HIV-infected patients (alone or with ganciclovir) ■ Treatment of acyclovir-resistant mucocutaneous herpes simplex virus (HSV) infections in immunocompromised patients.

## ACTION

■ Prevents viral replication by inhibiting viral DNA-polymerase and reverse transcriptase.

**Therapeutic Effects:** ■ Virustatic action against susceptible viruses including CMV.

## PHARMACOKINETICS

**Absorption:** IV administration results in complete bioavailability.

**Distribution:** Variable penetration into CSF. May concentrate in and be slowly released from bone.

**Metabolism and Excretion:** 80–90% excreted unchanged in urine.

**Half-life:** 3 hr (in patients with normal renal function); longer half-life of 90 hr may reflect release of drug from bone.

## CONTRAINDICATIONS AND PRECAUTIONS

**Contraindicated in:** ■ Hypersensitivity.

**Use Cautiously in:** ■ Renal impairment (dosage reduction required if CCr ≤1.4–1.6 ml/min/kg; see product information) ■ History of seizures ■ Pregnancy, lactation, or children (safety not established).

## ADVERSE REACTIONS AND SIDE EFFECTS*

■ **CNS:** SEIZURES, headache, anxiety, confusion, dizziness, fatigue, malaise, mental depression, weakness ■ **EENT:** conjunctivitis, eye pain, vision abnormalities ■ **Resp:** coughing, dyspnea ■ **CV:** chest pain, ECG abnormalities, edema, palpitations ■ **GI:** diarrhea, nausea, vomiting, abdominal pain, abnormal taste sensation, anorexia, constipation, dyspepsia ■ **GU:** renal failure, albuminuria, dysuria, nocturia, polyuria, urinary retention ■ **Derm:** increased sweating, pruritus, rash, skin ulceration ■ **F and E:** hypocalcemia, hypokalemia, hypomagnesemia, hyperphosphatemia, hypophosphatemia ■ **Hemat:** anemia, granulocytopenia, leukopenia ■ **Local:** pain/inflammation at injection site ■ **MS:** arthralgia, myalgia, back pain, involuntary muscle contraction ■ **Neuro:** ataxia, hypoesthesia, neuropathy, paresthesia, tremor ■ **Misc:** fever, chills, flu-like syndrome, lymphoma, sarcoma.

## INTERACTIONS

**Drug-Drug:** ■ Concurrent use with parenteral **pentamidine** may result in severe, life-threatening hypocalcemia ■ Risk of nephrotoxicity may be increased by concurrent use of other **nephrotoxic agents (amphotericin B, aminoglycosides).**

## ROUTE AND DOSAGE

- **IV (Adults):** *CMV retinitis*—60 mg/kg q 8 hr or 90 mg/kg q 12 hr for 2–3 wk, then 90–120 mg/kg/day as a single dose. Dosage reduction required for any degree of renal impairment; *HSV*—40 mg/kg q 8–12 hr for 2–3 wk or until healing occurs.

## AVAILABILITY

- *Injection:* 6000 mg/250 ml$^{Rx}$, 12,000 mg/500 ml$^{Rx}$.

## TIME/ACTION PROFILE

|    | ONSET | PEAK | DURATION |
|----|-------|------|----------|
| IV | rapid | end of infu-sion | 8–24 hr |

# NURSING IMPLICATIONS

## ASSESSMENT

- **CMV Retinitis:** Diagnosis of CMV retinitis should be determined by ophthalmoscopy before treatment with foscarnet. Ophthalmologic examinations should also be performed at the conclusion of induction and every 4 wk during maintenance therapy.
- ❑ Culture for CMV (urine, blood, throat) may be taken before administration. However, a negative CMV culture does not rule out CMV retinitis.
- **HSV Infections:** Assess lesions before and daily during therapy.
- *Lab Test Considerations:* Monitor serum creatinine before and 2–3 times weekly during induction therapy and at least once every 1–2 wk during maintenance therapy. Monitor 24-hr CCr before and periodically throughout therapy. If CCr drops below 0.4 ml/min/kg, foscarnet should be discontinued.
- ❑ Monitor serum calcium, magnesium, potassium, and phosphorus before and 2–3 times weekly during induction therapy and at least weekly during maintenance therapy. May cause decreased concentrations.
- ❑ May cause anemia, granulocytopenia, leukopenia, and thrombocytopenia. May cause elevated AST and ALT levels and abnormal A-G ratios.

## POTENTIAL NURSING DIAGNOSES

- Infection, risk for (Indications).

## IMPLEMENTATION

- **General:** Patient should be adequately hydrated with 750–1000 ml of 0.9% NaCl or D5W before first infusion to establish diuresis, then 750–1000 ml with 120 mg/kg of foscarnet or 500 ml with 40–60 mg/kg of foscarnet should be administered with each dose to prevent renal toxicity.
- **Intermittent Infusion:** May be administered via central line in standard 24 mg/ml solution undiluted. If administered via peripheral line, *must* be diluted to 12 mg/ml concentration with D5W or 0.9% NaCl to prevent vein irritation. Do not administer solution that is discolored or contains particulate matter. Use diluted solution within 24 hr.
- ❑ Dose is based on patient weight; excess solution may be discarded from bottle before administration to prevent overdosage.
- ❑ Patients who experience progression of CMV retinitis during maintenance therapy may be re-treated with induction therapy followed by maintenance therapy.
- *Rate:* Administer at a rate not to exceed 1 mg/kg/min. Doses of 40 or 60 mg/kg are infused over at least 1 hr; 90 mg/kg over 1.5–2 hr; and 90–120 mg/kg maintenance dose is infused over 2 hr.
- ❑ Infuse solution via infusion pump to ensure accurate infusion rate.
- **Y-Site Compatibility:** ◆ aldesleukin ◆ amikacin ◆ aminophylline ◆ ampicillin ◆ aztreonam ◆ benzquinamide ◆ cefazolin ◆ cefoperazone ◆ cefoxitin ◆ ceftazidime ◆ ceftizoxime ◆ ceftriaxone ◆ cefuroxime ◆ chloramphenicol ◆ cimetidine ◆ clindamycin ◆ dopamine ◆ erythromycin lactobionate ◆ fluconazole ◆ flucytosine ◆ furosemide ◆ gentamicin ◆ heparin ◆ hydrocortisone ◆ hydromorphone ◆ imipenen-cilastatin ◆ metoclopramide ◆ metronidazole ◆ miconazole ◆ morphine ◆ nafcillin ◆ oxacillin ◆ penicillin G potassium ◆ phenytoin ◆ piperacillin ◆ ranitidine ◆ ticarcillin/clavulanate ◆ tobramycin.
- **Y-Site Incompatibility:** Manufacturer recommends that foscarnet not be administered concurrently with other drugs or solutions in

the same IV catheter except D5W or 0.9% NaCl. ✦ acyclovir ✦ amphotericin B ✦ diazepam ✦ digoxin ✦ diphenhydramine ✦ dobutamine ✦ droperidol ✦ ganciclovir ✦ haloperidol ✦ leucovorin ✦ midazolam ✦ pentamidine ✦ prochlorperazine ✦ promethazine ✦ trimetrexate.

## PATIENT/FAMILY TEACHING

❑ Inform patient that foscarnet is not a cure for CMV retinitis. Progression of retinitis may continue in immunocompromised patients during and after therapy. Advise patients to have regular ophthalmologic exams.

❑ Advise patient to notify health care professional immediately if perioral tingling or numbness in the extremities or paresthesia occurs during or after infusion. If these signs of electrolyte imbalance occur during administration, infusion should be stopped and lab samples for serum electrolyte concentrations obtained immediately.

❑ Emphasize the importance of frequent follow-up exams to monitor renal function and electrolytes.

## EVALUATION

**Effectiveness of therapy can be demonstrated by:** ■ Management of the symptoms of CMV retinitis in patients with AIDS ■ Crusting over and healing of skin lesions in HSV infections.

---

## fosinopril, See ANGIOTENSIN-CONVERTING ENZYME (ACE) INHIBITORS.

---

## frovatriptan

(froe-va-**trip**-tan)
Frova

### CLASSIFICATION(S):
*Therapeutic: vascular headache suppressants*
*Pharmacologic: 5 HT₁ agonists*

**Pregnancy Category C**

## INDICATIONS

■ Acute treatment of migraine headache.

## ACTION

■ Acts as an agonist at specific 5-HT receptor sites in intracranial blood vessels and sensory trigeminal nerves. **Therapeutic Effects:** ■ Cranial vessel vasoconstriction with associated decrease in release of neuropeptides and resultant decrease in migraine headache.

## PHARMACOKINETICS

**Absorption:** 20–30% following oral administration.

**Distribution:** Unknown.

**Metabolism and Excretion:** Mostly metabolized by the liver (P450 1A2 enzyme system); some metabolites eliminated in urine, <10% excreted unchanged.

**Half-life:** 26 hr.

## CONTRAINDICATIONS AND PRECAUTIONS

**Contraindicated in:** ■ Hypersensitivity ■ History, symptoms or findings consistent with ❑ ischemic heart disease ❑ coronary artery vasospasm ❑ other significant underlying cardiovascular disease ■ Cerebrovascular syndromes including ❑ strokes of any type ❑ transient ischemic attacks ■ Uncontrolled hypertension ■ Hemiplegic or basilar migraine ■ Peripheral vascular disease, including ischemic bowel disease ■ Should not be used within 24 hr of any other 5-HT agonist or ergot-type compounds (dihydroergotamine) ■ Children <18 yr.

**Use Cautiously in:** ■ Elderly patients (may be more susceptible to adverse cardiovascular effects) ■ Pregnancy or lactation (safety not established).

**Exercise Extreme Caution in:** ■ Cardiovascular risk factors (hypertension, hypercholesterolemia, cigarette smoking, obesity, diabetes, strong family history, menopausal women or men >40 yr); use only if cardiovascular status has been evaluated and determined to be safe and first dose is administered under supervision.

## ADVERSE REACTIONS AND SIDE EFFECTS*

■ **CNS:** dizziness, drowsiness, fatigue ■ **CV:** CORONARY ARTERY VASOSPASM, MI, VENTRICULAR FIBRILLATION, VENTRICULAR TACHYCARDIA, chest pain, myocardial ischemia ■ **GI:** dry mouth, dyspepsia, nausea ■ **Derm:** flushing ■ **MS:** skeletal pain ■ **Neuro:** paresthesia ■ **Misc:** pain.

## INTERACTIONS

**Drug-Drug:** ■ Blood levels may be increased by **hormonal contraceptives** or **propranolol** ■ Blood levels may be decreased by **ergotamine** ■ Increased risk of serious vasospastic reactions with **dihydroergotamine** (concurrent use contraindicated).

## ROUTE AND DOSAGE

■ **PO (Adults):** 2.5 mg; if there has been initial relief, a second tablet may be taken after at least 2 hr (daily dose should not exceed 3 tablets and should not be used to treat more than 4 attacks/30 day period).

## AVAILABILITY

■ *Tablets:* 2.5 mg$^{Rx}$.

TIME/ACTION PROFILE (blood levels)

|  | ONSET | PEAK | DURATION |
|---|---|---|---|
| PO | unknown | 2–4 hr | unknown |

## NURSING IMPLICATIONS

### ASSESSMENT

❑ Assess pain location, intensity, duration, and associated symptoms (photophobia, phonophobia, nausea, vomiting) during migraine attack.

### POTENTIAL NURSING DIAGNOSES

■ Pain, acute (Indications).

### IMPLEMENTATION

■ **PO:** Tablets may be administered at any time after the headache starts.

### PATIENT/FAMILY TEACHING

■ **General Info:** Inform patient that frovatriptan should be used only during a migraine attack. It is meant to be used to relieve migraine attack but not to prevent or reduce the number of attacks.

❑ Instruct patient to administer frovatriptan as soon as symptoms appear, but it may be administered any time during an attack. If migraine symptoms return, a second dose may be used. Allow at least 2 hr between doses, and do not use more than 3 tablets in any 24-hr period.

❑ If dose does not relieve headache, additional frovatriptan doses are not likely to be effective; notify health care professional.

❑ Advise patient that lying down in a darkened room following frovatriptan administration may further help relieve headache.

❑ Caution patient not to use frovatriptan if she is pregnant, suspects she is pregnant, plans to become pregnant, or is breastfeeding. Adequate contraception should be used during therapy.

❑ May cause dizziness or drowsiness. Caution patient to avoid driving or other activities requiring alertness until response to medication is known.

❑ Advise patient to notify health care professional prior to next dose of frovatriptan if pain or tightness in the chest occurs during use. If pain is severe or does not subside, notify health care professional immediately. If wheezing; heart throbbing; swelling of eyelids, face, or lips; skin rash; skin lumps; or hives occur, notify health care professional immediately and do not take more frovatriptan without approval of health care professional. If feelings of tingling, heat, flushing, heaviness, pressure, drowsiness, dizziness, tiredness, or sickness develop, discuss with health care professional at next visit.

❑ Advise patient to avoid alcohol, which aggravates headaches, during frovatriptan use.

### EVALUATION

**Effectiveness of therapy can be demonstrated by:** ■ Relief of migraine attack.

---

## furosemide

(fur-**oh**-se-mide)

{Apo-Furosemide}, {Furoside}, Lasix, {Lasix Special}, {Myrosemide}, {Novosemide}, {Uritol}

### CLASSIFICATION(S):
**Therapeutic:** *diuretics*
**Pharmacologic:** *loop diuretics*

**Pregnancy Category C**

---

## INDICATIONS

■ Edema due to: ❏ CHF ❏ Hepatic or renal disease ■ Hypertension. **Unlabeled uses:** ■ Hypercalcemia of malignancy.

## ACTION

■ Inhibits the reabsorption of sodium and chloride from the loop of Henle and distal renal tubule ■ Increases renal excretion of water, sodium, chloride, magnesium, hydrogen, and calcium ■ May have renal and peripheral vasodilatory effects ■ Effectiveness persists in impaired renal function. **Therapeutic Effects:** ■ Diuresis and subsequent mobilization of excess fluid (edema, pleural effusions) ■ Decreased blood pressure.

## PHARMACOKINETICS

**Absorption:** 60–75% absorbed after oral administration ( ↓ in acute CHF); also absorbed from IM sites.

**Distribution:** Crosses placenta, enters breast milk.

**Protein Binding:** 91–97%.

**Metabolism and Excretion:** Some 30–40% metabolized by liver, some nonhepatic metabolism, some renal excretion as unchanged drug.

**Half-life:** 30–60 min ( ↑ in renal impairment and neonates, markedly ↑ in hepatic impairment).

## CONTRAINDICATIONS AND PRECAUTIONS

**Contraindicated in:** ■ Hypersensitivity ■ Cross-sensitivity with thiazides and sulfonamides may occur ■ Pre-existing electrolyte imbalance, hepatic coma, or anuria ■ Some liquid products may contain alcohol, avoid in patients with alcohol intolerance.

**Use Cautiously in:** ■ Severe liver disease (may precipitate hepatic coma; concurrent use with potassium-sparing diuretics may be necessary) ■ Electrolyte depletion ■ Geriatric patients (difficulty assessing hearing status; increased risk of hypotension) ■ Diabetes mellitus ■ Increasing azotemia ■ Pregnancy, lactation, or children (safety not established; has been used in children).

## ADVERSE REACTIONS AND SIDE EFFECTS*

■ **CNS:** dizziness, encephalopathy, headache, insomnia, nervousness ■ **EENT:** hearing loss, tinnitus ■ **CV:** hypotension ■ **GI:** constipation, diarrhea, dry mouth, dyspepsia, nausea, vomiting ■ **GU:** excessive urination ■ **Derm:** photosensitivity, rashes ■ **Endo:** hyperglycemia ■ **F and E:** dehydration, hypochloremia, hypokalemia, hypomagnesemia, hyponatremia, hypovolemia, metabolic alkalosis ■ **Hemat:** blood dyscrasias ■ **Metab:** hyperglycemia, hyperuricemia ■ **MS:** arthralgia, muscle cramps, myalgia ■ **Misc:** increased BUN.

## INTERACTIONS

**Drug-Drug:** ■ ↑ hypotension with **antihypertensives, nitrates,** or acute ingestion of **alcohol** ■ ↑ risk of hypokalemia with other **diuretics, piperacillin, amphotericin B, stimulant laxatives,** and **corticosteroids** ■ Hypokalemia may ↑ risk of **digoxin** toxicity ■ ↓ **lithium** excretion, may cause toxicity ■ ↑ risk of ototoxicity with **aminoglycosides** ■ May ↑ the effectiveness of **warfarin, thrombolytic agents,** or **anticoagulants**.

## ROUTE AND DOSAGE

■ **PO (Adults):** *Edema*—20–80 mg/day as a single dose initially, may repeat in 6–8 hr; may increase dose by 20–40 mg q 6–8 hr until desired response. Maintenance doses may be given once or twice daily or intermittently for 2–4 days/week (doses up to 2.5 g/day have been used in patients with CHF or renal disease). *Hypertension*—40 twice daily initially (when added to regimen, decrease dose of other antihypertensives by 50%); adjust further dosing based on response; *Hypercalcemia*—120 mg/day in 1–3 doses.

■ **PO (Children):** 2 mg/kg as a single dose; may be increased by 1–2 mg/kg q 6–8 hr (1–2 mg/kg/day initially, up to 5–6 mg/kg/day). Longer dosage intervals are recommended in neonates.

■ **IM, IV (Adults):** *Edema*—20–40 mg, may repeat in 2 hr and increase by 20 mg every 2 hr until response is obtained, maintenance dose may be given once-twice daily; *acute pulmonary edema*—40 mg, after 1 hr may give additional 80 mg (in CHF and renal failure, daily doses of up to 2.5 g have been used); *hypercalcemia*—80–100 mg, may repeat every 1–2 hr, titrate by response.)

■ **IM, IV (Children):** 1 mg/kg, may increase by 1 mg/kg q 2 hr (not to exceed 6 mg/kg).

## AVAILABILITY (generic available)

■ *Tablets:* 20 mg$^{Rx}$, 40 mg$^{Rx}$, 80 mg$^{Rx}$, {500 mg$^{Rx}$} ■ Cost: *Lasix*—20 mg$^{Rx}$ $21.12/100, 40 mg$^{Rx}$ $29.57/100, 80 mg$^{Rx}$ $23.91/50; *Generic*—20 mg$^{Rx}$ $19.00/100, 40 mg$^{Rx}$ $26.50/100, 80 mg$^{Rx}$ $35.90/100 ■ *Oral solution (10 mg/ml—orange flavor, 8 mg/ml—orange-pineapple flavor):* 8 mg/ml$^{Rx}$, 10 mg/ml$^{Rx}$ ■ Cost: 10 mg/ml$^{Rx}$ $10.40/60 ml ■ *Injection:* 10 mg/ml$^{Rx}$.

TIME/ACTION PROFILE (diuretic effect)

|  | ONSET | PEAK | DURATION |
|---|---|---|---|
| PO | 30–60 min | 1–2 hr | 6–8 hr |
| IM | 10–30 min | unknown | 4–8 hr |
| IV | 5 min | 30 min | 2 hr |

# NURSING IMPLICATIONS

## ASSESSMENT

❑ Assess fluid status during therapy. Monitor daily weight, intake and output ratios, amount and location of edema, lung sounds, skin turgor, and mucous membranes. Notify physician or other health care provider if thirst, dry mouth, lethargy, weakness, hypotension, or oliguria occurs.

❑ Monitor blood pressure and pulse before and during administration. Monitor frequency of prescription refills to determine compliance in patients treated for hypertension.

❑ Assess patients receiving digoxin for anorexia, nausea, vomiting, muscle cramps, paresthesia, and confusion. Patients taking digitalis glycosides are at increased risk of digitalis toxicity because of the potassium-depleting effect of the diuretic. Potassium supplements or potassium-sparing diuretics may be used concurrently to prevent hypokalemia.

❑ Assess patient for tinnitus and hearing loss. Audiometry is recommended for patients receiving prolonged high-dose IV therapy. Hearing loss is most common after rapid or high-dose IV administration in patients with decreased renal function or those taking other ototoxic drugs.

❑ Assess for allergy to sulfonamides.

■ *Lab Test Considerations:* Monitor electrolytes, renal and hepatic function, serum glucose, and uric acid levels before and peri-

odically throughout therapy. May cause ↓ serum potassium, calcium, and magnesium concentrations. May also cause ↑ BUN, serum glucose, creatinine, and uric acid levels.

## POTENTIAL NURSING DIAGNOSES

■ Fluid volume, excess (Side Effects).

## IMPLEMENTATION

■ **General:** Do not confuse furosemide with torsemide.

❑ Administer medication in the morning to prevent disruption of sleep cycle.

❑ IV is preferred over IM for parenteral administration.

■ **PO:** Administer orally with food or milk to minimize gastric irritation. Tablets may be crushed if patient has difficulty swallowing.

❑ Do not administer discolored solution or tablets.

■ **General:** When using furosemide for hypercalcemia, replace extracellular volume and sodium chloride to maintain fluid volume and increase calcium excretion effectively.

■ **Direct IV:** Administer undiluted.

■ *Rate:* Administer slowly over 1–2 min.

■ **Intermittent Infusion:** Dilute large doses in D5W, D10W, D20W, D5/0.9% NaCl, D5/LR, 0.9% NaCl, 3% NaCl, 1/6 M sodium lactate, or LR. Use reconstituted solution within 24 hr.

■ *Rate:* Administer at a rate not to exceed 4 mg/min in adults to prevent ototoxicity. Use an infusion pump to ensure accurate dosage.

■ **Syringe Compatibility:** ◆ bleomycin ◆ cisplatin ◆ cyclophosphamide ◆ fluorouracil ◆ heparin ◆ leucovorin calcium ◆ methotrexate ◆ mitomycin.

■ **Syringe Incompatibility:** ◆ doxapram ◆ doxorubicin ◆ droperidol ◆ metoclopramide ◆ milrinone ◆ vinblastine ◆ vincristine.

■ **Y-Site Compatibility:** ◆ allopurinol ◆ amifostone ◆ amikacin ◆ amphotericin B cholesteryl sulfate ◆ aztreonam ◆ bleomycin ◆ cefepime ◆ cisplatin ◆ cladribine ◆ cyclophosphamide ◆ cytarabine ◆ docetaxel ◆ doxorubicin liposome ◆ epinephrine ◆ etoposide ◆ fentanyl ◆ fludarabine ◆ fluorouracil ◆ foscarnet ◆ granisetron ◆ heparin ◆ hydrocortisone sodium succinate ◆ hydromorphone ◆ indomethacin

{ } = Available in Canada only.
*CAPITALS indicates life-threatening; underlines indicate most frequent.

◆ kanamycin ◆ leucovorin calcium ◆ linezolid ◆ lorazepam ◆ melphalan ◆ meropenem ◆ methotrexate ◆ mitomycin ◆ nitroglycerin ◆ norepinephrine ◆ paclitaxel ◆ piperacillin/tazobactam ◆ potassium chloride ◆ propofol ◆ ranitidine ◆ remifentanil ◆ sargramostim ◆ tacrolimus ◆ teniposide ◆ thiotepa ◆ tobramycin ◆ tolazoline ◆ vitamin B complex with C.

■ **Y-Site Incompatibility:** ◆ ciprofloxacin ◆ diltiazem ◆ droperidol ◆ esmolol ◆ filgrastim ◆ fluconazole ◆ gatifloxacin ◆ gemcitabine ◆ gentamicin ◆ hydralazine ◆ idarubicin ◆ levofloxacin ◆ metoclopramide ◆ midazolam ◆ milrinone ◆ netilmicin ◆ ondansetron ◆ quinidine gluconate ◆ thiopental ◆ vecuronium ◆ vinblastine ◆ vincristine ◆ vinorelbine.

## PATIENT/FAMILY TEACHING

■ **General Info:** Instruct patient to take furosemide as directed. Take missed doses as soon as possible; do not double doses.

❏ Caution patient to change positions slowly to minimize orthostatic hypotension. Caution patient that the use of alcohol, exercise during hot weather, or standing for long periods during therapy may enhance orthostatic hypotension.

❏ Instruct patient to consult health care professional regarding a diet high in potassium (see Appendix Q).

❏ Advise patient to consult health care professional before taking OTC medication or herbal products concurrently with this therapy.

❏ Instruct patient to notify health care professional of medication regimen before treatment or surgery.

❏ Caution patient to use sunscreen and protective clothing to prevent photosensitivity reactions.

❏ Advise patient to contact health care professional immediately if muscle weakness, cramps, nausea, dizziness, numbness, or tingling of extremities occurs.

❏ Advise patient taking *furosemide tablets* not to change brands when refilling prescription; bioavailability among brands is variable.

❏ Advise diabetic patients to monitor blood glucose closely; may cause increased blood glucose levels.

❏ Emphasize the importance of routine follow-up examinations.

■ **Hypertension:** Advise patients on antihypertensive regimen to continue taking medication even if feeling better. Furosemide controls but does not cure hypertension.

❏ Reinforce the need to continue additional therapies for hypertension (weight loss, exercise, restricted sodium intake, stress reduction, regular exercise, moderation of alcohol consumption, cessation of smoking).

## EVALUATION

**Effectiveness of therapy can be demonstrated by:** ■ Decrease in edema ❏ Decrease in abdominal girth ❏ Increase in urinary output ■ Decrease in blood pressure ■ Decrease in serum calcium when used to manage hypercalcemia.

# gabapentin

(ga-ba-**pen**-tin)

Neurontin

*CLASSIFICATION(S):*

**Therapeutic:** *analgesic adjuncts,
anticonvulsants*

**Pregnancy Category C**

## INDICATIONS

■ Partial seizures with and without secondary generalization (adjunct treatment) ■ Postherpetic neuralgia. **Unlabeled uses:** ■ Chronic pain ■ Prevention of migraine headache.

## ACTION

■ Mechanism of action is not known. May affect transport of amino acids across and stabilize neuronal membranes. **Therapeutic Effects:** ■ Decreased incidence of seizures ■ Decreased postherpetic pain.

## PHARMACOKINETICS

**Absorption:** Well absorbed after oral administration by active transport. At larger doses, transport becomes saturated and absorption decreases (bioavailability ranges from 60% for a 300-mg dose to 35% for a 1600-mg dose).
**Distribution:** Crosses blood-brain barrier; enters breast milk.
**Metabolism and Excretion:** Eliminated mostly by renal excretion of unchanged drug.
**Half-life:** 5–7 hr (normal renal function); up to 132 hr in anuria.

## CONTRAINDICATIONS AND PRECAUTIONS

**Contraindicated in:** ■ Hypersensitivity.
**Use Cautiously in:** ■ Renal insufficiency ( ↓ dose and/or ↑ dosing interval if CCr ≤60 ml/min) ■ Geriatric patients (because of age-related ↓ in renal function) ■ Pregnancy, lactation, or children <3 yr (safety not established).

## ADVERSE REACTIONS AND SIDE EFFECTS*

■ **CNS:** <u>confusion,</u>, <u>depression</u>, <u>drowsiness</u>, anxiety, concentration difficulties (children), dizziness, emotional lability (children), hostility,

hyperkinesia (children), malaise, vertigo, weakness ■ **EENT:** abnormal vision, nystagmus ■ **CV:** hypertension ■ **GI:** anorexia, flatulence, gingivitis ■ **MS:** arthralgia ■ **Neuro:** <u>ataxia</u>, altered reflexes, hyperkinesia, paresthesia ■ **Misc:** facial edema.

## INTERACTIONS

**Drug-Drug:** ■ **Antacids** may ↓ absorption of gabapentin ■ ↑ risk of CNS depression with other **CNS depressants,** including **alcohol, antihistamines, opioids,** and **sedative/hypnotics** ■ **Morphine** ↑ gabapentin levels and may ↑ risk of toxicity, dosage adjustments may be required.
**Drug-Natural Products:** ■ **Kava, valerian,** or **chamomile** can ↑ CNS depression.

## ROUTE AND DOSAGE

❑ **Epilepsy**

■ **PO (Adults and Children >12 yr):** 300 mg 3 times daily initially. Titration may be continued until desired (range is 900–1800 mg/day in 3 divided doses; doses should not be more than 12 hr apart). Doses up to 2400–3600 mg/day have been well tolerated.

■ **PO (Children ≥5–12 yr):** 10–15 mg/kg/day in 3 divided doses initially titrated upward over 3 days to 25–35 mg/kg/day in 3 divided doses; dosage interval should not exceed 12 hr (doses up to 50 mg/kg/day have been used).

■ **PO (Children 3–4 yrs):** 10–15 mg/kg/day in 3 divided doses initially titrated upward over 3 days to 40 mg/kg/day in 3 divided doses; dosage interval should not exceed 12 hr (doses up to 50 mg/kg/day have been used).

❑ **Renal Impairment**

■ **PO (Adults and Children >12 yr):** *CCr 30–60 ml/min*—300 mg twice daily; *CCr 15–30 ml/min*—300 mg once daily; *CCr <15 ml/min*—300 mg once every other day; further adjustments are based on clinical response.

❑ **Post-herpetic neuralgia**

■ **PO (Adults):** 300 mg once daily on first day, 300 mg twice daily on second day, then 300 mg three times/day on day 3, may then be titrated upward as needed up to 600 mg three times/day.

## AVAILABILITY (generic available)

■ *Capsules:* 100 mg^Rx, 300 mg^Rx, 400 mg^Rx ■ Cost: 100 mg $51.41/100, 300 mg $128.51/100, 400 mg $154.21/100 ■ *Tablets:* 600 mg^Rx, 800 mg^Rx ■ Cost: 600 mg $212.00/100, 800 mg $254.29/100 ■ *Oral solution (cool strawberry anise flavor):* 250 mg/5 ml^Rx.

TIME/ACTION PROFILE (blood levels)

|  | ONSET | PEAK | DURATION |
|---|---|---|---|
| PO | rapid | 2–4 hr | 8 hr |

# NURSING IMPLICATIONS

## ASSESSMENT

■ **Seizures:** Assess location, duration, and characteristics of seizure activity.
■ **Postherpetic Neuralgia & Chronic Pain:** Assess location, characteristics, and intensity of pain periodically during therapy.
■ *Lab Test Considerations:* May cause false-positive readings when testing for urinary protein with *Ames N-Multistix SG* dipstick test; use sulfosalicylic acid precipitation procedure.
❑ May cause leukopenia.

## POTENTIAL NURSING DIAGNOSES

■ Injury, risk for (Side Effects).

## IMPLEMENTATION

■ **PO:** May be administered without regard to meals.
❑ Gabapentin should be discontinued gradually over at least 1 wk. Abrupt discontinuation may cause increase in seizure frequency.

## PATIENT/FAMILY TEACHING

❑ Instruct patient to take medication exactly as directed. Patients on tid dosing should not exceed 12 hr between doses. Take missed doses as soon as possible; if less than 2 hr until next dose, take dose immediately and take next dose 1–2 hr later, then resume regular dosing schedule. Do not double doses. Do not discontinue abruptly; may cause increase in frequency of seizures.
❑ Advise patient not to take gabapentin within 2 hr of an antacid.

❑ Gabapentin may cause dizziness and drowsiness. Caution patient to avoid driving or activities requiring alertness until response to medication is known. Seizure patients should not resume driving until physician gives clearance based on control of seizure disorder.
❑ Advise female patient to notify health care professional if pregnancy is planned or suspected or if she intends to breastfeed or is breastfeeding an infant.
❑ Instruct patient to notify health care professional of medication regimen before treatment or surgery.
❑ Advise patient to carry identification describing disease process and medication regimen at all times.

## EVALUATION

**Effectiveness of therapy can be demonstrated by:** ■ Decrease in the frequency of or cessation of seizures ■ Decrease in postherpetic neuralgia pain ■ Decrease in intensity of chronic pain.

## galantamine
(ga-**lant**-a-meen)
Reminyl

### CLASSIFICATION(S):
*Therapeutic: anti-Alzheimer's agents*
*Pharmacologic: cholinergics (cholinesterase inhibitors)*

### Pregnancy Category B

## INDICATIONS

■ Treatment of mild to moderate dementia of the Alzheimer's type.

## ACTION

■ Enhances cholinergic function by reversible inhibition of cholinesterase. **Therapeutic Effects:** ■ Decreased dementia (temporary) associated with Alzheimer's disease ■ Does not alter the course of the disease.

## PHARMACOKINETICS

**Absorption:** Well absorbed (90%) following oral administration.
**Distribution:** Unknown.

**Metabolism and Excretion:** Mostly metabolized by the liver; 20% excreted unchanged in urine.

**Half-life:** 7 hr.

## CONTRAINDICATIONS AND PRECAUTIONS

**Contraindicated in:** ■ Hypersensitivity ■ Severe hepatic or renal impairment ■ Children or lactation (not recommended).

**Use Cautiously in:** ■ Patients with supraventricular cardiac conduction defects or concurrent use of drugs that may slow heart rate (increased risk of bradycardia) ■ History of ulcer disease/GI bleeding/concurrent NSAID use ■ Severe asthma or obstructive pulmonary disease ■ Mild to moderate renal impairment (avoid use if CCr <9 ml/min) ■ Mild to moderate hepatic impairment (cautious dose titration recommended) ■ Pregnancy (use only if potential benefit outweighs potential risk to fetus).

## ADVERSE REACTIONS AND SIDE EFFECTS*

■ **CNS:** fatigue, dizziness, headache, syncope ■ **CV:** bradycardia, chest pain ■ **GI:** anorexia, diarrhea, dyspepsia, flatulence, nausea, vomiting ■ **GU:** bladder outflow obstruction, incontinence ■ **Neuro:** tremor ■ **Misc:** weight loss.

## INTERACTIONS

**Drug-Drug:** ■ Will exaggerate neuromuscular blockade from **succinylcholine-type neuromuscular blocking agents** ■ May enhance the effects of other **cholinesterase inhibitors** or other **cholinergic agonists,** including **bethanechol** ■ May decrease the effectiveness of **anticholinergic medications** ■ Blood levels and effects may be increased by **ketoconazole, paroxetine, amitriptyline, fluvoxamine,** or **quinidine**.

**Drug-Natural Products:** ■ **Angel's trumpet, jimson weed,** and **scopolia** may antagonize cholinergic effects.

## ROUTE AND DOSAGE

■ **PO (Adults):** 4 mg twice daily initially, dose increments of 4 mg should be made at 4 wk intervals, up to 12 mg twice daily. Doses up to 16 mg twice daily have been used (range 16–32 mg/day).

## AVAILABILITY

■ *Tablets:* 4 mg^Rx, 8 mg^Rx, 12 mg^Rx ■ *Oral solution:* 4 mg/ml in 100 ml bottles^Rx.

TIME/ACTION PROFILE (antihcholinesterase activity)

| | ONSET | PEAK | DURATION |
|---|---|---|---|
| PO | unknown | 1 hr | 12 hr |

## NURSING IMPLICATIONS

### ASSESSMENT

❑ Assess cognitive function (memory, attention, reasoning, language, ability to perform simple tasks) periodically throughout therapy.

❑ Monitor heart rate periodically during therapy. May cause bradycardia.

### POTENTIAL NURSING DIAGNOSES

■ Thought processes, disturbed (Indications).

■ Injury, risk for (Indications).

### IMPLEMENTATION

■ **General:** Patient should be maintained on a stable dose for a minimum of 4 weeks prior to increasing dose.

❑ If dose has been interrupted for several days or longer, patient should be restarted at the lowest dose and the dose escalated to the current dose.

■ **PO:** Administer twice daily, preferrably with morning and evening meal. Administration with food, the use of antiemetic medications, and ensuring adequate fluid intake may decrease nausea and vomiting. Use pipette provided with oral solution to administer accurate amount.

### PATIENT/FAMILY TEACHING

❑ Emphasize the importance of taking galantamine daily, as directed. Instruct patient and/or caregiver in correct use of pipette if using oral solution. Missed doses should be skipped and regular schedule returned to the following day; do not double doses. Do not discontinue abruptly; although no increase in frequency of adverse events may occur, beneficial affects of galantamine are lost when the drug is discontinued.

❑ Caution patient and caregiver that galantamine may cause dizziness.

❑ Advise patient and caregiver to notify health care professional if nausea or vomiting persists beyond 7 days or if new symptoms occur or previously noted symptoms increase in severity.

❑ Advise patient and caregiver to notify health care professional of medication regimen prior to treatment or surgery.

❑ Emphasize the importance of follow-up exams to monitor progress.

## EVALUATION

**Clinical response to therapy can be evaluated by:** ■ Improvement in cognitive function (memory, attention, reasoning, language, ability to perform simple tasks) in patients with Alzheimer's disease.

---

# ganciclovir

(gan-**sye**-kloe-vir)

Cytovene, Vitrasert

*CLASSIFICATION(S):*
*Therapeutic: antivirals*

**Pregnancy Category C**

---

## INDICATIONS

■ **IV:** Treatment of cytomegalovirus (CMV) retinitis in immunocompromised patients, including HIV-infected patients (may be used with foscarnet) ■ Prevention of CMV infection in transplant patients at risk ■ **PO:** Maintenance treatment of stable CMV retinitis in immunocompromised patients after initial IV treatment and prevention of CMV retinitis in patients with advanced HIV infection.

## ACTION

■ CMV converts ganciclovir to its active form (ganciclovir phosphate) inside the host cell, where it inhibits viral DNA polymerase. **Therapeutic Effects:** ■ Antiviral effect directed preferentially against CMV-infected cells.

## PHARMACOKINETICS

**Absorption:** 5–9% absorbed after oral administration. IV administration results in complete bioavailability. Action of intravitreal implant is local.

**Distribution:** Widely distributed; enters CSF.

**Metabolism and Excretion:** 90% excreted unchanged by the kidneys.

**Half-life:** 2.9 hr (increased in renal impairment).

## CONTRAINDICATIONS AND PRECAUTIONS

**Contraindicated in:** ■ Hypersensitivity to ganciclovir or acyclovir.

**Use Cautiously in:** ■ Renal impairment (dosage reduction required if CCr <80 ml/min) ■ Geriatric patients (dosage reduction recommended) ■ Bone marrow depression or immunosuppression ■ Pregnancy, lactation, or children (safety not established).

## ADVERSE REACTIONS AND SIDE EFFECTS*

■ **CNS:** SEIZURES, abnormal dreams, coma, confusion, dizziness, drowsiness, headache, malaise, nervousness ■ **EENT:** retinal detachment; *intravitreal only*—decreased visual acuity, vitreous hemorrhage, hyphema, intraocular pressure spikes, lens opacities, macular abnormalities, optic nerve changes, uveitis ■ **Resp:** dyspnea ■ **CV:** arrhythmias, edema, hypertension, hypotension ■ **GI:** GI BLEEDING, abdominal pain, increased liver enzymes, nausea, vomiting ■ **GU:** gonadal suppression, hematuria, renal toxicity ■ **Derm:** alopecia, photosensitivity, pruritus, rash, urticaria ■ **Endo:** hypoglycemia ■ **Hemat:** neutropenia, thrombocytopenia, anemia, eosinophilia ■ **Local:** pain/phlebitis at IV site ■ **Neuro:** ataxia, tremor ■ **Misc:** fever.

## INTERACTIONS

**Drug-Drug:** ■ Increased risk of bone marrow depression with **antineoplastics, radiation therapy,** or **zidovudine** ■ Toxicity may be increased by **probenecid** ■ Increased risk of seizures with **imipenem/cilastatin** ■ Concurrent use of other **nephrotoxic drugs, cyclosporine,** or **amphotericin B** increases the risk of nephrotoxicity.

## ROUTE AND DOSAGE

■ **IV (Adults):** *Induction*—5 mg/kg q 12 hr for 14–21 days. *Maintenance regimen*—5 mg/kg/day or 6 mg/kg for 5 days of each week. If progression occurs, increase to q 12 hr regimen. *Prevention*—5 mg/kg q 12 hr for 7–14 days, then 5 mg/kg/day or 6 mg/kg for 5 days of each week.

- **PO (Adults):** *Maintenance regimen—* 1000 mg 3 times daily (with food) or 500 mg 6 times daily; *Prevention of CMV retinitis in advanced HIV infection—*1000 mg 3 times daily.
- **Intravitreal (Adults):** 4.5 mg implant.

## AVAILABILITY (generic available)

- *Capsules:* 250 mg^{Rx}, 500 mg^{Rx} ■ *Powder for injection:* 500 mg/vial^{Rx} ■ *Intravitreal insert:* 4.5 mg^{Rx}.

TIME/ACTION PROFILE (antiviral levels)

|  | ONSET | PEAK | DURATION |
|---|---|---|---|
| PO | rapid | 1.8–3 hr | 3–8 hr |
| IV | rapid | end of infusion | 12–24 hr |
| Intravitreal | rapid | unknown | 5–8 mo |

# NURSING IMPLICATIONS

## ASSESSMENT

- ❏ Diagnosis of CMV retinitis should be determined by ophthalmoscopy before treatment with ganciclovir.
- ❏ Culture for CMV (urine, blood, throat) may be taken before administration. However, a negative CMV culture does not rule out CMV retinitis. If symptoms do not respond after several weeks, resistance to ganciclovir may have occurred. Ophthalmologic exams should be performed weekly during induction and every 2 wk during maintenance or more frequently if the macula or optic nerve is threatened. Progression of CMV retinitis may occur during or after ganciclovir treatment.
- ❏ Assess for signs of infection (fever, chills, cough, hoarseness, lower back or side pain, sore throat, difficult or painful urination). Notify physician or other health care professional if these symptoms occur.
- ❏ Assess for bleeding (bleeding gums, bruising, petechiae; guaiac stools, urine, and emesis). Avoid IM injections and taking rectal temperatures. Apply pressure to venipuncture sites for 10 min.
- **Lab Test Considerations:** Monitor neutrophil and platelet count at least every 2 days during bid therapy and weekly thereafter. Granulocytopenia usually occurs during the first 2 wk of treatment but may occur anytime during therapy. Do not administer if neutrophil count <500/mm³ or platelet count <25,000/mm³. Recovery begins within 3–7 days of discontinuation of therapy.
- ❏ Monitor BUN and serum creatinine at least once every 2 wk throughout therapy.
- ❏ Monitor liver function tests (AST, ALT, serum bilirubin, alkaline phosphatase) periodically during therapy. May cause elevated levels.
- ❏ May cause a decrease in blood glucose.

## POTENTIAL NURSING DIAGNOSES

- ■ Infection, risk for (Indications, Patient/Family Teaching).

## IMPLEMENTATION

- **General:** Do not confuse Cytovene (ganciclovir) with Cytosar (cytarabine).
- ❏ Solution should be prepared in a biologic cabinet. Wear gloves, gown, and mask while handling medication. Discard IV equipment in specially designated containers.
- ❏ Do not administer subcut or IM; severe tissue irritation may result.
- **PO:** Administer capsules with food.
- **IV:** Observe infusion site for phlebitis. Rotate infusion site to prevent phlebitis.
- ❏ Maintain adequate hydration throughout therapy.
- **Intermittent Infusion:** Reconstitute 500 mg with 10 ml of sterile water for injection for a concentration of 50 mg/ml. Do not reconstitute with bacteriostatic water with parabens; precipitation will occur. Shake well to dissolve completely. Discard vial if particulate matter or discoloration occurs. Reconstituted solution is stable for 12 hr at room temperature; do not refrigerate.
- ❏ Dilute in 100 ml of D5W, 0.9% NaCl, Ringer's or LR for a concentration not exceeding 10 mg/ml. Once diluted for infusion, solution should be used within 24 hr. Refrigerate but do not freeze.
- **Rate:** Administer slowly, via infusion pump, over 1 hr using an in-line filter. Rapid administration may increase toxicity.
- **Y-Site Compatibility:** ◆ allopurinol ◆ amphotericin B cholesteryl sulfate ◆ cisplatin ◆

cyclophosphamide ♦ docetaxel ♦ doxorubicin liposome ♦ enalaprilat ♦ etoposide ♦ filgrastim ♦ fluconazole ♦ gatifloxacin ♦ granisetron ♦ linezolid ♦ melphalan ♦ methotrexate ♦ paclitaxel ♦ propofol ♦ remifentanil ♦ tacrolimus ♦ teniposide ♦ thiotepa.

■ **Y-Site Incompatibility:** ♦ aldesleukin ♦ amifostine ♦ aztreonam ♦ cytarabine ♦ doxorubicin ♦ fludarabine ♦ foscarnet ♦ gemcitabine ♦ ondansetron ♦ piperacillin/tazobactam ♦ sargramostim ♦ vinorelbine.

## PATIENT/FAMILY TEACHING

❑ Instruct patient to take ganciclovir with food, exactly as directed.

❑ Inform patient that ganciclovir is not a cure for CMV retinitis. Progression of retinitis may continue in immunocompromised patients during and after therapy. Advise patients to have regular ophthalmic exams at least every 6 wk. Duration of therapy for CMV prevention is based on the duration and degree of immunosuppression.

❑ Advise patient to notify health care professional if fever; chills; sore throat; other signs of infection; bleeding gums; bruising; petechiae; or blood in urine, stool, or emesis occurs. Caution patient to avoid crowds and persons with known infections. Instruct patient to use soft toothbrush and electric razor. Patient should be cautioned not to drink alcoholic beverages or take products containing aspirin or NSAIDs.

❑ Advise patient that ganciclovir may have teratogenic effects. A nonhormonal method of contraception should be used during and for at least 90 days after therapy.

❑ Caution patient to use sunscreen and protective clothing to prevent photosensitivity reactions.

❑ Emphasize the importance of frequent follow-up exams to monitor blood counts.

## EVALUATION

**Effectiveness of therapy can be demonstrated by:** ■ Management of the symptoms of CMV retinitis in immunocompromised patients ■ Prevention of CMV retinitis in transplant patients at risk.

---

## gatifloxacin, See FLUOROQUINOLONES.

---

# gefitinib
(je-**fit**-in-ib)
Iressa

## CLASSIFICATION(S):
**Therapeutic:** antineoplastics
**Pharmacologic:** enzyme inhibitors

## Pregnancy Category D

## INDICATIONS

■ Locally advanced or metastatic non-small cell lung cancer in patients who have not responded to platinum—or docetaxel-based chemotherapy.

## ACTION

■ Inhibits activation of kinases found in transmembrane cell surface receptors, including epidermal growth factor receptor (EGFR-TK). **Therapeutic Effects:** ■ Death of rapidly replicating cells, particularly malignant ones.

## PHARMACOKINETICS

**Absorption:** 60% absorbed following oral administration.

**Distribution:** Extensively distributed.

**Metabolism and Excretion:** Mostly metabolized by the liver (CYP 3A4 enzyme system); excreted in feces, <4% excreted in urine.

**Half-life:** 48 hr.

## CONTRAINDICATIONS AND PRECAUTIONS

**Contraindicated in:** ■ Hypersensitivity.

**Use Cautiously in:** ■ Idiopathic pulmonary fibrosis ( ↑ risk of pulmonary toxicity) ■ Concurrent use of strong inhibitors of the CYP 3A4 enzyme system (may increase risk of toxicity).

## ADVERSE REACTIONS AND SIDE EFFECTS*

■ **CNS:** weakness ■ **EENT:** aberrant eyelash, conjunctivitis, corneal erosion/ulcer, eye pain, ↓ vision ■ **CV:** peripheral edema ■ **Resp:** PULMONARY TOXICITY, dyspnea ■ **GI:** diarrhea, nausea, vomiting, anorexia, hepatotoxicity, mouth ulceration ■ **Derm:** acne, dry skin, rash, pruritus ■ **Metab:** weight loss ■ **Metab:** allergic reactions including ANGIOEDEMA.

## INTERACTIONS

**Drug-Drug:** ■ Strong inducers of the CYP 3A4 enzyme system, including **rifampin** and **phenytoin** ↓ blood levels and effects (consider ↑ dose of gefitinib to 500 mg/day) ■ Strong inhibitors of the CYP 3A4 enzyme system, including **ketoconazole** and **itraconazole** ↑ blood levels and effects (use with caution) ■ Absorption and efficacy may be ↓ by **drugs that** ↑ **gastric pH** including **cimetidine** and **ranitidine** ■ May ↑ the risk of bleeding with **warfarin**.

## ROUTE AND DOSAGE

■ **PO (Adults):** 250 mg once daily.

## AVAILABILITY

■ *Tablets:* 250 mg^Rx.

TIME/ACTION PROFILE

|    | ONSET | PEAK | DURATION |
|----|-------|------|----------|
| PO | unknown | unknown | unknown |

## NURSING IMPLICATIONS

### ASSESSMENT

❑ Assess for signs of pulmonary toxicity (dyspnea, cough, fever). If interstitial lung disease is confirmed, discontinue gefitinib and treat appropriately.

❑ Assess patient for eye symptoms such as pain during therapy. May require interruption of therapy and removal of aberrant eyelash. After symptoms and eye changes have resolved, may reinstate therapy.

■ *Lab Test Considerations:* Monitor liver function tests periodically. May cause ↑ transaminases, bilirubin, and alkaline phosphatase. Discontinue gefitinib if elevations are severe.

❑ Monitor for changes in prothrombin time and INR in patients taking warfarin. May cause ↑ levels.

### POTENTIAL NURSING DIAGNOSES

■ Diarrhea (Adverse Reactions).

■ Skin integrity, impaired (Side Effects).

■ Breathing pattern, ineffective (Adverse Reactions).

## IMPLEMENTATION

■ **PO:** Administer one tablet daily without regard to food.

❑ May interrupt therapy briefly (14 days) for patients with poorly tolerated diarrhea with dehydration or skin adverse reactions. Follow by restarting 250 mg dose.

## PATIENT/FAMILY TEACHING

❑ Instruct patient to take gefitinib as directed.

❑ Advise patient to notify health care professional promptly if severe persistent diarrhea, nausea, vomiting, or anorexia occur; if shortness of breath or cough occur or worsen; or eye irritation or other new symptoms develop.

❑ Instruct patient to notify health care professional if pregnancy is planned or suspected or if breastfeeding.

## EVALUATION

**Effectiveness of therapy can be demonstrated by:** ■ Decrease in size and spread of tumors in non-small cell lung cancer.

High Alert

## gemcitabine

(jem-**site**-a-been)

Gemzar

### CLASSIFICATION(S):

***Therapeutic:*** antineoplastics
***Pharmacologic:*** antimetabolites, nucleoside analogues

### Pregnancy Category D

## INDICATIONS

■ Pancreatic cancer (locally advanced or metastatic) ■ Inoperable locally advanced/metastatic non–small-cell lung cancer (with cisplatin).

## ACTION

■ Interferes with DNA synthesis (cell-cycle phase–specific). **Therapeutic Effects:** ■ Death of rapidly replicating cells, particularly malignant ones.

## PHARMACOKINETICS

**Absorption:** IV administration results in complete bioavailability.

**Distribution:** Unknown.

**Metabolism and Excretion:** Converted in cells to active diphosphate and triphosphate metabolites; these are excreted primarily by the kidneys.

**Half-life:** 32–94 min.

## CONTRAINDICATIONS AND PRECAUTIONS

**Contraindicated in:** ■ Hypersensitivity ■ Pregnancy or lactation.

**Use Cautiously in:** ■ History of cardiovascular disease ■ Impaired hepatic or renal function (increased risk of toxicity) ■ Patients with childbearing potential ■ Other chronic debilitating illness.

## ADVERSE REACTIONS AND SIDE EFFECTS*

■ **Resp:** PULMONARY TOXICITY, dyspnea, bronchospasm ■ **CV:** ARRHYTHMIAS, CEREBROVASCULAR ACCIDENT, MI, edema, hypertension ■ **GI:** HEPATOTOXICITY, diarrhea, nausea, stomatitis, transient elevation of hepatic transaminases, vomiting ■ **GU:** HEMOLYTIC UREMIC SYNDROME, hematuria, proteinuria ■ **Derm:** alopecia, rash ■ **Hemat:** anemia, leukopenia, thrombocytopenia ■ **Local:** injection site reactions ■ **Neuro:** paresthesias ■ **Misc:** flu-like symptoms, fever, anaphylactoid reactions.

## INTERACTIONS

**Drug-Drug:** ■ ↑ bone marrow depression with other **antineoplastics** or **radiation therapy** ■ May ↓ antibody response to **live virus vaccines** and ↑ risk of adverse reactions.

## ROUTE AND DOSAGE

Other regimens are used.

❑ **Pancreatic Cancer**

■ **IV (Adults):** 1000 mg/m² once weekly for 7 wk, followed by a week of rest. May be followed by cycles of once-weekly administration for 3 wk followed by a week of rest.

❑ **Non–Small-Cell Lung Cancer (with Cisplatin)**

■ **IV (Adults):** 1000 mg/m² on days 1, 8, and 15 of each 28-day cycle (cisplatin is also given on day 1) *or* 1250 mg/m² on days 1

and 8 of each 21-day cycle (cisplatin is also given on day 1).

## AVAILABILITY

■ *Powder for injection:* 200 mg in 10-ml vial^Rx, 1 g in 50-ml vial^Rx ■ Cost: 200 mg $117.95/10-ml vial, 1 g $589.90/50-ml vial.

TIME/ACTION PROFILE (effect on blood counts)

|  | ONSET | PEAK | DURATION |
|---|---|---|---|
| IV | unknown | unknown | unknown |

# NURSING IMPLICATIONS

## ASSESSMENT

❑ Monitor vital signs before and frequently during therapy.

❑ Monitor injection site during administration. Although gemcitabine is not considered a vesicant, local reactions may occur.

❑ Monitor for bone marrow depression. Assess for bleeding (bleeding gums, bruising, petechiae; guaiac stools, urine, and emesis) and avoid IM injections and taking rectal temperatures if platelet count is low. Apply pressure to venipuncture sites for 10 min. Assess for signs of infection during neutropenia. Anemia may occur. Monitor for increased fatigue, dyspnea, and orthostatic hypotension.

❑ Monitor intake and output, appetite, and nutritional intake. Mild to moderate nausea and vomiting occur frequently. Antiemetics may be used prophylactically.

■ *Lab Test Considerations:* Monitor CBC, including differential and platelet count, before each dose. Dose guidelines are based on the CBC. If the absolute granulocyte count is >1000 and platelet count is >100,000, the full dose may be administered. If the absolute granulocyte count is 500–999 or platelet count is 50,000–99,000, 75% of the dose may be given. If the absolute granulocyte count is <500 or the platelet count is <50,000, withhold further doses.

❑ Monitor hepatic and renal function before and periodically during therapy. May cause transient ↑ in serum AST, ALT, alkaline phosphatase, and bilirubin concentrations.

❑ May also cause ↑ BUN and serum creatinine concentrations, proteinuria, and hematuria.

## POTENTIAL NURSING DIAGNOSES
■ Infection, risk for (Adverse Reactions).

## IMPLEMENTATION
❑ **High Alert:** Fatalities have occurred with incorrect administration of chemotherapeutic agents. Before administering, clarify all ambiguous orders; double check single, daily, and course-of-therapy dose limits; have second practitioner independently double check original order, calculations and infusion pump settings.
■ **General:** Solution should be prepared in a biologic cabinet. Wear gloves, gown, and mask while handling IV medication. Discard IV equipment in specially designated containers.
■ **Intermittent Infusion:** To reconstitute, add 5 ml of 0.9% NaCl without preservatives to 200-mg vial or 25 ml of 0.9% NaCl to the 1-g vial of gemcitabine for a concentration of 40 mg/ml. Incomplete dissolution may result in concentrations greater than 40 mg/ml. May be further diluted with 0.9% NaCl for concentrations as low as 0.1 mg/ml. Solution is colorless to light straw color. Do not administer solutions that are discolored or contain particulate matter. Solution is stable for 24 hr at room temperature. Discard unused portions. Do not refrigerate; crystallization may occur.
■ **Rate:** Administer dose over 30 min. Infusions longer than 60 min have a greater incidence of toxicity.
■ **Y-Site Compatibility:** ◆ amifostine ◆ amikacin ◆ aminophylline ◆ ampicillin ◆ ampicillin/sulbactam ◆ aztreonam ◆ bleomycin ◆ bumetanide ◆ buprenorphine ◆ butorphanol ◆ calcium gluconate ◆ carboplatin ◆ carmustine ◆ cephazolin ◆ cefotetan ◆ cefoxitin ◆ ceftazidime ◆ ceftizoxime ◆ ceftriaxone ◆ cefuroxime ◆ chlorpromizine ◆ cimetidine ◆ ciprofloxacin ◆ cisplatin ◆ clindamycin ◆ cyclophosphamide ◆ cytarabine ◆ dactinomycin ◆ daunorubicin ◆ dexrazoxane ◆ diphenhydramine ◆ dobutamine ◆ docetaxel ◆ dopamine ◆ doxorubicin ◆ doxycycline ◆ droperidol ◆ enalaprilat ◆ etoposide ◆ etoposide phosphate ◆ famotidine ◆ floxuridine ◆ fluconazole ◆ fludarabine ◆ fluorouracil ◆ gatifloxacin ◆ gentamicin ◆ granisetron ◆ haloperidol ◆ heparin ◆ hydro-cortisone ◆ hydromorphone ◆ idarubicin ◆ ifosfamide ◆ leucoverin ◆ linezolid ◆ lorazepam ◆ mannitol ◆ meperidine ◆ mesna ◆ metoclopramide ◆ metronidazole ◆ minocycline ◆ mitoxantrone ◆ morphine ◆ nalbuphine ◆ netilmicin ◆ ofloxacin ◆ ondansetron ◆ paclitaxel ◆ plicamycin ◆ potassium chloride ◆ promethazine ◆ ranitidine ◆ sodium bicarbonate ◆ streptozocin ◆ teniposide ◆ thiotepa ◆ ticaricillin ◆ ticarcillin/clavulanate ◆ tobramycin ◆ topotecan ◆ trimethoprim/sulfamethoxazole ◆ vancomycin ◆ vinblastine ◆ vincristine ◆ vinorelbine ◆ zidovudine.
■ **Y-Site Incompatibility:** ◆ acyclovir ◆ amphotericin B ◆ cefoperazone ◆ cefotaxime ◆ furosemide ◆ ganciclovir ◆ imipenem-cilastatin ◆ irinotecan ◆ methotrexate ◆ methoprednisolone ◆ mitomycin ◆ piperacillin ◆ piperacillin/tazobactam ◆ prochlorperazine.

## PATIENT/FAMILY TEACHING
❑ Instruct patient to notify health care professional if fever; chills; sore throat; signs of infection; bleeding gums; bruising; petechiae; or blood in urine, stool, or emesis occurs. Caution patient to avoid crowds and persons with known infections. Instruct patient to use soft toothbrush and electric razor. Patient should be cautioned not to drink alcoholic beverages or take products containing aspirin or NSAIDs.
❑ Instruct patient to inspect oral mucosa for erythema and ulceration. If ulceration occurs, advise patient to use sponge brush and rinse mouth with water after eating and drinking. Stomatitis pain may require management with opioid analgesics.
❑ Instruct patient to notify health care professional if flu-like symptoms (fever, anorexia, headache, cough, chills, myalgia), swelling of the feet or legs, or shortness of breath occurs.
❑ Discuss with patient the possibility of hair loss. Explore methods of coping.
❑ Advise patient that this medication may have teratogenic effects. Contraception should be used during therapy.
❑ Instruct patient not to receive any vaccinations without advice of health care professional.

{ } = Available in Canada only.
\* CAPITALS indicates life-threatening; <u>underlines</u> indicate most frequent.

❏ Emphasize the need for periodic lab tests to monitor for side effects.

## EVALUATION

**Effectiveness of therapy can be demonstrated by:** ■ Palliative, symptomatic improvement in patients with pancreatic cancer ■ Decrease in size and spread of malignancy in lung cancer.

## gemfibrozil

(gem-**fye**-broe-zil)
Lopid

*CLASSIFICATION(S):*
*Therapeutic: lipid-lowering agents*
*Pharmacologic: fibric acid derivatives*

**Pregnancy Category C**

## INDICATIONS

■ Management of type II-b hyperlipidemia (decreased HDLs, increased LDLs, increased triglycerides) in patients who do not yet have clinical coronary artery disease and have failed therapy with diet, exercise, weight loss, or other agents (niacin, bile acid sequestrants).

## ACTION

■ Inhibits peripheral lipolysis ■ Decreases triglyceride production by the liver ■ Decreases production of the triglyceride carrier protein ■ Increases HDL. **Therapeutic Effects:** ■ Decreased plasma triglycerides and increased HDL.

## PHARMACOKINETICS

**Absorption:** Well absorbed after oral administration.

**Distribution:** Unknown.

**Metabolism and Excretion:** Some metabolism by the liver, 70% excreted by the kidneys (mostly unchanged), 6% excreted in feces.

**Half-life:** 1.3–1.5 hr.

## CONTRAINDICATIONS AND PRECAUTIONS

**Contraindicated in:** ■ Hypersensitivity ■ Primary biliary cirrhosis ■ Concurrent use of HMG-CoA reductase inhibitors.

**Use Cautiously in:** ■ Gallbladder disease ■ Liver disease ■ Severe renal impairment ■ Pregnancy, lactation, or children (safety not established).

## ADVERSE REACTIONS AND SIDE EFFECTS*

■ **CNS:** dizziness, headache ■ **EENT:** blurred vision ■ **GI:** <u>abdominal pain</u>, <u>diarrhea</u>, <u>epigastric pain</u>, flatulence, gallstones, heartburn, nausea, vomiting ■ **Derm:** alopecia, rashes, urticaria ■ **Hemat:** anemia, leukopenia ■ **MS:** myositis.

## INTERACTIONS

**Drug-Drug:** ■ May increase the effects of **warfarin** or **sulfonylurea oral hypoglycemic agents** ■ Concurrent use with **HMG-CoA reductase inhibitors** may increase the risk of rhabdomyolysis (avoid concurrent use) ■ May decrease the effect of **cyclosporine**.

## ROUTE AND DOSAGE

■ **PO (Adults):** 600 mg twice daily 30 min before breakfast and dinner.

## AVAILABILITY (generic available)

■ *Tablets:* 600 mg$^{Rx}$ ■ Cost: $84.22/60 ■ *Capsules:* {300 mg$^{Rx}$}.

TIME/ACTION PROFILE (triglyceride-VLDL–lowering effect)

| | ONSET | PEAK | DURATION |
|---|---|---|---|
| PO | 2–5 days | 4 wk | several mo |

## NURSING IMPLICATIONS

### ASSESSMENT

❏ Obtain patient's diet history, especially regarding fat and alcohol consumption.

■ *Lab Test Considerations:* Serum triglyceride and cholesterol levels should be monitored before and periodically throughout therapy. LDL and VLDL levels should be assessed before and periodically throughout therapy. Medication should be discontinued if paradoxical increase in lipid levels occurs.

❏ Liver function tests should be assessed before and periodically throughout therapy. May cause an increase in serum bilirubin, alkaline phosphatase, CK, LDH, AST, and ALT. If hepatic function tests rise significantly, therapy should be discontinued and not resumed.

❑ CBC and electrolytes should be evaluated every 3–6 mo and then yearly throughout course of therapy. May cause mild decrease in hemoglobin, hematocrit, and leukocyte counts. May cause a decrease in serum potassium concentrations.

❑ May cause slight increase in serum glucose.

## POTENTIAL NURSING DIAGNOSES

■ Noncompliance (Patient/Family Teaching).

## IMPLEMENTATION

■ **General:** Do not confuse Lopid (gemfibrozil) with Levbid (hyoscyamine).

■ **PO:** Administer 30 min before breakfast or dinner.

## PATIENT/FAMILY TEACHING

❑ Instruct patient to take medication exactly as directed, not to skip doses or double up on missed doses. If a dose is missed, take as soon as remembered unless almost time for next dose.

❑ Advise patient that this medication should be used in conjunction with dietary restrictions (fat, cholesterol, carbohydrates, alcohol), exercise, and cessation of smoking.

❑ Instruct patient to notify health care professional promptly if any of the following symptoms occur: severe stomach pains with nausea and vomiting, fever, chills, sore throat, rash, diarrhea, muscle cramping, general abdominal discomfort, or persistent flatulence.

## EVALUATION

**Effectiveness of therapy can be demonstrated by:** ■ Decrease in serum triglyceride and cholesterol levels and improved HDL to total cholesterol ratios. If response is not seen within 3 mo, medication is usually discontinued.

## gemifloxacin, See FLUOROQUINOLONES.

## gentamicin, See AMINOGLYCOSIDES.

## glimepiride, See HYPOGLYCEMIC AGENTS, ORAL.

## glipizide, See HYPOGLYCEMIC AGENTS, ORAL.

## glucagon
(**gloo**-ka-gon)
GlucaGen

**CLASSIFICATION(S):**
**Therapeutic:** hormones
**Pharmacologic:** pancreatics

**Pregnancy Category B**

## INDICATIONS

■ Acute management of severe hypoglycemia when administration of glucose is not feasible ■ Facilitation of radiographic examination of the GI tract. **Unlabeled uses:** ■ Antidote to: ❑ Beta blockers ❑ Calcium channel blockers.

## ACTION

■ Stimulates hepatic production of glucose from glycogen stores (glycogenolysis) ■ Relaxes the musculature of the GI tract (stomach, duodenum, small bowel, and colon), temporarily inhibiting movement ■ Has positive inotropic and chronotropic effects. **Therapeutic Effects:** ■ Increase in blood glucose ■ Relaxation of GI musculature, facilitating radiographic examination.

## PHARMACOKINETICS

**Absorption:** Well absorbed following IM and subcut administration.

**Distribution:** Unknown.

**Metabolism and Excretion:** Extensively metabolized by the liver, plasma, and kidneys.
**Half-life:** 8–18 min.

## CONTRAINDICATIONS AND PRECAUTIONS

**Contraindicated in:** ■ Hypersensitivity ■ Pheochromocytoma ■ Some products contain glycerin and phenol—avoid use in patients with hypersensitivities to these ingredients.

**Use Cautiously in:** ■ History suggestive of insulinoma or pheochromocytoma ■ Prolonged fasting, starvation, adrenal insufficiency or chronic hypoglycemia (low levels of releasable glucose) ■ When used to inhibit GI motility, use cautiously in geriatric patient with cardiac disease or diabetics ■ Pregnancy or lactation.

## ADVERSE REACTIONS AND SIDE EFFECTS*

■ **CV:** transient increase in heart rate and blood pressure ■ **GI:** <u>nausea</u>, <u>vomiting</u> ■ **Misc:** hypersensitivity reactions including <u>ANAPHYLAXIS</u>.

## INTERACTIONS

**Drug-Drug:** ■ Large doses may enhance the effect of **warfarin** ■ Negates the response to **insulin** or **oral hypoglycemic agents** ■ Hyperglycemic effect is intensified and prolonged by **epinephrine** ■ Patients on concurrent **beta blocker therapy** may have a greater increase in heart rate and blood pressure.

## ROUTE AND DOSAGE

❑ **Hypoglycemia**

■ **IV, IM, Subcut (Adults and Children ≥20–25 kg):** 1 mg; may be repeated in 15 min if necessary.

■ **IV, IM, Subcut (Children <20–25 kg or <6–8 yr):** 0.5 mg or 20–30 mcg/kg; may be repeated in 15 min if necessary.

❑ **Radiographic Examination of the GI Tract**

■ **IM, IV (Adults):** 0.25–2 mg; depending on location and duration of examination (0.5 mg IV or 2 mg IM for relaxation of stomach, for examination of the colon 2 mg IM 10 min before procedure).

❑ **Antidote (unlabeled)**

■ **IV (Adults):** *To beta blockers*—50–150 mcg (0.05–0.15 mg)/kg, followed by 1–5 mg/hr infusion. *To calcium channel blockers*—2 mg; additional doses determined by response.

## AVAILABILITY

■ ***Powder for injection:*** 1-mg^Rx vials as an emergency kit for low blood glucose and a diagnostic kit.

## TIME/ACTION PROFILE

| | ONSET | PEAK | DURATION |
|---|---|---|---|
| IM (hyperglycemic action) | within 10 min | 30 min | 60–90 min |
| IV (hyperglycemic action) | within 10 min | 5– min | 60–90 min |
| Subcut (hyperglycemic action) | within 10 min | 30–45 min | 60–90 min |
| IV (effect on GI musculature) | 45 sec (for 0.25–2-mg dose) | unknown | 9–17 min (0.25–0.5-mg dose); 22–25 min (2-mg dose) |
| IM (effect on GI musculature) | 8–10 min (1-mg dose); 4–7 min (2-mg dose) | unknown | 9–27 min (1-mg dose); 21–32 min (2-mg dose) |

# NURSING IMPLICATIONS

## ASSESSMENT

❑ Assess patient for signs of hypoglycemia (sweating, hunger, weakness, headache, dizziness, tremor, irritability, tachycardia, anxiety) prior to and periodically during therapy.

❑ Assess neurologic status throughout therapy. Institute safety precautions to protect patient from injury caused by seizures, falling, or aspiration. For insulin shock therapy, 0.5–1 mg is administered after 1 hr of coma; patient usually awakens in 10–25 min. If no response occurs, repeat the dose. Feed patient supplemental carbohydrates orally to replenish liver glycogen and prevent secondary hypoglycemia as soon as possible after awakening, especially pediatric patients.

❑ Assess nutritional status. Patients who lack liver glycogen stores (starvation, chronic hypoglycemia, adrenal insufficiency) will require glucose instead of glucagon.

❑ Assess for nausea and vomiting after administration of dose. Protect patients with depressed level of consciousness from aspiration by positioning on side; ensure that a suction unit is available. Notify physician if vomiting occurs; patient will require parenteral glucose to prevent recurrent hypoglycemia.

■ ***Lab Test Considerations:*** Monitor serum glucose levels throughout episode, during treatment, and for 3–4 hr after patient regains consciousness. Use of bedside finger-stick blood glucose determination methods is recommended for rapid results. Follow-up lab results may be ordered to validate finger-stick values, but do not delay treatment while awaiting lab results, as this could result in neurologic injury or death.

❏ Large doses of glucagon may cause a decrease in serum potassium concentrations.

## POTENTIAL NURSING DIAGNOSES

■ Injury, risk for (Indications).
■ Noncompliance (Patient/Family Teaching).

## IMPLEMENTATION

■ **General:** May be given subcut, IM, or IV. Reconstitute with diluent supplied in kit by manufacturer. Inspect solution prior to use; use only clear, water-like solution. Solution is stable for 48 hr if refrigerated, 24 hr at room temperature. Unmixed medication should be stored at room temperature.

❏ Administer supplemental carbohydrates IV or orally to facilitate increase of serum glucose levels.

■ **IV:** With doses >2 mg, use sterile water for injection instead of diluent supplied by manufacturer to minimize risk of thrombophlebitis, CNS toxicity, and myocardial depression from phenol preservative in diluent supplied by manufacturer. Use immediately after reconstituting. Final concentration should not exceed 1 mg/ml. Discard any unused portion.

■ **Direct IV:** Administer at a rate not exceeding 1 mg per min. May be administered through IV line containing D5W.

❏ May be given at the same time as a bolus of dextrose.

■ **Additive Incompatibility:** ♦ 0.9% NaCl ♦ potassium chloride ♦ calcium chloride.

## PATIENT/FAMILY TEACHING

■ **General Info:** Teach patient and family signs and symptoms of hypoglycemia. Instruct patient to take oral glucose as soon as symptoms of hypoglycemia occur—glucagon is reserved for episodes when patient is unable to swallow because of decreased level of consciousness.

■ **Home Care Issues:** Instruct family on correct technique to prepare, draw up, and administer injection. Health care professional must be contacted immediately after each dose for orders regarding further therapy or adjustment of insulin dose or diet.

❏ Advise family that patient should receive oral glucose when alertness returns.

❏ Instruct family to position patient on side until fully alert. Explain that glucagon may cause nausea and vomiting. Aspiration may occur if patient vomits while lying on back.

❏ Instruct patient to check expiration date monthly and to replace outdated medication immediately.

❏ Review hypoglycemic medication regimen, diet, and exercise programs.

❏ Patients with diabetes mellitus should carry a source of sugar (such as a packet of sugar or candy) and identification describing disease process and treatment regimen at all times.

## EVALUATION

**Effectiveness of therapy can be demonstrated by:** ■ Increase of serum glucose to normal levels with improved level of consciousness ■ Smooth muscle relaxation of the stomach, duodenum, and small and large intestine in patients undergoing radiologic examination of the GI tract.

## glyburide, See HYPOGLYCEMIC AGENTS, ORAL.

## glycopyrrolate

(glye-koe-**pye**-roe-late)
Robinul, Robinul-Forte

*CLASSIFICATION(S):*
***Therapeutic:*** antispasmodics
***Pharmacologic:*** anticholinergics

**Pregnancy Category B**

## INDICATIONS

■ Inhibits salivation and excessive respiratory secretions when given preoperatively ■ Reverses some of the secretory and vagal actions of cholinesterase inhibitors used to treat nondepolarizing neuromuscular blockade (cholinergic adjunct) ■ Adjunctive management of peptic ulcer disease.

## ACTION

■ Inhibits the action of acetylcholine at postganglionic sites located in smooth muscle, secretory glands, and the CNS (antimuscarinic activity) ■ Low doses decrease sweating, salivation, and respiratory secretions ■ Intermediate doses result in increased heart rate ■ Larger doses decrease GI and GU tract motility. **Therapeutic Effects:** ■ Decreased GI and respiratory secretions.

## PHARMACOKINETICS

**Absorption:** Incompletely absorbed after oral administration. Well absorbed after IM administration.

**Distribution:** Distribution not fully known. Does not significantly cross the blood-brain barrier or eye. Crosses the placenta.

**Metabolism and Excretion:** Eliminated primarily unchanged in the feces, via biliary excretion.

**Half-life:** 1.7 hr (0.6–4.6 hr).

## CONTRAINDICATIONS AND PRECAUTIONS

**Contraindicated in:** ■ Hypersensitivity ■ Narrow-angle glaucoma ■ Acute hemorrhage ■ Tachycardia secondary to cardiac insufficiency or thyrotoxicosis ■ Products containing benzyl alcohol should not be used in neonates ■ Children <12 yr (for management of peptic ulcer only).

**Use Cautiously in:** ■ Geriatric and very young patients (increased susceptibility to adverse reactions) ■ Patients who may have intra-abdominal infections ■ Prostatic hypertrophy ■ Chronic renal, hepatic, pulmonary, or cardiac disease ■ Pregnancy and lactation (safety not established).

## ADVERSE REACTIONS AND SIDE EFFECTS*

■ **CNS:** confusion, drowsiness ■ **EENT:** blurred vision, cycloplegia, dry eyes, mydriasis ■ **CV:** tachycardia, orthostatic hypotension, palpitations ■ **GI:** dry mouth, constipation ■ **GU:** urinary hesitancy, retention.

## INTERACTIONS

**Drug-Drug:** ■ Additive anticholinergic effects with other **anticholinergics,** including **antihistamines, tricyclic antidepressants, quinidine,** and **disopyramide** ■ May alter the absorption of other **orally administered drugs** by slowing motility of the GI tract ■ **Antacids** or **adsorbent antidiarrheal agents** decrease the absorption of anticholinergics ■ May increase GI mucosal lesions in patients taking oral **potassium chloride** tablets ■ Increased risk of adverse cardiovascular reactions with **cyclopropane** anesthesia ■ Concurrent use may decrease absorption of **ketoconazole** (administer 2 hr after ketoconazole).

## ROUTE AND DOSAGE

❑ **Control of Secretions during Surgery**
■ **IM (Adults):** 4.4 mcg/kg 30–60 min preop (not to exceed 0.1 mg).
■ **IM (Children):** 4.4–8.8 mcg/kg 30–60 min preop.

❑ **Cholinergic Adjunct**
■ **IV (Adults and Children):** 200 mcg for each 1 mg of neostigmine or 5 mg of pyridostigmine given at the same time.

❑ **Antiarrhythmic**
■ **IV (Adults):** 100 mcg, may be repeated q 2–3 min.
■ **IV (Children):** 4.4 mcg/kg (up to 100 mcg); may be repeated q 2–3 min.

❑ **Peptic Ulcer**
■ **PO (Adults):** 1–2 mg 2–3 times daily. An additional 2 mg may be given at bedtime; may be decreased to 1 mg twice daily (not to exceed 8 mg/day).
■ **IM, IV (Adults):** 100–200 mcg q 4 hr up to 4 times daily.

## AVAILABILITY (generic available)

■ *Tablets:* 1 mg$^{Rx}$, 2 mg$^{Rx}$ ■ *Injection:* 200 mcg (0.2 mg)/ml$^{Rx}$.

TIME/ACTION PROFILE (anticholinergic effects)

| | ONSET | PEAK | DURATION |
|---|---|---|---|
| PO | unknown | unknown | 8–12 hr |
| IM | 15–30 min | 30–45 min | 2–7 hr* |
| IV | 1 min | unknown | 2–7 hr* |

*Antisecretory effect lasts up to 7 hr; vagal blockade lasts 2–3 hr.

## NURSING IMPLICATIONS

### ASSESSMENT

❑ Assess heart rate, blood pressure, and respiratory rate before and periodically during parenteral therapy.

❑ Monitor intake and output ratios in geriatric or surgical patients; glycopyrrolate may cause urinary retention. Instruct patient to void before parenteral administration.

❑ Assess patient routinely for abdominal distention and auscultate for bowel sounds. If constipation becomes a problem, increasing fluids and adding bulk to the diet may help alleviate the constipating effects of the drug.

❑ Periodic intraocular pressure determinations should be made for patients receiving long-term therapy.

■ *Lab Test Considerations:* Antagonizes effects of pentagastrin and histamine during the gastric acid secretion test. Avoid administration for 24 hr preceding the test.

❑ May cause decreased uric acid levels in patients with gout or hyperuricemia.

■ *Toxicity and Overdose:* If overdosage occurs, neostigmine is the antidote.

### POTENTIAL NURSING DIAGNOSES

■ Oral mucous membrane, impaired (Side Effects).

■ Constipation (Side Effects).

### IMPLEMENTATION

■ **General:** Do not administer cloudy or discolored solution.

■ **PO:** Administer 30–60 min before meals to maximize absorption.

❑ Do not administer within 1 hr of antacids or antidiarrheal medications.

■ **IM:** May be administered undiluted or mixed and administered with D5W, D10W, or 0.9% NaCl.

■ **Direct IV:** May be given undiluted through Y-site injection.

■ *Rate:* Administer at a rate of 0.2 mg over 1–2 min.

■ **Syringe Compatibility:** ◆ benzquinamide ◆ chlorpromazine ◆ cimetidine ◆ codeine ◆ diphenhydramine ◆ droperidol ◆ hydromorphone ◆ hydroxyzine ◆ levorphanol ◆ lido-

caine ◆ meperidine ◆ midazolam ◆ morphine ◆ nalbuphine ◆ neostigmine ◆ oxymorphone ◆ prochlorperazine ◆ promethazine ◆ pyridostigmine ◆ ranitidine ◆ triflupromazine ◆ trimethobenzamide.

■ **Syringe Incompatibility:** ◆ chloramphenicol ◆ diazepam ◆ dimenhydrinate ◆ methohexital ◆ pentazocine ◆ pentobarbital ◆ secobarbital ◆ sodium bicarbonate ◆ thiopental.

■ **Solution Compatibility:** ◆ D5/0.45% NaCl ◆ D5W ◆ 0.9% NaCl ◆ Ringer's solution. Administer immediately after admixing.

■ **Additive Incompatibility:** ◆ methylprednisolone sodium succinate.

### PATIENT/FAMILY TEACHING

❑ Instruct patient to take glycopyrrolate exactly as directed and not to take more than the prescribed amount. Missed doses should be taken as soon as remembered if not just before next dose.

❑ Medication may cause drowsiness and blurred vision. Caution patient to avoid driving or other activities requiring alertness until response to the medication is known.

❑ Inform patient that frequent oral rinses, sugarless gum or candy, and good oral hygiene may help relieve dry mouth. Consult health care professional regarding use of saliva substitute if dry mouth persists for more than 2 wk.

❑ Advise patient to change positions slowly to minimize the effects of drug-induced orthostatic hypotension.

❑ Caution patient to avoid extremes of temperature. This medication decreases the ability to sweat and may increase the risk of heat stroke.

❑ Advise patient to notify health care professional immediately if eye pain or increased sensitivity to light occurs. Emphasize the importance of routine eye exams throughout therapy.

❑ Advise patient to consult health care professional before taking any OTC medications concurrently with this therapy.

### EVALUATION

**Effectiveness of therapy can be demonstrated by:** ■ Mouth dryness preoperatively ■

Reversal of cholinergic medications ■ Decrease in GI motility and pain in patients with peptic ulcer disease.

## granisetron
(gra-**nees**-e-tron)
Kytril

### CLASSIFICATION(S):
**Therapeutic:** antiemetics
**Pharmacologic:** 5 HT₃ antagonists

**Pregnancy Category B**

## INDICATIONS

■ Prevention of nausea and vomiting due to: ▢ emetogenic chemotherapy ▢ radiation therapy ■ Prevention and treatment of postoperative nausea and vomiting.

## ACTION

■ Blocks the effects of serotonin at receptor sites (selective antagonist) located in vagal nerve terminals and in the chemoreceptor trigger zone in the CNS. **Therapeutic Effects:** ■ Decreased incidence and severity of nausea and vomiting following emetogenic chemotherapy, radiation therapy or surgery.

## PHARMACOKINETICS

**Absorption:** 50% absorbed following oral administration.

**Distribution:** Distributes into erythrocytes; remainder of distribution is unknown.

**Metabolism and Excretion:** Mostly metabolized by the liver; 12% excreted unchanged in urine.

**Half-life:** *Patients with cancer*—8–9 hr (range 0.9–31.1 hr); *healthy volunteers*—4.9 hr (range 0.9–15.2 hr); *geriatric patients*—7.7 hr (range 2.6–17.7 hr).

## CONTRAINDICATIONS AND PRECAUTIONS

**Contraindicated in:** ■ Hypersensitivity.

**Use Cautiously in:** ■ Pregnancy or lactation (safety not established) ■ Children <2 yr (safe use of IV route not established) ■ Children <18 yr (safe use of PO route not established).

## ADVERSE REACTIONS AND SIDE EFFECTS*

■ **CNS:** <u>headache</u>, agitation, anxiety, CNS stimulation, drowsiness, weakness ■ **CV:** hypertension ■ **GI:** constipation, diarrhea, elevated liver enzymes, taste disorder ■ **Misc:** anaphylactoid reactions, fever.

## INTERACTIONS

**Drug-Drug:** ■ ↑ risk of extrapyramidal reactions with other **agents causing extrapyramidal reactions.**

## ROUTE AND DOSAGE

▢ **Prevention of Nausea and Vomiting Due to Emetogenic Chemotherapy**
■ **PO (Adults):** 1 mg twice daily; 1st dose given at least 60 min prior to chemotherapy and 2nd dose 12 hr later only on days when chemotherapy is administered; may also be given as 2 mg once daily at least 60 min prior to chemotherapy.
■ **IV (Adults and Children 2–16 yr):** 10 mcg/kg within 30 min prior to chemotherapy.

▢ **Prevention of Nausea and Vomiting Associated with Radiation Therapy**
■ **PO (Adults):** 2 mg taken once daily within 1 h of radiation therapy.

▢ **Prevention and Treatment of Postoperative Nausea and Vomiting**
■ **IV (Adults):** *Prevention*—1 mg prior to induction or anesthesia or just prior to reversal of anesthesia; *Treatment*—1 mg.

## AVAILABILITY

■ *Tablets:* 1 mgᴿˣ ■ Cost: $94.10/2 ■ *Oral solution (orange flavor):* 2 mg/10 ml in 30 ml bottlesᴿˣ ■ *Injection:* 1 mg/mlᴿˣ ■ Cost: $195.20.

TIME/ACTION PROFILE

|    | ONSET | PEAK | DURATION |
|----|-------|------|----------|
| PO | rapid | 60 min | 24 hr |
| IV | rapid | 30 min | up to 24 hr |

## NURSING IMPLICATIONS

### ASSESSMENT

▢ Assess patient for nausea, vomiting, abdominal distention, and bowel sounds prior to and following administration.

❏ Assess for extrapyramidal symptoms (involuntary movements, facial grimacing, rigidity, shuffling walk, trembling of hands) during therapy. This occurs rarely and is usually associated with concurrent use of other drugs known to cause this effect.

■ *Lab Test Considerations:* May cause ↑ AST and ALT levels.

## POTENTIAL NURSING DIAGNOSES

■ Nutrition, imbalanced: less than body requirements (Indications).

## IMPLEMENTATION

■ **General:** For chemotherapy or radiation granisetron is administered only on the day(s) chemotherapy or radiation is given. Continued treatment when not on chemotherapy or radiation therapy has not been found useful.

■ **PO:** Administer 1st dose up to 1 hr before chemotherapy or radiation therapy and 2nd dose 12 hr after the first.

❏ 2 tsp oral solution are equal to 2 mg granisetron.

■ **Direct IV:** May be administered undiluted or diluted in 20–50 ml of 0.9% NaCl or D5W. Solution should be prepared at time of administration but is stable for 24 hr at room temperature.

■ *Rate:* Administer undiluted granisetron over 30 sec or as a diluted solution over 5 min.

■ **Y-Site Compatibility:** ◆ acyclovir ◆ allopurinol ◆ amifostine ◆ amikacin ◆ aminophylline ◆ amphotericin B cholesteryl sulfate ◆ ampicillin ◆ ampicillin-sulbactam ◆ aztreonam ◆ bleomycin ◆ bumetanide ◆ buprenorphine ◆ butorphanol ◆ calcium gluconate ◆ carboplatin ◆ carmustine ◆ cefazolin ◆ cefepime ◆ cefoperazone ◆ cefotaxime ◆ cefotetan ◆ cefoxitin ◆ ceftazidime ◆ ceftizoxime ◆ ceftriaxone ◆ cefuroxime ◆ chlorpromazine ◆ cimetidine ◆ ciprofloxacin ◆ cisplatin ◆ cladribine ◆ clindamycin ◆ cyclophosphamide ◆ cytarabine ◆ dacarbazine ◆ dactinomycin ◆ daunorubicin ◆ dexamethasone ◆ diphenhydramine ◆ dobutamine ◆ docetaxel ◆ dopamine ◆ doxorubicin ◆ doxorubicin liposome ◆ doxycycline ◆ droperidol ◆ enalaprilat ◆ etoposide ◆ etoposide phosphate ◆ famotidine ◆ filgrastim ◆ floxuridine ◆ fluconazole ◆ fludarabine ◆ fluorouracil ◆ furosemide ◆ gatifloxacin ◆ ganciclovir ◆ gemcitabine ◆ gentamicin ◆ haloperidol ◆ heparin ◆ hydrocortisone ◆ hydromorphone ◆ idarubicin ◆ ifosfamide ◆ imipenem/cilastatin ◆ leucovorin ◆ linezolid ◆ lorazepam ◆ magnesium sulfate ◆ mechlorethamine ◆ melphalan ◆ meperidine ◆ mesna ◆ methotrexate ◆ methylprednisolone ◆ metoclopramide ◆ metronidazole ◆ miconazole ◆ minocycline ◆ mitomycin ◆ mitoxantrone ◆ morphine ◆ nalbuphine ◆ netilmicin ◆ ofloxacin ◆ paclitaxel ◆ piperacillin ◆ piperacillin-tazobactam ◆ plicamycin ◆ potassium chloride ◆ prochlorperazine ◆ promethazine ◆ propofol ◆ ranitidine ◆ sargramostim ◆ sodium bicarbonate ◆ streptozocin ◆ teniposide ◆ thiotepa ◆ ticarcillin ◆ ticarcillin/clavulanate ◆ tobramycin ◆ topotecan ◆ trimethoprim-sulfamethoxazole ◆ vancomycin ◆ vinblastine ◆ vincristine ◆ vinorelbine ◆ zidovudine.

■ **Y-Site Incompatibility:** ◆ amphotericin B.

■ **Additive Incompatibility:** Granisetron should not be admixed with other medications.

## PATIENT/FAMILY TEACHING

❏ Advise patient to notify health care professional immediately if involuntary movement of eyes, face, or limbs occurs.

## EVALUATION

**Effectiveness of therapy can be demonstrated by:** ■ Prevention of nausea and vomiting associated with emetogenic cancer chemotherapy or radiation therapy ■ Prevention and treatment of postoperative nausea and vomiting.

# GROWTH HORMONES

## somatropin (recombinant)

### (soe-ma-**troe**-pin)

Genotropin, Humatrope, Norditropin, Nutropin, Nutropin AQ, Nutropin Depot, Saizen, Serostim

## somatrem (recombinant)

### (**soe**-ma-trem)

Protropin

*CLASSIFICATION(S):*
*Therapeutic: hormones*
*Pharmacologic: growth hormones*

**Pregnancy Category B (Serostim only), C (all other trade names)**

## INDICATIONS

■ Growth failure in children due to chronic renal insufficiency ■ Growth failure in children due to deficiency of growth hormone (not Serostim) ■ Short stature associated with Turner's syndrome ■ Growth hormone deficiency in adults (Humatrope, Nutropin) ■ Short stature (Humatrope) ■ AIDS wasting or cachexia (Serostim only) ■ Increases spinal bone density in childhood–onset growth hormone–deficient patients (somatropin).

## ACTION

■ Produce growth (skeletal and cellular) ■ Metabolic actions include: ■ Increased protein synthesis ■ Increased carbohydrate metabolism ■ Lipid mobilization ■ Retention of sodium, phosphorus, and potassium ■ Somatropin has the same amino acid sequence as naturally occurring growth hormone; somatrem has 1 additional amino acid. Both are produced by recombinant DNA techniques. **Therapeutic Effects:** ■ Increased skeletal growth in children with growth hormone deficiency ■ Replacement of somatropin in deficient adults ■ Decreased wasting in patients with AIDS ■ Increased bone density in adult growth hormone–deficient patients.

## PHARMACOKINETICS

**Absorption:** Well absorbed.

**Distribution:** Localize to highly perfused organs (liver, kidneys).

**Metabolism and Excretion:** Broken down in renal cells to amino acids that are recirculated; some liver metabolism.

**Half-life:** *Subcut*—3.8 hr; *IM*—4.9 hr.

## CONTRAINDICATIONS AND PRECAUTIONS

**Contraindicated in:** ■ Closure of epiphyses ■ Active neoplasia ■ Hypersensitivity to *m*-cresol or glycerin (somatropin) or benzyl alcohol (somatrem) ■ Acute critical illness (therapy should not be initiated) ■ Prader-Willi syndrome with obesity and respiratory impairment (risk of fatal complications).

**Use Cautiously in:** ■ Growth hormone deficiency due to intracranial lesion ■ Coexisting adrenocorticotropic hormone (ACTH) deficiency ■ Diabetes (may cause insulin resistance) ■ Geriatric patients (↑ sensitivity, ↑ risk of adverse reactions ■ Thyroid dysfunction ■ Pregnancy or lactation (safety not established).

## ADVERSE REACTIONS AND SIDE EFFECTS*

■ **CV:** edema of the hands and feet ■ **Endo:** hyperglycemia, hypothyroidism, insulin resistance ■ **Local:** pain at injection site ■ **MS:** *Serostim only*—carpal tunnel syndrome, musculoskeletal pain.

## INTERACTIONS

**Drug-Drug:** ■ Excessive **corticosteroid** use (equivalent to 10–15 mg/m²/day) may ↓ response to somatropin.

## ROUTE AND DOSAGE

❏ **Somatropin (Protropin)**

■ **IM, Subcut (Children):** up to 0.3 mg (0.9 unit)/kg weekly; subcut route is preferred.

❏ **Somatropin (Genotropin)**

■ **Subcut (Children):** 0.16–0.24 mg/kg/wk divided in 6–7 daily doses.

■ **Subcut (Adults):** 0.04–0.8 mg/kg/wk divided in 6–7 daily doses.

❏ **Somatropin (Humatrope)**

■ **Subcut (Adults):** 0.018 unit/kg/day (up to 0.0375 unit/kg/day).

■ **IM, Subcut (Children):** 0.18 mg/kg (0.54 unit/kg)/wk given in divided doses on 3 alternating days or 6 times weekly (up to 0.3 mg/kg or 0.9 unit/kg/wk).

❏ **Somatropin (Nutropin/Nutropin AQ)**

■ **Subcut (Children):** *Growth hormone inadequacy*—0.3 mg/kg. *Chronic renal insufficiency*—0.35 mg/kg (1.05 units/kg)/wk given as daily injections. *Turner's syndrome*—≤0.375 mg/kg (1.125 units/kg)/wk in 3–7 divided doses.

■ **Subcut (Adults):** <0.006 mg/kg daily; may be increased to 0.025 mg/kg/day in patients <35 yrs or 0.0125 mg/kg in patients >35 yrs.

□ **Somatropin (Nutropin Depot)**

■ **Subcut (Children):** 1.5 mg/kg monthly (patients >15 kg will require more than one injection per dose) *or* 0.75 mg/kg twice monthly (patients >30 kg will require more than one injection per dose)

□ **Somatropin (Norditropin)**

■ **Subcut (Children):** 0.024–0.034 mg/kg 6–7 times weekly.

□ **Somatropin (Saizen)**

■ **Subcut, IM (Children):** 0.06 mg (0.18 unit/kg) 3 times weekly.

□ **Somatropin (Serostim)**

■ **Subcut (Adults):** >*55 kg*—6 mg once daily; *45–55 kg*—5 mg once daily; *35–45 kg*—4 mg once daily; <*35 kg*—0.1 mg/kg once daily.

**AVAILABILITY**

□ **Somatrem (Protropin)**

■*Powder for injection:* 5 mg (13 IU)/vial^Rx, 10 mg (26 IU)/vial^Rx.

□ **Somatropin/Genotropin**

■ *Powder for injection:* 1.5-mg intra-mix cartridge (delivers 1.3 mg)^Rx, 5.8-mg intra-mix cartridge (delivers 5 mg)^Rx, 5.8-mg intra-mix cartridge (delivers 5 mg) as Pen 5 system^Rx, 13.8-mg intra-mix cartridge (delivers 12 mg)^Rx, 13.8-mg intra-mix cartridge (delivers 12 mg) as Pen 12 system^Rx, MiniQuick system 0.2 mg^Rx, MiniQuick system 0.4 mg^Rx, MiniQuick system 0.6 mg^Rx, MiniQuick system 0.8 mg^Rx, MiniQuick system 1 mg^Rx, MiniQuick system 1.4 mg^Rx, MiniQuick system 1.6 mg^Rx, MiniQuick system 1.8 mg^Rx, MiniQuick system 2 mg^Rx.

□ **Humatrope**

■ *Powder for injection:* 5-mg/vial^Rx.

□ **Norditropin**

■ *Powder for injection:* 4-mg (12 units)/vial^Rx, 5-mg (13 units)/vial^Rx, 8-mg (24 units)/vial^Rx, 10-mg (26 units)/vial^Rx. ■ *Cartridges for injection (using Nordipen):* 5 mg/1.5 ml^Rx, 10 mg/1.5 ml^Rx, 15 mg/1.5ml^Rx.

□ **Nutropin**

■ *Powder for injection:* 5-mg (13 units)/vial^Rx, 10-mg (26 units)/vial^Rx.

□ **Nutropin AQ**

■ *Solution for injection (AQ):* 5 mg (15 units)/ml in 2-ml vial^Rx.

□ **Nutropin Depot**

■*Injectable suspension:* 13.5-mg single-use vial^Rx, 18-mg single-use vial^Rx, 22.5-mg single-use vial^Rx.

□ **Saizen**

■ *Powder for injection:* 5-mg (15 units)/vial^Rx, 6-mg (18 units)/vial^Rx.

□ **Serostim**

■ *Powder for injection:* 6-mg (15 units)/vial^Rx.

TIME/ACTION PROFILE (growth)

| | ONSET | PEAK | DURATION |
|---|---|---|---|
| IM, subcut | within 3 mo | unknown | 12–48 hr |

# NURSING IMPLICATIONS

## ASSESSMENT

■ **Growth Failure:** Monitor bone age annually and growth rate determinations, height, and weight every 3–6 mo during therapy.

■ **AIDS Wasting/Cachexia:** Re-evaluate treatment in patients who continue to lose weight in first 2 wk of treatment.

■ *Lab Test Considerations:* Monitor thyroid function prior to and during therapy. May decrease T⁴, radioactive iodine uptake, and thyroxine-binding capacity. Hypothyroidism necessitates concurrent thyroid replacement for growth hormone to be effective. Serum inorganic phosphorus, alkaline phosphatase, and parathyroid hormone may ↑ with somatropin therapy.

□ Monitor blood glucose periodically during therapy. Diabetic patients may require ↑ insulin dose.

□ Monitor for development of neutralizing antibodies if growth rate does not exceed 2.5 cm/6 mo.

□ Monitor alkaline phosphatase closely in patients with adult growth hormone deficiency.

## POTENTIAL NURSING DIAGNOSES

■ Body image, disturbed (Indications).

## IMPLEMENTATION

- **General:** Rotate injection sites with each injection.

- **Somatrem:** Reconstitute 5-mg vial with 1–5 ml and 10-mg vial with 1–10 ml of bacteriostatic water for injection, aiming the liquid against glass vial wall. Do not shake; swirl gently to dissolve. Solution is clear; do not use cloudy solutions. Discard vial after withdrawing dose.

- **Somatropin:** Reconstitute 5-mg vial with 1.5–5 ml of sterile water for injection provided by manufacturer (contains preservative *m* -cresol), aiming the liquid against glass vial wall. Do not shake; swirl gently to dissolve. Solution is clear; do not use solutions that are cloudy or contain a precipitate. Stable for 14 days when refrigerated; do not freeze.

- *Genotropin intra-mix:* Dissolve powder with solution provided with 2-chamber cartridge as directed. Gently tip cartridge upside down a few times until contents are completely dissolved. The 1.5-mg cartridge is stable following dilution for 24 hr if refrigerated. The 5.8-mg and 13.8-mg cartridges contain preservatives and are stable for 14 days if refrigerated.

- *Genotropin Pen:* Prepare and administer as directed in patient instruction insert. Store in the refrigerator.

- *Genotropin MiniQuick:* For single use only. Inject immediately after reconstitution; may be refrigerated for 24 hr after reconstitution. Follow directions on patient package insert for reconstitution and administration.

- *Humatrope:* Reconstitute each 5-mg vial with 1.5–5 ml of diluent provided. Stable for 14 days if refrigerated.

- *Norditropin:* Reconstitute each 4-mg or 8-mg vial with 2 ml of diluent. Use reconstituted vials within 14 days. If using cartridges for the Nordipen, each cartridge has a corresponding color-coded pen which is graduated to deliver the appropriate dose based on the concentration of norditropin in the cartridge. Color coding of cartridge and pen must match.

- *Nutropin/Nutropin AQ:* Reconstitute 5-mg vial with 1–5 ml and 10-mg vial with 1–10 ml of bacteriostatic water for injection. Reconstituted vials are stable for 14 days (Nutropin) or 28 days (Nutropin AQ) if refrigerated.

- *Saizen:* Reconstitute each 5-mg vial with 1–3 ml of bacteriostatic water for injection. Reconstituted vials are stable for 14 days if refrigerated. To use cool.click needle-free injector, wind the device to energize the spring, and draw medication into the Crystal Check nozzle. Using firm pressure at the injection site, hold the injector at a 90° angle and press the blue actuator button.

- *Serostim:* Reconstitute each vial with 1 ml of sterile water for injection. Use within 24 hr of reconstitution.

- **Subcut:** Injection volume for *somatropin* should not exceed 1 ml.

## PATIENT/FAMILY TEACHING

- Instruct patient and parents on correct procedure for reconstituting medication, site selection, technique for IM or subcut injection, and disposal of needles and syringes. Review dosage schedule. Somatropin injections should be at least 48 hr apart. Parents should report persistent pain or edema at injection site.

- Explain rationale for prohibition of use for increasing athletic performance. Administration to persons without growth hormone deficiency or after epiphyseal closure may result in acromegaly (coarsening of facial features; enlarged hands, feet, and internal organs; increased blood glucose; hypertension).

- Emphasize need for regular follow-up with endocrinologist to ensure appropriate growth rate, to evaluate lab work, and to determine bone age by x-ray exam.

- Assure parents and child that these dose forms are synthetic and therefore not capable of transmitting Creutzfeldt-Jakob disease, as was the original somatropin, which was extracted from human cadavers.

## EVALUATION

**Clinical response to therapy can be evaluated by:** ■ Child's attainment of adult height in growth failure secondary to pituitary growth hormone deficiency. Therapy is limited to period before closure of epiphyseal plates (approximately up to 14–15 yr in girls, 15–16 yr in boys) ■ Replacement of somatropin in deficient adults ■ Decreased wasting in patients with AIDS.

# guaifenesin

(gwye-**fen**-e-sin)

Anti-Tuss, {Benylin-E}, Breonesin, {Calmylin Expectorant}, Diabetic Tussin EX, Gee-Gee, Genatuss, GG-Cen, Glyate, Glycotuss, Glytuss, Guiatuss, Humibid Sprinkle, Hytuss, Hytuss-2X, Monafed, Mucinex, Mytussin, Naldecon Senior EX, Organidin NR, Pneumomist, {Resyl}, Robitussin, Scot-tussin Expectorant, Siltussin SA, Siltussin, Sinumist-SR Caplets, Tusibron, Tussin, Uni-tussin

### CLASSIFICATION(S):

**Therapeutic:** allergy, cold, and cough remedies, expectorants

**Pregnancy Category C**

## INDICATIONS

■ Coughs associated with viral upper respiratory tract infections.

## ACTION

■ Reduces viscosity of tenacious secretions by increasing respiratory tract fluid. **Therapeutic Effects:** ■ Mobilization and subsequent expectoration of mucus.

## PHARMACOKINETICS

**Absorption:** Well absorbed after oral administration.

**Distribution:** Unknown.

**Metabolism and Excretion:** Renally excreted as metabolites.

**Half-life:** Unknown.

## CONTRAINDICATIONS AND PRECAUTIONS

**Contraindicated in:** ■ Hypersensitivity ■ Some products contain alcohol and should be avoided in patients with known intolerance.

**Use Cautiously in:** ■ Cough lasting >1 wk or accompanied by fever, rash, or headache ■ Pregnancy (although safety has not been established, guaifenesin has been used without adverse effects) ■ Patients receiving disulfiram (liquid products may contain alcohol) ■ Diabetic patients (some products may contain sugar).

## ADVERSE REACTIONS AND SIDE EFFECTS*

■ **CNS:** dizziness, headache ■ **GI:** nausea, diarrhea, stomach pain, vomiting ■ **Derm:** rashes, urticaria.

## INTERACTIONS

**Drug-Drug:** ■ None significant.

## ROUTE AND DOSAGE

- ■ **PO (Adults):** 200–400 mg q 4 hr or 600–1200 mg q 12 hr as extended-release product (not to exceed 2400 mg/day).
- ■ **PO (Children 6–12 yr):** 100–200 mg q 4 hr or 600 mg q 12 hr as extended-release product (not to exceed 1200 mg/day).
- ■ **PO (Children 2–6 yr):** 50–100 mg q 4 hr (not to exceed 600 mg/day).

## AVAILABILITY (generic available)

■ *Syrup:* 100 mg/5 ml^OTC ■ Cost: $1.90/120 ml ■ *Oral solution:* 100 mg/5 mlRx, OTC, 200 mg/5 ml^OTC ■ *Capsules:* 200 mg^OTC ■ *Tablets:* 100 mg^OTC, 200 mg^Rx, ^OTC, 1200 mg^Rx ■ *Extended-release tablets (Mucinex):* 600 mg^Rx, 1200 mg^Rx ■ analgesics/antipyretics, antihistamines, decongestants, and cough suppressantsRx, OTC.

TIME/ACTION PROFILE (expectorant action)

|       | ONSET    | PEAK    | DURATION |
|-------|----------|---------|----------|
| PO    | 30 min   | unknown | 4–6 hr   |
| PO-ER | unknown  | unknown | 12 hr    |

# NURSING IMPLICATIONS

## ASSESSMENT

❑ Assess lung sounds, frequency and type of cough, and character of bronchial secretions periodically during therapy. Maintain fluid intake of 1500–2000 ml/day to decrease viscosity of secretions.

## POTENTIAL NURSING DIAGNOSES

■ Airway clearance, ineffective (Indications).

## IMPLEMENTATION

■ **PO:** Administer each dose of guaifenesin followed by a full glass of water to decrease viscosity of secretions.

❑ Sustained-release tablets should be swallowed whole; do not open, crush, break, or chew.

## PATIENT/FAMILY TEACHING

❑ Instruct patient to cough effectively. Patient should sit upright and take several deep breaths before attempting to cough.

❑ Inform patient that drug may occasionally cause dizziness. Avoid driving or other activities requiring alertness until response to drug is known.

❑ Advise patient to limit talking, stop smoking, maintain moisture in environmental air, and take some sugarless gum or hard candy to help alleviate the discomfort caused by a chronic nonproductive cough.

❑ Instruct patient to contact health care professional if cough persists longer than 1 wk or is accompanied by fever, rash, or persistent headache or sore throat.

## EVALUATION

**Effectiveness of therapy can be demonstrated by:** ■ Easier mobilization and expectoration of mucus from cough associated with upper respiratory infection.

## guanfacine

(**gwahn**-fa-seen)

Tenex

**CLASSIFICATION(S):**

**Therapeutic:** antihypertensives
**Pharmacologic:** centrally acting antiadrenergics

**Pregnancy Category B**

## INDICATIONS

■ Hypertension (with thiazide-type diuretics).

## ACTION

■ Stimulates CNS alpha$_2$-adrenergic receptors, producing a decrease in sympathetic outflow to heart, kidneys, and blood vessels. Result is decreased blood pressure and peripheral resistance, a slight decrease in heart rate, and no change in cardiac output. **Therapeutic Effects:** ■ Lowering of blood pressure.

## PHARMACOKINETICS

**Absorption:** Well absorbed (80%) following oral administration.

**Distribution:** Appears to be widely distributed.

**Metabolism and Excretion:** 50% metabolized by the liver, 50% excreted unchanged by the kidneys.

**Half-life:** 17 hr.

## CONTRAINDICATIONS AND PRECAUTIONS

**Contraindicated in:** ■ Hypersensitivity.

**Use Cautiously in:** ■ Severe coronary artery disease or recent myocardial infarction ■ Geriatric patients ( ↑ sensitivity, ↓ hepatic/cardiac/renal function) ■ Cerebrovascular disease ■ Severe renal or liver disease ■ Pregnancy, lactation, or children <12 yr (safety not established).

## ADVERSE REACTIONS AND SIDE EFFECTS*

■ **CNS:** <u>drowsiness</u>, <u>weakness</u>, depression, dizziness, fatigue, headache, insomnia ■ **EENT:** tinnitus ■ **Resp:** dyspnea ■ **CV:** bradycardia, chest pain, palpitations, rebound hypertension ■ **GI:** <u>constipation</u>, <u>dry mouth</u>, abdominal pain, nausea ■ **GU:** <u>impotence</u>.

## INTERACTIONS

**Drug-Drug:** ■ ↑ hypotension with other **antihypertensives, nitrates,** and acute ingestion of **alcohol** ■ ↑ CNS depression may occur with other **CNS depressants,** including **alcohol, antihistamines, opioid analgesics, tricyclic antidepressants,** and **sedative/hypnotics** ■ **NSAIDs** may ↓ effectiveness ■ **Adrenergics** may ↓ effectiveness.

## ROUTE AND DOSAGE

■ **PO (Adults):** 1 mg daily given at bedtime, may be increased if necessary at 3–4 wk intervals up to 2 mg/day; may also be given in 2 divided doses.

## AVAILABILITY (generic available)

■ **Tablets:** 1 mg$^{Rx}$, 2 mg$^{Rx}$ ■ Cost: 1 mg $120.60/100, 2 mg $165.33/100.

TIME/ACTION PROFILE (antihypertensive effect)

| | ONSET | PEAK | DURATION |
|---|---|---|---|
| PO (single dose) | unknown | 8–12 hr | 24 hr |
| PO (multiple doses) | within 1 wk | 1–3 mo | unknown |

# NURSING IMPLICATIONS

## ASSESSMENT

- ❑ Monitor blood pressure (lying and standing) and pulse frequently during initial dose adjustment and periodically during therapy. Report significant changes.
- ❑ Monitor frequency of prescription refills to determine adherence.
- ▪ *Lab Test Considerations:* May cause temporary, clinically insignificant ↑ in plasma growth hormone levels.
- ❑ May cause ↓ in urinary catecholamines and vanillylmandelic acid levels.

## POTENTIAL NURSING DIAGNOSES

- ▪ Injury, risk for (Side Effects).
- ▪ Noncompliance (Patient/Family Teaching).

## IMPLEMENTATION

- ▪ **PO:** Administer daily dose at bedtime to minimize daytime sedation.

## PATIENT/FAMILY TEACHING

- ❑ Emphasize the importance of continuing to take medication as directed, even if feeling well. Medication controls but does not cure hypertension. Instruct patient to take medication at the same time each day. Take missed doses as soon as remembered; do not double doses. If 2 or more doses are missed, consult health care professional. Do not discontinue abruptly; may cause sympathetic overstimulation (nervousness, anxiety, rebound hypertension, chest pain, tachycardia, increased salivation, nausea, trembling, stomach cramps, sweating, difficulty sleeping). These effects may occur 2–7 days after discontinuation, although rebound hypertension is rare and more likely to occur with high doses.

- ❑ Advise patient to make sure enough medication is available for weekends, holidays, and vacations. A written prescription may be kept in wallet in case of emergency.
- ❑ Encourage patient to comply with additional interventions for hypertension (weight reduction, low-sodium diet, smoking cessation, moderation of alcohol consumption, regular exercise, and stress management).
- ❑ Instruct patient and family on proper technique for blood pressure monitoring. Advise them to check blood pressure at least weekly and to report significant changes.
- ❑ May cause drowsiness or dizziness. Advise patient to avoid driving or other activities requiring alertness until response to the medication is known.
- ❑ Advise patient to consult health care professional before taking any OTC medications or herbal products, especially cough, cold, or allergy remedies.
- ❑ Caution patient to avoid alcohol and other CNS depressants while taking guanfacine.
- ❑ Advise patient to notify health care professional if dry mouth or constipation persists. Frequent mouth rinses, good oral hygiene, and sugarless gum or candy may minimize dry mouth. Increase in fluid and fiber intake and exercise may decrease constipation.
- ❑ Instruct patient to notify health care professional of medication regimen prior to treatment or surgery.
- ❑ Advise patient to notify health care professional if dizziness, prolonged drowsiness, fatigue, weakness, depression, headache, sexual dysfunction, mental depression, or sleep pattern disturbance occurs. Discontinuation may be required if drug-related mental depression occurs.
- ❑ Emphasize the importance of follow-up exams to evaluate effectiveness of medication.

## EVALUATION

**Effectiveness of therapy can be demonstrated by:** ▪ Decrease in blood pressure without excessive side effects.

---

{ } = Available in Canada only.
*CAPITALS indicates life-threatening; <u>underlines</u> indicate most frequent.

# halcinonide, See CORTICOSTEROIDS (TOPICAL/LOCAL).

# halobetasol, See CORTICOSTEROIDS (TOPICAL/LOCAL).

## haloperidol
(ha-loe-**per**-i-dole)
{Apo-Haloperidol}, Haldol, Haldol Decanoate, {Haldol LA}, {Novo-Peridol}, {Peridol}, {PMS Haloperidol}

### CLASSIFICATION(S):
**Therapeutic:** antipsychotics
**Pharmacologic:** butyrophenones

**Pregnancy Category C**

### INDICATIONS

■ Acute and chronic psychotic disorders including: ❏ shizophrenia ❏ manic states ❏ drug-induced psychoses ■ Also useful in managing aggressive or agitated patients ■ Tourette's syndrome ■ Severe behavioral problems in children which may be accompanied by: ❏ unprovoked, combative, explosive hyperexcitability ❏ hyperactivity accompanied by conduct disorders (short term use when other modalities have failed). **Unlabeled uses:** ■ Nausea and vomiting from surgery or chemotherapy.

### ACTION

■ Alters the effects of dopamine in the CNS ■ Also has anticholinergic and alpha-adrenergic blocking activity. **Therapeutic Effects:** ■ Diminished signs and symptoms of psychoses ■ Improved behavior in children with Tourette's syndrome or other behavioral problems.

### PHARMACOKINETICS

**Absorption:** Well absorbed following PO/IM administration. Decanoate salt is slowly absorbed and has a long duration of action.

**Distribution:** Concentrates in liver. Crosses placenta; enters breast milk.
**Protein Binding:** 90%.
**Metabolism and Excretion:** Mostly metabolized by the liver.
**Half-life:** 21–24 hr.

### CONTRAINDICATIONS AND PRECAUTIONS

**Contraindicated in:** ■ Hypersensitivity ■ Narrow-angle glaucoma ■ Bone marrow depression ■ CNS depression ■ Severe liver or cardiovascular disease ■ Some products contain tartrazine, sesame oil, or benzyl alcohol and should be avoided in patients with known intolerance or hypersensitivity.
**Use Cautiously in:** ■ Geriatric or debilitated patients (dosage reduction required) ■ Cardiac disease ■ Diabetes ■ Respiratory insufficiency ■ Prostatic hypertrophy ■ CNS tumors ■ Intestinal obstruction ■ Seizures ■ Pregnancy and lactation (safety not established).

### ADVERSE REACTIONS AND SIDE EFFECTS*

■ **CNS:** SEIZURES, extrapyramidal reactions, confusion, drowsiness, restlessness, tardive dyskinesia ■ **EENT:** blurred vision, dry eyes ■ **Resp:** respiratory depression ■ **CV:** hypotension, tachycardia ■ **GI:** constipation, dry mouth, anorexia, drug-induced hepatitis, ileus ■ **GU:** urinary retention ■ **Derm:** diaphoresis, photosensitivity, rashes ■ **Endo:** galactorrhea ■ **Hemat:** anemia, leukopenia ■ **Metab:** hyperpyrexia ■ **Misc:** NEUROLEPTIC MALIGNANT SYNDROME, hypersensitivity reactions.

### INTERACTIONS

**Drug-Drug:** ■ ↑ hypotension with **antihypertensives, nitrates,** or acute ingestion of **alcohol** ■ ↑ anticholinergic effects with **drugs having anticholinergic properties,** including **antihistamines, antidepressants, atropine, phenothiazines, quinidine,** and **disopyramide** ■ ↑ CNS depression with other **CNS depressants,** including **alcohol, antihistamines, opioid analgesics,** and **sedative/hypnotics** ■ Concurrent use with **epinephrine** may result in severe hypotension and tachycardia ■ May ↓ therapeutic effects of **levodopa** or **pergolide** ■ Acute encephalopathic syn-

---

{ } = Available in Canada only.
*CAPITALS indicates life-threatening; underlines indicate most frequent.

drome may occur when used with **lithium** ■ Dementia may occur with **methyldopa**.

**Drug-Natural Products:** ■ **Kava, valerian,** or **chamomile** can ↑ CNS depression.

## ROUTE AND DOSAGE

### �‣ Haloperidol

- **PO (Adults):** 0.5–5 mg 2–3 times daily. Patients with severe symptoms may require up to 100 mg/day.
- **PO (Geriatric Patients or Debilitated Patients):** 0.5–2 mg twice daily initially; may be gradually increased as needed.
- **PO (Children 3–12 yr or 15–40 kg):** 50 mcg/kg/day in 2–3 divided doses; may increase by 500 mcg (0.5 mg)/day q 5–7 days as needed (up to 75 mcg/kg/day for nonpsychotic disorders or Tourette's syndrome or 150 mcg/kg/day for psychoses).
- **IM (Adults):** 2–5 mg q 1–8 hr (not to exceed 100 mg/day).
- **IV (Adults):** 0.5–5 mg, may be repeated q 30 min (unlabeled).

### �‣ Haloperidol Decanoate

- **IM (Adults):** 10–15 times the previous daily PO dose but not to exceed 100 mg initially, given monthly (not to exceed 300 mg/mo).

## AVAILABILITY (generic available)

■ *Tablets:* 0.5 mg$^{Rx}$, 1 mg$^{Rx}$, 2 mg$^{Rx}$, 5 mg$^{Rx}$, 10 mg$^{Rx}$, 20 mg$^{Rx}$ ■ Cost: *Haldol*—1 mg $22.93/30, 2 mg $32.82/30; *generic*—1 mg $7.95/100, 2 mg $10.95/100 ■ *Oral concentrate:* 2 mg/ml$^{Rx}$ ■ *Haloperidol injection:* 5 mg/ml$^{Rx}$ ■ *Haloperidol decanoate injection:* 50 mg/ml$^{Rx}$, 100 mg/ml$^{Rx}$.

TIME/ACTION PROFILE (antipsychotic activity)

| | ONSET | PEAK | DURATION |
|---|---|---|---|
| PO | 2 hr | 2–6 hr | 8–12 hr |
| IM | 20–30 min | 30–45 min | 4–8 hr† |
| IM (decanoate) | 3–9 days | unknown | 1 mo |

†Effect may persist for several days.

## NURSING IMPLICATIONS

### ASSESSMENT

- ❑ Assess mental status (orientation, mood, behavior) prior to and periodically during therapy.
- ❑ Monitor blood pressure (sitting, standing, lying) and pulse prior to and frequently during the period of dosage adjustment. May cause QT interval changes on ECG.
- ❑ Observe patient carefully when administering medication, to ensure that medication is actually taken and not hoarded.
- ❑ Monitor intake and output ratios and daily weight. Assess patient for signs and symptoms of dehydration (decreased thirst, lethargy, hemoconcentration), especially in geriatric patients.
- ❑ Assess fluid intake and bowel function. Increased bulk and fluids in the diet help minimize constipating effects.
- ❑ Monitor patient for onset of akathisia (restlessness or desire to keep moving), which may appear within 6 hr of 1st dose and may be difficult to distinguish from psychotic agitation; benztropine may be used to differentiate. Observe closely for extrapyramidal side effects (*parkinsonian*—difficulty speaking or swallowing, loss of balance control, pill rolling, mask-like face, shuffling gait, rigidity, tremors; and *dystonic*—muscle spasms, twisting motions, twitching, inability to move eyes, weakness of arms or legs).
- ❑ Monitor for tardive dyskinesia (uncontrolled rhythmic movement of mouth, face, and extremities; lip smacking or puckering; puffing of cheeks; uncontrolled chewing; rapid or worm-like movements of tongue). Report immediately; may be irreversible.
- ❑ Monitor for development of neuroleptic malignant syndrome (fever, respiratory distress, tachycardia, seizures, diaphoresis, hypertension or hypotension, pallor, tiredness, severe muscle stiffness, loss of bladder control). Report symptoms immediately. May also cause leukocytosis, elevated liver function tests, elevated CPK.
- ■ **Lab Test Considerations:** Monitor CBC with differential and liver function tests periodically during therapy.

## POTENTIAL NURSING DIAGNOSES

- ■ Thought processes, disturbed (Indications).

## IMPLEMENTATION

- ■ **General:** Avoid skin contact with oral solution; may cause contact dermatitis.
- ■ **PO:** Administer with food or full glass of water or milk to minimize GI irritation.

- Use calibrated measuring device for accurate dosage. Do not dilute concentrate with coffee or tea; may cause precipitation. Should be given undiluted, but if necessary may dilute in at least 60 ml of liquid.
- **IM:** Inject slowly, using 2-in., 21-gauge needle into well-developed muscle via Z-track technique. Do not exceed 3 ml per injection site. Slight yellow color does not indicate altered potency. Keep patient recumbent for at least 30 min following injection to minimize hypotensive effects.
- **Direct IV:** May be administered undiluted for rapid control of acute psychosis or delirium.
- **Rate:** Administer at a rate of 5 mg/min.
- **Intermittent Infusion:** May be diluted in 30–50 ml of D5W.
- **Rate:** Infuse over 30 min.
- **Syringe Compatibility:** ◆ hydromorphone ◆ lorazepam ◆ sufentanil.
- **Syringe Incompatibility:** ◆ diphenhydramine ◆ heparin ◆ hydroxyzine ◆ ketorolac.
- **Y-Site Compatibility:** ◆ amifostine ◆ aztreonam ◆ cimetidine ◆ cisatracurium ◆ cladribine ◆ dobutamine ◆ docetaxel ◆ dopamine ◆ doxorubicin liposome ◆ etoposide phosphate ◆ famotidine ◆ fentanyl ◆ filgrastim ◆ fludarabine ◆ gatifloxacin ◆ gemcitabine ◆ granisetron ◆ hydromorphone ◆ lidocaine ◆ linezolid ◆ lorazepam ◆ melphalan ◆ methadone ◆ midazolam ◆ nitroglycerin ◆ norepinephrine ◆ ondansetron ◆ paclitaxel ◆ phenylephrine ◆ propofol ◆ remifentanil ◆ sufentanil ◆ tacrolimus ◆ teniposide ◆ theophylline ◆ thiotepa ◆ vinorelbine.
- **Y-Site Incompatibility:** ◆ allopurinol ◆ amphotericin B cholesteryl sulfate complex ◆ cefepime ◆ fluconazole ◆ foscarnet ◆ heparin ◆ piperacillin/tazobactam ◆ sargramostim.

## PATIENT/FAMILY TEACHING

- Advise patient to take medication as directed. Take missed doses as soon as remembered, with remaining doses evenly spaced throughout the day. May require several weeks to obtain desired effects. Do not increase dose or discontinue medication without consulting health care professional. Abrupt withdrawal may cause dizziness; nausea; vomiting; GI upset; trembling; or uncontrolled movements of mouth, tongue, or jaw.
- Inform patient of possibility of extrapyramidal symptoms and tardive dyskinesia. Caution patient to report symptoms immediately.
- Advise patient to change positions slowly to minimize orthostatic hypotension.
- May cause drowsiness. Caution patient to avoid driving or other activities requiring alertness until response to medication is known.
- Caution patient to avoid taking alcohol or other CNS depressants concurrently with this medication.
- Advise patient to use sunscreen and protective clothing when exposed to the sun to prevent photosensitivity reactions. Extremes of temperature should also be avoided, because this drug impairs body temperature regulation.
- Instruct patient to use frequent mouth rinses, good oral hygiene, and sugarless gum or candy to minimize dry mouth.
- Advise patient to notify health care professional of medication regimen prior to treatment or surgery.
- Instruct patient to notify health care professional promptly if weakness, tremors, visual disturbances, dark-colored urine or clay-colored stools, sore throat, or fever is noted.
- Emphasize the importance of routine follow-up exams.

## EVALUATION

**Effectiveness of therapy can be demonstrated by:** ■ Decrease in hallucinations, insomnia, agitation, hostility, and delusions ■ Decreased tics and vocalization in Tourette's syndrome ■ Improved behavior in children with severe behavioral problems. If no therapeutic effects are seen in 2–4 wk, dosage may be increased.

## haloprogin, See ANTIFUNGALS (TOPICAL).

## High Alert

# heparin
(**hep**-a-rin)
{Calcilean}, {Calciparine}, {Hepale-an}, {Heparin Leo}, Hep-Lock, Hep-Lock U/P

### CLASSIFICATION(S):
**Therapeutic:** anticoagulants
**Pharmacologic:** antithrombotics

### Pregnancy Category C

## INDICATIONS

■ Prophylaxis and treatment of various thromboembolic disorders including: ❑ Venous thromboembolism ❑ Pulmonary emboli ❑ Atrial fibrillation with embolization ❑ Acute and chronic consumptive coagulopathies ❑ Peripheral arterial thromboembolism ■ Used in very low doses (10–100 units) to maintain patency of IV catheters (heparin flush).

## ACTION

■ Potentiates the inhibitory effect of antithrombin on factor Xa and thrombin ■ In low doses, prevents the conversion of prothrombin to thrombin by its effects on factor Xa ■ Higher doses neutralize thrombin, preventing the conversion of fibrinogen to fibrin. **Therapeutic Effects:** ■ Prevention of thrombus formation ■ Prevention of extension of existing thrombi (full dose).

## PHARMACOKINETICS

**Absorption:** Well absorbed following subcut administration.
**Distribution:** Does not cross the placenta or enter breast milk.
**Protein Binding:** Very high (to low-density lipoproteins, globulins, and fibrinogen).
**Metabolism and Excretion:** Probably removed by the reticuloendothelial system (lymph nodes, spleen).
**Half-life:** 1–2 hr (increases with increasing dosage).

## CONTRAINDICATIONS AND PRECAUTIONS

**Contraindicated in:** ■ Hypersensitivity ■ Uncontrolled bleeding ■ Severe thrombocytopenia ■ Open wounds (full dose) ■ Products containing benzyl alcohol should not be used in premature infants.

**Use Cautiously in:** ■ Severe liver or kidney disease ■ Retinopathy (hypertensive or diabetic) ■ Untreated hypertension ■ Ulcer disease ■ Spinal cord or brain injury ■ History of congenital or acquired bleeding disorder ■ Malignancy ■ Women >60 yr (increased risk of bleeding) ■ May be used during pregnancy, but use with caution during the last trimester and in the immediate postpartum period.

**Exercise Extreme Caution in:** ■ Severe uncontrolled hypertension ■ Bacterial endocarditis, bleeding disorders ■ GI bleeding/ulceration/pathology ■ Hemorrhagic stroke ■ Recent CNS or ophthalmologic surgery ■ Active GI bleeding/ulceration ■ History of thrombocytopenia related to heparin.

## ADVERSE REACTIONS AND SIDE EFFECTS*

■ **GI:** drug-induced hepatitis ■ **Derm:** alopecia (long-term use), rashes, urticaria ■ **Hemat:** BLEEDING, anemia, thrombocytopenia ■ **Local:** pain at injection site ■ **MS:** osteoporosis (long-term use) ■ **Misc:** fever, hypersensitivity.

## INTERACTIONS

Heparin is frequently used concurrently or sequentially with other agents affecting coagulation. The risk of potentially serious interactions is greatest with full anticoagulation.

**Drug-Drug:** ■ Risk of bleeding may be increased by concurrent use of **drugs that affect platelet function,** including **aspirin, NSAIDs, clopidogrel, dipyridamole,** some **penicillins, ticlopidine, abciximab, eptifibitide, tirofiban,** and **dextran** ■ Risk of bleeding may be increased by concurrent use of **drugs that cause hypoprothrombinemia,** including **quinidine, cefamandole, cefmetazole, cefoperazone, cefotetan, plicamycin,** and **valproic acid** ■ Concurrent use of **thrombolytic agents** increases the risk of bleeding ■ Heparins affect the prothrombin time used in assessing the response to **warfarin** ■ **Digoxin, tetracyclines, nicotine,** and **antihistamines** may decrease the anticoagulant effect of heparin ■ **Streptokinase** may be followed by relative resistance to heparin.

**Drug-Natural Products:** ■ Increased risk of bleeding with **arnica, anise, chamomile, clove, dong quai, fever few, garlic, ginger,** and **Panax ginseng.**

## ROUTE AND DOSAGE

❑ **Therapeutic Anticoagulation**

■ **IV (Adults):** *Intermittent bolus*—10,000 units, followed by 5000–10,000 units q 4–6 hr. *Continuous infusion*—5000 units (35–70 units/kg), followed by 20,000–40,000 units infused over 24 hr (approx. 1000 units/hr or 15–18 units/kg/hr).

■ **IV (Children):** *Intermittent bolus*—50 units/kg, followed by 50–100 units/kg q 4 hr. *Continuous infusion*—50 units/kg, followed by 100 units/kg/4 hr or 20,000 units/m²/24 hr.

■ **Subcut (Adults):** 5000 units IV, followed by initial subcut dose of 10,000–20,000 units, then 8000–10,000 units q 8 hr or 15,000–20,000 units q 12 hr.

❑ **Prophylaxis of Thromboembolism**

■ **Subcut (Adults):** 5000 units q 8–12 hr (may be started 2 hr prior to surgery).

❑ **Cardiovascular Surgery**

■ **IV (Adults):** At least 150 units/kg (300 units/kg if procedure <60 min; 400 units/kg if >60 min).

❑ **"Flush"**

■ **IV (Adults and Children):** 10–100 units/ml solution to fill heparin lock set to needle hub; replace after each use.

## AVAILABILITY (generic available)

❑ **Heparin Sodium**

■ *Solution for injection:* 10 units/ml^Rx, 100 units/ml^Rx, 1000 units/ml^Rx, 5000 units/ml^Rx, 7500 units/ml^Rx, 10,000 units/ml^Rx, 20,000 units/ml^Rx, 40,000 units/ml^Rx ■ Cost: 1000 units/ml $1.10/ml, 5000 units/ml $1.44/ml ■ *Premixed solution:* 1000 units/500 ml^Rx, 2000 units/1000 ml^Rx, 12,500 units/250 ml^Rx, 25,000 units in 250 and 500 ml^Rx.

TIME/ACTION PROFILE (anticoagulant effect)

| | ONSET | PEAK | DURATION |
|---|---|---|---|
| Heparin subcut | 20–60 min | 2 hr | 8–12 hr |
| Heparin IV | immediate | 5–10 min | 2–6 hr |

## NURSING IMPLICATIONS

### ASSESSMENT

■ **General Info:** Assess patient for signs of bleeding and hemorrhage (bleeding gums; nosebleed; unusual bruising; black, tarry stools; hematuria; fall in hematocrit or blood pressure; guaiac-positive stools). Notify physician if these occur.

❑ Assess patient for evidence of additional or increased thrombosis. Symptoms will depend on area of involvement.

❑ Monitor patient for hypersensitivity reactions (chills, fever, urticaria). Report signs to physician.

■ **Subcut:** Observe injection sites for hematomas, ecchymosis, or inflammation.

■ *Lab Test Considerations:* Activated partial thromboplastin time (aPTT) and hematocrit should be monitored prior to and periodically throughout therapy. When *intermittent IV* therapy is used, draw aPTT levels 30 min before each dose during initial therapy and then periodically. During *continuous* administration, monitor aPTT levels every 4 hr during early therapy. For *subcut* therapy, draw blood 4–6 hr after injection.

❑ Monitor platelet count every 2–3 days throughout therapy. May cause mild thrombocytopenia, which appears on 4th day and resolves despite continued heparin therapy. Thrombocytopenia, which necessitates discontinuing medication, may develop on 8th day of therapy. Patients who have received a previous course of heparin may be at higher risk for severe thrombocytopenia for several months after the initial course.

❑ May cause prolonged prothrombin/time (PT) levels, elevations of serum thyroxine, T₃ resin and false-negative ¹²⁵I fibrinogen uptake tests.

❑ May cause decreased serum triglyceride and cholesterol levels and increased plasma free fatty acid concentrations.

❑ May also cause hyperkalemia and elevated AST and ALT levels.

■ *Toxicity and Overdose:* Protamine sulfate is the antidote. However, because of the short half-life, overdose can often be treated by withdrawing the drug.

## POTENTIAL NURSING DIAGNOSES

■ Tissue perfusion, ineffective (Indications).

■ Injury, risk for (Side Effects).

## IMPLEMENTATION

❏ **High Alert:** Unintended concomitant use of two heparin products (unfractionated heparin and LMW heparins) has resulted in serious harm or death. Review patients' recent (emergency department, operating room) and current medication administration records before administering any heparin or LMW heparin product. Dosage calculation and infusion pump programming errors have also occurred. Have second practitioner independently check original order, dose calculation and infusion pump settings. Do not confuse heparin with Hespan (hetastarch in sodium chloride). Do not confuse vials of heparin with vials of insulin.

■ **General:** Inform all personnel caring for patient of anticoagulant therapy. Venipunctures and injection sites require application of pressure to prevent bleeding or hematoma formation. IM injections of other medications should be avoided, because hematomas may develop.

❏ Dose of heparin should be checked with a second licensed personnel prior to administration.

❏ In patients requiring long-term anticoagulation, oral anticoagulant therapy should be instituted 4–5 days prior to discontinuing heparin therapy.

❏ Solution is colorless to slightly yellow.

■ **Subcut:** Administer deep into subcut tissue. Alternate injection sites between the left and right abdominal wall above the iliac crest. Inject entire length of needle at a 45° or 90° angle into a skin fold held between thumb and forefinger; hold skin fold throughout injection. Do not aspirate or massage. Rotate sites frequently. Do not administer IM because of danger of hematoma formation. Solution should be clear; do not inject solution containing particulate matter.

■ **Direct IV:** Loading dose usually precedes continuous infusion.

■ **Rate:** May be given undiluted over at least 1 min.

■ **Intermittent/Continuous Infusion:** Dilute in prescribed amount of 0.9% NaCl, D5W, or Ringer's solution for injection and give as a continuous or intermittent infusion. Ensure adequate mixing of heparin in solution by inverting container at least 6 times initially and periodically mixing during infusing.

■ **Rate:** Infusion may be administered over 4–24 hr. Use an infusion pump to ensure accuracy.

■ **Flush:** To prevent clot formation in intermittent infusion (heparin lock) sets, inject dilute heparin solution of 10–100 units/0.5–1 ml after each medication injection or every 8–12 hr. To prevent incompatibility of heparin with medication, flush lock set with sterile water or 0.9% NaCl for injection before and after medication is administered.

■ **Syringe Compatibility:** ◆ aminophylline ◆ amphotericin B ◆ ampicillin ◆ atropine ◆ bleomycin ◆ cefazolin ◆ cefoperazone ◆ cefotaxime ◆ cefoxitin ◆ chloramphenicol ◆ cimetidine ◆ cisplatin ◆ clindamycin ◆ cyclophosphamide ◆ diazoxide ◆ digoxin ◆ dimenhydrinate ◆ epinephrine ◆ fentanyl ◆ fluorouracil ◆ furosemide ◆ leucovorin ◆ lidocaine ◆ methotrexate ◆ metoclopramide ◆ mezlocillin ◆ mitomycin ◆ nafcillin ◆ naloxone ◆ neostigmine ◆ pancuronium ◆ penicillin G ◆ phenobarbital ◆ piperacillin ◆ succinylcholine ◆ trimethoprim/sulfamethoxazole ◆ verapamil ◆ vincristine.

■ **Syringe Incompatibility:** ◆ amikacin ◆ amiodarone ◆ chlorpromazine ◆ diazepam ◆ doxorubicin ◆ droperidol ◆ erythromycin lactobionate ◆ gentamicin ◆ haloperidol ◆ kanamycin ◆ meperidine ◆ methotrimeprazine ◆ netilmicin ◆ pentazocine ◆ promethazine ◆ streptomycin ◆ tobramycin ◆ triflupromazine ◆ vancomycin ◆ warfarin.

■ **Y-Site Compatibility:** ◆ acyclovir ◆ aldesleukin ◆ allopurinol ◆ amifostine ◆ aminophylline ◆ ampicillin ◆ ampicillin/sulbactam ◆ atracurium ◆ atropine ◆ aztreonam ◆ betamethasone ◆ bleomycin ◆ calcium gluconate ◆ cefazolin ◆ cefotetan ◆ ceftazidime ◆ ceftriaxone ◆ cephapirin ◆ chlordiazepoxide ◆ chlorpromazine ◆ cimetidine ◆ cisplatin ◆ cladribine ◆ clindamycin ◆ conjugated estrogens ◆ cyanocobalamin ◆ cyclophosphamide ◆ cytarabine ◆ dexamethasone ◆ digoxin ◆ diphenhydramine ◆ dopamine ◆ doxorubicin liposome ◆ edrophonium ◆ enalaprilat ◆ epinephrine ◆ erythromycin lactobionate ◆ esmolol ◆ ethacrynate ◆ famotidine ◆ fentanyl ◆ fluconazole ◆ fludarabine ◆ fluorouracil ◆ foscarnet ◆ furosemide ◆ hydralazine ◆ hydrocortisone ◆

hydromorphone ♦ insulin ♦ isoproterenol ♦ kanamycin ♦ leucovorin ♦ linezolid ♦ lidocaine ♦ lorazepam ♦ magnesium sulfate ♦ melphalan ♦ meperidine ♦ meropenem ♦ methotrexate ♦ methoxamine ♦ methyldopate ♦ methylergonovine ♦ metoclopramide ♦ metronidazole ♦ midazolam ♦ milrinone ♦ minocycline ♦ mitomycin ♦ morphine ♦ nafcillin ♦ neostigmine ♦ nitroglycerin ♦ nitroprusside ♦ norepinephrine ♦ ondansetron ♦ oxacillin ♦ oxytocin ♦ paclitaxel ♦ pancuronium ♦ penicillin G potassium ♦ pentazocine ♦ piperacillin ♦ piperacillin/tazobactam ♦ potassium chloride ♦ prednisolone ♦ procainamide ♦ prochlorperazine ♦ propofol ♦ propranolol ♦ pyridostigmine ♦ ranitidine ♦ remifentanil ♦ sargramostim ♦ scopolamine ♦ sodium bicarbonate ♦ streptokinase ♦ succinylcholine ♦ tacrolimus ♦ teniposide ♦ theophylline ♦ thiotepa ♦ ticarcillin ♦ ticarcillin/clavulanate ♦ tirofiban ♦ trimethobenzamide ♦ trimethophan camsylate ♦ vecuronium ♦ vinblastine ♦ vincristine ♦ warfarin ♦ zidovudine.

■ **Y-Site Incompatibility:** ♦ alatrofloxacin ♦ alteplase ♦ amiodarone ♦ amphotericin B cholesteryl sulfate ♦ ciprofloxacin ♦ diazepam ♦ doxycycline ♦ ergotamine tartrate ♦ filgrastim ♦ gatifloxacin ♦ gentamicin ♦ haloperidol ♦ idarubicin ♦ levofloxacin ♦ methotrimeprazine ♦ phenytoin ♦ tobramycin ♦ trifluoromazine ♦ vancomycin.

■ **Additive Compatibility:** It is recommended that heparin not be mixed in solution with other medications when given for anticoagulation, even those that are compatible, because changes in rate of heparin infusion may be required that would also affect admixtures. If heparin is added to an admixture, the following drugs are compatible: ♦ aminophylline ♦ amphotericin ♦ calcium gluconate ♦ cefepime ♦ cephapirin ♦ chloramphenicol ♦ clindamycin ♦ colistimethate ♦ dopamine ♦ erythromycin gluceptate ♦ fluconazole ♦ flumazenil ♦ furosemide ♦ lidocaine ♦ magnesium sulfate ♦ meropenem ♦ methyldopate ♦ methylprednisolone ♦ nafcillin ♦ octreotide ♦ potassium chloride ♦ prednisolone ♦ ranitidine ♦ sodium bicarbonate ♦ verapamil ♦ vitamin B complex ♦ vitamin B complex with C. Also compatible with TPN solutions or fat emulsion.

■ **Additive Incompatibility:** ♦ alteplase ♦ amikacin ♦ ciprofloxacin ♦ cytarabine ♦ daunorubicin ♦ erythromycin lactobionate ♦ gentamicin ♦ hyaluronidase ♦ kanamycin ♦ meperidine ♦ methadone ♦ morphine ♦ polymyxin B ♦ streptomycin.

## PATIENT/FAMILY TEACHING

■ **General Info:** Advise patient to report any symptoms of unusual bleeding or bruising to health care professional immediately.

❏ Instruct patient not to take medications containing aspirin or NSAIDs while on heparin therapy.

❏ Caution patient to avoid IM injections and activities leading to injury and to use a soft toothbrush and electric razor during heparin therapy.

❏ Advise patient to inform health care professional of medication regimen prior to treatment or surgery.

❏ Patients on anticoagulant therapy should carry an identification card with this information at all times.

## EVALUATION

**Clinical response to therapy can be evaluated by:** ■ Prolonged partial thromboplastin time (PTT) of 1.5–2.5 times the control, without signs of hemorrhage ■ Prevention of deep vein thrombosis and pulmonary emboli ■ Patency of IV catheters.

High Alert

# HEPARINS (LOW MOLECULAR WEIGHT)/HEPARINOIDS

**dalteparin**

(dal-**te**-pa-rin)
Fragmin

**enoxaparin**

(e-nox-a-**pa**-rin)
Lovenox

**fondaparinux**

(fon-da-**par**-i-nux)
Arixtra

**tinzaparin**

(tin-za-**pa**-rin)

Innohep

**CLASSIFICATION(S):**
**Therapeutic:** anticoagulants
**Pharmacologic:** antithrombotics

**Pregnancy Category B**

## INDICATIONS

■ Prevention of thromboembolic phenomena including deep vein thrombosis (DVT) and pulmonary emboli after abdominal surgery (not fondaparinux), knee/hip surgery or replacement ■ **Enoxaparin and dalteparin only:** Prevention of ischemic complications (with aspirin) in patients with ❏ unstable angina/non–Q–wave MI ❏ non–Q–wave MI ❏ **Enoxaparin only:** Treatment of DVT and prevention of DVT in patients at risk for thromboembolic complications due to severely restricted mobility during acute illness.

## ACTION

■ Potentiate the inhibitory effect of antithrombin on factor Xa and thrombin **Therapeutic Effects:** ■ Prevention of thrombus formation.

## PHARMACOKINETICS

**Absorption:** All agents are destroyed by enzymes in the GI tract, necessitating parenteral administration. Well absorbed after subcut administration (87% for dalteparin, 100% for fondaparinux and 92% for enoxaparin).

**Distribution:** *Fondaparinux*—Distributes mainly throughout the intravascular space; *others*—Unknown.

**Metabolism and Excretion:** *Dalteparin*—unknown; *enoxaparin*—weakly metabolized by the liver; renally eliminated; *fondaparinux*—eliminated mainly unchanged in urine; *tinzaparin*—partially metabolized, elimination is primarily renal.

**Half-life:** *Dalteparin*—2.1–2.3 hr (increased in renal insufficiency); *enoxaparin*—3–6 hr; *fondaparinux*—17–21 hr; *tinzaparin*—3.9 hr.

## CONTRAINDICATIONS AND PRECAUTIONS

**Contraindicated in:** ■ Hypersensitivity to specific agents or pork products; cross-sensitivity

may occur ■ Uncontrolled bleeding ■ Some products contain sulfites or benzyl alcohol and should be avoided in patients with known hypersensitivity or intolerance ■ Active major bleeding ■ Thrombocytopenia associated with the presence of antiplatelet antibodies associated with low-molecular-weight heparins ■ *Tinzaparin*—history of heparin-induced thrombocytopenia ■ *Dalteparin*—regional anesthesia during treatment for unstable angina/non–Q–wave MI ■ *Fondaparinux*—Severe renal impairment (CCr <30 ml/min; increased risk of bleeding) ■ Body weight <50 kg (markedly increased risk of bleeding)

**Use Cautiously in:** ■ Severe liver or kidney disease (adjust dose of enoxaparin if CCr <30 ml/min) ■ Mild-to-moderate renal impairment (fondaparinux) ■ Weight <45 kg (adjust dose of enoxaparin) ■ Retinopathy (hypertensive or diabetic) ■ Untreated hypertension ■ Geriatric patients (consider body size, age-related decreased in hepatic/renal/cardiovascular function and concurrent medications) ■ Recent history of ulcer disease ■ History of congenital or acquired bleeding disorder ■ Malignancy ■ Pregnancy, lactation, or children (safety not established).

**Exercise Extreme Caution in:** ■ Spinal/epidural anesthesia (increased risk of spinal/epidural hematomas, especially with concurrent NSAIDs, repeated or traumatic epidural puncture, or indwelling epidural catheter) ■ Severe uncontrolled hypertension ■ Bacterial endocarditis, bleeding disorders ■ GI bleeding/ulceration/pathology ■ Hemorrhagic stroke ■ Recent CNS or ophthalmologic surgery ■ Active GI bleeding/ulceration ■ History of thrombocytopenia related to heparin.

## ADVERSE REACTIONS AND SIDE EFFECTS*

■ **CNS:** dizziness, headache, insomnia ■ **CV:** edema ■ **GI:** constipation, nausea, reversible increase in liver enzymes, vomiting ■ **GU:** urinary retention ■ **Derm:** ecchymoses, pruritus, rash, urticaria ■ **Hemat:** BLEEDING, anemia, thrombocytopenia ■ **Local:** erythema at injection site, hematoma, irritation, pain ■ **Misc:** fever.

## INTERACTIONS

**Drug-Drug:** ■ Risk of bleeding may be ↑ by concurrent use of **warfarin** or **drugs that affect platelet function,** including **aspirin,**

NSAIDs, dipyridamole, some penicillins, clopidogrel, ticlopidine, abciximab, eftifibatide, tirofiban, thrombolytics and dextran.

**Drug-Natural Products:** ■ ↑ bleeding risk with **anise, arnica, chamomile, clove, feverfew, garlic, ginger, ginkgo, Panax ginseng,** and others.

## ROUTE AND DOSAGE

### ❑ Dalteparin

■ **Subcut (Adults):** *Prophylaxis of DVT before abdominal surgery*—2500 IU 1–2 hr before surgery, then once daily for 5–10 days; *prophylaxis of DVT in high-risk patients undergoing abdominal surgery*—5000 IU evening before surgery, then once daily for 5–10 days *or* 2500 IU 1–2 hr before surgery, another 2500 IU 12 hr later, then 5000 IU daily for 5–10 days; *prophylaxis of DVT in patients undergoing hip replacement surgery*—2500 IU within 2 hr before surgery, another 2500 IU evening of the day of surgery ≥6 hr after first dose, then 5000 IU daily for 5–10 days (if surgery is in the evening, omit second dose day of surgery) *or* 5000 IU evening before surgery, then 5000 IU daily for 5–10 days; *angina/non–Q-wave MI*—120 IU/kg (not to exceed 10,000 IU) q 12 hr with concurrent aspirin (75–165 mg/day); *systemic anticoagulation (unlabeled)*—200 IU/kg once daily or 100 IU/kg twice daily.

### ❑ Enoxaparin

■ **Subcut (Adults):** *DVT prophylaxis before knee/hip surgery*—30 mg twice daily starting within 24 hr postop and continued for 7–10 days or until ambulatory (up to 14 days); *DVT prophylaxis before following hip replacement*—40 mg subcut once daily, started 12 (±3) hours preop *or* 30 mg every 12 hr, started 12 to 24 hours postop, provided that hemostasis has been established at the wound site (may be continued for up to 3 wk after hospital discharge); *DVT prophylaxis before abdominal surgery*—40 mg once daily starting within 24 hr postop and continued for 7–10 days or until ambulatory (up to 14 days); *treatment of DVT/PE*—1 mg/kg q 12 hr or 1.5 mg/kg q 24 hr; *angina/non–Q-wave MI*—1 mg/kg q 12 hr (with aspirin 100–325 mg/day) for 2–8 days.

### ❑ Fondaparinux

■ **Subcut (Adults):** 2.5 mg once daily, starting 6–8 hr after surgery, continuing for 5–9 days (up to 11 days) following knee/hip replacement or continuing for 24 days following hip fracture surgery (up to 32 days).

### ❑ Tinzaparin

■ **Subcut (Adults):** *Treatment of deep vein thrombosis*—175 anti-Xa IU/kg once daily for at least 6 days and until adequate anticoagulation is achieved with warfarin; *prophylaxis of deep vein thrombosis*—3500 anti-Xa units (50 anti-Xa units/kg) once daily started 1-2 hr prior to surgery and continued for 5-10 days; *prophylaxis of deep vein thrombosis in patients undergoing orthopedic procedures*—75 anti-Xa units/kg daily starting 12-24 hr after surgery; doses of 4500 anti-Xa units 12 hr before surgery and following surgery have also been used. Prophylactic use is unlabeled.

## AVAILABILITY

### ❑ Dalteparin

■ *Solution for injection:* 2500 anti–factor Xa IU/0.2 ml^Rx, 5000 anti–factor Xa IU/0.2 ml^Rx ■ *Prefilled syringes:* 2500 IU ^Rx, 5000 IU ^Rx, 7500 IU ^Rx.

### ❑ Enoxaparin

■ *Solution for injection (prefilled syringes):* 30 mg/0.3 ml^Rx, 40 mg/0.4 ml, 60 mg/0.6 ml^Rx, 80 mg/0.8 ml^Rx, 100 mg/1 ml^Rx, 120 mg/0.8 ml^Rx, 150 mg/ml^Rx ■ Cost: 30 mg/0.3ml $183.50/10, 40 mg/0.4 ml $244.60/10, 60 mg/0.6ml $367.40/10, 80 mg/0.8 ml $489.80/10, 100 mg/1 ml $612.30/10 ■ *Solution for injection:* 30 mg/0.3 ml ampule^Rx, 300 mg/3 ml multi-dose vial^Rx ■ Cost: 300 mg/3 ml ampules $174.70/10.

### ❑ Fondaparinux

■ *Solution for subcut injection:* 2.5 mg/0.5 ml in prefilled syringes^Rx.

### ❑ Tinzaparin

■ *Solution for injection:* 20,000 anti-Xa units/ml in 2-ml vials.

TIME/ACTION PROFILE (anticoagulant effect)

| | ONSET | PEAK | DURATION |
|---|---|---|---|
| Dalteparin subcut | rapid | 4 hr | up to 24 hr |
| Enoxaparin subcut | unknown | unknown | 12 hr |
| Fondaparinux subcut | rapid | 3 hr | 24 hr |
| Tinzaparin subcut | rapid | 4–6 hr | 24 hr |

## NURSING IMPLICATIONS

### ASSESSMENT

- **General Info:** Assess for signs of bleeding and hemorrhage (bleeding gums; nosebleed; unusual bruising; black, tarry stools; hematuria; fall in hematocrit or blood pressure; guaiac-positive stools); bleeding from surgical site. Notify physician if these occur.
- Assess for evidence of additional or increased thrombosis. Symptoms depend on area of involvement. Monitor neurological status frequently for signs of neurological impairment. May require urgent treatment.
- Monitor for hypersensitivity reactions (chills, fever, urticaria). Report signs to physician.
- Monitor patients with epidural catheters frequently for signs and symptoms of neurologic impairment.
- **Subcut:** Observe injection sites for hematomas, ecchymosis, or inflammation.
- **Lab Test Considerations:** Monitor CBC, platelet count, and stools for occult blood periodically during therapy. If thrombocytopenia occurs, monitor closely. If hematocrit ↓ unexpectedly, assess patient for potential bleeding sites. In patients receiving *fondaparinux or tinazaparin*, if platelet count is <100,000/mm³, discontinue *fondaparinux or tinzaparin*.
- *Fondaparinux* is not accurately measured by prothrombin time (PT), activated thromboplastin time (aPTT), or international standards of heparin or low—molecular—weight heparins. If unexpected changes in coagulation parameters or major bleeding occurs, discontinue fondaparinux.
- Special monitoring of clotting times (aPTT) is not necessary. Patients receiving both *tinzaparin* and warfarin should have blood for PT/INR drawn just prior to the next scheduled dose of *tinzaparin*.
- May cause ↑ in AST and ALT levels.

- **Toxicity and Overdose:** For *enoxaparin* overdose, protamine sulfate 1 mg for each mg of *enoxaparin* should be administered by slow IV injection. For *dalteparin* overdose, protamine sulfate 1 mg for each 100 anti–factor Xa IU of *dalteparin* should be administered by slow IV injection. If the aPTT measured 2–4 hr after protamine administration remains prolonged, a 2nd infusion of protamine 0.5 mg/100 anti–factor Xa IU of *dalteparin* may be administered.

### POTENTIAL NURSING DIAGNOSES

- Tissue perfusion, ineffective (Indications).
- Injury, risk for (Side Effects).

### IMPLEMENTATION

- ❑ **High Alert:** Unintended concomitant use of two heparin products (unfractionated heparin and LMW heparins) has resulted in serious harm and death. Review patients' recent and current medication administration records before administering any heparin or LMW heparin product.
- **General:** Cannot be used interchangeably (unit for unit) with unfractionated heparin or other low-molecular-weight heparins.
- **Subcut:** Administer deep into subcut tissue. Alternate injection sites daily between the left and right anterolateral and left and right posterolateral abdominal wall, the upper thigh, or buttocks. Inject entire length of needle at a 45° or 90° angle into a skin fold held between thumb and forefinger; hold skin fold throughout injection. Do not aspirate or massage. Rotate sites frequently. Do not administer IM because of danger of hematoma formation. Solution should be clear; do not inject solution containing particulate matter.
- ❑ If excessive bruising occurs, ice cube massage of site before injection may lessen bruising.
- **Enoxaparin:** To avoid the loss of drug, do not expel the air bubble from the syringe before the injection.
- ❑ Per manufacturer's recommendations, to enhance absorption, only inject enoxaparin into left or right anterolateral or posterolateral abdominal wall.
- ❑ To minimize risk of bleeding after vascular instrumentation for unstable angina, recommended intervals between doses should be followed closely. Leave vascular access sheath in place for 6–8 hr after enoxaparin dose. Give next enoxaparin dose ≥6–8 hr

after sheath removal. Observe site for bleeding or hematoma formation.

■ **Fondaparinux:** Fondaparinux cannot be used interchangeably with heparin, low–molecular–weight heparins, or heparinoids as they differ in manufacturing process, anti-Xa and anti-IIa activity, units, and dosage. Each of these medications has its own instructions for use.

❑ Initial dose should be administered 6-8 hr after surgery. Administration before 6 hr after surgery has been associated with risk of major bleeding.

❑ Fondaparinux is provided in a single-dose prefilled syringe with an automatic needle protection system. Do not expel air bubble from prefilled syringe before injection to prevent loss of drug.

■ **Tinzaparin:** Tinzaparin should be administered daily for at least 6 days and until patient is adequately anticoagulated with warfarin (INR at least 2.0 for 2 consecutive days). Warfarin therapy should be started within 1–3 days of tinzaparin initiation.

❑ Solution is clear and colorless to slightly yellow; do not administer solutions that are discolored or contain particulate matter.

❑ Multiple dose vial contains benzyl alcohol; use with caution in pregnant women.

## PATIENT/FAMILY TEACHING

❑ Advise patient to report any symptoms of unusual bleeding or bruising, dizziness, itching, rash, fever, swelling, or difficulty breathing to health care professional immediately.

❑ Instruct patient not to take aspirin or NSAIDs without consulting health care professional while on therapy.

## EVALUATION

**Effectiveness of therapy can be demonstrated by:** ■ Prevention of DVT and pulmonary emboli ■ Treatment of DVT ■ Prevention of ischemic complications (with aspirin) in patients with unstable angina or non–Q-wave MI.

---

# HISTAMINE H₂ ANTAGONISTS

## cimetidine

(sye-**me**-ti-deen)

{Apo-Cimetidine}, {Novocimetine}, {Peptol}, Tagamet, Tagamet HB

## famotidine

(fa-**moe**-ti-deen)

Mylanta AR, Pepcid, Pepcid AC, Pepcid AC Acid Controller, {Pepcid RPD}

## nizatidine

(ni-**za**-ti-deen)

Axid, Axid AR

## ranitidine

(ra-**ni**-ti-deen)

Apo-Ranitidine, Zantac, {Zantac-C}, Zantac 75

## ranitidine bismuth citrate

(ra-**ni**-ti-deen**biss**-muth**sye**-trate)

Tritec

***CLASSIFICATION(S):***
***Therapeutic:*** *antiulcer agents*
***Pharmacologic:*** *histamine H2 antagonists*

**Pregnancy Category B, C (ranitidine bismuth citrate [with clarithromycin])**

---

## INDICATIONS

■ Short-term treatment of active duodenal ulcers and benign gastric ulcers ■ Prophylaxis of duodenal ulcers (at lower doses) ■ Management of GERD ■ Treatment and prevention of heartburn, acid indigestion, and sour stomach (OTC use) ■ **Cimetidine, famotidine, ranitidine:** Management of gastric hypersecretory states (Zollinger-Ellison syndrome) ■ **Cimetidine, famotidine, ranitidine IV:** Prevention and treatment of stress-induced upper GI bleeding in critically ill patients ■ **Ranitidine bismuth citrate:** With clarithromycin to eradicate *Helicobacter pylori* in the treatment of duodenal ulcers (should not be used alone to treat duodenal ulcers). **Unlabeled uses:** ■ Management of GI symptoms associated with the use of NSAIDs ■ Prevention of stress ulceration or aspiration pneumonitis ■ Prevention of acid inactivation of supplemental pancreatic enzymes in patients with pancreatic insufficiency ■ Management of urticaria.

## ACTION

■ Inhibits the action of histamine at the H$_2$-receptor site located primarily in gastric parietal cells, resulting in inhibition of gastric acid secretion ■ In addition, ranitidine bismuth citrate has some antibacterial action against *H. pylori*. **Therapeutic Effects:** ■ Healing and prevention of ulcers ■ Decreased symptoms of gastroesophageal reflux ■ Decreased secretion of gastric acid.

## PHARMACOKINETICS

**Absorption:** *Cimetidine*—well absorbed after oral and IM administration. *Famotidine*—40–45% absorbed after oral administration. *Nizatidine*—70–95% absorbed after oral administration. *Ranitidine*—50% absorbed after PO and IM administration. *Ranitidine bismuth citrate*—splits into ranitidine and bismuth in the GI tract; bismuth is not absorbed.

**Distribution:** All agents enter breast milk and cerebrospinal fluid.

**Metabolism and Excretion:** *Cimetidine*—30% metabolized by the liver; remainder is eliminated unchanged by the kidneys. *Famotidine*—up to 70% excreted unchanged by the kidneys, 30–35% metabolized by the liver. *Nizatidine*—60% excreted unchanged by the kidneys; some hepatic metabolism; at least 1 metabolite has histamine-blocking activity. *Ranitidine*—metabolized by the liver, mostly on first pass; 30% excreted unchanged by the kidneys after PO administration, 70–80% after parenteral administration.

**Half-life:** *Cimetidine*—2 hr; *famotidine*—2.5–3.5 hr; *nizatidine*—1.6 hr; *ranitidine*—1.7–3 hr (all are increased in renal impairment).

## CONTRAINDICATIONS AND PRECAUTIONS

**Contraindicated in:** ■ Hypersensitivity ■ Cross-sensitivity may occur ■ Some oral liquids contain alcohol and should be avoided in patients with known intolerance ■ Porphyria (ranitidine bismuth citrate only).

**Use Cautiously in:** ■ Renal impairment (more susceptible to adverse CNS reactions; increased dosage interval recommended for *cimetidine* if

renal impairment is severe, for *famotidine* if CCr <50 ml/min, for *nizatidine* if CCr <50 ml/min, and for *ranitidine* if CCr <50 ml/min; ranitidine bismuth citrate should not be used if CCr <25 ml/min) ■ Geriatric patients (more susceptible to adverse CNS reactions; dosage reduction recommended) ■ Pregnancy or lactation.

## ADVERSE REACTIONS AND SIDE EFFECTS*

■ **CNS:** <u>confusion</u>, dizziness, drowsiness, hallucinations, headache ■ **CV:** ARRHYTHMIAS ■ **GI:** altered taste, black tongue (ranitidine bismuth citrate only), constipation, dark stools (ranitidine bismuth citrate only), diarrhea, drug-induced hepatitis (nizatidine, cimetidine), nausea ■ **GU:** decreased sperm count, impotence ■ **Endo:** gynecomastia ■ **Hemat:** AGRANULOCYTOSIS, APLASTIC ANEMIA, anemia, neutropenia, thrombocytopenia ■ **Local:** pain at IM site ■ **Misc:** hypersensivity reactions, vaculitis.

## INTERACTIONS

**Drug-Drug:** ■ Cimetidine inhibits drug-metabolizing enzymes (cytochrome P450 pathway) in the liver; may lead to ↑ levels and toxicity with the following—some **benzodiazepines** (especially **chlordiazepoxide, diazepam,** and **midazolam**), some **beta blockers** (**labetalol, metoprolol, propranolol**), **caffeine, calcium channel blockers, carbamazepine, chloroquine, lidocaine, metronidazole, moricizine, pentoxifylline, phenytoin, propafenone, quinidine, quinine, metformin, sulfonylureas, tacrine theophylline, triamterene, tricyclic antidepressants, valproic acid,** and **warfarin.** ■ Famotidine, nizatidine, and ranitidine have a much smaller and less significant effect on the metabolism of other drugs ■ The effects of **succinylcholine, flecainide, procainamide, carmustine,** and **fluorouracil** are ↑ by cimetidine ■ All agents ↓ absorption of **ketoconazole** ■ **Antacids** and **sucralfate** ↓ absorption of all agents ■ **Clarithromycin** ↑ ranitidine levels.

## ROUTE AND DOSAGE

◘ **Cimetidine**

■ **PO (Adults):** *Short-term treatment of active ulcers*—300 mg 4 times daily *or* 800 mg at bedtime *or* 400–600 mg twice daily (not to exceed 2.4 g/day). *Duodenal ulcer prophylaxis*—300 mg twice daily *or* 400 mg at bedtime. *GERD*—800–1600 mg/day in divided doses. *Gastric hypersecretory conditions*—300–600 mg q 6 hr (up to 2400 mg/day). *OTC use*—up to 200 mg may be taken twice daily (not more than 2 wk) *or* 100 mg taken with a glass of water 0–30 min before food or beverages expected to cause symptoms.

■ **PO (Children):** *Short-term treatment of active ulcers*—20–40 mg/kg/day in 4 divided doses.

■ **IM, IV (Adults):** *Short-term treatment of active ulcers*—300 mg q 6 hr (not to exceed 2.4 g/day). *Continuous IV infusion*—900 mg infused over 24 hr (37.5 mg/hr); may be preceded by a 150-mg bolus dose. *Gastric hypersecretory conditions*—300–600 mg q 6 hr (up to 12 g/day have been used). *Prevention of aspiration pneumonitis*—300 mg IM 1 hr before anesthesia, then 300 mg IV q 4 hr until patient is conscious (unlabeled). *Prevention of upper GI bleeding in critically ill patients*—50 mg/hr.

■ **IM, IV (Children):** *Short-term treatment of active ulcers*—5–10 mg/kg q 6–8 hr.

❑ **Renal Impairment**

■ **IV, PO (Adults):** *Severely impaired renal function*—300 mg q 12 hr; *prevention of upper GI bleeding in critically ill patients if CCr <30 ml/min*—25 mg/hr.

■ **PO (Children):** 10–15 mg/kg/day.

❑ **Famotidine**

■ **PO (Adults):** *Short-term treatment of active ulcers*—40 mg/day at bedtime or 20 mg twice daily for up to 8 wk. *Duodenal ulcer prophylaxis*—20 mg once daily at bedtime. *GERD*—20 mg twice daily for up to 6 wk; up to 40 mg twice daily for up to 12 wk for esophagitis with erosions, ulcerations, and continuing symptoms. *Gastric hypersecretory conditions*—20 mg q 6 hr initially, up to 160 mg q 6 hr. *Prophylaxis of aspiration pneumonitis*—40 mg night before or morning of surgery (unlabeled). *OTC use*—10 mg for relief of symptoms; for prevention—10 mg 60 min before eating or take 10 mg as chewable tablet 15 minutes before heartburn-inducing foods or beverages (not to exceed 20 mg/24 hr for up to 2 wk).

■ **PO (Children 1–16 yr):** *Peptic ulcer*—0.5 mg/kg/day as a single bedtime dose or in divided doses twice daily (up to 40 mg daily); *GERD*—1—2 mg/kg/day in 2 divided doses for patients >10 kg or 3 divided doses for patients <10 kg (up to 40 mg twice daily).

■ **IV (Adults):** 20 mg q 12 hr.

❑ **Renal Impairment**

■ **PO (Adults):** *CCr <10 ml/min*—20 mg at bedtime or increase interval of usual dose to every 36–48 hr.

❑ **Nizatidine**

■ **PO (Adults):** *Short-term treatment of active ulcers*—300 mg once daily at bedtime or 150 mg twice daily. *Duodenal ulcer prophylaxis*—150 mg once daily at bedtime. *GERD*—150 mg twice daily. *OTC use*—75 mg 0–60 min before foods or beverages expected to cause symptoms.

❑ **Renal Impairment**

■ **PO (Adults):** *Short-term treatment of active ulcers*—*CCr 20–50 ml/min*—150 mg once daily; *CCr <20 ml/min*—150 mg every other day. *Duodenal ulcer prophylaxis*—*CCr 20–50 ml/min*—150 mg every other day; *CCr <20 ml/min*—150 mg every 3 days.

❑ **Ranitidine**

■ **PO (Adults):** *Short-term treatment of active ulcers*—150 mg twice daily *or* 300 mg once daily at bedtime. *Duodenal ulcer prophylaxis*—150 mg once daily at bedtime. *GERD*—150 mg twice daily. *Erosive esophagitis*—150 mg 4 times daily initially, then 150 mg twice daily as maintenance. *Gastric hypersecretory conditions*—150 mg twice daily initially; up to 6 g/day have been used. *OTC use*—75 mg when symptoms occur (up to twice daily).

■ **IV, IM (Adults):** 50 mg q 6–8 hr (not to exceed 400 mg/day). *Continuous IV infusion*—6.25 mg/hr. *Gastric hypersecretory conditions*—1 mg/kg/hr; may be increased by 0.5 mg/kg/hr (not to exceed 2.5 mg/kg/hr).

❑ **Renal Impairment**

■ **PO (Adults):** *CCr<50 ml/min*—150 mg q 24 hr; may be increased to 150 mg q 12 hr or more frequently if necessary; further reductions may be necessary if there is coexistent hepatic impairment.

### ❏ Ranitidine Bismuth Citrate

■ **PO (Adults):** 400 mg twice daily for 4 wk with clarithromycin 500 mg 3 times daily for first 2 wk.

## AVAILABILITY

### ❏ Cimetidine

■ *Tablets:* 100 mg$^{OTC}$, 200 mg$^{OTC}$, 300 mg$^{Rx}$, 400 mg$^{Rx}$, {600 mg$^{Rx}$}, 800 mg$^{Rx}$ ■ Cost: 200 mg $79.90/100, 300 mg $83.60/100, 400 mg $138.95/100, 800 mg $263.75/100 ■ *Oral liquid (mint-peach flavor):* 200 mg/5 ml$^{OTC}$, 300 mg/5 ml$^{Rx}$ ■ *Solution for injection:* 300 mg/2-ml vials$^{Rx}$, 300 mg/50 ml 0.9% NaCl$^{Rx}$.

### ❏ Famotidine

■ *Tablets:* 10 mg$^{OTC}$, 20 mg$^{Rx}$, 40 mg$^{Rx}$ ■ Cost: 10 mg $3.59/18, 20 mg $173.80/100, 40 mg $335.92/100 ■ *Orally disintegrating tablets (RPD) (mint flavor):* 20 mg$^{Rx}$, 40 mg$^{Rx}$ ■ *Chewable tablets with aspartame (mint flavor):* 10 mg$^{OTC}$ ■ *Oral suspension (cherry-banana-mint flavor):* 40 mg/5 ml$^{Rx}$ ■ *Solution for injection:* 10 mg/ml$^{Rx}$, 20 mg/50 ml 0.9% NaCl$^{Rx}$. ■ calcium carbonate and magnesium hydroxide$^{OTC}$ (Pepcid Complete, see Appendix B).

### ❏ Nizatidine

■ *Tablets:* 75 mg$^{OTC}$ ■ *Capsules:* 150 mg$^{Rx}$, 300 mg$^{Rx}$ ■ Cost: 150 mg $93.12/60, 300 mg $156.60/30.

### ❏ Ranitidine

■ *Tablets:* 75 mg$^{OTC}$, 150 mg$^{Rx}$, 300 mg$^{Rx}$ ■ Cost: 150 mg $113.90/60, 300 mg $103.39/30 ■ *Effervescent tablets (EFFERdose):* 75 mg$^{OTC}$, 150 mg$^{Rx}$ ■ *Effervescent granules (EFFERdose):* 150 mg/packet$^{Rx}$ ■ *Capsules (GELdose):* 150 mg$^{Rx}$, 300 mg$^{Rx}$ ■ *Syrup (peppermint flavor):* 15 mg/ml$^{Rx}$ ■ *Solution for injection:* 25 mg/ml in 2-, 10-, and 40-ml vials$^{Rx}$, 50 mg/100-ml containers$^{Rx}$.

### ❏ Ranitidine Bismuth Citrate

■ *Tablets:* 400 mg$^{Rx}$.

## TIME/ACTION PROFILE

| | ONSET | PEAK | DURATION |
|---|---|---|---|
| Cimetidine PO | 30 min | 45–90 min | 4–5 hr |
| Cimetidine IM, IV | 10 min | 30 min | 4–5 hr |
| Famotidine PO | within 60 min | 1–4 hr | 6–12 hr |
| Famotidine IV | within 60 min | 0.5–3 hr | 8–15 hr |
| Nizatidine PO | unknown | unknown | 8–12 hr |
| Ranitidine PO | unknown | 1–3 hr | 8–12 hr |
| Ranitidine IM | unknown | 15 min | 8–12 hr |
| Ranitidine IV | unknown | 15 min | 8–12 hr |

# NURSING IMPLICATIONS

## ASSESSMENT

❏ Assess patient for epigastric or abdominal pain and frank or occult blood in the stool, emesis, or gastric aspirate.

❏ Assess geriatric and debilitated patients routinely for confusion. Report promptly.

■ *Lab Test Considerations:* Monitor CBC with differential periodically throughout therapy.

❏ Antagonize effects of pentagastrin and histamine during gastric acid secretion testing. Avoid administration for 24 hr before the test.

❏ May cause false-negative results in skin tests using allergenic extracts. Histamine H₂ antagonists should be discontinued 24 hr before the test.

❏ May cause an increase in serum transaminases and serum creatinine.

❏ Serum prolactin concentration may be increased after IV bolus of *cimetidine*. May also cause decreased parathyroid concentrations.

❏ *Nizatidine* may cause elevated alkaline phosphatase concentrations or false-positive tests for urobilinogen.

❏ *Ranitidine* may cause false-positive results for urine protein; test with sulfosalicylic acid.

## POTENTIAL NURSING DIAGNOSES

■ Pain, acute (Indications).

## IMPLEMENTATION

- **General:** If antacids or sucralfate are used concurrently for relief of pain, avoid administration of antacids within 30 min–1 hr of the histamine H$_2$ antagonist and take sucralfate 2 hr after histamine H$_2$ antagonist; may decrease the absorption of histamine H$_2$ antagonists.
- **PO:** Administer with meals or immediately afterward and at bedtime to prolong effect.
- Doses administered once daily should be administered at bedtime to prolong effect.
- Cimetidine tablets have a characteristic odor.
- Shake oral suspension before administration. Discard unused suspension after 30 days.
- Remove foil from *ranitidine effervescent tablets or granules* and dissolve in 6–8 oz water before drinking.

### Cimetidine

- **Direct IV:** Dilute each 300 mg in 20 ml of 0.9% NaCl for injection.
- ***Rate:*** Administer over at least 5 min. Rapid administration may cause hypotension and arrhythmias.
- **Intermittent Infusion:** Dilute each 300 mg in 50 ml of 0.9% NaCl, D5W, D10W, D5/LR, D5/0.9% NaCl, D5/0.45% NaCl, D5/0.25% NaCl, Ringer's or LR, or sodium bicarbonate. Diluted solution is stable for 48 hr at room temperature. Refrigeration may cause cloudiness but will not affect potency. Do not use solution that is discolored or contains precipitate.
- ***Rate:*** Administer over 15–20 min.
- **Continuous Infusion:** Dilute cimetidine 900 mg in 100–1000 ml of compatible solution (see Intermittent Infusion).
- ***Rate:*** Usually infused at a rate of 37.5 mg/hr or greater but should be individualized.
- **Syringe Compatibility:** ◆ atropine ◆ butorphanol ◆ diazepam ◆ diphenhydramine ◆ doxapram ◆ droperidol ◆ fentanyl ◆ glycopyrrolate ◆ heparin ◆ hydromorphone ◆ hydroxyzine ◆ lorazepam ◆ meperidine ◆ midazolam ◆ morphine ◆ nafcillin ◆ nalbuphine ◆ penicillin G sodium ◆ pentazocine ◆ perphenazine ◆ prochlorperazine ◆ prochlorperazine edisylate ◆ promethazine ◆ scopolamine ◆ sodium

acetate ◆ sodium chloride ◆ sodium lactate ◆ sterile water.

- **Y-Site Compatibility:** ◆ acyclovir ◆ amifostine ◆ aminophylline ◆ atracurium ◆ aztreonam ◆ cisatracurium ◆ cisplatin ◆ cladribine ◆ cyclophosphamide ◆ cytarabine ◆ diltiazem ◆ docetaxel ◆ doxorubicin ◆ doxorubicin liposome ◆ enalaprilat ◆ esmolol ◆ etoposide phosphate ◆ filgrastim ◆ fluconazole ◆ fludarabine ◆ foscarnet ◆ gatifloxacin ◆ gemcitabine ◆ granisetron ◆ haloperidol ◆ heparin ◆ idarubicin ◆ inamrinone ◆ labetalol ◆ levofloxacin ◆ linezolid ◆ melphalan ◆ meropenem ◆ methotrexate ◆ midazolam ◆ milrinone ◆ ondansetron ◆ paclitaxel ◆ pancuronium ◆ piperacillin/tazobactam ◆ propofol ◆ remifentanil ◆ sargramostim ◆ tacrolimus ◆ teniposide ◆ theophylline ◆ thiotepa ◆ tolazoline ◆ topotecan ◆ vecuronium ◆ vinorelbine ◆ zidovudine.
- **Y-Site Incompatibility:** ◆ allopurinol ◆ amphotericin B cholesteryl sulfate ◆ cefepime ◆ indomethacin ◆ warfarin.

### Famotidine

- **Direct IV:** Dilute 2 ml (10 mg/ml solution) in 5 or 10 ml of 0.9% NaCl for injection.
- ***Rate:*** Administer over at least 2 min. Rapid administration may cause hypotension.
- **Intermittent Infusion:** Dilute each 20 mg in 100 ml of 0.9% NaCl, D5W, D10W, or LR for a concentration of 0.2 mg/ml. Diluted solution is stable for 48 hr at room temperature. Do not use solution that is discolored or contains a precipitate.
- ***Rate:*** Administer over 15–30 min.
- **Y-Site Compatibility:** ◆ acyclovir ◆ allopurinol ◆ amifostine ◆ aminophylline ◆ ampicillin ◆ ampicillin/sulbactam ◆ atropine ◆ aztreonam ◆ bretylium ◆ calcium gluconate ◆ cefazolin ◆ cefoperazone ◆ cefotaxime ◆ cefotetan ◆ cefoxitin ◆ ceftazidime ◆ ceftizoxime ◆ ceftriaxone ◆ cefuroxime ◆ chlorpromazine ◆ cisatracurium ◆ cisplatin ◆ cyclophosphamide ◆ cytarabine ◆ dextran 40 ◆ digoxin ◆ dobutamine ◆ docetaxel ◆ dopamine ◆ doxorubicin ◆ doxorubicin liposome ◆ droperidol ◆ enalaprilat ◆ epinephrine ◆ erythromycin lactobionate ◆ esmolol ◆ filgrastim ◆ fluconazole ◆ fludarabine ◆ folic acid ◆ gatifloxacin ◆ gemcitabine ◆ gentamicin ◆ granisetron ◆ haloperidol ◆ heparin ◆ hydrocortisone sodium

succinate ◆ hydromorphone ◆ inamrinone ◆ imipenem/cilastatin ◆ inamrinone ◆ insulin ◆ isoproterenol ◆ labetalol ◆ lidocaine ◆ linezolid ◆ lorazepam ◆ magnesium sulfate ◆ melphalan ◆ meperidine ◆ methylprednisolone ◆ metoclopramide ◆ midazolam ◆ morphine ◆ nafcillin ◆ nitroglycerin ◆ nitroprusside ◆ norepinephrine ◆ ondansetron ◆ oxacillin ◆ paclitaxel ◆ perphenazine ◆ phenylephrine ◆ phenytoin ◆ phytonadione ◆ piperacillin ◆ potassium chloride ◆ potassium phosphate ◆ procainamide ◆ propofol ◆ remifentanil ◆ sargramostim ◆ sodium bicarbonate ◆ teniposide ◆ theophylline ◆ thiamine ◆ thiotepa ◆ ticarcillin ◆ ticarcillin/clavulanate ◆ tirofiban ◆ verapamil ◆ vinorelbine.

■ **Y-Site Incompatibility:** ◆ alatrofloxacin ◆ amphotericin B cholesteryl sulfate ◆ cefepime ◆ piperacillin/tazobactam.

❑ **Ranitidine**

■ **Direct IV:** Dilute each 50 mg in 20 ml of 0.9% NaCl or D5W for injection.

■ **Rate:** Administer over at least 5 min. Rapid administration may cause hypotension and arrhythmias.

■ **Intermittent Infusion:** Dilute each 50 mg in 100 ml of 0.9% NaCl or D5W. Diluted solution is stable for 48 hr at room temperature. Do not use solution that is discolored or that contains precipitate.

■ **Rate:** Administer over 15–20 min.

■ **Continuous Infusion:** Add ranitidine to D5W for a concentration of 150 mg/250 ml (no greater than 2.5 mg/ml for Zollinger-Ellison patients).

■ **Rate:** Administer at a rate of 6.25 mg/hr. In patients with Zollinger-Ellison syndrome, start infusion at 1 mg/kg/hr. If gastric acid output is >10 mEq/hr or patient becomes symptomatic after 4 hr, adjust dose by 0.5 mg/kg/hr increments and remeasure gastric output.

■ **Syringe Compatibility:** ◆ atropine ◆ cyclizine ◆ dimenhydrinate ◆ diphenhydramine ◆ fentanyl ◆ glycopyrrolate ◆ hydromorphone ◆ meperidine ◆ metoclopramide ◆ morphine ◆ nalbuphine ◆ oxymorphone ◆ pentazocine ◆ perphenazine ◆ prochlorperazine ◆ promethazine ◆ scopolamine ◆ thiethylperazine.

■ **Syringe Incompatibility:** ◆ hydroxyzine ◆ methotrimeprazine ◆ midazolam ◆ pentobarbital ◆ phenobarbital.

■ **Y-Site Compatibility:** ◆ acyclovir ◆ aldesleukin ◆ amifostine ◆ aminophylline ◆ atracurium ◆ aztreonam ◆ bretylium ◆ cefepime ◆ cefoperazone ◆ cefoxitin ◆ ceftazidime ◆ ceftizoxime ◆ ciprofloxacin ◆ cisatracurium ◆ cisplatin ◆ cyclophosphamide ◆ cytarabine ◆ diltiazem ◆ dobutamine ◆ docetaxel ◆ dopamine ◆ doxorubicin ◆ doxorubicin liposome ◆ enalaprilat ◆ epinephrine ◆ esmolol ◆ etoposide phosphate ◆ fentanyl ◆ filgrastim ◆ fluconazole ◆ fludarabine ◆ foscarnet ◆ furosemide ◆ gatifloxacin ◆ gemcitabine ◆ granisetron ◆ heparin ◆ hydromorphone ◆ idarubicin ◆ labetalol ◆ linezolid ◆ lorazepam ◆ melphalan ◆ meperidine ◆ methotrexate ◆ midazolam ◆ milrinone ◆ morphine ◆ nitroglycerin ◆ norepinephrine ◆ ondansetron ◆ paclitaxel ◆ pancuronium ◆ piperacillin ◆ piperacillin/tazobactam ◆ procainamide ◆ remifentanil ◆ sargramostim ◆ tacrolimus ◆ teniposide ◆ theophylline ◆ thiopental ◆ thiotepa ◆ vecuronium ◆ vinorelbine ◆ warfarin ◆ zidovudine.

■ **Y-Site Incompatibility:** ◆ amphotericin B cholesteryl sulfate ◆ insulin

■ **Additive Compatibility:** ◆ amikacin ◆ amphotericin B cholesteryl sulfate ◆ chloramphenicol ◆ doxycycline ◆ furosemide ◆ gentamicin ◆ heparin ◆ insulin, regular ◆ lidocaine ◆ penicillin G sodium ◆ potassium chloride ◆ ticarcillin ◆ tobramycin ◆ vancomycin.

■ **Additive Incompatibility:** ◆ amphotericin B.

## PATIENT/FAMILY TEACHING

■ **General Info:** Instruct patient to take medication as directed for the full course of therapy, even if feeling better. Take missed doses as soon as remembered but not if almost time for next dose. Do not double doses.

❑ Advise patients taking OTC preparations not to take the maximum dose continuously for more than 2 wk without consulting health care professional. Notify health care professional if difficulty swallowing occurs or abdominal pain persists.

❑ Inform patient that smoking interferes with the action of histamine antagonists. Encourage patient to quit smoking or at least not to smoke after last dose of the day.

❑ May cause drowsiness or dizziness. Caution patient to avoid driving or other activities requiring alertness until response to the drug is known.

❑ Advise patient to avoid alcohol, products containing aspirin or NSAIDs, and foods that may cause an increase in GI irritation.

❑ Inform patient that increased fluid and fiber intake and exercise may minimize constipation.

❑ Advise patient to report onset of black, tarry stools; fever; sore throat; diarrhea; dizziness; rash; confusion; or hallucinations to health care professional promptly.

■ **Ranitidine Bismuth Citrate:** Inform patient that medication may temporarily cause stools and tongue to appear gray-black.

## EVALUATION

**Effectiveness of therapy can be demonstrated by:** ■ Decrease in abdominal pain ■ Prevention and treatment of gastric irritation and bleeding. Healing of duodenal ulcers can be seen by x-rays or endoscopy. Therapy is continued for at least 6 wk in treatment of ulcers but not usually longer than 8 wk ■ Decreased symptoms of esophageal reflux ■ Treatment of heartburn, acid indigestion, and sour stomach (OTC use) ■ Eradication of *H. pylori* in the treatment of duodenal ulcers (ranitidine and bismuth citrate only with anti-infectives).

## HMG-CoA REDUCTASE INHIBITORS

### atorvastatin
(a-**tore**-va-stat-in)
Lipitor

### fluvastatin
(**floo**-va-sta-tin)
Lescol

### lovastatin
(**loe**-va-sta-tin)
Altocor, Mevacor

### pravastatin
(**pra**-va-sta-tin)
Pravachol

### rosuvastatin
(roe-**soo**-va-sta-tin)
Crestor

### simvastatin
(**sim**-va-sta-tin)
Zocor

### CLASSIFICATION(S):
*Therapeutic: lipid-lowering agents*
*Pharmacologic: HMG-CoA reductase inhibitors*

### Pregnancy Category X

## INDICATIONS

■ Adjunct to dietary therapy in the management of primary hypercholesterolemia and mixed dyslipidemias ■ Reduction of lipids/cholesterol reduces the risk of MI and stroke sequelae (primary prevention and secondary prevention) and decreases the need for bypass procedures/angioplasty.

## ACTION

■ Inhibit an enzyme, 3-hydroxy-3-methylglutaryl-coenzyme A (HMG-CoA) reductase, which is responsible for catalyzing an early step in the synthesis of cholesterol. **Therapeutic Effects:** ■ Lowering of total and LDL cholesterol. Increase HDL and decrease VLDL cholesterol and triglycerides ■ Slowing of the progression of coronary artery disease with resultant decrease in MI/stroke and need for myocardial revascularization.

## PHARMACOKINETICS

**Absorption:** *Atorvastatin*—rapidly absorbed but undergoes extensive GI and hepatic metabolism, resulting in 14% bioavailability (30% for lipid-lowering activity); *fluvastatin*—98% absorbed after oral administration; *lovastatin, pravastatin*—poorly and variably absorbed after oral administration; *rosuvastatin*—20% absorbed following oral administration; *simvastatin*—85% absorbed but rapidly metabolized.

**Distribution:** *Atorvastatin*—probably enters breast milk. *Fluvastatin*—enters breast milk.

*Lovastatin*—crosses the blood-brain barrier and placenta. *Pravastatin*—enters hepatocytes, where action occurs; small amounts enter breast milk.

**Metabolism and Excretion:** All agents are extensively metabolized by the liver *atorvastatin, lovastatin* and *simvastatin* are metabolized by CYP3A4, most during first pass; excreted in bile and feces. Small amounts (*atorvastatin*—<2%; *fluvastatin*—5%; *pravastatin*—20%; *lovastatin*—10%; *rosuvastatin*—10% metabolized, 90% excreted in feces; *simvastatin*—13%) excreted unchanged by the kidneys. *Atorvastatin*—has 2 lipid-lowering metabolites.

**Half-life:** *Atorvastatin*—14 hr (lipid-lowering activity due to atorvastatin and its metabolites—20–30 hr); *fluvastatin*—1.2 hr; *lovastatin*—3 hr; *pravastatin*—1.3–2.7 hr; *rosuvastatin*—19 hr; *simvastatin*—unknown.

## CONTRAINDICATIONS AND PRECAUTIONS

**Contraindicated in:** ■ Hypersensitivity ■ Cross-sensitivity among agents may occur ■ Sepsis, acute hypotension, major surgery, trauma, severe metabolic disturbances, endocrine or electrolyte disorders, uncontrolled seizures ( ↑ risk of rhabdomyolysis; temporarily discontinue use until condition is resolved) ■ Active liver disease ■ Pregnancy or lactation ■ Concurrent use of gemfibrozil or azole antifungals

**Use Cautiously in:** ■ History of liver disease or significant alcohol use/abuse ■ *Rosuvastatin only*—patients with Asian ancestry (may have ↑ blood levels) ■ Renal impairment, advanced age or hypothyroidism ( ↑ risk of rhabdomyolysis) ■ Visual disturbances ■ Myopathy ■ Women of childbearing age ■ Children <8 yr (safety not established; some products approved for use in adults only).

## ADVERSE REACTIONS AND SIDE EFFECTS*

■ **CNS:** dizziness, headache, insomnia, weakness ■ **EENT:** rhinitis; *lovastatin*—blurred vision ■ **Resp:** bronchitis ■ **GI:** <u>abdominal cramps</u>, <u>constipation</u>, <u>diarrhea</u>, <u>flatus</u>, <u>heartburn</u>, altered taste, drug-induced hepatitis, dyspepsia, elevated liver enzymes, nausea, pancreatitis ■ **GU:** impotence ■ **Derm:** <u>rashes</u>, pruritus ■ **MS:** RHABDOMYOLYSIS, arthralgia, arthritis, myalgia, myositis ■ **Misc:** hypersensitivity reactions.

## INTERACTIONS

**Drug-Drug:** ■ Atorvastatin, lovastatin and simvastatin may interact with **CYP3A4 inhibitors** ■ Cholesterol-lowering effect may be ↑ with **bile acid sequestrants** ■ Bioavailability and effectiveness may be ↓ by **bile acid sequestrants** ■ Blood levels and the risk of myopathy are ↑ with **amiodarone, cyclosporine** and **gemfibrozil, clofibrate, erythromycin,** large doses of **niacin azole antifungal agents** and **ritonavir** (combined use with **clofibrate** or **gemfibrozil** contraindicated; temporary discontinuation recommended during azole antifungal therapy for all except rosuvastatin) ■ Atorvastatin and fluvastatin may slightly ↑ serum **digoxin** levels ■ Atorvastatin and rosuvastatin may ↑ levels of **hormonal contraceptives** ■ May increase effects of **warfarin** ■ **Rifampin** ↑ metabolism and may ↓ blood levels and effects of fluvastatin ■ **Isradipine** may ↓ the effectiveness of lovastatin ■ **Propranolol** ↓ blood levels of simvastatin ■ **Alcohol, cimetidine, ranitidine,** and **omeprazole** may ↑ fluvastatin levels ■ **Saquinavir** may ↑ blood levels and effects of atorvastatin, lovastatin and simvastatin ■ **Amprenavir** ↑ atrovastatin levels (consider fluvastatin, rosuvastatin or pravastatin) ■ **Antacids** ↓ absorption of rosuvastatin(administer 2 hr after rosuvastatin ■ **Cyclosporine** and **Gemfibrozil** ↑ levels and risk of toxicity of rosuvastatin(dosage adjustment required).

**Drug-Food:** ■ **Grapefruit juice** ↑ blood levels and increases risk of toxicity (for all except rosuvastatin) ■ **Food** enhances blood levels of lovastatin.

## ROUTE AND DOSAGE

❑ **Atorvastatin**
■ **PO (Adults):** 10—20 mg once daily initially (may start with 40 mg/day if LDL-C should be lowered by >45%); may be increased q 2–4 wk up to 80 mg/day.

❑ **Fluvastatin**
■ **PO (Adults):** 20 mg once daily at bedtime; may be increased to 40 mg once daily or 20 mg twice daily.

❑ **Lovastatin**
■ **PO (Adults):** *Immediate-release tablets*—20 mg once daily with evening meal. Increase at 4-wk intervals to a maximum of 80 mg/day in single or divided doses; *Extended–release tablets*—10-60 mg/day as a

single dose at bedtime. Dose should not exceed 20 mg/day if also receiving fibrates, cyclosporine or niacin.

■ **PO (Children /Adolescents 10-17 yr):** *Familial heterozygous hypercholesterolemia*—10-40 mg/day

❑ **Pravastatin**

■ **PO (Adults):** 10–40 mg once daily.

■ **PO (Children 14-18 yrs):** 40 mg once daily.

■ **PO (Children 8-13 yrs):** 20 mg once daily.

❑ **Rosuvastatin**

■ **PO (Adults):** 10 mg once daily initially (range 5–20 mg); dose may be adjusted at 2–4 wk intervals, some patients may require up to 40 mg/day; *concurrent cyclosporine therapy*—not to exceed 5 mg once daily; *concurrent gemfibrozil therapy*—not to exceed 10 mg once daily

❑ **Renal Impairment**

■ **PO (Adults):** *CCr <30 ml/min*—5 mg once daily intially, may be increased to but not exceed 10 mg/day.

❑ **Simvastatin**

■ **PO (Adults):** 5–10 mg once daily in the evening. *Geriatric patients, patients with LDL <190 mg/dl, or patients receiving cyclosporine*—5 mg/day initially. Increase at 4-wk intervals (not to exceed 10 mg/day in patients receiving cyclosporine) up to 40 mg/day.

## AVAILABILITY

❑ **Atorvastatin**

■ *Tablets:* 10 mg$^{Rx}$, 20 mg$^{Rx}$, 40 mg$^{Rx}$, 80 mg$^{Rx}$ ■ Cost: 10 mg $207.84/90, 20 mg $303.60/90, 40 mg $327.93/30, 80 mg $327.93/30.

❑ **Fluvastatin**

■ *Capsules:* 20 mg$^{Rx}$, 40 mg$^{Rx}$ ■ Cost: 20 mg $44.39/30, 40 mg $44.39/30.

❑ **Lovastatin**

■ *Immediate-release tablets:* 10 mg$^{Rx}$, 20 mg$^{Rx}$, 40 mg$^{Rx}$ ■ Cost: 10 mg $89.70/60, 20 mg $158.19/60, 40 mg $284.76/60 ■ *Extended-*

*release tablets:* 10 mg$^{Rx}$, 20 mg$^{Rx}$, 40 mg$^{Rx}$, 60 mg$^{Rx}$ ■ Niacin (Advicor).$^{Rx}$ See Appendix B.

❑ **Rosuvastatin**

■ *Tablets:* 5 mg$^{Rx}$, 10 mg$^{Rx}$, 20 mg$^{Rx}$, 40 mg$^{Rx}$.

❑ **Pravastatin**

■ *Tablets:* 10 mg$^{Rx}$, 20 mg$^{Rx}$, 40 mg$^{Rx}$, 80 mg$^{Rx}$ ■ Cost: 10 mg $250.30/90, 20 mg $250.30/90, 40 mg $391.19/90, 80 mg $419.88/90.

❑ **Simvastatin**

■ *Tablets:* 5 mg$^{Rx}$, 10 mg$^{Rx}$, 20 mg$^{Rx}$, 40 mg$^{Rx}$, 80 mg$^{Rx}$ ■ Cost: 5 mg $106.84/60, 10 mg $151.64/60, 20 mg $249.80/60, 40 mg $249.80/60, 80 mg $249.80/60.

TIME/ACTION PROFILE (cholesterol-lowering effect)

| | ONSET | PEAK | DURATION |
|---|---|---|---|
| Atorvastatin | unknown | unknown | 20–30 hr |
| Fluvastatin | 1–2 wk | 4–6 wk | unknown |
| Lovastatin | 2 wk | 4–6 wk | 6 wk* |
| Pravastatin | unknown | unknown | unknown |
| Rosuvastatin | unknown | 2–4 wk | unknown |
| Simvastatin | unknown | unknown | unknown |

*After discontinuation.

## NURSING IMPLICATIONS

### ASSESSMENT

❑ Obtain a dietary history, especially with regard to fat consumption.

❑ Ophthalmic exams are recommended before and yearly during therapy.

■ *Lab Test Considerations:* Evaluate serum cholesterol and triglyceride levels before initiating, after 4–6 wk of therapy, and periodically thereafter.

❑ Monitor liver function tests, including AST, before, at 6–12 wk after initiation of therapy or after dose elevation, and then every 6 mo. If AST levels ↑ to 3 times normal, HMG-CoA reductase inhibitor therapy should be discontinued. May also cause ↑ alkaline phosphatase and bilirubin levels.

❑ If patient develops muscle tenderness during therapy, monitor CPK levels. If CPK levels are markedly ↑ or myopathy occurs, therapy should be discontinued.

▫ May cause thyroid function test abnormalities.

## POTENTIAL NURSING DIAGNOSES

■ Noncompliance (Patient/Family Teaching).

## IMPLEMENTATION

■ **General:** Do not confuse Pravachol (pravastatin) with Prevacid (lansoprazole).

■ **PO:** Administer *lovastatin* with food. Administration on an empty stomach decreases absorption by approximately 30%. Initial once-daily dose is administered with the evening meal. Administer extended-release tablets at bedtime. Extended-release tablets should be swallowed whole, do not crush, break, or chew.

▫ Administer *fluvastatin, pravastatin,* and *simvastatin* once daily in the evening. May be administered without regard to food.

▫ If *fluvastatin,* or *pravastatin* is administered in conjunction with bile acid sequestrants (cholestyramine, colestipol), administer 1 hr before or at least 2 hr *(fluvastatin)* or 4 hr *(pravastatin)* after bile acid sequestrant.

## PATIENT/FAMILY TEACHING

▫ Instruct patient to take medication as directed and not to skip doses or double up on missed doses. Medication helps control but does not cure elevated serum cholesterol levels.

▫ Advise patient that this medication should be used in conjunction with diet restrictions (fat, cholesterol, carbohydrates, alcohol), exercise, and cessation of smoking.

▫ Instruct patient to notify health care professional if unexplained muscle pain, tenderness, or weakness occurs, especially if accompanied by fever or malaise.

▫ Advise patient to wear sunscreen and protective clothing to prevent photosensitivity reactions (rare).

▫ Instruct female patients to notify health care professional promptly if pregnancy is planned or suspected.

▫ Advise patient to notify health care professional of medication regimen before treatment or surgery.

▫ Emphasize the importance of follow-up exams to determine effectiveness and to monitor for side effects.

## EVALUATION

**Effectiveness of therapy can be demonstrated by:** ■ Decrease in serum LDL, VLDL, and total cholesterol levels ▫ Increase in HDL cholesterol levels ▫ Decrease in triglyceride levels ■ Slowing of the progression of coronary artery disease.

# hydralazine

(hye-**dral**-a-zeen)

Apresoline, {Novo-Hylazin}

*CLASSIFICATION(S):*

*Therapeutic: antihypertensives*

*Pharmacologic: vasodilators*

**Pregnancy Category C**

## INDICATIONS

■ Moderate to severe hypertension (with a diuretic). **Unlabeled uses:** ■ CHF unresponsive to conventional therapy with digoxin and diuretics.

## ACTION

■ Direct-acting peripheral arteriolar vasodilator. **Therapeutic Effects:** ■ Lowering of blood pressure in hypertensive patients and decreased afterload in patients with CHF.

## PHARMACOKINETICS

**Absorption:** Rapidly absorbed following oral administration; well absorbed from IM sites.

**Distribution:** Widely distributed. Crosses the placenta; enters breast milk in minimal concentrations.

**Metabolism and Excretion:** Mostly metabolized by the GI mucosa and liver.

**Half-life:** 2–8 hr.

## CONTRAINDICATIONS AND PRECAUTIONS

**Contraindicated in:** ■ Hypersensitivity ■ Some products contain tartrazine and should be avoided in patients with known intolerance.

**Use Cautiously in:** ■ Cardiovascular or cerebrovascular disease ■ Severe renal and hepatic disease ■ Pregnancy, lactation, or children (has been used safely during pregnancy).

## ADVERSE REACTIONS AND SIDE EFFECTS*

■ **CNS:** dizziness, drowsiness, headache ■ **CV:** tachycardia, angina, arrhythmias, edema, orthostatic hypotension ■ **GI:** diarrhea, nausea, vomiting ■ **Derm:** rashes ■ **F and E:** sodium retention ■ **MS:** arthralgias, arthritis ■ **Neuro:** peripheral neuropathy ■ **Misc:** drug-induced lupus syndrome.

## INTERACTIONS

**Drug-Drug:** ■ Additive hypotension with acute ingestion of **alcohol**, other **antihypertensives**, or **nitrates** ■ **MAO inhibitors** may exaggerate hypotension ■ May reduce the pressor response to **epinephrine** ■ **NSAIDs** may decrease antihypertensive response ■ **Beta blockers** decrease tachycardia from hydralazine (therapy may be combined for this reason) ■ **Metoprolol** and **propranolol** increase hydralazine levels ■ Increases blood levels of **metoprolol** and **propranolol**.

## ROUTE AND DOSAGE

■ **PO (Adults):** *Hypertension*—10 mg 4 times daily initially. After 2–4 days may increase to 25 mg 4 times daily for the rest of the 1st week; may then increase to 50 mg 4 times daily (up to 300 mg/day). Once maintenance dose is established, twice-daily dosing may be used. *CHF*—25–37.5 mg 4 times daily; may be increased up to 300 mg/day in 3–4 divided doses.

■ **PO (Children):** 0.75 mg/kg/day in 4 divided doses; may increase gradually to 7.5 mg/kg/day (200 mg/day) in 4 divided doses.

■ **IM, IV (Adults):** *Hypertension*—5–40 mg repeated as needed. *Eclampsia*—5 mg q 15–20 min; if no response after a total of 20 mg, consider an alternative agent.

■ **IM, IV (Children):** 1.7–3.5 mg/kg/day in 4–6 divided doses.

## AVAILABILITY (generic available)

■ *Tablets:* 10 mg^Rx, 25 mg^Rx, 50 mg^Rx, 100 mg^Rx ■ Cost: *Apresoline*—10 mg $29.84/100, 25 mg $39.84/100, 50 mg $68.22/100, 100 mg $83.84/100; *generic*—10 mg $3.43/100, 25

mg $5.92/100, 50 mg $7.24/100, 100 mg $8.51/100 ■ *Injection:* 20 mg/ml^Rx ■ hydrochlorothiazide and Reserpine^Rx. See Appendix B.

TIME/ACTION PROFILE (antihypertensive effect)

| | ONSET | PEAK | DURATION |
|---|---|---|---|
| PO | 45 min | 2 hr | 3–8 hr |
| IM | 10–30 min | 1 hr | 3–8 hr |
| IV | 10–20 min | 15–30 min | 3–8 hr |

# NURSING IMPLICATIONS

## ASSESSMENT

❑ Monitor blood pressure and pulse frequently during initial dosage adjustment and periodically throughout therapy. Report significant changes.

❑ Monitor frequency of prescription refills to determine adherence.

■ *Lab Test Considerations:* CBC, electrolytes, LE cell prep, and ANA titer should be monitored prior to and periodically during prolonged therapy.

❑ May cause a positive direct Coombs' test result.

## POTENTIAL NURSING DIAGNOSES

■ Tissue perfusion, ineffective (Indications).
■ Noncompliance (Patient/Family Teaching).

## IMPLEMENTATION

■ **General:** Do not confuse hydralazine with hydroxyzine.

❑ IM or IV route should be used only when drug cannot be given orally.

❑ May be administered concurrently with diuretics or beta blockers to permit lower doses and minimize side effects.

■ **PO:** Administer with meals consistently to enhance absorption.

❑ Pharmacist may prepare oral solution from hydralazine injection for patients with difficulty swallowing.

■ **Direct IV:** Administer undiluted. Use solution as quickly as possible after drawing through needle into syringe. Hydralazine changes color after contact with a metal filter.

{ } = Available in Canada only.
*CAPITALS indicates life-threatening; underlines indicate most frequent.

■ *Rate:* Administer at a rate of 10 mg over at least 1 min. Monitor blood pressure and pulse frequently after injection.

■ **Y-Site Compatibility:** ◆ heparin ◆ hydrocortisone sodium succinate ◆ potassium chloride ◆ verapamil ◆ vitamin B complex with C.

■ **Y-Site Incompatibility:** ◆ aminophylline ◆ ampicillin ◆ diazoxide ◆ furosemide.

■ **Solution Compatibility:** ◆ dextrose/saline combinations ◆ dextrose/Ringer's solution combinations ◆ D5/LR ◆ D5W ◆ D10W ◆ D10/LR ◆ 0.45% NaCl ◆ 0.9% NaCl ◆ Ringer's or LR.

## PATIENT/FAMILY TEACHING

❑ Emphasize the importance of continuing to take this medication, even if feeling well. Instruct patient to take medication at the same time each day; last dose of the day should be taken at bedtime. If a dose is missed, take as soon as remembered; do not double doses. If more than 2 doses in a row are missed, consult health care professional. Must be discontinued gradually to avoid sudden increase in blood pressure. Hydralazine controls but does not cure hypertension.

❑ Encourage patient to comply with additional interventions for hypertension (weight reduction, low-sodium diet, smoking cessation, moderation of alcohol intake, regular exercise, and stress management). Instruct patient and family on proper technique for blood pressure monitoring. Advise them to check blood pressure at least weekly and report significant changes.

❑ Patients should weigh themselves twice weekly and assess feet and ankles for fluid retention.

❑ May occasionally cause drowsiness. Advise patient to avoid driving or other activities requiring alertness until response to medication is known.

❑ Caution patient to avoid sudden changes in position to minimize orthostatic hypotension.

❑ Advise patient to consult health care professional before taking any cough, cold, or allergy remedies.

❑ Instruct patient to notify health care professional of medication prior to treatment or surgery.

❑ Advise patient to notify health care professional immediately if general tiredness; fever; muscle or joint aching; chest pain; skin rash;

sore throat; or numbness, tingling, pain, or weakness of hands and feet occurs. Vitamin B (pyridoxine) may be used to treat peripheral neuritis.

❑ Emphasize the importance of follow-up exams to evaluate effectiveness of medication.

## EVALUATION

**Effectiveness of therapy can be demonstrated by:** ■ Decrease in blood pressure without appearance of side effects ■ Decreased afterload in patients with CHF.

# hydrochlorothiazide, See DIURETICS (THIAZIDE).

High Alert

# hydrocodone
(hye-droe-**koe**-done)
Hycodan, {Robidone}, Tussigon (U.S. antitussive formulations contain homatropine)

### hydrocodone/acetaminophen
Anexsia, Bancap HC, Ceta-Plus, Co-Gesic, Dolacet, Duocet, Hydrocet, Hydrogesic, Hy-Phen, Lorcet, Lortab, Margesic-H, Norco, Oncet, Panacet, Stagesic, T-Gesic, Vanacet, Vicodin, Zydone

### hydrocodone/aspirin
Alor, Azdone, Damason-P, Lortab ASA, Panasal

### hydrocodone/ibuprofen
Vicoprofen

## CLASSIFICATION(S):
*Therapeutic: allergy, cold, and cough remedies (antitussive), nonopioid analgesics, opioid analgesics*

*Pharmacologic: opioid agonists/ nonopioid analgesic combinations*

**Schedule III (in combination)**

## Pregnancy Category C (with acetaminophen, or ibuprofen), UK (aspirin)

For information on the acetaminophen, aspirin, and ibuprofen components of these formulations, see the acetaminophen, aspirin, and ibuprofen monographs.

## INDICATIONS

■ Used mainly in combination with nonopioid analgesics (acetaminophen/aspirin/ibuprofen) in the management of moderate to severe pain ■ Antitussive (usually in combination products with decongestants).

## ACTION

■ Bind to opiate receptors in the CNS. Alter the perception of and response to painful stimuli while producing generalized CNS depression ■ Suppress the cough reflex via a direct central action. **Therapeutic Effects:** ■ Decrease in severity of moderate pain ■ Suppression of the cough reflex.

## PHARMACOKINETICS

**Absorption:** Well absorbed following oral administration.
**Distribution:** Unknown.
**Metabolism and Excretion:** Mostly metabolized by the liver.
**Half-life:** 3.8 hr.

## CONTRAINDICATIONS AND PRECAUTIONS

**Contraindicated in:** ■ Hypersensitivity to hydrocodone ■ Hypersensitivity to acetaminophen/ aspirin/ibuprofen (for combination products) ■ Aspirin- and ibuprofen-containing products should be avoided in patients with bleeding disorders or thrombocytopenia ■ Acetaminophen should be avoided in patients with severe hepatic or renal disease ■ Pregnancy or lactation (avoid chronic use) ■ Products containing alcohol, aspartame, saccharin, sugar, or tartrazine (FDC yellow dye #5) should be avoided in patients who have hypersensitivity or intolerance to these compounds.

**Use Cautiously in:** ■ Head trauma ■ Increased intracranial pressure ■ Severe renal, hepatic, or pulmonary disease ■ Hypothyroidism ■ Adrenal insufficiency ■ Alcoholism ■ Geriatric or debilitated patients (initial dosage reduction required; more prone to CNS depression, constipation) ■ Patients with undiagnosed abdominal pain ■ Prostatic hypertrophy.

## ADVERSE REACTIONS AND SIDE EFFECTS*

Noted for hydrocodone only; see acetaminophen/aspirin/ibuprofen monographs for specific information on individual components. ■ **CNS:** <u>confusion</u>, <u>sedation</u>, dysphoria, euphoria, floating feeling, hallucinations, headache, unusual dreams ■ **EENT:** blurred vision, diplopia, miosis ■ **Resp:** respiratory depression ■ **CV:** <u>hypotension</u>, bradycardia ■ **GI:** <u>constipation</u>, nausea, vomiting ■ **GU:** urinary retention ■ **Derm:** sweating ■ **Misc:** physical dependence, psychological dependence, tolerance.

## INTERACTIONS

**Drug-Drug:** ■ Use with extreme caution in patients receiving **MAO inhibitors** (may produce severe, unpredictable reactions—reduce initial dose of hydrocodone to 25% of usual dose) ■ Additive CNS depression with **alcohol, antihistamines,** and **sedative/hypnotics** ■ Administration of partial antagonist opioids (**buprenorphine, butorphanol, nalbuphine,** or **pentazocine**) may precipitate opioid withdrawal in physically dependent patients ■ **Buprenorphine** or **pentazocine** may decrease analgesia.

**Drug-Natural Products:** ■ Concomitant use of **kava, valerian, skullcap, chamomile,** or **hops** can increase CNS depression.

## ROUTE AND DOSAGE

■ **PO (Adults):** *Analgesic*—2.5–10 mg q 3–6 hr as needed; if using combination products, acetaminophen or aspirin dosage should not exceed 4 g/day; *Antitussive*—5 mg q 4–6 hr as needed.

■ **PO (Children):** *Analgesic*—0.15–0.2 mg/ kg q 3–6 hr.

## AVAILABILITY

❑ **Hydrocodone**

■*Hydrocodone tablets:* {5 mg (Hycodan)<sup>Rx</sup>} ■Cost: $77.82/100 ■*Hydrocodone syrup:* {5 mg/ml (Hycodan, Robidone)$^{Rx}$} ■ Cost: $71.56/480 ml.

❑ **Hydrocodone/Acetaminophen**

■ *Tablets:* 2.5 mg hydrocodone/500 mg acetaminophen (Lortab 2.5/500)$^{Rx}$, 5 mg hydrocodone/400 mg acetaminophen (Zydone)$^{Rx}$, 5 mg hydrocodone/500 mg acetaminophen (Anexsia 5/500, Co-Gesic, Dolacet, Hydrocet, HydrogesicHy-Phen, Lorcet, Lortab 5/500, Margesic -H, Panacet 5/500, Stagesic, T-Gesic,Vicodin,)$^{Rx}$, 7.5 mg hydrocodone/400 mg acetaminophen (Zydone)$^{Rx}$, 7.5 mg hydrocodone/500 mg acetaminophen (Lortab 7.5/500)$^{Rx}$, 7.5 mg hydrocodone/650 mg acetaminophen (Anexsia 7.5/650, Lorcet Plus)$^{Rx}$, 7.5 mg hydrocodone/750 mg acetaminophen (Vicodin ES)$^{Rx}$, 10 mg hydrocodone/325 mg acetaminophen(Norco)$^{Rx}$, 10 mg hydrocodone/500 mg acetaminophen (Lortab 10/500)$^{Rx}$, 10 mg hydrocodone/650 mg acetaminophen (Lorcet 10/650, Vicodin HP)$^{Rx}$, 10 mg hydrocodone/660 mg acetaminophen (Anexia 10/660)$^{Rx}$ ■ Cost: Lorcet-HD $40.94/100, Lorcet Plus $72.70/100, Lorcet 10/650 $111.82/100; Lortab 2.5/500 $77.82/100, Lortab 5/500 $64.20/100, Lortab 7.5/500 $77.82/100, Lortab 10/500 $72.84/100, Norco $68.23/100, Vicodin $52.23/100, Vicodin ES $60.24/100, Vicodin HP $78.84/100 ■ *Capsules:* 5 mg hydrocodone/500 mg acetaminophen (Bancap-HC, Dolacet, Hydrocet, Hydrogesic, Lorcet-HD, Margesic-H, Stagesic, T-Gesic, Zydone)$^{Rx}$ ■ *Elixir/oral solution:* 2.5 mg hydrocodone plus 167 mg acetaminophen/5 ml$^{Rx}$.

❑ **Hydrocodone/Aspirin**

■ *Tablets:* 5 mg hydrocodone/500 mg aspirin (Azdone, Damason-P, Lortab ASA, Panasal 5/500)$^{Rx}$ ■ antihistamines, caffeine, guaifenesin, decongestants$^{Rx}$. See Appendix B.

❑ **Hydrocodone/Ibuprofen**

■ *Tablets:* 7.5 mg hydrocodone/200 mg ibuprofen$^{Rx}$.

TIME/ACTION PROFILE (analgesic effect)

| | ONSET | PEAK | DURATION |
|---|---|---|---|
| PO | 10–30 min | 30–60 min | 4–6 hr |

# NURSING IMPLICATIONS

## ASSESSMENT

■ **General Info:** Assess blood pressure, pulse, and respirations before and periodically during administration. If respiratory rate is <10/min, assess level of sedation. Physical stimulation may be sufficient to prevent significant hypoventilation. Dose may need to be decreased by 25–50%. Initial drowsiness will diminish with continued use.

❑ Assess bowel function routinely. Prevention of constipation should be instituted with increased intake of fluids and bulk, and laxatives to minimize constipating effects. Stimulant laxatives should be administered routinely if opioid use exceeds 2–3 days, unless contraindicated.

■ **Pain:** Assess type, location, and intensity of pain prior to and 1 hr (peak) following administration. When titrating opioid doses, increases of 25–50% should be administered until there is either a 50% reduction in the patient's pain rating on a numerical or visual analogue scale or the patient reports satisfactory pain relief. A repeat dose can be safely administered at the time of the peak if previous dose is ineffective and side effects are minimal.

❑ An equianalgesic chart (see Appendix O) should be used when changing routes or when changing from one opioid to another.

❑ Prolonged use may lead to physical and psychological dependence and tolerance. This should not prevent patient from receiving adequate analgesia. Most patients who receive opioids for pain do not develop psychological dependence. If progressively higher doses are required, consider conversion to a stronger opioid.

■ **Cough:** Assess cough and lung sounds during antitussive use.

■ *Lab Test Considerations:* May cause increased plasma amylase and lipase concentrations.

■ *Toxicity and Overdose:* If an opioid antagonist is required to reverse respiratory depression or coma, naloxone (Narcan) is the antidote. Dilute the 0.4-mg ampule of naloxone in 10 ml of 0.9% NaCl and administer 0.5 ml (0.02 mg) by direct IV push every 2 min. For children and patients weighing <40 kg, dilute 0.1 mg of naloxone in 10 ml of 0.9% NaCl for a concentration of 10 mcg/ml and administer 0.5 mcg/kg every 2 min. Titrate dose to avoid withdrawal, seizures, and severe pain.

## POTENTIAL NURSING DIAGNOSES

- Pain, acute (Indications).
- Sensory perception, disturbed (visual, auditory) (Side Effects).
- Injury, risk for (Side Effects).

## IMPLEMENTATION

- *High Alert:* Accidental overdosage of opioid analgesics has resulted in fatalities. Before administering, clarify all ambiguous orders; have second practitioner independently check original order and dose calculations. Do not confuse hydrocodone with hydrocortisone. Do not confuse Lortab with Lorabid (loracarbef).

- **General:** Explain therapeutic value of medication prior to administration to enhance the analgesic effect.

- Regularly administered doses may be more effective than prn administration. Analgesic is more effective if given before pain becomes severe.

- Combination with nonopioid analgesics may have additive analgesic effects and permit lower doses. Maximum doses of nonopioid agents limit the titration of hydrocodone doses.

- Medication should be discontinued gradually after long-term use to prevent withdrawal symptoms.

- **PO:** May be administered with food or milk to minimize GI irritation.

## PATIENT/FAMILY TEACHING

- Advise patient to take medication exactly as directed and not to take more than the recommended amount. Severe and permanent liver damage may result from prolonged use or high doses of acetaminophen. Renal damage may occur with prolonged use of acetaminophen or aspirin. Doses of nonopioid agents should not exceed the maximum recommended daily dose.

- Instruct patient on how and when to ask for pain medication.

- May cause drowsiness or dizziness. Advise patient to call for assistance when ambulating or smoking. Caution patient to avoid driving or other activities requiring alertness until response to the medication is known.

- Advise patient to change positions slowly to minimize orthostatic hypotension.

- Caution patient to avoid concurrent use of alcohol or other CNS depressants with this medication.

- Encourage patient to turn, cough, and breathe deeply every 2 hr to prevent atelectasis.

- Advise patient that good oral hygiene, frequent mouth rinses, and sugarless gum or candy may decrease dry mouth.

## EVALUATION

**Effectiveness of therapy can be demonstrated by:** ■ Decrease in severity of pain without a significant alteration in level of consciousness or respiratory status ■ Suppression of nonproductive cough.

## hydrocortisone, See CORTICOSTEROIDS (SYSTEMIC), CORTICOSTEROIDS (TOPICAL/ LOCAL).

**High Alert**

# hydromorphone

(hye-droe-**mor**-fone)

Dilaudid, Dilaudid-HP, Hydrostat IR, PMS Hydromorphone

## CLASSIFICATION(S):

**Therapeutic:** *allergy, cold, and cough remedies (antitussives), opioid analgesics*

**Pharmacologic:** *opioid agonists*

**Schedule II**

**Pregnancy Category C**

## INDICATIONS

■ Moderate to severe pain (alone and in combination with nonopioid analgesics) ■ Antitussive (lower doses).

## ACTION

■ Binds to opiate receptors in the CNS ■ Alters the perception of and response to painful stimuli while producing generalized CNS depression ■ Suppresses the cough reflex via a direct central action. **Therapeutic Effects:** ■ Decrease in moderate to severe pain ■ Suppression of cough.

## PHARMACOKINETICS

**Absorption:** Well absorbed following oral, rectal, subcut, and IM administration.
**Distribution:** Widely distributed. Crosses the placenta; enters breast milk.
**Metabolism and Excretion:** Mostly metabolized by the liver.
**Half-life:** 2–4 hr.

## CONTRAINDICATIONS AND PRECAUTIONS

**Contraindicated in:** ■ Hypersensitivity ■ Some products contain bisulfites and should be avoided in patients with known hypersensitivity ■ Avoid chronic use during pregnancy or lactation.

**Use Cautiously in:** ■ Head trauma ■ Increased intracranial pressure ■ Severe renal, hepatic, or pulmonary disease ■ Hypothyroidism ■ Adrenal insufficiency ■ Alcoholism ■ Geriatric or debilitated patients (dosage reduction recommended) ■ Undiagnosed abdominal pain ■ Prostatic hypertrophy.

## ADVERSE REACTIONS AND SIDE EFFECTS*

■ **CNS:** confusion, sedation, dizziness, dysphoria, euphoria, floating feeling, hallucinations, headache, unusual dreams ■ **EENT:** blurred vision, diplopia, miosis ■ **Resp:** respiratory depression ■ **CV:** hypotension, bradycardia ■ **GI:** constipation, nausea, vomiting ■ **GU:** urinary retention ■ **Derm:** flushing, sweating ■ **Misc:** physical dependence, psychological dependence, tolerance.

## INTERACTIONS

**Drug-Drug:** ■ Exercise extreme caution with **MAO inhibitors** (may produce severe, unpredictable reactions—reduce initial dose of hydromorphone to 25% of usual dose) ■ Additive CNS depression with **alcohol, antidepressants, antihistamines,** and **sedative/hypnotics** ■ Administration of partial antagonists (**buprenorphine, butorphanol, nalbuphine,** or **pentazocine**) may precipitate opioid withdrawal in physically dependent patients ■ **Nalbuphine** or **pentazocine** may decrease analgesia.

**Drug-Natural Products:** ■ Concomitant use of **kava, valerian, skullcap, chamomile,** or **hops** can increase CNS depression.

## ROUTE AND DOSAGE

Doses depend on level of pain and tolerance.

❑ **Analgesic**

■ **PO (Adults ≥50 kg):** 4–8 mg q 3–4 hr initially (some patients may respond to doses as small as 2 mg initially).

■ **PO (Adults and Children <50 kg):** 0.06 mg/kg q 3–4 hr initially.

■ **IV, IM, Subcut (Adults ≥50 kg):** 1.5 mg q 3–4 hr as needed initially; may be increased.

■ **IV, IM, Subcut (Adults and Children <50 kg):** 0.015 mg/kg mg q 3–4 hr as needed initially; may be increased.

■ **IV (Adults):** *Continuous infusion (unlabeled)*—0.2–30 mg/hr depending on previous opioid use. An initial bolus of twice the hourly rate in mg may be given with subsequent "breakthrough" boluses of 50–100% of the hourly rate in mg.

■ **Rect (Adults):** 3 mg q 4–8 hr initially as needed.

❑ **Antitussive**

■ **PO (Adults):** 1 mg q 3–4 hr.

■ **PO (Children 6–12 yr):** 0.5 mg q 3–4 hr.

## AVAILABILITY (generic available)

■ *Tablets:* 1 mg^Rx, 2 mg^Rx, 3 mg^Rx, 4 mg^Rx, 8 mg^Rx ■ Cost: *Dilaudid*—2 mg $45.61/100, 4 mg $74.46/100, 8 mg $135.53/100; *generic*— 2 mg $37.18/100, 4 mg $61.35/100 ■ *Oral solution:* 5 mg/5 ml^Rx ■ *Injection:* 1 mg/ml^Rx, 2 mg/ml^Rx, 3 mg/ml^Rx, 4 mg/ml^Rx, 10 mg/ml^Rx ■ Cost: 1 mg/ml $23.75/25 ml, 2 mg/ml $10.63/20 ml ■ *Suppositories:* 3 mg^Rx ■ guaifenesin and alcohol (Dilaudid Cough Syrup)^Rx. See Appendix B.

TIME/ACTION PROFILE (analgesic effect)

|        | ONSET      | PEAK        | DURATION |
|--------|------------|-------------|----------|
| PO     | 30 min     | 90–120 min  | 4 hr     |
| Subcut | 15 min     | 30–90 min   | 4–5 hr   |
| IM     | 15 min     | 30–60 min   | 4–5 hr   |
| IV     | 10–15 min  | 15–30 min   | 2–3 hr   |
| Rect   | 15–30 min  | 30–90 min   | 4–5 hr   |

# NURSING IMPLICATIONS

## ASSESSMENT

- **General Info:** Assess blood pressure, pulse, and respirations before and periodically during administration. If respiratory rate is <10/min, assess level of sedation. Dose may need to be decreased by 25–50%. Initial drowsiness will diminish with continued use.

- ❏ Assess bowel function routinely. Prevention of constipation should be instituted with increased intake of fluids and bulk, and laxatives to minimize constipating effects. Stimulant laxatives should be administered routinely if opioid use exceeds 2–3 days, unless contraindicated.

- **Pain:** Assess type, location, and intensity of pain prior to and 1 hr following IM and 5 min (peak) following IV administration. When titrating opioid doses, increases of 25–50% should be administered until there is either a 50% reduction in the patient's pain rating on a numerical or visual analog scale or the patient reports satisfactory pain relief. A repeat dose can be safely administered at the time of the peak if previous dose is ineffective and side effects are minimal.

- ❏ Patients on a continuous infusion should have additional bolus doses provided every 15–30 min, as needed, for breakthrough pain. The bolus dose is usually set to the amount of drug infused each hour by continuous infusion.

- ❏ An equianalgesic chart (see Appendix O) should be used when changing routes or when changing from one opioid to another.

- ❏ Prolonged use may lead to physical and psychological dependence and tolerance. This should not prevent patient from receiving adequate analgesia. Most patients who receive hydromorphone for pain do not develop psychological dependence. Progressively higher doses may be required to relieve pain with long-term therapy.

- **Cough:** Assess cough and lung sounds during antitussive use.

- *Lab Test Considerations:* May increase plasma amylase and lipase concentrations.

- *Toxicity and Overdose:* If an opioid antagonist is required to reverse respiratory depression or coma, naloxone (Narcan) is the antidote. Dilute the 0.4-mg ampule of naloxone in 10 ml of 0.9% NaCl and administer 0.5 ml (0.02 mg) by direct IV push every 2 min. For children and patients weighing <40 kg, dilute 0.1 mg of naloxone in 10 ml of 0.9% NaCl for a concentration of 10 mcg/ml and administer 0.5 mcg every 2 min. Titrate dose to avoid withdrawal, seizures, and severe pain.

## POTENTIAL NURSING DIAGNOSES

- Pain, acute (Indications).

- Sensory perception, disturbed (visual, auditory) (Side Effects).

- Injury, risk for (Side Effects).

## IMPLEMENTATION

- ❏ *High Alert:* Accidental overdosage of opioid analgesics has resulted in fatalities. Before administering, clarify all ambiguous orders; have second practitioner independently check original order, dose calculations, and infusion pump settings. Do not confuse with meperidine or morphine; fatalities have occurred.

- **General:** Explain therapeutic value of medication prior to administration to enhance the analgesic effect.

- ❏ Regularly administered doses may be more effective than prn administration. Analgesic is more effective if given before pain becomes severe.

- ❏ Coadministration with nonopioid analgesics may have additive analgesic effects and permit lower opioid doses.

- ❏ Medication should be discontinued gradually after long-term use to prevent withdrawal symptoms.

- **PO:** May be administered with food or milk to minimize GI irritation.

- **Direct IV:** Dilute with at least 5 ml of sterile water or 0.9% NaCl for injection. Inspect solution for particulate matter. Slight yellow color does not alter potency. Store at room temperature.

- *Rate:* Administer slowly, at a rate not to exceed 2 mg over 3–5 min.

---

{ } = Available in Canada only.
*CAPITALS indicates life-threatening; <u>underlines</u> indicate most frequent.

❏ *High Alert:* Rapid administration may lead to increased respiratory depression, hypotension, and circulatory collapse.

■ **Syringe Compatibility:** ◆ atropine ◆ bupivacaine ◆ ceftazidime ◆ chlorpromazine ◆ cimetidine ◆ diphenhydramine ◆ fentanyl ◆ glycopyrrolate ◆ hydroxyzine ◆ lorazepam ◆ midazolam ◆ pentobarbital ◆ prochlorperazine ◆ promethazine ◆ ranitidine ◆ scopolamine ◆ thiethylperazine ◆ trimethobenzamide.

■ **Syringe Incompatibility:** ◆ ampicillin ◆ diazepam ◆ hyaluronidase ◆ phenobarbital ◆ phenytoin.

■ **Y-Site Compatibility:** ◆ acyclovir ◆ allopurinol ◆ amifostine ◆ amikacin ◆ aztreonam ◆ cefazolin ◆ cefepime ◆ cefoperazone ◆ cefotaxime ◆ cefoxitin ◆ ceftazidime ◆ ceftizoxime ◆ cefuroxime ◆ chloramphenicol ◆ cisatracurium ◆ cisplatin ◆ cladribine ◆ clindamycin ◆ cyclophosphamide ◆ cytarabine ◆ diltiazem ◆ dobutamine ◆ docetaxel ◆ dopamine ◆ doxorubicin ◆ doxorubicin liposome ◆ doxycycline ◆ erythromycin lactobionate ◆ etoposide ◆ famotidine ◆ fentanyl ◆ filgrastim ◆ fludarabine ◆ foscarnet ◆ furosemide ◆ gatifloxacin ◆ gemcitabine ◆ gentamicin ◆ granisetron ◆ heparin ◆ kanamycin ◆ labetalol ◆ linezolid ◆ lorazepam ◆ magnesium sulfate ◆ melphalan ◆ methotrexate ◆ metronidazole ◆ midazolam ◆ milrinone ◆ morphine ◆ nafcillin ◆ nitroglycerin ◆ norepinephrine ◆ ondansetron ◆ oxacillin ◆ paclitaxel ◆ penicillin G potassium ◆ piperacillin ◆ piperacillin/tazobactam ◆ propofol ◆ ranitidine ◆ remifentanil ◆ tacrolimus ◆ teniposide ◆ thiotepa ◆ ticarcillin ◆ tobramycin ◆ trimethoprim/sulfamethoxazole ◆ vancomycin ◆ vecuronium ◆ vinorelbine.

■ **Y-Site Incompatibility:** ◆ amphotericin B cholesteryl sulfate complex ◆ diazepam ◆ minocycline ◆ phenobarbital ◆ phenytoin ◆ sargramostim ◆ thiopental.

■ **Additive Compatibility:** ◆ ondansetron.

■ **Additive Incompatibility:** ◆ sodium bicarbonate ◆ thiopental.

■ **Solution Compatibility:** ◆ D5W ◆ D5/0.45% NaCl ◆ D5/0.9% NaCl ◆ D5/LR ◆ D5/Ringer's solution ◆ 0.45% NaCl ◆ 0.9% NaCl ◆ Ringer's and LR.

### PATIENT/FAMILY TEACHING

❏ Instruct patient on how and when to ask for pain medication.

❏ May cause drowsiness or dizziness. Advise patient to call for assistance when ambulat-

ing or smoking. Caution patient to avoid driving or other activities requiring alertness until response to medication is known.

❏ Advise patient to change positions slowly to minimize orthostatic hypotension.

❏ Instruct patient to avoid concurrent use of alcohol or other CNS depressants.

❏ Encourage patient to turn, cough, and breathe deeply every 2 hr to prevent atelectasis.

### EVALUATION

**Effectiveness of therapy can be demonstrated by:** ■ Decrease in severity of pain without a significant alteration in level of consciousness or respiratory status ■ Suppression of cough.

---

## hydroxocobalamin, See VITAMIN B₁₂ PREPARATIONS.

---

## hydroxychloroquine

(hye-drox-ee-**klor**-oh-kwin)

Plaquenil

**CLASSIFICATION(S):**

*Therapeutic: antimalarials, antirheumatics (DMARDs)*

**Pregnancy Category C**

### INDICATIONS

■ Suppression/chemoprophylaxis of malaria ■ Treatment of severe rheumatoid arthritis/systemic lupus erythematosus.

### ACTION

■ Inhibits protein synthesis in susceptible organisms by inhibiting DNA and RNA polymerase. **Therapeutic Effects:** ■ Death of plasmodia responsible for causing malaria ■ Also has anti-inflammatory properties.

### PHARMACOKINETICS

**Absorption:** Well absorbed (74%) following oral administation.

**Distribution:** Widely distributed; high concentrations in RBCs; crosses the placenta.

**Metabolism and Excretion:** Partially metabolized by the liver to active metabolites; partially excreted unchanged by the kidneys.

**Half-life:** 72–120 hr.

## CONTRAINDICATIONS AND PRECAUTIONS

**Contraindicated in:** ■ Hypersensitivity to hydroxychloroquine or chloroquine ■ Previous visual damage from hydroxychloroquine or chloroquine.

**Use Cautiously in:** ■ Concurrent use of hepatotoxic drugs ■ History of liver disease or alcoholism or renal impairment ■ Severe neurological disorders ■ Severe blood disorders ■ Retinal or visual field changes ■ G6PD deficiency ■ Psoriasis ■ Bone marrow depression ■ Obesity (determine dose by ideal body weight) ■ Pregnancy or lactation (avoid use unless treating/preventing malaria or treating amebic abscess) ■ Children (increased sensitivity to effects).

## ADVERSE REACTIONS AND SIDE EFFECTS*

■ **CNS:** SEIZURES, aggressiveness, anxiety, apathy, confusion, fatigue, headache, irritability, personality changes, psychoses ■ **EENT:** keratopathy, ototoxicity, retinopathy, tinnitus, visual disturbances ■ **CV:** ECG changes, hypotension ■ **GI:** abdominal cramps, anorexia, diarrhea, epigastric discomfort, nausea, vomiting ■ **Derm:** dermatoses ■ **Hemat:** AGRANULOCYTOSIS, APLASTIC ANEMIA, leukopenia, thrombocytopenia ■ **Neuro:** neuromyopathy, peripheral neuritis.

## INTERACTIONS

**Drug-Drug:** ■ May increase the risk of hepatotoxicity when administered with **hepatotoxic drugs** ■ May increase the risk of hematologic toxicity when administered with **penicillamine** ■ May increase risk of dermatitis when administered with other **agents having dermatologic toxicity** ■ May decrease serum titers of rabies antibody when given concurrently with **human diploid cell rabies vaccine** ■ **Urinary acidifiers** may increase renal excretion ■ May increase serum levels of **digoxin**.

## ROUTE AND DOSAGE

Antimalarial doses expressed as mg of base; antirheumatic doses expressed as mg of hydroxychloroquine sulfate (200 mg hydroxychloroquine sulfate = 155 mg of hydroxychloroquine base).

❏ **Malaria**

■ **PO (Adults):** *Suppression or chemoprophylaxis*—310 mg once weekly; start 1–2 wk prior to entering malarious area; continue for 4 wk after leaving area. *Treatment*—620 mg, then 310 mg at 6 hr, 24 hr, and 48 hr after initial dose.

■ **PO (Children):** *Suppression or chemoprophylaxis*—5 mg/kg once weekly; start 1–2 wk prior to entering malarious area; continue for 4 wk after leaving area. *Treatment*—10 mg/kg initially, then 5 mg/kg at 6 hr, 24 hr, and 48 hr after initial dose.

❏ **Rheumatoid Arthritis**

■ **PO (Adults):** 5 mg/kg initially, maintenance 200–400 mg/day.

❏ **Systemic Lupus Erythematosus**

■ **PO (Adults):** 5 mg/kg/day.

## AVAILABILITY

■ *Tablets:* 200 mg (155-mg base)$^{Rx}$ ■ Cost: $109.55/100.

TIME/ACTION PROFILE (blood levels)

| | ONSET | PEAK | DURATION |
|---|---|---|---|
| PO | rapid† | 1–2 hr | days–weeks |

†Onset of antirheumatic action may take 6 wk.

## NURSING IMPLICATIONS

### ASSESSMENT

■ **General Info:** Assess deep tendon reflexes periodically to determine muscle weakness. Therapy may be discontinued should this occur.

❏ Patients on prolonged high-dose therapy should have eye exams prior to and every 3–6 mo during therapy to detect retinal damage.

■ **Malaria or Lupus Erythematosus:** Assess patient for improvement in signs and symptoms of condition daily throughout course of therapy.

■ **Rheumatoid Arthritis:** Assess patient monthly for pain, swelling, and range of motion.

■ *Lab Test Considerations:* Monitor CBC and platelet count periodically throughout therapy. May cause decreased RBC, WBC, and platelet counts. If severe decreases occur that are not related to the disease process, hydroxychloroquine should be discontinued.

## POTENTIAL NURSING DIAGNOSES

■ Infection, risk for (Indications).

■ Pain, chronic (Indications).

## IMPLEMENTATION

■ **PO:** Administer with milk or meals to minimize GI distress.

❑ Tablets may be crushed and placed inside empty capsules for patients with difficulty swallowing. Contents of capsules may also be mixed with a teaspoonful of jam, jelly, or Jell-O prior to administration.

■ **Malaria Prophylaxis:** Hydroxychloroquine therapy should be started 2 wk prior to potential exposure and continued for 4–6 wk after leaving the malarious area.

## PATIENT/FAMILY TEACHING

❑ Instruct patient to take medication exactly as directed and continue full course of therapy even if feeling better. Missed doses should be taken as soon as remembered unless it is almost time for next dose. Do not double doses.

❑ Advise patients to avoid use of alcohol while taking hydroxychloroquine.

❑ Caution patient to keep hydroxychloroquine out of reach of children; fatalities have occurred with ingestion of 3 or 4 tablets.

❑ Explain need for periodic ophthalmic exams for patients on prolonged high-dose therapy. Advise patient that the risk of ocular damage may be decreased by the use of dark glasses in bright light. Protective clothing and sunscreen should also be used to reduce risk of dermatoses.

❑ Advise patient to notify health care professional promptly if sore throat, fever, unusual bleeding or bruising, blurred vision, visual changes, ringing in the ears, difficulty hearing, or muscle weakness occurs.

■ **Malaria Prophylaxis:** Review methods of minimizing exposure to mosquitoes with patients receiving hydroxychloroquine prophylactically (use repellent, wear long-sleeved shirt and long trousers, use screen or netting).

❑ Advise patient to notify health care professional if fever develops while traveling or within 2 mo of leaving an endemic area.

■ **Rheumatoid Arthritis:** Instruct patient to contact health care professional if no improvement is noticed within a few days. Treatment for rheumatoid arthritis may require up to 6 mo for full benefit.

## EVALUATION

**Effectiveness of therapy can be demonstrated by:** ■ Prevention or resolution of malaria ■ Improvement in signs and symptoms of rheumatoid arthritis ■ Improvement in symptoms of lupus erythematosus.

# hydroxyzine

(hye-**drox**-i-zeen)
{Apo-Hydroxyzine}, Atarax, Hyzine-50, {Multipax}, {Novohydroxyzin}, Vistaril

## CLASSIFICATION(S):

***Therapeutic:*** *antianxiety agents, antihistamines, sedative/hypnotics*

**Pregnancy Category C**

## INDICATIONS

■ Treatment of anxiety ■ Preoperative sedation ■ Antiemetic ■ Antipruritic ■ May be combined with opioid analgesics.

## ACTION

■ Acts as a CNS depressant at the subcortical level of the CNS ■ Has anticholinergic, antihistaminic, and antiemetic properties. **Therapeutic Effects:** ■ Sedation ■ Relief of anxiety ■ Decreased nausea and vomiting ■ Decreased allergic symptoms associated with release of histamine, including pruritus.

## PHARMACOKINETICS

**Absorption:** Well absorbed following PO/IM administration.

**Distribution:** Unknown.

**Metabolism and Excretion:** Completely metabolized by the liver; eliminated in the feces via biliary excretion.

**Half-life:** 3 hr.

## CONTRAINDICATIONS AND PRECAUTIONS

**Contraindicated in:** ■ Hypersensitivity ■ Pregnancy.

**Use Cautiously in:** ■ Severe hepatic dysfunction ■ Geriatric patients (dosage reduction recommended) ■ Labor (has been used safely) ■ Lactation (safety not established).

## ADVERSE REACTIONS AND SIDE EFFECTS*

■ **CNS:** drowsiness, agitation, ataxia, dizziness, headache, weakness ■ **Resp:** wheezing ■ **GI:** dry mouth, bitter taste, constipation, nausea ■ **GU:** urinary retention ■ **Derm:** flushing ■ **Local:** pain at IM site, abscesses at IM sites ■ **Misc:** chest tightness.

## INTERACTIONS

**Drug-Drug:** ■ Additive CNS depression with other **CNS depressants,** including **alcohol, antidepressants, antihistamines, opioid analgesics,** and **sedative/hypnotics** ■ Additive anticholinergic effects with other **drugs possessing anticholinergic properties,** including **antihistamines, antidepressants, atropine, haloperidol, phenothiazines, quinidine,** and **disopyramide.**
**Drug-Natural Products:** ■ Concomitant use of **kava, valerian, skullcap, chamomile,** or **hops** can increase CNS depression ■ Increased anticholinergic effects with **angel's trumpet, jimson weed,** and **scopolia.**

## ROUTE AND DOSAGE

■ **PO (Adults):** *Antianxiety, sedative/hypnotic*—25–100 mg single dose. *Antiemetic/antipruritic*—25–100 mg 3–4 times daily.
■ **PO (Children):** *Antianxiety, sedative/hypnotic*—0.6 mg/kg single dose. *Antiemetic, antipruritic*—0.5 mg/kg (15 mg/m²) q 6 hr.
■ **PO (Children 6–12 yr):** *Antiemetic, antipruritic*—12.5–25 mg q 6 hr as needed.
■ **PO (Children <6 yr):** *Antiemetic, antipruritic*—12.5 mg q 6 hr as needed.
■ **IM (Adults):** *Antianxiety*—50–100 mg q 4–6 hr. *Sedative/hypnotic*—50 mg single dose. *Antiemetic, adjunct to opioid analgesics*—25–100 mg.

■ **IM (Children):** *Antiemetic, adjunct to opioids*—1 mg/kg (30 mg/m²).

## AVAILABILITY (generic available)

■ *Tablets:* 10 mg$^{Rx}$, 25 mg$^{Rx}$, 50 mg$^{Rx}$, 100 mg$^{Rx}$ ■ Cost: *Atarax*—10 mg $65.24/100, 25 mg $98.84/100, 50 mg $121.92/100, 100 mg $144.82/100; *generic*—10 mg $8.01/100, 25 mg $12.24/100, 50 mg $13.82/100, 100 mg $95.82/100 ■ *Capsules:* {10 mg$^{Rx}$}, 25 mg$^{Rx}$, 50 mg$^{Rx}$, 100 mg$^{Rx}$ ■ Cost: *Vistaril*—25 mg $98.23/100, 50 mg $121.92/100, 100 mg $141.84/100; *generic*—25 mg $21.83/100, 50 mg $22.92/100, 100 mg $39.43/100 ■ *Syrup:* 10 mg/5 ml$^{Rx}$ ■ *Oral suspension:* 25 mg/5 ml$^{Rx}$ ■ *Injection:* 25 mg/ml$^{Rx}$, 50 mg/ml$^{Rx}$.

TIME/ACTION PROFILE (sedative, antiemetic, antipruritic effects)

|    | ONSET | PEAK | DURATION |
|----|-------|------|----------|
| PO | 15–30 min | 2–4 hr | 4–6 hr |
| IM | 15–30 min | 2–4 hr | 4–6 hr |

# NURSING IMPLICATIONS

## ASSESSMENT

■ **General Info:** Assess patient for profound sedation and provide safety precautions as indicated (side rails up, bed in low position, call bell within reach, supervision of ambulation and transfer).
■ **Anxiety:** Assess mental status, mood, and behavior.
■ **Nausea and Vomiting:** Assess degree of nausea and frequency and amount of emesis.
■ **Pruritus:** Assess degree of itching and character of involved skin.
■ *Lab Test Considerations:* May cause false-negative skin test results using allergen extracts. Discontinue hydroxyzine at least 72 hr before test.

## POTENTIAL NURSING DIAGNOSES

■ Anxiety (Indications).
■ Skin integrity, impaired (Indications).
■ Injury, risk for (Side Effects).

## IMPLEMENTATION

Do not confuse hydroxyzine with hydralazine or Atarax (hydroxyzine) with Ativan (lorazepam).

{ } = Available in Canada only.
*CAPITALS indicates life-threatening; underlines indicate most frequent.

■ **PO:** Tablets may be crushed and capsules opened and administered with food or fluids for patients having difficulty swallowing.

❑ Shake suspension well before administration.

■ **IM:** Administer *only* IM deep into well-developed muscle, preferably with Z-track technique. Injection is extremely painful. Do not use deltoid site. If must be administered to children, midlateral muscles of the thigh are preferred. Significant tissue damage, necrosis, and sloughing may result from subcut or intra-arterial injections. Hemolysis may result from IV injections. Rotate injection sites frequently.

■ **Syringe Compatibility:** ◆ atropine ◆ butorphanol ◆ chlorpromazine ◆ cimetidine ◆ codeine ◆ diphenhydramine ◆ doxapram ◆ droperidol ◆ fentanyl ◆ fluphenazine ◆ glycopyrrolate ◆ hydromorphone ◆ lidocaine ◆ meperidine ◆ methotrimeprazine ◆ metoclopramide ◆ midazolam ◆ morphine ◆ nalbuphine ◆ oxymorphone ◆ pentazocine ◆ perphenazine ◆ procaine ◆ prochlorperazine ◆ promethazine ◆ scopolamine ◆ sufentanil

■ **Syringe Incompatibility:** ◆ dimenhydrinate ◆ haloperidol ◆ heparin ◆ ketorolac ◆ pentobarbital ◆ ranitidine

## PATIENT/FAMILY TEACHING

❑ Instruct patient to take medication exactly as directed. Missed doses should be taken as soon as remembered unless it is almost time for next dose; do not double doses.

❑ May cause drowsiness or dizziness. Caution patient to avoid driving and other activities requiring alertness until response to medication is known.

❑ Advise patient to avoid concurrent use of alcohol or other CNS depressants with this medication.

❑ Inform patient that frequent mouth rinses, good oral hygiene, and sugarless gum or candy may help decrease dry mouth. If dry mouth persists for more than 2 wk, consult dentist about saliva substitute.

## EVALUATION

**Effectiveness of therapy can be demonstrated by:** ■ Decrease in anxiety ■ Relief of nausea and vomiting ■ Relief of pruritus ■ Sedation when used as a sedative/hypnotic.

# hyoscyamine

(hi-oh-**si**-a-meen)

Anaspaz, A-Spas S/L, Cystospaz, Cystospaz-M, Donnamar, ED-SPAZ, Gastrosed, Levsinex, Levsin, Levbid, L-hyoscyamine, NuLev

### CLASSIFICATION(S):

**Therapeutic:** *antispasmodics*
**Pharmacologic:** *anticholinergics*

**Pregnancy Category C**

## INDICATIONS

■ Control of gastric secretion, visceral spasm, hypermotility in spastic colitis, spastic bladder, pylorospasm, and related abdominal cramps ■ Decreases symptoms of various functional intestinal disorders including mild dysenteries, diverticulitis, infant colic, biliary and renal colic ■ Adjunctive therapy in peptic ulcer disease, irritable bowel syndrome, neurogenic bowel disturbances ■ Decreases pain and hypersecretion associated with pancreatitis ■ Relief of symptoms of acute rhinitis ■ Decreases rigidity and tremors associated with parkinsonism and controls related sialorrhea and hyperhidrosis. May also be used to manage anticholinesterase poisoning ■ Management of cystitis or renal colic ■ Management of some forms of heart block due to vagal activity ■ **IM, IV, Subcut:** Facilitation of diagnostic hypotonic duodenography; may also increase radiologic visibility of the kidneys ■ Preoperative administration decreases secretions and blocks bradycardia associated with some forms of anesthesia and related surgical agents.

## ACTION

■ Inhibits the muscarinic effect of acetylcholine in smooth muscle, secretory glands and the CNS. Small doses decrease salivary and bronchial secretions and decrease sweating; intermediate doses dilate the pupil, inhibit accommodation, increase heart rate (vagolytic action); large doses decrease GI and GU motility, further increase in dose decreases gastric acid secretion. **Therapeutic Effects:** ■ Decreased secretions with decreased GI and GU symptomatology ■ Increased heart rate.

## PHARMACOKINETICS

**Absorption:** Well absorbed; food does not affect absorption.
**Distribution:** Crosses the placenta and blood-brain barrier; enters breast milk.
**Metabolism and Excretion:** Excreted mostly unchanged by the kidneys.
**Half-life:** 3.5 hr.

## CONTRAINDICATIONS AND PRECAUTIONS

**Contraindicated in:** ■ Hypersensitivity ■ Narrow-angle glaucoma; synechiae ■ Tachycardia or unstable cardiovascular status ■ GI obstructive disease, paralytic ileus, intestinal atony, severe ulcerative colitis ■ Obstructive uropathy ■ Myasthenia gravis ■ Lactation ■ Products containing benzyl alcohol should not be used in newborn or immature infants ■ Some products contain alcohol, sulfites, or tartrazine and should be avoided in patients with known intolerance/hypersensitivity ■ Phenylketonuria (NuLev contains aspartame)

**Use Cautiously in:** ■ History of cardiovascular disease including CHF, arrhythmias, hypertension, tachycardia, or coronary artery disease ■ Renal disease or prostatic hypertrophy ■ Hepatic disease, early ileus, or reflux esophagitis ■ Automonic neuropathy ■ Hyperthyroidism ■ Geriatric patients (increased sensitivity) ■ Infants, small children, blondes, Down's syndrome, brain damage, or spastic paralysis (increased sensitivity) ■ Pregnancy (may cause fetal tachycardia; safety not established).

## ADVERSE REACTIONS AND SIDE EFFECTS*

■ **CNS:** confusion/excitement (especially in geriatric patients), dizziness, flushing, headache, insomnia, lightheadedness (IM, IV, subcut), nervousness ■ **EENT:** blurred vision, cycloplegia, increased intraocular pressure, mydriasis, photophobia ■ **CV:** palpitations, tachycardia ■ **GI:** dry mouth, altered taste perception, bloated feeling, constipation, nausea, paralytic ileus, vomiting ■ **GU:** impotence, urinary hesitancy/retention ■ **Derm:** decreased sweating, urticaria ■ **Local:** local irritation (IM, IV, subcut) ■ **Misc:** allergic reactions including ANAPHYLAXIS, fever (especially in children), suppression of lactation.

## INTERACTIONS

**Drug-Drug:** ■ Concurrent administration with **amantadine** increases anticholinergic side effects (may require dosage reduction) ■ Increases the effects of **atenolol** ■ Concurrent use with **phenothiazines** may result in decreased effect of phenothiazine and increased anticholinergic side effects (dosage reduction may be necessary) ■ Increased anticholinergic side effects with **tricyclic antidepressants**.

## ROUTE AND DOSAGE

■ **PO, SL (Adults):** 0.125–0.25 mg 3–4 times daily or 0.375–0.75 mg as sustained release form every 12 hr.
■ **PO (Children 2–<12 yr):** *orally disintegrating tablets (NuLev)*—0.0625–0.125 mg (1/2–1 tablet)every 4 hr, up to 6 times/day.
■ **PO (Children 34–36 kg):** 125–187 mcg every 4 hr as needed.
■ **PO (Children 22.7–33 kg):** 94–125 mcg every 4 hr as needed.
■ **PO (Children 13.6–22.6 kg):** 63 mcg every 4 hr as needed.
■ **PO (Children 9.1–13.5 kg):** 31.3 mcg every 4 hr as needed.
■ **PO (Children 6.8–9 kg):** 25 mcg every 4 hr as needed.
■ **PO (Children 4.5–6.7 kg):** 18.8 mcg every 4 hr as needed.
■ **PO (Children 3.4–4.4 kg):** 15.6 mcg every 4 hr as needed.
■ **PO (Children 2.3–3.3 kg):** 12.5 mcg every 4 hr as needed.
■ **IM, IV, Subcut (Adults):** *Gastrointestinal anticholinergic*—0.25–0.5 mg 3–4 times daily as needed; *preoperative prophylaxis of secretions*—0.5 mg or 0.005 mg/kg 30–60 min before anesthesia; *antiarrhythmic*—0.125 mg IV repeated as needed; *cholinergic adjunct (curariform block)*—0.2 mg for each 1 mg of neostigmine.
■ **IM, IV, Subcut (Children ≥2 yr):** *preoperative prophylaxis of secretions*—0.005 mg/kg 30–60 min before anesthesia.

## AVAILABILITY (generic available)

■ *Tablets:* 0.125 mg^Rx, 0.15 mg^Rx ■ Cost: *Levsin*—0.125 mg $22.99/30 ■ *Sublingual tablets:* 0.125 mg^Rx, 0.375 mg^Rx ■ Cost: *Levsin*

{ } = Available in Canada only.
*CAPITALS indicates life-threatening; underlines indicate most frequent.

*SL*—0.125 mg $15.51/100, 0.375 mg $52.95/ 100 ■ *Orally-disintegrating tablets (contains aspartame) (mint):* 0.125 mg$^{Rx}$ ■ Cost: *NuLev*—■ *Extended release tablets:* 0.375 mg$^{Rx}$ ■ *Timed release capsules:* 0.375 mg$^{Rx}$ ■ *Solution (drops) (orange):* 0.125 mg/ml$^{Rx}$ ■Cost: *Levsin*—$23.61/15 ml ■ *Elixir (orange):* 0.125 mg/5 ml$^{Rx}$ ■ *Injection:* 0.5 mg/ml$^{Rx}$.

TIME/ACTION PROFILE (GI effects)

| | ONSET | PEAK | DURATION |
|---|---|---|---|
| PO | 20–30 min | unknown | 4–6 hr |
| IM, IV, subcut | 2–3 min | unknown | 4–6 hr |

## NURSING IMPLICATIONS

### ASSESSMENT

❑ Assess vital signs and ECG tracings frequently during IV drug therapy. Report any significant changes in heart rate or blood pressure, or increased ventricular ectopy or angina to physician promptly.

❑ Monitor intake and output ratios in elderly or surgical patients because hyoscyamine may cause urinary retention.

❑ Assess patients routinely for abdominal distention and auscultate for bowel sounds. If constipation becomes a problem, increasing fluids and adding bulk to the diet may help alleviate constipation.

■ *Toxicity and Overdose:* If overdose occurs, physostigmine is the antidote.

### POTENTIAL NURSING DIAGNOSES

■ Cardiac output, decreased (Indications).

■ Oral mucous membrane, impaired (Side Effects).

■ Constipation (Side Effects).

### IMPLEMENTATION

■ **General:** Do not confuse Levbid (hyoscyamine) with Lithobid (lithium) Lopid (gemfibrozil) or Lorabid (loracarbef).

■ **PO:** Oral doses are usually given 30 min before meals.

■ **Direct IV:** Give IV undiluted or dilute in 10 ml of sterile water.

### PATIENT/FAMILY TEACHING

❑ Instruct patient to take exactly as directed. If a dose is missed, take as soon as remembered unless almost time for next dose. Do not double doses.

❑ May cause drowsiness. Caution patients to avoid driving or other activities requiring alertness until response to medication is known.

❑ Instruct patient that oral rinses, sugarless gum or candy, and frequent oral hygiene may help relieve dry mouth.

❑ Caution patients that hyoscyamine impairs heat regulation. Strenuous activity in a hot environment may cause heat stroke.

❑ Instruct patient to consult health care professional before taking any OTC medications concurrently with hyoscyamine.

❑ Inform male patients with benign prostatic hypertrophy that hyoscyamine may cause urinary hesitancy and retention. Changes in urinary stream should be reported to health care professional.

### EVALUATION

**Effectiveness of therapy can be demonstrated by:** ■ Increase in heart rate ■ Dryness of mouth ■ Reversal of muscarinic effects.

**High Alert**

# HYPOGLYCEMIC AGENTS, ORAL

**glimepiride**

(glye-**me**-pye-ride)

Amaryl

**glipizide**

(**glip**-i-zide)

Glucotrol, Glucotrol XL

**glyburide**

(**glye**-byoo-ride)

{Apo-Glyburide}, DiaBeta, {Euglucon}, {Gen-Glybe}, Glynase PresTab, Micronase, {Novo-Glyburide}, {Nu-Glyburide}

*CLASSIFICATION(S):*
*Therapeutic: antidiabetics*
*Pharmacologic: sulfonylureas*

**Pregnancy Category C (glimepiride and glipizide), B (glyburide)**

## INDICATIONS

■ Control of blood glucose in adult-onset non–insulin-dependent diabetes mellitus (type 2) when diet therapy fails. Require some pancreatic function.

## ACTION

■ Lower blood glucose by stimulating the release of insulin from the pancreas and increasing the sensitivity to insulin at receptor sites ■ May also decrease hepatic glucose production. **Therapeutic Effects:** ■ Lowering of blood glucose in diabetic patients.

## PHARMACOKINETICS

**Absorption:** All agents are well absorbed after oral administration.

**Distribution:** *Glyburide*—reaches high concentrations in bile and crosses the placenta.

**Protein Binding:** *Glimepiride*–99.5%, *glipizide* 99%, *glyburide* 99%.

**Metabolism and Excretion:** All agents are mostly metabolized by the liver. *Glimepiride*—converted to a metabolite with hypoglycemic activity.

**Half-life:** *Glimepiride*—5.3 hr (range 5–9.2 hr); *glipizide*—2.1–2.6 hr; *glyburide*—10 hr.

## CONTRAINDICATIONS AND PRECAUTIONS

**Contraindicated in:** ■ Hypersensitivity ■ Cross-sensitivity with sulfonamides (including thiazide diuretics) may occur ■ Insulin-dependent patients with diabetes ■ Diabetic coma or ketoacidosis ■ Severe renal, hepatic, thyroid, or other endocrine disease ■ Uncontrolled infection, serious burns, or trauma.

**Use Cautiously in:** ■ Severe cardiovascular or hepatic disease ■ Geriatric patients (increased sensitivity; lower initial doses recommended) ■ Severe renal disease (increased risk of hypoglycemia) ■ Infection, stress, or changes in diet may alter requirements for control of blood glucose ■ Impaired thyroid, pituitary, or adrenal function ■ Malnutrition, high fever, prolonged nausea, or vomiting ■ Pregnancy or lactation (safety not established; insulin recommended during pregnancy).

## ADVERSE REACTIONS AND SIDE EFFECTS*

■ **CNS:** dizziness, drowsiness, headache, weakness ■ **GI:** constipation, cramps, diarrhea, drug-induced hepatitis, heartburn, increased appetite, nausea, vomiting ■ **Derm:** photosensitivity, rashes ■ **Endo:** hypoglycemia ■ **F and E:** hyponatremia ■ **Hemat:** APLASTIC ANEMIA, agranulocytosis, leukopenia, pancytopenia, thrombocytopenia.

## INTERACTIONS

**Drug-Drug:** ■ Ingestion of **alcohol** may result in disulfiram-like reaction ■ Effectiveness may be decreased by concurrent use of **diuretics, corticosteroids, phenothiazines, oral contraceptives, estrogens, thyroid preparations, phenytoin, nicotinic acid, sympathomimetics,** and **isoniazid** ■ **Alcohol, androgens** (testosterone), **chloramphenicol, clofibrate, guanethidine, MAO inhibitors, NSAIDs** (except diclofenac), **salicylates, sulfonamides,** and **warfarin** may increase the risk of hypoglycemia ■ Concurrent use of **warfarin** may alter the response to both agents (increased effects of both initially, then decreased activity); close monitoring recommended during any changes in dosage ■ **Beta blockers** may alter the response to oral hypoglycemic agents (increase or decrease requirements; nonselective agents may cause prolonged hypoglycemia).

**Drug-Natural Products:** ■ **Glucosamine** may worsen blood glucose control ■ **Fenugreek, chromium,** and **coenzyme Q-10** may produce additive hypoglycemic effects.

## ROUTE AND DOSAGE

❑ **Glimepiride**

■ **PO (Adults):** 1–2 mg once daily initially; may increase q 1–2 wk up to 8 mg/day (usual range 1–4 mg/day).

■ **PO (Geriatric Patients):** 1 mg/day initially

❑ **Glipizide**

■ **PO (Adults):** 5 mg/day initially, increased as needed (range 2.5–40 mg/day); XL dosage form is given once daily. Doses >15 mg/day should be given as 2 divided doses.

■ **PO (Geriatric Patients):** 2.5 mg/day initially.

□ **Glyburide**

■ **PO (Adults):** *DiaBeta/Micronase (nonmicronized)*—2.5–5 mg once daily initially (range 1.25–20 mg/day). *Glynase PresTab (micronized)*—1.5–3 mg/day initially (range 0.75–12 mg/day; doses >6 mg/day should be given as divided doses). Increments should not exceed 1.5 mg/wk.

■ **PO (Geriatric Patients):** *DiaBeta/Micronase (nonmicronized)*—1.25–2.5 mg/day initially; may be increased by 2.5 mg/day weekly. *Glynase PresTab (micronized)*—0.75–3 mg/day; may be increased by 1.5 mg/day weekly.

## AVAILABILITY

□ **Glimepiride**

■ **Tablets:** 1 mg^Rx, 2 mg^Rx, 4 mg^Rx ■ Cost: 1 mg $26.46/100, 2 mg $42.87/100, 4 mg $80.87/100.

□ **Glipizide**

■ **Tablets:** 5 mg^Rx, 10 mg^Rx ■ Cost: 5 mg $34.60/100, 10 mg $69.10/100 ■ **Extended-release tablets:** 5 mg^Rx, 10 mg^Rx ■ Cost: 5 mg $35.77/100, 10 mg $70.80/100.

□ **Glyburide**

■ **Tablets:** 1.25 mg^Rx, 2.5 mg^Rx, 5 mg^Rx ■ Cost: *DiaBeta*—$19.68/100, 2.5 mg $38.58/100, 5 mg $70.80/100; *Micronase*—1.25 mg $28.70/100, 2.5 mg $47.96; 5 mg $81.09/100; *generic* 1.25 mg $16.40-18.35/100, 2.5 mg $30.60-31.05/100, 5 mg $53.00-58.85 ■ **Micronized tablets:** 1.5 mg^Rx, 3 mg^Rx, 6 mg^Rx ■ Cost: *Glynase PresTab*—1.5 mg $42.03/100, 3 mg $71.03/100, 6 mg $112.93; *generic*—1.5 mg $31.51-35.65/100, 3 mg $53.25-60.20/100, 6 mg $89.73/100.

TIME/ACTION PROFILE (hypoglycemic activity)

|  | ONSET | PEAK | DURATION |
|---|---|---|---|
| Glimepiride | unknown | 2–3 hr | 24 hr |
| Glipizide | 15–30 min | 1–2 hr | up to 24 hr |
| Glyburide | 45–60 min | 1.5–3 hr | 24 hr |

## NURSING IMPLICATIONS

### ASSESSMENT

□ Observe patient for signs and symptoms of hypoglycemic reactions (sweating, hunger, weakness, dizziness, tremor, tachycardia, anxiety).

□ Assess patient for allergy to sulfonamides.

■ **Lab Test Considerations:** Monitor serum glucose and glycosylated hemoglobin periodically throughout therapy to evaluate effectiveness of treatment.

□ Monitor CBC periodically throughout therapy. Report decrease in blood counts promptly.

□ May cause an increase in AST, LDH, BUN, and serum creatinine.

■ **Toxicity and Overdose:** Overdose is manifested by symptoms of hypoglycemia. Mild hypoglycemia may be treated with administration of oral glucose. Severe hypoglycemia should be treated with IV D50W followed by continuous IV infusion of more dilute dextrose solution at a rate sufficient to keep serum glucose at approximately 100 mg/dl.

## POTENTIAL NURSING DIAGNOSES

■ Nutrition, imbalanced: more than body requirements (Indications).

■ Noncompliance (Patient/Family Teaching).

## IMPLEMENTATION

□ **High Alert:** Accidental administration of oral hypoglycemic agents to non-diabetic adults and children has resulted in serious harm or death. Before administering, confirm that patient is diabetic. Several oral hypoglycemic agents are subject to sound-alike or look-alike confusion: Do not confuse glipizide with glyburide. Do not confuse Glucotrol with Glucotrol XL. Do not confuse micronase (glyburide) with Micro-K (potassium).

■ **General:** Patients stabilized on a diabetic regimen who are exposed to stress, fever, trauma, infection, or surgery may require administration of insulin.

□ To convert from other oral hypoglycemic agents, gradual conversion is not required. For insulin dosage of less than 20 units/day, change to oral hypoglycemic agents can be made without gradual dosage adjustment. Patients taking 20 or more units/day should convert gradually by receiving oral agent and a 25–30% reduction in insulin dose every day or every 2nd day with gradual insulin dosage reduction as tolerated. Monitor serum or urine glucose and ketones at least 3 times/day during conversion.

■ **PO:** May be administered once in the morning or divided into 2 doses. Administer most sulfonylureas with meals to ensure best diabetic control and to minimize gastric irritation. Do not administer after last meal of the day.

❑ *Glipizide* should be taken 30 min before a meal.

❑ *Nonmicronized glyburide* should not be taken with a meal high in fat. *Micronized glyburide* cannot be substituted for *nonmicronized glyburide.* Preparations are not equivalent.

❑ Tablets may be crushed and taken with fluids if patient has difficulty swallowing.

## PATIENT/FAMILY TEACHING

❑ Instruct patient to take medication at same time each day. If a dose is missed, take as soon as remembered unless almost time for next dose. Do not take if unable to eat.

❑ Explain to patient that this medication controls hyperglycemia but does not cure diabetes. Therapy is long term.

❑ Review signs of hypoglycemia and hyperglycemia with patient. If hypoglycemia occurs, advise patient to take a glass of orange juice or 2–3 tsp of sugar, honey, or corn syrup dissolved in water and notify health care professional.

❑ Encourage patient to follow prescribed diet, medication, and exercise regimen to prevent hypoglycemic or hyperglycemic episodes.

❑ Instruct patient in proper testing of serum glucose and ketones. These tests should be closely monitored during periods of stress or illness and health care professional notified if significant changes occur.

❑ May occasionally cause dizziness or drowsiness. Caution patient to avoid driving or other activities requiring alertness until response to medication is known.

❑ Caution patient to avoid other medications, especially aspirin and alcohol, while on this therapy without consulting health care professional.

❑ Concurrent use of alcohol may cause a disulfiram-like reaction (abdominal cramps, nausea, flushing, headaches, and hypoglycemia).

❑ Insulin is the recommended method of controlling blood glucose during pregnancy. Counsel female patients to use a form of contraception other than oral contraceptives and to notify health care professional promptly if pregnancy is planned or suspected.

❑ Caution patient to use sunscreen and protective clothing to prevent photosensitivity reactions.

❑ Advise patient to inform health care professional of medication regimen before treatment or surgery.

❑ Advise patient to carry a form of sugar (sugar packets, candy) and identification describing disease process and medication regimen at all times.

❑ Advise patient to notify health care professional promptly if unusual weight gain, swelling of ankles, drowsiness, shortness of breath, muscle cramps, weakness, sore throat, rash, or unusual bleeding or bruising occurs.

❑ Emphasize the importance of routine follow-up exams.

## EVALUATION

**Effectiveness of therapy can be demonstrated by:** ■ Control of blood glucose levels without the appearance of hypoglycemic or hyperglycemic episodes.

# ibandronate

(i-**ban**-dro-nate)

Boniva

## CLASSIFICATION(S):

**Therapeutic:** bone resorption inhibitors

**Pharmacologic:** biphosphonates

**Pregnancy Category C**

## INDICATIONS

■ Treatment/prevention of postmenopausal osteoporosis.

## ACTION

■ Inhibits resorption of bone by inhibiting ostoclast activity. **Therapeutic Effects:** ■ Reversal/prevention of progression of osteoporosis with decreased fractures.

## PHARMACOKINETICS

**Absorption:** 0.6% absorbed following oral administration (significantly decreased by food).

**Distribution:** Rapidly binds to bone.

**Protein Binding:** 90.9–99.5%

**Metabolism and Excretion:** 50–60% excreted in urine; unabsorbed drug is eliminated in feces.

**Half-life:** 10–60 hr.

## CONTRAINDICATIONS AND PRECAUTIONS

**Contraindicated in:** ■ Hypersensitivity ■ Uncorrected hypocalcemia ■ Inability to stand/sit upright for at least 60 min ■ CCr <30 ml/min.

**Use Cautiously in:** ■ Geriatric patients (consider age related decreases in body mass, renal and hepatic function, concurrent disease states and drug therapy) ■ Concurrent use of NSAIDs or aspirin ■ Pregnancy (use only if potential benefit outweighs risks to mother and fetus) ■ Lactation ■ Children <18 yr (safety not established).

## ADVERSE REACTIONS AND SIDE EFFECTS*

■ **GI:** <u>diarrhea</u>, <u>dyspepsia</u>, esophagitis, esophageal/gastric ulcer ■ **MS:** <u>pain in arms/legs</u>.

## INTERACTIONS

**Drug-Drug:** ■ Calcium- aluminum- magnesium- and iron- containing products, including **antacids** ↓ absorption (ibandronate should be taken 60 min before) ■ Concurrent use of NSAIDs including **aspirin,** may ↑ risk of gastric irritation.

**Drug-Food:** ■ Milk and other foods ↓ absorption.

## ROUTE AND DOSAGE

■ **PO (Adults):** 2.5 mg once daily.

## AVAILABILITY

■ **Tablets:** 2.5 mg^Rx.

TIME/ACTION PROFILE

| | ONSET | PEAK | DURATION |
|---|---|---|---|
| PO | unknown | 0.5–2 hr | 24 hr |

# NURSING IMPLICATIONS

## ASSESSMENT

■ **Osteoporosis:** Assess patients for low bone mass before and periodically during therapy.

■ **Lab Test Considerations:** Assess serum calcium before and periodically during therapy. Hypocalcemia and vitamin D deficiency should be treated before initiating ibandronate therapy.

❑ May cause ↓ total alkaline phosphatase levels.

❑ May cause hypercholesterolemia.

## POTENTIAL NURSING DIAGNOSES

■ Injury, risk for (Indications).

## IMPLEMENTATION

■ **PO:** Administer first thing in the morning with 6–8 oz plain water 30 min before other medications, beverages, or food.

## PATIENT/FAMILY TEACHING

❑ Instruct patient on the importance of taking exactly as directed, first thing in the morning, 60 min before other medications, beverages, or food. Ibandronate should be taken with 6–8 oz plain water (mineral water, orange juice, coffee, and other beverages decrease absorption). If a dose is missed, skip dose and resume the next morning; do not double doses or take later in the day. Do not discontinue without consulting health care professional.

❑ Caution patient to remain upright for 60 min following dose to facilitate passage to stomach and minimize risk of esophageal irritation.

❑ Advise patient to eat a balanced diet and consult health care professional about the need for supplemental calcium and vitamin D. Wait at least 60 min after administration before taking supplemental calcium and vitamin D.

❑ Encourage patient to participate in regular exercise and to modify behaviors that increase the risk of osteoporosis (stop smoking, reduce alcohol consumption).

❑ Advise female patient to notify health care professional if pregnancy is planned or suspected or if she is breastfeeding.

## EVALUATION

**Effectiveness of therapy can be demonstrated by:** ▪ Prevention of or decrease in the progression of osteoporosis in postmenopausal women.

---

# ibuprofen

(eye-byoo-**proe**-fen)

{Actiprofen}, Advil, Advil Migraine Liqui-Gels, {Apo-Ibuprofen}, Children's Advil, Children's Motrin, Excedrin IB, Genpril, Haltran, Junior Strength Advil, Menadol, Medipren, Midil Maximum Strength Cramp Formula, Motrin, Motrin Drops, Motrin IB, Motrin Junior Strength, Motrin Migraine Pain, {Novo-Profen}, Nu-Ibuprofen, Nuprin, PediaCare Children's Fever

## CLASSIFICATION(S):

**Therapeutic:** antipyretics, antirheumatics, nonopioid analgesics, nonsteroidal anti-inflammatory agents
**Pharmacologic:** nonopioid analgesics

---

**Pregnancy Category B (first trimester)**

## INDICATIONS

▪ Mild to moderate pain or dysmenorrhea ▪ Inflammatory disorders including: ❑ Rheumatoid arthritis ❑ Osteoarthritis ▪ Lowering of fever.

## ACTION

▪ Inhibits prostaglandin synthesis. **Therapeutic Effects:** ▪ Decreased pain and inflammation ▪ Reduction of fever.

## PHARMACOKINETICS

**Absorption:** Well absorbed from the GI tract.
**Distribution:** Does not enter breast milk in significant amounts.
**Protein Binding:** 99%.
**Metabolism and Excretion:** Mostly metabolized by the liver; small amounts (10%) excreted unchanged by the kidneys.
**Half-life:** 2–4 hr.

## CONTRAINDICATIONS AND PRECAUTIONS

**Contraindicated in:** ▪ Hypersensitivity ▪ Cross-sensitivity may exist with other NSAIDs, including aspirin ▪ Active GI bleeding or ulcer disease ▪ Chewable tablets contain aspartame and should not be used in patients with phenylketonuria.

**Use Cautiously in:** ▪ Severe cardiovascular, renal, or hepatic disease ▪ Geriatric patients ( ↑ risk of adverse reactions; ↓ initial dose recommended) ▪ Chronic alcohol use/abuse ▪ History of ulcer disease ▪ Pregnancy (use not recommended; has been associated with persistent pulmonary hypertension in infants) ▪ Lactation (has been used safely).

## ADVERSE REACTIONS AND SIDE EFFECTS*

▪ **CNS:** headache, dizziness, drowsiness, psychic disturbances ▪ **EENT:** amblyopia, blurred vision, tinnitus ▪ **CV:** arrhythmias, edema ▪ **GI:** GI BLEEDING, HEPATITIS, constipation, dyspepsia, nausea, vomiting, abdominal discomfort ▪ **GU:** cystitis, hematuria, renal failure ▪ **Derm:** rashes ▪ **Hemat:** blood dyscrasias, prolonged bleeding time ▪ **Misc:** allergic reactions including ANAPHYLAXIS.

## INTERACTIONS

**Drug-Drug:** ■ May limit the cardioprotective effects of low-dose **aspirin** ■ Concurrent use with **aspirin** may ↓ effectiveness of ibuprofen ■ Additive adverse GI side effects with **aspirin**, other **NSAIDs, corticosteroids**, or **alcohol** ■ Chronic use with **acetaminophen** may ↑ risk of adverse renal reactions ■ May ↓ effectiveness of **diuretics** or **antihypertensives** ■ May ↑ hypoglycemic effects of **insulin** or **oral hypoglycemic agents** ■ May slightly ↑ serum **digoxin** levels ■ May ↑ serum **lithium** levels and risk of toxicity ■ ↑ risk of toxicity from **methotrexate** ■ **Probenecid** ↑ risk of toxicity from ibuprofen ■ ↑ risk of bleeding with **cefamandole, cefotetan, cefoperazone, valproic acid, plicamycin, thrombolytic agents, warfarin,** and **drugs affecting platelet function** including **clopidogrel, ticlopidine, abciximab, eptifibatide,** or **tirofiban** ■ ↑ risk of adverse hematologic reactions with **antineoplastics** or **radiation therapy** ■ ↑ risk of nephrotoxicity with **cyclosporine**.

**Drug-Natural Products:** ■ ↑ bleeding risk with **anise, arnica, chamomile, clove, dong quai, fenugreek, feverfew, garlic, ginger, ginkgo, Panax ginseng, licorice,** and others.

## ROUTE AND DOSAGE

❑ **Analgesia**

■ **PO (Adults):** *Anti-inflammatory*—400–800 mg 3–4 times daily (not to exceed 3600 mg/day). *Analgesic/antidysmenorrheal/antipyretic*—200–400 mg q 4–6 hr (not to exceed 1200 mg/day).

■ **PO (Children 6 mo–12 yr):** *Anti-inflammatory*—20–40 mg/kg/day in 3–4 divided doses (not to exceed 50 mg/kg/day). *Antipyretic*—5 mg/kg for temperature <102.5°F (39.17°C) or 10 mg/kg for higher temperatures (not to exceed 40 mg/kg/day); may be repeated q 4–6 hr.

❑ **Pediatric OTC Dosing**

■ **PO (Children 11 yr—72–95 lb):** 300 mg q 6–8 hr.

■ **PO (Children 9–10 yr—60–71 lb):** 250 mg q 6–8 hr.

■ **PO (Children 6–8 yr—48–59 lb):** 200 mg q 6–8 hr.

■ **PO (Children 4–5 yr—36–47 lb):** 150 mg q 6–8 hr.

■ **PO (Children 2–3 yr—24–35 lb):** 100 mg q 6–8 hr.

## AVAILABILITY (generic available)

■ *Tablets:* 100 mg^OTC, 200 mg^OTC, 300 mg^Rx, 400 mg^Rx, 600 mg^Rx, 800 mg^Rx ■ Cost: 100 mg $2.98/100, 200 mg $4.32/100, 300 mg $5.82/100, 400 mg $9.45/100, 600 mg $29.08/100, 800 mg $41.67/100 ■ *Capsules (liqui-gels):* 200 mg^OTC ■ *Chewable tablets (fruit, grape, orange, and citrus flavor):* 50 mg^OTC, 100 mg^OTC ■ *Liquid (berry flavor):* 100 mg/5 ml^OTC ■ *Oral suspension (fruit, berry, grape flaovr):* 100 mg/5 ml^OTC, 100 mg/2.5 ml^OTC ■ *Pediatric drops (berry flavor):* 50 mg/1.25 ml^OTC ■ decongestants^OTC, hydrocodone (Vicoprofen)^Rx. See Appendix B.

TIME/ACTION PROFILE

| | ONSET | PEAK | DURATION |
|---|---|---|---|
| PO (analgesic) | 30 min | 1–2 hr | 4–6 hr |
| PO (anti-inflammatory) | 7 days | 1–2 wk | unknown |

# NURSING IMPLICATIONS

## ASSESSMENT

■ **General Info:** Patients who have asthma, aspirin-induced allergy, and nasal polyps are at increased risk for developing hypersensitivity reactions. Assess for rhinitis, asthma, and urticaria.

■ **Pain:** Assess pain (note type, location, and intensity) prior to and 1–2 hr following administration.

■ **Arthritis:** Assess pain and range of motion prior to and 1–2 hr following administration.

■ **Fever:** Monitor temperature; note signs associated with fever (diaphoresis, tachycardia, malaise).

■ *Lab Test Considerations:* BUN, serum creatinine, CBC, and liver function tests should be evaluated periodically in patients receiving prolonged courses of therapy.

❑ Serum potassium, BUN, serum creatinine, alkaline phosphatase, LDH, AST, and ALT tests may show ↑ levels. Blood glucose, hemoglobin, and hematocrit concentrations, leukocyte and platelet counts, and CCr may be ↓.

❑ May cause prolonged bleeding time, which may persist for <1 day following discontinuation of therapy.

## POTENTIAL NURSING DIAGNOSES

■ Pain, acute (Indications).
■ Mobility, impaired physical (Indications).

## IMPLEMENTATION

■ **General:** Administration in higher than recommended doses does not provide increased effectiveness but may cause increased side effects.
❑ Coadministration with opioid analgesics may have additive analgesic effects and may permit lower opioid doses.
■ **PO:** For rapid initial effect, administer 30 min before or 2 hr after meals. May be administered with food, milk, or antacids to decrease GI irritation. Tablets may be crushed and mixed with fluids or food; 800-mg tablet can be dissolved in water.
■ **Dysmenorrhea:** Administer as soon as possible after the onset of menses. Prophylactic treatment has not been shown to be effective.

## PATIENT/FAMILY TEACHING

❑ Advise patients to take ibuprofen with a full glass of water and to remain in an upright position for 15–30 min after administration.
❑ Instruct patient to take medication as directed. Take missed doses as soon as remembered but not if almost time for next dose. Do not double doses.
❑ May cause drowsiness or dizziness. Advise patient to avoid driving or other activities requiring alertness until response to medication is known.
❑ Caution patient to avoid the concurrent use of alcohol, aspirin, acetaminophen, or other OTC medications or herbal products without consulting health care professional.
❑ Advise patient to inform health care professional of medication regimen prior to treatment or surgery.
❑ Caution patient to wear sunscreen and protective clothing to prevent photosensitivity reactions.
❑ Instruct patients not to take OTC ibuprofen preparations for more than 10 days for pain or more than 3 days for fever, and to consult

health care professional if symptoms persist or worsen.

❑ Caution patient that use of ibuprofen with 3 or more glasses of alcohol per day may increase the risk of GI bleeding.

❑ Advise patient to consult health care professional if rash, itching, visual disturbances, tinnitus, weight gain, edema, black stools, persistent headache, or influenza-like syndrome (chills, fever, muscle aches, pain) occurs.

## EVALUATION

**Effectiveness of therapy can be demonstrated by:** ■ Decrease in severity of pain ■ Improved joint mobility. Partial arthritic relief is usually seen within 7 days, but maximum effectiveness may require 1–2 wk of continuous therapy. Patients who do not respond to one NSAID may respond to another ■ Reduction in fever.

# ibutilide
(eye-**byoo**-ti-lide)
Corvert

### CLASSIFICATION(S):
***Therapeutic:*** *antiarrhythmics (class III)*

### Pregnancy Category C

## INDICATIONS

■ Rapid conversion of recent-onset atrial flutter or fibrillation to normal sinus rhythm, including management of atrial flutter or fibrillation occurring within 1 wk of coronary artery bypass or cardiac valve surgery.

## ACTION

■ Activates slow inward current of sodium in cardiac tissue, resulting in delayed repolarization, prolonged action potential duration, and increased refractoriness ■ Mildly slows sinus rate and AV conduction. **Therapeutic Effects:** ■ Conversion to normal sinus rhythm.

## PHARMACOKINETICS

**Absorption:** IV administration results in complete bioavailability.
**Distribution:** Unknown.

**Metabolism and Excretion:** Highly metabolized by the liver, 1 metabolite is active; metabolites excreted by kidneys.

**Half-life:** 6 hr (2–12 hr).

## CONTRAINDICATIONS AND PRECAUTIONS

**Contraindicated in:** ■ Hypersensitivity.

**Use Cautiously in:** ■ CHF or left ventricular dysfunction (increased risk of more serious arrhythmias during infusion) ■ Pregnancy, lactation, or children <18 yr (safety not established).

## ADVERSE REACTIONS AND SIDE EFFECTS*

■ **CNS:** headache ■ **CV:** arrhythmias ■ **GI:** nausea.

## INTERACTIONS

**Drug-Drug:** ■ **Amiodarone, disopyramide, procainamide, quinidine,** and **sotalol** should not be given concurrently or within 4 hr because of additive effects on refractoriness ■ Proarrhythmic effects may increased by **phenothiazines, tricyclic** and **tetracyclic antidepressants,** some **antihistamines,** and **histamine H$_2$-receptor blocking agents;** concurrent use should be avoided.

## ROUTE AND DOSAGE

❏ **Atrial Fibrillation/Flutter**

■ **IV (Adults ≥60 kg):** 1 mg infusion; may be repeated 10 min after end of first infusion.

■ **IV (Adults <60 kg):** 0.01 mg/kg infusion; may be repeated 10 min after end of first infusion.

❏ **Atrial Fibrillation/Futter after Cardiac Surgery**

■ **IV (Adults ≥60 kg):** 0.5 mg infusion, may be repeated once.

■ **IV (Adults <60 kg):** 0.005 mg/kg infusion, may be repeated once.

## AVAILABILITY

■ *Solution for injection:* 0.1 mg/ml in 10-ml vial$^{Rx}$.

TIME/ACTION PROFILE (antiarrhythmic effect)

| | ONSET | PEAK | DURATION |
|---|---|---|---|
| IV | within 30–90 min | unknown | up to 24 hr |

## NURSING IMPLICATIONS

### ASSESSMENT

❏ Monitor ECG continuously throughout and for 4 hr after infusion or until QT interval normalizes. Discontinue if arrhythmia terminates or if sustained ventricular tachycardia, prolonged QT, or QT develops. Ibutilide may have proarrhythmic effects. These arrhythmias may be serious and potentially life threatening. Clinicians trained to treat ventricular arrhythmias, medications, and equipment (defibrillator/cardioverter) should be available during therapy and monitoring of patient.

### POTENTIAL NURSING DIAGNOSES

■ Cardiac output, decreased (Indications).

### IMPLEMENTATION

■ **General:** Oral antiarrhythmic therapy may be instituted 4 hr after ibutilide infusion.

■ **Intermittent Infusion:** May be administered undiluted or diluted in 50 ml of 0.9% NaCl or D5W for a concentration of approximately 0.017 mg/ml. Solution, diluted or undiluted, is stable for 24 hr at room temperature or 48 hr if refrigerated.

■ *Rate:* Administer over 10 min.

■ **Additive Incompatibility:** Information unavailable; do not admix with other solutions or medications.

### PATIENT/FAMILY TEACHING

❏ Inform patient of the purpose of ibutilide.

### EVALUATION

**Clinical response to therapy can be evaluated by:** ■ Conversion of recent-onset atrial flutter or fibrillation to normal sinus rhythm.

# idarubicin

(eye-da-**roo**-bi-sin)

Idamycin

**CLASSIFICATION(S):**
*Therapeutic:* antineoplastics
*Pharmacologic:* anthracyclines

**Pregnancy Category D**

## INDICATIONS

■ Acute myelogenous leukemia in adults (with other agents).

## ACTION

■ Inhibits nucleic acid synthesis. **Therapeutic Effects:** ■ Death of rapidly replicating cells, particularly malignant ones.

## PHARMACOKINETICS

**Absorption:** IV administration results in complete bioavailability.
**Distribution:** Rapidly distributed with extensive tissue binding. High degree of cellular uptake.
**Metabolism and Excretion:** Extensive hepatic and extrahepatic metabolism. One metabolite is active (idarubicinol). Primarily eliminated via biliary excretion.
**Half-life:** 22 hr (range 4–46 hr).

## CONTRAINDICATIONS AND PRECAUTIONS

**Contraindicated in:** ■ Pregnancy or lactation.
**Use Cautiously in:** ■ Children (safety not established) ■ Patients with childbearing potential ■ Active infection ■ Decreased bone marrow reserve ■ Geriatric patients ■ Other chronic debilitating illnesses ■ Hepatic impairment (dosage reduction may be required; avoid if bilirubin ≥5 mg/dl) ■ Renal impairment ■ Pre-existing cardiac disease ■ Previous daunorubicin or doxorubicin therapy.

## ADVERSE REACTIONS AND SIDE EFFECTS*

■ **CNS:** headache, mental status changes ■ **Resp:** pulmonary toxicity, pulmonary allergic reactions ■ **CV:** ARRHYTHMIAS, CARDIOTOXICITY, CHF ■ **GI:** abdominal cramps, diarrhea, mucositis, nausea, vomiting ■ **Derm:** alopecia, photosensitivity, rashes ■ **Endo:** gonadal suppression ■ **Hemat:** BLEEDING, anemia, leukopenia, thrombo-

cytopenia ■ **Local:** phlebitis at IV site ■ **Metab:** hyperuricemia ■ **Neuro:** peripheral neuropathy ■ **Misc:** fever.

## INTERACTIONS

**Drug-Drug:** ■ ↑ myelosuppression with other **antineoplastics** or **radiation therapy** ■ May ↓ antibody response to and increase risk of adverse reactions from **live-virus vaccines**.

## ROUTE AND DOSAGE

■ **IV (Adults):** 12 mg/m² daily for 3 days in combination with cytarabine.

## AVAILABILITY (generic available)

■ *Powder for injection:* 5-mg vials^Rx, 10-mg vials^Rx.

TIME/ACTION PROFILE (effects on blood counts)

|    | ONSET   | PEAK       | DURATION |
|----|---------|------------|----------|
| IV | Unknown | 10–14 days | 21 days  |

# NURSING IMPLICATIONS

## ASSESSMENT

❏ Monitor blood pressure, pulse, respiratory rate, and temperature frequently during administration. Report significant changes.

❏ Monitor for bone marrow depression. Assess for bleeding (bleeding gums, bruising, petechiae, guaiac stools, urine, and emesis) and avoid IM injections and taking rectal temperatures if platelet count is low. Apply pressure to venipuncture sites for 10 min. Assess for signs of infection during neutropenia. Anemia may occur. Monitor for increased fatigue, dyspnea, and orthostatic hypotension.

❏ Monitor intake and output ratios. Report significant discrepancies. Encourage fluid intake of 2000–3000 ml/day. Allopurinol and alkalinization of the urine may be used to decrease serum uric acid levels and to help prevent urate stone formation.

❏ Severe and protracted nausea and vomiting may occur as early as 1 hr after therapy and may last 24 hr. Parenteral antiemetics should be administered 30–45 min prior to therapy and routinely around the clock for the next 24 hr as indicated. Monitor amount of emesis; report emesis exceeding guidelines to prevent dehydration.

❑ Monitor for development of signs of myocardial toxicity manifested by life-threatening arrhythmias, cardiomyopathy, and CHF (peripheral edema, dyspnea, rales/crackles, weight gain). Chest x-ray, ECG, echocardiography, and radionuclide angiography determinations of ejection fraction should be monitored prior to and periodically during therapy.

❑ Assess injection site frequently for redness, irritation, or inflammation. May infiltrate painlessly. If extravasation occurs, infusion must be stopped and restarted elsewhere to avoid damage to subcut tissue. Treatment of extravasation includes rest and elevation of the extremity and application of intermittent ice packs (apply for 30 min immediately and 30 min qid for 3 days). If pain, erythema, or vesication persists longer than 48 hr, immediate plastic surgery may be warranted.

■ *Lab Test Considerations:* Monitor CBC, differential, and platelet count prior to and frequently during therapy. Nadirs of leukopenia and thrombocytopenia are 10–14 days, with recovery occurring 21 days after a dose.

❑ Monitor renal and hepatic function prior to and periodically during therapy. Idarubicin may cause hyperuricemia. May also cause transient ↑ in AST, ALT, LDH, serum alkaline phosphatase, and bilirubin.

## POTENTIAL NURSING DIAGNOSES

■ Infection, risk for (Adverse Reactions).
■ Nutrition, imbalanced: less than body requirements (Adverse Reactions).

## IMPLEMENTATION

■ **General:** Do not confuse Adriamycin (doxorubicin hydrochloride) with Idamycin (idarubicin).

❑ Solution should be prepared in a biologic cabinet. Wear gloves, gown, and mask while handling medication. Discard IV equipment in specially designated containers.

❑ See cytarabine monograph for specific information on administration of cytarabine with idarubicin.

■ **Direct IV:** Reconstitute 5-mg and 10-mg vials with 5 ml and 10 ml, respectively, of 0.9% NaCl (nonbacteriostatic) for injection for a concentration of 1 mg/ml. Vial contents are under pressure; use care when inserting needle.

❑ Reconstituted medication is stable for 72 hr at room temperature and 7 days if refrigerated.

■ *Rate:* Administer each dose slowly over 10–15 min through Y-site of a free-flowing infusion of 0.9% NaCl or D5W. Tubing may be attached to a butterfly needle and injected into a large vein.

■ **Syringe Incompatibility:** ◆ heparin.

■ **Y-Site Compatibility:** ◆ amifostine ◆ amikacin ◆ aztreonam ◆ cimetidine ◆ cyclophosphamide ◆ cytarabine ◆ diphenhydramine ◆ droperidol ◆ erythromycin lactobionate ◆ filgrastim ◆ gemcitabine ◆ granisetron ◆ imipenem/cilastatin ◆ magnesium sulfate ◆ mannitol ◆ melphalan ◆ metoclopramide ◆ potassium chloride ◆ ranitidine ◆ sargramostim ◆ thiotepa ◆ vinorelbine.

■ **Y-Site Incompatibility:** ◆ acyclovir ◆ allopurinol ◆ ampicillin/sulbactam ◆ cefazolin ◆ cefepime ◆ ceftazidime ◆ clindamycin ◆ dexamethasone ◆ etoposide ◆ furosemide ◆ gentamicin ◆ heparin ◆ hydrocortisone sodium succinate ◆ lorazepam ◆ meperidine ◆ methotrexate ◆ piperacillin/tazobactam ◆ sodium bicarbonate ◆ teniposide ◆ vancomycin ◆ vincristine.

## PATIENT/FAMILY TEACHING

❑ Instruct patient to notify health care professional promptly if fever; sore throat; signs of infection; bleeding gums; bruising; petechiae; blood in stools, urine, or emesis; increased fatigue; dyspnea; or orthostatic hypotension occurs. Caution patient to avoid crowds and persons with known infections. Instruct patient to use soft toothbrush and electric razor and to avoid falls. Caution patient not to drink alcoholic beverages or take medication containing aspirin or NSAIDs, as these may precipitate gastric bleeding.

❑ Instruct patient to report pain at injection site immediately.

❑ Instruct patient to inspect oral mucosa for erythema and ulceration. If ulceration occurs, advise patient to use sponge brush, rinse mouth with water after eating and drinking, and confer with health care professional if mouth pain interferes with eating.

Further courses of idarubicin should be withheld until recovery from mucositis, and subsequent doses should be decreased by 25%. Stomatitis pain may require treatment with opioid analgesics.

❏ Advise patient that this medication may have teratogenic effects. Contraception should be practiced during and for at least 4 mo after therapy is concluded.

❏ Instruct patient to notify health care professional immediately if irregular heartbeat, shortness of breath, or swelling of lower extremities occurs.

❏ Advise patient to wear sunscreen and protective clothing to prevent photosensitivity reactions.

❏ Discuss with patient the possibility of hair loss. Explore methods of coping.

❏ Instruct patient not to receive any vaccinations without advice of health care professional.

❏ Inform patient that urine may turn a reddish color.

❏ Emphasize the need for periodic lab tests to monitor for side effects.

## EVALUATION

**Effectiveness of therapy can be demonstrated by:** ■ Improvement of hematologic status in leukemias.

## ifosfamide

(**eye**-foss-fam-ide)

Ifex

### CLASSIFICATION(S):

**Therapeutic:** antineoplastics
**Pharmacologic:** alkylating agents

### Pregnancy Category D

## INDICATIONS

■ Germ cell testicular carcinoma (with other agents) ■ Used with mesna, which prevents ifosfamide-induced hemorrhagic cystitis.

## ACTION

■ Following conversion to active compounds, interferes with DNA replication and RNA transcription, ultimately disrupting protein synthesis (cell-cycle phase–nonspecific). **Therapeutic**

**Effects:** ■ Death of rapidly replicating cells, particularly malignant ones.

## PHARMACOKINETICS

**Absorption:** Administered IV only; inactive prior to conversion to metabolites.

**Distribution:** Excreted in breast milk.

**Metabolism and Excretion:** Metabolized by the liver to active antineoplastic compounds.

**Half-life:** 15 hr.

## CONTRAINDICATIONS AND PRECAUTIONS

**Contraindicated in:** ■ Hypersensitivity ■ Pregnancy or lactation.

**Use Cautiously in:** ■ Patients with childbearing potential ■ Active infections ■ Decreased bone marrow reserve ■ Geriatric patients ■ Other chronic debilitating illness ■ Impaired renal function ■ Children.

## ADVERSE REACTIONS AND SIDE EFFECTS*

■ **CNS:** CNS toxicity (somnolence, confusion, hallucinations, coma), cranial nerve dysfunction, disorientation, dizziness ■ **CV:** cardiotoxicity ■ **GI:** nausea, vomiting, anorexia, constipation, diarrhea, hepatotoxicity ■ **GU:** hemorrhagic cystitis, dysuria, sterility, renal toxicity ■ **Derm:** alopecia ■ **Hemat:** anemia, leukopenia, thrombocytopenia ■ **Local:** phlebitis ■ **Misc:** allergic reactions.

## INTERACTIONS

**Drug-Drug:** ■ ↑ myelosuppression with other **antineoplastics** or **radiation therapy** ■ Toxicity may be ↑ by **allopurinol** or **phenobarbital** ■ May ↓ antibody response to and ↑ risk of adverse reactions from **live-virus vaccines.**

## ROUTE AND DOSAGE

❏ **Other Regimens are Used.**

■ **IV (Adults):** 1.2 g/m²/day for 5 days; coadminister with mesna. May repeat cycle q 3 wk.

## AVAILABILITY

■ **Injection:** 1- and 3-g vials$^{Rx}$. ■ In a kit with mesna.

TIME/ACTION PROFILE (effects on blood counts)

| | ONSET | PEAK | DURATION |
|---|---|---|---|
| IV | unknown | 7–14 days | 21 days |

## NURSING IMPLICATIONS

### ASSESSMENT

❑ Monitor blood pressure, pulse, respiratory rate, and temperature frequently during administration. Report significant changes.

❑ Monitor urinary output frequently during therapy. Notify physician if hematuria occurs. To reduce the risk of hemorrhagic cystitis, fluid intake should be at least 3000 ml/day for adults and 1000–2000 ml/day for children. Mesna is given concurrently to prevent hemorrhagic cystitis.

❑ Monitor neurologic status. Ifosfamide should be discontinued if severe CNS symptoms (agitation, confusion, hallucinations, unusual tiredness) occur. Symptoms usually abate within 3 days of discontinuation of ifosfamide but may persist for longer; fatalities have been reported.

❑ Assess nausea, vomiting, and appetite. Weigh weekly. Premedication with an antiemetic may be used to minimize GI effects. Adjust diet as tolerated.

❑ Monitor for bone marrow depression. Assess for bleeding (bleeding gums, bruising, petechiae, guaiac stools, urine, and emesis) and avoid IM injections and taking rectal temperatures if platelet count is low. Apply pressure to venipuncture sites for 10 min. Assess for signs of infection during neutropenia. Anemia may occur. Monitor for increased fatigue, dyspnea, and orthostatic hypotension.

❑ **Lab Test Considerations:** Monitor CBC, differential, and platelet count prior to and periodically during therapy. Withhold dose and notify physician if WBC <2000/mm³ or platelet count is <50,000/mm³. Nadir of leukopenia and thrombocytopenia occurs within 7–14 days and usually recovers within 21 days of therapy.

❑ Urinalysis should be evaluated before each dose. Withhold dose and notify physician if

urinalysis shows >10 RBCs per high-power field.

❑ May cause ↑ in liver enzymes and serum bilirubin.

❑ Monitor AST, ALT, serum alkaline phosphatase, bilirubin, and LDH prior to and periodically during therapy. Ifosfamide may cause ↑ in liver enzymes and serum bilirubin.

❑ Monitor BUN, serum creatinine, phosphate, and potassium periodically during therapy.

## POTENTIAL NURSING DIAGNOSES

■ Infection, risk for (Side Effects).
■ Body image, disturbed (Side Effects).

## IMPLEMENTATION

■ **General:** Solution should be prepared in a biologic cabinet. Wear gloves, gown, and mask while handling IV medication. Discard IV equipment in specially designated containers.

■ **IV:** Prepare solution by diluting each 1-g vial with 20 ml of sterile water or bacteriostatic water for injection containing parabens. Use solution prepared without bacteriostatic water within 6 hr. Solution prepared with bacteriostatic water is stable for 1 wk at 30°C or 6 wk at 5°C.

■ **Intermittent Infusion:** May be further diluted to a concentration of 0.6 to 20 mg/ml in D5W, 0.9% NaCl, LR, or sterile water for injection.

■ **Rate:** Administer over at least 30 min.

■ **Syringe Compatibility:** ◆ epirubicin ◆ mesna.

■ **Continuous Infusion:** Has also been administered as a continuous infusion over 72 hr.

■ **Y-Site Compatibility:** ◆ allopurinol ◆ amifostine ◆ amphotericin B cholesteryl sulfate ◆ aztreonam ◆ doxorubicin liposome ◆ etoposide phosphate ◆ filgrastim ◆ fludarabine ◆ gatifloxacin ◆ gemcitabine ◆ granisetron ◆ linezolid ◆ melphalan ◆ ondansetron ◆ paclitaxel ◆ piperacillin/tazobactam ◆ propofol ◆ sargramostim ◆ sodium bicarbonate ◆ teniposide ◆ thiotepa ◆ topotecan ◆ vinorelbine.

■ **Y-Site Incompatibility:** ◆ cefepime ◆ methotrexate.

---

{ } = Available in Canada only.
*CAPITALS indicates life-threatening; <u>underlines</u> indicate most frequent.

■ **Additive Compatibility:** ◆ carboplatin ◆ cisplatin ◆ epirubicin ◆ etoposide ◆ fluorouracil ◆ mesna.

## PATIENT/FAMILY TEACHING

❑ Emphasize need for adequate fluid intake throughout therapy. Patient should void frequently to decrease bladder irritation from metabolites excreted by the kidneys. Notify health care professional immediately if hematuria is noted.

❑ Instruct patient to notify health care professional promptly if fever; chills; cough; hoarseness; sore throat; signs of infection; lower back or side pain; painful or difficult urination; bleeding gums; bruising; petechiae; blood in urine, stool, or emesis; or confusion occurs.

❑ Caution patient to avoid crowds and persons with known infections. Instruct patient to use soft toothbrush and electric razor and to avoid falls. Patients should also be cautioned not to drink alcoholic beverages or to take products containing aspirin or NSAIDs, as these may precipitate GI hemorrhage.

❑ Review with patient the need for contraception during therapy.

❑ Discuss with patient the possibility of hair loss. Explore methods of coping.

❑ Instruct patient not to receive any vaccinations without advice of health care professional; ifosfamide may decrease antibody response to and increase risk of adverse reactions from live-virus vaccines.

## EVALUATION

**Effectiveness of therapy can be demonstrated by:** ■ Decrease in size or spread of malignant germ cell testicular carcinoma.

---

High Alert

# imatinib

(i-**mat**-i-nib)

Gleevec

*CLASSIFICATION(S):*

***Therapeutic:*** *antineoplastics*
***Pharmacologic:*** *enzyme inhibitors*

**Pregnancy Category D**

## INDICATIONS

■ Chronic myeloid leukemia (CML) in blast crisis, accelerated phase, or in chronic phase after failure of interferon-alpha treatment ■ Kit (CD117) positive Metastatic/unresectable malignant gastrointestinal stomal tumors (GIST) ■ Pediatric patients with Philadelphia chromosome positive chronic myeloid leukemia after failure of bone marrow transplant or resistance to interferon-alpha.

## ACTION

■ Inhibits kinases which may be produced by malignant cell lines. **Therapeutic Effects:** ■ Inhibits production of malignant cell lines with decreased proliferation of leukemic cells in CML and malignant cells in GIST.

## PHARMACOKINETICS

**Absorption:** Well absorbed (98%) following oral administration.

**Distribution:** Unknown.

**Protein Binding:** 95%

**Metabolism and Excretion:** Mostly metabolized by the CYP3A4 enzyme system to N-demethyl imatinib, which is as active as imatinib. Excreted mostly in feces as metabolites. 5% excreted unchanged in urine.

**Half-life:** *Imatinib*—18 hr; *N-desmethyl imatinib*—40 hr.

## CONTRAINDICATIONS AND PRECAUTIONS

**Contraindicated in:** ■ Hypersensitivity ■ Pregnancy ■ Lactation.

**Use Cautiously in:** ■ Hepatic impairment (dosage reduction recommended if bilirubin >3 times normal or liver transaminases >5 times normal) ■ Geriatric patients (increased risk of edema) ■ Children <yr (safety not established).

## ADVERSE REACTIONS AND SIDE EFFECTS*

■ **CNS:** fatigue, headache, weakness ■ **Resp:** cough, dyspnea, epistaxis, nasopharyngitis, pneumonia ■ **GI:** HEPATOTOXICITY, abdominal pain, anorexia, constipation, diarrhea, dyspepsia, nausea, vomiting ■ **Derm:** petechiae, pruritus, skin rash ■ **F and E:** edema (including pleural effusion, pericardial infusion, anasarca, superficial edema and fluid retention), hypokalemia ■ **Hemat:** BLEEDING, NEUTROPENIA, THROMBOCYTOPENIA ■ **Metab:** weight gain ■ **MS:** arthralgia, muscle cramps, musculoskeletal pain, myalgia ■ **Misc:** fever, night sweats.

## INTERACTIONS

**Drug-Drug:** ■ Blood levels and effects are ↑ by concurrent **ketoconazole** ■ Blood levels and effects may be ↓ by **phenytoin** ■ ↑ blood levels of **simvastatin** ■ Imatinib inhibits the following enzyme systems: CYP2C9, CYP2D6, CYP3A4/5 and may be expected to alter the effects of other drugs metabolized by these systems.

## ROUTE AND DOSAGE

❑ **Chronic myeloid leukemia**

■ **PO (Adults):** *Chronic phase*—400 mg once daily, may be increased to 600 mg once daily; *accelerated phase or blast crisis*—600 mg once daily; may be increased to 800 mg/day given as 400 mg twice daily based on response and circumstances.

❑ **Hepatic Impairment**

■ **PO (Adults):** 300 mg once daily, may be increased to 400 mg once daily.

■ **PO (Children ≥ 3 yr):** 260 mg/m²/day; may be increased up to 340 mg/m²/day in 1–2 divided doses.

❑ **Hepatic Impairment**

■ **PO (Children):** 200 mg/m²/day; may be increased up to 260 mg/m²/day in 1–2 divided doses.

❑ **Gastrointestinal stromal tumors**

■ **PO (Adults):** 400 mg/day or 600 mg/day as a single dose.

## AVAILABILITY

■ *Tablets:* 100 mg^Rx, 400 mg^Rx ■Cost: 100 mg 2044.76/100, 400 mg 2453.70/30.

TIME/ACTION PROFILE (blood levels of imatinib)

| | ONSET | PEAK | DURATION |
|---|---|---|---|
| PO | unknown | 2–4 hr | 24 hr |

## NURSING IMPLICATIONS

### ASSESSMENT

❑ Monitor patient for fluid retention. Weigh regularly, and assess for signs of pleural effu-

sion, pericardial effusion, pulmonary edema, ascites (dyspnea, periorbital edema, swelling in feet and ankles, weight gain). Unexpected weight gain should be evaluated. Edema is usually managed with diuretics. General fluid retention is usually dose related, more common in accelerated phase or blast crisis, and is more common in the elderly. Treatment usually involves diuretics, supportive therapy, and interruption of imatinib.

❑ Monitor vital signs; may cause fever.

■ *Lab Test Considerations:* Monitor liver function before and monthly during treatment or when clinically indicated. May cause ↑ transamininases and bilirubin which usually lasts 1 wk and may require dose reduction or interruption. If bilirubin is >3 times the upper limit of normal or tramsaminases are >5 times the upper limit of normal withhold dose until bilirubin levels return to <1.5 times the upper limit of normal and transaminase levels to <2.5 times the upper limit of normal. Treatment may then be continued at reduced levels (patients on 400 mg/day should receive 300 mg/day and patients receiving 600 mg/day should receive 400 mg/day).

❑ Monitor CBC weekly for the first month, biweekly for the second month, and periodically during therapy. May cause neutropenia and thrombocytopenia, usually lasting 2–3 wk or 3–4 wk, respectively, and anemia. Usually requires dose reduction, but may require discontinuation. (see Implementation)

❑ May cause hypokalemia.

## POTENTIAL NURSING DIAGNOSES

■ Injury, risk for (Adverse Reactions).

## IMPLEMENTATION

❑ *High Alert:* Fatalities have occurred with incorrect administration of chemotherapeutic agents. Before administering, clarify all ambiguous orders; double check single, daily, and course-of-therapy dose limits; have second practitioner independently double check original order and dose calculations. Therapy should be initiated by physician experienced in the treatment of patients with chronic myeloid leukemia.

■ **General:** Patients requiring anticoagulation should receive low-molecular-weight or standard heparin, not warfarin.

❑ Treatment should be continued as long as patient continues to benefit.

■ **PO:** Administer with food and a full glass of water to minimize GI irritation.

❑ Tablets may be dispersed in water or apple juice (50 ml for the 100 mg and 100 ml for the 400 mg tablet) and stirred with a spoon for patients unable to swallow pills. Administer immediately after suspension.

❑ Patients receiving *chronic phase* treatment who develop an ANC <1.0 × 10⁹/L and/or platelets <50 × 10⁹L should stop imatinib until ANC ≥1.5 × 10⁹/L and platelets are ≥75 × 10⁹/L. Then resume imitinib treatment at 400 mg/day. If recurrence of decreased ANC and platelet levels occurs repeat dose reduction and resume at 300 mg/day when ANC and platelets are at above levels.

❑ Patients receiving accelerated phase and blast crisis treatment who develop an ANC <0.5 × 10⁹/L and/or platelets <10 × 10⁹/L should determine if cytopenia is related to leukemia via marrow aspirate or biopsy. If cytopenia is unrelated to leukemia, reduce dose to 400 mg/day. If cytopenia persists for 2 wks, reduce dose to 300 mg/day. If cytopenia persists for 4 wks and is still unrelated to leukemia, stop imatinib until ANC ≥1 × 10⁹/L and platelets are ≥20 × 10⁹/L. Then resume imatinib treatment at 300 mg/day.

## PATIENT/FAMILY TEACHING

❑ Explain purpose of imatinib to patient.

## EVALUATION

**Clinical response to therapy can be evaluated by:** ■ Decrease in production of leukemic cells in patients with CML and malignant cells in GIST.

---

# imipenem/cilastatin

(i-me-**pen**-em/sye-la-**stat**-in)
Primaxin

**CLASSIFICATION(S):**
**Therapeutic:** *anti-infectives*
**Pharmacologic:** *carbapenems*

**Pregnancy Category C**

---

## INDICATIONS

■ Treatment of: ❑ Lower respiratory tract infections ❑ Urinary tract infections ❑ Abdominal infections ❑ Gynecologic infections ❑ Skin and skin structure infections ❑ Bone and joint infections ❑ Bacteremia ❑ Endocarditis ❑ Polymicrobic infections.

## ACTION

■ Imipenem binds to the bacterial cell wall, resulting in cell death ■ Combination with cilastatin prevents renal inactivation of imipenem, resulting in high urinary concentrations ■ Imipenem resists the actions of many enzymes that degrade most other penicillins and penicillin-like anti-infectives. **Therapeutic Effects:** ■ Bactericidal action against susceptible bacteria. **Spectrum:** ■ Spectrum is broad ■ Active against most gram-positive aerobic cocci: ❑ *Streptococcus pneumoniae* ❑ Group A beta-hemolytic streptococci ❑ *Enterococcus* ❑ *Staphylococcus aureus* ■ Active against many gram-negative bacillary organisms: ❑ *Escherichia coli* ❑ *Klebsiella* ❑ *Acinetobacter* ❑ *Proteus* ❑ *Serratia* ❑ *Pseudomonas aeruginosa* ■ Also displays activity against: ❑ *Salmonella* ❑ *Shigella* ❑ *Neisseria gonorrhoeae* ❑ Numerous anaerobes.

## PHARMACOKINETICS

**Absorption:** Well absorbed after IM administration (imipenem 95%, cilastatin 75%). IV administration results in complete bioavailability.

**Distribution:** Widely distributed. Crosses the placenta; enters breast milk.

**Metabolism and Excretion:** *Imipenem and cilastatin*—70% excreted unchanged by the kidneys.

**Half-life:** *Imipenem and cilastatin*—1 hr (prolonged in renal impairment).

## CONTRAINDICATIONS AND PRECAUTIONS

**Contraindicated in:** ■ Hypersensitivity ■ Cross-sensitivity may occur with penicillins and cephalosporins.

**Use Cautiously in:** ■ Previous history of multiple hypersensitivity reactions ■ Seizure disorders ■ Geriatric patients ■ Renal impairment (dosage reduction required if CCr ≤70 ml/min/1.73 m²) ■ Pregnancy, lactation, or children (safety not established).

## ADVERSE REACTIONS AND SIDE EFFECTS*

■ **CNS:** SEIZURES, dizziness, somnolence ■ **CV:** hypotension ■ **GI:** PSEUDOMEMBRANOUS COLITIS, diarrhea, nausea, vomiting ■ **Derm:** rash, pruritus, sweating, urticaria ■ **Hemat:** eosinophilia ■ **Local:** phlebitis at IV site ■ **Misc:** allergic reaction including ANAPHYLAXIS, fever, superinfection.

## INTERACTIONS

**Drug-Drug:** ■ Do not admix with **aminoglycosides** (inactivation may occur) ■ **Probenecid** decreases renal excretion and increases blood levels ■ Increased risk of seizures with **ganciclovir** or **cyclosporine** (avoid concurrent use of ganciclovir).

## ROUTE AND DOSAGE

■ **IV (Adults):** *Mild infections*—250–500 mg q 6 hr. *Moderate infections*—500 mg q 6–8 hr *or* 1 g q 8 hr. *Serious infections*—500 mg q 6 hr to 1 g q 6–8 hr.

■ **IV (Children ≥3 mo [non-CNS infections]):** 15–25 mg/kg q 6 hr; higher doses have been used in older children with cystic fibrosis.

■ **IV (Children 4 wk–3 mo):** 25 mg/kg q 6 hr.

■ **IV (Children 1–4 wk):** 25 mg/kg q 8 hr.

■ **IV (Children <1 wk):** 25 mg/kg q 12 hr.

■ **IM (Adults):** 500–750 mg q 12 hr.

■ **IM (Children):** 10–15 mg/kg q 6 hr.

❑ **Renal Impairment**

■ **IV (Adults):** If dose for normal renal function is 1 g/day: *CCr 41–70 ml/min*—125–250 mg q 6–8 hr, *CCr 21–40 ml/min*—125–250 mg q 8–12 hr, *CCr 6–20 ml/min*—125–250 mg q 12 hr; **if dose for normal renal function is 1.5 g/day:** *CCr 41–70 ml/min*—125–250 mg q 6–8 hr, *CCr 21–40 ml/min*—125–250 mg q 8–12 hr, *CCr 6–20 ml/min*—125–250 mg q 12 hr; **if dose for normal renal function is 2 g/day:** *CCr 41–70 ml/min*—125–500 mg q 6–8 hr, *CCr 21–40 ml/min*—125–250 mg q 8–12 hr, *CCr 6–20 ml/min*—125–250 mg q 12 hr; **if dose for normal renal function is 3 g/day:** *CCr 41–70 ml/min*—250–500 mg q 6–8 hr, *CCr 21–40 ml/min*—250–500 mg q 6–8 hr, *CCr 6–20 ml/*

*min*—250–500 mg q 12 hr; **if dose for normal renal function is 4 g/day:** *CCr 41–70 ml/min*—250–750 mg q 6–8 hr, *CCr 21–40 ml/min*—250–500 mg q 6–8 hr, *CCr 6–20 ml/min*—250 –250 mg q 12 hr

## AVAILABILITY

■ ***Powder for IV injection:*** 250 mg imipenem/250 mg cilastatin[Rx], 500 mg imipenem/500 mg cilastatin[Rx] ■ Cost: 250 mg $397.15/25 vials, 500 mg $792.53/25 vials ■ ***Powder for IM injection:*** 500 mg imipenem/500 mg cilastatin[Rx], 750 mg imipenem/750 mg cilastatin[Rx].

TIME/ACTION PROFILE (blood levels)

| | ONSET | PEAK | DURATION |
|---|---|---|---|
| IM | rapid | 1–2 hr | 12 hr |
| IV | rapid | end of infusion | 6–8 hr |

# NURSING IMPLICATIONS

## ASSESSMENT

❑ Assess patient for infection (vital signs; appearance of wound, sputum, urine, and stool; WBC) at beginning of and throughout therapy.

❑ Obtain a history before initiating therapy to determine previous use of and reactions to penicillins. Persons with a negative history of penicillin sensitivity may still have an allergic response.

❑ Obtain specimens for culture and sensitivity before initiating therapy. First dose may be given before receiving results.

❑ Observe patient for signs and symptoms of anaphylaxis (rash, pruritus, laryngeal edema, wheezing). Discontinue the drug and notify the physician immediately if these occur. Have epinephrine, an antihistamine, and resuscitative equipment close by in the event of an anaphylactic reaction.

■ ***Lab Test Considerations:*** BUN, AST, ALT, LDH, serum alkaline phosphatase, bilirubin, and creatinine may be transiently increased.

❑ Hemoglobin and hematocrit concentrations may be decreased.

❑ May cause positive direct Coombs' test.

## POTENTIAL NURSING DIAGNOSES

■ Infection, risk for (Indications, Side Effects).

## IMPLEMENTATION

■ **General:** Do not confuse imipenem with omnipen.

■ **IM:** Reconstitute 500-mg vial with 2 ml and 750-mg vial with 3 ml of lidocaine without epinephrine. Shake well to form a suspension. Withdraw and inject entire contents of vial IM.

■ **Intermittent Infusion:** Reconstitute each 250- or 500-mg vial with 10 ml of compatible diluent and shake well. Transfer the resulting solution to not less than 100 ml of compatible diluent. Add an additional 10 ml to each previously reconstituted vial and shake well to ensure all medication is used. Transfer the remaining contents of the vial to the infusion container.

❏ Reconstitute 120-ml infusion bottles with 100 ml of a compatible diluent. Shake well until clear.

❏ *Compatible diluents* include 0.9% NaCl, D5W, D10W, D5/0.2% sodium bicarbonate, D5/0.9% NaCl, D5/0.45% NaCl, D5/0.225% NaCl, or mannitol 2.5%, 5%, or 10%. Solution may range from clear to yellow in color. Do not administer cloudy solutions. Solution is stable for 4 hr at room temperature and 24 hr if refrigerated.

■ *Rate:* Administer each 250- or 500-mg dose over 20–30 min and each 1-g dose over 40–60 min. Administer over 20–30 min for pediatric patients. Do not administer direct IV.

❏ Rapid infusion may cause nausea, vomiting, unusual tiredness or weakness, dizziness, or sweating. If these symptoms develop, slow infusion. Discontinuation of medication may be necessary.

■ **Y-Site Compatibility:** ◆ acyclovir ◆ aztreonam ◆ cisatracurium ◆ cefepime ◆ diltiazem ◆ docetaxel ◆ famotidine ◆ fludarabine ◆ foscarnet ◆ gatifloxacin ◆ granisetron ◆ idarubicin ◆ insulin ◆ linezolid ◆ melphalan ◆ methotrexate ◆ ondansetron ◆ propofol ◆ remifentanil ◆ tacrolimus ◆ teniposide ◆ thiotepa ◆ vinorelbine ◆ zidovudine.

■ **Y-Site Incompatibility:** ◆ allopurinol ◆ amphotericin B cholesterylsulfate ◆ fluconazole ◆ gemcitabine ◆ lorazepam ◆ meperidine ◆ midazolam ◆ sargramostim ◆ sodium bicarbonate.

■ **Additive Incompatibility:** May be inactivated if administered concurrently with aminoglycosides. If administered concurrently, administer in separate sites, if possible, at least 1 hr apart. If second site is unavailable, flush lines between medications.

## PATIENT/FAMILY TEACHING

❏ Advise patient to report the signs of superinfection (black, furry overgrowth on the tongue; vaginal itching or discharge; loose or foul-smelling stools) and allergy. Consult health care professional before treating with antidiarrheals.

❏ Caution patient to notify health care professional if fever and diarrhea occur, especially if stool contains blood, pus, or mucus. Advise patient not to treat diarrhea without consulting health care professional. May occur up to several weeks after discontinuation of medication.

## EVALUATION

**Clinical response to therapy can be evaluated by:** ■ Resolution of the signs and symptoms of infection. Length of time for complete resolution depends on the organism and site of infection.

# imipramine

(im-**ip**-ra-meen)

{Apo-Imipramine}, {Impril}, Norfranil, {Novopramine}, Tipramine, Tofranil, Tofranil PM

## CLASSIFICATION(S):

***Therapeutic:*** *antidepressants*
***Pharmacologic:*** *tricyclic antidepressants*

**Pregnancy Category C**

## INDICATIONS

■ Various forms of depression (with psychotherapy) ■ Enuresis in children. **Unlabeled uses:** ■ Adjunct in the management of chronic pain, incontinence (in adults), vascular headache prophylaxis, and cluster headache.

## ACTION

■ Potentiates the effect of serotonin and norepinephrine ■ Has significant anticholinergic properties. **Therapeutic Effects:** ■ Antidepressant action that develops slowly over several weeks.

## PHARMACOKINETICS

**Absorption:** Well absorbed from the GI tract. **Distribution:** Widely distributed. Probably crosses the placenta and enters breast milk. **Protein Binding:** 89–95%.

**Metabolism and Excretion:** Extensively metabolized by the liver, mostly on first pass; some conversion to active compounds. Undergoes enterohepatic recirculation and secretion into gastric juices.

**Half-life:** 8–16 hr.

## CONTRAINDICATIONS AND PRECAUTIONS

**Contraindicated in:** ■ Hypersensitivity ■ Cross-sensitivity with other antidepressants may occur ■ Narrow-angle glaucoma ■ Hypersensitivity to tartrazine or sulfites (in some preparations) ■ Pregnancy and lactation.

**Use Cautiously in:** ■ Geriatric patients (more susceptible to adverse reactions) ■ Pre-existing cardiovascular disease ■ Geriatric men with prostatic hyperplasia (more susceptible to urinary retention) ■ Seizures or history of seizure disorder.

## ADVERSE REACTIONS AND SIDE EFFECTS*

■ **CNS:** <u>drowsiness</u>, <u>fatigue</u>, agitation, confusion, hallucinations, insomnia ■ **EENT:** <u>blurred vision</u>, <u>dry eyes</u> ■ **CV:** ARRHYTHMIAS, <u>hypotension</u>, ECG changes ■ **GI:** <u>constipation</u>, <u>dry mouth</u>, nausea, paralytic ileus ■ **GU:** urinary retention ■ **Derm:** photosensitivity ■ **Endo:** gynecomastia ■ **Hemat:** blood dyscrasias.

## INTERACTIONS

**Drug-Drug:** ■ May cause hypotension, tachycardia, and potentially fatal reactions when used with **MAO inhibitors** (avoid concurrent use—discontinue 2 wk prior to imipramine) ■ Concurrent use with **SSRI antidepressants** may result in increased toxicity and should be avoided (**fluoxetine** should be stopped 5 wk before) ■ Concurrent use with **clonidine** may result in hypertensive crisis and should be avoided ■ Imipramine is metabolized in the liver by the cytochrome P450 2D6 enzyme and

its action may be affected by drugs that compete for metabolism by this enzyme including **other antidepressants, phenothiazines, carbamazepine, class 1C antiarrhythmics (propafenone, flecainide)**; when used concurrently, dosage reduction of one or the other or both may be necessary. Concurrent use of other drugs that inhibit the activity of the enzyme, including **cimetidine, quinidine, amiodarone,** and **ritonavir,** may result in increased effects of imipramine ■ May prevent the therapeutic response to **guanethidine** ■ Concurrent use with **levodopa** may result in delayed/decreased absorption of levodopa or hypertension ■ Blood levels and effects may be decreased by **rifamycins** ■ Concurrent use with **sparfloxacin** increases the risk of adverse cardiovascular reactions ■ Additive CNS depression with other CNS **depressants** including **alcohol, antihistamines, clonidine, opioid analgesics,** and **sedative/hypnotics** ■ **Barbiturates** may alter blood levels and effects ■ **Adrenergic** and **anticholinergic** side effects may be additive with other **agents having these properties** ■ **Phenothiazines** or **oral contraceptives** increase levels and may cause toxicity ■ **Cigarette smoking (nicotine)** may increase metabolism and alter effects.

**Drug-Natural Products:** ■ Concomitant use of **kava, valerian, skullcap, chamomile,** or **hops** can increase CNS depression ■ Increased anticholinergic effects with **angel's trumpet, jimson weed,** and **scopolia.**

## ROUTE AND DOSAGE

- ■ **PO (Adults):** 25–50 mg 3–4 times daily (not to exceed 300 mg/day); total daily dose may be given at bedtime.
- ■ **PO (Geriatric Patients):** 25 mg at bedtime initially, up to 100 mg/day in divided doses.
- ■ **PO (Children >12 yr):** *Antidepressant—* 25–50 mg/day in divided doses (not to exceed 100 mg/day).
- ■ **PO (Children 6–12 yr):** *Antidepressant—* 10–30 mg/day in 2 divided doses.
- ■ **PO (Children >6 yr):** *Enuresis—*25 mg once daily 1 hr before bedtime; increase if necessary by 25 mg at weekly intervals to 50 mg in children <12 yr, up to 75 mg in children >12 yr.

■ **IM (Adults):** Up to 100 mg/day in divided doses (not to exceed 300 mg/day).

## AVAILABILITY (generic available)

■ **Tablets:** 10 mg$^{Rx}$, 25 mg$^{Rx}$, 50 mg$^{Rx}$, {75 mg$^{Rx}$} ■Cost: *Tofranil*—10 mg $34.89/100, 25 mg $56.82/100, 50 mg $100.84/100; *generic*—10 mg $5.92/100, 25 mg $7.84/100, 50 mg $10.83/100 ■ **Capsules:** 75 mg$^{Rx}$, 100 mg$^{Rx}$, 125 mg$^{Rx}$, 150 mg$^{Rx}$ ■ **Injection:** 12.5 mg/ml$^{Rx}$.

TIME/ACTION PROFILE (antidepressant effect)

| | ONSET | PEAK | DURATION |
|---|---|---|---|
| PO, IM | hours | 2–6 wk | weeks |

# NURSING IMPLICATIONS

## ASSESSMENT

■ **General Info:** Monitor blood pressure and pulse rate prior to and during initial therapy.

❑ Monitor baseline and periodic ECGs in elderly patients or patients with heart disease and before increasing dosage with children treated for enuresis. May cause prolonged PR and QT intervals and may flatten T waves.

■ **Depression:** Assess mental status frequently. Confusion, agitation, and hallucinations may occur during initiation of therapy and may require dosage reduction. Monitor mood changes. Assess for suicidal tendencies, especially during early therapy. Restrict amount of drug available to patient.

■ **Enuresis:** Assess frequency of bedwetting throughout therapy.

■ **Pain:** Assess location, duration, and severity of pain periodically throughout therapy.

■ **Lab Test Considerations:** Assess leukocyte and differential blood counts and renal and hepatic functions prior to and periodically during prolonged or high-dose therapy.

❑ Serum levels may be monitored in patients who fail to respond to usual therapeutic dose. Therapeutic plasma concentration range for depression is 150–300 ng/ml.

❑ May cause alterations in blood glucose levels.

■ **Toxicity and Overdose:** Symptoms of acute overdose include disturbed concentration, confusion, restlessness, agitation, sei-zures, drowsiness, mydriasis, arrhythmias, fever, hallucinations, vomiting, and dyspnea.

❑ Treatment of overdose includes gastric lavage, activated charcoal, and a stimulant cathartic. Maintain respiratory and cardiac function (monitor ECG for at least 5 days) and temperature. Medications may include digoxin for CHF, antiarrhythmics, and anticonvulsants.

## POTENTIAL NURSING DIAGNOSES

■ Coping, ineffective (Indications).

■ Urinary elimination, impaired (Indications).

## IMPLEMENTATION

■ **General:** Do not confuse imipramine with desipramine.

❑ Dose increases should be made at bedtime because of sedation. Dose titration is a slow process; may take weeks to months. May be given as a single dose at bedtime to minimize sedation during the day.

■ **PO:** Administer medication with or immediately following a meal to minimize gastric irritation.

■ **IM:** May be slightly yellow or red in color. Crystals may develop if solution is cool; place ampule under warm running water for 1 min to dissolve.

## PATIENT/FAMILY TEACHING

■ **General Info:** Instruct patient to take medication exactly as directed. If a dose is missed, take as soon as possible unless almost time for next dose; if regimen is a single dose at bedtime, do not take in the morning because of side effects. Advise patient that drug effects may not be noticed for at least 2 wk. Abrupt discontinuation may cause nausea, vomiting, diarrhea, headache, trouble sleeping with vivid dreams, and irritability.

❑ May cause drowsiness and blurred vision. Caution patient to avoid driving and other activities requiring alertness until response to drug is known.

❑ Instruct patient to notify health care professional if visual changes occur. Inform patient that periodic glaucoma testing may be needed during long-term therapy.

❑ Caution patient to change positions slowly to minimize orthostatic hypotension.

❑ Advise patient to avoid alcohol or other CNS depressant drugs during therapy and for at least 3–7 days after therapy has been discontinued.

◻ Instruct patient to notify health care professional if urinary retention occurs or if dry mouth or constipation persists. Sugarless candy or gum may diminish dry mouth and an increase in fluid intake or bulk may prevent constipation. If symptoms persist, dose reduction or discontinuation may be necessary. Consult health care professional if dry mouth persists for more than 2 wk.

◻ Caution patient to use sunscreen and protective clothing to prevent photosensitivity reactions.

◻ Inform patient of need to monitor dietary intake, as possible increase in appetite may lead to undesired weight gain. Inform patient that increased amounts of riboflavin in the diet may be required; consult health care professional.

◻ Advise patient to notify health care professional of medication regimen prior to treatment or surgery.

◻ Therapy for depression is usually prolonged. Emphasize the importance of follow-up exams to evaluate progress.

■ **Children:** Inform parents that the side effects most likely to occur include nervousness, insomnia, unusual tiredness, and mild nausea and vomiting. Notify health care professional if these symptoms become pronounced.

◻ Advise parents to keep medication out of reach of children to prevent inadvertent overdose.

## EVALUATION

**Effectiveness of therapy can be demonstrated by:** ■ Increased sense of well-being ◻ Renewed interest in surroundings ◻ Increased appetite ◻ Improved energy level ◻ Improved sleep in patients treated for depression. Patient may require 2–6 wk of therapy before full therapeutic effects of medication are noticeable ■ Control of bedwetting in children >6 yr ■ Decrease in chronic neurogenic pain.

---

**High Alert**

# inamrinone
(in-**am**-ri-none)
Inocor

**CLASSIFICATION(S):**
*Therapeutic: inotropics*
*Pharmacologic: bipyridines*

**Pregnancy Category C**

## INDICATIONS

■ Short-term treatment of CHF unresponsive to digoxin, diuretics, and vasodilators.

## ACTION

■ Increases myocardial contractility ■ Decreases preload and afterload by a direct dilating effect on vascular smooth muscle. **Therapeutic Effects:** ■ Increased cardiac output (inotropic effect).

## PHARMACOKINETICS

**Absorption:** IV administration results in complete bioavailability.

**Distribution:** Unknown.

**Metabolism and Excretion:** 50% metabolized by the liver; 10–40% excreted unchanged by the kidneys.

**Half-life:** 3.6–5.8 hr (increased in CHF).

## CONTRAINDICATIONS AND PRECAUTIONS

**Contraindicated in:** ■ Hypersensitivity to inamrinone or bisulfites ■ Idiopathic hypertrophic subaortic stenosis.

**Use Cautiously in:** ■ Atrial fibrillation or flutter ■ Recent aggressive diuretic therapy (correct fluid and electrolyte disorders before administering inamrinone) ■ Thrombocytopenia (platelets <100,000/mm³) ■ Renal impairment (may require dosage adjustment) ■ Geriatric patients (age-related decline in renal function may require dosage adjustment) ■ Pregnancy, lactation, or children (safety not established).

---

## ADVERSE REACTIONS AND SIDE EFFECTS*

■ **Resp:** dyspnea ■ **CV:** <u>arrhythmias</u>, <u>hypotension</u> ■ **GI:** diarrhea, hepatotoxicity, nausea, vomiting ■ **F and E:** hypokalemia ■ **Hemat:** <u>thrombocytopenia</u> ■ **Misc:** <u>tachyphylaxis</u>, fever, hypersensitivity reactions.

## INTERACTIONS

**Drug-Drug:** ■ Inotropic effects may be additive with **digoxin** ■ Hypotension may be exaggerated by **disopyramide**.

## ROUTE AND DOSAGE

■ **IV (Adults):** 0.75 mg/kg loading dose; may be repeated in 30 min if necessary, then 5–10 mcg/kg/min infusion (total daily dose should not exceed 10 mg/kg).
■ **IV (Infants):** 3–4.5 mg/kg in divided doses followed by an infusion of 10 mcg/kg/min.
■ **IV (Neonates):** 3–4.5 mg/kg in divided doses followed by an infusion of 3–5 mcg/kg/min.

## AVAILABILITY

■ *Injection:* 5 mg/ml[Rx].

TIME/ACTION PROFILE (inotropic effect)

| | ONSET | PEAK | DURATION† |
|---|---|---|---|
| IV | 2–5 min | 10 min | 0.5–2 hr |

†After infusion is discontinued.

# NURSING IMPLICATIONS

## ASSESSMENT

❑ Monitor blood pressure, pulse, ECG, respiratory rate, cardiac index, pulmonary capillary wedge pressure, and central venous pressure frequently during administration. Notify physician promptly if hypotension occurs. Tachyphylaxis (rapid development of tolerance) commonly develops within the first 72 hr.
❑ Monitor intake and output and weigh daily. Assess for resolution of signs of CHF (peripheral edema, dyspnea, rales/crackles, weight gain). Fluid intake may need to be increased cautiously to ensure adequate cardiac filling pressure.
■ *Lab Test Considerations:* Platelet counts, serum electrolytes, liver enzymes, and renal function should be evaluated periodically throughout therapy. If platelet count is <150,000/mm³, notify physician promptly;

may require dose reduction. Increased liver enzymes may indicate hepatotoxicity. May cause decreased potassium levels.

## POTENTIAL NURSING DIAGNOSES

■ Cardiac output, decreased (Indications).
■ Activity intolerance (Indications).
■ Fluid volume, excess (Indications).

## IMPLEMENTATION

❑ *High Alert:* Intravenous vasoactive medications are inherently dangerous; fatalities have occurred from medication errors involving inamrinone. Before administering, have second practitioner check original order, dosage calculations and infusion pump settings. Do not confuse inamrinone with amiodarone.
■ **General:** Hypokalemia should be corrected before administration. Patients with atrial fibrillation/flutter may require digitalis glycoside therapy before treatment; inamrinone enhances atrioventricular conduction.
■ **Direct IV:** May be administered undiluted.
■ *Rate:* Administer loading dose over 2–3 min.
■ **Continuous Infusion:** Dilute inamrinone with 0.9% NaCl or 0.45% NaCl only, for a concentration of 1–3 mg/ml. Dilution with dextrose products may lead to decomposition of inamrinone, but may be administered through Y-tubing or directly into tubing of a running dextrose solution. Administer via infusion pump. Change tubing whenever concentration of solution is changed. Solution should be clear yellow. Use reconstituted solution within 24 hr of preparation.
■ *Rate:* Rate is titrated according to patient response.
■ **Syringe Compatibility:** ◆ propranolol ◆ verapamil.
■ **Y-Site Compatibility:** ◆ aminophylline ◆ atropine ◆ bretylium ◆ calcium chloride ◆ cimetidine ◆ digoxin ◆ dobutamine ◆ dopamine ◆ epinephrine ◆ famotidine ◆ hydrocortisone sodium succinate ◆ isoproterenol ◆ lidocaine ◆ methylprednisolone sodium succinate ◆ nitroglycerin ◆ nitroprusside ◆ norepinephrine ◆ phenylephrine ◆ potassium chloride ◆ propofol ◆ propranolol ◆ verapamil.
■ **Y-Site Incompatibility:** ◆ furosemide ◆ sodium bicarbonate.

## PATIENT/FAMILY TEACHING

❏ Advise patient to report any increase in dyspnea or chest pain, or the onset of hypersensitivity reactions, promptly.

❏ Advise patient to change positions slowly to minimize any drug-induced postural hypotension.

## EVALUATION

**Effectiveness of therapy can be demonstrated by:** ■ Increase in cardiac index and diuresis ❏ Decrease in pulmonary capillary wedge pressure, dyspnea, and edema.

## indapamide
(in-**dap**-a-mide)
{Lozide}, Lozol

### CLASSIFICATION(S):
**Therapeutic:** antihypertensives, diuretics
**Pharmacologic:** thiazide-like diuretics

### Pregnancy Category B

## INDICATIONS

■ Mild to moderate hypertension ■ Edema associated with CHF and other causes.

## ACTION

■ Increases excretion of sodium and water by inhibiting sodium reabsorption in the distal tubule ■ Promotes excretion of chloride, potassium, magnesium, and bicarbonate ■ May produce arteriolar dilation. **Therapeutic Effects:** ■ Lowering of blood pressure in hypertensive patients and diuresis with subsequent mobilization of edema.

## PHARMACOKINETICS

**Absorption:** Well absorbed from the GI tract after oral administration.

**Distribution:** Widely distributed.

**Metabolism and Excretion:** Mostly metabolized by the liver. Small amounts (7%) excreted unchanged by the kidneys.

**Half-life:** 14–18 hr.

## CONTRAINDICATIONS AND PRECAUTIONS

**Contraindicated in:** ■ Hypersensitivity ■ Cross-sensitivity with sulfonamides may occur ■ Anuria ■ Lactation.

**Use Cautiously in:** ■ Renal or severe hepatic impairment ■ Geriatric patients (increased sensitivity) ■ Pregnancy or children (safety not established).

## ADVERSE REACTIONS AND SIDE EFFECTS*

■ **CNS:** dizziness, drowsiness, lethargy ■ **CV:** arrhythmias, hypotension ■ **GI:** anorexia, cramping, nausea, vomiting ■ **Derm:** photosensitivity, rashes ■ **Endo:** hyperglycemia ■ **F and E:** <u>hypokalemia</u>, dehydration, hypochloremic alkalosis, hyponatremia, hypovolemia ■ **Metab:** <u>hyperuricemia</u> ■ **MS:** muscle cramps.

## INTERACTIONS

**Drug-Drug:** ■ Additive hypotension with other **antihypertensives, nitrates,** or acute ingestion of **alcohol** ■ Additive hypokalemia with **corticosteroids, amphotericin B, mezlocillin, piperacillin,** or **ticarcillin** ■ Decreases the excretion of **lithium**; may cause toxicity ■ Hypokalemia may increase risk of **digoxin** toxicity.

**Drug-Natural Products:** ■ **Licorice** and **stimulant laxative** herbs (**aloe, cascara sagrada, senna**) may increase risk of potassium depletion.

## ROUTE AND DOSAGE

■ **PO (Adults):** *Hypertension*—1.25–5 mg daily in the morning; may be increased at 4-wk intervals up to 5 mg/day. *Edema secondary to CHF*—2.5 mg daily in the morning; may be increased after 1 wk to 5 mg/day.

## AVAILABILITY (generic available)

■*Tablets:* 1.25 mg<sup>Rx</sup>, 2.5 mg<sup>Rx</sup> ■Cost: 1.25 mg $88.25/100, 2.5 mg $109.16/100; *generic*—1.25 mg $39.38/100, 2.5 mg $19.88/100.

TIME/ACTION PROFILE (antihypertensive effect)

| | ONSET | PEAK | DURATION |
|---|---|---|---|
| PO (single dose) | unknown | 24 hr | unknown |

PO (multiple 1–2 wk dose)     8–12 wk     up to 8 wk

## NURSING IMPLICATIONS

### ASSESSMENT

- ❏ Monitor blood pressure, intake and output, and daily weight and assess feet, legs, and sacral area for edema daily.
- ❏ Assess patient, especially if taking digoxin, for anorexia, nausea, vomiting, muscle cramps, paresthesia, and confusion; report signs of electrolyte imbalance. Patients taking digoxin have an increased risk of digitalis toxicity due to the potassium-depleting effect of the diuretic.
- ❏ Assess patient for allergy to sulfonamides.
- ■ *Lab Test Considerations:* Monitor electrolytes (especially potassium), blood glucose, BUN, serum creatinine, and uric acid levels periodically throughout therapy. May cause decreased potassium, sodium, and chloride concentrations. May increase serum glucose; diabetic patients may require increased oral hypoglycemic or insulin dosage. Increases uric acid level an average of 1.0 mg/100 ml; may precipitate an episode of gout.

### POTENTIAL NURSING DIAGNOSES

- ■ Fluid volume, excess (Indications).
- ■ Fluid volume, risk for deficit (Side Effects).

### IMPLEMENTATION

- ■ **General:** Administer in the morning to prevent disruption of sleep cycle.
- ■ **PO:** May be given with food or milk to minimize GI irritation.

### PATIENT/FAMILY TEACHING

- ■ **General Info:** Instruct patient to take this medication at the same time each day. If a dose is missed, take as soon as remembered but not just before next dose is due. Do not double doses. Advise patients using indapamide for hypertension to continue taking the medication even if feeling well. Indapamide controls but does not cure hypertension.
- ❏ Caution patient to change positions slowly to minimize orthostatic hypotension. This may be potentiated by alcohol.
- ❏ Advise patient to use sunscreen (avoid those containing PABA) and protective clothing when in the sun to prevent photosensitivity reactions.
- ❏ Instruct patient to follow a diet high in potassium (see Appendix Q).
- ❏ Advise patient to report muscle weakness, cramps, nausea, or dizziness to health care professional.
- ❏ Advise patient to consult health care professional before taking OTC medication concurrently with this therapy.
- ❏ Emphasize the importance of routine follow-up exams.
- ■ **Hypertension:** Instruct patient and family on proper technique of blood pressure monitoring. Advise them to check blood pressure at least weekly and to report significant changes.
- ❏ Encourage patient to comply with additional interventions for hypertension (weight reduction, low-sodium diet, regular exercise, smoking cessation, moderation of alcohol consumption, and stress management).

### EVALUATION

**Effectiveness of therapy can be demonstrated by:** ■ Control of hypertension ■ Decrease in edema secondary to CHF.

## indinavir

(in-**din**-a-veer)

Crixivan

*CLASSIFICATION(S):*
*Therapeutic: antiretrovirals*
*Pharmacologic: protease inhibitors*

**Pregnancy Category C**

### INDICATIONS

■ HIV infection (with other antiretrovirals). **Unlabeled uses:** ■ Prevention of HIV infection after known exposure (with other antiretrovirals).

### ACTION

■ Inhibits the action of HIV protease and prevents the cleavage of viral polyproteins. **Therapeutic Effects:** ■ Slowing of the progression of HIV infection and its sequelae.

## PHARMACOKINETICS

**Absorption:** Rapidly absorbed after oral administration.

**Distribution:** Unknown.

**Metabolism and Excretion:** Mostly metabolized by the liver; <20% excreted unchanged by the kidneys.

**Half-life:** 1.8 hr.

## CONTRAINDICATIONS AND PRECAUTIONS

**Contraindicated in:** ■ Hypersensitivity ■ Dehydration ■ Concurrent dihydroergotamine, ergotamine, midazolam, rifampin, triazolam, or St. John's wort.

**Use Cautiously in:** ■ Hepatic impairment (dosage reduction recommended in moderate to severe hepatic insufficiency caused by cirrhosis) ■ Hemophilia (increased risk of bleeding) ■ Diabetes mellitus ■ Pregnancy, lactation, or children (safety not established; breastfeeding not recommended in HIV-infected patients).

## ADVERSE REACTIONS AND SIDE EFFECTS*

■ **CNS:** dizziness, drowsiness, fatigue, headache, insomnia, weakness ■ **GI:** abdominal pain, acid regurgitation, altered taste, asymptomatic hyperbilirubinemia, diarrhea, nausea, vomiting ■ **GU:** nephrolithiasis ■ **Endo:** hyperglycemia ■ **F and E:** KETOACIDOSIS ■ **MS:** back pain, flank pain ■ **Misc:** redistribution of body fat.

## INTERACTIONS

**Drug-Drug:** ■ Concurrent use with **dihydroergotamine**, **ergotamine**, **midazolam**, **rifampin**, or **triazolam** is contraindicated because of ↑ risk of serious or life-threatening adverse reactions, including arrhythmias, excessive sedation, and vasoconstriction ■ **Rifampin** and **fluconazole** ↓ blood levels; concurrent use should be avoided ■ ↑ risk of myopathy with **lovastatin**, or **simvastatin** ■ ↑ blood levels of **rifabutin** (decrease dosage of rifabutin by 50%) and **hormonal contraceptives** ■ **Rifabutin, nevirapine,** and **efavirenz** ↓ indinavir levels; if concurrent rifabutin or efavirenz therapy is necessary, increase indinavir dose to 1000 mg q 8 hr ■ Blood levels are ↑ by **ketoconazole, itraconazole,** and **delavirdine** (decrease dose of indinavir to 600 mg

q 8 hr) ■ Alters absorption of **didanosine** ■ May ↑ blood levels and effects of **sildenafil**.

**Drug-Natural Products:** ■ **St. John's wort** significantly ↓ blood levels and effectiveness of **indinavir** (concurrent use is contraindicated).

**Drug-Food:** ■ **High-fat** or **high-protein meals** and **grapefruit juice** ↓ absorption.

## ROUTE AND DOSAGE

■ **PO (Adults):** 800 mg q 8 hr.

## AVAILABILITY

■ *Capsules:* 200 mg$^{Rx}$, 400 mg$^{Rx}$. ■ Cost: 100 mg $130.84/180,200 mg $523.35/360, 333 mg $326.56/135, 400 mg $523.25/180.

TIME/ACTION PROFILE (blood levels)

|    | ONSET | PEAK | DURATION |
|----|-------|------|----------|
| PO | rapid | 0.8 hr | 8 hr |

# NURSING IMPLICATIONS

## ASSESSMENT

❏ Assess patient for change in severity of symptoms of HIV infection and for symptoms of opportunistic infections throughout therapy.

■ *Lab Test Considerations:* Monitor viral load and CD4 cell count periodically during therapy.

❏ May cause hyperglycemia.

❏ May cause ↑ serum AST, ALT, total bilirubin, and amylase concentrations.

## POTENTIAL NURSING DIAGNOSES

■ Infection, risk for (Indications).

■ Noncompliance (Patient/Family Teaching).

## IMPLEMENTATION

■ **General:** Do not confuse indinavir with Denavir (penciclovir).

■ **PO:** Administer with water 1 hr before or 2 hr after a meal. May be taken with other liquids (skim milk, juice, coffee, tea) or a light meal (dry toast with jelly, coffee with skim milk and sugar, cornflakes with skim milk and sugar). Avoid high-fat, high-protein meals within 2 hr of indinavir.

❏ Patients on concurrent didanosine therapy should take didanosine and indinavir at least 1 hr apart.

## PATIENT/FAMILY TEACHING

- ❏ Emphasize the importance of taking indinavir exactly as directed, at evenly spaced times throughout day. Do not take more than prescribed amount and do not stop taking without consulting health care professional. Take missed doses as soon as remembered; do not double doses.
- ❏ Instruct patient that indinavir should not be shared with others.
- ❏ Instruct patient to store indinavir in original container with desiccant in bottle; indinavir is sensitive to moisture.
- ❏ Indinavir may cause kidney stones. Advise patient to drink at least 1.5 liters of water each day. Kidney stones may require 1–3 day interruption of therapy.
- ❏ Inform patient that indinavir may cause hyperglycemia. Advise patient to notify health care professional if increased thirst or hunger; unexplained weight loss; increased urination; fatigue; or dry, itchy skin occurs.
- ❏ Advise patient to avoid taking other medications (prescription, OTC, or natural products), without consulting health care professional.
- ❏ Advise patients concurrently taking didanosine that both medications must be taken on an empty stomach, 1 hr apart.
- ❏ Inform patient that indinavir does not cure AIDS and does not reduce the risk of transmission of HIV to others through sexual contact or blood contamination. Caution patient to use a condom and avoid sharing needles or donating blood to prevent spreading HIV to others.
- ❏ May cause drowsiness and dizziness. Advise patient to avoid driving and other activities requiring alertness until response to medication is known.
- ❏ Emphasize the importance of regular follow-up exams and blood counts to determine progress and monitor for side effects.

## EVALUATION

**Effectiveness of therapy can be demonstrated by:** ■ Delayed progression of AIDS and decreased opportunistic infections in patients with HIV ■ Improved CD4 cell count and decrease in viral load.

# indomethacin

(in-doe-**meth**-a-sin)

{Apo-Indomethacin}, {Indameth}, {Indocid}, Indocin, Indocin I.V., {Indocin PDA}, Indocin SR, Indochron E-R, {Novo-Methacin}, {Nu-Indo}

## CLASSIFICATION(S):

**Therapeutic:** antirheumatics, ductus arteriosus patency adjuncts (IV only), nonsteroidal anti-inflammatory agents

**Pregnancy Category B (first trimester)**

## INDICATIONS

■ **PO, Rect:** Inflammatory disorders including: ❏ Rheumatoid arthritis ❏ Gouty arthritis ❏ Osteoarthritis ❏ Ankylosing spondylitis ■ Generally reserved for patients who do not respond to less toxic agents ■ **IV:** Alternative to surgery in the management of patent ductus arteriosus in premature neonates.

## ACTION

■ Inhibits prostaglandin synthesis. **Therapeutic Effects:** ■ **PO, Rect:** Suppression of pain and inflammation ■ **IV:** Closure of patent ductus arteriosus.

## PHARMACOKINETICS

**Absorption:** Well absorbed after oral or rectal administration.

**Distribution:** Crosses the blood-brain barrier and the placenta. Enters breast milk.

**Protein Binding:** 99%.

**Metabolism and Excretion:** Mostly metabolized by the liver.

**Half-life:** 2.6–11 hr (prolonged in neonates—up to 60 hr, average range 12–21 hr).

## CONTRAINDICATIONS AND PRECAUTIONS

**Contraindicated in:** ■ Hypersensitivity ■ Known alcohol intolerance (suspension) ■ Cross-sensitivity may exist with other NSAIDs, including aspirin ■ Active GI bleeding ■ Ulcer disease ■ Proctitis or recent history of rectal bleeding.

**Use Cautiously in:** ■ Severe cardiovascular, renal, or hepatic disease ■ History of ulcer disease ■ Geriatric patients (increased risk of adverse reactions) ■ Pregnancy or lactation (not recommended during 2nd half of pregnancy) ■ Lactation.

## ADVERSE REACTIONS AND SIDE EFFECTS*

■ **CNS:** dizziness, drowsiness, headache, psychic disturbances ■ **EENT:** blurred vision, tinnitus ■ **CV:** arrhythmias, edema ■ **GI:** PO—DRUG-INDUCED HEPATITIS, GI BLEEDING, constipation, dyspepsia, nausea, vomiting, discomfort; *rectal*—rectal irritation, tenesmus ■ **GU:** cystitis, hematuria, renal failure ■ **Derm:** rashes ■ **F and E:** hyperkalemia ■ **Hemat:** blood dyscrasias, prolonged bleeding time ■ **Local:** phlebitis at IV site ■ **Misc:** allergic reactions including ANAPHYLAXIS.

## INTERACTIONS

**Drug-Drug:** ■ Concurrent use with **aspirin** may decrease effectiveness ■ Additive adverse GI effects with **aspirin**, other **NSAIDs, corticosteroids,** or **alcohol** ■ Chronic use of **acetaminophen** increases the risk of adverse renal reactions ■ May decrease effectiveness of **diuretics** or **antihypertensives** ■ May increase hypoglycemia from **insulins** or **oral hypoglycemic agents** ■ May increase risk of toxicity from **lithium** or **zidovudine** (concurrent use with zidovudine should be avoided) ■ Increases the risk of toxicity from **methotrexate** ■ **Probenecid** increases risk of toxicity from indomethacin ■ Increased risk of bleeding with **cefamandole, cefotetan, cefoperazone,** valproic acid, plicamycin, thrombolytic agents, warfarin, and **drugs affecting platelet function** including **clopidogrel, ticlopidine, abciximab, eptifibatide,** or **tirofiban** ■ Increased risk of adverse hematologic reactions with **antineoplastics** or **radiation therapy** ■ Increased risk of nephrotoxicity with **cyclosporine** ■ Concurrent use with **potassium-sparing diuretics** may result in hyperkalemia ■ May increase levels of **digitalis glycosides** and **aminoglycosides** in infants.

**Drug-Natural Products:** ■ Increased bleeding risk with **anise, arnica, chamomile, clove, dong quai, feverfew, garlic, ginger, ginkgo, Panax ginseng.**

## ROUTE AND DOSAGE
�‒ **Anti-inflammatory**

■ **PO (Adults):** *Antiarthritic*—25–50 mg 2–4 times daily *or* 75-mg extended-release capsule once or twice daily (not to exceed 200 mg or 150 mg of SR/day). A single bedtime dose of 100 mg may be used. *Antigout*—100 mg initially, followed by 50 mg 3 times daily for relief of pain, then decreased further.
■ **Rect (Adults):** 50 mg up to 4 times daily (not to exceed 200 mg/day by all routes).
■ **PO, Rect (Children):** 1.5–2.5 mg/kg/day in 3–4 divided doses (not to exceed 4 mg/kg/day or 150–200 mg/day).

�‒ **Closure of Patent Ductus Arteriosus**

■ **IV, PO (Neonates):** 0.2 mg/kg initially, then 2 subsequent doses at 12–24 hr intervals of 0.1 mg/kg if age <48 hr at time of initial dose; 0.2 mg/kg if 2–7 days at initial dose; 0.25 mg/kg if age >7 days at initial dose.

## AVAILABILITY (generic available)

■ *Capsules:* 25 mg$^{Rx}$, 50 mg$^{Rx}$ ■ Cost: *Indocin*—25 mg $61.24/100, 50 mg $103.29/100; generic—25 mg $19.84/100, 50 mg $23.34/100 ■ *Sustained-release capsules:* 75 mg$^{Rx}$ ■ Cost: *Indocin SR*—$121.42/60; *generic*—$60.22/60 ■ *Suppositories:* 50 mg$^{Rx}$, {100 mg$^{Rx}$} ■ *Oral suspension (fruit mint, pineapple coconut mint flavors):* 25 mg/5 ml$^{Rx}$ ■ *Powder for injection:* 1-mg vials$^{Rx}$.

TIME/ACTION PROFILE

| | ONSET | PEAK | DURATION |
|---|---|---|---|
| PO (analgesic) | 30 min | 0.5–2 hr | 4–6 hr |
| PO-ER (analgesic) | 30 min | unknown | 4–6 hr |
| PO (anti-inflammatory) | up to 7 days | 1–2 wk | unknown |
| PO-ER (anti-inflammatory) | up to 7 days | 1–2 wk | unknown |
| IV (closure of PDA) | up to 48 hr | unknown | unknown |

# NURSING IMPLICATIONS
## ASSESSMENT
■ **General Info:** Patients who have asthma, aspirin-induced allergy, and nasal polyps are

---

{ } = Available in Canada only.
*CAPITALS indicates life-threatening; underlines indicate most frequent.

at increased risk for developing hypersensitivity reactions. Monitor for rhinitis, asthma, and urticaria.

- **Arthritis:** Assess limitation of movement and pain—note type, location, and intensity before and 1–2 hr after administration.
- **Patent Ductus Arteriosus:** Monitor respiratory status and heart sounds routinely throughout therapy.
- ❑ Monitor intake and output. Fluid restriction is usually instituted throughout therapy.
- **Lab Test Considerations:** BUN, serum creatinine, CBC, serum potassium levels, and liver function tests should be evaluated periodically in patients receiving prolonged therapy.
- ❑ Serum potassium, BUN, serum creatinine, AST, and ALT tests may show increased levels. Blood glucose concentrations may be altered. Hemoglobin and hematocrit concentrations, leukocyte and platelet counts, and CCr may be decreased.
- ❑ Urine glucose and urine protein concentrations may be increased.
- ❑ Leukocyte and platelet count may be decreased. Bleeding time may be prolonged for several days after discontinuation.

## POTENTIAL NURSING DIAGNOSES

- Pain, acute (Indications).
- Mobility, impaired physical (Indications).

## IMPLEMENTATION

- **General:** If prolonged therapy is used, dose should be reduced to the lowest level that controls symptoms.
- **PO:** Administer after meals, with food, or with antacids to decrease GI irritation. Do not crush, break, or chew sustained-release capsules.
- ❑ Shake suspension before administration. Do not mix with antacid or any other liquid.
- **Direct IV:** Reconstitute with 1 or 2 ml of preservative-free 0.9% NaCl or preservative-free sterile water for a concentration of 0.1 mg/ml or 0.05 mg/ml, respectively. Reconstitute immediately before use and discard any unused solution. Do not dilute further or admix.
- **Rate:** Administer over 5–10 sec. Avoid extravasation, as solution is irritating to tissues.

- **Y-Site Compatibility:** ◆ furosemide ◆ insulin ◆ nitroprusside ◆ potassium chloride ◆ sodium bicarbonate.
- **Y-Site Incompatibility:** ◆ calcium gluconate ◆ cimetidine ◆ dobutamine ◆ dopamine ◆ gentamicin ◆ levofloxacin ◆ tobramycin ◆ tolazoline.
- **Rect:** Encourage patient to retain suppository for 1 hr after administration.

## PATIENT/FAMILY TEACHING

- **General Info:** Advise patient to take this medication with a full glass of water and to remain in an upright position for 15–30 min after administration.
- ❑ Instruct patient to take medication exactly as directed. Missed doses should be taken as soon as remembered if not almost time for next dose. Do not double doses.
- ❑ May cause drowsiness or dizziness. Advise patient to avoid driving or other activities requiring alertness until response to medication is known.
- ❑ Caution patient to avoid the concurrent use of alcohol, aspirin, other NSAIDs, acetaminophen, or other OTC medications without consulting health care professional.
- ❑ Caution patient to wear sunscreen and protective clothing to prevent photosensitivity reactions.
- ❑ Advise patient to inform health care professional of medication regimen before treatment or surgery.
- ❑ Instruct patient to notify health care professional if rash, itching, chills, fever, muscle aches, visual disturbances, weight gain, edema, abdominal pain, black stools, or persistent headache occurs.
- **Patent Ductus Arteriosus:** Explain to parents the purpose of medication and the need for frequent monitoring.

## EVALUATION

**Effectiveness of therapy can be demonstrated by:** ■ Decrease in severity of moderate pain ❑ Improved joint mobility. Partial arthritic relief is usually seen within 2 wk, but maximum effectiveness may require up to 1 mo of continuous therapy. Patients who do not respond to one NSAID may respond to another ■ Successful closure of patent ductus arteriosus.

# infliximab

(in-**flix**-i-mab)

Remicade

## CLASSIFICATION(S):

**Therapeutic:** antirheumatics (DMARDs), gastrointestinal anti-inflammatories

**Pharmacologic:** monoclonal antibodies

## Pregnancy Category C

## INDICATIONS

■ Active rheumatoid arthritis (moderate to severe, with methotrexate) ■ Active Crohn's disease (moderate to severe).

## ACTION

■ Neutralizes and prevents the activity of tumor necrosis factor-alpha (TNF-alpha), resulting in anti-inflammatory and antiproliferative activity. **Therapeutic Effects:** ■ Decreased pain and swelling, decreased rate of joint destruction and improved physical function in rheumatoid arthritis ■ Reduction and maintenance of closure of fistulae in Crohn's disease.

## PHARMACOKINETICS

**Absorption:** IV administration results in complete bioavailability.

**Distribution:** Predominantly distributed within the vascular compartment.

**Metabolism and Excretion:** Unknown.

**Half-life:** 9.5 days.

## CONTRAINDICATIONS AND PRECAUTIONS

**Contraindicated in:** ■ Hypersensitivity to infliximab, murine (mouse) proteins, or other components in the formulation ■ Lactation ■ CHF.

**Use Cautiously in:** ■ Patients being retreated after 2 yr without treatment (increased risk of adverse reactions) ■ History of tuberculosis or exposure (latent tuberculosis should be treated prior to infliximab therapy) ■ Geriatric patients ■ Pregnancy (use only if clearly needed) ■ Children (safety not established).

## ADVERSE REACTIONS AND SIDE EFFECTS*

■ **CNS:** fatigue, headache, anxiety, depression, dizziness, insomnia ■ **EENT:** conjunctivitis ■ **Resp:** upper respiratory tract infection, bronchitis, cough, dyspnea, laryngitis, pharyngitis, respiratory tract allergic reaction, rhinitis, sinusitis ■ **CV:** chest pain, hypertension, hypotension, tachycardia, CHF ■ **GI:** abdominal pain, nausea, vomiting, constipation, diarrhea, dyspepsia, flatulence, increased liver enzymes, intestinal obstruction, oral pain, tooth pain, ulcerative stomatitis ■ **GU:** dysuria, urinary frequency, urinary tract infection ■ **Derm:** acne, alopecia, dry skin, ecchymosis, eczema, erythema, flushing, hematoma, increased sweating, hot flushes, pruritus, urticaria, rash ■ **MS:** arthralgia, arthritis, back pain, involuntary muscle contractions, myalgia ■ **Neuro:** paresthesia ■ **Misc:** INFECTIONS (including reactivation tuberculosis and invasive fungal infections), fever, infusion reactions, chills, flu-like syndrome, herpes simplex, herpes zoster, hypersensitivity reactions, increased risk of lymphoma, lupus-like syndrome, moniliasis, pain, peripheral edema.

## INTERACTIONS

**Drug-Drug:** ■ None significant.

## ROUTE AND DOSAGE

❑ **Rheumatoid arthritis**

■ **IV (Adults):** 3 mg/kg followed by 3 mg/kg 2 and 6 wk after initial dose and then every 8 wk; dose may be adjusted in partial responders up to 10 mg/kg or treatment as often as every 4 wk (used with methotrexate).

❑ **Crohn's Disease**

■ **IV (Adults):** *Moderate-to-severe Crohn's disease*—5 mg/kg as a single infusion. *Fistulizing Crohn's disease*—5 mg/kg repeated 2 and 6 wk after initial infusion; maintenance dose of 5 mg/kg may be given q 8 wk.

## AVAILABILITY

■ *Powder for injection:* 100 mg/vial$^{Rx}$ ■ Cost: $611.33/vial.

---

{ } = Available in Canada only.
*CAPITALS indicates life-threatening; underlines indicate most frequent.

TIME/ACTION PROFILE (symptoms of Crohn's disease)

| | ONSET | PEAK | DURATION |
|---|---|---|---|
| IV | 1–2 wk | unknown | 12–48 wk† |

†After infusion.

## NURSING IMPLICATIONS

### ASSESSMENT

- **General Info:** Assess patient for infusion-related reactions (fever, chills, urticaria, pruritus) during and for 2 hr after infusion. Symptoms usually resolve when infusion is discontinued. Reactions are more common after 1st or 2nd infusion. Frequency of reactions may be reduced with immunosuppressant agents.
- ❑ Assess patient for latent tuberculosis with a tuberculin skin test prior to initiation of therapy. Treatment of latent tuberculosis should be initiated prior to therapy with infliximab.
- ❑ Observe patient for hypersensitivity reactions (urticaria, dyspnea, hypotension) throughout infusion. Discontinue infliximab if severe reaction occurs. Medications (antihistamines, acetaminophen, corticosteroids, epinephrine) and equipment should be readily available in the event of a severe reaction.
- **Rheumatoid Arthritis:** Assess patient for pain and range of motion prior to and periodically during therapy.
- **Crohn's Disease:** Assess patient for signs and symptoms of Crohn's disease before, throughout, and after therapy.
- **Lab Test Considerations:** May cause increase in positive ANA. Frequency may be decreased with baseline immunosuppressant therapy.

### POTENTIAL NURSING DIAGNOSES

- Pain, acute, chronic (Indications).
- Diarrhea (Indications).

### IMPLEMENTATION

- **Intermittent Infusion:** Calculate the total number of vials needed. Reconstitute each vial with 10 ml of sterile water for injection using a syringe with a 21-gauge needle or smaller. Direct stream to sides of vial. Do not use if vacuum is not present in vial. Gently swirl solution by rotating vial to dilute; do not shake. May foam on reconstitution; allow

to stand for 5 min. Solution is colorless to light yellow and opalescent; a few translucent particles may develop because infliximab is a protein. Do not use if opaque particles, discoloration, or other particles occur. Withdraw volume of total infliximab dose from infusion container containing 250 ml with 0.9% NaCl. Slowly add total dose of infliximab for a concentration ranging from 0.4 to 4 mg/ml. Mix gently. Infusion should begin within 3 hr of preparation. Solution is incompatible with polyvinyl chloride equipment. Prepare in glass infusion bottle or polypropylene or polyolefin bags. Do not reuse or store any portion of infusion solution.

- **Rate:** Administer over at least 2 hr through polyethylene-lined administration set with an in-line, sterile, nonpyrogenic, low protein-building filter with ≤1.2-micron pore size.
- **Y-Site Incompatibility:** Do not administer concurrently in the same line with any other agents.

### PATIENT/FAMILY TEACHING

- ❑ Advise patient that adverse reactions (myalgia, rash, fever, polyarthralgia, pruritus) may occur 3–12 days after delayed (>2 yr) retreatment with infliximab. Symptoms usually decrease or resolve within 1–3 days. Instruct patient to notify health care professional if symptoms occur.
- ❑ May cause dizziness. Caution patient to avoid driving or other activities requiring alertness until response to medication is known.

### EVALUATION

**Effectiveness of therapy can be demonstrated by:** ▪ Decreased pain and swelling with decreased rate of joint destruction in patients with rheumatoid arthritis ▪ Decrease in the signs and symptoms of Crohn's disease and a decrease in the number of draining enterocutaneous fistulas.

`High Alert`

# INSULINS
(**in**-su-lin)

**insulin aspart, rDNA origin**
Novolog

insulin lispro, rDNA origin
Humalog

insulin lispro/protamine insulin
lispro mixture, rDNA origin
Humalog 75/25, Humalog 50/50

regular insulin (insulin injection)
Humulin R, {Insulin-Toronto}, No-
volin R, Iletin II Regular, Velosulin
BR

NPH insulin (isophane insulin
suspension)
Humulin N, NPH Iletin II, {Novolin
ge NPH}, Novolin N

NPH/regular insulin mixtures
Humulin 50/50, Humulin 70/30,
Novolin 70/30

insulin zinc suspension (lente insulin)
Humulin L, Lente Iletin II, {Novo-
lin ge Lente}

insulin zinc suspension, extended
(ultralente insulin)
Humulin U Ultralente, {Novolin de
Ultralente}, Novolin U, Ultralente U

insulin glargine
Lantus

concentrated regular insulin
Regular (Concentrated) Iletin II U-
500

*CLASSIFICATION(S):*
*Therapeutic: antidiabetics, hor-
mones*
*Pharmacologic: pancreatics*

Pregnancy Category C (glargine),
B (all others)

See Appendix R for more information con-
cerning insulins.

## INDICATIONS

■ Treatment of insulin-dependent diabetes mellitus (type 1) ■ Management of non–insulin-dependent diabetes mellitus (type 2) unresponsive to treatment with diet and/or oral hypoglycemic agents ■ **Concentrated insulin U-500:** Only for use in patients with insulin requirements >200 units/day.

## ACTION

■ Lower blood glucose by increasing transport into cells and promoting the conversion of glucose to glycogen ■ Promote the conversion of amino acids to proteins in muscle and stimulate triglyceride formation ■ Inhibit the release of free fatty acids ■ Sources include pork, beef/pork combinations, semisynthetic, biosynthetic, and recombinant DNA. **Therapeutic Effects:** ■ Control of blood glucose in diabetic patients.

## PHARMACOKINETICS

**Absorption:** Rapidly absorbed from subcut administration sites. Absorption rate is determined by type of insulin, injection site, volume of injectate, and other factors.
**Distribution:** Widely distributed.
**Metabolism and Excretion:** Metabolized by liver, spleen, kidney, and muscle.
**Half-life:** 5–6 min (prolonged in patients with diabetes; biologic half-life is 1–1.5 hr).

## CONTRAINDICATIONS AND PRECAUTIONS

**Contraindicated in:** ■ Allergy or hypersensitivity to a particular type of insulin, preservatives, or other additives.
**Use Cautiously in:** ■ Stress, pregnancy, and infection (temporarily increase insulin requirements).

## ADVERSE REACTIONS AND SIDE EFFECTS*

■ **Derm:** urticaria ■ **Endo:** HYPOGLYCEMIA, rebound hyperglycemia (Somogyi effect) ■ **Local:** lipodystrophy, itching, lipohypertrophy, redness, swelling ■ **Misc:** allergic reactions including ANAPHYLAXIS.

## INTERACTIONS

**Drug-Drug:** ■ **Beta blockers** may block some of the signs and symptoms of hypoglycemia and delay recovery from hypoglycemia ■ **Thiazide diuretics, corticosteroids, diltiazem, dobutamine, thyroid preparations, estrogens, nicotine, protease inhibitor antiretrovirals,** and **rifampin** may increase insulin requirements ■ **Anabolic steroids (testosterone),** alcohol, clofibrate, guanethidine, MAO inhibitors, most NSAIDs, oral hypoglycemic agents, sulfinpyrazone, tetracyclines, phenylbutazone, and **warfarin** may decrease insulin requirements.

**Drug-Natural Products:** ■ **Glucosamine** may worsen blood glucose control ■ **Fenugreek, chromium,** and **coenzyme Q-10** may produce additive hypoglycemic effects.

### ROUTE AND DOSAGE

Dose depends on blood glucose, response, and many other factors.

❏ **Ketoacidosis—Regular Insulin Only**

■ **IV (Adults):** 0.1 unit/kg/hr as a continuous infusion.

■ **IV (Children):** Individualized on the basis of patient's weight.

❏ **Maintenance Therapy**

■ **Subcut (Adults and Children):** 0.5–1 unit/kg/day. *Adolescents during rapid growth*—0.8–1.2 units/kg/day.

### AVAILABILITY

■ *Insulin injection (regular insulin):* 100 units/ml^OTC ■Cost: $31.22/10 ml vial ■ *Regular (concentrated) insulin injection:* 500 units/ml^Rx ■ *Isophane insulin suspension (NPH insulin):* 100 units/ml^Rx ■ *NPH insulin/regular in suspension:* 70 units NPH/30 units regular in-sulin/ml (100 units/ml total)^OTC, 50 units NPH/50 units regular insulin/ml (100 units/ml total)^OTC ■Cost: $47.70/10 ml vial ■ *Insulin zinc suspension (lente):* 100 units/ml^OTC ■ *Insulin zinc suspension, extended (ultralente):* 100 units/ml^OTC ■*Insulin lispro:* 100 units/ml in 10-ml vials and 1.5-ml cartridges^Rx ■ *Insulin lispro 75/25:* protamine mix in 3 ml delivery device^Rx ■ *Insulin lispro 50/50:* protamine mix in 3 ml delivery device^Rx ■ *Insulin aspart(rDNA):* 100 units/ml cartridges and 10 ml vials^Rx ■ *Insulin glargine:* 100 units/ml in 5 ml vials^Rx, 10 ml vials^Rx, 3 ml cartridges^Rx.

### TIME/ACTION PROFILE (hypoglycemic effect)

| | ONSET | PEAK | DURATION |
|---|---|---|---|
| Insulin aspart subcut | 15 min | 1–3 hr | 3–5 hr |
| Insulin lispro subcut | 15 min | 30–90 min | 3–5 hr |
| Regular insulin IV | 10–30 min | 15–30 min | 30–60 min |
| Regular insulin subcut | 30–60 min | 2–4 hr | 5–7 hr |
| NPH subcut | 3–4 hr | 6–12 hr | 18–24 hr |
| Lente subcut | 1–3 hr | 8–12 hr | 18–28 hr |
| Insulin glargine subcut | 1.1 hr | 5 hr† | 24 hr |
| Ultralente subcut | 4–6 hr | 18–24 hr | 36 hr |
| 70%NPH/ 30%Regular Insulin mixture | 30 min | 4–8 hr | 24 hr |

†Small amounts of insulin glargine slowly released resulting in a relatively constant effect over time.

## NURSING IMPLICATIONS

### ASSESSMENT

❏ Assess patient for signs and symptoms of hypoglycemia (anxiety; chills; cold sweats; confusion; cool, pale skin; difficulty in concentration; drowsiness; excessive hunger; headache; irritability; nausea; nervousness; rapid pulse; shakiness; unusual tiredness or weakness) and hyperglycemia (drowsiness; flushed, dry skin; fruit-like breath odor; frequent urination; loss of appetite; tiredness; unusual thirst) periodically throughout therapy.

❏ Monitor body weight periodically. Changes in weight may necessitate changes in insulin dose.

■ *Lab Test Considerations:* May cause decreased serum inorganic phosphate, magnesium, and potassium levels.

❏ Monitor blood glucose and ketones every 6 hr throughout therapy, more frequently in ketoacidosis and times of stress. Glycosylated hemoglobin may also be monitored to determine effectiveness of therapy.

■ *Toxicity and Overdose:* Overdose is manifested by symptoms of hypoglycemia. Mild hypoglycemia may be treated by ingestion of oral glucose. Severe hypoglycemia is a life-threatening emergency; treatment consists of IV glucose, glucagon, or epinephrine. Recovery from hypoglycemia may be delayed due to the prolonged effect of subcut *insulin glargine.*

## POTENTIAL NURSING DIAGNOSES

■ Noncompliance (Patient/Family Teaching).

## IMPLEMENTATION

❏ *High Alert:* Medication errors involving insulins have resulted in serious patient harm and death. Clarify all ambiguous orders and do not accept orders using the abbreviation "u" for units, which can be misread as a zero or the numeral 4 and has resulted in tenfold overdoses. Insulins are available in different types and strengths and from different species. Check type, species source, dose, and expiration date with another licensed nurse. Do not interchange insulins without consulting physician or other health care professional. Do not confuse Lantus insulin with Lente insulin. Do not confuse regular **concentrated (U-500)** insulin with regular insulin.

■ **General:** Use *only* insulin syringes to draw up dose. The unit markings on the insulin syringe must match the insulin's units/ml. Special syringes for doses <50 units are available. Use *only* U-100 insulin syringes to draw up *insulin lispro* dose. Insulin syringe or OptiPen One can be used for administration of *insulin glargine.* Prior to withdrawing dose, rotate vial between palms to ensure uniform solution; do not shake.

❏ When mixing insulins, draw regular insulin or insulin lispro into syringe first to avoid contamination of regular insulin vial. *High Alert:* Do not mix *insulin glargine (Lantus)* with any other insulin or solution, or use syringes containing any other medicinal product or residue. If giving with a short acting insulin, use separate syringes and different injection sites. Solution should be clear and colorless with no particulate matter.

❏ Insulin should be stored in a cool place but does not need to be refrigerated. Store unopened vials and cartridges of *insulin glargine* in the refrigerator; do not freeze. If unable to refrigerate, the 10-ml vial can be kept in a cool place unrefrigerated for up to 28 days, and the 5-ml vial, up to 14 days. Once the cartridge is placed in an OptiPen One, do not refrigerate.

❏ Because of short duration of insulin lispro, supplementation with longer-acting insulin may be necessary to control blood glucose levels.

❏ When transferring from once-daily NPH human insulin or ultralente insulin to *insulin glargine*, the dose usually remains unchanged. When transferring from twice-daily NPH human insulin to insulin glargine, the initial dose of insulin glargine is usually reduced by 20%.

■ **Subcut:** Administer insulin lispro within 15 min before a meal.

❏ Administer *insulin glargine* subcut once daily at the same time each day. Do not administer IV.

❏ **IV:** Regular insulin is the *only* insulin that can be administered IV. Do not use if cloudy, discolored, or unusually viscous.

❏ *High Alert:* Regular (concentrated) insulin U-500 should not be given IV.

■ **Direct IV:** May be administered IV undiluted directly into vein or through Y-site.

■ *Rate:* Administer up to 50 units over 1 min.

■ **Continuous Infusion:** May be diluted in commonly used IV solutions as an infusion; however, insulin potency may be reduced by at least 20–80% by the plastic or glass container or tubing before reaching the venous system.

■ *Rate:* When administered as an infusion, rate should be ordered by physician, and infusion should be placed on an IV pump for accurate administration.

❏ Rate of administration should be decreased when serum glucose level reaches 250 mg/100 ml.

■ **Y-Site Compatibility:** ◆ amiodarone ◆ dobutamine ◆ esmolol ◆ heparin ◆ indomethacin ◆ midazolam ◆ milrinone ◆ oxytocin ◆ nitroglycerin ◆ nitroprusside ◆ potassium chloride ◆ propofol ◆ ritodrine ◆ sodium bicarbonate ◆ tacrolimus ◆ terbutaline

■ **Additive Compatibility:** May be added to total parenteral nutrition (TPN) solutions.

## PATIENT/FAMILY TEACHING

❑ Instruct patient on proper technique for administration. Include type of insulin, equipment (syringe, cartridge pens, alcohol swabs), storage, and place to discard syringes. Discuss the importance of not changing brands of insulin or syringes, selection and rotation of injection sites, and compliance with therapeutic regimen.

❑ Demonstrate technique for mixing insulins by drawing up regular insulin or insulin lispro first and rolling intermediate-acting insulin vial between palms to mix, rather than shaking (may cause inaccurate dose).

❑ Explain to patient that this medication controls hyperglycemia but does not cure diabetes. Therapy is long term.

❑ Instruct patient in proper testing of serum glucose and ketones. These tests should be closely monitored during periods of stress or illness and health care professional notified of significant changes.

❑ Emphasize the importance of compliance with nutritional guidelines and regular exercise as directed by health care professional.

❑ Advise patient to consult health care professional prior to using alcohol or other medications concurrently with insulin.

❑ Advise patient to notify health care professional of medication regimen prior to treatment or surgery.

❑ Advise patient to notify health care professional if nausea, vomiting, or fever develops, if unable to eat regular diet, or if blood glucose levels are not controlled.

❑ Instruct patient on signs and symptoms of hypoglycemia and hyperglycemia and what to do if they occur.

❑ Advise patient to notify health care professional if pregnancy is planned or suspected.

❑ Patients with diabetes mellitus should carry a source of sugar (candy, sugar packets) and identification describing their disease and treatment regimen at all times.

❑ Emphasize the importance of regular follow-up, especially during first few weeks of therapy.

## EVALUATION

**Effectiveness of therapy can be demonstrated by:** ■ Control of blood glucose levels without the appearance of hypoglycemic or hyperglycemic episodes.

# INTERFERONS, BETA
(in-ter-**feer**-on)

**interferon beta-1a**
AvonexRebif

**interferon beta-1b**
Betaseron,

## CLASSIFICATION(S):
**Therapeutic:** anti–multiple sclerosis agents
**Pharmacologic:** interferons

### Pregnancy Category C

## INDICATIONS
■ Multiple sclerosis.

## ACTION
■ Antiviral and immunoregulatory properties produced by interacting with specific receptor sites on cell surfaces may explain beneficial effects ■ Produced by recombinant DNA technology. **Therapeutic Effects:** ■ Reduce incidence of relapse (neurologic dysfunction) and slow physical disability.

## PHARMACOKINETICS
**Absorption:** Interferon beta-1b—50% absorbed following subcut administration.
**Distribution:** Unknown.
**Metabolism and Excretion:** Unknown.
**Half-life:** Interferon beta-1a—8.6 hr (subcut), 10 hr (IM); interferon beta-1b—8 min–4.3 hr.

## CONTRAINDICATIONS AND PRECAUTIONS
**Contraindicated in:** ■ Hypersensitivity to natural or recombinant interferon beta or human albumin.
**Use Cautiously in:** ■ Patients with a history of suicide attempt or depression ■ History of seizures ■ Cardiovascular disease ■ Patients with childbearing potential ■ Pregnancy, lactation, or children <18 yr (safety not established).

## ADVERSE REACTIONS AND SIDE EFFECTS*
■ CNS: SEIZURES, headache, weakness, anxiety, confusion, depersonalization, drowsiness, emotional lability, fainting, mental depression, sleep

disorders, suicidal ideation ▪ **EENT:** conjunctivitis, laryngitis, otitis ▪ **Resp:** dyspnea, upper respiratory tract infection ▪ **CV:** chest pain, edema, hypertension, palpitations, peripheral vascular disorders, tachycardia, vasodilation ▪ **GI:** constipation, diarrhea, dyspepsia, nausea, vomiting, abdominal pain, anorexia, elevated liver function studies, GI disorders ▪ **GU:** cystitis, ovarian cyst, pelvic pain ▪ **Derm:** sweating, alopecia, photosensitivity, phototoxicity ▪ **Endo:** menstrual disorders, breast pain, hypoglycemia, menorrhagia, spontaneous abortion ▪ **Hemat:** neutropenia, anemia, eosinophilia ▪ **Local:** injection-site reactions (increased with interferon beta-1b), injection site necrosis ▪ **Metab:** weight loss ▪ **MS:** myalgia, arthralgia, muscle spasm ▪ **Misc:** chills, fever, flu-like symptoms, pain, hypersensitivity reactions.

### INTERACTIONS

**Drug-Drug:** ▪ ↑ myelosuppression may occur with other myelosuppressives including **antineoplastic agents**.

**Drug-Natural Products:** ▪ Avoid concomitant use with immmunomodulating natural products such as **astragalus, echinacea**, and **melatonin**.

### ROUTE AND DOSAGE

❑ **Interferon Beta-1a**

▪ **IM (Adults):** *Avonex*—30 mcg once weekly.

▪ **Subcut (Adults):** *Rebif*—6.6 mcg three times weekly initially, increased over four weeks up to 44 mcg three times weekly.

❑ **Interferon Beta-1b**

▪ **Subcut (Adults):** *Betaseron*—0.25 mg (8 million IU) every other day.

### AVAILABILITY

❑ **Interferon Beta-1a (Avonex)**

▪ *Powder for injection:* 33 mcg (6.6 million IU/vial)$^{Rx}$. ▪ *Prefilled syringes:* 30 mcg/0.5 ml$^{Rx}$ ▪ *Pre-filled syringes (Rebif):* 22 mcg/0.5 ml$^{Rx}$, 44 mcg/0.5 ml$^{Rx}$.

❑ **Interferon Beta-1b**

▪ *Powder for injection (Betaseron):* 0.3 mg (9.6 million IU)/vial$^{Rx}$.

### TIME/ACTION PROFILE

| | ONSET | PEAK | DURATION |
|---|---|---|---|
| Interferon beta-1a IM* | within 12 hr | 48 hr | 4 days |
| Interferon beta-1b subcut† | rapid | 1–8 hr | unknown |

*Biologic response modifiers.
†Serum interferon levels.

## NURSING IMPLICATIONS

### ASSESSMENT

❑ Assess frequency of exacerbations of symptoms of multiple sclerosis periodically during therapy.

❑ Monitor patient for signs of depression during therapy. If depression occurs, notify physician or other health care professional immediately.

▪ *Lab Test Considerations:* Monitor hemoglobin, WBC, platelets, and blood chemistries including liver function tests prior to and periodically during therapy. Therapy may be temporarily discontinued if the absolute neutrophil count is <750/mm³, if AST or ALT exceeds 10 times the upper limit of normal, or if serum bilirubin exceeds 5 times the upper limit of normal. Once the absolute neutrophil count is >750/mm³ or the hepatic enzymes have returned to normal, therapy can be restarted at 50% of the original dose.

### POTENTIAL NURSING DIAGNOSES

▪ Knowledge, deficient, related to medication regimen (Patient/Family Teaching).

### IMPLEMENTATION

▪ **General:** Do not confuse products. Interferon beta-1a and interferon beta-1b are not interchangeable.

▪ **Interferon Beta-1a:** *Avonex:* Reconstitute with 1.1 ml of diluent and swirl gently to dissolve. Keep reconstituted solution in refrigerator; inject within 6 hr of reconstitution.

❑ *Rebif:* Administer subcut via pre-filled, single-use syringe at the same time (afternoon or evening) on the same days (Monday,

Wednesday, Friday) at least 48 hr apart each wk. Rotate sites with each injection to minimize risk of injection site reactions. Discard unused portions. Store in refrigerator.

■ **Interferon Beta-1b:** To reconstitute, inject 1.2 ml of diluent supplied into interferon beta-1b vial for a concentration of 0.25 mg (8 million IU)/ml. Swirl gently to dissolve completely; do not shake. Do not use solutions that are discolored or contain particulate matter. Keep reconstituted solution refrigerated; inject within 3 hr of reconstitution.

❏ Following reconstitution, withdraw 1 ml into a syringe with a 27-gauge needle and inject subcut into arm, abdomen, hip, or thigh. Discard unused portion; vials are for single dose only.

## PATIENT/FAMILY TEACHING

■ **Home Care Issues:** Instruct patient in correct technique for injection and care and disposal of equipment. Caution patient not to reuse needles or syringes and provide patient with a puncture-resistant container for disposal.

❏ Instruct patient to take medication as directed; do not change dose or schedule without consulting health care professional. Patients should receive a medication guide with each product.

❏ Inform patient that flu-like symptoms (fever, chills, myalgia, sweating, malaise) may occur during therapy. Acetaminophen may be used for relief of fever and myalgias.

❏ Caution patient to use sunscreen and wear protective clothes to prevent photosensitivity reactions.

❏ Advise patient to notify health care professional if pregnancy is planned or suspected. May cause spontaneous abortion.

## EVALUATION

**Effectiveness of therapy can be demonstrated by:** ■ Decrease in the frequency of relapse (neurologic dysfunction) in patients with relapsing-remitting multiple sclerosis.

# IODINE, IODIDE

**potassium iodide†**
Pima, SSKI, Thyro-Block

**sodium iodide**
Iodopen

**strong iodine solution**
Lugol's solution

## CLASSIFICATION(S):
*Therapeutic: antithyroid agents*
*Pharmacologic: iodine containing agents*

**Pregnancy Category A (potassium iodide), UK (others)**

†For more information on potassium iodide as a radiation protectant see *Potassium Iodide as a Thyroid Blocking Agent in Radiation Emergencies* at www.fda.gov.

## INDICATIONS

■ Adjunct with other antithyroid drugs in preparation for thyroidectomy ■ Treatment of thyrotoxic crisis ■ Radiation protectant following radiation emergencies or administration of radioactive iodine ■ Iodine replacement ■ As a supplement during long-term parenteral nutrition.

## ACTION

■ Rapidly inhibits the release and synthesis of thyroid hormones ■ Decreases the vascularity of the thyroid gland ■ Decreases thyroidal uptake of radioactive iodine following radiation emergencies or administration of radioactive isotopes of iodine ■ Iodine is a necessary component of thyroid hormone. **Therapeutic Effects:** ■ Control of hyperthyroidism ■ Decreased bleeding during thyroid surgery ■ Replacement/supplementation of iodine ■ Decreased incidence of thyroid cancer following radiation emergencies.

## PHARMACOKINETICS

**Absorption:** Converted in the GI tract and enters the circulation as iodine; also absorbed through skin and lungs; may also be obtained via recycling of iodothyronines.

**Distribution:** Concentrates in the thyroid gland and muscle; also found in skin, skeleton, breasts, and hair. Readily crosses the placenta; enters breast milk.

**Metabolism and Excretion:** Taken up by the thyroid gland, then eliminated via kidneys, liver, skin, lungs, and intestines.

**Half-life:** Unknown.

## CONTRAINDICATIONS AND PRECAUTIONS

**Contraindicated in:** ■ Hypersensitivity.

**Use Cautiously in:** ■ Tuberculosis ■ Bronchitis ■ Hyperkalemia ■ Impaired renal function ■ Pregnancy or lactation (although iodine is required during pregnancy, excess amounts may cause thyroid abnormalities/goiter in the newborn; excess use during lactation may cause skin rash or thyroid suppression in the infant).

## ADVERSE REACTIONS AND SIDE EFFECTS*

■ **GI:** diarrhea, GI irritation ■ **Derm:** acneiform eruptions ■ **Endo:** hypothyroidism, hyperthyroidism, thyroid hyperplasia ■ **F and E:** hyperkalemia (potassium iodide only) ■ **Misc:** hypersensitivity, iodism.

## INTERACTIONS

**Drug-Drug:** ■ Use with **lithium** may cause ↑ hypothyroidism ■ ↑ antithyroid effect of **methimazole** and **propylthiouracil** ■ ↑ hyperkalemia may result from combined use of potassium iodide with **potassium-sparing diuretics, ACE inhibitors, angiotensin II receptor antagonists** or **potassium supplements**.

## ROUTE AND DOSAGE

SSKI (saturated solution of potassium iodide) = 1 g potassium iodide/ml; Lugol's solution = iodine 50 mg/ml plus potassium iodide 100 mg/ml; sodium iodide =118 mcg sodium iodide (100 mcg iodide)/ml.

❑ **Preparation for Thyroidectomy**

■ **PO (Adults and Children):** *Strong iodine solution*—3–5 drops (0.1–0.3 ml) 3 times daily for 10 days prior to surgery. *Potassium iodide saturated solution* (SSKI)—1–5 drops (50–250 mg) 3 times daily for 10–14 days prior to surgery.

❑ **Hyperthyroidism**

■ **PO (Adults and Children):** *Strong iodine solution*—1 ml in water 3 times daily. *Potassium iodide saturated solution*—5 drops (250 mg) 3 times daily.

❑ **Radiation Protectant**

■ **PO (Adults >18 yr including pregnant or lactating women and adolescents approaching adult size):** 130 mg potassium iodide daily.

■ **PO (Children 3–18 yr):** 65 mg per day.

■ **PO (Children 1 mo–3 yr):** 32 mg per day.

■ **PO (Neonates):** 16 mg per day.

❑ **Replacement**

■ **PO (Adults):** *Strong iodine solution*—0.3–1 ml 3–4 times daily.

❑ **Nutritional Supplement**

■ **IV (Adults):** 1–2 mcg elemental iodide/kg/day added to parenteral nutrition. *Pregnant or lactating women*—2–3 mcg elemental iodide/kg/day added to parenteral nutrition.

■ **IV (Children):** 2–3 mcg elemental iodide/kg/day added to parenteral nutrition.

## AVAILABILITY

❑ **Potassium Iodide**

■ *Saturated solution (SSKI):* 1 g potassium iodide/ml in 30- and 240-ml bottles[Rx] ■ Cost: $56.31/240 ml, $12.10/30 ml ■ *Syrup:* 325 mg potassium iodide/5 ml[Rx] ■ *Tablets:* 130 mg[Rx] (available only through state and federal agencies).

❑ **Sodium Iodide**

■ *Solution for injection:* 100 mcg iodide (118 mg sodium iodide)/ml in 10-ml vials[Rx].

❑ **Strong Iodine Solution**

■ *Oral solution:* Iodine 50 mg/ml plus potassium iodide 100 mg/ml (5% iodine plus 10% potassium iodide) in 120-ml, pint, and gallon bottles[Rx].

TIME/ACTION PROFILE (effects on thyroid)

|    | ONSET | PEAK | DURATION |
|----|-------|------|----------|
| PO | 24 hr | 10–15 days | variable† |
| IV | rapid | unknown | unknown |

†Radiation protection lasts 24 hr.

# NURSING IMPLICATIONS

## ASSESSMENT

❑ Assess for signs and symptoms of iodism (metallic taste, stomatitis, skin lesions, cold symptoms, severe GI upset). Report these symptoms promptly to physician.

❑ Monitor response symptoms of hyperthyroidism (tachycardia, palpitations, nervousness, insomnia, diaphoresis, heat intolerance, tremors, weight loss).

❑ Monitor for hypersensitivity reaction (rash, pruritus, laryngeal edema, wheezing). Discontinue drug and notify physician immediately if these problems occur.

■ *Lab Test Considerations:* Monitor thyroid function before and periodically during therapy. May alter results of radionuclide thyroid imaging and may ↓ thyroidal uptake of $^{131}I$, $^{123}I$, and sodium pertechnetate$^{99m}Tc$ in thyroid uptake tests.

❑ Monitor serum potassium levels periodically during therapy. Monitor thyroid stimulating hormone (TSH) and free $T_4$ in neonates (within the first month of life) treated with potassium iodide for development of hypothyroidism. Thyroid hormone therapy should be instituted if hypothyroidism develops.

## POTENTIAL NURSING DIAGNOSES

■ Knowledge, deficient, related to medication regimen (Patient/Family Teaching).

## IMPLEMENTATION

■ **General:** Do not confuse iodine with Lodine (etodolac).

❑ For protection against inhaled radioiodines, administer potassium iodide prior to or immediately coincident with passage of the radioactive cloud, though a substantial protective effect lasts 3–4 hr after exposure.

■ **PO:** Mix solutions in a full glass of fruit juice, water, broth, formula, or milk. Administer after meals to minimize GI irritation.

❑ Solution is normally clear and colorless. Darkening upon standing does not affect potency of drug. Solutions that are brownish yellow should be discarded.

❑ Crystals may form, especially if refrigerated, but redissolve upon warming and shaking.

■ **IV:** Parenteral administration should be used only when oral administration is not possible.

■ **Continuous Infusion:** Sodium iodide is added to total parenteral nutrition solutions.

■ **Additive Compatibility:** ◆ amino acid solutions ◆ dextrose solutions ◆ electrolytes ◆ trace metals.

## PATIENT/FAMILY TEACHING

❑ Instruct patient to take medication as directed. Take missed doses as soon as possible but not just before next dose; do not double doses.

❑ Instruct patient to report suspected pregnancy to health care professional before therapy is initiated.

❑ Advise patient to consult health care professional about avoiding foods high in iodine (seafood, iodized salt, cabbage, kale, turnips) or potassium (see Appendix Q).

❑ Advise patient to consult health care professional before using OTC or herbal cold remedies. Some cold remedies use iodide as an expectorant.

■ **Hyperthyroidism:** Instruct patient to take medication as ordered. Missing a dose may precipitate hyperthyroidism.

■ **Nutritional Supplement:** Discuss the need for iodine in the body and identify food sources of iodine with patient.

## EVALUATION

**Effectiveness of therapy can be demonstrated by:** ■ Resolution of the symptoms of thyroid crisis ■ Decrease in size and vascularity of the gland before thyroid surgery. Use of iodides in the treatment of hyperthyroidism is usually limited to 2 wk ■ Protection of the thyroid gland from the effects of radioactive iodine ■ Prevention and treatment of iodine deficiency.

---

# ipratropium

(i-pra-**troe**-pee-um)

Atrovent

**CLASSIFICATION(S):**

*Therapeutic:* allergy, cold, and cough remedies, bronchodilators

*Pharmacologic:* anticholinergics

**Pregnancy Category B**

## INDICATIONS

■ **Inhaln:** Maintenance therapy of reversible airway obstruction due to COPD ■ **Intranasal:** Rhinorrhea associated with allergic and nonallergic perennial rhinitis (0.03% solution) or the common cold (0.06% solution). **Unla-**

**beled uses:** ■ **Inhaln:** Adjunctive management of bronchospasm caused by asthma.

## ACTION

■ **Inhaln:** Inhibits cholinergic receptors in bronchial smooth muscle, resulting in decreased concentrations of cyclic guanosine monophosphate (cGMP). Decreased levels of cGMP produce local bronchodilation ■ **Intranasal:** Local application inhibits secretions from glands lining the nasal mucosa. **Therapeutic Effects:** ■ **Inhaln:** Bronchodilation without systemic anticholinergic effects ■ **Intranasal:** Decreased rhinorrhea.

## PHARMACOKINETICS

**Absorption:** Minimal systemic absorption (2% for inhalation solution; 20% for inhalation aerosol; <20% following nasal use).
**Distribution:** Does not appear to cross the blood-brain barrier.
**Metabolism and Excretion:** Small amounts absorbed are metabolized by the liver.
**Half-life:** 2 hr.

## CONTRAINDICATIONS AND PRECAUTIONS

**Contraindicated in:** ■ Hypersensitivity to ipratropium, atropine, belladonna alkaloids, bromide or fluorocarbons ■ Peanut or soy allergy (inhaler contains soy lecithin) ■ Avoid use during acute bronchospasm.
**Use Cautiously in:** ■ Patients with bladder neck obstruction, prostatic hypertrophy, glaucoma, or urinary retention ■ Geriatric patients (may be more sensitive to effects) ■ Pregnancy, lactation, or children <5 yr (safety not established).

## ADVERSE REACTIONS AND SIDE EFFECTS*

■ **CNS:** dizziness, headache, nervousness ■ **EENT:** blurred vision, sore throat; *nasal only*—epistaxis, nasal dryness/irritation ■ **Resp:** bronchospasm, cough ■ **CV:** hypotension, palpitations ■ **GI:** GI irritation, nausea ■ **Derm:** rash ■ **Misc:** allergic reactions.

## INTERACTIONS

**Drug-Drug:** ■ Potential ↑ fluorocarbon toxicity when used with other **inhalation broncho**dilators having a fluorocarbon propellant ■ ↑ anticholinergic properties with other drugs having anticholinergic properties (antihistamines, phenothiazines, disopyramide).

## ROUTE AND DOSAGE

■ **Inhaln (Adults):** *Metered-dose inhaler*—1–4 inhalations 3–4 times daily (not to exceed 24 inhalations/24 hr or more frequently than q 4 hr). During initial therapy, up to 8 inhalations may be repeated. During acute exacerbations 6–8 inhalations q 3–4 hr using a spacer device may be needed. *Via nebulization*—250–500 mcg 3–4 times daily given q 6–8 hr as needed (up to 500 mcg q 4 hr).

■ **Inhaln (Children 5–12 yr):** *Metered dose inhaler*—1–2 inhalations q 6–8 hr as needed. *Via nebulization*—125–250 mcg 3–4 times daily given q 4–6 hr as needed.

■ **Intranasal (Adults and Children ≥12 yr):** *Perennial rhinitis*—2 sprays of 0.03% solution in each nostril 2–3 times daily (21 mcg/spray); *perennial rhinitis*—2 sprays of 0.06% solution in each nostril 3–4 times daily (42 mcg/spray) for up to 4 days.

## AVAILABILITY (generic available)

■ *Aerosol inhaler (contains soy lecithin):* 18 mcg/spray in 14-g canister (200 inhalations)[Rx] ■ **Cost:** *Atrovent*—$44.56/inhaler, $44.56/refill ■ *Inhalation solution:* {0.0125%[Rx]}, 0.02% in single-dose vials containing 500 mcg[Rx], {0.025%[Rx]} ■*Nasal spray:* 0.03% solution—21 mcg/spray in 30-ml bottle (345 sprays/bottle)[Rx], 0.06% solution—42 mcg/spray in 15-ml bottle (165 sprays)[Rx] ■ albuterol (Combivent, Duoneb)[Rx]. See Appendix B.

TIME/ACTION PROFILE (bronchodilation)

| | ONSET | PEAK | DURATION |
|---|---|---|---|
| Inhalation | 5–15 min | 1–2 hr | 3–4 hr (up to 8 hr) |
| Intranasal | 15 min | unknown | 6–12 hr |

# NURSING IMPLICATIONS

## ASSESSMENT

- **General Info:** Assess for allergy to atropine and belladonna alkaloids; patients with these allergies may also be sensitive to ipratropium. Assess for peanut or soy allergy (inhaler contains soy lecithin).
- **Inhaln:** Assess respiratory status (rate, breath sounds, degree of dyspnea, pulse) before administration and at peak of medication. Consult physician or other health care professional about alternative medication if severe bronchospasm is present; onset of action is too slow for patients in acute distress. If paradoxical bronchospasm (wheezing) occurs, withhold medication and notify physician or other health care professional immediately.
- **Nasal Spray:** Assess patient for rhinorrhea.

## POTENTIAL NURSING DIAGNOSES

- Airway clearance, ineffective (Indications).
- Activity intolerance (Indications).

## IMPLEMENTATION

- **General:** Do not confuse Atrovent with Alupent (metaproterenol). **Inhaln:** See Appendix F for administration of inhalation medications.
- ❑ When ipratropium is administered concurrently with other inhalation medications, administer adrenergic bronchodilators first, followed by ipratropium, then corticosteroids. Wait 5 min between medications.
- ❑ Solution for *nebulization* can be diluted with preservative-free 0.9% NaCl. Diluted solution should be used within 24 hr at room temperature or 48 hr if refrigerated. Solution can be mixed with preservative-free albuterol, cromolyn, or metaproterenol if used within 1 hr of mixing.

## PATIENT/FAMILY TEACHING

- **General Info:** Instruct patient in proper use of inhaler, nebulizer, or nasal spray and to take medication as directed. Take missed doses as soon as remembered unless almost time for the next dose; space remaining doses evenly during day. Do not double doses.
- ❑ Advise patient that rinsing mouth after using inhaler, good oral hygiene, and sugarless gum or candy may minimize dry mouth.

Health care professional should be notified if stomatitis occurs or if dry mouth persists for more than 2 wk.

- **Inhalation:** Caution patient not to exceed 12 doses within 24 hr. Patient should notify health care professional if symptoms do not improve within 30 min after administration of medication or if condition worsens.
- ❑ Explain need for pulmonary function tests prior to and periodically during therapy to determine effectiveness of medication.
- ❑ Caution patient to avoid spraying medication in eyes; may cause blurring of vision or irritation.
- ❑ Advise patient to inform health care professional if cough, nervousness, headache, dizziness, nausea, or GI distress occurs.
- **Nasal Spray:** Instruct patient in proper use of nasal spray. Clear nasal passages gently before administration. Do not inhale during administration, so medication remains in nasal passages. Prime pump initially with 7 actuations. If used regularly, no further priming is needed. If not used in 24 hr, prime with 2 actuations. If not used for >7 days, prime with 7 actuations.
- ❑ Advise patient to contact health care professional if symptoms do not improve within 1–2 wk or if condition worsens.

## EVALUATION

**Effectiveness of therapy can be demonstrated by:** ■ Decreased dyspnea ❑ Improved breath sounds ■ Decrease in rhinorrhea from perennial rhinitis or the common cold.

---

# irbesartan, See ANGIOTENSIN II RECEPTOR ANTAGONISTS.

---

# irinotecan

(eye-ri-noe-**tee**-kan)
Camptosar

### CLASSIFICATION(S):
**Therapeutic:** antineoplastics
**Pharmacologic:** enzyme inhibitors

### Pregnancy Category D

## INDICATIONS

■ Metastatic colorectalcancer (with 5-fluorouracil and leucovorin).

## ACTION

■ Interferes with DNA synthesis by inhibiting the enzyme topoisomerase. **Therapeutic Effects:** ■ Death of rapidly replicating cells, particularly malignant ones.

## PHARMACOKINETICS

**Absorption:** IV administration results in complete bioavailability.
**Distribution:** Unknown.
**Protein Binding:** *Irinotecan*—30–68%; *SN–38 (active metabolite)*—95%.
**Metabolism and Excretion:** Converted by the liver to SN–38, its active metabolite, which is also metabolized by the liver. Small amounts excreted by kidneys.
**Half-life:** 6 hr.

## CONTRAINDICATIONS AND PRECAUTIONS

**Contraindicated in:** ■ Hypersensitivity ■ Pregnancy or lactation.

**Use Cautiously in:** ■ Previous pelvic or abdominal irradiation or age ≥65 yr (increased risk of myelosuppression) ■ Presence of infection, underlying bone marrow depression, or concurrent chronic illness ■ History of prior pelvic/abdominal irradiation and serum bilirubin >1–2 mg/dl (initial dosage reduction recommended) ■ Geriatric patients (increased sensitivity to adverse effects; initiate at lower doses) ■ Previous severe myelosuppression or diarrhea (reinstitute at lower dose following resolution) ■ Patients with childbearing potential ■ Children (safety not established).

## ADVERSE REACTIONS AND SIDE EFFECTS*

■ **CNS:** dizziness, headache, insomnia, weakness ■ **EENT:** rhinitis ■ **Resp:** coughing, dyspnea ■ **CV:** edema, vasodilation ■ **GI:** DIARRHEA, ELEVATED LIVER ENZYMES, abdominal pain/cramping, anorexia, constipation, dyspepsia, flatulence, nausea, stomatitis, vomiting, abdominal enlargement, colonic ulceration ■ **Derm:** alopecia, rash, sweating ■ **F and E:** dehydration ■ **Hemat:** anemia, leukopenia, thrombocytopenia ■ **Local:** injection site reactions ■ **Metab:** weight loss ■ **MS:** back pain ■ **Misc:** chills, fever.

## INTERACTIONS

**Drug-Drug:** ■ Combination with **fluorouracil** may result in serious toxicity (dehydration, neutropenia, sepsis) ■ ↑ bone marrow depression may occur with other **antineoplastics** or **radiation therapy** ■ **Laxatives** should be avoided (diarrhea may be ↑) ■ **Diuretics** ↑ risk of dehydration (may discontinue during therapy) ■ **Dexamethasone** used as an antiemetic ↑ risk of hyperglycemia and lymphocytopenia ■ **Prochlorperazine** given on the same day as irinotecan ↑ risk of akathisia.
**Drug-Natural Products:** ■ **St. John's wort** ↑ increases levels and risk of toxicity.

## ROUTE AND DOSAGE

Other regimens are used; careful modification required for all levels of toxicity/tolerance.

❑ **Single Agent**

■ **IV (Adults):** *Weekly dosage schedule*—125 mg/m² once weekly for 4 wk, followed by a 2-wk rest period. Cycle may be repeated using doses which depend on patient tolerance and degree of toxicity encountered. *Once-every-3-wk schedule*—350 mg/m² once every 3 wk.

■ **IV (Geriatric Patients >70 yr):** Initiate at 300 mg/m² every 3 wk.

❑ **Hepatic Impairment**

■ **IV (Adults):** *Bilirubin 1–2 mg/dl and history of prior pelvic/abdominal irradiation—Weekly dosage schedule*—Initiate therapy at lower dose (100 mg/m²); once weekly for 4 wk, followed by a 2-wk rest period. Cycle may be repeated with dose adjusted as tolerated. *Once-every-3-wk schedule*—300 mg/m² once every 3 wk, dose adjusted as tolerated as low as 200 mg/m² and further adjusted in 50-mg increments.

❑ **As Part of Combination Therapy with Leucovorin and 5-Fluorouracil**

■ **IV (Adults):** *Regimen 1 (Bolus regimen)*—125 mg/m² once weekly for 4 wk, followed by a 2-wk rest period. Cycle may be repeated using doses that depend on patient tolerance and degree of toxicity encountered; *Regimen 2(Infusional regimen)*—180 mg/m² every 2 wk for 3 doses, followed by a 3-wk rest period. Cycle may be repeated using doses that depend on patient tolerance and degree of toxicity encountered.

## AVAILABILITY

■ *Solution for injection:* 20 mg/ml in 2–mlRx and 5-ml vials^Rx.

TIME/ACTION PROFILE (hematologic effects)

| | ONSET | PEAK | DURATION |
|---|---|---|---|
| IV | unknown | 21–29 days | 27–34 days |

## NURSING IMPLICATIONS

### ASSESSMENT

❑ Monitor vital signs frequently during administration.

❑ Monitor for bone marrow depression. Assess for bleeding (bleeding gums, bruising, petechiae, guaiac stools, urine, and emesis) and avoid IM injections and taking rectal temperatures if platelet count is low. Apply pressure to venipuncture sites for 10 min. Assess for signs of infection during neutropenia. Anemia may occur. Monitor for increased fatigue, dyspnea, and orthostatic hypotension.

❑ Monitor closely for the development of diarrhea. Two types may occur. The early type occurs within 24 hr of administration and may be preceded by cramps and sweating. Atropine 0.25–1 mg IV may be given to decrease symptoms. Potentially life-threatening diarrhea may occur more than 24 hr after a dose and may be accompanied by severe dehydration and electrolyte imbalance. Loperamide 4 mg initially, followed by 2 mg every 2 hr until diarrhea ceases for at least 12 hr (or 4 mg every 4 hr if given during sleeping hours) should be administered promptly to treat late-occurring diarrhea. Careful fluid and electrolyte replacement should be instituted to prevent complications. Subsequent doses should be delayed in patients with active diarrhea until diarrhea is resolved for 24 hr. If diarrhea is grade 2, 3, or 4, decrease subsequent doses of irinotecan.

❑ Nausea and vomiting are common. Pretreatment with dexamethasone 10 mg along with agents such as ondansetron or granisetron should be started on the same day as irinotecan at least 30 min before administration. Prochlorperazine may be used on subsequent days but may increase risk of akathisia if given on the same day as irinotecan.

❑ Assess IV site frequently for inflammation. Avoid extravasation. If extravasation occurs, infusion must be stopped and restarted in another vein to avoid damage to subcut tissue. Flushing site with sterile water and application of ice over the extravasated site are recommended.

■ *Lab Test Considerations:* Monitor CBC with differential and platelet count prior to each dose. Temporarily discontinue irinotecan if absolute neutrophil count is <500 cells/mm³ or if neutropenic fever occurs. Administration of a colony-stimulating factor may be considered if clinically significant decreases in WBC (<2000/mm³), neutrophil count (<1000/mm³), hemoglobin (<9 g/dl), or platelet count (<100,000 cells/mm³) occur.

❑ May cause ↑ serum alkaline phosphatase and AST concentrations.

## POTENTIAL NURSING DIAGNOSES

■ Infection, risk for (Adverse Reactions).

## IMPLEMENTATION

■ **General:** Solution should be prepared in a biologic cabinet. Wear gloves, gown, and mask while handling IV medication. Discard IV equipment in specially designated containers.

■ **Intermittent Infusion:** Dilute before infusion with D5W or 0.9% NaCl for a concentration of 0.12–1.1 mg/ml. Usual diluent is 500 ml of D5W. Solution is pale yellow. Do not administer solutions that are cloudy or contain particulate matter. Solution is stable for 24 hr at room temperature or 48 hr if refrigerated. To prevent microbial contamination, solutions should be used within 24 hr of dilution if refrigerated or 6 hr at room temperature. Do not refrigerate solutions diluted with 0.9% NaCl.

■ *Rate:* Administer dose over 90 min.

■ **Y-Site Incompatibility:** ✦ gemcitabine

■ **Additive Incompatibility:** Information unavailable. Do not admix with other solutions or medications.

## PATIENT/FAMILY TEACHING

❑ Instruct patient to report occurrence of diarrhea to health care professional immediately, especially if it occurs more than 24 hr after dose. Diarrhea may be accompanied by severe dehydration and electrolyte imbalance. It may be life-threatening and should be treated promptly.

❑ Instruct patient to notify health care professional promptly if fever; chills; sore throat; signs of infection; bleeding gums; bruising; petechiae; blood in urine, stool, or emesis occurs. Caution patient to avoid crowds and persons with known infections. Instruct patient to use soft toothbrush and electric razor. Caution patient not to drink alcoholic beverages or take products containing aspirin or other NSAIDs.

❑ Instruct patient to notify nurse of pain at injection site immediately.

❑ Instruct patient to notify health care professional if vomiting, fainting, or dizziness occurs.

❑ Discuss with patient possibility of hair loss. Explore methods of coping.

❑ Advise patient that this medication may have teratogenic effects. Contraception should be used during therapy.

❑ Instruct patient not to receive any vaccinations without consulting health care professional.

❑ Emphasize the need for periodic lab tests to monitor for side effects.

## EVALUATION

**Effectiveness of therapy can be demonstrated by:** ▪ Decrease in size and spread of malignancy.

---

# IRON SUPPLEMENTS

**carbonyl iron (100%)**

**(kar-bo-nileye-ern)**

Feosol, Icar

**ferrous fumarate (33% elemental iron)**

**(fer-usfyoo-ma-rate)**

Femiron, Feostat, Fumasorb, Fumerin, Hemocyte, Neo-Fer, {Nephro-Fer}, {Novofumar}, {Palafer}, Span-FF

**ferrous gluconate (12% elemental iron)**

**(fer-usgloo-koe-nate)**

{Apo-Ferrous Gluconate}, Fergon, Ferralet, {Fertinic}, {Novoferrogluc}, Simron

**ferrous sulfate (30% elemental iron)**

**(fer-ussul-fate)**

{Apo-Ferrous Sulfate}, ED-IN-SOL, Fe50, Feosol, Feratab, Fer-gen-sol, Fer-In-Sol, Fer-Iron, {Fero-Grad}, {Novoferrosulfa}, {PMS Ferrous Sulfate}, Slow FE

**iron dextran**

**(eye-erndex-tran)**

DexFerrum, InFeD

**iron polysaccharide**

**(eye-ern poll-ee-sak-a-ride)**

Hytinic, Niferex, Nu-Iron

**iron sucrose**

**(eye-ernsu-krose)**

Venofer

**sodium ferric gluconate complex**

**(so-dee-yumferr-icgloo-ko-nate)**

Ferrlecit

**CLASSIFICATION(S):**
**Therapeutic:** antianemics
**Pharmacologic:** iron supplements

**Pregnancy Category B (sodium ferric gluconate, iron sucrose), C (iron dextran)**

## INDICATIONS

▪ **PO:** Prevention/treatment of iron-deficiency anemia ▪ **IM, IV:** *Iron dextran*—Treatment/

---

prevention of iron-deficiency anemia in patients who cannot tolerate oral iron ■ *Sodium ferric gluconate complex, iron sucrose*—Treatment of iron deficiency in patients undergoing chronic hemodialysis who are concurrently receiving erythropoietin.

## ACTION

■ An essential mineral found in hemoglobin, myoglobin, and many enzymes ■ Parenteral iron enters the bloodstream and organs of the reticuloendothelial system (liver, spleen, bone marrow), where iron is separated out and becomes part of iron stores. **Therapeutic Effects:** ■ Prevention/treatment of iron deficiency.

## PHARMACOKINETICS

**Absorption:** 5–10% of dietary iron is absorbed. In deficiency states, this increases up to 30%. Therapeutically administered PO iron may be 60% absorbed; absorption is an active and passive transport process. Well absorbed following IM administration.

**Distribution:** Remains in the body for many months. Crosses the placenta; enters breast milk.

**Protein Binding:** ≥90%.

**Metabolism and Excretion:** Mostly recycled; small daily losses occurring via desquamation, sweat, urine, and bile.

**Half-life:** *Iron dextran, iron sucrose*—6 hr.

## CONTRAINDICATIONS AND PRECAUTIONS

**Contraindicated in:** ■ Primary hemochromatosis ■ Hemolytic anemias and other anemias not due to iron deficiency ■ Some products contain alcohol, tartrazine, or sulfites and should be avoided in patients with known intolerance or hypersensitivity ■ Concurrent oral iron therapy.

**Use Cautiously in:** ■ **PO:** Peptic ulcer ■ Ulcerative colitis or regional enteritis (condition may be aggravated) ■ Indiscriminate chronic use (may lead to iron overload) ■ **IM, IV:** Autoimmune disorders and arthritis (more susceptible to allergic reactions following IM, IV use) ■ Geriatric patients (lower initial dose may be recommended) ■ Lactation or children (safety of some parenteral products not established).

**Exercise Extreme Caution in:** ■ **IM, IV:** Patients with severe liver impairment ■ Geriatric patients (lower initial dose may be recom-

mended) ■ Lactation or children (safety of some parenteral products not established)

## ADVERSE REACTIONS AND SIDE EFFECTS*

■ **CNS:** *IM, IV*—SEIZURES , dizziness, headache, syncope ■ **CV:** *IM, IV*—hypotension, tachycardia ■ **GI:** nausea; *PO*—constipation, dark stools, diarrhea, epigastric pain, GI bleeding; *IM, IV*—taste disorder, vomiting ■ **Derm:** *IM, IV*—flushing, urticaria ■ **Local:** pain at IM site (iron dextran), phlebitis at IV site, skin staining at IM site (iron dextran) ■ **MS:** *IM, IV*—arthralgia, myalgia ■ **Misc:** *PO*—staining of teeth (liquid preparations); *IM, IV*—allergic reactions including ANAPHYLAXIS , fever, lymphadenopathy.

## INTERACTIONS

**Drug-Drug:** ■ **Tetracycline** and **antacids** ↑ oral absorption of iron by forming insoluble compounds ■ Oral iron supplements ↓ absorption of **Tetracyclines, fluoroquinolones,** and **penicillamine** (simultaneous administration should be avoided) ■ ↓ absorption of and may ↓ effects of **levodopa** and **methyldopa** ■ May ↓ efficacy of **levothyroxine** (concurrent administration should be avoided) ■ Concurrent administration of **cimetidine** may ↓ absorption ■ Doses of **ascorbic acid** ≥200 mg may ↑ absorption by ≥30% ■ **Chloramphenicol** and **vitamin E** may hematologic response to iron therapy.

**Drug-Food:** ■ Iron absorption is ↓ 33–50% by concurrent administration of food.

## ROUTE AND DOSAGE

❑ **Oral Iron Dosage for Iron Deficiency (mg elemental iron)**

■ **PO (Adults):** 100—200 mg/day (2–3 mg/kg/day) in 3 divided doses.

■ **PO (Children 2–12 yr or 15–30 kg):** 50–100 mg/day (1–1.5 mg/kg/day) in 3–4 divided doses.

■ **PO (Children 6 mo–2 yr):** Up to 6 mg/kg/day in 3–4 divided doses.

■ **PO (Infants):** 10–25 mg/day in 3–4 divided doses.

❑ **Carbonyl Iron**

■ **PO (Adults):** 50–100 mg 3 times daily.

❑ **Ferrous Fumarate**

■ **PO (Adults):** *Prophylactic*—200 mg/day. *Therapeutic*—200 mg 3–4 times daily. Controlled-release capsules may be given twice daily.

- **PO (Children):** *Prophylactic*—3 mg/kg/day. *Therapeutic*—3–6 mg/kg 3 times daily.

□ **Ferrous Gluconate**

- **PO (Adults):** *Prophylactic*—325 mg/day. *Therapeutic*—325–650 mg qid. Sustained-release capsules may be given twice daily.
- **PO (Children >2 yr):** *Prophylactic*—8 mg/kg/day. *Therapeutic*—16 mg/kg tid.

□ **Ferrous Sulfate**

- **PO (Adults):** *Prophylactic*—300–325 mg/day. *Therapeutic*—300 mg 2–4 times daily. Timed-release tablets may be given twice daily.
- **PO (Children):** *Prophylactic*—5 mg/kg/day. *Therapeutic*—10 mg/kg tid.

□ **Iron Dextran**

- **IV (Adults and Children):** Test dose of 0.5 ml (25 mg) is given prior to therapy.
- **IM, IV (Adults and Children >15 kg):** *Iron deficiency*—Total dose (ml) = 0.0442 (desired Hgb − actual Hgb) × lean body weight (kg) + (0.26 × lean body weight). Divided up and given in small daily doses until total is reached; not to exceed 100 mg/day. *Total dose IV infusion*—Total dose may be diluted and infused over 4–5 hr following a test dose of 10 drops (unlabeled).
- **IM, IV (Children 5–15 kg):** *Iron deficiency*—Total dose (ml) = 0.0442 (desired Hgb − actual Hgb) × weight (kg) + (0.26 × weight) (not to exceed 25 mg/day in children <5 kg; 50 mg/day in children <10 kg; or 100 mg/day in others).
- **IM, IV (Adults):** *Blood loss*—Dose (ml) = (Blood loss [ml] × hematocrit) ÷ 50.

□ **Iron Polysaccharide**

- **PO (Adults):** 50–100 mg 3 times daily.
- **PO (Children):** 4–6 mg/kg/day in 3 divided doses.
- **PO (Infants):** 1–2 mg/kg/day.
- **PO (Adults—Pregnant Women):** 30–60 mg/day.

□ **Iron Sucrose**

- **IV (Adults):** 100 mg (5 ml) during each dialysis session (up to 3 times weekly) for 10 doses (total 1000 mg); additional smaller doses may be necessary (no test dose needed).

□ **Sodium Ferric Gluconate Complex**

- **IV (Adults):** 10 ml (125 mg elemental iron) repeated during 8 sequential dialysis treatments to a total cumulative dose of 1 g.

**AVAILABILITY**

□ **Carbonyl Iron (100% Iron)**

- ***Tablets:*** 50 mg$^{OTC}$ ■ ***Oral suspension:*** 15 mg/1.25 ml in 118-ml bottles$^{OTC}$.

□ **Ferrous Fumarate (33% Elemental Iron)**

- ***Tablets:*** 63 mg$^{OTC}$, 195 mg$^{OTC}$, 200 mg$^{OTC}$, 324 mg$^{OTC}$, 325 mg$^{OTC}$ ■ ***Chewable tablets:*** 100 mg$^{OTC}$ ■ ***Controlled-release capsules:*** 325 mg$^{OTC}$ ■ ***Suspension (butterscotch flavor):*** 100 mg/5 ml$^{OTC}$, {300 mg/5 ml$^{OTC}$} ■ ***Drops:*** 45 mg/0.6 ml$^{OTC}$, {60 mg/1 ml$^{OTC}$}.

□ **Ferrous Gluconate (11.6% Elemental Iron)**

- ***Tablets:*** 300 mg$^{OTC}$, 320 mg$^{OTC}$, 325 mg$^{OTC}$ ■ ***Sustained-release tablets:*** 320 mg$^{OTC}$ ■ ***Soft gelatin capsules:*** 86 mg$^{OTC}$ ■ ***Elixir:*** 300 mg/5 ml$^{OTC}$ ■ ***Syrup:*** {300 mg/5 ml$^{OTC}$}.

□ **Ferrous Sulfate (20–30% Elemental Iron)**

- ***Tablets:*** 195 mg$^{OTC}$, 300 mg$^{OTC}$, 325 mg$^{OTC}$ ■ **Cost:** 324 mg $0.85/30 ■ ***Capsules:*** 150 mg$^{OTC}$, 250 mg$^{OTC}$ ■ ***Timed-release tablets:*** 525 mg$^{OTC}$ ■ ***Syrup:*** 90 mg/5 ml$^{OTC}$ ■ ***Elixir:*** 220 mg/5 ml$^{OTC}$ ■ ***Drops:*** 75 mg/0.6 ml$^{OTC}$, 125 mg/1 ml$^{OTC}$.

□ **Iron Dextran**

- ***Injection:*** 50 mg/ml$^{Rx}$.

□ **Iron Polysaccharide (mg Iron)**

- ***Capsules:*** 150 mg$^{OTC}$ ■ ***Elixir:*** 100 mg/5 ml$^{OTC}$ ■ ***Tablets:*** 50 mg$^{OTC}$.

□ **Iron Sucrose**

- ***Aqueous complex for injection:*** 20 mg/ml in 5 ml single-use vial (100 mg)$^{Rx}$.

---

{ } = Available in Canada only.
\* CAPITALS indicates life-threatening; <u>underlines</u> indicate most frequent.

## □ Sodium Ferric Gluconate Complex

■ *Injection:* 62.5 mg/5 ml in 5 ml ampules[Rx]
■ ascorbic acid, antacids, multiple vitamins, and other minerals[OTC]. See Appendix B.

TIME/ACTION PROFILE (effects on erythropoiesis)

|  | ONSET | PEAK | DURATION |
|---|---|---|---|
| PO | 4 days | 7–10 days | 2–4 mo |
| IM, IV | 4 days | 1–2 wk | wks–mos |

## NURSING IMPLICATIONS

### ASSESSMENT

□ Assess nutritional status and dietary history to determine possible cause of anemia and need for patient teaching.

□ Assess bowel function for constipation or diarrhea. Notify physician or other health care professional and use appropriate nursing measures should these occur.

■ **Iron Dextran, Iron Sucrose, and Sodium Ferric Gluconate Complex:** Monitor blood pressure and heart rate frequently following IV administration until stable. Rapid infusion rate may cause hypotension and flushing.

□ Assess patient for signs and symptoms of anaphylaxis (rash, pruritus, laryngeal edema, wheezing). Notify physician immediately if these occur. Keep epinephrine and resuscitation equipment close by in the event of an anaphylactic reaction.

■ *Lab Test Considerations:* Monitor hemoglobin, hematocrit, and reticulocyte values prior to and every 3 wk during the first 2 mo of therapy and periodically thereafter. Serum ferritin and iron levels may also be monitored to assess effectiveness of therapy.

□ Occult blood in stools may be obscured by black coloration of iron in stool. Guaiac test results may occasionally be false-positive. Benzidine test results are not affected by iron preparations.

■ **Iron Dextran:** Monitor hemoglobin, hematocrit, reticulocyte values, transferrin, ferritin, total iron-binding capacity, and plasma iron concentrations periodically during therapy. Serum ferritin levels peak in 7–9 days and return to normal in 3 wk. Serum iron determinations may be inaccurate for 1–2 wk after therapy with large doses; therefore, hemoglobin and hematocrit are used to gauge

initial response. Normal hemoglobin concentrations of 14.8 g/100 ml should be used for patients weighing >15 kg, while 12 g/100 ml should be used for patients weighing 15 kg or less.

□ May impart a brownish hue to blood drawn within 4 hr of administration. May cause false ↑ in serum bilirubin and false decrease in serum calcium values.

□ Prolonged PTT may be calculated when blood sample is anticoagulated with citrate dextrose solution; use sodium citrate instead.

■ **Iron Sucrose:** Monitor hemoglobin, hematocrit, serum ferritin, and transferritin saturation prior to and periodically during therapy. Transferrin saturation values increase rapidly after IV administration; therefore, serum iron values may be reliably obtained 48 hr after IV administration. Withhold iron therapy if evidence of iron overload occurs.

□ May cause ↑ liver enzymes.

■ *Toxicity and Overdose:* Early symptoms of overdose include stomach pain, fever, nausea, vomiting (may contain blood), and diarrhea. Late symptoms include bluish lips, fingernails, and palms; drowsiness; weakness; tachycardia; seizures; metabolic acidosis; hepatic injury; and cardiovascular collapse. Patient may appear to recover prior to the onset of late symptoms. Therefore, hospitalization continues for 24 hr after patient becomes asymptomatic to monitor for delayed onset of shock or GI bleeding. Late complications of overdose include intestinal obstruction, pyloric stenosis, and gastric scarring.

□ Treatment includes inducing emesis with syrup of ipecac. If patient is comatose or seizing, gastric lavage with sodium bicarbonate is performed. Deferoxamine is the antidote. Additional supportive treatments to maintain fluid and electrolyte balance and correction of metabolic acidosis are also indicated.

□ If signs of overdose occur during IV administration of iron sucrose, administration at a slower rate usually relieves symptoms.

### POTENTIAL NURSING DIAGNOSES

■ Activity intolerance (Indications).

### IMPLEMENTATION

■ **General:** Oral iron preparations should be discontinued prior to parenteral administration.

❑ Ferrlecit is for IV use only.

■ **PO:** Oral preparations are most effectively absorbed if administered 1 hr before or 2 hr after meals. If gastric irritation occurs, administer with meals. Take tablets and capsules with a full glass of water or juice. Do not crush or chew enteric-coated tablets and do not open capsules.

❑ Liquid preparations may stain teeth. Dilute in water or fruit juice, full glass (240 ml) for adults and $^1/_2$ glass (120 ml) for children, and administer with a straw or place drops at back of throat. Feosol elixir should be diluted in water only. Fer-In-Sol liquid or syrup may be diluted in water or fruit juice.

❑ Avoid using antacids, coffee, tea, dairy products, eggs, or whole-grain breads with or within 1 hr after administration of ferrous salts. Iron absorption is decreased by 33% if iron and calcium are given with meals. If calcium supplementation is needed, calcium carbonate does not decrease absorption of iron salts if supplements are administered between meals.

■ **Iron Dextran:** The 2-ml ampule may be used for IM or IV administration; the 10-ml multidose vial may be used only for IM administration.

❑ Prior to initial IM or IV dose, a test dose of 25 mg should be given by the same route as the dose will be given, to determine reaction. The IV test dose should be administered over 5 min. The IM dose should be administered in the same injection site and by same technique as the therapeutic dose. The remaining portion may be administered after 1 hr, if no adverse symptoms have occurred.

■ **IM:** Inject deeply via Z-track technique into upper outer quadrant of buttock, never into arm or other exposed areas. Use a 2–3 in., 19- or 20-gauge needle. Change needles between withdrawal from container and injection to minimize staining of subcut tissues. Stains are usually permanent.

■ **IV:** Following IV administration, patient should remain recumbent for at least 30 min to prevent orthostatic hypotension.

■ **Direct IV:** Administer undiluted.

■ *Rate:* Administer slowly at a rate of 50 mg (1 ml) over at least 1 min.

■ **Continuous Infusion:** May be diluted in 200–1000 ml of 0.9% NaCl or D5W; 0.9% NaCl is the preferred diluent; dilution in D5W increases incidence of pain and phlebitis.

■ *Rate:* Administer over 1–8 hr following a test dose of 10 drops/min for 10 min. Flush line with 10 ml of 0.9% NaCl at completion of infusion.

■ **Y-Site Incompatibility:** Discontinue other IV solutions during infusion.

■ **Additive Incompatibility:** Manufacturers recommend that iron dextran not be mixed with other solutions; however, iron dextran has been added to total parenteral nutrition solutions.

■ **Sodium Ferric Gluconate Complex:** Before initiating therapeutic doses, a test dose of 2 ml (25 mg of elemental iron) should be administered. Dilute test dose in 50 ml of 0.9% NaCl and administer IV over 60 min.

❑ To administer therapeutic dose of 10 ml (125 mg of elemental iron) dilute in 100 ml of 0.9% NaCl. Dialysis patients frequently require a cumulative dose of 1 g of elemental iron, administered over 8 sessions of sequential dialysis.

■ *Rate:* Administer over 1 hr.

■ **Iron Sucrose:** Do not administer iron sucrose concurrently with oral iron, as the absorption of oral iron is reduced.

❑ Each 5–ml vial contains 100 mg of elemental iron. Most patients require a minimum cumulative dose of 1000 mg of elemental iron, administered over 10 sequential dialysis sessions, to achieve a favorable hemoglobin or hematocrit response.

❑ Iron sucrose must only be administered IV directly into dialysis line, either by slow injection or by infusion. Solution is brown. Inspect for particulate matter or discoloration. Do not administer solutions that contain particulate matter or are discolored.

■ **Direct IV:** May be administered undiluted by slow injection into dialysis line.

■ *Rate:* Administer at a rate of 1 ml undiluted solution per minute, not to exceed one vial per injection. Discard any unused portion.

■ **Intermittent Infusion:** May also be administered via infusion, into dialysis line for hemodialysis patients. May reduce risk of hypotensive episodes. Each vial must be diluted in a maximum of 100 ml of 0.9% NaCl immediately prior to infusion. Unused diluted solution should be discarded.

- **Rate:** Infuse at a rate of 100 mg of iron over at least 15 min.

- **Additive Incompatibility:** Do not mix iron sucrose with other medications or add to parenteral nutrition solutions for IV infusion.

## PATIENT/FAMILY TEACHING

- **General Info:** Encourage patient to comply with medication regimen. Take missed doses as soon as remembered within 12 hr; otherwise, return to regular dosing schedule. Do not double doses.

- ❏ Advise patient that stools may become dark green or black and that this change is harmless.

- ❏ Instruct patient to follow a diet high in iron (see Appendix Q).

- ❏ Discuss with parents the risk of children's overdosing on iron. Medication should be stored in the original childproof container and kept out of reach of children. Do not refer to vitamins as candy. Medical help should be sought immediately if overdose is suspected, as death may occur. Parents should have syrup of ipecac at home but call pediatrician, emergency department, or poison control center for instructions before administering.

- **Iron Dextran:** Delayed reaction may occur 1–2 days after administration and last 3–4 days if IV route used, 3–7 days with IM route. Instruct patient to contact physician if fever, chills, malaise, muscle and joint aches, nausea, vomiting, dizziness, and backache occur.

## EVALUATION

**Clinical response to therapy can be evaluated by:** ■ Increase in hemoglobin, which may reach normal parameters after 1–2 mo of therapy. May require 3–6 mo for normalization of body iron stores ■ Increase in hemoglobin, hematocrit, and plasma iron levels with iron dextran. The diagnosis of iron-deficiency anemia should be reconfirmed if hemoglobin has not increased by 1 g/100 ml in 2 wk ■ Improvement in anemia of chronic renal failure.

## isoniazid
(eye-soe-**nye**-a-zid)
INH, {Isotamine}, Nydrazid, {PMS Isoniazid}, Laniazid

### CLASSIFICATION(S):
**Therapeutic:** antituberculars

### Pregnancy Category C

## INDICATIONS

■ First-line therapy of active tuberculosis, in combination with other agents ■ Prevention of tuberculosis in patients exposed to active disease (alone).

## ACTION

■ Inhibits mycobacterial cell wall synthesis and interferes with metabolism. **Therapeutic Effects:** ■ Bacteriostatic or bactericidal action against susceptible mycobacteria.

## PHARMACOKINETICS

**Absorption:** Well absorbed following PO/IM administration.

**Distribution:** Widely distributed; readily crosses the blood-brain barrier. Crosses the placenta; enters breast milk in concentrations equal to plasma.

**Metabolism and Excretion:** 50% metabolized by the liver at rates that vary widely among individuals; 50% excreted unchanged by the kidneys.

**Half-life:** 1–4 hr.

## CONTRAINDICATIONS AND PRECAUTIONS

**Contraindicated in:** ■ Hypersensitivity ■ Acute liver disease ■ Previous hepatitis from isoniazid.

**Use Cautiously in:** ■ History of liver damage or chronic alcohol ingestion ■ Black and Hispanic women, women in the postpartum period, or patients >50 yr (increased risk of drug-induced hepatitis) ■ Severe renal impairment (dosage reduction may be necessary) ■ Malnourished patients, patients with diabetes, or chronic alcoholics (increased risk of neuropathy) ■ Pregnancy and lactation (although safety is not established, isoniazid has been used with ethambutol to treat tuberculosis in pregnant women without harm to the fetus).

## ADVERSE REACTIONS AND SIDE EFFECTS*

■ **CNS:** psychosis, seizures ■ **EENT:** visual disturbances ■ **GI:** DRUG-INDUCED HEPATITIS, nausea, vomiting ■ **Derm:** rashes ■ **Endo:** gynecomastia ■ **Hemat:** blood dyscrasias ■ **Neuro:** peripheral neuropathy ■ **Misc:** fever.

## INTERACTIONS

**Drug-Drug:** ■ Additive CNS toxicity with other **antituberculars** ■ **BCG vaccine** may not be effective during isoniazid therapy ■ Isoniazid inhibits the metabolism of **phenytoin** ■ **Aluminum-containing antacids** may decrease absorption ■ Psychotic reactions and coordination difficulties may result with **disulfiram** ■ Concurrent administration of **pyridoxine** may prevent neuropathy ■ Increased risk of hepatotoxicity with other **hepatotoxic agents** including **alcohol** and **rifampin** ■ Isoniazid may decrease blood levels and effectiveness of **ketoconazole** ■ Concurrent use with **carbamazepine** increases carbamazepine blood levels and risk of hepatotoxicity.

**Drug-Food:** ■ Severe reactions may occur with ingestion of foods containing high concentrations of **tyramine** (see Appendix Q).

## ROUTE AND DOSAGE

■ **PO, IM (Adults):** 300 mg/day (5 mg/kg) *or* 15 mg/kg (up to 900 mg) 2–3 times weekly.

■ **PO, IM (Children):** 10–20 mg/kg/day (up to 300 mg/day) *or* 20–40 mg/kg (up to 900 mg) 2–3 times weekly.

## AVAILABILITY (generic available)

■ *Tablets:* 50 mg$^{Rx}$, 100 mg$^{Rx}$, 300 mg$^{Rx}$ ■ Cost: 100 mg $2.18/100, 300 mg $3.53/100 ■ *Syrup (orange, raspberry flavor):* 50 mg/5 ml$^{Rx}$ ■ *Injection:* 100 mg/ml$^{Rx}$ ■ rifampin (Rifamate)$^{Rx}$ or with rifampin and pyrazinamide (Rifater)$^{Rx}$. See Appendix B.

TIME/ACTION PROFILE (blood levels)

| | ONSET | PEAK | DURATION |
|----|-------|------|----------|
| PO | rapid | 1–2 hr | up to 24 hr |
| IM | rapid | 1–2 hr | up to 24 hr |

## NURSING IMPLICATIONS

### ASSESSMENT

❑ Mycobacterial studies and susceptibility tests should be performed prior to and periodically throughout therapy to detect possible resistance.

■ *Lab Test Considerations:* Hepatic function should be evaluated prior to and monthly throughout therapy. Increased AST, ALT, and serum bilirubin may indicate drug-induced hepatitis. Black and Hispanic women, postpartal women, and patients >50 yr are at highest risk. The risk is lower in children; therefore, liver function tests are usually ordered less frequently for children.

■ *Toxicity and Overdose:* If isoniazid overdosage occurs, treatment with pyridoxine (vitamin B) is instituted.

### POTENTIAL NURSING DIAGNOSES

■ Infection, risk for (Indications).
■ Noncompliance (Patient/Family Teaching).

### IMPLEMENTATION

■ **PO:** May be administered with food or antacids if GI irritation occurs, although antacids containing aluminum should not be taken within 1 hr of administration.

■ **IM:** Medication may cause discomfort at injection site. Massage site after administration and rotate injection sites.

❑ Solution may form crystals at low temperatures; crystals will redissolve upon warming to room temperature.

### PATIENT/FAMILY TEACHING

❑ Advise patient to take medication exactly as directed. If a dose is missed, take as soon as possible unless almost time for next dose; do not double up on missed doses. Emphasize the importance of continuing therapy even after symptoms have subsided. Therapy may be continued for 6 mo–2 yr.

❑ Advise patient to notify health care professional promptly if signs and symptoms of hepatitis (yellow eyes and skin, nausea, vomiting, anorexia, dark urine, unusual tiredness, or weakness) or peripheral neuritis (numbness, tingling, paresthesia) occur. Pyridoxine may be used concurrently to pre-

{ } = Available in Canada only.
*CAPITALS indicates life-threatening; underlines indicate most frequent.

vent neuropathy. Any changes in visual acuity, eye pain, or blurred vision should also be reported immediately.

❑ Caution patient to avoid the use of alcohol during this therapy, as this may increase the risk of hepatotoxicity. Ingestion of Swiss or Cheshire cheeses, fish (tuna, skipjack, and sardinella), and possibly tyramine-containing foods (see Appendix Q) should also be avoided, as they may result in redness or itching of the skin; hot feeling; rapid or pounding heartbeat; sweating; chills; cold, clammy feeling; headache; or light-headedness.

❑ Emphasize the importance of regular follow-up physical and ophthalmologic exams to monitor progress and to check for side effects.

## EVALUATION

**Effectiveness of therapy can be demonstrated by:** ■ Resolution of signs and symptoms of tuberculosis ❑ Negative sputum cultures ■ Prevention of activation of tuberculosis in persons known to have been exposed.

---

# ISOSORBIDE

**isosorbide dinitrate**

(eye-soe-**sor**-bide dye-**nye**-trate)
{Apo-ISDN}, {Cedocard-SR}, {Coronex}, Dilatrate-SR, ISDN, Iso-Bid, Isonate, Isorbid, Isordil, Isotrate, {Novosorbide}, Sorbitrate

**isosorbide mononitrate**

(eye-soe-**sor**-bide mo-noe-**nye**-trate)
Imdur, Ismo, Isotrate ER, Monoket

*CLASSIFICATION(S):*
*Therapeutic: antianginals*
*Pharmacologic: nitrates*

**Pregnancy Category C**

## INDICATIONS

■ Acute treatment of anginal attacks (SL only) ■ Prophylactic management of angina pectoris (dinitrate and mononitrate) ■ Treatment of chronic CHF (dinitrate).

## ACTION

■ Produce vasodilation (venous greater than arterial) ■ Decrease left ventricular end-diastolic pressure and left ventricular end-diastolic volume (preload). Net effect is reduced myocardial oxygen consumption ■ Increase coronary blood flow by dilating coronary arteries and improving collateral flow to ischemic regions. **Therapeutic Effects:** ■ Relief of anginal attacks and increase in cardiac output.

## PHARMACOKINETICS

**Absorption:** Well absorbed after PO and SL administration.

**Distribution:** Unknown.

**Metabolism and Excretion:** Mostly metabolized by the liver.

**Half-life:** *Isosorbide dinitrate*—50 min; *isosorbide mononitrate*—5 hr.

## CONTRAINDICATIONS AND PRECAUTIONS

**Contraindicated in:** ■ Hypersensitivity ■ Severe anemia ■ Concurrent use of sildenafil.

**Use Cautiously in:** ■ Head trauma or cerebral hemorrhage ■ Geriatric patients (start with lower doses) ■ Pregnancy (may compromise maternal/fetal circulation) ■ Children or lactation (safety not established).

## ADVERSE REACTIONS AND SIDE EFFECTS*

■ **CNS:** dizziness, headache, apprehension, weakness ■ **CV:** hypotension, tachycardia, paradoxic bradycardia, syncope ■ **GI:** abdominal pain, nausea, vomiting ■ **Misc:** cross-tolerance, flushing, tolerance.

## INTERACTIONS

**Drug-Drug:** ■ Concurrent use of **sildenafil** may result in significant and potentially fatal hypotension (concurrent use is contraindicated) ■ Additive hypotension with **antihypertensives**, acute ingestion of **alcohol, beta blockers, calcium channel blockers,** and **phenothiazines** ■ **Aspirin** may increase blood levels and effects ■ Effects may be antagonized by **dihydroergotamine.**

## ROUTE AND DOSAGE

❑ **Isosorbide Dinitrate**

■ **SL, Buccal (Adults):** *Acute attack of angina pectoris*—2.5–5 mg may be repeated q 5–10 min for 3 doses in 15–30 min. *Pro-*

*phylaxis of angina pectoris*—2.5–10 mg may be repeated q 2–3 hr or 15 mm prior to activities known to provoke angina.

■ **PO (Adults):** *Prophylaxis of angina pectoris*—5–20 mg initially. Usual maintenance dose is 10–40 mg q 6 hr or 40–80 mg q 8–12 hr as sustained-release form.

❑ **Isosorbide Mononitrate**

■ **PO (Adults):** *Ismo, Monoket*—20 mg twice daily (may start with 5 mg twice daily), 7 hr apart. *Imdur*—30–60 mg once daily; may increase to 120 mg once daily (up to 240 mg/day).

## AVAILABILITY (generic available)

❑ **Isosorbide Dinitrate**

■ *Sublingual tablets:* 2.5 mg$^{Rx}$, 5 mg$^{Rx}$, 10 mg$^{Rx}$ ■ Cost: *Isordil*—2.5 mg $27.70/100, 5 mg $29.63/100, 10 mg $34.61/100; *generic*— 2.5 mg $4.44–$9.69/100, 5 mg $5.06–$10.29/ 100 ■ *Tablets:* 2.5 mg$^{Rx}$, 5 mg$^{Rx}$, 10 mg$^{Rx}$, 20 mg$^{Rx}$, 30 mg$^{Rx}$, 40 mg$^{Rx}$ ■ Cost: *Isordil*—5 mg $29.75/100, 10 mg $33.29/100, 20 mg $53.71/ 100, 30 mg $60.40/100, 40 mg $65.51/100; *generic*—5 mg $2.96–$7.29/100, 10 mg $4.17–$7.69/100, 20 mg $4.31–$8.99/100, 30 mg $7.09/100 ■ *Extended-release tablets:* {20 mg$^{Rx}$}, 40 mg$^{Rx}$ ■ Cost: *generic*—$6.75– $17.60/100 ■ *Capsules:* 40 mg$^{Rx}$ ■ *Extended-release capsules:* 40 mg$^{Rx}$ ■ Cost: *Dilatrate-SR* $63.40/100.

❑ **Isosorbide Mononitrate**

■ *Tablets (ISMO, Monoket):* 10 mg$^{Rx}$, 20 mg$^{Rx}$ ■ Cost: *ISMO*—20 mg $80.40/100; *Monoket*—10 mg $76.36/100, 20 mg $80.38/ 100; *generic*—10 mg $65.45/100, 20 mg $53.36–$72.35/100 ■ *Extended-release tablets (Imdur, Isotrate ER):* 30 mg$^{Rx}$, 60 mg$^{Rx}$, 120 mg$^{Rx}$ ■ Cost: *Imdur*—30 mg $130.03/100, 60 mg $136.86/100, 120 mg $191.60/100, *Isotrate ER*—60 mg $117.41/ 100; *generic*—30 mg $111.55/100, 60 mg $116.11–$117.40/100.

TIME/ACTION PROFILE (cardiovascular effects)

| | ONSET | PEAK | DURATION |
|---|---|---|---|
| ISDN-SL | 2–5 min | unknown | 1–2 hr |
| ISDN-PO | 15–40 min | unknown | 4 hr |
| ISDN-PO-ER | 30 min | unknown | up to 12 hr |
| ISMN-PO | 30–60 min | unknown | 7 hr |
| ISMN-ER | unknown | unknown | 12 hr |

# NURSING IMPLICATIONS

## ASSESSMENT

❑ Assess location, duration, intensity, and precipitating factors of anginal pain.

❑ Monitor blood pressure and pulse routinely during period of dosage adjustment.

■ *Lab Test Considerations:* May cause falsely decreased serum cholesterol determinations.

❑ Excessive doses may increase methemoglobin concentrations.

❑ May cause increased urine vanillylmandelic acid (VMA) concentrations.

## POTENTIAL NURSING DIAGNOSES

■ Tissue perfusion, ineffective (Indications).

■ Activity intolerance (Indications).

## IMPLEMENTATION

❑ **Isosorbide Dinitrate**

■ **PO:** Administer 1 hr before or 2 hr after meals with a full glass of water for faster absorption.

❑ Extended-release tablets and capsules should be swallowed whole. Do not crush, break, or chew. **SL:** tablets should be held under tongue until dissolved.

❑ Avoid eating, drinking, or smoking until tablet is dissolved. Replace tablet if inadvertently swallowed.

❑ **Isosorbide Mononitrate**

■ **General:** Do not confuse Imdur with imuran, inderal, or K-Dur. Do not confuse Monoket with monopril (fosinopril).

■ **PO:** Medication should be taken on an empty stomach with a full glass of water.

## PATIENT/FAMILY TEACHING

❑ Instruct patient to take medication exactly as directed, even if feeling better. If a dose is missed, take as soon as remembered; doses of isosorbide dinitrate should be taken at least 2 hr apart (6 hr with extended-release preparations); daily doses of isosorbide mononitrate should be taken 7 hr apart. Do not double doses. Do not discontinue abruptly.

▢ Caution patient to make position changes slowly to minimize orthostatic hypotension.

▢ May cause dizziness. Caution patient to avoid driving or other activities requiring alertness until response to medication is known.

▢ Advise patient to avoid concurrent use of alcohol with this medication. Patients should also consult health care professional before taking OTC medications while taking isosorbide.

▢ Inform patient that headache is a common side effect that should decrease with continuing therapy. Aspirin or acetaminophen may be ordered to treat headache. Notify health care professional if headache is persistent or severe. Do not alter dose to avoid headache.

▢ Advise patient to notify health care professional if dry mouth or blurred vision occurs or if undigested extended-release isosorbide dinitrate tablets are found in stool.

## EVALUATION
**Effectiveness of therapy can be demonstrated by:** ▪ Decrease in frequency and severity of anginal attacks ▢ Increase in activity tolerance.

---

# isradipine
(is-**ra**-di-peen)
DynaCirc, DynaCirc CR

### CLASSIFICATION(S):
**Therapeutic:** antianginals, antihypertensives
**Pharmacologic:** calcium channel blockers

### Pregnancy Category C

## INDICATIONS
▪ Management of hypertension, angina pectoris, and vasospastic (Prinzmetal's) angina.

## ACTION
▪ Inhibits the transport of calcium into myocardial and vascular smooth muscle cells, resulting in inhibition of excitation-contraction coupling and subsequent contraction. **Therapeutic Effects:** ▪ Systemic vasodilation resulting in decreased blood pressure ▪ Coronary vasodilation

resulting in decreased frequency and severity of attacks of angina.

## PHARMACOKINETICS
**Absorption:** Well absorbed following oral administration but extensively metabolized, resulting in decreased bioavailability.
**Distribution:** Unknown.
**Protein Binding:** 95%.
**Metabolism and Excretion:** Completely metabolized by the liver.
**Half-life:** 8 hr.

## CONTRAINDICATIONS AND PRECAUTIONS
**Contraindicated in:** ▪ Hypersensitivity ▪ Sick sinus syndrome ▪ 2nd- or 3rd-degree AV block (unless an artificial pacemaker is in place) ▪ Blood pressure <90 mmHg.
**Use Cautiously in:** ▪ Severe hepatic impairment (dosage reduction recommended) ▪ Geriatric patients (dosage reduction recommended for most agents; increased risk of hypotension) ▪ Severe renal impairment ▪ History of serious ventricular arrhythmias or CHF ▪ Pregnancy, lactation, or children (safety not established).

## ADVERSE REACTIONS AND SIDE EFFECTS*
▪ **CNS:** abnormal dreams, anxiety, confusion, dizziness, drowsiness, headache, nervousness, psychiatric disturbances, weakness ▪ **EENT:** blurred vision, disturbed equilibrium, epistaxis, tinnitus ▪ **Resp:** cough, dyspnea ▪ **CV:** ARRHYTHMIAS, CHF, peripheral edema, bradycardia, chest pain, hypotension, palpitations, syncope, tachycardia ▪ **GI:** abnormal liver function studies, anorexia, constipation, diarrhea, dry mouth, dysgeusia, dyspepsia, nausea, vomiting ▪ **GU:** dysuria, nocturia, polyuria, sexual dysfunction, urinary frequency ▪ **Derm:** dermatitis, erythema multiforme, flushing, increased sweating, photosensitivity, pruritus/urticaria, rash ▪ **Endo:** gynecomastia, hyperglycemia ▪ **Hemat:** anemia, leukopenia, thrombocytopenia ▪ **Metab:** weight gain ▪ **MS:** joint stiffness, muscle cramps ▪ **Neuro:** paresthesia, tremor ▪ **Misc:** STEVENS-JOHNSON SYNDROME, gingival hyperplasia.

## INTERACTIONS
**Drug-Drug:** ▪ Additive hypotension may occur when used concurrently with **fentanyl,** other **antihypertensives, nitrates,** acute ingestion of **alcohol,** or **quinidine** ▪ Antihypertensive

effects may be decreased by concurrent use of NSAIDs ■ Concurrent use with **beta blockers, digoxin, disopyramide,** or **phenytoin** may result in bradycardia, conduction defects, or CHF.

## ROUTE AND DOSAGE

■ **PO (Adults):** 2.5 mg twice daily; may be increased q 2–4 wk by 5 mg/day (not to exceed 20 mg/day) *or* 5 mg once daily as CR tablets; may be increased q 2–4 wk by 5 mg/day (not to exceed 20 mg/day).

## AVAILABILITY

■ *Capsules:* 2.5 mg$^{Rx}$, 5 mg$^{Rx}$ ■ *Controlled-release tablets:* 5 mg$^{Rx}$, 10 mg$^{Rx}$.

TIME/ACTION PROFILE (cardiovascular effects†)

| | ONSET | PEAK | DURATION |
|---|---|---|---|
| PO | <2 hr | 2–3 hr | 12 hr |
| PO-CR | 2 hr | 8–10 hr | 24 hr |

†For single doses, maximal antihypertensive effect during chronic dosing may take 2–4 wk.

## NURSING IMPLICATIONS

### ASSESSMENT

❑ Monitor blood pressure and pulse prior to and periodically throughout therapy. Monitor ECG periodically in patients receiving prolonged therapy.
❑ Monitor intake and output ratios and daily weight. Assess patient for signs of CHF (peripheral edema, rales/crackles, dyspnea, weight gain, jugular venous distention).
■ **Angina:** Assess location, duration, intensity, and precipitating factors of patient's anginal pain.
■ *Lab Test Considerations:* Total serum calcium concentrations are not affected by calcium channel blockers.
❑ Monitor serum potassium periodically. Hypokalemia increases risk of arrhythmias; should be corrected.
❑ Monitor renal and hepatic functions periodically during long-term therapy. Several days of therapy may cause increase in hepatic enzymes, which return to normal upon discontinuation of therapy.

## POTENTIAL NURSING DIAGNOSES

■ Cardiac output, decreased (Side Effects).

## IMPLEMENTATION

■ **PO:** May be administered without regard to meals. May be administered with meals if GI irritation becomes a problem.
❑ Do not open, crush, break, or chew controlled-release tablets.

## PATIENT/FAMILY TEACHING

❑ Advise patient to take medication exactly as directed, even if feeling well. If a dose is missed, take as soon as possible unless almost time for next dose; do not double doses. May need to be discontinued gradually.
❑ Caution patient to change positions slowly to minimize orthostatic hypotension.
❑ May cause dizziness. Advise patient to avoid driving or other activities requiring alertness until response to the medication is known.
❑ Instruct patient to avoid concurrent use of alcohol or OTC medications without consulting health care professional.
❑ Caution patient to wear protective clothing and use sunscreen to prevent photosensitivity reactions.
❑ Advise patient to notify health care professional if irregular heartbeats, dyspnea, swelling of hands and feet, rash, pronounced dizziness, nausea, constipation, or hypotension occurs.
■ **Angina:** Instruct patient on concurrent nitrate or beta-blocker therapy to continue taking both medications as directed and to use SL nitroglycerin as needed for anginal attacks.
❑ Inform patient that anginal attacks may occur 30 min after administration because of reflex tachycardia. This is usually temporary and is not an indication for discontinuation.
❑ Advise patient to contact health care professional if chest pain does not improve, worsens after therapy, or occurs with diaphoresis or if shortness of breath or persistent headache occurs.
❑ Caution patient to discuss exercise restrictions with health care professional prior to exertion.

■ **Hypertension:** Encourage patient to comply with other interventions for hypertension (weight reduction, low-sodium diet, smoking cessation, moderation of alcohol consumption, regular exercise, and stress management). Medication controls but does not cure hypertension.

❑ Instruct patient and family in proper technique for monitoring BP. Advise patient to take BP weekly and to report significant changes to health care professional.

## EVALUATION

**Effectiveness of therapy can be demonstrated by:** ■ Decrease in blood pressure ■ Decrease in frequency and severity of anginal attacks ❑ Decrease in need for nitrate therapy ❑ Increase in activity tolerance and sense of well-being.

---

## itraconazole
(it-tra-**kon**-a-zole)
Sporanox

**CLASSIFICATION(S):**
**Therapeutic:** antifungals (systemic)

**Pregnancy Category C**

---

## INDICATIONS

■ **IV, PO:** ❑ Histoplasmosis ❑ Blastomycosis ❑ Aspergillosis ❑ Onychomycosis of the fingernail or toenail caused by *tinea unguium* in nonimmunocompromised patients (oral capsules only) ❑ Oropharyngeal lesophageal candidiasis ■ **IV:** Suspected fungal infections in febrile neutropenic patients.

## ACTION

■ Inhibits enzymes necessary for integrity of the fungal cell membrane. **Therapeutic Effects:** ■ Fungistatic effects against susceptible organisms. **Spectrum:** ■ Active against *Histoplasma capsulatum, Blastomyces dermatitidis, Cryptococcus neoformans, Aspergillus fumigatus, Trichophyton* spp., *Candida*, and *tinea unguium.*

## PHARMACOKINETICS

**Absorption:** Oral absorption is enhanced by food; IV administration results in complete bioavailability.

**Distribution:** Tissue concentrations are higher than plasma concentrations. Does not enter CSF; enters breast milk.

**Protein Binding:** *Itraconazole*—99.8%; *hydroxyitraconazole*—99.5%

**Metabolism and Excretion:** Mostly metabolized by the liver and excreted in feces. Hydroxyitraconazole, the major metabolite, has antifungal activity.

**Half-life:** 21 hr.

## CONTRAINDICATIONS AND PRECAUTIONS

**Contraindicated in:** ■ Hypersensitivity. Cross-sensitivity with other azole antifungals (**miconazole, ketoconazole**) may occur ■ Lactation ■ Concurrent **quinidine, dofetilide, pimozide, midazolam, triazolam, simvastatin,** or **lovastatin** ■ Severe renal impairment (CCr <30 ml/min) ■ CHF or other evidence of ventricular dysfunction.

**Use Cautiously in:** ■ Patients with hepatic impairment (dosage reduction may be required) ■ Patients with achlorhydria or hypochlorhydria (absorption will be decreased) ■ Pregnancy or children (safety not established).

## ADVERSE REACTIONS AND SIDE EFFECTS*

■ **CNS:** dizziness, drowsiness, fatigue, headache, malaise ■ **EENT:** tinnitus ■ **CV:** CHF, edema, hypertension ■ **GI:** HEPATOTOXICITY, nausea, abdominal pain, anorexia, diarrhea, flatulence, vomiting ■ **GU:** albuminuria, decreased libido, impotence ■ **Derm:** TOXIC EPIDERMAL NECROLYSIS, pruritus, rash ■ **Endo:** adrenal insufficiency ■ **F and E:** hypokalemia ■ **MS:** rhabdomyolysis ■ **Misc:** fever.

## INTERACTIONS

**Drug-Drug:** ■ Itraconazole is a potent inhibitor of the P450 3A hepatic enzyme, which can result in increased blood levels and effects of other drugs which are metabolized by this system ■ ↑ risk of potentially fatal arrhythmias with **quinidine, dofetilide,** or **pimozide** (concurrent use is contraindicated and may result in QTc prolongation, torsades de pointes, ventricular arrhythmias, and sudden death) ■ ↑ risk of excessive sedation with **midazolam** or **triazolam,** ↑ risk of adverse CNS reactions with **pimozide,** and ↑ risk of myopathy with **simvastatin** or **lovastatin** (concurrent use contraindicated) ■ May also ↑ blood levels and the risk of toxicity from **warfarin, ritonavir, indinavir, saquinavir, vinca alkaloids, busulfan, diazepam, felodipine, isradipine, nicardipine, nifedipine, nimodipine, cyclosporine vardenafil, tacrolimus, sildenafil methylprednisolone, digoxin,** and **quinidine** ▪ Absorption ↓ by **antacids, histamine H₂ blockers, sucralfate, gastric acid-pump inhibitors,** or other **agents that increase gastric pH,** including the buffer in **didanosine** (take 2 hr after itraconazole) ▪ **Phenytoin, phenobarbital, isoniazid, rifampin, rifabutin,** and **carbamazepine** ↑ metabolism and ↓ blood levels of itraconazole ( ↑ dosage may be necessary) ▪ Itraconazole ↓ metabolism and may ↑ effects of **phenytoin** and **oral hypoglycemic agents** ▪ If hypokalemia occurs, the risk of **digoxin** toxicity is ↑ ▪ Blood levels of itraconazole may be ↑ by **clarithromycin, erythromycin ritonavir,** and **indinavir.**

**Drug-Food:** ▪ **Food** increases absorption.

## ROUTE AND DOSAGE

❏ **Aspergillosis**

▪ **PO (Adults):** 200 mg once or twice daily for a minimum of 3 mo.

▪ **IV (Adults):** 200 mg twice daily for 4 doses, then 200 mg once daily.

❏ **Blastomycosis, Histoplasmosis**

▪ **PO (Adults):** 200 mg once daily; may be increased by 100 mg/day up to 200 mg twice daily.

▪ **IV (Adults):** 200 mg twice daily for 4 doses, then 200 mg once daily.

❏ **Onychomycosis**

▪ **PO (Adults):** *Toenail fungus with or without fingernail fungus*—200 mg/day for 12 consecutive wk. *Fingernail fungus*—200 mg twice daily for 1 wk, then 3 wk without therapy, then 200 mg twice daily an additional wk–6 mo.

❏ **Empiric Therapy for Suspected Fungal Infections in Febrile Neutropenic Patients**

▪ **IV (Adults):** 200 mg twice daily for 4 doses, then 200 mg once daily for 14 days.

❏ **Candidiasis**

▪ **PO (Adults):** *Oropharyngeal candidiasis*—200 mg (20 ml) daily for 1–2 wk. *Oropharyngeal candidiasis unresponsive to fluconazole*—100 mg (10 ml) twice daily for at least 2–4 wk. *Esophageal candidiasis*—100 mg (10 ml) once daily for at least 3 wk.

### AVAILABILITY

▪ *Capsules:* 100 mg<sup>Rx</sup> ▪ *Oral solution:* 10 mg/ml<sup>Rx</sup> ▪ *Injection:* 10 mg/ml in 25 ml ampules<sup>Rx</sup>.

TIME/ACTION PROFILE (blood levels)

| | ONSET | PEAK | DURATION |
|---|---|---|---|
| PO | rapid | 4 hr | 12–24 hr |
| IV | unknown | end of infusion | 12–24 hr |

# NURSING IMPLICATIONS

## ASSESSMENT

❏ Assess patient for signs and symptoms of infection (vital signs, lung sounds, sputum, WBC, oral and pharyngeal mucosa, nail beds) before and periodically during therapy.

❏ Specimens for culture should be taken before instituting therapy. Therapy may be started before results are obtained.

▪ *Lab Test Considerations:* Hepatic function tests should be monitored before and periodically during therapy, especially in patients with pre-existing hepatic function abnormalities. Discontinue itraconazole if abnormal values persist or worsen.

❏ Monitor serum potassium. May cause hypokalemia.

## POTENTIAL NURSING DIAGNOSES

▪ Infection, risk for (Indications).

▪ Noncompliance (Patient/Family Teaching).

## IMPLEMENTATION

▪ **General:** Do not interchange capsules and oral solution. Only oral solution is effective for oropharyngeal candidiasis.

- **Capsules:** Administer with a full meal to minimize nausea and vomiting and to increase absorption.
- Do not administer with antacids or other medications that may increase gastric pH; may decrease absorption of itraconazole.
- **Oral Solution:** Administer without food if possible. Swish solution in mouth vigorously, 10 ml at a time, for several seconds, then swallow.
- **Intermittent Infusion:** Add contents of 25–ml vial to 50–ml bag of 0.9% NaCl provided and mix gently. Do not use other diluents. Diluted solution is stable for 48 hr if refrigerated or at room temperature. Protect from light during storage; no protection is needed during administration.
- *Rate:* Using an infusion control device, administer 60 ml over 60 min. After infusion, flush line with 15-20 ml of 0.9% NaCl over 30 seconds to 15 min.

### PATIENT/FAMILY TEACHING

- Instruct patient to take medication as directed, even if feeling better. Doses should be taken at the same time each day.

- May occasionally cause drowsiness. Caution patient to avoid driving or other activities requiring alertness until response to medication is known.
- Instruct patient to notify health care professional if signs and symptoms of liver dysfunction (unusual fatigue, anorexia, nausea, vomiting, jaundice, dark urine, or pale stools) or CHF (dyspnea, peripheral edema, weight gain) occur. If signs of CHF occur, discontinue itraconazole and notify health care professional immediately.
- Advise patient to consult health care professional before taking any Rx, OTC, herbal medications concurrently with itraconazole.

### EVALUATION

**Effectiveness of therapy can be demonstrated by:** ■ Resolution of clinical and laboratory indications of fungal infections. Minimal treatment for systemic fungal infections is 3 mo. Inadequate period of treatment may lead to recurrence of active infection.

## kanamycin, See AMINOGLYCOSIDES.

## ketoconazole (systemic)†
(kee-toe-**koe**-na-zole)
Nizoral

*CLASSIFICATION(S):*
*Therapeutic: antifungals (systemic)*
**Pregnancy Category C**

†For topical use, see Antifungals (topical).

## INDICATIONS

■ Treatment of: ❏ Candidiasis (disseminated and mucocutaneous) ❏ Chromomycosis ❏ Coccidioidomycosis ❏ Histoplasmosis ❏ Paracoccidioidomycosis. **Unlabeled uses:** ■ Treatment of advanced prostate cancer ■ Treatment of Cushing's syndrome.

## ACTION

■ Disrupts fungal cell membrane ■ Interferes with fungal metabolism ■ Also inhibits the production of adrenal steroids. **Therapeutic Effects:** ■ Fungistatic or fungicidal action against susceptible organisms, depending on organism and site of infection. **Spectrum:** ■ Active against many pathogenic fungi, including: ❏ *Blastomyces* ❏ *Candida* ❏ *Coccidioides* ❏ *Cryptococcus* ❏ *Histoplasma* ❏ Many dermatophytes.

## PHARMACOKINETICS

**Absorption:** Absorption from the GI tract is pH dependent; increasing pH decreases absorption.

**Distribution:** Widely distributed. CNS penetration is unpredictable and minimal. Crosses the placenta; enters breast milk.

**Protein Binding:** 99%.

**Metabolism and Excretion:** Partially metabolized by the liver. Excreted in feces via biliary excretion.

**Half-life:** 8 hr.

## CONTRAINDICATIONS AND PRECAUTIONS

**Contraindicated in:** ■ Hypersensitivity ■ Pregnancy or lactation ■ Concurrent triazolam.

**Use Cautiously in:** ■ History of liver disease ■ Achlorhydria or hypochlorhydria ■ Alcoholism.

## ADVERSE REACTIONS AND SIDE EFFECTS*

■ **CNS:** dizziness, drowsiness ■ **EENT:** photophobia ■ **GI:** DRUG-INDUCED HEPATITIS, nausea, vomiting, abdominal pain, constipation, diarrhea, flatulence ■ **GU:** azoospermia, decreased male libido, menstrual irregularities, oligospermia ■ **Derm:** rashes ■ **Endo:** gynecomastia.

## INTERACTIONS

**Drug-Drug:** ■ Ketoconazole inhibits the hepatic P450 3A4 enzyme system, which results in ↓ metabolism and possibly ↑ effects and/or toxicity from **cyclosporine, tacrolimus, corticosteroids** (dosage reduction may be necessary), **calcium channel blockers,** sulfonylurea **oral hypoglycemic agents, quinidine, buspirone, clarithromycin, troleandomycin, erythromycin, cyclophosphamide, phenytoin, warfarin** ( ↑ risk of bleeding), **tamoxifen, tricyclic antidepressants, carbamazepine, nisoldipine, zolpidem, vinca alkaloids, ifosfamide,** some **benzodiazepines** (effect may persist for several days; use of triazolam is contraindicated), **alfentanil, fentanyl, sufentanil, donepezil, atorvastatin, lovastatin, simvastatin, amprenavir, indinavir** (dosage ↓ of indinavir recommended), **nelfinavir, ritonavir, saquinavir, quinidine, sildenafil** and **vardenafil** (dosage adjustments may be necessary) ■ May alter the effectiveness of **hormonal contraceptives** (alternative method of contraception recommended) ■ Drugs that ↑ gastric pH, including **antacids, histamine H₂ antagonists, didanosine** (chewable tablets, because of buffer), and **gastric acid–pump inhibitors** ↓ absorption (wait 2 hr before administration of ketoconazole) ■ **Sucralfate** and **isoniazid** also ↓ bioavailability ■ ↑ hepatotoxicity with other **hepatotoxic agents,** including **alcohol** ■ Disulfiram-like reaction may occur with **alcohol** ■ **Rifampin** or **isoniazid** may ↓ levels and

---

{ } = Available in Canada only.
*CAPITALS indicates life-threatening; underlines indicate most frequent.

effectiveness ■ May ↓ absorption and effectiveness of **theophylline**.

## ROUTE AND DOSAGE

■ **PO (Adults):** *Antifungal*—200–400 mg/day, single dose. *Prostate cancer*—400 mg 3 times daily (unlabeled).
■ **PO (Children >2 yr):** 3.3–6.6 mg/kg/day, single dose.

## AVAILABILITY (generic available)

■ ***Tablets:*** 200 mg$^{Rx}$ ■Cost: $59.99/14 ■ ***Oral suspension:*** {100 mg/5 ml$^{Rx}$}.

TIME/ACTION PROFILE (blood levels)

|    | ONSET | PEAK | DURATION |
|----|-------|------|----------|
| PO | rapid | 1–4 hr | 24 hr |

## NURSING IMPLICATIONS

### ASSESSMENT

❑ Assess patient for symptoms of infection prior to and periodically during therapy.
❑ Specimens for culture should be taken prior to instituting therapy. Therapy may be started before results are obtained.
■ **Lab Test Considerations:** Monitor hepatic function tests prior to and monthly for 3–4 mo and then periodically during therapy. May cause ↑ AST, ALT, serum alkaline phosphatase, and bilirubin concentrations. Ketoconazole should be discontinued if even minor abnormalities occur.
❑ May cause ↓ serum testosterone concentrations.

### POTENTIAL NURSING DIAGNOSES

■ Infection, risk for (Indications).
■ Noncompliance (Patient/Family Teaching).

### IMPLEMENTATION

■ **General:** Do not confuse Nizoral (ketoconazole) with Neoral (cyclosporine).
■ **PO:** Administer with meals or snacks to minimize nausea and vomiting.
❑ Shake suspension well prior to administration.
❑ Do not administer histamine H$_2$ antagonists or antacids within 2 hr of ketoconazole.
❑ For patients with achlorhydria, dissolve each tablet in 4 ml of aqueous solution of 0.2 N hydrochloric acid. Use a glass or plastic straw to avoid contact with teeth and follow

with a glass of water, swished in mouth and swallowed.

### PATIENT/FAMILY TEACHING

❑ Instruct patient to take medication as directed, at the same time each day, even if feeling better. Take missed doses as soon as remembered; if almost time for next dose, space missed dose and next dose 10–12 hr apart.
❑ May cause dizziness or drowsiness. Caution patient to avoid driving or other activities requiring alertness until response to medication is known.
❑ Advise patient to avoid taking OTC antacids within 2 hr of ketoconazole.
❑ Caution patient to wear sunglasses and to avoid prolonged exposure to bright light to prevent photophobic reactions.
❑ Advise patient to use a nonhormonal form of contraception during ketoconazole therapy.
❑ Advise patient to avoid concurrent use of alcohol while taking ketoconazole; may cause a disulfiram-like reaction (flushing, rash, peripheral edema, nausea, headache) and increase the risk of hepatotoxicity.
❑ Instruct patient to notify health care professional if abdominal pain, fever, or diarrhea becomes pronounced or if signs and symptoms of liver dysfunction (unusual fatigue, anorexia, nausea, vomiting, jaundice, dark urine, or pale stools) occur.

### EVALUATION

**Effectiveness of therapy can be demonstrated by:** ■ Resolution of clinical and laboratory indications of fungal infections ■ Minimal treatment for candidiasis is 1–2 wk and for other systemic mycoses is 6 mo ❑ Chronic mucocutaneous candidiasis usually requires maintenance therapy.

## ketoconazole, See ANTIFUNGALS (TOPICAL).

## ketoprofen

(kee-toe-**proe**-fen)

Actron, {Apo-Keto}, {Apo-Keto-E}, Orudis, {Orudis-E}, Orudis KT, {Orudis-SR}, Oruvail, {Rhodis}

## CLASSIFICATION(S):

**Therapeutic:** *antipyretics, antirheumatics, nonopioid analgesics, nonsteroidal anti-inflammatory agents*
**Pharmacologic:** *nonopioid analgesics*

### Pregnancy Category B (first trimester)

## INDICATIONS

■ Inflammatory disorders, including: ❑ Rheumatoid arthritis ❑ Osteoarthritis ■ Mild to moderate pain, including dysmenorrhea and fever.

## ACTION

■ Inhibits prostaglandin synthesis. **Therapeutic Effects:** ■ Suppression of pain and inflammation ■ Reduction of fever.

## PHARMACOKINETICS

**Absorption:** Well absorbed from the GI tract.
**Distribution:** Unknown.
**Protein Binding:** 99%.
**Metabolism and Excretion:** Mostly (60%) metabolized by the liver; some renal excretion.
**Half-life:** 2–4 hr.

## CONTRAINDICATIONS AND PRECAUTIONS

**Contraindicated in:** ■ Hypersensitivity ■ Cross-sensitivity may exist with other NSAIDs, including aspirin ■ Active GI bleeding ■ Ulcer disease ■ Some products contain tartrazine and should be avoided in patients with known intolerance.
**Use Cautiously in:** ■ Severe cardiovascular, renal, or hepatic disease ■ History of ulcer disease ■ Renal impairment (dosage reduction suggested) ■ Extended-release product should not be used in geriatric patients, patients of small stature, or patients with renal impairment ■ Chronic alcohol use/abuse ■ Pregnancy, lactation, or children (safety not established; avoid use during 2nd half of pregnancy).

## ADVERSE REACTIONS AND SIDE EFFECTS*

■ **CNS:** drowsiness, headache, dizziness ■ **EENT:** blurred vision, tinnitus ■ **CV:** edema ■

**GI:** DRUG-INDUCED HEPATITIS, GI BLEEDING, constipation, diarrhea, dyspepsia, nausea, vomiting, anorexia, discomfort, flatulence ■ **GU:** cystitis, hematuria, renal failure ■ **Derm:** photosensitivity, rashes ■ **Endo:** gynecomastia ■ **Hemat:** blood dyscrasias, prolonged bleeding time ■ **MS:** myalgia ■ **Misc:** allergic reactions including ANAPHYLAXIS, fever.

## INTERACTIONS

**Drug-Drug:** ■ **Aspirin** alters distribution, metabolism, and excretion of ketoprofen (concurrent use not recommended) ■ Additive adverse GI effects with other **NSAIDs, corticosteroids,** or **alcohol** ■ Chronic use with **acetaminophen** may increase the risk of adverse renal reactions ■ May decrease the effectiveness of **diuretics** or **antihypertensives** ■ May increase the hypoglycemic effects of **insulin** or sulfonylurea **oral hypoglycemic agents** ■ May increase serum **lithium** levels and increase the risk of toxicity ■ Increases the risk of toxicity from **methotrexate** ■ **Probenecid** increases risk of toxicity from ketoprofen (concurrent use not recommended) ■ Increased risk of bleeding with **cefamandole, cefotetan, cefoperazone, valproic acid, plicamycin, thrombolytic agents, clopidogrel, ticlopidine, eptifibatide, tirofiban,** or **anticoagulants** ■ Increased risk of adverse hematologic reactions with **antineoplastics** or **radiation therapy** ■ Increased risk of nephrotoxicity with **cyclosporine.**

**Drug-Natural Products:** ■ Increased bleeding risk with **anise, arnica, chamomile, clove, dong quai, feverfew, garlic, ginger, ginkgo, Panax ginseng.**

## ROUTE AND DOSAGE

■ **PO (Adults):** *Anti-inflammatory*—150–300 mg/day in 3–4 divided doses or 150–200 mg once daily as extended-release product. *Analgesic*—25–50 mg q 6–8 hr. *OTC analgesic/antipyretic*—12.5 mg q 4–6 hr; if relief is not obtained 1 hr after first dose, an additional dose may be given. An initial dose of 25 mg may be used (not to exceed 25 mg/4–6 hr or 75 mg/24 hr).

---

{ } = Available in Canada only.
* CAPITALS indicates life-threatening; underlines indicate most frequent.

## AVAILABILITY (generic available)

■ *Tablets:* 12.5 mg$^{OTC}$ ■ *Capsules:* 25 mg$^{Rx}$, 50 mg$^{Rx}$, 75 mg$^{Rx}$ ■ *Extended-release capsules:* 100 mg$^{Rx}$, 150 mg$^{Rx}$, 200 mg$^{Rx}$ ■ Cost: 100 mg $181.48/100, 150 mg $220.58/100, 200 mg $249.08/100.

### TIME/ACTION PROFILE

|  | ONSET | PEAK | DURATION |
|---|---|---|---|
| PO (analgesic) | within 60 min | 1 hr | 4–6 hr |
| PO (anti-inflammatory) | few days–1 wk | unknown | up to 24 hr (SR products) |

# NURSING IMPLICATIONS

## ASSESSMENT

■ **General Info:** Patients who have asthma, aspirin-induced allergy, and nasal polyps are at increased risk for developing hypersensitivity reactions. Assess for rhinitis, wheezing, and urticaria.

■ **Arthritis:** Assess pain and range of motion prior to and 1 hr following administration.

■ **Pain:** Assess pain (note type, location, and intensity) prior to and 1 hr following administration.

■ **Fever:** Monitor temperature; note signs associated with fever (diaphoresis, tachycardia, malaise).

■ *Lab Test Considerations:* BUN, serum creatinine, CBC, and liver function tests should be evaluated periodically in patients receiving prolonged courses of therapy.

❑ Serum potassium, BUN, serum creatinine, alkaline phosphatase, LDH, AST, and ALT tests may show increased levels. Blood glucose, hemoglobin and hematocrit concentrations, leukocyte and platelet counts, and CCr may be decreased.

❑ May prolong bleeding time by 3–4 min.

❑ May alter results of urine albumin, bilirubin, 17-ketosteroid, and 17-hydroxycorticosteroid determinations.

## POTENTIAL NURSING DIAGNOSES

■ Pain, acute (Indications).

■ Mobility, impaired physical (Indications).

## IMPLEMENTATION

■ **General:** Do not confuse Oruvail (ketoprofen) with Elavil (amitriptyline).

❑ Administration in higher-than-recommended doses does not provide increased effectiveness but may cause increased side effects.

❑ Coadministration with opioid analgesics may have additive analgesic effects and may permit lower opioid doses.

❑ Analgesic is more effective if given before pain becomes severe.

■ **PO:** For rapid initial effect, administer 30 min before or 2 hr after meals. Capsules may be administered with food, milk, or antacids containing aluminum hydroxide and magnesium hydroxide to decrease GI irritation.

❑ Extended-release capsules should be swallowed whole; do not open or chew.

■ **Dysmenorrhea:** Administer as soon as possible after the onset of menses. Prophylactic treatment has not been proved effective.

## PATIENT/FAMILY TEACHING

❑ Advise patient to take this medication with a full glass of water and to remain in an upright position for 15–30 min after administration.

❑ Instruct patient to take medication exactly as directed. If a dose is missed, it should be taken as soon as remembered but not if almost time for the next dose. Do not double doses.

❑ May cause drowsiness or dizziness. Advise patient to avoid driving or other activities requiring alertness until response to medication is known.

❑ Caution patient to avoid the concurrent use of alcohol, aspirin, acetaminophen, or other OTC medications without consulting health care professional.

❑ Advise patient to inform health care professional of medication regimen prior to treatment or surgery.

❑ Caution patient to wear sunscreen and protective clothing to prevent photosensitivity reactions.

❑ Instruct patients not to take OTC ketoprofen preparations for more than 10 days for pain or more than 3 days for fever and to consult health care professional if symptoms persist or worsen.

❑ Caution patient that use of ketoprofen with 3 or more glasses of alcohol may increase risk of GI bleeding.

❑ Advise patient to consult health care professional if rash, itching, visual disturbances, tinnitus, weight gain, edema, black stools, persistent headache, or influenza-like syndrome (chills, fever, muscle aches, pain) occurs.

## EVALUATION

**Effectiveness of therapy can be demonstrated by:** ■ Improved joint mobility ■ Decrease in severity of pain. Improvement in arthritis may be seen in a few days to 1 wk; 1–2 wk may be required for maximum effectiveness. Patients who do not respond to one NSAID may respond to another ■ Reduction of fever.

# ketorolac†
(kee-**toe**-role-ak)
Toradol

## CLASSIFICATION(S):

**Therapeutic:** nonsteroidal anti-inflammatory agents, nonopioid analgesics
**Pharmacologic:** pyrroziline carboxylic acid

## Pregnancy Category C

†See Appendix C for ophthalmic use.

## INDICATIONS

■ Short-term management of pain (not to exceed 5 days total for all routes combined).

## ACTION

■ Inhibits prostaglandin synthesis, producing peripherally mediated analgesia ■ Also has antipyretic and anti-inflammatory properties. **Therapeutic Effects:** ■ Decreased pain.

## PHARMACOKINETICS

**Absorption:** Rapidly and completely absorbed following all routes of administration.
**Distribution:** Enters breast milk in low concentrations.
**Metabolism and Excretion:** <50% metabolized by the liver. Ketorolac and its metabolites are excreted primarily by the kidneys (92%); 6% excreted in feces.

**Half-life:** 4.5 hr (range 3.8–6.3 hr; increased in geriatric patients and patients with impaired renal function).

## CONTRAINDICATIONS AND PRECAUTIONS

**Contraindicated in:** ■ Hypersensitivity ■ Cross-sensitivity with other NSAIDs may exist ■ Labor, delivery or lactation ■ Pre- or perioperative use ■ Known alcohol intolerance (injection only).
**Use Cautiously in:** ■ History of GI bleeding ■ Renal impairment (dosage reduction may be required) ■ Cardiovascular disease ■ Pregnancy and children (use not recommended during 2nd half of pregnancy).

## ADVERSE REACTIONS AND SIDE EFFECTS*

■ **CNS:** <u>drowsiness</u>, abnormal thinking, dizziness, euphoria, headache ■ **Resp:** asthma, dyspnea ■ **CV:** edema, pallor, vasodilation ■ **GI:** GI BLEEDING, abnormal taste, diarrhea, dry mouth, dyspepsia, GI pain, nausea ■ **GU:** oliguria, renal toxicity, urinary frequency ■ **Derm:** pruritus, purpura, sweating, urticaria ■ **Hemat:** prolonged bleeding time ■ **Local:** injection site pain ■ **Neuro:** paresthesia ■ **Misc:** allergic reactions including, <u>anaphylaxis</u>.

## INTERACTIONS

**Drug-Drug:** ■ Concurrent use with **aspirin** may decrease effectiveness ■ Additive adverse GI effects with **aspirin**, other **NSAIDs, potassium supplements, corticosteroids,** or **alcohol** ■ Chronic use with **acetaminophen** may increase the risk of adverse renal reactions ■ May decrease the effectiveness of **diuretics** or **antihypertensives** ■ May increase serum **lithium** levels and increase the risk of toxicity ■ Increases the risk of toxicity from **methotrexate** ■ Increased risk of bleeding with **cefamandole, cefotetan, cefoperazone, valproic acid, clopidogrel, ticlopidine, tirofiban, eptifibatide, plicamycin, thrombolytic agents,** or **anticoagulants** ■ Increased risk of adverse hematologic reactions with **antineoplastics** or **radiation therapy** ■ May increase the risk of nephrotoxicity from **cyclosporine** ■ **Probenecid** increases ketorolac blood levels and the risk of adverse reactions (concurrent use should be avoided).

{ } = Available in Canada only.
* CAPITALS indicates life-threatening; <u>underlines</u> indicate most frequent.

**Drug-Natural Products:** ■ Increased bleeding risk with **anise, arnica, chamomile, clove, dong quai, feverfew, garlic, ginger, ginkgo, Panax ginseng.**

## ROUTE AND DOSAGE

Oral therapy is indicated only as a continuation of parenteral therapy; parenteral therapy should not exceed 20 doses/5 days. Total duration of therapy by all routes should not exceed 5 days.

■ **PO (Adults <65 yr):** 20 mg initially, followed by 10 mg q 4–6 hr as needed (not to exceed 40 mg/day).

■ **PO (Adults ≥65 yr, <50 kg, or with renal impairment):** 10 mg q 4–6 hr as needed (not to exceed 40 mg/day).

■ **IM (Adults <65 yr):** *Single dose*—60 mg. *Multiple dosing*—30 mg q 6 hr (not to exceed 120 mg/day).

■ **IM (Adults ≥65 yr, <50 kg, or with renal impairment):** *Single dose*—30 mg. *Multiple dosing*—15 mg q 6 hr (not to exceed 60 mg/day).

■ **IV (Adults <65 yr):** *Single dose*—30 mg. *Multiple dosing*—30 mg q 6 hr (not to exceed 120 mg/day).

■ **IV (Adults ≥65 yr, <50 kg, or with renal impairment):** *Single dose*—15 mg. *Multiple dosing*—15 mg q 6 hr (not to exceed 60 mg/day).

## AVAILABILITY

■ *Tablets:* 10 mg$^{Rx}$ ■Cost: $19.00/20 ■ *Injection:* 15 mg/ml in 1-ml preloaded syringes$^{Rx}$, 30 mg/ml in 1- and 2-ml preloaded syringes$^{Rx}$.

TIME/ACTION PROFILE (analgesic effects)

| | ONSET | PEAK | DURATION |
|---|---|---|---|
| PO | unknown | 2–3 hr | 4–6 hr or longer |
| IM, IV | 10 min | 1–2 hr | 6 hr or longer |

## NURSING IMPLICATIONS

### ASSESSMENT

■ **General Info:** Patients who have asthma, aspirin-induced allergy, and nasal polyps are at increased risk for developing hypersensitivity reactions. Assess for rhinitis, asthma, and urticaria.

■ **Pain:** Assess pain (note type, location, and intensity) prior to and 1–2 hr following administration.

■ *Lab Test Considerations:* Liver function tests, especially AST and ALT, should be evaluated periodically in patients receiving prolonged courses of therapy. May cause increased levels.

❑ May cause prolonged bleeding time that may persist for 24–48 hr following discontinuation of therapy.

❑ May cause increased BUN, serum creatinine, or potassium concentrations.

## POTENTIAL NURSING DIAGNOSES

■ Pain, acute (Indications).

## IMPLEMENTATION

■ **General:** Do not confuse Toradol (ketorolac) with Torecan (thiethylperazine) or tramadol (Ultram).

❑ Administration in higher-than-recommended doses does not provide increased effectiveness but may cause increased side effects. Duration of ketorolac therapy, by all routes combined, should not exceed 5 days.

❑ Coadministration with opioid analgesics may have additive analgesic effects and may permit lower opioid doses.

■ **PO:** Ketorolac therapy should always be given initially by the IM or IV route. Oral therapy should be used *only* as a continuation of parenteral therapy.

■ **Direct IV:** Administer undiluted.

■ *Rate:* Administer over at least 15 sec.

■ **Syringe Compatibility:** ◆ sufentanil.

■ **Syringe Incompatibility:** ◆ haloperidol ◆ hydroxyzine ◆ meperidine ◆ morphine ◆ nalbuphine ◆ prochlorperazine ◆ promethazine ◆ thiethylperazine.

■ **Y-Site Compatibility:** ◆ alatrofloxacin ◆ sufentanil.

■ **Solution Compatibility:** ◆ D5/0.9% NaCl ◆ D5W ◆ Ringer's injection ◆ lactated Ringer's injection ◆ 0.9% NaCl.

## PATIENT/FAMILY TEACHING

❑ Instruct patient on how and when to ask for pain medication.

❑ Instruct patient to take medication exactly as directed. If dose is missed, it should be taken as soon as remembered if not almost time for next dose. Do not double doses.

❑ May cause drowsiness or dizziness. Advise patient to avoid driving or other activities requiring alertness until response to the medication is known.

❑ Caution patient to avoid the concurrent use of alcohol, aspirin, NSAIDs, acetaminophen, or other OTC medications without consulting health care professional.

❑ Advise patient to inform health care professional of medication regimen prior to treatment or surgery.

❑ Advise patient to consult health care professional if rash, itching, visual disturbances, tinnitus, weight gain, edema, black stools, persistent headache, or influenza-like syndrome (chills, fever, muscle aches, pain) occurs.

## EVALUATION

**Effectiveness of therapy can be demonstrated by:** ▪ Decrease in severity of pain. Patients who do not respond to one NSAID may respond to another.

## High Alert

# labetalol
(la-**bet**-a-lole)
Normodyne, Trandate

**CLASSIFICATION(S):**
**Therapeutic:** antianginals, antihypertensives
**Pharmacologic:** beta blockers

**Pregnancy Category C**

## INDICATIONS
■ Management of hypertension.

## ACTION
■ Blocks stimulation of beta$_1$ (myocardial)- and beta$_2$ (pulmonary, vascular, and uterine)-adrenergic receptor sites ■ Also has alpha$_1$-adrenergic blocking activity, which may result in more orthostatic hypotension. **Therapeutic Effects:** ■ Decreased blood pressure.

## PHARMACOKINETICS
**Absorption:** Well absorbed but rapidly undergoes extensive first-pass hepatic metabolism, resulting in 25% bioavailability.
**Distribution:** Some CNS penetration; crosses the placenta.
**Metabolism and Excretion:** Undergoes extensive hepatic metabolism.
**Half-life:** 3–8 hr.

## CONTRAINDICATIONS AND PRECAUTIONS
**Contraindicated in:** ■ Uncompensated CHF ■ Pulmonary edema ■ Cardiogenic shock ■ Bradycardia or heart block.
**Use Cautiously in:** ■ Renal impairment ■ Hepatic impairment ■ Geriatric patients (increased sensitivity to beta blockers; initial dosage reduction recommended) ■ Pulmonary disease (including asthma) ■ Diabetes mellitus (may mask signs of hypoglycemia) ■ Thyrotoxicosis (may mask symptoms) ■ Patients with a history of severe allergic reactions (intensity of reactions may be increased) ■ Pregnancy, lactation, or children (safety not established; may cause

fetal/neonatal bradycardia, hypotension, hypoglycemia, or respiratory depression).

## ADVERSE REACTIONS AND SIDE EFFECTS*
■ **CNS:** fatigue, weakness, anxiety, depression, dizziness, drowsiness, insomnia, memory loss, mental status changes, nightmares ■ **EENT:** blurred vision, dry eyes, nasal stuffiness ■ **Resp:** bronchospasm, wheezing ■ **CV:** ARRHYTHMIAS, BRADYCARDIA, CHF, PULMONARY EDEMA, orthostatic hypotension ■ **GI:** constipation, diarrhea, nausea ■ **GU:** impotence, decreased libido ■ **Derm:** itching, rashes ■ **Endo:** hyperglycemia, hypoglycemia ■ **MS:** arthralgia, back pain, muscle cramps ■ **Neuro:** paresthesia ■ **Misc:** drug-induced lupus syndrome.

## INTERACTIONS
**Drug-Drug:** ■ **General anesthesia, IV,** and **verapamil** may cause additive myocardial depression ■ Additive bradycardia may occur with **digoxin** ■ Additive hypotension may occur with other **antihypertensives,** acute ingestion of **alcohol,** or **nitrates** ■ Concurrent **thyroid** administration may decrease effectiveness ■ May alter the effectiveness of **insulin** or **oral hypoglycemic agents** (dosage adjustments may be necessary) ■ May decrease the effectiveness of **adrenergic bronchodilators** and **theophylline** ■ May decrease the beneficial beta cardiovascular effects of **dopamine** or **dobutamine** ■ Use cautiously within 14 days of **MAO inhibitor therapy** (may result in hypertension) ■ Effects may be increased by **propranolol** or **cimetidine** ■ Concurrent **NSAIDs** may decrease antihypertensive action.

## ROUTE AND DOSAGE
■ **PO (Adults):** 100 mg twice daily initially, may be increased by 100 mg twice daily q 2–3 days as needed (usual range 400–800 mg/day in 2–3 divided doses; doses up to 1.2–2.4 g/day have been used).
■ **IV (Adults):** 20 mg (0.25 mg/kg) initially, additional doses of 40–80 mg may be given q 10 min as needed (not to exceed 300 mg total dose) *or* 2 mg/min infusion (range 50–300 mg total dose required).

## AVAILABILITY (generic available)

■ *Tablets:* 100 mg$^{Rx}$, 200 mg$^{Rx}$, 300 mg$^{Rx}$ ■ Cost: 100 mg $48.00/100, 200 mg $68.10/100, 300 mg $90.59/100 ■ *Injection:* 5 mg/ml$^{Rx}$.

TIME/ACTION PROFILE (cardiovascular effects)

|  | ONSET | PEAK | DURATION |
|---|---|---|---|
| PO | 20 min–2 hr | 1–4 hr | 8–12 hr |
| IV | 2–5 min | 5 min | 16–18 hr |

# NURSING IMPLICATIONS

## ASSESSMENT

❑ Monitor blood pressure and pulse frequently during dose adjustment and periodically during therapy. Assess for orthostatic hypotension when assisting patient up from supine position.

❑ Check frequency of refills to determine compliance.

❑ Patients receiving *labetalol IV* must be supine during and for 3 hr after administration. Vital signs should be monitored every 5–15 min during and for several hours after administration.

❑ Monitor intake and output ratios and daily weight. Assess patient routinely for evidence of fluid overload (peripheral edema, dyspnea, rales/crackles, fatigue, weight gain, jugular venous distention).

■ *Lab Test Considerations:* May cause increased BUN, serum lipoprotein, potassium, triglyceride, and uric acid levels.

❑ May cause increased ANA titers.

❑ May cause increase in blood glucose levels.

❑ May cause increased serum alkaline phosphatase, LDH, AST, and ALT levels. Discontinue if jaundice or laboratory signs of hepatic function impairment occur.

■ *Toxicity and Overdose:* Monitor patients receiving beta blockers for signs of overdose (bradycardia, severe dizziness or fainting, severe drowsiness, dyspnea, bluish fingernails or palms, seizures). Notify physician or other health care professional immediately if these signs occur.

❑ Glucagon has been used to treat bradycardia and hypotension.

## POTENTIAL NURSING DIAGNOSES

■ Cardiac output, decreased (Side Effects).

■ Noncompliance (Patient/Family Teaching).

## IMPLEMENTATION

❑ *High Alert:* IV vasoactive medications are inherently dangerous. Before administering intravenously, have second practitioner independently check original order, dosage calculations, and infusion pump settings. Do not confuse labetolol with Lamictil.

■ **General:** Discontinuation of concurrent clonidine should take place gradually, with beta blocker discontinued first. Then, after several days, discontinue clonidine.

■ **PO:** Take apical pulse prior to administering. If <50 bpm or if arrhythmia occurs, withhold medication and notify physician or other health care professional.

❑ Administer with meals or directly after eating to enhance absorption.

■ **Direct IV:** Administer undiluted.

■ *Rate:* Administer slowly over 2 min.

■ **Continuous Infusion:** Add 200 mg to 160 ml of diluent (1 mg/1 ml solution) or 200 mg to 250 ml of diluent (2 mg/3 ml solution). Compatible diluents include D5W, 0.9% NaCl, D5/0.25% NaCl, D5/0.9% NaCl, D5/Ringer's solution, D5/LR, Ringer's and LR.

■ *Rate:* Administer at a rate of 2 mg/min and titrate for desired response. Infuse via infusion pump to ensure accurate dosage.

■ **Y-Site Compatibility:** ◆ amikacin ◆ aminophylline ◆ amiodarone ◆ ampicillin ◆ butorphanol ◆ calcium gluconate ◆ cefazolin ◆ ceftazidine ◆ ceftizoxime ◆ chloramphenicol ◆ cimetidine ◆ clindamycin ◆ diltiazem ◆ dobutamine ◆ dopamine ◆ enalaprilat ◆ epinephrine ◆ erythromycin lactobionate ◆ esmolol ◆ famotidine ◆ fentanyl ◆ gatifloxacin ◆ gentamicin ◆ hydromorphone ◆ lidocaine ◆ linezolid ◆ lorazepam ◆ magnesium sulfate ◆ meperidine ◆ metronidazole ◆ midazolam ◆ milrinone ◆ morphine ◆ nitroglycerin ◆ nitroprusside ◆ norepinephrine ◆ oxacillin ◆ penicillin G potassium ◆ piperacillin ◆ potassium chloride ◆ potassium phosphate ◆ propofol ◆ ranitidine ◆ sodium acetate ◆ tobramycin ◆ trimethoprim/sulfamethoxazole ◆ vancomycin ◆ vecuronium.

■ **Y-Site Incompatibility:** ◆ amphotericin B cholesteryl sulfate complex ◆ cefoperazone ◆ ceftriaxone ◆ nafcillin ◆ tobramycin ◆ warfarin.

■ **Additive Incompatibility:** ◆ sodium bicarbonate.

## PATIENT/FAMILY TEACHING

■ **General Info:** Instruct patient to take medication exactly as directed, at the same time each day, even if feeling well; do not skip or double up on missed doses. If a dose is missed, it should be taken as soon as possible up to 8 hr before next dose. Abrupt withdrawal may precipitate life-threatening arrhythmias, hypertension, or myocardial ischemia.

❑ Advise patient to make sure enough medication is available for weekends, holidays, and vacations. A written prescription may be kept in wallet in case of emergency.

❑ Teach patient and family how to check pulse and blood pressure. Instruct them to check pulse daily and blood pressure biweekly. Advise patient to hold dose and contact health care professional if pulse is <50 bpm or blood pressure changes significantly.

❑ May cause drowsiness or dizziness. Caution patients to avoid driving or other activities that require alertness until response to the drug is known. Caution patients receiving labetalol IV to call for assistance during ambulation or transfer.

❑ Advise patients to make position changes slowly to minimize orthostatic hypotension, especially during initiation of therapy or when dose is increased. Patients taking oral labetalol should be especially cautious when drinking alcohol, standing for long periods, or exercising, and during hot weather, because orthostatic hypotension is enhanced.

❑ Caution patient that this medication may increase sensitivity to cold.

❑ Instruct patient to consult health care professional before taking any OTC medications, especially cold preparations, concurrently with this medication.

❑ Patients with diabetes should closely monitor blood glucose, especially if weakness, malaise, irritability, or fatigue occurs. Medication may mask tachycardia and increased blood pressure as signs of hypoglycemia, but dizziness and sweating may still occur.

❑ Advise patient to notify health care professional if slow pulse, difficulty breathing, wheezing, cold hands and feet, dizziness, light-headedness, confusion, depression, rash, fever, sore throat, unusual bleeding, or bruising occurs.

❑ Instruct patient to inform health care professional of medication regimen prior to treatment or surgery.

❑ Advise patient to carry identification describing disease process and medication regimen at all times.

■ **Hypertension:** Reinforce the need to continue additional therapies for hypertension (weight loss, sodium restriction, stress reduction, regular exercise, moderation of alcohol consumption, and smoking cessation). Medication controls but does not cure hypertension.

## EVALUATION

**Effectiveness of therapy can be demonstrated by:** ■ Decrease in blood pressure.

# lactulose

**(lak**-tyoo-lose)
Cephulac, Cholac, Chronulac, Constilac, Constulose, Duphalac, Enulose, Evalose, Heptalac, Kritalose, {Lactulax}, Lactulose PSE, Portalac

## CLASSIFICATION(S):
**Therapeutic:** *laxatives*
**Pharmacologic:** *osmotics*

### Pregnancy Category B

## INDICATIONS

■ Treatment of chronic constipation in adults and geriatric patients ■ Adjunct in the management of portal-systemic (hepatic) encephalopathy (PSE).

## ACTION

■ Increases water content and softens the stool ■ Lowers the pH of the colon, which inhibits the diffusion of ammonia from the colon into the blood, thereby reducing blood ammonia levels.

**Therapeutic Effects:** ■ Relief of constipation ■ Decreased blood ammonia levels with improved mental status in PSE.

## PHARMACOKINETICS

**Absorption:** Less than 3% absorbed after oral administration.

**Distribution:** Unknown.

**Metabolism and Excretion:** Absorbed lactulose is excreted unchanged in the urine. Unabsorbed lactulose is metabolized by colonic bacteria to lactic, acetic, and formic acids.

**Half-life:** Unknown.

## CONTRAINDICATIONS AND PRECAUTIONS

**Contraindicated in:** ■ Patients on low-galactose diets.

**Use Cautiously in:** ■ Diabetes mellitus ■ Excessive or prolonged use (may lead to dependence) ■ Pregnancy, lactation, or children (safety not established).

## ADVERSE REACTIONS AND SIDE EFFECTS*

■ **GI:** belching, cramps, distention, flatulence, diarrhea ■ **Endo:** hyperglycemia (diabetic patients).

## INTERACTIONS

**Drug-Drug:** ■ Should not be used with other **laxatives** in the treatment of hepatic encephalopathy (leads to inability to determine optimal dose of lactulose) ■ **Anti-infectives** may diminish effectiveness in treatment of hepatic encephalopathy.

## ROUTE AND DOSAGE

❑ **Constipation**

■ **PO (Adults):** 15–30 ml/day up to 60 ml/day as liquid or 10–20 g as powder for oral solution (up to 40 g /day has been used)

■ **PO (Children):** 7.5 ml daily (unlabeled).

❑ **PSI**

■ **PO (Adults):** 30–45 ml 3–4 times/day; may be given q 1–2 hr initially to induce laxation.

■ **PO (Infants):** 2.5–10 ml daily in divided doses (unlabeled).

■ **PO (Children and Adolescents):** 40–90 ml daily in divided doses (unlabeled).

■ **Rect (Adults):** 300 ml diluted and administered as a retention enema q 4–6 hr.

## AVAILABILITY (generic available)

■ *Syrup (cola flavor):* 10 g lactulose/15 ml$^{Rx}$ ■ Cost: $10.94/100 ■ *Single-use packets (Kristalose):* 10 g$^{Rx}$, 20 g$^{Rx}$.

TIME/ACTION PROFILE (relief of constipation)

| | ONSET | PEAK | DURATION |
|---|---|---|---|
| PO | 24–48 hr | unknown | unknown |

# NURSING IMPLICATIONS

## ASSESSMENT

■ **General Info:** Assess patient for abdominal distention, presence of bowel sounds, and normal pattern of bowel function.

❑ Assess color, consistency, and amount of stool produced.

■ **PSI:** Assess mental status (orientation, level of consciousness) before and periodically throughout course of therapy.

■ *Lab Test Considerations:* Decreases blood ammonia concentrations by 25–50%.

❑ May cause increased blood glucose levels in diabetic patients.

❑ Monitor serum electrolytes periodically when used chronically. May cause diarrhea with resulting hypokalemia and hypernatremia.

## POTENTIAL NURSING DIAGNOSES

■ Constipation (Indications).

## IMPLEMENTATION

■ **General:** When used in hepatic encephalopathy, dosage should be adjusted until patient averages 2–3 soft bowel movements per day. During initial therapy, 30–45 ml may be given hourly to induce rapid laxation.

❑ Darkening of solution does not alter potency.

■ **PO:** Mix with fruit juice, water, milk, or carbonated citrus beverage to improve flavor. Administer with a full glass (240 ml) of water or juice. May be administered on an empty stomach for more rapid results.

❑ Dissolve single dose packets (Kristalose) in 4 oz of water. Solution should be colorless to slightly pale yellow.

■ **Rect:** To administer enema, use rectal balloon catheter. Mix 300 ml of lactulose with 700 ml of water or 0.9% NaCl. Enema should be retained for 30–60 min. If inadvertently evacuated, may repeat administration.

## PATIENT/FAMILY TEACHING

❏ Encourage patients to use other forms of bowel regulation, such as increasing bulk in the diet, increasing fluid intake, and increasing mobility. Normal bowel habits are individualized and may vary from 3 times/day to 3 times/wk.

❏ Caution patients that this medication may cause belching, flatulence, or abdominal cramping. Health care professional should be notified if this becomes bothersome or if diarrhea occurs.

## EVALUATION

**Effectiveness of therapy can be demonstrated by:** ▪ Passage of a soft, formed bowel movement, usually within 24–48 hr ▪ Clearing of confusion, apathy, and irritation and improved mental status in PSI. Improvement may occur within 2 hr after enema and 24–48 hr after oral administration.

# lamivudine
(la-**mi**-vyoo-deen)
Epivir, Epivir HBV, 3TC

*CLASSIFICATION(S):*
*Therapeutic: antiretrovirals, antivirals*
*Pharmacologic: nucleoside reverse transcriptase inhibitors*

**Pregnancy Category C**

## INDICATIONS

▪ HIV infection (with other antiretrovirals) ▪ Chronic hepatitis B infection. **Unlabeled uses:** ▪ Part of HIV-postexposure prophylaxis with zidovudine and indinavir.

## ACTION

▪ After intracellular conversion to its active form (lamivudine-5-triphosphate), inhibits viral DNA synthesis by inhibiting the enzyme reverse transcriptase. **Therapeutic Effects:** ▪ Slows the progression of HIV infection and decreases the occurrence of its sequelae ▪ Increases CD4 cell counts and decreases viral load ▪ Protec-

tion from liver damage caused by chronic hepatitis B infection; decreases viral load.

## PHARMACOKINETICS

**Absorption:** Well absorbed after oral administration (86% in adults, 66% in infants and children).

**Distribution:** Distributes into the extravascular space. Some penetration into CSF; remainder of distribution unknown.

**Metabolism and Excretion:** Mostly excreted unchanged in urine; <5% metabolized by the liver.

**Half-life:** *Adults*—3.7 hr; *children*—2 hr.

## CONTRAINDICATIONS AND PRECAUTIONS

**Contraindicated in:** ▪ Hypersensitivity ▪ Lactation.

**Use Cautiously in:** ▪ Impaired renal function (increased dosing interval/decreased dose recommended if CCr <50 ml/min) ▪ Women, prolonged exposure, obesity, history of liver disease (increased risk of lactic acidosis and severe hepatomegaly with steatosis) ▪ Coinfection with hepatitis B (hepatitis may recur after discontinuation of lamivudine) ▪ Geriatric patients (dosage reduction may be necessary) ▪ Pregnancy or children <3 mo (safety not established).

**Exercise Extreme Caution in:** ▪ Pediatric patients with a history of pancreatitis (use only if no alternative).

## ADVERSE REACTIONS AND SIDE EFFECTS*

Noted for combination of lamivudine plus zidovudine. ▪ **CNS:** SEIZURES, fatigue, headache, insomnia, malaise, depression, dizziness ▪ **Resp:** cough ▪ **GI:** HEPATOMEGALY WITH STEATOSIS, PANCREATITIS (↑ in pediatric patients), anorexia, diarrhea, nausea, vomiting, abdominal discomfort, abnormal liver function studies, dyspepsia ▪ **Derm:** alopecia, erythema multiforme, rashes, urticaria ▪ **Endo:** hyperglycemia ▪ **F and E:** lactic acidosis ▪ **Hemat:** anemia, neutropenia, pure red cell aplasia ▪ **MS:** musculoskeletal pain, arthralgia, muscle weakness, myalgia, rhabdomyolysis ▪ **Neuro:** neuropathy ▪ **Misc:** hypersensitivity reactions including ANAPHYLAXIS and STEVENS-JOHNSON SYNDROME.

## INTERACTIONS

**Drug-Drug:** ▪ **Trimethoprim/sulfamethoxazole** ↑ lamivudine blood levels (dosage alteration may be necessary in renal impairment) ▪ ↑ risk of pancreatitis with concurrent use of other **drugs causing pancreatitis** ▪ ↑ risk of neuropathy with concurrent use of other **drugs causing neuropathy** ▪ Combination therapy with **tenofovir** and **abacavir** may lead to virologic nonresponse and should not be used.

## ROUTE AND DOSAGE

❑ **HIV infection**

▪ **PO (Adults and Children >12 yr and ≥50 kg):** 150 mg twice daily.
▪ **PO (Adults <50 kg):** 2 mg/kg twice daily.
▪ **PO (Children 3 mo–12 yr):** 4 mg/kg twice daily (up to 150 mg twice daily).

❑ **Renal Impairment**

▪ **PO (Adults):** *CCr 30–49 ml/min*—150 mg once daily; *CCr 15–29 ml/min*—150 mg first dose, then 10 mg once daily; *CCr 5–14 ml/min*—150 mg first dose, then 50 mg once daily; *CCr <5 ml/min*—50 mg first dose, then 25 mg once daily.

❑ **Chronic Hepatitis B**

▪ **PO (Adults):** 100 mg once daily.

❑ **Renal Impairment**

▪ **PO (Adults):** *CCr 30–49 ml/min*—100 mg first dose, then 50 mg once daily; *CCr 15–29 ml/min*—100 mg first dose, then 25 mg once daily; *CCr 5–14 ml/min*—35 mg first dose, then 15 mg once daily; *CCr <5 ml/min*—35 mg first dose, then 10 mg once daily.
▪ **PO (Children 2–17 yr):** 3 mg/kg once daily (up to 100 mg/day).

## AVAILABILITY

❑ **Epivir**

▪ *Tablets:* 150 mg$^{Rx}$, 300 mg$^{Rx}$ ▪Cost: 150 mg $86.22/60 ▪ *Oral solution (strawberry-banana flavor):* 10 mg/ml in 240-ml bottles$^{Rx}$ ▪ Cost: 10 mg/ml $80.92/240 ml.

❑ **Epivir HBV**

▪ *Tablets:* 100 mg$^{Rx}$ ▪ Cost: $303.40/60 ▪ *Oral solution (strawberry-banana flavor):* 5 mg/ml in 240 ml bottlesRx ▪ Cost: $60.67/240 ml ▪ zidovudine (Combivir$^{Rx}$); zidovudine and abacavir (Trizivir$^{Rx}$). See Appendix B.

## TIME/ACTION PROFILE (blood levels)

| | ONSET | PEAK | DURATION |
|---|---|---|---|
| PO | unknown | 0.9 hr† | 12 hr |

†On an empty stomach; peak levels occur at 3.2 hr if lamivudine is taken with food. Food does not affect total amount of drug absorbed.

# NURSING IMPLICATIONS

## ASSESSMENT

▪ **HIV:** Assess patient for change in severity of symptoms of HIV infection and for symptoms of opportunistic infection during therapy.
❑ Monitor patient for signs and symptoms of peripheral neuropathy (tingling, burning, numbness, or pain in hands or feet); may be difficult to differentiate from peripheral neuropathy of severe HIV disease. May require discontinuation of therapy.
❑ Assess patient, especially pediatric patients, for signs of pancreatitis (nausea, vomiting, abdominal pain) periodically during therapy. May require discontinuation of therapy.
▪ **Chronic Hepatitis B Infection:** Monitor signs of hepatitis (jaundice, fatigue, anorexia, pruritus) during therapy.
▪ *Lab Test Considerations:*
❑ Monitor viral load and CD4 levels before and periodically during therapy.
❑ Monitor serum amylase, lipase, and triglycerides periodically during therapy. Elevated serum levels may indicate pancreatitis and require discontinuation.
❑ Monitor liver function. May cause elevated levels of AST, ALT, CPK, bilirubin, and alkaline phosphatase, which usually resolve after interruption of therapy. Lactic acidosis may occur with hepatic toxicity causing hepatic steatosis; may be fatal, especially in women.
❑ May rarely cause neutropenia and anemia.

## POTENTIAL NURSING DIAGNOSES

▪ Infection, risk for (Indications).

## IMPLEMENTATION

▪ **General:** Do not confuse lamivudine with lamontrigine. Do not confuse Epivir tablets and oral solution with Epivir-HBV tablets and oral solutions. Epivir Tablets and Oral Solution contain a higher dose of the same active ingredient (lamivudine) than in Epivir-HBV Tablets and Oral Solution. Epivir-HBV was developed for patients with hepatitis B and should not be used for patients dually infected with HIV and hepatitis B; use may lead to lamivudine-resistant HIV due to sub-therapeutic dose.

■ **PO:** May be administered without regard to food.

## PATIENT/FAMILY TEACHING

❑ Instruct patient to take lamivudine as directed, every 12 hr. Explain the difference between Epivir and Epivir-HBV to patients. Emphasize the importance of compliance with full course of therapy, not taking more than the prescribed amount, and not discontinuing without consulting health care professional. Take missed doses as soon as possible unless almost time for next dose. Do not double doses. Caution patient not to share medication with others.

❑ Inform patient that lamivudine does not cure HIV disease or prevent associated or opportunistic infections. Lamivudine does not reduce the risk of transmission of HIV to others through sexual contact or blood contamination. Caution patient to use a condom during sexual contact and avoid sharing needles or donating blood to prevent spreading HIV to others. Advise patient that the long-term effects of lamivudine are unknown at this time.

❑ Instruct patient to notify health care professional promptly if signs of peripheral neuropathy or pancreatitis occur.

❑ Advise patient not to take other OTC or prescription medications or herbal products without consulting health care professional.

❑ Emphasize the importance of regular follow-up exams and blood tests to determine progress and monitor for side effects.

## EVALUATION

**Effectiveness of therapy can be demonstrated by:** ■ Slowing of the progression of HIV infection and its sequelae ■ Decrease in viral load and improvement in CD4 levels in patients with advanced HIV infection ■ Protection from liver damage caused by chronic hepatitis B infection; decreases viral load.

# lamotrigine
(la-**moe**-tri-jeen)
Lamictal

## CLASSIFICATION(S):
*Therapeutic: anticonvulsants*

## Pregnancy Category C

## INDICATIONS

■ Adjunct treatment of partial seizures in adults with epilepsy ■ Lennox-Gastaut syndrome ■ Conversion to monotherapy in adults with partial seizures receiving a single enzyme-inducing antiepileptic drug ■ Maintenance treatment of bipolar disorder.

## ACTION

■ Stabilizes neuronal membranes by inhibiting sodium transport. **Therapeutic Effects:** ■ Decreased incidence of seizures ■ Delayed time to recurrence of mood episodes.

## PHARMACOKINETICS

**Absorption:** 98% absorbed following oral administration.

**Distribution:** Enters breast milk. Highly bound to melanin-containing tissues (eyes, pigmented skin).

**Metabolism and Excretion:** Mostly metabolized by the liver to inactive metabolites; 10% excreted unchanged by the kidneys.

**Half-life:** 25.4 hr (during chronic therapy of lamotrigine alone).

## CONTRAINDICATIONS AND PRECAUTIONS

**Contraindicated in:** ■ Hypersensitivity ■ Lactation.

**Use Cautiously in:** ■ Patients with reduced renal function (lower maintenance doses may be required) ■ Patients with impaired cardiac function ■ Patients with impaired hepatic function ■ Pregnancy or children <16 yr (safety not established as monotherapy; may be used in patients 2–16 yr with Lennox-Gastaut syndrome).

## ADVERSE REACTIONS AND SIDE EFFECTS*

■ **CNS:** <u>ataxia</u>, <u>dizziness</u>, <u>headache</u>, behavior changes, depression, drowsiness, insomnia, tremor ■ **EENT:** blurred vision, double vision, rhinitis ■ **GI:** <u>nausea</u>, <u>vomiting</u> ■ **GU:** vaginitis ■ **Derm:** <u>photosensitivity</u>, <u>rash</u> ■ **MS:** arthralgia ■ **Misc:** allergic reactions including Stevens-Johnson syndrome.

## INTERACTIONS

**Drug-Drug:** ■ Concurrent use with **carbamazepine** may result in ↓ levels of lamotrigine and ↑ levels of an active metabolite of carbamazepine ■ Lamotrigine levels are ↓ by concurrent use of **phenobarbital, phenytoin,** or **primidone** ■ Concurrent use with **valproic acid** results in a twofold ↑ in lamotrigine levels and a ↓ in valproic acid level (lamotrigine dose should be ↓ by at least 50%).

## ROUTE AND DOSAGE

◻ **Epilepsy**

### In combination with Other Antiepileptic Agents

■ **PO (Adults >12 yr):** *Patients taking carbamazepine, phenobarbital, phenytoin, or primidone*—50 mg daily as a single dose for first 2 wk, then 50 mg twice daily for next 2 wk; then increase by 100 mg/day on a weekly basis to maintenance dose of 150–250 mg twice daily (not to exceed 500 mg/day). *Patients taking carbamazepine, phenobarbital, phenytoin, or primidone with valproic acid*—25 mg every other day for first 2 wk, then 25 mg once daily for next 2 wk; then increase by 25–50 mg/day every 1–2 wk to maintenance dose of 50–75 mg twice daily (not to exceed 200 mg/day).

■ **PO (Children 2–12 yr):** *Patients taking carbamazepine, phenobarbital, phenytoin, or primidone*—0.6 mg/kg/day in 2 divided doses (rounded down to nearest 5 mg) for first 2 wk, then 1.2 mg/kg in 2 divided doses (rounded down to nearest 5 mg) for next 2 wk; then increase by 1.2 mg/kg/day (rounded down to nearest 5 mg) q 1–2 wk to maintenance dose of 5–15 mg/kg day (not to exceed 400 mg/day in 2 divided doses). *Patients taking carbamazepine, phenobarbital, phenytoin, or primidone with valproic acid*—0.15 mg/kg/day in 1–2 divided doses (rounded down to nearest 5 mg) for first 2 wk; if initial calculated dose is 2.5–5 mg/

day, then initial dose should be 5 mg every other day for 2 wk). Then 0.3 mg/kg in 1–2 divided doses (rounded down to nearest 5 mg) for next 2 wk; then increase by 0.3 mg/kg/day (rounded down to nearest 5 mg) q 1–2 wk to maintenance dose of 1–5 mg/kg day (not to exceed 200 mg/day in 1–2 divided doses).

### Conversion to Monotherapy

■ **PO (Adults ≥16 yr):** 50 mg/day for 2 wk, then 50 mg twice daily for 2 wk, then increase by 100 mg/day q 1–2 wk to maintenance dose of 300–500 mg/day in 2 divided doses; when target level is reached, decrease other antiepileptic by 20% weekly over 4 wk.

◻ **Bipolar disorder**

### Escalation regimen

■ **PO (Adults):** *Patients not taking cabamazepine, valproate or other enzyme-inducing drugs*—25 mg/day for 2 wk, then 50 mg/day for 2 wk, then 100 mg/day for 1 wk, then 200 mg/day; *Patients taking valproate*—25 mg every other day for 2 wk, then 25 mg/day for 2 wk, then 50 mg/day for one wk, then 100 mg/day; *Patients taking cabamazepine (or other enzyme inducers), but not taking valporate* 50 mg/day for 2 wk, then 100 mg/day (in divided doses) for 2 wk, then 200 mg/day (in divided doses) for one wk, then 300 mg/day (in divided doses) for one week, then up to 400 mg/day (in divided doses).

### Dosage adjustment following discontinuation of other psychotropics

■ **PO (Adults):** *Following discontinuation of other psychotropics*—maintain previous dose; *following discontinuation of valproate*—100 mg/day, then increase to 150 mg/day for one wk, then 200 mg/day; *following discontinuation of carbamazepine or other enzyme-inducers*—400 mg/day for one wk, then 300 mg/day for one wk, then 200 mg/day.

## AVAILABILITY

■ *Tablets:* 25 mg[Rx], 100 mg[Rx], 150 mg[Rx], 200 mg[Rx] ■ *Chewable dispersible tablets:* 2 mg[Rx], 5 mg[Rx], 25 mg[Rx].

TIME/ACTION PROFILE (blood levels)

| | ONSET | PEAK | DURATION |
|---|---|---|---|
| PO | unknown | 1.4–4.8 hr | unknown |

# NURSING IMPLICATIONS

## ASSESSMENT

- **General Info:** Assess patient for skin rash frequently during therapy. Discontinue lamotrigine at first sign of rash; may be life-threatening. Stevens-Johnson syndrome or toxic epidermal necrolysis may develop. Rash usually occurs during the initial 2–8 wk of therapy and is more frequent in patients taking multiple antiepileptic agents, especially valproic acid, and much more frequent in patients <16 yr.
- **Seizures:** Assess location, duration, and characteristics of seizure activity.
- **Bipolar disorders:** Assess mood, ideation, and behaviors frequently. Initiate suicide precautions if indicated.
- *Lab Test Considerations:* Lamotrigine plasma concentrations may be monitored periodically during therapy, especially in patients concurrently taking other anticonvulsants. Therapeutic plasma concentration range has not been established.

## POTENTIAL NURSING DIAGNOSES

- Skin integrity, risk for impaired (Adverse Reactions).
- Injury, risk for (Side Effects).

## IMPLEMENTATION

- **General:** Do not confuse lamotrigine (Lamictal) with terbinafine (Lamisil), maprotiline (Ludiomil), diphenoxylate/atropine (Lomotil) or lamivudine (Epivir).
- **PO:** May be administered without regard to meals.
- Lamotrigine should be discontinued gradually over at least 2 wk, unless safety concerns require a more rapid withdrawal. Abrupt discontinuation may cause increase in seizure frequency.
- **Chewable/Dispersible Tablets:** May be swallowed whole, chewed, or dispersed in water or dispersed in fruit juice. If chewed, follow with water or fruit juice to aid in swallowing.

## PATIENT/FAMILY TEACHING

- Instruct patient to take medication exactly as directed. Take missed doses as soon as possible unless almost time for next dose. Do not double doses. Do not discontinue abruptly; may cause increase in frequency of seizures.
- Advise patient to notify health care professional immediately if skin rash occurs or if frequency of seizures increases.
- May cause dizziness, drowsiness, and blurred vision. Caution patient to avoid driving or activities requiring alertness until response to medication is known. Do not resume driving until physician gives clearance based on control of seizure disorder.
- Caution patient to wear sunscreen and protective clothing to prevent photosensitivity reactions.
- Advise patient to notify health care professional if pregnancy is planned or suspected or if patient intends to breastfeed or is breastfeeding.
- Instruct patient to notify health care professional of medication regimen prior to treatment or surgery.
- Advise patient to carry identification at all times describing disease process and medication regimen.

## EVALUATION

**Effectiveness of therapy can be demonstrated by:** ■ Decrease in the frequency of or cessation of seizures ■ Decreased incidence of mood swings in bipolar disorders.

---

# lansoprazole

(lan-**soe**-pra-zole)
Prevacid

*CLASSIFICATION(S):*
*Therapeutic: antiulcer agents*
*Pharmacologic: proton-pump inhibitors*

**Pregnancy Category B**

---

{ } = Available in Canada only.
*CAPITALS indicates life-threatening; <u>underlines</u> indicate most frequent.

## INDICATIONS

■ Erosive esophagitis ■ Duodenal ulcers (with or without anti-infectives for *Helicobacter pylori*) ■ Active benign gastric ulcer ■ Short-term treatment of symptomatic GERD ■ Healing and risk reduction of NSAID-associated gastric ulcer ■ Pathologic hypersecretory conditions, including Zollinger-Ellison syndrome.

## ACTION

■ Binds to an enzyme in the presence of acidic gastric pH, preventing the final transport of hydrogen ions into the gastric lumen. **Therapeutic Effects:** ■ Diminished accumulation of acid in the gastric lumen, with lessened acid reflux ■ Healing of duodenal ulcers and esophagitis.

## PHARMACOKINETICS

**Absorption:** 80% absorbed after oral administration.
**Distribution:** Unknown.
**Protein Binding:** 97%.
**Metabolism and Excretion:** Extensively metabolized by the liver to inactive compounds. Converted intracellularly to at least two other antisecretory compounds.
**Half-life:** Less than 2 hr (increased in geriatric patients and patients with impaired hepatic function).

## CONTRAINDICATIONS AND PRECAUTIONS

**Contraindicated in:** ■ Hypersensitivity.
**Use Cautiously in:** ■ Geriatric patients (maintenance dose should not exceed 30 mg/day unless additional acid suppression is required) ■ Severe hepatic impairment (not to exceed 30 mg/day in these patients) ■ Pregnancy, lactation, or children <1 yr (safety not established).

## ADVERSE REACTIONS AND SIDE EFFECTS*

■ **CNS:** dizziness, headache ■ **GI:** diarrhea, abdominal pain, nausea ■ **Derm:** rash.

## INTERACTIONS

**Drug-Drug:** ■ Sucralfate ↓ absorption of lansoprazole (take 30 min before sucralfate) ■ May ↓ absorption of drugs requiring acid pH, including **ketoconazole, itraconazole, ampicillin esters, iron salts,** and **digoxin.** ■ May ↑ risk of bleeding with warfarin (monitor INR/PT).

## ROUTE AND DOSAGE

■ **PO (Adults):** *Short-term treatment of duodenal ulcer*—15 mg once daily for 4 wk; *H. pylori eradication to reduce the risk of duodenal ulcer recurrence*—30 mg twice daily with clarithromycin 500 mg twice daily and amoxicillin 1000 mg twice daily for 10–14 days (triple therapy) or 30 mg three times daily with 1000 mg amoxicillin three times daily for 14 days (dual therapy); *maintenance of healed duodenal ulcers*—15 mg once daily; *short-term treatment of gastric ulcers/healing of NSAID-associated gastric ulcer*—30 mg once daily for up to 8 wk; *risk reduction of NSAID-associated gastric ulcer*—15 mg once daily for up to 12 wk; *short-term treatment of symptomatic GERD*—15 mg once daily for up to 8 wk; *short-term treatment of erosive esophagitis*—30 mg once daily for up to 8 wk (8 additional weeks may be necessary); *maintenance of healing of erosive esophagitis*—15 mg once daily; *pathologic hypersecretory conditions*—60 mg once daily intially, up to 90 mg twice daily (daily dose >120 mg should be given in divided doses).
■ **PO (Children 1–11 yr and >30 kg):** *GERD/esophagitis*—30 mg once daily for up to 12 wk.
■ **PO (Children 1–11 yr and ≤ 30 kg):** *GERD/esophagitis*—15 mg once daily for up to 12 wk.

## AVAILABILITY

■ *Delayed-release capsules:* 15 mg$^{Rx}$, 30 mg$^{Rx}$ ■ **Cost:** 15 mg $125.92/30; 30 mg $427.70/100 ■ *Delayed-release orally disintegrated tablets (SoluTabs):* 15 mg$^{Rx}$, 30 mg$^{Rx}$ ■ *Delayed-release oral suspension packets:* 15 mg$^{Rx}$, 30 mg$^{Rx}$ ■ amoxicillin and clarithromycin as part of a compliance package (Prevpac)$^{Rx}$. See Appendix B.

TIME/ACTION PROFILE (acid suppression)

|    | ONSET | PEAK | DURATION |
|----|-------|------|----------|
| PO | rapid | unknown | more than 24 hr |

# NURSING IMPLICATIONS

## ASSESSMENT

❏ Assess patient routinely for epigastric or abdominal pain and for frank or occult blood in stool, emesis, or gastric aspirate.

- **Lab Test Considerations:** May cause abnormal liver function tests, including increased AST, ALT, alkaline phosphatase, LDH, and bilirubin.
- ❑ May cause ↑ serum creatinine and ↑ or ↓ electrolyte levels.
- ❑ May alter RBC, WBC, and platelet levels.
- ❑ May also cause ↑ gastrin levels, abnormal A/G ratio, hyperlipidemia, and ↑ or ↓ cholesterol.
- ❑ Monitor INR and prothrombin time in patients taking warfarin.

## POTENTIAL NURSING DIAGNOSES

- Pain, acute (Indications).

## IMPLEMENTATION

Do not confuse Prevacid (lansoprazole) with Pravachol (pravastatin).

- **PO:** Administer before meals. Capsules may be opened and sprinkled on 1 tbsp of applesauce, pudding, cottage cheese, or yogurt and swallowed immediately for patients with difficulty swallowing. Do not crush or chew capsule contents.
- ❑ Orally disintegrating tablets may be placed on tongue, allowed to disintegrate and swallowed with or without water.
- ❑ Oral suspension may be prepared by emptying packet into 2 tbsp of water. Do not use other liquids or foods. Stir well and drink immediately. If material remains in glass, add water and drink immediately. Do not administer oral suspension through enteral tubes.
- ❑ For patients with an NG tube, capsules may be opened and intact granules may be mixed in 40 ml of apple, cranberry, grape, orange, pineapple, prune, or V8 vegetable juice and injected through the NG tube into stomach. Flush NG tube with additional apple juice to clear tube. If administered via jejunostomy tube, lansoprazole should be prepared as a suspension with 2.5 ml of 4.2% sodium bicarbonate and 2.5 ml water.
- ❑ Antacids may be used concurrently.

## PATIENT/FAMILY TEACHING

- ❑ Instruct patient to take medication as directed for the full course of therapy, even if feeling better.

- ❑ Advise patient to avoid alcohol, products containing aspirin or NSAIDs, and foods that may cause an increase in GI irritation.
- ❑ May occasionally cause dizziness. Caution patient to avoid driving and other activities that require alertness until response to medication is known.
- ❑ Advise patient to report onset of black, tarry stools; diarrhea; or abdominal pain to health care professional promptly.

## EVALUATION

**Effectiveness of therapy can be demonstrated by:** ■ Decrease in abdominal pain or prevention of gastric irritation and bleeding. Healing of duodenal ulcers can be seen on x-ray examination or endoscopy. Therapy is continued for at least 2–4 wk. Therapy for pathologic hypersecretory conditions may be long term ■ Healing in patients with erosive esophagitis. Therapy is continued for up to 8 wk, and an additional 8-wk course may be used for patients who do not heal in 8 wk or whose ulcer recurs.

## leflunomide

(le-**flu**-noe-mide)

Arava

### CLASSIFICATION(S):

**Therapeutic:** antirheumatics (DMARDs)

**Pharmacologic:** immune response modifiers

### Pregnancy Category X

## INDICATIONS

- Rheumatoid arthritis (disease-modifying agent).

## ACTION

- Inhibits an enzyme required for pyrimidine synthesis; has antiproliferative and anti-inflammatory effects. **Therapeutic Effects:** ■ Decreased pain and inflammation, slowed structural progression and improved physical function.

## PHARMACOKINETICS

**Absorption:** Tablets are 80% absorbed following oral administration; rapidly converted to the M1 metabolite, which is responsible for pharmacologic activity.

**Distribution:** Crosses the placenta.

**Protein Binding:** 99%.

**Metabolism and Excretion:** Extensively metabolized with metabolites excreted in urine (43%) and feces (48%). Also undergoes biliary recycling.

**Half-life:** 14–18 days.

## CONTRAINDICATIONS AND PRECAUTIONS

**Contraindicated in:** ■ Hypersensitivity ■ Women who are or may become pregnant ■ Compromised immune function, including bone marrow dysplasia or severe uncontrolled infection ■ Concurrent vaccination with live vaccines ■ Children <18 yr ■ Lactation.

**Use Cautiously in:** ■ Renal insufficiency ■ Women with childbearing potential ■ Men attempting to father a child.

**Exercise Extreme Caution in:** ■ Significant hepatic impairment, including positive serology for hepatitis B or C

## ADVERSE REACTIONS AND SIDE EFFECTS*

■ **CNS:** headache, dizziness, weakness ■ **Resp:** bronchitis, increased cough, pharyngitis, pneumonia, respiratory infection, rhinitis, sinusitis ■ **CV:** chest pain, hypertension ■ **GI:** diarrhea, nausea, abdominal pain, abnormal liver enzymes/hepatotoxicity, anorexia, dyspepsia, gastroenteritis, mouth ulcers, vomiting ■ **GU:** urinary tract infection ■ **Derm:** alopecia, rash, dry skin, eczema, pruritus ■ **F and E:** hypokalemia ■ **Metab:** weight loss ■ **MS:** arthralgia, back pain, joint disorder, leg cramps, synovitis, tenosynovitis ■ **Neuro:** paresthesia ■ **Misc:** allergic reactions, flu syndrome, infection, pain.

## INTERACTIONS

**Drug-Drug:** ■ **Cholestyramine** and **activated charcoal** cause a rapid and significant ↓ in blood levels of active metabolite ■ Concurrent use of **methotrexate** and other **hepatotoxic drugs** ↑ risk of hepatotoxicity ■ Concurrent administration of **rifampin** ↑ blood levels of the active metabolite ■ May ↑ risk of bleeding with **warfarin.**

## ROUTE AND DOSAGE

■ **PO (Adults):** *Loading dose*—100 mg daily for 3 days; *maintenance dosing*—20 mg/day (if intolerance occurs, dose may be decreased to 10 mg/day).

## AVAILABILITY

■ **Tablets:** 10 mg^Rx, 20 mg^Rx, 100 mg^Rx ■Cost: 10 mg $272.46/30, 20 mg $272.46/30, 100 mg $141.33/3.

TIME/ACTION PROFILE (antirheumatic effect)

| | ONSET | PEAK | DURATION |
|---|---|---|---|
| PO | 1 mo | 3–6 mo | wks–mos† |

†Due to persistence of active metabolite.

# NURSING IMPLICATIONS

## ASSESSMENT

❏ Assess range of motion and degree of swelling and pain in affected joints before and periodically during therapy.

■ **Lab Test Considerations:** Monitor liver function throughout therapy. ALT should be assessed at baseline, then monthly during initial 6 mo of therapy, then every 6–8 wks. If given concurrently with methotrexate, monitor ALT, AST, and serum albumin monthly. May cause ↑ ALT and AST, which are usually reversible with reduction in dose or discontinuation, but may be fatal. If ALT is 2–3 times the upper limit of normal, reduce dose to 10 mg/day and continue therapy. Monitor closely after dose reduction; plasma levels may not decrease for several weeks due to long half-life. If ALT elevation of 2–3 times the upper limit of normal persists despite dose reduction or if ALT >3 times the upper limit of normal occurs, discontinue leflunomide and administer cholestyramine (see Toxicity and Overdose). Monitor closely and readminister cholestyramine as indicated.

❏ Monitor CBC with platelets monthly for 6 mo following initiation of therapy and every 6–8 wks thereafter. If used with methotrexate or other immunosuppressive therapy continue monitoring monthly. If bone marrow depression occurs, discontinue leflunomide and begin decreasing levels with cholestyramine (see Implementation).

❑ May rarely cause elevations of alkaline phosphatase and bilirubin.

■ *Toxicity and Overdose:* If overdose or significant toxicity occurs, cholestyramine 8 g 3 times a day for 24 hr, or activated charcoal orally or via nasogastric tube, 50 g every 6 hr for 24 hr, is recommended to accelerate elimination.

## POTENTIAL NURSING DIAGNOSES

■ Mobility, impaired physical (Indications).
■ Pain, acute (Indications).

## IMPLEMENTATION

■ **PO:** Initiate therapy with loading dose of 100 mg/day for 3 days, followed by 20 mg/day dose. May decrease to 10 mg/day if not well tolerated.

■ **Drug Elimination Procedure:** Recommended to achieve nondectable plasma levels <0.02 mg/L after stopping treatment with leflunomide. Administer cholestyramine 8 g 3 times daily for 11 days. (Days do not need to be consecutive unless rapid lowering of levels is desired.) Verify plasma levels <0.02 mg/L by 2 separate tests at least 14 days apart. If plasma levels >0.02 mg/L, consider additional cholestyramine treatment. Plasma levels may take up to 2 yr to reach nondetectable levels without drug elimination procedure.

## PATIENT/FAMILY TEACHING

❑ Instruct patient to take leflunomide exactly as directed.

❑ May cause dizziness. Caution patient to avoid driving or other activities requiring alertness until response to medication is known.

❑ Caution patients of childbearing age that leflunomide has teratogenic effects. Women wishing to become pregnant must undergo the drug elimination procedure (see Implementation) and verify that the M1 metabolite plasma levels are <0.02 mg/L. Men wishing to father a child should also take cholestyramine 8 g 3 times daily for 11 days to minimize any possible risk.

❑ Advise patient to consult health care professional prior to taking other medications or herbal products concurrently with leflunomide. Aspirin, NSAIDs, or low-dose corticosteroids may be continued during therapy, but other agents for treatment of rheumatoid arthritis may require discontinuation.

❑ Discuss the possibility of hair loss with patient. Explore methods of coping.

❑ Instruct patient to avoid vaccinations with live vaccines during and following therapy without consulting health care professional.

## EVALUATION

**Effectiveness of therapy can be demonstrated by:** ■ Decrease in signs and symptoms of rheumatoid arthritis and slowing of structural damage as evidenced by x-ray erosions and joint narrowings ❑ Improved physical function.

---

# lepirudin (rDNA)
(le-**peer**-yoo-din)
Refludan

## CLASSIFICATION(S):
*Therapeutic: anticoagulants*
*Pharmacologic: thrombin inhibitors*

### Pregnancy Category B

## INDICATIONS

■ Management of thromboembolic disease and prevention of its complications in patients who have experienced heparin-induced thrombocytopenia.

## ACTION

■ Acts as an anticoagulant by inhibiting the action of thrombin ■ Produced by recombinant DNA technology. **Therapeutic Effects:** ■ Anticoagulation with prevention of thromboembolic complications.

## PHARMACOKINETICS

**Absorption:** IV administration results in complete bioavailability.

**Distribution:** Distributes mainly to extracellular fluids.

**Metabolism and Excretion:** Metabolized by release of amino acids caused by breakdown of drug; 48% excreted unchanged in urine.

**Half-life:** 1.3 hr.

---

## CONTRAINDICATIONS AND PRECAUTIONS

**Contraindicated in:** ■ Hypersensitivity
**Use Cautiously in:** ■ Recent puncture of large vessels/organ biopsy ■ Vessel/organ anomaly ■ Recent CVA, stroke, intracerebral surgery or other neuroaxial procedure ■ Severe uncontrolled hypertension ■ Severe renal impairment (CCr <15 ml/min) ■ Bacterial endocarditis ■ Hemorrhagic diatheses ■ Recent major surgery ■ Recent major bleeding ■ Severe liver impairment ■ Moderate renal impairment (reduced bolus and maintenance infusion rate recommended if CCr 15<50 ml/min) ■ Pregnancy, lactation or children (safety not established).

## ADVERSE REACTIONS AND SIDE EFFECTS*

■ **Hemat:** BLEEDING ■ **Misc:** allergic reactions including ANAPHYLAXIS.

## INTERACTIONS

**Drug-Drug:** ■ Increased risk of bleeding with **thrombolytic agents, NSAIDs, valproic acid, plicamycin, cefamonadole, cefotetan, cefoperazone,** platelet aggregation inhibitors including **aspirin, dipyridamole, clopidogrel, ticlopidine, tirofiban,** and **eptifibatide.**

## ROUTE AND DOSAGE

■ **IV (Adults):** 0.4 mg/kg (not to exceed 44 mg) as a bolus over 15–20 sec, followed by 0.15 mg/kg/hr (not to exceed 16.5 mg/hr) initially, further adjustments made on the basis of laboratory assessment (aPTT) but should not exceed infusion rate of 0.21 mg/kg/hr without checking for coagulation abnormalities.

❑ **Renal Impairment**
■ **IV (Adults):** 0.2 mg/kg as a bolus over 15–20 sec, then if *CCr 45–60 ml/min*—0.075 mg/kg/hr; if *CCr 30–44 ml/min*—0.045 mg/kg/hr; if *CCr 15–29 ml/min*—0.0225 mg/kg/hr.

## AVAILABILITY

■ *Powder for injection:* 50 mg/vial[Rx].

TIME/ACTION PROFILE (anticoagulant effect)

| | ONSET | PEAK | DURATION |
|---|---|---|---|
| IV | within 30–90 min | unknown | up to 24 hr |

## NURSING IMPLICATIONS

### ASSESSMENT

■ **General Info:** Assess patient for signs of bleeding and hemorrhage (bleeding gums, nosebleed, unusual bruising, black tarry stools, hematuria, fall in hematocrit or blood pressure, guaiac-positive stools). Notify physician if these occur.

❑ Monitor patient for hypersensitivity reactions (chills, fever, urticaria). Report signs to physician.

■ *Lab Test Considerations:* Dosage is adjusted according to aPTT ratio (patient aPTT at a given time over aPTT reference value, usually median of laboratory normal range for aPTT). Target range for aPTT ratio during treatment should be 1.5–2.5.

❑ Determine baseline aPTT prior to therapy; therapy should not be started in patients with an aPTT ratio of >2.5.

❑ First aPTT should be drawn 4 hr after initiation of therapy, then at least daily during therapy. More frequent monitoring is required in patients with serious liver injury or renal impairment.

❑ If aPTT ratio is out of target range, confirm ratio before modifying dose, unless clinically necessitated. If the confirmed ratio is above the target range, stop infusion for 2 hr. Restart infusion at 50% of previous dose without bolus and determine aPTT ratio in 4 hr.

❑ If confirmed ratio is below target range, increase infusion in steps of 20% and determine ratio in 4 hr.

■ *Toxicity and Overdose:* If life-threatening bleeding occurs and excessive plasma levels of lepirudin are suspected, immediately stop infusion, determine aPTT and other coagulation levels, determine hemoglobin and prepare for blood transfusion. No specific antidote for lepirudin is available.

### POTENTIAL NURSING DIAGNOSES

■ Tissue perfusion, ineffective (Indications).
■ Injury, risk for (Side Effects).

### IMPLEMENTATION

■ **General:** Inform all personnel caring for patient of anticoagulant therapy. Venipunctures and injection sites require application of pressure to prevent bleeding or hematoma formation. IM injections of other medications should be avoided, as hematomas may develop.

❑ In patients scheduled to receive coumadin derivatives for oral anticoagulation, lepirudin dose should be gradually decreased to reach an aPTT ratio just above 1.5 before initiating oral anticoagulant therapy.

■ **Direct IV:** Reconstitute each vial with 1 ml of sterile water for injection or 0.9% NaCl. Shake gently. Clear, colorless solution should be obtained within a few seconds to 3 min. Do not use solutions that are cloudy or contain particulate matter. Transfer contents of vial into a 10-ml syringe and dilute to a total volume of 10 ml with sterile water for injection, 0.9% NaCl, or D5W, for a concentration of 5 mg/ml.

■ *Rate:* Administer slowly over 15–20 sec.

■ **Continuous Infusion:** Reconstitute 2 vials with 1 mg each using sterile water for injection or 0.9% NaCl. Transfer the contents into an infusion bag containing 500 ml or 250 ml of 0.9% NaCl or D5W for concentrations of 0.2 mg/ml or 0.4 mg/ml, respectively. Solution is stable for 24 hr at room temperature. Warm to room temperature before administering. Discard unused solution.

■ *Rate:* Infuse at a rate of 0.15 mg/kg/hr. Use an infusion pump to ensure accuracy.

■ **Additive Incompatibility:** Do not admix with other drugs.

## PATIENT/FAMILY TEACHING

■ **General Info:** Advise patient to report any symptoms of unusual bleeding or bruising to health care professional immediately.

❑ Caution patient to avoid IM injections and activities leading to injury and to use a soft toothbrush and electric razor during therapy.

## EVALUATION

**Clinical response to therapy can be evaluated by:** ■ Range of aPTT ratio from 1.5–2.5, without signs of hemorrhage ■ Treatment and prevention of thromboembolic disease and its sequelae.

## letrozole
(**let**-roe-zole)

Femara

### CLASSIFICATION(S):
**Therapeutic:** antineoplastics
**Pharmacologic:** aromatase inhibitors

### Pregnancy Category D

## INDICATIONS

■ First-line treatment of postmenopausal women with hormone receptor positive or hormone receptor unknown metastatic or advanced breast cancer ■ Advanced breast cancer in postmenopausal patients with disease progression despite antiestrogen therapy.

## ACTION

■ Inhibits the enzyme aromatase, which is partially responsible for conversion of precursors to estrogen. **Therapeutic Effects:** ■ Lowers levels of circulating estrogen, which may halt progression of estrogen-sensitive breast cancer.

## PHARMACOKINETICS

**Absorption:** Rapidly and completely absorbed.
**Distribution:** Unknown.
**Metabolism and Excretion:** Mostly metabolized by the liver.
**Half-life:** 2 days.

## CONTRAINDICATIONS AND PRECAUTIONS

**Contraindicated in:** ■ Hypersensitivity ■ Pregnancy.
**Use Cautiously in:** ■ Severe hepatic impairment ■ Lactation or children (safety not established).

## ADVERSE REACTIONS AND SIDE EFFECTS*

■ **CNS:** anxiety, depression, dizziness, drowsiness, fatigue, headache, vertigo, weakness ■ **Resp:** coughing, dyspnea, pleural effusion ■ **CV:** chest pain, edema, hypertension ■ **GI:** <u>nausea</u>, abdominal pain, anorexia, constipation, diarrhea, dyspepsia, vomiting ■ **Derm:** alopecia, hot flashes, increased sweating, pruritus, rash ■ **F and E:** hypercalcemia ■ **Metab:** hypercholesterolemia, weight gain ■ **MS:** <u>musculoskeletal pain</u>, arthralgia, fractures.

## INTERACTIONS

**Drug-Drug:** ■ None significant.

## ROUTE AND DOSAGE

■ **PO (Adults):** 2.5 mg daily.

## AVAILABILITY

■ *Tablets:* 2.5 mg$^{Rx}$ ■ **Cost:** $187.20/30.

TIME/ACTION PROFILE (effect on lowering of serum estradiol levels)

| | ONSET | PEAK | DURATION |
|---|---|---|---|
| PO | unknown | 2–3 days | unknown |

## NURSING IMPLICATIONS

### ASSESSMENT

❑ Assess patient for pain and other side effects periodically throughout therapy.
■ *Lab Test Considerations:* May cause elevated GTT cholesterol levels.

### POTENTIAL NURSING DIAGNOSES

■ Pain, acute (Side Effects).

### IMPLEMENTATION

■ **PO:** May be taken without regard to food.

### PATIENT/FAMILY TEACHING

❑ Instruct patient to take medication as directed.
❑ Inform patient of potential for adverse reactions and advise her to notify health care professional if side effects are problematic.

### EVALUATION

**Effectiveness of therapy can be demonstrated by:** ■ Slowing of disease progression in women with advanced breast cancer.

---

# leucovorin calcium

(loo-koe-**vor**-in)

citrovorum factor, folinic acid, Wellcovorin

## CLASSIFICATION(S):

*Therapeutic: antidotes (for methotrexate), vitamins*
*Pharmacologic: folic acid analogues*

**Pregnancy Category C**

---

## INDICATIONS

■ Minimizes hematologic effects of high-dose methotrexate therapy (leucovorin rescue) ■ Advanced colorectal carcinoma (with 5–fluorouracil) ■ Management of overdoses/prevention of toxicity from folic acid antagonists (pyrimethamine, trimethoprim, trimetrexate) ■ Folic acid deficiency (megaloblastic anemia) unresponsive to oral replacement.

## ACTION

■ The reduced form of folic acid that serves as a cofactor in the synthesis of DNA and RNA.
**Therapeutic Effects:** ■ Reversal of toxic effects of folic acid antagonists ■ Reversal of folic acid deficiency.

## PHARMACOKINETICS

**Absorption:** Well absorbed (38%)following PO administration. Bioavailability decreases with larger doses. Oral absorption is saturated at doses >25 mg.

**Distribution:** Widely distributed. Concentrates in the CNS and liver.

**Metabolism and Excretion:** Extensively converted to tetrahydrofolic derivatives, including 5-methyltetrahydrofolate, a major storage form.

**Half-life:** 3.5 hr.

## CONTRAINDICATIONS AND PRECAUTIONS

**Contraindicated in:** ■ Hypersensitivity ■ Preparations containing benzyl alcohol should not be used in neonates.

**Use Cautiously in:** ■ Undiagnosed anemia (may mask the progression of pernicious anemia) ■ Pregnancy and lactation (safety not established but has been used safely to treat megaloblastic anemia in pregnancy) ■ **Coadministration with high-dose methotrexate requires crucial timing of dosing and knowledge of methotrexate levels** ■ Ascites ■ Renal failure ■ Dehydration ■ Pleural effusions ■ Urine pH <7.

## ADVERSE REACTIONS AND SIDE EFFECTS*

■ **Hemat:** thrombocytosis (intra-arterial methotrexate only) ■ **Misc:** allergic reactions (rash, urticaria, wheezing).

## INTERACTIONS

**Drug-Drug:** ■ May ↓ anticonvulsant effect of **barbiturates, phenytoin,** or **primidone** ■ High doses of the liquid contain significant **al-**

cohol and may cause ↑ CNS depression when used with **CNS depressants**. ■ Concurrent use with **trimethoprim/sulfamethoxazole** may result in ↓ anti-infective efficacy and poor therapeutic outcome when used to treat *Pneumocystis carinii* pneumonia in HIV patients ■ May ↑ therapeutic effects and toxicity of **fluorouracil**; therapy may be combined for this purpose.

## ROUTE AND DOSAGE

❑ **High-Dose Methotrexate—Leucovorin Rescue. Must start within 24 hr of methotrexate.**

■ **PO, IM, IV (Adults and Children):** *Normal methotrexate elimination*—10 mg/m² q 6 hr (1st dose IV/IM, then change to PO) until methotrexate level is <5 × 10⁻⁸ M (0.05 micromolar). Larger doses/longer duration may be required in patients with aciduria, ascites, dehydration, renal impairment, GI obstruction, pleural/peritoneal effusions. Dose of leucovorin should be determined on the basis of plasma methotrexate levels.

❑ **Advanced Colorectal Cancer**

■ **IV (Adults):** 200 mg/m² followed by 5-fluorouracil 370 mg/m² or leucovorin 20 mg/m² is followed by 5-fluorouracil 425 mg/m². Regimen is given daily for 5 days q 4–5 wk.

❑ **Prevention of Hematologic Toxicity from Trimetrexate**

■ **PO, IV (Adults and Children):** 20 mg/m² q 6 hr continued for 72 hr after last trimetrexate dose (oral doses should be rounded up to the next 25 mg); both trimetrexate and leucovorin doses require adjustment for hematologic toxicity.

❑ **Prevention of Hematologic Toxicity from Pyrimethamine**

■ **PO, IV (Adults and Children):** 5–15 mg/ day.

❑ **Inadvertent Overdose of Folic Acid Antagonists**

■ **IM, IV (Adults and Children):** *Methotrexate–large doses*—75 mg IV followed by 12 mg IM q 6 hr for 4 doses; *methotrexate–average doses*—6–12 mg IM q 6 hr for 4 doses; *other folic acid antagonists*—amount equal in mg to folic acid antagonist.

❑ **Megaloblastic Anemia**

■ **PO, IM, IV (Adults and Children):** Up to 1 mg/day (up to 6 mg/day for dihydrofolate reductase deficiency).

## AVAILABILITY (generic available)

■ *Tablets:* 5 mg^Rx, 10 mg^Rx, 15 mg^Rx, 25 mg^Rx ■ *Solution for injection:* 3 mg/ml in 1-ml ampules^Rx, 5 mg/ml^Rx ■ *Powder for injection:* 50, 100, and 350-mg vials^Rx.

TIME/ACTION PROFILE (serum folate levels)

|    | ONSET | PEAK | DURATION |
|----|-------|------|----------|
| PO | 20–30 min | unknown | 3–6 hr |
| IM | 10–20 min | unknown | 3–6 hr |
| IV | <5 min | unknown | 3–6 hr |

# NURSING IMPLICATIONS

## ASSESSMENT

■ **General Info:** Assess patient for nausea and vomiting secondary to methotrexate therapy or folic acid antagonists (pyrimethamine and trimethoprim) overdose. Parenteral route may be necessary to ensure that patient receives dose.

❑ Monitor for development of allergic reactions (rash, urticaria, wheezing). Notify physician if these occur.

■ **Megaloblastic Anemia:** Assess degree of weakness and fatigue.

■ *Lab Test Considerations:* **Leucovorin rescue:** Monitor serum methotrexate levels to determine dosage and effectiveness of therapy. Leucovorin calcium levels should be equal to or greater than methotrexate level. Rescue continues until serum methotrexate level is <5 × 10M.

❑ Monitor CCr and serum creatinine prior to and every 24 hr during therapy to detect methotrexate toxicity. An increase >50% over the pretreatment concentration at 24 hr is associated with severe renal toxicity.

❑ Monitor urine pH every 6 hr during therapy; pH should be maintained >7 to decrease nephrotoxic effects of high-dose methotrexate. Sodium bicarbonate or acetazolamide may be ordered to alkalinize urine.

❑ *Megaloblastic anemia*—Monitor plasma folic acid levels, hemoglobin, hematocrit, and reticulocyte count prior to and periodically during therapy.

**POTENTIAL NURSING DIAGNOSES**

■ Injury, risk for (Indications).

■ Nutrition, imbalanced: less than body requirements (Indications).

**IMPLEMENTATION**

■ **General:** Do not confuse folinic acid (leucovorin calcium) with folic acid. Do not confuse leucovorin with leukeran (chlorambucil) or leukine (sargramostim).

❑ Make sure leucovorin calcium is available before administering high-dose methotrexate. Administration must be initiated within 24 hr of methotrexate therapy.

❑ Administer as soon as possible after toxic dose of folic acid antagonists (pyrimethamine and trimethoprim). Effectiveness of therapy begins to decrease 1 hr after overdose.

■ **PO:** Parenteral therapy should be used in patients with GI toxicity, with nausea and vomiting, or with doses >25 mg.

■ **IM:** IM route is preferred for treatment of megaloblastic anemia. Ampules of leucovorin calcium injection for IM use do not require reconstitution.

■ **Direct IV:** To reconstitute 50-mg vial of leucovorin calcium for injection, add 5 ml of bacteriostatic water or sterile water for injection for a concentration of 10 mg/ml. Use 10-ml diluent for 100-mg vial. The 350-mg vial should be reconstituted with 17 ml of diluent for a concentration of 20 mg/ml. If dose is >10 mg/m², do not use product containing benzyl alcohol. Use immediately if reconstituted with sterile water for injection. Stable for 7 days when reconstituted with bacteriostatic water.

■ *Rate:* Rate should not exceed 160 mg/min (16 ml of 10 mg/ml solution per min).

■ **Intermittent Infusion:** May be diluted in 100–500 ml of D5W, D10W, 0.9% NaCl, Ringer's or LR. Stable for 24 hr.

■ **Y-Site Compatibility:** ◆ amifostine ◆ aztreonam ◆ bleomycin ◆ cefepime ◆ cisplatin ◆ cladribine ◆ cyclophosphamide ◆ docetaxel ◆ doxorubicin ◆ doxorubicin liposome ◆ etoposide phosphate ◆ filgrastim ◆ fluconazole ◆ fluorouracil ◆ furosemide ◆ gatifloxacin ◆ gemcitabine ◆ granisetron ◆ heparin ◆ linezolid ◆ methotrexate ◆ metoclopramide ◆ mito-

mycin ◆ piperacillin/tazobactam ◆ tacrolimus ◆ teniposide ◆ thiotepa ◆ vinblastine ◆ vincristine.

■ **Y-Site Incompatibility:** ◆ amphotericin B cholesteryl sulfate complex ◆ droperidol ◆ foscarnet ◆ sodium bicarbonate.

**PATIENT/FAMILY TEACHING**

■ **General Info:** Explain purpose of medication to patient. Emphasize need to take exactly as ordered. Advise patient to contact health care professional if a dose is missed.

■ **Leucovorin Rescue:** Instruct patient to drink at least 3 liters of fluid each day during leucovorin rescue.

■ **Folic Acid Deficiency:** Encourage patient to eat a diet high in folic acid (meat proteins; bran; dried beans; and green, leafy vegetables).

**EVALUATION**

**Effectiveness of therapy can be demonstrated by:** ■ Reversal of bone marrow and GI toxicity in patients receiving methotrexate or in overdose of folic acid antagonists ■ Increased sense of well-being and increased production of normoblasts in patients with megaloblastic anemia.

# leuprolide

(loo-**proe**-lide)

Eligard, Lupron, Lupron Depot, Lupron Depot-PED, Lupron Depot-3 Month, Viadur

*CLASSIFICATION(S):*

*Therapeutic:* antineoplastics

*Pharmacologic:* hormones, gonadotropin-releasing hormones

**Pregnancy Category X**

**INDICATIONS**

■ **Injection, depot or implant:** Advanced prostate cancer in patients who are unable to tolerate orchiectomy or estrogen therapy (may be used in combination with flutamide or bicalutamide) ❑ Management of central precocious puberty (CPP) ■ **3.75-mg depot only:** Endometriosis ❑ Uterine fibroids (with iron therapy).

## ACTION

■ A synthetic analogue of luteinizing hormone–releasing hormone (LHRH) ■ Initially causes a transient increase in testosterone; however, with continuous administration, testosterone levels are decreased ■ Reduces gonadotropins, testosterone, and estradiol. **Therapeutic Effects:** ■ Decreased testosterone levels and resultant decrease in spread of prostate cancer ■ Reduction of pain/lesions in endometriosis ■ Decreased growth of fibroids ■ Delayed puberty.

## PHARMACOKINETICS

**Absorption:** Rapidly and almost completely absorbed following subcut administration. More slowly absorbed following IM administration of depot form; consistent levels maintained following implant.

**Distribution:** Unknown.

**Metabolism and Excretion:** Unknown.

**Half-life:** 3 hr.

## CONTRAINDICATIONS AND PRECAUTIONS

**Contraindicated in:** ■ Intolerance to synthetic analogues of LHRH (GnRH) ■ Pregnancy or lactation (depot form).

**Use Cautiously in:** ■ Hypersensitivity to benzyl alcohol (results in induration and erythema at subcut site).

## ADVERSE REACTIONS AND SIDE EFFECTS*

■ **CNS:** dizziness, headache, syncope; *depot*—drowsiness, personality disorder; *subcut*—anxiety, blurred vision, lethargy, memory disorder, mood swings; *implant*—insomnia ■ **EENT:** blurred vision; *subcut*—hearing disorder ■ **Resp:** hemoptysis; *depot*—epistaxis, throat nodules; *subcut*—cough, pleural rub, pulmonary fibrosis, pulmonary infiltrate ■ **CV:** MI, PULMONARY EMBOLI, angina, arrhythmias; *depot*—vasodilation; *subcut*—transient ischemic attack/stroke; *implant*—edema ■ **GI:** anorexia, diarrhea, dysphagia, nausea, vomiting; *depot*—gingivitis; *subcut*—GI BLEEDING, hepatic dysfunction, peptic ulcer, rectal polyps, taste disorders ■ **GU:** decreased testicular size, dysuria, incontinence, testicular pain; *depot*—cervix disorder; *subcut*—bladder spasm, penile swelling, prostate pain, urinary obstruction ■ **Derm:** *de-*

*pot*—hair growth, rash; *subcut*—dry skin, hair loss, pigmentation, skin cancer, skin lesions ■ **Endo:** breast swelling, breast tenderness, diabetes ■ **F and E:** hypercalcemia, lower extremity edema ■ **Local:** burning, itching, swelling at injection site; *implant*—pain ■ **Hemat:** *implant*—anemia ■ **Metab:** *depot*—hyperuricemia, increased bone density ■ **MS:** fibromyalgia, transient increase in bone pain (prostate cancer only); *subcut*—ankylosing spondylitis, joint pain, pelvic fibrosis, temporal bone pain ■ **Neuro:** *subcut*—peripheral neuropathy ■ **Misc:** hot flashes, chills, decreased libido, fever; *depot*—body odor, epistaxis.

## INTERACTIONS

**Drug-Drug:** ■ ↑ antineoplastic effects with **antiandrogens (megestrol, flutamide).**

## ROUTE AND DOSAGE

❑ **Prostate Cancer**
■ **Subcut (Adults):** 1 mg/day, 7.5 mg once monthly, 22.5 mg every 3 mo or 30 mg every 4 mo.
■ **IM (Adults):** 7.5 mg once monthly *or* 22.5 mg every 3 mo.
■ **Implant: (Adults):** one implant (72 mg) every 12 months.

❑ **Endometriosis/Fibroids**
■ **IM (Adults):** 3.75 mg once monthly, or 11.25 every 3 mo, or 30 mg every 4 mo.

❑ **Central Precocious Puberty (CPP)**
■ **Subcut (Children):** 50 mcg/kg/day, may be increased by 10 mcg/kg/day as required.
■ **IM (Children >37.5 kg):** 15 mg q 4 wk.
■ **IM (Children 25–37.5 kg):** 11.25 mg q 4 wk.
■ **IM (Children ≤25 kg):** 7.5 mg q 4 wk.

## AVAILABILITY (generic available)

■ *Solution for injection:* 5 mg/ml in 2.8-ml vial[Rx] ■ *Lyophilized microspheres for depot injection:* 3.75-mg single-use vial[Rx], 7.5-mg single-use vial[Rx] ■ *Lyophilized microspheres for pediatric depot injection:* 7.5 mg[Rx], 11.25 mg[Rx], 15-mg single-use kits[Rx] ■ *Lyophilized microspheres for 3-mo depot injection:* 22.5-mg single-use kits[Rx] ■ *Lyophilized microspheres for 4-mo depot injection:* 30 mg[Rx] ■ *Polymeric matrix in-*

*jectable formulation for subcut use:* 7.5 mg^Rx, 22.5 mg^Rx, 30 mg^Rx ■ *Implant:* 72 mg^Rx.

TIME/ACTION PROFILE (effect on hormone levels)

| | ONSET† | PEAK‡ | DURATION§ |
|---|---|---|---|
| Subcut | within 1st week | 2–4 wk | 4–12 wk |
| IM | within 1st week | 2–4 wk | 4–12 wk |
| IM-depot | within 1st week | 2–4 wk | 4–12 wk |
| implant | 3 days | 2 wk | 12 mos |

†Initial transient increase in testosterone and estradiol levels.
‡Maximum decline in testosterone and estradiol levels.
§Restoration of normal pituitary–gonadal function; in amenorrheic patients, normal menses usually returns 60–90 days after treatment is discontinued.

# NURSING IMPLICATIONS

## ASSESSMENT

- **Prostate Cancer:** Assess patient for an increase in bone pain, especially during the first few weeks of therapy. Monitor patients with vertebral metastases for increased back pain and decreased sensory/motor function.
- ❑ Monitor intake and output ratios; assess for bladder distention in patients with urinary tract obstruction during initiation of therapy.
- **Fibroids:** Assess patient for severity of symptoms (bloating, pelvic pain, pressure, excessive vaginal bleeding) periodically during therapy.
- **Endometriosis:** Assess patient for endometrial pain prior to and periodically during therapy.
- **CPP:** Prior to therapy, diagnosis of CPP should be confirmed by onset of secondary sex characteristics in girls <8 yr or boys <9 yr; a complete physical and endocrinologic examination, including height, weight, hand and wrist x-ray; total sex steroid level (estradiol or testosterone); adrenal steroid level; beta human chorionic gonadotropin level; GnRH stimulation test; and computerized tomography of the head must be performed. These parameters are monitored after 1–2 mo and every 6–12 mo during therapy.
- ❑ Assess patient for signs of precocious puberty (menses, breast development, testicular growth) periodically during therapy. Dose is

increased until no progression of the disease is noted either clinically or by lab test parameters, then usually maintained throughout therapy. Discontinuation of therapy should be considered before age 11 in girls and age 12 in boys.

- **Lab Test Considerations:** Initially ↑, then ↓ luteinizing hormone (LH) and follicle-stimulating hormone (FSH). This leads to castration levels of testosterone in boys 2–4 wk after initial increase in concentrations.
- ❑ Monitor testosterone, prostatic acid phosphate, and prostate-specific antigen (PSA) levels to evaluate response to therapy. Transient ↑ in levels may occur during the 1st month of therapy for prostate cancer.
- ❑ May cause ↑ BUN, serum calcium, uric acid, hypoproteinemia, LDH, alkaline phosphatase, AST, hyperglycemia, hyperlipidemia, hyperphosphatemia, WBC, PT, or PTT. May also cause ↓ platelets and serum potassium.

## POTENTIAL NURSING DIAGNOSES

- Sexual dysfunction (Side Effects).

## IMPLEMENTATION

- **Subcut, IM:** Use syringe supplied by manufacturer. Rotate sites.
- ❑ Leuprolide depot is *only* for IM injection.
- ❑ *Monthly formulation:* To reconstitute a single vial, use a 22-gauge needle; withdraw 1 ml of diluent and inject into vial to mix. To mix 2 or more vials, withdraw 0.5 ml and inject into each vial for a total volume of 1 ml. Shake each vial well; suspension will appear milky. Withdraw entire contents of all vials into syringe and inject immediately. Patients may store medication at room temperature.
- ❑ *4-mo subcut formulation (Eligard):* Assemble the Eligard kit and reconstitute solution using syringes provided, as directed by manufacturer. Mix in syringes as directed by manufacturer, do not shake. Solution must reach room temperature before administration and must be administered within 30 min of mixing, or be discarded. Solution is light tan to tan in color.
- ❑ *3-mo IM formulation:* For single IM injection, reconstitute lyphosized microspheres using a 23-gauge needle; withdraw 1.5 ml of diluent and inject into vial. Shake well until

suspension is uniformly milky. Withdraw entire contents and inject immediately.

❑ Store at room temperature; stable for 24 hr following reconstitution.

❑ *12-mo implant:* Implant is inserted in the inner aspect of the upper arm and provides continuous release of leuprolide for 12 mo. At the end of 12 mo, implant must be removed; a new implant may be inserted for continuous therapy.

## PATIENT/FAMILY TEACHING

■ **General Info:** Advise patient that medication may cause hot flashes. Notify health care professional if these become bothersome.

■ **Prostate Cancer:** Instruct patient and family on subcut injection technique. Review patient insert provided with leuprolide patient-administration kit.

❑ Instruct patient to take medication exactly as directed. If a dose is missed, take as soon as remembered unless not remembered until next day.

❑ Advise patient that bone pain may increase at initiation of therapy. This will resolve with time. Patient should discuss with health care professional use of analgesics to control pain.

❑ Instruct patient to notify health care professional promptly if difficulty urinating, weakness, or numbness occurs.

■ **Endometriosis:** Advise patient to use a form of contraception other than oral contraceptives during therapy. Inform patient that amenorrhea is expected but does not guarantee contraception.

■ **Central Precocious Puberty:** Instruct patient and family on the proper technique for subcut injection. Emphasize the importance of administering the medication at the same time each day. Rotate injection sites periodically.

❑ Inform patient and parents that if injections are not given daily, pubertal process may be reactivated.

❑ Advise patient and parents that during the first 2 mo of therapy patient may experience a light menstrual flow or spotting. Health care professional should be notified if this continues beyond 2nd mo.

❑ Instruct patient and parents to notify health care professional immediately if irritation at the injection site or unusual signs or symptoms occur.

## EVALUATION

**Effectiveness of therapy can be demonstrated by:** ■ Decrease in the spread of prostate cancer ■ Decrease in lesions and pain in endometriosis ■ Resolution of the signs of CCP ■ Improvement in preoperative hematologic parameters in patients with anemia from uterine fibroids.

# levalbuterol
(leev-al-**byoo**-ter-ole)
Xopenex

### CLASSIFICATION(S):
*Therapeutic:* bronchodilators
*Pharmacologic:* adrenergics

### Pregnancy Category C

## INDICATIONS

■ Bronchospasm due to reversible airway disease (short-term control agent).

## ACTION

■ Binds to beta-adrenergic receptors in airway smooth muscle leading to activation of adenyl-cyclase and increased levels of cyclic-3', 5'-adenosine monophosphate (cAMP). Increases in cAMP activate kinases, which inhibit the phosphorylation of myosin and decrease intracellular calcium. Decreased intracellular calcium relaxes smooth muscle airways. **Therapeutic Effects:** ■ Relaxation of airway smooth muscle with subsequent bronchodilation ■ Relatively selective for beta (pulmonary) receptors.

## PHARMACOKINETICS

**Absorption:** Some absorption occurs following inhalation.

**Distribution:** Unknown.

**Metabolism and Excretion:** Unknown.

**Half-life:** Unknown.

## CONTRAINDICATIONS AND PRECAUTIONS

**Contraindicated in:** ■ Hypersensitivity.

**Use Cautiously in:** ■ Cardiovascular disorders (including coronary insufficiency, hypertension, and arrhythmias) ■ History of seizures ■ Hyperthyroidism ■ Diabetes mellitus ■ Unusual sensitivity to adrenergic amines ■ Pregnancy, lactation, or children <6 yr (safety not established). **Exercise Extreme Caution in:** ■ Concurrent use or use within 2 weeks of **tricyclic antidepressants** or **MAO inhibitors** (may increase the risk of adverse cardiovascular reactions).

## ADVERSE REACTIONS AND SIDE EFFECTS*

■ **CNS:** anxiety, dizziness, headache, nervousness ■ **Resp:** increased cough, paradoxical bronchospasm, turbinate edema ■ **CV:** tachycardia ■ **GI:** dyspepsia ■ **Endo:** hyperglycemia ■ **F and E:** hypokalemia ■ **Neuro:** tremor.

## INTERACTIONS

**Drug-Drug:** ■ Concurrent use or use within 2 weeks of **tricyclic antidepressants** or **MAO inhibitors** may ↑ risk of adverse cardiovascular reactions (use with extreme caution). ■ **Beta blockers** block the beneficial pulmonary effects of adrenergic bronchodilators (choose cardioselective beta blockers if necessary and with caution) ■ May ↑ risk of hypokalemia from **potassium-losing diuretics** ■ May ↓ serum **digoxin** levels ■ May ↑ risk of arrhythmias with **hydrocarbon inhalation anesthetics** or **cocaine**.

**Drug-Natural Products:** ■ Use with caffeine-containing herbs (**guarana, tea, coffee**) ↑ stimulant effect.

## ROUTE AND DOSAGE

- ■ **Inhaln (Adults):** 0.63 mg via nebulization three times daily (every 6–8 hr); may be increased to 1.25 mg three times daily (every 6–8 hr).
- ■ **Inhaln (Children 6–11 yr):** 0.31 mg three times daily (not exceed 0.63 mg three times daily).

## AVAILABILITY

■ *Inhalation solution:* 0.31 mg/vial$^{Rx}$ in green foil pouch containing 12 vials, 0.63 mg/vial$^{Rx}$ in yellow foil pouch containing 12 vials, 1.25 mg/vial$^{Rx}$ in red foil pouch containing 12 vials.

TIME/ACTION PROFILE (bronchodilation)

| | ONSET | PEAK | DURATION |
|---|---|---|---|
| Inhalation | rapid | 30 min | 6–8 hr |

# NURSING IMPLICATIONS

## ASSESSMENT

- ❏ Assess lung sounds, pulse, and blood pressure before administration and during peak of medication. Note amount, color, and character of sputum produced. Closely monitor patients on higher dose for adverse effects.
- ❏ Monitor pulmonary function tests before initiating therapy and periodically during course to determine effectiveness of medication.
- ❏ Observe for paradoxical bronchospasm (wheezing). If condition occurs, withhold medication and notify physician or other health care provider immediately.
- ■ *Lab Test Considerations:* May cause ↑ serum glucose and ↓ serum potassium.

## POTENTIAL NURSING DIAGNOSES

- ■ Airway clearance, ineffective (Indications).

## IMPLEMENTATION

**Inhaln:** Allow at least 1 min between inhalations of aerosol medication.

- ❏ For nebulization, levalbuterol solution does not require dilution prior to administration. Once the foil pouch is opened, vials must be used within 2 weeks; open vials may be stored for 1 week. Discard vial if solution is not clear.

## PATIENT/FAMILY TEACHING

- ❏ Instruct patient in the proper use of the nebulizer (see Appendix F) and to take levalbuterol exactly as directed. Caution patient not to exceed recommended dose; may cause adverse effects, paradoxical bronchospasm, or loss of effectiveness of medication.
- ❏ Advise patient to consult health care professional before taking any OTC medications or alcohol concurrently with this therapy. Caution patient to also avoid smoking and other respiratory irritants.
- ❏ Instruct patient to contact health care professional immediately if shortness of breath is not relieved by medication or is accompa-

nied by diaphoresis, dizziness, palpitations, or chest pain.

◻ Advise patients to use levalbuterol first if using other inhalation medications, and allow 5 min to elapse before administering other inhalant medications unless otherwise directed.

◻ Advise patient to rinse mouth with water after each inhalation dose to minimize dry mouth.

◻ Instruct patient to notify health care professional if no response to the usual dose of levalbuterol.

### EVALUATION

**Effectiveness of therapy can be demonstrated by:** ■ Prevention or relief of bronchospasm.

---

# levetiracetam
(le-ve-teer-**a**-se-tam)

Keppra

**CLASSIFICATION(S):**
**Therapeutic:** anticonvulsants

**Pregnancy Category C**

---

### INDICATIONS

■ Partial onset seizures in adults (adjunct).

### ACTION

■ Appears to inhibit burst firing without affecting normal neuronal excitability and may selectively prevent hypersynchronization of epileptiform burst firing and propagation of seizure activity **Therapeutic Effects:** ■ Decreased incidence and severity of seizures.

### PHARMACOKINETICS

**Absorption:** Rapidly and completely absorbed following oral administration.

**Distribution:** Unknown.

**Metabolism and Excretion:** 66% excreted unchanged by the kidneys; some metabolism by the liver (metabolites inactive).

**Half-life:** 7.1 hr (increased in renal impairment).

### CONTRAINDICATIONS AND PRECAUTIONS

**Contraindicated in:** ■ Hypersensitivity
**Use Cautiously in:** ■ Geriatric patients (renal elimination decreased; dosage reduction may be necessary) ■ Renal impairment (dosage reduction recommended if CCr ≤ 80 ml/minr.

### ADVERSE REACTIONS AND SIDE EFFECTS*

■ **CNS:** dizziness, fatigue/somnolence, <u>weakness</u>, behavioral abnormalities ■ **Neuro:** coordination difficulties.

### INTERACTIONS

**Drug-Drug:** ■ None noted.

### ROUTE AND DOSAGE

◻ **Hepatic Impairment**
■ **PO (Adults):** 500 mg twice daily initially; may be increased by 1000 mg/day at 2 wk intervals up to 3000 mg/day.
◻ **Renal Impairment**
■ **PO (Adults):** *CCr 50–80 ml/min*—500–1000 mg q 12 hr initially; *CCr 30–50 ml/min*—250–750 mg q 12 hr initially; *CCr <30 ml/min*—250–500 mg q 12 hr initially.

### AVAILABILITY

■ **Tablets:** 250 mg$^{Rx}$, 500 mg$^{Rx}$, 750 mg$^{Rx}$. ■ **Oral solution (grape-flavored):** 100 mg/ml in 16–oz bottles$^{Rx}$.

TIME/ACTION PROFILE (blood levels)

| | ONSET | PEAK | DURATION |
|---|---|---|---|
| PO | rapid | 1–1.5 hr† | 12 hr |

†1 hr in the fasting state, 1.5 hr when taken with food.

## NURSING IMPLICATIONS

### ASSESSMENT

◻ Do not confuse Keppra with Kaletra, an antiretroviral.
◻ Assess location, duration, and characteristics of seizure activity.
◻ Assess patient for CNS adverse effects throughout therapy. These adverse effects are categotized as somnolence and fatigue

(asthenia), coordination difficulties (ataxia, abnormal gait, or incoordination), and behavioral abnormalities (agitation, hostility, anxiety, apathy, emotional lability, depersonalization, depression) and usually occur during the first 4 wk of therapy.

■ *Lab Test Considerations:* May cause ↓ RBC and WBC and abnormal liver function tests.

### POTENTIAL NURSING DIAGNOSES

■ Injury, risk for (Side Effects).

### IMPLEMENTATION

■ **PO:** May be administered without regard to meals.
❏ Discontinue gradually to minimize the risk of increase in seizure frequency.

### PATIENT/FAMILY TEACHING

❏ Instruct patient to take medication as directed. Take missed doses as soon as possible unless almost time for next dose. Do not double doses. Do not discontinue abruptly; may cause increase in frequency of seizures.
❏ May cause dizziness and somnolence. Caution patient to avoid driving or activities requiring alertness until response to medication is known. Do not resume driving until physician gives clearance based on control of seizure disorder.
❏ Advise patient to notify health care professional if pregnancy is planned or suspected.
❏ Instruct patient to notify health care professional of medication regimen prior to treatment or surgery.
❏ Advise patient to carry identification describing disease process and medication regimen at all times.

### EVALUATION

**Effectiveness of therapy can be demonstrated by:** ■ Decrease in the frequency of or cessation of seizures.

---

## levobupivacaine, See EPIDURAL LOCAL ANESTHETICS.

---

## levodopa
(**lee**-voe-doe-pa)
Dopar, Larodopa, L -dopa

---

## carbidopa/levodopa
(**kar**-bi-doe-pa/**lee**-voe-doe-pa)
Sinemet, Sinemet CR

### CLASSIFICATION(S):
*Therapeutic: antiparkinson agents*
*Pharmacologic: dopamine agonists*

**Pregnancy Category, UK (levodopa), C (carbidopa/levodopa)**

### INDICATIONS

■ Parkinson's disease ■ Not useful for drug-induced extrapyramidal reactions.

### ACTION

■ Levodopa is converted to dopamine in the CNS, where it serves as a neurotransmitter ■ Carbidopa, a decarboxylase inhibitor, prevents peripheral destruction of levodopa. **Therapeutic Effects:** ■ Relief of tremor and rigidity in Parkinson's syndrome.

### PHARMACOKINETICS

**Absorption:** Well absorbed following oral administration.

**Distribution:** Widely distributed. *Levodopa*—enters the CNS in small concentrations. *Carbidopa*—does not cross the blood-brain barrier but does cross the placenta. Both enter breast milk.

**Metabolism and Excretion:** *Levodopa*—mostly metabolized by the GI tract and liver. *Carbidopa*—30% excreted unchanged by the kidneys.

**Half-life:** *Levodopa*—1 hr; *carbidopa*—1–2 hr.

### CONTRAINDICATIONS AND PRECAUTIONS

**Contraindicated in:** ■ Hypersensitivity ■ Narrow-angle glaucoma ■ MAO inhibitor therapy ■ Malignant melanoma ■ Undiagnosed skin lesions ■ Lactation ■ Some products contain tartrazine and should be avoided in patients with known hypersensitivity.

**Use Cautiously in:** ■ History of cardiac, psychiatric, or ulcer disease ■ Pregnancy or children <18 yr (safety not established).

## ADVERSE REACTIONS AND SIDE EFFECTS*

■ **CNS:** involuntary movements, anxiety, dizziness, hallucinations, memory loss, psychiatric problems ■ **EENT:** blurred vision, mydriasis ■ **GI:** nausea, vomiting, anorexia, dry mouth, hepatotoxicity ■ **Derm:** melanoma ■ **Hemat:** hemolytic anemia, leukopenia ■ **Misc:** darkening of urine or sweat.

## INTERACTIONS

**Drug-Drug:** ■ Use with **MAO inhibitors** may result in hypertensive reactions ■ ↑ risk of arrhythmias with **inhalation hydrocarbon anesthetics** (especially **halothane**; if possible discontinue 6–8 hr before anesthesia) ■ **Phenothiazines, haloperidol, papaverine, phenytoin,** and **reserpine** may ↓ effect of levodopa ■ Large doses of **pyridoxine** may ↓ beneficial effects of levodopa ■ Concurrent use with **methyldopa** may alter the effectiveness of levodopa and ↑ risk of CNS side effects ■ ↑ hypotension may result with concurrent **antihypertensives** ■ **Anticholinergics** may ↓ absorption of levodopa ■ ↑ risk of adverse reactions with **selegilene** or **cocaine.**

**Drug-Natural Products:** ■ **Kava** may ↓ levodopa effectiveness.

**Drug-Food:** ■ Ingestion of foods containing large amounts of **pyridoxine** may ↓ effect of levodopa.

## ROUTE AND DOSAGE

❑ **Levodopa**

■ **PO (Adults):** 250 mg 2–4 times daily; may increase by 100–750 mg q 3–7 days until desired effect is achieved (not to exceed 8 g/day).

❑ **Carbidopa/Levodopa**

Tablets contain 10/100, 25/100, 25/250 mg.

■ **PO (Adults):** *Patients not currently receiving levodopa*—10 mg carbidopa/100 mg levodopa 3–4 times daily or 25 mg carbidopa/100 mg levodopa 3 times daily; may be increased every 1–2 days until desired effect is achieved. *Conversion from levodopa alone (<1.5 g/day)*—25 mg carbidopa/100 mg levodopa 3–4 times daily; may be increased every 1–2 days until desired effect is achieved. *Conversion from levodopa alone*

*(>1.5 g/day)*—25 mg carbidopa/250 mg levodopa 3–4 times daily; may be increased every 1–2 days until desired effect is achieved.

❑ **Carbidopa/Levodopa Extended-Release**

Extended-release (ER) tablets contain 25/100 or 50/200 of carbidopa and levodopa, respectively.

■ **PO (Adults):** *Patients not currently receiving levodopa*—50 mg carbidopa/200 mg levodopa twice daily (minimum of 6 hr apart) initially. *Conversion from levodopa alone*—initiate therapy at 25% of the daily dose of levodopa; for moderate disease start with 50 mg carbidopa/200 mg levodopa twice daily. *Conversion from standard carbidopa/levodopa*—initiate therapy with at least 10% more levodopa content/day (may need up to 30% more) given at 4–8 hr intervals while awake. Allow 3 days between dosage changes; some patients may require larger doses and shorter dosing intervals.

## AVAILABILITY

❑ **Levodopa**

■ *Tablets:* 100 mg^{Rx}, 250 mg^{Rx}, 500 mg^{Rx} ■ *Capsules:* 100 mg^{Rx}, 250 mg^{Rx}, 500 mg^{Rx}.

❑ **Carbidopa/Levodopa**

■ *Tablets:* 10 mg carbidopa/100 mg levodopa^{Rx}, 25 mg carbidopa/100 mg levodopa^{Rx}, 25 mg carbidopa/250 mg levodopa^{Rx} ■ Cost: 10 mg/100 mg $82.69/100, 25 mg/100 mg $93.36/100, 25 mg/250 mg $118.79/100 ■ *Extended-release tablets:* 25 mg carbidopa/100 mg levodopa^{Rx}, 50 mg carbidopa/200 mg levodopa^{Rx} ■ entacapone (StalevoRx. See Appendix B).

TIME/ACTION PROFILE (antiparkinson effects)

| | ONSET | PEAK | DURATION |
|---|---|---|---|
| Carbidopa | unknown | unknown | 5–24 hr |
| Levodopa | 10–15 min | unknown | 5–24 hr or more |
| Carbidopa/levodopa sustained release | unknown | 2 hr | 12 hr |

## NURSING IMPLICATIONS

### ASSESSMENT

❑ Assess parkinsonian symptoms (akinesia, rigidity, tremors, pill rolling, shuffling gait, mask-like face, twisting motions, and drooling) during therapy. "On-off phenomenon" may cause symptoms to appear or improve suddenly.

❑ Assess blood pressure and pulse frequently during period of dose adjustment.

■ *Lab Test Considerations:* May cause false-positive test results in Coombs' test, serum and urine uric acid, serum gonadotropin, urine norepinephrine, and urine protein concentrations.

❑ Dipstick for urine ketones may reveal false-positive results.

❑ Monitor hepatic and renal function and CBC periodically in patients on long-term therapy. May cause ↑ BUN, AST, ALT, bilirubin, alkaline phosphatase, LDH, and serum protein-bound iodine concentrations.

■ *Toxicity and Overdose:* Assess for signs of toxicity (involuntary muscle twitching, facial grimacing, spasmodic eye winking, exaggerated protrusion of tongue, behavioral changes). Consult physician or other health care professional if symptoms occur.

### POTENTIAL NURSING DIAGNOSES

■ Mobility, impaired physical (Indications).

■ Injury, risk for (Indications).

### IMPLEMENTATION

■ **General:** Do not confuse levodopa with methyldopa.

❑ In the carbidopa/levodopa combination, the number following the drug name represents the milligrams of each respective drug.

❑ Wait 8 hr after last levodopa dose before switching patient to carbidopa/levodopa. Carbidopa reduces the need for levodopa by 75%. Administering carbidopa shortly after a full dose of levodopa may result in toxicity.

❑ In preoperative patients or patients who are NPO, confer with physician or other health care professional about continuing medication administration.

■ **PO:** Administer food shortly after medication to minimize gastric irritation; taking food before or concurrently may retard levodopa's effects but may be necessary to minimize GI irritation. If patient has difficulty swallowing, confer with pharmacist.

❑ Controlled-release tablets may be administered as whole or half tablets, but they should not be crushed or chewed.

### PATIENT/FAMILY TEACHING

❑ Instruct patient to take this drug as directed. Take missed doses as soon as remembered, unless next scheduled dose is within 2 hr; do not double doses.

❑ Explain that gastric irritation may be decreased by eating food shortly after taking medications but that high-protein meals may impair levodopa's effects. Dividing the daily protein intake among all the meals may help ensure adequate protein intake and drug effectiveness. Do not drastically alter diet during levodopa therapy without consulting health care professional.

❑ May cause drowsiness or dizziness. Advise patient to avoid driving and other activities that require alertness until response to drug is known.

❑ Caution patient to change positions slowly to minimize orthostatic hypotension. Health care professional should be notified if orthostatic hypotension occurs.

❑ Instruct patient that frequent rinsing of mouth, good oral hygiene, and sugarless gum or candy may decrease dry mouth.

❑ Caution patient to monitor skin lesions for any changes. Health care professional should be notified promptly because carbidopa/levodopa may activate malignant melanoma.

❑ Advise patient to confer with health care professional before taking OTC medications, especially cold remedies. Patients receiving only levodopa should avoid multivitamins. Large amounts of vitamin B (pyridoxine) may interfere with the action of levodopa.

❑ Inform patient that harmless darkening of urine or sweat may occur.

❑ Advise patient to notify health care professional if palpitations, urinary retention, involuntary movements, behavioral changes, severe nausea and vomiting, or new skin lesions occur. Dosage reduction may be required.

### EVALUATION

**Effectiveness of therapy can be demonstrated by:** ■ Resolution of parkinsonian signs and symptoms. Therapeutic effects usually become evident after 2–3 wk of therapy but may require up to 6 mo. Patients who take this medication for several years may experience a decrease in the effectiveness of this drug. Effectiveness may sometimes be restored after a "drug holiday."

## levofloxacin, See FLUOROQUINOLONES.

## levonorgestrel, See CONTRACEPTIVES, HORMONAL.

## levothyroxine, See THYROID PREPARATIONS.

**High Alert**

# LIDOCAINE

**lidocaine (parenteral)**

**(lye**-doe-kane)

LidoPen, Xylocaine, {Xylocard}

**lidocaine (local anesthetic)**
Dilocaine, Lidoject, Nervocaine, Octocaine, Xylocaine

**lidocaine (mucosal)**
Anestacon, Xylocaine Viscous

**lidocaine patch**
Lidoderm

**lidocaine (topical)**
DermaFlex, ELA-Max, Solarcaine Aloe Extra Burn Relief, Xylocaine, Zilactin-L

*CLASSIFICATION(S):*
*Therapeutic: anesthetics—topical/ local, antiarrhythmics (class IB)*

**Pregnancy Category B**

## INDICATIONS

■ **IV:** Ventricular arrhythmias ■ **IM:** Self-injected or when IV unavailable (during transport to hospital facilities) ■ **Local:** Infiltration/mucosal/ topical anesthetic ■ **Patch:** Pain due to postherpetic neuralgia.

## ACTION

■ **IV, IM:** Suppresses automaticity and spontaneous depolarization of the ventricles during diastole by altering the flux of sodium ions across cell membranes with little or no effect on heart rate ■ **Local:** Produces local anesthesia by inhibiting transport of ions across neuronal membranes, thereby preventing initiation and conduction of normal nerve impulses. **Therapeutic Effects:** ■ Control of ventricular arrhythmias ■ Local anesthesia.

## PHARMACOKINETICS

**Absorption:** Well absorbed after administration into the deltoid muscle; some absorption follows local use.

**Distribution:** Widely distributed. Concentrates in adipose tissue. Crosses the blood-brain barrier and placenta.

**Metabolism and Excretion:** Mostly metabolized by the liver.

**Half-life:** Biphasic—initial phase, 7–30 min; terminal phase, 90–120 min.

## CONTRAINDICATIONS AND PRECAUTIONS

Applies mainly to systemic use.

**Contraindicated in:** ■ Hypersensitivity; crosssensitivity may occur ■ Advanced AV block.

**Use Cautiously in:** ■ Liver disease, CHF, patients weighing <50 kg, and geriatric patients (reduce bolus and/or maintenance dose) ■ Respiratory depression, shock, or heart block ■ Pregnancy or lactation (safety not established).

## ADVERSE REACTIONS AND SIDE EFFECTS*

Applies mainly to systemic use. ■ **CNS:** SEIZURES, confusion, drowsiness, dizziness, nervousness, tremor ■ **EENT:** *mucosal use*—decreased or absent gag reflex ■ **CV:** CARDIAC ARREST, arrhythmias, bradycardia, hypotension ■ **GI:** nausea, vomiting ■ **Local:** stinging, burning, contact dermatitis, erythema ■ **Misc:** allergic reactions, including ANAPHYLAXIS.

## INTERACTIONS

Applies mainly to systemic use.

**Drug-Drug:** ■ ↑ cardiac depression and toxicity with **phenytoin**, amiodarone, **quinidine**, **procainamide**, or **propranolol** ■ **Cimetidine** and **beta blockers** may ↓ metabolism and ↑ risk of toxicity.

## ROUTE AND DOSAGE

❑ **Antiarrhythmic**

■ **IV (Adults):** 50–100 mg (1 mg/kg) bolus (may be repeated in 5 min), then 1–4 mg/min (20–50 mcg/kg/min) infusion (up to 4.5 mg/kg or 300 mg in 1 hr).

■ **IV (Children):** 1 mg/kg bolus; may be repeated after 5 min (not to exceed 3 mg/kg), followed by 30 mcg/kg/min infusion (range 20–50 mcg/kg/min).

■ **IM (Adults and Children ≥50 kg):** 300 mg (4.5 mg/kg); may be repeated in 60–90 min.

❑ **Local**

■ **Infiltration: (Adults and Children):** Infiltrate affected area as needed (increased amount and frequency of use increases likelihood of systemic absorption and adverse reactions).

■ **Topical (Adults):** Apply as needed (not to exceed 35 g/day as cream).

■ **Mucosal: (Adults):** *For anesthetizing oral surfaces*—20 mg as 2 sprays/quadrant (not to exceed 30 mg/quadrant) may be used. 15 ml of the viscous solution may be used q 3 hr for oral or pharyngeal pain. *For anesthetizing the female urethra*—3–5 ml of the jelly or 20 mg as 2% solution may be used. *For anesthetizing the male urethra*—5–10 ml of the jelly or 5–15 ml of 2% solution may be used before catheterization or 30 ml of jelly before cystoscopy or similar procedures. Topical solutions may be used to anesthetize mucous membranes of the larynx, trachea, or esophagus.

■ **Patch: (Adults):** Up to 3 patches may be applied once for up to 12 hr in any 24 hr period; consider smaller areas of application in geriatric or debilitated patients.

## AVAILABILITY (generic available)

■ *Autoinjector for IM injection:* 300 mg/3 ml[Rx] ■ *Direct IV injection:* 10 mg/ml (1%)[Rx], 20 mg/ml (2%)[Rx] ■ *For IV admixture:* 40 mg/ml (4%)[Rx], 100 mg/ml (10%)[Rx], 200 mg/ml (20%)[Rx] ■ *Premixed solution for IV infusion:* 2 mg/ml (0.2%)[Rx], 4 mg/ml (0.4%)[Rx], 8 mg/ml (0.8%)[Rx] ■ *Injection for local infiltration/nerve block:* 0.5%[Rx], 1%[Rx], 1.5%[Rx], 2%[Rx], 4%[Rx], 5%[Rx] ■ epinephrine for local infiltration[Rx]

■ *Cream:* 4% [OTC] ■ *Gel:* 0.5%[OTC], 2.5%[OTC] ■ *Jelly:* 2%[Rx] ■ *Liquid:* 5%[Rx] ■ *Ointment:* 5%[Rx] ■ *Patch:* 5% patch ■ *Solution:* 4%[Rx] ■ *Spray:* 10%[Rx] ■ *Viscous solution:* 2%[Rx] ■ prilocaine (as EMLA cream); with epinephrine for iontophoretic dermal delivery (Numby Stuff).

TIME/ACTION PROFILE (IV, IM = antiarrhythmic effects; local = anesthetic effects)

| | ONSET | PEAK | DURATION |
|---|---|---|---|
| IV | immediate | immediate | 10–20 min (up to several hours after continuous infusion) |
| IM | 5–15 min | 20–30 min | 60–90 min |
| Local | rapid | unknown | 1–3 hr |

# NURSING IMPLICATIONS

## ASSESSMENT

■ **Antiarrhythmic:** Monitor ECG continuously and blood pressure and respiratory status frequently during administration.

■ **Anesthetic:** Assess degree of numbness of affected part.

■ *Lab Test Considerations:* Serum electrolyte levels should be monitored periodically during prolonged therapy.

❑ IM administration may cause increased CPK levels.

■ *Toxicity and Overdose:* Serum lidocaine levels should be monitored periodically during prolonged or high-dose therapy. Therapeutic serum lidocaine levels range from 1.5 to 5 mcg/ml.

❑ Signs and symptoms of toxicity include confusion, excitation, blurred or double vision, nausea, vomiting, ringing in ears, tremors, twitching, seizures, difficulty breathing, severe dizziness or fainting, and unusually slow heart rate.

❑ If symptoms of overdose occur, stop infusion and monitor patient closely.

## POTENTIAL NURSING DIAGNOSES

- Cardiac output, decreased (Indications).
- Pain, acute (Indications).

## IMPLEMENTATION

- ▢ **High Alert:** Lidocaine is readily absorbed through mucous membranes. Inadvertent overdosage of lidocaine jelly and spray has resulted in patient harm or death from neurologic and/or cardiac toxicity. Do not exceed recommended dosages.
- **Throat Spray:** Ensure that gag reflex is intact before allowing patient to drink or eat.
- **IM:** IM injections are recommended only when ECG monitoring is not available and benefits outweigh risks. Administer IM injections only into deltoid muscle while frequently aspirating to prevent IV injection.
- **IV:** Only 1% and 2% solutions are used for direct IV injection.
- **Direct IV:** Administer undiluted IV loading dose of 1 mg/kg at a rate of 25–50 mg over 1 min. May repeat dose after 5 min. Follow by IV infusion. Do not use lidocaine with preservatives or other medications, such as epinephrine, for IV injection.
- **Continuous Infusion:** To prepare for IV infusion, add 1 g lidocaine to 250, 500, or 1000 ml of D5W. Solution is stable for 24 hr. Other compatible solutions include D5/LR, D5/0.45% NaCl, D5/0.9% NaCl, 0.45% NaCl, 0.9% NaCl, and LR.
- **Rate:** Administer via infusion pump for accurate dose at a rate of 1–4 mg/min.
- **Y-Site Compatibility:** ◆ alteplase ◆ amiodarone ◆ cefazolin ◆ ciprofloxacin ◆ cisatracurium ◆ diltiazem ◆ dobutamine ◆ dopamine ◆ enalaprilat ◆ etomidate ◆ famotidine ◆ gatifloxacin ◆ haloperidol ◆ heparin ◆ inamrinone ◆ labetalol ◆ levofloxacin ◆ linezolid ◆ meperidine ◆ morphine ◆ nitroglycerin ◆ nitroprusside ◆ potassium chloride ◆ propofol ◆ remifentanil ◆ streptokinase ◆ theophylline ◆ tirofiban ◆ vitamin B complex with C ◆ warfarin.
- **Y-Site Incompatibility:** ◆ amphotericin B cholesteryl sulfate ◆ thiopental.
- **Infiltration:** Lidocaine with epinephrine may be used to minimize systemic absorption and prolong local anesthesia.

- **Topical:** Apply *ELA-Max* 30 min. prior to a needlestick.

## PATIENT/FAMILY TEACHING

- **General Info:** May cause drowsiness and dizziness. Advise patient to call for assistance during ambulation and transfer.
- **IM:** Available in LidoPen Auto-Injector for use outside the hospital setting. Advise patient to telephone health care professional immediately if symptoms of a heart attack occur. Do not administer unless instructed by health care professional. To administer, remove safety cap and place back end on thickest part of thigh or deltoid muscle. Press hard until needle prick is felt. Hold in place for 10 sec, then massage area for 10 sec. Do not drive after administration unless absolutely necessary.
- **Topical:** Apply *Lidoderm Patch* to intact skin to cover the most painful area. Patch may be cut to smaller sizes with scissors before removing release liner. Clothing may be worn over patch. If irritation or burning sensation occurs during application, remove patch until irritation subsides. Wash hands after application; avoid contact with eyes. Dispose of used patch to avoid access by children or pets.

## EVALUATION

**Effectiveness of therapy can be demonstrated by:** ■ Decrease in ventricular arrhythmias ■ Local anesthesia.

## lidocaine/prilocaine

(**lye**-doe-kane/**pri**-loe-kane)
EMLA

### CLASSIFICATION(S):

*Therapeutic: anesthetics—topical/local*

### Pregnancy Category B

## INDICATIONS

- Produces local anesthesia prior to minor painful procedures including: ▢ Insertion of cannulae or needles ▢ Arterial/venous/lumbar puncture ❑ Intramuscular injections ❑ Dermal procedures ❑ Laser treatments ❑ Circumcision ■ When applied to genital mucous membranes in preparation for superficial minor surgery or as preparation for infiltration anesthesia.

## ACTION

■ Produces local anesthesia by inhibiting transport of ions across neuronal membranes, thereby preventing initiation and conduction of normal nerve impulses. Combination of two anesthetics is applied as a system consisting of a cream under an occlusive dressing. Active drug is released into the dermal and epidermal skin layers, resulting in accumulation of local anesthetic in the regions of dermal pain receptors and nerve endings. **Therapeutic Effects:** ■ Anesthetic action localized to the area of the application.

## PHARMACOKINETICS

**Absorption:** Small amounts are systemically absorbed during 4-hr placement of EMLA system.

**Distribution:** Small amounts absorbed are widely distributed and cross the placenta and blood-brain barrier.

**Metabolism and Excretion:** *Lidocaine—* mostly metabolized by the liver. *Prilocaine—* metabolized by the liver and kidneys.

**Half-life:** *Lidocaine—*7–30 min first phase, 90–120 min terminal phase: *Prilocaine—*10–50 min.

## CONTRAINDICATIONS AND PRECAUTIONS

**Contraindicated in:** ■ Hypersensitivity to lidocaine, prilocaine, or any other amide-type local anesthetic ■ Hypersensitivity to any other product in the formulation ■ Should not be applied to middle ear ■ Congenital or idiopathic methemoglobinemia ■ Infants <6 mo who are receiving methemoglobin-inducing agents.

**Use Cautiously in:** ■ Repeated use or use on large areas of skin (more likely to result in systemic absorption) ■ Geriatric, acutely ill, or debilitated patients ■ Severe liver disease ■ Any conditions associated with methemoglobinemia (including glucose-6-phosphate dehydrogenase deficiency) ■ Neonates and children <20 kg or 37 weeks gestation (area/duration of treatment should be limited) ■ Lactation.

## ADVERSE REACTIONS AND SIDE EFFECTS*

■ **Local:** blanching, redness, alteration in temperature sensation, edema, itching, rash ■ **Misc:** allergic reactions including ANAPHYLAXIS.

## INTERACTIONS

**Drug-Drug:** ■ Concurrent use with class I antiarrhythmics including **tocainide** and **mexiletine** may result in adverse cardiovascular effects ■ Concurrent use with other **local anesthetics** may result in additive toxicity ■ Concurrent use with **sulfonamides** in children increases the risk of methemoglobinemia (avoid concurrent use in children <12 mo).

## ROUTE AND DOSAGE

■ **Topical (Adults and Children):** *Minor dermal procedures including venipuncture and IV cannulation—*2.5 g ($^1/_2$ of the 5-g tube) applied to 20–25 cm² (2 in. by 2 in.) area of skin, covered with an occlusive dressing or one anesthetic disc applied for at least 1 hr. *Major dermal procedures including split-thickness skin graft harvesting—* 2 g/10 cm² area of skin, covered with an occlusive dressing for at least 2 hr. *Adult male genital skin—*as an adjunct prior to local anesthetic infiltration, apply a thick layer (1 g/10 cm²) to skin surface for 15 min; local infiltration anesthesia should be performed immediately after removal of cream. *Adult female genital mucous membranes—*apply a thick layer (5–log) for 5–10 min.

■ **Topical (Children 7–12 yr and >20 kg):** Dose should not exceed 20 g over more than 200 cm² for more than 4 hr.

■ **Topical (Children 1–6 yr and >10 kg):** Dose should not exceed 10 g over more than 100 cm² for more than 4 hr.

■ **Topical (Children 3 mo–12 mo and >5 kg):** Dose should not exceed 2 g over more than 20 cm² for more than 4 hr.

■ **Topical (Children 0–3 mo or <5 kg):** Dose should not exceed 1 g over more than 10 cm² for more than 1 hr.

## AVAILABILITY

■ *Cream:* 2.5% lidocaine with 2.5% prilocaine in 5- and 30-g tubes^Rx ■ *Anesthetic disc:* 2.5% lidocaine with 2.5% prilocaine in a topical adhesive system (1 g/10 cm²)^Rx.

TIME/ACTION PROFILE (local anesthesia)

| | ONSET | PEAK | DURATION† |
|---|---|---|---|
| Top | 15 min | 3 hr | 1–2 hr |

†Following removal of occlusive dressing.

## NURSING IMPLICATIONS

### ASSESSMENT

- Assess application site for open wounds. Apply only to intact skin.
- Assess application site for anesthesia following removal of system and prior to procedure.

### POTENTIAL NURSING DIAGNOSES

- Pain, acute (Indications).

### IMPLEMENTATION

- **Topical:** When used for minor dermal procedures (venipuncture, IV cannulation, arterial puncture, lumbar puncture), apply the 2.5-g tube of cream ($\frac{1}{2}$ of the 5-g tube) to each 2 in. by 2 in. area of skin in a *thick* layer at the site of the impending procedure. Remove the center cutout piece from an occlusive dressing (supplied with the 5-g tube) and peel the paper liner from the paper-framed dressing. Cover the lidocaine/prilocaine cream so that there is a *thick* layer of cream underneath the occlusive dressing. Do not spread out or rub in the cream. Smooth the dressing edges carefully and ensure it is secure to avoid leakage. Remove the paper frame and mark the time of application on the occlusive dressing. Lidocaine/prilocaine cream must be applied *at least 1 hr* before the start of a minor dermal procedure (venipuncture, IV cannulation). Anesthesia may be more profound with 90 min–2 hr application. Remove the occlusive dressing and wipe off the lidocaine/prilocaine cream. Clean the entire area with antiseptic solution and prepare the patient for the procedure.
- For major dermal procedures (skin graft harvesting), follow the same procedure using larger amounts of lidocaine/prilocaine cream and the appropriate-size occlusive dressing. Lidocaine/prilocaine cream must be applied *at least 2 hr* before major dermal procedures.

- The anesthetic disc is applied by taking hold of the aluminum flap at the corner and bending it backward. Then take hold of the corner of the beige-colored anesthetic disc layer and pull the two layers apart. Do not touch the white round disc containing the lidocaine/prilocaine cream. Place on area to be anesthesized and press firmly around the edges to ensure good adhesion to the skin; do not press the center of the disc. Mark the time of application with a ballpoint pen on the border of the disc. Apply *at least 1 hr* prior to painful procedure. Remove the disc and wipe off the lidocaine/prilocaine cream. Clean the entire area with antiseptic solution and prepare the patient for the procedure.

### PATIENT/FAMILY TEACHING

- Explain the purpose of cream and occlusive dressing to patient and parents. Inform the patient that lidocaine/prilocaine cream may block all sensations in the treated skin. Caution patient to avoid trauma to the area from scratching, rubbing, or exposure to extreme heat or cold temperatures until all sensation has returned.
- **Home Care Issues:** Instruct patient or parent in proper application. Provide a diagram of location for application.

### EVALUATION

**Clinical response to therapy can be evaluated by:** ■ Anesthesia in the area of application.

## lindane
(**lin**-dane)
gamma benzene hexachloride, {GBH}, G-Well, {Hexit}, {PMS Lindane}, Scabene

### CLASSIFICATION(S):
**Therapeutic:** *pediculocides, scabicides*

**Pregnancy Category B**

## INDICATIONS

■ Second-line treatment of parasitic arthropod infestation (scabies and head, body, and crab lice) for use only in patients who are intolerant to or do not respond to less toxic agents.

## ACTION

■ Causes seizures and death in parasitic arthropods. **Therapeutic Effects:** ■ Cure of infestation by parasitic arthropods.

## PHARMACOKINETICS

**Absorption:** Significant systemic absorption (9–13%) occurs slowly with topical application.

**Distribution:** Stored in fat.

**Metabolism and Excretion:** Metabolized by the liver.

**Half-life:** 18 hr (infants and children).

## CONTRAINDICATIONS AND PRECAUTIONS

**Contraindicated in:** ■ Hypersensitivity ■ Areas of skin rash, abrasion, or inflammation (absorption is increased) ■ History of seizures ■ Lactation ■ Children ≤2 yr (increased risk of CNS toxicity).

**Use Cautiously in:** ■ Pregnancy (do not exceed recommended dose; do not use >2 courses of therapy) ■ Children ≤10 yr, geriatric patients, patients <50 kg, patients with skin conditions (increased risk of systemic absorption and CNS side effects).

## ADVERSE REACTIONS AND SIDE EFFECTS*

All adverse reactions except dermatologic are signs of systemic absorption and toxicity. ■ **CNS:** CNS TOXICITY ■ **CV:** tachycardia ■ **GI:** nausea, vomiting ■ **Derm:** contact dermatitis (repeated application), local irritation.

## INTERACTIONS

**Drug-Drug:** ■ Concurrent use of **medications that lower seizure threshold** (may ↑ risk of seizures) ■ Simultaneous topical use of **skin, scalp,** or **hair** products may increase systemic absorption.

## ROUTE AND DOSAGE

❏ **Scabies**

■ **Topical (Adults and Children):** 1% cream or lotion applied to all skin surfaces from neck to toes; may require a 2nd treatment 1 wk later.

■ **Topical (Children 2–10 yr):** 1% lotion applied to all skin surfaces from neck to toes; may require a 2nd treatment 1 wk later.

❏ **Head Lice or Crab Lice**

■ **Topical (Adults):** 15–30 ml (up to 60 ml) of shampoo; may require a 2nd treatment 1 wk later.

■ **Topical (Children 2–10 yr):** 15–30 ml of shampoo; may require a 2nd treatment 1 wk later.

## AVAILABILITY (generic available)

■ **Lotion:** 1%ᴿˣ ■ Cost: *generic*—$3.90/60 ml ■ **Shampoo:** 1%ᴿˣ ■ Cost: *generic*—$4.12/60 ml.

TIME/ACTION PROFILE (antiparasitic action)

| | ONSET | PEAK | DURATION |
|---|---|---|---|
| Top | rapid | rapid | 190 min |

# NURSING IMPLICATIONS

## ASSESSMENT

❏ Assess skin and hair for signs of infestation before and after treatment.

❏ Examine family members and close contacts for infestation. When used in treatment of pediculosis pubis or scabies, sexual partners should receive concurrent prophylactic therapy.

## POTENTIAL NURSING DIAGNOSES

■ Skin integrity, risk for impaired (Indications).

## IMPLEMENTATION

■ **General:** Due to serious side effects, no more than 2 oz may be dispensed at a time and no refills are allowed.

■ **Topical:** When applying medication to another person, wear gloves to prevent systemic absorption.

❏ Do not apply to open wounds (scratches, cuts, sores on skin or scalp) to minimize systemic absorption. Avoid contact with the eyes. If eye contact occurs, flush thoroughly with water and notify physician or other health care professional.

❏ Institute appropriate isolation techniques.

■ **Lotion:** Instruct patient to bathe with soap and water. Dry skin well and allow to cool before application. Apply lotion in amount sufficient to cover entire body surface with a thin film from neck down (60 ml for an adult). Leave medication on for 8–12 hr, then remove by washing. If rash, burning, or itching develops, wash off medication and notify physician or other health care professional.

■ **Shampoo:** Use a sufficient amount of shampoo to wet hair and scalp (30 ml for short hair, 45 ml for medium hair, 60 ml for long hair). Rub thoroughly into hair and scalp and leave in place for 4 min. Then use enough water to work up a good lather; follow with thorough rinsing and drying. If applied in shower or bath, do not let shampoo run down on other parts of body or into water in which patient is sitting. When hair is dry, use fine-toothed comb to remove remaining nits or nit shells. Shampoo may also be used on combs and brushes to prevent spread of infestation.

### PATIENT/FAMILY TEACHING

■ **General Info:** Instruct patient on application technique and provide with a medication guide. Patient should repeat therapy only at the recommendation of health care professional. Discuss hygienic measures to prevent and to control infestation. Discuss potential for infectious contacts with patient. Explain why household members should be examined and sexual partners treated simultaneously.

❑ Instruct patient to wash all recently worn clothing and used bed linens and towels in very hot water or to dry clean to prevent reinfestation or spreading.

❑ Instruct patient not to apply other oils or creams during therapy; these increase the absorption of lindane and may lead to toxicity.

❑ Explain to patient that itching may persist after treatment; consult health care professional about use of topical hydrocortisone or systemic antihistamines.

❑ Advise patient that eyelashes can be treated by applying petroleum jelly 3 times/day for 1 wk.

■ **Shampoo:** Advise patient that shampoo should not be used as a regular shampoo in the absence of infestation. Emphasize need to avoid contact with eyes.

■ **Children:** Advise parents to monitor young children closely for evidence of CNS toxicity (seizures, dizziness, clumsiness, fast heartbeat, muscle cramps, nervousness, restlessness, irritability, nausea, vomiting) during and immediately after treatment.

### EVALUATION

**Effectiveness of therapy can be demonstrated by:** ■ Resolution of signs of infestation with scabies or lice.

## linezolid

(li-**nez**-o-lid)

Zyvox

*CLASSIFICATION(S):*
*Therapeutic: anti-infectives*
*Pharmacologic: oxazolidinones*

**Pregnancy Category C**

### INDICATIONS

■ Treatment of: ❑ Infections caused by vancomycin-resistant *Enterococcus faecium* ❑ Nosocomial pneumonia caused by *Staphylococcus aureus* (methicillin-susceptible and -resistant strains) ❑ Complicated skin/skin structure infections caused by *Staphylococcus aureus* (methicillin-susceptible and -resistant strains), *Streptococcus pyogenes* or *Streptococcus agalactiae* (including diabetic foot infections) ❑ Uncomplicated skin/skin structure infections caused by *Staphylococcus aureus* (methicillin-susceptible and -resistant strains), *Streptococcus pyogenes* ❑ Community-acquired pneumonia caused by *Streptococcus pneumoniae* (penicillin-susceptible strains only) or *Staphylococcus aureus* (methicillin-susceptible strains only).

### ACTION

■ Inhibits bacterial protein synthesis at the level of the 23S ribosome of the 50S subunit. **Therapeutic Effects:** ■ Bactericidal action against streptococci; bacteriostatic action against enterococci and staphylococci.

## PHARMACOKINETICS

**Absorption:** Rapidly and extensively (100%) absorbed following oral administration.

**Distribution:** Readily distributes to well-perfused tissues.

**Metabolism and Excretion:** 65% metabolized, mostly by the liver; 30% excreted unchanged by the kidneys.

**Half-life:** 6.4 hr.

## CONTRAINDICATIONS AND PRECAUTIONS

**Contraindicated in:** ■ Hypersensitivity ■ Phenylketonuria (suspension contains aspartame).

**Use Cautiously in:** ■ Thrombocytopenia, concurrent use of antiplatelet agents or bleeding diathesis (platelet counts should be monitored more frequently) ■ Pregnancy or lactation or children (safety not established).

## ADVERSE REACTIONS AND SIDE EFFECTS*

■ **CV:** headache, insomnia ■ **GI:** PSEUDOMEMBRANOUS COLITIS, diarrhea, increased liver function tests, nausea, taste alteration, vomiting ■ **Hemat:** thrombocytopenia ■ **Neuro:** optic neuropathy, peripheral neuropathy.

## INTERACTIONS

**Drug-Drug:** ■ Linezolid has monoamine oxidase inhibitory properties; response to **indirect-acting sympathomimetics, vasopressors,** or **dopaminergic agents** may be ↑. Initial doses of **adrenergics** such as **dopamine** or **epinephrine** should be ↓ and carefully titrated.

**Drug-Food:** ■ Because of monoamine oxidase inhibitory properties, consumption of large amounts of foods or beverages containing tyramine should be avoided ( ↑ risk of pressor response. See Appendix Q).

## ROUTE AND DOSAGE

❑ **Vancomycin-resistant *Enterococcus faecium* infections.**

■ **PO, IV (Adults):** 600 mg every 12 hr for 14–28 days.

■ **PO, IV (Children birth-11 yr):** (in the first week of life, pre-term neonates may initially receive 10 mg/kg every 12 hr).

❑ **Pneumonia, complicated skin/skin structure infections**

■ **PO, IV (Adults):** 600 mg every 12 hr for 10–14 days.

■ **PO, IV (Children birth-11 yr):** 10 mg/kg every 8 hr for 10–14 days (in the first week of life, pre-term neonates may initially receive 10 mg/kg every 12 hr).

❑ **Uncomplicated skin/skin structure infections**

■ **PO (Adults):** 400 mg q 12 hr for 10–14 days.

■ **PO, IV (Children 5-11 yr):** 10 mg/kg every 12 hr for 10–14 days.

■ **PO, IV (Children <5 yr):** 10 mg/kg every 8 hr for 10–14 days (in the first week of life, pre-term neonates may initially receive 10 mg/kg every 12 hr).

## AVAILABILITY

■ *Oral suspension: (orange):* 100 mg/5 ml[Rx] ■ *Tablets:* 400 mg[Rx], 600 mg[Rx] ■ *Solution for injection:* 200 mg/100 ml bag[Rx], 400 mg/200 ml bag[Rx], 600 mg/300 ml bag[Rx].

TIME/ACTION PROFILE

|    | ONSET | PEAK | DURATION |
|----|-------|------|----------|
| PO | rapid | 1–2 hr | 12 hr |
| IV | rapid | end of infusion | 12 hr |

# NURSING IMPLICATIONS

## ASSESSMENT

■ **General Info:** Assess patient for infection (vital signs; appearance of wound, sputum, urine, and stool; WBC) at beginning of and throughout therapy.

❑ Obtain specimens for culture and sensitivity prior to initiating therapy. First dose may be given before receiving.

■ **Pseudomembranous Colitis:** Assess bowel status (bowel sounds, frequency and consistency of stools, presence of blood in stools) throughout therapy.

■ *Lab Test Considerations:* May cause thrombocytopenia. Monitor platelet count in patients who are at risk for increased bleeding, who have pre-existing thrombocytopenia, who receive concurrent medications that may decrease platelet count, or who may require >2 weeks of therapy.

❑ May cause ↑ AST, ALT, LDH, alkaline phosphatase and BUN.

## POTENTIAL NURSING DIAGNOSES

■ Infection, risk for (Indications).

## IMPLEMENTATION

■ **General:** Dosage adjustment is not necessary when switching from IV to oral dose.

■ **PO:** May be administered with or without food.

❑ Before using gently invert 3–5 times to mix; do not shake. Store at room temperature.

■ **Intermittent Infusion:** Injection is administered in single- and ready-to-use infusion bags. Do not administer infusion containing particulate matter.

■ *Rate:* Administer over 30–120 minutes. Do not use bag in series connections. Flush line before and after infusion.

■ **Y-Site Compatibility:** ◆ acyclovir ◆ alfentanil ◆ amikacin ◆ aminophylline ◆ ampicillin ◆ ampicillin/sulbactam ◆ aztreonam ◆ bretylium ◆ buprenorphine ◆ butorphanol ◆ calcium gluconate ◆ carboplatin ◆ cefazolin ◆ cefoperazone ◆ cefotetan ◆ cefoxitin ◆ ceftazidime ◆ ceftizoxime ◆ ceftriaxone ◆ cefuroxime ◆ cimetidine ◆ ciprofloxacin ◆ cisatracurium ◆ cisplatin ◆ clindamycin ◆ cyclophosphamide ◆ cyclosporine ◆ cytarabine ◆ D5/0.45% NaCl ◆ D5/0.9% NaCl ◆ D5W ◆ digoxin ◆ diphenhydramine ◆ dobutamine ◆ dopamine ◆ doxorubicin ◆ doxycycline ◆ droperidol ◆ enalaprilat ◆ esmolol ◆ etoposide phosphate ◆ famotidine ◆ fentanyl ◆ fluconazole ◆ fluorouracil ◆ furosemide ◆ ganciclovir ◆ gemcitabine ◆ granisetron ◆ haloperidol ◆ heparin ◆ hydrocortisone ◆ hydromorphone ◆ ifosfamide ◆ imipenem/cilastatin ◆ labetalol ◆ lactated Ringer's injection. ◆ leucovorin ◆ levofloxacin ◆ lidocaine ◆ lorazepam ◆ magnesium sulfate ◆ mannitol ◆ meperidine ◆ meropenem ◆ mesna ◆ methotrexate ◆ methylprednisolone ◆ metoclopramide ◆ metronidazole ◆ midazolam ◆ minocycline ◆ mitoxantrone ◆ morphine ◆ nalbuphine ◆ naloxone ◆ nitroglycerin ◆ ofloxacin ◆ ondansetron ◆ paclitaxel ◆ pentobarbital ◆ phenobarbital ◆ piperacillin ◆ piperacillin/tazobactam ◆ potassium chloride ◆ prochlorperazine ◆ promethazine ◆ propranolol ◆ ranitidine ◆ remifentanil ◆ Ringer's injection ◆ sodium bicarbonate ◆ 0.9% NaCl ◆ sufentanil ◆ theophylline ◆ ticarcillin ◆ tobramycin ◆ trimethoprim/sulfamethoxazole ◆ vancomycin ◆ vecuronium ◆ verapamil ◆ vincristine ◆ zidovudine.

■ **Y-Site Incompatibility:** ◆ amphotericin B ◆ chlorpromazine ◆ diazepam ◆ erythromycin lactobionate ◆ pentamidine ◆ phenytoin.

## PATIENT/FAMILY TEACHING

❑ Advise patients taking oral linezolid to take as directed. Take missed doses as soon as remembered unless almost time for next dose; do not double dose.

❑ Instruct patient to avoid large quantities of foods or beverages containing tyramine (See Appendix Q). May cause hypertensive response.

❑ Instruct patient to notify health care professional if patient has a history of hypertension and before patient takes other medications or herbal products, especially cold remedies, decongestants, or antidepressants.

❑ Advise patient to notify health care professional if no improvement is seen in a few days.

## EVALUATION

**Clinical response to therapy can be evaluated by:** ■ Resolution of signs and symptoms of infection. Length of time for complete resolution depends on organism and site of infection.

# liothyronine, See THYROID PREPARATIONS.

# liotrix, See THYROID PREPARATIONS.

# lisinopril, See ANGIOTENSIN-CONVERTING ENZYME (ACE) INHIBITORS.

# lithium
(lith-ee-um)

{Carbolith}, {Duralith}, Eskalith, Eskalith-CR, {Lithizine}, Lithobid, Lithonate, Lithotabs

**CLASSIFICATION(S):**
*Therapeutic:* antimanics

**Pregnancy Category D**

## INDICATIONS

■ Bipolar affective disorders (treatment of acute manic episodes and prophylaxis against recurrence).

## ACTION

■ Alters cation transport in nerve and muscle ■ May also influence reuptake of neurotransmitters. **Therapeutic Effects:** ■ Prevents/decreases incidence of acute manic episodes.

## PHARMACOKINETICS

**Absorption:** Completely absorbed after oral administration.
**Distribution:** Widely distributed into many tissues and fluids; CSF levels are 50% of plasma levels. Crosses the placenta; enters breast milk.
**Metabolism and Excretion:** Excreted almost entirely unchanged by the kidneys.
**Half-life:** 20–27 hr.

## CONTRAINDICATIONS AND PRECAUTIONS

**Contraindicated in:** ■ Hypersensitivity ■ Severe cardiovascular or renal disease ■ Dehydrated or debilitated patients ■ Should be used only where therapy, including blood levels, may be closely monitored ■ Some products contain alcohol or tartrazine and should be avoided in patients with known hypersensitivity or intolerance ■ Pregnancy or lactation.
**Use Cautiously in:** ■ Geriatric patients (initial dosage reduction recommended) ■ Any degree of cardiac, renal, or thyroid disease ■ Diabetes mellitus ■ Children (safety not established).

## ADVERSE REACTIONS AND SIDE EFFECTS*

■ **CNS:** SEIZURES, fatigue, headache, impaired memory, ataxia, confusion, dizziness, drowsiness, psychomotor retardation, restlessness, stupor ■ **EENT:** aphasia, blurred vision, dysarthria, tinnitus ■ **CV:** ARRHYTHMIAS, ECG changes, edema, hypotension ■ **GI:** abdominal pain, anorexia, bloating, diarrhea, nausea, dry mouth,

metallic taste ■ **GU:** polyuria, glycosuria, nephrogenic diabetes insipidus, renal toxicity ■ **Derm:** acneiform eruption, folliculitis, alopecia, diminished sensation, pruritus ■ **Endo:** hypothyroidism, goiter, hyperglycemia, hyperthyroidism ■ **F and E:** hyponatremia ■ **Hemat:** leukocytosis ■ **Metab:** weight gain ■ **MS:** muscle weakness, hyperirritability, rigidity ■ **Neuro:** tremors.

## INTERACTIONS

**Drug-Drug:** ■ May prolong the action of **neuromuscular blocking agents** ■ ↑ risk of neurologic toxicity with **haloperidol** or **molindone** ■ **Diuretics, methyldopa, probenecid, fluoxetine,** and **NSAIDs** may ↑ risk of toxicity ■ Blood levels may be ↑ by **ACE inhibitors** ■ Lithium may ↓ effects of **chlorpromazine** ■ **Chlorpromazine** may mask early signs of lithium toxicity ■ Hypothyroid effects may be additive with **potassium iodide** or **antithyroid agents** ■ **Aminophylline, phenothiazines,** and **drugs containing large amounts of sodium** ↑ renal elimination and ↓ effectiveness ■ **Psyllium** can ↓ **lithium** levels.

**Drug-Natural Products:** ■ Caffeine-containing herbs (**cola nut, guarana, mate, tea, coffee**) may ↓ **lithium** serum levels and efficacy.

**Drug-Food:** ■ Large changes in **sodium** intake may alter the renal elimination of lithium. ↑ sodium intake will ↑ renal excretion.

## ROUTE AND DOSAGE

Precise dosing is based on serum lithium levels. 300 mg lithium carbonate contains 8–12 mEq lithium.

■ **PO (Adults and children ≥12 yr):** *Tablets/capsules*—300–600 mg 3 times daily initially; usual maintenance dose is 300 mg 3–4 times daily. *Slow-release capsules*—200–300 mg 3 times daily initially; increased up to 1800 mg/day in divided doses. Usual maintenance dose is 300–400 mg 3 times daily. *Extended-release tablets*—450–900 mg twice daily *or* 300–600 mg 3 times daily initially; usual maintenance dose is 450 mg twice daily *or* 300 mg 3 times daily.

■ **PO (Children <12 yr):** 15–20 mg (0.4–0.5 mEq)/kg/day in 2–3 divided doses; dosage may be adjusted weekly.

## AVAILABILITY (generic available)

- **Capsules:** 150 mg[Rx], 300 mg[Rx], 600 mg[Rx] ∎
Cost: *Eskalith*—300 mg $20.35/100;
*generic*—$9.38/90 ∎ **Tablets:** 300 mg[Rx] ∎ *Extended-release tablets:* 300 mg[Rx], 450 mg[Rx]
- **Slow-release capsules:** 150 mg[Rx], 300 mg[Rx] ∎ **Syrup:** 300 mg (8 mEq lithium)/5 ml[Rx].

TIME/ACTION PROFILE (antimanic effects)

| | ONSET | PEAK | DURATION |
|---|---|---|---|
| PO, PO–ER | 5–7 days | 10–21 days | days |

# NURSING IMPLICATIONS

## ASSESSMENT

- ❑ Assess mood, ideation, and behaviors frequently. Initiate suicide precautions if indicated.
- ❑ Monitor intake and output ratios. Report significant changes in totals. Unless contraindicated, fluid intake of at least 2000–3000 ml/day should be maintained. Weight should also be monitored at least every 3 mo.
- ∎ **Lab Test Considerations:** Evaluate renal and thyroid function, WBC with differential, serum electrolytes, and glucose periodically during therapy.
- ∎ **Toxicity and Overdose:** Monitor serum lithium levels twice weekly during initiation of therapy and every 2–3 mo during chronic therapy. Draw blood samples in the morning immediately before next dose. Therapeutic levels range from 0.5 to 1.5 mEq/L.
- ❑ Assess patient for signs and symptoms of lithium toxicity (vomiting, diarrhea, slurred speech, decreased coordination, drowsiness, muscle weakness, or twitching). If these occur, report before administering next dose.

## POTENTIAL NURSING DIAGNOSES

- ∎ Thought processes, disturbed (Indications).
- ∎ Violence, for self-directed (Indications).
- ∎ Violence, risk for other-directed (Indications).
- ∎ Noncompliance (Patient/Family Teaching).

## IMPLEMENTATION

- ∎ **General:** Do not confuse Lithobid (lithium) with Levbid (hyoscyamine).
- ∎ **PO:** Administer with food or milk to minimize GI irritation. Extended-release preparations should be swallowed whole; do not break, crush, or chew.

## PATIENT/FAMILY TEACHING

- ❑ Instruct patient to take medication as directed, even if feeling well. Take missed doses as soon as remembered unless within 2 hr of next dose (6 hr if extended release).
- ❑ Lithium may cause dizziness or drowsiness. Caution patient to avoid driving or other activities requiring alertness until response to medication is known.
- ❑ Low sodium levels may predispose patient to toxicity. Advise patient to drink 2000–3000 ml fluid each day and eat a diet with consistent and moderate sodium intake. Excessive amounts of coffee, tea, and cola should be avoided because of diuretic effect. Avoid activities that cause excess sodium loss (heavy exertion, exercise in hot weather, saunas). Notify health care professional of fever, vomiting, and diarrhea, which also cause sodium loss.
- ❑ Advise patient that weight gain may occur. Review principles of a low-calorie diet.
- ❑ Instruct patient to consult health care professional before taking OTC medications or herbal products concurrently with this therapy.
- ❑ Advise patient to use contraception and to consult health care professional if pregnancy is suspected.
- ❑ Review side effects and symptoms of toxicity with patient. Instruct patient to stop medication and report signs of toxicity to health care professional promptly.
- ❑ Explain to patients with cardiovascular disease or over 40 yr of age the need for ECG evaluation before and periodically during therapy. Patient should inform health care professional if fainting, irregular pulse, or difficulty breathing occurs.
- ❑ Emphasize the importance of periodic lab tests to monitor for lithium toxicity.

## EVALUATION

**Effectiveness of therapy can be demonstrated by:** ■ Resolution of the symptoms of mania (hyperactivity, pressured speech, poor judgment, need for little sleep) ■ Decreased incidence of mood swings in bipolar disorders ■ Improved affect in unipolar disorders. Improvement in condition may require 1–3 wk.

## lomefloxacin, See FLUOROQUINOLONES.

# loperamide

(loe-**per**-a-mide)

Diar-aid Caplets, Imodium, Imodium A-D, Kaopectate II Caplets, Maalox Antidiarrheal Caplets, Neo-Diaral, Pepto Diarrhea Control

*CLASSIFICATION(S):*
*Therapeutic: antidiarrheals*

**Pregnancy Category B**

## INDICATIONS

■ Adjunctive therapy of acute diarrhea ■ Chronic diarrhea associated with inflammatory bowel disease ■ Decreases the volume of ileostomy drainage.

## ACTION

■ Inhibits peristalsis and prolongs transit time by a direct effect on nerves in the intestinal muscle wall ■ Reduces fecal volume, increases fecal viscosity and bulk while diminishing loss of fluid and electrolytes. **Therapeutic Effects:** ■ Relief of diarrhea.

## PHARMACOKINETICS

**Absorption:** Not well absorbed following oral administration.

**Distribution:** Unknown. Does not cross the blood-brain barrier.

**Protein Binding:** 97%.

**Metabolism and Excretion:** Metabolized partially by the liver, undergoes enterohepatic recirculation; 30% eliminated in the feces. Minimal excretion in the urine.

**Half-life:** 10.8 hr.

## CONTRAINDICATIONS AND PRECAUTIONS

**Contraindicated in:** ■ Hypersensitivity ■ Patients in whom constipation must be avoided ■ Abdominal pain of unknown cause, especially if associated with fever ■ Alcohol intolerance (liquid only).

**Use Cautiously in:** ■ Hepatic dysfunction ■ Geriatric patients ■ Pregnancy, lactation, or children <2 yr (safety not established).

## ADVERSE REACTIONS AND SIDE EFFECTS*

■ **CNS:** drowsiness, dizziness ■ **GI:** constipation, abdominal pain/distention/discomfort, dry mouth, nausea, vomiting ■ **Misc:** allergic reactions.

## INTERACTIONS

**Drug-Drug:** ■ Additive CNS depression with other **CNS depressants,** including **alcohol, antihistamines, opioid analgesics,** and **sedative/hypnotics** ■ Additive anticholinergic properties with other **drugs having anticholinergic properties,** including **antidepressants** and **antihistamines.**

**Drug-Natural Products:** ■ **Kava, valerian, skullcap, chamomile,** or **hops** can increase CNS depression.

## ROUTE AND DOSAGE

■ **PO (Adults):** 4 mg initially, then 2 mg after each loose stool. Maintenance dose usually 4–8 mg/day in divided doses (not to exceed 8 mg/day for OTC use or 16 mg/day for Rx use).

■ **PO (Children 9–11 yr or 30–47 kg):** 2 mg initially; then 1 mg after each loose stool (not to exceed 6 mg/24 hr; OTC use should not exceed 2 days).

■ **PO (Children 6–8 yr or 24–30 kg):** 1 mg initially, then 1 mg after each loose stool (not to exceed 4 mg/24 hr; OTC use should not exceed 2 days).

## AVAILABILITY (generic available)

■ *Tablets:* 2 mg^OTC ■ Cost: $3.56/12 ■ *Capsules:* 2 mg^Rx ■ *Liquid:* 1 mg/5 ml^OTC ■ Cost: $5.60/120 ml ■ simethicone (Immodium Advanced^OTC, see Appendix B).

TIME/ACTION PROFILE (relief of diarrhea)

| | ONSET | PEAK | DURATION |
|---|---|---|---|
| PO | 1 hr | 2.5–5 hr | 10 hr |

## NURSING IMPLICATIONS

### ASSESSMENT

❑ Assess frequency and consistency of stools and bowel sounds prior to and throughout therapy.
❑ Assess fluid and electrolyte balance and skin turgor for dehydration.

### POTENTIAL NURSING DIAGNOSES

▪ Diarrhea (Indications).
▪ Injury, risk for (Side Effects).

### IMPLEMENTATION

▪ **PO:** Administer with clear fluids to help prevent dehydration, which may accompany diarrhea.

### PATIENT/FAMILY TEACHING

❑ Instruct patient to take medication exactly as directed. Do not take missed doses, and do not double doses. In acute diarrhea, medication may be ordered after each unformed stool. Advise patient not to exceed the maximum number of doses.
❑ May cause drowsiness. Advise patient to avoid driving or other activities requiring alertness until response to drug is known.
❑ Advise patient that frequent mouth rinses, good oral hygiene, and sugarless gum or candy may relieve dry mouth.
❑ Caution patient to avoid using alcohol and other CNS depressants concurrently with this medication.
❑ Instruct patient to notify health care professional if diarrhea persists or if fever, abdominal pain, or distention occurs.

### EVALUATION

**Effectiveness of therapy can be demonstrated by:** ▪ Decrease in diarrhea ❑ In acute diarrhea, treatment should be discontinued if no improvement is seen in 48 hr ❑ In chronic diarrhea, if no improvement has occurred after

at least 10 days of treatment with maximum dose, loperamide is unlikely to be effective.

# lopinavir/ritonavir
(loe-**pin**-a-veer/ri-**toe**-na-veer)
Kaletra

## CLASSIFICATION(S):
***Therapeutic:*** *antiretrovirals*
***Pharmacologic:*** *protease inhibitors, metabolic inhibitors*

### Pregnancy Category C

### INDICATIONS

▪ HIV infection (with other antiretrovirals).

### ACTION

▪ **Lopinavir:** Inhibits HIV viral protease ▪ **Ritonavir:** Although ritonavir has antiretroviral activity of its own (inhibits the action of HIV protease and prevents the cleavage of viral polyproteins), it is combined with lopinavir to inhibit the metabolism of lopinavir thus increasing its plasma levels. **Therapeutic Effects:** ▪ Increased CD4 cell counts and decreased viral load with subsequent slowed progression of HIV infection and its sequelae.

### PHARMACOKINETICS

**Absorption:** Well absorbed following oral administration; food enhances absorption.

**Distribution:** *Ritonavir*—poor CNS penetration.

**Protein Binding:** *Lopinavir*—98–99% bound to plasma proteins.

**Metabolism and Excretion:** *Lopinavir*—completey metabolized in the liver by cytochrome P450 3A (CY P450 P3A); ritonavir is a potent inhibitor of this enzyme. *Ritonavir*—highly metabolized by the liver (by CY P450 P3A and CY P2D6 enzymes); one metabolite has antiretroviral activity; 3.5% excreted unchanged in urine.

**Half-life:** *Lopinavir*—5–6 hr *Ritonavir*—3–5 hr.

## CONTRAINDICATIONS AND PRECAUTIONS

**Contraindicated in:** ■ Hypersensitivity ■ Concurrent use of dihydroergotamine, ergotamine, ergonovine, flecainide, methylergonovine, midazolam, pimozide, propafenone, amiodaroneand triazolam, which are highly dependent on CY P3A or CY P2D6 for metabolism and for which increased blood levels may result in serious and/or life-threatening events ■ Concurrent use with simastatin, lovastatin, St. John's wort (hypericum perforatum) is not recommended ■ Hypersensitivity or intolerance to alcohol or castor oil (present in capsules and liquid).

**Use Cautiously in:** ■ Known alcohol intolerance (oral solution contains alcohol) ■ Concurrent use with atorvastatin (may increase risk of rhabdomyolysis) ■ Concurrent use of antiarrhythmics including lidocaine and quinidine (therapeutic blood level monitoring recommended) ■ Concurrent use of anticonvulsants including carbamazepine, phenobarbital or phenytoin (may decrease effectiveness of lopinavir) ■ Concurrent use of dihydropyridine calcium channel blockers including felodipine, nifedipine and nicardipine (clinical monitoring recommended due to increased levels of calcium channel blocker) ■ Impaired hepatic function, history of hepatitis (for ritonavir content) ■ Pregnancy or lactation (safety not established; breastfeeding not recommended in HIV-infected patients)

**Exercise Extreme Caution in:** ■ Concurrent use with sildenafil should be undertaken with extreme caution and may result in hypotension, syncope, visual changes and prolonged erection.

## ADVERSE REACTIONS AND SIDE EFFECTS*

■ **CNS:** headache, insomnia, weakness ■ **GI:** diarrhea( ↑ in children), abdominal pain, nausea, pancreatitis, taste aversion (in children), vomiting( ↑ in children) ■ **Derm:** rash.

## INTERACTIONS

**Drug-Drug:** ■ Concurrent use of **flecainide, amiodarone, propafenone, dihydroergotamine, ergonovine, ergotamine, methylergonovine, pimozide, midazolam,** and **triazolam,** is contraindicated because of the risk of potentially serious, life-threatening drug interactions ■ Concurrent use with **sildenafil** should be undertaken with extreme caution and

may result in hypotension, syncope, visual changes and prolonged erection (dosage reduction of sildenafil to 25 mg every 48 hr with monitoring recommended) ■ Concurrent use with **rifampin** ↓ effectiveness of antiretroviral therapy and should not be undertaken ■ Should not be used concurrently with **simvastatin** or **lovastatin** due to ↑ risk of rhabdomyolysis; similar risk exists for **atorvastatin;** use lowest possible dose with careful monitoring ■ Concurrent use with **efavirenz** or **nevirapine** ↓ lopinavir/ritonavir levels and effectiveness; dosage increase may be necessary ■ **Delavirdine** ↑ lopinavir levels ■ ↑ levels of **lidocaine** and **quinidine** (blood level monitoring recommended) ■ Concurrent use of anticonvulsants including **carbamazepine, phenobarbital,** or **phenytoin** may ↓ effectiveness of lopinavir ■ ↑ levels ofdihydropyridine calcium channel blockers including **felodipine, nifedipine,** and **nicardipine** (clinical monitoring recommended) ■ May alter levels and effectiveness of **warfarin** ■ ↑ levels of **clarithromycin** (dosage reduction recommended for patients with CCr ≤60 ml/min ■ ↑ blood levels of **itraconazole** and **ketoconazole** (high antifungaldoses not recommended) ■ ↑ levels of **rifabutin** (dosage reduction recommended) ■ ↓ blood levels of **atovaquone** (may require dosage increase) ■ **Dexamethasone** ↓ blood levels and may ↓ effectiveness of lopinavir ■ Oral solution contains alcohol may produce intolerance when administered with **disulfiram** or **metronidazole** ■ May ↑ levels and risk of toxicity with immunosuppressant including **cyclosporine** or **tacrolimus** (blood level monitoring recommended) ■ May ↓ levels and effects of **methadone** (dosage of **methadone** may need to be ↑ ) ■ May ↓ levels and contraceptive efficacy of some estrogen-based **hormonal contraceptives** including **ethinyl estradiol** (alternative or additional methods of contraception recommended).

**Drug-Natural Products:** ■ Concurrent use with **St. John's wort** may ↓ levels and beneficial effect of lopinavir/ritonavir.

## ROUTE AND DOSAGE

■ **PO (Adults and Children >40 kg):** 400/100 mg (3 capsules or 5 ml oral solution) twice daily.

■ **PO (Children 15–40 kg):** 10 mg/kg lopinavir content twice daily.

- **PO (Children 7–15 kg):** 12 mg/kg lopinavir content twice daily.
- **With concurrent efavirenz or nevirapine**
- **PO (Adults and Children >40 kg):** 533/133 mg (4 capsules or 6.5 ml oral solution) twice daily.
- **PO (Children 15–50 kg):** 11 mg/kg lopinavir content twice daily.
- **PO (Children 7–15 kg):** 13 mg/kg lopinavir content twice daily.

## AVAILABILITY

- ***Capsules:*** 133.3 mg lopinavir/33 mg ritonavir ▪ Cost: 133.3 mg/33.3 mg, $703.50/180 ▪ ***Oral solution (cotton candy or vanilla):*** 80 mg lopinavir/20 mg ritonavir per ml (contains 42.4% alcohol) in 60-ml bottles ▪ Cost: 80 mg/20 mg per ml $351.75/160 ml.

TIME/ACTION PROFILE (blood levels)

| | ONSET | PEAK | DURATION |
|---|---|---|---|
| Lopinavir PO | rapid | 4 hr | 12 hr |
| Ritonavir PO | rapid | 4 hr* | 12 hr |

*Non-fasting.

# NURSING IMPLICATIONS

## ASSESSMENT

- ❏ Do not confuse Kaletra with Keppra, an antiseizure medication.
- ❏ Assess patient for change in severity of HIV symptoms and for symptoms of opportunistic infections during therapy.
- ❏ Assess patient for signs of pancreatitis (nausea, vomiting, abdominal pain, increased serum lipase or amylase) periodically during therapy. May require discontinuation of therapy.
- ▪ ***Lab Test Considerations:*** Monitor viral load and CD4 counts regularly during therapy.
- ❏ Monitor triglyceride and cholesterol levels prior to initiating therapy and periodically during therapy.
- ❏ May cause hyperglycemia.
- ❏ May cause ↑ serum AST, ALT, GGT, and total bilirubin concentrations.

## POTENTIAL NURSING DIAGNOSES

- ▪ Infection, risk for (Indications).
- ▪ Noncompliance (Patient/Family Teaching).

## IMPLEMENTATION

- ▪ **General:** Do not confuse with Retrovir (zidovudine) or ritonavir (Norvir).
- ❏ Patients taking concurrent didanosine should take didanosine 1 hr before or 2 hr after taking lopinavir/ritonavir.
- ▪ **PO:** Administer with food to enhance absorption.
- ❏ Oral solution is light yellow to orange.
- ❏ Capsules and oral solution are stable if refrigerated until expiration date on label or 2 months at room temperature.

## PATIENT/FAMILY TEACHING

- ❏ Emphasize the importance of taking lopinavir/ritonavir as directed, at evenly spaced times throughout day. Do not take more than prescribed amount, and do not stop taking this or other antiretrovirals without consulting health care professional. Take missed doses as soon as remembered; do not double doses.
- ❏ Instruct patient that lopinavir/ritonavir should not be shared with others.
- ❏ Advise patient to avoid taking other medications, RX, OTC, or herbal products, especially St. John's wort, without consulting health care professional.
- ❏ Inform patient that lopinavir/ritonavir does not cure AIDS or prevent associated or opportunistic infections. Lopinavir/ritonavir does not reduce the risk of transmission of HIV to others through sexual contact or blood contamination. Caution patient to use a condom during sexual contact and to avoid sharing needles or donating blood to prevent spreading the AIDS virus to others. Advise patient that the long-term effects of lopinavir/ritonavir are unknown at this time.
- ❏ Inform patient that lopinavir/ritonavir may cause hyperglycemia. Advise patient to notify health care professional if increased thirst or hunger; unexplained weight loss; or increased urination occurs.

□ Advise patients taking oral contraceptives to use a nonhormonal method of birth control during lopinavir/ritonavir therapy.

□ Caution patients taking sildenafil of increased risk of sildenafil-associated side effects (hypotension, visual changes, sustained erection). Notify health care professional promptly if these occur.

□ Inform patient that redistribution and accumulation of body fat may occur causing central obesity, dorsocervical fat enlargement (buffalo hump), peripheral wasting, breast enlargement, and cushingoid appearance. The cause and long-term effects are not known.

□ Instruct patient to notify health care professional if pregnancy is planned or suspected of if breastfeeding an infant.

□ Emphasize the importance of regular follow-up exams and blood counts to determine progress and monitor for side effects.

### EVALUATION

**Effectiveness of therapy can be demonstrated by:** ■ Delayed progression of AIDS and decreased opportunistic infections in patients with HIV ■ Decrease in viral load and improvement in CD4 cell counts.

## loracarbef, See CEPHALOSPORINS—SECOND GENERATION.

## loratadine
(lor-**a**-ta-deen)
Alavert, Claritin, Claritin Reditabs

*CLASSIFICATION(S):*
*Therapeutic: antihistamines*

**Pregnancy Category B**

### INDICATIONS

■ Relief of symptoms of seasonal allergies ■ Management of chronic idiopathic urticaria ■ Management of hives.

### ACTION

■ Blocks peripheral effects of histamine released during allergic reactions. **Therapeutic Effects:** ■ Decreased symptoms of allergic reactions (nasal stuffiness; red, swollen eyes, itching).

### PHARMACOKINETICS

**Absorption:** Rapidly absorbed after oral administration (80%).
**Distribution:** Unknown.
**Protein Binding:** *Loratadine*—97%; *descarboethoxyloratadine*—73–77%.
**Metabolism and Excretion:** Rapidly and extensively metabolized during first pass through the liver. Much is converted to descarboethoxyloratadine, an active metabolite.
**Half-life:** *Loratadine*—7.8–11 hr; *descarboethoxyloratadine*—20 hr.

### CONTRAINDICATIONS AND PRECAUTIONS

**Contraindicated in:** ■ Hypersensitivity ■ Lactation.
**Use Cautiously in:** ■ Patients with hepatic impairment or CCr <30 ml/min ( ↓ dose to 10 mg every other day) ■ Patients receiving drugs known to affect hepatic metabolism of drugs ■ Geriatric patients ( ↑ risk of adverse reactions) ■ Pregnancy or children <2 yr (safety not established).

### ADVERSE REACTIONS AND SIDE EFFECTS*

■ **CNS:** confusion, drowsiness (rare), paradoxical excitation ■ **EENT:** blurred vision ■ **GI:** dry mouth, GI upset ■ **Derm:** photosensitivity, rash ■ **Metab:** weight gain.

### INTERACTIONS

**Drug-Drug:** ■ The following interactions may occur, but are less likely to occur with loratidine that with more sedating antihistamines ■ **MAO inhibitors** may intensify and prolong effects of antihistamines ■ ↑ CNS depression may occur with other **CNS depressants,** including **alcohol, antidepressants, opioid analgesics,** and **sedative/hypnotics.**
**Drug-Natural Products:** ■ **Kava, valerian, skullcap, chamomile,** or **hops** can ↑ CNS depression.

### ROUTE AND DOSAGE

■ **PO (Adults and Children ≥6 yr):** 10 mg once daily.
■ **PO (Children ≥2–5 yr):** 5 mg once daily.
□ **Renal Impairment**

- **PO (Adults):** *CCr <30 ml/min*—10 mg every other day.
- ❏ **Hepatic Impairment**
- **PO (Adults):** 10 mg every other day

## AVAILABILITY

■ *Rapidly disintegrating tablets (mint):* 10 mg^OTC ■ *Tablets:* 10 mgOTC, {10 mg^Rx} ■ *Syrup:* 5 mg/5 ml^OTC ■ pseudoephedrine (Claritin-D) OTC. See Appendix B.

TIME/ACTION PROFILE (antihistaminic effects)

| | ONSET | PEAK | DURATION |
|---|---|---|---|
| PO | 1–3 hr | 8–12 hr | >24 hr |

## NURSING IMPLICATIONS

### ASSESSMENT
- ❏ Assess allergy symptoms (rhinitis, conjunctivitis, hives) before and periodically during therapy.
- ❏ Assess lung sounds and character of bronchial secretions. Maintain fluid intake of 1500–2000 ml/day to decrease viscosity of secretions.
- ■ **Lab Test Considerations:** May cause false-negative result on allergy skin testing.

### POTENTIAL NURSING DIAGNOSES
- ■ Airway clearance, ineffective (Indications).
- ■ Injury, risk for (Adverse Reactions).

### IMPLEMENTATION
- ■ **PO:** Administer once daily.
- ❏ For rapidly disintegrating tablets (*Alavert, Claritin Reditabs*)—place on tongue. Tablet disintegrates rapidly. May be taken with or without water.

### PATIENT/FAMILY TEACHING
- ❏ Instruct patient to take medication exactly as directed.
- ❏ May cause dizziness or drowsiness. Caution patient to avoid driving or other activities requiring alertness until response to medication is known.
- ❏ Caution patient to use sunscreen and protective clothing to prevent photosensitivity reactions.
- ❏ Advise patient to avoid taking alcohol or other CNS depressants concurrently with this drug.
- ❏ Advise patient that good oral hygiene, frequent rinsing of mouth with water, and sugarless gum or candy may minimize dry mouth. Patient should notify dentist if dry mouth persists >2 wk.
- ❏ Instruct patient to contact health care professional immediately if dizziness, fainting, or fast or irregular heartbeat occurs or if symptoms persist.

### EVALUATION
**Effectiveness of therapy can be demonstrated by:** ■ Decrease in allergic symptoms ■ Management of hives.

## lorazepam
(lor-**az**-e-pam)
{Apo-Lorazepam}, Ativan, {Novo-Lorazem}, {Nu-Loraz}

### CLASSIFICATION(S):
**Therapeutic:** *anesthetic adjuncts, antianxiety agents, sedative/hypnotics*
**Pharmacologic:** *benzodiazepines*

**Schedule IV**

**Pregnancy Category D**

### INDICATIONS
■ Adjunct in the management of anxiety or insomnia ■ Preoperative sedation ■ Decreases preoperative anxiety and provides amnesia. **Unlabeled uses:** ■ **IV:** Antiemetic prior to chemotherapy ■ Management of status epilepticus.

### ACTION
■ Depresses the CNS, probably by potentiating GABA, an inhibitory neurotransmitter. **Therapeutic Effects:** ■ Sedation ■ Decreased anxiety ■ Decreased seizures.

### PHARMACOKINETICS
**Absorption:** Well absorbed following oral administration. Rapidly and completely absorbed

{ } = Available in Canada only.
*CAPITALS indicates life-threatening; underlines indicate most frequent.

following IM administration. Sublingual absorption is more rapid than oral and is similar to IM.
**Distribution:** Widely distributed. Crosses the blood-brain barrier. Crosses the placenta; enters breast milk.
**Metabolism and Excretion:** Highly metabolized by the liver.
**Half-life:** 10–20 hr.

## CONTRAINDICATIONS AND PRECAUTIONS

**Contraindicated in:** ■ Hypersensitivity ■ Cross-sensitivity with other benzodiazepines may exist ■ Comatose patients or those with pre-existing CNS depression ■ Uncontrolled severe pain ■ Narrow-angle glaucoma ■ Pregnancy and lactation.
**Use Cautiously in:** ■ Severe hepatic/renal/pulmonary impairment ■ Myasthenia gravis ■ History of suicide attempt or drug abuse ■ Geriatric or debilitated patients (dosage reduction recommended) ■ Hypnotic use should be short-term.

## ADVERSE REACTIONS AND SIDE EFFECTS*

■ **CNS:** <u>dizziness</u>, <u>drowsiness</u>, <u>lethargy</u>, hangover, headache, mental depression, paradoxical excitation ■ **EENT:** blurred vision ■ **Resp:** respiratory depression ■ **CV:** *rapid IV use only—* APNEA, CARDIAC ARREST, bradycardia, hypotension ■ **GI:** constipation, diarrhea, nausea, vomiting ■ **Derm:** rashes ■ **Misc:** physical dependence, psychological dependence, tolerance.

## INTERACTIONS

**Drug-Drug:** ■ Additive CNS depression with other **CNS depressants** including **alcohol, antihistamines, antidepressants, opioid analgesics,** and other **sedative/hypnotics** including other benzodiazepines ■ May decrease the efficacy of **levodopa** ■ **Smoking** may increase metabolism and decrease effectiveness ■ **Probenecid** may decrease metabolism of lorazepam, enhancing its actions.
**Drug-Natural Products:** ■ Concomitant use of **kava, valerian, skullcap, chamomile,** or **hops** can increase CNS depression.

## ROUTE AND DOSAGE

■ **PO (Adults):** *Anxiety*—1–3 mg 2–3 times daily (up to 10 mg/day). *Insomnia*—2–4 mg at bedtime.

■ **PO (Geriatric Patients or Debilitated Patients):** *Anxiety*—0.5–2 mg/day in divided doses initially. *Insomnia*—0.25–1 mg initially, increased as needed.
■ **IM (Adults):** *Preoperative sedation*—50 mcg (0.05 mg)/kg 2 hr before surgery (not to exceed 4 mg).
■ **IV (Adults):** *Preoperative sedation*—44 mcg (0.044 mg)/kg (not to exceed 2 mg) 15–20 min before surgery. *Operative amnestic effect*—up to 50 mcg/kg (not to exceed 4 mg). *Antiemetic*—2 mg 30 min prior to chemotherapy; may be repeated q 4 hr as needed (unlabeled). *Anticonvulsant*—50 mcg (0.05 mg)/kg, up to 4 mg; may be repeated after 10–15 min (not to exceed 8 mg/12 hr; unlabeled).

## AVAILABILITY (generic available)

■ *Tablets:* 0.5 mg$^{Rx}$, 1 mg$^{Rx}$, 2 mg$^{Rx}$ ■ Cost: *Ativan*—0.5 mg $80.55/100, 1 mg $104.90/100r, 2 mg $152.91/100; *generic*—0.5 mg $66.94/100, 1 mg $85.23/100, 2 mg $134.2/100 ■ *Concentrated solution:* 2 mg/ml$^{Rx}$ ■ *Injection:* 2 mg/ml$^{Rx}$, 4 mg/ml$^{Rx}$.

TIME/ACTION PROFILE (sedation)

|  | ONSET | PEAK | DURATION |
|---|---|---|---|
| PO | 15–45 min | 1–6 hr | up to 48 hr |
| IM | 15–30 min | 1–2 hr† | up to 48 hr |
| IV | rapid | 15–20 min | up to 48 hr |

†Amnestic response.

# NURSING IMPLICATIONS

## ASSESSMENT

■ **Anxiety:** Assess degree and manifestations of anxiety prior to and periodically throughout therapy.
❑ Prolonged high-dose therapy may lead to psychological or physical dependence. Restrict amount of drug available to patient.
■ **Status Epilepticus:** Assess location, duration, characteristics, and frequency of seizures.
■ *Lab Test Considerations:* Patients on high-dose therapy should receive routine evaluation of renal, hepatic, and hematologic function.

## POTENTIAL NURSING DIAGNOSES

■ Anxiety (Indications).
■ Injury, risk for (Indications, Side Effects).

## IMPLEMENTATION

- **General:** Do not confuse Ativan (lorazepam) with Atarax (hydroxyzine).
- Following parenteral administration, keep patient supine for at least 8 hr and observe closely.
- **PO:** Tablet may also be given sublingually (unlabeled) for more rapid onset.
- **IM:** Administer IM doses deep into muscle mass at least 2 hr before surgery for optimum effect.
- **Direct IV:** Dilute immediately before use with an equal amount of sterile water, D5W, or 0.9% NaCl for injection. Do not use if solution is colored or contains a precipitate.
- **Rate:** Administer direct IV, through Y-site at a rate of 2 mg over 1 min. Rapid IV administration may result in apnea, hypotension, bradycardia, or cardiac arrest.
- **Y-Site Compatibility:** ◆ acyclovir ◆ alatrofloxacin ◆ albumin ◆ allopurinol ◆ amifostine ◆ amikacin ◆ amphotericin B cholesteryl sulfate ◆ atracurium ◆ bumetanide ◆ cefepime ◆ cefmetazole ◆ ciprofloxacin ◆ cisatracurium ◆ cisplatin ◆ cladribine ◆ clonidine ◆ cyclophosphamide ◆ cytarabine ◆ dexamethasone sodium phosphate ◆ diltiazem ◆ dobutamine ◆ docetaxel ◆ dopamine ◆ doxorubicin ◆ doxorubicin liposome ◆ epinephrine ◆ erythromycin lactobionate ◆ etomidate ◆ etoposide ◆ famotidine ◆ fentanyl ◆ filgrastim ◆ fluconazole ◆ fludarabine ◆ fosphenytoin ◆ furosemide ◆ gatifloxacin ◆ gentamicin ◆ granisetron ◆ haloperidol ◆ heparin ◆ hydrocortisone sodium succinate ◆ hydromorphone ◆ labetalol ◆ levofloxacin ◆ linezolid ◆ melphalan ◆ methotrexate ◆ metronidazole ◆ midazolam ◆ milrinone ◆ morphine ◆ nitroglycerin ◆ norepinephrine ◆ paclitaxel ◆ pancuronium ◆ piperacillin ◆ piperacillin/tazobactam ◆ potassium chloride ◆ propofol ◆ ranitidine ◆ remifentanil ◆ tacrolimus ◆ teniposide ◆ thiotepa ◆ trimethoprim/sulfamethoxazole ◆ vancomycin ◆ vecuronium ◆ vinorelbine ◆ zidovudine.
- **Y-Site Incompatibility:** ◆ aldesleukin ◆ aztreonam ◆ floxacillin ◆ idarubicin ◆ imipenem/cilastatin ◆ omeprazole ◆ ondansetron ◆ sargramostim ◆ sufentanil.

## PATIENT/FAMILY TEACHING

- Instruct patient to take medication exactly as directed and not to skip or double up on missed doses. If medication is less effective after a few weeks, check with health care professional; do not increase dose. Abrupt withdrawal may cause tremors, nausea, vomiting, and abdominal and muscle cramps.
- May cause drowsiness or dizziness. Advise patient to avoid driving or other activities requiring alertness until response to medication is known.
- Caution patient to avoid taking alcohol or other CNS depressants concurrently with this medication.
- Instruct patient to contact health care professional immediately if pregnancy is planned or suspected.
- Emphasize the importance of follow-up exams to determine effectiveness of the medication.

## EVALUATION

**Effectiveness of therapy can be demonstrated by:** ■ Increase in sense of well-being ❑ Decrease in subjective feelings of anxiety without excessive sedation ■ Reduction of preoperative anxiety ■ Postoperative amnesia ■ Improvement in sleep patterns. Need for continued therapy should be re-evaluated regularly. Minimum effective dose should be used.

**losartan, See ANGIOTENSIN II RECEPTOR ANTAGONISTS.**

**lovastatin, See HMG-CoA REDUCTASE INHIBITORS.**

# MAGNESIUM AND ALUMINUM SALTS

### magaldrate

(**mag**-al-drate)

{Losopan}, Lowsium, Riopan, {Riopan Extra Strength}

### magnesium hydroxide/aluminum hydroxide

(mag-**nee**-zhum hye-**drox**-ide/ a-**loo**-mi-num hye-**drox**-ide)

Alamag, {Diovol}, {Diovol Ex}, {Gelusil}, {Gelusil Extra Strength}, Maalox, Maalox TC, Mintox, Mylanta Double Strength, {Neutralca-S}, Rulox, Rulox No. 1, Rulox No. 2

## CLASSIFICATION(S):

**Therapeutic:** antiulcer agents
**Pharmacologic:** antacids

**Pregnancy Category UK**

## INDICATIONS

■ Treat peptic ulcer pain and promote healing of duodenal and gastric ulcers ■ Useful in a variety of GI complaints, including: ▫ Hyperacidity ▫ Indigestion ▫ GERD ▫ Heartburn.

## ACTION

■ Neutralize gastric acid following dissolution in gastric contents ■ Inactivate pepsin if pH is raised to ≥4. **Therapeutic Effects:** ■ Neutralization of gastric acid with healing of ulcers and decrease in associated pain.

## PHARMACOKINETICS

**Absorption:** During routine use, antacids are nonabsorbable. With chronic use, 15–30% of magnesium and smaller amounts of aluminum may be absorbed.

**Distribution:** Small amounts absorbed are widely distributed, cross the placenta, and appear in breast milk. Aluminum concentrates in the CNS.

**Metabolism and Excretion:** Excreted by the kidneys.

**Half-life:** Unknown.

## CONTRAINDICATIONS AND PRECAUTIONS

**Contraindicated in:** ■ Severe abdominal pain of unknown cause, especially if accompanied by fever ■ Anuria (magnesium only) ■ Products containing tartrazine or sugar in patients with known intolerance.

**Use Cautiously in:** ■ Antacids containing magnesium in patients with any degree of renal insufficiency.

## ADVERSE REACTIONS AND SIDE EFFECTS*

■ **GI:** *aluminum salts*—constipation; *magnesium salts*—diarrhea ■ **F and E:** *magnesium salts*—hypermagnesemia; *aluminum salts*—hypophosphatemia.

## INTERACTIONS

**Drug-Drug:** ■ Magnesium and aluminum salts change the absorptive characteristics of many **orally administered drugs** ■ Destroy coating of **enteric-coated drugs,** causing premature release into the stomach and resulting in altered absorption or side effects ■ Absorption of **tetracyclines, phenothiazines, ketoconazole, itraconazole** (take antacids 2 hr later), **iron salts, fluoroquinolones,** and **isoniazid** may be decreased ■ If urine pH is increased by large doses, **salicylate** blood levels may be decreased and **quinidine, flecainide,** and **amphetamine** levels may be increased.

## ROUTE AND DOSAGE

Dosages vary, depending on concentration of ingredients in product chosen. Generally 5–30 ml or 1–2 tablets are given 1–3 hr after meals and at bedtime. In the early healing phase of peptic ulcer, more frequent administration may be necessary.

▫ **Peptic Ulcer Disease**

■ **PO (Adults):** *Uncomplicated duodenal/ gastric ulcers*—administer 1 and 3 hr after meals and at bedtime. Additional doses may be used for recurring symptoms; continue for 4–6 wk for duodenal ulcers and until healing is complete for gastric ulcers.

{ } = Available in Canada only.
*CAPITALS indicates life-threatening; underlines indicate most frequent.

### ❑ Esophageal Reflux

- **PO (Adults):** *Acute management*—antacid suspension q 30–60 min. *Maintenance*— administer 1 and 3 hr after meals and at bedtime; additional doses may be used for recurring symptoms.

### ❑ GI Bleeding/Stress Ulceration

- **PO (Adults):** Administer q 1 hr or as needed to maintain pH of nasogastric aspirate >3.5.

### ❑ Prevention of Anesthesia-Induced GI Aspiration

- **PO (Adults):** Antacid suspension given 30 min prior to general anesthesia.

### AVAILABILITY (generic available)

### ❑ Magaldrate

- *Liquid:* 540 mg/5 ml^OTC ■ *Suspension:* 540 mg/5 ml^OTC.

### ❑ Magnesium Hydroxide/Aluminum Hydroxide

- *Chewable Tablets:* 200 mg aluminum hydroxide/200 mg magnesium hydroxide^OTC, 400 mg aluminum hydroxide/400 mg magnesium hydroxide^OTC ■ *Suspension:* 200 mg aluminum hydroxide/225 mg magnesium hydroxide/5 ml^OTC, 300 mg aluminum hydroxide/600 mg magnesium hydroxide/5 ml^OTC ■ simethicone^OTC. See Appendix B.

TIME/ACTION PROFILE (effect on gastric pH)

| | ONSET | PEAK | DURATION |
|---|---|---|---|
| Aluminum PO | slightly delayed | 30 min | 30 min–1 hr (empty stomach); 3 hr (after meals) |
| Magnesium PO | immediate | 30 min | 30 min–1 hr (empty stomach); 3 hr (after meals) |

## NURSING IMPLICATIONS

### ASSESSMENT

- **Antacid:** Assess for heartburn and indigestion as well as location, duration, character, and precipitating factors of gastric pain.
- *Lab Test Considerations:* Monitor serum phosphate, potassium, and calcium levels periodically during chronic use. May cause increased serum calcium and decreased serum phosphate concentrations.
- ❑ May cause increased serum gastrin and systemic and urinary pH.
- ❑ Antagonize effects of pentagastrin and histamine during gastric acid secretion testing. Avoid administration for 24 hr preceding the test.

### POTENTIAL NURSING DIAGNOSES

- Pain, acute (Indications).

### IMPLEMENTATION

- **General:** Magnesium and aluminum are combined as antacids to balance the constipating effects of aluminum with the laxative effects of magnesium.
- **PO:** To prevent tablets from entering small intestine in undissolved form, they must be chewed thoroughly before swallowing. Follow with ½ glass of water.
- ❑ Shake suspensions well before administration.
- ❑ For an antacid effect, administer 1–3 hr after meals and at bedtime.

### PATIENT/FAMILY TEACHING

- ❑ Caution patient to consult health care professional before taking antacids for more than 2 wk if problem is recurring, if relief is not obtained, or if symptoms of gastric bleeding (black, tarry stools; coffee-ground emesis) occur.
- ❑ Advise patient not to take this medication within 2 hr of taking other medications.
- ❑ Some antacids contain large amounts of sodium. Caution patient on sodium-restricted diet to check sodium content when on long-term high-dose therapy.

### EVALUATION

**Effectiveness of therapy can be demonstrated by:** ■ Relief of gastric pain and irritation.

---

**magnesium salicylate, See SALICYLATES.**

# MAGNESIUM SALTS (ORAL)

**magnesium chloride (12% Mg; 9.8 mEq Mg/g)**

(mag-**nee**-zhum **klor**-ide)
Chloromag, Slo-Mag

**magnesium citrate (16.2% Mg; 4.4 mEq Mg/g)**

(mag-**nee**-zhum**si**-trate)
Citrate of Magnesia, Citroma, {Citromag}

**magnesium gluconate (5.4% Mg; 4.4 mEq/g)**

Almoate, Magtrate, Magonate

**magnesium hydroxide (41.7% Mg; 34.3 mEq Mg/g)**

(mag-**nee**-zhum hye-**drox**-ide)
Phillips Magnesia Tablets, Phillips Milk of Magnesia, MOM

**magnesium oxide (60.3% Mg; 49.6 mEq Mg/g)**

(mag-**nee**-zhum **ox**-ide)
Mag-Ox 400, Maox, Uro-Mag

**CLASSIFICATION(S):**

*Therapeutic: mineral and electrolyte replacements/supplements, laxatives*
*Pharmacologic: salines*

**Pregnancy Category UK**

## INDICATIONS

■ Treatment/prevention of hypomagnesemia ■ As a: ❑ Laxative ❑ Bowel evacuant in preparation for surgical/radiographic procedures ■ Milk of Magnesia has also been used as an antacid.

## ACTION

■ Essential for the activity of many enzymes ■ Play an important role in neurotransmission and muscular excitability ■ Are osmotically active in GI tract, drawing water into the lumen and causing peristalsis. **Therapeutic Effects:** ■ Replacement in deficiency states ■ Evacuation of the colon.

## PHARMACOKINETICS

**Absorption:** Up to 30% may be absorbed orally.
**Distribution:** Widely distributed. Cross the placenta and are present in breast milk.
**Metabolism and Excretion:** Excreted primarily by the kidneys.
**Half-life:** Unknown.

## CONTRAINDICATIONS AND PRECAUTIONS

**Contraindicated in:** ■ Hypermagnesemia ■ Hypocalcemia ■ Anuria ■ Heart block ■ Active labor or within 2 hr of delivery (unless used for preterm labor).
**Use Cautiously in:** ■ Any degree of renal insufficiency.

## ADVERSE REACTIONS AND SIDE EFFECTS*

■ **GI:** <u>diarrhea</u> ■ **Derm:** flushing, sweating.

## INTERACTIONS

**Drug-Drug:** ■ Potentiates **neuromuscular blocking agents** ■ May decrease absorption of **fluoroquinolones, nitrofurantoin,** and **tetracyclines** and **penicillamine.**

## ROUTE AND DOSAGE

❑ **Prevention of Deficiency (in mg of Magnesium)**

■ **PO (Adults and Children >10 yr):** *Adolescent and adult men—270–400* mg/day; *adolescent and adult women—280–300* mg/day; *pregnant women—320* mg/day; *breastfeeding women—340–355* mg/day.
■ **PO (Children 7–10 yr):** 170 mg/day.
■ **PO (Children 4–6 yr):** 120 mg/day.
■ **PO (Children birth–3 yr):** 40–80 mg/day.

❑ **Treatment of Deficiency (expressed as mg of Magnesium)**

■ **PO (Adults):** 200–400 mg/day in 3–4 divided doses.
■ **PO (Children 6–11 yr):** 3–6 mg/kg/day in 3–4 divided doses.

❑ **Laxative**

■ **PO (Adults):** *Magnesium citrate*—240 ml; *magnesium hydroxide (Milk of Magnesia)*—30–60 ml single or divided dose or 10–20 ml as concentrate.

■ **PO (Children 6–12 yr):** *Magnesium citrate*—100 ml; *magnesium hydroxide (Milk of Magnesia)*—15–30 ml single or divided dose.

■ **PO (Children 2–5 yr):** *magnesium hydroxide (Milk of Magnesia)*—5–15 ml single or divided dose.

## AVAILABILITY

❑ **Magnesium Chloride**

■ *Sustained-release tablets:* 535 mg (64 mg magnesium)$^{OTC}$ ■ *Enteric-coated tablets:* 833 mg (100 mg magnesium)$^{OTC}$.

❑ **Magnesium Citrate**

■ *Oral solution:* 240-, 296-, and 300-ml bottles (77 mEq magnesium/100 ml)$^{OTC}$.

❑ **Magnesium gluconate**

■ *Tablets:* 500 mg$^{OTC}$ ■ *Liquid:* 54 mg/5 ml$^{OTC}$.

❑ **Magnesium Hydroxide**

■ *Liquid:* 400 mg/5 ml (164 mg magnesium/5 ml)$^{OTC}$ ■ *Concentrated liquid:* 800 mg/5 ml (328 mg magnesium/5 ml)$^{OTC}$ ■ *Chewable tablets:* 300 mg (130 mg magnesium)$^{OTC}$, 600 mg (260 mg magnesium)$^{OTC}$.

❑ **Magnesium Oxide**

■ *Tablets:* 400 mg (241.3 mg magnesium)$^{OTC}$ ■ *Capsules:* 140 mg (84.5 mg magnesium)$^{OTC}$.

TIME/ACTION PROFILE (laxative effect)

| | ONSET | PEAK | DURATION |
|---|---|---|---|
| PO | 3–6 hr | unknown | unknown |

# NURSING IMPLICATIONS

## ASSESSMENT

■ **Laxative:** Assess patient for abdominal distention, presence of bowel sounds, and usual pattern of bowel function.

❑ Assess color, consistency, and amount of stool produced.

■ **Antacid:** Assess for heartburn and indigestion as well as location, duration, character, and precipitating factors of gastric pain.

## POTENTIAL NURSING DIAGNOSES

■ Constipation (Indications).

## IMPLEMENTATION

■ **PO:** To prevent tablets entering small intestine in undissolved form, they must be chewed thoroughly before swallowing. Follow with ½ glass of water.

❑ *Magnesium citrate:* Refrigerate solutions to ensure they retain potency and palatability. May be served over ice. Magnesium citrate in an open container will lose carbonation upon standing; this will not affect potency but may reduce palatability.

❑ *Magnesium hydroxide:* Shake solution well before administration.

■ **Antacid:** Administer 1–3 hr after meals and at bedtime.

❑ Powder and liquid forms are considered more effective than tablets.

■ **Laxative:** Administer on empty stomach for more rapid results. Follow all oral laxative doses with a full glass of liquid to prevent dehydration and for faster effect. Do not administer at bedtime or late in the day.

## PATIENT/FAMILY TEACHING

■ **General Info:** Advise patient not to take this medication within 2 hr of taking other medications, especially fluoroquinolones, nitrofurantoin, and tetracyclines.

■ **Antacids:** Caution patient to consult health care professional before taking antacids for more than 2 wk if problem is recurring, if relief is not obtained, or if symptoms of gastric bleeding (black, tarry stools; coffee-ground emesis) occur.

■ **Laxatives:** Advise patient that laxatives should be used only for short-term therapy. Long-term therapy may cause electrolyte imbalance and dependence.

❑ Encourage patient to use other forms of bowel regulation, such as increasing bulk in the diet, fluid intake, and mobility. Normal bowel habits are individualized; frequency of bowel movement may vary from 3 times/day to 3 times/wk.

❑ Advise patient to notify health care professional if unrelieved constipation, rectal bleeding, or symptoms of electrolyte imbalance (muscle cramps or pain, weakness, dizziness) occur.

## EVALUATION

**Effectiveness of therapy can be demonstrated by:** ■ Relief of gastric pain and irritation ■ Passage of a soft, formed bowel movement, usually within 3–6 hr ■ Prevention and treatment of magnesium deficiency.

**High Alert**

# magnesium sulfate (IV) (9.9% Mg; 8.1 mEq Mg/g)

(mag-**nee**-zhum**sul**-fate)

### CLASSIFICATION(S):

*Therapeutic:* mineral and electrolyte replacements/supplements
*Pharmacologic:* minerals/electrolytes

**Pregnancy Category D**

## INDICATIONS

■ Treatment/prevention of hypomagnesemia ■ Anticonvulsant in severe eclampsia or preeclampsia. **Unlabeled uses:** ■ Preterm labor ■ Treatment of Torsades de pointes.

## ACTION

■ Essential for the activity of many enzymes ■ Plays an important role in neurotransmission and muscular excitability. **Therapeutic Effects:** ■ Replacement in deficiency states ■ Resolution of eclampsia.

## PHARMACOKINETICS

**Absorption:** IV administration results in complete bioavailability; well absorbed from IM sites.
**Distribution:** Widely distributed. Crosses the placenta and is present in breast milk.
**Metabolism and Excretion:** Excreted primarily by the kidneys.
**Half-life:** Unknown.

## CONTRAINDICATIONS AND PRECAUTIONS

**Contraindicated in:** ■ Hypermagnesemia ■ Hypocalcemia ■ Anuria ■ Heart block ■ Active labor or within 2 hr of delivery (unless used for preterm labor).

**Use Cautiously in:** ■ Any degree of renal insufficiency.

## ADVERSE REACTIONS AND SIDE EFFECTS*

■ **CNS:** drowsiness ■ **Resp:** decreased respiratory rate ■ **CV:** arrhythmias, bradycardia, hypotension ■ **GI:** diarrhea ■ **Derm:** flushing, sweating ■ **Metab:** hypothermia.

## INTERACTIONS

**Drug-Drug:** ■ Potentiate **neuromuscular blocking agents**.

## ROUTE AND DOSAGE

❑ **Treatment of Deficiency (expressed as mg of Magnesium)**
■ **IM (Adults):** *Severe deficiency*—250 mg/kg over 4 hr; *mild deficiency*—1 g q 6 hr for 4 doses.
■ **IV (Adults):** *Severe deficiency*—5 g.
❑ **Eclampsia/Pre-eclampsia**
■ **IV, IM (Adults):** 4–5 g by IV infusion, concurrently with up to 5 g IM in each buttock; then 4–5 g IM q 4 hr *or* 4 g by IV infusion followed by 1–2 g/hr continuous infusion (not to exceed 40 g/day or 20 g/48 hr in the presence of severe renal insufficiency).
❑ **Part of Parenteral Nutrition**
■ **IV (Adults):** 4–24 mEq/day.
■ **IV (Children):** 0.25–0.5 mEq/kg/day.

## AVAILABILITY (generic available)

■ *Injection:* 10%[Rx], 12.5%[Rx], 25%[Rx], 50%[Rx].

TIME/ACTION PROFILE (anticonvulsant effect)

|    | ONSET | PEAK | DURATION |
|----|-------|------|----------|
| IM | 60 min | unknown | 3–4 hr |
| IV | immediate | unknown | 30 min |

# NURSING IMPLICATIONS

## ASSESSMENT

■ **Hypomagnesemia/Anticonvulsant:** Monitor pulse, blood pressure, respirations, and ECG frequently throughout administration of parenteral magnesium sulfate. Respirations should be at least 16/min before each dose.

❏ Monitor neurologic status before and throughout therapy. Institute seizure precautions. Patellar reflex (knee jerk) should be tested before each parenteral dose of magnesium sulfate. If response is absent, no additional doses should be administered until positive response is obtained.

❏ Monitor newborn for hypotension, hyporeflexia, and respiratory depression if mother has received magnesium sulfate.

❏ Monitor intake and output ratios. Urine output should be maintained at a level of at least 100 ml/4 hr.

■ *Lab Test Considerations:* Serum magnesium levels and renal function should be monitored periodically throughout administration of parenteral magnesium sulfate.

## POTENTIAL NURSING DIAGNOSES

■ Injury, risk for (Indications, Side Effects).

## IMPLEMENTATION

❏ *High Alert:* Accidental overdosage of IV magnesium has resulted in serious patient harm and death. Have second practitioner independently double check original order, dosage calculations, and infusion pump settings. Do not confuse milligram (mg), gram (g), or milliequivalent (mEq) dosages.

■ **IM:** Administer deep IM into gluteal sites. Administer subsequent injections in alternate sides.

❏ Use 25–50% concentrations for adults, 20% concentrations for children <14 yr.

■ **Direct IV:** Administer 10% solution undiluted.

■ *Rate:* Administer at a rate of 1.5 ml of a 10% solution (or its equivalent) over 1 min.

■ **Continuous Infusion:** When given as an anticonvulsant, dilute 4 g in 250 ml of D5W or 0.9% NaCl.

❏ When given for hypomagnesemia, may dilute 5 g in 1000 ml of D5W, 0.9% NaCl, or Ringer's or LR.

■ *Rate:* When given as an anticonvulsant, administer at a rate not to exceed 3 ml/min.

❏ When given for hypomagnesemia, administer slowly over 3 hr.

❏ Use infusion pump to accurately regulate rate.

■ **Y-Site Compatibility:** ◆ acyclovir ◆ aldesleukin ◆ amifostine ◆ amikacin ◆ ampicillin ◆ aztreonam ◆ cefazolin ◆ cefoperazone ◆ cefo-

taxime ◆ cefoxitin ◆ cephalothin ◆ cephapirin ◆ chloramphenicol ◆ clindamycin ◆ dobutamine ◆ doxycycline ◆ enalaprilat ◆ erythromycin lactobionate ◆ esmolol ◆ famotidine ◆ fludarabine ◆ gatifloxacin ◆ gentamicin ◆ granisetron ◆ heparin ◆ hydrocortisone sodium succinate ◆ hydromorphone ◆ idarubicin ◆ insulin ◆ kanamycin ◆ labetalol ◆ linezolid ◆ meperidine ◆ metronidazole ◆ minocycline ◆ morphine ◆ nafcillin ◆ ondansetron ◆ oxacillin ◆ paclitaxel ◆ penicillin G potassium ◆ piperacillin ◆ piperacillin/tazobactam ◆ potassium chloride ◆ sargramostim ◆ thiotepa ◆ ticarcillin ◆ tobramycin ◆ trimethoprim/sulfamethoxazole ◆ vancomycin ◆ vitamin B complex with C.

■ **Y-Site Incompatibility:** ◆ alatrofloxacin ◆ cefepime.

## PATIENT/FAMILY TEACHING

❏ Explain purpose of medication to patient and family.

## EVALUATION

**Effectiveness of therapy can be demonstrated by:** ■ Normal serum magnesium concentrations ■ Control of seizures associated with toxemias of pregnancy.

---

# mannitol

(**man**-i-tol)
Osmitrol, Resectisol

### CLASSIFICATION(S):
**Therapeutic:** *diuretics*
**Pharmacologic:** *osmotic diuretics*

### Pregnancy Category C

## INDICATIONS

■ **IV:** Adjunct in the treatment of: ❏ Acute oliguric renal failure ❏ Edema ❏ Increased intracranial or intraocular pressure ❏ Toxic overdose ■ **GU irrigant:** During transurethral procedures (2.5–5% solution only).

## ACTION

■ Increases the osmotic pressure of the glomerular filtrate, thereby inhibiting reabsorption of water and electrolytes ■ Causes excretion of: ■ Water ■ Sodium ■ Potassium ■ Chloride ■ Calcium ■ Phosphorus ■ Magnesium ■ Urea ■ Uric acid. **Therapeutic Effects:** ■ Mobilization of excess fluid in oliguric renal failure or edema ■ Reduction of intraocular or intracranial pressure ■ Increased urinary excretion of toxic materials ■ Decreased hemolysis when used as an irrigant after transurethral prostatic resection.

## PHARMACOKINETICS

**Absorption:** IV administration produces complete bioavailability. Some absorption may follow use as a GU irrigant.

**Distribution:** Confined to the extracellular space; does not usually cross the blood-brain barrier or eye.

**Metabolism and Excretion:** Excreted by the kidneys; minimal liver metabolism.

**Half-life:** 100 min.

## CONTRAINDICATIONS AND PRECAUTIONS

**Contraindicated in:** ■ Hypersensitivity ■ Anuria ■ Dehydration ■ Active intracranial bleeding.

**Use Cautiously in:** ■ Pregnancy and lactation (safety not established).

## ADVERSE REACTIONS AND SIDE EFFECTS*

■ **CNS:** confusion, headache ■ **EENT:** blurred vision, rhinitis ■ **CV:** transient volume expansion, chest pain, CHF, pulmonary edema, tachycardia ■ **GI:** nausea, thirst, vomiting ■ **GU:** renal failure, urinary retention ■ **F and E:** dehydration, hyperkalemia, hypernatremia, hypokalemia, hyponatremia ■ **Local:** phlebitis at IV site.

## INTERACTIONS

**Drug-Drug:** ■ Hypokalemia increases the risk of **digoxin** toxicity.

## ROUTE AND DOSAGE

■ **IV (Adults):** *Edema, oliguric renal failure*—50–100 g as a 5–25% solution; may precede with a test dose of 0.2 g/kg over 3–5 min. *Reduction of intracranial/intraocular pressure*—0.25–2 g/kg as 15–25% solution over 30–60 min (500 mg/kg may be sufficient in small or debilitated patients). *Diuresis in drug intoxications*—50–200 g as a 5–25% solution titrated to maintain urine flow of 100–500 ml/hr.

■ **IV (Children):** *Edema, oliguric renal failure*—0.25–2 g/kg (60 g/m²) as a 15–20% solution over 2–6 hr; may precede with a test dose of 0.2 g/kg over 3–5 min. *Reduction of intracranial/intraocular pressure*—1–2 g/kg (30–60 g/m²) as a 15–20% solution over 30–60 min (500 mg/kg may be sufficient in small or debilitated patients). *Diuresis in drug intoxications*—up to 2 g/kg (60 g/m²) as a 5–10% solution.

## AVAILABILITY (generic available)

■ *IV injection:* 5%^Rx, 10%^Rx, 15%^Rx, 20%^Rx ■ *GU irrigant:* 5%^Rx ■ sorbitol for GU irrigation^Rx.

TIME/ACTION PROFILE (diuretic effect)

|    | ONSET | PEAK | DURATION |
|----|-------|------|----------|
| IV | 30–60 min | 1 hr | 6–8 hr |

# NURSING IMPLICATIONS

## ASSESSMENT

■ **General Info:** Monitor vital signs, urine output, CVP, and pulmonary artery pressures (PAP) before and hourly throughout administration. Assess patient for signs and symptoms of dehydration (decreased skin turgor, fever, dry skin and mucous membranes, thirst) or signs of fluid overload (increased CVP, dyspnea, rales/crackles, edema).

❑ Assess patient for anorexia, muscle weakness, numbness, tingling, paresthesia, confusion, and excessive thirst. Report signs of electrolyte imbalance.

■ **Increased Intracranial Pressure:** Monitor neurologic status and intracranial pressure readings in patients receiving this medication to decrease cerebral edema.

■ **Increased Intraocular Pressure:** Monitor for persistent or increased eye pain or decreased visual acuity.

■ *Lab Test Considerations:* Renal function and serum electrolytes should be monitored routinely throughout course of therapy.

## POTENTIAL NURSING DIAGNOSES

■ Fluid volume, excess (Indications).
■ Fluid volume, risk for deficit (Side Effects).

{ } = Available in Canada only.
*CAPITALS indicates life-threatening; underlines indicate most frequent.

## IMPLEMENTATION

- **General:** Observe infusion site frequently for infiltration. Extravasation may cause tissue irritation and necrosis.
- ▢ Do not administer electrolyte-free mannitol solution with blood. If blood must be administered simultaneously with mannitol, add at least 20 mEq NaCl to each liter of mannitol.
- ▢ Confer with physician regarding placement of an indwelling Foley catheter (except when used to decrease intraocular pressure).
- **IV:** Administer by IV infusion undiluted. If solution contains crystals, warm bottle in hot water and shake vigorously. Do not administer solution in which crystals remain undissolved. Cool to body temperature. Use an in-line filter for 15%, 20%, and 25% infusions.
- **Test Dose:** Administer over 3–5 min to produce a urine output of 30–50 ml/hr. If urine flow does not increase, administer 2nd test dose. If urine output is not at least 30–50 ml/hr for 2–3 hr after 2nd test dose, patient should be re-evaluated.
- **Oliguria:** Administration rate should be titrated to produce a urine output of 30–50 ml/hr. Administer child's dose over 2–6 hr.
- **Increased Intracranial Pressure:** Infuse dose over 30–60 min in adults and children.
- **Intraocular Pressure:** Administer dose over 30 min. When used preoperatively, administer 60–90 min before surgery.
- **Y-Site Compatibility:** ◆ amifostine ◆ aztreonam ◆ fludarabine ◆ fluorouracil ◆ gatifloxacin ◆ idarubicin ◆ linezolid ◆ melphalan ◆ ondansetron ◆ paclitaxel ◆ piperacillin/tazobactam ◆ sargramostim ◆ teniposide ◆ thiotepa ◆ vinorelbine.
- **Y-Site Incompatibility:** ◆ cefepime ◆ filgrastim.
- **Irrigation:** Add contents of two 50-ml vials of 25% mannitol to 900 ml of sterile water for injection for a 2.5% solution for irrigation. Use only clear solutions.

## PATIENT/FAMILY TEACHING

- ▢ Explain purpose of therapy to patient.

## EVALUATION

**Effectiveness of therapy can be demonstrated by:** ▪ Urine output of at least 30–50 ml/hr or an increase in urine output in accordance with parameters set by physician ▪ Reduction in intracranial pressure ▪ Reduction of intraocular pressure ▪ Excretion of certain toxic substances ▪ Irrigation during transurethral prostate resection.

# MAST CELL STABILIZERS

## cromolyn†
## (kroe-moe-lin)
Intal, NasalCrom, {Rynacrom}

## nedocromil†
## (ne-doe-kroe-mil)
Tilade

### CLASSIFICATION(S):
**Therapeutic:** antiasthmatics, allergy, cold, and cough remedies
**Pharmacologic:** mast cell stabilizers

### Pregnancy Category B

†For ophthalmic use, see Appendix C.

## INDICATIONS

▪ Prophylaxis (long-term control) of allergic disorders including rhinitis and asthma ▪ Prevention of exercise-induced bronchospasm.

## ACTION

▪ Prevents the release of histamine and slow-reacting substance of anaphylaxis (SRS-A) from sensitized mast cells. **Therapeutic Effects:** ▪ Decreased frequency and intensity of allergic reactions.

## PHARMACOKINETICS

**Absorption:** *Cromolyn*—Poorly absorbed; action is local. Small amounts may reach systemic circulation after inhalation. *Nedocromil*—90% of the inhaled dose is swallowed; 2.5–3% of swallowed drug is absorbed. Inhaled drug that reaches the lung is completely absorbed (total bioavailability is 6–9%).

**Distribution:** Because only small amounts are absorbed, distribution of these agents is not known. They do not cross biologic membranes well, and their action is primarily local.

**Metabolism and Excretion:** Small amounts absorbed are excreted unchanged in bile and urine.

**Half-life:** *Cromolyn*—80 min; *nedocromil*—1.5–2.3 hr.

## CONTRAINDICATIONS AND PRECAUTIONS

**Contraindicated in:** ■ Hypersensitivity ■ Acute attacks of asthma (inhalation products).

**Use Cautiously in:** ■ *Cromolyn*—Children <2 yr (safety not established) ■ *Nedocromil*—Children <12 yr (safety not established) ■ Will not relieve and may worsen acute attacks of bronchospasm (inhalation) ■ Pregnancy and lactation (safety not established).

## ADVERSE REACTIONS AND SIDE EFFECTS*

■ **CNS:** headache ■ **EENT:** *intranasal*—nasal irritation, sneezing ■ **Resp:** *inhalation*—irritation of the throat and trachea, bronchospasm, cough ■ **GI:** unpleasant taste ■ **Derm:** erythema, rash, urticaria ■ **Misc:** allergic reactions including ANAPHYLAXIS or worsening of conditions being treated.

## INTERACTIONS

**Drug-Drug:** ■ None significant.

## ROUTE AND DOSAGE

### ❏ Cromolyn

■ **Inhaln (Adults and Children ≥2 yr):** 20-mg inhaler capsules or nebulizer solution (for children 2–5 yr use nebulizer) or 2 sprays (0.8 mg/spray) as aerosol 4 times daily. For prevention of bronchospasm, use 2 aerosol sprays 10–15 min before exposure to known precipitating situation.

■ **Intranasal (Adults and Children ≥2 yr):** 1 spray (5.2 mg/spray) each nostril 3–4 times daily (up to 6 times daily).

### ❏ Nedocromil

■ **Inhaln (Adults and Children ≥6 yr):** 2 sprays (1.75 mg/spray) 4 times daily; decrease to 2–3 times daily as allowed. For prevention of bronchospasm, use 2 sprays up to 30 min before exposure to known precipitating situation (unlabeled).

## AVAILABILITY

### ❏ Cromolyn

■ *Capsules for inhalation:* 20 mg[Rx] ■ *Solution for nebulization:* 10 mg/ml[Rx] ■ Cost: $49.72/60 2 ml cartridges ■ *Aerosol spray for inhalation:* 800 mcg/spray in 8.1-g (112 sprays) or 14.2-g (≥200 sprays) containers[Rx] ■ *Nasal solution:* 40 mg/ml (5.2 mg/spray) in 13-ml (≥100 sprays) or 26-ml (≥200 sprays) containers[OTC] ■ *Nasal insufflation:* {10 mg/cartridge[Rx]}.

### ❏ Nedocromil

■ *Aerosol for inhalation:* 1.75 mg/spray in 16.2-g canister (at least 112 inhalations)[Rx].

TIME/ACTION PROFILE (effects on symptoms)

| | ONSET | PEAK | DURATION |
|---|---|---|---|
| Cromolyn—inhalation | <1 wk | 2–4 wk | unknown |
| Cromolyn—nasal | <1 wk | 2–4 wk | unknown |
| Nedocromil—inhalation | within 2 wk | unknown | unknown |

## NURSING IMPLICATIONS

### ASSESSMENT

■ **Inhaln:** Evaluate pulmonary function testing before initiating therapy in asthmatics.

❏ Assess lung sounds and respiratory function before and periodically during therapy.

■ **Intranasal:** Assess for symptoms of rhinitis (stuffiness, rhinorrhea).

### POTENTIAL NURSING DIAGNOSES

■ Airway clearance, ineffective (Indications).

### IMPLEMENTATION

■ **General:** Reduction in dose of other asthma medications may be possible after 2–4 wk of therapy. **Inhaln:** Medication should be used prophylactically, not during acute asthma attacks or status asthmaticus.

❏ Pretreatment with bronchodilator may be required to increase delivery of inhalation product.

{ } = Available in Canada only.
*CAPITALS indicates life-threatening; underlines indicate most frequent.

- Do not use solution that is cloudy or contains a precipitate. Compatible with acetylcysteine, albuterol, epinephrine, isoetharine, isoproterenol, preservative-free ipratropium, metaproterenol, and terbutaline solutions for up to 60 min.
- Incompatible with bitolterol.

## PATIENT/FAMILY TEACHING

- **General Info:** Medication must be used routinely and not more frequently than prescribed. Take missed doses as soon as remembered and space other doses at regular intervals. Do not double doses. Do not discontinue therapy without consulting health care professional, or exacerbation of symptoms may occur.
- Instruct patient not to discontinue concurrent corticosteroid or bronchodilator therapy without consulting health care professional.
- If cromolyn is prescribed before contact with known allergen or exercise, explain that it should be administered 10–15 min, and no earlier than 60 min, in advance.
- **Inhaln:** Inform patient that *Intal* capsules for inhalation are to be used for Spinhaler or Halermatic devices only.
- Instruct patient in the proper use of the metered-dose inhaler. See Appendix F for instructions.
- Advise patient that gargling and rinsing the mouth after each dose helps to decrease dryness of mouth, throat irritation, and hoarseness.
- Caution patient to notify health care professional if asthmatic symptoms do not improve within 4 wk, worsen, or recur.
- **Intranasal:** Instruct patient to clear nasal passages before administration and to inhale through nose during administration.

## EVALUATION

**Therapeutic effects, observable within 2–4 wk after beginning therapy, are demonstrated by:** ■ Reduction in symptoms of asthma ■ Prevention of exercise-induced bronchospasm ■ Decrease in the symptoms of rhinitis.

---

## meclizine
(**mek**-li-zeen)

Antivert, Antrizine, {Bonamine}, Bonine, Dramamine Less Drowsy Formula, Meni-D, Vergon

### CLASSIFICATION(S):
***Therapeutic:*** *antiemetics, antihistamines*

### Pregnancy Category B

## INDICATIONS

■ Management/prevention of: □ Motion sickness □ Vertigo.

## ACTION

■ Has central anticholinergic, CNS depressant, and antihistaminic properties ■ Decreases excitability of the middle ear labyrinth and depresses conduction in middle ear vestibular-cerebellar pathways. **Therapeutic Effects:** ■ Decreased motion sickness ■ Decreased vertigo from vestibular pathology.

## PHARMACOKINETICS

**Absorption:** Absorbed after oral administration.
**Distribution:** Unknown.
**Metabolism and Excretion:** Unknown.
**Half-life:** 6 hr.

## CONTRAINDICATIONS AND PRECAUTIONS

**Contraindicated in:** ■ Hypersensitivity ■ Pregnancy.
**Use Cautiously in:** ■ Prostatic hypertrophy ■ Narrow-angle glaucoma ■ Geriatric (increased sensitivity; increased risk of adverse reactions) ■ Children or lactation (safety not established).

## ADVERSE REACTIONS AND SIDE EFFECTS*

■ **CNS:** <u>drowsiness</u>, fatigue ■ **EENT:** blurred vision ■ **GI:** dry mouth.

## INTERACTIONS

**Drug-Drug:** ■ Additive CNS depression with other **CNS depressants,** including **alcohol,** other **antihistamines, opioid analgesics,** and **sedative/hypnotics** ■ Additive anticholinergic effects with other **drugs possessing anticholinergic properties,** including some **antihistamines, antidepressants, atropine, haloperidol, phenothiazines, quinidine,** and **disopyramide.**

## ROUTE AND DOSAGE

■ **PO (Adults):** *Motion sickness*—25–50 mg 1 hr before exposure; may repeat in 24 hr. *Vertigo*—25–100 mg/day in divided doses.

## AVAILABILITY

■ *Tablets:* 12.5 mg$^{Rx}$, 25 mg$^{Rx}$, $^{OTC}$, 50 mg$^{Rx}$ ■ Cost: 12.5 mg $4.09/100, 25 mg $5.40/100, 50 mg $6.99/100 ■ *Chewable tablets:* 25 mg$^{Rx}$, $^{OTC}$ ■ *Capsules:* 15 mg$^{OTC}$, 25 mg$^{Rx}$, 30 mg$^{OTC}$.

TIME/ACTION PROFILE (antihistaminic effects)

|  | ONSET | PEAK | DURATION |
|---|---|---|---|
| PO | 1 hr | unknown | 8–24 hr |

# NURSING IMPLICATIONS

## ASSESSMENT

■ **General Info:** Assess patient for level of sedation after administration.

■ **Motion Sickness:** Assess patient for nausea and vomiting before and 60 min after administration.

■ **Vertigo:** Assess degree of vertigo periodically in patients receiving meclizine for labyrinthitis.

■ *Lab Test Considerations:* May cause false-negative results in skin tests using allergen extracts. Discontinue meclizine 72 hr before testing.

## POTENTIAL NURSING DIAGNOSES

■ Injury, risk for (Side Effects).

## IMPLEMENTATION

■ **PO:** Administer oral doses with food, water, or milk to minimize GI irritation. Chewable tablet may be chewed or swallowed whole.

## PATIENT/FAMILY TEACHING

■ **General Info:** Instruct patient to take meclizine exactly as directed. If a dose is missed, take as soon as possible unless almost time for next dose. Do not double doses.

❏ May cause drowsiness. Caution patient to avoid driving or other activities requiring alertness until response to the medication is known.

❏ Advise patient that frequent mouth rinses, good oral hygiene, and sugarless gum or candy may decrease dryness of mouth.

❏ Caution patient to avoid concurrent use of alcohol and other CNS depressants with this medication.

■ **Motion Sickness:** When used as prophylaxis for motion sickness, advise patient to take medication at least 1 hr before exposure to conditions that may cause motion sickness.

## EVALUATION

**Effectiveness of therapy can be demonstrated by:** ■ Prevention and relief of symptoms in motion sickness ■ Prevention and treatment of vertigo due to vestibular pathology.

# medroxyprogesterone, See CONTRACEPTIVES, HORMONAL.

# medroxyprogesterone†

(me-**drox**-ee-proe-jess-te-rone)
Amen, Curretab, Cycrin, Depo-Provera, Provera

## CLASSIFICATION(S):

*Therapeutic: antineoplastics, contraceptive hormones*
*Pharmacologic: hormones, progestins*

### Pregnancy Category X

†For contraceptive use see Contraceptives, Hormonal monograph.

## INDICATIONS

■ To decrease endometrial hyperplasia in postmenopausal women receiving concurrent estrogen (0.625 mg/day conjugated estrogens) ■ Treatment of secondary amenorrhea and abnormal uterine bleeding caused by hormonal imbalance ■ **IM:** Treatment of advanced unresponsive endometrial or renal carcinoma. **Unlabeled uses:** ■ Obesity-hypoventilation (pickwickian) syndrome ■ sleep apnea ■ hypersomnolence.

## ACTION

■ A synthetic form of progesterone—actions include secretory changes in the endometrium, increases in basal body temperature, histologic changes in vaginal epithelium, relaxation of uterine smooth muscle, mammary alveolar tissue growth, pituitary inhibition, and withdrawal bleeding in the presence of estrogen. **Therapeutic Effects:** ■ Decreased endometrial hyperplasia in postmenopausal women receiving concurrent estrogen (combination with estrogen decreases vasomotor symptoms and prevents osteoporosis) ■ Restoration of hormonal balance with control of uterine bleeding ■ Management of endometrial or renal cancer ■ Prevention of pregnancy.

## PHARMACOKINETICS

**Absorption:** 0.6–10% absorbed after oral administration.
**Distribution:** Enters breast milk.
**Metabolism and Excretion:** Metabolized by the liver.
**Half-life:** *1st phase*—52 min; *2nd phase*—230 min; *biological*—14.5 hr.

## CONTRAINDICATIONS AND PRECAUTIONS

**Contraindicated in:** ■ Hypersensitivity ■ Hypersensitivity to parabens (IM suspension only) ■ Pregnancy ■ Missed abortion ■ Thromboembolic disease ■ Cerebrovascular disease ■ Severe liver disease ■ Breast or genital cancer ■ Porphyria.
**Use Cautiously in:** ■ History of liver disease ■ Renal disease ■ Cardiovascular disease ■ Seizure disorders ■ Mental depression ■ Lactation (when used as a contraceptive, wait until 6 wk after delivery if breastfeeding).

## ADVERSE REACTIONS AND SIDE EFFECTS*

■ **CNS:** depression ■ **EENT:** retinal thrombosis ■ **CV:** PULMONARY EMBOLISM, thromboembolism, thrombophlebitis ■ **GI:** drug-induced hepatitis, gingival bleeding ■ **GU:** cervical erosions ■ **Derm:** chloasma, melasma, rashes ■ **Endo:** amenorrhea, breakthrough bleeding, breast tenderness, changes in menstrual flow, galactorrhea, hyperglycemia, spotting ■ **F and E:** edema ■ **Misc:** allergic reactions including ANAPHYLAXIS and ANGIOEDEMA, weight gain, weight loss.

## INTERACTIONS

**Drug-Drug:** ■ May decrease the effectiveness of **bromocriptine** when used concurrently for galactorrhea/amenorrhea ■ Contraceptive effectiveness may be decreased by **carbamazepine, phenobarbital, phenytoin, rifampin,** or **rifabutin** ■ **Aminoglutethimide** may decrease oral absorption.

## ROUTE AND DOSAGE

❏ **Postmenopausal Women Receiving Concurrent Estrogen**

■ **PO (Adults):** 2.5–5 mg daily concurrently with 0.625 mg conjugated estrogens (monophasic regimen) *or* 5 mg daily on days 15–28 of the cycle with 0.625 mg conjugated estrogens taken daily throughout cycle (biphasic regimen).

❏ **Secondary Amenorrhea**

■ **PO (Adults):** 5–10 mg/day for 5–10 days; start at any time in cycle.

❏ **Dysfunctional Uterine Bleeding/Induction of Menses**

■ **PO (Adults):** 5–10 mg/day for 5–10 days, starting on day 16 or day 21 of menstrual cycle.

❏ **Renal or Endometrial Carcinoma**

■ **IM (Adults):** 400–1000 mg, may be repeated weekly; if improvement occurs, attempt to decrease dosage to 400 mg monthly.

## AVAILABILITY (generic available)

■ *Tablets:* 2.5 mg$^{Rx}$, 5 mg$^{Rx}$, 10 mg$^{Rx}$, {100 mg$^{Rx}$} ■ Cost: *Provera*—2.5 mg $52.86/100, 5 mg $79.79/100; *generic*—2.5 mg $26.93/100, 5 mg $49.44/100 ■ *Suspension for depot injection:* {50 mg/ml$^{Rx}$}, {100 mg/ml$^{Rx}$}, 150 mg/ml$^{Rx}$, 400 mg/ml$^{Rx}$ ■ conjugated estrogens as Prempro (single combination tablet of 0.626 mg conjugated estrogens plus 2.5 or 5 mg medroxyprogesterone) or Premphase (0.625 mg conjugated estrogens tablet for 14 days followed by combination tablet of 0.625 mg conjugated estrogens plus 5 mg medroxyprogesterone for days 15–28) in convenience packages$^{Rx}$. See Appendix B.

TIME/ACTION PROFILE (IM = antineoplastic effects)

| | ONSET | PEAK | DURATION |
|---|---|---|---|
| PO | unknown | unknown | unknown |
| IM | wks–mos | mo | unknown† |

†Contraceptive effect lasts 3 mo.

# NURSING IMPLICATIONS

## ASSESSMENT

- **General Info:** Monitor blood pressure periodically throughout therapy.
- Assess patient's usual menstrual history. Administration of drug may begin on any day of cycle in patients with amenorrhea and on day 16 or 21 of cycle in patients with dysfunctional bleeding.
- Monitor intake and output ratios and weekly weight. Report significant discrepancies or steady weight gain.
- **Lab Test Considerations:** Monitor hepatic function before and periodically throughout therapy.
- May cause increased alkaline phosphatase levels. May decrease pregnanediol excretion concentrations.
- May cause increased serum LDL concentrations or decreased HDL concentrations.
- May alter thyroid hormone assays.

## POTENTIAL NURSING DIAGNOSES

- Sexual dysfunction (Indications).
- Tissue perfusion, ineffective (Side Effects).

## IMPLEMENTATION

- **General:** Do not confuse Provera (medroxyprogesterone) with Covera (verapamil).
- Only the 150 mg/ml vial should be used for contraception.
- **IM:** Shake vial vigorously before preparing IM dose. Administer deep IM.
- In patients with cancer, IM dose may initially be required weekly. Once stabilized, IM dose may be required only monthly.

## PATIENT/FAMILY TEACHING

- Explain the dosage schedule. Instruct patient to take medication at the same time each day. If a dose is missed, patient should make up dose as soon as remembered, but do not double doses.
- Advise patients receiving medroxyprogesterone for menstrual dysfunction to anticipate withdrawal bleeding 3–7 days after discontinuing medication.
- Review patient package insert (PPI) with patient. Emphasize the importance of notifying health care professional if the following side effects occur: visual changes, sudden weakness, incoordination, difficulty with speech, headache, leg or calf pain, shortness of breath, chest pain, changes in vaginal bleeding pattern, yellow skin, swelling of extremities, depression, or rash. Patients receiving medroxyprogesterone for cancer may not receive PPI.
- Advise patient to keep a 1-mo supply of medroxyprogesterone available at all times.
- Instruct patient in correct method of monthly breast self-examination. Increased breast tenderness may occur.
- Advise patient that gingival bleeding may occur. Instruct patient to use good oral hygiene and to receive regular dental care and examinations.
- Instruct patient to notify health care professional if menstrual period is missed or if pregnancy is suspected. Patient should not attempt conception for 3 mo after discontinuing medication in order to decrease risk to fetus.
- Medroxyprogesterone may cause melasma (brown patches of discoloration) on face when patient is exposed to sunlight. Advise patient to avoid sun exposure and to wear sunscreen or protective clothing when outdoors.
- Emphasize the importance of routine follow-up physical exams, including blood pressure; breast, abdomen, and pelvic exams; and Papanicolaou smears every 6–12 mo.

## EVALUATION

**Effectiveness of therapy can be demonstrated by:** ■ Regular menstrual periods ■ Decrease in endometrial hyperplasia in postmenopausal women receiving concurrent estrogen ■ Control of the spread of endometrial or renal cancer.

# megestrol
(me-**jess**-trole)
Megace

**CLASSIFICATION(S):**
**Therapeutic:** antineoplastics, hormones
**Pharmacologic:** progestins

**Pregnancy Category D (tablets), X (suspension)**

## INDICATIONS

■ Palliative treatment of endometrial and breast carcinoma, either alone or with surgery or radiation (tablets only) ■ Treatment of anorexia, weight loss, and cachexia associated with AIDS (oral suspension only).

## ACTION

■ Antineoplastic effect may result from inhibition of pituitary function. **Therapeutic Effects:** ■ Regression of tumor ■ Increased appetite and weight gain in patients with AIDS.

## PHARMACOKINETICS

**Absorption:** Well absorbed from the GI tract.
**Distribution:** Unknown.
**Protein Binding:** ≥90%.
**Metabolism and Excretion:** Completely metabolized by the liver.
**Half-life:** 38 hr (range 13–104 hr).

## CONTRAINDICATIONS AND PRECAUTIONS

**Contraindicated in:** ■ Hypersensitivity ■ Pregnancy, missed abortion, or lactation ■ Undiagnosed vaginal bleeding ■ Severe liver disease ■ Suspension contains alcohol and should be avoided in patients with known intolerance.
**Use Cautiously in:** ■ Diabetes ■ Mental depression ■ Renal disease ■ History of thrombophlebitis ■ Cardiovascular disease ■ Seizure disorders.

## ADVERSE REACTIONS AND SIDE EFFECTS*

■ **CV:** THROMBOEMBOLISM, edema ■ **GI:** GI irritation ■ **Derm:** alopecia ■ **Endo:** asymptomatic adrenal suppression (chronic therapy) ■ **Hemat:** thrombophlebitis ■ **MS:** carpal tunnel syndrome.

## INTERACTIONS

**Drug-Drug:** ■ None significant.

## ROUTE AND DOSAGE

■ **PO (Adults):** *Breast carcinoma*—160 mg/day single dose or divided doses; *endometrial/ovarian carcinoma*—40–320 mg/day in divided doses; *anorexia associated with AIDS*—800 mg day; may decrease to 400 mg/day after 1 mo (range 400–800 mg/day).

## AVAILABILITY (generic available)

■ *Tablets:* 20 mg^Rx, 40 mg^Rx ■ Cost: 20 mg $75.68/100, 40 mg $134.96/100 ■ *Oral suspension (lemon-lime flavor):* 40 mg/ml^Rx ■ Cost: 40 mg/ml $166.59/240 ml.

TIME/ACTION PROFILE (antineoplastic activity)

|     | ONSET   | PEAK | DURATION |
| --- | ------- | ---- | -------- |
| PO  | wk–mos  | 2 mo | unknown  |

# NURSING IMPLICATIONS

## ASSESSMENT

■ **General Info:** Assess patient for swelling, pain, or tenderness in legs. Report these signs of deep vein thrombophlebitis.
■ **Anorexia:** Monitor weight, appetite, and nutritional intake in patients with AIDS.

## POTENTIAL NURSING DIAGNOSES

■ Knowledge, deficient, related to medication regimen (Patient/Family Teaching).

## IMPLEMENTATION

■ **General:** Because of high dose, suspension is most convenient form for patients with AIDS.
■ **PO:** May be administered with meals if GI irritation becomes a problem.

## PATIENT/FAMILY TEACHING

❏ Instruct patient to take medication exactly as directed; do not skip or double up on missed doses. Missed doses may be taken as long as it is not right before next dose. Gradually decrease dose prior to discontinuation.
❏ Advise patient to report to health care professional any unusual vaginal bleeding or signs of deep vein thrombophlebitis.
❏ Advise patient that this medication may have teratogenic effects. Contraception should be used during therapy and for at least 4 mo after therapy is completed.

❑ Discuss with patient the possibility of hair loss. Explore methods of coping.

## EVALUATION

**Effectiveness of therapy can be demonstrated by:** ■ Slowing or arresting the spread of endometrial or breast malignancy. Therapeutic effects usually occur within 2 mo of initiating therapy ■ Increased appetite and weight gain in patients with AIDS.

---

# meloxicam
(me-**lox**-i-kam)
Mobic

## CLASSIFICATION(S):
*Therapeutic: nonsteroidal anti-inflammatory agents*
*Pharmacologic: nonopioid analgesics*

**Pregnancy Category C**

---

## INDICATIONS
■ Relief of signs and symptoms of osteoarthritis.

## ACTION
■ Inhibit prostaglandin synthesis, probably by inhibiting the enzyme cyclooxygenase. **Therapeutic Effects:** ■ Decreased pain and inflammation associated with osteoarthritis ■ Also decreases fever.

## PHARMACOKINETICS
**Absorption:** Well absorbed following oral administration.
**Distribution:** Unknown.
**Protein Binding:** 99.4.%.
**Metabolism and Excretion:** Mostly metabolized to inactive metabolites by the liver via the P450 enzyme system; metabolites are excreted in urine and feces.
**Half-life:** 20.1 hr.

## CONTRAINDICATIONS AND PRECAUTIONS
**Contraindicated in:** ■ Hypersensitivity ■ Cross-sensitivity may occur with other NSAIDs, including aspirin ■ Severe renal impairment (CCr ≤15

ml/min) ■ Concurrent use of aspirin (increased risk of adverse reactions).
**Use Cautiously in:** ■ Dehydration (correct deficits before initiating therapy) ■ Impaired renal function, heart failure, liver dysfunction, geriatric patients (≥65 yr), concurrent ACE inhibitor or diuretic therapy (increased risk of reversible renal dysfunction) ■ Coagulation disorders or concurrent anticoagulant therapy (may increase risk of bleeding) ■ Pregnancy, lactation, or children <18 yr (safety not established; avoid use late in pregnancy).

## ADVERSE REACTIONS AND SIDE EFFECTS*
■ **CV:** edema ■ **GI:** GI BLEEDING, abnormal liver function tests, diarrhea, dyspepsia, nausea ■ **Derm:** pruritus ■ **Hemat:** anemia, leukopenia, thrombocytopenia.

## INTERACTIONS
**Drug-Drug:** ■ May decrease the antihypertensive effects of **ACE inhibitors** ■ May decrease the diuretic effects of **furosemide** or **thiazide diuretics** ■ Concurrent use with **aspirin** increases meloxicam blood levels and may increase risk of adverse reactions ■ Concurrent use with **cholestyramine** decreases blood levels ■ Increases plasma **lithium** levels (close monitoring recommended when meloxicam is introduced or withdrawn) ■ May increase the risk of bleeding with **anticoagulants,** including **warfarin.**

## ROUTE AND DOSAGE
■ **PO (Adults):** 7.5 mg once daily; some patients may require 15 mg/day.

## AVAILABILITY
■ *Tablets:* 7.5 mg.

TIME/ACTION PROFILE

| | ONSET | PEAK* | DURATION |
|---|---|---|---|
| PO | unknown | 5–6 hr | 24 hr |

*Blood levels.

# NURSING IMPLICATIONS

## ASSESSMENT
■ **General Info:** Patients who have asthma, aspirin-induced allergy, and nasal polyps are

at increased risk for developing hypersensitivity reactions. Assess for rhinitis, asthma, and urticaria.

- **General Info:** Assess pain and range of motion prior to and 1–2 hr following administration.

- *Lab Test Considerations:* BUN, serum creatinine, CBC, and liver function tests should be evaluated periodically in patients receiving prolonged courses of therapy. May cause anemia, thrombocytopenia, leukopenia, and abnormal liver or renal function tests.

□ Bleeding time may be prolonged.

## POTENTIAL NURSING DIAGNOSES

- Pain, acute (Indications).
- Mobility, impaired physical (Indications).

## IMPLEMENTATION

- **General:** Administration in higher than recommended doses does not provide increased effectiveness but may cause increased side effects.

- **PO:** May be administered without regard to food.

## PATIENT/FAMILY TEACHING

□ Advise patient to take this medication with a full glass of water and to remain in an upright position for 15–30 min after administration.

□ Instruct patient to take medication exactly as directed. If a dose is missed, it should be taken as soon as remembered but not if almost time for the next dose. Do not double doses.

□ Caution patient to avoid the concurrent use of alcohol, aspirin, acetaminophen, or other OTC medications without consulting health care professional.

□ Advise patient to inform health care professional of medication regimen prior to treatment or surgery.

□ Advise patient to consult health care professional if rash, itching, visual disturbances, weight gain, edema, black stools, or signs of hepatotoxicity (nausea, fatigue, lethargy, jaundice, upper right quadrant tenderness, flu-like symptoms) occur.

## EVALUATION

**Effectiveness of therapy can be demonstrated by:** ■ Relief of pain ■ Improved joint mobility. Patients who do not respond to one NSAID may respond to another.

# melphalan

(**mel**-fa-lan)
Alkeran, L-PAM, phenylalanine mustard

## CLASSIFICATION(S):
**Therapeutic:** antineoplastics
**Pharmacologic:** alkylating agents

**Pregnancy Category D**

## INDICATIONS

■ Alone or with other therapies for □ Multiple myeloma □ Ovarian cancer. **Unlabeled uses:** ■ Breast cancer ■ Prostate cancer ■ Testicular carcinoma ■ Chronic myelogenous leukemia ■ Osteogenic sarcoma.

## ACTION

■ Inhibits DNA and RNA synthesis by alkylation (cell-cycle phase–nonspecific). **Therapeutic Effects:** ■ Death of rapidly replicating cells, particularly malignant ones ■ Also has immunosuppressive properties.

## PHARMACOKINETICS

**Absorption:** Incompletely and variably absorbed following oral administration.

**Distribution:** Rapidly distributed throughout total body water.

**Protein Binding:** ≤30%.

**Metabolism and Excretion:** Rapidly metabolized in the bloodstream. Small amounts (10%) excreted unchanged by the kidneys.

**Half-life:** 1.5 hr.

## CONTRAINDICATIONS AND PRECAUTIONS

**Contraindicated in:** ■ Hypersensitivity to melphalan or chlorambucil ■ Pregnancy or lactation.

**Use Cautiously in:** ■ Patients with childbearing potential ■ Active infections ■ Decreased bone marrow reserve ■ Geriatric patients or patients with other chronic debilitating illnesses ■ Impaired renal function (dose reduction recommended if BUN ≥30 mg/dl) ■ Children (safety not established).

## ADVERSE REACTIONS AND SIDE EFFECTS*

■ **Resp:** bronchopulmonary dysplasia, pulmonary fibrosis ■ **GI:** diarrhea, hepatitis, nausea, stomatitis, vomiting ■ **GU:** infertility ■ **Derm:** alopecia, pruritus, rashes ■ **Endo:** menstrual irregularities ■ **Hemat:** leukopenia, thrombocytopenia, anemia ■ **Metab:** hyperuricemia ■ **Misc:** allergic reactions, including ANAPHYLAXIS (more common after IV use).

## INTERACTIONS

**Drug-Drug:** ■ ↑ bone marrow depression with other **antineoplastics** or **radiation therapy** ■ May ↓ antibody response to **live-virus vaccines** and ↑ risk of adverse reactions ■ May ↑ the risk of pulmonary toxicity with **carmustine** ■ Concurrent IV use with **cyclosporine** may ↑ risk of renal failure ■ Risk of enterocolitis may be ↑ with concurrent **nalidixic acid**.

## ROUTE AND DOSAGE

❏ **Multiple Myeloma**

■ **PO (Adults):** 150 mcg (0.15 mg)/kg/day for 7 days, followed by 3-wk rest, then 50 mcg (0.05 mg)/kg/day maintenance dose *or* 100–150 mcg/kg/day or 250 mg (0.25 mg)/kg/day for 4 days followed by 2–4-wk rest, then 2–4 mg/day maintenance dose *or* 7 mg/m² *or* 250 mcg (0.25 mg)/kg daily for 5 days q 5–6 wk.

■ **IV (Adults):** 16 mg/m² q 2 wk for 4 doses, then q 4 wk.

❏ **Ovarian Carcinoma**

■ **PO (Adults):** 200 mcg (0.2 mg)/kg/day for 5 days q 4–5 wk.

## AVAILABILITY

■ *Tablets:* 2 mg$^{Rx}$ ■ *Powder for injection:* 50 mg$^{Rx}$.

TIME/ACTION PROFILE (effects on blood counts)

| | ONSET | PEAK | DURATION |
|---|---|---|---|
| PO | 5 days | 2–3 wk | 5–6 wk |

## NURSING IMPLICATIONS

### ASSESSMENT

❏ Assess for signs of infection (fever, chills, sore throat, cough, hoarseness, lower back or side pain, difficult or painful urination). Notify physician if these symptoms occur.

❏ Assess for bleeding (bleeding gums, bruising, petechiae, guaiac stools, urine, and emesis). Avoid IM injections and taking rectal temperatures. Apply pressure to venipuncture sites for 10 min.

❏ May cause nausea and vomiting. Monitor intake and output, appetite, and nutritional intake. Prophylactic antiemetics may be used. Adjust diet as tolerated.

❏ Monitor for symptoms of gout (increased uric acid, joint pain, edema). Encourage patient to drink at least 2 L of fluid per day. Allopurinol may be given to decrease uric acid levels.

❏ Anemia may occur. Monitor for increased fatigue and dyspnea.

❏ Assess patient for allergy to chlorambucil. Patients may have cross-sensitivity.

■ *Lab Test Considerations:* Monitor CBC and differential weekly during therapy. The nadir of leukopenia occurs in 2–3 wk. Notify physician if leukocyte count is <3000/mm³. The nadir of thrombocytopenia occurs in 2–3 wk. Notify physician if platelet count is <100,000/mm³. Recovery of leukopenia and thrombocytopenia occurs in 5–6 wk.

❏ Monitor liver function studies (AST, ALT, LDH, bilirubin) and renal function studies (BUN, creatinine) prior to and periodically during therapy to detect hepatotoxicity and nephrotoxicity.

❏ May cause ↑ uric acid. Monitor periodically during therapy.

❏ May cause ↑ 5-hydroxyindoleacetic acid (5-HIAA) concentrations as a result of tumor breakdown.

## POTENTIAL NURSING DIAGNOSES

■ Injury, risk for (Side Effects).

■ Infection, risk for (Side Effects).

---

{ } = Available in Canada only.
*CAPITALS indicates life-threatening; underlines indicate most frequent.

## IMPLEMENTATION

- **General:** Solution should be prepared in a biologic cabinet. Wear gloves, gown, and mask while handling medication. Discard IV equipment in specially designated container.
- If solution contacts skin or mucosa, immediately wash skin or mucosa with soap and water.
- **PO:** May be ordered in divided doses or as a single daily dose.
- **Intermittent Infusion:** Reconstitute with 10 ml of diluent supplied for a concentration of 5 mg/ml and shake vigorously until solution is clear. Dilute dose immediately with 0.9% NaCl for a concentration of ≤0.45 mg/ml. Administer within 60 min of reconstitution.
- *Rate:* Administer over at least 15 min.
- **Y-Site Compatibility:** ◆ acyclovir ◆ amikacin ◆ aminophylline ◆ ampicillin ◆ aztreonam ◆ bleomycin ◆ bumetanide ◆ buprenorphine ◆ butorphanol ◆ calcium gluconate ◆ carboplatin ◆ carmustine ◆ cefazolin ◆ cefepime ◆ cefoperazone ◆ cefotaxime ◆ cefotetan ◆ ceftazidime ◆ ceftizoxime ◆ ceftriaxone ◆ cefuroxime ◆ cimetidine ◆ cisplatin ◆ clindamycin ◆ cyclophosphamide ◆ cytarabine ◆ dacarbazine ◆ dactinomycin ◆ daunorubicin ◆ diphenhydramine ◆ doxorubicin ◆ doxycycline ◆ droperidol ◆ enalaprilat ◆ etoposide ◆ famotidine ◆ floxuridine ◆ fluconazole ◆ fludarabine ◆ fluorouracil ◆ furosemide ◆ ganciclovir ◆ gentamicin ◆ haloperidol ◆ heparin ◆ hydrocortisone ◆ hydromorphone ◆ idarubicin ◆ ifosfamide ◆ imipenem/cilastatin ◆ lorazepam ◆ mannitol ◆ mechlorethamine ◆ meperidine ◆ mesna ◆ methotrexate ◆ metoclopramide ◆ metronidazole ◆ minocycline ◆ mitomycin ◆ mitoxantrone ◆ morphine ◆ nalbuphine ◆ netilmicin ◆ ondansetron ◆ pentostatin ◆ piperacillin ◆ plicamycin ◆ potassium chloride ◆ prochlorperazine edisylate ◆ promethazine ◆ ranitidine ◆ sodium bicarbonate ◆ streptozocin ◆ teniposide ◆ thiotepa ◆ ticarcillin ◆ ticarcillin/clavulanate ◆ tobramycin ◆ trimethoprim/sulfamethoxazole ◆ vancomycin ◆ vinblastine ◆ vincristine ◆ vinorelbine ◆ zidovudine.
- **Y-Site Incompatibility:** ◆ amphotericin B ◆ chlorpromazine.

## PATIENT/FAMILY TEACHING

- Instruct patient to take melphalan exactly as directed, even if nausea and vomiting occur.

If vomiting occurs shortly after dose is taken, consult health care professional. If a dose is missed, do not take at all.
- Advise patient to notify physician if fever; chills; dyspnea; persistent cough; sore throat; signs of infection; bleeding gums; bruising; petechiae; or blood in urine, stool, or emesis occurs. Caution patient to avoid crowds and persons with known infections. Instruct patient to use soft toothbrush and electric razor. Caution patient not to drink alcoholic beverages or take products containing aspirin or other NSAIDs.
- Instruct patient to notify health care professional if rash, itching, joint pain, or swelling occurs.
- Instruct patient to inspect oral mucosa for redness and ulceration. If ulceration occurs, advise patient to use sponge brush and to rinse mouth with water after eating and drinking. Consult physician if pain interferes with eating. Stomatitis pain may require treatment with opioid analgesics.
- Advise patient that although fertility may be decreased, contraception should be used during melphalan therapy because of potential teratogenic effects on the fetus.
- Instruct patient not to receive any vaccinations without advice of health care professional.
- Emphasize need for periodic lab tests to monitor for side effects.

## EVALUATION

**Effectiveness of therapy can be demonstrated by:** ■ Decrease in size and spread of malignant tissue.

---

**High Alert**

# meperidine

(me-**per**-i-deen)

Demerol, pethidine

### CLASSIFICATION(S):

*Therapeutic:* opioid analgesics

*Pharmacologic:* opioid agonists

**Schedule II**

**Pregnancy Category C**

# INDICATIONS

■ Moderate or severe pain (alone or with nonopioid agents) ■ Anesthesia adjunct ■ Analgesic during labor ■ Preoperative sedation. **Unlabeled uses:** ■ Rigors.

# ACTION

■ Binds to opiate receptors in the CNS. Alters the perception of and response to painful stimuli, while producing generalized CNS depression. **Therapeutic Effects:** ■ Decrease in severity of pain.

# PHARMACOKINETICS

**Absorption:** 50% from the GI tract; well absorbed from IM sites. Oral and parenteral doses are not equal.

**Distribution:** Widely distributed. Crosses the placenta; enters breast milk.

**Protein Binding:** High.

**Metabolism and Excretion:** Mostly metabolized by the liver; some converted to normeperidine, which may accumulate and cause seizures. 5% excreted unchanged by the kidneys.

**Half-life:** 3–5 hr (prolonged in impaired renal or hepatic function).

# CONTRAINDICATIONS AND PRECAUTIONS

**Contraindicated in:** ■ Hypersensitivity ■ Hypersensitivity to bisulfites (some injectable products) ■ Pregnancy or lactation (chronic use) ■ Recent (14–21 days) MAO inhibitor therapy.

**Use Cautiously in:** ■ Head trauma ■ Increased intracranial pressure ■ Severe renal, hepatic, or pulmonary disease ■ Hypothyroidism ■ Adrenal insufficiency ■ Alcoholism ■ Geriatric or debilitated patients (dosage reduction suggested) ■ Undiagnosed abdominal pain or prostatic hyperplasia ■ Labor (respiratory depression may occur in the newborn) ■ Patients with renal impairment, or extensive burns ■ High dose or prolonged therapy (>600 mg/day or >2 days; increased risk of CNS stimulation and seizures due to accumulation of normeperidine) ■ Children (increased risk of seizures due to accumulation of normeperidine).

# ADVERSE REACTIONS AND SIDE EFFECTS*

■ **CNS:** SEIZURES, confusion, sedation, dysphoria, euphoria, floating feeling, hallucinations, headache, unusual dreams ■ **EENT:** blurred vision, diplopia, miosis ■ **Resp:** respiratory depression ■ **CV:** hypotension, bradycardia ■ **GI:** constipation, nausea, vomiting ■ **GU:** urinary retention ■ **Derm:** flushing, sweating ■ **Misc:** physical dependence, psychological dependence, tolerance.

# INTERACTIONS

**Drug-Drug:** ■ Use with extreme caution in patients receiving **MAO inhibitors** or **procarbazine** (may cause fatal reaction—contraindicated within 14–21 days of MAO inhibitor therapy) ■ ↑ CNS depression with **alcohol, antihistamines,** and **sedative/hypnotics** ■ Administration of **agonist/antagonist opioid analgesics** may precipitate opioid withdrawal in physically dependent patients ■ **Nalbuphine** or **pentazocine** may ↓ analgesia ■ **Protease inhibitor antiretrovirals** may ↑ effects and adverse reactions (concurrent use should be avoided ■ **Phenytoin** ↑ metabolism and may ↓ effects ■ **Chlorpromazine** and **thioridazine** may ↑ the risk of adverse reactions (concurrent use should be avoided).

**Drug-Natural Products:** ■ Concomitant use of **kava, valerian,** or **chamomile** can ↓ CNS depression.

# ROUTE AND DOSAGE

■ **PO, IM, Subcut (Adults):** *Analgesia*—50–150 mg q 3–4 hr. *Analgesia during labor*—50–100 mg IM or subcut when contractions become regular; may repeat q 1–3 hr. *Preoperative sedation*—50–100 mg IM or subcut 30–90 min before anesthesia.

■ **PO, IM, Subcut (Children):** *Analgesia*—1–1.8 mg/kg q 3–4 hr (should not exceed 100 mg/dose). *Preoperative sedation*—1–2.2 mg/kg 30–90 min before anesthesia (not to exceed adult dose).

■ **IV (Adults):** 15–35 mg/hr as a continuous infusion; *PCA*—10 mg initially; with a range Of 1–5 mg/incremental dose, recommended lockout interval is 6–10 min (minimum 5 min).

## AVAILABILITY (generic available)

■ *Tablets:* 50 mg$^{Rx}$, 100 mg$^{Rx}$ ■ Cost: 50 mg $99.04/100, 100 mg $188.37/100 ■ *Syrup (banana flavor):* 50 mg/5 ml$^{Rx}$ ■ *Injection:* {10 mg/ml$^{Rx}$}, 25 mg/ml$^{Rx}$, 50 mg/ml$^{Rx}$, 75 mg/ml$^{Rx}$, 100 mg/ml$^{Rx}$ ■ promethazine (Mepergan) and atropine$^{Rx}$. See Appendix B.

TIME/ACTION PROFILE (analgesia)

|        | ONSET      | PEAK      | DURATION |
|--------|-----------|-----------|----------|
| PO     | 15 min    | 60 min    | 2–4 hr   |
| IM     | 10–15 min | 30–50 min | 2–4 hr   |
| Subcut | 10–15 min | 40–60 min | 2–4 hr   |
| IV     | immediate | 5–7 min   | 2–4 hr   |

# NURSING IMPLICATIONS

## ASSESSMENT

❏ Assess type, location, and intensity of pain prior to and 1 hr following PO, subcut, and IM doses and 5 min (peak) following IV administration. When titrating opioid doses, increases of 25–50% should be administered until there is either a 50% reduction in the patient's pain rating on a numerical or visual analog scale or the patient reports satisfactory pain relief. A repeat dose can be safely administered at the time of the peak if previous dose is ineffective and side effects are minimal.

❏ An equianalgesic chart (see Appendix O) should be used when changing routes or when changing from one opioid to another.

❏ Assess blood pressure, pulse, and respirations before and periodically during administration. If respiratory rate is <10/min, assess level of sedation. Dose may need to be decreased by 25–50%. Initial drowsiness will diminish with continued use.

❏ Assess bowel function routinely. Prevention of constipation should be instituted with increased intake of fluids and bulk and with laxatives to minimize constipating effects. Stimulant laxatives should be administered routinely if opioid use exceeds 2–3 days, unless contraindicated.

❏ Prolonged use may lead to physical and psychological dependence and tolerance. This should not prevent patient from receiving adequate analgesia. Most patients who receive meperidine for pain do not develop psychological dependence. Progressively higher doses may be required to relieve pain with long-term therapy.

❏ Monitor patients on chronic or high-dose therapy for CNS stimulation (restlessness, irritability, seizures) due to accumulation of normeperidine metabolite. Risk of toxicity increases with doses >600 mg/24 hr, chronic administration (>2 days), and renal impairment.

■ *Lab Test Considerations:* May increase plasma amylase and lipase concentrations.

■ *Toxicity and Overdose:* If an opioid antagonist is required to reverse respiratory depression or coma, naloxone (Narcan) is the antidote. Dilute the 0.4-mg ampule of naloxone in 10 ml of 0.9% NaCl and administer 0.5 ml (0.02 mg) by direct IV push every 2 min. For children and patients weighing <40 kg, dilute 0.1 mg of naloxone in 10 ml of 0.9% NaCl for a concentration of 10 mcg/ml and administer 0.5 mcg/kg every 2 min. Titrate dose to avoid withdrawal, seizures, and severe pain. In patients receiving meperidine chronically, naloxone may precipitate seizures by eliminating the CNS depressant effects of meperidine, allowing the convulsant activity of normeperidine to predominate. Monitor patient closely.

## POTENTIAL NURSING DIAGNOSES

■ Pain, acute (Indications).

■ Sensory perception, disturbed (visual, auditory) (Side Effects).

■ Injury, risk for (Side Effects).

## IMPLEMENTATION

❏ *High Alert:* Accidental overdosage of opioid analgesics has resulted in fatalities. Before administering, clarify all ambiguous orders; have second practitioner independently check original order, dose calculations, and infusion pump settings. Do not confuse with morphine or hydromorphone; fatalities have occurred.

■ **General:** Explain therapeutic value of medication prior to administration to enhance the analgesic effect.

❏ Regularly administered doses may be more effective than prn administration. Analgesic is more effective if given before pain becomes severe.

❏ Coadministration with nonopioid analgesics may have additive analgesic effects and permit lower doses.

□ Oral dose is <50% as effective as parenteral. When changing to oral administration, dose may need to be increased (see Appendix O).

□ Medication should be discontinued gradually after long-term use to prevent withdrawal symptoms.

□ May be administered via PCA pump.

■ **PO:** Doses may be administered with food or milk to minimize GI irritation. Syrup should be diluted in half-full glass of water.

■ **IM:** Administration of repeated subcut doses may cause local irritation.

■ **Direct IV:** Dilute to a concentration of 10 mg/ml with sterile water or 0.9% NaCl for injection.

□ *High Alert:* Administer slowly. Rapid administration may lead to increased respiratory depression, hypotension, and circulatory collapse.

■ **Continuous Infusion:** Dilute to a concentration of 1 mg/ml with D5W, D10W, dextrose/saline combinations, dextrose/Ringer's or lactated Ringer's injection combinations, 0.45% NaCl, 0.9% NaCl, or Ringer's or LR. Administer via infusion pump.

■ **Syringe Compatibility:** ◆ atropine ◆ chlorpromazine ◆ cimetidine ◆ dimenhydrinate ◆ diphenhydramine ◆ droperidol ◆ glycopyrrolate ◆ hydroxyzine ◆ ketamine ◆ metoclopramide ◆ midazolam ◆ ondansetron ◆ perphenazine ◆ prochlorperazine ◆ promethazine ◆ ranitidine ◆ scopolamine.

■ **Syringe Incompatibility:** ◆ heparin ◆ pentobarbital.

■ **Y-Site Compatibility:** ◆ amifostine ◆ amikacin ◆ ampicillin ◆ ampicillin/sulbactam ◆ atenolol ◆ aztreonam ◆ bumetanide ◆ cefazolin ◆ cefotaxime ◆ cefotetan ◆ cefoxitin ◆ ceftazidime ◆ ceftizoxime ◆ ceftriaxone ◆ cefuroxime ◆ chloramphenicol ◆ cisatracurium ◆ cladribine ◆ clindamycin ◆ dexamethasone ◆ diltiazem ◆ diphenhydramine ◆ dobutamine ◆ docetaxel ◆ dopamine ◆ doxycycline ◆ droperidol ◆ erythromycin lactobionate ◆ etoposide phosphate ◆ famotidine ◆ filgrastim ◆ fluconazole ◆ fludarabine ◆ gatifloxacin ◆ gemcitabine ◆ gentamicin ◆ granisetron ◆ heparin ◆ hydrocortisone sodium succinate ◆ insulin ◆ kanamycin ◆ labetalol ◆ lidocaine ◆ linezolid ◆ magnesium sulfate ◆ melphalan ◆

methyldopate ◆ methylprednisolone ◆ metoclopramide ◆ metoprolol ◆ metronidazole ◆ ondansetron ◆ oxacillin ◆ oxytocin ◆ paclitaxel ◆ penicillin G potassium ◆ piperacillin ◆ piperacillin/tazobactam ◆ potassium chloride ◆ propofol ◆ propranolol ◆ ranitidine ◆ remifentanil ◆ sargramostim ◆ teniposide ◆ thiotepa ◆ ticarcillin ◆ ticarcillin/clavulanate ◆ tobramycin ◆ trimethoprim/sulfamethoxazole ◆ vancomycin ◆ verapamil ◆ vinorelbine.

■ **Y-Site Incompatibility:** ◆ allopurinol ◆ amphotericin B cholesteryl sulfate ◆ cefepime ◆ cefoperazone ◆ doxorubicin liposome ◆ idarubicin ◆ imipenem/cilastatin ◆ minocycline.

## PATIENT/FAMILY TEACHING

□ Instruct patient on how and when to ask for pain medication.

□ Instruct patient to take meperidine as directed. If dose is less effective after a few weeks, do not increase dose without consulting health care professional.

□ May cause drowsiness or dizziness. Advise patient to call for assistance when ambulating or smoking. Caution patient to avoid driving or other activities requiring alertness until response to medication is known.

□ Advise patient to change positions slowly to minimize orthostatic hypotension.

□ Instruct patient to avoid concurrent use of alcohol or other CNS depressants.

□ Advise ambulatory patients that nausea and vomiting may be decreased by lying down.

□ Encourage patient to turn, cough, and breathe deeply every 2 hr to prevent atelectasis.

## EVALUATION

**Effectiveness of therapy can be demonstrated by:** ■ Decrease in severity of pain without a significant alteration in level of consciousness or respiratory status.

## mesalamine
(me-**sal**-a-meen)
Asacol, Canasa, Pentasa, Rowasa, {Salofalk}

{ } = Available in Canada only.
*CAPITALS indicates life-threatening; underlines indicate most frequent.

## INDICATIONS

■ Inflammatory bowel diseases including: ❑ Ulcerative colitis ❑ Proctitis ❑ Proctosigmoiditis.

## ACTION

■ Locally acting anti-inflammatory action in the colon, where activity is probably due to inhibition of prostaglandin synthesis. **Therapeutic Effects:** ■ Reduction in the symptoms of inflammatory bowel disease.

## PHARMACOKINETICS

**Absorption:** 28% absorbed following oral administration; 10–30% absorbed from the colon, depending on retention time, following rectal administration.
**Distribution:** Unknown.
**Metabolism and Excretion:** Some metabolism occurs, site unknown; mostly eliminated unchanged in the feces.
**Half-life:** 12 hr PO (range 2–15 hr); 0.5–1.5 hr rectal.

## CONTRAINDICATIONS AND PRECAUTIONS

**Contraindicated in:** ■ Hypersensitivity reactions to sulfonamides, salicylates, mesalamine, or sulfasalazine ■ Cross-sensitivity with furosemide, sulfonylurea hypoglycemic agents, or carbonic anhydrase inhibitors may exist ■ G6PD deficiency ■ Hypersensitivity to bisulfites (mesalamine enema only) ■ Urinary tract or intestinal obstruction ■ Porphyria.
**Use Cautiously in:** ■ Severe hepatic or renal impairment ■ Pregnancy (safety not established) ■ Lactation (safety not established).

## ADVERSE REACTIONS AND SIDE EFFECTS*

■ **CNS:** <u>headache</u>, dizziness, malaise, weakness ■ **EENT:** pharyngitis, rhinitis ■ **CV:** pericarditis ■ **GI:** diarrhea, eructation (PO), flatulence, nausea, vomiting ■ **GU:** interstitial nephritis, pancreatitis, renal failure ■ **Derm:** hair loss, rash ■ **Local:** anal irritation (enema, suppository) ■ **MS:** back pain ■ **Misc:** ANAPHYLAXIS, acute intolerance syndrome, fever.

## INTERACTIONS

**Drug-Drug:** ■ May ↓ metabolism and increase effects/toxicity of **mercaptopurine** or **thioguanine**.

## ROUTE AND DOSAGE

■ **PO (Adults):** 800 mg 3 times daily for 6 wk as delayed-release tablets *or* 1 g 4 times daily as extended-release capsules.
■ **Rect (Adults):** 4-g enema (60 ml) at bedtime, retained for 8 hr for 3–6 wk *or* 500-mg suppository twice daily for 2 wk, may be increased to three times daily if necessary.

## AVAILABILITY

■*Delayed-release tablets:* {250 mg$^{Rx}$}, 400 mg$^{Rx}$, {500 mg$^{Rx}$} ■Cost: 250 mg $130.06/240, 400 mg $90.54/100 ■ *Extended-release capsules:* 250 mg$^{Rx}$ ■ *Extended-release tablets:* {250 mg$^{Rx}$}, {500 mg$^{Rx}$} ■ *Suppositories:* 500 mg$^{Rx}$ ■*Rectal suspension:* 4 g/60 ml$^{Rx}$.

TIME/ACTION PROFILE (clinical improvement)

|  | ONSET | PEAK | Duration |
|---|---|---|---|
| PO | unknown | unknown | 6–8 hr |
| Rectal | 3–21 days | unknown | 24 hr |

# NURSING IMPLICATIONS

## ASSESSMENT

■ **General Info:** Assess patient for allergy to sulfonamides and salicylates. Patients allergic to sulfasalazine may take mesalamine or olsalazine without difficulty, but therapy should be discontinued if rash or fever occurs.
❑ Monitor intake and output ratios. Fluid intake should be sufficient to maintain a urine output of at least 1200–1500 ml daily to prevent crystalluria and stone formation.
■ **Inflammatory Bowel Disease:** Assess abdominal pain and frequency, quantity, and consistency of stools at the beginning of and during therapy.
■ *Lab Test Considerations:* Monitor urinalysis, BUN, and serum creatinine prior to and periodically during therapy. Mesalamine may cause renal toxicity.
❑ Mesalamine may cause ↑ AST and ALT levels, serum alkaline phosphatase, GGTP, LDH, amylase, and lipase.

## POTENTIAL NURSING DIAGNOSES

- Pain, acute (Indications).
- Diarrhea (Indications).

## IMPLEMENTATION

- **General:** Do not confuse Asacol (mesalamine) with Os-Cal (calcium carbonate).
- **PO:** Administer before meals and at bedtime with a full glass of water. Tablets should be swallowed whole; do not break the outer coating, which is designed to remain intact. Intact or partially intact tablets may occasionally be found in the stool. If this occurs repeatedly, advise patient to notify health care professional.
- **Rect:** Patient should empty bowel prior to administration of rectal dose forms.
- ❑ Avoid excessive handling of *suppository*. Remove foil wrapper and insert pointed end first into rectum with gentle pressure. Suppository should be retained for 1–3 hr or more for maximum benefit.
- ❑ Administer 60-ml retention enema once daily at bedtime. Solution should be retained for approximately 8 hr. Prior to administration of *rectal suspension*, shake bottle well and remove the protective cap. Have patient lie on left side with the lower leg extended and the upper leg flexed for support or place the patient in knee-chest position. Gently insert the applicator tip into the rectum, pointing toward the umbilicus. Squeeze the bottle steadily to discharge most of the preparation.

## PATIENT/FAMILY TEACHING

- **General Info:** Instruct patient on the correct method of administration. Advise patient to take medication as directed, even if feeling better. If a dose is missed, it should be taken as soon as remembered unless almost time for next dose.
- ❑ May cause dizziness. Caution patient to avoid driving or other activities that require alertness until response to medication is known.
- ❑ Advise patient to notify health care professional if skin rash, sore throat, fever, mouth sores, unusual bleeding or bruising, wheezing, fever, or hives occur.

- ❑ Instruct patient to notify health care professional if symptoms do not improve after 1–2 mo of therapy.
- ❑ Instruct patient to notify health care professional if symptoms worsen or do not improve. If symptoms of acute intolerance (cramping, acute abdominal pain, bloody diarrhea, fever, headache, rash) occur, discontinue therapy and notify health care professional immediately.
- ❑ Inform patient that proctoscopy and sigmoidoscopy may be required periodically during treatment to determine response.
- **Rect:** Instruct patient to use *rectal suspension* at bedtime and retain suspension all night for best results.
- ❑ Advise patient not to change brands of mesalamine without consulting health care professional.

## EVALUATION

**Clinical response to therapy can be evaluated by:** ■ Decrease in diarrhea and abdominal pain ■ Return to normal bowel pattern in patients with inflammatory bowel disease. Effects may be seen within 3–21 days. The usual course of therapy is 3–6 wk ■ Maintenance of remission in patients with inflammatory bowel disease.

---

## mesna

**(mes**-na)
Mesnex, {Uromitexan}

### CLASSIFICATION(S):
***Therapeutic:*** *antidotes*
***Pharmacologic:*** *ifosfamide detoxifying agents*

### Pregnancy Category B

---

## INDICATIONS

■ Prevention of ifosfamide-induced hemorrhagic cystitis (see Ifosfamide monograph). **Unlabeled uses:** ■ May also prevent hemorrhagic cystitis from cyclophosphamide.

---

{ } = Available in Canada only.
*CAPITALS indicates life-threatening; underlines indicate most frequent.

## ACTION

■ Binds to the toxic metabolites of ifosfamide in the kidneys. **Therapeutic Effects:** ■ Prevents hemorrhagic cystitis from ifosfamide.

## PHARMACOKINETICS

**Absorption:** IV administration results in complete bioavailability; 45–79% absorbed after oral administration. Following IV with PO dosing increases systemic exposure.

**Distribution:** Unknown.

**Metabolism and Excretion:** Rapidly converted to mesna disulfide, then back to mesna in the kidneys, where it binds to toxic metabolites of ifosfamide (18–26% excreted as free mesna in urine after IV and PO dosing).

**Half-life:** *Mesna*—0.36 hr (IV); 1.2—8.3 hr (IV followed by PO); *mesna disulfide*—1.17 hr.

## CONTRAINDICATIONS AND PRECAUTIONS

**Contraindicated in:** ■ Hypersensitivity to mesna or other thiol (rubber) compounds.

**Use Cautiously in:** ■ Pregnancy or lactation (safety not established).

## ADVERSE REACTIONS AND SIDE EFFECTS*

■ **CNS:** dizziness, drowsiness, headache ■ **GI:** anorexia, diarrhea, nausea, unpleasant taste, vomiting ■ **Derm:** flushing ■ **Local:** injection site reactions ■ **Misc:** flu-like symptoms.

## INTERACTIONS

**Drug-Drug:** ■ None significant.

## ROUTE AND DOSAGE

■ **IV (Adults):** Give a dose of mesna equal to 20% of the ifosfamide dose at the same time as ifosfamide and 4 and 8 hr after.

■ **PO, IV (Adults):** Give a dose of IV mesna equal to 20% of the ifosfamide dose at the same time as ifosfamide; then give PO mesna equal to 40% of the ifosfamide dose 2 and 6 hours after ifosfamide (total mesna dose is 100% of ifosfamide dose).

## AVAILABILITY

■ *Tablets:* 400 mg^Rx ■ *Injection:* 100 mg/ml in 2-, 4-, and 10-ml ampules^Rx ■ In a kit with ifosfamide.

TIME/ACTION PROFILE (detoxifying action)

| | ONSET | PEAK | DURATION |
|---|---|---|---|
| PO, IV | rapid | unknown | 4 hr |

# NURSING IMPLICATIONS

## ASSESSMENT

❑ Monitor for development of hemorrhagic cystitis in patients receiving ifosfamide.

■ *Lab Test Considerations:* Causes a false-positive result when testing urinary ketones.

## POTENTIAL NURSING DIAGNOSES

■ Knowledge, deficient, related to medication regimen (Patient/Family Teaching).

## IMPLEMENTATION

■ **General:** Initial IV bolus is to be given at time of ifosfamide administration.

■ **PO:** If second and third doses are given orally, administer 2 and 6 hours after IV dose.

❑ If PO mesna is vomited within 2 hr of administration, repeat dose or use IV mesna.

■ **Intermittent Infusion:** 2nd IV dose is given 4 hr later, 3rd dose is given 8 hr after initial dose. This schedule must be repeated with each subsequent dose of ifosfamide. Dilute 2-, 4-, and 10-ml ampules, containing a concentration of 100 mg/ml in 8 ml, 16 ml, or 50 ml, respectively, of D5W, 0.9% NaCl, D5/0.9% NaCl, D5/0.2% NaCl, D5/0.33% NaCl, or LR, for a final concentration of 20 mg/ml. Refrigerate to store. Use within 6 hr. Discard unused solution. Administer over 15–30 min or as a continuous infusion.

■ **Syringe Compatibility:** ◆ ifosfamide.

■ **Y-Site Compatibility:** ◆ allopurinol ◆ amifostine ◆ aztreonam ◆ cefepime ◆ docetaxel ◆ doxorubicin liposome ◆ etoposide ◆ filgrastim ◆ fludarabine ◆ gatifloxacin ◆ gemcitabine ◆ granisetron ◆ linezolid ◆ melphalan ◆ methotrexate ◆ ondansetron ◆ paclitaxel ◆ piperacillin/tazobactam ◆ sargramostim ◆ sodium bicarbonate ◆ teniposide ◆ thiotepa ◆ vinorelbine.

■ **Y-Site Incompatibility:** ◆ amphotericin B cholesteryl complex.

■ **Additive Compatibility:** ◆ cyclophosphamide ◆ ifosfamide.

■ **Additive Incompatibility:** ◆ carboplatin ◆ cisplatin.

## PATIENT/FAMILY TEACHING

❑ Inform patient that unpleasant taste may occur during administration.

❑ Advise patient to notify health care professional if nausea, vomiting, or diarrhea persists or is severe.

## EVALUATION

**Effectiveness of therapy can be demonstrated by:** ■ Prevention of hemorrhagic cystitis associated with ifosfamide therapy.

## mestranol/norethindrone, See CONTRACEPTIVES, HORMONAL.

## metaproterenol

(met-a-proe-**ter**-e-nole)
Alupent

**CLASSIFICATION(S):**
**Therapeutic:** bronchodilators
**Pharmacologic:** adrenergics

**Pregnancy Category C**

## INDICATIONS

■ Treatment/prevention of bronchospasm due to reversible airway disease (a short-term control agent).

## ACTION

■ Results in the accumulation of cyclic adenosine monophosphate (cAMP) at beta-adrenergic receptors ■ Produces bronchodilation ■ Inhibits the release of mediators of immediate hypersensitivity reactions from mast cells ■ Relatively selective for beta$_2$(pulmonary)-adrenergic receptor sites, with less effect on beta$_1$(cardiac)-adrenergic receptors. **Therapeutic Effects:** ■ Bronchodilation.

## PHARMACOKINETICS

**Absorption:** Small amounts may be systemically absorbed following inhalation, but rapidly undergo extensive metabolism.
**Distribution:** Unknown.
**Metabolism and Excretion:** Extensively metabolized by the liver and other tissues.

**Half-life:** Unknown.

## CONTRAINDICATIONS AND PRECAUTIONS

**Contraindicated in:** ■ Hypersensitivity to adrenergic amines ■ Selected products may contain bisulfites, alcohol (in some oral liquid preparations), or fluorocarbons (in some inhalers) and should be avoided in patients with known hypersensitivity or intolerance.

**Use Cautiously in:** ■ Cardiac disease ■ Hypertension ■ Hyperthyroidism ■ Diabetes ■ Glaucoma ■ Elderly patients (more susceptible to adverse reactions; may require dosage reduction) ■ Excessive use may lead to tolerance and paradoxical bronchospasm (inhaler) ■ Pregnancy (near term), lactation, and children <12 yr (safety not established).

## ADVERSE REACTIONS AND SIDE EFFECTS*

■ **CNS:** nervousness, restlessness, tremor, headache, insomnia ■ **Resp:** PARADOXICAL BRONCHOSPASM (excessive use of inhalers) ■ **CV:** angina, arrhythmias, hypertension, tachycardia ■ **GI:** nausea, vomiting ■ **Endo:** hyperglycemia.

## INTERACTIONS

**Drug-Drug:** ■ Concurrent use with other **adrenergics (sympathomimetic)** will have additive adrenergic side effects ■ Use with **MAO inhibitors** may lead to hypertensive crisis ■ **Beta blockers** may negate therapeutic effect.

**Drug-Natural Products:** ■ Use with caffeine-containing herbs (**cola nut, guarana, mate, tea, coffee**) increases stimulant effect.

## ROUTE AND DOSAGE

■ **Inhaln (Adults >12 yr):** *Metered-dose inhaler*—2–3 inhalations q 3–4 hr (not to exceed 12 inhalations/day). *IPPB*—0.2–0.3 ml of 5% solution or 2.5 ml of 0.4–0.6% solution for nebulization 3–4 times daily (not to exceed q 4 hr use).

## AVAILABILITY (generic available)

■ *Inhalation aerosol:* 650 mcg/spray (100 inhalations/5 ml)$^{Rx}$, {750 mcg/spray (100 inhalations/5 ml)$^{Rx}$} ■ *Inhalation solution:* 0.4%$^{Rx}$, 0.6%$^{Rx}$, 5%$^{Rx}$.

---

{ } = Available in Canada only.
*CAPITALS indicates life-threatening; underlines indicate most frequent.

TIME/ACTION PROFILE (bronchodilation)

| | ONSET | PEAK | DURATION |
|---|---|---|---|
| Inhaln-aerosol | within 1 min | 1 hr | 1–5 hr |
| Inhaln-IPPB | 5–30 min | unknown | 2–6 hr |

# NURSING IMPLICATIONS

## ASSESSMENT

- **Bronchodilator:** Assess lung sounds, respiratory pattern, pulse, and blood pressure before administration and during peak of medication. Note amount, color, and character of sputum produced. Report abnormal findings.
- Monitor pulmonary function tests before initiating therapy and periodically throughout course to determine effectiveness of medication.
- Observe for paradoxical bronchospasm (wheezing). If condition occurs, withhold medication and notify physician or other health care provider immediately.
- Observe patient for drug tolerance and rebound bronchospasm. Patients requiring more than 3 inhalation treatments in 24 hr should be under close supervision. If minimal or no relief is seen after 3–5 inhalation treatments within 6–12 hr, further treatment with aerosol alone is not recommended.
- **Lab Test Considerations:** May cause decreased serum potassium concentrations, which are usually transient and dose related; rarely occurs at recommended doses and is more pronounced with frequent use of high doses.
- **Toxicity and Overdose:** Symptoms of overdose include persistent agitation, chest pain or discomfort, decreased blood pressure, dizziness, hyperglycemia, hypokalemia, seizures, tachyarrhythmias, persistent trembling, and vomiting.
- Treatment includes discontinuing beta-adrenergic agonists and symptomatic, supportive therapy. Cardioselective beta-adrenergic blocking agents are used cautiously, as they may induce bronchospasm.

## POTENTIAL NURSING DIAGNOSES

- Airway clearance, ineffective (Indications).

## IMPLEMENTATION

- **General:** Do not confuse Alupent (metaproterenol) with Atrovent (ipratropium).
- **Inhaln:** For IPPB administration, dilute each dose in 2.5 ml of 0.9% NaCl. Do not use if solution is brown or darker than slightly yellow, pinkish, or if it contains a precipitate.

## PATIENT/FAMILY TEACHING

- **General Info:** Instruct patient to take medication exactly as directed. If on a scheduled dosing regimen, take a missed dose as soon as possible; space remaining doses at regular intervals. Do not double doses. Caution patient not to exceed recommended dose; may cause adverse effects, paradoxical bronchospasm, or loss of effectiveness of medication.
- Instruct patient to contact health care professional immediately if shortness of breath is not relieved by medication or is accompanied by diaphoresis, dizziness, palpitations, or chest pain.
- Advise patient to consult health care professional before taking any OTC medications or alcoholic beverages concurrently with this therapy. Caution patient also to avoid smoking and other respiratory irritants.
- **Inhaln:** Review correct administration technique (aerosolization, IPPB, metered-dose inhaler) with patient. See Appendix F for administration with metered-dose inhaler. Wait 1–5 min before administering next dose. Mouthpiece should be washed after each use.
- Do not spray inhaler near eyes.
- Instruct patient to save inhaler; refill canisters may be available.
- Advise patient to use bronchodilator first if using other inhalation medications, and allow 5 min to elapse before administering other inhalant medications, unless otherwise directed.
- Advise patient to rinse mouth with water after each inhalation dose to minimize dry mouth.
- Advise patient to maintain adequate fluid intake (2000–3000 ml/day) to help liquefy tenacious secretions.
- Instruct patient to notify health care professional if contents of one canister are used up in less than 2 wk.

## EVALUATION
**Effectiveness of therapy can be demonstrated by:** ▪ Prevention or relief of bronchospasm ▪ Increase in ease of breathing ▪ Prevention of exercise-induced asthma.

# metaxalone
(me-**tax**-a-lone)
Skelaxin

## CLASSIFICATION(S):
**Therapeutic:** skeletal muscle relaxants (centrally acting)

**Pregnancy Category UK**

## INDICATIONS
▪ Muscle spasm associated with acute painful musculoskeletal conditions (with rest and physical therapy).

## ACTION
▪ Skeletal muscle relaxation, probably as a result of CNS depression. **Therapeutic Effects:**
▪ Skeletal muscle relaxation.

## PHARMACOKINETICS
**Absorption:** Well absorbed following oral administration.
**Distribution:** Unknown.
**Metabolism and Excretion:** Mostly metabolized by the liver; metabolites excreted in urine.
**Half-life:** 2–3 hr.

## CONTRAINDICATIONS AND PRECAUTIONS
**Contraindicated in:** ▪ Hypersensitivity ▪ Significant hepatic/renal impairment ▪ History of drug-induced hemolytic anemia or other anemia.
**Use Cautiously in:** ▪ History of seizures ▪ Pregnancy, lactation, or children ≤12 yr (safety not established; use only in pregnancy/lactation if possible benefits outweigh potential risks).

## ADVERSE REACTIONS AND SIDE EFFECTS*
▪ **CNS:** <u>drowsiness</u>, <u>dizziness</u>, confusion, headache, irritability, nervousness ▪ **GI:** <u>nausea</u>, anorexia, dry mouth, GI upset, vomiting ▪ **GU:** urinary retention.

## INTERACTIONS
**Drug-Drug:** ▪ ↑ CNS depression with other **CNS depressants** including **alcohol, antihistamines, opioid analgesics,** and **sedative/ hypnotics.**
**Drug-Natural Products:** ▪ Concomitant use of **kava, valerian,** or **chamomile** can ↑ CNS depression.

## ROUTE AND DOSAGE
▪ **PO (Adults):** 800 mg 3–4 times daily.

## AVAILABILITY
▪ **Tablets:** 400 mg$^{Rx}$, 800 mg$^{Rx}$ ▪ Cost: $400 mg 89.11/100.

TIME/ACTION PROFILE

|  | ONSET | PEAK | DURATION |
|----|----|----|----|
| PO | 1 hr | 2 hr | 4–6 hr |

# NURSING IMPLICATIONS

## ASSESSMENT
❑ Assess patient for pain, muscle stiffness, and range of motion before and periodically during therapy.
▪ **Lab Test Considerations:** Monitor hepatic function tests closely in patients with pre-existing liver damage.
❑ May cause false-positive Benedict's tests.

## POTENTIAL NURSING DIAGNOSES
▪ Pain, acute (Indications).
▪ Mobility, impaired bed (Indications).
▪ Injury, risk for (Side Effects).

## IMPLEMENTATION
▪ **General:** Provide safety measures as indicated. Supervise ambulation and transfer of patients.
▪ **PO:** Administer 3–4 times daily.

## PATIENT/FAMILY TEACHING
❑ Instruct patient to take medication as directed. Take missed doses within 1 hr; if not, return to regular dosing schedule. Do not double doses.

---

{ } = Available in Canada only.
*CAPITALS indicates life-threatening; <u>underlines</u> indicate most frequent.

- ❑ Encourage patient to comply with additional therapies prescribed for muscle spasm (rest, physical therapy, heat).
- ❑ Medication may cause dizziness, drowsiness, and blurred vision. Advise patient to avoid driving and other activities requiring alertness until response to drug is known.
- ❑ Instruct patient to make position changes slowly to minimize orthostatic hypotension.
- ❑ Advise patient to avoid concurrent use of alcohol and other CNS depressants while taking this medication.
- ❑ Instruct patient to notify health care professional if skin rash or yellowish discoloration of the skin or eyes occurs.
- ❑ Emphasize the importance of routine follow-up exams to monitor progress.

## EVALUATION

**Effectiveness of therapy can be demonstrated by:** ■ Decreased musculoskeletal pain and muscle spasticity ❑ Increased range of motion.

---

## metformin
(met-**for**-min)
Glucophage, Glucophage XR, {Novo-Metformin}

**CLASSIFICATION(S):**
**Therapeutic:** antidiabetics
**Pharmacologic:** biguanides

**Pregnancy Category B**

---

## INDICATIONS

■ Management of type 2 diabetes mellitus; may be used with diet, insulin, or sulfonylurea oral hypoglycemics.

## ACTION

■ Decreases hepatic glucose production ■ Decreases intestinal glucose absorption ■ Increases sensitivity to insulin. **Therapeutic Effects:** ■ Maintenance of blood glucose.

## PHARMACOKINETICS

**Absorption:** 50–60% absorbed after oral administration.
**Distribution:** Enters breast milk in concentrations similar to plasma.

**Metabolism and Excretion:** Eliminated almost entirely unchanged by the kidneys.
**Half-life:** 17.6 hr.

## CONTRAINDICATIONS AND PRECAUTIONS

**Contraindicated in:** ■ Hypersensitivity ■ Metabolic acidosis ■ Dehydration, sepsis, hypoxemia, hepatic impairment, excessive alcohol use (acute or chronic) ■ Renal dysfunction (serum creatinine >1.5 mg/dl in men or >1.4 mg/dl in women) ■ Radiographic studies requiring IV iodinated contrast media (withhold metformin) ■ CHF.

**Use Cautiously in:** ■ Concurrent renal disease ■ Geriatric/debilitated patients ( ↓ doses may be required; avoid in patients >80 yr unless renal function is normal) ■ Chronic alcohol use/abuse ■ Serious medical conditions (MI, stroke) ■ Patients undergoing stress (infection, surgical procedures) ■ Hypoxia ■ Pituitary deficiency or hyperthyroidism ■ Pregnancy, lactation, or children <10 yr (safety not established; extended release for use in patients >17 yr only).

## ADVERSE REACTIONS AND SIDE EFFECTS*

■ **GI:** abdominal bloating, diarrhea, nausea, vomiting, unpleasant metallic taste ■ **Endo:** hypoglycemia ■ **F and E:** LACTIC ACIDOSIS ■ **Misc:** decreased vitamin $B_{12}$ levels.

## INTERACTIONS

**Drug-Drug:** ■ Acute or chronic **alcohol** ingestion or **iodinated contrast media** ↑ risk of lactic acidosis ■ **Amiloride, digoxin, morphine, procainamide, quinidine, ranitidine, triamterene, trimethoprim, calcium channel blockers,** and **vancomycin** may compete for elimination pathways with metformin. Altered responses may occur ■ **Cimetidine** and **furosemide** may ↑ effects of metformin ■ **Nifedipine** ↑ absorption and effects.
**Drug-Natural Products:** ■ **Glucosamine** may worsen blood glucose control ■ **Fenugreek, chromium,** and **coenzyme Q-10** may produce ↑ hypoglycemic effects.

## ROUTE AND DOSAGE

■ **PO (Adults and children >17 yr):** 500 mg twice daily; may increase by 500 mg at weekly intervals up to 2000 mg/day. If doses >2000 mg/day are required, give in 3 divided doses (not to exceed 2500 mg/day) or 850 mg once daily; may increase by 850 mg at 2-wk intervals (in divided doses) up to 2550 mg/day in divided doses (up to 850 mg 3 times daily); *Extended-release tablets—* 500 mg once daily with evening meal, may increase by 500 mg at weekly intervals up to 2000 mg once daily. If 2000 mg once daily is inadequate, 1000 mg twice daily may be used.

■ **PO (Children >10 yr):** 500 mg twice daily, may be increased by 500 mg/day at 1–wk intervals, up to 2000 mg/day in 2 divided doses.

## AVAILABILITY (generic available)

■ *Tablets:* 500 mg^{Rx}, 850 mg^{Rx}, 1000 mg^{Rx} ■ Cost: 500 mg $78.26/100, 850 mg $133.04/100, 1000 mg $161.22/100 ■ *Extended-release tablets (Glucophage XR):* 500 mg^{Rx}, 750 mg^{Rx} ■ with glyburide (Glucovance^{Rx}).

TIME/ACTION PROFILE (control of blood glucose)

| | ONSET | PEAK | DURATION |
|---|---|---|---|
| PO | several days | 2–4 wk | 12 hr (24 hr for extended release tablets) |

# NURSING IMPLICATIONS

## ASSESSMENT

❏ Observe patient for signs and symptoms of hypoglycemic reactions (abdominal pain, sweating, hunger, weakness, dizziness, headache, tremor, tachycardia, anxiety) when combined with oral sulfonylureas.

❏ Patients who have been well controlled on metformin who develop illness or laboratory abnormalities should be assessed for ketoacidosis or lactic acidosis. Assess serum electrolytes, ketones, glucose, and, if indicated, blood pH, lactate, pyruvate, and metformin levels. If either form of acidosis is present, discontinue metformin immediately and treat acidosis.

■ *Lab Test Considerations:* Serum glucose and glycosylated hemoglobin should be monitored periodically throughout therapy to evaluate effectiveness of therapy. May cause false-positive results for urine ketones.

❏ Blood glucose concentrations should be monitored routinely by patient and every 3 mo by health care professional to determine effectiveness of therapy.

❏ Assess renal function before initiating and at least annually throughout therapy. Discontinue metformin if renal impairment occurs.

❏ Monitor serum folic acid and vitamin B$_{12}$ every 1–2 yr in long-term therapy. Metformin may interfere with absorption.

## POTENTIAL NURSING DIAGNOSES

■ Nutrition, imbalanced: more than body requirements (Indications).

■ Noncompliance (Patient/Family Teaching).

## IMPLEMENTATION

■ **General:** Patients stabilized on a diabetic regimen who are exposed to stress, fever, trauma, infection, or surgery may require administration of insulin. Withhold metformin and reinstitute after resolution of acute episode.

❏ Metformin therapy should be temporarily discontinued in patients requiring surgery involving restricted intake of food and fluids. Resume metformin when oral intake has resumed and renal function is normal.

❏ Withhold metformin before or at the time of studies requiring IV administration of iodinated contrast media and for 48 hr after study.

■ **PO:** Administer metformin with meals to minimize GI effects.

❏ XR tablets must be swallowed whole; do not crush or chew.

## PATIENT/FAMILY TEACHING

❏ Instruct patient to take metformin at the same time each day, exactly as directed. If a dose is missed, take as soon as possible unless almost time for next dose. Do not double doses.

❏ Explain to patient that metformin helps control hyperglycemia but does not cure diabetes. Therapy is usually long term.

❑ Encourage patient to follow prescribed diet, medication, and exercise regimen to prevent hyperglycemic or hypoglycemic episodes.

❑ Review signs of hypoglycemia and hyperglycemia with patient. If hypoglycemia occurs, advise patient to take a glass of orange juice or 2–3 tsp of sugar, honey, or corn syrup dissolved in water, and notify health care professional.

❑ Instruct patient in proper testing of blood glucose and urine ketones. These tests should be monitored closely during periods of stress or illness and health care professional notified if significant changes occur.

❑ Explain to patient the risk of lactic acidosis and the potential need for discontinuation of metformin therapy if a severe infection, dehydration, or severe or continuing diarrhea occurs or if medical tests or surgery is required. Symptoms of lactic acidosis (chills, diarrhea, dizziness, low blood pressure, muscle pain, sleepiness, slow heartbeat or pulse, dyspnea, or weakness) should be reported to health care professional immediately.

❑ Caution patient to avoid taking other prescription or OTC medications or alcohol during metformin therapy without consulting health care professional.

❑ Insulin is the recommended method of controlling blood glucose during pregnancy. Counsel female patients to use a form of contraception other than oral contraceptives and to notify health care professional promptly if pregnancy is planned or suspected.

❑ Inform patient that metformin may cause an unpleasant or metallic taste that usually resolves spontaneously.

❑ Inform patients taking XR tablets that inactive ingredients resembling XR tablet may appear in stools.

❑ Advise patient to inform health care professional of medication regimen before treatment or surgery.

❑ Advise patient to carry a form of sugar (sugar packets, candy) and identification describing disease process and medication regimen at all times.

❑ Advise patient to report the occurrence of diarrhea, nausea, vomiting, and stomach pain or fullness to health care professional.

❑ Emphasize the importance of routine follow-up exams and regular testing of blood glucose, glycosylated hemoglobin, renal function, and hematologic parameters.

## EVALUATION

**Effectiveness of therapy can be demonstrated by:** ▪ Control of blood glucose levels without the appearance of hypoglycemic or hyperglycemic episodes. Control may be achieved within a few days, but full effect of therapy may be delayed for up to 2 wk. If patient has not responded to metformin after 4 wk of maximum dose therapy, an oral sulfonylurea may be added. If satisfactory results are not obtained with 1–3 mo of concurrent therapy, oral agents may be discontinued and insulin therapy instituted.

---

**High Alert**

# methadone

**(meth**-a-done)
Dolophine, Methadose

### CLASSIFICATION(S):
***Therapeutic:*** *opioid analgesics*
***Pharmacologic:*** *opioid agonists*

**Schedule II**

**Pregnancy Category C**

---

## INDICATIONS

▪ Severe pain ▪ Suppresses withdrawal symptoms in opioid detoxification.

## ACTION

▪ Binds to opiate receptors in the CNS ▪ Alters the perception of and response to painful stimuli, while producing generalized CNS depression. **Therapeutic Effects:** ▪ Decrease in severity of pain ▪ Suppression of withdrawal symptoms during detoxification and maintenance from heroin and other opioids.

## PHARMACOKINETICS

**Absorption:** Well absorbed from all sites (50% absorbed following oral administration).

**Distribution:** Widely distributed. Crosses the placenta; enters breast milk.

**Protein Binding:** High.

**Metabolism and Excretion:** Mostly metabolized by the liver; some metabolites are active and may accumulate with chronic administration.

**Half-life:** 15–25 hr; increases with chronic use.

## CONTRAINDICATIONS AND PRECAUTIONS

**Contraindicated in:** ■ Hypersensitivity ■ Known alcohol intolerance (some oral solutions) ■ Pregnancy or lactation (chronic use) ■ Concurrent MAO inhibitor therapy.

**Use Cautiously in:** ■ Head trauma ■ Increased intracranial pressure ■ Severe renal, hepatic, or pulmonary disease ■ Hypothyroidism ■ Adrenal insufficiency ■ Alcoholism ■ Geriatric or debilitated patients (dosage reduction suggested) ■ Undiagnosed abdominal pain ■ Prostatic hypertrophy or ureteral stricture.

## ADVERSE REACTIONS AND SIDE EFFECTS*

■ **CNS:** <u>confusion</u>, <u>sedation</u>, dizziness, dysphoria, euphoria, floating feeling, hallucinations, headache, unusual dreams ■ **EENT:** blurred vision, diplopia, miosis ■ **Resp:** respiratory depression ■ **CV:** <u>hypotension</u>, bradycardia ■ **GI:** <u>constipation</u>, nausea, vomiting ■ **GU:** urinary retention ■ **Derm:** flushing, sweating ■ **Misc:** physical dependence, psychological dependence, tolerance.

## INTERACTIONS

**Drug-Drug:** ■ Use with extreme caution in patients receiving **MAO inhibitors** (may result in severe, unpredictable reactions—reduce initial dose of methadone to 25% of usual dose) ■ Additive CNS depression with **alcohol, antihistamines,** and **sedative/hypnotics** ■ Concurrent **nevirapine** decreases blood levels and may induce withdrawal ■ Administration of **agonist/antagonist opioids** may precipitate opioid withdrawal in physically dependent patients ■ **Nalbuphine** or **pentazocine** may decrease analgesia ■ **Phenytoin** and **rifampin** may increase metabolism and decrease analgesia ■ **Fluvoxamine** may increase CNS depression; with **fluvoxamine,** opioid withdrawal may occur ■ May increase blood levels and effects of **desipramine.**

**Drug-Natural Products:** ■ Concomitant use of **kava, valerian, skullcap, chamomile,** or **hops** can increase CNS depression.

## ROUTE AND DOSAGE

Larger doses may be required for analgesia during chronic therapy; interval may be decreased/dosage increased if pain recurs.

■ **PO (Adults and Children ≥50 kg):** *Analgesic*—20 mg q 6–8 hr. *Opioid detoxification*—15–40 mg once daily or amount needed to prevent withdrawal. Dosage may be decreased q 1–2 days; maintenance dose is determined on an individual basis.

■ **PO (Adults and Children <50 kg):** *Analgesic*—0.2 mg/kg q 6–8 hr.

■ **IM, Subcut (Adults and Children ≥50 kg):** *Analgesic*—10 mg q 6–8 hr. *Opioid detoxification*—15–40 mg once daily or amount needed to prevent withdrawal. Dosage may be decreased q 1–2 days; maintenance dose is determined on an individual basis.

■ **IM, Subcut (Adults and Children <50 kg):** 0.1 mg/kg mg q 6–8 hr.

## AVAILABILITY (generic available)

■ *Tablets:* 5 mg$^{Rx}$, 10 mg$^{Rx}$ ■ *Dispersible tablets (diskettes):* 40 mg (available only to licensed detoxification/maintenance programs)$^{Rx}$ ■ *Oral solution:* 5 mg/5 ml$^{Rx}$, 10 mg/5 ml$^{Rx}$ ■ *Oral concentrate:* 10 mg/ml$^{Rx}$.

TIME/ACTION PROFILE (analgesic effect)

|  | ONSET | PEAK | DURATION |
|---|---|---|---|
| PO | 30–60 min | 90–120 min | 4–12 hr |
| IM, subcut | 10–20 min | 60–120 min | 4–6 hr |

# NURSING IMPLICATIONS

## ASSESSMENT

■ **Pain:** Assess type, location, and intensity of pain prior to and 1–2 hr (peak) following administration. When titrating opioid doses, increases of 25–50% should be administered until there is either a 50% reduction in the patient's pain rating on a numeric or visual analogue scale or the patient reports satisfactory pain relief. A repeat dose can be safely administered at the time of the peak if previous dose is ineffective and side effects are minimal. Cumulative effects of this medication may require periodic dosage adjustments.

❑ Doses of methadone for patients on methadone maintenance prevent only withdrawal symptoms; *no analgesia is provided.* Additional opioid doses are required for treatment of pain.

❑ An equianalgesic chart (see Appendix O) should be used when changing routes or when changing from one opioid to another.

❑ Assess blood pressure, pulse, and respirations before and periodically during administration. If respiratory rate is <10/min, assess level of sedation. Dose may need to be decreased by 25–50%. Initial drowsiness will diminish with continued use.

❑ Assess bowel function routinely. Prevention of constipation should be instituted with increased intake of fluids and bulk and with laxatives to minimize constipating effects. Stimulant laxatives should be administered routinely if opioid use exceeds 2–3 days, unless contraindicated.

❑ Prolonged use may lead to physical and psychological dependence and tolerance. This should not prevent patient from receiving adequate analgesia. Most patients who receive methadone for pain do not develop psychological dependence. Progressively higher doses may be required to relieve pain with long-term therapy.

■ **Opioid Detoxification:** Assess patient for signs of opioid withdrawal (irritability, runny nose and eyes, abdominal cramps, body aches, sweating, loss of appetite, shivering, unusually large pupils, trouble sleeping, weakness, yawning). Methadone maintenance is undertaken only by federally approved treatment centers. This does not preclude maintenance for addicts hospitalized for other conditions and who require temporary maintenance during their care.

■ *Lab Test Considerations:* May increase plasma amylase and lipase levels.

■ *Toxicity and Overdose:* If an opioid antagonist is required to reverse respiratory depression or coma, naloxone (Narcan) is the antidote. Dilute the 0.4-mg ampule of naloxone in 10 ml of 0.9% NaCl and administer 0.5 ml (0.02 mg) by direct IV push every 2 min. For children and patients weighing <40 kg, dilute 0.1 mg of naloxone in 10

ml of 0.9% NaCl for a concentration of 10 mcg/ml and administer 0.5 mcg/kg every 2 min. Titrate dose to avoid withdrawal, seizures, and severe pain.

## POTENTIAL NURSING DIAGNOSES

■ Pain, acute (Indications).

■ Sensory perception, disturbed (visual, auditory) (Side Effects).

■ Injury, risk for (Side Effects).

## IMPLEMENTATION

❑ *High Alert:* Accidental overdosage of opioid analgesics has resulted in fatalities. Before administering, clarify all ambiguous orders; have second practitioner independently check original order and dose calculations.

■ **General:** Explain therapeutic value of medication prior to administration to enhance the analgesic effect.

❑ Regularly administered doses may be more effective than prn administration. Analgesic is more effective if administered before pain becomes severe. For patients in chronic severe pain, the oral solution containing 5 or 10 mg/5 ml is recommended on a fixed dosage schedule.

❑ Coadministration with nonopioid analgesics may have additive analgesic effects and may permit lower doses.

❑ Medication should be discontinued gradually after long-term use to prevent withdrawal symptoms.

❑ Diskettes (dispersible tablets) are to be dissolved and used for detoxification and maintenance treatment only.

■ **PO:** Doses may be administered with food or milk to minimize GI irritation.

❑ Dilute each dose of 10 mg/ml oral concentrate with at least 30 ml of water or other liquid prior to administration.

■ **Subcut, IM:** IM is the preferred parenteral route for repeated doses. Subcut administration may cause tissue irritation.

## PATIENT/FAMILY TEACHING

❑ Instruct patient on how and when to ask for pain medication.

❑ Instruct patient to take methadone exactly as directed. If dose is less effective after a few weeks, do not increase dose without consulting health care professional.

- May cause drowsiness or dizziness. Advise patient to call for assistance when ambulating or smoking and to avoid driving or other activities requiring alertness until response to medication is known.
- Advise patient to change positions slowly to minimize orthostatic hypotension.
- Caution patient to avoid concurrent use of alcohol or other CNS depressants with this medication.
- Encourage patient to turn, cough, and breathe deeply every 2 hr to prevent atelectasis.

## EVALUATION

**Effectiveness of therapy can be demonstrated by:** ■ Decrease in severity of pain without a significant alteration in level of consciousness or respiratory status ■ Prevention of withdrawal symptoms in detoxification from heroin and other opioid analgesics.

## methimazole
(meth-**im**-a-zole)
Tapazole

*CLASSIFICATION(S):*
*Therapeutic: antithyroid agents*

**Pregnancy Category D**

## INDICATIONS

■ Palliative treatment of hyperthyroidism ■ Used as an adjunct to control hyperthyroidism in preparation for thyroidectomy or radioactive iodine therapy.

## ACTION

■ Inhibits the synthesis of thyroid hormones. **Therapeutic Effects:** ■ Decreased signs and symptoms of hyperthyroidism.

## PHARMACOKINETICS

**Absorption:** Rapidly absorbed following oral administration.

**Distribution:** Crosses the placenta and enters breast milk in high concentrations.

**Metabolism and Excretion:** Mostly metabolized by the liver; <10% eliminated unchanged by the kidneys.

**Half-life:** 3–5 hr.

## CONTRAINDICATIONS AND PRECAUTIONS

**Contraindicated in:** ■ Hypersensitivity ■ Lactation.

**Use Cautiously in:** ■ Patients with decreased bone marrow reserve ■ Patients >40 yr (increased risk of agranulocytosis) ■ Pregnancy (may be used cautiously; however, thyroid problems may occur in the fetus).

## ADVERSE REACTIONS AND SIDE EFFECTS*

■ **CNS:** drowsiness, headache, vertigo ■ **GI:** diarrhea, drug-induced hepatitis, loss of taste, nausea, parotitis, vomiting ■ **Derm:** rash, skin discoloration, urticaria ■ **Hemat:** AGRANULOCYTOSIS, anemia, leukopenia, thrombocytopenia ■ **MS:** arthralgia ■ **Misc:** fever, lymphadenopathy.

## INTERACTIONS

**Drug-Drug:** ■ Additive bone marrow depression with **antineoplastics** or **radiation therapy** ■ Antithyroid effect may be decreased by **potassium iodide** or **amiodarone** ■ Increased risk of agranulocytosis with **phenothiazines** ■ May alter response to **warfarin** and **digoxins.**

## ROUTE AND DOSAGE

- **PO (Adults):** *Thyrotoxic crisis*—15–20 mg q 4 hr during the first 24 hr (with other interventions). *Hyperthyroidism*—15–60 mg/day as a single dose or divided doses for 6–8 wk. *Maintenance*—5.30 mg/kg as a single dose or 2 divided doses.
- **PO (Children):** *Initial*—400 mcg (0.4 mg)/kg/day in single dose or 2 divided doses. *Maintenance*—200 mcg/kg/day in single dose or 2 divided doses.

## AVAILABILITY

- *Tablets:* 5 mg$^{Rx}$, 10 mg$^{Rx}$.

TIME/ACTION PROFILE (effect on thyroid function)

| | ONSET | PEAK | DURATION |
|---|---|---|---|
| PO | 1 wk | 4–10 wk | wks |

# NURSING IMPLICATIONS

## ASSESSMENT

- ❏ Monitor response for symptoms of hyperthyroidism or thyrotoxicosis (tachycardia, palpitations, nervousness, insomnia, fever, diaphoresis, heat intolerance, tremors, weight loss, diarrhea).
- ❏ Assess patient for development of hypothyroidism (intolerance to cold, constipation, dry skin, headache, listlessness, tiredness, or weakness). Dosage adjustment may be required.
- ❏ Assess patient for skin rash or swelling of cervical lymph nodes. Treatment may be discontinued if this occurs.
- ■ *Lab Test Considerations:* Thyroid function studies should be monitored prior to therapy, monthly during initial therapy, and every 2–3 mo throughout therapy.
- ❏ WBC and differential counts should be monitored periodically throughout therapy. Agranulocytosis may develop rapidly; it usually occurs during the first 2 mo and is more common in patients over 40 yr and those receiving >40 mg/day. This necessitates discontinuation of therapy.
- ❏ May cause increased AST, ALT, LDH, alkaline phosphatase, serum bilirubin, and prothrombin time.

## POTENTIAL NURSING DIAGNOSES

- ■ Noncompliance (Patient/Family Teaching).

## IMPLEMENTATION

- ■ **PO:** Administer at same time in relation to meals every day. Food may either increase or decrease absorption.

## PATIENT/FAMILY TEACHING

- ❏ Instruct patient to take medication exactly as directed, around the clock. If a dose is missed, take as soon as remembered; take both doses together if almost time for next dose; check with health care professional if more than 1 dose is missed. Consult health care professional prior to discontinuing medication.
- ❏ Instruct patient to monitor weight 2–3 times weekly. Notify health care professional of significant changes.
- ❏ May cause drowsiness. Caution patient to avoid driving or other activities requiring alertness until response to medication is known.
- ❏ Advise patient to consult health care professional regarding dietary sources of iodine (iodized salt, shellfish).
- ❏ Advise patient to report sore throat, fever, chills, headache, malaise, weakness, yellowing of eyes or skin, unusual bleeding or bruising, rash, or symptoms of hyperthyroidism or hypothyroidism promptly.
- ❏ Instruct patient to consult health care professional before taking any OTC medications.
- ❏ Advise patient to carry identification describing medication regimen at all times.
- ❏ Advise patient to notify health care professional of medication regimen prior to treatment or surgery.
- ❏ Emphasize the importance of routine exams to monitor progress and to check for side effects.

## EVALUATION

**Effectiveness of therapy can be demonstrated by:** ■ Decrease in severity of symptoms of hyperthyroidism (lowered pulse rate and weight gain) ■ Return of thyroid function studies to normal ■ May be used as short-term adjunctive therapy to prepare patient for thyroidectomy or radiation therapy or may be used in treatment of hyperthyroidism. Treatment from 6 mo to several years may be necessary, usually averaging 1 yr.

---

# methocarbamol
(meth-oh-**kar**-ba-mole)
Carbacot, Robaxin

## CLASSIFICATION(S):

*Therapeutic: skeletal muscle relaxants (centrally acting)*

**Pregnancy Category C**

## INDICATIONS

■ Adjunctive treatment of muscle spasm associated with acute painful musculoskeletal conditions (with rest and physical therapy).

## ACTION

■ Skeletal muscle relaxation, probably as a result of CNS depression. **Therapeutic Effects:** ■ Skeletal muscle relaxation.

## PHARMACOKINETICS

**Absorption:** Rapidly absorbed from the GI tract.

**Distribution:** Widely distributed. Crosses the placenta; enters breast milk in small amounts.

**Metabolism and Excretion:** Metabolized by the liver.

**Half-life:** 1–2 hr.

## CONTRAINDICATIONS AND PRECAUTIONS

**Contraindicated in:** ■ Hypersensitivity ■ Hypersensitivity to polyethylene glycol (parenteral only) ■ Renal impairment (parenteral form).

**Use Cautiously in:** ■ Pregnancy, lactation, and children (safety not established) ■ Seizure disorders (parenteral form).

## ADVERSE REACTIONS AND SIDE EFFECTS*

■ **CNS:** SEIZURES (IV, IM only), dizziness, drowsiness, light-headedness ■ **EENT:** blurred vision, nasal congestion ■ **CV:** *IV*—bradycardia, hypotension ■ **GI:** anorexia, GI upset, nausea ■ **GU:** brown, black, or green urine ■ **Derm:** flushing (IV only), pruritus, rashes, urticaria ■ **Local:** pain at IM site, phlebitis at IV site ■ **Misc:** allergic reactions including ANAPHYLAXIS (IM, IV use only), fever.

## INTERACTIONS

**Drug-Drug:** ■ Additive CNS depression with other **CNS depressants,** including **alcohol, antihistamines, opioid analgesics,** and **sedative/hypnotics.**

**Drug-Natural Products:** ■ Concomitant use of **kava, valerian, skullcap, chamomile,** or **hops** can increase CNS depression.

## ROUTE AND DOSAGE

■ **PO (Adults):** 1.5 g qid initially (up to 8 g/day) for 2–3 days, then 4–4.5 g/day in 3–6 divided doses; may be followed by maintenance dosing of 750 mg q 4 hr or 1 g 4 times daily or 1.5 g 3 times daily.

■ **IM, IV (Adults):** 1–3 g/day for not more than 3 days; course may be repeated after a 48-hr rest.

## AVAILABILITY (generic available)

■ *Tablets:* 500 mg$^{Rx}$, 750 mg$^{Rx}$ ■ Cost: *Robaxin*—500 mg $65.30/100, 750 mg $93.34/100; *generic*—500 mg $14.93/100, 750 mg $15.92/100 ■ *Injection:* {100 mg/ml in 10-ml ampules$^{Rx}$}, 100 mg/ml in 10-ml vials$^{Rx}$ ■ aspirin (Robaxisal)$^{Rx}$. See Appendix B.

TIME/ACTION PROFILE (skeletal muscle relaxation)

|     | ONSET | PEAK | DURATION |
| --- | --- | --- | --- |
| PO | 30 min | 2 hr | unknown |
| IM | rapid | unknown | unknown |
| IV | immediate | end of infusion | unknown |

# NURSING IMPLICATIONS

## ASSESSMENT

❑ Assess patient for pain, muscle stiffness, and range of motion before and periodically throughout therapy.

❑ Monitor pulse and blood pressure every 15 min during parenteral administration.

❑ Assess patient for allergic reactions (skin rash, asthma, hives, wheezing, hypotension) after parenteral administration. Keep epinephrine and oxygen on hand in the event of a reaction.

❑ Monitor IV site. Injection is hypertonic and may cause thrombophlebitis. Avoid extravasation.

■ *Lab Test Considerations:* Monitor renal function periodically during prolonged parenteral therapy (>3 days), because polyethylene glycol 300 vehicle is nephrotoxic.

❑ May cause falsely increased urinary 5-hydroxyindoleacetic acid (5-HIAA) and vanillylmandelic acid (VMA) determinations.

{ } = Available in Canada only.
* CAPITALS indicates life-threatening; underlines indicate most frequent.

## POTENTIAL NURSING DIAGNOSES

- Pain, acute (Indications).
- Mobility, impaired physical (Indications).
- Injury, risk for (Side Effects).

## IMPLEMENTATION

- **General:** Provide safety measures as indicated. Supervise ambulation and transfer of patients.
- **PO:** May be administered with food to minimize GI irritation. Tablets may be crushed and mixed with food or liquids to facilitate swallowing. For administration via NG tube, crush tablet and suspend in water or saline.
- **IM:** Do not administer subcut. IM injections should contain no more than 5 ml (500 mg) at a time in the gluteal region.
- **Direct IV:** Administer undiluted.
- *Rate:* Administer at a rate of 3 ml (300 mg) over 1 min.
- **Intermittent Infusion:** Dilute each dose in no more than 250 ml of 0.9% NaCl or D5W for injection. Do not refrigerate after dilution.
- Have patient remain recumbent during and for at least 10–15 min after infusion to avoid orthostatic hypotension.

## PATIENT/FAMILY TEACHING

- Advise patient to take medication exactly as directed. Missed doses should be taken within 1 hr; if not, return to regular dosing schedule. Do not double doses.
- Encourage patient to comply with additional therapies prescribed for muscle spasm (rest, physical therapy, heat).
- May cause dizziness, drowsiness, and blurred vision. Advise patient to avoid driving and other activities requiring alertness until response to drug is known.
- Instruct patient to change positions slowly to minimize orthostatic hypotension.
- Advise patient to avoid concurrent use of alcohol and other CNS depressants.
- Inform patient that urine may turn black, brown, or green, especially if left standing.
- Instruct patient to notify health care professional if skin rash, itching, fever, or nasal congestion occurs.
- Emphasize the importance of routine follow-up exams to monitor progress.

## EVALUATION

**Effectiveness of therapy can be demonstrated by:** ■ Decreased musculoskeletal pain and muscle spasticity ❏ Increased range of motion.

High Alert

# methotrexate

(meth-o-**trex**-ate)

amethopterin, Folex, Folex PFS, Rheumatrex, Trexall

### CLASSIFICATION(S):

*Therapeutic: antineoplastics, antirheumatics (DMARDs), immunosuppressants*
*Pharmacologic: antimetabolites*

### Pregnancy Category X

## INDICATIONS

■ Alone or with other treatment modalities in the treatment of: ❏ Trophoblastic neoplasms (choriocarcinoma, chorioadenoma destruens, hydatidiform mole) ❏ Leukemias ❏ Breast carcinoma ❏ Head carcinoma ❏ Neck carcinoma ❏ Lung carcinoma ■ Treatment of severe psoriasis and rheumatoid arthritis unresponsive to conventional therapy ■ Treatment of mycosis fungoides (cutaneous T-cell lymphoma).

## ACTION

■ Interferes with folic acid metabolism. Result is inhibition of DNA synthesis and cell reproduction (cell-cycle S-phase–specific) ■ Also has immunosuppressive activity. **Therapeutic Effects:** ■ Death of rapidly replicating cells, particularly malignant ones, and immunosuppression.

## PHARMACOKINETICS

**Absorption:** Small doses are well absorbed from the GI tract. Larger doses incompletely absorbed.
**Distribution:** Actively transported across cell membranes, widely distributed. Does not reach therapeutic concentrations in the CSF. Crosses placenta; enters breast milk in low concentrations. Absorption in children is variable (23–95%) and dose-dependent.
**Metabolism and Excretion:** Excreted mostly unchanged by the kidneys.

**Half-life:** *Low dose*—3–10 hr; *high dose*—8—15 hr (increased in renal impairment).

## CONTRAINDICATIONS AND PRECAUTIONS

**Contraindicated in:** ■ Hypersensitivity ■ Pregnancy or lactation ■ Products containing benzyl alcohol should not be used in neonates.

**Use Cautiously in:** ■ Renal impairment (CCr must be ≥60 ml/min prior to therapy) ■ Patients with childbearing potential ■ Active infections ■ Decreased bone marrow reserve ■ Geriatric patients or patients with other chronic debilitating illnesses.

## ADVERSE REACTIONS AND SIDE EFFECTS*

■ **CNS:** arachnoiditis (IT use only), dizziness, drowsiness, headaches, malaise ■ **EENT:** blurred vision, dysarthria transient blindness ■ **Resp:** PULMONARY FIBROSIS, interstitial pneumonitis ■ **GI:** anorexia, hepatotoxicity, nausea, stomatitis, vomiting ■ **GU:** infertility ■ **Derm:** alopecia, painful plaque erosions (during psoriasis treatment), photosensitivity, pruritus, rashes, skin ulceration, urticaria ■ **Hemat:** APLASTIC ANEMIA, anemia, leukopenia, thrombocytopenia ■ **Metab:** hyperuricemia ■ **MS:** osteonecrosis, stress fracture ■ **Misc:** nephropathy, chills, fever, soft tissue necrosis.

## INTERACTIONS

**Drug-Drug:** ■ The following drugs may ↑ hematologic toxicity of methotrexate: high-dose **salicylates, NSAIDs, oral hypoglycemic agents (sulfonylureas), phenytoin, tetracyclines, probenecid, trimethoprim/sulfamethoxazole, pyrimethamine,** and **chloramphenicol** ■ ↑ hepatotoxicity with other **hepatotoxic drugs** including **azathioprine, sulfasalazine,** and **retinoids** ■ ↑ nephrotoxicity with other **nephrotoxic drugs** ■ ↑ bone marrow depression with other **antineoplastics** or **radiation therapy** ■ **Radiation therapy** ↑ risk of soft tissue necrosis and osteonecrosis ■ May ↓ antibody response to **live-virus vaccines** and ↑ risk of adverse reactions ■ ↑ risk of neurologic reactions with **acyclovir** (IT methotrexate only) ■ **Asparaginase** may ↓ effects of methotrexate.

**Drug-Natural Products:** ■ Concomitant use with **echinacea** and **melatonin** may interfere with immunosuppression ■ **Caffeine** may ↓ efficacy of methotrexate, similar effect may occur with **guarana**.

## ROUTE AND DOSAGE

### ❏ Trophoblastic Neoplasms

■ **PO, IM (Adults):** 15–30 mg/day for 5 days; repeat after 1 or more weeks for 3–5 courses.

### ❏ Breast Cancer

■ **IV (Adults):** 40 mg/m² on days 1 and 8 (with other agents; many regimens are used).

### ❏ Leukemia

■ **PO (Adults):** *Induction*—3.3 mg/m²/day, usually with prednisone.

■ **PO, IM (Adults):** *Maintenance*—20–30 mg/m² twice weekly.

■ **IV (Adults):** 2.5 mg/kg q 2 wk.

■ **IT (Adults):** 12 mg/m² or 15 mg.

■ **IT (Children ≥3 yr):** 12 mg.

■ **IT (Children 2 yr):** 10 mg.

■ **IT (Children 1 yr):** 8 mg.

■ **IT (Children <1 yr):** 6 mg.

### ❏ Osteosarcoma

■ **IV (Adults):** 12 g/m² as a 4-hr infusion followed by leucovorin rescue, usually as part of a combination chemotherapeutic regimen (or increase dose until peak serum methotrexate level is $1 \times 10^{-3}$ M/L but not to exceed 15 g/m²; 12 courses are given starting 4 wk after surgery and repeated at scheduled intervals.

### ❏ Psoriasis

Therapy may be preceded by a 5–10-mg test dose.

■ **PO (Adults):** 2.5–5 mg q 12 hr for 3 doses *or* q 8 hr for 4 doses once weekly (not to exceed 30 mg/wk).

■ **PO, IM, IV (Adults):** 10–25 mg/weekly (not to exceed 30 mg/wk).

### ❏ Arthritis

Therapy may be preceded by a 5–10-mg test dose in adults.

- **PO (Adults):** 7.5 mg weekly (2.5 mg q 12 hr for 3 doses or single dose, not to exceed 20 mg/wk); when response is obtained, dosage should be decreased.
- **PO (Children):** 10 mg/m² once weekly initially, may be increased up to 20–30 mg/m²; however, response may be better if doses >20 mg/m² are given IM or subcut.

### □ Mycosis Fungoides

- **PO, IM, Subcut (Adults):** 5–50 mg once weekly; if response is poor, dose may be changed to 15–37.5 mg twice weekly.
- **IM (Adults):** 50 mg once weekly or 25 mg twice weekly.

### AVAILABILITY (generic available)

- **Tablets:** 2.5 mg^Rx, 5 mg^Rx, 7.5 mg^Rx, 10 mg^Rx, 15 mg^Rx ■ Cost: *Rheumatrex*—2.5 mg $89.39/20; *generic*—2.5 mg $61.00/20 ■ *Injection:* 2.5 mg/ml^Rx, 25 mg/ml^Rx, 20 mg^Rx, 50 mg^Rx, 100 mg^Rx, 250 mg^Rx, 1 g^Rx ■ *Preservative-free injection:* 25 mg/ml^Rx.

TIME/ACTION PROFILE (effects on blood counts)

| | ONSET | PEAK | DURATION |
|---|---|---|---|
| PO, IM, IV | 4–7 days | 7–14 days | 21 days |

## NURSING IMPLICATIONS

### ASSESSMENT

- **General Info:** Monitor blood pressure, pulse, and respiratory rate periodically during administration. Report significant changes.
- □ Monitor for abdominal pain, diarrhea, or stomatitis. Report occurrence; therapy may need to be discontinued.
- □ Monitor for bone marrow depression. Assess for bleeding (bleeding gums, bruising, petechiae, guaiac stools, urine, and emesis) and avoid IM injections and taking rectal temperatures if platelet count is low. Apply pressure to venipuncture sites for 10 min. Assess for signs of infection during neutropenia. Anemia may occur. Monitor for increased fatigue, dyspnea, and orthostatic hypotension.
- □ Monitor intake and output ratios and daily weights. Report significant changes in totals.
- □ Monitor for symptoms of pulmonary toxicity, which may manifest early as a dry, nonproductive cough.

- □ Monitor for symptoms of gout (increased uric acid, joint pain, edema). Encourage patient to drink at least 2 L of fluid each day. Allopurinol and alkalinization of urine may be used to decrease uric acid levels.
- □ Assess nutritional status. Administering an antiemetic prior to and periodically during therapy and adjusting diet as tolerated may help maintain fluid and electrolyte balance and nutritional status.
- **IT:** Assess for development of nuchal rigidity, headache, fever, confusion, drowsiness, dizziness, weakness, or seizures.
- **Rheumatoid Arthritis:** Assess patient for pain and range of motion prior to and periodically during therapy.
- **Psoriasis:** Assess skin lesions prior to and periodically during therapy.
- **Lab Test Considerations:** Monitor CBC and differential prior to and frequently during therapy. The nadir of leukopenia and thrombocytopenia occurs in 7–14 days. Leukocyte and thrombocyte counts usually recover 7 days after the nadirs. Notify physician of any sudden drop in values.
- □ Monitor renal (BUN and creatinine) and hepatic function (AST, ALT, bilirubin, and LDH) prior to and routinely during therapy. Urine pH should be monitored prior to high-dose methotrexate therapy and every 6 hr during leucovorin rescue. Urine pH should be kept above 7.0 to prevent renal damage.
- □ May cause ↑ serum uric acid concentrations, especially during initial treatment of leukemia and lymphoma.
- **Toxicity and Overdose:** Monitor serum methotrexate levels every 12–24 hr during high-dose therapy until levels are <5 × 10 M. This monitoring is essential to plan correct leucovorin dose and determine duration of rescue therapy.
- □ With high-dose therapy, patient must receive leucovorin rescue within 24–48 hr to prevent fatal toxicity. In cases of massive overdose, hydration and urinary alkalization may be required to prevent renal tubule damage. Monitor fluid and electrolyte status. Intermittent hemodialysis using a high-flux dialyzer may be used for clearance until levels are <0.05 micromolar.

### POTENTIAL NURSING DIAGNOSES

- Infection, risk for (Adverse Reactions).

- Nutrition, imbalanced: less than body requirements (Adverse Reactions).

**IMPLEMENTATION**

- **High Alert:** Fatalities have occurred with chemotherapeutic agents. Before administering, clarify all ambiguous orders; double check single, daily, and course-of-therapy dose limits; have second practitioner independently double check original order, calculations and infusion pump settings. Methotrexate for non-oncologic use is given at a much lower dose and frequency—often just once a week. Do not confuse non-oncologic dosing regimens with dosing regimens for cancer patients.

- **General:** Solutions for injection should be prepared in a biologic cabinet. Wear gloves, gown, and mask while handling medication. Discard equipment in specially designated containers (see Appendix M).

- **Direct IV:** Reconstitute each vial with 25 ml of 0.9% NaCl for a concentration no greater than 25 mg/ml. Use sterile preservative-free diluents for high-dose regimens to prevent complications from large amounts of benzyl alcohol. Do not use preparations that are discolored or that contain a precipitate. Reconstitute immediately before use. Discard unused portion.

- **Rate:** Administer at a rate of 10 mg/min into Y-site of a free-flowing IV.

- **Intermittent/Continuous Infusion:** May also be diluted in D5W, D5/0.9% NaCl, or 0.9% NaCl and infused as intermittent or continuous infusion.

- **Rate:** Administration rates of 4–20 mg/hr have been used.

- **Syringe Compatibility:** ♦ bleomycin ♦ cisplatin ♦ cyclophosphamide ♦ doxapram ♦ doxorubicin ♦ fluorouracil ♦ furosemide ♦ heparin ♦ leucovorin ♦ mitomycin ♦ vinblastine ♦ vincristine.

- **Syringe Incompatibility:** ♦ droperidol.

- **Y-Site Compatibility:** ♦ allopurinol ♦ amifostine ♦ amphotericin B cholesteryl sulfate ♦ asparaginase ♦ aztreonam ♦ bleomycin ♦ cefepime ♦ ceftriaxone ♦ cimetidine ♦ cisplatin ♦ cyclophosphamide ♦ cytarabine ♦ daunorubicin ♦ diphenhydramine ♦ doxorubicin ♦

doxorubicin liposome ♦ etoposide ♦ etoposide phosphate ♦ famotidine ♦ filgrastim ♦ fludarabine ♦ fluorouracil ♦ furosemide ♦ ganciclovir ♦ gatifloxacin ♦ granisetron ♦ heparin ♦ hydromorphone ♦ imipenem/cilastatin ♦ leucovorin ♦ linezolid ♦ lorazepam ♦ melphalan ♦ mesna ♦ methylprednisolone sodium succinate ♦ metoclopramide ♦ mitomycin ♦ morphine ♦ ondansetron ♦ oxacillin ♦ paclitaxel ♦ piperacillin/tazobactam ♦ prochlorperazine ♦ ranitidine ♦ sargramostim ♦ teniposide ♦ thiotepa ♦ vinblastine ♦ vincristine ♦ vinorelbine.

- **Y-Site Incompatibility:** ♦ chlorpromazine ♦ gemcitabine ♦ idarubicin ♦ ifosfamide ♦ midazolam ♦ nalbuphine ♦ promethazine ♦ propofol.

- **Additive Compatibility:** ♦ cyclophosphamide ♦ cytarabine ♦ fluorouracil ♦ mercaptopurine ♦ ondansetron ♦ sodium bicarbonate ♦ vincristine.

- **IT:** Reconstitute preservative-free methotrexate with preservative-free 0.9% NaCl, Elliot's B solution, or patient's CSF to a concentration of 1 mg/ml. May be administered via lumbar puncture or Ommaya reservoir. To prevent bacterial contamination, use immediately.

**PATIENT/FAMILY TEACHING**

- Instruct patient to take medication as directed. If a dose is missed, it should be omitted. Consult health care professional if vomiting occurs shortly after a dose is taken.

- Instruct patient to notify health care professional promptly if fever; chills; cough; hoarseness; sore throat; signs of infection; lower back or side pain; painful or difficult urination; bleeding gums; bruising; petechiae; blood in stools, urine, or emesis; increased fatigue; dyspnea; or orthostatic hypotension occurs. Caution patient to avoid crowds and persons with known infections. Instruct patient to use soft toothbrush and electric razor and to avoid falls. Caution patient not to drink alcoholic beverages or take medication containing aspirin or other NSAIDs; may precipitate gastric bleeding.

- Instruct patient to inspect oral mucosa for erythema and ulceration. If ulceration occurs, advise patient to use sponge brush and to rinse mouth with water after eating and drinking. Topical therapy may be used if mouth pain interferes with eating. Stomatitis pain may require treatment with opioid analgesics.

❑ Instruct patient to avoid the use of OTC drugs or herbal products without first consulting health care professional.

❑ Advise patient that this medication may have teratogenic effects. Contraception should be used during therapy and for at least 3 mo for men and 1 ovulatory cycle for women after completion of therapy.

❑ Discuss the possibility of hair loss with patient. Explore methods of coping.

❑ Instruct patient not to receive any vaccinations without advice of health care professional.

❑ Caution patient to use sunscreen and protective clothing to prevent photosensitivity reactions.

❑ Emphasize the need for periodic lab tests to monitor for side effects.

## EVALUATION

**Effectiveness of therapy can be demonstrated by:** ■ Improvement of hematopoietic values in leukemia ❑ Decrease in symptoms of meningeal involvement in leukemia ■ Decrease in size and spread of non-Hodgkin's lymphomas and other solid cancers ■ Resolution of skin lesions in severe psoriasis ■ Decreased joint pain and swelling ❑ Improved mobility in patients with rheumatoid arthritis ■ Regression of lesions in mycosis fungoides.

# methyldopa
(meth-ill-**doe**-pa)

Aldomet, {Apo-Methyldopa}, {Dopamet}, {Novamedopa}, {Nu-Medopa}

## CLASSIFICATION(S):
**Therapeutic:** antihypertensives
**Pharmacologic:** centrally acting antiadrenergics

## Pregnancy Category B

## INDICATIONS

■ Management of moderate to severe hypertension (with other agents).

## ACTION

■ Stimulates CNS alpha-adrenergic receptors, producing a decrease in sympathetic outflow to heart, kidneys, and blood vessels. Result is decreased blood pressure and peripheral resistance, a slight decrease in heart rate, and no change in cardiac output. **Therapeutic Effects:** ■ Lowering of blood pressure.

## PHARMACOKINETICS

**Absorption:** 50% absorbed from the GI tract. Parenteral form, methyldopate hydrochloride, is slowly converted to methyldopa.

**Distribution:** Crosses the blood-brain barrier. Crosses the placenta; small amounts enter breast milk.

**Metabolism and Excretion:** Partially metabolized by the liver, partially excreted unchanged by the kidneys.

**Half-life:** 1.7 hr.

## CONTRAINDICATIONS AND PRECAUTIONS

**Contraindicated in:** ■ Hypersensitivity ■ Active liver disease ■ Oral suspension contains alcohol and bisulfites and should be avoided in patients with known intolerance.

**Use Cautiously in:** ■ Previous history of liver disease ■ Geriatric patients (increased risk of adverse reactions) ■ Pregnancy (has been used safely) ■ Lactation.

## ADVERSE REACTIONS AND SIDE EFFECTS*

■ **CNS:** <u>sedation</u>, decreased mental acuity, depression ■ **EENT:** nasal stuffiness ■ **CV:** MYOCARD-ITIS, bradycardia, edema, orthostatic hypotension ■ **GI:** DRUG-INDUCED HEPATITIS, diarrhea, dry mouth ■ **GU:** impotence ■ **Hemat:** eosinophilia, hemolytic anemia ■ **Misc:** fever.

## INTERACTIONS

**Drug-Drug:** ■ Additive hypotension with other **antihypertensives,** acute ingestion of **alcohol, anesthesia,** and **nitrates** ■ **Amphetamines, barbiturates, tricyclic antidepressants, NSAIDs,** and **phenothiazines** may decrease antihypertensive effect of methyldopa ■ Increased effects and risk of psychoses with **haloperidol** ■ Excess sympathetic stimulation may occur with concurrent use of **MAO inhibitors** or other **adrenergics** ■ May increase the effects of **tolbutamide** ■ May increase **lithium** toxicity ■ Additive hypotension and CNS toxicity with **levodopa** ■ Additive CNS depression may occur with **alcohol, antihistamines, sedative/hypnotics,** some **antidepressants,** and **opioid analgesics** ■ Concurrent use with **nonselective beta blockers** may rarely cause paradoxical hypertension.

## ROUTE AND DOSAGE

- **PO (Adults):** 250–500 mg 2–3 times daily (not to exceed 500 mg/day if used with other agents); may be increased q 2 days as needed; usual maintenance dose is 500 mg–2 g/day (not to exceed 3 g/day).
- **PO (Children):** 10 mg/kg/day (300 mg/m²/day); may be increased q 2 days up to 65 mg/kg/day in divided doses (not to exceed 3 g/day).
- **IV (Adults):** 250–500 mg q 6 hr (up to 1 g q 6 hr).
- **IV (Children):** 5–10 mg/kg q 6 hr; up to 65 mg/kg/day in divided doses (not to exceed 3 g/day).

## AVAILABILITY (generic available)

■ *Tablets:* 125 mg$^{Rx}$, 250 mg$^{Rx}$, 500 mg$^{Rx}$ ■ Cost: *Aldomet*—125 mg $29.85/100, 250 mg $38/100, 500 mg $69.44/100; *generic*—125 mg $9.75/100, 250 mg $12.50/100, 500 mg $22.50/100 ■ *Oral suspension (orange-pineapple flavor, contains bisulfites):* 250 mg/5 ml$^{Rx}$ ■ *Injection:* 250 mg/5 ml in 5- and 10-ml vials$^{Rx}$ ■ hydrochlorothiazide (Aldoril)$^{Rx}$ or chlorothiazide (Aldoclor)$^{Rx}$. See Appendix B.

TIME/ACTION PROFILE (antihypertensive effect)

|     | ONSET | PEAK | DURATION |
|-----|-------|------|----------|
| PO  | 12–24 hr | 4–6 hr | 24–48 hr |
| IV  | 4–6 hr | unknown | 10–16 hr |

## NURSING IMPLICATIONS

### ASSESSMENT

- ❑ Monitor blood pressure and pulse frequently during initial dosage adjustment and periodically throughout therapy. Report significant changes.
- ❑ Monitor frequency of prescription refills to determine compliance.

- ❑ Monitor intake and output ratios and weight and assess for edema daily, especially at beginning of therapy. Report weight gain or edema; sodium and water retention may be treated with diuretics.
- ❑ Assess patient for depression or other alterations in mental status. Notify physician or other health care professional promptly if these symptoms develop.
- ❑ Monitor temperature during therapy. Drug fever may occur shortly after initiation of therapy and may be accompanied by eosinophilia and hepatic function changes. Monitor hepatic function test if unexplained fever occurs.
- ■ *Lab Test Considerations:* Renal and hepatic function and CBC should be monitored before and periodically throughout therapy.
- ❑ Monitor direct Coombs' test before and after 6 and 12 mo of therapy. May cause a positive direct Coombs' test, rarely associated with hemolytic anemia.
- ❑ May cause increased BUN, serum creatinine, potassium, sodium, prolactin, uric acid, AST, ALT, alkaline phosphatase, and bilirubin concentrations.
- ❑ May cause prolonged prothrombin times.
- ❑ May interfere with serum creatinine and AST measurements.

## POTENTIAL NURSING DIAGNOSES

- ■ Injury, risk for (Side Effects).
- ■ Noncompliance (Patient/Family Teaching).

## IMPLEMENTATION

- ■ **General:** Do not confuse methyldopa with levodopa or L-dopa.
- ❑ Fluid retention and expanded volume may cause tolerance to develop within 2–3 mo after initiation of therapy. Diuretics may be added to regimen at this time to maintain control.
- ❑ Dosage increases should be made with the evening dose to minimize drowsiness.
- ❑ When changing from IV to oral forms, dosage should remain consistent.
- ■ **PO:** Shake suspension before administration.
- ■ **Intermittent Infusion:** Dilute in 100 ml of D5W, 0.9% NaCl, D5/0.9% NaCl, 5% sodium bicarbonate, or Ringer's solution.

{ } = Available in Canada only.
*CAPITALS indicates life-threatening; underlines indicate most frequent.

■ **Rate:** Infuse slowly over 30–60 min.

■ **Y-Site Compatibility:** ◆ esmolol ◆ heparin ◆ meperidine ◆ morphine ◆ theophylline.

**PATIENT/FAMILY TEACHING**

❏ Emphasize the importance of continuing to take this medication, even if feeling well. Instruct patient to take medication at the same time each day; last dose of the day should be taken at bedtime. If a dose is missed, take as soon as remembered but not if almost time for next dose. Do not double doses.

❏ Encourage patient to comply with additional interventions for hypertension (weight reduction, low-sodium diet, smoking cessation, moderation of alcohol consumption, regular exercise, and stress management). Methyldopa controls but does not cure hypertension.

❏ Instruct patient and family on proper technique for monitoring blood pressure. Advise them to check blood pressure at least weekly and to report significant changes.

❏ Inform patient that urine may darken or turn red-black when left standing.

❏ May cause drowsiness. Advise patient to avoid driving or other activities requiring alertness until response to medication is known. Drowsiness usually subsides after 7–10 days of continuous use.

❏ Caution patient to avoid sudden changes in position to decrease orthostatic hypotension.

❏ Advise patient that frequent mouth rinses, good oral hygiene, and sugarless gum or candy may minimize dry mouth. Notify health care professional if dry mouth continues for >2 wk.

❏ Caution patient to avoid concurrent use of alcohol or other CNS depressants.

❏ Advise patient to consult health care professional before taking any cough, cold, or allergy remedies.

❏ Advise patient to notify health care professional of medication regimen before treatment or surgery.

❏ Instruct patient to notify health care professional if fever, muscle aches, or flu-like syndrome occurs.

**EVALUATION**

**Effectiveness of therapy can be demonstrated by:** ■ Decrease in blood pressure without appearance of side effects.

# methylergonovine

(meth-ill-er-goe-**noe**-veen)

Methergine

**CLASSIFICATION(S):**

**Therapeutic:** oxytocic

**Pharmacologic:** ergot alkaloids

**Pregnancy Category C**

## INDICATIONS

■ Prevention and treatment of postpartum or postabortion hemorrhage caused by uterine atony or subinvolution.

## ACTION

■ Directly stimulates uterine and vascular smooth muscle. **Therapeutic Effects:** ■ Uterine contraction.

## PHARMACOKINETICS

**Absorption:** Well absorbed following oral or IM administration.

**Distribution:** Unknown. Enters breast milk in small quantities.

**Metabolism and Excretion:** Probably metabolized by the liver.

**Half-life:** 30–120 min.

## CONTRAINDICATIONS AND PRECAUTIONS

**Contraindicated in:** ■ Hypersensitivity ■ Should not be used to induce labor.

**Use Cautiously in:** ■ Hypertensive or eclamptic patients (more susceptible to hypertensive and arrhythmogenic side effects) ■ Severe hepatic or renal disease ■ Sepsis.

**Exercise Extreme Caution in:** ■ Third stage of labor.

## ADVERSE REACTIONS AND SIDE EFFECTS*

■ **CNS:** dizziness, headache ■ **EENT:** tinnitus ■ **Resp:** dyspnea ■ **CV:** HYPOTENSION, arrhythmias, chest pain, hypertension, palpitations ■ **GI:** nausea, vomiting ■ **GU:** cramps ■ **Derm:** diaphoresis ■ **Misc:** allergic reactions.

## INTERACTIONS

**Drug-Drug:** ■ Excessive vasoconstriction may result when used with heavy cigarette smoking (**nicotine**) or other **vasopressors** such as **dopamine.**

## ROUTE AND DOSAGE

- **PO (Adults):** 200–400 mcg (0.4–0.6 mg) q 6–12 hr for 2–7 days.
- **IM, IV (Adults):** 200 mcg (0.2 mg) q 2–4 hr for up to 5 doses.

### AVAILABILITY

- **Tablets:** 200 mcg (0.2 mg)$^{Rx}$ ■ **Injection:** 200 mcg (0.2 mg)/ml in 1-ml ampules$^{Rx}$.

TIME/ACTION PROFILE (effects on uterine contractions)

|    | ONSET | PEAK | DURATION |
|----|-------|------|----------|
| PO | 5–15 min | unknown | 3 hr |
| IM | 2–5 min | unknown | 3 hr |
| IV | immediate | unknown | 45 min–3 hr |

## NURSING IMPLICATIONS

### ASSESSMENT

- ❑ Monitor blood pressure, heart rate, and uterine response frequently during medication administration. Notify physician or other health care professional promptly if uterine relaxation becomes prolonged or if character of vaginal bleeding changes.
- ❑ Assess for signs of ergotism (cold, numb fingers and toes, chest pain, nausea, vomiting, headache, muscle pain, weakness).
- ■ **Lab Test Considerations:** If no response to methylergonovine, calcium levels may need to be assessed. Effectiveness of medication is decreased with hypocalcemia.
- ❑ May cause decreased serum prolactin levels.

### POTENTIAL NURSING DIAGNOSES

- ■ Pain, acute (Side Effects).

### IMPLEMENTATION

- ■ **IV:** IV administration is used for emergencies only. Oral and IM routes are preferred.
- ■ **Direct IV:** May be given undiluted or diluted in 5 ml of 0.9% NaCl and administered through Y-site. Do not add to IV solutions. Do not mix in syringe with any other drug. Refrigerate; stable for storage at room temperature for 60 days; deteriorates with age. Use only solution that is clear and colorless and that contains no precipitate.

- ■ **Rate:** Administer at a rate of 0.2 mg over at least 1 min.
- ■ **Y-Site Compatibility:** ◆ heparin ◆ hydrocortisone sodium succinate ◆ potassium chloride ◆ vitamin B complex with C.

### PATIENT/FAMILY TEACHING

- ❑ Instruct patient to take medication as directed; do not skip or double up on missed doses. If a dose is missed, omit it and return to regular dosage schedule.
- ❑ Advise patient that medication may cause menstrual-like cramps.
- ❑ Caution patient to avoid smoking, because nicotine constricts blood vessels.
- ❑ Instruct patient to notify health care professional if infection develops, as this may cause increased sensitivity to the medication.

### EVALUATION

**Effectiveness of therapy can be demonstrated by:** ■ Contractions that maintain uterine tone and prevent postpartum hemorrhage.

## methylphenidate

(meth-ill-**fen**-i-date)

Concerta, Metadate CD, Metadate ER, Methylin, Methylin SR, {PMS-Methylphenidate}, {Riphenidate}, Ritalin, Ritalin LA, Ritalin-SR

### CLASSIFICATION(S):

**Therapeutic:** central nervous system stimulants

**Schedule II**

**Pregnancy Category C**

### INDICATIONS

■ Treatment of ADHD (adjunct) ■ Symptomatic treatment of narcolepsy. **Unlabeled uses:** ■ Management of some forms of refractory depression.

### ACTION

■ Produces CNS and respiratory stimulation with weak sympathomimetic activity. **Therapeutic Effects:** ■ Increased attention span in ADHD ■

Increased motor activity, mental alertness, and diminished fatigue in narcoleptic patients.

## PHARMACOKINETICS

**Absorption:** Well absorbed after oral administration; absorption of sustained or extended-release tablet (SR) is delayed and provides continuous release. *Metadate CD, Concerta, Ritalin LA*—provides initial rapid release followed by a second continuous release (biphasic release).

**Distribution:** Unknown.

**Metabolism and Excretion:** Mostly metabolized (80%) by the liver.

**Half-life:** 1–3 hr.

## CONTRAINDICATIONS AND PRECAUTIONS

**Contraindicated in:** ■ Hypersensitivity ■ Hyperexcitable states ■ Hyperthyroidism ■ Patients with psychotic personalities or suicidal or homicidal tendencies ■ Glaucoma ■ Motor tics ■ Concurrent use or use within 14 days of MAO inhibitors.

**Use Cautiously in:** ■ History of cardiovascular disease ■ Hypertension ■ Diabetes mellitus ■ Geriatric or debilitated patients ■ Continual use (may result in psychological or physical dependence) ■ Seizure disorders (may lower seizure threshold) ■ Concerta product should be used cautiously in patients with esophageal motility disorders (may increase the risk of obstruction) ■ Pregnancy or lactation (safety not established).

## ADVERSE REACTIONS AND SIDE EFFECTS*

■ **CNS:** hyperactivity, insomnia, restlessness, tremor, dizziness, headache, irritability ■ **EENT:** blurred vision ■ **CV:** hypertension, palpitations, tachycardia, hypotension ■ **GI:** anorexia, constipation, cramps, diarrhea, dry mouth, metallic taste, nausea, vomiting ■ **Derm:** rashes ■ **Neuro:** akathisia, dyskinesia ■ **Misc:** fever, hypersensitivity reactions, physical dependence, psychological dependence, suppression of weight gain (children), tolerance.

## INTERACTIONS

**Drug-Drug:** ■ ↑ sympathomimetic effects with other **adrenergics,** including **vasoconstrictors** and **decongestants** ■ Use with **MAO inhibitors** or **vasopressors** may result in hypertensive crisis (concurrent use or use within

14 days of MAO inhibitors is contraindicated) ■ May antagonize the hypotensive effect of **guanethidine** ■ Metabolism of **warfarin, anticonvulsants,** and **tricyclic antidepressants** may be ↓ and effects ↑ ■ Avoid concurrent use with **pimozide** (may mask cause of tics) ■ Concurrent use with intrathecal **clonidine** may result in serious adverse reactions.

**Drug-Natural Products:** ■ Use with caffeine-containing herbs (**guarana, tea, coffee**) ↑ stimulant effect.

**Drug-Food:** ■ Excessive use of **caffeine**-containing foods or beverages (**coffee, cola, tea**) may cause ↑ CNS stimulation.

## ROUTE AND DOSAGE

■ **PO (Adults):** 5–20-mg 2–3 times daily as prompt-release tablets. When maintenance dose is determined, may change to extended-release formulation

■ **PO (Children >6 yr):** *Prompt release tablets*—0.3 mg/kg/dose or 2.5–5 mg before breakfast and lunch; increase by 5–10 mg at weekly intervals (not to exceed 60 mg/day or 2 mg/kg/day). When maintenance dose is determined, may change to extended-release formulation. *Ritalin SR, Metadate ER*—may be used in place of the Prompt-release tablets when the 8-hour dosage corresponds to the titrated 8-hour dosage of the Prompt-release tablets; *Ritalin LA*—can be used in place of twice-daily regimen given once daily at same total dose, or in place of SR product at same dose; *Concerta (patients who have not taken methylphenidate previously)*— 18 mg once daily in the morning initially, may be titrated as needed up to 54 mg/day. *Concerta (patients are currently taking other forms of methylphenidate)*—18 mg once daily in the morning if previous dose was 5 mg 2–3 times daily or 20-mg daily as SR product, 36 mg once daily in the morning if previous dose was 10 mg 2–3 times daily or 40 mg daily as SR product, 54 mg once daily in the morning if previous dose was 15 mg 2–3 times daily or 60 mg once daily as SR product. *Metadate CD*—20 mg once daily. Dosage may be adjusted in weekly 20-mg increments to a maximum of 60 mg/day taken once daily in the morning.

## AVAILABILITY (generic available)

■ *Prompt-release tablets:* {5 mg^Rx, 10 mg^Rx, 20 mg^Rx} ■ Cost: *Ritalin*—5 mg $43.48/

100, 10 mg $61.98/100, 20 mg $89.12/100; *generic*—5 mg $33.40/100, 10 mg $47.70/ 100, 20 mg $68.25/100 ■ *Extended-release tablets (Metadate ER):* {10 mg$^{Rx}$, 20 mg$^{Rx}$} ■Cost: 10 mg $93.09/100, 20 mg $88.65/100 ■ *Extended-release tablets (other):* {10 mg$^{Rx}$, 20 mg$^{Rx}$} ■ *Extended-release tablets (Concerta):* {18 mg$^{Rx}$, 27 mg$^{Rx}$, 36 mg$^{Rx}$ 54 mg$^{Rx}$} ■ Cost: 54 mg $256.25/100, 18 mg $231.25/100, 36 mg $243.75/100 ■ *Extended-release tablets:* {10 mg$^{Rx}$, 20 mg$^{Rx}$} ■ Cost: *Ritalin SR*—$138.42/100; *generic*—$89.26/100 ■ *Extended-release capsules (Metadate CD):* {20 mg$^{Rx}$} ■ Cost: $34.68/30 ■ *Extended-release capsules (Ritalin LA):* {20 mg$^{Rx}$, 30 mg$^{Rx}$, 40 mg$^{Rx}$}.

TIME/ACTION PROFILE (CNS stimulation)

| | ONSET | PEAK | DURATION |
|---|---|---|---|
| PO | unknown | 1–3 hr | 4–6 hr |
| PO-ER | unknown | unknown | up to 8 hr† |

†depends on formulation

## NURSING IMPLICATIONS

### ASSESSMENT

■ **General Info:** Monitor blood pressure, pulse, and respiration before administering and periodically during therapy.

❑ Monitor growth, both height and weight, in children on long-term therapy.

❑ May produce a false sense of euphoria and well-being. Provide frequent rest periods and observe patient for rebound depression after the effects of the medication have worn off.

❑ Methylphenidate has high dependence and abuse potential. Tolerance to medication occurs rapidly; do not increase dose.

❑ **ADHD:** Assess children for attention span, impulse control, and interactions with others. Therapy may be interrupted at intervals to determine whether symptoms are sufficient to continue therapy.

❑ **Narcolepsy:** Observe and document frequency of episodes.

■ *Lab Test Considerations:* Monitor CBC, differential, and platelet count periodically in patients receiving prolonged therapy.

### POTENTIAL NURSING DIAGNOSES

■ Thought processes, disturbed (Side Effects).

### IMPLEMENTATION

■ **PO:** Administer with or after a meal. Sustained-release tablets should be swallowed whole; do not crush, break, or chew. Medate CD and Ritalin LA capsules may be opened and sprinkled on cool applesauce; entire mixture should be ingested immediately and followed by a drink of water. Do not store for future use.

### PATIENT/FAMILY TEACHING

■ **General Info:** Instruct patient to take medication as directed. If a dose is missed, take the remaining doses for that day at regularly spaced intervals; do not double doses. Take the last dose before 6 PM to minimize the risk of insomnia. Instruct patient not to alter dose without consulting health care professional. Abrupt cessation of high doses may cause extreme fatigue and mental depression.

❑ Advise patient to check weight 2–3 times weekly and report weight loss to health care professional.

❑ May cause dizziness or blurred vision. Caution patient to avoid driving or activities requiring alertness until response to medication is known.

❑ Inform patient and/or parents that shell of Concerta tablet may appear in the stool. This is no cause for concern.

❑ Advise patient to avoid using caffeine-containing beverages concurrently with this therapy.

❑ Advise patient to notify health care professional if nervousness, insomnia, palpitations, vomiting, skin rash, or fever occurs.

❑ Inform patient that health care professional may order periodic holidays from the drug to assess progress and to decrease dependence.

❑ Emphasize the importance of routine follow-up exams to monitor progress.

■ **ADHD:** Advise parents to notify school nurse of medication regimen.

## EVALUATION

**Effectiveness of therapy can be demonstrated by:** ■ Decreased frequency of narcoleptic symptoms ■ Improved attention span and social interactions in ADHD.

## methylprednisolone, See CORTICOSTEROIDS (SYSTEMIC), CORTICOSTEROIDS (TOPICAL/LOCAL).

## metoclopramide
(met-oh-**kloe**-pra-mide)
{Apo-Metoclop}, Clopra, {Emex}, {Maxeran}, Octamide, Octamide-PFS, Reclomide, Reglan

**CLASSIFICATION(S):**
**Therapeutic:** antiemetics

**Pregnancy Category B**

## INDICATIONS

■ Prevention of chemotherapy-induced emesis ■ Treatment of postsurgical and diabetic gastric stasis ■ Facilitation of small bowel intubation in radiographic procedures ■ Management of esophageal reflux ■ Treatment and prevention of postoperative nausea and vomiting when nasogastric suctioning is undesirable. **Unlabeled uses:** ■ Treatment of hiccups ■ Adjunct management of migraine headaches.

## ACTION

■ Blocks dopamine receptors in chemoreceptor trigger zone of the CNS ■ Stimulates motility of the upper GI tract and accelerates gastric emptying. **Therapeutic Effects:** ■ Decreased nausea and vomiting ■ Decreased symptoms of gastric stasis ■ Easier passage of nasogastric tube into small bowel.

## PHARMACOKINETICS

**Absorption:** Well absorbed from the GI tract, from rectal mucosa, and from IM sites.

**Distribution:** Widely distributed into body tissues and fluids. Crosses blood-brain barrier and placenta. Enters breast milk in concentrations greater than plasma.

**Metabolism and Excretion:** Partially metabolized by the liver; 25% eliminated unchanged in the urine.

**Half-life:** 2.5–5 hr.

## CONTRAINDICATIONS AND PRECAUTIONS

**Contraindicated in:** ■ Hypersensitivity ■ Possible GI obstruction or hemorrhage ■ History of seizure disorders ■ Pheochromocytoma ■ Parkinson's disease.

**Use Cautiously in:** ■ History of depression ■ Diabetes (may alter response to insulin) ■ Pregnancy and lactation (safety not established) ■ Children and geriatric patients (increased incidence of extrapyramidal reactions).

## ADVERSE REACTIONS AND SIDE EFFECTS*

■ **CNS:** <u>drowsiness</u>, <u>extrapyramidal reactions</u>, <u>restlessness</u>, anxiety, depression, irritability, tardive dyskinesia ■ **CV:** arrhythmias (supraventricular tachycardia, bradycardia), hypertension, hypotension ■ **GI:** constipation, diarrhea, dry mouth, nausea ■ **Endo:** gynecomastia.

## INTERACTIONS

**Drug-Drug:** ■ Additive CNS depression with other **CNS depressants,** including **alcohol, antidepressants, antihistamines, opioid analgesics,** and **sedative/hypnotics** ■ May increase absorption and risk of toxicity from **cyclosporine** ■ May affect the GI absorption of other **orally administered drugs** as a result of effect on GI motility ■ May exaggerate hypotension during **general anesthesia** ■ Increased risk of extrapyramidal reactions with agents such as **haloperidol** or **phenothiazines** ■ **Opioids** and **anticholinergics** may antagonize the GI effects of metoclopramide ■ Use cautiously with **MAO inhibitors** (causes release of catecholamines) ■ May increase neuromuscular blockade from **succinylcholine** ■ May decrease the effectiveness of **levodopa**.

## ROUTE AND DOSAGE

❑ **Prevention of Chemotherapy-Induced Vomiting**

■ **IV (Adults):** 1–2 mg/kg 30 min before chemotherapy. Additional doses of 1–2 mg/kg may be given q 2 hr for 2 doses, then q 3 hr for 3 additional doses. May also be given as 3 mg/kg before chemotherapy, followed by 0.5 mg/kg/hr for 8 hr (unlabeled).

- **Facilitation of Small Bowel Intubation**
- **IV (Adults):** 10 mg.
- **IV (Children 6–14 yr):** 2.5–5 mg (dose should not exceed 0.5 mg/kg).
- **IV (Children <6 yr):** 0.1 mg/kg.
- **Diabetic Gastroparesis**
- **PO (Adults):** 10 mg 30 min before meals and at bedtime.
- **Gastroesophageal Reflux**
- **PO (Adults):** 10–15 mg 30 min before meals and at bedtime (not to exceed 0.5 mg/kg/day). A single dose of 20 mg may be given preventively. Some patients may respond to doses as small as 5 mg.
- **Postoperative Nausea/Vomiting**
- **IM (Adults):** 10–20 mg.
- **Treatment of Hiccups**
- **PO, IM (Adults):** 10–20 mg 4 times daily PO; may be preceded by a single 10-mg dose IM (unlabeled).

## AVAILABILITY (generic available)

■ *Tablets:* 5 mg$^{Rx}$, 10 mg$^{Rx}$ ■ Cost: *Reglan*—5 mg $50.91/100, 10 mg $80.26/100; *generic*— 5 mg $29.77/100, 10 mg $21.12/100 ■ *Concentrated solution:* 10 mg/ml$^{Rx}$ ■ *Syrup (apricot-peach flavor):* 5 mg/5 ml$^{Rx}$ ■ *Injection:* 5 mg/ml$^{Rx}$.

TIME/ACTION PROFILE (effects on peristalsis)

| | ONSET | PEAK | DURATION |
|----|----|----|----|
| PO | 30–60 min | unknown | 1–2 hr |
| IM | 10–15 min | unknown | 1–2 hr |
| IV | 1–3 min | immediate | 1–2 hr |

## NURSING IMPLICATIONS

### ASSESSMENT

- Assess patient for nausea, vomiting, abdominal distention, and bowel sounds before and after administration.
- Assess patient for extrapyramidal side effects (*parkinsonian*—difficulty speaking or swallowing, loss of balance control, pill rolling, mask-like face, shuffling gait, rigidity, tremors; and *dystonic*—muscle spasms, twisting motions, twitching, inability to move eyes, weakness of arms or legs) periodically throughout course of therapy. May occur weeks to months after initiation of therapy and are reversible on discontinuation. Dystonic reactions may occur within minutes of IV infusion and stop within 24 hr of discontinuation of metoclopramide. May be treated with 50 mg of IM diphenhydramine or diphenhydramine 1 mg/kg IV may be administered prophylactically 15 min before metoclopramide IV infusion.
- Monitor for tardive dyskinesia (uncontrolled rhythmic movement of mouth, face, and extremities; lip smacking or puckering; puffing of cheeks; uncontrolled chewing; rapid or worm-like movements of tongue). Usually occurs after a year or more of continued therapy. Report immediately; may be irreversible.
- Assess patient for signs of depression periodically throughout therapy.
- *Lab Test Considerations:* May alter hepatic function test results.
- May cause increased serum prolactin and aldosterone concentrations.

## POTENTIAL NURSING DIAGNOSES

- Nutrition, imbalanced: less than body requirements (Indications).
- Injury, risk for (Side Effects).

## IMPLEMENTATION

- **PO:** Administer doses 30 min before meals and at bedtime.
- **IM:** For prevention of postoperative nausea and vomiting, inject IM near the end of surgery.
- **Rect:** Suppositories may be made by pharmacist. Administer 1 suppository 30–60 min before each meal and at bedtime.
- **Direct IV:** Administer IV dose 30 min before administration of chemotherapeutic agent.
- *Rate:* Doses may be given slowly over 1–2 min. Rapid administration causes a transient but intense feeling of anxiety and restlessness followed by drowsiness.
- **Intermittent Infusion:** May be diluted for IV infusion in 50 ml of D5W, 0.9% NaCl, D5/0.45% NaCl, Ringer's solution, or LR. Diluted

solution is stable for 48 hr if protected from light or 24 hr under normal light.

■ *Rate:* Infuse slowly over at least 15 min.

■ **Syringe Compatibility:** ◆ bleomycin ◆ butorphanol ◆ chlorpromazine ◆ cisplatin ◆ cyclophosphamide ◆ cytarabine ◆ dexamethasone ◆ diphenhydramine ◆ doxorubicin ◆ droperidol ◆ fentanyl ◆ fluorouracil ◆ heparin ◆ hydrocortisone ◆ leucovorin ◆ lidocaine ◆ magnesium sulfate ◆ meperidine ◆ methotrimeprazine ◆ methylprednisolone sodium succinate ◆ midazolam ◆ mitomycin ◆ morphine ◆ ondansetron ◆ prochlorperazine ◆ ranitidine ◆ vinblastine ◆ vincristine.

■ **Y-Site Compatibility:** ◆ acyclovir ◆ aldesleukin ◆ amifostine ◆ aztreonam ◆ bleomycin ◆ ciprofloxacin ◆ cisatracurium ◆ cisplatin ◆ cladribine ◆ cyclophosphamide ◆ cytarabine ◆ diltiazem ◆ docetaxel ◆ doxorubicin ◆ droperidol ◆ etoposide ◆ famotidine ◆ filgrastim ◆ fluconazole ◆ fludarabine ◆ fluorouracil ◆ foscarnet ◆ gatifloxacin ◆ gemcitabine ◆ granisetron ◆ heparin ◆ idarubicin ◆ leucovorin ◆ levofloxacin ◆ linezolid ◆ melphalan ◆ meperidine ◆ meropenem ◆ methotrexate ◆ mitomycin ◆ morphine ◆ ondansetron ◆ paclitaxel ◆ piperacillin/tazobactam ◆ remifentanil ◆ sargramostim ◆ sufentanil ◆ tacrolimus ◆ teniposide ◆ thiotepa ◆ topotecan ◆ vinblastine ◆ vincristine ◆ vinorelbine ◆ zidovudine.

■ **Y-Site Incompatibility:** ◆ amphotericin B cholesteryl sulfate complex ◆ cefepime ◆ doxorubicin liposome ◆ furosemide ◆ propofol.

### PATIENT/FAMILY TEACHING

❑ Instruct patient to take metoclopramide exactly as directed. If a dose is missed, take as soon as remembered if not almost time for next dose.

❑ May cause drowsiness. Caution patient to avoid driving or other activities requiring alertness until response to medication is known.

❑ Advise patient to avoid concurrent use of alcohol and other CNS depressants while taking this medication.

❑ Advise patient to notify health care professional immediately if involuntary movement of eyes, face, or limbs occurs.

### EVALUATION

**Effectiveness of therapy can be demonstrated by:** ■ Prevention or relief of nausea and vomiting ■ Decreased symptoms of gastric stasis ■ Facilitation of small bowel intubation ■ Decreased symptoms of esophageal reflux.

---

# metolazone
(me-**tole**-a-zone)
Mykrox, Zaroxolyn

### CLASSIFICATION(S):
**Therapeutic:** *antihypertensives, diuretics*
**Pharmacologic:** *thiazide-like diuretics*

### Pregnancy Category B

## INDICATIONS

■ Mild to moderate hypertension ■ Edema associated with CHF or the nephrotic syndrome (Zaroxolyn only).

## ACTION

■ Increases excretion of sodium and water by inhibiting sodium reabsorption in the distal tubule ■ Promotes excretion of chloride, potassium, magnesium, and bicarbonate ■ May produce arteriolar dilation. **Therapeutic Effects:** ■ Lowering of blood pressure in hypertensive patients ■ Diuresis with subsequent mobilization of edema. Effect may continue in renal impairment.

## PHARMACOKINETICS

**Absorption:** Absorption is more rapid and more complete with prompt tablet (Mykrox). Absorption is more variable with extended tablet (Zaroxolyn).
**Distribution:** Unknown.
**Metabolism and Excretion:** Excreted mainly unchanged by the kidneys.
**Half-life:** *Extended tablet*—8 hr; *prompt tablet*—14 hr.

## CONTRAINDICATIONS AND PRECAUTIONS

**Contraindicated in:** ■ Hypersensitivity ■ Cross-sensitivity with other sulfonamides may exist ■ Anuria ■ Lactation.
**Use Cautiously in:** ■ Severe hepatic impairment ■ Geriatric patients (increased sensitivity) ■ Pregnancy or children (safety not established; children may be more susceptible to diuretic and hypokalemic effects).

## ADVERSE REACTIONS AND SIDE EFFECTS*

■ **CNS:** drowsiness, lethargy ■ **CV:** chest pain, hypotension, palpitations ■ **GI:** anorexia, bloating, cramping, drug-induced hepatitis, nausea, vomiting ■ **Derm:** photosensitivity, rashes ■ **Endo:** hyperglycemia ■ **F and E:** hypokalemia, dehydration, hypercalcemia, hypochloremic alkalosis, hypomagnesemia, hyponatremia, hypophosphatemia, hypovolemia ■ **Hemat:** blood dyscrasias ■ **Metab:** hyperuricemia ■ **MS:** muscle cramps ■ **Misc:** chills, pancreatitis.

## INTERACTIONS

**Drug-Drug:** ■ Additive hypotension with **nitrates,** acute ingestion of **alcohol,** or other **antihypertensives** ■ Additive hypokalemia with **corticosteroids, amphotericin B, mezlocillin, piperacillin,** or **ticarcillin** ■ May increase the risk of **digoxin** toxicity ■ Decreases the excretion of **lithium**; may cause toxicity ■ May decrease the effectiveness of **methenamine** ■ **Stimulant laxatives** (including **aloe, cascara sagrada, senna**) may increase risk of potassium depletion.

**Drug-Food:** ■ **Food** may increase extent of absorption.

## ROUTE AND DOSAGE

❑ **Mykrox**

■ **PO (Adults):** *Hypertension*—0.5–1 mg/day.

❑ **Zaroxolyn**

■ **PO (Adults):** *Hypertension*—2.5–5 mg/day; *edema*—5–20 mg/day.

## AVAILABILITY

■ *Mykrox tablets:* 0.5 mg$^{Rx}$ ■ Cost: $85.24/100 ■ *Zaroxolyn tablets:* 2.5 mg$^{Rx}$, 5 mg$^{Rx}$, 10 mg$^{Rx}$ ■ Cost: 2.5 mg $97.44/100, 5 mg $93.18/100, 10 mg $87.81/100.

TIME/ACTION PROFILE (diuretic effect†)

|  | ONSET | PEAK | DURATION |
|---|---|---|---|
| PO | 1 hr | 2 hr | 12–24 hr |

†Full antihypertensive effect may take days–weeks.

## NURSING IMPLICATIONS

### ASSESSMENT

■ **General Info:** Monitor blood pressure, intake and output, and daily weight, and assess feet, legs, and sacral area for edema daily.

❑ Assess patient, especially if taking digoxin, for anorexia, nausea, vomiting, muscle cramps, paresthesia, and confusion. Notify physician or other health care professional if these signs of electrolyte imbalance occur. Patients taking digoxin are at risk of digoxin toxicity because of the potassium-depleting effect of the diuretic.

❑ Assess patient for allergy to sulfonamides.

■ **Hypertension:** Monitor blood pressure before and periodically throughout therapy.

❑ Monitor frequency of prescription refills to determine compliance.

■ *Lab Test Considerations:* Monitor electrolytes (especially potassium), blood glucose, BUN, and serum creatinine and uric acid levels before and periodically throughout therapy.

❑ May cause increase in serum and urine glucose in diabetic patients.

❑ May cause an increase in serum bilirubin, calcium, creatinine, and uric acid, and a decrease in serum magnesium, potassium, and sodium and urinary calcium concentrations.

❑ May cause decreased serum protein-bound iodine (PBI) concentrations.

❑ May cause increased serum cholesterol, low-density lipoprotein, and triglyceride concentrations.

### POTENTIAL NURSING DIAGNOSES

■ Fluid volume, excess (Indications).
■ Fluid volume, risk for deficit (Side Effects).

### IMPLEMENTATION

■ **General:** Administer in the morning to prevent disruption of sleep cycle.

❑ Intermittent dose schedule may be used for continued control of edema.

❑ Extended (Zaroxolyn) and prompt (Mykrox) metolazone tablets are not equal. Do not substitute.

{ } = Available in Canada only.
*CAPITALS indicates life-threatening; underlines indicate most frequent.

- **PO:** May give with food or milk to minimize GI irritation.

## PATIENT/FAMILY TEACHING

- **General Info:** Instruct patient to take this medication at the same time each day. If a dose is missed, take as soon as remembered but not just before next dose is due. Do not double doses.
- Instruct patient to monitor weight biweekly and notify health care professional of significant changes.
- Caution patient to change positions slowly to minimize orthostatic hypotension. This may be potentiated by alcohol.
- Advise patient to use sunscreen and protective clothing in the sun to prevent photosensitivity reactions.
- Instruct patient to discuss dietary potassium requirements with health care professional (see Appendix Q).
- Instruct patient to notify health care professional of medication regimen before treatment or surgery.
- Advise patient to report muscle weakness, cramps, nausea, vomiting, diarrhea, or dizziness to health care professional.
- Emphasize the importance of routine follow-up exams.
- **Hypertension:** Advise patient to continue taking the medication even if feeling better. Medication controls but does not cure hypertension.
- Encourage patient to comply with additional interventions for hypertension (weight reduction, low-sodium diet, regular exercise, smoking cessation, moderation of alcohol consumption, and stress management).
- Instruct patient and family in correct technique for monitoring weekly blood pressure.
- Advise patient to consult health care professional before taking OTC medication, especially cough or cold preparations, concurrently with this therapy.

## EVALUATION

**Effectiveness of therapy can be demonstrated by:** ■ Decrease in blood pressure ■ Increase in urine output ■ Decrease in edema.

**High Alert**

# metoprolol

(me-**toe**-proe-lole)
{Betaloc}, {Betaloc Durules}, {Lopresor}, {Lopresor SR}, Lopresor, {Novometoprol}, Toprol-XL

## CLASSIFICATION(S):

**Therapeutic:** antianginals, antihypertensives
**Pharmacologic:** beta blockers

### Pregnancy Category C

## INDICATIONS

■ Hypertension ■ Angina pectoris ■ Prevention of MI and decreased mortality in patients with recent MI ■ Management of stable, symptomatic (class II or III) heart failure due to ischemic, hypertensive or cardiomyopathc origin (may be used with ACE inhibitors, diuretics and/or digoxin; Toprol XL 25 mg only). **Unlabeled uses:** ■ Ventricular arrhythmias/tachycardia ■ Migraine prophylaxis ■ Tremors ■ Aggressive behavior ■ Drug-induced akathisia ■ Anxiety.

## ACTION

■ Blocks stimulation of $beta_1$(myocardial)-adrenergic receptors. Does not usually affect $beta_2$(pulmonary, vascular, uterine)-adrenergic receptor sites. **Therapeutic Effects:** ■ Decreased blood pressure and heart rate ■ Decreased frequency of attacks of angina pectoris ■ Decreased rate of cardiovascular mortality and hospitalization in patients with heart failure.

## PHARMACOKINETICS

**Absorption:** Well absorbed after oral administration.

**Distribution:** Crosses the blood-brain barrier, crosses the placenta; small amounts enter breast milk.

**Metabolism and Excretion:** Mostly metabolized by the liver.

**Half-life:** 3–7 hr.

## CONTRAINDICATIONS AND PRECAUTIONS

**Contraindicated in:** ■ Uncompensated CHF ■ Pulmonary edema ■ Cardiogenic shock ■ Bradycardia or heart block.

Use Cautiously in: ■ Renal impairment ■ Hepatic impairment ■ Geriatric patients (increased sensitivity to beta blockers; initial dosage reduction recommended) ■ Pulmonary disease (including asthma; beta₁ selectivity may be lost at higher doses) ■ Diabetes mellitus (may mask signs of hypoglycemia) ■ Thyrotoxicosis (may mask symptoms) ■ Patients with a history of severe allergic reactions (intensity of reactions may be increased) ■ Pregnancy, lactation, or children (safety not established; all agents cross the placenta and may cause fetal/neonatal bradycardia, hypotension, hypoglycemia, or respiratory depression).

## ADVERSE REACTIONS AND SIDE EFFECTS*

■ **CNS:** fatigue, weakness, anxiety, depression, dizziness, drowsiness, insomnia, memory loss, mental status changes, nervousness, nightmares ■ **EENT:** blurred vision, stuffy nose ■ **Resp:** bronchospasm, wheezing ■ **CV:** BRADYCARDIA, CHF, PULMONARY EDEMA, hypotension, peripheral vasoconstriction ■ **GI:** constipation, diarrhea, drug-induced hepatitis, dry mouth, flatulence, gastric pain, heartburn, increased liver function studies, nausea, vomiting ■ **GU:** impotence, decreased libido, urinary frequency ■ **Derm:** rashes ■ **Endo:** hyperglycemia, hypoglycemia ■ **MS:** arthralgia, back pain, joint pain ■ **Misc:** drug-induced lupus syndrome.

## INTERACTIONS

**Drug-Drug:** ■ **General anesthesia, IV phenytoin,** and **verapamil** may cause ↑ myocardial depression ■ ↑ bradycardia may occur with **digoxin** ■ ↑ hypotension may occur with other **antihypertensives,** acute ingestion of **alcohol,** or **nitrates** ■ Concurrent use with **amphetamines, cocaine, ephedrine, epinephrine, norepinephrine, phenylephrine,** or **pseudoephedrine** may result in unopposed alpha-adrenergic stimulation (excessive hypertension, bradycardia) ■ Concurrent administration of **thyroid** medication may ↓ effectiveness ■ May alter the effectiveness of **insulins** or **oral hypoglycemic agents** (dosage adjustments may be necessary) ■ May ↓ the effectiveness of **theophylline** ■ May ↓ beneficial beta₁-cardiovascular effects of **dopamine** or **dobutamine** ■ Use cautiously within

14 days of **MAO inhibitor** therapy (may result in hypertension).

## ROUTE AND DOSAGE

■ **PO (Adults):** *Antihypertensive/antianginal*—100 mg/day as a single dose or 2 divided doses; may be increased q 7 days as needed up to 450 mg/day (for angina, give in divided doses). Extended-release products are given once daily. *MI*—25–50 mg (starting 15 min after last IV dose) q 6 hr for 48 hr, then 100 mg twice daily for a minimum of 3 mo. *Heart failure*—12.5–25 mg once daily, can be doubled every 2 wk up to 200 mg/day. *Migraine prevention*—50–100 mg 2–4 times daily (unlabeled).
■ **IV (Adults):** *MI*—5 mg q 2 min for 3 doses, followed by oral dosing.

## AVAILABILITY

■ *Tablets:* 50 mg^Rx, 100 mg^Rx ■ Cost: *Lopressor*—50 mg $80.45/100, 100 mg $120.79/100; *generic*—50 mg $43.50/100, 100 mg $65.40/100 ■ *Extended-release tablets (succinate; Toprol XL):* 25 mg^Rx, 50 mg^Rx, 100 mg^Rx, 200 mg^Rx ■ *Extended-release tablets (tartrate):* 100 mg^Rx ■ *Injection:* 1 mg/ml^Rx ■ hydrochlorothiazide (Lopressor HCT)^Rx. See Appendix B.

TIME/ACTION PROFILE (cardiovascular effects)

| | ONSET | PEAK | DURATION |
|---|---|---|---|
| PO† | 15 min | unknown | 6–12 hr |
| PO–ER | unknown | 6–12 hr | 24 hr |
| IV | immediate | 20 min | 5–8 hr |

†Maximal effects on BP (chronic therapy) may not occur for 1 wk. Hypotensive effects may persist for up to 4 wk after discontinuation.

# NURSING IMPLICATIONS

## ASSESSMENT

❑ Monitor blood pressure, ECG, and pulse frequently during dose adjustment and periodically during therapy.
❑ Monitor vital signs and ECG every 5–15 min during and for several hours after parenteral administration. If heart rate <40 bpm, especially if cardiac output is also decreased, administer atropine 0.25–0.5 mg IV.

- Monitor intake and output ratios and daily weights. Assess routinely for signs and symptoms of CHF (dyspnea, rales/crackles, weight gain, peripheral edema, jugular venous distention).

- **Angina:** Assess frequency and characteristics of anginal attacks periodically during therapy.

- *Lab Test Considerations:* May cause ↑ BUN, serum lipoprotein, potassium, triglyceride, and uric acid levels.

- May cause ↑ ANA titers.

- May cause ↑ in blood glucose levels.

- May cause ↑ serum alkaline phosphatase, LDH, AST, and ALT levels.

## POTENTIAL NURSING DIAGNOSES

- Cardiac output, decreased (Side Effects).
- Noncompliance (Patient/Family Teaching).

## IMPLEMENTATION

- *High Alert:* IV vasoactive medications are inherently dangerous. Before administering intravenously, have second practitioner independently check original order and dosage calculations. Do not confuse metoprolol with misoprostol.

- **PO:** Take apical pulse before administering. If <50 bpm or if arrhythmia occurs, withhold medication and notify physician or other health care professional.

- Administer metoprolol with meals or directly after eating.

- Extended-release tablets should be swallowed whole; do not crush, break, or chew.

- **Direct IV:** May be administered by injecting 5 mg rapidly at 2-min intervals for 3 doses. Oral therapy should begin 15 min after last IV dose.

- **Y-Site Compatibility:** ◆ alteplase ◆ meperidine ◆ morphine.

- **Y-Site Incompatibility:** ◆ amphotericin B cholesteryl sulfate.

## PATIENT/FAMILY TEACHING

- **General Info:** Instruct patient to take medication as directed, at the same time each day, even if feeling well; do not skip or double up on missed doses. Take missed doses as soon as possible up to 8 hr before next dose. Abrupt withdrawal may precipitate life-threatening arrhythmias, hypertension, or myocardial ischemia.

- Teach patient and family how to check pulse daily and blood pressure biweekly and to report significant changes to health care professional.

- May cause drowsiness. Caution patient to avoid driving or other activities that require alertness until response to the drug is known.

- Advise patient to change positions slowly to minimize orthostatic hypotension.

- Caution patient that this medication may increase sensitivity to cold.

- Instruct patient to consult health care professional before taking any OTC medications or herbal products, especially cold preparations, concurrently with this medication. Patients on antihypertensive therapy should also avoid excessive amounts of caffeinated coffee, tea, and cola.

- Diabetics should closely monitor blood glucose, especially if weakness, malaise, irritability, or fatigue occurs. Medication does not block sweating as a sign of hypoglycemia.

- Advise patient to notify health care professional if slow pulse, difficulty breathing, wheezing, cold hands and feet, dizziness, light-headedness, confusion, depression, rash, fever, sore throat, unusual bleeding, or bruising occurs.

- Instruct patient to inform health care professional of medication regimen before treatment or surgery.

- Advise patient to carry identification describing disease process and medication regimen at all times.

- **Hypertension:** Reinforce the need to continue additional therapies for hypertension (weight loss, sodium restriction, stress reduction, regular exercise, moderation of alcohol consumption, and smoking cessation). Medication controls but does not cure hypertension.

## EVALUATION

**Effectiveness of therapy can be demonstrated by:** ■ Decrease in blood pressure ■ Reduction in frequency of anginal attacks ❑ Increase in activity tolerance ■ Prevention of MI.

## metronidazole
(me-troe-**ni**-da-zole)

{Apo-Metronidazole}, Flagyl, Flagyl ER, Metric 21, MetroCream, MetroGel, MetroGel-Vaginal, MetroLotion, Metro IV, Metryl, {Nidagel}, Noritate, {Novonidazol}, Protostat, {Trikacide}

## CLASSIFICATION(S):

**Therapeutic:** *anti-infectives, antiprotozoals, antiulcer agents*

**Pregnancy Category B**

## INDICATIONS

■ **PO, IV:** Treatment of the following anaerobic infections: ❑ Intra-abdominal infections (may be used with a cephalosporin) ❑ Gynecologic infections ❑ Skin and skin structure infections ❑ Lower respiratory tract infections ❑ Bone and joint infections ❑ CNS infections ❑ Septicemia ❑ Endocarditis ■ **IV:** Perioperative prophylactic agent in colorectal surgery ■ **PO:** Amebicide in the management of amebic dysentery, amebic liver abscess, and trichomoniasis ❑ Treatment of peptic ulcer disease caused by *Helicobacter pylori* ■ **Topical:** Treatment of acne rosacea ■ **Vag:** Management of bacterial vaginosis. **Unlabeled uses:** ■ Treatment of giardiasis ■ Treatment of anti-infective associated pseudomembranous colitis.

## ACTION

■ Disrupts DNA and protein synthesis in susceptible organisms. **Therapeutic Effects:** ■ Bactericidal, trichomonacidal, or amebicidal action. **Spectrum:** ■ Most notable for activity against anaerobic bacteria, including: ❑ *Bacteroides* ❑ *Clostridium* ■ In addition, is active against: ❑ *Trichomonas vaginalis* ❑ *Entamoeba histolytica* ❑ *Giardia lamblia* ❑ *H. pylori* ❑ *Clostridium difficile.*

## PHARMACOKINETICS

**Absorption:** 80% absorbed after oral administration. Minimal absorption after topical or vaginal application.

**Distribution:** Widely distributed into most tissues and fluids, including CSF. Crosses the placenta and enters fetal circulation rapidly; enters breast milk in concentrations equal to plasma levels.

**Metabolism and Excretion:** Partially metabolized by the liver (30–60%), partially excreted unchanged in the urine, 6–15% eliminated in the feces.

**Half-life:** 6–8 hr.

## CONTRAINDICATIONS AND PRECAUTIONS

**Contraindicated in:** ■ Hypersensitivity ■ Hypersensitivity to parabens (topical only) ■ First trimester of pregnancy.

**Use Cautiously in:** ■ History of blood dyscrasias ■ History of seizures or neurologic problems ■ Severe hepatic impairment (dosage reduction suggested) ■ Pregnancy (although safety not established, has been used to treat trichomoniasis in 2nd- and 3rd-trimester pregnancy—but not as single-dose regimen) ■ Lactation (if needed, use single dose and interrupt nursing for 24 hr thereafter) ■ Children (safe use of IV form not established; safety of oral form for infections other than amebiasis in children not established).

## ADVERSE REACTIONS AND SIDE EFFECTS*

■ **CNS:** SEIZURES, <u>dizziness, headache</u> ■ **EENT:** tearing (topical only) ■ **GI:** <u>abdominal pain, anorexia, nausea,</u> diarrhea, dry mouth, furry tongue, glossitis, unpleasant taste, vomiting ■ **Derm:** rashes, urticaria; *topical only*—burning, mild dryness, skin irritation, transient redness ■ **Hemat:** leukopenia ■ **Local:** phlebitis at IV site ■ **Neuro:** peripheral neuropathy ■ **Misc:** superinfection.

## INTERACTIONS

**Drug-Drug:** ■ **Cimetidine** may decrease the metabolism of metronidazole ■ **Phenobarbital** increases metabolism and may decrease effectiveness ■ Metronidazole increases the effects of **warfarin** ■ Disulfiram-like reaction may occur with **alcohol** ingestion ■ May cause acute psychosis and confusion with **disulfiram** ■ Increased risk of leukopenia with **fluorouracil** or **azathioprine.**

## ROUTE AND DOSAGE

■ **PO (Adults):** *Anaerobic infections*—7.5 mg/kg q 6 hr (not to exceed 4 g/day). *Trichomoniasis*—250 mg q 8 hr for 7 days *or* single 2-g dose *or* 1 g bid for 1 day. *Amebia-*

---

{ } = Available in Canada only.
\* CAPITALS indicates life-threatening; <u>underlines</u> indicate most frequent.

*sis*—500–750 mg q 8 hr for 5–10 days. *H. pylori*—250 mg 4 times daily *or* 500 mg twice daily for 1–2 wk (with other agents). *Bacterial vaginoses*—750 mg once daily as ER tablets for 7 days.

■ **PO (Children):** *Trichomoniasis*—5 mg/kg q 8 hr for 7–10 days. *Amebiasis*—11.6–16.7 mg/kg q 8 hr for 5–10 days (not to exceed 750 mg/dose).

■ **IV (Adults):** *Anaerobic infections*—Initial dose 15 mg/kg, then 7.5 mg/kg q 6–8 hr *or* 500 mg q 6–8 hr (not to exceed 4 g/day). *Perioperative prophylaxis*—Initial dose 15 mg/kg 1 hr before surgery, then 7.5 mg/kg 6 and 12 hr later. *Amebiasis*—500–750 mg q 8 hr for 5–10 days.

■ **Topical (Adults):** *Acne rosacea*—apply thin film to affected area bid.

■ **Vag (Adults):** *Bacterial vaginosis*—One applicatorful (0.75% gel) 2 times daily for 5 days.

## AVAILABILITY (generic available)

■ *Tablets:* 250 mg$^{Rx}$, 500 mg$^{Rx}$ ■ Cost: *Flagyl*—250 mg $198.05/50, 500 mg $346.37/50; *generic*—250 mg $23.13/50, 500 mg $23.13/50 ■ with bismuth subsalicylate and tetracycline in a compliace package (Helidac); with clarithromycin and omeprazole in a compliance package (Losec 1-2-3M) ■ *Extended-release (ER) tablets:* 750 mg$^{Rx}$ ■ Cost: *Flagyl ER*—$171.00/30 ■ *Capsules:* 375 mg$^{Rx}$, {500 mg$^{Rx}$} ■ Cost: *Flagyl*—$117.45/50 ■ *Powder for injection:* 500-mg vials$^{Rx}$ ■ *Premixed injection:* 500 mg/100 ml$^{Rx}$ RTU (ready to use) ■ *Topical gel:* 0.75%$^{Rx}$ in 28.4-g tubes ■ *Topical cream:* 0.75% in 28.4-g tubes$^{Rx}$ ■ *Topical lotion:* 0.75% in 59-ml bottle$^{Rx}$ ■ *Vaginal gel:* 0.75% (37.5 mg/5 g applicatorful) in 70-g tubes$^{Rx}$ ■ Cost: $36.05 ■ bismuth subsalicylate tablets and tetracycline capsules (Helidac$^{Rx}$) as part of a compliance package. See Appendix B.

TIME/ACTION PROFILE (PO, IV = blood levels; topical = improvement in rosacea)

|  | ONSET | PEAK | DURATION |
|---|---|---|---|
| PO | rapid | 1–3 hr | 8 hr |
| PO-ER | rapid | unknown | up to 24 hr |
| IV | rapid | end of infusion | 6–8 hr |
| Topical | 3 wk | 9 wk | 12 hr |
| Vaginal | unknown | 6–12 hr | 12 hr |

## NURSING IMPLICATIONS

### ASSESSMENT

■ **General Info:** Assess patient for infection (vital signs; appearance of wound, sputum, urine, and stool; WBC) at beginning of and throughout therapy.

❑ Obtain specimens for culture and sensitivity before initiating therapy. First dose may be given before receiving results.

❑ Monitor neurologic status during and after IV infusions. Inform physician if numbness, paresthesia, weakness, ataxia, or seizures occur.

❑ Monitor intake and output and daily weight, especially for patients on sodium restriction. Each 500 mg of Flagyl IV for dilution contains 5 mEq of sodium; each 500 mg of Flagyl RTU contains 14 mEq of sodium.

■ **Giardiasis:** Monitor three stool samples taken several days apart, beginning 3–4 wk after treatment.

■ *Lab Test Considerations:* May alter results of serum AST, ALT, and LDH tests.

### POTENTIAL NURSING DIAGNOSES

■ Infection, risk for (Indications).

■ Diarrhea (Indications).

### IMPLEMENTATION

■ **PO:** Administer with food or milk to minimize GI irritation. Tablets may be crushed for patients with difficulty swallowing.

■ **Intermittent Infusion:** Flagyl IV RTU is prediluted and ready to use (5 mg/ml). Prefilled plastic minibags should not be used in series connections; air embolism may result. Crystals may form during refrigeration but will dissolve when warmed to room temperature.

❑ Preparation of Flagyl IV requires a specific process. Do not use aluminum needles or hubs; color will turn orange/rust. Add 4.4 ml of sterile or bacteriostatic sterile water, or 0.9% or bacteriostatic 0.9% NaCl for injection (100 mg/ml). Solution should be clear, pale yellow-green. Do not use cloudy or precipitated solution. Dilute further to at least 8 mg/ml with 0.9% NaCl, D5W, or LR. Neutralize solution with 5 mEq sodium bicarbonate for each 500 mg. Mix thoroughly. Carbon dioxide gas will be generated and may require venting. Do not refrigerate. Stable for 24 hr at room temperature.

■ *Rate:* Administer IV doses as a slow infusion, each single dose over 1 hr.

■ **Y-Site Compatibility:** ◆ acyclovir ◆ allopurinol ◆ amifostine ◆ cefepime ◆ cisatracurium ◆ clarithromycin ◆ cyclophosphamide ◆ diltiazem ◆ docetaxel ◆ dopamine ◆ doxorubicin liposome ◆ enalaprilat ◆ esmolol ◆ etoposide ◆ fluconazole ◆ foscarnet ◆ gatifloxacin ◆ gemcitabine ◆ granisetron ◆ heparin ◆ hydromorphone ◆ labetalol ◆ linezolid ◆ lorazepam ◆ magnesium sulfate ◆ melphalan ◆ meperidine ◆ methylprednisolone ◆ midazolam ◆ morphine ◆ perphenazine ◆ piperacillin/tazobactam ◆ remifentanil ◆ sargramostim ◆ tacrolimus ◆ teniposide ◆ theophylline ◆ thiotepa ◆ vinorelbine.

■ **Y-Site Incompatibility:** Manufacturer recommends discontinuing primary IV during metronidazole infusion. ◆ amphotericin B cholesteryl sulfate ◆ aztreonam ◆ filgrastim

■ **Additive Incompatibility:** Do not admix with other medications.

■ **Topical:** Cleanse affected area before application. Apply and rub in a thin film twice daily, morning and evening. Avoid contact with eyes.

## PATIENT/FAMILY TEACHING

❏ Instruct patient to take medication exactly as directed with evenly spaced times between doses, even if feeling better. Do not skip doses or double up on missed doses. If a dose is missed, take as soon as remembered if not almost time for next dose.

❏ Advise patients treated for trichomoniasis that sexual partners may be asymptomatic sources of reinfection and should be treated concurrently. Patient should also refrain from intercourse or use a condom to prevent reinfection.

❏ Caution patient to avoid intake of alcoholic beverages or preparations containing alcohol during and for at least 1 day after treatment with metronidazole, including vaginal gel. May cause a disulfiram-like reaction (flushing, nausea, vomiting, headache, abdominal cramps).

❏ May cause dizziness or light-headedness. Caution patient to avoid driving or other activities requiring alertness until response to medication is known.

❏ Inform patient that medication may cause an unpleasant metallic taste.

❏ Advise patient not to take OTC medications concurrently without consulting health care professional.

❏ Advise patient that frequent mouth rinses, good oral hygiene, and sugarless gum or candy may minimize dry mouth. Notify health care professional if dry mouth persists for more than 2 wk.

❏ Advise patient to inform health care professional if pregnancy is suspected before taking this medication.

❏ Inform patient that medication may cause urine to turn dark.

❏ Advise patient to consult health care professional if no improvement in a few days or if signs and symptoms of superinfection (black, furry overgrowth on tongue; vaginal itching or discharge; loose or foul-smelling stools) develop.

■ **Vag:** Instruct patient in correct technique for intravaginal instillation. Advise patient to avoid intercourse during treatment with vaginal gel.

■ **Topical:** Instruct patient on correct technique for application of topical gel. Cosmetics may be used after application of gel.

## EVALUATION

**Effectiveness of therapy can be demonstrated by:** ■ Resolution of the signs and symptoms of infection. Length of time for complete resolution depends on organism and site of infection ❏ Significant results should be seen within 3 wk of application of topical gel. Application may be continued for 9 wk.

## miconazole, See ANTIFUNGALS (TOPICAL), ANTIFUNGALS (VAGINAL).

High Alert

# midazolam
(mid-**ay**-zoe-lam)
Versed

**CLASSIFICATION(S):**

**Therapeutic:** *antianxiety agents, sedative/hypnotics*
**Pharmacologic:** *benzodiazepines*

**Schedule IV**

**Pregnancy Category D**

## INDICATIONS

■ **PO:** Preprocedural sedation and anxiolysis in pediatric patients ■ **IM, IV:** Preoperative sedation/anxiolysis/amnesia ■ **IV:** Provides sedation/anxiolysis/amnesia during therapeutic, diagnostic, or radiographic procedures (conscious sedation) ❑ Aids in the induction of anesthesia and as part of balanced anesthesia ❑ As a continuous infusion, provides sedation of mechanically ventilated patients during anesthesia or in a critical care setting.

## ACTION

■ Acts at many levels of the CNS to produce generalized CNS depression ■ Effects may be mediated by GABA, an inhibitory neurotransmitter. **Therapeutic Effects:** ■ Short-term sedation ■ Postoperative amnesia.

## PHARMACOKINETICS

**Absorption:** Rapidly absorbed following oral administration; undergoes substantial intestinal and first-pass hepatic metabolism. Well absorbed following IM administration; IV administration results in complete bioavailability.

**Distribution:** Crosses the blood-brain barrier and placenta.

**Protein Binding:** 97%.

**Metabolism and Excretion:** Almost exclusively metabolized by the liver, resulting in conversion to hydroxymidazolam, an active metabolite, and 2 other inactive metabolites (metabolized by cytochrome P450 3A4 enzyme system); metabolites are excreted in urine.

**Half-life:** 1–12 hr (increased in renal impairment or CHF).

## CONTRAINDICATIONS AND PRECAUTIONS

**Contraindicated in:** ■ Hypersensitivity ■ Cross-sensitivity with other benzodiazepines may occur ■ Shock ■ Comatose patients or those with pre-existing CNS depression ■ Uncontrolled severe pain ■ Products containing benzyl alcohol should not be used in neonates ■ Pregnancy ■ Acute narrow-angle glaucoma.

**Use Cautiously in:** ■ Pulmonary disease ■ CHF ■ Renal impairment ■ Severe hepatic impairment ■ Obese pediatric patients (calculate dose on the basis of ideal body weight) ■ Geriatric or debilitated patients (especially patients >70 yr) more susceptible to cardiorespiratory depressant effects; dosage reduction required ■ Lactation (safety not established).

## ADVERSE REACTIONS AND SIDE EFFECTS*

■ **CNS:** agitation, drowsiness, excess sedation, headache ■ **EENT:** blurred vision ■ **Resp:** APNEA, LARYNGOSPASM, RESPIRATORY DEPRESSION, bronchospasm, coughing ■ **CV:** CARDIAC ARREST, arrhythmias ■ **GI:** hiccups, nausea, vomiting ■ **Derm:** rashes ■ **Local:** phlebitis at IV site, pain at IM site.

## INTERACTIONS

**Drug-Drug:** ■ ↑ CNS depression with **alcohol, antihistamines, opioid analgesics,** and other **sedative/hypnotics** (↓ midazolam dose by 30–50% if used concurrently) ■ ↑ risk of hypotension with **antihypertensives,** acute ingestion of **alcohol,** or **nitrates** ■ Midazolam is metabolized by the cytochrome P450 3A4 enzyme system; drugs that induce or inhibit this system may be expected to alter the effects of midazolam ■ **Carbamazepine, phenytoin, rifampin, rifabutin,** and **phenobarbital** ↓ levels of midazolam ■ The following agents ↓ midazolam metabolism and may ↑ its effects: **erythromycin, cimetidine, ranitidine, diltiazem, verapamil, fluconazole, itraconazole,** and **ketoconazole.**

**Drug-Natural Products:** ■ Concomitant use of **kava, valerian,** or **chamomile** can ↑ CNS depression.

**Drug-Food:** ■ **Grapefruit juice** ↓ metabolism and may ↑ effects of midazolam.

## ROUTE AND DOSAGE

Dosage must be individualized, taking caution to reduce dosage in geriatric patients and in those who are already sedated.

❑ **Preoperative Sedation/Anxiolysis/Amnesia**

■ **PO (Children 6 mo–16 yr):** *Older (6–16 yr), more cooperative patients*—0.25–0.5 mg/kg; *younger, less cooperative patients*—may require up to 1 mg/kg (dose should not exceed 20 mg); *patients with cardiac/respiratory compromise or concurrent CNS depressants*—0.25 mg/kg.

■ **IM (Adults Otherwise Healthy and <60 yr):** 70–80 mcg/kg 1 hr before surgery (usual dose 5 mg).

■ **IM (Adults ≥60 yr, Debilitated or Chronically Ill):** 20–30 mcg/kg 1 hr before surgery (usual dose 1–3 mg).

■ **IM (Children):** 100–150 mcg (0.01–0.15 mg)/kg up to 500 mcg (0.5 mg)/kg; not to exceed 10 mg/dose.

❑ **Conscious Sedation for Short Procedures**

■ **IV (Adults and Children Otherwise Healthy >12 yr and <60 yr):** 1–1.5 mg initially; dosage may be increased further as needed. Total doses >3.5 mg are rarely needed (reduce dose by 30% if other CNS depressants are used). Maintenance doses of 25% of the dose required for initial sedation may be given as necessary.

■ **IV (Geriatric Patients ≥60 yr, Debilitated or Chronically Ill):** 1–2.5 mg initially; dosage may be increased further as needed. Total doses >5 mg are rarely needed (reduce dose by 50% if other CNS depressants are used). Maintenance doses of 25% of the dose required for initial sedation may be given as necessary.

❑ **Conscious Sedation for Short Procedures or Prior to Anesthesia**

■ **IV (Children 6–12 yr):** 50–100 mcg/kg (not to exceed 600 mcg/kg [or 6 mg] total dose).

■ **IV (Children 6 mo–5 yr):** 25–50 mcg/kg initially; up to 400 mcg/kg total dose may be required (not to exceed 10 mg total dose).

❑ **Induction of Anesthesia (Adjunct)**

May give additional dose of 25% of initial dose if needed.

■ **IV (Adults Otherwise Healthy and <55 yr):** 300–350 mcg/kg initially (up to 600 mcg/kg total). If patient is premedicated, initial dose should be further reduced.

■ **IV (Geriatric Patients >55 yr):** 150–300 mcg/kg as initial dose. If patient is premedicated, initial dose should be further reduced.

■ **IV (Adults—Debilitated):** 150–250 mcg/kg initial dose. If patient is premedicated, initial dose should be further reduced.

❑ **Sedation in Critical Care Settings**

■ **IV (Adults):** 10–50 mcg/kg (0.5–4 mg in most adults) initially if a loading dose is required; may repeat q 10–15 min until desired effect is obtained; may be followed by infusion at 20–100 mcg/kg/hr (1–7 mg/hr in most adults).

■ **IV (Children):** *Intubated patients only—*50–200 mcg/kg initially as a loading dose; follow with infusion at 60–120 mcg/kg/min (1–2 mcg/kg/min).

■ **IV (Neonates >32 wk):** *Intubated patients only—*60 mcg/kg/hr (1 mcg/kg/min).

■ **IV (Neonates <32 wk):** *Intubated patients only—*30 mcg/kg/hr (0.5 mcg/kg/min).

**AVAILABILITY (generic available)**

■ *Injection:* 1 mg/ml[Rx], 5 mg/ml[Rx] ■ *Syrup (cherry flavor):* 2 mg/ml[Rx].

TIME/ACTION PROFILE (sedation)

|     | ONSET | PEAK | DURATION |
| --- | --- | --- | --- |
| IM | 15 min | 30–60 min | 2–6 hr |
| IV | 1.5–5 min | rapid | 2–6 hr |

# NURSING IMPLICATIONS

## ASSESSMENT

❑ Assess level of sedation and level of consciousness throughout and for 2–6 hr following administration.

❑ Monitor blood pressure, pulse, and respiration continuously during IV administration. Oxygen and resuscitative equipment should be immediately available.

■ *Toxicity and Overdose:* If overdose occurs, monitor pulse, respiration, and blood pressure continuously. Maintain patent airway and assist ventilation as needed. If hypotension occurs, treatment includes IV fluids, repositioning, and vasopressors.

❑ The effects of midazolam can be reversed with flumazenil (Romazicon).

## POTENTIAL NURSING DIAGNOSES

- Breathing pattern, ineffective (Adverse Reactions).
- Injury, risk for (Side Effects).

## IMPLEMENTATION

◻ **High Alert:** Accidental overdosage of oral midazolam syrup to children has resulted in serious harm and death. Do not accept orders prescribed by volume (5 mL or 1 tsp); instead, request dosage be expressed in milligrams. Have second practitioner independently check original order and dose calculations. Midazolam syrup should only be administered by health care professionals authorized to administer conscious sedation. Do not confuse Versed (midazolam) with VePesid (etoposide).

- **PO:** To use the *Press-in Bottle Adaptor (PIBA),* remove the cap and push bottle adaptor into neck of bottle. Close bottle tightly with cap. Solution is a clear red to purplish-red cherry-flavored syrup. Then remove cap and insert tip of oral dispenser in bottle adaptor. Push the plunger completely down toward tip of oral dispenser and insert firmly into bottle adaptor. Turn entire unit (bottle and oral dispenser) upside down. Pull plunger out slowly until desired amount of medication is withdrawn into oral dispenser. Turn entire unit right side up and slowly remove oral dispenser from the bottle. Tip of dispenser may be covered with tip of cap until time of use. Close bottle with cap after each use.

◻ Dispense directly into mouth. Do not mix with any liquid prior to dispensing.

- **IM:** Administer IM doses deep into muscle mass.

- **Direct IV:** Administer undiluted or diluted with D5W, 0.9% NaCl, or lactated Ringer's injection through Y-site.

◻ When administered concurrently with opioid analgesics, dose should be reduced by 30–50%.

- **Rate:** Administer each dose slowly over at least 2 min. Monitor IV site closely to avoid extravasation. Titrate dose to patient response. Rapid injection, especially in neonates, has caused severe hypotension.

- **Continuous Infusion:** Dilute 5 mg/ml to a concentration of 0.5 mg/ml with 0.9% NaCl or D5W.

- **Rate:** Usual infusion rate is 0.02–0.1 mg/kg/hr (1–7 mg/hr). Titrate to desired level of sedation. Assess sedation at regular intervals and adjust rate up or down by 25–50% as needed. Dose should also be decreased by 10–25% every few hours to find minimum effective infusion rate, which prevents accumulation of midazolam and provides more rapid recovery upon termination.

◻ In pediatric patients, rate of 0.06–0.12 mg/kg/hr (1–2 mcg/kg/min) can be increased or decreased by 25% based on assessment of sedation.

◻ In neonates, rate of 0.03 mg/kg/hr (0.5 mcg/kg/min) is used for neonates <32 weeks and rate of 0.06 mg/kg/hr (1 mcg/kg/min) is used for neonates >32 weeks of age.

- **Syringe Compatibility:** alfentanil ◆ atracurium ◆ atropine ◆ buprenorphine ◆ butorphanol ◆ chlorpromazine ◆ cimetidine ◆ diphenhydramine ◆ droperidol ◆ fentanyl ◆ glycopyrrolate ◆ hydromorphone ◆ hydroxyzine ◆ meperidine ◆ metoclopramide ◆ morphine ◆ nalbuphine ◆ ondansetron ◆ promethazine ◆ scopolamine ◆ sufentanil ◆ thiethylperazine ◆ trimethobenzamide.

- **Syringe Incompatibility:** ◆ prochlorperazine ◆ ranitidine.

- **Y-Site Compatibility:** ◆ alatrofloxacin ◆ amikacin ◆ amiodarone ◆ atracurium ◆ calcium gluconate ◆ cefazolin ◆ cefotaxime ◆ cimetidine ◆ ciprofloxacin ◆ cisatracurium ◆ clindamycin ◆ digoxin ◆ diltiazem ◆ dopamine ◆ epinephrine ◆ erythromycin lactobionate ◆ esmolol ◆ etomidate ◆ famotidine ◆ fentanyl ◆ fluconazole ◆ gatifloxacin ◆ gentamicin ◆ haloperidol ◆ heparin ◆ hydromorphone ◆ insulin ◆ labetalol ◆ linezolid ◆ lorazepam ◆ methylprednisolone ◆ metronidazole ◆ morphine ◆ nitroglycerin ◆ nitroprusside ◆ norepinephrine ◆ pancuronium ◆ piperacillin ◆ potassium chloride ◆ ranitidine ◆ remifentanil ◆ sufentanil ◆ theophylline ◆ tobramycin ◆ vancomycin ◆ vecuronium.

- **Y-Site Incompatibility:** ◆ albumin ◆ amphotericin B cholesteryl sulfate ◆ ampicillin ◆ bumetanide ◆ butorphanol ◆ ceftazidime ◆ cefuroxime ◆ clonidine ◆ floxacillin ◆ foscarnet ◆ fosphenytoin ◆ furosemide ◆ hydrocortisone ◆ imipenem/cilastatin ◆ methotrexate ◆ nafcillin ◆ omeprazole ◆ sodium bicarbonate ◆ thiopental ◆ trimethoprim/sulfamethoxazole.

## PATIENT/FAMILY TEACHING

❑ Inform patient that this medication will decrease mental recall of the procedure.
❑ May cause drowsiness or dizziness. Advise patient to request assistance prior to ambulation and transfer and to avoid driving or other activities requiring alertness for 24 hr following administration.
❑ Instruct patient to inform health care professional prior to administration if pregnancy is suspected.
❑ Advise patient to avoid alcohol or other CNS depressants for 24 hr following administration of midazolam.

## EVALUATION

**Effectiveness of therapy can be demonstrated by:** ■ Sedation during and amnesia following surgical, diagnostic, and radiologic procedures ■ Sedation and amnesia for mechanically ventilated patients in a critical care setting.

# mifepristone
(mi-fe-**priss**-tone)
Mifeprex

*CLASSIFICATION(S):*
*Therapeutic: abortifacients*
*Pharmacologic: antiprogestational agents*

**Pregnancy Category UK**

## INDICATIONS

■ Medical termination of intrauterine pregnancy through 49-day pregnancy.

## ACTION

■ Antagonizes endometrial and myometrial effects of progesterone ■ Sensitizes the myometrium to contraction-inducing activity of prostaglandins. **Therapeutic Effects:** ■ Termination of pregnancy.

## PHARMACOKINETICS

**Absorption:** Rapidly absorbed following oral administration (69% bioavailability).
**Distribution:** Unknown.

**Protein Binding:** 98%.
**Metabolism and Excretion:** Mostly metabolized by the liver (cytochrome CYP450 3A4 [CYP450 3A4] enzyme system).
**Half-life:** 18 hr.

## CONTRAINDICATIONS AND PRECAUTIONS

**Contraindicated in:** ■ Presence of an intrauterine device (IUD) ■ Confirmed or suspected ectopic pregnancy ■ Undiagnosed adnexal mass ■ Chronic adrenal failure ■ Concurrent long-term corticosteroid therapy ■ Bleeding disorders or concurrent anticoagulant therapy ■ Inherited porphyrias.

**Use Cautiously in:** ■ Chronic medical conditions such as cardiovascular, hypertensive, hepatic, renal, or respiratory disease (safety and efficacy not established) ■ Women >35 yrs old or who smoke ≥10 cigarettes/day.

## ADVERSE REACTIONS AND SIDE EFFECTS*

■ **CNS:** dizziness, fainting, headache, weakness ■ **GI:** abdominal pain, diarrhea, nausea, vomiting ■ **GU:** uterine bleeding, uterine cramping, ruptured ectopic pregnancy, pelvic pain.

## INTERACTIONS

**Drug-Drug:** ■ Blood levels and therapeutic effectiveness may be ↑ by **ketoconazole, itraconazole, and erythromycin** ■ Blood levels and effects may be ↓ by **rifampin, dexamethasone, phenytoin, phenobarbital,** and **carbamazepine** ■ Mifepristone may ↓ metabolism and ↑ effects of other **drugs metabolized by the CYP 450 3A4 enzyme system,** including **some agents used during general anesthesia.**

**Drug-Natural Products:** ■ Blood levels and effects may be ↓ by St. John's wort.
**Drug-Food:** ■ Blood levels and effects may be ↑ by **grapefruit juice.**

## ROUTE AND DOSAGE

■ **PO (Adults):** *Day 1*—600 mg (given as three 200 mg tablets) as a single dose, followed on *day 3* by 400 mcg misoprostol (Cytotec), unless abortion has occurred and has been confirmed by clinical or ultrasonographic examination (see misoprostol monograph).

## AVAILABILITY

- **Tablets:** 200 mg.

TIME/ACTION PROFILE (termination of pregnancy)

|  | ONSET | PEAK | DURATION |
|---|---|---|---|
| PO | unknown | within 2 days | unknown |

# NURSING IMPLICATIONS

## ASSESSMENT

- ❏ Determine duration of pregnancy. Pregnancy is dated from the first day of the last menstrual period in a presumed 28-day cycle with ovulation occuring at mid-cycle and can be determined by menstrual history and clinical examination; use ultrasound if duration is uncertain or if ectopic pregnancy is suspected.
- ❏ Assess amount of bleeding and cramping during treatment. Determine if termination is complete on day 14.
- ■ **Lab Test Considerations:** Decrease in hemoglobin, hematocrit, and RBCs may occur in women who bleed heavily.
- ❏ Changes in quantitative human chorionic gonadotropin (hCG) levels are not accurate until at least 10 days after mifepristone administration; complete termination of pregnancy must be confirmed by clinical examination.

## POTENTIAL NURSING DIAGNOSES

- ■ Pain, acute (Side Effects).

## IMPLEMENTATION

- ■ **General:** Mifepristone should be administered only by health care professionals that have read and understood the prescribing information, are able to assess gestational age of an embryo and diagnose ectopic pregnancies, and who are able to provide surgical intervention in cases of incomplete abortion or severe bleeding.
- ❏ Any IUD should be removed prior to mifepristone adminstration.
- ❏ Measures to prevent rhesus immunization, similar to those of surgical abortion, should be taken.

- ■ **PO:** On *day 1*, after the patient has read the Medication Guide and signed the Patient Agreement, administer three 200 mg tablets as a single dose. On *day 3*, unless abortion has occurred and been confirmed by clinical examination or ultrasound, administer two 200 mcg tablets of misoprostol. On *day 14*, confirm that termination of pregnancy has occurred by clinical examination or ultrasound.

## PATIENT/FAMILY TEACHING

- ❏ Advise patient of the treatment and its effects. Patients must be given a copy of the Medication Guide and Patient Agreement. Patient must understand the necessity of completing the treatment schedule of three office visits (day 1, day 3, and day 14).
- ❏ Inform patient that vaginal bleeding and uterine cramping will probably occur and that prolonged or heavy vaginal bleeding is not proof of complete expulsion. Bleeding or spotting occurs for an average of 9–16 days; but may continue for more than 30 days. Advise patient that if the treatment fails, there is a risk of fetal malformation; medical abortion failures are managed by surgical termination.
- ❏ Instruct patient in the steps to take in an emergency situation, including precise instructions and a telephone number to call if she has problems or concerns.
- ❏ May cause dizziness or fainting. Caution patient to avoid driving or other activities requiring alertness until response to medication is known.
- ❏ Caution patient that pregnancy can occur following termination of pregnancy and before resumption of normal menses. Contraception can be initiated as soon as pregnancy termination is confirmed, or before sexual intercourse is resumed.
- ❏ Advise patient to notify health care professional if she smokes at least 10 cigarettes a day.

## EVALUATION

**Clinical response to therapy can be evaluated by:** ■ Termination of an intrauterine pregnancy of less than 49 days in duration.

# miglitol

(**mi**-gli-tole)
Glyset

**CLASSIFICATION(S):**
**Therapeutic:** antidiabetics
**Pharmacologic:** alpha-glucosidase inhibitors

**Pregnancy Category B**

## INDICATIONS

■ Management of non–insulin-dependent diabetes mellitus (type 2) in conjunction with dietary therapy; may be used concurrently with sulfonylurea oral hypoglycemic agents.

## ACTION

■ Lowers blood glucose by inhibiting the enzyme alpha-glucosidase in the GI tract, resulting in delayed glucose absorption. **Therapeutic Effects:** ■ Lowering of blood glucose in diabetic patients, especially postprandial hyperglycemia.

## PHARMACOKINETICS

**Absorption:** Completely absorbed at lower doses (25 mg); 50–70% absorbed at higher doses (100 mg).

**Distribution:** Distributes primarily into extracellular fluid; small amounts enter breast milk.

**Metabolism and Excretion:** Not metabolized; action is primarily local in the GI tract; amounts that are absorbed are excreted mostly unchanged in urine.

**Half-life:** 2 hr.

## CONTRAINDICATIONS AND PRECAUTIONS

**Contraindicated in:** ■ Hypersensitivity ■ Diabetic ketoacidosis ■ Inflammatory bowel disease or other chronic intestinal conditions resulting in impaired absorption or predisposition to obstruction ■ Lactation.

**Use Cautiously in:** ■ Patients with fever, infection, trauma, or stress (may cause hyperglycemia requiring alternate therapy) ■ Renal impairment (use not recommended if creatinine

>2 mg/dl) ■ Pregnancy or children (safety not established).

## ADVERSE REACTIONS AND SIDE EFFECTS*

■ **GI:** <u>abdominal pain</u>, <u>diarrhea</u>, <u>flatulence</u> ■ **Hemat:** low serum iron.

## INTERACTIONS

**Drug-Drug:** ■ May decrease absorption of **ranitidine** and **propranolol** ■ Effects may be decreased by **intestinal adsorbents** (such as **charcoal**) and **digestive enzyme products**; concurrent use should be avoided.

**Drug-Food:** ■ Concurrent **carbohydrates** may increase diarrhea.

## ROUTE AND DOSAGE

■ **PO (Adults):** 25 mg 3 times daily; may begin with 25 mg once daily; may be increased up to 100 mg 3 times daily.

## AVAILABILITY

■ **Tablets:** 25 mg$^{Rx}$, 50 mg$^{Rx}$, 100 mg$^{Rx}$ ■ Cost: 25 mg $48.75/100, 50 mg $57.50/100, 100 mg $65.84/100.

TIME/ACTION PROFILE (effect on glucose absorption)

|    | ONSET | PEAK | DURATION |
|----|-------|------|----------|
| PO | rapid | within 1 hr | unknown |

# NURSING IMPLICATIONS

## ASSESSMENT

❑ Observe patient for signs and symptoms of hypoglycemic reactions (sweating, hunger, weakness, dizziness, tremor, tachycardia, anxiety), especially when taking concurrently with other oral hypoglycemic agents.

■ *Lab Test Considerations:* Serum glucose and glycosylated hemoglobin levels should be monitored periodically throughout therapy to evaluate effectiveness of therapy.

■ *Toxicity and Overdose:* Symptoms of overdose are transient increase in flatulence, diarrhea, and abdominal discomfort. Miglitol alone does not cause hypoglycemia; however, other concurrently administered hypoglycemic agents may produce hypoglycemia requiring treatment. Mild hypoglycemia may be treated with administration of oral glucose.

## POTENTIAL NURSING DIAGNOSES

- Nutrition, imbalanced: more than body requirements (Indications).
- Noncompliance (Patient/Family Teaching).

## IMPLEMENTATION

- **General:** Patients stabilized on a diabetic regimen who are exposed to stress, fever, trauma, infection, or surgery may require administration of insulin.
- Does not cause hypoglycemia when taken while fasting but may increase hypoglycemic effect of other hypoglycemic agents.
- **PO:** Administer miglitol 3 times daily with the first bite of each meal. Dose may be started lower and increased gradually to minimize GI effects.

## PATIENT/FAMILY TEACHING

- Instruct patient to take miglitol at the same time each day, exactly as directed.
- Explain to patient that miglitol helps control hyperglycemia but does not cure diabetes. Therapy is usually long term.
- Encourage patient to follow prescribed diet, medication, and exercise regimen to prevent hyperglycemic or hypoglycemic episodes.
- Review signs of hypoglycemia and hyperglycemia with patient. If hypoglycemia occurs, advise patient to take a glass of orange juice, 2–3 tsp of sugar, honey, or corn syrup dissolved in water, and notify health care professional.
- Instruct patient in proper testing of blood glucose or urine ketones. These tests should be monitored closely during periods of stress or illness and health care professional notified of significant changes.
- Insulin is the recommended method of controlling blood glucose during pregnancy. Counsel female patients to use a form of contraception other than oral contraceptives and to notify health care professional promptly if pregnancy is planned or suspected.
- Advise patient to inform health care professional of medication regimen prior to treatment or surgery.
- Advise patient to carry a form of oral glucose (dextrose, D-glucose) and identification de-

scribing disease process and medication regimen at all times.
- Emphasize the importance of routine follow-up exams and regular testing of blood glucose and glycosylated hemoglobin.

## EVALUATION

**Effectiveness of therapy can be demonstrated by:** ■ Control of blood glucose levels without the appearance of hypoglycemic or hyperglycemic episodes.

---

**High Alert**

# milrinone

(**mill**-ri-none)
Primacor

**CLASSIFICATION(S):**
**Therapeutic:** inotropics

**Pregnancy Category C**

---

## INDICATIONS

■ Short-term treatment of CHF unresponsive to conventional therapy with digoxin, diuretics, and vasodilators.

## ACTION

■ Increases myocardial contractility ■ Decreases preload and afterload by a direct dilating effect on vascular smooth muscle. **Therapeutic Effects:** ■ Increased cardiac output (inotropic effect).

## PHARMACOKINETICS

**Absorption:** IV administration results in complete bioavailability.
**Distribution:** Unknown.
**Metabolism and Excretion:** 80–90% excreted unchanged by the kidneys.
**Half-life:** 2.3 hr (increased in renal impairment).

## CONTRAINDICATIONS AND PRECAUTIONS

**Contraindicated in:** ■ Hypersensitivity ■ Severe aortic or pulmonic valvular heart disease ■ Hypertrophic subaortic stenosis (may increase outflow tract obstruction).
**Use Cautiously in:** ■ History of arrhythmias, electrolyte abnormalities, abnormal digoxin levels, or insertion of vascular catheters (in-

creased risk of ventricular arrhythmias) ■ Renal impairment (reduced infusion rate recommended if CCr is <50 ml/min) ■ Pregnancy, lactation, or children (safety not established).

## ADVERSE REACTIONS AND SIDE EFFECTS*

■ **CNS:** headache, tremor ■ **CV:** VENTRICULAR ARRHYTHMIAS, angina pectoris, chest pain, hypotension, supraventricular arrhythmias ■ **CV:** skin rash ■ **GI:** liver function abnormalities ■ **F and E:** hypokalemia ■ **Hemat:** thrombocytopenia.

## INTERACTIONS

**Drug-Drug:** ■ None significant.

## ROUTE AND DOSAGE

■ **IV (Adults):** *Loading dose*—50 mcg/kg followed by *infusion* at 0.50 mcg/kg/min (range 0.375–0.75 mcg/kg/min).

## AVAILABILITY

■ *Injection:* 1 mg/ml in 10- and 20-ml vials and 5-ml preloaded syringes[Rx].

TIME/ACTION PROFILE (hemodynamic effects)

| | ONSET | PEAK | DURATION |
|---|---|---|---|
| IV | 5–15 min | unknown | 3–6 hr |

## NURSING IMPLICATIONS

### ASSESSMENT

❑ Monitor heart rate and blood pressure continuously during administration. Milrinone should be slowed or discontinued if blood pressure drops excessively.

❑ Monitor intake and output and daily weight. Assess patient for resolution of signs and symptoms of CHF (peripheral edema, dyspnea, rales/crackles, weight gain) and improvement in hemodynamic parameters (increase in cardiac output and cardiac index, decrease in pulmonary capillary wedge pressure). Correct effects of previous aggressive diuretic therapy to allow for optimal filling pressure.

❑ Monitor ECG continuously during infusion. Arrhythmias are common and may be life threatening. The risk of ventricular arrhyth-

mias is increased in patients with a history of arrhythmias, electrolyte abnormalities, abnormal digoxin levels, or insertion of vascular catheters.

■ *Lab Test Considerations:* Monitor electrolytes and renal function frequently during administration. Hypokalemia should be corrected prior to administration to decrease the risk of arrhythmias.

❑ Monitor platelet count during therapy.

■ *Toxicity and Overdose: High Alert:* Overdose manifests as hypotension. Dose should be decreased or discontinued. Supportive measures may be necessary.

## POTENTIAL NURSING DIAGNOSES

■ Cardiac output, decreased (Indications).

## IMPLEMENTATION

❑ *High Alert:* Accidental overdose of milrinone can cause patient harm or death. Have second practitioner independently check original order, dosage calculations, and infusion pump settings.

■ **Direct IV:** Loading dose may be administered undiluted.

■ *Rate:* Administer the loading dose over 10 min.

■ **Continuous Infusion:** The 20-mg vial may be diluted with 180 ml of diluent for a concentration of 100 mcg/ml, with 113 ml of diluent for a concentration of 150 mcg/ml, or with 80 ml of diluent for a concentration of 200 mcg/ml. Compatible diluents include 0.45% NaCl, 0.9% NaCl, and D5W. Do not use solutions that are discolored or contain particulate matter.

■ *Rate:* Infusion rate is titrated according to hemodynamic and clinical response.

■ **Syringe Compatibility:** ◆ atropine ◆ calcium chloride ◆ digoxin ◆ epinephrine ◆ lidocaine ◆ morphine ◆ propranolol ◆ sodium bicarbonate ◆ verapamil.

■ **Syringe Incompatibility:** ◆ furosemide.

■ **Y-Site Compatibility:** ◆ atracurium ◆ bumetanide ◆ calcium gluconate ◆ cimetidine ◆ digoxin ◆ diltiazem ◆ dobutamine ◆ dopamine ◆ epinephrine ◆ fentanyl ◆ heparin ◆ hydromorphone ◆ insulin ◆ isoproterenol ◆ labetalol ◆ lorazepam ◆ magnesium sulfate ◆ midazolam ♦ morphine ♦ nitroglycerine ♦ nitroprusside ♦ norepinephrine ♦ pancuronium ♦ potassium chloride ♦ propofol ♦ propranolol ♦ quinidine gluconate. ♦ ranitidine ♦ rocuronium ♦ sodium bicarbonate ♦ theophylline ♦ thiopental ♦ torsemide ♦ vecuronium ■ **Y-Site Incompatibility:** ♦ furosemide ♦ procainamide.

### PATIENT/FAMILY TEACHING

❑ Inform patient and family of reasons for administration. Milrinone is not a cure but is a temporary measure to control the symptoms of CHF.

### EVALUATION

**Clinical response to therapy can be evaluated by:** ■ Decrease in the signs and symptoms of CHF ❑ Improvement in hemodynamic parameters.

---

## minocycline, See TETRACYCLINES.

---

## mirtazapine

(meer-**taz**-a-peen)
Remeron, Remeron Soltabs

### CLASSIFICATION(S):
**Therapeutic:** antidepressants
**Pharmacologic:** tetracyclic antidepressants

### Pregnancy Category C

### INDICATIONS

■ Depression (with psychotherapy).

### ACTION

■ Potentiates the effects of norepinephrine and serotonin. **Therapeutic Effects:** ■ Antidepressant action, which may develop only over several weeks.

### PHARMACOKINETICS

**Absorption:** Well absorbed but rapidly metabolized, resulting in 50% bioavailability.
**Distribution:** Unknown.
**Protein Binding:** 85%.
**Metabolism and Excretion:** Extensively metabolized by the liver (P450 2D6, 1A2 and 3A

enzymes involved); metabolites excreted in urine (75%) and feces (15%).
**Half-life:** 20–40 hr.

### CONTRAINDICATIONS AND PRECAUTIONS

**Contraindicated in:** ■ Hypersensitivity ■ Concurrent MAO inhibitor therapy.

**Use Cautiously in:** ■ History of seizures ■ History of suicide attempt ■ History of mania/hypomania ■ Geriatric patients or patients with hepatic or renal impairment (may need lower doses) ■ Pregnancy, lactation, or children (safety not established).

### ADVERSE REACTIONS AND SIDE EFFECTS*

■ **CNS:** <u>drowsiness</u>, abnormal dreams, abnormal thinking, agitation, anxiety, apathy, confusion, dizziness, malaise, weakness ■ **EENT:** sinusitis ■ **Resp:** dyspnea, increased cough ■ **CV:** edema, hypotension, vasodilation ■ **GI:** <u>constipation</u>, <u>dry mouth</u>, <u>increased appetite</u>, abdominal pain, anorexia, elevated liver enzymes, nausea, vomiting ■ **GU:** urinary frequency ■ **Derm:** pruritus, rash ■ **F and E:** increased thirst ■ **Hemat:** AGRANULOCYTOSIS ■ **Metab:** <u>weight gain</u>, hypercholesterolemia, increased triglycerides ■ **MS:** arthralgia, back pain, myalgia ■ **Neuro:** hyperkinesia, hypesthesia, twitching ■ **Misc:** flu-like syndrome.

### INTERACTIONS

**Drug-Drug:** ■ May cause hypertension, seizures, and death when used with **MAO inhibitors**; do not use within 14 days of MAO inhibitor therapy ■ ↑ CNS depression with other **CNS depressants**, including **alcohol** and **benzodiazepines** ■ **Drugs affecting P450 enzymes CYP2D6, CYP1A2,** and **CYP3A4** may alter the effects of mirtazapine.

**Drug-Natural Products:** ■ Concomitant use of **kava, valerian, skullcap, chamomile,** or **hops** can ↑ CNS depression ■ ↑ risk of serotonergic side effects including serotonin syndrome with **St. John's wort** and **SAMe.**

### ROUTE AND DOSAGE

■ **PO (Adults):** 15 mg/day as a single bedtime dose initially; may be increased q 1–2 wk up to 45 mg/day.

## AVAILABILITY (generic available)

■ *Tablets:* 15 mg$^{Rx}$, 30 mg$^{Rx}$, 45 mg$^{Rx}$ ■ Cost: 15 mg $83.15/30, 30 mg $85.65/30, 45 mg $87.30/30 ■ *Orally disintegrating tablets:* 15 mg$^{Rx}$, 30 mg$^{Rx}$, 45 mg$^{Rx}$ ■ Cost: 15 mg $72.11/30, 30 mg $74.28/30, 45 mg $79.12/30.

TIME/ACTION PROFILE (antidepressant effect)

|     | ONSET   | PEAK             | DURATION |
| --- | ------- | ---------------- | -------- |
| PO  | 1–2 wk  | 6 wk or more     | unknown  |

## NURSING IMPLICATIONS

### ASSESSMENT

❑ Assess mental status frequently. Assess for suicidal tendencies, especially during early therapy. Restrict amount of drug available to patient.

❑ Monitor blood pressure and pulse rate periodically during initial therapy. Report significant changes.

❑ Monitor for seizure activity in patients with a history of seizures or alcohol abuse. Institute seizure precautions.

■ *Lab Test Considerations:* Assess CBC and hepatic function before and periodically during therapy.

### POTENTIAL NURSING DIAGNOSES

■ Coping, ineffective (Indications).
■ Anxiety (Indications).

### IMPLEMENTATION

■ **General:** May be given as a single dose at bedtime to minimize excessive drowsiness or dizziness.

❑ May be taken without regard to food. For orally disintegrating tablets, do not attempt to push through foil backing; with dry hands, peal back backing and remove tablet. Immediately place tablet on tongue; tablet will dissolve in seconds, then swallow with saliva. Administration with liquid is not necessary.

### PATIENT/FAMILY TEACHING

❑ Instruct patient to take mirtazapine exactly as directed. If a dose is missed, take as soon as remembered; if almost time for next dose, skip missed dose and return to regular schedule. If single bedtime dose regimen is used, do not take missed dose in morning, but consult health care professional. Do not discontinue abruptly; gradual dosage reduction may be required.

❑ May cause drowsiness and dizziness. Caution patient to avoid driving and other activities requiring alertness until response to drug is known.

❑ Caution patient to change positions slowly to minimize orthostatic hypotension.

❑ Advise patient to avoid alcohol or other CNS depressant drugs during and for at least 3–7 days after therapy has been discontinued.

❑ Advise patient to notify health care professional if dry mouth, urinary retention, or constipation occurs. Frequent rinses, good oral hygiene, and sugarless candy or gum may diminish dry mouth. An increase in fluid intake, fiber, and exercise may prevent constipation.

❑ Inform patient of need to monitor dietary intake. Increase in appetite may lead to undesired weight gain.

❑ Advise patient to consult health care professional before taking any OTC cold remedies or herbal products with this medication.

❑ Advise patient to notify health care professional of medication regimen before treatment or surgery.

❑ Therapy for depression may be prolonged. Emphasize the importance of follow-up exam to monitor effectiveness and side effects.

### EVALUATION

**Effectiveness of therapy can be demonstrated by:** ■ Resolution of the symptoms of depression: ❑ Increased sense of well-being ❑ Renewed interest in surroundings ❑ Increased appetite ❑ Improved energy level ❑ Improved sleep ❑ Therapeutic effects may be seen within 1 wk, although several wk are usually necessary before improvement is observed.

## misoprostol
(mye-soe-**prost**-ole)
Cytotec

**CLASSIFICATION(S):**
**Therapeutic:** *antiulcer agents, cytoprotective agents*
**Pharmacologic:** *prostaglandins*

**Pregnancy Category X**

## INDICATIONS

■ Prevention of gastric mucosal injury from NSAIDs, including aspirin, in high-risk patients (geriatric patients, debilitated patients, or those with a history of ulcers) ■ With mifepristone for termination of pregnancy. **Unlabeled uses:** ■ Treatment of duodenal ulcers.

## ACTION

■ Acts as a prostaglandin analogue, decreasing gastric acid secretion (antisecretory effect) and increasing the production of protective mucus (cytoprotective effect) ■ Causes uterine contractions. **Therapeutic Effects:** ■ Prevention of gastric ulceration from NSAIDs ■ With mifepristone terminates pregnancy of less than 49 days.

## PHARMACOKINETICS

**Absorption:** Well absorbed following oral administration and rapidly converted to its active form (misoprostol acid).
**Distribution:** Unknown.
**Protein Binding:** 85%.
**Metabolism and Excretion:** Undergoes some metabolism and is then excreted by the kidneys.
**Half-life:** 20–40 min.

## CONTRAINDICATIONS AND PRECAUTIONS

**Contraindicated in:** ■ Hypersensitivity to prostaglandins ■ Pregnancy or lactation (when used to prevent NSAID-induced gastric injury).
**Use Cautiously in:** ■ Patients with childbearing potential ■ Children <18 yr (safety not established).
**Exercise Extreme Caution in:** ■ When used for cervical ripening (unlabeled use) may cause uterine rupture; risk factors are late trimester pregnancy, previous cesarian section or uterine surgery or ≥ 5 previous pregnancies.

## ADVERSE REACTIONS AND SIDE EFFECTS*

■ **CNS:** headache ■ **GI:** abdominal pain, diarrhea, constipation, dyspepsia, flatulence, nausea, vomiting ■ **GU:** miscarriage, menstrual disorders.

## INTERACTIONS

**Drug-Drug:** ■ Increased risk of diarrhea with **magnesium-containing antacids.**

## ROUTE AND DOSAGE

■ **PO (Adults):** *Antiulcer*—200 mcg 4 times daily with or after meals and at bedtime, *or* 400 mcg twice daily, with the last dose at bedtime. If intolerance occurs, dosage may be decreased to 100 mcg 4 times daily. *Termination of Pregnancy*—400 mcg single dose two days after mifepristone if abortion has not occurred.

## AVAILABILITY (generic available)

■ *Tablets:* 100 mcg (0.1 mg)^Rx, 200 mcg (0.2 mg)^Rx ■ Cost: 100 mcg $48.26/60, 200 mcg $70.28/60 ■ 50 mg diclofenac/200 mcg misoprostol and 75 mg diclofenac/200 mcg misoprostol (Arthrotec)^Rx. See Appendix B.

TIME/ACTION PROFILE (effect on gastric acid secretion)

|    | ONSET | PEAK | DURATION |
|----|-------|------|----------|
| PO | 30 min | unknown | 3–6 hr |

# NURSING IMPLICATIONS

## ASSESSMENT

❏ Assess patient routinely for epigastric or abdominal pain and for frank or occult blood in the stool, emesis, or gastric aspirate.
❏ Assess women of childbearing age for pregnancy. Misoprostol is usually begun on 2nd or 3rd day of menstrual period following a negative pregnancy test result.

## POTENTIAL NURSING DIAGNOSES

■ Pain, acute (Indications).

## IMPLEMENTATION

■ **General:** Do not confuse Cytotec (misoprostol) with Cytoxan (cyclophosphamide).
❏ Misoprostol therapy should be started at the onset of treatment with NSAIDs.
■ **PO:** Administer medication with meals and at bedtime to reduce severity of diarrhea.
❏ Antacids may be administered before or after misoprostol for relief of pain. Avoid those

containing magnesium, because of increased diarrhea with misoprostol.

## PATIENT/FAMILY TEACHING

❑ Instruct patient to take medication as directed for the full course of therapy, even if feeling better. Take missed doses as soon as possible unless almost time for next dose; do not double doses. Emphasize that sharing of this medication may be dangerous.

❑ Inform patient that misoprostol will cause spontaneous abortion. Women of childbearing age must be informed of this effect through verbal and written information and must use contraception throughout therapy. If pregnancy is suspected, the woman should stop taking misoprostol and immediately notify her health care professional.

❑ Inform patient that diarrhea may occur. Health care professional should be notified if diarrhea persists for more than 1 wk. Also advise patient to report onset of black, tarry stools or severe abdominal pain.

❑ Advise patient to avoid alcohol and foods that may cause an increase in GI irritation.

## EVALUATION

**Effectiveness of therapy can be demonstrated by:** ■ The prevention of gastric ulcers in patients receiving chronic NSAID therapy.

---

## mitomycin

(mye-toe-**mye**-sin)

MitoExtra, Mutamycin

### CLASSIFICATION(S):

**Therapeutic:** *antineoplastics*
**Pharmacologic:** *antitumor antibiotics*

### Pregnancy Category UK

---

## INDICATIONS

■ Used with other agents in the management of disseminated adenocarcinoma of the stomach or pancreas. **Unlabeled uses:** ■ Palliative treatment of: ❑ Carcinoma of the colon or breast ❑ Head and neck tumors ❑ Advanced biliary, lung, and cervical squamous cell carcinomas.

## ACTION

■ Primarily inhibits DNA synthesis by causing cross-linking; also inhibits RNA and protein synthesis (cell-cycle phase–nonspecific but is most active in S and G phases). **Therapeutic Effects:** ■ Death of rapidly replicating cells, particularly malignant ones.

## PHARMACOKINETICS

**Absorption:** IV administration results in complete bioavailability.

**Distribution:** Widely distributed, concentrates in tumor tissue. Does not enter CSF.

**Metabolism and Excretion:** Mostly metabolized by the liver. Small amounts (<10%) excreted unchanged by the kidneys and in bile.

**Half-life:** 50 min.

## CONTRAINDICATIONS AND PRECAUTIONS

**Contraindicated in:** ■ Hypersensitivity ■ Pregnancy or lactation.

**Use Cautiously in:** ■ Patients with childbearing potential ■ Active infections ■ Decreased bone marrow reserve ■ Geriatric patients or patients with other chronic debilitating illnesses ■ Impaired liver function ■ History of pulmonary problems.

## ADVERSE REACTIONS AND SIDE EFFECTS*

■ **Resp:** PULMONARY TOXICITY ■ **CV:** edema ■ **GI:** nausea, vomiting, anorexia, stomatitis ■ **GU:** infertility, renal failure ■ **Derm:** alopecia, desquamation ■ **Hemat:** leukopenia, thrombocytopenia, anemia ■ **Local:** phlebitis at IV site ■ **Misc:** HEMOLYTIC UREMIC SYNDROME, fever, prolonged malaise.

## INTERACTIONS

**Drug-Drug:** ■ Additive bone marrow depression with other **antineoplastics** or **radiation therapy** ■ May decrease antibody response to **live-virus vaccines** and increase the risk of adverse reactions ■ Concurrent or sequential use with **vinca alkaloids** may result in respiratory toxicity.

## ROUTE AND DOSAGE

■ **IV (Adults):** 20 mg/m² every 6–8 wk.

## AVAILABILITY

■ *Injection:* 5-mg, 20-mg, and 40-mg vials^Rx ■ Cost: 5 mg $128.05/1, 20 mg $434.60/1, 40 mg $915.00/1.

TIME/ACTION PROFILE (effects on blood counts)

|    | ONSET | PEAK | DURATION |
|----|-------|------|----------|
| IV | 3–8 wk | 4–8 wk | up to 3 mo |

## NURSING IMPLICATIONS

### ASSESSMENT

◻ Monitor vital signs periodically during administration.

◻ Monitor for bone marrow depression. Assess for bleeding (bleeding gums, bruising, petechiae, guaiac stools, urine, and emesis) and avoid IM injections and taking rectal temperatures if platelet count is low. Apply pressure to venipuncture sites for 10 min. Assess for signs of infection during neutropenia. Anemia may occur. Monitor for increased fatigue, dyspnea, and orthostatic hypotension.

◻ Monitor intake and output, appetite, and nutritional intake. Nausea and vomiting usually occur within 1–2 hr. Vomiting may stop within 3–4 hr; nausea may persist for 2–3 days. Antiemetics may be administered prophylactically. Adjust diet as tolerated to help maintain fluid and electrolyte balance and nutritional status.

◻ Assess respiratory status and chest x-ray examination prior to and periodically throughout course of therapy. Cough, bronchospasm, hemoptysis, or dyspnea usually occurs after several doses and may be indicative of pulmonary toxicity, which may be life threatening.

◻ Monitor for potentially fatal hemolytic uremic syndrome in patients receiving long-term therapy. Symptoms include microangiopathic hemolytic anemia, thrombocytopenia, renal failure, and hypertension.

■ *Lab Test Considerations:* Monitor CBC with differential, platelet count, and observation for fragmented RBCs on peripheral blood smears prior to and periodically

throughout therapy and for several months following therapy.

◻ The nadirs of leukopenia and thrombocytopenia occur in 4–8 wk. Notify physician if leukocyte count is <4000/mm³ or if platelet count is <150,000/mm³ or is progressively declining. Recovery from leukopenia and thrombocytopenia occurs within 10 wk after cessation of therapy. Myelosuppression is cumulative and may be irreversible. Repeat courses of therapy are held until leukocyte count is >4000/mm³ and platelet count is >100,000/mm³.

◻ Monitor liver function studies (AST, ALT, LDH, bilirubin) and renal function studies (BUN, creatinine) prior to and periodically throughout therapy to detect hepatotoxicity and nephrotoxicity. Notify physician if creatinine is >1.7 mg/dl.

### POTENTIAL NURSING DIAGNOSES

■ Injury, risk for (Side Effects).

■ Infection, risk for (Side Effects).

■ Body image, disturbed (Side Effects).

### IMPLEMENTATION

■ **General:** Solution should be prepared in a biologic cabinet. Wear gloves, gown, and mask while handling medication. Discard equipment in designated containers.

◻ Ensure patency of IV. Extravasation may cause severe tissue necrosis. If patient complains of discomfort at IV site, discontinue immediately and restart infusion at another site. Promptly notify physician of extravasation.

■ **Direct IV:** Reconstitute 5-mg vial with 10 ml and 10-mg vial with 40 ml of sterile water for injection. Shake the vial; may need to stand at room temperature for additional time to dissolve. Final solution is blue-gray. Reconstituted solution is stable for 7 days at room temperature, 14 days if refrigerated.

■ *Rate:* May be administered IV push over 5–10 min through free-flowing IV of 0.9% NaCl or D5W.

■ **Y-Site Compatibility:** ◆ amifostine ◆ bleomycin ◆ cisplatin ◆ cyclophosphamide ◆ doxorubicin ◆ droperidol ◆ fluorouracil ◆ furosemide ◆ granisetron ◆ heparin ◆ leucovorin ◆ melphalan ◆ methotrexate ◆ metoclopramide ◆ ondansetron ◆ teniposide ◆ thiotepa ◆ vinblastine ◆ vincristine.

■ **Y-Site Incompatibility:** ◆ aztreonam ◆ cefepime ◆ etoposide ◆ filgrastim ◆ gemcitabine ◆ piperacillin/tazobactam ◆ sargramostim ◆ topotecan ◆ vinorelbine.

## PATIENT/FAMILY TEACHING

❑ Instruct patient to notify health care professional promptly if fever; chills; cough; hoarseness; sore throat; signs of infection; lower back or side pain; painful or difficult urination; bleeding gums; bruising; petechiae; blood in stools, urine, or emesis; increased fatigue; dyspnea; or orthostatic hypotension occurs. Caution patient to avoid crowds and persons with known infections. Instruct patient to use soft toothbrush and electric razor and to avoid falls. Caution patient not to drink alcoholic beverages or take medication containing aspirin or NSAIDs; may precipitate gastric bleeding.

❑ Instruct patient to notify health care professional if decreased urine output, edema in lower extremities, shortness of breath, skin ulceration, or persistent nausea occurs.

❑ Instruct patient to inspect oral mucosa for redness and ulceration. If ulceration occurs, advise patient to use sponge brush and rinse mouth with water after eating and drinking. Topical agents may be used if pain interferes with eating. Stomatitis pain may require treatment with opioid analgesics.

❑ Discuss with patient the possibility of hair loss. Explore coping strategies.

❑ Advise patient that, although mitomycin may cause infertility, contraception during therapy is necessary because of teratogenic effects.

❑ Instruct patient not to receive any vaccinations without advice of health care professional.

❑ Emphasize need for periodic lab tests to monitor for side effects.

## EVALUATION

**Effectiveness of therapy can be demonstrated by:** ■ Decrease in size and spread of malignant tissue.

# mitoxantrone
(mye-toe-**zan**-trone)
Novantrone

## CLASSIFICATION(S):
**Therapeutic:** antineoplastics
**Pharmacologic:** antitumor antibiotics

**Pregnancy Category D**

## INDICATIONS

■ Acute nonlymphocytic leukemia (ANLL) in adults (with other antineoplastics) ■ Initial chemotherapy for patients with pain associated with advanced hormone-refractory prostate cancer ■ Secondary (chronic) progressive, progressive relapsing, or worsening relapsing-remitting multiple sclerosis (MS). **Unlabeled uses:** ■ Breast cancer, liver cancer, and non-Hodgkin's lymphoma.

## ACTION

■ Inhibits DNA synthesis (cell-cycle phase–nonspecific). **Therapeutic Effects:** ■ Death of rapidly replicating cells, particularly malignant ones ■ Decreased pain in patients with advanced prostate cancer ■ Decreased disability and slowed progression of MS.

## PHARMACOKINETICS

**Absorption:** IV administration results in complete bioavailability.
**Distribution:** Widely distributed; limited penetration of CSF.
**Metabolism and Excretion:** Mostly eliminated by hepatobiliary clearance; <10% excreted unchanged by the kidneys.
**Half-life:** 5.8 days.

## CONTRAINDICATIONS AND PRECAUTIONS

**Contraindicated in:** ■ Hypersensitivity ■ Pregnancy or lactation.

**Use Cautiously in:** ■ Previous cardiac disease ■ Patients with childbearing potential ■ Active infections ■ Depressed bone marrow reserve ■ Previous mediastinal radiation ■ Geriatric patients or patients with other chronic debilitating illness ■ Children (safety not established) ■ Impaired hepatobiliary function or decreased blood counts (dosage reduction required).

## ADVERSE REACTIONS AND SIDE EFFECTS*

■ **CNS:** SEIZURES, headache ■ **EENT:** blue-green sclera, conjunctivitis ■ **Resp:** cough, dyspnea ■ **CV:** CARDIOTOXICITY, arrhythmias, ECG changes ■ **GI:** abdominal pain, diarrhea, hepatic toxicity, nausea, stomatitis, vomiting ■ **GU:** blue-green urine, gonadal suppression, renal failure ■ **Derm:** alopecia, rashes ■ **Hemat:** anemia, leukopenia, secondary leukemia, thrombocytopenia ■ **Metab:** hyperuricemia ■ **Misc:** fever, hypersensitivity reactions.

## INTERACTIONS

**Drug-Drug:** ■ ↑ bone marrow depression with other **antineoplastics** or **radiation therapy** ■ Risk of cardiomyopathy ↑ by previous **anthracycline antineoplastics (daunorubicin, doxorubicin, idarubicin)** or **mediastinal radiation** ■ May ↓ antibody response to **live-virus vaccines** and ↑ risk of adverse reactions.

## ROUTE AND DOSAGE

❑ **Acute Nonlymphatic Leukemia**

■ **IV (Adults):** *Induction*—12 mg/m²/day for 3 days (usually given with cytosine arabinoside 100 mg/m²/day for 7 days); if incomplete remission occurs, a 2nd induction may be given. *Consolidation*—12 mg/m²/day for 2 days (usually given with cytosine arabinoside 100 mg/m²/day for 5 days), given 6 wk after induction with another course 4 wk later.

❑ **Advanced Prostate Cancer**

■ **IV (Adults):** 12–14 mg/m² single dose as a short infusion (with corticosteroids).

❑ **Multiple Sclerosis**

■ **IV (Adults):** 12 mg/m² q 3 mo.

## AVAILABILITY

■ *Injection:* 2 mg/ml in 10-, 12.5-, and 15-ml vials[Rx].

TIME/ACTION PROFILE (effects on blood counts)

|  | ONSET | PEAK | DURATION |
|---|---|---|---|
| IV | unknown | 10 days | 21 days |

# NURSING IMPLICATIONS

## ASSESSMENT

■ **General Info:** Monitor for hypersensitivity reaction (rash, urticaria, bronchospasm, tachycardia, hypotension). If these occur, stop infusion and notify physician. Keep epinephrine, an antihistamine, and resuscitation equipment close by in the event of an anaphylactic reaction.

❑ Monitor for bone marrow depression. Assess for bleeding (bleeding gums, bruising, petechiae, guaiac stools, urine, and emesis) and avoid IM injections and taking rectal temperatures if platelet count is low. Apply pressure to venipuncture sites for 10 min. Assess for signs of infection during neutropenia. Anemia may occur. Monitor for increased fatigue, dyspnea, and orthostatic hypotension.

❑ Monitor intake and output, appetite, and nutritional intake. Assess patient for nausea and vomiting. Antiemetics may be administered prophylactically. Adjust diet as tolerated to help maintain fluid and electrolyte balance and nutritional status.

❑ Monitor chest x-ray, ECG, echocardiography, and radionuclide angiography to determine ejection fraction prior to and periodically during therapy. May cause cardiotoxicity, especially in patients who have received daunorubicin or doxorubicin. Assess for rales/crackles, dyspnea, edema, jugular vein distention, ECG changes, arrhythmias, and chest pain.

❑ Monitor for symptoms of gout (increased uric acid levels and joint pain and swelling). Encourage patient to drink at least 2 L of fluid per day. Allopurinol may be given to decrease serum uric acid levels.

❑ Assess patients for signs of CHF (dysphea, peripheral edema/rales/crackles). Potentially fatal CHF may occur during or for months or years after therapy. Risk is greater in patients receiving a cumulative dose >140 mg/m².

■ **Multiple sclerosis:** Assess frequency of exacerbations of symptoms of multiple sclerosis periodically during therapy.

■ *Lab Test Considerations:* Monitor CBC with differential and platelet count prior to and periodically during therapy. The nadir of leukopenia usually occurs within 10 days, and recovery usually occurs within 21 days.

❑ Monitor liver function studies (AST, ALT, LDH, bilirubin) and renal function studies

(BUN, creatinine) prior to and periodically during therapy to detect hepatotoxicity and nephrotoxicity.

❑ May cause ↑ uric acid concentrations. Monitor periodically during therapy.

## POTENTIAL NURSING DIAGNOSES

- Injury, risk for (Side Effects).
- Infection, risk for (Side Effects).
- Body image, disturbed (Side Effects).

## IMPLEMENTATION

- **General:** Solution should be prepared in a biologic cabinet. Wear gloves, gown, and mask while handling medication. Discard equipment in designated containers.
- ❑ Avoid contact with skin. Use Luer-Lok tubing to prevent accidental leakage. If contact with skin occurs, immediately wash skin with soap and water.
- ❑ Clean all spills with an aqueous solution of calcium hypochlorite. Mix solution by adding 5.5 parts (per weight) of calcium hypochlorite to 13 parts water.
- **IV:** Monitor IV site. If extravasation occurs, discontinue IV and restart at another site. Mitoxantrone is not a vesicant.
- **Direct IV:** Dilute dark blue mitoxantrone solution in at least 50 ml of 0.9% NaCl or D5W. Discard unused solution appropriately.
- **Rate:** Administer slowly over at least 3 min into the tubing of a free-flowing IV of 0.9% NaCl or D5W.
- **Intermittent Infusion:** May be further diluted in D5W, 0.9% NaCl, or D5/0.9% NaCl and used immediately.
- **Y-Site Compatibility:** ◆ allopurinol ◆ amifostine ◆ etoposide ◆ etoposide phosphate ◆ filgrastim ◆ fludarabine ◆ gatifloxacin ◆ gemcitabine ◆ granisetron ◆ linezolid ◆ melphalan ◆ ondansetron ◆ sargramostim ◆ teniposide ◆ thiotepa ◆ vinorelbine.
- **Y-Site Incompatibility:** ◆ amphotericin B cholesteryl sulfate ◆ aztreonam ◆ cefepime ◆ doxorubicin liposome ◆ paclitaxel ◆ piperacillin/tazobactam ◆ propofol.
- **Additive Compatibility:** ◆ cyclophosphamide ◆ cytarabine ◆ etoposide ◆ fluorouracil ◆ hydrocortisone sodium succinate ◆ potassium chloride.

- **Additive Incompatibility:** heparin.

## PATIENT/FAMILY TEACHING

- ❑ Instruct patient to notify health care professional promptly if fever; chills; cough; hoarseness; sore throat; signs of infection; lower back or side pain; painful or difficult urination; bleeding gums; bruising; petechiae; blood in stools, urine, or emesis; increased fatigue; dyspnea; or orthostatic hypotension occurs. Caution patient to avoid crowds and persons with known infections. Instruct patient to use soft toothbrush and electric razor and to avoid falls. Caution patient not to drink alcoholic beverages or take medication containing aspirin or NSAIDS; may precipitate gastric bleeding.
- ❑ Instruct patient to notify health care professional if abdominal pain, yellow skin, cough, diarrhea, or decreased urine output occurs.
- ❑ Inform patient that medication may cause the urine and sclera to turn blue-green.
- ❑ Instruct patient to inspect oral mucosa for redness and ulceration. If mouth sores occur, advise patient to use sponge brush and rinse mouth with water after eating and drinking. Topical agents may be used if pain interferes with eating. Stomatitis pain may require treatment with opioid analgesics.
- ❑ Discuss with patient the possibility of hair loss. Explore coping strategies.
- ❑ Advise patient that, although mitoxantrone may cause infertility, contraception during therapy is necessary because of possible teratogenic effects.
- ❑ Instruct patient not to receive any vaccinations without advice of health care professional.
- ❑ Emphasize need for periodic lab tests to monitor for side effects.

## EVALUATION

**Effectiveness of therapy can be demonstrated by:** ■ Decrease in the production and spread of leukemic cells ■ Decreased pain in patients with prostate cancer ■ Decrease in the frequency of relapse (neurologic dysfunction) in patients with relapsing-remitting multiple sclerosis.

**moexipril, See ANGIOTENSIN-CONVERTING ENZYME (ACE) INHIBITORS.**

**mometasone, See CORTICOSTEROIDS (NASAL), CORTICOSTEROIDS (TOPICAL/LOCAL).**

# MONOAMINE OXIDASE (MAO) INHIBITORS

**phenelzine**

**(fen**-el-zeen)

Nardil

**tranylcypromine**

(tran-ill-**sip**-roe-meen)

Parnate

*CLASSIFICATION(S):*

*Therapeutic: antidepressants*
*Pharmacologic: monamine oxidase (MAO) inhibitors*

**Pregnancy Category C**

## INDICATIONS

■ Treatment of neurotic or atypical depression, usually in conjunction with psychotherapy, in patients who may not tolerate other modes of therapy (tricyclic antidepressants, SSRIs, or electroconvulsive therapy).

## ACTION

■ Inhibit the enzyme monoamine oxidase, resulting in an accumulation of various neurotransmitters (dopamine, epinephrine, norepinephrine, and serotonin) in the body. **Therapeutic Effects:** ■ Improved mood in depressed patients.

## PHARMACOKINETICS

**Absorption:** All are well absorbed from the GI tract.

**Distribution:** All cross the placenta and probably enter breast milk.

**Metabolism and Excretion:** All are mostly metabolized by the liver.

**Half-life:** Unknown.

## CONTRAINDICATIONS AND PRECAUTIONS

**Contraindicated in:** ■ Hypersensitivity ■ Liver disease ■ Severe renal disease ■ Cerebrovascular disease ■ Pheochromocytoma ■ CHF ■ History of headache ■ Concurrent meperidine, concurrent SSRI antidepressants, nefazodone, or trazodone administration.

**Use Cautiously in:** ■ Patients who may be suicidal or have a history of drug dependency ■ Symptomatic cardiovascular disease ■ Hyperthyroidism ■ Seizure disorders ■ Geriatric patients (increased risk of adverse reactions) ■ Pregnancy, lactation, or children (safety not established).

**Exercise Extreme Caution in:** ■ Surgery (should be discontinued several weeks before surgery if possible because of increased risk of unpredictable reactions).

## ADVERSE REACTIONS AND SIDE EFFECTS*

■ CNS: SEIZURES , dizziness, headache, insomnia, restlessness, weakness, confusion, drowsiness ■ EENT: blurred vision, glaucoma, nystagmus ■ CV: HYPERTENSIVE CRISIS , arrhythmias, orthostatic hypotension, edema ■ GI: diarrhea, abdominal pain, anorexia, constipation, dry mouth, nausea, vomiting ■ GU: dysuria, urinary incontinence, urinary retention ■ Derm: rashes ■ Endo: hypoglycemia ■ MS: arthralgia.

## INTERACTIONS

**Drug-Drug:** ■Serious, potentially fatal adverse reactions may occur with concurrent use of other **antidepressants (SSRIs, nefazodone, trazodone), carbamazepine, cyclobenzaprine, maprotiline, furazolidone, procarbazine,** or **selegiline.** Avoid using within 2 wk of each other (wait 5 wk from end of **fluoxetine** therapy) ■Hypertensive crisis may occur with **amphetamines, methyldopa, levodopa, dopamine, epinephrine, norepinephrine, guanethidine, guanadrel, reserpine,** or **vasoconstrictors** ■Hypertension or hypotension, coma, seizures, and death may occur with **opioids** (avoid use of **meperidine** within 14–21 days of MAO inhibitor therapy—decrease initial dose of other agents to 25% of usual dose) ■ Concurrent use with **dextromethorphan** may produce hypertension, excitation, and hyperpyrexia; similar effects may occur with **tryptophan** (avoid concurrent use of tryptophan or initiate in very small doses) ■ Hypertension may occur with concurrent use of **buspirone**; avoid using within 10 days of each other ■ Excess CNS stimulation and hypertension may occur with **methylphenidate** ■ Additive hypotension may occur with **antihypertensives** or **spinal anesthesia** ■ Additive hypoglycemia may occur with **insulins** or **oral hypoglycemic agents** ■ **Doxapram** may increase pressor response.

**Drug-Natural Products:** ■ Serious, potentially fatal adverse effects (serotonin syndrome) may occur with concomitant use of **St. John's wort** and **SAMe** ■ Hypertensive crises may occur with large amounts of **caffeine**-containing herbs (**cola nut, guarana, malt, coffee, tea**) ■ Insomnia, headache, tremor, hypomania may occur with **ginseng.**

**Drug-Food:** ■ Hypertensive crisis may occur with ingestion of foods containing high concentrations of **tyramine** (see Appendix Q) ■ Consumption of foods or beverages with high **caffeine** content increases the risk of hypertension and arrhythmias.

## ROUTE AND DOSAGE

### ❏ Phenelzine

■ **PO (Adults):** 15 mg 3 times daily; increase to 60–90 mg/day in divided doses, then gradually reduce to smallest effective dose (15 mg/day or every other day).

■ **PO (Geriatric Patients):** 15 mg/day initially, with slow dose titration.

### ❏ Tranylcypromine

■ **PO (Adults):** 30 mg/day in 2 divided doses (morning and afternoon); after 2 wk can increase by 10 mg/day, at 1–3 wk intervals, up to 60 mg/day.

■ **PO (Geriatric Patients):** 2.5–5 mg/day initially; increase every 3–4 days up to 45 mg/day.

## AVAILABILITY

### ❏ Phenelzine

■ *Tablets:* 15 mg^Rx.

### ❏ Tranylcypromine

■ *Tablets:* 10 mg^Rx.

TIME/ACTION PROFILE (antidepressant effect)

| | ONSET | PEAK | DURATION |
|---|---|---|---|
| Phenelzine | 1–4 wk | 2–6 wk | 2 wk |
| Tranylcypromine | 2 days–3 wk | 2–3 wk | 3–5 days |

## NURSING IMPLICATIONS

### ASSESSMENT

❏ Assess mental status, mood changes, and anxiety level frequently. Assess for suicidal tendencies, especially during early therapy. Restrict amount of drug available to patient.

❏ Monitor blood pressure and pulse rate before and frequently throughout therapy. Report significant changes promptly.

❏ Monitor intake and output ratios and daily weight. Assess patient for peripheral edema and urinary retention.

■ *Lab Test Considerations:* Assess hepatic function periodically during prolonged or high-dose therapy.

❏ Monitor serum glucose closely in diabetic patients; hypoglycemia may occur.

■ *Toxicity and Overdose:* Concurrent ingestion of tyramine-rich foods and many medications may result in a life-threatening hypertensive crisis. Signs and symptoms of hypertensive crisis include chest pain, tachycardia, severe headache, nausea and vomiting, photosensitivity, and enlarged pupils. Treatment includes IV phentolamine.

❏ Symptoms of overdose include anxiety, irritability, tachycardia, hypertension or hypotension, respiratory distress, dizziness, drowsiness, hallucinations, confusion, seizures, fever, and diaphoresis. Treatment includes induction of vomiting or gastric lavage and supportive therapy as symptoms arise.

### POTENTIAL NURSING DIAGNOSES

■ Coping, ineffective (Indications).
■ Noncompliance (Patient/Family Teaching).

### IMPLEMENTATION

■ **General:** Do not administer these medications in the evening because the psychomotor stimulating effects may cause insomnia or other sleep disturbances.

- **PO:** Tablets may be crushed and mixed with food or fluids for patients with difficulty swallowing.

### PATIENT/FAMILY TEACHING

- Instruct patient to take medication exactly as directed. If a dose is missed, take if remembered within 2 hr; otherwise, omit and return to regular dosage schedule. Medication should not be abruptly discontinued as withdrawal symptoms (nausea, vomiting, malaise, nightmares, agitation, psychosis, seizures) may occur.
- Caution patient to avoid alcohol, CNS depressants, OTC drugs, and foods or beverages containing tyramine (see Appendix Q) during and for at least 2 wk after therapy has been discontinued; they may precipitate a hypertensive crisis. Contact health care professional immediately if symptoms of hypertensive crisis develop.
- May cause dizziness or drowsiness. Caution patient to avoid driving and other activities requiring alertness until response to medication is known.
- Caution patient to change positions slowly to minimize orthostatic hypotension. Geriatric patients are at increased risk for this side effect.
- Advise patient to notify health care professional if dry mouth, urinary retention, or constipation occurs. Frequent rinses, good oral hygiene, and sugarless candy or gum may diminish dry mouth. An increase in fluid intake, fiber, and exercise may prevent constipation.
- Instruct patient to notify health care professional of severe headache, palpitations, chest or throat tightness, sweating, dizziness, neck stiffness, nausea, or vomiting.
- Advise patient to notify health care professional of medication regimen before treatment or surgery. If possible, therapy should be discontinued at least 2 wk before surgery.
- Instruct patient to carry identification describing medication regimen at all times.
- Emphasize the importance of participation in psychotherapy if recommended by health care professional and follow-up exams to evaluate progress. Ophthalmic testing should also be done periodically during long-term therapy.

### EVALUATION

**Effectiveness of therapy can be demonstrated by:** ■ Improved mood in depressed patients □ Decreased anxiety □ Increased appetite □ Improved energy level □ Improved sleep □ Patients may require 1–4 wk of therapy before therapeutic effects of medication are seen.

---

# montelukast
(mon-te-**loo**-kast)
Singulair

## CLASSIFICATION(S):
**Therapeutic:** *allergy, cold, and cough remedies, bronchodilators*
**Pharmacologic:** *leukotriene antagonists*

### Pregnancy Category B

---

### INDICATIONS

■ Prevention and chronic treatment of asthma ■ Management of seasonal allergic rhinitis.

### ACTION

■ Antagonizes the effects of leukotrienes, which mediate the following: ■ Airway edema ■ Smooth muscle constriction ■ Altered cellular activity ■ Result is decreased inflammatory process, which is part of asthma and allergic rhinitis. **Therapeutic Effects:** ■ Decreased frequency and severity of acute asthma attacks ■ Decreased severity of allergic rhinitis.

### PHARMACOKINETICS

**Absorption:** Rapidly absorbed (63–73%) following oral administration.
**Distribution:** Unknown.
**Protein Binding:** 99%.
**Metabolism and Excretion:** Mostly metabolized by the liver (by P450 3A4 and 2C9 enzyme systems); metabolites eliminated in feces via bile; negligible renal excretion.
**Half-life:** 2.7–5.5 hr.

### CONTRAINDICATIONS AND PRECAUTIONS

**Contraindicated in:** ■ Hypersensitivity ■ Lactation.
**Use Cautiously in:** ■ Acute attacks of asthma ■ Phenylketonuria (chewable tablets contain aspartame) ■ Hepatic impairment (may need low-

er doses) ∎ Reduction of corticosteroid therapy (may increase the risk of eosinophilic conditions) ∎ Pregnancy, lactation, or children <2 yr (safety not established).

## ADVERSE REACTIONS AND SIDE EFFECTS*

∎ **CNS:** fatigue, headache, weakness ∎ **EENT:** otitis (children), sinusitis (children) ∎ **Resp:** cough ∎ **GI:** abdominal pain, diarrhea (children), dyspepsia, nausea (children), increased liver enzymes ∎ **Derm:** rash ∎ **Misc:** eosinophilic conditions (including CHURG-STRAUSS SYNDROME), fever.

## INTERACTIONS

**Drug-Drug:** ∎ Drugs which induce the CYP450 enzyme system (**phenobarbital** and **rifampin**) may decrease the effects of montelukast.

## ROUTE AND DOSAGE

∎ **PO (Adults and Children ≥15 yr):** 10 mg once daily.
∎ **PO (Children 6–14 yr):** 5 mg once daily (as chewable tablet).
∎ **PO (Children 2–5 yr):** 4 mg once daily (as chewable tablet).
∎ **PO (Children 12–23 mo):** *Asthma only—* 4 mg once daily (as oral granules).

## AVAILABILITY

∎ *Tablets:* 10 mg$^{Rx}$ ∎ *Chewable tablets (cherry flavor):* 4 mg$^{Rx}$, 5 mg$^{Rx}$ ∎Cost: 4 mg $79.26/30; 5 mg $79.26/30; 10 mg $79.26/30 ∎ *Oral granules:* 4 mg/packet in 30-packet cartons$^{Rx}$ ∎ Cost: $89.54/carton.

TIME/ACTION PROFILE (improved symptoms of asthma)

| | ONSET | PEAK† | DURATION |
|---|---|---|---|
| PO (swallow) | within 24 hr | 3–4 hr | 24 hr |
| PO (chew) | within 24 hr | 2–2.5 hr | 24 hr |

†Blood levels.

# NURSING IMPLICATIONS

## ASSESSMENT

❏ Assess lung sounds and respiratory function prior to and periodically throughout therapy

❏ Assess allergy symptoms (rhinitis, conjunctivitis, hives) before and periodically throughout therapy.
∎ *Lab Test Considerations:* May cause ↑ AST and ALT concentrations.

## POTENTIAL NURSING DIAGNOSES

∎ Airway clearance, ineffective (Indications).

## IMPLEMENTATION

∎ **General:** Doses of inhaled corticosteroids may be gradually decreased with supervision of health care professional; do not discontinue abruptly.
∎ **PO:** For asthma, administer once daily in the evening. For allergic rhinitis, may be administered at any time of day.
❏ Administer granules directly into mouth or mixed in a spoonful of cold or room temperature foods (use only applesauce, mashed carrots, rice, or ice cream). Do not open packet until ready to use. After opening packet, administer full dose within 15 min. Do not store mixture. Discard unused portion. Do not dissolve granules in fluid, but fluid may be taken following administration. Granules may be administered without regard to meals.

## PATIENT/FAMILY TEACHING

❏ Instruct patient to take medication daily in the evening, even if not experiencing symptoms of asthma. Do not double doses. Do not discontinue therapy without consulting health care professional.
❏ Instruct patient not to discontinue or reduce other asthma medications without consulting health care professional.
❏ Advise patient that montelukast is not used to treat acute asthma attacks, but may be continued during an acute exacerbation. Patient should carry rapid-acting therapy for bronchospasm at all times. Advise patient to notify health care professional if more than the maximum number of short-acting bronchodilator treatments prescribed for a 24-hr period are needed.

## EVALUATION

**Effectiveness of therapy can be demonstrated by:** ∎ Prevention of and reduction in symptoms of asthma ■ Decrease in severity of allergic rhinitis.

## moricizine
(more-**i**-sizz-een)
Ethmozine

**CLASSIFICATION(S):**
**Therapeutic:** antiarrhythmics (class IA)

**Pregnancy Category B**

### INDICATIONS

■ Life-threatening ventricular arrhythmias, including sustained ventricular tachycardia.

### ACTION

■ Suppresses abnormal automaticity and prolongs PR interval and QRS duration by blocking fast sodium channel in myocardial tissue ■ Also has membrane-stabilizing and local anesthetic properties. **Therapeutic Effects:** ■ Suppression of life-threatening arrhythmias.

### PHARMACOKINETICS

**Absorption:** Well absorbed but rapidly metabolized after oral administration.

**Distribution:** Enters breast milk.

**Protein Binding:** 95%.

**Metabolism and Excretion:** Extensively metabolized; <1% excreted unchanged in the urine. Metabolites may be active.

**Half-life:** 1.5–3.5 hr.

### CONTRAINDICATIONS AND PRECAUTIONS

**Contraindicated in:** ■ Hypersensitivity ■ Cardiogenic shock ■ 2nd- or 3rd-degree AV block or bundle branch block (unless a pacemaker has been placed).

**Use Cautiously in:** ■ Electrolyte disturbances ■ Severe renal or hepatic impairment (initial dosage reduction may be necessary) ■ CHF ■ Pregnancy, lactation, or children (safety not established).

**Exercise Extreme Caution in:** ■ Sick sinus syndrome.

### ADVERSE REACTIONS AND SIDE EFFECTS*

■ **CNS:** dizziness, fatigue, headache, nervousness, sleep disorders, weakness ■ **EENT:** blurred vision ■ **Resp:** dyspnea ■ **CV:** ARRHYTHMIAS, chest pain, CHF, palpitations ■ **GI:** nausea, diarrhea, dry mouth, dyspepsia, vomiting ■ **Derm:** sweating ■ **MS:** musculoskeletal pain ■ **Neuro:** paresthesia ■ **Misc:** drug fever.

### INTERACTIONS

**Drug-Drug:** ■ Decreases blood levels of **theophylline** ■ **Cimetidine** increases blood levels of moricizine.

### ROUTE AND DOSAGE

■ **PO (Adults):** 600–900 mg/day given q 8 hr; within this range, dosage may be adjusted by 150 mg/day every 3 days as required and tolerated. Some patients may tolerate q 12 hr dosing (not to exceed 900 mg/day).

### AVAILABILITY

■ **Tablets:** 200 mg^Rx, 250 mg^Rx, 300 mg^Rx ■ Cost: 200 mg $114.86/100, 250 mg $137.14/100, 300 mg $156.13/100.

TIME/ACTION PROFILE (arrhythmia suppression)

|  | ONSET | PEAK | DURATION |
|---|---|---|---|
| PO | unknown | 0.5–2 hr | 8–12 hr |

## NURSING IMPLICATIONS

### ASSESSMENT

❑ Monitor ECG or Holter monitor before and periodically throughout therapy. May cause PR and QT prolongation.
❑ Monitor blood pressure and pulse periodically during therapy.
❑ Monitor intake and output ratios and daily weight. Assess patient for signs of CHF (peripheral edema, rales/crackles, dyspnea, weight gain, jugular venous distention).
■ **Lab Test Considerations:** Renal, pulmonary, and hepatic function, and CBC should be evaluated periodically in patients receiving long-term therapy.

### POTENTIAL NURSING DIAGNOSES

■ Cardiac output, decreased (Indications).

# IMPLEMENTATION

■ **General:** Do not confuse Ethmozine (morizocine) with Erythrocin (erythromycin).

❑ Moricizine therapy should be initiated in a hospital with facilities for cardiac rhythm monitoring.

❑ Previous antiarrhythmic therapy should be withdrawn 1–2 half-lives before starting moricizine.

❑ Dosage adjustments should be at least 3 days apart because of the long half-life of moricizine.

❑ Pre-existing hypokalemia, hyperkalemia, or hypomagnesemia should be corrected before instituting therapy.

■ **PO:** Tablets are usually administered every 8 hr. Total daily dose may be divided and administered every 12 hr for greater compliance, but risk of adverse reactions is greater with higher single dose.

## PATIENT/FAMILY TEACHING

❑ Instruct patient to take medication around the clock exactly as directed, even if feeling better. Missed doses should be taken as soon as remembered if within 6 hr; omit if remembered later. Gradual dosage reduction may be necessary.

❑ May cause dizziness or visual disturbances. Caution patient to avoid driving and other activities requiring alertness until response to medication is known.

❑ Advise patient to notify health care professional of medication regimen before treatment or surgery.

❑ Instruct patient to notify health care professional if chest pain, shortness of breath, fever, or diaphoresis occurs.

❑ Advise patient to carry identification describing disease process and medication regimen at all times.

❑ Emphasize the importance of follow-up exams to monitor progress.

## EVALUATION

**Effectiveness of therapy can be demonstrated by:** ■ Decrease in frequency of ventricular arrhythmias.

---

High Alert

# morphine

(mor-feen)

Astramorph, Astramorph PF, Avinza, Duramorph, {Epimorph}, Infumorph, Kadian, {M-Eslon}, {Morphine H.P.}, {Morphitec}, {M.O.S.}, {M.O.S.-S.R.}, MS, MS Contin, {MS●IR}, MSIR, MSO₄, OMS Concentrate, Oramorph SR, RMS, Roxanol, Roxanol Rescudose, Roxanol-T, {Statex}

## CLASSIFICATION(S):

**Therapeutic:** opioid analgesics
**Pharmacologic:** opioid agonists

**Schedule II**

**Pregnancy Category C**

## INDICATIONS

■ Severe pain ■ Pulmonary edema ■ Pain associated with MI.

## ACTION

■ Binds to opiate receptors in the CNS. Alters the perception of and response to painful stimuli while producing generalized CNS depression. **Therapeutic Effects:** ■ Decrease in severity of pain.

## PHARMACOKINETICS

**Absorption:** Variably absorbed (about 30%) following oral administration. More reliably absorbed from rectal, subcut, and IM sites.

**Distribution:** Widely distributed. Crosses the placenta; enters breast milk in small amounts.

**Metabolism and Excretion:** Mostly metabolized by the liver.

**Half-life:** 2–3 hr.

## CONTRAINDICATIONS AND PRECAUTIONS

**Contraindicated in:** ■ Hypersensitivity ■ Some products contain tartrazine, bisulfites, or alcohol and should be avoided in patients with known hypersensitivity.

---

**Use Cautiously in:** ■ Head trauma ■ Increased intracranial pressure ■ Severe renal, hepatic, or pulmonary disease ■ Hypothyroidism ■ Adrenal insufficiency ■ History of substance abuse ■ Geriatric or debilitated patients (dosage reduction suggested) ■ Undiagnosed abdominal pain ■ Prostatic hypertrophy ■ Patients undergoing procedures that rapidly decrease pain (cordotomy, radiation); long-acting agents should be discontinued 24 hr before and replaced with short-acting agents ■ Pregnancy or lactation (avoid chronic use; has been used during labor but may cause respiratory depression in the newborn).

## ADVERSE REACTIONS AND SIDE EFFECTS*

■ **CNS:** <u>confusion</u>, <u>sedation</u>, dizziness, dysphoria, euphoria, floating feeling, hallucinations, headache, unusual dreams ■ **EENT:** blurred vision, diplopia, miosis ■ **Resp:** RESPIRATORY DE-PRESSION ■ **CV:** <u>hypotension</u>, bradycardia ■ **GI:** <u>constipation</u>, nausea, vomiting ■ **GU:** urinary retention ■ **Derm:** flushing, itching, sweating ■ **Misc:** physical dependence, psychological dependence, tolerance.

## INTERACTIONS

**Drug-Drug:** ■ Use with **extreme caution** in patients receiving **MAO inhibitors** within 14 days prior (may result in unpredictable, severe reactions— ↓ initial dose of morphine to 25% of usual dose) ■ ↑ CNS depression with **alcohol, sedative/hypnotics, clomipramine, barbiturates, tricyclic antidepressants,** and **antihistamines** ■ Administration of **partial-antagonist opioid analgesics** may precipitate opioid withdrawal in physically dependent patients ■ **Buprenorphine, nalbuphine, butorphanol,** or **pentazocine** may ↓ analgesia ■ May ↑ the anticoagulant effect of **warfarin** ■ **Cimetidine** ↓ metabolism and may ↑ effects.

**Drug-Natural Products:** ■ Concomitant use of **kava, valerian, skullcap, chamomile,** or **hops** can ↑ CNS depression.

## ROUTE AND DOSAGE

Larger doses may be required during chronic therapy.

■ **PO, Rect (Adults ≥50 kg):** *Usual starting dose for moderate to severe pain in opioid-naive patients*—30 mg q 3–4 hr initially *or* once 24-hr opioid requirement is determined, convert to controlled, extended *or* sustained-release morphine by administering total daily oral morphine dose every 24 hr (as *Kadian* or *Avinza* ), 50% of the total daily oral morphine dose every 12 hr (as *Oramorph SR, Kadian, MS Contin* ), or 33% of the total daily oral morphine dose every 8 hr (as *MS Contin* ). See equianalgesic chart, Appendix O. *Avinza* dose should not exceed 1600 mg/day because of fumaric acid in formulation.

■ **PO, Rect (Adults and Children <50 kg):** *Usual starting dose for moderate to severe pain in opioid-naive patients*—0.3 mg/kg q 3–4 hr initially.

■ **IM, IV, Subcut (Adults ≥50 kg):** *Usual starting dose for moderate to severe pain in opioid-naive patients*—4–10 mg q 3–4 hr. *MI—8–15 mg, for very severe pain additional smaller doses may be given every 3–4 hr*

■ **IM, IV, Subcut (Adults and Children <50 kg):** *Usual starting dose for moderate to severe pain in opioid-naive patients*—0.1 mg/kg q 3–4 hr.

■ **IV, Subcut (Adults):** *Continuous infusion*—0.8–10 mg/hr; may be preceded by a bolus of 15 mg (infusion rates vary greatly; up to 400 mg/hr have been used).

■ **Epidural (Adults):** *Intermittent injection*—5 mg/day (initially); if relief is not obtained at 60 min, 1–2 mg increments may be made; (total dose not to exceed 10 mg/day. *Continuous infusion*—2–4 mg/24 hr; may increase by 1–2 mg/day (up to 30 mg/day).

■ **IT (Adults):** 0.2–1 mg.

## AVAILABILITY (generic available)

■ *Soluble tablets:* 10 mg<sup>Rx</sup>, 15 mg<sup>Rx</sup>, 30 mg<sup>Rx</sup> ■ *Tablets:* 15 mg<sup>Rx</sup>, 30 mg<sup>Rx</sup> ■ Cost: *MSIR*—15 mg $18.32/100, 30 mg $31.22/100 ■ *Extended (controlled, sustained)-release tablets:* 15 mg<sup>Rx</sup>, 30 mg<sup>Rx</sup>, 60 mg<sup>Rx</sup>, 100 mg<sup>Rx</sup>, 200 mg<sup>Rx</sup> ■ Cost: *MS Contin*—15 mg $99.63/100, 30 mg $189.34/100, 60 mg $369.44/100, 100 mg $546.99/100, 200 mg $1001.71/100; *Oramorph SR*—15 mg $90.03/100, 30 mg $171.09/100, 60 mg $333.83/100, 100 mg $511.24/100 ■ *Sustained-release capsules (Kadian):* 10 mg<sup>Rx</sup>, 20 mg<sup>Rx</sup>, 30 mg<sup>Rx</sup>, 50 mg<sup>Rx</sup>, {60 mg<sup>Rx</sup>}, 100 mg<sup>Rx</sup> ■ Cost: *Kadian*—20 mg $105.49/60, 30 mg $119.00/60, 50 mg $223.05/60, 60 mg $227.39/60, 100 mg

$383.80/60 ■ *Extended-release capsules (Avinza):* 30 mg$^{Rx}$, 60 mg$^{Rx}$, 90 mg$^{Rx}$, 120 mg$^{Rx}$ ■Cost: *Avinza*—30 mg $231.00/100, 60 mg $445.00/100, 90 mg $675.00/100, 120 mg $790.00/100 ■ *Oral solution (Roxanol-T—20 mg/ml fruit and mint flavor; also unflavored):* 10 mg/5 ml$^{Rx}$, 20 mg/5 ml$^{Rx}$, 100 mg/5 ml$^{Rx}$, {2 mg/ml$^{Rx}$}, {4 mg/ml$^{Rx}$}, 20 mg/ml (concentrate)$^{Rx}$ ■ Cost: *Roxanol*—20 mg/ml $20.76/30 ml ■*Rectal suppositories:* 5 mg$^{Rx}$, 10 mg$^{Rx}$, 20 mg$^{Rx}$, 30 mg$^{Rx}$ ■ *Solution for IM, subcut, IV injection:* 1 mg/ml$^{Rx}$, 2 mg/ml$^{Rx}$, 4 mg/ml$^{Rx}$, 5 mg/ml$^{Rx}$, 8 mg/ml$^{Rx}$, 10 mg/ml$^{Rx}$, 15 mg/ml$^{Rx}$, 25 mg/ml$^{Rx}$, 50 mg/ml$^{Rx}$ ■ *Solution for epidural, IV injection (preservative-free):* 0.5 mg/ml$^{Rx}$, 1 mg/ml$^{Rx}$ ■ *Solution for epidural or IT use (continuous microinfusion device; preservative-free):* 10 mg/ml in 20-ml vial$^{Rx}$, 25 mg/ml in 20-ml vial$^{Rx}$ ■ *Solution for IV injection (PCA device):* 1 mg/ml$^{Rx}$, 2 mg/ml$^{Rx}$, 3 mg/ml$^{Rx}$, 5 mg/ml$^{Rx}$.

TIME/ACTION PROFILE (analgesia)

| | ONSET | PEAK | DURATION |
|---|---|---|---|
| PO | unknown | 60–120 min | 4–5 hr |
| PO-ER, SR | unknown | variable | 8–24 hr |
| IM | 10–30 min | 30–60 min | 4–5 hr |
| Subcut | 20 min | 50–90 min | 4–5 hr |
| Rect | unknown | 20–60 min | 4–5 hr |
| IV | rapid | 20 min | 4–5 hr |
| Epidural | 6–30 min | unknown | up to 24 hr |
| IT | rapid (min) | unknown | up to 24 hr |

# NURSING IMPLICATIONS

## ASSESSMENT

❑ Assess type, location, and intensity of pain prior to and 1 hr following PO, subcut, IM, and 20 min (peak) following IV administration. When titrating opioid doses, increases of 25–50% should be administered until there is either a 50% reduction in the patient's pain rating on a numerical or visual analogue scale or the patient reports satisfactory pain relief. When titrating doses of short-acting morphine, a repeat dose can be safely administered at the time of the peak if previous dose is ineffective and side effects are minimal.

❑ Patients on a continuous infusion should have additional bolus doses provided every 15–30 min, as needed, for breakthrough pain. The bolus dose is usually set to the amount of drug infused each hour by continuous infusion.

❑ Patients taking sustained-release morphine may require additional short-acting opioid doses for breakthrough pain. Doses should be equivalent to 10–20% of 24 hr total and given every 2 hr as needed.

❑ An equianalgesic chart (see Appendix O) should be used when changing routes or when changing from one opioid to another.

❑ **High Alert:** Assess level of consciousness, blood pressure, pulse, and respirations before and periodically during administration. If respiratory rate is <10/min, assess level of sedation. Physical stimulation may be sufficient to prevent significant hypoventilation. Subsequent doses may need to be decreased by 25–50%. Initial drowsiness will diminish with continued use.

❑ Prolonged use may lead to physical and psychological dependence and tolerance. This should not prevent patient from receiving adequate analgesia. Most patients who receive morphine for pain do not develop psychological dependence. Progressively higher doses may be required to relieve pain with long-term therapy.

❑ Assess bowel function routinely. Institute prevention of constipation with increased intake of fluids and bulk and with laxatives to minimize constipating effects. Administer stimulant laxatives routinely if opioid use exceeds 2–3 days, unless contraindicated.

■ *Lab Test Considerations:* May ↑ plasma amylase and lipase levels.

■ *Toxicity and Overdose:* If an opioid antagonist is required to reverse respiratory depression or coma, naloxone (Narcan) is the antidote. Dilute the 0.4-mg ampule of naloxone in 10 ml of 0.9% NaCl and administer 0.5 ml (0.02 mg) by direct IV push every 2 min. For children and adults weighing <40 kg, dilute 0.1 mg of naloxone in 10 ml of 0.9% NaCl for a concentration of 10 mcg/ml and administer 0.5 mcg/kg every 2

{ } = Available in Canada only.
*CAPITALS indicates life-threatening; <u>underlines</u> indicate most frequent.

min. Titrate dose to avoid withdrawal, seizures, and severe pain.

## POTENTIAL NURSING DIAGNOSES

■ Pain, acute (Indications).

■ Sensory perception, disturbed (visual, auditory) (Side Effects).

■ Injury, risk for (Side Effects).

## IMPLEMENTATION

❑ **High Alert:** Do not confuse morphine with hydromorphone or meperidine—errors have resulted in death. Other errors associated with morphine include overdose and infusion pump miscalculations. Consider patients' previous analgesic use and current requirements, but clarify doses that greatly exceed normal range. Have second practitioner independently check original order, dose calculations and infusion pump settings.

■ **General:** Explain therapeutic value of medication prior to administration to enhance the analgesic effect.

❑ Regularly administered doses may be more effective than prn administration. Analgesic is more effective if given before pain becomes severe.

❑ Coadministration with nonopioid analgesics may have additive analgesic effects and may permit lower doses.

❑ When transferring from other opioids or other forms of morphine to extended-release tablets, administer a total daily dose of oral morphine equivalent to previous daily dose (see Appendix O) and divided every 8 hr (MS Contin), every 12 hr (Kadian, MS Contin, Oramorph SR), every 24 hr (Kadian or Avinza).

❑ Morphine should be discontinued gradually to prevent withdrawal symptoms after long-term use.

■ **PO:** Doses may be administered with food or milk to minimize GI irritation.

❑ Administer solution with properly calibrated measuring device; may be diluted in a glass of fruit juice just prior to administration to improve taste.

❑ Extended-release and controlled-release tablets should be swallowed whole; do not crush, break, or chew.

❑ *Kadian and Avinza* capsules may be opened and the pellets sprinkled onto applesauce immediately prior to administration. Patients should rinse mouth and swallow to assure ingestion of entire dose. Pellets should not be chewed, crushed, or dissolved. *Kadian* capsules may also be opened and sprinkled on approximately 10 ml of water and flushed while swirling through a pre-wetted 16 French gastrostomy tube fitted with a funnel at the port end. Additional water should be used to tranfer and flush any remaining pellets. *Kadian* should not be administered via a nasogastric tube.

■ **Rect:** *MS Contin* and *Oramorph SR* have been administered rectally.

■ **IM, Subcut:** Use IM route for repeated doses, because morphine is irritating to subcut tissues.

■ **IV:** Solution is colorless; do not administer discolored solution.

■ **Direct IV:** Dilute with at least 5 ml of sterile water or 0.9% NaCl for injection.

■ *Rate:* **High Alert:** Administer 2.5–15 mg over 4–5 min. Rapid administration may lead to increased respiratory depression, hypotension, and circulatory collapse.

■ **Continuous Infusion:** May be added to D5W, D10W, 0.9% NaCl, 0.45% NaCl, Ringer's or LR, dextrose/saline solution, or dextrose/Ringer's or LR in a concentration of 0.1–1 mg/ml or greater for continuous infusion.

■ *Rate:* Administer via infusion pump to control the rate. Dose should be titrated to ensure adequate pain relief without excessive sedation, respiratory depression, or hypotension. May be administered via patient-controlled analgesia (PCA) pump.

■ **Syringe Compatibility:** ♦ atropine ♦ benzquinamide ♦ bupivacaine ♦ cimetidine ♦ dimenhydrinate ♦ diphenhydramine ♦ droperidol ♦ glycopyrrolate ♦ hydroxyzine ♦ ketamine ♦ metoclopramide ♦ midazolam ♦ milrinone ♦ ondansetron ♦ perphenazine ♦ ranitidine ♦ scopolamine.

■ **Y-Site Compatibility:** ♦ allopurinol ♦ amifostine ♦ amikacin ♦ aminophylline ♦ amiodarone ♦ ampicillin ♦ ampicillin/sulbactam ♦ atenolol ♦ atracurium ♦ atropine ♦ aztreonam ♦ bumetanide ♦ calcium chloride ♦ cefazolin ♦ cefoperazone ♦ cefotaxime ♦ cefotetan ♦ cefoxitin ♦ ceftazidime ♦ ceftizoxime ♦ ceftriaxone ♦ cefuroxime ♦ chloramphenicol ♦ cisatracurium ♦ cisplatin ♦ cladribine ♦ clindamycin ♦ cyclophosphamide ♦ cytarabine ♦

dexamethasone sodium phosphate ◆ diazepam ◆ digoxin ◆ diltiazem ◆ diphenhydramine ◆ dobutamine ◆ docetaxel ◆ dopamine ◆ doxorubicin ◆ doxycycline ◆ enalaprilat ◆ epinephrine ◆ erythromycin lactobionate ◆ esmolol ◆ etomidate ◆ etoposide ◆ famotidine ◆ filgrastim ◆ fluconazole ◆ fludarabine ◆ foscarnet ◆ gatifloxacin ◆ gemcitabine ◆ gentamicin ◆ granisetron ◆ heparin ◆ hydrocortisone sodium succinate ◆ insulin ◆ kanamycin ◆ ketorolac ◆ labetalol ◆ levofloxacin ◆ lidocaine ◆ linezolid ◆ lorazepam ◆ magnesium sulfate ◆ melphalan ◆ meropenem ◆ methotrexate ◆ methotrimeprazine ◆ methyldopate ◆ methylprednisolone ◆ metoclopramide ◆ metoprolol ◆ metronidazole ◆ midazolam ◆ milrinone ◆ nafcillin ◆ nitroglycerin ◆ nitroprusside ◆ norepinephrine ◆ ondansetron ◆ oxacillin ◆ oxytocin ◆ paclitaxel ◆ pancuronium ◆ phenobarbital ◆ penicillin G potassium ◆ piperacillin ◆ piperacillin/tazobactam ◆ potassium chloride ◆ propranolol ◆ ranitidine ◆ scopolamine ◆ sodium bicarbonate ◆ tacrolimus ◆ teniposide ◆ thiotepa ◆ ticarcillin ◆ ticarcillin/clavulanate ◆ tobramycin ◆ trimethoprim/sulfamethoxazole ◆ vancomycin ◆ vecuronium ◆ vinorelbine ◆ vitamin B complex with C ◆ warfarin ◆ zidovudine.

■ **Y-Site Incompatibility:** ◆ alatrofloxacin ◆ amphotericin B cholesteryl sulfate ◆ cefepime ◆ doxorubicin liposome ◆ minocycline ◆ phenytoin ◆ sargramostim.

## PATIENT/FAMILY TEACHING

❑ Instruct patient how and when to ask for pain medication.

❑ **High Alert:** Instruct family not to administer PCA doses to the sleeping patient. Overmedication, sedation, and respiratory depression can result.

❑ May cause drowsiness or dizziness. Caution patient to call for assistance when ambulating or smoking and to avoid driving or other activities requiring alertness until response to medication is known.

❑ Advise patient to change positions slowly to minimize orthostatic hypotension.

❑ Caution patient to avoid concurrent use of alcohol or other CNS depressants with this medication.

❑ Encourage patients who are immobilized or on prolonged bedrest to turn, cough, and breathe deeply every 2 hr to prevent atelectasis.

■ **Home Care Issues:** *High Alert:* Explain to patient and family how and when to administer morphine and how to care for infusion equipment properly.

❑ Emphasize the importance of aggressive prevention of constipation with the use of morphine.

## EVALUATION

**Effectiveness of therapy can be demonstrated by:** ■ Decrease in severity of pain without a significant alteration in level of consciousness or respiratory status ■ Decrease in symptoms of pulmonary edema.

## moxifloxacin, See FLUOROQUINOLONES.

## mupirocin
(myoo-**peer**-oh-sin)
Bactroban, Bactroban Nasal

*CLASSIFICATION(S):*
*Therapeutic: anti-infectives*

**Pregnancy Category B**

## INDICATIONS

■ **Topical:** Treatment of: ❑ Impetigo ❑ Secondarily infected traumatic skin lesions (up to 10 cm in length or 100 cm² area) caused by *Staphylococcus aureus* and *Streptococcus pyogenes* ■ **Intranasal:** Eradicates nasal colonization with methicillin-resistant *S. aureus*.

## ACTION

■ Inhibits bacterial protein synthesis. **Therapeutic Effects:** ■ Inhibition of bacterial growth and reproduction. **Spectrum:** ■ Greatest activity against gram-positive organisms, including: ❑ *S. aureus* ❑ Beta-hemolytic streptococci ■ Resolution of impetigo ■ Eradication of *S. aureus* carrier state.

{ } = Available in Canada only.
*CAPITALS indicates life-threatening; underlines indicate most frequent.

## PHARMACOKINETICS

**Absorption:** Minimal systemic absorption.

**Distribution:** Remains in the stratum corneum after topical use for prolonged periods of time (72 hr).

**Metabolism and Excretion:** Metabolized in the skin, removed by desquamation.

**Half-life:** Unknown.

## CONTRAINDICATIONS AND PRECAUTIONS

**Contraindicated in:** ■ Hypersensitivity to mupirocin or polyethylene glycol.

**Use Cautiously in:** ■ Pregnancy or lactation (safety not established).

## ADVERSE REACTIONS AND SIDE EFFECTS*

■ **CNS:** *nasal only*—headache ■ **EENT:** *nasal only*—cough, itching, pharyngitis, rhinitis, upper respiratory tract congestion ■ **GI:** nausea; *nasal only*—altered taste ■ **Derm:** *topical only*—burning, itching, pain, stinging.

## INTERACTIONS

**Drug-Drug:** ■ Nasal mupirocin should not be used concurrently with other **nasal products.**

## ROUTE AND DOSAGE

■ **Topical (Adults and Children ≥2 mo):** Apply 3 times daily.

■ **Intranasal (Adults and Children ≥12 yr):** Apply half of the contents of a single-use nasal ointment tube to each nostril twice daily for 5 days.

## AVAILABILITY

■ *Ointment:* 2% in 22-g tubes^Rx, {2% in 15- and 30-g tubes^OTC} ■ Cost: $21.85/15 g ■ *Cream:* 2% in 15- and 30-g tubes^Rx ■ Cost: $29.10/15 g ■ *Nasal ointment:* 2% in 1-g single-use tubes^Rx.

TIME/ACTION PROFILE (anti-infective effect)

| | ONSET | PEAK | DURATION |
|---|---|---|---|
| Nasal | unknown | unknown | 12 hr |
| Topical† | unknown | 3–5 days | 72 hr |

†Resolution of lesions.

## NURSING IMPLICATIONS

### ASSESSMENT

❑ Assess lesions before and daily during therapy.

### POTENTIAL NURSING DIAGNOSES

■ Skin integrity, impaired (Indications).

■ Infection, risk for (Indications, Patient/Family Teaching).

### IMPLEMENTATION

■ **Topical:** Wash affected area with soap and water and dry thoroughly. Apply a small amount of mupirocin to the affected area 3 times daily and rub in gently. Treated area may be covered with gauze if desired.

■ **Nasal:** Apply one half of the ointment from the single-use tube to each nostril twice daily (morning and evening) for 5 days. After application, close nostrils by pressing together and releasing sides of the nose repeatedly for 1 min.

### PATIENT/FAMILY TEACHING

■ **General Info:** Instruct patient on the correct application of mupirocin. Advise patient to apply medication exactly as directed for the full course of therapy. If a dose is missed, apply as soon as possible unless almost time for next dose.

■ **Topical:** Teach patient and family appropriate hygienic measures to prevent spread of impetigo.

❑ Instruct parents to notify school nurse for screening and prevention of transmission.

❑ Patient should consult health care professional if symptoms have not improved in 3–5 days.

### EVALUATION

**Effectiveness of therapy can be demonstrated by:** ■ Healing of skin lesions. If no clinical response is seen in 3–5 days, condition should be re-evaluated ■ Eradication of methicillin-resistant *S. aureus* carrier state in patients and health care workers during institutional outbreaks.

## muromonab-CD3
(myoo-roe-**moe**-nab CD3)
Orthoclone OKT3

## INDICATIONS

■ Acute renal allograft rejection reactions in transplant patients that have occurred despite conventional antirejection therapy ■ Acute corticosteroid-resistant hepatic or cardiac allograft rejection reactions.

## ACTION

■ A purified immunoglobulin antibody that acts as an immunosuppressant by interfering with normal T-cell function. **Therapeutic Effects:** ■ Reversal of graft rejection in transplant patients.

## PHARMACOKINETICS

**Absorption:** Administered IV only, resulting in complete bioavailability.
**Distribution:** Unknown.
**Metabolism and Excretion:** Eliminated by binding to T lymphocytes.
**Half-life:** 18 hr.

## CONTRAINDICATIONS AND PRECAUTIONS

**Contraindicated in:** ■ Hypersensitivity to muromonab-CD3, murine (mouse) proteins, or polysorbate ■ Previous muromonab therapy ■ Fluid overload ■ Fever >37.8°C or 100°F ■ Chickenpox or recent exposure to chickenpox ■ Herpes zoster.

**Use Cautiously in:** ■ Active infections ■ Depressed bone marrow reserve ■ Chronic debilitating illnesses ■ CHF ■ Pregnancy, lactation, or children <2 yr (safety not established).

## ADVERSE REACTIONS AND SIDE EFFECTS*

■ **CNS:** tremor, aseptic meningitis, dizziness ■ **Resp:** PULMONARY EDEMA, dyspnea, shortness of breath, wheezing ■ **CV:** chest pain ■ **GI:** diarrhea, nausea, vomiting ■ **Misc:** CYTOKINE RELEASE SYNDROME, INFECTIONS, chills, fever, hypersensitivity reactions, increased risk of lymphoma.

## INTERACTIONS

**Drug-Drug:** ■ Additive immunosuppression with other **immunosuppressives** ■ Concurrent **prednisone** and **azathioprine** dosages should be reduced during muromonab therapy (increased risk of infection and lymphoproliferative disorders) ■ **Cyclosporine** should be reduced or discontinued during muromonab-CD3 therapy (increased risk of infection and lymphoproliferative disorders) ■ Increased risk of adverse CNS reactions with **indomethacin** ■ May decrease the antibody response to and increase the risk of adverse reactions from **live-virus vaccines.**

**Drug-Natural Products:** ■ Concommitant use with **astragalus, echinacea,** and **melatonin** may interfere with immunosuppression.

## ROUTE AND DOSAGE

■ **IV (Adults):** 5 mg/day for 10–14 days (pretreatment with corticosteroids, acetaminophen, and/or antihistamines recommended).
■ **IV (Children):** 0.1 mg (100 mcg)/kg/day for 10–14 days.

## AVAILABILITY

■ *Solution for injection:* 1 mg/ml in 5-ml ampules^Rx.

TIME/ACTION PROFILE (noted as levels of circulating CD3-positive T cells)

| | ONSET | PEAK | DURATION |
|---|---|---|---|
| IV | mins | 2–7 days | 1 wk |

# NURSING IMPLICATIONS

## ASSESSMENT

❏ Assess for fluid overload (monitor weight and intake and output, assess for edema and rales/crackles). Notify physician if patient has experienced 3% or more weight gain in the previous week. Chest x-ray examination should be obtained within 24 hr before beginning therapy. Fluid-overloaded patients are at high risk of developing pulmonary edema. Monitor vital signs and breath sounds closely.

❏ Assess for cytokine release syndrome (CRS), usually manifested by high fever and chills, headache, tremor, nausea and vomiting, chest pain, muscle and joint pain, generalized weakness, shortness of breath, dizziness, abdominal pain, malaise, diarrhea, and trembling of hands, but may occasionally cause a severe, life-threatening, shock-like reaction. The severity of this reaction is greatest with initial dose. Reaction occurs within 30–48 hr and may persist for up to 6 hr. Acetaminophen and antihistamines may be used to treat early reactions. Patient temperature should be maintained below 37.8°C (100°F) at administration of each dose. Manifestations of CRS may be prevented or minimized by pretreatment with methylprednisolone sodium succinate 8 mg/kg IV given 1–4 hr before 1st dose of muromonab-CD3. Hydrocortisone 100 mg IV may also be given 30 min after the 1st and possibly 2nd dose to control respiratory side effects. Serious symptoms of CRS may require oxygen, IV fluids, corticosteroids, vasopressors, antihistamines, and intubation.

❏ Monitor for signs of anaphylactic or hypersensitivity reactions at each dose. Resuscitation equipment should be readily available.

❏ Monitor for infection (fever, chills, rash, sore throat, purulent discharge, dysuria). Notify physician immediately if these symptoms occur; may necessitate discontinuation of therapy.

❏ Monitor for development of aseptic meningitis. Onset is usually within 3 days of beginning therapy. Assess for fever, headache, nuchal rigidity, and photophobia.

■ **Lab Test Considerations:** Monitor CBC with differential and platelet count before and periodically throughout therapy.

❏ Monitor assays of T cells (CD3, CD4, CD8); target CD3 is <25 cells/mm$^3$ or plasma levels as determined by ELISA daily; target levels should be ≥800 ng/ml.

❏ Monitor BUN, serum creatinine, and hepatic enzymes (AST, ALT, alkaline phosphatase, bilirubin), especially during the first 1–3 days of therapy. May cause transient increases.

## POTENTIAL NURSING DIAGNOSES

■ Infection, risk for (Side Effects).

■ Fluid volume, excess (Side Effects).

## IMPLEMENTATION

■ **General:** Physician will reduce dosage of corticosteroids and azathioprine and discontinue cyclosporine during 10–14-day course

of muromonab-CD3. Cyclosporine may be resumed 3 days before end of therapy.

❏ Initial dose is administered during hospitalization; patient should be monitored closely for 48 hr. Subsequent doses may be administered on outpatient basis.

❏ Keep medication refrigerated at 2–8°C. Do not shake vial. Solution may contain a few fine translucent particles that do not affect potency. Discard unused portion.

■ **Direct IV:** Draw solution into syringe via low-protein-binding 0.2- or 0.22-micrometer filter to ensure removal of translucent protein particles that may be present. Discard filter and attach 20-gauge needle for IV administration.

■ **Rate:** Administer IV push over <1 min. Do not administer as an infusion.

■ **Compatibility:** Do not admix; do not administer in IV line containing other medications. If line must be used for other medications, flush with 0.9% NaCl before and after muromonab-CD3.

## PATIENT/FAMILY TEACHING

❏ Explain purpose of medication to patient. Inform patient of possible initial-dose side effects, which are markedly reduced in subsequent doses. Explain that patient will need to resume lifelong therapy with other immunosuppressive drugs after completion of muromonab-CD3 course.

❏ Inform patient of potential for CRS. Describe reportable symptoms.

❏ Advise patient to notify health care professional at first sign of rash, urticaria, tachycardia, dyspnea, or difficulty swallowing.

❏ May cause dizziness. Caution patient to avoid driving or other activities requiring alertness until response is known.

❏ Instruct patient not to receive any vaccinations and to avoid contact with persons receiving oral polio vaccine without advice of health care professional.

## PATIENT/FAMILY TEACHING

❏ Instruct patient to continue to avoid crowds and persons with known infections, as this drug also suppresses the immune system.

## EVALUATION

**Effectiveness of therapy can be demonstrated by:** ■ Reversal of the symptoms of acute organ rejection.

# mycophenolate

(mye-koe-**fee**-noe-late)
CellCept

**CLASSIFICATION(S):**
**Therapeutic:** immunosuppressants

**Pregnancy Category C**

## INDICATIONS

■ Prevention of rejection in allogenic renal, hepatic, and cardiac transplantation (used concurrently with cyclosporine and corticosteroids).

## ACTION

■ Inhibits the enzyme inosine monophosphate dehydrogenase, which is involved in purine synthesis. This inhibition results in suppression of T- and B-lymphocyte proliferation. **Therapeutic Effects:** ■ Prevention of kidney transplant rejection.

## PHARMACOKINETICS

**Absorption:** Following oral and IV administration, mycophenolate is rapidly hydrolyzed to mycophenolic acid (MPA), its active metabolite.
**Distribution:** Unknown.
**Protein Binding:** MPA—97%.
**Metabolism and Excretion:** MPA is extensively metabolized; <1% excreted unchanged in urine. Some enterohepatic recirculation of MPA occurs.
**Half-life:** MPA—17.9 hr.

## CONTRAINDICATIONS AND PRECAUTIONS

**Contraindicated in:** ■ Hypersensitivity ■ Pregnancy or lactation.
**Use Cautiously in:** ■ Active serious pathology of the GI tract (including history of ulcer disease or GI bleeding) ■ Phenylketonuria (oral suspension contains aspartame) ■ Severe chronic renal impairment (dosage not to exceed 1 g twice daily if CCr <25 ml/min/1.73 m²) ■ Delayed graft function following transplantation (observe for increased toxicity) ■ Patients with childbearing potential ■ Children (safety not established).

## ADVERSE REACTIONS AND SIDE EFFECTS*

■ **GI:** GI BLEEDING, diarrhea, vomiting ■ **Hemat:** leukopenia ■ **Misc:** sepsis, increased risk of malignancy.

## INTERACTIONS

**Drug-Drug:** ■ Combined use with **azathioprine** is not recommended (effects unknown) ■ **Acyclovir** and **ganciclovir** compete with MPA for renal excretion and, in patients with renal failure, may ↑ each other's toxicity ■ **Magnesium and aluminum hydroxide** antacids ↓ the absorption of MPA (avoid simultaneous administration) ■ **Cholestyramine** and **colestipol** ↓ the absorption of MPA (avoid concurrent use) ■ Toxicity may be ↑ by **salicylates** ■ May interfere with the action of **oral contraceptives** (additional contraceptive method should be used) ■ May ↓ the antibody response to and ↑ risk of adverse reactions from **live-virus vaccines,** although influenza vaccine may be useful.
**Drug-Food:** ■ When administered with food, peak blood levels of MPA are significantly ↓.

## ROUTE AND DOSAGE

❑ **Renal Transplantation**
■ **PO, IV (Adults):** 1 g twice daily; IV can be started ≤24 hr after transplantation and switched to PO as soon as possible (IV not recommended for ≥14 days).

❑ **Hepatic Transplantation**
■ **PO, IV (Adults):** 1 g twice daily IV, or 1.5 g twice daily PO.

❑ **Cardiac Transplantation**
■ **PO, IV (Adults):** 1.5 g twice daily; IV may be started ≤24 hr after transplantation and switched to PO as soon as possible (IV not recommended for ≥14 days).

❑ **Renal Impairment**
■ **PO, IV (Adults):** GFR <25 ml/min—daily dose should not exceed 2 g.

## AVAILABILITY

■ **Capsules:** 250 mg^Rx ■ **Tablets:** 250 mg^Rx, 500 mg^Rx ■ **Oral suspension (fruit flavor):** 200 mg/ml in 225 ml bottles^Rx ■ **Powder for injection:** 500 mg/20 ml vial^Rx.

---

{ } = Available in Canada only.
*CAPITALS indicates life-threatening; underlines indicate most frequent.

TIME/ACTION PROFILE (blood levels of MPA)

| | ONSET | PEAK | DURATION |
|---|---|---|---|
| PO | rapid | 0.8–1.3 hr | N/A |

# NURSING IMPLICATIONS

## ASSESSMENT

❏ Assess for symptoms of organ rejection throughout therapy.

■ *Lab Test Considerations:* Monitor CBC with differential weekly during the 1st mo, twice monthly for the 2nd and 3rd mo of therapy, and then monthly during the 1st yr. Neutropenia occurs most frequently from 31–180 days post-transplant. If ANC is <1000/mm$^3$, dose should be reduced or discontinued.

❏ Monitor hepatic and renal status and electrolytes periodically during therapy. May cause ↑ serum alkaline phosphatase, AST, ALT, LDH, and creatinine. May also cause hypercalcemia, hypocalcemia, hyperuricemia, hyperlipidemia, hypoglycemia, and hypoproteinemia.

## POTENTIAL NURSING DIAGNOSES

■ Infection, risk for (Adverse Reactions).

## IMPLEMENTATION

■ **General:** The initial dose of mycophenolate should be given within 72 hr of transplant.

❏ Women of childbearing years should have a negative serum or urine pregnancy test within 1 wk prior to initiation of therapy.

■ **PO:** Administer on an empty stomach, 1 hr before or 2 hr after meals. Capsules should be swallowed whole; do not open, crush, or chew. Mycophenolate may be teratogenic; contents of capsules should not be inhaled or come in contact with skin or mucous membranes.

❏ Do not administer mycophenolate concurrently with antacids containing magnesium or aluminum.

■ **IV:** IV route should only be used for patients unable to take oral medication and should be switched to oral dose form as soon as patient can tolerate capsules or tablets.

■ **Intermittent Infusion:** Reconstitute each vial with 14 ml of D5W. Shake gently to dissolve. Solution is slightly yellow; discard if solution is discolored or contains particulate matter. Dilute contents of 2 vials (1-g dose) further with 140 ml of D5W or 3 vials (1.5-g dose) with 210 ml of D5W for a concentration of 6 mg/ml. Solution is stable for 4 hr.

■ *Rate:* Administer via slow IV infusion over 2 hr.

■ **Y-Site Incompatibility:** Do not admix or administer mycophenolate in same catheter as other medications.

## PATIENT/FAMILY TEACHING

❏ Instruct patient to take medication as directed, at the same time each day. Do not skip or double up on missed doses. Do not discontinue without consulting health care professional.

❏ Reinforce the need for lifelong therapy to prevent transplant rejection. Review symptoms of rejection for the transplanted organ, and stress need to notify health care professional immediately if signs of rejection or infection occur.

❏ Inform female patients of the importance of simultaneously using two reliable forms of contraception, unless abstinence is the chosen method, prior to beginning, during, and for 6 wk following discontinuation of therapy.

❏ Advise patient to avoid contact with persons with contagious diseases.

❏ Inform patient of the increased risk of lymphoma and other malignancies. Advise patient to use sunscreen and wear protective clothing to decrease risk of skin cancer.

❏ Advise patient to consult health care professional prior to taking other medications concurrently with mycophenolate.

❏ Emphasize the importance of routine follow-up laboratory tests.

## EVALUATION

**Effectiveness of therapy can be demonstrated by:** ■ Prevention of rejection of transplanted organs.

# nabumetone

(na-**byoo**-me-tone)

Relafen

*CLASSIFICATION(S):*

*Therapeutic: antirheumatics, nonsteroidal anti-inflammatory agents*

**Pregnancy Category C**

## INDICATIONS

■ Symptomatic management of rheumatoid arthritis and osteoarthritis.

## ACTION

■ Inhibits prostaglandin synthesis. **Therapeutic Effects:** ■ Suppression of pain and inflammation.

## PHARMACOKINETICS

**Absorption:** Nabumetone (a prodrug) is 80% absorbed after oral administration; 35% is rapidly converted to 6-methoxy-2-naphthylacetic acid (6-MNA), which is the active drug.

**Distribution:** Unknown.

**Protein Binding:** >99%.

**Metabolism and Excretion:** 6-MNA is metabolized by the liver to inactive compounds.

**Half-life:** 24 hr (increased in severe renal impairment).

## CONTRAINDICATIONS AND PRECAUTIONS

**Contraindicated in:** ■ Hypersensitivity ■ Use with other NSAIDs, including aspirin; cross-sensitivity may occur ■ Active GI bleeding or ulcer disease.

**Use Cautiously in:** ■ Severe cardiovascular, renal, or hepatic disease ■ History of ulcer disease ■ Pregnancy, lactation, or children (safety not established; avoid using during 2nd half of pregnancy).

## ADVERSE REACTIONS AND SIDE EFFECTS*

■ **CNS:** agitation, anxiety, confusion, depression, dizziness, drowsiness, fatigue, headache, insomnia, malaise, weakness ■ **EENT:** abnormal vision, tinnitus ■ **Resp:** dyspnea, hypersensitivity pneumonitis ■ **CV:** edema, fluid retention, vasculitis ■ **GI:** GI BLEEDING, abdominal pain, diarrhea, abnormal liver function tests, anorexia, constipation, dry mouth, dyspepsia, flatulence, gastritis, gastroenteritis, increased appetite, nausea, stomatitis, vomiting ■ **GU:** albuminuria, azotemia, interstitial nephritis ■ **Derm:** increased sweating, photosensitivity, pruritus, rash ■ **Hemat:** prolonged bleeding time ■ **Metab:** weight gain ■ **Neuro:** paresthesia, tremor ■ **Misc:** allergic reactions including ANAPHYLAXIS, ANGIONEUROTIC EDEMA.

## INTERACTIONS

**Drug-Drug:** ■ Additive adverse GI effects with **aspirin, other NSAIDs, potassium supplements, corticosteroids,** or **alcohol** ■ Chronic use with **acetaminophen** may increase the risk of adverse renal reactions ■ May decrease the effectiveness of **diuretics** or **antihypertensives** ■ May increase the hypoglycemic effects of **insulins** or **oral hypoglycemic agents** ■ Increases the risk of toxicity from **methotrexate** ■ Increased risk of bleeding with **cefotetan, cefoperazone, valproic acid, plicamycin, anticoagulants, ticlopidine, clopidogrel, eptifibatide, tirofiban,** or **thrombolytic agents** ■ Increased risk of adverse hematologic reactions with **antineoplastics** or **radiation therapy** ■ Concurrent use with **cyclosporine** may increase the risk of renal toxicity.

## ROUTE AND DOSAGE

■ **PO (Adults):** 1000 mg/day as a single dose or divided dose twice daily; may be increased up to 2000 mg/day; use lowest effective dose during chronic therapy.

## AVAILABILITY

■ *Tablets:* 500 mg$^{Rx}$, 750 mg$^{Rx}$ ■ Cost: 500 mg $140.65/100, 750 mg $166.10/100.

TIME/ACTION PROFILE (analgesia/anti-inflammatory effects)

| | ONSET | PEAK | DURATION |
|---|---|---|---|
| PO | 1–2 days | few days–2 wk | 12–24 hr |

## NURSING IMPLICATIONS

### ASSESSMENT

□ Patients who have asthma, aspirin-induced allergy, and nasal polyps are at increased risk for developing hypersensitivity reactions. Monitor for rhinitis, asthma, and urticaria.

□ Assess pain and range of motion before and periodically throughout therapy.

■ *Lab Test Considerations:* BUN, serum creatinine, CBC, and liver function tests should be evaluated periodically in patients receiving prolonged courses of therapy.

□ Serum potassium, BUN, serum creatinine, alkaline phosphatase, LDH, AST, and ALT tests may show increased levels. Blood glucose, hemoglobin, and hematocrit concentrations, leukocyte and platelet counts, and CCr may be decreased.

□ May cause prolonged bleeding time.

### POTENTIAL NURSING DIAGNOSES

■ Pain, acute (Indications).

■ Mobility, impaired physical (Indications).

### IMPLEMENTATION

■ **General:** Administration in higher than recommended doses does not provide increased effectiveness but may cause increased side effects.

■ **PO:** Administer with meals or antacids to decrease GI irritation and increase absorption.

### PATIENT/FAMILY TEACHING

□ Advise patient to take this medication with a full glass of water and to remain in an upright position for 15–30 min after administration.

□ Instruct patient to take medication exactly as directed. If a dose is missed, it should be taken as soon as remembered but not if almost time for the next dose. Do not double doses.

□ May cause drowsiness, dizziness, or visual disturbances. Advise patient to avoid driving or other activities requiring alertness until response to the medication is known.

□ Advise patient to use sunscreen and protective clothing to prevent photosensitivity reactions.

□ Caution patient to avoid the concurrent use of alcohol, aspirin, acetaminophen, or other OTC medications without consulting health care professional.

□ Advise patient to inform health care professional of medication regimen before treatment or surgery.

□ Advise patient to consult health care professional if rash, itching, visual disturbances, tinnitus, weight gain, edema, black stools, persistent headache, or influenza-like syndrome (chills, fever, muscle aches, pain) occurs.

### EVALUATION

**Effectiveness of therapy can be demonstrated by:** ■ Decreased pain and improved joint mobility. Partial arthritic relief is usually seen within 1 wk, but maximum effectiveness may require 2 wk or more of continuous therapy. Patients who do not respond to one NSAID may respond to another.

---

# nadolol
(**nay**-doe-lole)
Corgard, {Syn-Nadolol}

*CLASSIFICATION(S):*
*Therapeutic: antianginals, antihypertensives*
*Pharmacologic: beta blockers*

**Pregnancy Category C**

---

### INDICATIONS

■ Management of hypertension ■ Management of angina pectoris. **Unlabeled uses:** ■ Arrhythmias ■ Migraine prophylaxis ■ Tremors (essential, lithium-induced, parkinsonian) ■ Aggressive behavior ■ Antipsychotic-associated akathisia ■ Situational anxiety ■ Esophageal varices ■ Reduction of intraocular pressure.

### ACTION

■ Blocks stimulation of beta$_1$ (myocardial) and beta$_2$ (pulmonary, vascular, and uterine) receptor sites. **Therapeutic Effects:** ■ Decreased heart rate and blood pressure.

### PHARMACOKINETICS

**Absorption:** 30% absorbed after oral administration.

**Distribution:** Minimal penetration of the CNS. Crosses the placenta and enters breast milk.

**Metabolism and Excretion:** 70% excreted unchanged by the kidneys.
**Half-life:** 10–24 hr (increased in renal impairment).

## CONTRAINDICATIONS AND PRECAUTIONS

**Contraindicated in:** ■ Uncompensated CHF ■ Pulmonary edema ■ Cardiogenic shock ■ Bradycardia or heart block.

**Use Cautiously in:** ■ Renal impairment (CCr <50 ml/min) ■ Hepatic impairment ■ Geriatric patients (increased sensitivity to beta blockers; initial dosage reduction recommended) ■ Pulmonary disease (including asthma) ■ Diabetes mellitus (may mask signs of hypoglycemia) ■ Thyrotoxicosis (may mask symptoms) ■ Patients with a history of severe allergic reactions (intensity of reactions may be increased) ■ Pregnancy, lactation, or children (safety not established; crosses the placenta and may cause fetal/neonatal bradycardia, hypotension, hypoglycemia, or respiratory depression).

## ADVERSE REACTIONS AND SIDE EFFECTS*

■ **CNS:** fatigue, weakness, anxiety, depression, dizziness, drowsiness, insomnia, memory loss, mental status changes, nightmares ■ **EENT:** blurred vision, dry eyes, nasal stuffiness ■ **Resp:** bronchospasm, wheezing ■ **CV:** ARRHYTHMIAS, BRADYCARDIA, CHF, PULMONARY EDEMA, orthostatic hypotension, peripheral vasoconstriction ■ **GI:** constipation, diarrhea, nausea ■ **GU:** impotence, decreased libido ■ **Derm:** itching, rashes ■ **Endo:** hyperglycemia, hypoglycemia ■ **MS:** arthralgia, back pain, muscle cramps ■ **Neuro:** paresthesia ■ **Misc:** drug-induced lupus syndrome.

## INTERACTIONS

**Drug-Drug:** ■ **General anesthesia, IV phenytoin, diltiazem,** and **verapamil** may cause additive myocardial depression ■ Additive bradycardia may occur with **digoxin** ■ Additive hypotension may occur with other **antihypertensives,** acute ingestion of **alcohol,** or **nitrates** ■ Concurrent use with **amphetamines, cocaine, ephedrine, epinephrine, norepinephrine, phenylephrine,** or **pseudoephedrine** may result in unopposed alpha-adrenergic stimulation (excessive hypertension, bradycardia) ■ Concurrent use with **clonidine** increases hypotension and bradycardia ■ Concurrent **thyroid** administration may decrease effectiveness ■ May alter the effectiveness of **insulins** or **oral hypoglycemic agents** (dosage adjustments may be necessary) ■ May decrease the effectiveness of **theophylline** ■ May decrease the beneficial beta cardiovascular effects of **dopamine** or **dobutamine** ■ Use cautiously within 14 days of **MAO inhibitor therapy** (may result in hypertension) ■ Concurrent **NSAIDs** may decrease antihypertensive action.

## ROUTE AND DOSAGE

■ **PO (Adults):** *Antianginal*—40 mg once daily initially; may increase by 40–80 mg/day q 3–7 days as needed (up to 240 mg/day). *Antihypertensive*—40 mg once daily initially; may increase by 40–80 mg/day q 7 days as needed (up to 320 mg/day).

❑ **Renal Impairment**
■ **PO (Adults):** *CCr 31–50 ml/min*—increase dosing interval to 24–36 hr; *CCr 10–30 ml/min*—increase dosing interval to 24–48 hr; *CCr <10 ml/min*—increase dosing interval to 40–60 hr.

## AVAILABILITY (generic available)

■ *Tablets:* 20 mg$^{Rx}$, 40 mg$^{Rx}$, 80 mg$^{Rx}$, 120 mg$^{Rx}$, 160 mg$^{Rx}$ ■ Cost: *Corgard*—20 mg $130.72/100, 40 mg $153.25/100, 80 mg $210.13/100, 120 mg $273.86/100, 160 mg $304.60/100; *generic*—20 mg $84.42/100, 40 mg $95.84/100, 80 mg $141.61/100, 120 mg $169.96/100, 160 mg $179.47/100 ■ bendroflumethiazide (Corzide$^{Rx}$). See Appendix B.

TIME/ACTION PROFILE (anithypertensive effects)

| | ONSET | PEAK | DURATION |
|---|---|---|---|
| PO† | up to 5 days | 6–9 days | 24 hr |

†With chronic dosing.

## NURSING IMPLICATIONS

### ASSESSMENT

■ **General Info:** Monitor blood pressure and pulse frequently during dose adjustment and periodically during therapy. Assess for orthostatic hypotension when assisting patient up from supine position.

❑ Monitor intake and output ratios and daily weight. Assess patient routinely for evidence of fluid overload (peripheral edema, dyspnea, rales/crackles, fatigue, weight gain, jugular venous distention).

■ **Hypertension:** Check frequency of refills to determine compliance.

■ **Angina:** Assess frequency and characteristics of angina periodically during therapy.

■ *Lab Test Considerations:* May cause increased BUN, serum lipoprotein, potassium, triglyceride, and uric acid levels.

❑ May cause increased ANA titers.

❑ May cause increase in blood glucose levels.

■ *Toxicity and Overdose:* Monitor patients receiving beta blockers for signs of overdose (bradycardia, severe dizziness or fainting, severe drowsiness, dyspnea, bluish fingernails or palms, seizures). Notify physician or other health care professional immediately if these signs occur.

## POTENTIAL NURSING DIAGNOSES

■ Cardiac output, decreased (Side Effects).

■ Noncompliance (Patient/Family Teaching).

## IMPLEMENTATION

■ **General:** Discontinuation of concurrent clonidine should be done gradually, with beta blocker discontinued first; then, after several days, discontinue clonidine.

■ **PO:** Take apical pulse before administering. If <50 bpm or if arrhythmia occurs, withhold medication and notify physician or other health care professional.

❑ May be administered with food or on an empty stomach.

❑ Tablets may be crushed and mixed with food.

## PATIENT/FAMILY TEACHING

■ **General Info:** Instruct patient to take medication exactly as directed, at the same time each day, even if feeling well; do not skip or double up on missed doses. Take missed doses as soon as possible up to 8 hr before next dose. Abrupt withdrawal may precipitate life-threatening arrhythmias, hypertension, or myocardial ischemia.

❑ Advise patient to ensure that enough medication is available for weekends, holidays, and vacations. A written prescription may be kept in wallet for emergencies.

❑ Teach patient and family how to check pulse and blood pressure. Instruct them to check pulse daily and blood pressure biweekly. Advise patient to hold dose and contact health care professional if pulse is <50 bpm or if blood pressure changes significantly.

❑ May cause drowsiness or dizziness. Caution patients to avoid driving or other activities that require alertness until response to the drug is known.

❑ Advise patients to make position changes slowly to minimize orthostatic hypotension, especially during initiation of therapy or when dose is increased.

❑ Caution patient that this medication may increase sensitivity to cold.

❑ Instruct patient to consult health care professional before taking any OTC medications, especially cold preparations, concurrently with this medication.

❑ Patients with diabetes should closely monitor blood glucose, especially if weakness, malaise, irritability, or fatigue occurs. Medication may mask some signs of hypoglycemia, but dizziness and sweating may still occur.

❑ Advise patient to notify health care professional if slow pulse, difficulty breathing, wheezing, cold hands and feet, dizziness, confusion, depression, rash, fever, sore throat, unusual bleeding, or bruising occurs.

❑ Instruct patient to inform health care professional of medication regimen before treatment or surgery.

❑ Advise patient to carry identification describing disease process and medication regimen at all times.

■ **Hypertension:** Reinforce the need to continue additional therapies for hypertension (weight loss, sodium restriction, stress reduction, regular exercise, moderation of alcohol consumption, and smoking cessation). Medication controls but does not cure hypertension.

■ **Angina:** Caution patient to avoid overexertion with decrease in chest pain.

## EVALUATION

**Effectiveness of therapy can be demonstrated by:** ■ Decrease in blood pressure ■ Reduction in frequency of angina ❑ Increase in activity tolerance. May require up to 5 days before therapeutic effects are seen.

## nafarelin
(na-**fare**-e-lin)
Synarel

**CLASSIFICATION(S):**
**Therapeutic:** hormones
**Pharmacologic:** gonadotropin-releasing hormones

**Pregnancy Category X**

### INDICATIONS

■ Management of endometriosis ■ Management of central precocious puberty (gonadotropin-dependent) in children.

### ACTION

■ Acts as a synthetic analog of gonadotropin-releasing hormone (GnRH). Initially increases pituitary production of luteinizing hormone (LH) and follicle-stimulating hormone (FSH), which cause ovarian steroid production. Chronic administration leads to decreased production of gonadotropins. Endometriotic lesions are sensitive to ovarian hormones. **Therapeutic Effects:** ■ Reduction in lesions and associated pain in endometriosis ■ Arrest and regression of puberty in children with central precocious puberty.

### PHARMACOKINETICS

**Absorption:** Well absorbed following intranasal administration.
**Distribution:** Unknown.
**Metabolism and Excretion:** 20–40% excreted in feces; 3% excreted unchanged by the kidneys.
**Half-life:** 3 hr.

### CONTRAINDICATIONS AND PRECAUTIONS

**Contraindicated in:** ■ Hypersensitivity to GnRH, its analogues, or sorbitol ■ Pregnancy or lactation.
**Use Cautiously in:** ■ Rhinitis.

### ADVERSE REACTIONS AND SIDE EFFECTS*

■ **CNS:** <u>emotional instability</u>, <u>headaches</u>, depression, insomnia ■ **EENT:** <u>nasal irritation</u> ■ **CV:** edema ■ **GU:** <u>vaginal dryness</u> ■ **Derm:** <u>acne</u>, hirsutism, seborrhea ■ **Endo:** <u>cessation of menses</u>, <u>impaired fertility</u>, <u>reduced breast size</u> ■ **MS:** decreased bone density, myalgia ■ **Misc:** <u>decreased libido</u>, <u>hot flashes</u>, hypersensitivity reactions, weight gain.

### INTERACTIONS

**Drug-Drug:** ■ Concurrent **topical nasal decongestants** may reduce absorption of nafarelin (administer decongestant at least 2 hr after nafarelin).

### ROUTE AND DOSAGE

■ **Intranasal (Adults):** *Endometriosis*—1 spray (200 mcg) in 1 nostril in the morning and 1 spray in the other nostril in the evening (400 mcg/day). May be increased to 1 spray in each nostril in the morning and evening (800 mcg/day).
■ **Intranasal (Children):** *Central precocious puberty*—2 sprays in each nostril in the morning and in the evening (1600 mcg/day); may be increased up to 1800 mcg/day (3 sprays in alternating nostrils 3 times daily).

### AVAILABILITY

■ *Nasal spray:* 2 mg/ml 10-ml bottle (200 mcg/spray)[Rx] ■ Cost: $453.36/10 ml.

TIME/ACTION PROFILE (decreased ovarian steroid production)

| | ONSET | PEAK | DURATION |
|---|---|---|---|
| Intranasal | within 4 wk | 3–4 wk | 3–6 mo† |

†Relief of symptoms of endometriosis following discontinuation.

## NURSING IMPLICATIONS

### ASSESSMENT

■ **Endometriosis:** Assess patient for endometriotic pain periodically throughout therapy.
■ **Central Precocious Puberty:** Prior to therapy, a complete physical and endocrinologic examination including height, weight, hand and wrist x-ray, total sex steroid level (estra-

diol or testosterone), adrenal steroid level, beta human chorionic gonadotropin level, GnRH stimulation test, pelvic/adrenal/testicular ultrasound, and CT of the head must be performed. These parameters are monitored after 6–8 wk and every 3–6 mo during therapy.

❑ Assess patient for signs of precocious puberty (menses, breast development, testicular growth) periodically throughout therapy.

❑ Nafarelin is discontinued when the onset of normal puberty is desired. Monitor the onset of normal puberty and assess menstrual cycle, reproductive function, and final adult height.

## POTENTIAL NURSING DIAGNOSES

■ Pain, acute (Indications).

■ Sexual dysfunction (Indications, Side Effects).

## IMPLEMENTATION

■ **Endometriosis:** Treatment should be started between days 2 and 4 of the menstrual cycle and continued for up to 6 mo.

## PATIENT/FAMILY TEACHING

■ **General Info:** Instruct patient on the correct technique for nasal spray: The head should be tilted back slightly; wait 30 sec between sprays.

❑ Advise patient to consult health care professional if rhinitis occurs during therapy. If a topical decongestant is needed, do not use decongestant until 2 hr after nafarelin dosing. If possible, avoid sneezing during and immediately after nafarelin dose.

■ **Endometriosis:** Inform patient that 1 spray should be administered into 1 nostril in the morning and 1 spray into the other nostril in the evening for the 400 mcg/day dose. If dose is increased to 800 mcg/day, administer 1 spray to each nostril (2 sprays) morning and evening; 1 bottle should provide a 30-day supply at the 400 mcg/day dose.

❑ Advise patient to use a form of contraception other than oral contraceptives during therapy. Inform patient that amenorrhea is expected. Instruct patient to notify health care professional if regular menstruation persists or if successive doses are missed.

❑ Advise patient that medication may cause hot flashes. Notify health care professional if these become bothersome.

■ **Central Precocious Puberty:** Instruct patient on correct timing and number of sprays. The 1600 mcg/day dose is achieved by 2 sprays to each nostril in the morning (4 sprays) and 2 sprays to each nostril in the evening (4 sprays), for a total of 8 sprays. The 1800 mcg/day dose is achieved by 3 sprays into alternating nostrils 3 times per day, for a total of 9 sprays. Inform patient and parents that if doses are not taken as directed, pubertal process may be reactivated. One bottle should provide a 7-day supply at the 1600 mcg/day dose.

❑ Advise patient and parents that during 1st mo of therapy some signs of puberty (vaginal bleeding, breast enlargement) may occur. These should resolve after the 1st mo of therapy. If these signs persist after the 2nd mo of therapy, notify health care professional.

## EVALUATION

**Clinical response to therapy can be evaluated by:** ■ Reduction in lesions and associated pain in endometriosis ■ Resolution of the signs of precocious puberty.

## nafcillin, See PENICILLINS, PENICILLINASE RESISTANT.

## naftifine, See ANTIFUNGALS (TOPICAL).

| High Alert |

## nalbuphine

(**nal**-byoo-feen)

Nubain

*CLASSIFICATION(S):*
***Therapeutic:*** *opioid analgesics*
***Pharmacologic:*** *opioid agonists/ analgesics*

**Pregnancy Category C**

## INDICATIONS

■ Moderate to severe pain ■ Also provides: ❑ Analgesia during labor ❑ Sedation before surgery ❑ Supplement to balanced anesthesia.

## ACTION

■ Binds to opiate receptors in the CNS ■ Alters the perception of and response to painful stimuli while producing generalized CNS depression ■ In addition, has partial antagonist properties, which may result in opioid withdrawal in physically dependent patients. **Therapeutic Effects:** ■ Decreased pain.

## PHARMACOKINETICS

**Absorption:** Well absorbed after IM and subcut administration.

**Distribution:** Probably crosses the placenta and enters breast milk.

**Metabolism and Excretion:** Mostly metabolized by the liver and eliminated in the feces via biliary excretion. Minimal amounts excreted unchanged by the kidneys.

**Half-life:** 5 hr.

## CONTRAINDICATIONS AND PRECAUTIONS

**Contraindicated in:** ■ Hypersensitivity to nalbuphine or bisulfites ■ Patients who are physically dependent on opioids and have not been detoxified (may precipitate withdrawal).

**Use Cautiously in:** ■ Head trauma ■ Increased intracranial pressure ■ Severe renal, hepatic, or pulmonary disease ■ Hypothyroidism ■ Adrenal insufficiency ■ Alcoholism ■ Geriatric or debilitated patients (dosage reduction suggested) ■ Undiagnosed abdominal pain ■ Prostatic hypertrophy ■ Patients who have recently received opioid agonists ■ Pregnancy (has been used during labor but may cause respiratory depression in the newborn) ■ Lactation or children (safety not established).

## ADVERSE REACTIONS AND SIDE EFFECTS*

■ **CNS:** <u>dizziness</u>, <u>headache</u>, <u>sedation</u>, confusion, dysphoria, euphoria, floating feeling, hallucinations, unusual dreams ■ **EENT:** blurred vision, diplopia, miosis (high doses) ■ **Resp:** respiratory depression ■ **CV:** hypertension, orthostatic hypotension, palpitations ■ **GI:** <u>dry mouth</u>, <u>nausea</u>, <u>vomiting</u>, constipation, ileus ■ **GU:** urinary urgency ■ **Derm:** <u>clammy feeling</u>, sweating ■ **Misc:** physical dependence, psychological dependence, tolerance.

## INTERACTIONS

**Drug-Drug:** ■ Use with extreme caution in patients receiving **MAO inhibitors** (may result in unpredictable, severe reactions—reduce initial dose of nalbuphine to 25% of usual dose) ■ Additive CNS depression with **alcohol, antihistamines,** and **sedative/hypnotics** ■ May precipitate withdrawal in patients who are physically dependent on **opioid agonists** ■ Avoid concurrent use with other **opioid analgesic agonists** (may diminish analgesic effect).

**Drug-Natural Products:** ■ Concomitant use of **kava, valerian, skullcap, chamomile,** or **hops** can increase CNS depression.

## ROUTE AND DOSAGE

❑ **Analgesia**

■ **IM, Subcut, IV (Adults):** Usual dose is 10 mg q 3–6 hr (single dose not to exceed 20 mg; total daily dose not to exceed 160 mg).

❑ **Supplement to Balanced Anesthesia**

■ **IV (Adults):** *Initial*—0.3–3 mg/kg over 10–15 min. *Maintenance*—0.25–0.5 mg/kg as needed.

## AVAILABILITY (generic available)

■*Injection:* 10 mg/ml in 1- and 10-ml vials[Rx], 20 mg/ml in 1- and 10-ml vials and 1-ml preloaded syringes[Rx].

TIME/ACTION PROFILE (analgesia)

|  | ONSET | PEAK | DURATION |
|---|---|---|---|
| IM | <15 min | 60 min | 3–6 hr |
| Subcut | <15 min | unknown | 3–6 hr |
| IV | 2–3 min | 30 min | 3–6 hr |

# NURSING IMPLICATIONS

## ASSESSMENT

❑ Assess type, location, and intensity of pain before and 1 hr after IM or 30 min (peak) after IV administration. When titrating opioid doses, increases of 25–50% should be administered until there is either a 50% reduction in the patient's pain rating on a numeric or visual analogue scale or the patient reports satisfactory pain relief. A repeat dose can be safely administered at the time of the peak if previous dose is ineffective and side effects are minimal. Patients requiring doses higher than 20 mg should be converted to an opioid agonist. Nalbuphine is not recommended for prolonged use or as first-line therapy for acute or cancer pain.

◻ An equianalgesic chart (see Appendix O) should be used when changing routes or when changing from one opioid to another.

◻ Assess blood pressure, pulse, and respirations before and periodically during administration. If respiratory rate is <10/min, assess level of sedation. Physical stimulation may be sufficient to prevent significant hypoventilation. Dose may need to be decreased by 25–50%. Nalbuphine produces respiratory depression, but this does not markedly increase with increased doses.

◻ Assess previous analgesic history. Antagonistic properties may induce withdrawal symptoms (vomiting, restlessness, abdominal cramps, and increased blood pressure and temperature) in patients physically dependent on opioids.

◻ Although this drug has a low potential for dependence, prolonged use may lead to physical and psychological dependence and tolerance. This should not prevent patient from receiving adequate analgesia. Most patients who receive nalbuphine for pain do not develop psychological dependence. If tolerance develops, changing to an opioid agonist may be required to relieve pain.

■ *Lab Test Considerations:* May cause increased serum amylase and lipase concentrations.

■ *Toxicity and Overdose:* If an opioid antagonist is required to reverse respiratory depression or coma, naloxone (Narcan) is the antidote. Dilute the 0.4-mg ampule of naloxone in 10 ml of 0.9% NaCl and administer 0.5 ml (0.02 mg) by direct IV push every 2 min. For children and patients weighing <40 kg, dilute 0.1 mg of naloxone in 10 ml of 0.9% NaCl for a concentration of 10 mcg/ml and administer 0.5 mcg/kg every 2 min. Titrate dose to avoid withdrawal, seizures, and severe pain.

## POTENTIAL NURSING DIAGNOSES

■ Pain, acute (Indications).

■ Injury, risk for (Side Effects).

■ Sensory perception, disturbed (visual, auditory) (Side Effects).

## IMPLEMENTATION

◻ *High Alert:* Accidental overdosage of opioid analgesics has resulted in fatalities. Before administering, clarify all ambiguous orders; have second practitioner independently check original order, dose calculations, and infusion pump settings.

■ **General:** Explain therapeutic value of medication before administration to enhance the analgesic effect.

◻ Regularly administered doses may be more effective than prn administration. Analgesic is more effective if administered before pain becomes severe.

◻ Coadministration with nonopioid analgesics may have additive effects and permit lower opioid doses.

■ **IM:** Administer deep into well-developed muscle. Rotate sites of injections.

■ **Direct IV:** May give IV undiluted.

■ **Rate:** Administer slowly, each 10 mg over 3–5 min.

■ **Syringe Compatibility:** ◆ atropine ◆ cimetidine ◆ diphenhydramine ◆ droperidol ◆ glycopyrrolate ◆ hydroxyzine ◆ lidocaine ◆ midazolam ◆ prochlorperazine ◆ ranitidine ◆ scopolamine ◆ trimethobenzamide.

■ **Syringe Incompatibility:** ◆ diazepam ◆ ketorolac ◆ pentobarbital.

■ **Y-Site Compatibility:** ◆ amifostine ◆ aztreonam ◆ filgrastim ◆ fludarabine ◆ gatifloxacin ◆ linezolid ◆ melphalan ◆ paclitaxel ◆ teniposide ◆ thiotepa ◆ vinorelbine.

■ **Y-Site Incompatibility:** ◆ cefepime ◆ methotrexate ◆ nafcillin ◆ piperacillin/tazobactam ◆ sargramostim ◆ sodium bicarbonate.

## PATIENT/FAMILY TEACHING

◻ Instruct patient on how and when to ask for pain medication.

◻ May cause drowsiness or dizziness. Advise patient to call for assistance when ambulating and to avoid driving or other activities requiring alertness until response to the medication is known.

◻ Caution patient to change positions slowly to minimize orthostatic hypotension.

◻ Advise patient that frequent mouth rinses, good oral hygiene, and sugarless gum or candy may decrease dry mouth.

◻ Encourage patient to turn, cough, and breathe deeply every 2 hr to prevent atelectasis.

❑ Advise patient to avoid concurrent use of alcohol or other CNS depressants with this medication.

## EVALUATION

**Effectiveness of therapy can be demonstrated by:** ■ Decrease in severity of pain without significant alteration in level of consciousness or respiratory status.

# naloxone
(nal-**ox**-one)
Narcan

### CLASSIFICATION(S):
**Therapeutic:** antidotes (for opioids)
**Pharmacologic:** opioid antagonists

### Pregnancy Category B

## INDICATIONS

■ Reversal of CNS depression and respiratory depression because of suspected opioid overdosage. **Unlabeled uses:** ■ Management of refractory circulatory shock.

## ACTION

■ Competitively blocks the effects of opioids, including CNS and respiratory depression, without producing any agonist (opioid-like) effects. **Therapeutic Effects:** ■ Reversal of signs of opioid excess.

## PHARMACOKINETICS

**Absorption:** Well absorbed after IM or subcut administration.
**Distribution:** Rapidly distributed to tissues. Crosses the placenta.
**Metabolism and Excretion:** Metabolized by the liver.
**Half-life:** 60–90 min (up to 3 hr in neonates).

## CONTRAINDICATIONS AND PRECAUTIONS

**Contraindicated in:** ■ Hypersensitivity.
**Use Cautiously in:** ■ Cardiovascular disease ■ Patients physically dependent on opioids (may precipitate severe withdrawal) ■ Pregnancy (may cause withdrawal in mother and fetus if mother is opioid dependent) ■ Lactation (safety not established) ■ Neonates of opioid-dependent mothers.

## ADVERSE REACTIONS AND SIDE EFFECTS*

■ **CV:** hypertension, hypotension, ventricular fibrillation, ventricular tachycardia ■ **GI:** nausea, vomiting.

## INTERACTIONS

**Drug-Drug:** ■ Can precipitate withdrawal in patients physically dependent on **opioid analgesics** ■ Larger doses may be required to reverse the effects of **buprenorphine, butorphanol, nalbuphine, pentazocine,** or **propoxyphene** ■ Antagonizes postoperative **opioid analgesics**.

## ROUTE AND DOSAGE

❑ **Postoperative Opioid-Induced Respiratory Depression**

■ **IV (Adults):** 0.02–0.2 mg q 2–3 min until response obtained; repeat q 1–2 hr if needed.

■ **IV (Children):** 5–10 mcg; may repeat q 2–3 min until response obtained. Additional doses may be given q 1–2 hr if needed.

■ **IM, IV, Subcut (Neonates):** 10 mcg (0.01 mg)/kg; may repeat q 2–3 min until response obtained. Additional doses may be given q 1–2 hr if needed.

❑ **Opioid-Induced Respiratory Depression during Chronic (>1 wk) Opioid Use**

■ **IV, IM, Subcut (Adults >40 kg):** 20–40 mcg (0.02–0.04 mg) given as small, frequent (q min) boluses or as an infusion titrated to improve respiratory function without reversing analgesia.

■ **IV, IM, Subcut (Adults and Children <40 kg):** 0.5–2 mcg/kg given as small, frequent (q min) boluses or as an infusion titrated to improve respiratory function without reversing analgesia.

❑ **Overdose of Opioids**

■ **IV, IM, Subcut (Adults):** *Patients not suspected of being opioid dependent*—0.4 mg (10 mcg/kg); may repeat q 2–3 min (IV route is preferred). Some patients may require up to 2 mg. *Patients suspected to be opioid dependent*—Initial dose should be decreased to 0.1–0.2 mg q 2–3 min. May also be given by IV infusion at rate adjusted to patient's response.

- **IV, IM, Subcut (Children):** 10 mcg (0.01 mg)/kg q 2–3 min; if no response occurs, dose may be increased to 100 mcg (0.1 mg)/kg.

## AVAILABILITY (generic available)

- *Injection:* 0.4 mg/ml$^{Rx}$ ■ *Neonatal injection:* 0.02 mg/ml$^{Rx}$ ■ pentazocine (Talwin NX)$^{Rx}$. See Appendix B.

TIME/ACTION PROFILE (reversal of opioid effects)

|  | ONSET | PEAK | DURATION |
|---|---|---|---|
| IV | 1–2 min | unknown | 45 min |
| IM, subcut | 2–5 min | unknown | >45 min |

# NURSING IMPLICATIONS

## ASSESSMENT

- ❑ Monitor respiratory rate, rhythm, and depth; pulse, ECG, blood pressure; and level of consciousness frequently for 3–4 hr after the expected peak of blood concentrations. After a moderate overdose of a short half-life opioid, physical stimulation may be enough to prevent significant hypoventilation. The effects of some opioids may last longer than the effects of naloxone, and repeat doses may be necessary.
- ❑ Patients who have been receiving opioids for >1 wk are extremely sensitive to the effects of naloxone. Dilute and administer carefully.
- ❑ Assess patient for level of pain after administration when used to treat postoperative respiratory depression. Naloxone decreases respiratory depression but also reverses analgesia.
- ❑ Assess patient for signs and symptoms of opioid withdrawal (vomiting, restlessness, abdominal cramps, increased blood pressure, and temperature). Symptoms may occur within a few minutes to 2 hr. Severity depends on dose of naloxone, the opioid involved, and degree of physical dependence.
- ❑ Lack of significant improvement indicates that symptoms are caused by a disease process or other non-opioid CNS depressants not affected by naloxone.

- *Toxicity and Overdose:* Naloxone is a pure antagonist with no agonist properties and minimal toxicity.

## POTENTIAL NURSING DIAGNOSES

- Breathing pattern, ineffective (Indications).
- Coping, ineffective (Indications).
- Pain, acute.

## IMPLEMENTATION

- **General:** Larger doses of naloxone may be necessary when used to antagonize the effects of buprenorphine, butorphanol, nalbuphine, pentazocine, and propoxyphene.
- ❑ Resuscitation equipment, oxygen, vasopressors, and mechanical ventilation should be available to supplement naloxone therapy as needed.
- **Direct IV:** Administer undiluted for *suspected opioid overdose.*
- ❑ For patients with *opioid-induced respiratory depression,* dilute 0.4 mg of naloxone in 10 ml of sterile water or 0.9% NaCl for injection.
- ❑ For children or others weighing <40 kg, dilute 0.1 mg of naloxone in 10 ml of sterile water or 0.9% NaCl for injection for a concentration of 10 mcg/ml.
- *Rate:* Administer at a rate of 0.1–0.4 mg over 15 seconds in patients with *suspected opioid overdose.*
- ❑ For patients who develop *opioid-induced respiratory depression,* administer dilute solution of 0.4 mg/10 ml at a rate of 0.5 ml (0.02 mg) by direct IV push every 2 min. Titrate dose to avoid withdrawal and severe pain. Excessive dose in postoperative patients may cause excitement, pain, hypotension, hypertension, pulmonary edema, ventricular tachycardia and fibrillation, and seizures.
- ❑ For children and others weighing <40 kg, administer 10 mcg/ml solution at a rate of 0.5 mcg/kg every 1–2 min. Titrate dose to avoid withdrawal, seizures, and severe pain.
- **Continuous Infusion:** Dilute in D5W or 0.9% NaCl for injection. Naloxone 2 mg in 500 ml equals a concentration of 4 mcg/ml. Mixture is stable for 24 hr; discard unused solution.
- *Rate:* Titrate dose according to patient response. Supplemental doses administered subcut or IM, or a continuous infusion may provide longer-lasting effects.

❑ Doses should be titrated carefully in postoperative patients to avoid interference with control of postoperative pain.

■ **Syringe Compatibility:** ◆ heparin ◆ ondansetron

■ **Y-Site Compatibility:** ◆ gatifloxacin ◆ linezolid ◆ propofol

■ **Y-Site Incompatibility:** ◆ amphotericin B cholesteryl sulfate.

■ **Additive Incompatibility:** Incompatible with preparations containing bisulfite, sulfite, and solutions with an alkaline pH.

### PATIENT/FAMILY TEACHING

❑ As medication becomes effective, explain purpose and effects of naloxone to patient.

### EVALUATION

**Clinical response to therapy can be evaluated by:** ■ Adequate ventilation ❑ Alertness without significant pain or withdrawal symptoms.

---

# nandrolone decanoate

**(nan**-dro-lone dek-a-**noe**-ate)
Deca-Durabolin, Hybolin Decanoate, Kabolin

### CLASSIFICATION(S):
**Therapeutic:** antianemics, hormones
**Pharmacologic:** anabolic steroids

**Schedule III**

**Pregnancy Category X**

---

### INDICATIONS

■ Treatment of anemia associated with renal insufficiency.

### ACTION

■ Stimulates erythropoietin production and may have a direct stimulant action on bone marrow. **Therapeutic Effects:** ■ Increased hemoglobin and RBC volume.

### PHARMACOKINETICS

**Absorption:** Well absorbed following IM administration.

**Distribution:** Unknown.

**Metabolism and Excretion:** Unknown.

**Half-life:** Unknown.

### CONTRAINDICATIONS AND PRECAUTIONS

**Contraindicated in:** ■ Hypersensitivity ■ Pregnancy or lactation ■ Some products contain sesame oil and should be avoided in patients with known hypersensitivity ■ Advanced breast cancer with associated hypercalcemia ■ Breast cancer in males ■ Severe hepatic impairment ■ Hypercalcemia ■ Nephrosis or nephrotic phase of nephritis ■ Prostate cancer.

**Use Cautiously in:** ■ Cardiac or hepatic impairment ■ Coronary artery disease or history of MI ■ Diabetes mellitus ■ Benign prostatic hyperplasia ■ Children ■ Geriatric patients.

### ADVERSE REACTIONS AND SIDE EFFECTS*

■ **CNS:** insomnia ■ **CV:** edema ■ **GI:** abdominal fullness, diarrhea, hepatic dysfunction ■ **GU:** changes in libido, impotence, prostatic hyperplasia ■ **Derm:** acne ■ **Endo:** <u>virilism in women and prepubertal men</u> ■ **F and E:** hypercalcemia ■ **MS:** muscle cramps ■ **Misc:** chills.

### INTERACTIONS

**Drug-Drug:** ■ Increased risk of hepatotoxicity with other **hepatotoxic agents** ■ Increased risk of bleeding with **warfarin, NSAIDs,** and **salicylates.**

### ROUTE AND DOSAGE

■ **IM (Adults and Children ≥14 yr):** *Women*—50–100 mg q wk; *men*—100–200 mg q wk.

■ **IM (Children 2–13 yr):** 25–50 mg q 3–4 wk.

### AVAILABILITY (generic available)

■ *Injection:* 100 mg/ml in 2 ml vial^Rx, 200 mg/ml in 1 ml vial^Rx ■ Cost: *Deca-Durabolin*—100 mg/ml in 2 ml vial: $290.16/10; 200 mg/ml in 1 ml vial: $695.18/25.

---

{ } = Available in Canada only.
*CAPITALS indicates life-threatening; <u>underlines</u> indicate most frequent.

TIME/ACTION PROFILE (blood levels)

| | ONSET | PEAK | DURATION |
|---|---|---|---|
| IM | unknown | 3–6 days | unknown |

## NURSING IMPLICATIONS

### ASSESSMENT

□ Monitor response for symptoms of anemia (fatigue, dyspnea, pallor).

■ *Lab Test Considerations:* Monitor CBC periodically throughout therapy.

### POTENTIAL NURSING DIAGNOSES

■ Activity intolerance (Indications).

### IMPLEMENTATION

■ **IM:** Inject deeply into gluteal muscle.

### PATIENT/FAMILY TEACHING

□ Explain the purpose of the medication to patient.

□ Instruct patient to report signs of edema or excessive virilism to health care professional.

□ Emphasize the importance of periodic lab tests to monitor progress and need for medication.

### EVALUATION

**Effectiveness of therapy can be demonstrated by:** ■ Increased hemoglobin and RBC volume.

---

## naproxen

(na-**prox**-en)

Aleve, Anaprox, Anaprox DS, {Apo-Napro-Na}, Apo-Napro-Na DS, {Apo-Naproxen}, EC-Naprosyn, Naprelan, Napron X, Naprosyn, {Naprosyn-E}, {Naprosyn-SR}, {Naxen}, {Novo-Naprox}, {Novo-Naprox Sodium DS}, {Nu-Naprox}, {Synflex}, {Synflex DS}

### CLASSIFICATION(S):

*Therapeutic: nonopioid analgesics, nonsteroidal anti-inflammatory agents, antipyretics*

**Pregnancy Category B (first trimester)**

---

## INDICATIONS

■ Mild to moderate pain ■ Dysmenorrhea ■ Fever ■ Inflammatory disorders, including: □ Rheumatoid arthritis □ Osteoarthritis.

## ACTION

■ Inhibits prostaglandin synthesis. **Therapeutic Effects:** ■ Decreased pain ■ Reduction of fever ■ Suppression of inflammation.

## PHARMACOKINETICS

**Absorption:** Completely absorbed from the GI tract. Sodium salt (Anaprox) is more rapidly absorbed.

**Distribution:** Crosses the placenta; enters breast milk in low concentrations.

**Protein Binding:** >99%.

**Metabolism and Excretion:** Mostly metabolized by the liver.

**Half-life:** 10–20 hr.

## CONTRAINDICATIONS AND PRECAUTIONS

**Contraindicated in:** ■ Hypersensitivity ■ Cross-sensitivity may occur with other NSAIDs, including aspirin ■ Active GI bleeding ■ Ulcer disease.

**Use Cautiously in:** ■ Severe cardiovascular, renal, or hepatic disease ■ History of ulcer disease ■ Chronic alcohol use/abuse ■ Pregnancy, lactation or children <2 yr (safety not established; avoid using during second half of pregnancy).

## ADVERSE REACTIONS AND SIDE EFFECTS*

■ **CNS:** dizziness, drowsiness, headache ■ **EENT:** tinnitus ■ **Resp:** dyspnea ■ **CV:** edema, palpitations, tachycardia ■ **GI:** DRUG-INDUCED HEPATITIS, GI BLEEDING, constipation, dyspepsia, nausea, anorexia, diarrhea, discomfort, flatulence, vomiting ■ **GU:** cystitis, hematuria, renal failure ■ **Derm:** photosensitivity, rashes, sweating ■ **Hemat:** blood dyscrasias, prolonged bleeding time ■ **Misc:** allergic reactions including ANAPHYLAXIS.

## INTERACTIONS

**Drug-Drug:** ■ Concurrent use with **aspirin** decreases naproxen blood levels and may decrease effectiveness ■ Increased risk of bleeding with **anticoagulants, thrombolytic agents, eptifibatide, tirofiban, cefotetan, cefoperazone, valproic acid, clopidogrel, ticlopidine,** and **plicamycin** ■ Additive adverse GI side effects with **aspirin, corticosteroids,** and other **NSAIDs** ■ **Probenecid** increases blood levels and may increase toxicity ■ Increased risk of photosensitivity with other **photosensitizing agents** ■ May increase the risk of toxicity from **methotrexate, antineoplastics,** or **radiation therapy** ■ May increase serum levels and risk of toxicity from **lithium** ■ Increased risk of adverse renal effects with **cyclosporine** or chronic use of **acetaminophen** ■ May decrease response to **antihypertensives** or **diuretics** ■ May increase risk of hypoglycemia with **insulin** or **oral hypoglycemic agents.**

**Drug-Natural Products:** ■ Increased anticoagulant effect and bleeding risk with **anise, arnica, chamomile, clove, dong quai, fenugreek, feverfew, garlic, ginger, ginkgo, Panax ginseng, licorice,** and others.

## ROUTE AND DOSAGE

275 mg naproxen sodium is equivalent to 250 mg naproxen.

### ❏ Anti-inflammatory/Analgesic/Antidysmenorrheal

■ **PO (Adults):** *Naproxen*—250–500 mg bid (up to 1.5 g/day). *Delayed-release naproxen*—375–500 mg twice daily. *Naproxen sodium*—275–550 mg twice daily (up to 1.65 g/day).

■ **PO (Children >2 yr):** 5 mg/kg/day twice daily as naproxen suspension.

### ❏ Antigout

■ **PO (Adults):** *Naproxen*—750 mg naproxen initially, then 250 mg q 8 hr. *Naproxen sodium*—825 mg initially, then 275 mg q 8 hr.

### ❏ OTC Use (naproxen sodium)

■ **PO (Adults):** 200 mg q 8–12 hr or 400 mg followed by 200 mg q 12 hr (not to exceed 600 mg/24 hr).

■ **PO (Geriatric Patients >65 yr):** Not to exceed 200 mg q 12 hr.

## AVAILABILITY

### ❏ Naproxen

■ *Tablets (Naprosyn, {Apo-Naproxen, Naxen, Novo-Naprox, Nu-Naprox}):* {125 mg$^{Rx}$}, 250 mg$^{Rx}$, 375 mg$^{Rx}$, 500 mg$^{Rx}$ ■ Cost: 250 mg \$83.72/100, 375 mg \$110.76/100, 500 mg \$135.20/100 ■ *Controlled-release tablets (Naprelan):* 375 mg$^{Rx}$, 500 mg$^{Rx}$ ■ *Delayed-release tablets (EC-Naprosyn, Naprosyn-E):* {250 mg$^{Rx}$}, 375 mg$^{Rx}$, 500 mg$^{Rx}$ ■ *Extended-release tablets (Naprosyn-SR):* {750 mg$^{Rx}$} ■ *Oral suspension (Naprosyn):* 25 mg/ml$^{Rx}$ ■ Cost: 25 mg/ml \$38.23/500 ml ■ *Suppositories (Naprosyn, Naxen):* {500 mg$^{Rx}$.}

### ❏ Naproxen Sodium

■ *Tablets (Aleve, Anaprox, Anaprox DS, Apo-Napro-Na, Novo-Naprox Sodium, Novo-Naprox Sodium DS, Synaflex, Synaflex DS):* 220 mg$^{OTC}$, 275 mg$^{Rx}$, 550 mg$^{Rx}$ ■ Cost: 275 mg \$71.51/100, 550 mg \$116.05/100.

## TIME/ACTION PROFILE

| | ONSET | PEAK | DURATION |
|---|---|---|---|
| PO (analgesic) | 1 hr | unknown | 8–12 hr |
| PO (anti-inflammatory) | 14 days | 2–4 wk | unknown |

## NURSING IMPLICATIONS

### ASSESSMENT

■ **General Info:** Patients who have asthma, aspirin-induced allergy, and nasal polyps are at increased risk for developing hypersensitivity reactions. Assess for rhinitis, asthma, and urticaria.

■ **Pain:** Assess pain (note type, location, and intensity) prior to and 1–2 hr following administration.

■ **Arthritis:** Assess pain and range of motion prior to and 1–2 hr following administration.

■ **Fever:** Monitor temperature; note signs associated with fever (diaphoresis, tachycardia, malaise).

■ *Lab Test Considerations:* BUN, serum creatinine, CBC, and liver function tests should be evaluated periodically in patients receiving prolonged courses of therapy.

❏ Serum potassium, BUN, serum creatinine, alkaline phosphatase, LDH, AST, and ALT tests may show increased levels. Blood glucose, hemoglobin, and hematocrit concentrations, leukocyte and platelet counts, and CCr may be decreased.

❏ Bleeding time may be prolonged up to 4 days following discontinuation of therapy.

❏ May alter test results for urine 5-HIAA and urine steroid determinations.

## POTENTIAL NURSING DIAGNOSES

■ Pain, acute (Indications).

■ Mobility, impaired physical (Indications).

## IMPLEMENTATION

■ **General:** Administration in higher than recommended doses does not provide increased effectiveness but may cause increased side effects.

❏ Coadministration with opioid analgesics may have additive analgesic effects and may permit lower opioid doses.

❏ Analgesic is more effective if given before pain becomes severe.

■ **PO:** For rapid initial effect, administer 30 min before or 2 hr after meals. May be administered with food, milk, or antacids to decrease GI irritation. Food slows but does not reduce the extent of absorption. Do not mix suspension with antacid or other liquid prior to administration.

■ **Dysmenorrhea:** Administer as soon as possible after the onset of menses. Prophylactic treatment has not been shown to be effective.

## PATIENT/FAMILY TEACHING

❏ Advise patient to take this medication with a full glass of water and to remain in an upright position for 15–30 min after administration.

❏ Instruct patient to take medication exactly as directed. If a dose is missed, it should be taken as soon as remembered but not if almost time for the next dose. Do not double doses.

❏ May cause drowsiness or dizziness. Advise patient to avoid driving or other activities requiring alertness until response to the medication is known.

❏ Caution patient to avoid the concurrent use of alcohol, aspirin, acetaminophen, or other OTC medications without consulting health care professional. Use of naproxen with 3 or more glasses of alcohol per day may increase risk of GI bleeding.

❏ Advise patient to inform health care professional of medication regimen prior to treatment or surgery.

❏ Caution patient to wear sunscreen and protective clothing to prevent photosensitivity reactions.

❏ Instruct patients not to take OTC naproxen preparations for more than 3 days for fever and to consult health care professional if symptoms persist or worsen.

❏ Advise patient to consult health care professional if rash, itching, visual disturbances, tinnitus, weight gain, edema, black stools, persistent headache, or influenza-like syndrome (chills, fever, muscle aches, pain) occurs.

## EVALUATION

**Effectiveness of therapy can be demonstrated by:** ■ Relief of pain ■ Improved joint mobility. Partial arthritic relief is usually seen within 2 wk, but maximum effectiveness may require 2–4 wk of continuous therapy. Patients who do not respond to one NSAID may respond to another ■ Reduction of fever.

## naratriptan

(nar-a-**trip**-tan)

Amerge

### CLASSIFICATION(S):

**Therapeutic:** vascular headache suppressants

**Pharmacologic:** 5 HT₁ agonists

### Pregnancy Category C

## INDICATIONS

■ Acute treatment of migraine headache.

## ACTION

■ Acts as an agonist at specific 5-HT₁ receptor sites in intracranial blood vessels and sensory trigeminal nerves. **Therapeutic Effects:** ■ Cranial vessel vasoconstriction with resultant decrease in migraine headache.

## PHARMACOKINETICS

**Absorption:** Well absorbed (70%) following oral administration.

**Distribution:** Unknown.

**Metabolism and Excretion:** 60% excreted unchanged in urine; 30% metabolized by the liver.
**Half-life:** 6 hr (increased in renal impairment).

## CONTRAINDICATIONS AND PRECAUTIONS

**Contraindicated in:** ■ Hypersensitivity ■ Geriatric patients ■ Ischemic cardiovascular, cerebrovascular, or peripheral vascular syndromes ■ History of significant cardiovascular disease ■ Uncontrolled hypertension ■ Severe renal impairment (CCr <15 ml/min) ■ Severe hepatic impairment ■ Should not be used within 24 hr of other 5-HT$_1$ agonists or ergot-type compounds (dihydroergotamine).

**Use Cautiously in:** ■ Mild to moderate renal or hepatic impairment (dose should not exceed 2.5 mg/24 hr; initial dose should be decreased) ■ Pregnancy, lactation, or children (safety not established).

**Exercise Extreme Caution in:** ■ Cardiovascular risk factors (hypertension, hypercholesterolemia, cigarette smoking, obesity, diabetes, strong family history, menopausal women or men >40 yr); use only if cardiovascular status has been evaluated and determined to be safe and 1st dose is administered under supervision.

## ADVERSE REACTIONS AND SIDE EFFECTS*

■ **CNS:** dizziness, drowsiness, malaise/fatigue ■ **CV:** CORONARY ARTERY VASOSPASM, MI, VENTRICULAR FIBRILLATION, VENTRICULAR TACHYCARDIA, myocardial ischemia ■ **GI:** nausea ■ **Neuro:** paresthesia ■ **Misc:** pain/pressure sensation in throat/neck.

## INTERACTIONS

**Drug-Drug:** ■ Concurrent use with **SSRI antidepressants** may result in weakness, hyper-reflexia, and incoordination ■ **Cigarette smoking** increases the metabolism of naratriptan ■ Blood levels and effects are increased by **hormonal contraceptives** ■ Avoid concurrent use (within 24 hr of each other) with **ergot-containing drugs (dihydroergotamine)** may result in prolonged vasospastic reactions ■ Avoid concurrent (within 2 wk) use with **MAO inhibitors**; produces increased systemic exposure and risk of adverse reactions to naratriptan ■ Serotonin syndrome may occur with **sibutramine**.
**Drug-Natural Products:** ■ Increased risk of serotinergic side effects including serotonin syndrome with **St. John's wort** and **SAMe.**

## ROUTE AND DOSAGE

■ **PO (Adults):** 1 or 2.5 mg; dose may be repeated in 4 hr if response is inadequate (not to exceed 5 mg/24 hr or treatment of more than 4 headaches/mo).

## AVAILABILITY

■ *Tablets:* 1 mg$^{Rx}$, 2.5 mg$^{Rx}$ ■ Cost: 1 mg $150.70/9, 2.5 mg $150.70/9.

TIME/ACTION PROFILE (decreased migraine pain)

| | ONSET | PEAK | DURATION |
|---|---|---|---|
| PO | 30–60 min | 2–3 hr† | up to 24 hr |

†3–4 hr during migraine attack.

# NURSING IMPLICATIONS

## ASSESSMENT

❑ Assess pain location, character, intensity, and duration and associated symptoms (photophobia, phonophobia, nausea, vomiting) during migraine attack.

## POTENTIAL NURSING DIAGNOSES

■ Pain, acute (Indications).

## IMPLEMENTATION

■ **PO:** Tablets may be administered at any time after the headache starts.

## PATIENT/FAMILY TEACHING

❑ Inform patient that naratriptan should be used only during a migraine attack. It is meant to be used for relief of migraine attacks but not to prevent or reduce the number of attacks.

❑ Instruct patient to administer naratriptan as soon as symptoms of a migraine attack appear, but it may be administered any time during an attack. If migraine symptoms return, a 2nd dose may be used. Allow at least 4 hr between doses, and do not use more than 2 tablets in any 24-hr period. Do not use to treat more than 4 headaches per month.

❏ Advise patient that lying down in a darkened room following naratriptan administration may further help relieve headache.

❏ Caution patient not to use naratriptan if she is pregnant, suspects she is pregnant, or plans to become pregnant. Adequate contraception should be used during therapy.

❏ Advise patient to notify health care professional prior to next dose of naratriptan if pain or tightness in the chest occurs during use. If pain is severe or does not subside, notify health care professional immediately. If wheezing; heart throbbing; swelling of eyelids, face, or lips; skin rash; skin lumps; or hives occur, notify health care professional immediately and do not take more naratriptan without approval of health care professional. If feelings of tingling, heat, flushing, heaviness, pressure, drowsiness, dizziness, tiredness, or sickness develop, discuss with health care professional at next visit.

❏ Instruct patient not to take additional naratriptan if no response is seen with initial dose without consulting health care professional. There is no evidence that 5 mg provides greater relief than 2.5-mg dose. Additional naratriptan doses are not likely to be effective, and alternative medications, as previously discussed with health care professional, may be used.

❏ Naratriptan may cause dizziness or drowsiness. Caution patient to avoid driving or other activities requiring alertness until response to medication is known.

❏ Advise patient to avoid alcohol, which aggravates headaches, during naratriptan use.

## EVALUATION

**Effectiveness of therapy can be demonstrated by:** ■ Relief of migraine attack.

## nateglinide
(na-**teg**-li-nide)
Starlix

**CLASSIFICATION(S):**
**Therapeutic:** antidiabetics
**Pharmacologic:** meglitinides

**Pregnancy Category C**

## INDICATIONS

■ As monotherapy and as an adjunct to diet and exercise to improve glycemic control in patients with type 2 diabetes. In addition, may be used concomitantly with metformin to improve glycemic control.

## ACTION

■ Stimulates the release of insulin from pancreatic beta cells by closing potassium channels, which results in the opening of calcium channels in beta cells. This is followed by release of insulin. Requires functioning pancreatic beta cells. **Therapeutic Effects:** ■ Lowering of blood glucose.

## PHARMACOKINETICS

**Absorption:** Well absorbed (73%) following oral administration; absorption is rapid.

**Distribution:** Unknown.

**Protein Binding:** 98%.

**Metabolism and Excretion:** Mostly metabolized by the liver (cytochrome P2 C9 and P3 A4 [CYP2 C9 and CYP3 A4] enzyme systems); 16% excreted unchanged in urine.

**Half-life:** 1.5 hr.

## CONTRAINDICATIONS AND PRECAUTIONS

**Contraindicated in:** ■ Hypersensitivity ■ Pregnancy or lactation (insulin recommended to control diabetes during pregnancy) ■ Diabetic ketoacidosis ■ Type 1 diabetes.

**Use Cautiously in:** ■ Geriatric patients, malnourished patients, patients with pituitary or adrenal insufficiency (increased susceptibility to hypoglycemia) ■ Strenuous physical exercise, insufficient caloric intake (increased risk of hypoglycemia) ■ Autonomic neuropathy (hypoglycemia may be masked) ■ Moderate to severe liver impairment ■ Fever, infection, trauma, or surgery (may lead to transient loss of glycemic control; insulin may be required) ■ Children (safety not established).

## ADVERSE REACTIONS AND SIDE EFFECTS*

■ **CNS:** dizziness ■ **Resp:** bronchitis, coughing, upper respiratory infection ■ **GI:** diarrhea ■ **Endo:** HYPOGLYCEMIA ■ **MS:** arthropathy, back pain ■ **Misc:** flu symptoms.

## INTERACTIONS

**Drug-Drug:** ■ Concurrent use with **beta blockers** may mask hypoglycemia ■ **Alcohol**, combination with other **antidiabetics, NSAIDs, MAO inhibitors, nonselective beta blockers** may increase the risk of hypoglycemia ■ Hypoglycemic effects may be decreased by **thiazide diuretics, corticosteroids, thyroid supplements,** or **sympathomimetic (adrenergic) agents**.

**Drug-Food:** ■ Blood levels and effects are significantly decreased when administered prior to a **liquid meal**.

## ROUTE AND DOSAGE

■ **PO (Adults):** 120 mg three times daily before meals; patients who are approaching glycemic control may be started at 60 mg three times daily.

## AVAILABILITY

■ *Tablets:* 60 mg^Rx, 120 mg^Rx.

TIME/ACTION PROFILE (effect on blood glucose)

| | ONSET | PEAK | DURATION |
|---|---|---|---|
| PO | within 20 min | 1 hr | 4 hr |

# NURSING IMPLICATIONS

## ASSESSMENT

❑ Observe patient for signs and symptoms of hypoglycemic reactions (sweating, hunger, weakness, dizziness, tremor, tachycardia, anxiety).

■ *Lab Test Considerations:* Monitor serum glucose and HbA$_{1c}$ periodically throughout therapy to evaluate effectiveness of treatment.

❑ May cause increased uric acid levels.

■ *Toxicity and Overdose:* Overdose is manifested by symptoms of hypoglycemia. Mild hypoglycemia may be treated with administration of oral glucose. Severe hypoglycemia should be treated with IV D50W followed by continuous IV infusion of more dilute dextrose solution at a rate sufficient to keep serum glucose at approximately 100 mg/dl.

## POTENTIAL NURSING DIAGNOSES

■ Nutrition, imbalanced: more than body requirements (Indications).

■ Noncompliance (Patient/Family Teaching).

## IMPLEMENTATION

■ **General:** Patients stabilized on a diabetic regimen who are exposed to stress, fever, trauma, infection, or surgery may require administration of insulin.

■ **PO:** Administer 1–30 min prior to meals.

❑ May be administered concurrently with metformin.

## PATIENT/FAMILY TEACHING

❑ Instruct patient to take medication at same time each day. If a dose is missed, take as soon as remembered unless almost time for next dose. Do not take if unable to eat.

❑ Explain to patient that this medication controls hyperglycemia but does not cure diabetes. Therapy is long term.

❑ Review signs of hypoglycemia and hyperglycemia with patient. If hypoglycemia occurs, advise patient to take a glass of orange juice or 2–3 tsp of sugar, honey, or corn syrup dissolved in water and notify health care professional.

❑ Encourage patient to follow prescribed diet, medication, and exercise regimen to prevent hypoglycemic or hyperglycemic episodes.

❑ Instruct patient in proper testing of serum glucose and ketones. These tests should be closely monitored during periods of stress or illness and health care professional notified if significant changes occur.

❑ May occasionally cause dizziness. Caution patient to avoid driving or other activities requiring alertness until response to medication is known.

❑ Caution patient to avoid other medications, especially aspirin and alcohol, while on this therapy without consulting health care professional.

❑ Insulin is the recommended method of controlling blood glucose during pregnancy. Counsel female patients to use a form of contraception other than oral contraceptives and to notify health care professional promptly if pregnancy is planned or suspected.

❏ Advise patient to inform health care professional of medication regimen prior to treatment or surgery.

❏ Advise patient to carry a form of sugar (sugar packets, candy) and identification describing disease process and medication regimen at all times.

❏ Emphasize the importance of routine follow-up exams.

## EVALUATION

**Effectiveness of therapy can be demonstrated by:** ■ Control of blood glucose levels without the appearance of hypoglycemic or hyperglycemic episodes.

# nedocromil, See MAST CELL STABILIZERS.

# nefazodone
(neff-**a**-zoe-done)
Serzone

*CLASSIFICATION(S):*
*Therapeutic:* antidepressants

**Pregnancy Category C**

## INDICATIONS

■ Major depression (in conjunction with psychotherapy).

## ACTION

■ Inhibits the reuptake of serotonin and norepinephrine by neurons ■ Antagonizes alpha$_1$-adrenergic receptors. **Therapeutic Effects:** ■ Antidepressant action, which may develop only over several weeks.

## PHARMACOKINETICS

**Absorption:** Well absorbed but undergoes extensive and variable first-pass hepatic metabolism (bioavailability about 20%).
**Distribution:** Widely distributed; enters the CNS.
**Protein Binding:** ≥99%.
**Metabolism and Excretion:** Extensively metabolized. One metabolite (hydroxynefazodone) has antidepressant activity.

**Half-life:** *Nefazodone*—2–4 hr; *hydroxynefazodone*—1.5–4 hr.

## CONTRAINDICATIONS AND PRECAUTIONS

**Contraindicated in:** ■ Hypersensitivity ■ Concurrent MAO inhibitor therapy ■ Active liver disease or baseline elevated serum transaminases.

**Use Cautiously in:** ■ Geriatric patients (initiate therapy at lower doses) ■ History of suicide attempt or drug abuse ■ Underlying cardiovascular or cerebrovascular disease ■ History of mania ■ Pregnancy, lactation, or children <18 yr (safety not established).

## ADVERSE REACTIONS AND SIDE EFFECTS*

■ **CNS:** <u>dizziness</u>, <u>insomnia</u>, <u>somnolence</u>, agitation, confusion, weakness ■ **EENT:** abnormal vision, blurred vision, eye pain, tinnitus ■ **Resp:** dyspnea ■ **CV:** bradycardia, hypotension ■ **GI:** HEPATIC FAILURE, HEPATOTOXICITY, <u>constipation</u>, <u>dry mouth</u>, <u>nausea</u>, gastroenteritis ■ **GU:** impotence ■ **Derm:** rashes ■ **Hemat:** decreased hematocrit.

## INTERACTIONS

**Drug-Drug:** ■ Serious, potentially fatal reactions may occur during concurrent use with **MAO inhibitors** (do not use concurrently or within 2 wk of MAO inhibitors; discontinue nefazodone at least 7 days before starting MAO inhibitor therapy) ■ ↑ CNS depression with other CNS depressants including **alcohol, antihistamines, opioid analgesics,** and **sedative/hypnotics** ■ May ↑ blood levels and effects of **alprazolam** or **triazolam** ■ May increase serum **digoxin** levels ■ Additive hypotension may occur with **antihypertensives, nitrates,** or acute ingestion of **alcohol** ■ May ↑ risk of myopathy with **HMG-CoA reductase inhibitors.**

**Drug-Natural Products:** ■ ↑ risk of serotinergic side effects including serotonin syndrome with **St. John's wort** and **SAMe** ■ **Kava, valerian,** or **chamomile** can ↑ CNS depression.

## ROUTE AND DOSAGE

■ **PO (Adults):** 100 mg twice daily initially; may be increased weekly up to 600 mg/day in 2 divided doses.

- **PO (Geriatric Patients):** 50 mg twice daily initially; may be increased weekly as tolerated.

## AVAILABILITY

- *Tablets:* 50 mg$^{Rx}$, 100 mg$^{Rx}$, 150 mg$^{Rx}$, 200 mg$^{Rx}$, 250 mg$^{Rx}$ ■ Cost: 50 mg $85.61/60, 100 mg $87.67/60, 150 mg $89.32/60, 200 mg $91.00/60, 250 mg $92.69/60.

TIME/ACTION PROFILE (antidepressant action)

| | ONSET | PEAK | DURATION |
|---|---|---|---|
| PO | days–wks | several wk | unknown |

## NURSING IMPLICATIONS

### ASSESSMENT

- ❏ Assess mental status and mood changes. Inform physician or other health care professional if patient demonstrates significant increase in anxiety, nervousness, or insomnia.
- ❏ Assess suicidal tendencies, especially in early therapy. Restrict amount of drug available to patient.
- ❏ Monitor blood pressure and pulse before and periodically during therapy.
- ❏ Monitor liver function tests prior to and routinely during therapy. Obtain LFTs at first sign of hepatic dysfunction (nausea, vomiting, abdominal pain, fatigue, anorexia, dark urine).
- ■ *Lab Test Considerations:* May cause decrease in hematocrit and leukopenia.
- ❏ Monitor liver function periodically. If serum AST or ALT levels are >3 times the upper limit of normal discontinue nefazodone.
- ❏ May also cause hypercholesterolemia and hypoglycemia.

### POTENTIAL NURSING DIAGNOSES

- ■ Coping, ineffective (Indications).
- ■ Injury, risk for (Side Effects).

### IMPLEMENTATION

- ■ **General:** Do not confuse Serozone (nefazodone) with Seroquel (quetiapine).
- ■ **PO:** Administer doses twice daily.

### PATIENT/FAMILY TEACHING

- ❏ Instruct patient to take medication as directed. Several weeks may be required to obtain a full antidepressant response. Once response is obtained, therapy should be continued for at least 6 mo. If a dose is missed, take as soon as possible unless almost time for next dose. Do not double doses.
- ❏ May cause drowsiness or dizziness. Caution patient to avoid driving or other activities requiring alertness until response to the drug is known.
- ❏ Advise patient to make position changes slowly to minimize orthostatic hypotension.
- ❏ Caution patient to avoid taking alcohol or other CNS depressant drugs during therapy and not to take other prescription, OTC medications, or herbal products without consulting health care professional.
- ❏ Advise patient to notify health care professional immediately if signs of liver dysfunction (jaundice, anorexia, GI complaints, malaise) occur.
- ❏ Inform patient that frequent mouth rinses, good oral hygiene, and sugarless gum or candy may minimize dry mouth. If dry mouth persists for more than 2 wk, consult health care professional regarding use of saliva substitute.
- ❏ Instruct female patient to inform health care professional if pregnancy is planned or suspected or if breastfeeding.
- ❏ Instruct patient to notify health care professional of signs of allergy (rash, hives) or if agitation, blurred or other changes in vision, confusion, dizziness, unsteadiness, difficult or frequent urination, difficulty concentrating, or memory problems occur.
- ❏ Emphasize the importance of follow-up examinations to monitor progress. Encourage patient participation in psychotherapy.

### EVALUATION

**Effectiveness of therapy can be demonstrated by:** ■ Increased sense of well-being ❏ Renewed interest in surroundings. May require several weeks of therapy to obtain full response. Need for therapy should be periodically reassessed. Therapy is usually continued for 6 mo or more.

# nelfinavir

(nell-**finn**-a-veer)
Viracept

**CLASSIFICATION(S):**
**Therapeutic:** antiretrovirals
**Pharmacologic:** protease inhibitors

**Pregnancy Category B**

## INDICATIONS

■ HIV infection (with other antiretrovirals).

## ACTION

■ Inhibits HIV protease and prevents cleavage of viral polyproteins. **Therapeutic Effects:** ■ Increased CD4 cell count and decreased viral load ■ Slowed progression of HIV infection with less sequelae.

## PHARMACOKINETICS

**Absorption:** Well absorbed after oral administration.
**Distribution:** Unknown.
**Protein Binding:** >98%.
**Metabolism and Excretion:** Mostly metabolized (CYP 3A4 enzyme system) and excreted in feces as metabolites (78%) or unchanged drug (22%); minimal renal excretion.
**Half-life:** 3.5–5 hr.

## CONTRAINDICATIONS AND PRECAUTIONS

**Contraindicated in:** ■ Hypersensitivity ■ Concurrent amiodarone, ergot derivatives, midazolam, quinidine, rifampin, pimozide, simvastatin, lovastatin, rifampin, St. John's wort, or triazolam ■ Lactation (breastfeeding should be avoided by HIV-infected patients).
**Use Cautiously in:** ■ Hemophiliacs ( ↑ risk of bleeding) ■ Diabetes mellitus (may exacerbate condition) ■ Hepatic impairment.

## ADVERSE REACTIONS AND SIDE EFFECTS*

■ **CNS:** SEIZURES, anxiety, depression, dizziness, drowsiness, emotional lability, headache, hyperkinesia, insomnia, malaise, migraine headache, sleep disorders, suicidal ideation, weakness ■ **EENT:** acute iritis, pharyngitis, rhinitis, sinusitis ■ **Resp:** dyspnea ■ **GI:** diarrhea, anorexia, dyspepsia, elevated liver function studies, epigastric pain, flatulence, GI bleeding, hepatitis, nausea, oral ulcerations, pancreatitis, vomiting ■ **GU:** nephrolithiasis, sexual dysfunction ■ **Derm:** pruritus, rash, sweating, urticaria ■ **Endo:** hyperglycemia ■ **F and E:** dehydration ■ **Hemat:** anemia, leukopenia, thrombocytopenia ■ **Metab:** hyperlipidemia, hyperuricemia ■ **MS:** arthralgia, arthritis, back pain , myalgia, myopathy ■ **Neuro:** myasthenia, paresthesia ■ **Misc:** allergic reactions, fever, redistribution of body fat.

## INTERACTIONS

**Drug-Drug:** ■ Concurrent **amiodarone, dihydroergotamine, ergotamine, methylergonovine, ergonovine, midazolam, simvastatin, lovastatin, pimozide, quinidine,** or **triazolam** should be avoided; nelfinavir inhibits the action of the CYP3A4 enzyme system and concurrent use may result in excess sedation, vasoconstriction, rhabdomyolysis, or serious cardiac arrhythmias ■ Since nelfinavir is also metabolized by the CYP3A4 enzyme system, potent inducers of the enzyme such as **rifampin** may ↓ blood levels of nelfinavir and promote resistance to its effects; concurrent use should be avoided. ■ ↓ metabolism and may ↑ effects of **rifabutin** (dosage of rifabutin should be ↓ by 50%), **carbamazepine, phenobarbital,** or **phenytoin** (concurrent use with rifampin should be avoided) ■ Plasma levels and effectiveness may be ↑ by **ketoconazole, indinavir, delavirdine,** or **ritonavir** ■ May ↓ levels of **methadone**; dosage of methadone may need to be ↑ ■ ↑ plasma levels of **indinavir, saquinavir, cyclosporine tacrolimus, sirolimus,** and **azithromycin** ■ ↑ levels and effects of **sildenafil** (sildenafil dose should not exceed 25 mg in 48 hr) ■ ↑ levels and risk of toxicity from **atorvastatin** (use lowest dose of atorvastatin or consider fluvastatin) ■ Blood levels may be ↓ by **nevirapine** ■ Should not be given at the same time as **didanosine** ■ May ↓ plasma levels and effectiveness of **hormonal contraceptives** or **delavirdine.**

**Drug-Natural Products:** ■ **St. John's wort** induces metabolism of nelfinavir, decreasing blood levels and may promote resistance to its effects.

**Drug-Food:** ■ **Food** ↑ absorption.

## ROUTE AND DOSAGE

- **PO (Adults and Children >13 yr):** 750 mg 3 times daily *or* 1250 mg twice daily.
- **PO (Children 2–13 yr):** 20–30 mg/kg 3 times daily (not to exceed 750 mg 3 times daily).

### AVAILABILITY

- *Tablets:* 250 mg$^{Rx}$, 625 mg$^{Rx}$ ■ Cost: $628.61/270 ■ *Oral powder:* 50 mg nelfinavir/1 g powder (1 g powder/level scoopful).

TIME/ACTION PROFILE (plasma levels)

| | ONSET | PEAK | DURATION |
|---|---|---|---|
| PO | rapid | 2–4 hr | 8 hr |

# NURSING IMPLICATIONS

## ASSESSMENT

- ❏ Assess patient for change in severity of HIV symptoms and opportunistic infections throughout therapy.
- ■ *Lab Test Considerations:* Monitor viral load and CD4 cell counts regularly during therapy. May cause hyperglycemia. May cause up arrow serum AST, ALT, total bilirubin, alkaline phosphatase, LDH, and CPK concentrations. May cause anemia, leukopenia, thrombocytopenia, hyperlipidemia, and hyperuricemia.

## POTENTIAL NURSING DIAGNOSES

- ■ Infection, risk for (Indications).
- ■ Noncompliance (Patient/Family Teaching).

## IMPLEMENTATION

- ■ **General:** Do not confuse nelfinavir (Viracept) with nevirapine (Viramune).
- ■ **PO:** Administer with a meal.
- ❏ Oral powder may be mixed with a small amount of water, milk, formula, soy formula, soy milk, or dietary supplements. Do not mix with acid, food, or juice (orange juice, apple juice, applesauce); results in a bitter taste. Do not reconstitute powder with water in its original container. Once mixed, the entire contents must be consumed to obtain the full dose. Mixture is stable for up to 6 hr if refrigerated.

## PATIENT/FAMILY TEACHING

- ❏ Emphasize the importance of taking nelfinavir exactly as directed at evenly spaced times throughout the day. Do not take more than prescribed amount and do not stop taking without consulting health care professional. Take missed doses as soon as remembered; do not double doses.
- ❏ Instruct patient that nelfinivir should not be shared with others.
- ❏ Advise patient to avoid taking other Rx, OTC, or herbal products, without consulting health care professional.
- ❏ Inform patient that nelfinavir does not cure AIDS or prevent associated or opportunistic infections. Nelfinavir does not reduce the risk of transmission of HIV to others through sexual contact or blood contamination. Caution patient to avoid sexual contact or to use a condom and to avoid sharing needles or donating blood to prevent spreading the AIDS virus to others. Advise patient that the long-term effects of nelfinavir are unknown at this time.
- ❏ Inform patient that nelfinavir may cause hyperglycemia. Advise patient to notify health care professional if increased thirst or hunger; unexplained weight loss; increased urination; fatigue; or dry, itchy skin occurs.
- ❏ Advise patient that if diarrhea occurs, it can usually be controlled with OTC antidiarrheals, such as loperamide, which slow GI motility.
- ❏ Advise patient taking oral contraceptives to use a nonhormonal method of birth control during nelfinavir therapy.
- ❏ Emphasize the importance of regular follow-up and blood counts to determine progress and monitor for side effects.

### EVALUATION

**Effectiveness of therapy can be demonstrated by:** ■ Delayed progression of AIDS and decreased opportunistic infections in patients with HIV ■ Improvement in CD4 cell count and decrease in viral load.

## neomycin, See AMINOGLYCOSIDES.

---

## neostigmine

(nee-oh-**stig**-meen)

Prostigmin

**CLASSIFICATION(S):**
**Therapeutic:** antimyasthenics
**Pharmacologic:** cholinergics

**Pregnancy Category C**

### INDICATIONS

■ Improvement in muscle strength in symptomatic treatment of myasthenia gravis ■ Prevention and treatment of postoperative bladder distention and urinary retention or ileus ■ Reversal of nondepolarizing neuromuscular blockers.

### ACTION

■ Inhibits the breakdown of acetylcholine so that it accumulates and has a prolonged effect ■ Effects include miosis, increased intestinal and skeletal muscle tone, bronchial and ureteral constriction, bradycardia, increased salivation, lacrimation, and sweating. **Therapeutic Effects:** ■ Improved muscular function in patients with myasthenia gravis, improved bladder-emptying in patients with urinary retention, or reversal of nondepolarizing neuromuscular blockers.

### PHARMACOKINETICS

**Absorption:** Poorly absorbed following oral administration, necessitating large oral doses compared with parenteral doses.

**Distribution:** Probably does not cross the placenta or enter breast milk.

**Metabolism and Excretion:** Metabolized by plasma cholinesterases and the liver.

**Half-life:** PO, IV—40–60 min; IM—50–90 min.

### CONTRAINDICATIONS AND PRECAUTIONS

**Contraindicated in:** ■ Hypersensitivity ■ Mechanical obstruction of the GI or GU tract.

**Use Cautiously in:** ■ History of asthma ■ Ulcer disease ■ Cardiovascular disease ■ Epilepsy ■ Hyperthyroidism ■ Pregnancy (may cause uterine irritability after IV administration near term; newborns may display muscle weakness) ■ Lactation.

### ADVERSE REACTIONS AND SIDE EFFECTS*

■ **CNS:** SEIZURES, dizziness, weakness ■ **EENT:** lacrimation, miosis ■ **Resp:** bronchospasm, excess secretions ■ **CV:** bradycardia, hypotension ■ **GI:** abdominal cramps, diarrhea, excess salivation, nausea, vomiting ■ **Derm:** sweating, rashes.

### INTERACTIONS

**Drug-Drug:** ■ Action may be antagonized by **drugs possessing anticholinergic properties,** including **antihistamines, antidepressants, atropine, haloperidol, phenothiazines, quinidine,** and **disopyramide** ■ Prolongs action of **depolarizing muscle-relaxing agents (succinylcholine, decamethonium).**

### ROUTE AND DOSAGE

❏ **Myasthenia Gravis**

■ **PO (Adults):** 15 mg q 3–4 hr initially; increase at daily intervals until optimal response is achieved. Usual maintenance dose is 150 mg/day (up to 375 mg/day may be needed).

■ **PO (Children):** 2 mg/kg/day (60 mg/m$^2$) in 6–8 divided doses.

■ **Subcut, IM (Adults):** 0.5 mg.

■ **Subcut, IM (Children):** 10–40 mcg/kg q 2–3 hr; may give with 10 mcg/kg atropine.

❏ **Bladder Atony, Abdominal Distention: Prevention**

■ **IM, Subcut (Adults):** 250 mcg q 4–6 hr for 2–3 days.

❏ **Bladder Atony, Abdominal Distention: Treatment**

■ **IM, Subcut (Adults):** 500 mcg as needed; may repeat q 3 hr for 5 doses after bladder has been emptied for bladder atony.

❏ **Antidote for Nondepolarizing Neuro-muscular Blockers**

■ **IV (Adults):** 0.5–2 mg slowly; pretreat with 0.6–1.2 mg atropine IV (may be repeated to a total dose of 5 mg).

■ **IV (Children):** 40 mcg/kg with 20 mcg/kg atropine.

### AVAILABILITY (generic available)

■ **Tablets:** 15 mg$^{Rx}$ ■ **Injection:** 1:1000 in 10-ml vials$^{Rx}$, 1:2000 in 1-ml ampules and 10-ml vials$^{Rx}$, 1:4000 in 1-ml ampules$^{Rx}$ ■ **In** *combination with:* atropine (Neostigmine Methylsulfate Min-I-Mix)$^{Rx}$.

TIME/ACTION PROFILE (cholinergic effects, increased muscle tone)

|     | ONSET | PEAK | DURATION |
|-----|-------|------|----------|
| PO  | 45–75 min | unknown | 2–4 hr |
| IM  | 10–30 min | 20–30 min | 2–4 hr |
| IV  | 10–30 min | 20–30 min | 2–4 hr |

## NURSING IMPLICATIONS

### ASSESSMENT

- **General Info:** Assess pulse, respiratory rate, and blood pressure prior to administration. Report significant changes in heart rate.
- **Myasthenia Gravis:** Assess neuromuscular status, including vital capacity, ptosis, diplopia, chewing, swallowing, hand grasp, and gait, prior to administering and at peak effect. Patients with myasthenia gravis may be advised to keep a daily record of their condition and the effects of this medication.
- ❑ Assess patient for overdosage and underdosage or resistance. Both have similar symptoms (muscle weakness, dyspnea, dysphagia), but symptoms of overdosage usually occur within 1 hr of administration, whereas underdosage symptoms occur 3 or more hr after administration. Overdosage (cholinergic crisis) symptoms may also include increased respiratory secretions and saliva, bradycardia, nausea, vomiting, cramping, diarrhea, and diaphoresis. A Tensilon test (edrophonium chloride) may be used to distinguish between overdosage and underdosage.
- **Postoperative Ileus:** Monitor abdominal status (assess for distention, auscultate bowel sounds). A rectal tube may be inserted to facilitate expulsion of flatus.
- **Postoperative Urinary Retention:** Assess for bladder distention. Monitor intake and output. If patient is unable to void within 1 hr of neostigmine administration, consider catheterization.
- **Antidote to Nondepolarizing Neuromuscular Blocking Agents:** Monitor reversal of effects of neuromuscular blocking agents with a peripheral nerve stimulator. Recovery usually occurs consecutively in the following muscles: diaphragm, intercostal muscles, muscles of the glottis, abdominal muscles, limb muscles, muscles of mastication, and levator muscles of the eyelids. Closely observe the patient for residual muscle weakness and respiratory distress throughout the recovery period. Maintain airway patency and ventilation until recovery of normal respiration occurs.

- *Toxicity and Overdose:* If overdose occurs, atropine is the antidote.

### POTENTIAL NURSING DIAGNOSES

- Mobility, impaired physical (Indications).
- Breathing pattern, ineffective (Indications).

### IMPLEMENTATION

- **General:** Oral and parenteral doses are not interchangeable.
- ❑ When used as an antidote to nondepolarizing neuromuscular blocking agents, atropine may be used prior to or concurrently with neostigmine to prevent or treat bradycardia.
- **PO:** Administer with food or milk to minimize side effects. For patients who have difficulty chewing, neostigmine may be taken 30 min before meals.
- **Direct IV:** Administer doses undiluted. May be given through Y-site of an IV of D5W, 0.9% NaCl, Ringer's solution, or LR.
- *Rate:* Administer each 0.5 mg over 1 min.
- **Syringe Compatibility:** ◆ glycopyrrolate ◆ heparin ◆ pentobarbital ◆ thiopental.
- **Y-Site Compatibility:** ◆ heparin ◆ hydrocortisone sodium succinate ◆ potassium chloride ◆ vitamin B complex with C.

### PATIENT/FAMILY TEACHING

- ❑ Instruct patient to take medication exactly as directed. Do not skip or double up on missed doses. Patients with a history of dysphagia should have a nonelectric or battery-operated backup alarm clock to remind them of exact dosage time. Patients with dysphagia may not be able to swallow the medication if the dose is not taken exactly on time. Taking the dose late may result in myasthenic crisis. Taking the dose early may result in cholinergic crisis. Patients with myasthenia gravis must continue this regimen as lifelong therapy.

{ } = Available in Canada only.
*CAPITALS indicates life-threatening; underlines indicate most frequent.

❑ Instruct patient with myasthenia gravis to space activities to avoid fatigue.

❑ Advise patient to carry identification describing disease and medication regimen at all times.

## EVALUATION

**Effectiveness of therapy can be demonstrated by:** ■ Relief of ptosis and diplopia ❑ Improved chewing, swallowing, extremity strength, and breathing without the appearance of cholinergic symptoms in myasthenia gravis ■ Relief or prevention of postoperative gastrointestinal ileus ■ Relief of nonobstructive postoperative urinary retention ■ Reversal of nondepolarizing neuromuscular blocking agents in general anesthesia.

---

**High Alert**

# nesiritide

(ne-**sir**-i-tide)
Natrecor

### CLASSIFICATION(S):
**Therapeutic:** none assigned
**Pharmacologic:** vasodilators (human B-type natriuretic peptide)

### Pregnancy Category C

---

## INDICATIONS

■ Treatment of acutely decompensated CHF in patients who have dyspnea at rest or with minimal activity; has been used with digoxin, diuretics, and ACE inhibitors.

## ACTION

■ Binds to guanyl cyclase receptors in vascular smooth muscle and endothelial cells, producing increased intracellular guanosine $3'5'$-cyclic monophosphate (cGMP) and smooth muscle cell relaxation. cGMP acts as a "second messenger" to dilate veins and arteries. **Therapeutic Effects:** ■ Dose-dependent reduction in pulmonary capillary wedge pressure (PCWP) and systemic arterial pressure in patients with heart failure and resultant decrease in dyspnea.

## PHARMACOKINETICS

**Absorption:** IV administration results in complete bioavailability.
**Distribution:** Unknown.

**Metabolism and Excretion:** Cleared from circulation by binding to cell surface clearance receptors resulting in cellular internalization and proteolysis, proteolytic breakdown by endopeptidases, and renal filtration.
**Half-life:** 18 min.

## CONTRAINDICATIONS AND PRECAUTIONS

**Contraindicated in:** ■ Hypersensitivity ■ Cardiogenic shock ■ systolic blood pressure <90 mm Hg ■ Low cardiac filling pressure, significant valvular stenosis, restrictive/subtractive cardiomyopathy, constrictive pericarditis/cardiac tamponade, or other conditions in which cardiac output is dependent on venous return.

**Use Cautiously in:** ■ Heart failure where renal function is dependent on activity of the renin/angiotensin/aldosterone system (may cause azotemia) ■ BP <100 mm Hg (increased risk of hypotension) ■ Geriatric patients (some may be more sensitive to effects) ■ Pregnancy, lactation, or children (safety not established).

## ADVERSE REACTIONS AND SIDE EFFECTS*

■ **CNS:** anxiety, confusion, dizziness, headache, insomnia, drowsiness ■ **EENT:** amblyopia ■ **Resp:** APNEA, cough, hemoptysis ■ **CV:** hypotension, arrhythmias, bradycardia ■ **GI:** abdominal pain, nausea, vomiting ■ **GU:** increased creatinine ■ **Derm:** itching, rash, sweating ■ **Hemat:** anemia ■ **Local:** injection site reactions ■ **MS:** back pain, leg cramps ■ **Neuro:** paresthesia, tremor ■ **Misc:** fever.

## INTERACTIONS

**Drug-Drug:** ■ None reported.

## ROUTE AND DOSAGE

■ **IV (Adults):** 2 mcg/kg bolus followed by 0.01 mcg/kg/min as a continuous infusion.

## AVAILABILITY

■ *Lyophilized powder for injection (requires reconstitution:* 1.5 mg/vial[Rx].

TIME/ACTION PROFILE (effects on cardiovascular parameters)

| | ONSET | PEAK | DURATION |
|---|---|---|---|
| IV | 15 min | 1 hr | 60 min† |

†longer with higher than recommended doses.

# NURSING IMPLICATIONS

## ASSESSMENT

❏ Monitor blood pressure, pulse, ECG, respiratory rate, cardiac index, PCWP, and central venous pressure frequently during administration. May cause hypotension, especially in patients with a BP <100 mm Hg. Reduce dose or discontinue nesiritide if patient develops hypotension. Use IV fluids and changes in body position to support blood pressure if symptomatic hypotension occurs. Nesiritide may be restarted at a dose reduced by 30% with no bolus administration once patient is stabilized. Hypotension may be prolonged for hours, requiring a period of monitoring prior to restarting administration.

❏ Monitor intake and output and weigh daily. Assess for decrease in signs of CHF (dyspnea, rales/crackles, peripheral edema, weight gain).

■ *Lab Test Considerations:* Monitor BUN and serum creatinine. May cause elevations in serum creatinine.

## POTENTIAL NURSING DIAGNOSES

■ Cardiac output, decreased (Indications).

■ Activity intolerance (Indications).

■ Fluid volume, excess (Indications).

## IMPLEMENTATION

❏ *High Alert:* Intravenous vasoactive medications have an increased potential for causing harm. Have second practitioner independently check original order, dosage calculations, and infusion pump settings. Administer only in settings where blood pressure can be closely monitored.

■ **IV:** Reconstitute 1.5-mg vial of nesiritide by adding 5 ml of diluent removed from a pre-filled 250-ml plastic IV bag containing preservative-free D5W, 0.9% NaCl, D5/0.45% NaCl, or D5/0.2% NaCl. Do not shake vial; rock gently so all surfaces including stopper are in contact with diluent to ensure complete reconstitution. Use only clear, colorless solutions containing no particulate matter. Withdraw entire content of reconstituted vial and add to 250-ml plastic IV bag for a concentration of 6 mcg/ml. Invert IV bag several times to ensure complete mixing of solution. Use reconstituted solution within 24 hrs.

❏ Prime the IV tubing with an infusion of 25 ml prior to connecting to the patient's vascular access port and prior to administering bolus or infusion. Flush catheter between administration of nesiritide and other medications. Do not administer through a central heparin-coated catheter, as nesiritide binds to heparin. Concomitant administration of a heparin infusion through a separate catheter is acceptable.

■ **Direct IV:** After preparation of infusion bag, withdraw bolus volume from infusion bag. To calculate amount: bolus volume = 0.33 × patient weight (kg). Do not use a higher dose than the recommended 2-mcg/kg dose.

■ *Rate:* Administer bolus over 60 seconds through a port in the IV tubing.

■ **Intermittent Infusion:** Immediately follow bolus with infusion. To calculate infusion: infusion flow rate (ml/hr = 0.1 × patient weight (kg). Do not increase dose more frequently than every 3 hr to a maximum dose of 0.3 mcg/kg/min.

■ *Rate:* Infuse at a flow rate of 0.1 ml/kg/hr for a dose of 0.01 mcg/kg/min.

■ **Y-Site Incompatibility:** ◆ bumetanide ◆ enalaprilat ◆ ethacrynic acid ◆ furosemide ◆ heparin ◆ hydralazine ◆ insulin.

## PATIENT/FAMILY TEACHING

❏ Explain purpose of nesiritide to patient and family.

## EVALUATION

**Effectiveness of therapy can be demonstrated by:** ■ Improvement in dyspnea and reduction in mean PCWP in patients with decompensated CHF.

# netilmicin, See AMINOGLYCOSIDES.

# nevirapine
(ne-**veer**-a-peen)
Viramune

---

*CLASSIFICATION(S):*
**Therapeutic:** *antiretrovirals*
**Pharmacologic:** *non-nucleoside reverse transcriptase inhibitors*

**Pregnancy Category C**

---

## INDICATIONS

■ Management of HIV infection in combination with a nucleoside analogue.

## ACTION

■ Binds to the enzyme reverse transcriptase, which results in disruption of DNA synthesis. **Therapeutic Effects:** ■ Slowed progression of HIV infection and decreased occurrence of sequelae.

## PHARMACOKINETICS

**Absorption:** >90% absorbed after oral administration.

**Distribution:** Crosses the placenta and enters breast milk; enters CSF in levels that are 45% of those in plasma.

**Metabolism and Excretion:** Mostly metabolized by the liver; minor amounts excreted unchanged in urine.

**Half-life:** 25–30 hr (during multiple dosing).

## CONTRAINDICATIONS AND PRECAUTIONS

**Contraindicated in:** ■ Hypersensitivity ■ Concurrent ketoconazole.

**Use Cautiously in:** ■ Hepatic or renal impairment ■ Pregnancy, lactation, or children (safety not established; breastfeeding not recommended in HIV-infected patients).

## ADVERSE REACTIONS AND SIDE EFFECTS*

Seen during combination therapy. ■ **CNS:** <u>headache</u> ■ **GI:** HEPATOXICITY, <u>elevated liver enzyme levels</u>, nausea, abdominal pain, diarrhea, hepatitis, ulcerative stomatitis ■ **Derm:** RASH (MAY PROGRESS TO TOXIC EPIDERMAL NECROLYSIS) ■ **Hemat:** granulocytopenia (increased in children) ■ **MS:** myalgia ■ **Neuro:** paresthesia, peripheral neuropathy ■ **Misc:** STEVENS-JOHNSON SYNDROME, <u>fever</u>.

## INTERACTIONS

**Drug-Drug:** ■ Nevirapine induces the hepatic P450 enzyme system and can affect the behavior of drugs metabolized by this system ■ Significantly decreases **ketoconazole** levels (concurrent use is contraindicated) ■ May induce **methadone** withdrawal within 2 weeks of starting therapy in patients physically dependent on methadone ■ May decrease plasma levels and effectiveness of protease inhibitors, antiretrovirals, **indinavir, saquinavir,** and **hormonal contraceptives** (concurrent use of hormonal contraceptives should be avoided) ■ May alter blood levels and effectiveness of **rifampin** or **rifabutin** (use together only with careful monitoring) ■ **Cimetidine** and **macrolide anti-infectives** increase nevirapine levels.

## ROUTE AND DOSAGE

■ **PO (Adults):** 200 mg daily for the first 2 wk, then 200 mg twice daily (in combination with a nucleoside analog antiretroviral).

■ **PO (Children ≥8 yr):** 4 mg/kg once daily for first 2 wk, then 4 mg/kg twice daily.

■ **PO (Children 2 mo–8 yr):** 4 mg/kg once daily for first 2 wk, then 7 mg/kg twice daily.

## AVAILABILITY

■ *Tablets:* 200 mg$^{Rx}$ ■ *Oral suspension:* 50 mg/5 ml$^{Rx}$.

TIME/ACTION PROFILE (blood levels)

| | ONSET | PEAK | DURATION |
|---|---|---|---|
| PO | rapid | 4 hr | 12 hr |

# NURSING IMPLICATIONS

## ASSESSMENT

❑ Assess patient for change in severity of HIV symptoms and for symptoms of opportunistic infections throughout therapy.

❑ Assess patient for rash, especially during 1st mo of therapy. If rash is severe or accompanied by systemic symptoms, therapy must be discontinued immediately.

■ *Lab Test Considerations:* Monitor viral load and CD4 cell count regularly during therapy.

❑ May cause elevated serum AST and ALT concentrations; monitor closely, especially in the first 6 mo of therapy. If moderate to severe liver function test abnormalities occur, nevirapine doses should be held until levels return to normal. Discontinue if liver function abnormalities recur when therapy is resumed.

## POTENTIAL NURSING DIAGNOSES

- Infection, risk for (Indications).
- Noncompliance (Patient/Family Teaching).

## IMPLEMENTATION

- **General:** Do not confuse nevirapine (Viramune) with nelfinavir (Viracept).
- **PO:** May be administered with or without food.
- If therapy is interrupted for more than 7 days, restart therapy at 200 mg daily for 14 days, then increase dose to 200 mg twice daily.

## PATIENT/FAMILY TEACHING

- Emphasize the importance of taking nevirapine exactly as directed, at evenly spaced times throughout day. Do not take more than prescribed amount and do not stop taking without consulting health care professional. If a dose is missed, take as soon as remembered; do not double doses.
- Instruct patient that nevirapine should not be shared with others.
- Advise patient to avoid taking other medications, prescription or OTC, without consulting health care professional.
- Inform patient that nevirapine does not cure AIDS or prevent associated or opportunistic infections. Nevirapine does not reduce the risk of transmission of HIV to others through sexual contact or blood contamination. Caution patient to use a condom and avoid sharing needles or donating blood to prevent spreading the AIDS virus to others. Advise patient that the long-term effects of nevirapine are unknown at this time.
- Advise patients taking oral contraceptives to use a nonhormonal method of birth control during nevirapine therapy.
- Advise patient not to take other medications concurrently without consulting health care professional.
- Instruct patient to notify health care professional immediately if rash occurs.
- Emphasize the importance of regular follow-up exams and blood counts to determine progress and monitor for side effects.

## EVALUATION

**Effectiveness of therapy can be demonstrated by:** ■ Delayed progression of AIDS and decreased opportunistic infections in patients with HIV ■ Decrease in viral load and increase in CD4 cell counts.

# niacin

**(nye**-a-sin)
Edur-Acin, Nia-Bid, Niac, Niacels, Niacor, Niaspan, Nicobid, Nico-400, Nicolar, Nicotinex, nicotinic acid, {Novo-Niacin}, Slo-Niacin, vitamin B

## niacinamide

(nye-a-**sin**-a-mide)
nicotinamide

### CLASSIFICATION(S):
**Therapeutic:** lipid-lowering agents, vitamins
**Pharmacologic:** water soluble vitamins

### Pregnancy Category C

## INDICATIONS

■ Treatment and prevention of niacin deficiency (pellagra) ■ Adjunctive therapy in certain hyperlipidemias (niacin only).

## ACTION

■ Required as coenzymes (for lipid metabolism, glycogenolysis, and tissue respiration) ■ Large doses decrease lipoprotein and triglyceride synthesis by inhibiting the release of free fatty acids from adipose tissue and decreasing hepatic lipoprotein synthesis (niacin only) ■ Cause peripheral vasodilation in large doses (niacin only). **Therapeutic Effects:** ■ Decreased blood lipids (niacin only) ■ Supplementation in deficiency states.

## PHARMACOKINETICS

**Absorption:** Well absorbed following oral administration.

**Distribution:** Widely distributed following conversion to niacinamide. Enters breast milk.

**Metabolism and Excretion:** Amounts required for metabolic processes are converted to niacinamide. Large doses of niacin are excreted unchanged in the urine.

**Half-life:** 45 min.

## CONTRAINDICATIONS AND PRECAUTIONS

**Contraindicated in:** ■ Hypersensitivity to niacin ■ Some products may contain tartrazine and should be avoided in patients with known hypersensitivity ■ Alcohol intolerance (Nicotinex only).

**Use Cautiously in:** ■ Liver disease ■ Arterial bleeding ■ History of peptic ulcer disease ■ Gout ■ Glaucoma ■ Diabetes mellitus.

## ADVERSE REACTIONS AND SIDE EFFECTS*

Adverse reactions and side effects refer to IV administration or doses used to treat hyperlipidemias. ■ **CNS:** nervousness, panic ■ **EENT:** blurred vision, loss of central vision, proptosis, toxic amblyopia ■ **CV:** orthostatic hypotension ■ **GI:** HEPATOTOXICITY (ER oral form only), GI upset, bloating, diarrhea, dry mouth, flatulence, heartburn, hunger pains, nausea, peptic ulceration ■ **Derm:** flushing of the face and neck, pruritus, burning, dry skin, hyperpigmentation, increased sebaceous gland activity, rashes, stinging or tingling of skin ■ **Metab:** glycosuria, hyperglycemia, hyperuricemia.

## INTERACTIONS

**Drug-Drug:** ■ Increased risk of myopathy with concurrent use of **HMG-CoA reductase inhibitors** ■ Additive hypotension with ganglionic blocking agents (**guanethidine, guanadrel**) ■ Large doses may decrease the uricosuric effects of **probenecid** or **sulfinpyrazone**.

## ROUTE AND DOSAGE

■ **PO (Adults and Children):** *Dietary supplement*—10–20 mg/day. *Dietary deficiency*—Up to 500 mg/day in divided doses. *Hyperlipidemias–Niacin only*—100–500 mg/day initially; increase slowly up to 1–2 g tid (up to 8 g/day).

■ **PO (Children 7–10 yr):** *Prevention of deficiency*—13 mg/day.

■ **PO (Children 4–6 yr):** *Prevention of deficiency*—12 mg/day.

■ **PO (Children birth–3 yr):** *Prevention of deficiency*—5–9 mg/day.

## AVAILABILITY

❑ **Niacin**

■ *Tablets:* 25 mg$^{OTC}$, 50 mg$^{OTC}$, 100 mg$^{OTC}$, 125 mg$^{OTC}$, 250 mg$^{OTC}$, 400 mg$^{OTC}$, 500 mg$^{Rx, OTC}$ ■ *Extended-release tablets:* 125 mg$^{Rx, OTC}$, 250 mg$^{Rx, OTC}$, 400 mg$^{OTC}$, 500 mg$^{Rx, OTC}$, 750 mg$^{Rx, OTC}$, 1000 mg$^{OTC}$ ■ Cost: 500 mg $53.47/100, 750 mg $68.92/100, 1000 mg $92.83/100 ■ *Extended-release capsules:* 125 mg$^{Rx, OTC}$, 250 mg$^{Rx, OTC}$, 300 mg$^{Rx, OTC}$, 400 mg$^{Rx, OTC}$, 500 mg$^{Rx, OTC}$ ■ *Elixir:* 50 mg/5 ml in pints and gallons$^{OTC}$ ■ Lovastatin (Advicor) see Appendix B.

❑ **Niacinamide**

■ *Tablets:* 50 mg$^{OTC}$, 100 mg$^{OTC}$, 125 mg$^{OTC}$, 250 mg$^{OTC}$, 500 mg$^{Rx, OTC}$.

TIME/ACTION PROFILE (effects on blood lipids)

| | ONSET | PEAK | DURATION |
|---|---|---|---|
| PO (cholesterol) | several days | unknown | unknown |
| PO (triglycerides) | several hr | unknown | unknown |

# NURSING IMPLICATIONS

## ASSESSMENT

■ **Vitamin Deficiency:** Assess patient for signs of niacin deficiency (*pellagra*—dermatitis, stomatitis, glossitis, anemia, nausea and vomiting, confusion, memory loss, and delirium) prior to and periodically throughout therapy.

■ **Hyperlipidemia:** Obtain a diet history, especially with regard to fat consumption.

■ *Lab Test Considerations:* Serum glucose and uric acid levels and hepatic function tests should be monitored periodically during prolonged high-dose therapy. Notify physician or other health care professional if AST, ALT, or LDH becomes elevated. May increase prothrombin times and decrease serum albumin.

❑ High-dose therapy may cause elevated serum glucose and uric acid levels.

❑ When niacin is used as a lipid-lowering agent, serum cholesterol and triglyceride levels should be monitored prior to and periodically throughout course of therapy.

## POTENTIAL NURSING DIAGNOSES

- Nutrition, imbalanced: less than body requirements (Indications).
- Noncompliance (Patient/Family Teaching).

## IMPLEMENTATION

- **General:** Because of infrequency of single B-vitamin deficiencies, combinations are commonly administered.
- **PO:** Administer with meals or milk to minimize GI irritation.
- Timed-release tablets and capsules should be swallowed whole, without crushing, breaking, or chewing. Use calibrated measuring device to ensure accurate dosage of solution.

## PATIENT/FAMILY TEACHING

- **General Info:** Inform patient that cutaneous flushing and a sensation of warmth, especially in the face, neck, and ears; itching or tingling; and headache may occur within the first 2 hr after taking the drug. These effects are usually transient and subside with continued therapy. If flushing is distressing or persistent, aspirin 300 mg given 30 min before each dose or slow upward titration of dose may decrease flushing.
- Advise patient to change positions slowly to minimize orthostatic hypotension.
- Instruct patients taking long-term extended-release niacin to report signs of hepatotoxicity (darkening of urine, light gray–colored stool, loss of appetite, severe stomach pain, yellow eyes or skin) to health care professional.
- Emphasize the importance of follow-up examinations to evaluate progress.
- **Vitamin Deficiency:** Encourage patient to comply with dietary recommendations of health care professional. Explain that the best source of vitamins is a well-balanced diet with foods from the four basic food groups.
- Foods high in niacin include meats, eggs, milk, and dairy products; little is lost during ordinary cooking.
- Patients self-medicating with vitamin supplements should be cautioned not to exceed RDA. The effectiveness of megadoses for

treatment of various medical conditions is unproved and may cause side effects.

- **Hyperlipidemia:** Advise patient that this medication should be used in conjunction with dietary restrictions (fat, cholesterol, carbohydrates, alcohol), exercise, and cessation of smoking.

## EVALUATION

**Effectiveness of therapy can be demonstrated by:** ■ Prevention and treatment of niacin deficiency ■ Decrease in serum cholesterol and triglyceride levels.

## nicardipine
(nye-**kar**-di-peen)
Cardene, Cardene SR, Cardene IV

### CLASSIFICATION(S):
**Therapeutic:** antianginals, antihypertensives
**Pharmacologic:** calcium channel blockers

**Pregnancy Category C**

## INDICATIONS

■ Management of: □ Hypertension □ Angina pectoris □ Vasospastic (Prinzmetal's) angina. **Unlabeled uses:** ■ Management of CHF.

## ACTION

■ Inhibits the transport of calcium into myocardial and vascular smooth muscle cells, resulting in inhibition of excitation-contraction coupling and subsequent contraction. **Therapeutic Effects:** ■ Systemic vasodilation resulting in decreased blood pressure ■ Coronary vasodilation resulting in decreased frequency and severity of attacks of angina.

## PHARMACOKINETICS

**Absorption:** Well absorbed following oral administration but extensively metabolized, resulting in decreased bioavailability.
**Distribution:** Unknown.
**Metabolism and Excretion:** Mostly metabolized by the liver; ≤10% excreted unchanged by kidneys.

**Half-life:** 2–4 hr.

## CONTRAINDICATIONS AND PRECAUTIONS

**Contraindicated in:** ■ Hypersensitivity ■ Sick sinus syndrome ■ 2nd- or 3rd-degree AV block (unless an artificial pacemaker is in place) ■ BP <90 mmHg ■ Advanced aortic stenosis.

**Use Cautiously in:** ■ Severe hepatic impairment (dosage reduction recommended) ■ Geriatric patients (dosage reduction/slower IV infusion rates recommended for most agents; increased risk of hypotension) ■ Severe renal impairment (dosage reduction may be necessary) ■ History of serious ventricular arrhythmias or CHF ■ Pregnancy, lactation, or children (safety not established).

## ADVERSE REACTIONS AND SIDE EFFECTS*

■ **CNS:** abnormal dreams, anxiety, confusion, dizziness, drowsiness, headache, jitteriness, nervousness, psychiatric disturbances, weakness ■ **EENT:** blurred vision, disturbed equilibrium, epistaxis, tinnitus ■ **Resp:** cough, dyspnea, shortness of breath ■ **CV:** ARRHYTHMIAS, CHF, peripheral edema, bradycardia, chest pain, hypotension, palpitations, syncope, tachycardia ■ **GI:** abnormal results in liver function studies, anorexia, constipation, diarrhea, dry mouth, dysgeusia, dyspepsia, nausea, vomiting ■ **GU:** dysuria, nocturia, polyuria, sexual dysfunction, urinary frequency ■ **Derm:** dermatitis, erythema multiforme, flushing, increased sweating, photosensitivity, pruritus/urticaria, rash ■ **Endo:** gynecomastia, hyperglycemia ■ **Hemat:** anemia, leukopenia, thrombocytopenia ■ **Metab:** weight gain ■ **MS:** joint stiffness, muscle cramps ■ **Neuro:** paresthesia, tremor ■ **Misc:** STEVENS-JOHNSON SYNDROME, gingival hyperplasia.

## INTERACTIONS

**Drug-Drug:** ■ Additive hypotension may occur when used concurrently with **fentanyl,** other **antihypertensives, nitrates,** acute ingestion of **alcohol,** or **quinidine** ■ Antihypertensive effects may be decreased by concurrent use of **NSAIDs** ■ Concurrent use with **beta blockers, digoxin, disopyramide,** or **phenytoin** may result in bradycardia, conduction defects, or CHF ■ **Cimetidine** and **propranolol** may decrease metabolism and increase the risk of toxicity ■ May decrease the metabolism of and increase the risk of toxicity from **cyclospo-**rine, **prazosin, quinidine,** or **carbamazepine.**

**Drug-Food:** ■ **Grapefruit juice** increases serum levels and effect.

## ROUTE AND DOSAGE

■ **PO (Adults):** 20 mg 3 times daily, may increase q 3 days (range 20–40 mg 3 times daily); or 30 mg twice daily as sustained-release form (up to 60 mg twice daily).

■ **IV (Adults):** *To replace PO use*—0.5–2.2 mg/hr continuous infusion. *For acute hypertensive episodes*—5 mg/hr titrated as needed (up to 15 mg/hr).

## AVAILABILITY (generic available)

■ *Capsules:* 20 mg$^{Rx}$, 30 mg$^{Rx}$ ■ Cost: 20 mg $42.42/100, 30 mg $68.10/100 ■ *Sustained-release capsules:* 30 mg$^{Rx}$, 45 mg$^{Rx}$, 60 mg$^{Rx}$ ■ Cost: 30 mg $41.92/60, 45 mg $66.55/60, 60 mg $79.68/60 ■ *Injection:* 2.5 mg/ml in 10-ml amps$^{Rx}$.

TIME/ACTION PROFILE (cardiovascular effects)

|  | ONSET | PEAK | DURATION |
|---|---|---|---|
| PO | 20 min | 0.5–2 hr | 8 hr |
| PO-ER | unknown | unknown | 12 hr |
| IV | within min | 45 min | 50 hr† |

†Following discontinuation.

# NURSING IMPLICATIONS

## ASSESSMENT

■ **General Info:** Monitor blood pressure and pulse prior to therapy, during dosage titration, and periodically throughout therapy. Monitor ECG periodically during prolonged therapy.

❑ Monitor intake and output ratios and daily weight. Assess for signs of CHF (peripheral edema, rales/crackles, dyspnea, weight gain, jugular venous distention).

■ **Angina:** Assess location, duration, intensity, and precipitating factors of patient's anginal pain.

■ *Lab Test Considerations:* Total serum calcium concentrations are not affected by calcium channel blockers.

❑ Monitor serum potassium periodically. Hypokalemia increases risk of arrhythmias; should be corrected.

- Monitor renal and hepatic functions periodically during long-term therapy. Several days of therapy may cause increase in hepatic enzymes, which return to normal upon discontinuation of therapy.

## POTENTIAL NURSING DIAGNOSES

- Cardiac output, decreased (Indications).
- Pain, acute (Indications).

## IMPLEMENTATION

- **General:** Do not confuse nicardipine with nifedipine or nimodipine. Do not confuse Cardene (nicardipine) with Cardura (doxazosin), codeine, or Cardizem (diltiazem).
- To transfer from IV nicardipine infusion to oral therapy with other antihypertensive, start oral therapy simultaneously with discontinuation of nicardipine infusion. If transferring to oral nicardipine therapy, administer first dose of a 3-times-a-day regimen 1 hr prior to discontinuation of infusion.
- Dosage adjustments of nicardipine should be made no more frequently than every 3 days.
- **PO:** May be administered without regard to meals. May be administered with meals if GI irritation becomes a problem.
- Do not open, crush, break, or chew sustained-release capsules.
- **Continuous Infusion:** Dilute each 25-mg ampule with 240 ml of D5W, D5/0.45% NaCl, D5/0.9% NaCl, D5/potassium chloride 40 mEq, 0.45% NaCl, or 0.9% NaCl for a concentration of 0.1 mg/ml. Stable for 24 hr at room temperature.
- *Rate:* Administer via slow infusion. Titrate rate according to blood pressure response. Continuous infusions of 0.5 mg/hr, 1.2 mg/hr, and 2.2 mg/hr produce average plasma concentrations equal to a 20-mg, 30-mg, and 40-mg oral dose, respectively, given every 8 hr at steady state.
- **Y-Site Compatibility:** ◆ diltiazem ◆ dobutamine ◆ dopamine ◆ epinephrine ◆ fentanyl ◆ gatifloxacin ◆ hydromorphone ◆ labetalol ◆ linezolid ◆ lorazepam ◆ midazolam ◆ milrinone ◆ morphine ◆ nitroglycerin ◆ norepinephrine ◆ ranitidine ◆ vecuronium.
- **Y-Site Incompatibility:** ◆ furosemide ◆ heparin ◆ thiopental.

## PATIENT/FAMILY TEACHING

- **General Info:** Advise patient to take medication exactly as directed, even if feeling well. If a dose is missed, take as soon as possible unless almost time for next dose; do not double doses. May need to be discontinued gradually.
- Instruct patient on technique for monitoring pulse. Instruct patient to contact health care professional if heart rate is <50 bpm.
- Caution patient to change positions slowly to minimize orthostatic hypotension.
- May cause drowsiness or dizziness. Advise patient to avoid driving or other activities requiring alertness until response to the medication is known.
- Instruct patient to avoid concurrent use of alcohol or OTC medications, especially cold preparations, without consulting health care professional.
- Advise patient to notify health care professional if irregular heartbeat, dyspnea, swelling of hands and feet, pronounced dizziness, nausea, constipation, or hypotension occurs or if headache is severe or persistent.
- Caution patient to wear protective clothing and to use sunscreen to prevent photosensitivity reactions.
- **Angina:** Instruct patient on concurrent nitrate or beta-blocker therapy to continue taking both medications as directed and to use SL nitroglycerin as needed for anginal attacks.
- Advise patient to contact health care professional if chest pain does not improve, worsens after therapy, or occurs with diaphoresis; if shortness of breath; or if persistent headache occurs.
- Caution patient to discuss exercise restrictions with health care professional prior to exertion.
- **Hypertension:** Encourage patient to comply with other interventions for hypertension (weight reduction, low-sodium diet, smoking cessation, moderation of alcohol consumption, regular exercise, and stress management). Medication controls but does not cure hypertension.
- Instruct patient and family in proper technique for monitoring blood pressure. Advise

patient to take blood pressure weekly and to report significant changes to health care professional.

## EVALUATION

**Effectiveness of therapy can be demonstrated by:** ■ Decrease in blood pressure ■ Decrease in frequency and severity of anginal attacks □ Decrease in need for nitrate therapy □ Increase in activity tolerance and sense of well-being.

---

# NICOTINE

(**nik**-o-teen)

**nicotine chewing gum**
Nicorette

**nicotine inhaler**
Nicotrol Inhaler

**nicotine lozenge**
Commit

**nicotine nasal spray**
Nicotrol NS

**nicotine transdermal**
Clear Nicoderm CQ, Habitrol, Nicoderm CQ, Nicotrol, Nicotrol TD

## CLASSIFICATION(S):
**Therapeutic:** smoking deterrants

## Pregnancy Category X (gum), D (transdermal)

---

## INDICATIONS

■ Adjunct therapy (with behavior modification) in the management of nicotine withdrawal in patients desiring to give up cigarette smoking.

## ACTION

■ Provides a source of nicotine during controlled withdrawal from cigarette smoking. **Therapeutic Effects:** ■ Lessened sequelae of nicotine withdrawal (irritability, insomnia, somnolence, headache, and increased appetite).

## PHARMACOKINETICS

**Absorption:** *Chewing gum, lozenge*—Slowly absorbed from buccal mucosa during chewing/sucking. *Inhaler*—50% of 4-mg dose is sys-temically absorbed; absorption from buccal mucosa is slow, most of nicotine released from inhaler is deposited in the mouth. *Nasal spray*—93% absorbed from nasal mucosa. *Transdermal*—68% of nicotine released from the system is absorbed through the skin (Nicoderm).

**Distribution:** Enters breast milk freely; crosses the placenta.

**Metabolism and Excretion:** Mostly metabolized by the liver. Small amounts are metabolized by kidneys and lungs; 10–20% excreted unchanged by kidneys.

**Half-life:** 1–2 hr.

## CONTRAINDICATIONS AND PRECAUTIONS

**Contraindicated in:** ■ Severe cardiovascular disease ■ Temporomandibular joint disease (gum only) ■ Children ■ Pregnancy or lactation ■ Phenylketonuria (gum lozenge contains aspartame) ■ Continued smoking ■ Hypersensitivity to menthol (inhaler only).

**Use Cautiously in:** ■ Cardiovascular disease including hypertension ■ Diabetes mellitus ■ Pheochromocytoma ■ Peripheral vascular diseases ■ Skin disorders (transdermal only) ■ Dental disorders (gum only) ■ History of chronic nasal disorders (nasal spray only) ■ Esophagitis, pharyngitis, or stomatitis (gum only) ■ Hyperthyroidism ■ Lactation (potential for adverse effects in the newborn) ■ Peptic ulcer disease ■ Hepatic disease ■ Patients <50 kg or who smoke <10 cigarettes/day (use lower initial dose) ■ Women with childbearing potential.

## ADVERSE REACTIONS AND SIDE EFFECTS*

■ **CNS:** headache, insomnia, abnormal dreams, dizziness, drowsiness, impaired concentration, nervousness, weakness ■ **EENT:** sinusitis; *gum*—pharyngitis; *nasal spray*—nasopharyngeal irritation, rhinitis, sneezing, watering eyes, eye irritation; *inhaler*—local mouth/throat irritation ■ **Resp:** *Nasal spray, inhaler*—bronchospasm/increased cough ■ **CV:** tachycardia, atrial fibrillation, chest pain, hypertension ■ **GI:** abdominal pain, abnormal taste, constipation, diarrhea, dry mouth, dyspepsia, nausea, vomiting; *gum*—belching, increased appetite, increased salivation, oral injury, sore mouth, hiccups ■ **Derm:** *transdermal*—burning at patch site, erythema, pruritus, cutaneous hypersensitivity, rash, sweating ■ **Endo:** dysmenorrhea ■ **MS:** arthralgia, back pain, myalgia; *gum*—jaw muscle ache ■ **Neuro:** paresthesia ■ **Misc:** allergy, pain.

## INTERACTIONS

**Drug-Drug:** ■ **Hydrocarbons** and **constituents of cigarette smoke** ↑ metabolism and ↓ effects of several medications. These effects are gradually reversed during smoking cessation ■ **Insulin** requirements may ↓ during smoking cessation ■ Effects of **acetaminophen, furosemide, caffeine, imipramine, oxazepam, pentazocine, propranolol,** or other **beta blockers, adrenergic antagonists (prazosin, labetalol),** and **theophylline** may be ↑ during smoking cessation because of decreased metabolism; dosage ↑ at cessation may be necessary ■ Doses of **isoproterenol** or **phenylephrine** may need to be ↑ because of lower levels of circulating catecholamines at cessation of smoking ■ Concurrent treatment with **bupropion** may cause treatment-emergent hypertension.

## ROUTE AND DOSAGE

■ **Transdermal (Adults):** *Habitrol*—21 mg/day for 4–8 wk, 14 mg/day for 2–4 wk, then 7 mg/day for 2–4 wk (8–16 wk total); system is worn 24 hr. *Nicoderm CQ*—21 mg/day for 6 wk, 14 mg/day for 2 wk, then 7 mg/day for 2 wk (10 wk total); system is worn 24 hr. *Nicotrol*—15 mg (1 patch)/day for 6 wk; system is removed at bedtime (worn 16 hr/day).

■ **Transdermal (Adults, Adolescents, or Children <100 Pounds Who Smoke <10 Cigarettes/Day or Who Have Underlying Cardiovascular Disease):** *Habitrol*—14 mg/day for 4–8 wk, then 7 mg/day for 2–4 wk (6–8 wk total); system is worn 24 hr. *Nicoderm CQ*—14 mg/day for 6 wk, then 7 mg/day for 2 wk (8 wk total).

■ **Gum: (Adults):** If patient smokes <25 cigarettes/day start with 2 mg gum, if patient smokes ≥ 25 cigarettes/day start with 4 mg gum (not to exceed 24 pieces gum/day); then one piece of gum every 1–2 hr for 6 weeks, then one piece of gum every 2–4 hr for 2 weeks, then one piece of gum every 4–8 hr for 2 weeks, then discontinue.

■ **Lozenge: (Adults):** If first cigarette is desired >30 min after awakening, start with 2 mg lozenge, if first cigarette is desired <30 min after awakening, start with 4 mg lozenge; then one lozenge every 1–2 hr (not to exceed 20 lozenges/day or more than 5 lozenges in 6 hr) for 6 weeks, then one lozenge every 2–4 hr for 2 weeks, then one lozenge every 4–8 hr for 2 weeks, then discontinue.

■ **Intranasal (Adults):** One spray in each nostril 1–2 times/hr (up to 5 times/hr) or 40 times/day (not to exceed 3 mo).

■ **Inhaln (Adults):** Patients are encouraged to use at least 6 cartridges/day for first 3–6 wk, with additional cartridges as necessary (up to 16/day) for 12 wk. Patients are self-titrated to level of nicotine they require (usual usage 6–16 cartridges/day) followed by gradual withdrawal over 6–12 wk. Each cartridge should be used as 80 deep inhalations over 20 min.

## AVAILABILITY (generic available)

■ *Chewing gum (Nicorette) (mint and orange flavor):* 2 mg^OTC, 4 mg^OTC ■ Cost: 2 mg $27.51/48, 4 mg $30.96/48 ■ *Inhalation (Nicotrol Inhaler):* each system contains 42 cartridges containing 10 mg of nicotine (deliver 4 mg)^Rx ■ *Lozenge:* 2 mg^OTC, 4 mg^OTC ■ *Nasal spray (Nicotrol NS):* 10 mg/ml (0.5 mg/spray) in 10-ml bottles (100 doses)^Rx, 4 mg^Rx ■ *Transdermal patch (Habitrol):* 7 mg/day^Rx, 14 mg/day^Rx, 21 mg/day^Rx, ^OTC ■ *Transdermal patch (Nicotrol):* 15 mg/day^OTC ■ *Transdermal patch (Nicoderm CQ):* 7 mg/day^OTC, 14 mg/day^OTC, 21 mg/day^OTC ■ *Transdermal patch (Prostep):* 11 mg/day^OTC, 22 mg/day^OTC.

TIME/ACTION PROFILE (nicotine blood levels)

| | ONSET | PEAK | DURATION |
|---|---|---|---|
| Gum (Nicorette) | rapid | 15–30 min | unknown |
| Inhaler (Nicotrol) | slow | 15 min after end of inhalation | unknown |
| Nasal spray (Nicotrol NS) | rapid | 4–15 min | unknown |
| Transdermal (Nicoderm CQ) | rapid | 2–4 hr | unknown |

| Transdermal (Habitrol) | rapid | 6–12 hr | unknown |

## NURSING IMPLICATIONS

### ASSESSMENT

- **General Info:** Prior to therapy, assess smoking history (number of cigarettes smoked daily, smoking patterns, nicotine content of preferred brand, degree to which patient inhales smoke).
- ❏ Assess patient for symptoms of smoking withdrawal (irritability, drowsiness, fatigue, headache, nicotine craving) periodically during nicotine replacement therapy (NRT).
- ❏ Evaluate progress in smoking cessation periodically during therapy.
- **Gum:** Assess patient for history of temporomandibular joint pain or dysfunction.
- ***Toxicity and Overdose:*** Monitor for nausea, vomiting, diarrhea, increased salivation, abdominal pain, headache, dizziness, auditory and visual disturbances, weakness, dyspnea, hypotension, and irregular pulse.

### POTENTIAL NURSING DIAGNOSES

- Coping, ineffective (Indications).

### IMPLEMENTATION

- **Gum:** Protect gum from light; exposure to light causes gum to turn brown. **Transdermal:** Determine whether patch is to be worn for 16 or 24 hr. *Nicotrol* system should be applied upon awakening and removed at bedtime.
- **Nasal Spray:** Regular use of the spray during the 1st wk of therapy may help patient adjust to irritant effects of the spray.

### PATIENT/FAMILY TEACHING

- **General Info:** Explain to patient the necessity of immediate cessation of smoking upon initiation and throughout therapy.
- ❏ Encourage patient to participate in a smoking cessation program while using this product.
- ❏ Review the patient instruction sheet enclosed in the package.
- ❏ Instruct patient in proper method of disposal of unit. Emphasize need to keep out of the reach of children.
- ❏ Nicotine in any form can be harmful to a pregnant woman and/or the fetus. Assist patient in determining risk/benefit of NRT and

harm to the fetus versus the likelihood of stopping smoking without NRT.
- ❏ Emphasize the importance of regular visits to health care professional to monitor progress of smoking cessation.
- **Gum:** Explain purpose of nicotine gum to patient. The patient should chew 1 piece of gum whenever a craving for nicotine occurs or according to a fixed schedule (every 1–2 hr while awake) as directed. The gum should be chewed slowly until a tingling sensation is felt (about 15 chews). Then, patient should stop chewing and store the gum between the cheek and gums until the tingling sensation disappears (about 1 min). The process of stopping, then resuming chewing should be repeated for approximately 30 min. Rapid, vigorous chewing may result in side effects similar to those of smoking too many cigarettes (headache, dizziness, nausea, increased salivation, heartburn, and hiccups).
- ❏ Inform patient that the gum has a slight tobacco/pepper-like taste. Many patients initially find it unpleasant and slightly irritating to the mouth. This usually resolves after several days of therapy.
- ❏ Advise patient to carry gum at all times during therapy.
- ❏ Advise patient to avoid eating or drinking acidic beverages (coffee, juices, wine, soft drinks) for 15 min before and during chewing of nicotine gum; these interfere with buccal absorption of nicotine.
- ❏ The gum usually can be chewed by denture wearers. Contact dentist if the gum adheres to bridgework.
- ❏ Use of the gum may be discontinued when 1–2 pieces/day are sufficient to control the craving for nicotine. Gradual reduction of dose over 2–3 mo can be accomplished by decreasing daily dose by 1 or more every 4–7 days, decreasing chewing time with each piece from 30 min to 10–15 min for 4–7 days, and then decreasing number of pieces per day; substituting one or more pieces of sugarless gum for pieces of nicotine gum; increasing number of doses substituted every 4–7 days; replacing 4-mg dose with 2-mg dose; or applying any of these suggestions. The duration of treatment is limited to 6 mo because physical and psychological dependence can occur. Discontinuing the gum too soon may result in withdrawal symptoms

(anxiety, irritability, GI distress, headache, drowsiness, or tobacco craving).

❏ Instruct patient not to swallow gum.

❏ Dispose of the gum by wrapping in wrapper to prevent ingestion by children and animals. Call the poison control center, emergency department, or health care professional immediately if a child ingests the gum.

❏ Emphasize the need to discontinue the gum and to inform health care professional if pregnancy occurs.

■ **Transdermal:** Instruct patient in application and use of patch. Apply patch at the same time each day. Keep patch in sealed pouch until ready to apply. Apply to clean, dry skin of upper arm or torso free of oil, hair, scars, cuts, burns, or irritation. Press patch firmly in place with palm for 10 sec, making sure there is good contact, especially around the edges. Keep patch in place during showering, bathing, or swimming; replace patches that have fallen off. Wash hands with plain water after handling patches; soap will increase absorption of nicotine. Do not trim or cut patch. Alternate application sites. Dispose of used patches by folding adhesive sides together and replacing in protective pouch or aluminum foil; keep out of reach of children.

❏ Advise patient that redness, itching, and burning at application site usually subside within 1 hr. Instruct patient to notify health care professional and not apply new patch if signs of allergic reaction (urticaria, generalized rash, hives) or persistent local skin reactions (severe erythema, pruritus, edema) occur.

❏ May cause drowsiness or dizziness. Caution patient to avoid driving or other activities requiring alertness until response to medication is known.

■ **Nasal Spray:** Instruct patient in proper use of spray. Tilt head back slightly. Do not sniff, swallow, or inhale through nose as spray is being administered. Dose should be used for 8 wk, then discontinued over 4–6 wk.

❏ Discontinue nasal spray by using ½ dose (1 spray at a time), using the spray less frequently, skipping a dose by not using every hour, or setting a planned stop date for use of the spray.

❏ Patients who fail to stop smoking should be given a therapy holiday before another attempt.

❏ Instruct patient to replace childproof cap after using and before disposal.

■ **Inhalation:** Inhalation regimens should consist of frequent, continuous puffing for 20 minutes.

■ **Lozenge:** Instruct patient to place lozenge in mouth and allow it to slowly dissolve (20–30 min). Minimize swallowing; advise patient not to chew or swallow lozenge. May cause a warm tingling sensation in mouth. Advise patient to occasionally move lozenge from side to side of mouth until completely dissolved. Instruct patient not to eat or drink 15 min before or while lozenge is in mouth. For best chances of quitting, use at least 9 lozenges/day during 1st 6 wks. Do not use more than 1 lozenge at a time or use continuously one after the another; may cause hiccoughs, heartburn, and other side effects. Lozenge should not be used after 12 wks without consulting health care professional.

### EVALUATION

**Effectiveness of therapy can be demonstrated by:** ■ Smoking cessation ■ Decrease in nicotine withdrawal symptoms in patients participating in NRT in a supervised smoking cessation program. Therapy with nicotine gum and inhalation is limited to 6 mo; most patients begin a gradual withdrawal after 3 mo of therapy. Nicotine transdermal and inhalation should be discontinued if patient is unable to stop smoking by 4th wk of therapy, as patient is unlikely to quit on that attempt. Therapy with nicotine transdermal should not be used for longer than 20 wk. Treatment with nasal spray for longer than 3 mo has not been shown to improve outcome.

## nifedipine

(nye-**fed**-i-peen)

Adalat, Adalat CC, {Apo-Nifed}, Nifedical XL, {Novo-Nifedin}, {Nu-Nifed}, Procardia, Procardia XL

## CLASSIFICATION(S):

**Therapeutic:** antianginals, antihypertensives
**Pharmacologic:** calcium channel blockers

**Pregnancy Category C**

## INDICATIONS

■ Management of: ▫ Hypertension (extended-release only) ▫ Angina pectoris ▫ Vasospastic (Prinzmetal's) angina. **Unlabeled uses:** ■ Prevention of migraine headache ■ Management of CHF or cardiomyopathy.

## ACTION

■ Inhibits calcium transport into myocardial and vascular smooth muscle cells, resulting in inhibition of excitation-contraction coupling and subsequent contraction. **Therapeutic Effects:** ■ Systemic vasodilation, resulting in decreased blood pressure ■ Coronary vasodilation, resulting in decreased frequency and severity of attacks of angina.

## PHARMACOKINETICS

**Absorption:** Well absorbed after oral administration, but large amounts are rapidly metabolized (primarily by CYP 3A4 enzyme system), resulting in decreased bioavailability (45–70%); bioavailability is increased (80%) with long-acting (CC, PA, XL) forms.
**Distribution:** Unknown.
**Protein Binding:** 92–98%.
**Metabolism and Excretion:** Mostly metabolized by the liver.
**Half-life:** 2–5 hr.

## CONTRAINDICATIONS AND PRECAUTIONS

**Contraindicated in:** ■ Hypersensitivity ■ Sick sinus syndrome ■ 2nd- or 3rd-degree AV block (unless an artificial pacemaker is in place) ■ Blood pressure <90 mmHg ■ Coadministration with grapefruit juice.
**Use Cautiously in:** ■ Severe hepatic impairment ( ↓ dose recommended) ■ History of porphyria ■ Geriatric patients ( ↓ dose recommended; increased risk of hypotension) ■ Severe renal impairment ( ↓ dose may be necessary) ■ History of serious ventricular arrhythmias or CHF ■ Pregnancy, lactation, or children (safety not established).

## ADVERSE REACTIONS AND SIDE EFFECTS*

■ **CNS:** headache, abnormal dreams, anxiety, confusion, dizziness, drowsiness, jitteriness, nervousness, psychiatric disturbances, weakness ■ **EENT:** blurred vision, disturbed equilibrium, epistaxis, tinnitus ■ **Resp:** cough, dyspnea, shortness of breath ■ **CV:** ARRHYTHMIAS, CHF, peripheral edema, bradycardia, chest pain, hypotension, palpitations, syncope, tachycardia ■ **GI:** abnormal liver function studies, anorexia, constipation, diarrhea, dry mouth, dysgeusia, dyspepsia, nausea, vomiting ■ **GU:** dysuria, nocturia, polyuria, sexual dysfunction, urinary frequency ■ **Derm:** flushing, dermatitis, erythema multiforme, increased sweating, photosensitivity, pruritus/urticaria, rash ■ **Endo:** gynecomastia, hyperglycemia ■ **Hemat:** anemia, leukopenia, thrombocytopenia ■ **Metab:** weight gain ■ **MS:** joint stiffness, muscle cramps ■ **Neuro:** paresthesia, tremor ■ **Misc:** STEVENS-JOHNSON SYNDROME, gingival hyperplasia.

## INTERACTIONS

**Drug-Drug:** ■ Additive hypotension may occur when used concurrently with **fentanyl,** other **antihypertensives, nitrates,** acute ingestion of **alcohol,** or **quinidine** ■ Antihypertensive effects may be decreased by concurrent use of **NSAIDs** ■ May increase serum levels and risk of toxicity from **digoxin** ■ Concurrent use with **beta blockers, digoxin, disopyramide,** or **phenytoin** may result in bradycardia, conduction defects, or CHF ■ **Cimetidine** and **propranolol** may decrease metabolism and increase the risk of toxicity ■ May decrease the metabolism of and increase the risk of toxicity from **cyclosporine, prazosin, quinidine,** or **carbamazepine.**
**Drug-Food:** ■ **Grapefruit juice** increases serum levels and effect; coadministration should be avoided.

## ROUTE AND DOSAGE

■ **PO (Adults):** 10–30 mg 3 times daily (not to exceed 180 mg/day), *or* 10–20 mg twice daily as PA form, *or* 30–90 mg once daily as sustained-release (CC, XL) form (not to exceed 90–120 mg/day).

## AVAILABILITY (generic available)

■ *Capsules:* {5 mg$^{Rx}$}, 10 mg$^{Rx}$, 20 mg$^{Rx}$ ■ Cost: *Procardia*—10 mg $74.59/100, 20 mg $134.20/100; *generic*—10 mg $49.75–59.95/

100, 20 mg $109.91/100 ■ *Tablets:* {10 mg$^{Rx}$} ■ *Extended-release tablets (Adalat CC, Nifedical XL, Procardia XL):* {10 mg$^{Rx}$}, {20 mg$^{Rx}$}, 30 mg$^{Rx}$, 60 mg$^{Rx}$, 90 mg$^{Rx}$ ■ Cost: *Adalat CC*—30 mg $129.94/100, 60 mg $231.47/100, 90 mg $263.54/100; *Procardia XL*—30 mg $151.63/100, 60 mg $262.40/100, 90 mg $302.75/100.

TIME/ACTION PROFILE

|  | ONSET | PEAK | DURATION |
| --- | --- | --- | --- |
| PO | 20 min | unknown | 6–8 hr |
| PO–PA | unknown | 4 hr | 12 hr |
| PO–CC, PA, XL | unknown | 6 hr | 24 hr |

# NURSING IMPLICATIONS

## ASSESSMENT

■ **General Info:** Monitor blood pressure and pulse before therapy, during dose titration, and periodically during therapy. Monitor ECG periodically during prolonged therapy.
❑ Monitor intake and output ratios and daily weight. Assess for signs of CHF (peripheral edema, rales/crackles, dyspnea, weight gain, jugular venous distention).
❑ Patients receiving digoxin concurrently with nifedipine should have routine tests of serum digoxin levels and be monitored for signs and symptoms of digoxin toxicity.
■ **Angina:** Assess location, duration, intensity, and precipitating factors of patient's anginal pain.
■ *Lab Test Considerations:* Total serum calcium concentrations are not affected by calcium channel blockers.
❑ Monitor serum potassium periodically. Hypokalemia increases risk of arrhythmias; should be corrected.
❑ Monitor renal and hepatic functions periodically during long-term therapy. Several days of therapy may cause increase in hepatic enzymes, which return to normal upon discontinuation of therapy.
❑ Nifedipine may cause positive ANA and direct Coombs' test results.

## POTENTIAL NURSING DIAGNOSES

■ Cardiac output, decreased (Indications).

■ Pain, acute (Indications).

## IMPLEMENTATION

■ **PO:** May be administered without regard to meals. May be administered with meals if GI irritation becomes a problem.
❑ Do not open, crush, break, or chew extended-release tablets. Empty tablets that appear in stool are not significant.
❑ Avoid administration with grapefruit juice.
❑ Sublingual use is not recommended due to serious adverse drug reactions.

## PATIENT/FAMILY TEACHING

■ **General Info:** Advise patient to take medication exactly as directed, even if feeling well. Take missed doses as soon as possible unless almost time for next dose; do not double doses. May need to be discontinued gradually.
❑ Instruct patient on technique for monitoring pulse. Instruct patient to contact health care professional if heart rate is <50 bpm.
❑ Caution patient to change positions slowly to minimize orthostatic hypotension.
❑ May cause drowsiness or dizziness. Advise patient to avoid driving or other activities requiring alertness until response to the medication is known.
❑ Instruct patient on importance of maintaining good dental hygiene and seeing dentist frequently for teeth cleaning to prevent tenderness, bleeding, and gingival hyperplasia (gum enlargement).
❑ Instruct patient to avoid concurrent use of alcohol or OTC medications and natural/herbal products, especially cold preparations, without consulting health care professional.
❑ Advise patient to notify health care professional if irregular heartbeat, dyspnea, swelling of hands and feet, pronounced dizziness, nausea, constipation, or hypotension occurs or if headache is severe or persistent.
❑ Caution patient to wear protective clothing and use sunscreen to prevent photosensitivity reactions.
■ **Angina:** Instruct patient on concurrent nitrate or beta-blocker therapy to continue taking both medications as directed and use SL nitroglycerin as needed for anginal attacks.

❑ Inform patient that anginal attacks may occur 30 min after administration because of reflex tachycardia. This is usually temporary and is not an indication for discontinuation.

❑ Advise patient to contact health care professional if chest pain does not improve, worsens after therapy, or occurs with diaphoresis; if shortness of breath occurs; or if persistent headache occurs.

❑ Caution patient to discuss exercise restrictions with health care professional before exertion.

■ **Hypertension:** Encourage patient to comply with other interventions for hypertension (weight reduction, low-sodium diet, smoking cessation, moderation of alcohol consumption, regular exercise, and stress management). Medication controls but does not cure hypertension.

❑ Instruct patient and family in proper technique for monitoring blood pressure. Advise patient to take blood pressure weekly and to report significant changes to health care professional.

## EVALUATION

**Effectiveness of therapy can be demonstrated by:** ■ Decrease in blood pressure ■ Decrease in frequency and severity of anginal attacks ❑ Decrease in need for nitrate therapy ❑ Increase in activity tolerance and sense of well-being.

## nilutamide
(nye-**loot**-a-mide)
{Anandron}, Nilandron

### CLASSIFICATION(S):
**Therapeutic:** antineoplastics
**Pharmacologic:** antiandrogens

### Pregnancy Category C

## INDICATIONS

■ Management of metastatic prostate cancer (with surgical castration).

## ACTION

■ Blocks the effects of androgen (testosterone) at the cellular level. **Therapeutic Effects:** ■ Decreased spread of prostate cancer.

## PHARMACOKINETICS

**Absorption:** Rapidly and completely absorbed following oral administration.
**Distribution:** Unknown.
**Metabolism and Excretion:** Extensively metabolized by the liver; two metabolites have antiandrogenic activity; <2% excreted unchanged in urine.
**Half-life:** 41–49 hr.

## CONTRAINDICATIONS AND PRECAUTIONS

**Contraindicated in:** ■ Hypersensitivity ■ Severe hepatic impairment ■ Severe respiratory insufficiency.
**Use Cautiously in:** ■ History of liver disease or alcoholism ■ History of respiratory problems ■ Pregnancy, lactation, or children (safety not established).

## ADVERSE REACTIONS AND SIDE EFFECTS*

■ **CNS:** dizziness ■ **EENT:** impaired adaptation to darkness, abnormal vision ■ **Resp:** interstitial pneumonitis ■ **CV:** hypertension ■ **GI:** HEPATOTOXICITY, constipation, hepatitis, increased liver enzymes, nausea ■ **Derm:** hot flashes, hair loss, sweating.

## INTERACTIONS

**Drug-Drug:** ■ May increase the effects of **warfarin, phenytoin,** and **theophylline** ■ May cause **alcohol** intolerance.

## ROUTE AND DOSAGE

■ **PO (Adults):** 300 mg once daily for 30 days; then 150 mg once daily.

## AVAILABILITY

■ *Tablets:* 150 mg$^{Rx}$, {100 mg$^{Rx}$}.

TIME/ACTION PROFILE (antiandrogenic effects)

|     | ONSET | PEAK    | DURATION |
|-----|-------|---------|----------|
| PO  | rapid | unknown | 24 hr    |

## NURSING IMPLICATIONS

### ASSESSMENT

❑ Patients should have a chest x-ray prior to initiation of therapy. Assess patient for symptoms of interstitial pneumonitis (dyspnea or worsening of pre-existing dyspnea). If symptoms occur, nilutamide should be discontinued until cause can be determined. Pneumonitis usually occurs during the first 3 mo of therapy and is almost always reversible when treatment is discontinued.

■ *Lab Test Considerations:* Monitor hepatic function prior to and every 3 mo throughout therapy. If AST or ALT is elevated more than 2–3 times normal, treatment should be discontinued.

❑ May cause hyperglycemia; increased serum alkaline phosphatase, BUN, and creatinine; and leukopenia.

## POTENTIAL NURSING DIAGNOSES
■ Injury, risk for (Side Effects).

## IMPLEMENTATION
■ **PO:** May be taken without regard to food.

## PATIENT/FAMILY TEACHING
❑ Instruct patient to take nilutamide exactly as directed. If a dose is missed, take as soon as possible unless almost time for next dose. Do not double doses.

❑ Caution patient that adaptation to darkness may be impaired and may cause difficulty driving at night or through tunnels. Wearing tinted glasses may minimize this effect.

❑ Advise patient to notify physician immediately if dark urine, fatigue, abdominal pain, yellow eyes or skin, or unexplained GI symptoms occur. Hepatotoxicity usually resolves when nilutamide is discontinued but may be progressive and fatal; requires immediate medical attention.

## EVALUATION
**Effectiveness of therapy can be demonstrated by:** ■ Decrease in the spread of prostate cancer.

---

## nimodipine
(nye-**moe**-di-peen)
Nimotop

### CLASSIFICATION(S):
*Therapeutic: subarachnoid hemorrhage therapy agents*

*Pharmacologic: calcium channel blockers*

**Pregnancy Category C**

---

## INDICATIONS
■ Management of subarachnoid hemorrhage.

## ACTION
■ Inhibits the transport of calcium into vascular smooth muscle cells, resulting in inhibition of excitation-contraction coupling and subsequent contraction ■ Potent peripheral vasodilator.
**Therapeutic Effects:** ■ Prevention of vascular spasm after subarachnoid hemorrhage, resulting in decreased neurologic impairment.

## PHARMACOKINETICS
**Absorption:** Well absorbed following oral administration but extensively metabolized, resulting in decreased bioavailability.
**Distribution:** Crosses the blood-brain barrier; remainder of distribution unknown.
**Protein Binding:** >95%.
**Metabolism and Excretion:** Mostly metabolized by the liver; ≤10% excreted unchanged by kidneys.
**Half-life:** 1–2 hr.

## CONTRAINDICATIONS AND PRECAUTIONS
**Contraindicated in:** ■ Hypersensitivity ■ Sick sinus syndrome ■ 2nd- or 3rd-degree AV block (unless an artificial pacemaker is in place) ■ BP <90 mmHg.
**Use Cautiously in:** ■ Severe hepatic impairment (dosage reduction recommended) ■ Geriatric patients (dosage reduction recommended; increased risk of hypotension) ■ Severe renal impairment ■ History of serious ventricular arrhythmias or CHF ■ Pregnancy, lactation, or children (safety not established).

## ADVERSE REACTIONS AND SIDE EFFECTS*
■ **CNS:** abnormal dreams, anxiety, confusion, dizziness, drowsiness, headache, nervousness, psychiatric disturbances, weakness ■ **EENT:** blurred vision, disturbed equilibrium, epistaxis, tinnitus ■ **Resp:** cough, dyspnea ■ **CV:** ARRHYTHMIAS , CHF , bradycardia, chest pain, hypotension,

palpitations, peripheral edema, syncope, tachycardia ■ **GI:** abnormal liver function studies, anorexia, constipation, diarrhea, dry mouth, dysgeusia, dyspepsia, nausea, vomiting ■ **GU:** dysuria, nocturia, polyuria, sexual dysfunction, urinary frequency ■ **Derm:** dermatitis, erythema multiforme, flushing, increased sweating, photosensitivity, pruritus/urticaria, rash ■ **Endo:** gynecomastia, hyperglycemia ■ **Hemat:** anemia, leukopenia, thrombocytopenia ■ **Metab:** weight gain ■ **MS:** joint stiffness, muscle cramps ■ **Neuro:** paresthesia, tremor ■ **Misc:** STEVENS-JOHNSON SYNDROME, gingival hyperplasia.

## INTERACTIONS

**Drug-Drug:** ■ Additive hypotension may occur when used concurrently with **fentanyl,** other **antihypertensives, nitrates,** acute ingestion of **alcohol,** or **quinidine** ■ Concurrent use with **beta blockers, digoxin, disopyramide,** or **phenytoin** may result in bradycardia, conduction defects, or CHF.

**Drug-Natural Products:** ■ **Grapefruit juice** increases serum levels and effect.

## ROUTE AND DOSAGE

■ **PO (Adults):** 60 mg q 4 hr for 21 days; therapy should be started within 96 hr of subarachnoid hemorrhage.

❏ **Hepatic Impairment**

■ **PO (Adults):** 30 mg q 4 hr for 21 days; therapy should be started within 96 hr of subarachnoid hemorrhage.

## AVAILABILITY

■ **Capsules:** 30 mg^Rx ■ Cost: $203.19/30.

TIME/ACTION PROFILE (vasodilation)

| | ONSET | PEAK | DURATION |
|---|---|---|---|
| PO | unknown | 1 hr | 4 hr |

## NURSING IMPLICATIONS

### ASSESSMENT

❏ Assess patient's neurologic status (level of consciousness, movement) prior to and periodically following administration.

❏ Monitor blood pressure and pulse prior to therapy and periodically throughout therapy.

❏ Monitor intake and output ratios and daily weight. Assess for signs of CHF (peripheral edema, rales/crackles, dyspnea, weight gain, jugular venous distention).

■ **Lab Test Considerations:** Total serum calcium concentrations are not affected by calcium channel blockers.

❏ Monitor serum potassium periodically. Hypokalemia increases risk of arrhythmias; should be corrected.

❏ Monitor renal and hepatic functions periodically. Several days of therapy may cause increase in hepatic enzymes, which return to normal upon discontinuation of therapy.

❏ May occasionally cause decreased platelet count.

## POTENTIAL NURSING DIAGNOSES

■ Tissue perfusion, ineffective (Indications).

## IMPLEMENTATION

■ **General:** Do not confuse nimodipine with nicardipine or nifedipine.

❏ Begin administration within 96 hr of subarachnoid hemorrhage and continue every 4 hr for 21 consecutive days.

■ **PO:** If patient is unable to swallow capsule, make a hole in both ends of the capsule with a sterile 18-gauge needle and extract the contents into a syringe. Empty contents into water or nasogastric tube and flush with 30 ml normal saline.

## PATIENT/FAMILY TEACHING

■ **General Info:** Advise patient to take medication exactly as directed, even if feeling well. If a dose is missed, take as soon as possible unless almost time for next dose; do not double doses. May need to be discontinued gradually.

❏ Caution patient to change positions slowly to minimize orthostatic hypotension.

❏ May cause drowsiness or dizziness. Advise patient to avoid driving or other activities requiring alertness until response to the medication is known.

❏ Instruct patient to avoid concurrent use of alcohol or OTC medications, especially cold preparations, without consulting health care professional.

❏ Advise patient to notify health care professional if irregular heartbeats, dyspnea, swelling of hands and feet, pronounced dizziness, nausea, constipation, or hypotension occurs or if headache is severe or persistent.

❏ Caution patient to wear protective clothing and use sunscreen to prevent photosensitivity reactions.

## EVALUATION

**Effectiveness of therapy can be demonstrated by:** ■ Improvement in neurologic deficits due to vasospasm following subarachnoid hemorrhage.

## nisoldipine

(nye-**sole**-di-peen)

Sular

### CLASSIFICATION(S):

**Therapeutic:** antihypertensives
**Pharmacologic:** calcium channel blockers

### Pregnancy Category C

## INDICATIONS

■ Management of hypertension.

## ACTION

■ Inhibits the transport of calcium into vascular smooth muscle cells, resulting in inhibition of vasoconstriction and dilation of arterioles. **Therapeutic Effects:** ■ Systemic vasodilation, resulting in decreased blood pressure.

## PHARMACOKINETICS

**Absorption:** Well absorbed (87%) following oral administration but rapidly and extensively metabolized in the gut wall, resulting in 5% bioavailability.
**Distribution:** Unknown.
**Metabolism and Excretion:** Highly metabolized CYP3A4 enzyme system.
**Half-life:** 7–12 hr.

## CONTRAINDICATIONS AND PRECAUTIONS

**Contraindicated in:** ■ Hypersensitivity ■ Cross-sensitivity with calcium channel blockers may occur ■ Concurrent phenytoin use.
**Use Cautiously in:** ■ CHF/left ventricular dysfunction ■ Hepatic impairment (dosage reduction may be necessary) ■ Geriatric patients (dosage reduction may be necessary) ■ Coronary artery disease (may precipitate angina) ■ Pregnancy, lactation, or children (safety not established).

## ADVERSE REACTIONS AND SIDE EFFECTS*

■ **CNS:** headache, dizziness ■ **EENT:** pharyngitis, sinusitis ■ **CV:** peripheral edema, chest pain, hypotension, palpitations ■ **GI:** nausea ■ **Derm:** rash ■ **Endo:** gynecomastia.

## INTERACTIONS

**Drug-Drug:** ■ Additive hypotension may occur with other **antihypertensives,** acute ingestion of **alcohol,** or **nitrates** ■ Antihypertensive effects may be decreased by concurrent use of **NSAIDs** ■ **Phenytoin** or **other CYP3A4 inducers** decrease blood levels and effectiveness (avoid concurrent use).
**Drug-Food:** ■ **Grapefruit juice** significantly increases blood levels and effects of nisoldipine; concurrent ingestion should be avoided ■ Blood levels are increased by concurrent ingestion of a **high-fat meal** and should be avoided.

## ROUTE AND DOSAGE

■ **PO (Adults):** 20 mg/day as a single dose initially; may be increased by 10 mg/day q 7 days, up to 60 mg/day (usual range 20–40 mg/day).

## AVAILABILITY

■ *Extended-release tablets:* 10 mg^Rx, 20 mg^Rx, 30 mg^Rx, 40 mg^Rx ■ Cost: 10 mg $96.38/100, 20 mg $96.38/100, 30 mg $96.38/100, 40 mg $96.38/100.

TIME/ACTION PROFILE (antihypertensive effects)

| | ONSET | PEAK | DURATION |
|---|---|---|---|
| PO | unknown | 6–12 hr | 24 hr |

## NURSING IMPLICATIONS

### ASSESSMENT

❑ Monitor blood pressure and pulse prior to therapy, during dosage titration, and periodically throughout therapy. Monitor ECG periodically during prolonged therapy.
❑ Monitor intake and output ratios and daily weight. Assess for signs of CHF (peripheral edema, rales/crackles, dyspnea, weight gain, jugular venous distention).

■ *Lab Test Considerations:* Total serum calcium concentrations are not affected by calcium channel blockers.

## POTENTIAL NURSING DIAGNOSES

■ Cardiac output, decreased (Indications).

## IMPLEMENTATION

■ **PO:** Avoid administration within 1 hr of high-fat meals or grapefruit products.
❑ Do not crush, break, or chew tablets.

## PATIENT/FAMILY TEACHING

❑ Advise patient to take medication exactly as directed, even if feeling well. If a dose is missed, take as soon as possible unless almost time for next dose; do not double doses. May need to be discontinued gradually.
❑ Encourage patient to comply with other interventions for hypertension (weight reduction, low-sodium diet, smoking cessation, moderation of alcohol consumption, regular exercise, and stress management). Medication controls but does not cure hypertension.
❑ Instruct patient and family in proper technique for monitoring blood pressure. Advise patient to take blood pressure weekly and to report significant changes to health care professional.
❑ Caution patient to change positions slowly to minimize orthostatic hypotension.
❑ May cause dizziness. Advise patient to avoid driving or other activities requiring alertness until response to the medication is known.
❑ Instruct patient to avoid concurrent use of alcohol or OTC medications, especially cold preparations, without consulting health care professional.
❑ Advise patient to notify health care professional if irregular heartbeat, dyspnea, swelling of hands and feet, pronounced dizziness, nausea, constipation, or hypotension occurs or if headache is severe or persistent.

## EVALUATION

**Effectiveness of therapy can be demonstrated by:** ■ Decrease in blood pressure.

## nitazoxanide

(nit-a-**zox**-a-nide)
Alinia

## INDICATIONS

■ Treatment of diarrhea due to *Cryptosporidium parvum* and *Giardia lamblia* in children ages 1–11.

## ACTION

■ Interferes with electron transfer reaction necessary for anaerobic energy metabolism of offending organisms. **Therapeutic Effects:** ■ Antiprotozoal action resulting in decreased diarrhea.

## PHARMACOKINETICS

**Absorption:** Following oral administration, nitazoxanide is rapidly converted to tizoxanide which is the active metabolite; tizoxanide is further metabolized.
**Distribution:** Unknown.
**Protein Binding:** >99%.
**Metabolism and Excretion:** *Tizoxanide*—excreted in urine, bile, and feces; inactive metabolites excreted in urine, bile, and feces.
**Half-life:** Unknown.

## CONTRAINDICATIONS AND PRECAUTIONS

**Contraindicated in:** ■ Hypersensitivity.
**Use Cautiously in:** ■ Hepatic and/or renal impairment ■ Diabetics (contains 1.48 g sucrose/5 ml) ■Children <1 yr or >11 yr; adults, pregnancy or lactation (safety not established).

## ADVERSE REACTIONS AND SIDE EFFECTS*

■ **CNS:** dizziness ■ **EENT:** yellow eye discoloration ■ **GI:** abdominal pain, diarrhea, vomiting ■ **GU:** discolored urine ■ **Derm:** pruritus, sweating ■ **Misc:** fever.

## INTERACTIONS

**Drug-Drug:** ■ May interact with other **highly protein-bound drugs** by competing for binding sites.

## ROUTE AND DOSAGE

■ **PO (Children 4–11 yr):** 200 mg (10 ml) every 12 hr for 3 days.

- **PO (Children 1–4 yr):** 100 mg (5 ml) every 12 hr for 3 days.

## AVAILABILITY

- **Oral suspension (strawberry):** 100 mg/5 ml in 60 ml bottle^Rx.

TIME/ACTION PROFILE (blood levels)

| | ONSET | PEAK | DURATION |
|---|---|---|---|
| PO | unknown† | 1–4 hr | 12 hr |

†Onset of antidiarrheal activity is 24–48 hr.

## NURSING IMPLICATIONS

### ASSESSMENT

- Assess frequency and consistency of stools and bowel sounds before and during therapy.
- Assess fluid and electrolyte balance and skin turgor for dehydration.

### POTENTIAL NURSING DIAGNOSES

- Diarrhea (Indications).

### IMPLEMENTATION

- **PO:** Administer with food. Keep container tightly closed and shake well before each administration. Suspension may be stored at room temperature for 7 days; discard unused portion.

### PATIENT/FAMILY TEACHING

- Explain to parents administration of medication and monitoring of condition.

### EVALUATION

**Effectiveness of therapy can be demonstrated by:** ■ Resolution of symptoms: no watery stools, no more than 2 soft stools within the past 24 hr and no unformed stools within the past 48 hr.

---

# nitrofurantoin

(nye-troe-fyoor-**an**-toyn)

{Apo-Nitrofurantoin}, Furadantin, Macrobid, Macrodantin

*CLASSIFICATION(S):*
*Therapeutic: anti-infectives*

---

**Pregnancy Category B**

## INDICATIONS

■ Urinary tract infections caused by susceptible organisms; not effective in systemic bacterial infections ■ Chronic suppressive therapy of urinary tract infections.

## ACTION

■ Interferes with bacterial enzymes. **Therapeutic Effects:** ■ Bactericidal or bacteriostatic action against susceptible organisms. **Spectrum:** ■ Many gram-negative and some gram-positive organisms, specifically: ❏ *Citrobacter* ❏ *Corynebacterium* ❏ *Enterobacter* ❏ *Escherichia coli* ❏ *Klebsiella* ❏ *Neisseria* ❏ *Salmonella* ❏ *Shigella* ❏ *Staphylococcus aureus* ❏ *Staphylococcus epidermidis* ❏ *Enterococcus.*

## PHARMACOKINETICS

**Absorption:** Readily absorbed after oral administration. Absorption is slower but more complete with macrocrystals (Macrodantin).
**Distribution:** Crosses placenta; enters breast milk.
**Metabolism and Excretion:** Partially metabolized by the liver; 30–50% excreted unchanged by the kidneys.
**Half-life:** 20 min (increased in renal impairment).

## CONTRAINDICATIONS AND PRECAUTIONS

**Contraindicated in:** ■ Hypersensitivity ■ Hypersensitivity to parabens (suspension) ■ Oliguria or anuria ■G6PD deficiency ■Infants <1 mo and pregnancy near term (increased risk of hemolytic anemia in newborn).
**Use Cautiously in:** ■ Patients with diabetes or debilitated patients (neuropathy may be more common) ■ Geriatric patients (increased risk of hepatic/pulmonary reactions) ■ Pregnancy and lactation (safety not established but has been used safely in pregnant women; breastfeeding may cause hemolysis in G6PD-deficient infants).

## ADVERSE REACTIONS AND SIDE EFFECTS*

■ **CNS:** dizziness, drowsiness, headache ■ **EENT:** nystagmus ■ **Resp:** pneumonitis ■ **CV:**

---

chest pain ■ **GI:** PSEUDOMEMBRANOUS COLITIS, <u>anorexia</u>, <u>nausea</u>, <u>vomiting</u>, abdominal pain, diarrhea, drug-induced hepatitis ■ **GU:** rust/brown discoloration of urine ■ **Derm:** photosensitivity ■ **Hemat:** blood dyscrasias, hemolytic anemia ■ **Neuro:** peripheral neuropathy ■ **Misc:** <u>hypersensitivity reactions</u>.

## INTERACTIONS

**Drug-Drug:** ■ **Probenecid** and **sulfinpyrazone** prevent high urinary concentrations; may ↓ effectiveness ■ **Antacids** may decrease absorption ■ ↑ risk of neurotoxicity with **neurotoxic drugs** ■ ↑ risk of hepatotoxicity with **hepatotoxic drugs** ■ ↑ risk of pneumonitis with **drugs having pulmonary toxicity.**

## ROUTE AND DOSAGE

■ **PO (Adults):** *Treatment of active infection*—50–100 mg q 6–8 hr *or* 100 mg q 12 hr as extended-release product. *Chronic suppression*—50–100 mg single evening dose.

■ **PO (Children >1 mo):** *Treatment of active infection*—0.75–1.75 mg/kg q 6 hr. *Chronic suppression*—1 mg/kg/day as a single dose at bedtime (unlabeled).

## AVAILABILITY (generic available)

■ *Tablets:* 50 mg$^{Rx}$, 100 mg$^{Rx}$ ■ *Oral suspension:* 25 mg/5 ml$^{Rx}$ ■ *Capsules:* 25 mg$^{Rx}$, 50 mg$^{Rx}$, 100 mg$^{Rx}$ ■ Cost: *Macrodantin*—25 mg $83.18/100, 50 mg $109.53/100, 100 mg $186.01/100 ■ *Extended-release capsules:* 100 mg$^{Rx}$ ■ Cost: *Macrobid*—100 mg $144.91/100.

TIME/ACTION PROFILE (urine levels)

|    | ONSET | PEAK | DURATION |
|----|-------|------|----------|
| PO | unknown | 30 min | 6–12 hr |

# NURSING IMPLICATIONS

## ASSESSMENT

❑ Assess for signs and symptoms of urinary tract infection (frequency, urgency, pain, and burning on urination; fever; cloudy or foul-smelling urine) before and periodically during therapy.

❑ Obtain specimens for culture and sensitivity before and during drug administration.

❑ Monitor intake and output ratios. Report significant discrepancies in totals.

■ *Lab Test Considerations:* Monitor CBC routinely with patients on prolonged therapy.

❑ May cause ↑ serum glucose, bilirubin, alkaline phosphatase, BUN, and creatinine.

## POTENTIAL NURSING DIAGNOSES

■ Infection, risk for (Indications).

## IMPLEMENTATION

■ **PO:** Administer with food or milk to minimize GI irritation, to delay and increase absorption, to increase peak concentration, and to prolong duration of therapeutic concentration in the urine.

❑ Do not crush tablets or open capsules.

❑ Administer liquid preparations with calibrated measuring device. Shake well before administration. Oral suspension may be mixed with water, milk, fruit juices, or infant formula. Rinse mouth with water after administration of oral suspension to avoid staining teeth.

## PATIENT/FAMILY TEACHING

❑ Instruct patient to take medication around the clock, as directed. Take missed doses as soon as remembered and space next dose 2–4 hr apart. Do not skip or double up on missed doses.

❑ May cause dizziness or drowsiness. Caution patient to avoid driving or other activities requiring alertness until response to medication is known.

❑ Inform patient that medication may cause a rust-yellow to brown discoloration of urine, which is not significant.

❑ Advise patient to notify health care professional if fever, chills, cough, chest pain, dyspnea, skin rash, numbness or tingling of the fingers or toes, or intolerable GI upset occurs. Signs of superinfection (milky, foul-smelling urine; perineal irritation; dysuria) should also be reported.

❑ Instruct patient to notify health care professional if fever and diarrhea develop, especially if stool contains blood, pus, or mucus. Advise patient not to treat diarrhea without consulting health care professional.

❑ Instruct patient to consult health care professional if no improvement is seen within a few days after initiation of therapy.

## EVALUATION

**Effectiveness of therapy can be demonstrated by:** ■ Resolution of the signs and symptoms of infection. Therapy should be continued for a minimum of 7 days and for at least 3 days after the urine has become sterile ■ Decrease in the frequency of infections in chronic suppressive therapy.

# nitroglycerin
(nye-tro-**gli**-ser-in)

**extended-release capsules**
Nitrocot, NitroglynE-R, Nitro-par, Nitro-Time

**extended-release tablets**
Nitrong

**extended-release buccal tablets**
Nitrogard, {Nitrogard SR}

**intravenous**
Nitro-Bid IV, Tridil

**translingual spray**
Nitrolingual

**ointment**
Nitro-Bid, Nitrol

**sublingual**
Nitrostat, NitroQuick

**transdermal system**
Deponit, Minitran, Nitrek, Nitrodisc, Nitro-Dur, Transderm-Nitro

*CLASSIFICATION(S):*
*Therapeutic: antianginals*
*Pharmacologic: nitrates*

**Pregnancy Category C**

## INDICATIONS

■ Acute (**translingual and SL**) and long-term prophylatic (**oral, buccal, transdermal**) management of angina pectoris ■ **PO:** Adjunct treatment of CHF ■ **IV:** Adjunct treatment of acute MI ■ Production of controlled hypotension during surgical procedures ■ Treatment of CHF associated with acute MI ■ Production of controlled hypotension during surgical procedures. **Unlabeled uses:** ■ Management of chronic CHF.

## ACTION

■ Increases coronary blood flow by dilating coronary arteries and improving collateral flow to ischemic regions ■ Produces vasodilation (venous greater than arterial) ■ Decreases left ventricular end-diastolic pressure and left ventricular end-diastolic volume (preload) ■ Reduces myocardial oxygen consumption. **Therapeutic Effects:** ■ Relief or prevention of anginal attacks ■ Increased cardiac output ■ Reduction of blood pressure.

## PHARMACOKINETICS

**Absorption:** Well absorbed after oral, buccal, and sublingual administration. Also absorbed through skin. Orally administered nitroglycerin is rapidly metabolized, leading to decreased bioavailability.

**Distribution:** Unknown.

**Metabolism and Excretion:** Undergoes rapid and almost complete metabolism by the liver; also metabolized by enzymes in bloodstream.

**Half-life:** 1–4 min.

## CONTRAINDICATIONS AND PRECAUTIONS

**Contraindicated in:** ■ Hypersensitivity ■ Severe anemia ■ Pericardial tamponade ■ Constrictive pericarditis ■ Alcohol intolerance (large IV doses only) ■ Concurrent use of sildenafil.

**Use Cautiously in:** ■ Head trauma or cerebral hemorrhage ■ Glaucoma ■ Hypertrophic cardiomyopathy ■ Severe liver impairment ■ Malabsorption or hypermotility (PO) ■ Hypovolemia (IV) ■ Normal or decreased pulmonary capillary wedge pressure (IV) ■ Cardioversion (remove transdermal patch before procedure) ■ Pregnancy (may compromise maternal/fetal circulation) ■ Children or lactation (safety not established).

{ } = Available in Canada only.
*CAPITALS indicates life-threatening; underlines indicate most frequent.

## ADVERSE REACTIONS AND SIDE EFFECTS*

■ **CNS:** dizziness, headache, apprehension, restlessness, weakness ■ **EENT:** blurred vision ■ **CV:** hypotension, tachycardia, syncope ■ **GI:** abdominal pain, nausea, vomiting ■ **Derm:** contact dermatitis (transdermal or ointment) ■ **Misc:** alcohol intoxication (large IV doses only), cross-tolerance, flushing, tolerance.

## INTERACTIONS

**Drug-Drug:** ■ Concurrent use of nitrates in any form with **sildenafil** increases the risk of serious and potentially fatal hypotension; concurrent use is contraindicated. ■ Additive hypotension with **antihypertensives,** acute ingestion of **alcohol, beta blockers, calcium channel blockers, haloperidol,** or **phenothiazines** ■ **Agents having anticholinergic properties (tricyclic antidepressants, antihistamines, phenothiazines)** may decrease absorption of lingual, sublingual, or buccal nitroglycerin.

## ROUTE AND DOSAGE

■ **SL (Adults):** 0.3–0.6 mg; may repeat q 5 min for 15 min for acute attack. **Lingual Spray (Adults):** 1–2 sprays; may be repeated q 5 min for 15 min.
■ **Buccal (Adults):** 1 mg q 5 hr; dosage and frequency may be increased as needed.
■ **PO (Adults):** *Extended-release capsules—* 2.5–9 mg q 8–12 hr. *Extended-release tablets—*1.3–6.5 mg q 8–12 hr.
■ **IV (Adults):** 5 mcg/min; increase by 5 mcg/min q 3–5 min to 20 mcg/min, then increase by 10–20 mcg/min q 3–5 min (dosing determined by hemodynamic parameters).
■ **Transdermal (Adults):** *Ointment*—(1 in. = 15 mg) 1–2 in. q 8 hr (up to 5 in. q 4 hr). *Transdermal patch*—0.1–0.6 mg/hr, up to 0.8 mg/hr. Patch should be worn 12–14 hr/day.

## AVAILABILITY (generic available)

■ *Extended-release tablets:* 2.6 mg$^{Rx}$, 6.5 mg$^{Rx}$, 9 mg$^{Rx}$ ■ *Extended-release capsules:* 2.5 mg$^{Rx}$, 6.5 mg$^{Rx}$, 9 mg$^{Rx}$ ■ *Sublingual tablets:* 0.3 mg$^{Rx}$, 0.4 mg$^{Rx}$, 0.6 mg$^{Rx}$ ■ Cost: *NitroQuick*—0.3 mg $6.82/100, 0.4 mg $6.82/100, 0.6 mg $6.82/100; *Nitrostat*—0.3 mg $9.09/100, 0.4 mg $9.09/100, 0.6 mg $9.09/100 ■ *Translingual spray:* 0.4 mg/spray in 14.5-g canister (200 doses)$^{Rx}$ ■ *Extended-release buccal tablets:* 1 mg$^{Rx}$, 2

mg$^{Rx}$, 3 mg$^{Rx}$, {5 mg$^{Rx}$} ■ *Transdermal systems:* 0.1 mg/hr$^{Rx}$, 0.2 mg/hr$^{Rx}$, 0.3 mg/hr$^{Rx}$, 0.4 mg/hr$^{Rx}$, 0.6 mg/hr$^{Rx}$, 0.8 mg/hr$^{Rx}$ ■ *Transdermal ointment:* 2%$^{Rx}$ ■ *Injection:* 0.5 mg/ml$^{Rx}$, 5 mg/ml$^{Rx}$ ■ *Injection solution:* 25 mg/250 ml$^{Rx}$, 50 mg/250 ml$^{Rx}$, 50 mg/500 ml$^{Rx}$, 100 mg/250 ml$^{Rx}$, 200 mg/500 ml$^{Rx}$.

TIME/ACTION PROFILE (cardiovascular effects)

| | ONSET | PEAK | DURATION |
|---|---|---|---|
| SL | 1–3 min | unknown | 30–60 min |
| Buccal-ER | unknown | unknown | 5 hr |
| PO-ER | 40–60 min | unknown | 8–12 hr |
| TD-Oint | 20–60 min | unknown | 4–8 hr |
| TD-Patch | 40–60 min | unknown | 8–24 hr |
| IV | immediate | unknown | several min |

# NURSING IMPLICATIONS

## ASSESSMENT

❑ Assess location, duration, intensity, and precipitating factors of patient's anginal pain.
❑ Monitor blood pressure and pulse before and after administration. Patients receiving IV nitroglycerin require continuous ECG and blood pressure monitoring. Additional hemodynamic parameters may be monitored.
■ *Lab Test Considerations:* May cause increased urine catecholamine and urine vanillylmandelic acid concentrations.
❑ Excessive doses may cause increased methemoglobin concentrations.
❑ May cause falsely elevated serum cholesterol levels.

## POTENTIAL NURSING DIAGNOSES

■ Pain, acute (Indications).
■ Tissue perfusion, ineffective (Indications).

## IMPLEMENTATION

■ **PO:** Administer dose 1 hr before or 2 hr after meals with a full glass of water for faster absorption. Sustained-release preparations should be swallowed whole; do not crush, break, or chew. **SL:** Tablet should be held under tongue until dissolved. Avoid eating, drinking, or smoking until tablet is dissolved. **Buccal:** Place tablet under upper lip or between cheek and gum. Onset of action may be increased by touching the tablet with the tongue or by drinking hot liquids.

- **IV:** Doses must be diluted and administered as an infusion. Standard infusion sets made of polyvinyl chloride (PVC) plastic may absorb up to 80% of the nitroglycerin in solution. Use glass bottles only and special tubing provided by manufacturer.
- **Continuous Infusion:** Dilute in D5W or 0.9% NaCl in a concentration of 25–40 mcg/ml, dependent upon patient's fluid tolerance. Solution is stable for 48 hr at room temperature. Solution is not explosive either before or after dilution.
- *Rate:* Administer via infusion pump to ensure accurate rate. Titrate rate according to patient response.
- **Y-Site Compatibility:** ◆ alatrofloxacin ◆ amiodarone ◆ amphotericin B cholesteryl sulfate complex ◆ atracurium ◆ cisatracurium ◆ diltiazem ◆ dobutamine ◆ dopamine ◆ epinephrine ◆ esmolol ◆ famotidine ◆ fentanyl ◆ fluconazole ◆ furosemide ◆ gatifloxacin ◆ haloperidol ◆ heparin ◆ hydralazine ◆ hydromorphone ◆ inamrinone ◆ insulin ◆ labetalol ◆ lidocaine ◆ linezolid ◆ lorazepam ◆ midazolam ◆ morphine ◆ norepinephrine ◆ nitroprusside ◆ pancuronium ◆ propofol ◆ ranitidine ◆ remifentanil ◆ streptokinase ◆ tacrolimus ◆ theophylline ◆ thiopental ◆ vecuronium ◆ warfarin.
- **Y-Site Incompatibility:** ◆ alteplase ◆ levofloxacin.
- **Additive Incompatibility:** Manufacturer recommends that nitroglycerin not be admixed with other medications.
- **Topical:** Sites of topical application should be rotated to prevent skin irritation. Remove patch or ointment from previous site before application.
- ❏ Doses may be increased to the highest dose that does not cause symptomatic hypotension.
- ❏ Apply ointment by using dose-measuring application papers supplied with ointment. Squeeze ointment onto measuring scale printed on paper. Use paper to spread ointment onto nonhairy area of skin (chest, abdomen, thighs; avoid distal extremities) in a thin, even layer, covering a 2–3-in. area. Do not allow ointment to come in contact with hands. Do not massage or rub in ointment;

this will increase absorption and interfere with sustained action. Apply occlusive dressing if ordered.

- ❏ Transdermal patches may be applied to any hairless site (avoid distal extremities or areas with cuts or calluses). Apply firm pressure over patch to ensure contact with skin, especially around edges. Apply a new dosage unit if the first one becomes loose or falls off. Units are waterproof and not affected by showering or bathing. Do not cut or trim system to adjust dosage. Do not alternate between brands of transdermal products; dosage may not be equivalent. Remove patches before cardioversion or defibrillation to prevent patient burns. Patch may be worn for 12–14 hr and removed for 10–12 hr at night to prevent development of tolerance.

## PATIENT/FAMILY TEACHING

- **General Info:** Instruct patient to take medication exactly as directed, even if feeling better. If a dose is missed, take as soon as remembered unless next dose is scheduled within 2 hr (6 hr with extended-release preparations). Do not double doses. Do not discontinue abruptly; gradual dosage reduction may be necessary to prevent rebound angina.
- ❏ Caution patient to change positions slowly to minimize orthostatic hypotension. First dose should be taken while in a sitting or reclining position, especially in geriatric patients.
- ❏ Advise patient to avoid concurrent use of alcohol with this medication. Patient should also consult health care professional before taking OTC medications while taking nitroglycerin.
- ❏ Inform patient that headache is a common side effect that should decrease with continuing therapy. Aspirin or acetaminophen may be ordered to treat headache. Notify health care professional if headache is persistent or severe.
- ❏ Advise patient to notify health care professional if dry mouth or blurred vision occurs.
- **Acute Anginal Attacks:** Advise patient to sit down and use medication at first sign of attack. Relief usually occurs within 5 min. Dose may be repeated if pain is not relieved in 5–10 min. Call health care professional or

go to nearest emergency room if anginal pain is not relieved by 3 tablets in 15 min.

- **SL:** Inform patient that tablets should be kept in original glass container or in specially made metal containers, with cotton removed to prevent absorption. Tablets lose potency in containers made of plastic or cardboard or when mixed with other capsules or tablets. Exposure to air, heat, and moisture also causes loss of potency. Instruct patient not to open bottle frequently, handle tablets, or keep bottle of tablets next to body (i.e., shirt pocket) or in automobile glove compartment. Advise patient that tablets should be replaced 6 mo after opening to maintain potency.
- **Lingual Spray:** Instruct patient to lift tongue and spray dose under tongue.

## EVALUATION

**Effectiveness of therapy can be demonstrated by:** ■ Decrease in frequency and severity of anginal attacks ❑ Increase in activity tolerance. During long-term therapy, tolerance may be minimized by intermittent administration in 12–14 hr or 10–12 hr off intervals ■ Controlled hypotension during surgical procedures.

---

## nitroprusside

(nye-troe-**pruss**-ide)

Nitropress

**CLASSIFICATION(S):**
**Therapeutic:** antihypertensives
**Pharmacologic:** vasodilators

**Pregnancy Category C**

---

## INDICATIONS

■ Hypertensive crises ■ Controlled hypotension during anesthesia ■ Cardiac pump failure or cardiogenic shock (alone or with dopamine).

## ACTION

■ Produces peripheral vasodilation by a direct action on venous and arteriolar smooth muscle. **Therapeutic Effects:** ■ Rapid lowering of blood pressure ■ Decreased cardiac preload and afterload.

## PHARMACOKINETICS

**Absorption:** IV administration results in complete bioavailability.
**Distribution:** Unknown.
**Metabolism and Excretion:** Rapidly metabolized in RBCs and tissues to cyanide and subsequently by the liver to thiocyanate.
**Half-life:** 2 min.

## CONTRAINDICATIONS AND PRECAUTIONS

**Contraindicated in:** ■ Hypersensitivity ■ Decreased cerebral perfusion.

**Use Cautiously in:** ■ Renal disease (increased risk of thiocyanate accumulation) ■ Hepatic disease (increased risk of cyanide accumulation) ■ Geriatric patients (increased sensitivity) ■ Hypothyroidism ■ Hyponatremia ■ Vitamin B deficiency ■ Pregnancy or lactation (safety not established).

## ADVERSE REACTIONS AND SIDE EFFECTS*

■ **CNS:** dizziness, headache, restlessness ■ **EENT:** blurred vision, tinnitus ■ **CV:** dyspnea, hypotension, palpitations ■ **GI:** abdominal pain, nausea, vomiting ■ **F and E:** acidosis ■ **Local:** phlebitis at IV site ■ **Misc:** CYANIDE TOXICITY, thiocyanate toxicity.

## INTERACTIONS

**Drug-Drug:** ■ Increased hypotensive effect with **ganglionic blocking agents, general anesthetics,** and other **antihypertensives** ■ **Estrogens** and **sympathomimetics** may decrease the response to nitroprusside.

## ROUTE AND DOSAGE

- **IV (Adults and Children):** 0.3 mcg/kg/min initially; may be increased as needed up to 10 mcg/kg/min (usual dose is 3 mcg/kg/min; not to exceed 10 min of therapy at 10 mcg/kg/min infusion rate).

## AVAILABILITY (generic available)

- **Powder for injection:** 50 mg/vial[Rx].

TIME/ACTION PROFILE (hypotensive effect)

|  | ONSET | PEAK | DURATION |
|---|---|---|---|
| IV | immediate | rapid | 1–10 min |

# NURSING IMPLICATIONS

## ASSESSMENT

❏ Monitor blood pressure, heart rate, and ECG frequently throughout therapy; continuous monitoring is preferred. Consult physician for parameters. Monitor for rebound hypertension following discontinuation of nitroprusside.

❏ Pulmonary capillary wedge pressure (PCWP) may be monitored in patients with MI or CHF.

■ *Lab Test Considerations:* May cause decrease in bicarbonate concentrations, P $CO_2$, and pH.

❏ May cause increased lactate concentrations.

❏ May cause increased serum cyanide and thiocyanate concentrations.

❏ Monitor serum methemoglobin concentrations in patients receiving >10 mg/kg and exhibiting signs of impaired oxygen delivery despite adequate cardiac output and arterial P $CO_2$ (blood is chocolate brown without change on exposure to air). Treatment of methemoglobinemia is 1–2 mg/kg of methylene blue IV administered over several minutes.

■ *Toxicity and Overdose:* If severe hypotension occurs, drug effects are quickly reversed, within 1–10 min, by decreasing rate or temporarily discontinuing infusion. May place patient in Trendelenburg position to maximize venous return.

❏ Plasma thiocyanate levels should be monitored daily in patients receiving prolonged infusions at a rate >3 mcg/kg/min or 1 mcg/kg/min in patients with anuria. Thiocyanate levels should not exceed 1 millimole/liter.

❏ Signs and symptoms of thiocyanate toxicity include tinnitus, toxic psychoses, hyperreflexia, confusion, weakness, seizures, and coma.

❏ Cyanide toxicity may manifest as lactic acidosis, hypoxemia, tachycardia, altered consciousness, seizures, and characteristic breath odor similar to almonds.

❏ Acute treatment of cyanide toxicity includes 4–6 mg/kg of *sodium nitrite* (as a 3% solution) over 2–4 min. This acts as a buffer for cyanide by converting 10% of hemoglobin to methemoglobin. If administration of sodium nitrite is delayed, inhalation of crushed ampule (vaporole, aspirole) of *amyl nitrite* for 15–30 sec of every minute should be started until sodium nitrite is running. Following completion of sodium nitrite infusion, administer *sodium thiosulfate* 150–200 mcg/kg (available as 25% and 50% solutions). This will convert cyanide to thiocyanate, which may then be eliminated. If required, entire regimen may be repeated in 2 hr at 50% of the initial doses.

## POTENTIAL NURSING DIAGNOSES

■ Tissue perfusion, ineffective (Indications).

## IMPLEMENTATION

■ **General:** If infusion of 10 mcg/kg/min for 10 min does not produce adequate reduction in blood pressure, manufacturer recommends nitroprusside be discontinued.

❏ May be administered in left ventricular CHF concurrently with an inotropic agent (dopamine, dobutamine) when effective doses of nitroprusside restore pump function and cause excessive hypotension.

■ **Continuous Infusion:** Reconstitute each 50 mg with 2–3 ml of D5W for injection without preservatives. Dilute further in 250–1000 ml of D5W for concentrations of 200–500 mcg/ml. Do not use other diluents for reconstitution or infusion. Wrap infusion bottle in aluminum foil to protect from light; administration set tubing need not be covered. Amber plastic bags do not offer sufficient protection from light; wrap must be opaque. Freshly prepared solution has a slight brownish tint; discard if solution is dark brown, orange, blue, green, or dark red. Solution must be used within 24 hr of preparation.

❏ Avoid extravasation.

■ *Rate:* Administer via infusion pump to ensure accurate dosage rate.

■ **Y-Site Compatibility:** ◆ atracurium ◆ diltiazem ◆ dobutamine ◆ dopamine ◆ enalaprilat ◆ esmolol ◆ famotidine ◆ heparin ◆ inamrinone ◆ indomethacin ◆ insulin ◆ labetalol ◆ lidocaine ◆ midazolam ◆ morphine ◆ nitroglycerin ◆ pancuronium ◆ tacrolimus ◆ theophylline ◆ vecuronium.

■ **Additive Incompatibility:** Do not admix with other medications.

**PATIENT/FAMILY TEACHING**

❑ Advise patient to report the onset of tinnitus, dyspnea, dizziness, headache, or blurred vision immediately.

**EVALUATION**

**Effectiveness of therapy can be demonstrated by:** ■ Decrease in blood pressure without the appearance of side effects ■ Treatment of cardiac pump failure or cardiogenic shock.

## nizatidine, See HISTAMINE H₂ ANTAGONISTS.

## norethindrone, See CONTRACEPTIVES, HORMONAL.

## norfloxacin, See FLUOROQUINOLONES.

## norgestimate/ethinyl estradiol, See CONTRACEPTIVES, HORMONAL.

## norgestrel, See CONTRACEPTIVES, HORMONAL.

## nortriptyline
(nor-**trip**-ti-leen)
Aventyl, Pamelor

*CLASSIFICATION(S):*
*Therapeutic:* antidepressants
*Pharmacologic:* tricyclic antidepressants

**Pregnancy Category UK**

**INDICATIONS**

■ Treatment of various forms of depression (with psychotherapy). **Unlabeled uses:** ■ Management of chronic neurogenic pain.

**ACTION**

■ Potentiates the effect of serotonin and norepinephrine ■ Has significant anticholinergic properties. **Therapeutic Effects:** ■ Antidepressant action that develops slowly over several weeks.

**PHARMACOKINETICS**

**Absorption:** Well absorbed after oral administration.

**Distribution:** Widely distributed. Enters breast milk in small amounts; probably crosses the placenta.

**Protein Binding:** 92%.

**Metabolism and Excretion:** Extensively metabolized by the liver, much of it on its first pass. Some is converted to active compounds. Undergoes enterohepatic recirculation and secretion into gastric juices.

**Half-life:** 18–28 hr.

**CONTRAINDICATIONS AND PRECAUTIONS**

**Contraindicated in:** ■ Hypersensitivity ■ Narrow-angle glaucoma ■ Alcohol intolerance (solution only) ■ Pregnancy and lactation.

**Use Cautiously in:** ■ Geriatric patients (more susceptible to adverse reactions; dosage reduction recommended) ■ Pre-existing cardiovascular disease ■ Geriatric men with prostatic hyperplasia (more susceptible to urinary retention) ■ History of seizures ■ Asthma.

**ADVERSE REACTIONS AND SIDE EFFECTS\***

■ **CNS:** drowsiness, fatigue, lethargy, agitation, confusion, extrapyramidal reactions, hallucinations, headache, insomnia ■ **EENT:** blurred vision, dry eyes, dry mouth ■ **CV:** ARRHYTHMIAS, hypotension, ECG changes ■ **GI:** constipation, nausea, paralytic ileus, unpleasant taste ■ **GU:** urinary retention ■ **Derm:** photosensitivity ■ **Endo:** gynecomastia ■ **Hemat:** blood dyscrasias ■ **Metab:** weight gain.

**INTERACTIONS**

**Drug-Drug:** ■ May cause hypertension, hyperpyrexia, seizures, and death when used with **MAO inhibitors** (avoid concurrent use—discontinue 2 wk before starting nortriptyline) ■ May prevent the therapeutic response to most **antihypertensives** ■ Hypertensive crisis may occur with **clonidine** ■ Additive CNS depression with other **CNS depressants,** including **alcohol, antihistamines, opioid analgesics,**

and **sedative/hypnotics** ∎ Adrenergic effects may be additive with other **adrenergic agents,** including **vasoconstrictors** and **decongestants** ∎Additive anticholinergic effects with other **drugs possessing anticholinergic properties,** including **antihistamines, antidepressants, atropine, haloperidol, phenothiazines, quinidine,** and **disopyramide** ∎ **Cimetidine, fluoxetine,** or **hormonal contraceptives** increase blood levels and risk of toxicity ∎ Increased risk of agranulocytosis with **antithyroid agents.**

**Drug-Natural Products:** ∎ Concomitant use of **kava, valerian, skullcap, chamomile,** or **hops** can increase CNS depression ∎ **St. John's wort** may decrease serum concentrations and efficacy ∎ Increased anticholinergic effects with **angel's trumpet, jimson weed,** and **scopolia.**

## ROUTE AND DOSAGE

∎ **PO (Adults):** 25 mg 3–4 times daily, up to 150 mg/day.
∎ **PO (Geriatric Patients):** 30–50 mg/day in divided doses.
∎ **PO (Children >12 yr):** 25–50 mg/day or 1–3 mg/kg/day in divided doses initially.
∎ **PO (Children 6–12 yr):** 10–20 mg/day or 1–3 mg/kg/day in divided doses.

## AVAILABILITY (generic available)

∎ *Capsules:* 10 mg^Rx, 25 mg^Rx, 50 mg^Rx, 75 mg^Rx ∎Cost: *Aventyl*—10 mg $52.24/100, 25 mg $63.34/100, 75 mg $75.83/100; *Pamelor*—10 mg $63.50/100, 25 mg $116.83/100, 50 mg $222.24/100, 75 mg $281.73/100; *generic*—10 mg $43.45/100, 25 mg $82.24/100, 50 mg $141.27/100, 75 mg $229.95/100 ∎ *Oral solution:* 10 mg/5 ml^Rx.

TIME/ACTION PROFILE (antidepressant effect)

| | ONSET | PEAK | DURATION |
|---|---|---|---|
| PO | 2–3 wk | 6 wk | unknown |

## NURSING IMPLICATIONS

### ASSESSMENT

∎ **General Info:** Monitor mental status and affect. Assess for suicidal tendencies, especially during early therapy. Restrict amount of drug available to patient.

❑ Monitor blood pressure and pulse rate before and during initial therapy. Report significant decreases in blood pressure or a sudden increase in pulse rate.

❑ Monitor baseline and periodic ECGs in geriatric patients or patients with heart disease. May cause prolonged PR and QT intervals and may flatten T waves.

∎ **Pain:** Assess type, location, and severity of pain before and periodically throughout therapy.

∎ *Lab Test Considerations:* Assess leukocyte and differential blood counts, liver function, and serum glucose periodically. May cause elevated serum bilirubin and alkaline phosphatase. May cause bone marrow depression. Serum glucose may be increased or decreased.

❑ Serum levels may be monitored in patients who fail to respond to usual therapeutic dose. Therapeutic plasma concentration range is 50–150 ng/ml.

❑ May cause alterations in blood glucose levels.

∎ *Toxicity and Overdose:* Symptoms of acute overdose include disturbed concentration, confusion, restlessness, agitation, seizures, drowsiness, mydriasis, arrhythmias, fever, hallucinations, vomiting, and dyspnea.

❑ Treatment of overdose includes gastric lavage, activated charcoal, and a stimulant cathartic. Maintain respiratory and cardiac function (monitor ECG for at least 5 days) and temperature. Medications may include digoxin for CHF, antiarrhythmics, and anticonvulsants.

## POTENTIAL NURSING DIAGNOSES

∎ Coping, ineffective (Indications).
∎ Injury, risk for (Side Effects).

## IMPLEMENTATION

∎ **General:** Do not confuse nortriptyline with desipramine.

∎ **PO:** Administer medication with meals to minimize gastric irritation.

❑ May be given as a single dose at bedtime to minimize sedation during the day. Dose increases should be made at bedtime because of sedation.

## PATIENT/FAMILY TEACHING

❑ Instruct patient to take medication exactly as directed. If a dose is missed, take as soon as possible unless almost time for next dose; if regimen is a single dose at bedtime, do not take in the morning because of side effects. Advise patient that drug effects may not be noticed for at least 2 wk. Abrupt discontinuation may cause nausea, vomiting, diarrhea, headache, trouble sleeping with vivid dreams, and irritability.

❑ May cause drowsiness and blurred vision. Caution patient to avoid driving and other activities requiring alertness until response to drug is known.

❑ Instruct patient to notify health care professional if visual changes occur. Inform patient that periodic glaucoma testing may be required during long-term therapy.

❑ Caution patient to make position changes slowly to minimize orthostatic hypotension. (This side effect is less pronounced with this medication than with other tricyclic antidepressants.)

❑ Advise patient to avoid alcohol or other CNS depressant drugs during therapy and for at least 3–7 days after therapy has been discontinued.

❑ Instruct patient to notify health care professional if urinary retention occurs or if dry mouth or constipation persists. Sugarless candy or gum may diminish dry mouth, and an increase in fluid intake or bulk may prevent constipation. If symptoms persist, dose reduction or discontinuation may be necessary. Consult health care professional if dry mouth persists for more than 2 wk.

❑ Caution patient to use sunscreen and protective clothing to prevent photosensitivity reactions.

❑ Inform patient of need to monitor dietary intake. Increase in appetite may lead to undesired weight gain.

❑ May have teratogenic effects. Instruct patient to notify health care professional immediately if pregnancy is planned or suspected.

❑ Advise patient to notify health care professional of medication regimen before treatment or surgery.

❑ Therapy for depression is usually prolonged. Emphasize the importance of follow-up exams and participation in prescribed psychotherapy.

## EVALUATION

**Effectiveness of therapy can be demonstrated by:** ■ Increased sense of well-being ❑ Renewed interest in surroundings ❑ Increased appetite ❑ Improved energy level ❑ Improved sleep ■ Decrease in severity of chronic neurogenic pain. Patients may require 2–6 wk of therapy before full therapeutic effects of medication are seen.

# nystatin
(nye-**stat**-in)
Mycostatin, {Nadostine}, Nilstat, Nystex, {PMS-Nystatin}

## CLASSIFICATION(S):
**Therapeutic:** antifungals (topical/local)

### Pregnancy Category B

For other nystatin dosage forms, see antifungals (topical) and antifungals (vaginal).

## INDICATIONS

■ **Lozenges, oral suspension:** Local treatment of oropharyngeal candidiasis ■ Treatment of intestinal candidiasis.

## ACTION

■ Binds to fungal cell membrane, allowing leakage of cellular contents. **Therapeutic Effects:** ■ Fungistatic or fungicidal action. **Spectrum:** ■ Active against most pathogenic *Candida* species, including *C. albicans*.

## PHARMACOKINETICS

**Absorption:** Poorly absorbed; action is primarily local.
**Distribution:** Unknown.
**Metabolism and Excretion:** Excreted unchanged in the feces after oral administration.
**Half-life:** Unknown.

## CONTRAINDICATIONS AND PRECAUTIONS

**Contraindicated in:** ■ Hypersensitivity ■ Some products may contain ethyl alcohol or benzyl alcohol—avoid use in patients who may be hypersensitive to or intolerant of these additives.

**Use Cautiously in:** ■ Denture wearers (dentures require soaking in nystatin suspension) ■ Children <5 yr (lozenges, pastilles, troches).

## ADVERSE REACTIONS AND SIDE EFFECTS*

■ **GI:** diarrhea, nausea, stomach pain (large doses), vomiting.

## INTERACTIONS

**Drug-Drug:** ■ None significant.

## ROUTE AND DOSAGE

■ **PO (Adults and Children):** 400,000–600,000 units 4 times daily as oral suspension or 200,000–400,000 units 4–5 times daily as pastilles (lozenges).
■ **PO (Infants):** 200,000 units 4 times daily.
■ **PO (Infants, Premature and Low Birth Weight):** 100,000 units 4 times daily.

## AVAILABILITY (generic available)

■ *Oral suspension:* 100,000 units/ml in 5-, 60-, and 480-ml containers^Rx ■ Cost: *Mycostatin*— $28.20/60 ml; *generic*—60 ml $8.23/60 ml ■ *Oral pastilles (lozenges, troches):* 200,000 units/troche^Rx ■ *Powder for oral suspension:* ⅛ tsp = 500,000 units in 50-, 150-, and 500-million, 1-, 2-, and 5-billion-unit containers^Rx ■ *Oral tablets:* 500,000 units^Rx ■ Cost: *Mycostatin*—$72.93/100; *generic*—$48.96/100.

TIME/ACTION PROFILE (antifungal effects)

| | ONSET | PEAK | DURATION |
|---|---|---|---|
| Top | rapid | unknown | 2 hr† |

†Maintenance of saliva levels required to inhibit growth of *Candida* species after oral dissolution of 2 lozenges.

## NURSING IMPLICATIONS

### ASSESSMENT

❏ Inspect oral mucous membranes before and frequently throughout therapy. Increased irritation of mucous membranes may indicate need to discontinue medication.

### POTENTIAL NURSING DIAGNOSES

■ Skin integrity, risk for impaired (Indications).
■ Infection, risk for (Indications).

### IMPLEMENTATION

■ **PO:** Suspension should be administered by placing ½ of dose in each side of mouth. Patient should hold suspension in mouth or swish throughout mouth for several minutes before swallowing, then gargle and swallow. Use calibrated measuring device for liquid doses. Shake well before administration.
❏ To prepare oral solution from powder, add ⅛ tsp (approximately 500,000 units) to 120 ml of water and stir well. Prepare immediately before use; contains no preservatives.
❏ Lozenges (pastilles) should be allowed to dissolve slowly and completely in mouth; do not chew or swallow whole. Nystatin vaginal tablets can be administered orally for treatment of oral candidiasis.

### PATIENT/FAMILY TEACHING

❏ Instruct patient to take medication as directed. If a dose is missed, take as soon as remembered but not if almost time for next dose. Do not double doses. Therapy should be continued for at least 2 days after symptoms subside.
❏ Advise patient to report increased irritation of mucous membranes or lack of therapeutic response to health care professional.

### EVALUATION

**Effectiveness of therapy can be demonstrated by:** ■ Decrease in stomatitis ❏ To prevent relapse after oral therapy, therapy should be continued for 48 hr after symptoms have disappeared and cultures are negative ❏ Therapy for a period of 2 wk is usually sufficient, but more prolonged therapy may be necessary.

**nystatin, See also ANTIFUNGALS (TOPICAL), ANTIFUNGALS (VAGINAL).**

## octreotide

(ok-**tree**-oh-tide)
Sandostatin, Sandostatin LAR

*CLASSIFICATION(S):*
*Therapeutic: antidiarrheals, hormones*

**Pregnancy Category B**

### INDICATIONS

■ Treatment of severe diarrhea and flushing episodes in patients with GI endocrine tumors, including metastatic carcinoid tumors and vasoactive intestinal peptide tumors (VIPomas). **Unlabeled uses:** ■ Relief of symptoms and suppressed tumor growth in patients with pituitary tumors associated with acromegaly ■ Management of diarrhea in AIDS patients or patients with fistulas.

### ACTION

■ Suppresses secretion of serotonin and gastroenterohepatic peptides ■ Increases absorption of fluid and electrolytes from the GI tract and increases transit time ■ Decreases levels of serotonin metabolites ■ Also suppresses growth hormone, insulin, and glucagon. **Therapeutic Effects:** ■ Control of severe flushing and diarrhea associated with GI endocrine tumors.

### PHARMACOKINETICS

**Absorption:** Well absorbed following subcut administration and IM administration of depot form.
**Distribution:** Unknown.
**Protein Binding:** 65%.
**Metabolism and Excretion:** 32% excreted unchanged in urine.
**Half-life:** 1.5 hr.

### CONTRAINDICATIONS AND PRECAUTIONS

**Contraindicated in:** ■ Hypersensitivity.
**Use Cautiously in:** ■ Gallbladder disease (increased risk of stone formation) ■ Renal impairment (dosage reduction may be necessary) ■ Hyperglycemia or hypoglycemia (changes in blood glucose may occur) ■ Fat malabsorption

(may be aggravated) ■ Pregnancy or lactation (safety not established).

### ADVERSE REACTIONS AND SIDE EFFECTS*

■ **CNS:** dizziness, drowsiness, fatigue, headache, weakness ■ **EENT:** visual disturbances ■ **CV:** edema, orthostatic hypotension, palpitations ■ **GI:** abdominal pain, cholelithiasis, diarrhea, fat malabsorption, nausea, vomiting ■ **Derm:** flushing ■ **Endo:** hyperglycemia, hypoglycemia ■ **Local:** injection-site pain.

### INTERACTIONS

**Drug-Drug:** ■ May alter requirements for **insulin** or **oral hypoglycemic agents** ■ May reduce blood levels of **cyclosporine**.

### ROUTE AND DOSAGE

❑ **Carcinoid Tumors**

■ **Subcut, IV (Adults):** *Sandostatin*—100–600 mcg/day in 2–4 divided doses during first 2 wk of therapy (range 50–1500 mcg/day).
■ **IM (Adults):** *Sandostatin LAR*—20 mg q 4 wk for 2 mo; dosage may be further adjusted.

❑ **VIPomas**

■ **Subcut, IV (Adults):** *Sandostatin*—200–300 mcg/day in 2–4 divided doses during first 2 wk of therapy (range 150–750 mcg/day).
■ **IM (Adults):** *Sandostatin LAR*—20 mg q 2 wk for 2 mo; dosage may be further adjusted.

❑ **Suppression of Growth Hormone (Acromegaly)**

■ **Subcut, IV (Adults):** *Sandostatin*—50–100 mcg 2–3 times daily.
■ **IM (Adults):** *Sandostatin LAR*—20 mg q 4 wk for 3 mo, then adjusted on the basis of growth hormone levels.

❑ **Antidiarrheal (AIDS Patients)**

■ **Subcut, IV (Adults):** 100–1800 mcg/day (unlabeled).

### AVAILABILITY

■ *Injection:* 0.05 mg/ml in 1-ml ampules[Rx], 0.1 mg/ml in 1-ml ampules[Rx], 0.2 mg/ml in 5-

ml vials^Rx, 0.5 mg/ml in 1-ml ampules^Rx, 1 mg/ml in 5-ml vials^Rx ■ Cost: 50 mcg/ml 5-ml vial $121.44/20 vials, 100 mcg/ml 5-ml vial $235.54/20 vials, 200 mcg/ml 5-ml vial $121.41/vial, 500 mcg/ml 1-ml vial $1136.08/20 vials, 1 mg/ml 5-ml vial $597.43/vial ■ *Depot injection:* 10 mg^Rx, 20 mg^Rx, 30 mg^Rx ■ Cost: 10 mg $1368.75/injection, 20 mg $1368.75/injection, 30 mg $2053.12/injection.

TIME/ACTION PROFILE (control of symptoms)

| | ONSET | PEAK | DURATION |
|---|---|---|---|
| Subcut, IV | unknown | unknown | up to 12 hr |
| IM (LAR) | unknown | 2 wk | up to 4 wk |

## NURSING IMPLICATIONS

### ASSESSMENT

- ❑ Assess frequency and consistency of stools and bowel sounds throughout therapy.
- ❑ Monitor pulse and blood pressure prior to and periodically throughout therapy.
- ❑ Assess patient's fluid and electrolyte balance and skin turgor for dehydration.
- ❑ Monitor diabetic patients for signs of hypoglycemia. May require reduction in requirements for insulin and sulfonylureas and treatment with diazoxide.
- ❑ Assess patient for gallbladder disease; assess for pain and monitor ultrasound examinations of gallbladder and bile ducts prior to and periodically throughout prolonged therapy.
- ■ *Lab Test Considerations:* Monitor 5-HIAA (urinary 5-hydroxyindoleacetic acid), plasma serotonin, and plasma substance P in patients with carcinoid; plasma vasoactive intestinal peptide (VIP) in patients with VIPoma; and free $T_4$ and serum glucose concentrations prior to and periodically throughout therapy in all patients taking octreotide.
- ❑ Monitor quantitative 72-hr fecal fat and serum carotene determinations periodically for possible drug-induced aggravations of fat malabsorption.
- ❑ May cause a slight increase in liver enzymes.
- ❑ May cause decreased serum thyroxine ($T_4$) concentrations.

### POTENTIAL NURSING DIAGNOSES

- ■ Diarrhea (Indications).

## IMPLEMENTATION

- ■ **General:** Do not use solution that is discolored or contains particulate matter. Ampules should be refrigerated but may be stored at room temperature for the days they will be used. Discard unused solution.
- ■ **Subcut:** Administer the smallest volume needed to achieve required dose to prevent pain at injection site. Rotate injection sites; avoid multiple injections in same site within short periods of time. Preferred injection sites are the hip, thigh, or abdomen.
- ❑ Administer injections between meals and at bedtime to avoid GI side effects.
- ❑ Allow medication to reach room temperature prior to injection to minimize local reactions at injection site.
- ■ **IM:** Mix IM solution by adding diluent included in kit. Administer immediately after mixing into the gluteal muscle. Avoid using deltoid site due to pain of injection.
- ❑ Patients with carcinoid tumors and VIPomas should continue to receive subcut dose for 2 wk following switch to IM depot form to maintain therapeutic level.
- ■ **Direct IV:** Bolus injections have been used under emergency conditions.
- ■ *Rate:* Administer over 3 min.
- ■ **Intermittent Infusion:** Dilute in 50–200 ml of 0.9% NaCl or D5W.
- ■ *Rate:* Administer over 15–30 min.

### PATIENT/FAMILY TEACHING

- ■ **General Info:** May cause dizziness, drowsiness, or visual disturbances. Caution patient to avoid driving or other activities requiring alertness until response to medication is known.
- ❑ Advise patient to change positions slowly to minimize orthostatic hypotension.
- ■ **Home Care Issues:** Instruct patients administering octreotide at home on correct technique for injection, storage, and disposal of equipment.
- ❑ Instruct patient to administer octreotide exactly as directed. If a dose is missed, administer as soon as possible, then return to regular schedule. Do not double doses.

### EVALUATION

**Effectiveness of therapy can be demonstrated by:** ■ Decrease in severity of diarrhea and improvement of electrolyte imbalances in patients with carcinoid or VIP-secreting tumors ■ Relief of symptoms and suppressed tumor growth in patients with pituitary tumors associated with acromegaly ■ Management of diarrhea in patients with AIDS.

## ofloxacin, See FLUOROQUINOLONES.

## olanzapine
(oh-**lan**-za-peen)
Zyprexa, Zyprexa Zydis

*CLASSIFICATION(S):*
*Therapeutic: antipsychotics*
*Pharmacologic: thienobenzodiazepines*

**Pregnancy Category C**

### INDICATIONS

■ Psychotic disorders including ❑ Acute manic episodes associated with bipolar disorder (may be used with lithium or valproate) ❑ long-term treatment/maintenance of schizophrenia. **Unlabeled uses:** ■ Management of anorexia nervosa.

### ACTION

■ Antagonizes dopamine and serotonin type 2 in the CNS ■ Also has anticholinergic, antihistaminic, and anti–alpha$_1$-adrenergic effects. **Therapeutic Effects:** ■ Decreased manifestations of psychoses.

### PHARMACOKINETICS

**Absorption:** Well absorbed but rapidly metabolized by first-pass effect, resulting in 60% bioavailability. Conventional tablets and orally disintegrating tablets are bioequivalent.

**Distribution:** Extensively distributed.

**Protein Binding:** 93%.

**Metabolism and Excretion:** Highly metabolized (mostly by the hepatic P450 CYP 1A2 system); 7% excreted unchanged in urine.

**Half-life:** 21–54 hr.

### CONTRAINDICATIONS AND PRECAUTIONS

**Contraindicated in:** ■ Hypersensitivity ■ Lactation ■ **Orally disintegrating tablets only:** Phenylketonuria (orally disintegrating tablets contain aspartame).

**Use Cautiously in:** ■ Patients with hepatic impairment ■ Geriatric patients (may require smaller doses) ■ Cardiovascular or cerebrovascular disease ■ History of seizures ■ History of attempted suicide ■ Prostatic hypertrophy ■ Narrow-angle glaucoma ■ History of paralytic ileus ■ Pregnancy or children <18 yr (safety not established).

### ADVERSE REACTIONS AND SIDE EFFECTS*

■ **CNS:** NEUROLEPTIC MALIGNANT SYNDROME , SEIZURES , agitation, dizziness, headache, restlessness, sedation, weakness, dystonia, insomnia, mood changes, personality disorder, speech impairment, tardive dyskinesia ■ **EENT:** amblyopia, rhinitis, increased salivation, pharyngitis ■ **Resp:** cough, dyspnea ■ **CV:** orthostatic hypotension, tachycardia, chest pain ■ **GI:** constipation, dry mouth, abdominal pain, increased appetite, nausea ■ **GU:** decreased libido, urinary incontinence ■ **Derm:** photosensitivity ■ **Endo:** diabetes mellitus, goiter ■ **F and E:** increased thirst ■ **Metab:** weight gain, weight loss ■ **MS:** hypertonia, joint pain ■ **Neuro:** tremor ■ **Misc:** fever, flu-like syndrome.

### INTERACTIONS

**Drug-Drug:** ■ Effects may be ↓ by concurrent **carbamazepine, omeprazole,** or **rifampin** ■ ↑ hypotension may occur with **antihypertensives** ■ ↑ CNS depression may occur with concurrent use of **alcohol** or other **CNS depressants** ■ May antagonize the effects of **levodopa** or other **dopamine agonists.**

### ROUTE AND DOSAGE

■ **PO (Adults—Most Patients):** *Schizophrenia*—5–10 mg/day initially; may increase at weekly intervals by 5 mg/day (not to exceed 20 mg/day). *Bipolar mania*—10–15 mg/day initially; may increase every 24 hr by 5 mg/day (not to exceed 20 mg/day).

{ } = Available in Canada only.
*CAPITALS indicates life-threatening; underlines indicate most frequent.

■ **PO (Adults—Debilitated or Non-smoking Female Patients ≥65 yr):** Initiate therapy at 5 mg/day.

## AVAILABILITY

■ **Tablets:** 2.5 mg$^{Rx}$, 5 mg$^{Rx}$, 7.5 mg$^{Rx}$, 10 mg$^{Rx}$, 15 mg$^{Rx}$ ■ Cost: 2.5 mg $311.21/60, 5 mg $367.57/60, 7.5 mg $405.32/60, 10 mg $558.72/60, 15 mg $838.08/60 ■ **Orally disintegrating tablets (Zydis):** 5 mg$^{Rx}$, 10 mg$^{Rx}$, 15 mg$^{Rx}$, 20 mg$^{Rx}$ ■ Cost: 10 mg $315.10/30.

TIME/ACTION PROFILE (antipsychotic effects)

| | ONSET | PEAK | DURATION |
|---|---|---|---|
| PO | unknown | 1 wk | unknown |

## NURSING IMPLICATIONS

### ASSESSMENT

■ **General Info:** Assess mental status (orientation, mood, behavior) before and periodically during therapy.

❑ Monitor blood pressure (sitting, standing, lying), ECG, pulse, and respiratory rate before and frequently during the period of dose adjustment.

❑ Observe patient carefully when administering medication to ensure that medication is actually taken and not hoarded.

❑ Assess fluid intake and bowel function. Increased bulk and fluids in the diet may help minimize constipation.

❑ Monitor patient for onset of akathisia (restlessness or desire to keep moving) and extrapyramidal side effects (*parkinsonian*—difficulty speaking or swallowing, loss of balance control, pill rolling, mask-like face, shuffling gait, rigidity, tremors; and *dystonic*—muscle spasms, twisting motions, twitching, inability to move eyes, weakness of arms or legs) every 2 mo during therapy and 8–12 wk after therapy has been discontinued. Report these symptoms if they occur, as reduction in dosage or discontinuation of medication may be necessary. Trihexyphenidyl or diphenhydramine may be used to control symptoms.

❑ Monitor for tardive dyskinesia (uncontrolled rhythmic movement of mouth, face, and extremities; lip smacking or puckering; puffing of cheeks; uncontrolled chewing; rapid or worm-like movements of tongue). Report immediately; may be irreversible.

❑ Monitor for development of neuroleptic malignant syndrome (fever, respiratory distress, tachycardia, seizures, diaphoresis, hypertension or hypotension, pallor, tiredness, severe muscle stiffness, loss of bladder control). Notify physician or other health care professional immediately if these symptoms occur.

■ **Lab Test Considerations:** Evaluate CBC, liver function tests, and ocular examinations periodically during therapy. May cause ↓ platelets. May cause ↑ bilirubin, AST, ALT, GGT, CPK, and alkaline phosphatase.

## POTENTIAL NURSING DIAGNOSES

■ Thought processes, disturbed (Indications).
■ Noncompliance (Patient/Family Teaching).

## IMPLEMENTATION

■ **General:** Do not confuse Zyprexa (olanzapine) with Celexa (citalopram) or Zyrtec (cetirizine).

■ **PO:** May be administered without regard to meals.

❑ For orally disintegrating tablets, peel back foil on blister, do not push tablet through foil. Using dry hands, remove from foil and place entire tablet in mouth. Tablet will disintegrate with or without liquid.

### PATIENT/FAMILY TEACHING

❑ Advise patient to take medication as directed and not to skip doses or double up on missed doses. May need to discontinue gradually.

❑ Inform patient of possibility of extrapyramidal symptoms and tardive dyskinesia. Instruct patient to report these symptoms immediately to health care professional.

❑ Advise patient to change positions slowly to minimize orthostatic hypotension.

❑ Medication may cause drowsiness. Caution patient to avoid driving or other activities requiring alertness until response to the medication is known.

❑ Caution patient to avoid taking alcohol or other CNS depressants concurrently with this medication.

❑ Advise patient to use sunscreen and protective clothing when exposed to the sun. Extremes of temperature (exercise, hot weather, hot baths or showers) should also be avoided because this drug impairs body temperature regulation.

- ❑ Instruct patient to use frequent mouth rinses, good oral hygiene, and sugarless gum or candy to minimize dry mouth. Consult health care professional if dry mouth continues for >2 wk.
- ❑ Advise patient to notify health care professional of medication regimen before treatment or surgery.
- ❑ Instruct patient to notify health care professional promptly if sore throat, fever, unusual bleeding or bruising, rash, weakness, tremors, visual disturbances, dark-colored urine, or clay-colored stools occur.
- ❑ Emphasize the importance of routine follow-up exams and continued participation in psychotherapy as indicated.

### EVALUATION

**Effectiveness of therapy can be demonstrated by:** ■ Decrease in excitable, paranoic, or withdrawn behavior.

## olmesartan, See ANGIOTENSIN II RECEPTOR ANTAGONISTS.

## olsalazine

(ole-**sal**-a-zeen)

Dipentum

**CLASSIFICATION(S):**

**Therapeutic:** gastrointestinal anti-inflammatories

**Pregnancy Category C**

### INDICATIONS

■ Ulcerative colitis (when patients cannot tolerate sulfasalazine).

### ACTION

■ Locally acting anti-inflammatory action in the colon, where activity is probably due to inhibition of prostaglandin synthesis. **Therapeutic Effects:** ■ Reduction in the symptoms of inflammatory bowel disease.

### PHARMACOKINETICS

**Absorption:** Acts locally in colon, where 98–99% is converted to mesalamine (5-aminosalicylic acid).

**Distribution:** Action is primarily local and remains in the colon.

**Metabolism and Excretion:** 2% absorbed into systemic circulation is rapidly metabolized; mostly eliminated as mesalamine in the feces.

**Half-life:** 0.9 hr.

### CONTRAINDICATIONS AND PRECAUTIONS

**Contraindicated in:** ■ Hypersensitivity reactions to salicylates ■ Cross-sensitivity with furosemide, sulfonylurea hypoglycemic agents, or carbonic anhydrase inhibitors may exist ■ G6PD deficiency ■ Urinary tract or intestinal obstruction ■ Children <2 yr (safe use not established) ■ Porphyria.

**Use Cautiously in:** ■ Severe hepatic or renal impairment ■ Pregnancy ■ Geriatric patients (consider decrease in body mass, hepatic/renal/cardiac function, intercurrent illness and drug therapies ■ Renal impairment (increased risk of renal tubular damage) ■ Lactation (safety not established).

### ADVERSE REACTIONS AND SIDE EFFECTS*

■ **CNS:** ataxia, confusion, dizziness, drowsiness, headache, mental depression, psychosis, restlessness ■ **GI:** diarrhea, abdominal pain, anorexia, exacerbation of colitis, drug-induced hepatitis, nausea, vomiting ■ **Derm:** itching, rash ■ **Hemat:** blood dyscrasias.

### INTERACTIONS

**Drug-Drug:** ■ May ↓ metabolism and increase effects/toxicity of **mercaptopurine** or **thioguanine**.

### ROUTE AND DOSAGE

■ **PO (Adults):** 500 mg twice daily.

### AVAILABILITY

■ **Capsules:** 250 mg[Rx].

TIME/ACTION PROFILE (levels)

| | ONSET | PEAK | Duration |
|---|---|---|---|
| PO | unknown | 1 hr; 4–8 hr | 12 hr |

# NURSING IMPLICATIONS

## ASSESSMENT

- **General Info:** Assess patient for allergy to sulfonamides and salicylates. Patients allergic to sulfasalazine may take mesalamine or olsalazine without difficulty, but therapy should be discontinued if rash or fever occur.
- Monitor intake and output ratios. Fluid intake should be sufficient to maintain a urine output of at least 1200–1500 ml daily to prevent crystalluria and stone formation.
- **Inflammatory Bowel Disease:** Assess abdominal pain and frequency, quantity, and consistency of stools at the beginning of and throughout therapy.
- *Lab Test Considerations:* Monitor urinalysis, BUN, and serum creatinine prior to and periodically during therapy.
- Olsalazine may cause ↑ AST and ALT levels. Monitor CBC prior to and every 3–6 mo during prolonged therapy. Discontinue olsalazine if blood dyscrasias occur.

## POTENTIAL NURSING DIAGNOSES

- Pain, acute (Indications).
- Diarrhea (Indications).

## IMPLEMENTATION

- **PO:** Administer with food in evenly divided doses every 12 hr.

## PATIENT/FAMILY TEACHING

- Instruct patient to take medication as directed, even if feeling better. Take missed doses as soon as remembered unless almost time for next dose.
- May cause dizziness. Caution patient to avoid driving or other activities that require alertness until response to medication is known.
- Advise patient to notify health care professional if skin rash, sore throat, fever, mouth sores, unusual bleeding or bruising, wheezing, fever, or hives occurs.
- Instruct patient to notify health care professional if symptoms do not improve after 1–2 mo of therapy.
- Instruct patient to notify health care professional if symptoms worsen or do not improve. If symptoms of acute intolerance (cramping, acute abdominal pain, bloody diarrhea, fever, headache, rash) occur, discontinue therapy and notify health care professional immediately.
- Inform patient that proctoscopy and sigmoidoscopy may be required periodically during treatment to determine response.

## EVALUATION

**Clinical response to therapy can be evaluated by:** ■ Decrease in diarrhea and abdominal pain ■ Return to normal bowel pattern in patients with inflammatory bowel disease. Effects may be seen within 3–21 days. The usual course of therapy is 3–6 wk ■ Maintenance of remission in patients with inflammatory bowel disease ■ Decrease in pain and inflammation, and increase in mobility in patients with rheumatoid arthritis.

---

# omalizumab
(o-ma-**liz**-u-mab)
Xolair

## CLASSIFICATION(S):
*Therapeutic:* antiasthmatics
*Pharmacologic:* monoclonal antibodies

### Pregnancy Category B

---

## INDICATIONS

- Moderate to severe asthma not controlled by inhaled corticosteroids.

## ACTION

- Inhibits binding of IgE to receptors on mast cells and eosinophils; preventing the release of mediators of the allergic response. Also decreases amount of IgE receptors on basophils. **Therapeutic Effects:** ■ Decreased incidence of exacerbations of asthma.

## PHARMACOKINETICS

**Absorption:** 62% absorbed slowly from subcut sites.
**Distribution:** Enters breast milk.

**Metabolism and Excretion:** Degraded similarly to IgG via binding degradation, reticuloendothelial system and the liver.
**Half-life:** 26 days.

## CONTRAINDICATIONS AND PRECAUTIONS

**Contraindicated in:** ■ Hypersensitivity ■ Acute bronchospasm.

**Use Cautiously in:** ■ Chronic use of inhaled corticosteroids ■ Pregnancy, lactation, or children <12 yr (safety not established, use in pregnancy only if clearly needed.

## ADVERSE REACTIONS AND SIDE EFFECTS*

■ **Local:** injection site reactions ■ **Misc:** allergic reactions including ANAPHYLAXIS, ↑ risk of malignancy.

## INTERACTIONS

**Drug-Drug:** ■ None noted.

## ROUTE AND DOSAGE

■ **Subcut (Adults and Children >12 yr):** 150–375 mg every 2–4 wk (determined by pretreatment serum IgE level and body weight).

## AVAILABILITY

■ **Sterile powder for subcut injection (requires reconstitution:** 150 mg/vial.

TIME/ACTION PROFILE (effects on IgE levels)

| | ONSET | PEAK | DURATION |
|---|---|---|---|
| Subcut | within 1 hr | unknown | up to 1 yr |

# NURSING IMPLICATIONS

## ASSESSMENT

❑ Assess lung sounds and respiratory function prior to and periodically during therapy.
❑ Assess allergy symptoms (rhinitis, conjunctivitis, hives) before and periodically throughout therapy.
❑ Assess for allergic reactions (urticaria, tongue and/or throat edema) within 2 hr of first or subsequent injections. Observe patient following injection. Epinephrine, di-phenhydramine, and corticosteroids should be available in case of anaphylaxis.
❑ Monitor for injection site reactions (bruising, redness, warmth, burning, stinging, itching, hives, pain, induration, mass, inflammation). Usually occur within 1 hr of injection, last <8 days, and decrease in frequency with subsequent dosing.
■ **Lab Test Considerations:** Serum IgE levels will ↑ following administration and may persist for up to 1 year following discontinuation. Serum total IgE levels obtained <1 year following discontinuation may not reflect steady state free IgE levels and should not be used to reassess the dosing regimen.

## POTENTIAL NURSING DIAGNOSES

■ Airway clearance, ineffective.

## IMPLEMENTATION

■ **General:** Doses of inhaled corticosteroids may be gradually decreased with supervision of health care professional; do not discontinue abruptly.
■ **Subcut:** To reconstitute draw 1.4 ml of sterile water for injection into a 3-cc syringe with a 1-inch 18-gauge needle. With the vial upright on a flat surface, inject the sterile water into vial. Keep vial upright and gently swirl for approximately 1 min to evenly wet powder. Do not shake. Lyophilized omalizumab takes 15–20 min to dissolve. Gently swirl vial for 5–10 seconds every 5 min to dissolve any remaining particles. Solution should be clear or slightly opalescent and may have small bubbles or foam around edge of vial. Do not use if particles are visible or if contents do not dissolve completely within 40 min. Invert vial for 15 seconds to allow solution to drain toward stopper. Solution may be somewhat viscous. In order to obtain full 1.2 ml dose, all of solution must be withdrawn from the vial using a new 3-cc syringe with an 18-gauge needle, before expelling any air or excess solution from syringe. Administer within 8 hr if refrigerated or within 4 hr if stored at room temperature. Discard unused solution.
❑ Replace the 18-gauge needle with a 25-gauge needle for subcut injection. Because solution is slightly viscous, injection may take 5–10

---

{ } = Available in Canada only.
*CAPITALS indicates life-threatening; underlines indicate most frequent.

seconds to administer. Divide doses >150 mg into 2 injection sites.

## PATIENT/FAMILY TEACHING

❏ Explain purpose of medication to patient. Inform patient that they may not see immediate results from omalizumab therapy.

❏ Instruct patient not to discontinue or reduce other asthma medications, especially inhaled corticosteroids, without consulting health care professional.

## EVALUATION

**Effectiveness of therapy can be demonstrated by:** ▪ Decreased incidence of exacerbations of asthma.

## omeprazole

(o-**mep**-ra-zole)

{Losec}, Prilosec

### CLASSIFICATION(S):

**Therapeutic:** antiulcer agents
**Pharmacologic:** proton-pump inhibitors

### Pregnancy Category C

## INDICATIONS

▪ GERD ▪ Duodenal ulcers (with or without anti-infectives for *Helicobacter pylori*) ▪ Pathologic hypersecretory conditions, including Zollinger-Ellison syndrome ▪ OTC: Heartburn occuring ≥ twice/wk.

## ACTION

▪ Binds to an enzyme on gastric parietal cells in the presence of acidic gastric pH, preventing the final transport of hydrogen ions into the gastric lumen. **Therapeutic Effects:** ▪ Diminished accumulation of acid in the gastric lumen with lessened gastroesophageal reflux ▪ Healing of duodenal ulcers.

## PHARMACOKINETICS

**Absorption:** Rapidly absorbed following oral administration.
**Distribution:** Good distribution into gastric parietal cells.
**Protein Binding:** 95%.
**Metabolism and Excretion:** Extensively metabolized by the liver.

**Half-life:** 0.5–1 hr (increased in liver disease).

## CONTRAINDICATIONS AND PRECAUTIONS

**Contraindicated in:** ▪ Hypersensitivity.

**Use Cautiously in:** ▪ Liver disease (dosage reduction may be necessary) ▪ Pregnancy, lactation, or children <2 yr (safety not established).

## ADVERSE REACTIONS AND SIDE EFFECTS*

▪ **CNS:** dizziness, drowsiness, fatigue, headache, weakness ▪ **CV:** chest pain ▪ **GI:** <u>abdominal pain</u>, acid regurgitation, constipation, diarrhea, flatulence, nausea, vomiting ▪ **Derm:** itching, rash ▪ **Misc:** allergic reactions.

## INTERACTIONS

**Drug-Drug:** ▪ Omperazole is metabolized by the CYP450 enzyme system and may compete with other agents metabolized by this system ▪ ↓ metabolism and may ↑ effects of **diazepam, flurazepam, triazolam, cyclosporine, disulfiram, phenytoin,** and **warfarin** ▪ May interfere with absorption of drugs requiring acidic gastric pH, including esters of **ampicillin, iron salts, digoxin, cyanocobalamine,** and **ketoconazole** ▪ Has been used safely with **antacids** ▪ May increase the risk of bleeding with **warfarin** (monitor INR/PT).

## ROUTE AND DOSAGE

▪ **PO (Adults):** *GERD*—20 mg once daily. *Duodenal ulcers associated with* H. pylori—40 mg daily in the morning with clarithromycin for 2 wk, then 20 mg once daily for 2 wk *or* 20 mg twice daily with clarithromycin 500 mg twice daily and amoxicillin 1000 mg twice daily for 10 days (if ulcer is present at beginning of therapy, continue omeprazole 20 mg daily for 18 more days); has also been used with clarithromycin and metronidazole. *Gastric ulcer*—40 mg once daily for 4–6 wk. *Gastric hypersecretory conditions*—60 mg once daily initially; may be increased up to 120 mg 3 times daily (doses >80 mg/day should be given in divided doses); *OTC*—20 mg once daily for up to 14 days.

▪ **PO (Children >2 yr and <20 kg):** 10 mg once daily.

- **PO (Children >2 yr and ≥20 kg):** 20 mg once daily.

## AVAILABILITY (generic available)

- **Delayed-release capsules:** 10 mg$^{Rx}$, 20 mg$^{Rx}$, $^{OTC}$, 40 mg$^{Rx}$ ■ Cost: 10 mg $119.06/30, 20 mg $429.98/100, 40 mg $190.70/30 ■ metronidazole and clarithromycin in a compliance package (Losec 1-2-3 M); with amoxicillin and clarithromycin in a compliance package (Losec 1-2-3-A) (in Canada only; see Appendix B).

TIME/ACTION PROFILE (antisecretory effects)

|     | ONSET | PEAK | DURATION |
|-----|-------|------|----------|
| PO  | within 1 hr | within 2 hr | 72–96 hr |

## NURSING IMPLICATIONS

### ASSESSMENT

- ❑ Assess patient routinely for epigastric or abdominal pain and frank or occult blood in the stool, emesis, or gastric aspirate.
- ■ **Lab Test Considerations:** Monitor CBC with differential periodically during therapy.
- ❑ May cause ↑ AST, ALT, alkaline phosphatase, and bilirubin.
- ❑ May cause serum gastrin concentrations to ↑ during first 1–2 wk of therapy. Levels return to normal after discontinuation of omeprazole.
- ❑ Monitor INR and prothrombin time in patients taking warfarin.

### POTENTIAL NURSING DIAGNOSES

- ■ Pain, acute (Indications).

### IMPLEMENTATION

- ■ **General:** Do not confuse Prilosec (omeprazole) with Prinivil (lisinopril).
- ■ **PO:** Administer doses before meals, preferably in the morning. Capsules should be swallowed whole; do not crush or chew. Capsules may be opened and sprinkled on cool applesauce; entire mixture should be ingested immediately and followed by a drink of water. Do not store for future use.
- ❑ May be administered concurrently with antacids.

### PATIENT/FAMILY TEACHING

- ❑ Instruct patient to take medication as directed for the full course of therapy, even if feeling better. Take missed doses as soon as remembered but not if almost time for next dose. Do not double doses.
- ❑ May cause occasional drowsiness or dizziness. Caution patient to avoid driving or other activities requiring alertness until response to medication is known.
- ❑ Advise patient to avoid alcohol, products containing aspirin or NSAIDs, and foods that may cause an increase in GI irritation.
- ❑ Advise patient to report onset of black, tarry stools; diarrhea; abdominal pain; or persistent headache to health care professional promptly.

### EVALUATION

**Effectiveness of therapy can be demonstrated by:** ■ Decrease in abdominal pain or prevention of gastric irritation and bleeding. Healing of duodenal ulcers can be seen on x-ray examination or endoscopy ■ Decrease in symptoms of GERD. Therapy is continued for 4–8 wk after initial episode.

## ondansetron
(on-**dan**-se-tron)
Zofran

### CLASSIFICATION(S):
**Therapeutic:** antiemetics
**Pharmacologic:** 5 HT$_3$ antagonists

### Pregnancy Category B

### INDICATIONS

■ Prevention of nausea and vomiting associated with chemotherapy or radiation therapy ■ **IM, IV:** Prevention and treatment of postoperative nausea and vomiting.

### ACTION

■ Blocks the effects of serotonin at 5-HT$_3$–receptor sites (selective antagonist) located in vagal nerve terminals and the chemoreceptor trigger zone in the CNS. **Therapeutic Effects:** ■ Decreased incidence and severity of nausea and vomiting following chemotherapy or surgery.

## PHARMACOKINETICS

**Absorption:** IV administration results in complete bioavailability; 50% absorbed following oral administration.

**Distribution:** Unknown.

**Metabolism and Excretion:** Extensively metabolized by the liver; 5% excreted unchanged by the kidneys.

**Half-life:** 3.5–5.5 hr.

## CONTRAINDICATIONS AND PRECAUTIONS

**Contraindicated in:** ■ Hypersensitivity ■ Orally disintegrating tablets contain aspartame and should not be used in patients with phenylketonuria.

**Use Cautiously in:** ■ Liver impairment (daily dose not to exceed 8 mg) ■ Abdominal surgery (may mask ileus) ■ Pregnancy, lactation, or children ≤3 yr (safety not established).

## ADVERSE REACTIONS AND SIDE EFFECTS*

■ **CNS:** <u>headache</u>, dizziness, drowsiness, fatigue, weakness ■ **GI:** <u>constipation</u>, <u>diarrhea</u>, abdominal pain, dry mouth, increased liver enzymes ■ **Neuro:** extrapyramidal reactions.

## INTERACTIONS

**Drug-Drug:** ■ May be affected by **drugs altering the activity of liver enzymes.**

## ROUTE AND DOSAGE

■ **PO (Adults and Children ≥12 yr):** *Prevention of chemotherapy-induced nausea/vomiting*—8 mg 30 min prior to chemotherapy and repeated 8 hr later; 8 mg q 12 hr may be given for 1–2 days following chemotherapy. *Prevention of radiation-induced nausea/vomiting*—8 mg 1–2 hr prior to radiation; may be repeated q 8 hr, depending on type, location, and extent of radiation. *Prevention of postoperative nausea/vomiting*—16 mg 1 hr before induction of anesthesia.

■ **PO (Children 4–11 yr):** *Prevention of chemotherapy-induced nausea/vomiting*—4 mg 30 min prior to chemotherapy and repeated 4 and 8 hr later; 4 mg q 8 hr may be given for 1–2 days following chemotherapy.

■ **IV (Adults):** *Prevention of chemotherapy-induced nausea/vomiting*—0.15 mg/kg 15–30 min prior to chemotherapy, repeated 4 and 8 hr later, or 32-mg single dose 30 min prior to chemotherapy (lower doses have been used).

■ **IM, IV (Adults):** *Prevention of postoperative nausea/vomiting*—4 mg before induction of anesthesia or postoperatively.

■ **IV (Children 4–18 yr):** *Prevention of chemotherapy-induced nausea/vomiting*—0.15 mg/kg 15–30 min prior to chemotherapy, repeated 4 and 8 hr later.

■ **IV (Children 2–12 yr and ≤40 kg):** *Prevention of postoperative nausea/vomiting*—0.15 mg/kg.

■ **IV (Children >40 kg):** *Prevention of postoperative nausea/vomiting*—4 mg.

❏ **Hepatic Impairment**

■ **PO, IM, IV (Adults):** Not to exceed 8 mg/day.

## AVAILABILITY

■ *Orally disintegrating tablets (contain aspartame):* 4 mg<sup>Rx</sup>, 8 mg<sup>Rx</sup> ■ Cost: 4 mg $520.73/30, 8 mg $867.36/30 ■ *Tablets:* 4 mg<sup>Rx</sup>, 8 mg<sup>Rx</sup>, 24 mg<sup>Rx</sup> ■ Cost: 4 mg $52.08/3, 8 mg $86.72/3, 24 mg $86.72/1 ■ *Oral solution (strawberry flavor):* 4 mg/5 ml<sup>Rx</sup> ■ Cost: $176.89/50 ml ■ *Injection:* 2 mg/ml in 2- and 20-ml vials<sup>Rx</sup> ■ Cost: $128.24/5 vials ■ *Premixed injection:* 32 mg/50 ml single-dose containers<sup>Rx</sup>.

TIME/ACTION PROFILE (antiemetic effect)

| | ONSET | PEAK | DURATION |
|---|---|---|---|
| PO, IV | rapid | 15–30 min | 4 hr–8 hr |
| IM | rapid | 40 min | unknown |

# NURSING IMPLICATIONS

## ASSESSMENT

❏ Assess patient for nausea, vomiting, abdominal distention, and bowel sounds prior to and following administration.

❏ Assess patient for extrapyramidal effects (involuntary movements, facial grimacing, rigidity, shuffling walk, trembling of hands) periodically during therapy.

■ *Lab Test Considerations:* May cause transient ↑ in serum bilirubin, AST, and ALT levels.

## POTENTIAL NURSING DIAGNOSES

- Nutrition, imbalanced: less than body requirements (Indications).
- Diarrhea (Side Effects).
- Constipation (Side Effects).

## IMPLEMENTATION

- **General:** Do not confuse Zofran (ondansetron) with Zosyn (piperacillin/tazobactam).
- ❏ First dose is administered prior to emetogenic event.
- **PO:** For orally disintegrating tablets, do not attempt to push through foil backing; with dry hands, peel back backing and remove tablet. Immediately place tablet on tongue; tablet will dissolve in seconds, then swallow with saliva. Administration of liquid is not necessary.
- **Direct IV:** Administer undiluted immediately before induction of anesthesia or postoperatively if nausea and vomiting occur shortly after surgery.
- *Rate:* Administer over at least 30 sec and preferably over 2–5 min.
- **Intermittent Infusion:** Dilute doses for prevention of nausea and vomiting associated with chemotherapy in 50 ml of D5W, 0.9% NaCl, D5/0.9% NaCl, D5/0.45% NaCl. Solution is clear and colorless. Stable for 7 days at room temperature following dilution.
- *Rate:* Administer each dose as an IV infusion over 15 min.
- **Syringe Compatibility:** ◆ alfentanil ◆ atropine ◆ fentanyl ◆ glycopyrrolate ◆ meperidine ◆ metoclopramide ◆ midazolam ◆ morphine ◆ naloxone ◆ neostigmine ◆ propofol
- **Syringe Incompatibility:** ◆ droperidol
- **Y-Site Compatibility:** ◆ alatrofloxacin ◆ aldesleukin ◆ amifostine ◆ amikacin ◆ aztreonam ◆ bleomycin ◆ carboplatin ◆ carmustine ◆ cefazolin ◆ cefotaxime ◆ cefoxitin ◆ ceftazidime ◆ ceftizoxime ◆ cefuroxime ◆ chlorpromazine ◆ cimetidine ◆ cisatracurium ◆ cisplatin ◆ cladribine ◆ clindamycin ◆ cyclophosphamide ◆ cytarabine ◆ dacarbazine ◆ dactinomycin ◆ daunorubicin ◆ dexamethasone sodium phosphate ◆ diphenhydramine ◆ dopamine ◆ doxorubicin ◆ doxorubicin liposome ◆ doxycycline ◆ droperidol ◆ etoposide ◆ etoposide phosphate ◆ famotidine ◆ filgrastim ◆

floxuridine ◆ fluconazole ◆ fludarabine ◆ gatifloxacin ◆ gemcitabine ◆ gentamicin ◆ haloperidol ◆ heparin ◆ hydrocortisone sodium succinate ◆ hydrocortisone sodium phosphate ◆ hydromorphone ◆ ifosfamide ◆ imipenem/cilastatin ◆ linezolid ◆ magnesium sulfate ◆ mannitol ◆ mechlorethamine ◆ melphalan ◆ meperidine ◆ mesna ◆ methotrexate ◆ metoclopramide ◆ mitomycin ◆ mitoxantrone ◆ morphine ◆ paclitaxel ◆ pentostatin ◆ piperacillin/tazobactam ◆ potassium chloride ◆ promethazine ◆ prochlorperazine edisylate ◆ ranitidine ◆ remifentanil ◆ sodium acetate ◆ streptozocin ◆ teniposide ◆ thiotepa ◆ ticarcillin ◆ ticarcillin/clavulanate ◆ topotecan ◆ vancomycin ◆ vinblastine ◆ vincristine ◆ vinorelbine ◆ zidovudine.

- **Y-Site Incompatibility:** ◆ acyclovir ◆ allopurinol ◆ aminophylline ◆ amphotericin B ◆ amphotericin B cholesteryl sulfate ◆ ampicillin ◆ ampicillin/sulbactam ◆ cefepime ◆ cefoperazone ◆ furosemide ◆ ganciclovir ◆ lorazepam ◆ methylprednisolone sodium succinate ◆ piperacillin ◆ sargramostim ◆ sodium bicarbonate.

## PATIENT/FAMILY TEACHING

- ❏ Instruct patient to take ondansetron as directed.
- ❏ Advise patient to notify health care professional immediately if involuntary movement of eyes, face, or limbs occurs.

## EVALUATION

**Effectiveness of therapy can be demonstrated by:** ■ Prevention of nausea and vomiting associated with initial and repeat courses of emetogenic cancer chemotherapy ■ Prevention of postoperative nausea and vomiting ■ Prevention of nausea and vomiting due to radiation therapy.

## oprelvekin

(o-**prell**-ve-kin)

Neumega

*CLASSIFICATION(S):*

*Therapeutic:* colony-stimulating factors

---

---

*Pharmacologic: interleukins, thrombopoetic growth factors*

**Pregnancy Category C**

---

## INDICATIONS

■ Prevention of severe thrombocytopenia and reduction of the need for platelet transfusions following myelosuppressive chemotherapy in patients with nonmyeloid malignancies at risk for thrombocytopenia.

## ACTION

■ Stimulates production of megakaryocytes and platelets. **Therapeutic Effects:** ■ Increased platelet count.

## PHARMACOKINETICS

**Absorption:** >80% absorbed following subcut administration.
**Distribution:** Unknown.
**Metabolism and Excretion:** Appears to be mostly metabolized, with metabolites eliminated by kidneys.
**Half-life:** 6.9 hr.

## CONTRAINDICATIONS AND PRECAUTIONS

**Contraindicated in:** ■ Hypersensitivity ■ Lactation.
**Use Cautiously in:** ■ Any condition in which sodium and water retention would pose problems (CHF, renal disease) ■ Pre-existing pericardial effusion or ascites (may be exacerbated) ■ History of atrial arrhythmias (especially if receiving cardiac medications or previous doxorubicin therapy) ■ Pre-existing papilledema or tumors of the CNS ■ Pregnancy or children (safety not established).

## ADVERSE REACTIONS AND SIDE EFFECTS*

These effects occurred in patients who had recently received myelosuppressive chemotherapy. ■ **CNS:** dizziness, headache, insomnia, nervousness, weakness ■ **EENT:** conjunctival hemorrhage, blurred vision, papilledema, pharyngitis, rhinitis ■ **Resp:** cough, dyspnea, pleural effusions ■ **CV:** atrial fibrillation, edema, palpitations, syncope, tachycardia, vasodilation ■ **GI:** anorexia, constipation, diarrhea, dyspepsia, mucositis, nausea, oral moniliasis, vomiting, abdominal pain ■ **Derm:** alopecia, ecchymoses, rash ■ **F and E:** sodium and water retention ■

**Local:** injection-site reactions ■ **MS:** bone pain, myalgia ■ **Misc:** chills, fever, infection, pain.

## INTERACTIONS

**Drug-Drug:** ■ None significant.

## ROUTE AND DOSAGE

■ **Subcut (Adults):** 50 mcg/kg once daily for 10–21 days.

## AVAILABILITY

■ *Powder for injection:* 5-mg vial$^{Rx}$.

TIME/ACTION PROFILE (increase in platelet count)

| | ONSET | PEAK | DURATION |
|---|---|---|---|
| Subcut | 5–9 days | unknown | 7–14 days† |

†Counts continue to rise for 7 days following discontinuation and then return to baseline by 14 days.

# NURSING IMPLICATIONS

## ASSESSMENT

❑ Assess patient for signs of fluid retention (dyspnea on exertion, peripheral edema) during therapy. Fluid retention is a common side effect that usually resolves within several days following discontinuation of oprelvekin.

■ *Lab Test Considerations:* Monitor platelet count prior to and periodically during therapy, especially at expected nadir. Therapy is continued until postnadir platelet count is ≥50,000 cells/ml.

❑ CBC should be monitored prior to and at regular intervals during therapy. Decrease in hemoglobin concentration, hematocrit, and RBC count may occur because of increased plasma volume (dilutional anemia); usually begins within 3–5 days of therapy and is reversible within a week of discontinuation of therapy.

❑ Monitor electrolyte concentrations in patients receiving chronic diuretic therapy. Hypokalemia may be fatal.

❑ May cause an increase in plasma fibrinogen.

## POTENTIAL NURSING DIAGNOSES

■ Fluid volume, excess (Side Effects).

## IMPLEMENTATION

■ **General:** Therapy should be started within 6–24 hr after completion of chemotherapy and continued for 10–21 days.

❏ Treatment should be discontinued at least 2 days prior to next planned chemotherapy cycle.

■ **Subcut:** Reconstitute with 1 ml of sterile water for injection without preservatives for a concentration of 5 mg/ml. Direct diluent to sides of vial and swirl gently. Solution is clear and colorless. Do not administer solutions that are discolored or contain particulate matter. Do not shake or agitate vigorously. Do not freeze. Do not reuse vials. Administer within 3 hr of reconstitution as a single injection in abdomen, hip, thigh, or upper arm.

### PATIENT/FAMILY TEACHING

❏ Instruct patient in proper technique for preparation and administration of medication. Provide a puncture-resistant container for disposal of needles.

❏ May cause transient blurred vision or dizziness. Caution patient to avoid driving or other activities requiring alertness until response to medication is known.

❏ Advise patient to notify health care professional if pregnancy is planned or suspected.

❏ Inform patient of side effects and advise patient to notify health care professional if chest pain, shortness of breath, fatigue, blurred vision, or irregular heartbeat persists.

### EVALUATION

**Effectiveness of therapy can be demonstrated by:** ■ Increase in postnadir platelet count to ≥50,000 cells/ml.

---

## orphenadrine

(or-**fenn**-a-dreen)

Antiflex, Banflex, {Disipal}, Flexoject, Flexon, Mio-Rel, Myolin, Myotrol, Norflex, Orfro, Orphenate

### CLASSIFICATION(S):

**Therapeutic:** *skeletal muscle relaxants (centrally acting)*
**Pharmacologic:** *diphenhydramine analogues*

---

**Pregnancy Category C**

### INDICATIONS

■ Adjunct to rest and physical therapy in the treatment of muscle spasm associated with acute painful musculoskeletal conditions ■ Adjunct therapy of Parkinson's disease (Canadian labeling only).

### ACTION

■ Skeletal muscle relaxation, probably due to CNS depression. **Therapeutic Effects:** ■ Skeletal muscle relaxation, with decreased discomfort.

### PHARMACOKINETICS

**Absorption:** Readily absorbed after oral and IM administration; IV administration results in complete bioavailability.

**Distribution:** Unknown.

**Metabolism and Excretion:** Mostly metabolized by the liver.

**Half-life:** 14 hr.

### CONTRAINDICATIONS AND PRECAUTIONS

**Contraindicated in:** ■ Hypersensitivity ■ Bladder neck obstruction, prostatic hypertrophy, glaucoma, myasthenia gravis, peptic ulcer disease, GI obstruction.

**Use Cautiously in:** ■ Underlying cardiovascular disease ■ Impaired renal function ■ Pregnancy, lactation, or children (safety not established).

### ADVERSE REACTIONS AND SIDE EFFECTS*

■ **CNS:** CNS excitation, confusion, dizziness, drowsiness ■ **EENT:** blurred vision, dry eyes ■ **CV:** orthostatic hypotension, tachycardia ■ **GI:** constipation, dry mouth ■ **GU:** urinary retention.

### INTERACTIONS

**Drug-Drug:** ■ Concurrent use of other **anticholinergics** increases the risk of anticholinergic side effects ■ Increased risk of CNS depression with other **CNS depressants** including **alcohol, antihistamines, antidepres-**

---

sants, **sedative/hypnotics**, or **opioid analgesics**.

**Drug-Natural Products:** ■ **Kava, valerian, skullcap, chamomile,** or **hops** can increase CNS depression.

## ROUTE AND DOSAGE
❑ **Skeletal muscle relaxation**
- ■ **PO (Adults):** 100 mg twice daily.
- ■ **IV, IM (Adults):** 60 mg q 12 hr.
❑ **Adjunctive therapy of Parkinson's disease**
- ■ **PO (Adults):** 50 mg 3 times daily (lower doses if used with other agents).

## AVAILABILITY (generic available)
■ *Tablets:* {50 mg$^{otc}$} ■ *Extended-release tablets:* 100 mg$^{Rx}$ ■ Cost: $68.49/30 ■ *Injection:* 30 mg/ml$^{Rx}$.

TIME/ACTION PROFILE (skeletal muscle effects)

|       | ONSET       | PEAK    | DURATION |
|-------|-------------|---------|----------|
| PO-ER | within 1 hr | 6–8 hr  | 12 hr    |
| IM    | 5 min       | 30 min  | 12 hr    |
| IV    | immediate   | unknown | 12 hr    |

# NURSING IMPLICATIONS

## ASSESSMENT
- ■ **Skeletal Muscle Relaxant:** Assess patient for pain, muscle stiffness, and range of motion before and periodically throughout therapy.
- ■ **Parkinson's Disease:** Assess parkinsonian and extrapyramidal symptoms (restlessness or desire to keep moving, rigidity, tremors, pill rolling, mask-like face, shuffling gait, muscle spasms, twisting motions, difficulty speaking or swallowing, loss of balance control) prior to and throughout therapy.
- ■ *Lab Test Considerations:* Monitor CBC and renal and hepatic function tests periodically during prolonged therapy.

## POTENTIAL NURSING DIAGNOSES
- ■ Pain, acute (Indications).
- ■ Mobility, impaired physical (Indications).
- ■ Injury, risk for (Side Effects).

## IMPLEMENTATION
- ■ **General:** Do not confuse Norflex (orphenadrine) with norfloxacin (Noroxin).

❑ Provide safety measures as indicated. Supervise ambulation and transfer of patients.
- ■ **PO:** Do not break, crush or chew extended-release tablets.
- ■ **Direct IV:** May be administered undiluted.

## PATIENT/FAMILY TEACHING
- ❑ Advise patient to take medication exactly as directed. Missed doses should be taken within 1 hr; if not, return to regular dosing schedule. Do not double doses.
- ❑ Encourage patient to comply with additional therapies prescribed for muscle spasm (rest, physical therapy, heat).
- ❑ Medication may cause dizziness, drowsiness, and blurred vision. Advise patient to avoid driving and other activities requiring alertness until response to drug is known.
- ❑ Instruct patient to make position changes slowly to minimize orthostatic hypotension.
- ❑ Advise patient to avoid concurrent use of alcohol and other CNS depressants while taking this medication.
- ❑ Emphasize the importance of routine follow-up exams to monitor progress.

## EVALUATION
**Effectiveness of therapy can be demonstrated by:** ■ Decreased musculoskeletal pain and muscle spasticity ❑ Increased range of motion ■ Decrease in tremors and rigidity and an improvement in gait and balance.

# oseltamivir
(o-sel-**tam**-i-vir)
Tamiflu

*CLASSIFICATION(S):*
*Therapeutic: antivirals*
*Pharmacologic: neuramidase inhibitors*

**Pregnancy Category C**

## INDICATIONS
■ Uncomplicated acute illness due to influenza infection in adults and children >1 yr who have had symptoms for ≤2 days ■ Prevention of influenza in patients ≥13 yrs.

## ACTION

- Inhibits the enzyme neuramidase, which may alter virus particle aggregation and release. **Therapeutic Effects:** ▪ Reduced duration of flu-related symptoms.

## PHARMACOKINETICS

**Absorption:** Rapidly absorbed from the GI tract and converted by the liver to the active form, oseltamivir carboxylate. 75% reaches systemic circulation as the active drug.
**Distribution:** Unknown.
**Metabolism and Excretion:** Rapidly metabolized by the liver to oseltamivir carboxylate, the active drug. Oseltamivir is >99% excreted unchanged in urine.
**Half-life:** *Oseltamivir carboxylate*—6–10 hr.

## CONTRAINDICATIONS AND PRECAUTIONS

**Contraindicated in:** ▪ Hypersensitivity.
**Use Cautiously in:** ▪ Pregnancy and lactation (safety not established; use only if potential benefits outweigh possible risks) ▪ Children <18 yr (safety not established).

## ADVERSE REACTIONS AND SIDE EFFECTS*

▪ **CNS:** insomnia, vertigo ▪ **Resp:** bronchitis ▪ **GI:** nausea, vomiting.

## INTERACTIONS

**Drug-Drug:** ▪ None significant.

## ROUTE AND DOSAGE

❑ **Treatment of Influenza**
▪ **PO (Adults and Children >40 kg):** 75 mg twice daily for 5 days.
▪ **PO (Children 23–40 kg):** 60 mg twice daily.
▪ **PO (Children 15–23 kg):** 45 mg twice daily.
▪ **PO (Children ≤15 kg and ≥1 yr):** 30 mg twice daily.
❑ **Renal Impairment**
▪ **PO (Adults):** *CCr <30 ml/min*—75 mg once daily for 5 days.
❑ **Influenza Prevention**
▪ **PO (Adults and Children ≥13 yrs):** 75 mg once daily for at least 7 days.

❑ **Renal Impairment**
▪ **PO (Adults and Children ≥13 yrs):** *CCr 10–30 ml/min*—75 mg every other day.

## AVAILABILITY

▪ *Capsules:* 75 mg$^{Rx}$ ▪ *Oral suspension (tutti-frutti flavor):* 12 mg/min in 60–ml bottle$^{Rx}$.

TIME/ACTION PROFILE (blood levels)

|    | ONSET | PEAK | DURATION |
|----|-------|------|----------|
| PO | unknown | unknown | 12 hr |

# NURSING IMPLICATIONS

## ASSESSMENT

❑ Monitor influenza symptoms (sudden onset of fever, cough, headache, fatigue, muscular weakness, sore throat). Additional supportive treatment may be indicated to treat symptoms.

## POTENTIAL NURSING DIAGNOSES

▪ Infection, risk for (Indications).

## IMPLEMENTATION

- ▪ **General:** Treatment with oseltamivir should be started as soon as possible from the first sign of flu symptoms.
- ▪ **PO:** May be administered with food or milk to minimize GI irritation. To prepare oral solution, tap closed bottle to loosen powder. Add total amount of water for constitution and shake closed bottle for 15 seconds. Remove childproof cap and push bottle adaptor into neck of bottle. Close bottle with childproof top tightly, assuring proper seating of bottle adaptor and childproof status. Shake well before use. Use within 10 days of constitution.

## PATIENT/FAMILY TEACHING

❑ Instruct patient to take oseltamivir as soon as influenza symptoms appear and to continue to take it as directed for the full course of therapy, even if feeling better. Take missed doses as soon as remembered unless within 2 hr of next dose. Do not double doses.

{ } = Available in Canada only.
*CAPITALS indicates life-threatening; underlines indicate most frequent.

- Caution patient that oseltamivir should not be shared with anyone, even if they have the same symptoms.
- Advise patient that oseltamivir is not a substitute for a flu shot. Patients should receive annual flu shot according to immunization guidelines.
- Advise patient to consult health care professional before taking other medications concurrently with oseltamivir.

## EVALUATION

**Clinical response to therapy can be evaluated by:** ■ Reduction of the duration of flu symptoms.

## oxacillin, See PENICILLINS, PENICILLINASE RESISTANT.

# oxaprozin

(ox-a-**proe**-zin)

Daypro

## CLASSIFICATION(S):

**Therapeutic:** antirheumatics, nonsteroidal anti-inflammatory agents

**Pregnancy Category B, C (first trimester), UK (second and third trimester)**

## INDICATIONS

■ Rheumatoid arthritis and osteoarthritis.

## ACTION

■ Inhibits prostaglandin synthesis. **Therapeutic Effects:** ■ Suppression of pain and inflammation.

## PHARMACOKINETICS

**Absorption:** Well absorbed following oral administration (80%); 35% is rapidly converted to an active metabolite.

**Distribution:** Unknown.

**Protein Binding:** 99.9%.

**Metabolism and Excretion:** The active metabolite is metabolized by the liver to inactive compounds.

**Half-life:** 42–50 hr.

## CONTRAINDICATIONS AND PRECAUTIONS

**Contraindicated in:** ■ Hypersensitivity ■ Cross-sensitivity may exist with other NSAIDs, including aspirin ■ Active GI bleeding or ulcer disease.

**Use Cautiously in:** ■ Severe cardiovascular or hepatic disease ■ Renal impairment (lower initial dose may be necessary) ■ History of ulcer disease ■ Geriatric patients (dosage adjustments may be necessary due to age-related decrease in renal function) ■ Pregnancy, lactation, or children (safety not established; not recommended for use during the second half of pregnancy).

## ADVERSE REACTIONS AND SIDE EFFECTS*

■ **CNS:** agitation, anxiety, confusion, depression, dizziness, drowsiness, fatigue, headache, insomnia, malaise, weakness ■ **EENT:** abnormal vision, tinnitus ■ **Resp:** dyspnea, hypersensitivity pneumonitis ■ **CV:** edema, vasculitis ■ **GI:** GI BLEEDING, abdominal pain, diarrhea, dyspepsia, abnormal liver function tests, anorexia, cholestatic jaundice, constipation, dry mouth, duodenal ulcer, flatulence, gastritis, increased appetite, nausea, stomatitis, vomiting ■ **GU:** albuminuria, azotemia, interstitial nephritis ■ **Derm:** increased sweating, photosensitivity, pruritus, rash ■ **Hemat:** prolonged bleeding time ■ **Metab:** weight gain ■ **Neuro:** paresthesia, tremor ■ **Misc:** allergic reactions including ANAPHYLAXIS, ANGIONEUROTIC EDEMA

## INTERACTIONS

**Drug-Drug:** ■ ↑ adverse GI effects and toxicity with **aspirin**, other **NSAIDs, potassium supplements, corticosteroids,** or **alcohol** ■ Chronic use with **acetaminophen** may ↑ risk of adverse renal reactions ■ May ↓ effectiveness of **diuretics** or **antihypertensive** therapy ■ May ↑ hypoglycemic effects of **insulin** or **oral hypoglycemic agents** ■ ↑ risk of toxicity from **methotrexate** ■ ↑ risk of bleeding with **cefotetan, cefoperazone, plicamycin, thrombolytic agents, anticoagulants, ticlopidine, clopidogrel, eptifibatide,** or **tirofiban** ■ ↑ risk of adverse hematologic reactions with **antineoplastics** or **radiation therapy.**

**Drug-Natural Products:** ■ ↑ anticoagulant effect and bleeding risk with **arnica, chamomile, clove, feverfew, garlic, ginger, ginkgo, Panax ginseng, licorice,** and others.

## ROUTE AND DOSAGE

■ **PO (Adults):** 1200 mg once daily; onset may be more rapid with an initial 1800-mg dose. Patients with low body weight, mild disease, or renal impairment may be started at 600 mg/day (not to exceed 1800 mg/day or 26 mg/kg/day). Daily doses >1200 mg should be given in 2–3 divided doses. Consideration should be given to decreasing dose to lowest effective amount.

## AVAILABILITY (generic available)

■ *Tablets:* 600 mg$^{Rx}$ ■ Cost: 600 mg *Daypro*—$181.79/100; *generic*—$181.54/100.

TIME/ACTION PROFILE (antirheumatic action)

| | ONSET | PEAK | DURATION |
|---|---|---|---|
| PO | within 7 days | unknown | unknown |

## NURSING IMPLICATIONS

### ASSESSMENT

❑ Patients who have asthma, aspirin-induced allergy, and nasal polyps are at increased risk for developing hypersensitivity reactions. Monitor for rhinitis, asthma, and urticaria.

❑ Assess pain and range of motion prior to and periodically throughout therapy.

■ *Lab Test Considerations:* May cause prolonged bleeding time, which may persist for up to 2 wk following discontinuation of therapy.

❑ Evaluate BUN, serum creatinine, CBC, and liver function tests periodically in patients receiving prolonged therapy. Serum potassium, BUN, serum creatinine, alkaline phosphatase, LDH, AST, and ALT tests may show ↑ levels. Blood glucose, hemoglobin, and hematocrit concentrations, leukocyte and platelet counts, and CCr may be ↓.

### POTENTIAL NURSING DIAGNOSES

■ Pain, acute (Indications).

### IMPLEMENTATION

■ **General:** Administration in higher than recommended doses does not provide increased effectiveness but may cause increased side effects.

■ **PO:** Administer with food or antacids to decrease GI irritation.

### PATIENT/FAMILY TEACHING

❑ Advise patient to take this medication with a full glass of water and to remain in an upright position for 15–30 min after administration.

❑ Instruct patient to take medication exactly as directed. Take missed doses as soon as remembered but not if almost time for the next dose. Do not double doses.

❑ May cause drowsiness and dizziness. Advise patient to avoid driving or other activities requiring alertness until response to the medication is known.

❑ Caution patient to avoid the concurrent use of alcohol, aspirin, acetaminophen, or other OTC medications or herbal products without consulting health care professional.

❑ Advise patient to notify health care professional of medication regimen prior to treatment or surgery. Oxaprozin should be discontinued 2 wk prior to surgery.

❑ Caution patient to use sunscreen and protective clothing to prevent photosensitivity reactions.

❑ Advise patient to consult health care professional if rash, itching, visual disturbances, tinnitus, weight gain, edema, black stools, persistent headache, or influenza-like syndrome (chills, fever, muscle aches, pain) occurs.

### EVALUATION

**Effectiveness of therapy can be demonstrated by:** ■ Decreased pain and improved joint mobility. Maximum effectiveness may require 2 wk or more of continuous therapy. Patients who do not respond to one NSAID may respond to another.

## oxazepam

(ox-**az**-e-pam)
{Apo-Oxazepam}, {Novoxapam},
Serax

---

{ } = Available in Canada only.
*CAPITALS indicates life-threatening; <u>underlines</u> indicate most frequent.

## INDICATIONS

■ Management of anxiety ■ Symptomatic treatment of alcohol withdrawal.

## ACTION

■ Depresses the CNS, probably by potentiating GABA, an inhibitory neurotransmitter. **Therapeutic Effects:** ■ Decreased anxiety ■ Diminished symptoms of alcohol withdrawal.

## PHARMACOKINETICS

**Absorption:** Well absorbed following oral administration. Absorption is slower than with other benzodiazepines.

**Distribution:** Widely distributed. Crosses the blood-brain barrier. May cross the placenta and enter breast milk.

**Metabolism and Excretion:** Metabolized by the liver to inactive compounds.

**Protein Binding:** 97%.

**Half-life:** 5–15 hr.

## CONTRAINDICATIONS AND PRECAUTIONS

**Contraindicated in:** ■ Hypersensitivity ■ Cross-sensitivity with other benzodiazepines may exist ■ Comatose patients or those with pre-existing CNS depression ■ Uncontrolled severe pain ■ Narrow-angle glaucoma ■ Pregnancy and lactation ■ Some products contain tartrazine and should be avoided in patients with known intolerance.

**Use Cautiously in:** ■ Hepatic dysfunction ■ History of suicide attempt or drug abuse ■ Geriatric/debilitated patients (initial dosage reduction recommended) ■ Severe chronic obstructive pulmonary disease ■ Myasthenia gravis.

## ADVERSE REACTIONS AND SIDE EFFECTS*

■ **CNS:** <u>dizziness</u>, <u>drowsiness</u>, confusion, hangover, headache, impaired memory, mental depression, paradoxical excitation, slurred speech ■ **EENT:** blurred vision ■ **Resp:** respiratory

depression ■ **CV:** tachycardia ■ **GI:** constipation, diarrhea, drug-induced hepatitis, nausea, vomiting ■ **GU:** urinary problems ■ **Derm:** rashes ■ **Hemat:** leukopenia ■ **Misc:** physical dependence, psychological dependence, tolerance.

## INTERACTIONS

**Drug-Drug:** ■ Additive CNS depression with other **CNS depressants,** including **alcohol, antihistamines, antidepressants, opioid analgesics,** and other **sedative/hypnotics** (including other benzodiazepines) ■ May decrease the therapeutic effectiveness of **levodopa** ■ **Hormonal contraceptives** or **phenytoin** may decrease effectiveness ■ **Theophylline** may decrease sedative effects of oxazepam.

**Drug-Natural Products:** ■ Concomitant use of **kava, valerian, skullcap, chamomile,** or **hops** can increase CNS depression.

## ROUTE AND DOSAGE

■ **PO (Adults):** *Antianxiety agent*—10–30 mg 3–4 times daily. *Sedative/hypnotic/ management of alcohol withdrawal*—15–30 mg 3–4 times daily.

■ **PO (Geriatric Patients):** 5 mg 1–2 times daily initially or 10 mg 3 times daily; may be increased as needed.

## AVAILABILITY (generic available)

■ *Capsules:* 10 mg[Rx], 15 mg[Rx], 30 mg[Rx] ■Cost: *Serax*—10 mg $92.75/100, 15 mg $121.25/100, 30 mg $169.21/100; *generic*—10 mg $75.31/100, 15 mg $94.70/100, 30 mg $136.98/100 ■ *Tablets:* {10 mg[Rx]}, 15 mg[Rx], {30 mg[Rx]} ■Cost: *Serax*—15 mg $131.24/100.

TIME/ACTION PROFILE (sedation)

| | ONSET | PEAK | DURATION |
|---|---|---|---|
| PO | 45–90 min | unknown | 6–12 hr |

# NURSING IMPLICATIONS

## ASSESSMENT

❑ Assess patient for anxiety and level of sedation (ataxia, dizziness, slurred speech) periodically throughout therapy.

❑ Prolonged high-dose therapy may lead to psychological or physical dependence. Restrict the amount of drug available to patient.

■ **Lab Test Considerations:** Monitor CBC and liver function tests periodically during prolonged therapy.

❑ May cause decreased thyroidal uptake of sodium iodide $^{123}$I and $^{131}$I.

## POTENTIAL NURSING DIAGNOSES

■ Anxiety (Indications).

■ Injury, risk for (Side Effects).

## IMPLEMENTATION

■ **General:** Medication should be tapered at the completion of therapy. Sudden cessation of medication may lead to withdrawal (insomnia, irritability, nervousness, tremors).

■ **PO:** Administer with food if GI irritation becomes a problem.

## PATIENT/FAMILY TEACHING

❑ Instruct patient to take oxazepam exactly as directed. Missed doses should be taken within 1 hr; if remembered later, omit and return to regular dosing schedule. Do not double or increase doses. If dose is less effective after a few weeks, notify health care professional.

❑ May cause drowsiness or dizziness. Caution patient to avoid driving or other activities requiring alertness until response to medication is known.

❑ Advise patient to avoid the use of alcohol and to consult health care professional prior to the use of OTC preparations that contain antihistamines or alcohol.

❑ Advise patient to inform health care professional if pregnancy is planned or suspected.

❑ Advise patient to notify health care professional of medication regimen prior to treatment or surgery.

❑ Emphasize the importance of follow-up exams to monitor effectiveness of medication.

## EVALUATION

**Effectiveness of therapy can be demonstrated by:** ■ Decreased sense of anxiety ❑ Increased ability to cope ■ Prevention or relief of acute agitation, tremor, and hallucinations during alcohol withdrawal.

# oxcarbazepine

(ox-kar-**baz**-e-peen)
Trileptal

## CLASSIFICATION(S):
**Therapeutic:** anticonvulsants
**Pharmacologic:** carbamazepine analogues

### Pregnancy Category C

## INDICATIONS

■ Monotherapy or adjunctive therapy of partial seizures in adults with epilepsy ■ Adjunctive therapy of partial seizures in patients 4–16 yr with epilepsy. **Unlabeled uses:** ■ Management of trigeminal neuralgia.

## ACTION

■ Blocks sodium channels in neural membranes, stabilizing hyperexcitable states, inhibiting repetitive neuronal firing, and decreasing propagation of synaptic impulses. **Therapeutic Effects:** ■ Decreased incidence of seizures.

## PHARMACOKINETICS

**Absorption:** Rapidly absorbed after oral administration and rapidly converted to the active 10-hydroxy metabolite (MHD).

**Distribution:** Enters breast milk in significant amounts.

**Metabolism and Excretion:** Extensively converted to MHD, which is then primarily excreted by the kidneys.

**Half-life:** *Oxcarbazepine*—2 hr; *MHD*—9 hr.

## CONTRAINDICATIONS AND PRECAUTIONS

**Contraindicated in:** ■ Hypersensitivity; cross-sensitivity with carbamazepine may occur ■ Lactation.

**Use Cautiously in:** ■ Renal impairment (dosage reduction recommended if CCR <30 ml/min) ■ Pregnancy (use only if potential benefit justifies the potential risk to the fetus) ■ Children <4 yr (safety not established).

## ADVERSE REACTIONS AND SIDE EFFECTS*

■ **CNS:** dizziness/vertigo, drowsiness/fatigue, headache, cognitive symptoms ■ **EENT:** abnormal vision, diplopia, nystagmus ■ **GI:** abdominal pain, dyspepsia, nausea, vomiting, thirst ■ **Derm:** acne, rash, urticaria ■ **F and E:** hyponatremia ■ **Neuro:** ataxia, gait disturbances, tremor ■ **Misc:** allergic reactions, lymphadenopathy.

## INTERACTIONS

**Drug-Drug:** ■ Oxcarbazepine may inhibit the CYP 2C19 enzyme system and would be expected to alter the effects of other drugs that are metabolized by this system. Oxcarbazepine and MHD induce the P450 3A4/5 enzyme systems and would be expected to alter the effects of other drugs that are metabolized by this system. This may result in decreased levels and effectiveness of **hormonal contraceptives, felodipine, isradipine, nicardipine, nifedipine,** and **nimodipine.** In addition, oxcarbazepine itself is metabolized by cytochrome P450 system and other **drugs that alter the activity of this system** ■ Additive CNS depression may occur with other CNS depressants, including **alcohol, antihistamines, antidepressants, sedative/hypnotics,** and **opioid analgesics** ■ **Carbamazepine, phenobarbital, phenytoin, valproic acid,** and **verapamil** decrease levels ■ May increase serum levels and effects of **phenytoin** (dosage reduction of phenytoin may be required).

## ROUTE AND DOSAGE

■ **PO (Adults):** *Adjunctive therapy*—300 mg twice daily; may be increased by up to 600 mg/day at weekly intervals up to 1200 mg/day (up to 2400 mg/day may be needed). *conversion to monotherapy*—300 mg twice daily; may be increased by 600 mg/day at weekly intervals, whereas other antiepileptic drugs are tapered over 3–6 wk; dosage of oxcarbazepine should be increased up to 2400 mg/day over a period of 2–4 wk. *initiation of monotherapy*—300 mg twice daily, increase by 300 mg/day every third day, up to 1200 mg/day.

■ **PO (Children 4–16 yr):** *Adjunctive therapy*—4–5 mg/kg twice daily (up to 600 mg/day), increased over 2 wk to achieve 900 mg/day in patients 20–29 kg, 1200 mg/day in patients 29.1–39 kg and 1800 mg/day in patients >39 kg (range 6–51 mg/kg/day).

❑ **Renal Impairment**

■ **PO (Adults):** *CCr<30 ml/min*—Initiate therapy at 300 mg/day and increase slowly to achieve desired response.

## AVAILABILITY

■ **Tablets:** 150 mg$^{Rx}$, 300 mg$^{Rx}$, 600 mg$^{Rx}$ ■ Cost: 150 mg $96.21/100, 300 mg $175.70/100, 600 mg $322.94/100 ■ **Oral suspension:** 60 mg/ml in 250-ml bottle$^{Rx}$.

TIME/ACTION PROFILE (blood levels)

| | ONSET | PEAK | DURATION |
|---|---|---|---|
| PO 12 hr | PO | rapid | 4.5 hr† |

†Steady-state levels of MHD are reached after 2–3 days during twice-daily dosing.

# NURSING IMPLICATIONS

## ASSESSMENT

■ **Seizures:** Assess frequency, location, duration, and characteristics of seizure activity. Hyponatremia may increase frequency and severity of seizures.

❑ Monitor patient for CNS changes. May manifest as cognitive symptoms (psychomotor slowing, difficulty with concentration, speech or language problems), somnolence or fatigue, or coordination abnormalties (ataxia, gait disturbances).

■ **Lab Test Considerations:** Monitor ECG and serum electrolytes before and periodically during therapy. May cause hyponatremia. Usually occurs during the first 3 mo of therapy. May require dose reduction, fluid restriction, or discontinuation of therapy. Sodium levels return to normal within a few days of discontinuation.

## POTENTIAL NURSING DIAGNOSES

■ Injury, risk for (Indications, Side Effects).

## IMPLEMENTATION

■ **General:** Implement seizure precautions as indicated.

■ **PO:** Administer twice daily with or without food.

## PATIENT/FAMILY TEACHING

■ **General Info:** Instruct patient to take oxcarbazepine in equally spaced doses, exactly as directed. If a dose is missed, take as soon as possible but not just before next dose; do not double doses. Notify health care professional if more than one dose is missed. Medication should be gradually discontinued to prevent seizures.

- ❑ May cause dizziness, drowsiness, or CNS changes. Advise patients to avoid driving or other activities requiring alertness until response to medication is known. Do not resume driving until physician gives clearance based on control of seizure disorder.
- ❑ Advise patient not to take alcohol or other CNS depressants concurrently with this medication.
- ❑ Advise female patients to use an additional nonhormonal method of contraception during therapy and until next menstrual period. Instruct patient to notify health care professional if pregnancy is planned or suspected.
- ❑ Instruct patient to notify health care professional of medication regimen before treatment or surgery.
- ❑ Advise patients to carry identification describing disease and medication regimen at all times.

### EVALUATION

**Effectiveness of therapy can be demonstrated by:** ■ Absence or reduction of seizure activity.

## oxiconazole, See ANTIFUNGALS (TOPICAL).

## OXYBUTYNIN

**oxybutynin (oral)**

(ox-i-**byoo**-ti-nin)

Ditropan, Ditropan XL

**oxybutynin (transdermal)**

Oxytrol

### CLASSIFICATION(S):

**Therapeutic:** *urinary tract antispasmodics*
**Pharmacologic:** *anticholinergics*

**Pregnancy Category B**

### INDICATIONS

■ Urinary symptoms that may be associated with neurogenic bladder including: ❑ Frequent urination ❑ Urgency ❑ Nocturia ❑ Incontinence ■ Overactive bladder.

### ACTION

■ Inhibits the action of acetylcholine at postganglionic receptors ■ Has direct spasmolytic action on smooth muscle, including smooth muscle lining the GU tract, without affecting vascular smooth muscle. **Therapeutic Effects:** ■ Increased bladder capacity ■ Delayed desire to void ■ Decreased urge incontinence, urinary urgency, and frequency and decreased number of urinary accidents associated with overactive bladder.

### PHARMACOKINETICS

**Absorption:** Rapidly absorbed following oral administration, but undergoes extensive first-pass metabolism; XL tablets provide extended release. Transdermal absorption occurs by passive diffusion through intact skin and bypasses the first-pass effect.

**Distribution:** Widely distributed.

**Metabolism and Excretion:** Extensively metabolized by the liver (CYP 3A4 enzyme system). One metabolite is pharmacologically active; metabolites are renally excreted with negligable excretion of unchanged drug.

**Half-life:** 7–8 hr.

### CONTRAINDICATIONS AND PRECAUTIONS

**Contraindicated in:** ■ Hypersensitivity ■ Uncontrolled narrow angle-glaucoma ■ Intestinal obstruction or atony ■ Toxic megacolon ■ Paralytic ileus ■ Severe colitis ■ Myasthenia gravis ■ Acute hemorrhage with shock ■ Obstructive uropathy.

**Use Cautiously in:** ■ Hepatic/renal impairment ■ Lactation (may be inhibited) ■ Bladder outflow obstruction ■ Cardiovascular disease ■ Reflux esophagitis or gastrointestinal osbstructive disorders ■ Geriatric patients (increased risk of adverse reactions) ■ Pregnancy or children <5 yr (safety not established).

## ADVERSE REACTIONS AND SIDE EFFECTS*

■ **CNS:** dizziness, drowsiness, hallucinations, insomnia, weakness ■ **EENT:** blurred vision, cycloplegia, increased intraocular pressure, mydriasis, photophobia ■ **CV:** palpitations, tachycardia ■ **GI:** bloated feeling, constipation, dry mouth, nausea, vomiting ■ **GU:** impotence, urinary hesitancy, urinary retention ■ **Derm:** decreased sweating, urticaria, *transdermal only:* application site reactions ■ **Endo:** suppressed lactation ■ **Metab:** hyperthermia ■ **Misc:** allergic reactions, fever, hot flashes.

## INTERACTIONS

**Drug-Drug:** ■ ↑ anticholinergic effects with other **agents having anticholinergic properties,** including **amantadine, antidepressants, phenothiazines, disopyramide,** and **haloperidol** ■ Additive CNS depression with other **CNS depressants,** including **alcohol, antihistamines, antidepressants, opioids,** and **sedative/hypnotics** ■ May ↑ serum levels and risk of toxicity from **nitrofurantoin** ■ May decrease effectiveness of **levodopa** ■ May ↑ absorption of **atenolol** ■ Concurrent use with **haloperidol** may result in tardive dyskinesia, worsening of schizophrenia, and decreased haloperidol levels ■ May ↑ serum **digoxin** (slow-dissolution tablets) levels ■ Concurrent use of **drugs that cause esophagitis** including **doxycycline** and **biphosphonates** may exacerbate esophagitis.

**Drug-Natural Products:** ■ ↑ anticholinergic effects with **angel's trumpet, jimson weed,** and **scopolia.**

## ROUTE AND DOSAGE

■ **PO (Adults):** 5 mg 2–3 times daily (not to exceed 5 mg 4 times daily) or 10–15 mg once daily as XL tablets
■ **PO (Children >5 yr):** 5 mg 2–3 times daily (not to exceed 15 mg/day).
■ **Transdermal (Adults):** One 3.9 mg system applied twice weekly (every 3–4 days).

## AVAILABILITY (generic available)

■ *Tablets:* 5 mg[Rx] ■ Cost: *Ditropan*—5 mg $83.94/100; *generic*—5 mg $12.60/100 ■ *Extended release tablets:* 5 mg[Rx], 10 mg[Rx], 15 mg[Rx] ■ Cost: 5 mg $256.25/100, 10 mg $278.75/100, 15 mg $308.75/100 ■ *Syrup:* 5 mg/5 ml[Rx] ■ Cost: $90.96/480 ml ■ *Transdermal system:* 39 cm² system containing 36 mg

oxybutynin delivering 3.9 mg/day[Rx] ■ Cost: $87.88/8 patches.

TIME/ACTION PROFILE (urinary spasmolytic effect)

| | ONSET | PEAK | DURATION |
|---|---|---|---|
| PO | 30–60 min | 3–6 hr | 6–10 hr (up to 24 hr with XL tablet) |
| Transdermal | within 24 hr | 36 hr | 3–4 days |

# NURSING IMPLICATIONS

## ASSESSMENT

❑ Monitor voiding pattern and intake and output ratios, and assess abdomen for bladder distention prior to and periodically during therapy. Catheterization may be used to assess postvoid residual. Cystometry, to diagnose type of bladder dysfunction, is usually performed prior to prescription of oxybutynin.

## POTENTIAL NURSING DIAGNOSES

■ Urinary elimination, impaired (Indications).
■ Pain, acute (Indications).

## IMPLEMENTATION

■ **General:** Do not confuse Ditropan (oxybutynin) with diazepam.
■ **PO:** May be administered on an empty stomach or with meals or milk to prevent gastric irritation. **Transdermal:** Apply patch on same two days each week (Sunday/Wednesday, Monday/Thursday) to hip, abdomen, or buttock in an area that is clean, dry, and without irritation. Patch should be worn continuously.

## PATIENT/FAMILY TEACHING

❑ Instruct patient to take oxybutinin as directed. Take missed doses as soon as remembered unless almost time for next dose.
❑ May cause drowsiness or blurred vision. Advise patient to avoid driving and other activities requiring alertness until response to medication is known.
❑ Advise patient to avoid concurrent use of alcohol and other CNS depressants while taking this medication.
❑ Instruct patient that frequent rinsing of mouth, good oral hygiene, and sugarless gum or candy may decrease dry mouth.

Health care professional should be notified if mouth dryness persists >2 wk.

❑ Inform patient that oxybutynin decreases the body's ability to perspire. Avoid strenuous activity in a warm environment because overheating may occur.

❑ Advise patient to wear sunglasses when out in bright sunlight; increased sensitivity to light may occur.

❑ Advise patient to notify health care professional if urinary retention occurs or if constipation persists. Discuss methods of preventing constipation, such as increasing dietary bulk, increasing fluid intake, and increasing mobility.

❑ Discuss need for continued medical follow-up. Periodic cystometry may be used to evaluate effectiveness. Ophthalmic exams should be performed periodically to detect glaucoma, especially in patients over 40 yr of age.

■ **Transdermal:** Instruct patient on correct application and disposal of patch. Open pouch by tearing along arrows; apply immediately. Apply ½ patch to skin by removing ½ protective cover and applying firmly to skin. Apply second half by bending in half and rolling patch onto skin while removing protective liner. Press patch firmly in place.

❑ Remove slowly; fold in half, sticky sides together, and discard. Wash site with mild soap and water or a small amount of baby oil.

## EVALUATION

**Effectiveness of therapy can be demonstrated by:** ■ Relief of bladder spasm and associated symptoms (frequency, urgency, nocturia, and incontinence) in patients with a neurogenic bladder.

---

| High Alert |
| --- |

# oxycodone
(ox-i-**koe**-done)

Endocodone, M-Oxy, Oxycontin, OxyFAST, OxyIR, Percolone, Roxicodone, Roxicodone SR, {Supeudol}

---

**oxycodone/acetaminophen†**
{Endocet}, {Oxycocet}, Percocet, {Percocet}, Roxicet, Roxilox, Tylox

**oxycodone/aspirin†**
{Endodan}, {Oxycodan}, Percodan, Percodan-Demi, Roxiprin

## CLASSIFICATION(S):
**Therapeutic:** opioid analgesics
**Pharmacologic:** opioid agonists, opioid agonists/nonopioid analgesic combinations

### Schedule II

### Pregnancy Category C (oxycodone alone)

†See also acetaminophen and salicylates monographs.

## INDICATIONS
■ Moderate to severe pain.

## ACTION
■ Bind to opiate receptors in the CNS ■ Alter the perception of and response to painful stimuli, while producing generalized CNS depression. **Therapeutic Effects:** ■ Decreased pain.

## PHARMACOKINETICS
**Absorption:** Well absorbed from the GI tract.
**Distribution:** Widely distributed. Cross the placenta; enter breast milk.
**Metabolism and Excretion:** Mostly metabolized by the liver.
**Half-life:** 2–3 hr.

## CONTRAINDICATIONS AND PRECAUTIONS
**Contraindicated in:** ■ Hypersensitivity ■ Pregnancy or lactation (avoid chronic use) ■ Some products contain alcohol or bisulfites and should be avoided in patients with known intolerance or hypersensitivity.
**Use Cautiously in:** ■ Head trauma ■ Increased intracranial pressure ■ Severe renal, hepatic, or pulmonary disease ■ Hypothyroidism ■ Adrenal insufficiency ■ Alcoholism ■ Geriatric or debilitated patients (initial dosage reduction recom-

---

{ } = Available in Canada only.
*CAPITALS indicates life-threatening; underlines indicate most frequent.

mended) ■ Undiagnosed abdominal pain ■ Prostatic hypertrophy.

## ADVERSE REACTIONS AND SIDE EFFECTS*

■ **CNS:** confusion, sedation, dizziness, dysphoria, euphoria, floating feeling, hallucinations, headache, unusual dreams ■ **EENT:** blurred vision, diplopia, miosis ■ **Resp:** RESPIRATORY DE-PRESSION ■ **CV:** orthostatic hypotension ■ **GI:** constipation, dry mouth, nausea, vomiting ■ **GU:** urinary retention ■ **Derm:** flushing, sweating ■ **Misc:** physical dependence, psychological dependence, tolerance.

## INTERACTIONS

**Drug-Drug:** ■Use with caution in patients receiving **MAO inhibitors** (may result in unpredictable reactions—decrease initial dose of oxycodone to 25% of usual dose) ■ ↑ CNS depression with **alcohol, antihistamines,** and **sedative/hypnotics** ■ Administration of **partial-antagonist opioid analgesics** may precipitate withdrawal in physically dependent patients ■ **Nalbuphine, buprenorphine,** or **pentazocine** may decrease analgesia.

**Drug-Natural Products:** ■ Concomitant use of **kava, valerian,** or **chamomile** can ↑ CNS depression.

## ROUTE AND DOSAGE

Larger doses may be required during chronic therapy. Consider cumulative effects of additional acetaminophen/aspirin; if toxic levels are exceeded, change to pure oxycodone product.

■ **PO (Adults ≥50 kg):** 5–10 mg q 3–4 hr initially, as needed. Controlled-release tablets (Oxycontin) may be given q 12 hr after careful consideration as to dose, indication, and previous analgesic use/abuse history.

■ **PO (Adults <50 kg or Children 6–12 years):** 1.25 mg every 6 hr as needed or 0.2 mg/kg q 3–4 hr initially, as needed.

■ **PO (Children >12):** 2.5 mg every 6 hr as needed.

■ **Rect (Adults):** 10–40 mg 3–4 times daily initially, as needed.

## AVAILABILITY (generic available)

❏ **Oxycodone**

■ **Tablets:** 5 mg (Percolone, Roxicodone, Supeudol)$^{Rx}$ ■ Cost: *Percolone*—68.75/100; *Roxicodone*—$42.49/100; *generic*—$30.60–41.05/100 ■ **Immediate-release capsules:**

5 mg (OxyIR)$^{Rx}$ ■ **Controlled-release tablets:** 10 mg$^{Rx}$, 20 mg$^{Rx}$, 40 mg$^{Rx}$, 80 mg (Oxycontin, Roxicodone SR)$^{Rx}$, 160 mg (Oxycontin) ■ Cost: *Oxycontin*—10 mg $129.21/100, 20 mg $247.28/100, 40 mg $438.75/100, 80 mg $825.01/100; 160 mg $1555.71/100. *Roxicodone SR*— ■ **Oral solution (burgundy cherry):** 5 mg/5 ml in 500-ml bottle (Roxicodone)$^{Rx}$ ■Cost: $41.65/500 ml ■ **Concentrated oral solution:** 20 mg/ml in 30-ml bottle with dropper (Roxicodone Intensol, Oxy-FAST)$^{Rx}$ ■Cost: *Roxicodone Intensol*—$40.56/30 ml; *OxyFAST*—$40.78/30 ml.

❏ **Oxycodone/Acetaminophen**

■ **Tablets:** {2.5 mg oxycodone with 325 mg acetaminophen (Percocet 2.5)$^{Rx}$}, 5 mg oxycodone with 325 mg acetaminophen (Endocet, Oxycet, Percocet, Roxicet)$^{Rx}$, 7.5 mg oxycodone with 500 mg acetaminophen (Percocet 7.5/500)$^{Rx}$, 7.5 mg oxycodone with 325 mg acetaminophen (Percocet 7.5/325)$^{Rx}$, 10 mg oxycodone with 650 mg acetaminophen (Percocet 10/650)$^{Rx}$, 10 mg oxycodone with 325 mg acetaminophen (Percocet 10/325)$^{Rx}$ ■Cost: *Endocet*—$31.05/100, *Percocet 5*—$114.31/100, *Roxicet*—$31.04/100, ■ **Capsules:** 5 mg oxycodone with 500 mg acetaminophen (Roxilox, Tylox)$^{Rx}$ ■ Cost: *Roxilox*—$57.72/100; *Tylox*—$99.96/100 ■ **Caplets:** 5 mg oxycodone with 500 mg acetaminophen (Roxicet 5/500)$^{Rx}$ ■Cost: $57.60/100 ■ **Oral solution (mint):** 5 mg oxycodone with 325 mg acetaminophen/5 ml (Roxicet Solution) in 500-ml bottles$^{Rx}$ ■ Cost: $37.37/500 ml.

❏ **Oxycodone/Aspirin**

■ **Tablets:** 2.44 mg oxycodone with 325 mg aspirin (Percodan-Demi)$^{Rx}$, 4.88 mg oxycodone with 325 mg aspirin (Endodan, Oxycodan, Percodan, Roxiprin)$^{Rx}$.

TIME/ACTION PROFILE (analgesic effects)

| | ONSET | PEAK | DURATION |
|---|---|---|---|
| PO | 10–15 min | 60–90 min | 3–6 hr |
| PO-CR | 10–15 min | 3 hr | 12 hr |

# NURSING IMPLICATIONS

## ASSESSMENT

❏ Assess type, location, and intensity of pain prior to and 1 hr (peak) after administration. When titrating opioid doses, increases of 25–50% should be administered until there is either a 50% reduction in the patient's pain rating on a numerical or visual analogue scale or the patient reports satisfactory pain relief. A repeat dose can be safely administered at the time of the peak if previous dose is ineffective and side effects are minimal.

❏ Patients taking controlled-release tablets may require additional short-acting opioid doses for breakthrough pain. Doses should be equivalent to 10–20% of 24 hr total and given every 2 hr as needed.

❏ An equianalgesic chart (see Appendix O) should be used when changing routes or when changing from one opioid to another.

❏ Assess blood pressure, pulse, and respirations before and periodically during administration. If respiratory rate is <10/min, assess level of sedation. Physical stimulation may be sufficient to prevent significant hypoventilation. Dose may need to be decreased by 25–50%. Initial drowsiness will diminish with continued use.

❏ Prolonged use may lead to physical and psychological dependence and tolerance. This should not prevent patient from receiving adequate analgesia. Most patients who receive oxycodone for pain do not develop psychological dependence. Progressively higher doses may be required to relieve pain with long-term therapy.

❏ Assess bowel function routinely. Prevention of constipation should be instituted with increased intake of fluids and bulk, and laxatives to minimize constipating effects. Stimulant laxatives should be administered routinely if opioid use exceeds 2–3 days, unless contraindicated.

■ *Lab Test Considerations:* May ↑ plasma amylase and lipase levels.

■ *Toxicity and Overdose:* If an opioid antagonist is required to reverse respiratory depression or coma, naloxone (Narcan) is the antidote. Dilute the 0.4-mg ampule of naloxone in 10 ml of 0.9% NaCl and administer 0.5 ml (0.02 mg) by direct IV push every 2 min. For children and patients weighing <40 kg, dilute 0.1 mg of naloxone in 10 ml of 0.9% NaCl for a concentration of 10 mcg/ml and administer 0.5 mcg/kg every 2

min. Titrate dose to avoid withdrawal, seizures, and severe pain.

## POTENTIAL NURSING DIAGNOSES

■ Pain, acute (Indications).
■ Sensory perception, disturbed (visual, auditory) (Side Effects).
■ Injury, risk for (Side Effects).

## IMPLEMENTATION

❏ *High Alert:* Accidental overdosage of opioid analgesics has resulted in fatalities. Before administering, clarify all ambiguous orders; have second practitioner independently check original order and dose calculations. Do not confuse oxycodone with OxyContin. Do not confuse Percocet with Percodan.

■ **General:** Regularly administered doses may be more effective than prn administration. Analgesic is more effective if given before pain becomes severe.

❏ Coadministration with nonopioid analgesics may have additive analgesic effects and may permit lower doses. Medication should be discontinued gradually after long-term use to prevent withdrawal symptoms.

■ **PO:** May be administered with food or milk to minimize GI irritation.

❏ Administer solution with properly calibrated measuring device.

❏ Controlled-release tablets should be swallowed whole; do not crush, break, or chew. Taking broken, chewed, or crushed controlled-release tablets leads to rapid release and absorption of a potentially fatal dose of oxycodone.

■ **Controlled Release:** Dose should be based on 24-hr opioid requirement determined with short-acting opioids then converted to controlled-release form.

## PATIENT/FAMILY TEACHING

❏ Instruct patient on how and when to ask for pain medication. Caution patient not to increase the dose of controlled-release oxycodone without consulting health care professional.

❏ Caution patient that controlled-release oxycodone is a potential drug of abuse. Medication should be protected from theft and never given to anyone other than the individual for whom it was prescribed.

❑ Medication may cause drowsiness or dizziness. Advise patient to call for assistance when ambulating or smoking. Caution patient to avoid driving and other activities requiring alertness until response to medication is known.

❑ Advise patients taking Oxycontin tablets that empty matrix tablets may appear in stool.

❑ Advise patient to make position changes slowly to minimize orthostatic hypotension.

❑ Advise patient to avoid concurrent use of alcohol or other CNS depressants with this medication.

❑ Encourage patient to turn, cough, and breathe deeply every 2 hr to prevent atelectasis.

## EVALUATION

**Effectiveness of therapy can be demonstrated by:** ■ Decrease in severity of pain without a significant alteration in level of consciousness or respiratory status.

---

**High Alert**

# oxymorphone
(ox-i-**mor**-fone)
Numorphan

### CLASSIFICATION(S):
**Therapeutic:** opioid analgesics
**Pharmacologic:** opioid agonists

### Schedule II

### Pregnancy Category UK

## INDICATIONS

■ Management of moderate to severe pain ■ Supplement in balanced anesthesia.

## ACTION

■ Binds to opiate receptors in the CNS ■ Alters the perception of and response to painful stimuli, while producing generalized CNS depression. **Therapeutic Effects:** ■ Decrease in pain.

## PHARMACOKINETICS

**Absorption:** Well absorbed following IM, subcut, or rectal administration.

**Distribution:** Widely distributed; crosses placenta, enters breast milk.

**Metabolism and Excretion:** Mostly metabolized by the liver.

**Half-life:** 2.6–4 hr.

## CONTRAINDICATIONS AND PRECAUTIONS

**Contraindicated in:** ■ Hypersensitivity ■ Pregnancy or lactation (avoid chronic use) ■ Children <12 yr.

**Use Cautiously in:** ■ Head trauma ■ Increased intracranial pressure ■ Severe renal, hepatic, or pulmonary disease ■ Hypothyroidism ■ Adrenal insufficiency ■ Alcoholism ■ Geriatric or debilitated patients (initial dosage reduction recommended) ■ Undiagnosed abdominal pain ■ Prostatic hypertrophy.

## ADVERSE REACTIONS AND SIDE EFFECTS*

■ **CNS:** confusion, sedation, dizziness, dysphoria, euphoria, floating feeling, hallucinations, headache, unusual dreams ■ **EENT:** blurred vision, diplopia, miosis ■ **Resp:** RESPIRATORY DEPRESSION ■ **CV:** orthostatic hypotension ■ **GI:** constipation, dry mouth, nausea, vomiting ■ **GU:** urinary retention ■ **Derm:** flushing, sweating ■ **Misc:** physical dependence, psychological dependence, tolerance.

## INTERACTIONS

**Drug-Drug:** ■ Use with caution in patients receiving **MAO inhibitors** (may result in unpredictable reactions—decrease initial dose of oxymorphone to 25% of usual dose) ■ ↑ CNS depression with **alcohol, antihistamines,** and **sedative/hypnotics** ■ Administration of **partial-antagonist opioid analgesics** may precipitate withdrawal in physically dependent patients ■ **Nalbuphine, buprenorphine,** or **pentazocine** ↓ analgesia.

**Drug-Natural Products:** ■ Concomitant use of **kava, valerian,** or **chamomile** can ↑ CNS depression.

## ROUTE AND DOSAGE

Larger doses may be required during chronic therapy.

■ **Subcut, IM (Adults):** 1–1.5 mg q 3–6 hr as needed. *Analgesia during labor*—0.5–1 mg.

■ **IV (Adults):** 0.5 mg q 3–6 hr as needed; increase as needed.

- **Rect (Adults):** 5 mg q 4–6 hr as needed.

## AVAILABILITY

- *Injection:* 1 mg/ml in 1-ml ampules<sup>Rx</sup>, 1.5 mg/ml in 1-ml ampules and 10-ml vials<sup>Rx</sup> ■ Cost: 1 mg/ml $29.50/10-ml vial, 1.5 mg/ml $34.50/10-ml vial ■ *Suppositories:* 5 mg<sup>Rx</sup> ■ Cost: $29.19/6.

TIME/ACTION PROFILE (analgesic effects)

|        | ONSET      | PEAK       | DURATION |
|--------|------------|------------|----------|
| IM     | 10–15 min  | 30–90 min  | 3–6 hr   |
| IV     | 5–10 min   | 15–30 min  | 3–6 hr   |
| Subcut | 10–20 min  | unknown    | 3–4 hr   |
| Rect   | 15–30 min  | 120 min    | 3–6 hr   |

# NURSING IMPLICATIONS

## ASSESSMENT

- ❏ Assess type, location, and intensity of pain prior to and 1 hr following IM and 15–30 min (peak) following IV administration. When titrating opioid doses, increases of 25–50% should be administered until there is either a 50% reduction in the patient's pain rating on a numerical or visual analog scale or the patient reports satisfactory pain relief. A repeat dose can be safely administered at the time of the peak if previous dose is ineffective and side effects are minimal.

- ❏ An equianalgesic chart (see Appendix O) should be used when changing routes or when changing from one opioid to another.

- ❏ Assess blood pressure, pulse, and respirations before and periodically during administration. If respiratory rate is <10/min, assess level of sedation. Physical stimulation may be sufficient to prevent significant hypoventilation. Dose may need to be decreased by 25–50%. Initial drowsiness will diminish with continued use.

- ❏ Prolonged use may lead to physical and psychological dependence and tolerance. This should not prevent patient from receiving adequate analgesia. Most patients who receive oxymorphone for pain do not develop psychological dependence. Progressively higher doses may be required to relieve pain with long-term therapy.

- ❏ Assess bowel function routinely. Prevention of constipation should be instituted with increased intake of fluids and bulk, and laxatives. Stimulant laxatives should be administered routinely if opioid use exceeds 2–3 days, unless contraindicated.

- ■ *Lab Test Considerations:* May ↑ plasma amylase and lipase levels.

- ■ *Toxicity and Overdose:* If an opioid antagonist is required to reverse respiratory depression or coma, naloxone (Narcan) is the antidote. Dilute the 0.4-mg ampule of naloxone in 10 ml of 0.9% NaCl and administer 0.5 ml (0.02 mg) by direct IV push every 2 min. For children and patients weighing <40 kg, dilute 0.1 mg of naloxone in 10 ml of 0.9% NaCl for a concentration of 10 mcg/ml and administer 0.5 mcg/kg every 2 min. Titrate dose to avoid withdrawal, seizures, and severe pain.

## POTENTIAL NURSING DIAGNOSES

- ■ Pain, acute (Indications).
- ■ Sensory perception, disturbed (visual, auditory) (Side Effects).
- ■ Injury, risk for (Side Effects).

## IMPLEMENTATION

- ❏ *High Alert:* Accidental overdosage of opioid analgesics has resulted in fatalities. Before administering, clarify all ambiguous orders; have second practitioner independently check original order, dose calculations, and infusion pump settings.

- ■ **General:** Explain therapeutic value of medication prior to administration to enhance the analgesic effect.

- ❏ Regularly administered doses may be more effective than prn administration. Analgesic is more effective if given before pain becomes severe.

- ❏ Coadministration with nonopioid analgesics may have additive analgesic effects and may permit lower doses.

- ❏ Medication should be discontinued gradually after long-term use to prevent withdrawal symptoms.

- ■ **Rect:** Suppositories should be stored in the refrigerator.

- **Direct IV:** Administer undiluted over 2–3 min.

## PATIENT/FAMILY TEACHING

❏ Instruct patient on how and when to ask for pain medication.

❏ Medication may cause drowsiness or dizziness. Advise patient to call for assistance when ambulating or smoking. Caution patient to avoid driving and other activities requiring alertness until response to medication is known.

❏ Advise patient to make position changes slowly to minimize orthostatic hypotension.

❏ Advise patient to avoid concurrent use of alcohol or other CNS depressants with this medication.

❏ Encourage patient to turn, cough, and breathe deeply every 2 hr to prevent atelectasis.

## EVALUATION

**Effectiveness of therapy can be demonstrated by:** ■ Decrease in severity of pain without a significant alteration in level of consciousness or respiratory status.

---

## oxytocin

(ox-i-**toe**-sin)
Pitocin, Syntocinon

**CLASSIFICATION(S):**
**Therapeutic:** hormones
**Pharmacologic:** oxytocics

**Pregnancy Category X (intranasal), UK (IV, IM)**

## INDICATIONS

■ **IV:** Induction of labor at term ■ Facilitation of uterine contractions at term ■ Facilitation of threatened abortion ■ Postpartum control of bleeding after expulsion of the placenta ■ **Intranasal:** Used to promote milk letdown in lactating women. **Unlabeled uses:** ■ Evaluation of fetal competence (fetal stress test).

## ACTION

■ Stimulates uterine smooth muscle, producing uterine contractions similar to those in spontaneous labor ■ Stimulates mammary gland smooth muscle, facilitating lactation ■ Has vaso-

pressor and antidiuretic effects. **Therapeutic Effects:** ■ Induction of labor (IV) ■ Milk letdown (intranasal).

## PHARMACOKINETICS

**Absorption:** Well absorbed from the nasal mucosa.

**Distribution:** Widely distributed in extracellular fluid. Small amounts reach fetal circulation.

**Metabolism and Excretion:** Rapidly metabolized by liver and kidneys.

**Half-life:** 3–9 min.

## CONTRAINDICATIONS AND PRECAUTIONS

**Contraindicated in:** ■ Hypersensitivity ■ Anticipated nonvaginal delivery ■ Pregnancy (intranasal).

**Use Cautiously in:** ■ First and second stages of labor.

## ADVERSE REACTIONS AND SIDE EFFECTS*

Maternal adverse reactions are noted for IV use only. ■ **CNS:** *maternal*— COMA, SEIZURES, *fetal*— INTRACRANIAL HEMORRHAGE ■ **Resp:** *fetal*— ASPHYXIA, hypoxia ■ **CV:** *maternal*—hypotension; *fetal*— arrhythmias ■ **F and E:** *maternal*—hypochloremia, hyponatremia, water intoxication ■ **Misc:** *maternal*—increased uterine motility, painful contractions, abruptio placentae, decreased uterine blood flow, hypersensitivity.

## INTERACTIONS

**Drug-Drug:** ■ Severe hypertension may occur if oxytocin follows administration of **vasopressors** ■ Concurrent use with **cyclopropane** anesthesia may result in excessive hypotension.

## ROUTE AND DOSAGE

❏ **Induction/Stimulation of Labor**

■ **IV (Adults):** 0.5–2 milliunits/min; increase by 1–2 milliunits/min q 15–60 min until pattern established (usually 5–6 milliunits/min; maximum 20 milliunits/min), then decrease dose.

❏ **Postpartum Hemorrhage**

■ **IV (Adults):** 10 units infused at 20–40 milliunits/min.

■ **IM (Adults):** 10 units after delivery of placenta.

□ **Incomplete/Inevitable Abortion**

■ **IV (Adults):** 10 units at a rate of 20–40 milliunits/min.

□ **Promotion of Milk Letdown**

■ **Intranasal (Adults):** 1 spray in 1 or both nostrils 2–3 min before breastfeeding or pumping breasts.

□ **Fetal Stress Test**

■ **IV (Adults):** 0.5 milliunits/min; may be doubled q 20 min until 3 moderate contractions occur in one 10-min period (usually 5–6 milliunits/min) to a maximum of 20 milliunits/min with maternal/fetal monitoring.

## AVAILABILITY (generic available)

■ *Solution for injection:* 10 units/ml in 0.5- and 1-ml ampules^Rx, 1-ml prefilled syringes^Rx, 1-ml and 10-ml vials^Rx ■ *Nasal spray:* 40 units/ml in 2- and 5-ml containers^Rx.

TIME/ACTION PROFILE (IV = uterine contractions; intranasal = milk letdown)

|  | ONSET | PEAK | DURATION |
|---|---|---|---|
| IV | immediate | unknown | 1 hr |
| IM | 3–5 min | unknown | 30–60 min |
| Intranasal | few min | unknown | 20 min |

# NURSING IMPLICATIONS

## ASSESSMENT

□ Fetal maturity, presentation, and pelvic adequacy should be assessed prior to administration of oxytocin for induction of labor.

□ Assess character, frequency, and duration of uterine contractions; resting uterine tone; and fetal heart rate frequently throughout administration. If contractions occur <2 min apart and are >50–65 mm Hg on monitor, if they last 60–90 sec or longer, or if a significant change in fetal heart rate develops, stop infusion and turn patient on her left side to prevent fetal anoxia. Notify physician or other health care professional immediately.

□ Monitor maternal blood pressure and pulse frequently and fetal heart rate continuously throughout administration.

□ This drug occasionally causes water intoxication. Monitor patient for signs and symptoms (drowsiness, listlessness, confusion, headache, anuria) and notify physician or other health care professional if they occur.

■ *Lab Test Considerations:* Monitor maternal electrolytes. Water retention may result in hypochloremia or hyponatremia.

## POTENTIAL NURSING DIAGNOSES

■ Knowledge, deficient, related to medication regimen (Patient/Family Teaching).

## IMPLEMENTATION

■ **General:** Do not confuse Pitocin (oxytocin) with Pitressin (vasopressin).

□ Do not administer oxytocin simultaneously by more than one route.

■ **Continuous Infusion:** Rotate infusion container to ensure thorough mixing. Store solution in refrigerator, but do not freeze.

□ Infuse via infusion pump for accurate dosage. Oxytocin should be connected via Y-site injection to an IV of 0.9% NaCl for use during adverse reactions.

□ Magnesium sulfate should be available if needed for relaxation of the myometrium.

■ **Induction of Labor:** Dilute 1 ml (10 units) in 1 L of compatible infusion fluid for a concentration of 10 milliunits/ml.

■ *Rate:* Begin infusion at 0.5–2 milliunits/min (0.05–0.2 ml); increase in increments of 1–2 milliunits/min at 15–30-min intervals until contractions simulate normal labor.

■ **Postpartum Bleeding:** For control of postpartum bleeding, dilute 1–4 ml (10–40 units) in 1 L of compatible infusion fluid (10–40 milliunits/ml).

■ *Rate:* Begin infusion at a rate of 20–40 milliunits/min to control uterine atony. Adjust rate as indicated.

■ **Incomplete or Inevitable Abortion:** For incomplete or inevitable abortion, dilute 1 ml (10 units) in 500 ml of compatible infusion fluid for a concentration of 20 milliunits/ml.

■ *Rate:* Infuse at a rate of 20–40 milliunits/min.

■ **Y-Site Compatibility:** ◆ heparin ◆ hydrocortisone sodium succinate ◆ insulin ◆ meperidine ◆ morphine ◆ potassium chloride ◆ vitamin B complex with C.

---

{ } = Available in Canada only.
*CAPITALS indicates life-threatening; <u>underlines</u> indicate most frequent.

■ **Solution Compatibility:** ◆ dextrose/Ringer's or lactated Ringer's combinations ◆ dextrose/saline combinations ◆ Ringer's or lactated Ringer's injection ◆ D5W ◆ D10W ◆ 0.45% NaCl ◆ 0.9% NaCl. **Intranasal:** Hold squeeze bottle upright while patient is in sitting position. Patient should clear nasal passages prior to administration.

## PATIENT/FAMILY TEACHING

■ **General Info:** Advise patient to expect contractions similar to menstrual cramps after administration has started.

■ **Nasal Spray:** Advise patient to administer nasal spray 2–3 min prior to planned breastfeeding. Patient should notify health care professional if milk drips from non-nursed breast or if uterine cramps occur.

## EVALUATION

**Effectiveness of therapy can be demonstrated by:** ■ Onset of effective contractions ■ Increase in uterine tone ■ Effective letdown reflex.

## paclitaxel
(**pak**-li-tax-el)
Onxol, Taxol

*CLASSIFICATION(S):*
*Therapeutic: antineoplastics*
*Pharmacologic: taxoids*

Pregnancy Category D

### INDICATIONS

■ Advanced ovarian cancer (with cisplatin) ■ Non–small cell lung cancer when potentially curative surgery or radiation therapy is not an option ■ Metastatic ovarian cancer unresponsive to other therapy ■ Metastatic breast cancer unresponsive to other therapy ■ Node-positive breast cancer when administered sequentially to standard combination chemotherapy ■ Treatment of AIDS-related Kaposi's sarcoma.

### ACTION

■ Interferes with the normal cellular microtubule function that is required for interphase and mitosis. **Therapeutic Effects:** ■ Death of rapidly replicating cells, particularly malignant ones.

### PHARMACOKINETICS

**Absorption:** IV administration results in complete bioavailability.
**Distribution:** Unknown.
**Metabolism and Excretion:** Probably highly metabolized by the liver.
**Half-life:** 5.3–17.4 hr.

### CONTRAINDICATIONS AND PRECAUTIONS

**Contraindicated in:** ■ Hypersensitivity to paclitaxel or to castor oil (vehicle contains polyoxyethylated castor oil) ■ Known alcohol intolerance ■ Pregnancy or lactation ■ WBC ≤1500/mm³ in patients with ovarian or breast cancer ■ WBC ≤1000/mm³ in patients with AIDS-related Kaposi's sarcoma.
**Use Cautiously in:** ■ Severe hepatic impairment ■ Geriatric patients (may have increased risk of neuropathy and cardiovascular events) ■ Childbearing potential ■ Active infection ■ De-

creased bone marrow reserve ■ Chronic debilitating illnesses ■ Children (safety not established).

### ADVERSE REACTIONS AND SIDE EFFECTS*

■ **CNS:** abnormal ECG, malaise, weakness ■ **CV:** bradycardia, hypotension ■ **GI:** <u>diarrhea</u>, <u>nausea</u>, <u>vomiting</u>, abnormal liver function tests, stomatitis ■ **Derm:** <u>alopecia</u>, maculopapular rash, pruritus, radiation recall reactions ■ **Hemat:** <u>anemia</u>, <u>leukopenia</u>, <u>thrombocytopenia</u> ■ **MS:** arthralgia, <u>myalgia</u> ■ **Neuro:** <u>peripheral neuropathy</u> ■ **Misc:** hypersensitivity reactions including ANAPHYLAXIS and STEVENS-JOHNSON SYNDROME, TOXIC EPIDERMAL NECROLYSIS.

### INTERACTIONS

**Drug-Drug:** ■ **Ketoconazole** may ↓ metabolism and ↑ risk of serious toxicity; concurrent use should be undertaken with caution; **cyclosporine, doxorubicin, felodipine, diazepam,** and **midazolam** may also ↓ metabolism and ↑ toxicity ■ ↑ risk of myelosuppression with other **antineoplastics** or **radiation therapy** ■ **Phenobarbital** and **carbamazepine** may ↓ blood levels and effectiveness ■ Concurrent **radiation** increases the risk of radiation pneumonitis ■ Myelosuppression ↑ when given after **cisplatin** ■ May ↑ levels and toxicity of **doxorubicin** ■ May ↓ antibody response to and ↑ risk of adverse reactions from **live-virus vaccines.**

### ROUTE AND DOSAGE

Many other regimens are used.

❑ **Ovarian Carcinoma**
■ **IV (Adults):** *First-line therapy*—175 mg/m² over 3 hr every 3 wk, or 135 mg/m² over 24 hr every 3 wk, followed by cisplatin; *after failure of first-line therapy*—135 mg/m² or 175 mg/m² over 3 hr every 3 wk.

❑ **Breast Carcinoma**
■ **IV (Adults):** *Adjuvant treatment of node-positive breast cancer*—175 mg/m² over 3 hr every 3 wk for 4 courses sequentially to doxorubicin-containing combination chemotherapy (Taxol only); *progression of metastatic disease or relapse within 6 mo of*

*adjuvant therapy*—175 mg/m² over 3 hr every 3 wk.

□ **Non-Small Cell Lung Cancer**

■ **IV (Adults):** 135 mg/m² over 24 hr every 3 wk, followed by cisplatin.

□ **AIDS-Related Kaposi's Sarcoma**

■ **IV (Adults):** 135 mg/m² q 3 wk or 100 mg/m² q 2 wk (dosage reduction/adjustment may be necessary in patients with advanced HIV infection).

## AVAILABILITY (generic available)

■ *Concentrate for injection:* 30 mg/5-ml vials^Rx, 100 mg/16.7-ml vials^Rx, 150 mg/25-ml vials^Rx, 300 mg/50-ml vials^Rx ■ Cost: 6 mg/ml $182.63/5 ml, $608.76/16.7 ml, $1826.25/50 ml.

TIME/ACTION PROFILE (effect on WBCs)

| | ONSET | PEAK | DURATION |
|---|---|---|---|
| IV | unknown | 11 days | 3 wk |

# NURSING IMPLICATIONS

## ASSESSMENT

□ Monitor vital signs frequently, especially during first hr of 24-hr infusion.

□ Monitor for hypersensitivity reactions continuously during the first 30 min and frequently thereafter. These occur frequently (19%), usually during the first 10 min of paclitaxel infusion, after the first or second dose. Pretreatment is recommended for **all** patients and should include dexamethasone 20 mg PO (10 mg for patients with advanced HIV disease) 12 and 6 hours prior to paclitaxel, diphenhydramine 50 mg IV 30–60 min prior to paclitaxel, and cimetidine 300 mg or ranitidine 50 mg IV 30–60 min prior to paclitaxel. Most common manifestations are dyspnea, hypotension, and chest pain. If these occur, stop infusion and notify physician. Treatment may include bronchodilators, epinephrine, antihistamines, and corticosteroids. Keep these agents and resuscitative equipment close by in the event of an anaphylactic reaction. Other manifestations of hypersensitivity reactions include flushing and rash.

□ Monitor cardiovascular status especially during first hr of infusion. Hypotension and bradycardia are common but usually do not require treatment. Continuous ECG monitoring is recommended only for patients with serious underlying conduction abnormalities.

□ Monitor for bone marrow depression. Assess for bleeding (bleeding gums, bruising, petechiae, guaiac stools, urine, and emesis) and avoid IM injections and taking rectal temperatures if platelet count is low. Apply pressure to venipuncture sites for 10 min. Assess for signs of infection during neutropenia. Anemia may occur. Monitor for increased fatigue, dyspnea, and orthostatic hypotension. Granulocyte-colony stimulating factor (G-CSF) may be used if necessary.

□ Assess for development of peripheral neuropathy. If severe symptoms occur, subsequent dosage should be reduced by 20%.

□ Monitor intake and output, appetite, and nutritional intake. Paclitaxel causes nausea and vomiting in 60% of patients. Prophylactic antiemetics may be used. Adjust diet as tolerated to help maintain fluid and electrolyte balance and nutritional status.

□ Assess patient for arthralgia and myalgia, which usually begin 2–3 days after therapy and resolve within 5 days. Pain is usually relieved by nonopioid analgesics but may be severe enough to require treatment with opioid analgesics.

■ *Lab Test Considerations:* Monitor CBC and differential prior to and periodically during therapy. The nadir of leukopenia occurs in 11 days, with recovery by days 15–21. Notify physician if the leukocyte count is <1500/mm³ (1000/mm³ in AIDS-related Kaposi's sarcoma) or if the platelet count is <100,000/mm³. Subsequent doses are usually held until leukocyte count is >1500/mm³ (1000/mm³ in AIDS-related Kaposi's sarcoma) and platelet count is >100,000/mm³.

□ Monitor liver function studies (AST, ALT, LDH, bilirubin) prior to and periodically during therapy to detect hepatotoxicity.

□ May cause ↑ serum triglycerides.

## POTENTIAL NURSING DIAGNOSES

■ Infection, risk for (Adverse Reactions).

■ Injury, risk for (Adverse Reactions).

## IMPLEMENTATION

■ **General:** Do not confuse Taxol (paclitaxel) with Taxotere (docetaxel). Do not confuse paclitaxel with Paxil (paroxitine).

- **Continuous Infusion:** Paclitaxel must be diluted prior to injection. Dilute contents of 5-ml (30-mg) vials to a concentration of 0.3–1.2 mg/ml with the following diluents: 0.9% NaCl, D5W, D5/0.9% NaCl, or dextrose in Ringer's solution. Although haziness in the solution is normal, inspect for particulate matter or discoloration before use. Use an in-line filter of not >0.22-micron pore size. Solutions are stable for 27 hr at room temperature and lighting. Do not use PVC containers or administration sets.

- ***Rate:*** Dose for *breast cancer or AIDS-related Kaposi's sarcoma* is administered over 3 hr. Dose for *ovarian cancer* is administered as a 24-hr infusion.

- **Y-Site Compatibility:** ♦ acyclovir ♦ amikacin ♦ aminophylline ♦ ampicillin/sulbactam ♦ bleomycin ♦ butorphanol ♦ calcium chloride ♦ carboplatin ♦ cefepime ♦ cefotetan ♦ ceftazidime ♦ ceftriaxone ♦ cimetidine ♦ cisplatin ♦ cladribine ♦ cyclophosphamide ♦ cytarabine ♦ dacarbazine ♦ diphenhydramine ♦ doxorubicin ♦ droperidol ♦ etoposide ♦ etoposide phosphate ♦ famotidine ♦ floxuridine ♦ fluconazole ♦ fluorouracil ♦ furosemide ♦ ganciclovir ♦ gatifloxacin ♦ gemcitabine ♦ gentamicin ♦ granisetron ♦ haloperidol ♦ heparin ♦ hydrocortisone ♦ hydromorphone ♦ ifosfamide ♦ linezolid ♦ lorazepam ♦ magnesium sulfate ♦ mannitol ♦ meperidine ♦ mesna ♦ methotrexate ♦ metoclopramide ♦ morphine ♦ nalbuphine ♦ ondansetron ♦ pentostatin ♦ potassium chloride ♦ prochlorperazine edisylate ♦ propofol ♦ ranitidine ♦ sodium bicarbonate ♦ thiotepa ♦ topotecan ♦ vancomycin ♦ vinblastine ♦ vincristine ♦ zidovudine.

- **Y-Site Incompatibility:** ♦ amphotericin B ♦ amphotericin B cholesteryl sulfate ♦ chlorpromazine ♦ doxorubicin liposome ♦ methylprednisolone sodium succinate ♦ mitoxantrone.

## PATIENT/FAMILY TEACHING

- Instruct patient to notify health care professional promptly if fever; chills; cough; hoarseness; sore throat; signs of infection; lower back or side pain; painful or difficult urination; bleeding gums; bruising; petechiae; blood in stools, urine, or emesis; increased fatigue; dyspnea; or orthostatic hypotension occurs. Caution patient to avoid crowds and persons with known infections. Instruct patient to use soft toothbrush and electric razor and to avoid falls. Caution patient not to drink alcoholic beverages or to take medication containing aspirin or NSAIDs; may precipitate gastric bleeding.

- Instruct patient to notify health care professional if abdominal pain, yellow skin, weakness, paresthesia, gait disturbances, or joint or muscle aches occur.

- Instruct patient to inspect oral mucosa for redness and ulceration. If mouth sores occur, advise patient to use a sponge brush and rinse mouth with water after eating and drinking. Stomatitis usually resolves in 5–7 days.

- Discuss with patient the possibility of hair loss. Complete hair loss usually occurs between days 14 and 21 and is reversible after discontinuation of therapy. Explore coping strategies.

- Advise patient to use a nonhormonal method of contraception.

- Instruct patient not to receive any vaccinations without advice of health care professional.

- Emphasize the need for periodic lab tests to monitor for side effects.

## EVALUATION

**Effectiveness of therapy can be demonstrated by:** ■ Decrease in size or spread of malignancy.

---

# palonosetron

(pa-lone-**o**-se-tron)
Aloxi

### CLASSIFICATION(S):
***Therapeutic:*** antiemetics
***Pharmacologic:*** 5 HT$_3$ antagonists

**Pregnancy Category B**

## INDICATIONS

■ Prevention of acute and delayed nausea and vomiting caused by moderate or highly emetogenic chemotherapy.

---

{ } = Available in Canada only.
*CAPITALS indicates life-threatening; <u>underlines</u> indicate most frequent.

## ACTION

■ Blocks the effects of serotonin at receptor sites (selective antagonist) located in vagal nerve terminals and in the chemoreceptor trigger zones in the CNS. **Therapeutic Effects:** ■ Decreased incidence and severity of nausea and vomiting following emetogenic chemotherapy.

## PHARMACOKINETICS

**Absorption:** IV administration results in complete bioavailability.
**Distribution:** Unknown.
**Metabolism and Excretion:** 50% metabolized; 40% excreted unchanged in urine.
**Half-life:** 40 hr.

## CONTRAINDICATIONS AND PRECAUTIONS

**Contraindicated in:** ■ Hypersensitivity; cross-sensitivity with other 5–HT$_3$ antagonists may occur ■ Lactation.
**Use Cautiously in:** ■ Hereditary or acquired QTc prolongation, hypokalemia, hypomagnesemia, concurrent diuretic or antiarrhythmic therapy or history of high cumulative anthracycline therapy (may increase risk of arrhythmias) ■ Pregnancy or children (safety not established).

## ADVERSE REACTIONS AND SIDE EFFECTS*

■ **CNS:** dizziness, headache ■ **GI:** constipation, diarrhea.

## INTERACTIONS

**Drug-Drug:** ■ Concurrent **diuretic** or **antiarrhythmic** therapy or history of high cumulative **anthracycline** therapy may ↑ risk of arrhythmias.

## ROUTE AND DOSAGE

■ **IV (Adults):** 0.25 mg 30 min before start of chemotherapy.

## AVAILABILITY

■ *Solution for IV injection:* 0.25 mg/5 ml vials[Rx].

TIME/ACTION PROFILE

| | ONSET | PEAK | DURATION |
|---|---|---|---|
| IV | within 30 min | unknown | 7 days |

## NURSING IMPLICATIONS

### ASSESSMENT

❑ Assess patient for nausea, vomiting, abdominal distention, and bowel sounds prior to and following administration.
■ *Lab Test Considerations:* May cause transient ↑ in serum bilirubin, AST, and ALT levels.

### POTENTIAL NURSING DIAGNOSES

■ Nutrition, imbalanced: less than body requirements (Indications).
■ Diarrhea (Side Effects).
■ Constipation (Side Effects).

### IMPLEMENTATION

■ **General:** First dose is administered prior to emetogenic event.
❑ Repeated dose within a 7-day period is not recommended.
■ **Direct IV:** Administer dose undiluted 30 min prior to chemotherapy. Flush line prior to and after administration with 0.9% NaCl. Do not administer solutions that are discolored or contain particulate matter.
■ *Rate:* Administer over 30 seconds.
■ **Y-Site Incompatibility:** Do not mix with other drugs.

### PATIENT/FAMILY TEACHING

❑ Inform patient of purpose of medication.
❑ Advise patient to notify health care professional if nausea or vomiting occurs.

### EVALUATION

**Effectiveness of therapy can be demonstrated by:** ■ Prevention of nausea and vomiting associated with initial and repeat courses of emetogenic cancer chemotherapy.

## pamidronate
(pa-**mid**-roe-nate)
Aredia

### CLASSIFICATION(S):
*Therapeutic: bone resorption inhibitors*
*Pharmacologic: biphosphonates, hypocalcemics*

### Pregnancy Category D

## INDICATIONS

■ Moderate to severe hypercalcemia associated with malignancy ■ Osteolytic bone lesions associated with multiple myeloma or breast cancer ■ Moderate to severe Paget's disease.

## ACTION

■ Inhibits resorption of bone. **Therapeutic Effects:** ■ Decreased serum calcium ■ Decreased skeletal destruction in multiple myeloma or breast cancer ■ Decreased skeletal complications in Paget's disease.

## PHARMACOKINETICS

**Absorption:** IV administration results in complete bioavailability.

**Distribution:** Rapidly absorbed by bone. Reaches high concentrations in bone, liver, spleen, teeth, and tracheal cartilage. Approximately 50% of a dose is retained by bone and then slowly released.

**Metabolism and Excretion:** 50% is excreted unchanged in the urine.

**Half-life:** Elimination half-life from plasma is biphasic—1st phase 1.6 hr, 2nd phase 27.2 hr. Elimination half-life from bone is 300 days.

## CONTRAINDICATIONS AND PRECAUTIONS

**Contraindicated in:** ■ Hypersensitivity to pamidronate, other biphosphonates, or mannitol.

**Use Cautiously in:** ■ Underlying cardiovascular disease, especially CHF (initiate saline hydration cautiously) ■ Renal impairment (dosage reduction recommended) ■ Pregnancy, lactation, or children (safety not established).

## ADVERSE REACTIONS AND SIDE EFFECTS*

■ **CNS:** fatigue ■ **EENT:** conjunctivitis, blurred vision, eye pain/inflammation, rhinitis ■ **Resp:** rales ■ **CV:** arrhythmias, hypertension, syncope, tachycardia ■ **GI:** <u>nausea</u>, abdominal pain, anorexia, constipation, vomiting ■ **F and E:** <u>hypocalcemia</u>, <u>hypokalemia</u>, <u>hypomagnesemia</u>, <u>hypophosphatemia</u>, fluid overload ■ **Hemat:** <u>leukopenia</u>, anemia ■ **Local:** <u>phlebitis at injection site</u> ■ **Metab:** hypothyroidism ■ **MS:** <u>muscle stiffness</u>, bone pain ■ **Misc:** <u>fever</u>, <u>generalized pain</u>.

## INTERACTIONS

**Drug-Drug:** ■ Hypokalemia and hypomagnesemia may ↑ risk of **digoxin** toxicity ■ **Calcium** and **vitamin D** will antagonize the beneficial effects of pamidronate.

## ROUTE AND DOSAGE

Single doses should not exceed 90 mg.

❑ **Hypercalcemia of Malignancy**

■ **IV (Adults):** *Moderate hypercalcemia—* 30–90 mg; may be repeated after 7 days.

❑ **Osteolytic Lesions from Multiple Myeloma**

■ **IV (Adults):** 90 mg monthly.

❑ **Osteolytic Lesions from Metastatic Breast Cancer**

■ **IV (Adults):** 90 mg q 3–4 wk.

❑ **Paget's Disease**

■ **IV (Adults):** 90–180 mg/treatment; may be given as 30 mg daily for 3 days up to 30 mg/wk for 6 wk. Single doses of 60–90 mg may also be effective.

## AVAILABILITY (generic available)

■ *Injection:* 30 mg/vial^Rx, 60 mg/vial^Rx, 90 mg/vial^Rx ■ Cost: 30 mg $1119.44/4 vials, 90 mg $839.60/vial.

TIME/ACTION PROFILE (effect on serum calcium)

|    | ONSET | PEAK | DURATION |
|----|-------|------|----------|
| IV | 24 hr | 7 days | unknown |

# NURSING IMPLICATIONS

## ASSESSMENT

❑ Monitor intake/output ratios and blood pressure frequently during therapy. Assess for signs of fluid overload (edema, rales/crackles).

❑ Monitor symptoms of hypercalcemia (nausea, vomiting, anorexia, weakness, constipation, thirst, and cardiac arrhythmias).

❑ Observe for evidence of hypocalcemia (paresthesia, muscle twitching, laryngospasm, and Chvostek's or Trousseau's sign). Protect

symptomatic patients by elevating and padding side rails; keep bed in low position.
- ❑ Monitor IV site for phlebitis (pain, redness, swelling). Symptomatic treatment should be used if this occurs.
- ❑ Assess for bone pain. Treatment with nonopioid or opioid analgesics may be necessary.
- ■ **Lab Test Considerations:** Monitor serum electrolytes (including calcium, phosphate, potassium, and magnesium), hemoglobin, and creatinine closely. Monitor CBC and platelet count during the first 2 wk of therapy.

## POTENTIAL NURSING DIAGNOSES
- ■ Pain, acute (Indications, Side Effects).
- ■ Injury, risk for (Indications).

## IMPLEMENTATION
- ■ **General:** Vigorous saline hydration, maintaining a urine output of 2000 ml/24 hr, should be undertaken concurrently with pamidronate therapy. Initiate saline hydration cautiously in patients with underlying cardiovascular disease, especially CHF.
- ❑ Patients with severe hypercalcemia should be started at the 90-mg dose.
- ■ **IV:** Reconstitute by adding 10 ml of sterile water for injection to each vial for a concentration of 30 mg/10 ml, 60 mg/ml, or 90 mg/ml. Allow drug to dissolve before withdrawing. Solution is stable for 24 hr if refrigerated.
- ■ **Hypercalcemia:** Dilute further in 1000 ml of 0.45% NaCl, 0.9% NaCl, or D5W. Solution is stable for 24 hr at room temperature.
- ■ **Rate:** Administer 60-mg infusion over at least 4 hr and 90-mg infusion over 24 hr.
- ■ **Multiple Myeloma:** Dilute reconstituted solution in 500 ml of 0.45% NaCl, 0.9% NaCl, or D5W.
- ■ **Rate:** Administer over 4 hr.
- ■ **Paget's Disease:** Dilute reconstituted solution in 500 ml of 0.45% NaCl, 0.9% NaCl, or D5W.
- ■ **Rate:** Administer over 4 hr.
- ■ **Additive Incompatibility:** Calcium-containing solutions, such as Ringer's solution.

## PATIENT/FAMILY TEACHING
- ❑ Advise patient to report signs of hypercalcemic relapse (bone pain, anorexia, nausea, vomiting, thirst, lethargy) or eye problems (pain, inflammation, blurred vision, conjunctivitis) to health care professional promptly.
- ❑ Advise patient to notify nurse of pain at the infusion site.
- ❑ Encourage patient to comply with dietary recommendations. Diet should contain adequate amounts of calcium and vitamin D.
- ❑ Advise patient to notify health care professional if bone pain is severe or persistent.
- ❑ Emphasize the need for keeping follow-up exams to monitor progress, even after medication is discontinued, to detect relapse.

## EVALUATION
**Effectiveness of therapy can be demonstrated by:** ■ Lowered serum calcium levels ■ Decreased pain from lytic lesions.

# pancrelipase
(pan-kre-**li**-pase)
Cotazym, {Cotazym-65 B}, Cotazym E.C.S. 8, Cotazym E.C.S. 20, Cotazym-S, Creon 10, Creon 25, Enzymase-16, Ilozyme, Ku-Zyme HP, Lipram-PN16, Lipram-CR20, Lipram-UL12, Lipram-PN10, Lipram-UL18, Lipram,-UL20, Pancoate, Pancrease, Pancrease MT 4, Pancrease MT 10, Pancrease MT 16, Pancrease MT 20, Pancrebarb MS-8, Protilase, Ultrase MT 12, Ultrase MT 20, Viokase, Zymase

## CLASSIFICATION(S):
**Therapeutic:** *digestive agents*
**Pharmacologic:** *pancreatic enzymes*

## Pregnancy Category C

## INDICATIONS
- ■ Pancreatic insufficiency associated with: ❑ Chronic pancreatitis ❑ Pancreatectomy ❑ Cystic fibrosis ❑ GI bypass surgery ❑ Ductal obstruction secondary to tumor.

## ACTION
- ■ Contains lipolytic, amylolytic, and proteolytic activity. **Therapeutic Effects:** ■ Increased digestion of fats, carbohydrates, and proteins in the GI tract.

## PHARMACOKINETICS
**Absorption:** Unknown.
**Distribution:** Unknown.
**Metabolism and Excretion:** Unknown.
**Half-life:** Unknown.

## CONTRAINDICATIONS AND PRECAUTIONS
**Contraindicated in:** ■ Hypersensitivity to hog proteins.
**Use Cautiously in:** ■ Pregnancy or lactation (safety not established).

## ADVERSE REACTIONS AND SIDE EFFECTS*
■ **EENT:** nasal stuffiness ■ **Resp:** dyspnea, shortness of breath, wheezing ■ **GI:** <u>abdominal pain</u> (high doses only), <u>diarrhea</u>, <u>nausea</u>, <u>stomach cramps</u>, oral irritation ■ **GU:** hematuria ■ **Derm:** hives, rash ■ **Metab:** hyperuricemia ■ **Misc:** allergic reactions.

## INTERACTIONS
**Drug-Drug:** ■ Antacids (**calcium carbonate** or **magnesium hydroxide**) may decrease effectiveness of pancrelipase ■ May decrease the absorption of concurrently administered **iron supplements**.
**Drug-Food:** ■ **Alkaline foods** destroy coating on enteric-coated products.

## ROUTE AND DOSAGE
■ **PO (Adults):** 1–3 capsule(s) before or with meals; dosage may be increased as needed (up to 8 capsules may be needed), *or* 1–2 delayed-release capsule(s), *or* 0.7 g powder.
■ **PO (Children):** 1–3 capsule(s) before or with meals; dosage may be increased as needed, *or* 1–2 delayed-release capsule(s), *or* 0.7 g powder.

## AVAILABILITY (generic available)
■ *Capsules:* 8000 units lipase/30,000 units protease and amylase^Rx ■ *Delayed-release capsules:* 4000 units lipase/12,000 units protease and amylase^Rx, 4000 units lipase/25,000 units protease/20,000 units amylase^Rx, 5000 units lipase/20,000 units protease and amylase^Rx, {8000 units lipase/30,000 units protease and amylase^Rx}, 10,000 units lipase/30,000 units protease and amylase^Rx, 12,000 units lipase/24,000 units protease and amylase^Rx, 12,000 units lipase/39,000 units protease and amylase^Rx, 16,000 units lipase/48,000 units protease and amylase^Rx, {20,000 units lipase/55,000 units protease and amylase^Rx}, 20,000 units lipase/65,000 units protease and amylase^Rx, 24,000 units lipase/78,000 units protease and amylase^Rx ■ *Powder:* 16,800 units lipase/70,000 units protease and amylase^Rx.

TIME/ACTION PROFILE (digestant effects)

| | ONSET | PEAK | DURATION |
|----|-------|------|----------|
| PO | rapid | unknown | unknown |

# NURSING IMPLICATIONS

## ASSESSMENT
❑ Assess patient's nutritional status (height, weight, skin-fold thickness, arm muscle circumference, and lab values) prior to and periodically throughout therapy.
❑ Monitor stools for high fat content (steatorrhea). Stools will be foul-smelling and frothy.
❑ Assess patient for allergy to pork; sensitivity to pancrelipase may exist.
■ *Lab Test Considerations:* May cause elevated serum and urine uric acid concentrations.

## POTENTIAL NURSING DIAGNOSES
■ Nutrition, imbalanced: less than body requirements (Indications).

## IMPLEMENTATION
■ **PO:** Administer immediately before or with meals and snacks.
❑ Capsules may be opened and sprinkled on foods. Capsules filled with enteric-coated beads should not be chewed (sprinkle on soft foods that can be swallowed without chewing, such as applesauce or Jell-O).
❑ Pancrelipase is destroyed by acid. Concurrent sodium bicarbonate or aluminum-containing antacids may be used with nonenteric-coated preparations to neutralize gastric pH. Enteric-coated beads are designed to withstand the acid pH of the stomach. These medications should not be chewed or mixed with alkaline foods prior to ingestion or coating will be destroyed.

{ } = Available in Canada only.
*CAPITALS indicates life-threatening; <u>underlines</u> indicate most frequent.

## PATIENT/FAMILY TEACHING

❑ Encourage patients to comply with diet recommendations of health care professional (generally high-calorie, high-protein, low-fat). Dosage should be adjusted for fat content of diet. Usually 300 mg of pancrelipase is necessary to digest every 17 g of dietary fat. If a dose is missed, it should be omitted.

❑ Instruct patient not to chew tablets and to swallow them quickly with plenty of liquid to prevent mouth and throat irritation. Patient should be sitting upright to enhance swallowing. Eating immediately after taking medication helps further ensure that the medication is swallowed and does not remain in contact with mouth and esophagus for a prolonged period. Patient should avoid sniffing powdered contents of capsules, as sensitization of nose and throat may occur (nasal stuffiness or respiratory distress).

❑ Instruct patient to notify health care professional if joint pain, swelling of legs, gastric distress, or rash occurs.

## EVALUATION

**Effectiveness of therapy can be demonstrated by:** ■ Improved nutritional status in patients with pancreatic insufficiency ❑ Normalization of stools in patients with steatorrhea.

**High Alert**

# pancuronium

(pan-cure-**oh**-nee-yum)
Pavulon

## CLASSIFICATION(S):

**Therapeutic:** neuromuscular blocking agents—nondepolarizing

**Pregnancy Category C**

## INDICATIONS

■ Induction of skeletal muscle paralysis and facilitation of intubation after induction of anesthesia in surgical procedures ■ Facilitation of compliance during mechanical ventilation.

## ACTION

■ Prevents neuromuscular transmission by blocking the effect of acetylcholine at the myoneural junction. Has no analgesic or anxiolytic properties. **Therapeutic Effects:** ■ Skeletal muscle paralysis.

## PHARMACOKINETICS

**Absorption:** Following IV administration, absorption is essentially complete.

**Distribution:** Rapidly distributes into extracellular fluid; small amounts cross the placenta.

**Metabolism and Excretion:** Excreted mostly unchanged by the kidneys; small amounts are eliminated in bile.

**Half-life:** 2 hr.

## CONTRAINDICATIONS AND PRECAUTIONS

**Contraindicated in:** ■ Hypersensitivity ■ Hypersensitivity to bromides ■ Products containing benzyl alcohol should be avoided in neonates.

**Use Cautiously in:** ■ Patients with underlying cardiovascular disease (increased risk of arrhythmias) ■ Dehydration or electrolyte abnormalities (should be corrected) ■ Situations in which histamine release would be problematic ■ Fractures or muscle spasm ■ Geriatric patients or patients with impaired renal function (decreased elimination) ■ Hyperthermia (increased duration/intensity of paralysis) ■ Patients with significant hepatic impairment (altered response) ■ Shock ■ Extensive burns (may be more resistant to effects of cisatracurium) ■ Low plasma pseudocholinesterase levels (may be seen in association with anemia, dehydration, cholinesterase inhibitors/insecticides, severe liver disease, pregnancy, or hereditary predisposition) ■ Obese patients ■ Pregnancy, lactation, or children (safety not established for some agents; most agents have been used safely in pregnant women undergoing cesarean section; selected agents have been used safely in children).

**Exercise Extreme Caution in:** ■ Patients with neuromuscular diseases such as myasthenia gravis (small test dose may be used to assess response).

## ADVERSE REACTIONS AND SIDE EFFECTS*

■ **Resp:** bronchospasm ■ **CV:** hypertension, tachycardia ■ **GI:** excessive salivation ■ **Derm:** rash ■ **Misc:** allergic reactions including ANAPHYLAXIS.

## INTERACTIONS

**Drug-Drug:** ■ Intensity and duration of paralysis may be prolonged by pretreatment with **succinylcholine, general anesthesia** (inhalation), **aminoglycosides, vancomycin, tetracyclines, polymyxin B, colistin, clindamycin, lidocaine,** and other **local anesthetics, lithium, quinidine, procainamide, beta blockers, potassium-losing diuretics,** or **magnesium** ■ **Inhalation anesthetics** including **enflurane, isoflurane, halothane, desflurane,** and **sevoflurane** may enhance effects ■ Higher infusion rates may be required and duration of action may be shortened in patients receiving long-term **carbamazepine** or **phenytoin.**

## ROUTE AND DOSAGE

■ **IV (Adults and Children >1 mo):** 40–100 mcg/kg initially; incremental doses of 10 mcg/kg may be given q 20–60 min to maintain paralysis. *Provision of relaxation to allow mechanical ventilation*—15 mcg/kg.

## AVAILABILITY

■ *Injection:* 1 mg/ml in 10-ml vials$^{Rx}$, 2 mg/ml in 2- and 5-ml ampules$^{Rx}$.

TIME/ACTION PROFILE (neuromuscular blockade)

|   | ONSET | PEAK | DURATION |
|---|-------|------|----------|
| IV | 30–45 sec | 3–4.5 min | 35–45 min |

## NURSING IMPLICATIONS

### ASSESSMENT

❏ Assess respiratory status continuously throughout therapy with neuromuscular blocking agents. These medications should be used only to facilitate intubation or in patients already intubated.

❏ Neuromuscular response should be monitored with a peripheral nerve stimulator intraoperatively. Paralysis is initially selective and usually occurs sequentially in the following muscles: levator muscles of eyelids, muscles of mastication, limb muscles, abdominal muscles, muscles of the glottis, intercostal muscles, and the diaphragm. Recovery of muscle function usually occurs in reverse order.

❏ Monitor ECG, heart rate, and blood pressure throughout administration.

❏ Observe the patient for residual muscle weakness and respiratory distress during the recovery period.

❏ Monitor infusion site frequently. If signs of tissue irritation or extravasation occur, discontinue and restart in another vein.

■ *Toxicity and Overdose:* If overdose occurs, use peripheral nerve stimulator to determine the degree of neuromuscular blockade. Maintain airway patency and ventilation until recovery of normal respirations occurs.

❏ Administration of anticholinesterase agents (neostigmine, pyridostigmine) may be used to antagonize the action of neuromuscular blocking agents once the patient has demonstrated some spontaneous recovery from neuromuscular block. Atropine is usually administered prior to or concurrently with anticholinesterase agents to counteract the muscarinic effects.

❏ Administration of fluids and vasopressors may be necessary to treat severe hypotension or shock.

## POTENTIAL NURSING DIAGNOSES

■ Breathing pattern, ineffective (Indications).

■ Communication, impaired verbal (Side Effects).

■ Fear (Side Effects).

## IMPLEMENTATION

❏ *High Alert:* Unintended administration of a neuromuscular blocking agent instead of administration of the intended medication or administration of a neuromuscular blocking agent in the absence of ventilatory support has resulted in serious harm or death. Confusing similarities in packaging and insufficiently controlled access to these medications are often implicated in these medication errors. Store these products in a separate, locked container.

■ **General:** Dose is titrated to patient response.

❏ Neuromuscular blocking agents have *no* effect on consciousness or pain threshold. Ad-

{ } = Available in Canada only.
*CAPITALS indicates life-threatening; <u>underlines</u> indicate most frequent.

equate anesthesia/analgesia should *always* be used when neuromuscular blocking agents are used as an adjunct to surgical procedures or when painful procedures are performed. Benzodiazepines and/or analgesics should be administered concurrently when prolonged neuromuscular blocker therapy is used for ventilator patients, because patient is awake and able to feel all sensations.

❏ If eyes remain open throughout prolonged administration, protect corneas with artificial tears.

❏ Store pancuronium in refrigerator. To prevent absorption by plastic, pancuronium should not be stored in plastic syringes. May be administered in plastic syringes.

❏ Most neuromuscular blocking agents are incompatible with barbiturates and sodium bicarbonate. Do not admix.

■ **Direct IV:** Incremental doses may be administered every 20–60 min as needed. Dose is titrated to patient response.

■ **Intermittent Infusion:** May be diluted in 0.9% NaCl, D5W, D5/0.9% NaCl, and LR injection. Solution is stable for 48 hr.

■ *Rate:* Titrate rate according to patient response.

■ **Syringe Compatibility:** ◆ heparin.

■ **Y-Site Compatibility:** ◆ aminophylline ◆ cefazolin ◆ cefuroxime ◆ cimetidine ◆ dobutamine ◆ dopamine ◆ epinephrine ◆ esmolol ◆ etomidate ◆ fentanyl ◆ fluconazole ◆ gentamicin ◆ heparin ◆ hydrocortisone sodium succinate ◆ isoproterenol ◆ levofloxacin ◆ lorazepam ◆ midazolam ◆ morphine ◆ nitroglycerin ◆ nitroprusside ◆ ranitidine ◆ trimethoprim/sulfamethoxazole ◆ vancomycin.

■ **Y-Site Incompatibility:** ◆ diazepam ◆ thiopental.

## PATIENT/FAMILY TEACHING

❏ Explain all procedures to patient receiving neuromuscular blocker therapy without general anesthesia, because consciousness is not affected by neuromuscular blocking agents alone.

❏ Reassure patient that communication abilities will return as the medication wears off.

## EVALUATION

**Effectiveness of therapy can be demonstrated by:** ■ Adequate suppression of the twitch response when tested with peripheral nerve stimulation and subsequent muscle paralysis ■ Improved compliance during mechanical ventilation.

# pantoprazole
(pan-**toe**-pra-zole)
Protonix, Protonix I.V.

*CLASSIFICATION(S):*
*Therapeutic: antiulcer agents*
*Pharmacologic: gastric acid pump inhibitors*

**Pregnancy Category B**

## INDICATIONS

■ Erosive esophagitis associated with GERD ■ Decrease relapse rates of daytime and nighttime heartburn symptoms on patients with GERD ■ Pathologic gastric hypersecretory conditions.

## ACTION

■ Binds to an enzyme in the presence of acidic gastric pH, preventing the final transport of hydrogen ions into the gastric lumen. **Therapeutic Effects:** ■ Diminished accumulation of acid in the gastric lumen, with lessened acid reflux ■ Healing of duodenal ulcers and esophagitis ■ Decreased acid secretion in hypersecretory conditions.

## PHARMACOKINETICS

**Absorption:** Tablet is enteric-coated; absorption occurs only after tablet leaves the stomach.

**Distribution:** Unknown.

**Protein Binding:** 98%.

**Metabolism and Excretion:** Mostly metabolized by the liver via the cytochrome P450 (CYP) system; inactive metabolites are excreted in urine (71%) and feces (18%).

**Half-life:** 1 hr.

## CONTRAINDICATIONS AND PRECAUTIONS

**Contraindicated in:** ■ Hypersensitivity ■ Lactation.

**Use Cautiously in:** ■ Pregnancy or children (safety not established).

## ADVERSE REACTIONS AND SIDE EFFECTS*

■ **CNS:** headache ■ **GI:** abdominal pain, diarrhea, eructation, flatulence ■ **Endo:** hyperglycemia.

## INTERACTIONS

**Drug-Drug:** ■ May alter the bioavailability and effects of **drugs for which absorption is pH dependent** ■ May ↑ risk of bleeding with **warfarin** (monitor INR/PT).

## ROUTE AND DOSAGE

■ **PO (Adults):** *GERD*—40 mg once daily; *Gastric hypersecretory conditions*—40 mg twice daily, up to 120 mg twice daily.
■ **IV (Adults):** *GERD*—40 mg once daily for 7–10 days. *Gastric hypersecretory conditions*—80 mg q 12 hr (up to 240 mg/day).

## AVAILABILITY

■ *Delayed-release tablets:* 20 mg^Rx, 40 mg^Rx ■ Cost: 20 mg $281.88/90, 40 mg $281.88/90 ■ *Powder for injection:* 40 mg/vial^Rx ■ Cost: $600.00/25 vials.

TIME/ACTION PROFILE (effect on acid secretion)

|  | ONSET† | PEAK | DURATION† |
|---|---|---|---|
| PO, IV | 2.5 hr | unknown | 1 wk |

†Onset = 51% inhibition; duration = return to normal following discontinuation.

## NURSING IMPLICATIONS

### ASSESSMENT

❑ Assess patient routinely for epigastric or abdominal pain and for frank or occult blood in stool, emesis, or gastric aspirate.
■ **Lab Test Considerations:** May cause abnormal liver function tests, including ↑ AST, ALT, alkaline phosphatase, and bilirubin.

### POTENTIAL NURSING DIAGNOSES

■ Pain, acute (Indications).

### IMPLEMENTATION

■ **General:** Patients receiving pantoprazole IV should be converted to PO dosing as soon as possible.

■ **PO:** May be administered with or without food. Do not break, crush, or chew tablets.
❑ Antacids may be used concurrently.
■ **Intermittent Infusion:** Reconstitute with 0.9% NaCl. Dilute further with 100 ml of D5W, 0.9% NaCl, or LR for a concentration of 0.4 mg/ml. Administer through filter provided to remove precipitates that may form when solution is mixed. If in-line filter is used, position below y-site closest to patient.
■ *Rate:* Administer over 15 min at a rate of <3 mg/min.
■ **Y-Site Incompatibility:** Administer through a dedicated line or flush line before and after administration. Do not administer in line with other solutions.

### PATIENT/FAMILY TEACHING

❑ Instruct patient to take medication as directed for the full course of therapy, even if feeling better.
❑ Advise patient to avoid alcohol, products containing aspirin or NSAIDs, and foods that may cause an increase in GI irritation.
❑ Advise patient to report onset of black, tarry stools; diarrhea; or abdominal pain to health care professional promptly.

### EVALUATION

**Effectiveness of therapy can be demonstrated by:** ■ Healing in patients with erosive esophagitis. Therapy is continued for up to 8 wk.

# paricalcitol, See VITAMIN D COMPOUNDS.

# paroxetine
(par-**ox**-e-teen)
Paxil, Paxil CR

### CLASSIFICATION(S):
*Therapeutic: antianxiety agents, antidepressants*
*Pharmacologic: selective serotonin reuptake inhibitors (SSRIs)*

**Pregnancy Category C**

## INDICATIONS

■ Treatment of: ❑ Depression ❑ Panic disorder ❑ OCD ❑ Social anxiety disorder ❑ Generalized anxiety disorder ❑ Post-traumatic stress disorder ■ Generalized anxiety disorder (often in conjunction with psychotherapy).

## ACTION

■ Inhibits neuronal reuptake of serotonin in the CNS, thus potentiating the activity of serotonin; has little effect on norepinephrine or dopamine. **Therapeutic Effects:** ■ Antidepressant action ■ Decreased frequency of panic attacks, OCD, or anxiety ■ Improvement in manifestations of post-traumatic stress disorder.

## PHARMACOKINETICS

**Absorption:** Well absorbed (50–100%) following oral administration. Controlled-release tablets are enteric-coated and control medication release over 4–5 hr.

**Distribution:** Widely distributed throughout body fluids and tissues, including the CNS; enters breast milk.

**Protein Binding:** 95%.

**Metabolism and Excretion:** Highly metabolized by the liver (partly by P450 2D6 enzyme system); 2% excreted unchanged in urine.

**Half-life:** 21 hr.

## CONTRAINDICATIONS AND PRECAUTIONS

**Contraindicated in:** ■ Hypersensitivity ■ Concurrent MAO inhibitor therapy (may result in serious, potentially fatal reactions).

**Use Cautiously in:** ■ Severe renal or hepatic impairment, geriatric or debilitated patients (start with smaller doses; daily dose should not be >40 mg) ■ History of mania ■ History or risk of suicide attempt ■ Pregnancy, lactation, or children (safety not established).

## ADVERSE REACTIONS AND SIDE EFFECTS*

■ **CNS:** <u>anxiety</u>, <u>dizziness</u>, <u>drowsiness</u>, <u>headache</u>, <u>insomnia</u>, <u>weakness</u>, agitation, amnesia, confusion, emotional lability, hangover, impaired concentration, malaise, mental depression, syncope ■ **EENT:** blurred vision, rhinitis ■ **Resp:** cough, pharyngitis, respiratory disorders, yawning ■ **CV:** chest pain, edema, hypertension, palpitations, postural hypotension, tachycardia, vasodilation ■ **GI:** <u>constipation</u>, <u>diarrhea</u>, <u>dry mouth</u>, <u>nausea</u>, abdominal pain, decreased appetite, dyspepsia, flatulence, increased appetite, taste disturbances, vomiting ■ **GU:** <u>ejaculatory disturbance</u>, decreased libido, genital disorders, urinary disorders, urinary frequency ■ **Derm:** <u>sweating</u>, photosensitivity, pruritus, rash ■ **Metab:** weight gain, weight loss ■ **MS:** back pai , myalgia, myasthenia, myopathy ■ **Neuro:** <u>tremor</u>, myoclonus, paresthesia ■ **Misc:** chills, fever.

## INTERACTIONS

**Drug-Drug:** ■ Serious, potentially fatal reactions (hyperthermia, rigidity, myoclonus, autonomic instability, with fluctuating vital signs and extreme agitation, which may proceed to delirium and coma) may occur with concurrent **MAO inhibitor** therapy. MAO inhibitors should be stopped at least 14 days prior to paroxetine therapy. Paroxetine should be stopped at least 14 days prior to MAO inhibitor therapy ■ May ↓ metabolism and ↑ effects of certain **drugs that are metabolized by the liver,** including other **antidepressants, phenothiazines, class IC antiarrhythmics, procyclidine,** and **quinidine.** Concurrent use should be undertaken with caution ■ **Cimetidine** ↑ blood levels ■ **Phenobarbital** and **phenytoin** may ↓ effectiveness ■ Concurrent use with **alcohol** is not recommended ■ May ↓ the effectiveness of **digoxin** ■ Concurrent use with **tryptophan** may result in headache, nausea, sweating, and dizziness ■ May ↑ risk of bleeding with **warfarin** without altering INR time ■ Concurrent use with **5-HT₁ agonist vascular headache suppressants (frovatriptan, naratriptan, rizatriptan, sumatriptan, zolmitriptan)** may result in weakness, hyperreflexia, and incoordination.

**Drug-Natural Products:** ■ ↑ risk of serotinergic side effects including serotonin syndrome with **St. John's wort** and **SAMe.**

## ROUTE AND DOSAGE

❑ **Depression**

■ **PO (Adults):** 20 mg as a single dose in the morning; may be increased by 10 mg/day at weekly intervals (range 20–50 mg). *Controlled-release tablets*—25 mg once daily initially. May increase at weekly intervals by 1.25 mg, up to 62.5 mg/day.

■ **PO (Geriatric Patients or Debilitated Patients):** 10 mg/day initially; may be slowly increased (not to exceed 40 mg/day). *Con-*

*trolled-release tablets*—12.5 mg once daily initially; may be titrated up to 50 mg/day.

❑ **Obsessive-Compulsive Disorder**

■ **PO (Adults):** 20 mg/day initially; increase by 10 mg/day q wk up to 40 mg (range 40–60 mg/day).

❑ **Panic Disorder**

■ **PO (Adults):** 10 mg/day initially; increase by 10 mg/day q wk up to 40 mg (range 10–60 mg/day).

❑ **Social Anxiety Disorder**

■ **PO (Adults):** 20 mg/day.

❑ **Generalized anxiety disorder**

■ **PO (Adults):** 20 mg once daily initially; increase by 10 mg/day q wk up to 50 mg (range 20–50 mg/day).

❑ **Post-traumatic Stress Disorder**

■ **PO (Adults):** 20 mg/day initially, may be increased by 10 mg/day at weekly intervals up to 50 mg/day.

❑ **Hepatic Impairment**

■ **PO (Adults):** *Severe hepatic impairment*—10 mg/day initially; may be slowly increased (not to exceed 40 mg/day). *Controlled-release tablets*—12.5 mg once daily initially; may be titrated up to 50 mg/day.

❑ **Renal Impairment**

■ **PO (Adults):** *Severe renal impairment*—10 mg/day initially; may be slowly increased (not to exceed 40 mg/day). *Controlled-release tablets*—12.5 mg once daily initially; may be titrated up to 50 mg/day.

## AVAILABILITY (generic available)

■ *Paroxetine hydrochloride tablets:* 10 mg<sup>Rx</sup>, 20 mg<sup>Rx</sup>, 30 mg<sup>Rx</sup>, 40 mg<sup>Rx</sup> ■ Cost: 10 mg $77.94/30, 20 mg $81.32/30, 30 mg $83.78/30, 40 mg $88.50/30 ■ *Paroxetine hydrochloride-controlled-release tablets:* 12.5 mg<sup>Rx</sup>, 25 mg<sup>Rx</sup>, 37.5 mg<sup>Rx</sup> ■ *Paroxetine hydrochloride oral suspension (orange flavor):* 10 mg/5 ml<sup>Rx</sup> ■ Cost: 10 mg/5 ml $129.68/250-ml bottle ■ *Paroxetine mesylate tablets:* 10 mg<sup>Rx</sup>, 20 mg<sup>Rx</sup>, 30 mg<sup>Rx</sup>, 40 mg<sup>Rx</sup>.

**TIME/ACTION PROFILE** (antidepressant action)

| | ONSET | PEAK | DURATION |
|---|---|---|---|
| PO | 1–4 wk | unknown | unknown |

# NURSING IMPLICATIONS

## ASSESSMENT

■ **General Info:** Monitor appetite and nutritional intake. Weigh weekly. Notify physician or other health care professional of continued weight loss. Adjust diet as tolerated to support nutritional status.

■ **Depression:** Monitor mood changes. Inform physician or other health care professional if patient demonstrates significant increase in anxiety, nervousness, or insomnia.

❑ Assess for suicidal tendencies, especially during early therapy. Restrict amount of drug available to patient.

■ **OCD:** Assess patient for frequency of obsessive-compulsive behaviors. Note degree to which these thoughts and behaviors interfere with daily functioning.

■ **Panic Attacks:** Assess frequency and severity of panic attacks.

■ **Social Anxiety Disorder:** Assess frequency and severity of episodes of anxiety.

■ **Post-traumatic Stress Disorder:** Assess manifestations of post-traumatic stress disorder periodically during therapy.

■ *Lab Test Considerations:* Monitor CBC and differential periodically during therapy. Report leukopenia or anemia.

## POTENTIAL NURSING DIAGNOSES

■ Coping, ineffective (Indications).
■ Injury, risk for (Side Effects).

## IMPLEMENTATION

■ **General:** Do not confuse paroxetine (Paxil) with paclitaxel (Taxol).

❑ Periodically reassess dose and continued need for therapy.

■ **PO:** Administer as a single dose in the morning. May administer with food to minimize GI irritation. Controlled-release tablets should be swallowed whole. Do not crush, break, or chew.

## PATIENT/FAMILY TEACHING

❏ Instruct patient to take paroxetine as directed. Take missed doses as soon as possible and return to regular dosing schedule. Do not double doses. Caution patient to consult health care professional before discontinuing paroxetine. Daily doses should be decreased slowly. Abrupt withdrawal may cause dizziness, sensory disturbances, agitation, anxiety, nausea, and sweating.

❏ May cause drowsiness or dizziness. Caution patient to avoid driving and other activities requiring alertness until response to the drug is known.

❏ Advise patient to avoid alcohol or other CNS-depressant drugs during therapy and to consult with health care professional before taking other medications or herbal products with paroxetine.

❏ Inform patient that frequent mouth rinses, good oral hygiene, and sugarless gum or candy may minimize dry mouth. If dry mouth persists for more than 2 wk, consult health care professional regarding use of saliva substitute.

❏ Advise patient to wear sunscreen and protective clothing to prevent photosensitivity reactions.

❏ Instruct female patient to inform health care professional if pregnancy is planned or suspected or if she is breastfeeding.

❏ Advise patient to notify health care professional if headache, weakness, nausea, anorexia, anxiety, or insomnia persists.

❏ Emphasize the importance of follow-up exams to monitor progress. Encourage patient participation in psychotherapy.

## EVALUATION

**Effectiveness of therapy can be demonstrated by:** ■ Increased sense of well-being ❏ Renewed interest in surroundings. May require 1–4 wk of therapy to obtain antidepressant effects ■ Decrease in obsessive-compulsive behaviors ■ Decrease in frequency and severity of panic attacks ■ Decrease in frequency and severity of episodes of anxiety ■ Improvement in manifestations of post-traumatic stress disorder.

---

## pegaspargase
(peg-ass-**par**-jase)

Oncaspar, PEG-L-asparaginase

### CLASSIFICATION(S):
**Therapeutic:** antineoplastics
**Pharmacologic:** enzymes

**Pregnancy Category C**

## INDICATIONS

■ Treatment (usually with other agents) of acute lymphoblastic leukemia (ALL) in patients who have had a previous hypersensitivity reaction to native asparaginase.

## ACTION

■ Consists of L-asparaginase bound to polyethylene glycol (PEG). This compound depletes asparagine, which leukemic cells cannot synthesize. Normal cells are able to produce their own asparagine and are less susceptible to the effects of asparaginase. Binding to PEG renders asparaginase less antigenic and therefore less likely to induce hypersensitivity reactions. **Therapeutic Effects:** ■ Death of leukemic cells.

## PHARMACOKINETICS

**Absorption:** IV administration results in complete bioavailability.
**Distribution:** Unknown.
**Metabolism and Excretion:** Metabolized by serum proteases and in the reticuloendothelial system.
**Half-life:** 5.7 days (less in patients with previous hypersensitivity to native L-asparaginase).

## CONTRAINDICATIONS AND PRECAUTIONS

**Contraindicated in:** ■ Pancreatitis or history of pancreatitis ■ History of previous hemorrhagic reaction to asparaginase therapy ■ Previous hypersensitivity reactions to pegaspargase.
**Use Cautiously in:** ■ History of previous hypersensitivity reactions to other drugs ■ Patients with childbearing potential ■ Pregnancy or lactation (safety not established).

## ADVERSE REACTIONS AND SIDE EFFECTS*

■ **CNS:** SEIZURES, headache, malaise ■ **GI:** PANCREATITIS, abdominal pain, abnormal liver function tests, anorexia, diarrhea, lip edema, nausea, vomiting ■ **Derm:** jaundice ■ **Endo:** hyperglycemia ■ **F and E:** peripheral edema ■ **Hemat:**

decreased fibrinogen, disseminated intra-vascular coagulation, hemolytic anemia, increased thromboplastin, leukopenia, pancytopenia, thrombocytopenia ■ **Local:** injection site hypersensitivity, injection site pain, thrombosis ■ **MS:** arthralgia, myalgia, pain in extremities ■ **Neuro:** paresthesia ■ **Misc:** chills, hypersensitivity reactions, night sweats.

## INTERACTIONS

**Drug-Drug:** ■ May alter response to **anticoagulants** or **antiplatelet agents** ■ May alter the response to other **drugs that are metabolized by the liver.**

## ROUTE AND DOSAGE

■ **IM, IV (Adults up to 21 yr, and Children with Body Surface Area ≥0.6 m²):** 2500 IU/m² q 14 days (usually in combination with other agents).

■ **IM, IV (Children with Body Surface Area <0.6 m²):** 82.5 IU/kg q 14 days (usually in combination with other agents).

## AVAILABILITY

■ **Injection:** 750 IU/ml^Rx.

TIME/ACTION PROFILE (hematologic effects)

| | ONSET | PEAK | DURATION |
|---|---|---|---|
| IV | rapid | unknown | 14 days |

## NURSING IMPLICATIONS

### ASSESSMENT

❏ Assess patient for previous hypersensitivity reactions to native L-asparaginase. Monitor for hypersensitivity reaction (urticaria, diaphoresis, facial swelling, joint pain, hypotension, bronchospasm). Epinephrine and resuscitation equipment should be readily available. Reaction may occur up to 2 hr after administration.

❏ Monitor for development of bone marrow depression. Assess for fever, sore throat, and signs of infection. Monitor platelet count throughout therapy. Assess for bleeding (bleeding gums, bruising, petechiae, guaiac test stools, urine, and emesis). Avoid giving IM injections and taking rectal temperatures. Apply pressure to venipuncture sites for 10 min. Anemia may occur. Monitor for increased fatigue, dyspnea, and orthostatic hypotension.

❏ Monitor patient frequently for signs of pancreatitis (nausea, vomiting, abdominal pain).

❏ Assess nausea, vomiting, and appetite. Weigh patient weekly. Prophylactic antiemetics may be used prior to administration.

■ **Lab Test Considerations:** Monitor CBC prior to and periodically throughout therapy. May alter coagulation studies. Fibrinogen may be decreased; PT and partial thromboplastin time (PTT) may be increased.

❏ Monitor serum amylase frequently to detect pancreatitis.

❏ Monitor blood glucose; may cause hyperglycemia.

❏ May cause elevated BUN and serum creatinine.

❏ Hepatotoxicity may be manifested by increased AST, ALT, or bilirubin. Liver function tests usually return to normal after therapy.

❏ May cause decreased serum calcium.

❏ May cause elevated serum and urine uric acid and hyponatremia.

## POTENTIAL NURSING DIAGNOSES

■ Infection, risk for (Adverse Reactions).

## IMPLEMENTATION

■ **General:** Do not confuse pegaspargase with asparaginase.

❏ IM is the preferred route because of a lower incidence of adverse reactions.

❏ Solutions should be prepared in a biologic cabinet. Wear gloves, gown, and mask while handling medication. Discard equipment in specially designated containers.

■ **IM:** Limit single injection volume to 2 ml. If volume of injection is >2 ml, use multiple injection sites.

■ **Intermittent Infusion:** Dilute each dose in 100 ml of 0.9% NaCl or D5W. Do not shake or agitate. Do not use if solution is cloudy or has formed a precipitate.

❏ Use only 1 dose per vial; do not re-enter the vial. Discard unused portions.

❏ Keep refrigerated but do not freeze. Freezing destroys activity but does not change the appearance of pegaspargase.

■ **Rate:** Administer over 1–2 hr via Y-site through an infusion that is already running.

■ **Additive Incompatibility:** Information unavailable. Do not admix with other medications or solutions.

## PATIENT/FAMILY TEACHING

❏ Inform patient of the possibility of hypersensitivity reactions, including anaphylaxis.

❏ Advise patient that concurrent use of other medications may increase the risk of bleeding and the toxicity of pegaspargase. Consult health care professional before taking any other medications, including OTC drugs.

❏ Instruct patient to notify health care professional if abdominal pain, severe nausea and vomiting, jaundice, fever, chills, sore throat, bleeding or bruising, excess thirst or urination, or mouth sores occur. Caution patient to avoid crowds and persons with known infections. Instruct patient to use soft toothbrush, electric razor, and to be especially careful to avoid falls. Patients should also be cautioned not to drink alcoholic beverages or take medications containing aspirin or NSAIDs because these may precipitate gastric bleeding.

❏ Instruct patient not to receive any vaccinations without advice of health care professional. Advise parents that this may alter child's immunization schedule.

❏ Emphasize the need for periodic lab tests to monitor for side effects.

## EVALUATION

**Effectiveness of therapy can be demonstrated by:** ■ Improvement of hematologic status in patients with leukemia.

## pegfilgrastim

(peg-fil-**gra**-stim)

Neulasta

### CLASSIFICATION(S):

**Therapeutic:** colony-stimulating factors

### Pregnancy Category C

## INDICATIONS

■ To decrease the incidence of infection (febrile neutropenia) in patients with nonmyeloid malignancies receiving myelosuppressive antineoplastics associated with a high risk of febrile neutropenia.

## ACTION

■ Filgrastim is a glycoprotein that binds to and stimulates neutrophils to divide and differentiate. Also activates mature neutrophils. Binding to a polyethylene glycol molecule prolongs its effects. **Therapeutic Effects:** ■ Decreased incidence of infection in patients who are neutropenic from chemotherapy.

## PHARMACOKINETICS

**Absorption:** Well absorbed following subcut administration.

**Distribution:** Unknown.

**Metabolism and Excretion:** Unknown.

**Half-life:** 15–80 hr.

## CONTRAINDICATIONS AND PRECAUTIONS

**Contraindicated in:** ■ Hypersensitivity to filgrastim or *Escherichia coli*-derived proteins.

**Use Cautiously in:** ■ Patients with sickle cell disease (increased risk of sickle cell crisis) ■ Concurrent use of lithium ■ Malignancy with myeloid characteristics ■ Pregnancy, lactation, or children (safety not established; 6-mg fixed dose should not be used in infants, children, and smaller adolescents weighing <45 kg; use in pregnancy only if potential benefits to mother justifies potential risk to the fetus).

## ADVERSE REACTIONS AND SIDE EFFECTS*

■ **Resp:** ADULT RESPIRATORY DISTRESS SYNDROME (ARDS) ■ **GI:** SPLENIC RUPTURE ■ **Hemat:** SICKLE CELL CRISIS, leukocytosis ■ **MS:** medullary bone pain ■ **Misc:** allergic reaction including ANAPHYLAXIS.

## INTERACTIONS

**Drug-Drug:** ■ Simultaneous use with **antineoplastics** may have adverse effects on rapidly proliferating neutrophils; avoid use for 24 hr before and 24 hr following chemotherapy ■ **Lithium** may potentiate the release of neutrophils; concurrent use should be undertaken cautiously.

## ROUTE AND DOSAGE

■ **Subcut (Adults):** 6 mg per chemotherapy cycle.

## AVAILABILITY

■ *Solution for subcut injection:* 6 mg/0.6 ml in prefilled syringes[Rx].

TIME/ACTION PROFILE

| | ONSET | PEAK | DURATION |
|---|---|---|---|
| Subcut | unknown | unknown | unknown |

## NURSING IMPLICATIONS

### ASSESSMENT

❏ Assess patient for bone pain throughout therapy. Pain is usually mild to moderate and controllable with nonopioid analgesics, but may require opioid analgesics.

❏ Assess patient periodically for signs of ARDS (fever, lung infiltration, respiratory distress). If ARDS occurs, treat condition and discontinue pegfilgrastim and/or withold until symptoms resolve.

■ *Lab Test Considerations:* Obtain CBC and platelet count before chemotherapy. Monitor hematocrit and platelet count regularly.

❏ May cause elevated LDH, alkaline phosphatase, and uric acid.

### POTENTIAL NURSING DIAGNOSES

■ Infection, risk for (Indications).

■ Pain, acute (Side Effects).

### IMPLEMENTATION

■ **General:** Pegfilgrastim should not be administered between 14 and 24 days after administration of cytotoxic chemotherapy.

❏ Keep patients with sickle cell disease receiving pegfilgrastim well hydrated and monitor for sickle cell crisis.

■ **Subcut:** Administer subcut once per chemotherapy cycle. Do not administer solutions that are discolored or contain particulate matter. Do not shake. Store refrigerated; may be allowed to reach room temperature for a maximum of 48 hr, but protect from light.

❏ Supplied in prefilled syringes. Following administration, activate UltraSafe Needle Guard to prevent needle sticks by placing hands behind needle, grasping guard with one hand, and sliding guard forward until needle is completely covered and guard clicks into place. If audible click is not heard, guard may not be completely activated. Dispose of by placing entire prefilled syringe with guard activated into puncture-proof container.

### PATIENT/FAMILY TEACHING

❏ Advise patient to notify health care professional immediately if signs of allergic reaction (shortness of breath, hives, rash, pruritus, laryngeal edema) or signs of splenic rupture (left upper abdominal or shoulder tip pain) occur.

❏ Emphasize the importance of compliance with therapy and regular monitoring of blood counts.

■ **Home Care Issues:** Instruct patient on correct disposal technique for home administration. Caution patient not to reuse needle, syringe, or drug product. Provide patient with a puncture-proof container for disposal of prefilled syringe.

### EVALUATION

**Effectiveness of therapy can be demonstrated by:** ■ Decreased incidence of infection in patients who receive bone-marrow–depressing antineoplastics.

# penbutolol

(pen-**byoo**-toe-lole)
Levatol

*CLASSIFICATION(S):*
*Therapeutic: antihypertensives*
*Pharmacologic: beta blockers*

**Pregnancy Category C**

## INDICATIONS

■ Management of hypertension.

## ACTION

■ Blocks stimulation of beta$_1$(myocardial) and beta$_2$(pulmonary, vascular, and uterine) -adrenergic receptor sites ■ Also has intrinsic sympathomimetic activity (ISA), which may produce less bradycardia. **Therapeutic Effects:** ■ Decreased heart rate and blood pressure.

## PHARMACOKINETICS

**Absorption:** Well absorbed after oral administration.

**Distribution:** Moderate CNS penetration; crosses the placenta.

**Protein Binding:** 80–98%.

**Metabolism and Excretion:** Mostly metabolized by the liver.

**Half-life:** 5 hr.

## CONTRAINDICATIONS AND PRECAUTIONS

**Contraindicated in:** ■ Uncompensated CHF ■ Pulmonary edema ■ Cardiogenic shock ■ Bradycardia or heart block.

**Use Cautiously in:** ■ Renal impairment ■ Hepatic impairment (lower doses may be necessary) ■ Pulmonary disease (including asthma) ■ Diabetes mellitus (may mask signs of hypoglycemia) ■ Thyrotoxicosis (may mask symptoms) ■ Patients with a history of severe allergic reactions (intensity of reactions may be increased) ■ Geriatric patients (increased sensitivity to beta blockers; initial dosage reduction recommended) ■ Pregnancy, lactation, or children (safety not established; all agents cross the placenta and may cause fetal/neonatal bradycardia, hypotension, hypoglycemia, or respiratory depression).

## ADVERSE REACTIONS AND SIDE EFFECTS*

■ **CNS:** <u>fatigue</u>, <u>weakness</u>, anxiety, depression, dizziness, drowsiness, insomnia, memory loss, mental status changes, nervousness, nightmares ■ **EENT:** blurred vision, dry eyes, nasal stuffiness ■ **Resp:** bronchospasm, wheezing ■ **CV:** ARRHYTHMIAS, BRADYCARDIA, CHF, PULMONARY EDEMA, orthostatic hypotension, peripheral vasoconstriction ■ **GI:** constipation, diarrhea, nausea ■ **GU:** <u>impotence</u>, decreased libido ■ **Derm:** itching, rashes ■ **Endo:** hyperglycemia, hypoglycemia ■ **MS:** arthralgia, back pain, muscle cramps ■ **Neuro:** paresthesia ■ **Misc:** drug-induced lupus syndrome.

## INTERACTIONS

**Drug-Drug:** ■ **General anesthesia, IV phenytoin,** and **verapamil** may cause additive myocardial depression ■ Additive bradycardia may occur with **digoxin** ■ Additive hypotension may occur with other **antihypertensives,** acute ingestion of **alcohol,** or **nitrates** ■ Concurrent use with **amphetamines, cocaine,** ephedrine, epinephrine, norepinephrine, phenylephrine, or pseudoephedrine may result in unopposed alpha-adrenergic stimulation (excessive hypertension, bradycardia) ■ Concurrent administration of **thyroid preparations** decreases effectiveness ■ May alter the effectiveness of **insulins** or **oral hypoglycemic agents** (dosage adjustments may be necessary) ■ May decrease the effectiveness of **beta-adrenergic bronchodilators** and **theophylline** ■ May decrease the beneficial beta$_1$-cardiovascular effects of **dopamine** or **dobutamine** ■ Use cautiously within 14 days of **MAO inhibitors** (may result in hypertension) ■ Concurrent **NSAIDs** may decrease antihypertensive action.

## ROUTE AND DOSAGE

■ **PO (Adults):** 20 mg once daily.

## AVAILABILITY

■ *Tablets:* 20 mg$^{Rx}$ ■ Cost: $143.65/100.

TIME/ACTION PROFILE (cardiovascular effects)

| | ONSET | PEAK | DURATION |
|---|---|---|---|
| PO | 1 hr | 1.5–3 hr† | Up to 24 hr |

†After single dose; full effect not seen until several weeks of therapy.

# NURSING IMPLICATIONS

## ASSESSMENT

■ **General Info:** Monitor blood pressure and pulse frequently during dosage adjustment period and periodically throughout therapy. Assess for orthostatic hypotension when assisting patient up from supine position.

❑ Monitor intake and output ratios and daily weight. Assess patient routinely for evidence of fluid overload (peripheral edema, dyspnea, rales/crackles, fatigue, weight gain, jugular venous distention).

■ *Lab Test Considerations:* May cause increased BUN, serum lipoprotein, potassium, triglyceride, and uric acid levels.

❑ May cause increased ANA titers.

❑ May cause increase in blood glucose levels.

## POTENTIAL NURSING DIAGNOSES

■ Cardiac output, decreased (Side Effects).

■ Noncompliance (Patient/Family Teaching).

## IMPLEMENTATION

- **General:** Take apical pulse before administering. If <50 bpm or if arrhythmia occurs, withhold medication and notify physician or other health care professional.
- **PO:** May be administered with food or on an empty stomach.

## PATIENT/FAMILY TEACHING

- **General Info:** Instruct patient to take medication exactly as directed, at the same time each day, even if feeling well; do not skip or double up on missed doses. If a dose is missed, it should be taken as soon as possible up to 8 hr before next dose. Abrupt withdrawal may precipitate life-threatening arrhythmias, hypertension, or myocardial ischemia.
- Advise patient to make sure that enough medication is available for weekends, holidays, and vacations. A written prescription may be kept in wallet in case of emergency.
- Teach patient and family how to check pulse and blood pressure. Instruct them to check pulse daily and blood pressure biweekly. Advise patient to hold dose and contact health care professional if pulse is <50 bpm or if blood pressure changes significantly.
- May cause drowsiness or dizziness. Caution patient to avoid driving or other activities that require alertness until response to the drug is known.
- Advise patient to change positions slowly to minimize orthostatic hypotension, especially during initiation of therapy or on dose increase.
- Caution patient that this medication may increase sensitivity to cold.
- Instruct patient to consult health care professional before taking any OTC medications, especially cold preparations, concurrently with this medication.
- Diabetics should closely monitor blood glucose, especially if weakness, malaise, irritability, or fatigue occurs. Medication may mask tachycardia and increased blood pressure as signs of hypoglycemia, but dizziness and sweating may still occur.
- Advise patient to notify health care professional if slow pulse, difficulty breathing, wheezing, cold hands and feet, dizziness, confusion, depression, rash, fever, sore throat, unusual bleeding, or bruising occurs.
- Instruct patient to inform health care professional of medication regimen before treatment or surgery.
- Advise patient to carry identification describing disease process and medication regimen at all times.
- **Hypertension:** Reinforce the need to continue additional therapies for hypertension (weight loss, sodium restriction, stress reduction, regular exercise, moderation of alcohol consumption, and smoking cessation). Medication controls but does not cure hypertension.

## EVALUATION

**Effectiveness of therapy can be demonstrated by:** ■ Decrease in blood pressure. Maximum antihypertensive effects are usually seen by the end of week 2. Full effects of lower doses may not be seen for 4–6 wk.

# PENICILLINS
(pen-i-**sill**-ins)

**penicillin G**
Pfizerpen

**penicillin V**
{Apo-Pen VK}, Beepen-VK, {Nadopen-V}, {Novo-Pen-VK}, {Pen-Vee}, Pen-Vee K, {PVF K}, Veetids

**procaine penicillin G**
{Ayercillin}, Wycillin

**benzathine penicillin G**
Bicillin L-A, {Megacillin}, Permapen

## CLASSIFICATION(S):
***Therapeutic:*** *anti-infectives*
***Pharmacologic:*** *penicillins*

## Pregnancy Category B

## INDICATIONS

■ Treatment of a wide variety of infections including: ❏ Pneumococcal pneumonia ❏ Streptococcal pharyngitis ❑ Syphilis ❑ Gonorrhea strains ■ Treatment of enterococcal infections (requires the addition of an aminoglycoside) ■ Prevention of rheumatic fever ■ Should not be used as a single agent to treat anthrax. **Unlabeled uses:** ■ Treatment of Lyme disease, prevention of recurrent *S. pneumoniae septicemia* in children with sickle-cell disease.

## ACTION

■ Bind to bacterial cell wall, resulting in cell death. **Therapeutic Effects:** ■ Bactericidal action against susceptible bacteria. **Spectrum:** ■ Active against: ❑ Most gram-positive organisms, including many streptococci (*Streptococcus pneumoniae*, group A beta-hemolytic streptococci), staphylococci (non–penicillinase-producing strains), and *Bacillus anthracis* ❑ Some gram-negative organisms, such as *Neisseria meningitidis* and *N. gonorrhoeae* (only penicillin susceptible strains) ❑ Some anaerobic bacteria and spirochetes including *Borellia burgdorferi*.

## PHARMACOKINETICS

**Absorption:** Variably absorbed from the GI tract. *Penicillin V*—resists acid degradation in the GI tract. *Procaine and benzathine penicillin*—IM absorption is delayed and prolonged and results in sustained therapeutic blood levels.

**Distribution:** Widely distributed, although CNS penetration is poor in the presence of uninflamed meninges. Cross the placenta and enter breast milk.

**Protein Binding:** 60%.

**Metabolism and Excretion:** Minimally metabolized by the liver, excreted mainly unchanged by the kidneys.

**Half-life:** 30–60 min.

## CONTRAINDICATIONS AND PRECAUTIONS

**Contraindicated in:** ■ Previous hypersensitivity to penicillins (cross-sensitivity may exist with cephalosporins) ■ Hypersensitivity to procaine or benzathine (procaine and benzathine preparations only) ■ Some products may contain tartrazine and should be avoided in patients with known hypersensitivity.

**Use Cautiously in:** ■ Geriatric patients (consider decreased body mass, age-related decrease in renal/hepatic/cardiac function, intercurrent diseases and drug therapy) ■ Severe renal insufficiency (dosage reduction recommended) ■ Pregnancy (although safety not established, has been used safely) ■ Lactation.

## ADVERSE REACTIONS AND SIDE EFFECTS*

■ **CNS:** SEIZURES ■ **GI:** diarrhea, epigastric distress, nausea, vomiting, pseudomembranous colitis ■ **GU:** interstitial nephritis ■ **Derm:** rashes, urticaria ■ **Hemat:** eosinophilia, hemolytic anemia, leukopenia ■ **Local:** pain at IM site, phlebitis AT IV SITE ■ **Misc:** allergic reactions including ANAPHYLAXIS and SERUM SICKNESS, superinfection.

## INTERACTIONS

**Drug-Drug:** ■ Penicillin V may ↓ effectiveness of oral contraceptive agents ■ **Probenecid** ↓ renal excretion and ↑ blood levels of penicillin (therapy may be combined for this purpose) ■ **Neomycin** may ↓ absorption of penicillin V ■ Concurrent use with **methotrexate** ↓ methotrexate elimination and ↑ risk of serious toxicity.

## ROUTE AND DOSAGE

1 mg = 1600 units.

### ❑ Penicillin G

■ **IM, IV (Adults):** *Most infections*—1–5 million units q 4–6 hr.

■ **IM, IV (Children):** 8333–16,667 units/kg q 4 hr; 12,550–25,000 units/kg q 6 hr; up to 250,000 units/kg/day in divided doses, some infections may require up to 300,000 units/kg/day.

■ **IV (Infants >7 days):** 75,000 units/kg/day in divided doses every 8 hr; *meningitis*—200,000–300,000 units/kg/day in divided doses q 6 hr.

■ **IV (Infants <7 days):** 50,000 units/kg/day in divided doses q 12 hr; *Streptococcus B meningitis*—100,000–150,000 units/kg/day in divided doses.

### ❑ Penicillin V

■ **PO (Adults and Children ≥12 yr):** *Most infections*—125–500 mg q 6–8 hr. *Rheumatic fever prevention*—125–250 mg q 12 hr.

■ **PO (Children <12 yr):** *Lyme disease*—50 mg/kg/day in 4 divided doses (unlabeled); prevention of *S. pneumoniae* sepsis in children with sickle cell disease—125 mg twice daily.

□ **Benzathine Penicillin G**

■ **IM (Adults):** *Streptococcal infections/erysipeloid*—1.2 million units single dose. *Primary, secondary, and early latent syphilis*—2.4 million units single dose. *Tertiary and late latent syphilis (not neurosyphilis)*—2.4 million units once weekly for 3 wk. *Prevention of rheumatic fever*—1.2 million units q 3–4 wk.

■ **IM (Children >27 kg):** *Streptococcal infections/erysipeloid*—900,000–1.2 million units (single dose). *Primary, secondary, and early latent syphilis*—up to 2.4 million units single dose. *Late latent or latent syphilis of undetermined duration*—50,000 units/kg weekly for 3 wk. *Prevention of rheumatic fever*—1.2 million units q 2–3 wk.

■ **IM (Children <27 kg):** *Streptococcal infections/erysipeloid*—300,000–600,000 units single dose. *Primary, secondary, and early latent syphilis*—up to 2.4 million units single dose. *Late latent or latent syphilis of undetermined duration*—50,000 units/kg weekly for 3 wk. *Prevention of rheumatic fever*—1.2 million units q 2–3 wk.

□ **Procaine Penicillin G**

■ **IM (Adults):** *Moderate or severe infections*—600,000–1.2 million units/day, single dose or 2 divided doses. *Neurosyphilis*—2.4 million units/day with 500 mg probenecid PO 4 times daily for 10–14 days.

■ **IM (Children):** *Congenital syphilis*—50,000 units/kg/day for 10–14 days.

**AVAILABILITY (generic available)**

□ **Penicillin G Potassium**

■ *Powder for injection:* 1 million units/vial^Rx, 5 million units/vial^Rx, 20 million units/vial^Rx ■ *Premixed (frozen) solution for injection:* 1 million units/50 ml^Rx, 2 million units/50 ml^Rx, 3 million units/50 ml^Rx.

□ **Penicillin V Potassium**

■ *Tablets:* 400,000 units (250 mg)^Rx, 800,000 units (500 mg)^Rx ■ Cost: *generics*—250 mg $6.51/100, 500 mg $23.01/100 ■ *Oral solution:* 200,000 units (125 mg)/5 ml^Rx, 400,000 units (250 mg)/5 ml^Rx ■ Cost: *Veetids*—125

mg/5 ml $3.64/200 ml, 250 mg/5 ml $4.02/200 ml.

□ **Procaine Penicillin G**

■ *Suspension for IM injection:* 600,000 units/dose in 1-ml prefilled syringes^Rx, 1,200,000 units/dose in 2-ml prefilled syringes^Rx, 2,400,000 units/dose in 4-ml prefilled syringes^Rx.

□ **Benzathine Penicillin G**

■ *Suspension for IM injection:* 300,000 units/ml in 10-ml vials and 1-ml prefilled syringes^Rx, 600,000 units/ml in 1-, 2-, and 4-ml prefilled syringes^Rx.

TIME/ACTION PROFILE (blood levels)

| | ONSET | PEAK | DURATION |
|---|---|---|---|
| Penicillin PO | rapid | 0.5–1 hr | 4–6 hr |
| Penicillin G IM | rapid | 0.25–0.5 hr | 4–6 hr |
| Benzathine penicillin IM | delayed | 12–24 hr | 3 wk |
| Procaine penicillin IM | delayed | 1–4 hr | 12 hr |
| Penicillin G IV | rapid | end of infusion | 4–6 hr |

# NURSING IMPLICATIONS

## ASSESSMENT

□ Assess for infection (vital signs; appearance of wound, sputum, urine, and stool; WBC) at beginning of and during therapy.

□ Obtain a history to determine previous use of and reactions to penicillins or cephalosporins. Persons with a negative history of penicillin sensitivity may still have an allergic response.

□ Obtain specimens for culture and sensitivity before initiating therapy. First dose may be given before receiving results.

□ Observe patient for signs and symptoms of anaphylaxis (rash, pruritus, laryngeal edema, wheezing). Discontinue drug and notify physician or other health care professional immediately if these symptoms occur. Keep epinephrine, an antihistamine, and resuscitation equipment close by in case of an anaphylactic reaction.

■ *Lab Test Considerations:* May cause positive direct Coombs' test results.

❏ Hyperkalemia may develop after large doses of penicillin G potassium.

❏ Monitor serum sodium concentrations in patient with hypertension or CHF. Hypernatremia may develop after large doses of penicillin sodium.

❏ May cause ↑ AST, ALT, LDH, and serum alkaline phosphatase concentrations.

❏ May cause leukopenia and neutropenia, especially with prolonged therapy or hepatic impairment.

## POTENTIAL NURSING DIAGNOSES

■ Infection, risk for (Indications, Side Effects).

■ Noncompliance (Patient/Family Teaching).

## IMPLEMENTATION

■ **General:** Do not confuse penicillin with penicillamine. Do not confuse penicillin G potassium with penicillin G procaine.

■ **PO:** Administer around the clock. Penicillin V may be administered without regard for meals.

❏ Use calibrated measuring device for liquid preparations. Solution is stable for 14 days if refrigerated.

■ **IV, IM:** Reconstitute according to manufacturer's directions with sterile water for injection, D5W, or 0.9% NaCl.

■ **IM:** Shake medication well before injection. Inject penicillin deep into a well-developed muscle mass at a slow, consistent rate to prevent blockage of the needle. Massage well. Accidental injury near or into a nerve can result in severe pain and dysfunction.

❏ Penicillin G potassium or sodium may be diluted with lidocaine (without epinephrine) 1% or 2% to minimize pain from IM injection.

❏ Never give penicillin G benzathine or penicillin G procaine suspensions IV. May cause embolism or toxic reactions.

■ **IV:** Change IV sites every 48 hr to prevent phlebitis.

❏ Administer slowly and observe patient closely for signs of hypersensitivity.

■ **Intermittent Infusion:** Doses of 3 million units or less should be diluted in at least 50 ml of D5W or 0.9% NaCl; doses of more than 3 million units should be diluted with 100 ml.

■ *Rate:* Infuse over 1–2 hr in adults or 15–30 min in children.

■ **Continuous Infusion:** Doses of 10 million units or more may be diluted in 1 or 2 L.

■ *Rate:* Infuse over 24 hr.

❏ **Penicillin G Potassium**

■ **Y-Site Compatibility:** ◆ acyclovir ◆ amiodarone ◆ cyclophosphamide ◆ diltiazem ◆ enalaprilat ◆ esmolol ◆ fluconazole ◆ foscarnet ◆ heparin ◆ hydromorphone ◆ labetalol ◆ magnesium sulfate ◆ meperidine ◆ morphine ◆ perphenazine ◆ potassium chloride ◆ tacrolimus ◆ theophylline ◆ verapamil ◆ vitamin B complex with C.

■ **Y-Site Incompatibility:** If aminoglycosides and penicillins must be administered concurrently, administer in separate sites at least 1 hr apart.

■ **Additive Incompatibility:** Incompatible with aminoglycosides; do not admix.

❏ **Penicillin G Sodium**

■ **Y-Site Incompatibility:** If aminoglycosides and penicillins must be administered concurrently, administer in separate sites at least 1 hr apart.

■ **Additive Incompatibility:** Incompatible with aminoglycosides; do not admix.

## PATIENT/FAMILY TEACHING

❏ Instruct patient to take medication around the clock and to finish drug completely as directed, even if feeling better. Advise patient that sharing this medication may be dangerous.

❏ Advise patient to report signs of superinfection (black, furry overgrowth on tongue; vaginal itching or discharge; loose or foul-smelling stools) and allergy.

❏ Instruct patient to notify health care professional if fever and diarrhea develop, especially if stool contains blood, pus, or mucus. Advise patient not to treat diarrhea without consulting health care professional.

❏ Instruct patient to notify health care professional if symptoms do not improve.

❏ Advise patient taking oral contraceptives to use an additional nonhormonal method of contraception during therapy with penicillin V and until next menstrual period.

❏ Patient with an allergy to penicillin should be instructed to always carry an identification card with this information.

## EVALUATION

**Clinical response to therapy can be evaluated by:** ■ Resolution of signs and symptoms of infection. Length of time for complete resolution depends on the organism and site of infection ■ Prevention of rheumatic fever.

# PENICILLINS, PENICILLINASE RESISTANT

### cloxacillin

(klox-a-**sill**-in)

{Apo-Cloxi}, Cloxapen, {Novo-Cloxin}, {Nu-Cloxi}, {Orbenin}

### dicloxacillin

(dye-klox-a-**sill**-in)

Dycill, Dynapen, Pathocil

### nafcillin

(naf-**sill**-in)

Nallpen, Unipen

### oxacillin

(ox-a-**sill**-in)

Bactocill

### CLASSIFICATION(S):

**Therapeutic:** anti-infectives
**Pharmacologic:** penicillinase resistant

**Pregnancy Category B**

## INDICATIONS

■ Treatment of the following infections due to penicillinase-producing staphylococci: ❏ Respiratory tract infections ❏ Sinusitis ❏ Skin and skin structure infections ■ **Nafcillin, oxacillin:** Are also used to treat: ❏ Bone and joint infections ❏ Urinary tract infections ❏ Endocarditis ❏ Septicemia ❏ Meningitis.

## ACTION

■ Bind to bacterial cell wall, leading to cell death. Resist the action of penicillinase, an enzyme capable of inactivating penicillin. **Therapeutic Effects:** ■ Bactericidal action. Spec-

trum: ■ Active against most gram-positive aerobic cocci but less so than penicillin ■ Spectrum is notable for activity against: ❏ Penicillinase-producing strains of *Staphylococcus aureus* ❏ *Staphylococcus epidermidis* ■ Not active against methicillin-resistant staphylococci.

## PHARMACOKINETICS

**Absorption:** *Cloxacillin*—Moderately absorbed (37–60%) following oral administration. *Dicloxacillin*—Rapidly but incompletely (35–76%) absorbed from the GI tract. *Nafcillin*—Poorly and erratically absorbed from the GI tract; well absorbed from IM sites. *Oxacillin*—Rapidly but incompletely absorbed from the GI tract; well absorbed from IM sites.

**Distribution:** *Cloxacillin, dicloxacillin*—Widely distributed; penetration into CSF is minimal; cross the placenta and enter breast milk. *Nafcillin, oxacillin*—Widely distributed; penetration into CSF is minimal but sufficient in the presence of inflamed meninges; cross the placenta and enter breast milk.

**Metabolism and Excretion:** *Cloxacillin*—Some metabolism by the liver (9–22%) and some renal excretion of unchanged drug (30–45%). *Dicloxacillin*—Some metabolism by the liver (6–10%) and some renal excretion of unchanged drug (60%); small amounts eliminated in the feces via the bile. *Nafcillin, oxacillin*—Partially metabolized by the liver (nafcillin 60%, oxacillin 49%), partially excreted unchanged by the kidneys.

**Half-life:** *Cloxacillin*—0.5–1.1 hr (increased in severe hepatic and renal dysfunction); *dicloxacillin*—0.5–1 hr (increased in severe hepatic and renal dysfunction); *nafcillin*—0.5–1.5 hr (increased in renal impairment); *oxacillin*—0.3–0.8 hr (increased in severe hepatic impairment).

## CONTRAINDICATIONS AND PRECAUTIONS

**Contraindicated in:** ■ Hypersensitivity to penicillins (cross-sensitivity with cephalosporins may exist).

**Use Cautiously in:** ■ Severe renal or hepatic impairment ■ Pregnancy or lactation (safety not established).

{ } = Available in Canada only.
*CAPITALS indicates life-threatening; underlines indicate most frequent.

## ADVERSE REACTIONS AND SIDE EFFECTS*

■ **CNS:** SEIZURES (high doses) ■ **GI:** PSEUDOMEM-BRANOUS COLITIS, diarrhea, nausea, drug-induced hepatitis, vomiting ■ **GU:** interstitial nephritis (increased with nafcillin, oxacillin) ■ **Derm:** rashes, urticaria ■ **Hemat:** blood dyscrasias ■ **Local:** pain at IM sites, phlebitis at IV sites ■ **Misc:** allergic reactions including ANAPHYLAXIS and SERUM SICKNESS, superinfection.

## INTERACTIONS

**Drug-Drug:** ■ **Probenecid** decreases renal excretion and increases blood levels ■ May alter the effect of **warfarin.**

**Drug-Food:** ■ **Food** and **acidic juices** decrease absorption.

## ROUTE AND DOSAGE

### ❏ Cloxacillin

■ **PO (Adults and Children >20 kg):** 250–500 mg q 6 hr.
■ **PO (Children >1 mo and <20 kg):** 6.25–12.5 mg/kg q 6 hr.

### ❏ Dicloxacillin

■ **PO (Adults and Children ≥40 kg):** 125–250 mg q 6 hr (up to 6 g/day).
■ **PO (Children <40 kg):** 3.125–6.25 mg/kg q 6 hr (up to 25 mg/kg q 6 hr in cystic fibrosis patients).

### ❏ Nafcillin

Parenteral nafcillin contains 2.9 mEq sodium/g.
■ **PO (Adults):** 250–1000 mg q 4–6 hr.
■ **PO (Children and Infants):** *Most infections*—6.25–12.5 mg/kg q 6 hr. *Pharyngitis*—250 mg q 8 hr.
■ **PO (Neonates):** 10 mg/kg q 6–8 hr.
■ **IM (Adults):** 500 mg q 4–6 hr.
■ **IM (Children and Infants):** 25 mg/kg q 12 hr.
■ **IM (Neonates):** 10 mg/kg q 12 hr.
■ **IV (Adults):** 500–1500 mg q 4–6 hr.
■ **IV (Children, Infants, and Neonates):** *Most infections*—10–20 mg/kg q 4 hr or 20–40 mg/kg q 8 hr (up to 200 mg/kg/day).
■ **IM, IV (Neonates ≥2 kg):** *Meningitis*—50 mg/kg q 8 hr for the first 7 days of life, then 50 mg/kg q 6 hr.
■ **IM, IV (Neonates <2 kg):** *Meningitis*—25–50 mg/kg q 12 hr for the first 7 days of life, then 50 mg/kg q 8 hr.

### ❏ Oxacillin

Injection contains 2.5–3.1 mEq sodium/g.
■ **PO (Adults and Children ≥40 kg):** 500–1000 mg q 4–6 hr.
■ **PO (Children <40 kg):** 12.5–25 mg/kg q 6 hr.
■ **IM, IV (Adults and Children ≥40 kg):** 250–2000 mg q 4–6 hr (up to 20 g/day).
■ **IM, IV (Children <40 kg):** 12.5–25 mg/kg q 6 hr *or* 16.7 mg/kg q 4 hr.
■ **IM, IV (Neonates and Premature Infants):** *Most infections*—6.25 mg/kg q 6 hr.
■ **IM, IV (Neonates ≥2 kg):** *Meningitis*—50 mg/kg q 8 hr for the first 7 days of life, then 50 mg/kg q 6 hr.
■ **IM, IV (Neonates <2 kg):** *Meningitis*—25–50 mg/kg q 12 hr for the first 7 days of life, then 50 mg/kg q 8 hr.

## AVAILABILITY (generic available)

### ❏ Cloxacillin

■ *Capsules:* 250 mg$^{Rx}$, 500 mg$^{Rx}$ ■ *Oral solution:* 125 mg/5 ml$^{Rx}$ ■ *Powder for injection:* {250-mg}, {500-mg}, {and 2-g vials$^{Rx}$.}

### ❏ Dicloxacillin

■ *Capsules:* 125 mg$^{Rx}$, 250 mg$^{Rx}$, 500 mg$^{Rx}$ ■ *Oral suspension:* 62.5 mg/5 ml$^{Rx}$.

### ❏ Nafcillin

■ *Tablets:* 500 mg$^{Rx}$ ■ *Capsules:* 250 mg$^{Rx}$ ■ *Powder for injection:* 1-, 2-, and 10-g vials$^{Rx}$.

### ❏ Oxacillin

■ *Capsules:* 250 mg$^{Rx}$, 500 mg$^{Rx}$ ■ *Oral solution:* 250 mg/5 ml$^{Rx}$ ■ *Powder for injection:* 250-mg, 500-mg, 2-g, 4-g, and 10-g vials$^{Rx}$.

TIME/ACTION PROFILE (blood levels)

| | ONSET | PEAK | DURATION |
|---|---|---|---|
| Cloxacillin PO | 30 min | 30–120 min | 6 hr |
| Dicloxacillin PO | 30 min | 30–120 min | 6 hr |
| Nafcillin PO, IM | 30 min | 60–120 min | 4–6 hr |
| Nafcillin IV | rapid | end of infusion | 4–6 hr |
| Oxacillin PO | rapid | 30–60 min | 4–6 hr |
| Oxacillin IM | rapid | 30 min | 4–6 hr |
| Oxacillin IV | rapid | end of infusion | 4–6 hr |

# NURSING IMPLICATIONS

## ASSESSMENT

❑ Assess patient for infection (vital signs; appearance of wound, sputum, urine, and stool; WBC) at beginning of and throughout therapy.

❑ Obtain a history before initiating therapy to determine previous use of and reactions to penicillins or cephalosporins. Persons with a negative history of penicillin sensitivity may still have an allergic response.

❑ Obtain specimens for culture and sensitivity prior to initiating therapy. First dose may be given before receiving results.

❑ Observe patient for signs and symptoms of anaphylaxis (rash, pruritus, laryngeal edema, wheezing, abdominal pain). Discontinue the drug and notify the physician or other health care professional immediately if these occur. Keep epinephrine, an antihistamine, and resuscitation equipment close by in the event of an anaphylactic reaction.

❑ Assess vein for signs of irritation and phlebitis. Change IV site every 48 hr to prevent phlebitis.

■ *Lab Test Considerations:* May cause leukopenia and neutropenia, especially with prolonged therapy or hepatic impairment.

❑ May cause positive direct Coombs' test result.

❑ May cause elevations in AST, ALT, LDH, and serum alkaline phosphatase concentrations.

## POTENTIAL NURSING DIAGNOSES

■ Infection, risk for (Indications, Side Effects).

■ Noncompliance (Patient/Family Teaching).

## IMPLEMENTATION

■ **PO:** Administer around the clock on an empty stomach at least 1 hr before or 2 hr after meals. Take with a full glass of water; acidic juices may decrease absorption of penicillins.

❑ Use calibrated measuring device for liquid preparations. Shake well. Solution is stable for 14 days if refrigerated.

❑ **Nafcillin**

■ **IV, IM:** To reconstitute, add 3.4 ml to each 1-g vial or 6.8 ml to each 2-g vial, for a concentration of 250 mg/ml. Stable for 2–7 days if refrigerated.

■ **Direct IV:** Dilute reconstituted solution with 15–30 ml of sterile water, 0.45% NaCl, or 0.9% NaCl for injection.

■ *Rate:* Administer over 5–10 min.

■ **Intermittent Infusion:** Dilute to a concentration of 2–40 mg/ml with sterile water for injection, 0.9% NaCl, D5W, D10W, D5/0.25% NaCl, D5/0.45% NaCl, D5/0.9% NaCl, D5/LR, Ringer's or LR. Stable for 24 hr at room temperature, 96 hr if refrigerated.

■ *Rate:* Infuse over at least 30–60 min to avoid vein irritation.

■ **Y-Site Compatibility:** ◆ acyclovir ◆ atropine ◆ cyclophosphamide ◆ diazepam ◆ enalaprilat ◆ esmolol ◆ famotidine ◆ fentanyl ◆ fluconazole ◆ foscarnet ◆ hydromorphone ◆ levofloxacin ◆ magnesium sulfate ◆ morphine ◆ perphenazine ◆ propofol ◆ theophylline ◆ zidovudine.

■ **Y-Site Incompatibility:** ◆ droperidol ◆ insulin ◆ labetalol ◆ midazolam ◆ nalbuphine ◆ pentazocine ◆ verapamil. If penicillins and aminoglycosides must be administered concurrently, administer at separate sites.

❑ **Oxacillin**

■ **IV, IM:** To reconstitute for IM or IV use, add 1.4 ml of sterile water for injection to each 250-mg vial, 2.7 ml to each 500-mg vial, 5.7 ml to each 1-g vial, 11.5 ml to each 2-g vial, and 23 ml to each 4-g vial, for a concentration of 250 mg/1.5 ml. Stable for 3 days at room temperature or 7 days if refrigerated.

■ **Direct IV:** Further dilute each reconstituted 250-mg or 500-mg vial with 5 ml of sterile water or 0.9% NaCl for injection, 10 ml for each 1-g vial, 20 ml for each 2-g vial, and 40 ml for each 4-g vial.

■ *Rate:* Administer slowly over 10 min.

■ **Intermittent Infusion:** Dilute to a concentration of 0.5–40 mg/ml with 0.9% NaCl, D5W, D5/0.9% NaCl, or LR.

■ *Rate:* May be infused for up to 6 hr.

■ **Y-Site Compatibility:** ◆ acyclovir ◆ cyclophosphamide ◆ diltiazem ◆ famotidine ◆ fluconazole ◆ foscarnet ◆ heparin ◆ hydrocortisone sodium succinate ◆ hydromorphone ◆ labetalol ◆ magnesium sulfate ◆ meperidine ◆

methotrexate ◆ morphine ◆ perphenazine ◆ potassium chloride ◆ tacrolimus ◆ vitamin B complex with C ◆ zidovudine.

■ **Y-Site Incompatibility:** ◆ sodium bicarbonate ◆ verapamil. If penicillins and aminoglycosides must be administered concurrently, administer at separate sites.

## PATIENT/FAMILY TEACHING

❑ Instruct patient to take medication around the clock and to finish the drug completely as directed, even if feeling better. Missed doses should be taken as soon as remembered. Advise patient that sharing of this medication may be dangerous.

❑ Advise patient to report signs of superinfection (black, furry overgrowth on the tongue; vaginal itching or discharge; loose or foul-smelling stools) and allergy.

❑ Instruct patient to notify health care professional if fever and diarrhea develop, especially if stool contains blood, pus, or mucus. Advise patient not to treat diarrhea without consulting health care professional.

❑ Instruct patient to notify health care professional if symptoms do not improve.

## EVALUATION

**Clinical response to therapy can be evaluated by:** ■ Resolution of the signs and symptoms of infection. Length of time for complete resolution depends on the organism and site of infection.

## pentamidine
(pen-**tam**-i-deen)
NebuPent, Pentam 300, {Pentacarinat}, {Pneumopent}

### CLASSIFICATION(S):
***Therapeutic:*** *antiprotozoals*

### Pregnancy Category C

## INDICATIONS

■ **IV:** Treatment of *Pneumocystis carinii* pneumonia (PCP) ■ **Inhaln:** Prevention of PCP in AIDS or HIV-positive patients who have had PCP or who have a peripheral CD4 lymphocyte count of ≤200/mm³. **Unlabeled uses:** ■ **Inhaln:** Treatment of PCP.

## ACTION

■ Appears to disrupt DNA or RNA synthesis in protozoa ■ Also has a direct toxic effect on pancreatic islet cells. **Therapeutic Effects:** ■ Death of susceptible protozoa.

## PHARMACOKINETICS

**Absorption:** Minimal systemic absorption occurs following inhalation.

**Distribution:** Widely and extensively distributed but does not cross the blood-brain barrier. Concentrates in liver, kidneys, lungs, and spleen, with prolonged storage in some tissues.

**Metabolism and Excretion:** 1–30% excreted unchanged by the kidneys. Remainder of metabolic fate unknown.

**Half-life:** 6.4–9.4 hr (increased in renal impairment).

## CONTRAINDICATIONS AND PRECAUTIONS

**Contraindicated in:** ■ History of previous anaphylactic reaction to pentamidine.

**Use Cautiously in:** ■ Hypotension ■ Hypertension ■ Hypoglycemia ■ Hyperglycemia ■ Hypocalcemia ■ Leukopenia ■ Thrombocytopenia ■ Anemia ■ Renal impairment (dosage reduction required) ■ Diabetes mellitus ■ Liver impairment ■ Cardiovascular disease ■ Bone marrow depression, previous antineoplastic therapy, or radiation therapy ■ Pregnancy or lactation (safety not established during pregnancy; breastfeeding not recommended).

## ADVERSE REACTIONS AND SIDE EFFECTS*

For parenteral form, unless otherwise indicated. ■ **CNS:** anxiety, headache, confusion, dizziness, hallucinations ■ **EENT:** *inhalation—* burning in throat ■ **Resp:** *inhalation—*bronchospasm, cough ■ **CV:** ARRHYTHMIAS, HYPOTENSION ■ **GI:** PANCREATITIS, abdominal pain, anorexia, drug-induced hepatitis, nausea, unpleasant metallic taste, vomiting ■ **GU:** nephrotoxicity ■ **Derm:** pallor, rash ■ **Endo:** HYPOGLYCEMIA, hyperglycemia ■ **F and E:** hyperkalemia, hypocalcemia ■ **Hemat:** anemia, leukopenia, thrombocytopenia ■ **Local: IV:** phlebitis, pruritus, urticaria at IV site. **IM:** sterile abscesses at IM sites ■ **Misc:** allergic reactions including ANAPHYLAXIS, STEVENS-JOHNSON SYNDROME, chills, fever.

## INTERACTIONS

Interactions listed for parenteral administration.

**Drug-Drug:** ■ Concurrent use with **erythromycin IV** may increase the risk of potentially fatal arrhythmias ■ Additive nephrotoxicity with other **nephrotoxic agents,** including **aminoglycosides, amphotericin B,** and **vancomycin** ■ Additive bone marrow depression with **antineoplastics** or previous **radiation therapy** ■ Increased risk of pancreatitis with **didanosine** ■ Increased risk of nephrotoxicity, hypocalcemia, and hypomagnesemia with **foscarnet.**

## ROUTE AND DOSAGE

■ **IV (Adults and Children):** 4 mg/kg once daily for 14–21 days (longer treatment may be required in AIDS patients; some patients may respond to 3 mg/kg/day).

■ **Inhaln (Adults):** *NebuPent, Pentacarinat*—300 mg q 4 wk, using a Respirgard II jet nebulizer (150 mg q 2 wk has also been used). *Pneumopent*—60 mg q 24–72 hr for 5 doses over a 2-wk period, then q 2 wk using a Fisoneb ultrasonic nebulizer.

■ **Inhaln (Children >5 yr):** *NebuPent, Pentacarinat*—300 mg q 4 wk, using a Respirgard II jet nebulizer (for patients who cannot tolerate trimethoprim/sulfamethoxazole; unlabeled).

## AVAILABILITY (generic available)

■ *Injection:* 300 mg/vial^Rx ■ *Solution for aerosol use (NebuPent, Pentacarinat):* 300 mg/vial^Rx ■ *Solution for aerosol use (Pneumopent):* {60 mg/vial^Rx}.

TIME/ACTION PROFILE (blood levels)

|  | ONSET | PEAK | DURATION |
| --- | --- | --- | --- |
| IV | unknown | end of infu-sion | 24 hr |
| Inhaln | unknown | unknown | unknown |

## NURSING IMPLICATIONS

### ASSESSMENT

■ **General Info:** Assess patient for infection (vital signs, sputum, WBC) and monitor respiratory status (rate, character, lung sounds, dyspnea, sputum) at beginning of and throughout therapy.

❑ Obtain specimens for culture and sensitivity prior to initiating therapy. First dose may be given before receiving results.

■ **IV, IM:** Monitor blood pressure frequently during and following IM or IV administration of pentamidine. Patient should be lying down during administration. Sudden, severe hypotension may occur following a single dose. Resuscitation equipment should be immediately available.

❑ Assess patient for signs of hypoglycemia (anxiety; chills; diaphoresis; cold, pale skin; headache; increased hunger; nausea; nervousness; shakiness) and hyperglycemia (drowsiness; flushed, dry skin; fruit-like breath odor; increased thirst; increased urination; loss of appetite), which may occur up to several months after therapy is discontinued.

❑ Pulse and ECG should be monitored prior to and periodically during course of therapy. Fatalities due to cardiac arrhythmias, tachycardia, and cardiotoxicity have been reported.

■ **Inhaln:** A tuberculin skin test, chest x-ray, and sputum culture should be performed prior to administration to rule out tuberculosis.

■ *Lab Test Considerations: IM, IV*—Blood glucose concentrations should be monitored prior to, daily during, and for several months following therapy. Severe hypoglycemia and permanent diabetes mellitus have occurred.

❑ Monitor BUN and serum creatinine prior to and daily during therapy to monitor for nephrotoxicity. Concentrations may be increased.

❑ Monitor CBC and platelet count prior to and every 3 days during therapy. Pentamidine may cause leukopenia, anemia, and thrombocytopenia.

❑ May cause elevated serum bilirubin, alkaline phosphatase, AST, and ALT concentrations. These liver function tests should be monitored prior to and every 3 days during therapy.

❑ Serum calcium and magnesium concentrations should be monitored prior to and every

---

{ } = Available in Canada only.

*CAPITALS indicates life-threatening; underlines indicate most frequent.

3 days during therapy, as pentamidine may cause hypocalcemia and hypomagnesemia.

❑ May cause elevated serum potassium concentrations.

## POTENTIAL NURSING DIAGNOSES

■ Infection, risk for (Indications, Side Effects).

## IMPLEMENTATION

■ **General:** Pentamidine must be given on a regular schedule for the full course of therapy. If a dose is missed, administer as soon as remembered. If almost time for the next dose, skip the missed dose and return to the regular schedule. Do not double doses.

■ **IM:** Dilute 300 mg of pentamidine with 3 ml of sterile water for injection for a concentration of 100 mg/ml. IM administration should be used only for patients with adequate muscle mass and given deep IM via Z-track technique. May cause sterile abscesses.

■ **Intermittent Infusion:** To reconstitute, add 3–5 ml of sterile water for injection or D5W to each 300-mg vial for a concentration of 100, 75, or 60 mg/ml, respectively. Withdraw dose and dilute further in 50–250 ml of D5W. Solution is stable for 48 hr at room temperature. Discard unused portions.

■ **Rate:** Administer slowly over 1–2 hr.

■ **Y-Site Compatibility:** ◆ diltiazem ◆ gatifloxacin ◆ zidovudine.

■ **Y-Site Incompatibility:** ◆ aldesleukin ◆ cefazolin ◆ cefoperazone ◆ cefotaxime ◆ cefoxitin ◆ ceftazidime ◆ ceftriaxone ◆ fluconazole ◆ foscarnet ◆ linezolid.

■ **Inhaln:** If using inhalation bronchodilator, administer bronchodilator 5–10 min prior to pentamidine administration.

❑ Administer in a well-ventilated area.

❑ Administration with patient in supine or recumbent position appears to provide a more uniform distribution of pentamidine.

❑ *NebuPent* or *Pentacarinat:* Dilute 300 or 600 mg (for prophylaxis or treatment, respectively) in 6 ml of sterile water for injection. Place reconstituted solution into Respirgard II nebulizer. Do not dilute with 0.9% NaCl or admix with other medications, as solution will form a precipitate. Do not use Respirgard II nebulizer for other medications.

❑ Administer inhalation dose through nebulizer until chamber is empty, approximately 30–45 min.

❑ *Pneumopent:* Remove rubber stopper and set upside down on a clean surface for use later. Add 3–5 ml of sterile water for inhalation or preservative-free water for injection to vial and replace rubber stopper. Do not use tap water or 0.9% NaCl. Powder should dissolve immediately; if not, shake gently to mix. Solution should be clear and colorless; do not use if cloudy. Solution is stable for 24 hr at room temperature or 48 hr if refrigerated. Place entire reconstituted contents into Fisoneb ultrasonic nebulizer.

❑ Administer with the flow rate of the nebulizer at the midflow mark over approximately 15 min until the chamber is empty.

## PATIENT/FAMILY TEACHING

■ **General Info:** Inform patient of the importance of completing the full course of pentamidine therapy, even if feeling better.

■ **IV:** Instruct patient to notify health care professional promptly if fever; sore throat; signs of infection; bleeding of gums; unusual bruising; petechiae; or blood in stool, urine, or emesis occurs. Caution patient to avoid crowds and persons with known infections. Instruct patient to use soft toothbrush and electric razor and to avoid falls. Patient should not be given IM injections or rectal thermometers. Patient should be cautioned not to drink alcoholic beverages or take medication containing aspirin or NSAIDs, as these may precipitate gastric bleeding.

❑ Caution patient to make position changes slowly to minimize orthostatic hypotension.

■ **Inhaln:** Advise patient that an unpleasant metallic taste may occur with pentamidine administration but is not significant.

❑ Inform patients who continue to smoke that bronchospasm and coughing during therapy are more likely.

## EVALUATION

**Clinical response to therapy can be evaluated by:** ■ Prevention or resolution of the signs and symptoms of PCP in HIV-positive patients.

## pentoxifylline

(pen-tox-**if**-i-lin)

Trental

*CLASSIFICATION(S):*

*Therapeutic: blood viscosity reducing agents*

**Pregnancy Category C**

### INDICATIONS

■ Management of symptomatic peripheral vascular disease (intermittent claudication).

### ACTION

■ Increases the flexibility of RBCs by increasing levels of cyclic adenosine monophosphate (cAMP) ■ Decreases blood viscosity by inhibiting platelet aggregation and decreasing fibrinogen. **Therapeutic Effects:** ■ Increased blood flow.

### PHARMACOKINETICS

**Absorption:** Well absorbed following oral administration.

**Distribution:** Bound to RBC membrane. Enters breast milk.

**Metabolism and Excretion:** Metabolized by RBCs and the liver.

**Half-life:** 25–50 min.

### CONTRAINDICATIONS AND PRECAUTIONS

**Contraindicated in:** ■ Hypersensitivity ■ Intolerance to other xanthine derivatives (caffeine and theophylline).

**Use Cautiously in:** ■ Coronary artery or cerebrovascular disease ■ Renal disease (lower doses may be used) ■ Geriatric patients (increased risk of adverse reactions) ■ Pregnancy, lactation, or children (safety not established).

### ADVERSE REACTIONS AND SIDE EFFECTS*

■ **CNS:** agitation, dizziness, drowsiness, headache, insomnia, nervousness ■ **EENT:** blurred vision ■ **Resp:** dyspnea ■ **CV:** angina, arrhythmias, edema, flushing, hypotension ■ **GI:** abdominal discomfort, belching, bloating, diarrhea, dyspepsia, flatus, nausea, vomiting ■ **Neuro:** tremor.

### INTERACTIONS

**Drug-Drug:** ■ Additive hypotension may occur with **antihypertensives** and **nitrates** ■ May increase the risk of bleeding with **warfarin, heparin, aspirin, NSAIDs, cefoperazone, cefotetan, plicamycin, valproic acid, clopidogrel, ticlopidine, eptifibatide, tirofiban,** or **thrombolytic agents** ■ May increase the risk of **theophylline** toxicity ■ **Smoking** may decrease the beneficial effects of pentoxifylline.

**Drug-Natural Products:** ■ Increased bleeding risk with **anise, arnica, asafoetida, chamomile, clove, dong quai, fenugreek, feverfew, garlic, ginger, ginkgo, Panax ginseng, licorice,** and others.

### ROUTE AND DOSAGE

■ **PO (Adults):** 400 mg 3 times daily; if GI or CNS side effects occur, decrease dose to 400 mg twice daily.

### AVAILABILITY (generic available)

■ *Controlled-release tablets:* 400 mg$^{Rx}$ ■ Cost: $68.64/100 ■ *Extended-release tablets:* 400 mg$^{Rx}$.

TIME/ACTION PROFILE (improvement in blood flow)

|  | ONSET | PEAK | DURATION |
|---|---|---|---|
| PO | 2–4 wk | 8 wk | 8 hr |

## NURSING IMPLICATIONS

### ASSESSMENT

❑ Assess patient for intermittent claudication prior to and periodically throughout therapy.

❑ Monitor blood pressure periodically in patients on concurrent antihypertensive therapy.

### POTENTIAL NURSING DIAGNOSES

■ Pain, acute (Indications).

■ Activity intolerance (Indications).

{ } = Available in Canada only.
*CAPITALS indicates life-threatening; underlines indicate most frequent.

## IMPLEMENTATION

- **PO:** Administer with meals to minimize GI irritation. Tablets should be swallowed whole; do not crush, break, or chew.
- ◻ If GI and CNS side effects occur, decrease dose to twice daily. Discontinue if side effects persist.

## PATIENT/FAMILY TEACHING

- ◻ Instruct patient to take medication exactly as directed. If a dose is missed, it should be taken as soon as remembered unless almost time for next dose. Consult health care professional before discontinuing medication, because several weeks of therapy may be required before effects are seen.
- ◻ May cause dizziness and blurred vision. Caution patient to avoid driving and other activities requiring alertness until response to medication is known.
- ◻ Advise patient to avoid smoking, because nicotine constricts blood vessels.
- ◻ Instruct patient to notify health care professional if nausea, vomiting, GI upset, drowsiness, dizziness, or headache persists.

## EVALUATION

**Effectiveness of therapy can be demonstrated by:** ■ Relief from cramping in calf muscles, buttocks, thighs, and feet during exercise ◻ Improvement in walking endurance. Therapeutic effects may be seen in 2–4 wk, but therapy should be continued for ≥8 wk.

## pergolide

(**per**-goe-lide)

Permax

### CLASSIFICATION(S):

**Therapeutic:** antiparkinson agents
**Pharmacologic:** dopamine agonists

### Pregnancy Category B

## INDICATIONS

- ■ Management of Parkinson's disease in conjunction with levodopa/carbidopa.

## ACTION

- ■ Acts as a dopamine agonist, directly stimulating postsynaptic dopaminergic receptors in the CNS. **Therapeutic Effects:** ■ Continued relief of symptoms of Parkinson's disease at a lower dosage of levodopa/carbidopa.

## PHARMACOKINETICS

**Absorption:** Well absorbed following oral administration.

**Distribution:** Unknown.

**Protein Binding:** 90%.

**Metabolism and Excretion:** Highly metabolized by the liver. Metabolites are excreted by the kidneys.

**Half-life:** Unknown.

## CONTRAINDICATIONS AND PRECAUTIONS

**Contraindicated in:** ■ Hypersensitivity to pergolide or ergot derivatives ■ Lactation (may inhibit lactation).

**Use Cautiously in:** ■ Arrhythmias ■ History of psychiatric disorders ■ Pregnancy or children (safety not established).

## ADVERSE REACTIONS AND SIDE EFFECTS*

- ■ **CNS:** drowsiness, dyskinesia, hallucinations, confusion, insomnia ■ **EENT:** rhinitis ■ **Resp:** dyspnea ■ **CV:** orthostatic hypotension, arrhythmias (atrial premature contractions, sinus tachycardia), hypertension, palpitations ■ **GI:** constipation, nausea, abdominal pain, diarrhea, dry mouth, dyspepsia.

## INTERACTIONS

**Drug-Drug:** ■ **Phenothiazines, metoclopramide, reserpine,** or **haloperidol** may decrease effectiveness by antagonizing the effects of dopamine ■ Additive hypotension may occur with **antihypertensives.**

## ROUTE AND DOSAGE

- ■ **PO (Adults):** 50 mcg/day for 2 days; increase by 100–150 mcg/day every 3rd day for 12 days, then may increase by 250 mcg/day every 3rd day until optimal response is obtained. Usual dose is 1 mg 3 times daily (not to exceed 5 mg/day). Usually given in 3 divided doses.

## AVAILABILITY

- ■ **Tablets:** 50 mcg (0.05 mg)$^{Rx}$, 250 mcg (0.25 mg)$^{Rx}$, 1 mg$^{Rx}$ ■ Cost: 0.05 mg $35.60/30, 0.25 mg $188.18/100, 1 mg $417.09/100.

TIME/ACTION PROFILE (antiparkinson effects)

| | ONSET | PEAK | DURATION |
|---|---|---|---|
| PO | unknown | unknown | unknown |

## NURSING IMPLICATIONS

### ASSESSMENT

❑ Assess patient for signs and symptoms of Parkinson's disease (tremor, muscle weakness and rigidity, ataxic gait) prior to and during therapy.

❑ Assess patient for confusion or hallucinations. Notify physician or other health care professional if these occur.

❑ Monitor ECG and blood pressure frequently during dose adjustment and periodically during therapy.

### POTENTIAL NURSING DIAGNOSES

■ Mobility, impaired physical (Indications).

■ Injury, risk for (Indications, Side Effects).

### IMPLEMENTATION

■ **PO:** An attempt to reduce the dose of levodopa/carbidopa may be made cautiously during pergolide therapy.

❑ Administer with meals to minimize nausea; usually resolves with continued therapy.

### PATIENT/FAMILY TEACHING

❑ Instruct patient to take medication as directed. Take missed doses as soon as remembered if not almost time for next dose. Do not double doses. Consult health care professional before reducing dose or discontinuing medication.

❑ May cause drowsiness. Caution patient to avoid driving or other activities requiring alertness until response to medication is known.

❑ Advise patient to change positions slowly to minimize orthostatic hypotension. Initial dose may be administered at bedtime to minimize this effect.

❑ Inform patient that frequent mouth rinses, good oral hygiene, and sugarless gum or candy may minimize dry mouth. Advise patient to consult health care professional if dry mouth persists for longer than 2 wk.

### EVALUATION

**Effectiveness of therapy can be demonstrated by:** ■ Improved response to levodopa/carbidopa in patients with Parkinson's disease.

## perindopril, See ANGIOTENSIN-CONVERTING ENZYME (ACE) INHIBITORS.

## permethrin

(per-**meth**-rin)

Acticin, Elimite, Nix

**CLASSIFICATION(S):**

**Therapeutic:** *pediculocides*

**Pregnancy Category B**

### INDICATIONS

■ **1% lotion:** Eradication of *Pediculus humanus capitis* (head lice and their eggs) ❑ Prevention of infestation of head lice during epidemics ■ **5% cream:** Eradication of *Sarcoptes scabiei* (scabies).

### ACTION

■ Causes repolarization and paralysis in lice by disrupting sodium transport in normal nerve cells. **Therapeutic Effects:** ■ Death of parasites.

### PHARMACOKINETICS

**Absorption:** Small amounts (<2%) systemically absorbed. Remains on hair for 10 days.

**Distribution:** Unknown.

**Metabolism and Excretion:** Rapidly inactivated by enzymes.

**Half-life:** Unknown.

### CONTRAINDICATIONS AND PRECAUTIONS

**Contraindicated in:** ■ Hypersensitivity to permethrin, pyrethrins (insecticides or veterinary pesticides), chrysanthemums, or isopropyl alcohol.

**Use Cautiously in:** ■ Pregnancy or lactation ■ Children <2 yr (1% lotion) ■ Children <2 mo (5% cream).

## ADVERSE REACTIONS AND SIDE EFFECTS*

■ **Derm:** burning, itching, rash, redness, stinging, swelling ■ **Neuro:** numbness, tingling.

## INTERACTIONS

**Drug-Drug:** ■ No significant interactions.

## ROUTE AND DOSAGE

❏ **Head Lice (Treatment and Prevention)**
■ **Topical (Adults and Children >2 yr):** 1% lotion applied to the hair, left on for 10 min, then rinsed, for 1 application.

❏ **Scabies**
■ **Topical (Adults and Children):** Massage 5% cream into all skin surfaces. Leave on for 8–14 hr, then wash off.
■ **Topical (Infants >2 mo):** Massage 5% cream into hairline, scalp, neck, temple, and forehead. Leave on for 8–14 hr, then wash off.

## AVAILABILITY (generic available)

■ *Liquid cream rinse (lotion):* 1% in 60-ml containers^OTC ■ *Cream:* 5% in 60-g tube^Rx ■ Cost: *Elimite*—$26.99/60 g; *Acticin*—$23.62/60 g.

TIME/ACTION PROFILE (pediculocidal action)

| | ONSET | PEAK | DURATION |
|---|---|---|---|
| Topical | 10 min | unknown | 14 days |

# NURSING IMPLICATIONS

## ASSESSMENT

■ **Head Lice:** Assess scalp for presence of lice and their ova (nits) prior to and 1 wk after application of permethrin.
■ **Scabies:** Assess skin for scabies prior to and following therapy.

## POTENTIAL NURSING DIAGNOSES

■ Home maintenance, impaired (Indications).
■ Self-care deficit, bathing/hygiene (Indications).

## IMPLEMENTATION

■ **Topical:** For topical application only.

## PATIENT/FAMILY TEACHING

■ **General Info:** Instruct patient to notify health care professional if scalp itching, numbness, redness, or rash occurs.
❏ Instruct patient to avoid getting Elimite cream in eyes. If this occurs, eyes should be flushed thoroughly with water. Health care professional should be contacted if eye irritation persists.
❏ Advise patient that others residing in the home should also be checked for lice.
❏ Instruct patient on methods of preventing reinfestation. All clothes, including outdoor apparel and household linens, should be machine-washed using very hot water and dried for at least 20 min in a hot dryer. Dry-clean nonwashable clothes. Brushes and combs should be soaked in hot (130°F), soapy water for 5–10 min. Remind patient that brushes and combs should not be shared. Wigs and hairpieces should be shampooed. Rugs and upholstered furniture should be vacuumed. Toys should be washed in hot, soapy water. Items that cannot be washed should be sealed in a plastic bag for 2 wk.
❏ If patient is a child, instruct parents to notify school nurse or day care center so that classmates and playmates can be checked.
■ **Head Lice:** Instruct patient to wash hair with regular shampoo, rinse, and towel dry. Each container holds enough medication for one treatment. Shake the container well. Thoroughly wet scalp and hair with the lotion. The patient should use as much of the solution as needed to coat entire head of hair, then discard remainder of solution. Allow lotion to remain on hair for 10 min, then thoroughly rinse hair and towel dry with a clean towel. Comb hair with a fine-toothed comb to remove dead lice and eggs (not necessary but may be desired for cosmetic effects). Products are available for removal of nits (Rid Lice Egg Loosener Gel® Step 2). Schools usually require children to be nit-free prior to returning to school.
❏ Explain to patient that permethrin will protect from reinfestation for 2 wk. These effects continue even when the patient resumes regular shampooing.
■ **Scabies:** Instruct patient to massage thoroughly into the skin from head to soles of feet. Treat infants on the hairline, neck, scalp, temple, and forehead. Remove the

cream by washing after 8–14 hr. Usually 30 g (¹/₂ tube) is sufficient for adults. One application is curative.

## EVALUATION

**Effectiveness of therapy can be demonstrated by:** ■ The absence of lice and eggs 1 wk after therapy. A second application is indicated if lice are detected at this time ❏ Prevention of infestation of head lice during epidemics ■ Eradication of scabies following one application ■ If resistance to permethrin develops, malathion may be used.

---

# phenazopyridine

(fen-az-oh-**peer**-i-deen)

Azo-Standard, Baridium, Geridium, {Phenazo}, Prodium, Pyridiate, Pyridium, Pyridium Plus, Urodine, Urogesic, UTI Relief

## CLASSIFICATION(S):

**Therapeutic:** nonopioid analgesics
**Pharmacologic:** urinary tract analgesics

## Pregnancy Category B

---

## INDICATIONS

■ Provides relief from the following urinary tract symptoms, which may occur in association with infection or following urologic procedures: ❏ Pain ❏ Itching ❏ Burning ❏ Urgency ❏ Frequency.

## ACTION

■ Acts locally on the urinary tract mucosa to produce analgesic or local anesthetic effects ■ Has no antimicrobial activity. **Therapeutic Effects:** ■ Diminished urinary tract discomfort.

## PHARMACOKINETICS

**Absorption:** Appears to be well absorbed following oral administration.
**Distribution:** Unknown. Small amounts cross the placenta.
**Metabolism and Excretion:** Rapidly excreted unchanged in the urine.
**Half-life:** Unknown.

## CONTRAINDICATIONS AND PRECAUTIONS

**Contraindicated in:** ■ Hypersensitivity ■ Glomerulonephritis ■ Severe hepatitis, uremia, or renal failure ■ Renal insufficiency ■ G6PD deficiency.
**Use Cautiously in:** ■ Hepatitis ■ Pregnancy or lactation (safety not established).

## ADVERSE REACTIONS AND SIDE EFFECTS*

■ **CNS:** headache, vertigo ■ **GI:** hepatotoxicity, nausea ■ **GU:** <u>bright-orange urine</u>, renal failure ■ **Derm:** rash ■ **Hemat:** hemolytic anemia, methemoglobinemia.

## INTERACTIONS

**Drug-Drug:** ■ None significant.

## ROUTE AND DOSAGE

■ **PO (Adults):** 200 mg 3 times daily for 2 days.
■ **PO (Children):** 4 mg/kg 3 times daily for 2 days.

## AVAILABILITY (generic available)

■ **Tablets:** 95 mg^OTC, 100 mg^Rx, {100 mg^OTC}, {200 mg^OTC}, 200 mg^Rx ■ Cost: 100 mg^Rx $45.09/100, 200 mg^Rx $83.28/100.

TIME/ACTION PROFILE (urinary analgesia)

| | ONSET | PEAK | DURATION |
|---|---|---|---|
| PO | unknown | 5–6 hr | 6–8 hr |

# NURSING IMPLICATIONS

## ASSESSMENT

❏ Assess patient for urgency, frequency, and pain on urination prior to and throughout therapy.
■ **Lab Test Considerations:** Renal function should be monitored periodically during course of therapy.
❏ Interferes with urine tests based on color reactions (glucose, ketones, bilirubin, steroids, protein).

## POTENTIAL NURSING DIAGNOSES

■ Pain, acute (Indications).
■ Urinary elimination, impaired (Indications).

---

{ } = Available in Canada only.
*CAPITALS indicates life-threatening; <u>underlines</u> indicate most frequent.

## IMPLEMENTATION

■ **General:** Medication should be discontinued after pain or discomfort is relieved (usually 2 days for treatment of urinary tract infection). Concurrent antibiotic therapy should continue for full prescribed duration.

■ **PO:** Administer medication with or following meals to decrease GI irritation. Do not crush, break, or chew tablet.

## PATIENT/FAMILY TEACHING

❑ Instruct patient to take medication exactly as directed. If a dose is missed, take as soon as remembered unless almost time for next dose.

❑ Advise patient that while phenazopyridine administration is stopped once pain or discomfort is relieved, concurrent antibiotic therapy must be continued for full duration of therapy. Do not save unused portion of phenazopyridine without consulting health care professional.

❑ Inform patient that drug causes reddish-orange discoloration of urine that may stain clothing or bedding. Sanitary napkin may be worn to avoid clothing stains. May also cause staining of soft contact lenses.

❑ Instruct patient to notify health care professional if rash, skin discoloration, or unusual tiredness occurs.

## EVALUATION

**Effectiveness of therapy can be demonstrated by:** ■ Decrease in pain and burning on urination.

---

## phenelzine, See MONOAMINE OXIDASE (MAO) INHIBITORS.

---

# phenobarbital

(fee-noe-**bar**-bi-tal)

{Ancalixir}, Luminal, Solfoton

### CLASSIFICATION(S):

**Therapeutic:** anticonvulsants, sedative/hypnotics

**Pharmacologic:** barbiturates

### Schedule IV

### Pregnancy Category D

## INDICATIONS

■ Anticonvulsant in tonic-clonic (grand mal), partial, and febrile seizures in children ■ Preoperative sedative and in other situations in which sedation may be required ■ Hypnotic (short-term). **Unlabeled uses:** ■ Prevention/treatment of hyperbilirubinemia.

## ACTION

■ Produces all levels of CNS depression ■ Depresses the sensory cortex, decreases motor activity, and alters cerebellar function ■ Inhibits transmission in the nervous system and raises the seizure threshold ■ Capable of inducing (speeding up) enzymes in the liver that metabolize drugs, bilirubin, and other compounds. **Therapeutic Effects:** ■ Anticonvulsant activity ■ Sedation.

## PHARMACOKINETICS

**Absorption:** Absorption is slow but relatively complete (70–90%).

**Distribution:** Unknown.

**Metabolism and Excretion:** 75% metabolized by the liver, 25% excreted unchanged by the kidneys.

**Half-life:** 2–6 days.

## CONTRAINDICATIONS AND PRECAUTIONS

**Contraindicated in:** ■ Hypersensitivity ■ Comatose patients or those with pre-existing CNS depression ■ Uncontrolled severe pain ■ Lactation ■ Known alcohol intolerance (elixir only).

**Use Cautiously in:** ■ Hepatic dysfunction ■ Severe renal impairment ■ History of suicide attempt or drug abuse ■ Geriatric patients (initial dosage reduction recommended) ■ Hypnotic use should be short-term. Chronic use may lead to dependence ■ Pregnancy (chronic use results in drug dependency in the infant; may result in coagulation defects and fetal malformation; acute use at term may result in respiratory depression in the newborn).

## ADVERSE REACTIONS AND SIDE EFFECTS*

■ **CNS:** <u>hangover</u>, delirium, depression, drowsiness, excitation, lethargy, vertigo ■ **Resp:** respiratory depression; *IV*—LARYNGOSPASM, bronchospasm ■ **CV:** *IV*—hypotension ■ **GI:** constipation, diarrhea, nausea, vomiting ■ **Derm:** photosensitivity, rashes, urticaria ■ **Local:** phlebitis at IV site ■ **MS:** arthralgia, myalgia, neuralgia ■

**Misc:** hypersensitivity reactions including ANGIOEDEMA and SERUM SICKNESS, physical dependence, psychological dependence.

## INTERACTIONS

**Drug-Drug:** ■ Additive CNS depression with other **CNS depressants**, including **alcohol, antihistamines, opioid analgesics,** and other **sedative/hypnotics** ■ May induce hepatic enzymes that metabolize other drugs, decreasing their effectiveness, including **hormonal contraceptives, warfarin, chloramphenicol, cyclosporine, dacarbazine, corticosteroids, tricyclic antidepressants, felodipine, clonazepam, carbamazepine, verapamil, theophylline, metronidazole, griseofulvin,** and **quinidine** ■ May increase the risk of hepatic toxicity of **acetaminophen** ■ **MAO inhibitors, valproic acid,** or **divalproex** may decrease the metabolism of phenobarbital, increasing sedation ■ **Rifampin** may increase metabolism of and decrease effects of phenobarbital ■ May increase the risk of hematologic toxicity with **cyclophosphamide.**

**Drug-Natural Products:** ■ Concomitant use of **kava, valerian, skullcap, chamomile,** or **hops** can increase CNS depression ■ **St. John's wort** may decrease effects.

## ROUTE AND DOSAGE

■ **PO (Adults):** *Anticonvulsant*—60–250 mg/day as a single dose or 2–3 divided doses. *Sedative*—30–120 mg/day in 2–3 divided doses. *Hypnotic*—100–320 mg at bedtime. *Hyperbilirubinemia*—30–60 mg 3 times daily.

■ **PO (Children):** *Anticonvulsant*—1–6 mg/kg/day, single dose or divided doses. *Sedative*—2 mg/kg (60 mg/m²) 3 times daily. *Hyperbilirubinemia*—1–4 mg/kg 3 times daily.

■ **PO, IM, IV (Children):** *Preoperative sedative*—1–3 mg/kg 60–90 min preop.

■ **PO, IM (Neonates):** *Hyperbilirubinemia*—5–10 mg/kg/day.

■ **IM, IV (Adults):** *Sedative*—30–120 mg/day in 2–3 divided doses. *Preoperative sedative*—130–200 mg 90 min preop. *Hypnotic*—100–325 mg at bedtime.

■ **IV (Adults):** *Anticonvulsant*—100–320 mg as needed initially (total of 600 mg/24-hr period). *Status epilepticus*—10–20 mg/kg.

■ **IV (Children):** *Anticonvulsant*—10–20 mg/kg initially, followed by 1–6 mg/kg/day. *Status epilepticus*—15–20 mg/kg.

## AVAILABILITY (generic available)

■ *Tablets:* 8 mg^Rx, 15 mg^Rx, 30 mg^Rx, 60 mg^Rx, 100 mg^Rx ■ Cost: *generic*—15 mg $4.82/100, 30 mg $8.23/100, 60 mg $9.54/100, 100 mg $10.82/100 ■ *Capsules:* 15 mg^Rx ■ *Elixir:* 20 mg/5 ml^Rx ■ *Injection:* 30 mg/ml in 1-ml prefilled syringes^Rx, 60 mg/ml in 1-ml prefilled syringes^Rx, 65 mg/ml in 1-ml vials^Rx, 130 mg/ml in 1-ml prefilled syringes, 1-ml vials, and 1-ml ampules^Rx ■ phenytoin^Rx. See Appendix B.

TIME/ACTION PROFILE (sedation†)

|  | ONSET | PEAK | DURATION |
|---|---|---|---|
| PO | 30–60 min | unknown | >6 hr |
| IM, subcut | 10–30 min | unknown | 4–6 hr |
| IV | 5 min | 30 min | 4–6 hr |

†Full anticonvulsant effects occur after 2–3 wk of chronic dosing unless a loading dose has been used.

# NURSING IMPLICATIONS

## ASSESSMENT

■ **General Info:** Monitor respiratory status, pulse, and blood pressure frequently in patients receiving phenobarbital IV. Equipment for resuscitation and artificial ventilation should be readily available. Respiratory depression is dose-dependent.

❑ Prolonged therapy may lead to psychological or physical dependence. Restrict amount of drug available to patient, especially if depressed, suicidal, or with a history of addiction.

■ **Seizures:** Assess location, duration, and characteristics of seizure activity.

■ **Sedation:** Assess level of consciousness and anxiety when used as a preoperative sedative.

❑ Assess postoperative patients for pain. Phenobarbital may increase sensitivity to painful stimuli.

■ *Lab Test Considerations:* Patients on prolonged therapy should have hepatic and renal function and CBC evaluated periodically.

❏ Serum folate concentrations should be monitored periodically during therapy because of increased folate requirements of patients on long-term anticonvulsant therapy with phenobarbital.

❏ May cause decreased serum bilirubin concentrations in neonates, in patients with congenital nonhemolytic unconjugated hyperbilirubinemia, and in epileptics.

■ *Toxicity and Overdose:* Serum phenobarbital levels may be monitored when used as an anticonvulsant. Therapeutic blood levels are 10–40 mcg/ml. Symptoms of toxicity include confusion, drowsiness, dyspnea, slurred speech, and staggering.

## POTENTIAL NURSING DIAGNOSES

■ Injury, risk for (Indications, Side Effects).

## IMPLEMENTATION

■ **General:** Do not confuse phenobarbital with pentobarbital.

❏ Supervise ambulation and transfer of patients following administration. Remove cigarettes. Side rails should be raised and call bell within reach at all times. Keep bed in low position. Institute seizure precautions.

❏ When changing from phenobarbital to another anticonvulsant, gradually decrease phenobarbital dose while concurrently increasing dose of replacement medication to maintain anticonvulsant effects.

■ **PO:** Tablets may be crushed and mixed with food or fluids (do not administer dry) for patients with difficulty swallowing. Oral solution may be taken undiluted or mixed with water, milk, or fruit juice. Use calibrated measuring device for accurate measurement of liquid doses.

■ **IM:** Injections should be given deep into the gluteal muscle to minimize tissue irritation. Do not inject >5 ml into any one site, because of tissue irritation.

■ **IV:** Doses may require 15–30 min to reach peak concentrations in the brain. Administer minimal dose and wait for effectiveness before administering 2nd dose to prevent cumulative barbiturate-induced depression.

■ **Direct IV:** Reconstitute sterile powder for IV dose with a minimum of 3 ml of sterile water for injection. Dilute further with 10 ml of sterile water. Do not use solution that is not absolutely clear within 5 min after reconstitution or that contains a precipitate. Discard powder or solution that has been exposed to air for longer than 30 min.

❏ Solution is highly alkaline; avoid extravasation, which may cause tissue damage and necrosis. If extravasation occurs, injection of 5% procaine solution into affected area and application of moist heat may be ordered.

■ *Rate:* Administer each 60 mg over at least 1 min. Titrate slowly for desired response. Rapid administration may result in respiratory depression.

■ **Y-Site Compatibility:** ◆ enalaprilat ◆ gatifloxacin ◆ levofloxacin ◆ linezolid ◆ meropenem ◆ propofol ◆ sufentanil.

■ **Y-Site Incompatibility:** ◆ hydromorphone.

## PATIENT/FAMILY TEACHING

❏ Advise patient to take medication exactly as directed. If a dose is missed, take as soon as remembered if not almost time for next dose; do not double doses.

❏ Advise patients on prolonged therapy not to discontinue medication without consulting health care professional. Abrupt withdrawal may precipitate seizures or status epilepticus.

❏ Medication may cause daytime drowsiness. Caution patient to avoid driving and other activities requiring alertness until response to medication is known. Do not resume driving until physician gives clearance based on control of seizure disorder.

❏ Caution patient to avoid taking alcohol or other CNS depressants concurrently with this medication.

❏ Advise female patients using oral contraceptives to use an additional nonhormonal contraceptive during therapy and until next menstrual period. Instruct patient to contact health care professional immediately if pregnancy is planned or suspected.

❏ Advise patient to notify health care professional if fever, sore throat, mouth sores, unusual bleeding or bruising, nosebleeds, or petechiae occur.

## EVALUATION

**Effectiveness of therapy can be demonstrated by:** ■ Decrease or cessation of seizure activity without excessive sedation. Several weeks may be required to achieve maximum anticonvulsant effects ■ Preoperative sedation ■

Improvement in sleep patterns ∎ Decrease in serum bilirubin levels.

## phentolamine
(fen-**tole**-a-meen)
Regitine, {Rogitine}

### CLASSIFICATION(S):
***Therapeutic:*** *agents for pheochromocytoma*
***Pharmacologic:*** *alpha-adrenergic blockers*

### Pregnancy Category C

## INDICATIONS

∎ **IV:** Control of blood pressure during surgical removal of a pheochromocytoma ∎ **IV, Infiltration:** Prevention and treatment of dermal necrosis and sloughing following extravasation of norepinephrine, phenylephrine, or dopamine. **Unlabeled uses:** ∎ **IM, IV:** Treatment of hypertension associated with pheochromocytoma or adrenergic (sympathetic) excess, such as administration of phenylephrine, tyramine-containing foods in patients on MAO inhibitor therapy, or clonidine withdrawal.

## ACTION

∎ Produces incomplete and short-lived blockade of alpha-adrenergic receptors located primarily in smooth muscle and exocrine glands ∎ Induces hypotension by direct relaxation of vascular smooth muscle and by alpha blockade. **Therapeutic Effects:** ∎ Reduction of blood pressure in situations in which hypertension is due to adrenergic (sympathetic) excess ∎ When infiltrated locally, reverses vasoconstriction caused by norepinephrine or dopamine.

## PHARMACOKINETICS

**Absorption:** Well absorbed following IM administration.

**Distribution:** Unknown.

**Metabolism and Excretion:** 10% excreted unchanged by kidneys.

**Half-life:** Unknown.

## CONTRAINDICATIONS AND PRECAUTIONS

**Contraindicated in:** ∎ Hypersensitivity ∎ Coronary or cerebral arteriosclerosis ∎ Renal impairment.

**Use Cautiously in:** ∎ Peptic ulcer disease ∎ Geriatric patients (more susceptible to hypotensive effects; dosage reduction recommended) ∎ Pregnancy or lactation (safety not established).

## ADVERSE REACTIONS AND SIDE EFFECTS*

With parenteral use. ∎ **CNS:** CEREBROVASCULAR SPASM, dizziness, weakness ∎ **EENT:** nasal stuffiness ∎ **CV:** HYPOTENSION, MI, angina, arrhythmias, tachycardia ∎ **GI:** abdominal pain, diarrhea, nausea, vomiting, aggravation of peptic ulcer ∎ **Derm:** flushing.

## INTERACTIONS

**Drug-Drug:** ∎ Antagonizes the effects of **alpha-adrenergic stimulants** ∎ May decrease the pressor response to **ephedrine** or **phenylephrine** ∎ Severe hypotension may occur with concurrent use of **epinephrine** or **methoxamine** ∎ Use with **guanethidine** or **guanadrel** may result in exaggerated hypotension and bradycardia ∎ Decreases peripheral vasoconstriction from high doses of **dopamine**.

## ROUTE AND DOSAGE

❏ **Hypertension Associated with Pheochromocytoma—Before/During Surgery**
∎ **IV (Adults):** 5 mg given 1–2 hr preop, repeated as necessary. May be infused at a rate of 0.5–1 mg/min during surgery.
∎ **IV, IM (Children):** 1 mg or 0.1 mg/kg (3 mg/m²) given 1–2 hr preop, repeated IV as necessary during surgery.

❏ **Prevention of Dermal Necrosis During Infusion of Norepinephrine, Phenylephrine, or Dopamine**
∎ **IV (Adults):** Add 10 mg phentolamine to every 1000 ml of fluid containing norepinephrine.

❏ **Treatment of Dermal Necrosis Following Extravasation of Norepinephrine, Phenylephrine, or Dopamine**
∎ **Infiltrate (Adults):** 5–10 mg.

■ **Infiltrate (Children):** 0.1–0.2 mg/kg (up to 10 mg).

## AVAILABILITY (generic available)

■ *Powder for injection:* 5 mg/vial$^{Rx}$.

TIME/ACTION PROFILE (alpha-adrenergic blockade)

|    | ONSET     | PEAK   | DURATION   |
|----|-----------|--------|------------|
| IM | unknown   | 20 min | 30–45 min  |
| IV | immediate | 2 min  | 15–30 min  |

# NURSING IMPLICATIONS

## ASSESSMENT

❏ Monitor blood pressure, pulse, and ECG every 2 min until stable during IV administration. If hypotensive crisis occurs, epinephrine is contraindicated and may cause paradoxic further decrease in blood pressure; norepinephrine may be used.

## POTENTIAL NURSING DIAGNOSES

■ Tissue perfusion, ineffective (Indications).

■ Injury, risk for (Indications).

## IMPLEMENTATION

■ **General:** Patient should remain supine throughout parenteral administration.

■ **IV:** Reconstitute each 5 mg with 1 ml of sterile water for injection or 0.9% NaCl. Discard unused solution.

■ *Rate:* Inject each 5 mg over 1 min.

■ **Continuous Infusion:** Dilute 5–10 mg in 500 ml of D5W.

■ *Rate:* Titrate infusion rate according to patient response.

❏ May also add 10 mg to every 1000 ml of fluid containing norepinephrine for prevention of dermal necrosis and sloughing. Does not affect pressor effect of norepinephrine.

■ **Syringe Compatibility:** ◆ papaverine.

■ **Y-Site Compatibility:** ◆ amiodarone.

■ **Additive Compatibility:** ◆ dobutamine ◆ norepinephrine.

■ **Infiltration:** Dilute 5–10 mg of phentolamine in 10 ml of 0.9% NaCl. For children, use 0.1–0.2 mg/kg up to a maximum of 10 mg. Infiltrate site of extravasation promptly. Must be given within 12 hr of extravasation to be effective.

## PATIENT/FAMILY TEACHING

❏ Advise patient to change positions slowly to minimize orthostatic hypotension.

❏ Instruct patient to notify health care professional if chest pain occurs during IV infusion.

## EVALUATION

**Clinical response to therapy can be evaluated by:** ■ Decrease in blood pressure ■ Prevention of dermal necrosis and sloughing in extravasation of norepinephrine, dopamine, and phenylephrine.

# PHENYTOIN/FOSPHENYTOIN

## phenytoin

## (**fen**-i-toyn)

Dilantin, diphenylhydantoin, DPH, Phenytek

## fosphenytoin

## (foss-**fen**-i-toyn)

Cerebyx

## CLASSIFICATION(S):

***Therapeutic:*** *antiarrhythmics (class IB), anticonvulsants*

***Pharmacologic:*** *hydantoins*

**Pregnancy Category C (phenytoin), D (fosphenytoin)**

## INDICATIONS

■ **Phenytoin:** Treatment/prevention of tonic-clonic (grand mal) seizures and complex partial seizures ■ **Fosphenytoin:** ❏ Short-term (<5 day) management of seizures when oral phenytoin use is not feasible ❏ Treatment/prevention of seizures during neurosurgery. **Unlabeled uses:** ■ **Phenytoin:** As an antiarrhythmic, particularly for arrhythmias associated with cardiac glycoside toxicity ■ Management of painful syndromes, including trigeminal neuralgia.

## ACTION

■ Limit seizure propagation by altering ion transport ■ Antiarrhythmic properties as a result of improvement in AV conduction ■ May also decrease synaptic transmission ■ Fosphenytoin is rapidly converted to phenytoin, which is responsible for its pharmacologic effects. **Thera-**

**peutic Effects:** ▪ Diminished seizure activity ▪ Control of arrhythmias ▪ Decreased pain.

## PHARMACOKINETICS

**Absorption:** *Phenytoin*—Absorbed slowly from the GI tract. Bioavailability differs between extended and prompt release products. *Fosphenytoin*—Rapidly converted to phenytoin following IV administration and completely absorbed following IM administration.

**Distribution:** Distribute into CSF and other body tissues and fluids. Enter breast milk; cross the placenta, achieving similar maternal/fetal levels. Preferentially distribute into fatty tissue.

**Metabolism and Excretion:** Mostly metabolized by the liver; minimal amounts excreted in the urine.

**Half-life:** *Fosphenytoin*—15 min; *phenytoin*—22 hr (longer at higher blood levels).

## CONTRAINDICATIONS AND PRECAUTIONS

**Contraindicated in:** ▪ Hypersensitivity ▪ Hypersensitivity to propylene glycol (phenytoin injection only) ▪ Alcohol intolerance (phenytoin injection and liquid only) ▪ Sinus bradycardia, sinoatrial block, 2nd- or 3rd-degree heart block, or Stokes-Adams syndrome.

**Use Cautiously in:** ▪ Hepatic or renal disease (increased risk of adverse reactions; dosage reduction recommended for hepatic impairment) ▪ Geriatric patients or those with severe cardiac or respiratory disease (parenteral use—increased risk of serious adverse reactions, especially with IV phenytoin) ▪ Obese patients (initial dose of IV phenytoin should be based on ideal body weight + 1.33 times excess weight) ▪ Pregnancy (safety not established; may result in fetal hydantoin syndrome if used chronically or hemorrhage in the newborn if used at term) ▪ Lactation (safety not established).

## ADVERSE REACTIONS AND SIDE EFFECTS*

Most listed are for chronic use of phenytoin. ▪ **CNS:** <u>ataxia</u>, agitation, cerebral edema, coma, dizziness, drowsiness, dysarthria, dyskinesia, extrapyramidal syndrome, headache, nervousness, weakness ▪ **EENT:** <u>diplopia</u>, <u>nystagmus</u>, tinnitus ▪ **CV:** <u>hypotension</u> (increased with IV phenytoin), tachycardia, vasodilation ▪ **GI:** <u>gingival hyperplasia</u>, <u>nausea</u>, altered taste, anorexia, constipation, drug-induced hepatitis, dry mouth, vomiting, weight loss ▪ **GU:** pink, red, reddish-brown discoloration of urine ▪ **Derm:** <u>hypertrichosis</u>, <u>rashes</u>, exfoliative dermatitis, pruritus ▪ **F and E:** hypocalcemia ▪ **Hemat:** AGRANULOCYTOSIS, APLASTIC ANEMIA, leukopenia, megaloblastic anemia, thrombocytopenia ▪ **MS:** back pain, osteomalacia, pelvic pain ▪ **Misc:** allergic reactions including STEVENS-JOHNSON SYNDROME, fever, lymphadenopathy.

## INTERACTIONS

**Drug-Drug:** ▪ **Phenylbutazone, disulfiram,** acute ingestion of **alcohol, amiodarone, isoniazid, chloramphenicol, influenza vaccine, sulfonamides, fluoxetine, benzodiazepines, omeprazole, itraconazole, ketoconazole, fluconazole, miconazole, estrogens, halothane, methylphenidate, phenothiazines, salicylates, tolbutamide, trazodone, felbamate,** and **cimetidine** may increase phenytoin blood levels ▪ **Barbiturates, carbamazepine, reserpine,** chronic ingestion of **alcohol,** and may decrease phenytoin blood levels ▪ Phenytoin may alter the effects of **felbamate, corticosteroids, doxycycline, rifampin, quinidine, methadone, cyclosporine,** and **estrogens** ▪ IV phenytoin and **dopamine** may cause additive hypotension ▪ Additive CNS depression with other **CNS depressants,** including **alcohol, antihistamines, antidepressants, opioid analgesics,** and **sedative/hypnotics** ▪ **Antacids** may decrease absorption of orally administered phenytoin ▪ May decrease the effectiveness of **streptozocin** or **theophylline** ▪ Additive cardiac depression may occur with **propranolol** or **lidocaine** ▪ **Calcium** and **sucralfate** decrease phenytoin absorption ▪ Initially phenytoin will increase the effects of **warfarin** in patients stabilized on **warfarin** therapy; this is followed by a decreased response to **warfarin** (monitoring of response to **warfarin** recommended during initiation and maintenance of phenytoin with appropriate adjustments made).

**Drug-Food:** ▪ Phenytoin may decrease absorption of **folic acid** ▪ Concurrent administration of **enteral tube feedings** may decrease phenytoin absorption.

## ROUTE AND DOSAGE

### ▫ Fosphenytoin

All doses are expressed as phenytoin sodium equivalents (PE).

▪ **IV (Adults and Children):** *Status epilepticus*—5–20 mg PE/kg.

▪ **IV, IM (Adults and Children):** *Nonemergent and maintenance dosing*—10–20 mg PE/kg (loading dose); 4–6 mg PE/kg/day (maintenance dose).

### ▫ Phenytoin (Used as an anticonvulsant)

IM administration should be a last resort. Dosage should be increased by 50% over previously established daily oral dosage.

▪ **PO (Adults):** Loading dose 1 g or 20 mg/kg as extended capsules in 3–4 divided doses at 2-hr intervals or as 400 mg, then 300 mg q 2 hr for 2 doses; maintenance dose 300–400 mg/day. May be given once daily as extended capsules (Dilantin Kapseals) or in 3 divided doses; usual maximum dose 600 mg/day.

▪ **PO (Geriatric Patients):** 3 mg/kg/day in divided doses.

▪ **PO (Children):** Initially 5 mg/kg/day; maintenance dose 4–8 mg/kg/day (250 mg/m²) in 2–3 divided doses (not to exceed 300 mg/day).

▪ **IV (Adults):** 15–20 mg/kg. Rate not to exceed 25–50 mg/min, followed by 100 mg q 6–8 hr.

▪ **IV (Children):** 15–20 mg/kg (250 mg/m²) at 1–3 mg/kg/min.

### ▫ Phenytoin (Used as an antiarrhythmic)

▪ **IV (Adults):** 50–100 mg q 10–15 min until arrhythmia is abolished, 15 mg/kg have been given, or toxicity occurs.

### ▫ Phenytoin (Used as an antineuralgic)

▪ **PO (Adults):** 200–600 mg/day in divided doses.

## AVAILABILITY

### ▫ Fosphenytoin

▪ *Injection:* 150 mg (100 mg phenytoin equivalent) in 2-ml vials^Rx, 750 mg (500 mg phenytoin equivalent) in 10-ml vials^Rx.

### ▫ Phenytoin

▪ *Chewable tablets:* 50 mg^Rx ▪ *Oral suspension:* 30 mg/5 ml^Rx, 125 mg/5 ml^Rx ▪ *Prompt-release capsules:* 30 mg^Rx, 100 mg^Rx ▪ *Extended capsules:* 30 mg^Rx, 100 mg^Rx ▪ Cost: 30 mg $24.41/100; 100 mg $28.30/100 ▪ *Injection:* 50 mg/ml in 2- and 5-ml ampules^Rx, 2- and 5-ml vials^Rx, and 2-ml prefilled syringes^Rx. ▪ phenobarbital^Rx. See Appendix B.

TIME/ACTION PROFILE (anticonvulsant effect)

| | ONSET† | PEAK | DURATION |
|---|---|---|---|
| Fosphenytoin IM | unknown | 30 min | up to 24 hr |
| Fosphenytoin IV | 15–45 min | 15–60 min | up to 24 hr |
| Phenytoin PO | 2–24 hr (1 wk) | 1.5–3 hr | 6–12 hr |
| Phenytoin PO-ER | 2–24 hr (1 wk) | 4–12 hr | 12–36 hr |
| Phenytoin IV | 1–2 hr (1 wk) | rapid | 12–24 hr |
| Phenytoin IM | unknown (erratic) | erratic | 12–24 hr |

†() = time required for onset of action without a loading dose.

## NURSING IMPLICATIONS

### ASSESSMENT

▪ **Seizures:** Assess location, duration, frequency, and characteristics of seizure activity. EEG may be monitored periodically throughout therapy.

▪ **Arrhythmias:** Monitor ECG continuously during treatment of arrhythmias.

▪ **Neuralgia:** Assess pain (location, duration, intensity, precipitating factors) prior to and periodically throughout therapy.

▪ **Phenytoin:** Assess oral hygiene. Vigorous oral cleaning beginning within 10 days of initiation of phenytoin therapy may help control gingival hyperplasia.

▫ Assess patient for phenytoin hypersensitivity syndrome (fever, skin rash, lymphadenopathy). Rash usually occurs within the first 2 wk of therapy. Hypersensitivity syndrome usually occurs at 3–8 wk but may occur up to 12 wk after initiation of therapy. May lead to renal failure, rhabdomyolysis, or hepatic necrosis; may be fatal.

- **Fosphenytoin:** Monitor blood pressure, ECG, and respiratory function continuously during administration of fosphenytoin and throughout period when peak serum plasma occurs (10–20 min following infusion).
- Observe patient for development of rash. Fosphenytoin should be discontinued at the first sign of skin reactions. Serious adverse reactions such as exfoliative, purpuric, or bullous rashes or the development of lupus erythematosus, Stevens-Johnson syndrome, or toxic epidermal necrolysis preclude further use of phenytoin or fosphenytoin. If less serious skin eruptions (measles-like or scarlatiniform) occur, fosphenytoin may be resumed after complete clearing of the rash. If rash reappears, further use of fosphenytoin or phenytoin should be avoided.
- **Lab Test Considerations:** *Phenytoin:* CBC and platelet count, serum calcium, albumin, urinalysis, and hepatic and thyroid function tests should be monitored prior to and monthly for the first several months, then periodically throughout therapy.
- May cause increased serum alkaline phosphatase, GTT, and glucose levels.
- Serum folate concentrations should be monitored periodically during prolonged therapy.
- **Toxicity and Overdose:** *Phenytoin:* Serum phenytoin levels should be routinely monitored. Therapeutic blood levels are 10–20 mcg/ml in patients with normal serum albumin and renal function. In patients with altered protein binding (neonates, patients with renal failure, hypoalbuminemia, acute trauma), free phenytoin serum concentrations should be monitored. Therapeutic serum free phenytoin levels are 0.8–2 mcg/ml.
- Progressive signs and symptoms of phenytoin toxicity include nystagmus, ataxia, confusion, nausea, slurred speech, and dizziness.

## POTENTIAL NURSING DIAGNOSES

- Injury, risk for (Indications).
- Oral mucous membrane, impaired (Side Effects).

## IMPLEMENTATION

- **General:** Do not confuse fosphenytoin (Cerebyx) with celecoxib (Celebrex) or with citalopram (Celexa).

- Implement seizure precautions.
- When transferring from phenytoin to another anticonvulsant, dosage adjustments are made gradually over several weeks
- When substituting *fosphenytoin* for oral *phenytoin* therapy, the same total daily dose may be given as a single dose. Unlike parenteral phenytoin, fosphenytoin may be given safely by the IM route.
- The anticonvulsant effect of fosphenytoin is not immediate. Additional measures (including parenteral benzodiazepines) are usually required in the immediate management of status epilepticus. Loading dosage of *fosphenytoin* should be followed with the institution of maintenance anticonvulsant therapy.
- **PO:** Administer with or immediately after meals to minimize GI irritation. Shake liquid preparations well before pouring. Use a calibrated measuring device for accurate dosage. Chewable tablets must be crushed or chewed well before swallowing. Capsules may be opened and mixed with food or fluids for patients with difficulty swallowing. To prevent direct contact of alkaline drug with mucosa, have patient swallow some liquid first, follow with mixture of medication, then follow with a full glass of water or milk or with food.
- If patient is receiving enteral tube feedings, 2 hr should elapse between feeding and phenytoin administration. If phenytoin is administered via nasogastric tube, flush tube with 2–4 oz water before and after administration.
- Do not interchange chewable phenytoin tablets with phenytoin sodium capsules, because they are not bioequivalent.
- Capsules labeled "extended" may be used for once-a-day dosage (Dilantin Kapseals only); those labeled "prompt" may result in toxic serum levels if used for once-a-day dosage.

- **Phenytoin**
  - **IV:** Slight yellow color will not alter solution potency. If refrigerated, may form precipitate, which dissolves after warming to room temperature. Discard solution that is not clear.
  - To prevent precipitation and minimize local venous irritation, follow infusion with 0.9%

{ } = Available in Canada only.
*CAPITALS indicates life-threatening; underlines indicate most frequent.

NaCl. Avoid extravasation; phenytoin is caustic to tissues.

- **Direct IV:** Administer at a rate not to exceed 50 mg over 1 min (25 mg/min [may be as low as 5–10 mg/min] in patients who may develop hypotension, patients who are on sympathomimetic medication, patients with cardiovascular disease, or geriatric patients; 1–3 mg/kg/min in neonates). Rapid administration may result in severe hypotension, cardiovascular collapse, or CNS depression.
- **Intermittent Infusion:** Administer by mixing with no more than 50 ml of 0.9% NaCl in a concentration of 1–10 mg/ml. Administer immediately following admixture. Use tubing with a 0.45- to 0.22-micron in-line filter.
- ***Rate:*** Complete infusion within 1 hr at a rate not to exceed 50 mg/min. Monitor cardiac function and blood pressure throughout infusion.
- **Y-Site Compatibility:** ◆ esmolol ◆ famotidine ◆ fluconazole ◆ foscarnet ◆ tacrolimus.
- **Y-Site Incompatibility:** ◆ ciprofloxacin ◆ diltiazem ◆ enalaprilat ◆ gatifloxacin ◆ hydromorphone ◆ linezolid ◆ potassium chloride ◆ sufentanil ◆ vitamin B complex with C.
- **Additive Incompatibility:** Do not admix with other solutions or medications, especially dextrose, because precipitation will occur.

### ◘ Fosphenytoin

- **Direct IV:** Dilute fosphenytoin in D5W or 0.9% NaCl for a concentration of 1.5–25 mg PE/kg. May be refrigerated for up to 48 hours.
- ***Rate:*** Administer at a rate of <150 mg PE/min to minimize risk of hypotension.
- **Y-Site Compatibility:** ◆ lorazepam
- **Y-Site Incompatibility:** ◆ midazolam
- **Additive Incompatibility:** Information unavailable. Do not admix with other solutions or medications.

### PATIENT/FAMILY TEACHING

- **General Info:** May cause drowsiness or dizziness. Caution patient to avoid driving or other activities requiring alertness until response to medication is known. Do not resume driving until physician gives clearance based on control of seizure disorder.
- ◘ Advise patient to carry identification at all times describing disease process and medication regimen.
- ◘ Advise patient to notify health care professional if skin rash, severe nausea or vomiting, drowsiness, slurred speech, unsteady gait, swollen glands, bleeding or tender gums, yellow skin or eyes, joint pain, fever, sore throat, unusual bleeding or bruising, or persistent headache occurs.
- ◘ Emphasize the importance of routine exams to monitor progress. Patient should have routine physical exams, especially monitoring skin and lymph nodes, and EEG testing.
- **Phenytoin:** Instruct patient to take medication exactly as directed, at the same time each day. If a dose is missed from a once-a-day schedule, take as soon as possible and return to regular dosing schedule. If taking several doses a day, take missed dose as soon as possible within 4 hr of next scheduled dose; do not double doses. Consult health care professional if doses are missed for 2 consecutive days. Abrupt withdrawal may lead to status epilepticus.
- ◘ Caution patient to avoid taking alcohol or OTC medications concurrently with phenytoin without consulting health care professional.
- ◘ Instruct patient on importance of maintaining good dental hygiene and seeing dentist frequently for teeth cleaning to prevent tenderness, bleeding, and gingival hyperplasia. Institution of oral hygiene program within 10 days of initiation of phenytoin therapy may minimize growth rate and severity of gingival enlargement. Patients under 23 yr of age and those taking doses >500 mg/day are at increased risk for gingival hyperplasia.
- ◘ Advise patient that brands of phenytoin may not be equivalent. Check with health care professional if brand or dosage form is changed.
- ◘ Inform patient that phenytoin may color urine pink, red, or reddish brown, but color change is not significant.
- ◘ Advise diabetic patients to monitor blood glucose carefully and to notify health care professional of significant changes.
- ◘ Instruct patient to notify health care professional of medication regimen prior to treatment or surgery.
- ◘ Advise patient not to take phenytoin within 2–3 hr of antacids or antidiarrheals.
- ◘ Advise female patients to use an additional nonhormonal method of contraception dur-

ing therapy and until next menstrual period. Instruct patient to notify health care professional if pregnancy is planned or suspected.

## EVALUATION

**Effectiveness of therapy can be demonstrated by:** ■ Decrease or cessation of seizures without excessive sedation ■ Suppression of arrhythmias ■ Relief of pain due to neuralgia.

---

## phosphate/biphosphate

(**foss**-fate/bye-**foss**-fate)

Fleet Enema, Fleet Phospho-Soda, Visicol

### CLASSIFICATION(S):
**Therapeutic:** laxatives (saline)

**Pregnancy Category C (Visicol)**

---

## INDICATIONS

■ Preparation of the bowel prior to surgery or radiologic studies ■ Intermittent treatment of chronic constipation ■ **Visicol:** Cleansing of the bowel as a preparation for colonoscopy in adults 18 years of age or older.

## ACTION

■ Osmotically active in the lumen of the GI tract ■ Produces laxative effect by causing water retention and stimulation of peristalsis ■ Stimulates motility and inhibits fluid and electrolyte absorption from the small intestine. **Therapeutic Effects:** ■ Relief of constipation ■ Emptying of the bowel.

## PHARMACOKINETICS

**Absorption:** 1–20% of rectally administered sodium and phosphate may be absorbed; some absorption follows oral administration.
**Distribution:** Unknown.
**Metabolism and Excretion:** Excreted by the kidneys.
**Half-life:** Unknown.

## CONTRAINDICATIONS AND PRECAUTIONS

**Contraindicated in:** ■ Hypersensitivity ■ Abdominal pain, nausea, or vomiting, especially when associated with fever or other signs of an acute abdomen ■ Severe renal or cardiovascular disease ■ Intestinal obstruction ■ Pregnancy (at term) ■ *Visicol*—CHF, ascites, unstable angina, acute colitis, toxic megacolon, or hypomotility syndrome.

**Use Cautiously in:** ■ Excessive or chronic use (may lead to dependence) ■ Renal or cardiovascular disease, dehydration, or concurrent use of diuretics or other drugs known to alter electrolytes (correct abnormalities prior to administration) ■ Pregnancy (may cause sodium retention and edema) ■ *Visicol tablets*—use cautiously within 3 mos of MI, cardiac surgery, in patients with acute exacerbations of inflammatory bowel disease.

## ADVERSE REACTIONS AND SIDE EFFECTS*

■ **CNS:** *Visicol*—dizziness, headache ■ **CV:** ARRHYTHMIAS ■ **GI:** cramping, nausea, colonic aphtous ulcerations; *Visicol*—abdominal bloating, abdominal pain, vomiting ■ **F and E:** hyperphosphatemia, hypocalcemia, hypokalmemia, sodium retention.

## INTERACTIONS

**Drug-Drug:** ■ *Visicol*—Concurrently administered oral medications may not be absorbed due to rapid peristalsis and diarrhea

## ROUTE AND DOSAGE

Each Fleet Enema contains 4.4 g sodium/118 ml. Each 20 ml of Fleet Phospho-Soda oral solution contains 96.4 mEq sodium.

■ **PO (Adults):** 20–30 ml Phospho-Soda; *Visicol*—evening before colonoscopy: 3 tablets every 15 min (with at least 8 oz of water), last dose will be 2 tablets (total of 20 tablets), on morning of colonoscopy starting 3–5 hr before procedure, 3 tablets every 15 min (with at least 8 oz of clear liquids), last dose will be 2 tablets (total of 20 tablets); should not be repeated in less than 7 days.

■ **PO (Children):** 5–15 ml Phospho-Soda.

■ **Rect (Adults and Children >12 yr):** 118 ml Fleet Enema.

■ **Rect (Children >2 yr):** $^{1}/_{2}$ of the adult dose.

## AVAILABILITY (generic available)

■ *Oral solution:* 18 g sodium phosphate and 48 g sodium biphosphate/100 ml in 45-, 90-, and 237-ml containers^OTC ■ *Enema:* 7 g sodium phosphate and 19 g sodium biphosphate/118 ml in 67.5- and 133-ml containers^OTC ■ *Tablets (Visicol):* 2 g (40 tablets/bottle)^Rx.

TIME/ACTION PROFILE (laxative effect)

|  | ONSET | PEAK | DURATION |
|---|---|---|---|
| PO | 0.5–3 hr | unknown | unknown |
| Rect | 2–5 min | unknown | unknown |

## NURSING IMPLICATIONS

### ASSESSMENT

❑ Assess patient for fever, abdominal distention, presence of bowel sounds, and usual pattern of bowel function.
❑ Assess color, consistency, and amount of stool produced.
❑ May rarely cause arrhythmias. Monitor patients with underlying cardiovascular disease, renal disease, bowel perforation, misuse, or overdose.
■ *Lab Test Considerations:* May cause increased serum sodium and phosphorus levels, decreased serum calcium and potassium levels, and acidosis. Electrolyte changes are transient, self-limiting, do not require treatment, and are not usually associated with adverse clinical events.

### POTENTIAL NURSING DIAGNOSES

■ Constipation (Indications).

### IMPLEMENTATION

■ **General:** Do not administer at bedtime or late in the day.
■ **PO:** Administer on an empty stomach for more rapid results. Mix dose in at least ½ glass cold water. May be followed by carbonated beverage or fruit juice to improve flavor.
❑ See Route and Dose section for dosing of Visicol. Undigested Visicol tablets may appear in the stool or be visualized during colonoscopy.
■ **Rect:** Position patient on left side with knee slightly flexed. Insert prelubricated tip about 2 in. into rectum, aiming toward the umbilicus. Gently squeeze bottle until empty. Discontinue if resistance is met, because perfo-

ration may occur if contents are forced into rectum.

### PATIENT/FAMILY TEACHING

❑ Advise patient that laxatives should be used only for short-term therapy. Long-term therapy may cause electrolyte imbalance and dependence.
❑ Caution patient on sodium restriction that this product has a high sodium content.
❑ Advise patient not to take oral form of this medication within 2 hr of other medications.
❑ Encourage patient to use other forms of bowel regulation, such as increasing bulk in the diet, fluid intake, and mobility. Normal bowel habits may vary from 3 times/day to 3 times/wk.
❑ Advise patient to notify health care professional if unrelieved constipation, rectal bleeding, or symptoms of electrolyte imbalance (muscle cramps or pain, weakness, dizziness, and so forth) occur.

### EVALUATION

**Effectiveness of therapy can be demonstrated by:** ■ Soft, formed bowel movement ■ Evacuation of the bowel.

## phytonadione

(fye-toe-na-**dye**-one)
AquaMEPHYTON, Mephyton, vitamin K

### CLASSIFICATION(S):
**Therapeutic:** *antidotes, vitamins*
**Pharmacologic:** *fat-soluble vitamins*

### Pregnancy Category UK

### INDICATIONS

■ Prevention and treatment of hypoprothrombinemia, which may be associated with: ❑ Excessive doses of oral anticoagulants ❑ Salicylates ❑ Certain anti-infective agents ❑ Nutritional deficiencies ❑ Prolonged total parenteral nutrition ■ Prevention of hemorrhagic disease of the newborn.

### ACTION

■ Required for hepatic synthesis of blood coagulation factors II (prothrombin), VII, IX, and

X. **Therapeutic Effects:** ■ Prevention of bleeding due to hypoprothrombinemia.

## PHARMACOKINETICS

**Absorption:** Well absorbed following oral, IM, or subcut administration. Oral absorption requires presence of bile salts. Some vitamin K is produced by bacteria in the GI tract.
**Distribution:** Crosses the placenta; does not enter breast milk.
**Metabolism and Excretion:** Rapidly metabolized by the liver.
**Half-life:** Unknown.

## CONTRAINDICATIONS AND PRECAUTIONS

**Contraindicated in:** ■ Hypersensitivity ■ Hypersensitivity or intolerance to benzyl alcohol (injection only).
**Use Cautiously in:** ■ Impaired liver function.
**Exercise Extreme Caution in:** ■ Severe life-threatening reactions have occured following IV administration; use other routes unless risk is justified.

## ADVERSE REACTIONS AND SIDE EFFECTS*

■ **GI:** gastric upset, unusual taste ■ **Derm:** flushing, rash, urticaria ■ **Hemat:** hemolytic anemia ■ **Local:** erythema, pain at injection site, swelling ■ **Misc:** allergic reactions, hyperbilirubinemia (large doses in very premature infants), kernicterus.

## INTERACTIONS

**Drug-Drug:** ■ Large doses will counteract the effect of **warfarin** ■ Large doses of **salicylates** or broad-spectrum **anti-infectives** may increase vitamin K requirements ■ **Bile acid sequestrants, mineral oil,** and **sucralfate** may decrease vitamin K absorption from the GI tract.

## ROUTE AND DOSAGE

IV use of phytonadione should be reserved for emergencies.

❏ **Treatment of Hypoprothrombinemia**

■ **PO, Subcut, IM, IV (Adults):** 2.5–10 mg; repeat PO in 12–48 hr if necessary or in 6–8 hr after parenteral dose (up to 25–50 mg;

smaller doses have been used to partially reverse the effects of warfarin).

■ **PO, Subcut, IM, IV (Children):** 5–10 mg.
■ **PO, IM, Subcut, IV (Infants):** 1–2 mg.

❏ **Prevention of Hypoprothrombinemia during Total Parenteral Nutrition**

■ **IM, IV (Adults):** 5–10 mg once weekly.
■ **IM, IV (Children):** 2–5 mg once weekly.

❏ **Prevention of Hemorrhagic Disease of Newborn**

■ **IM (Neonates):** 0.5–1 mg, within 1 hr of birth. May be repeated in 2–3 wk if mother received previous anticonvulsant/anticoagulant/anti-infective/antitubercular therapy. 1–5 mg may be given IM to mother 12–24 hr before delivery.

❏ **Treatment of Hemorrhagic Disease of Newborn**

■ **IM, Subcut (Neonates):** 1 mg.

## AVAILABILITY

■ *Tablets:* 5 mg$^{Rx}$ ■ *Injection (aqueous colloid solution):* 2 mg/ml in 0.5-ml ampules$^{Rx}$ ■ *Injection (aqueous dispersion):* 10 mg/ml in 1-ml ampules and 2.5- and 5-ml vials$^{Rx}$.

TIME/ACTION PROFILE

| | ONSET | PEAK† | DURATION‡ |
|---|---|---|---|
| PO | 6–12 hr | unknown | unknown |
| IM, subcut | 1–2 hr | 3–6 hr | 12–14 hr |
| IV | 1–2 hr | 3–6 hr | 12 hr |

†Control of hemorrhage.
‡Normal PT achieved.

# NURSING IMPLICATIONS

## ASSESSMENT

❏ Monitor for frank and occult bleeding (guaiac stools, Hematest urine, and emesis). Monitor pulse and blood pressure frequently; notify physician immediately if symptoms of internal bleeding or hypovolemic shock develop. Inform all personnel of patient's bleeding tendency to prevent further trauma. Apply pressure to all venipuncture sites for at least 5 min; avoid unnecessary IM injections.

■ *Lab Test Considerations:* Prothrombin time (PT) should be monitored prior to and throughout vitamin K therapy to determine response to and need for further therapy.

## POTENTIAL NURSING DIAGNOSES

■ Nutrition, imbalanced: less than body requirements (Indications).
■ Tissue perfusion, ineffective (Indications).

## IMPLEMENTATION

■ **General:** The parenteral route is preferred for phytonadione therapy but, because of severe, potentially fatal hypersensitivity reactions, IV vitamin K is not recommended.
❑ Administration of whole blood or plasma may also be required in severe bleeding because of the delayed onset of this medication.
❑ Phytonadione is an antidote for warfarin overdose but does not counteract the anticoagulant activity of heparin.
■ **Direct IV:** May be administered undiluted.
■ *Rate:* If IV administration is unavoidable, administer very slowly, at a rate not to exceed 1 mg/min.
■ **Intermittent Infusion:** May also be diluted in 0.9% NaCl, D5W, or D5/0.9% NaCl.
■ *Rate:* If IV administration is unavoidable, administer very slowly, at a rate not to exceed 1 mg/min.
■ **Y-Site Compatibility:** ◆ ampicillin ◆ epinephrine ◆ famotidine ◆ heparin ◆ hydrocortisone sodium succinate ◆ potassium chloride ◆ tolazoline ◆ vitamin B complex with C.
■ **Y-Site Incompatibility:** ◆ dobutamine.

## PATIENT/FAMILY TEACHING

❑ Instruct patient to take this medication as ordered. If a dose is missed, take as soon as remembered unless almost time for next dose. Notify health care professional of missed doses.
❑ Cooking does not destroy substantial amounts of vitamin K. Patient should not drastically alter diet while taking vitamin K. See Appendix Q for foods high in vitamin K.
❑ Caution patient to avoid IM injections and activities leading to injury. Use a soft toothbrush, do not floss, and shave with an electric razor until coagulation defect is corrected.
❑ Advise patient to report any symptoms of unusual bleeding or bruising (bleeding gums; nosebleed; black, tarry stools; hematuria; excessive menstrual flow).
❑ Patients receiving vitamin K therapy should be cautioned not to take OTC medications without advice of health care professional.
❑ Advise patient to inform health care professional of medication regimen prior to treatment or surgery.
❑ Advise patient to carry identification at all times describing disease process.
❑ Emphasize the importance of frequent lab tests to monitor coagulation factors.

## EVALUATION

**Effectiveness of therapy can be demonstrated by:** ■ Prevention of spontaneous bleeding or cessation of bleeding in patients with hypoprothrombinemia secondary to impaired intestinal absorption or oral anticoagulant, salicylate, or anti-infective therapy ■ Prevention of hemorrhagic disease in the newborn.

## pilocarpine (oral)†
(pye-loe-**kar**-peen)
Salagen

*CLASSIFICATION(S):*
*Therapeutic: none assigned*
*Pharmacologic: cholinergics*

**Pregnancy Category C**

†For ophthalmic use of pilocarpine, see Appendix C.

## INDICATIONS

■ Management of xerostomia, which may occur as a consequence of radiation therapy for cancer of the head and neck ■ Treatment of dry mouth in patients with Sjögren's syndrome.

## ACTION

■ Stimulates cholinergic receptors, resulting in primarily muscarinic action, including stimulation of exocrine glands ■ Other effects include: ■ Increased sweating, gastric secretions ■ Increased bronchial secretions ■ Increased tone and motility of the urinary tract, gallbladder, and biliary duct smooth muscle. **Therapeutic Effects:** ■ Increased salivary gland secretion.

## PHARMACOKINETICS

**Absorption:** Well absorbed after oral administration.

**Distribution:** Unknown.

**Metabolism and Excretion:** Inactivated at neuronal synapses and in plasma. Some unchanged pilocarpine and metabolites are excreted in urine.

**Half-life:** *After 5-mg dose for 2 days*—0.8 hr; *after 10-mg dose for 2 days*—1.3 hr.

## CONTRAINDICATIONS AND PRECAUTIONS

**Contraindicated in:** ■ Hypersensitivity ■ Uncontrolled asthma ■ Angle-closure glaucoma ■ Iritis.

**Use Cautiously in:** ■ History of pulmonary disease (asthma, bronchitis, or chronic obstructive pulmonary disease) ■ Biliary tract disease or cholelithiasis ■ Cardiovascular disease ■ Retinal disease ■ Nephrolithiasis ■ History of psychiatric or cognitive disorders ■ Pregnancy, lactation, or children (safety not established).

## ADVERSE REACTIONS AND SIDE EFFECTS*

■ **CNS:** dizziness, headache, weakness ■ **EENT:** amblyopia, epistaxis, rhinitis ■ **CV:** edema, hypertension, tachycardia ■ **GI:** <u>nausea</u>, <u>vomiting</u>, dyspepsia, dysphagia ■ **GU:** urinary frequency ■ **Derm:** <u>flushing</u>, <u>sweating</u> ■ **Neuro:** tremors ■ **Misc:** chills, voice change.

## INTERACTIONS

**Drug-Drug:** ■ Concurrent use of **anticholinergics** will decrease the effectiveness of pilocarpine ■ Concurrent use of **bethanechol** or **ophthalmic cholinergics** may result in additive cholinergic effects ■ Concurrent use with **beta blockers** may increase the risk of adverse cardiovascular reactions (conduction disturbances).

**Drug-Natural Products:** ■ **Angel's trumpet, jimson weed,** and **scopolia** may antagonize cholinergic effects.

## ROUTE AND DOSAGE

❏ **Head and Neck Cancer Patients**

■ **PO (Adults):** 5 mg 3 times daily; may be increased to 10 mg 3 times daily.

❏ **Patients with Sjögren's Syndrome**

■ **PO (Adults):** 5 mg 4 times daily.

## AVAILABILITY

■ *Tablets:* 5 mg^Rx ■ Cost: $127.60/100.

TIME/ACTION PROFILE

| | ONSET | PEAK | DURATION |
|---|---|---|---|
| PO | 20 min | 1 hr | 3–5 hr |

## NURSING IMPLICATIONS

### ASSESSMENT

❏ Assess oral mucosa for dryness and ulceration periodically throughout therapy.

### POTENTIAL NURSING DIAGNOSES

■ Oral mucous membrane, impaired (Indications).

### IMPLEMENTATION

■ **PO:** Use lowest dose that is tolerated and effective for maintenance.

### PATIENT/FAMILY TEACHING

❏ Instruct patient to take medication exactly as directed.

❏ Caution patient that pilocarpine may cause visual changes, especially at night; avoid driving or other activities requiring alertness until effects of medication are known.

❏ Advise patient to drink adequate daily fluids (1500–2000 ml/day), especially if sweating occurs. Less than adequate fluid intake may lead to dehydration.

### EVALUATION

**Effectiveness of therapy can be demonstrated by:** ■ Increased salivary gland secretion in patients with xerostomia ■ Decrease in dry mouth in patients with Sjögren's syndrome. Full effects in cancer patients may not be seen for up to 12 weeks or 6 weeks in patients with Sjögren's syndrome.

## pindolol
(**pin**-doe-lole)

{Novo-Pindol}, {Syn-Pindolol}, Visken

**CLASSIFICATION(S):**
**Therapeutic:** antihypertensives
**Pharmacologic:** beta blockers

**Pregnancy Category B**

## INDICATIONS

■ Management of hypertension. **Unlabeled uses:** ■ Management of angina pectoris.

## ACTION

■ Blocks stimulation of beta$_1$ (myocardial) and beta$_2$ (pulmonary, vascular, and uterine) -adrenergic receptor sites ■ Has intrinsic sympathomimetic activity (ISA), which may produce less bradycardia. **Therapeutic Effects:** ■ Decreased heart rate and blood pressure.

## PHARMACOKINETICS

**Absorption:** Well absorbed following oral administration.
**Distribution:** Moderate CNS penetration. Crosses the placenta; enters breast milk.
**Metabolism and Excretion:** Partially metabolized by the liver; 50% excreted unchanged by the kidneys.
**Half-life:** 3–4 hr.

## CONTRAINDICATIONS AND PRECAUTIONS

**Contraindicated in:** ■ Uncompensated CHF ■ Pulmonary edema ■ Cardiogenic shock ■ Bradycardia or heart block.
**Use Cautiously in:** ■ Renal impairment ■ Hepatic impairment ■ Geriatric patients (increased sensitivity to beta blockers; initial dosage reduction recommended) ■ Pulmonary disease (including asthma) ■ Diabetes mellitus (may mask signs of hypoglycemia) ■ Thyrotoxicosis (may mask symptoms) ■ Patients with a history of severe allergic reactions (intensity of reactions may be increased) ■ Pregnancy, lactation, or children (safety not established; may cause fetal/neonatal bradycardia, hypotension, hypoglycemia, or respiratory depression).

## ADVERSE REACTIONS AND SIDE EFFECTS*

■ **CNS:** fatigue, weakness, anxiety, depression, dizziness, drowsiness, insomnia, memory loss, mental status changes, nervousness, nightmares ■ **EENT:** blurred vision, dry eyes, nasal stuffiness ■ **Resp:** bronchospasm, wheezing ■ **CV:** ARRHYTHMIAS, BRADYCARDIA, CHF, PULMONARY EDEMA, orthostatic hypotension, peripheral vasoconstriction ■ **GI:** constipation, diarrhea, nausea ■ **GU:** impotence, decreased libido ■ **Derm:** itching, rashes ■ **Endo:** hyperglycemia, hypoglycemia ■ **MS:** arthralgia, back pain, muscle cramps ■ **Neuro:** paresthesia ■ **Misc:** drug-induced lupus syndrome.

## INTERACTIONS

**Drug-Drug:** ■ **General anesthesia, IV phenytoin,** and **verapamil** may cause additive myocardial depression ■ Additive bradycardia may occur with **digoxin** ■ Additive hypotension may occur with other **antihypertensives,** acute ingestion of **alcohol,** or **nitrates** ■ Concurrent use with **amphetamines, cocaine, ephedrine, epinephrine, norepinephrine, phenylephrine,** or **pseudoephedrine** may result in unopposed alpha-adrenergic stimulation (excessive hypertension, bradycardia) ■ Concurrent **thyroid preparations** administration may decrease effectiveness ■ May alter the effectiveness of **insulin** or **oral hypoglycemic agents** (dosage adjustments may be necessary) ■ May decrease the effectiveness of **beta-adrenergic bronchodilators** and **theophylline** ■ May decrease the beneficial beta cardiovascular effects of **dopamine** or **dobutamine** ■ Use cautiously within 14 days of **MAO inhibitors** (may result in hypertension) ■ Concurrent **NSAIDs** may decrease antihypertensive action.

## ROUTE AND DOSAGE

■ **PO (Adults):** 5 mg twice daily initially; may be increased by 10 mg/day q 2–3 wk as needed (up to 45–60 mg/day).

## AVAILABILITY (generic available)

■ **Tablets:** 5 mg$^{Rx}$, 10 mg$^{Rx}$, {15 mg$^{Rx}$} ■ Cost: *Visken*—5 mg $98.71/100, 10 mg $101.20/100; *generic*—5 mg $59.98–69.30/100, 10 mg $79.51–$93.52/100.

TIME/ACTION PROFILE (cardiovascular effects)

| | ONSET | PEAK | DURATION |
|---|---|---|---|
| PO | 7 days | 2 wk | 8–24 hr |

# NURSING IMPLICATIONS

## ASSESSMENT

- **General Info:** Monitor blood pressure and pulse frequently during dosage adjustment period and periodically throughout therapy. Assess for orthostatic hypotension when assisting patient up from supine position.
- Monitor intake and output ratios and daily weight. Assess patient routinely for evidence of fluid overload (peripheral edema, dyspnea, rales/crackles, fatigue, weight gain, jugular venous distention).
- **Angina:** Assess frequency and characteristics of anginal attacks periodically throughout therapy.
- *Lab Test Considerations:* May cause increased BUN, serum lipoprotein, potassium, triglyceride, and uric acid levels.
- May cause increased ANA titers.
- May cause increase in blood glucose levels.

## POTENTIAL NURSING DIAGNOSES

- Cardiac output, decreased (Side Effects).
- Noncompliance (Patient/Family Teaching).

## IMPLEMENTATION

- **General:** Do not confuse pindolol and parlodel or Plendil (felodipine).
- **PO:** Take apical pulse prior to administering. If <50 bpm or if arrhythmia occurs, withhold medication and notify physician or other health care professional.
- May be administered with food or on an empty stomach.

## PATIENT/FAMILY TEACHING

- **General Info:** Instruct patient to take medication exactly as directed, at the same time each day, even if feeling well; do not skip or double up on missed doses. If a dose is missed, it should be taken as soon as possible up to 4 hr before next dose. Abrupt withdrawal may precipitate life-threatening arrhythmias, hypertension, or myocardial ischemia.
- Advise patient to make sure enough medication is available for weekends, holidays, and vacations. A written prescription may be kept in wallet in case of emergency.

- Teach patient and family how to check pulse and blood pressure. Instruct them to check pulse daily and blood pressure biweekly. Advise patient to hold dose and contact health care professional if pulse is <50 bpm or blood pressure changes significantly.
- May cause drowsiness or dizziness. Caution patients to avoid driving or other activities that require alertness until response to the drug is known.
- Advise patients to change positions slowly to minimize orthostatic hypotension, especially during initiation of therapy or when dose is increased.
- Caution patient that this medication may increase sensitivity to cold.
- Instruct patient to consult health care professional before taking any OTC medications, especially cold preparations, concurrently with this medication.
- Patients with diabetes should closely monitor blood glucose, especially if weakness, malaise, irritability, or fatigue occurs. Medication may mask tachycardia and increased blood pressure as signs of hypoglycemia, but dizziness and sweating may still occur.
- Advise patient to notify health care professional if slow pulse, difficulty breathing, wheezing, cold hands and feet, dizziness, confusion, depression, rash, fever, sore throat, unusual bleeding or bruising occurs.
- Instruct patient to inform health care professional of medication regimen prior to treatment or surgery.
- Advise patient to carry identification describing disease process and medication regimen at all times.
- **Hypertension:** Reinforce the need to continue additional therapies for hypertension (weight loss, sodium restriction, stress reduction, regular exercise, moderation of alcohol consumption, and smoking cessation). Medication controls but does not cure hypertension.
- **Angina:** Caution patient to avoid overexertion with decrease in chest pain.

## EVALUATION

**Effectiveness of therapy can be demonstrated by:** ■ Decrease in blood pressure ■

Reduction in frequency of anginal attacks ❏ Increase in activity tolerance.

## pioglitazone
(pi-o-**glit**-a-zone)
Actos

*CLASSIFICATION(S):*
*Therapeutic: antidiabetics (oral)*
*Pharmacologic: thiazolidinediones*

**Pregnancy Category C**

### INDICATIONS

■ Management of type 2 diabetes mellitus; may also be used with a sulfonylurea, metformin, or insulin when the combination of diet, exercise, and metformin does not achieve glycemic control.

### ACTION

■ Improves sensitivity to insulin by acting as an agonist at receptor sites involved in insulin responsiveness and subsequent glucose production and utilization ■ Requires insulin for activity. **Therapeutic Effects:** ■ Decreased insulin resistance, resulting in glycemic control without hypoglycemia.

### PHARMACOKINETICS

**Absorption:** Well absorbed following oral administration.
**Distribution:** Unknown.
**Protein Binding:** >99% bound to plasma proteins. Active metabolites are also highly (>99%) bound.
**Metabolism and Excretion:** Extensively metabolized by the liver; at least two metabolites have pharmacologic activity. Minimal renal excretion of unchanged drug.
**Half-life:** *Pioglitazone*—3–7 hr; *total pioglitazone (pioglitazone plus metabolites)*—16–24 hr.

### CONTRAINDICATIONS AND PRECAUTIONS

**Contraindicated in:** ■ Hypersensitivity ■ Diabetic ketoacidosis ■ Clinical evidence of active liver disease or increased ALT (>2.5 times upper limit of normal) ■ Pregnancy or lactation (not recommended for use during pregnancy or lactation; insulin should be used) ■ Children

<18 yr or type 1 diabetes (requires insulin for activity).
**Use Cautiously in:** ■ Edema ■ CHF (avoid use in moderate to severe CHF) ■ Hepatic impairment ■ Women with childbearing potential (may restore ovulation and risk of pregnancy).

### ADVERSE REACTIONS AND SIDE EFFECTS*

■ **CV:** edema ■ **Hemat:** anemia.

### INTERACTIONS

**Drug-Drug:** ■ May ↓ efficacy of **hormonal contraceptives** ■ Pioglitazone is metabolized by the CYP450 3A4 enzyme system. Concurrent use of drugs that alter the activity of this system may result in drug-drug interactions ■ **Ketoconazole** may ↑ effects of pioglitazone. Concurrent use with **insulin** may ↑ risk of CHF (consider predisposing factors).
**Drug-Natural Products:** ■ **Glucosamine** may worsen blood glucose control ■ **Chromium** and **coenzyme Q-10** may produce ↑ hypoglycemic effects.

### ROUTE AND DOSAGE

■ **PO (Adults):** 15–30 mg once daily, may be increased to 45 mg/day if needed. Doses greater than 30 mg have not been evaluated in combination with insulin and other antidiabetics.

### AVAILABILITY

■ *Tablets:* 15 mg$^{Rx}$, 30 mg$^{Rx}$, 45 mg$^{Rx}$ ■ Cost: 15 mg $92.30/30, 30 mg $142.24/30, 45 mg $160.31/30.

TIME/ACTION PROFILE (effects on blood glucose)

| | ONSET | PEAK | DURATION |
|---|---|---|---|
| PO | 30 min | 2–4 hr | 24 hr |

## NURSING IMPLICATIONS

### ASSESSMENT

❏ Observe patient taking concurrent insulin for signs and symptoms of hypoglycemic reactions (sweating, hunger, weakness, dizziness, tremor, tachycardia, anxiety).
■ *Lab Test Considerations:* Monitor serum glucose and Hb A$_{1c}$ periodically during therapy to evaluate effectiveness of treatment.

❑ Monitor CBC with differential periodically during therapy. May cause ↓ in hemoglobin and hematocrit, usually during the first 4–12 wk of therapy; then levels stabilize.

❑ Monitor serum ALT levels before starting therapy, every 2 months during the first 12 months of therapy, and periodically thereafter or if jaundice or symptoms of hepatic dysfunction occur. Pioglitazone should not be started in patients with active liver disease or ALT levels >2.5 times the upper limit of normal. Patients with mild ALT ↑ should have more frequent monitoring. If ALT ↑ to >3 times the upper limit of normal, recheck ALT promptly. Discontinue pioglitazone if ALT remains >3 times normal.

❑ May cause transient ↑ in CPK levels.

## POTENTIAL NURSING DIAGNOSES

■ Nutrition, imbalanced: more than body requirements (Indications).

■ Noncompliance (Patient/Family Teaching).

## IMPLEMENTATION

■ **General:** Patients stabilized on a diabetic regimen who are exposed to stress, fever, trauma, infection, or surgery may require administration of insulin.

■ **PO:** May be administered with or without meals.

## PATIENT/FAMILY TEACHING

❑ Instruct patient to take medication exactly as directed. If dose for 1 day is missed, do not double dose the next day.

❑ Explain to patient that this medication controls hyperglycemia but does not cure diabetes. Therapy is long-term.

❑ Review signs of hypoglycemia and hyperglycemia with patient. If hypoglycemia occurs, advise patient to take a glass of orange juice or 2–3 tsp of sugar, honey, or corn syrup dissolved in water and notify health care professional.

❑ Encourage patient to follow prescribed diet, medication, and exercise regimen to prevent hypoglycemic or hyperglycemic episodes.

❑ Instruct patient in proper testing of serum glucose and ketones. These tests should be closely monitored during periods of stress or illness, and health care professional should be notified if significant changes occur.

❑ Advise patient to notify health care professional immediately if signs of hepatic dysfunction (nausea, vomiting, abdominal pain, fatigue, anorexia, dark urine, jaundice) or CHF (edema, shortness of breath, rapid weight gain) occur.

❑ Insulin is the preferred method of controlling blood glucose during pregnancy. Counsel female patients that higher doses of oral contraceptives or a form of contraception other than oral contraceptives may be required and to notify health care professional promptly if pregnancy is planned or suspected.

❑ Advise patient to inform health care professional of medication regimen before treatment or surgery.

❑ Advise patient to carry a form of sugar (sugar packets, candy) and identification describing disease process and medication regimen at all times.

❑ Emphasize the importance of routine follow-up exams.

## EVALUATION

**Effectiveness of therapy can be demonstrated by:** ■ Control of blood glucose levels.

# piperacillin/tazobactam
(pi-**per**-a-sill-in/tay-zoe-**bak**-tam)
Zosyn

## piperacillin
(pi-**per**-a-sill-in)
Pipracil

*CLASSIFICATION(S):*
*Therapeutic: anti-infectives*
*Pharmacologic: extended spectrum penicillins*

**Pregnancy Category B**

## INDICATIONS

■ **Piperacillin:** Treatment of serious infections due to susceptible organisms, including: ❑ Skin and skin structure infections ❑ Bone and joint infections ❑ Septicemia ❑ Respiratory tract infections ❑ Intra-abdominal infections ❑ Gynecologic and urinary tract infections ■ Combination with an aminoglycoside may be synergistic against *Pseudomonas* ■ Has been combined with other antibiotics in the treatment of infections in immunosuppressed patients ■ Perioperative prophylactic anti-infective in abdominal, genitourinary, and head and neck surgery ■ **Piperacillin/Tazobactam:** ❑ Appendicitis ❑ Skin and skin structure infections ❑ Gynecologic infections ❑ Pneumonia caused by piperacillin-resistant, beta-lactamase–producing bacteria.

## ACTION

■ **Piperacillin:** Binds to bacterial cell wall membrane, causing cell death. Spectrum is extended compared with other penicillins ■ **Tazobactam:** Inhibits beta-lactamase, an enzyme that can destroy penicillins. **Therapeutic Effects:** ■ Death of susceptible bacteria. **Spectrum:** ■ **Piperacillin:** Spectrum similar to penicillin but greatly extended, including several important gram-negative aerobic pathogens, notably ❑ *Pseudomonas aeruginosa* ❑ *Escherichia coli* ❑ *Proteus mirabilis* ❑ *Providencia rettgeri* ❑ *Neisseria gonorrhoeae* ■ Also active against some anaerobic bacteria, including ❑ *Bacteroides* ■ Not active against penicillinase-producing staphylococci or beta-lactamase–producing ❑ Enterobacteriaceae ■ **Piperacillin/Tazobactam:** Active against piperacillin-resistant, beta-lactamase–producing ❑ *Bacteroides fragilis* ❑ *E. coli* ❑ *Staphylococcus aureus* ❑ *Haemophilus influenzae.*

## PHARMACOKINETICS

**Absorption:** Piperacillin is well absorbed (80%) from IM sites.
**Distribution:** Widely distributed. Enter CSF well only when meninges are inflamed. Cross the placenta and enter breast milk in low concentrations.
**Metabolism and Excretion:** Piperacillin is mostly (90%) excreted unchanged by the kidneys; 10% excreted in bile. Piperacillin/tazobactam is 80% renally excreted.
**Half-life:** 0.7–1.2 hr.

## CONTRAINDICATIONS AND PRECAUTIONS

**Contraindicated in:** ■ Hypersensitivity to penicillins or tazobactam (cross-sensitivity with cephalosporins may occur).

**Use Cautiously in:** ■ Renal impairment (dosage reduction or increased interval recommended if CCr <40 ml/min) ■ Sodium restriction ■ Pregnancy and lactation (safety not established).

## ADVERSE REACTIONS AND SIDE EFFECTS*

■ **CNS:** SEIZURES (higher doses), confusion, lethargy ■ **CV:** arrhythmias, CHF ■ **GI:** PSEUDOMEMBRANOUS COLITIS, diarrhea, drug-induced hepatitis, nausea ■ **GU:** hematuria (children only), interstitial nephritis ■ **Derm:** rashes, urticaria ■ **F and E:** hypokalemia, hypernatremia ■ **Hemat:** bleeding, blood dyscrasias, increased bleeding time ■ **Local:** pain at IM site, phlebitis at IV site ■ **Metab:** metabolic alkalosis ■ **Misc:** hypersensitivity reactions, including ANAPHYLAXIS and SERUM SICKNESS, superinfection.

## INTERACTIONS

**Drug-Drug:** ■ **Probenecid** ↓ renal excretion and ↑ blood levels ■ May alter excretion of **lithium** ■ **Potassium-losing diuretics, corticosteroids,** or **amphotericin B** may ↑ risk of hypokalemia ■ ↑ risk of hepatotoxicity with other **hepatotoxic agents** ■ May ↓ half-life of **aminoglycosides** in patients with renal impairment.

## ROUTE AND DOSAGE

Contains 1.85 mEq sodium/g of piperacillin.

❑ **Piperacillin**

■ **IM, IV (Adults):** *Most infections*—3–4 g q 4–6 hr (up to 24 g/day). *Complicated urinary tract infections*—3–4 g q 6–8 hr. *Uncomplicated urinary tract infections*—1.5–2 g q 6 hr *or* 3–4 g q 12 hr.
■ **IM, IV (Neonates ≥2 kg):** *Meningitis*—50 mg/kg q 8 hr for the first 7 days of life, then 50 mg/kg q 6 hr.
■ **IM, IV (Neonates <2 kg):** *Meningitis*—50 mg/kg q 12 hr for the first 7 days of life, then 50 mg/kg q 8 hr.

❑ **Renal Impairment**

■ **IM, IV (Adults):** *CCr 20–40 ml/min*—3–4 g q 8 hr; *CCr <20 ml/min*—3– 4 g q 12 hr.

❑ **Piperacillin/Tazobactam**

(dosage expressed as combined piperacillin tazobactam content)

■ **IV (Adults):** 3.375–4.5 g q 6 hr.
❑ **Renal Impairment**

- **IV (Adults):** *CCr 20–40 ml/min*—2.25–3.375 g q 6 hr; *CCr <20 ml/min*—2.25 g q 6–8 hr.

## AVAILABILITY

□ **Piperacillin**

■ *Powder for injection:* 2-, 3-, and 4-g vials and infusion bottles<sup>Rx</sup>, 40-g bulk vials<sup>Rx</sup>.

□ **Piperacillin/Tazobactam**

■ *Powder for injection:* 2-g piperacillin/0.25-g tazobactam vials and 50-ml premixed frozen containers<sup>Rx</sup>, 3-g piperacillin/0.375-g tazobactam vials and 50-ml premixed frozen containers<sup>Rx</sup>, 4-g piperacillin/0.5-g tazobactam vials and 50- ml premixed frozen containers<sup>Rx</sup>.

TIME/ACTION PROFILE (piperacillin blood levels)

|    | ONSET | PEAK | DURATION |
|----|-------|------|----------|
| IM | rapid | 30–50 min | 4–6 hr |
| IV | rapid | end of infusion | 4–6 hr |

# NURSING IMPLICATIONS

## ASSESSMENT

□ Assess patient for infection (vital signs; appearance of wound, sputum, urine, and stool; WBC) at beginning of and during therapy.

□ Obtain a history before initiating therapy to determine previous use of and reactions to penicillins or cephalosporins. Persons with a negative history of penicillin sensitivity may still have an allergic response.

□ Obtain specimens for culture and sensitivity prior to initiating therapy. First dose may be given before receiving results.

□ Observe patient for signs and symptoms of anaphylaxis (rash, pruritus, laryngeal edema, wheezing). Discontinue the drug and notify the physician or other health care professional immediately if these occur. Keep epinephrine, an antihistamine, and resuscitation equipment close by in the event of an anaphylactic reaction.

■ *Lab Test Considerations:* Evaluate renal and hepatic function, CBC, serum potassium,

and bleeding times prior to and routinely during therapy.

□ May cause positive direct Coombs' test result.

□ May cause ↑ BUN, creatinine, AST, ALT, serum bilirubin, alkaline phosphatase, and LDH.

□ May cause leukopenia and neutropenia, especially with prolonged therapy or hepatic impairment.

□ May cause prolonged prothrombin and partial thromboplastin time.

□ *Piperacillin* may cause elevated serum sodium and decreased serum potassium concentrations.

□ *Piperacillin/tazobactam* may also cause ↓ hemoglobin and hematocrit and thrombocytopenia, eosinophilia, leukopenia, and neutropenia. It also may cause proteinuria; hematuria; pyuria; hyperglycemia; ↓ total protein or albumin; and abnormalities in sodium, potassium, and calcium levels.

## POTENTIAL NURSING DIAGNOSES

■ Infection, risk for (Indications, Side Effects).

## IMPLEMENTATION

■ **General:** Do not confuse Zosyn (piperacillin/tazobactam) with Zofran (ondansetron).

■ **IM:** To constitute for IM use, add 4 ml of sterile water, bacteriostatic water, 0.9% NaCl for injection, or 0.5 or 1% lidocaine hydrochloride injection (without epinephrine) to each 2-g vial, 6 ml to each 3-g vial, and 8 ml to each 4-g vial for a concentration of 1 g/2.5 ml.

□ Inject deep into a well-developed muscle mass and massage well. IM injections should not exceed 2 g at each site.

□ **Piperacillin**

■ **IV:** Reconstitution for IV use with at least 5 ml of sterile water for injection, 0.9% NaCl, or bacteriostatic water. Shake well until dissolved. Reconstituted solution is stable for 24 hr at room temperature and 7 days if refrigerated.

□ Change IV sites every 48 hr to prevent phlebitis.

■ **Direct IV:** Inject slowly, over 3–5 min, to minimize vein irritation.

■ **Intermittent Infusion:** Dilute in at least 50 ml of 0.9% NaCl, D5W, D5/0.9% NaCl, or LR.

■ **Rate:** Administer over 20–30 min for adults and 30 min for children.

■ **Y-Site Compatibility:** ◆ acyclovir ◆ allopurinol ◆ amifostine ◆ aztreonam ◆ ciprofloxacin ◆ cyclophosphamide ◆ diltiazem ◆ docetaxel ◆ doxorubicin liposome ◆ enalaprilat ◆ esmolol ◆ etoposide ◆ famotidine ◆ fludarabine ◆ foscarnet ◆ granisetron ◆ heparin ◆ hydromorphone ◆ labetalol ◆ linezolid ◆ lorazepam ◆ magnesium sulfate ◆ melphalan ◆ meperidine ◆ midazolam ◆ morphine ◆ perphenazine ◆ propofol ◆ ranitidine ◆ remifentanil ◆ tacrolimus ◆ teniposide ◆ theophylline ◆ thiotepa ◆ verapamil ◆ zidovudine.

■ **Y-Site Incompatibility:** If aminoglycosides and penicillins must be administered concurrently, administer in separate sites at least 1 hr apart. ◆ amphotericin B cholesteryl sulfate ◆ filgrastim ◆ fluconazole ◆ gatifloxacin ◆ gemcitabine ◆ ondansetron ◆ sargramostim ◆ vinorelbine.

❑ **Piperacillin/Tazobactam**

■ **Intermittent Infusion:** Reconstitute with 5 ml of 0.9% NaCl, sterile or bacteriostatic water for injection, or D5W. Do not use LR—incompatible. Shake well until dissolved. Dilute further in at least 50 ml of diluent. Discard any unused solution after 24 hr at room temperature or 48 hr if refrigerated.

■ **Rate:** Administer over at least 30 min.

■ **Y-Site Compatibility:** ◆ aminophylline ◆ aztreonam ◆ bleomycin ◆ bumetanide ◆ buprenorphine ◆ butorphanol ◆ calcium gluconate ◆ carboplatin ◆ carmustine ◆ cefepime ◆ cimetidine ◆ clindamycin ◆ cyclophosphamide ◆ cytarabine ◆ diphenhydramine ◆ docetaxel ◆ dopamine ◆ enalaprilat ◆ etoposide ◆ floxuridine ◆ fluconazole ◆ fludarabine ◆ fluorouracil ◆ furosemide ◆ granisetron ◆ heparin ◆ hydrocortisone ◆ hydromorphone ◆ ifosfamide ◆ leucovorin calcium ◆ linezolid ◆ lorazepam ◆ magnesium sulfate ◆ mannitol ◆ meperidine ◆ mesna ◆ methotrexate ◆ methylprednisolone sodium succinate ◆ metoclopramide ◆ metronidazole ◆ morphine ◆ ondansetron ◆ plicamycin ◆ potassium chloride ◆ ranitidine ◆ remifentanil ◆ sargramostim ◆ sodium bicarbonate ◆ thiotepa ◆ trimethoprim/sulfamethoxazole ◆ vinblastine ◆ vincristine ◆ zidovudine.

■ **Y-Site Incompatibility:** ◆ acyclovir ◆ alatrofloxacin ◆ amphotericin B ◆ amphotericin B cholesteryl sulfate ◆ chlorpromazine ◆ cisplatin ◆ dacarbazine ◆ daunorubicin ◆ dobutamine ◆ doxorubicin ◆ doxorubicin liposome ◆ doxycycline ◆ droperidol ◆ famotidine ◆ ganciclovir ◆ gatifloxacin ◆ gemcitabine ◆ haloperidol ◆ idarubicin ◆ minocycline ◆ mitomycin ◆ mitoxantrone ◆ nalbuphine ◆ prochlorperazine edisylate ◆ promethazine ◆ streptozocin

## PATIENT/FAMILY TEACHING

❑ Advise patient to report the signs of superinfection (black, furry overgrowth on the tongue; vaginal itching or discharge; loose or foul-smelling stools) and allergy.

❑ Caution patient to notify health care professional if fever and diarrhea occur, especially if stool contains blood, pus, or mucus. Advise patient not to treat diarrhea without consulting health care professional. May occur up to several weeks after discontinuation of medication.

## EVALUATION

**Clinical response to therapy can be evaluated by:** ■ Resolution of the signs and symptoms of infection. Length of time for complete resolution depends on the organism and site of infection.

## pirbuterol
(peer-**byoo**-ter-ole)
Maxair

**CLASSIFICATION(S):**
**Therapeutic:** bronchodilators
**Pharmacologic:** adrenergics

**Pregnancy Category C**

## INDICATIONS

■ Management of reversible airway disease due to intermittent asthma or COPD quick-relief agent).

## ACTION

■ Results in the accumulation of cyclic adenosine monophosphate (cAMP) at beta-adrenergic receptors ■ Produces bronchodilation ■ Inhibits the release of mediators of immediate hypersensitivity reactions from mast cells ■ Relatively selective for beta$_2$ (pulmonary)-adrenergic receptor sites with less effect on beta$_1$ (cardiac)-adrenergic receptors. **Therapeutic Effects:** ■ Bronchodilation.

## PHARMACOKINETICS

**Absorption:** Minimal systemic absorption occurs following inhalation.

**Distribution:** Unknown.

**Metabolism and Excretion:** Metabolized by the liver.

**Half-life:** 2 hr.

## CONTRAINDICATIONS AND PRECAUTIONS

**Contraindicated in:** ■ Hypersensitivity to adrenergic amines ■ Known hypersensitivity or intolerance to fluorocarbons.

**Use Cautiously in:** ■ Cardiac disease ■ Hypertension ■ Hyperthyroidism ■ Diabetes ■ Glaucoma ■ Elderly patients (more susceptible to adverse reactions; may require dosage reduction) ■ Excessive use may lead to tolerance and paradoxical bronchospasm (inhaler) ■ Pregnancy (near term), lactation, and children <2 yr (safety not established).

## ADVERSE REACTIONS AND SIDE EFFECTS*

■ **CNS:** nervousness, restlessness, tremor, headache, insomnia ■ **Resp:** PARADOXICAL BRONCHOSPASM ■ **CV:** angina, arrhythmias, hypertension, tachycardia ■ **GI:** nausea, vomiting ■ **Endo:** hyperglycemia.

## INTERACTIONS

**Drug-Drug:** ■ Concurrent use with other **adrenergics** will have ↑ adrenergic side effects ■ Use with **MAO inhibitors** may lead to hypertensive crisis ■ **Beta blockers** may ↓ therapeutic effect.

**Drug-Natural Products:** ■ Use with caffeine-containing herbs (**cola nut, guarana, mate, tea, coffee**) ↑ stimulant effect.

## ROUTE AND DOSAGE

■ **Inhaln (Adults):** 1–2 inhalations q 4–6 hr (not to exceed 12 inhalations/day).

## AVAILABILITY

■ *Inhalation aerosol:* 200 mcg/spray (≥300 inhalations/25.6-g canister)$^{Rx}$ ■ Cost: $63.78/ 14-g canister, $50.52/25.6-g canister.

TIME/ACTION PROFILE (bronchodilation)

|  | ONSET | PEAK | DURATION |
|---|---|---|---|
| Inhaln | within 5 min | 1.5 hr | 6–8 hr |

# NURSING IMPLICATIONS

## ASSESSMENT

❏ Assess lung sounds, respiratory pattern, pulse, and blood pressure before administration and during peak of medication. Note amount, color, and character of sputum produced, and report abnormal findings.

❏ Monitor pulmonary function tests before initiating therapy and periodically during therapy to determine effectiveness.

❏ Observe for paradoxical bronchospasm (wheezing). If condition occurs, withhold medication and notify physician or other health care professional immediately.

❏ Observe patient for drug tolerance and rebound bronchospasm. Patients requiring more than 3 inhalation treatments in 24 hr should be under close supervision. If minimal or no relief is seen after 3–5 inhalation treatments within 6–12 hr, further treatment with aerosol alone is not recommended.

## POTENTIAL NURSING DIAGNOSES

■ Airway clearance, ineffective (Indications).

## IMPLEMENTATION

**Inhaln:** When pirbuterol is used concurrently with corticosteroid or ipratropium inhalations, administer bronchodilator first and other medications 5 min apart to prevent toxicity from inhaled fluorocarbon propellants.

## PATIENT/FAMILY TEACHING

❏ Instruct patient to take medication as directed. If on a scheduled dosing regimen, take a missed dose as soon as possible; space remaining doses at regular intervals. Do not double doses. Caution patient not to exceed recommended dose; may cause adverse effects, paradoxical bronchospasm, or loss of effectiveness of medication.

❑ Instruct patient to contact health care professional immediately if shortness of breath is not relieved by medication or is accompanied by diaphoresis, dizziness, palpitations, or chest pain.

❑ Advise patient to consult health care professional before taking any OTC medications, herbal products, or alcoholic beverages concurrently with this therapy. Caution patient also to avoid smoking and other respiratory irritants.

■ **Inhaln:** Review correct administration technique with patient. See Appendix F for administration with metered-dose inhaler. Wait 1–5 min before administering next dose. Mouthpiece should be washed after each use.

❑ Advise patient to use bronchodilator first if using other inhalation medications, and allow 5 min to elapse before administering other inhalant medications, unless otherwise directed.

❑ Advise patient to rinse mouth with water after each inhalation dose to minimize dry mouth.

❑ Advise patient to maintain adequate fluid intake (2000–3000 ml/day) to help liquefy tenacious secretions.

❑ Advise patient to consult health care professional if respiratory symptoms are not relieved or worsen after treatment or if chest pain, headache, severe dizziness, palpitations, nervousness, or weakness occurs.

❑ Instruct patient to notify health care professional if contents of one canister are used up in less than 2 wk.

## EVALUATION

**Effectiveness of therapy can be demonstrated by:** ■ Prevention or relief of bronchospasm ■ Increase in ease of breathing.

# piroxicam
(peer-**ox**-i-kam)
{Apo-Piroxicam}, Feldene, {Novo-Pirocam}, {Nu-Pirox}, {PMS-Piroxicam}

## CLASSIFICATION(S):
**Therapeutic:** antirheumatics, nonsteroidal anti-inflammatory agents

## Pregnancy Category C

## INDICATIONS

■ Management of inflammatory disorders, including: ❑ Rheumatoid arthritis ❑ Osteoarthritis. **Unlabeled uses:** ■ Management of dysmenorrhea.

## ACTION

■ Inhibits prostaglandin synthesis. **Therapeutic Effects:** ■ Suppression of pain and inflammation.

## PHARMACOKINETICS

**Absorption:** Well absorbed from the GI tract.

**Distribution:** Unknown. Enters breast milk in small amounts.

**Metabolism and Excretion:** Mostly metabolized by the liver. Minimal amounts excreted unchanged by the kidneys.

**Half-life:** 50 hr.

## CONTRAINDICATIONS AND PRECAUTIONS

**Contraindicated in:** ■ Hypersensitivity ■ Cross-sensitivity may exist with other NSAIDs, including aspirin ■ Active GI bleeding or ulcer disease ■ Lactation.

**Use Cautiously in:** ■ Severe cardiovascular or hepatic disease ■ History of ulcer disease ■ Renal impairment (dosage reduction recommended) ■ Pregnancy or children (safety not established; avoid use during 2nd half of pregnancy).

## ADVERSE REACTIONS AND SIDE EFFECTS*

■ **CNS:** drowsiness, headache, dizziness ■ **EENT:** blurred vision, tinnitus ■ **CV:** edema ■ **GI:** DRUG-INDUCED HEPATITIS, GI BLEEDING, discomfort, dyspepsia, nausea, vomiting, anorexia, constipation, diarrhea, flatulence ■ **GU:** renal failure ■ **Derm:** rashes ■ **Hemat:** blood dyscrasias, prolonged bleeding time ■ **Misc:** allergic reactions including ANAPHYLAXIS.

## INTERACTIONS

**Drug-Drug:** ■ Concurrent use with **aspirin** decreases piroxicam blood levels and may decrease effectiveness ■ Increased risk of bleeding with **anticoagulants, cefoperazone, cefotetan, heparin, ticlopidine, clopidogrel, eptifibatide, tirofiban, thrombolytic agents, valproic acid,** or **plicamycin** ■ Additive adverse GI side effects with **aspirin, corticosteroids,** and other **NSAIDs** ■ **Probenecid** increases blood levels and may increase toxicity ■ May decrease response to **antihypertensives** or **diuretics** ■ May increase serum levels and risk of toxicity from **lithium** ■ May increase risk of hypoglycemia from **insulin** or **oral hypoglycemic agents** ■ Increased risk of adverse renal effects with **gold compounds, cyclosporine,** or chronic use of **acetaminophen** ■ May increase the risk of hematologic toxicity from **antineoplastics** or **radiation therapy.**

**Drug-Natural Products:** ■ Increased anticoagulant effect and bleeding risk with **anise, arnica, chamomile, clove, dong quai, fenugreek, feverfew, garlic, ginger, ginkgo, Panax ginseng, licorice,** and others.

## ROUTE AND DOSAGE

- **PO (Adults):** *Anti-inflammatory*—10–20 mg/day; may be given as single dose or 2 divided doses. *Antidysmenorrheal*—40 mg initially, then 20 mg/day.
- **PO (Geriatric Patients):** 10 mg/day initially.

## AVAILABILITY (generic available)

■ *Capsules:* 10 mg^Rx, 20 mg^Rx ■ Cost: *Feldene*—10 mg $147.09/100, 20 mg $297.93/100; *generic*—$129.14/100, 20 mg $244.83/100 ■ *Suppositories:* {10 mg^Rx}, {20 mg^Rx}.

TIME/ACTION PROFILE

| | ONSET | PEAK | DURATION |
|---|---|---|---|
| PO (analgesic effect) | 1 hr | unknown | 48–72 hr |
| PO (anti-inflammatory effect) | 7–12 days | 2–3 wk† | unknown |

†May take up to 12 wk.

## NURSING IMPLICATIONS

### ASSESSMENT

- **General Info:** Patients who have asthma, aspirin-induced allergy, and nasal polyps are at increased risk for developing hypersensitivity reactions. Monitor for rhinitis, asthma, and urticaria.
- **Arthritis:** Assess pain and range of motion prior to and 1–2 hr following administration.
- *Lab Test Considerations:* Bleeding time may be prolonged for up to 2 wk following discontinuation of therapy.
  - ❑ May cause decreased hemoglobin, hematocrit, leukocyte, and platelet counts.
  - ❑ Monitor liver function tests periodically during therapy. May cause elevated serum alkaline phosphatase, LDH, AST, and ALT concentrations.
  - ❑ Monitor BUN, serum creatinine, and electrolytes periodically during therapy. May cause increased BUN, serum creatinine, and electrolyte concentrations and decreased urine electrolyte concentrations.

### POTENTIAL NURSING DIAGNOSES

- Pain, acute (Indications).
- Mobility, impaired physical (Indications).

### IMPLEMENTATION

- **General:** Administration in higher than recommended doses does not provide increased effectiveness but may cause increased side effects.
- **PO:** Administer after meals or with food or an antacid containing aluminum or magnesium to minimize gastric irritation. Administer as soon as possible after the onset of menses. Prophylactic use has not been proved effective.

### PATIENT/FAMILY TEACHING

- ❑ Advise patient to take this medication with a full glass of water and to remain in an upright position for 15–30 min after administration.
- ❑ Instruct patient to take medication exactly as directed. If a dose is missed, it should be taken as soon as remembered but not if almost time for the next dose. Do not double doses.

❑ May cause drowsiness or dizziness. Advise patient to avoid driving or other activities requiring alertness until response to the medication is known.

❑ Caution patient to avoid the concurrent use of alcohol, aspirin, acetaminophen, or other OTC medications without consulting health care professional.

❑ Advise patient to inform health care professional of medication regimen prior to treatment or surgery.

❑ Caution patient to use sunscreen and protective clothing to prevent photosensitivity reaction (rare).

❑ Advise patient to consult health care professional if rash, itching, visual disturbances, tinnitus, weight gain, edema, black stools, persistent headache, or influenza-like syndrome (chills, fever, muscle aches, pain) occurs.

### EVALUATION

**Effectiveness of therapy can be demonstrated by:** ■ Decreased pain and improved joint mobility. Partial arthritic relief is usually seen within 2 wk, but maximum effectiveness may require up to 12 wk of continuous therapy. Patients who do not respond to one NSAID may respond to another.

# plicamycin

(plye-ka-**mye**-sin)

Mithramycin, Mithracin

### CLASSIFICATION(S):

**Therapeutic:** antineoplastics, hypocalcemics
**Pharmacologic:** antitumor antibiotics

### Pregnancy Category X

## INDICATIONS

■ Treatment of advanced unresponsive testicular carcinoma ■ Management of hypercalcemia and hypercalciuria associated with malignancy.

## ACTION

■ Forms a complex with DNA that subsequently inhibits RNA synthesis ■ Antagonizes the action of vitamin D and inhibits the action of parathyroid hormone on osteoclasts. **Therapeutic Ef-**fects:** ■ Death of rapidly replicating cells, particularly malignant ones ■ Lowering of serum calcium.

## PHARMACOKINETICS

**Absorption:** Administered IV only, resulting in complete bioavailability.

**Distribution:** Appears to concentrate in the liver, renal tubule, and bone surface. Crosses the blood-brain barrier.

**Metabolism and Excretion:** Excreted primarily by the kidneys.

**Half-life:** Unknown.

## CONTRAINDICATIONS AND PRECAUTIONS

**Contraindicated in:** ■ Hypersensitivity ■ Bleeding disorders ■ Depressed bone marrow reserve ■ Hypocalcemia ■ Severe renal or liver disease ■ Pregnancy or lactation.

**Use Cautiously in:** ■ Active infections ■ Other chronic debilitating illnesses ■ Renal or hepatic impairment (dosage reduction required) ■ Patients with childbearing potential ■ Children (safety not established).

## ADVERSE REACTIONS AND SIDE EFFECTS*

■ **CNS:** dizziness, drowsiness, fatigue, headache, irritability, malaise, mental depression, nervousness, weakness ■ **EENT:** epistaxis ■ **GI:** anorexia, diarrhea, drug-induced hepatitis, nausea, stomatitis, vomiting ■ **GU:** gonadal suppression, renal failure ■ **Derm:** facial flushing, rashes ■ **F and E:** <u>hypocalcemia</u>, hypokalemia, hypophosphatemia, rebound hypercalcemia ■ **Hemat:** BLEEDING, <u>thrombocytopenia</u>, anemia, leukopenia ■ **Local:** phlebitis at IV site ■ **Misc:** fever.

## INTERACTIONS

**Drug-Drug:** ■ Additive myelosuppression with other **antineoplastics** or **radiation therapy** ■ Increased risk of bleeding with **aspirin, warfarin, thrombolytic agents, heparin** and other **heparin-like agents, some cephalosporins, NSAIDs** (including **aspirin, ticlopidine, clopidogrel, tirofiban, eptifibatide, sulfinpyrazone, valproic acid,** or **dextran**) ■ Increased risk of hepatotoxicity with other **hepatotoxic agents** ■ Increased risk of renal toxicity with other **nephrotoxic agents.**

**Drug-Natural Products:** ■ Increased anticoagulant effect and bleeding risk with **anise,**

arnica, chamomile, clove, dong quai, fenugreek, feverfew, garlic, ginger, ginkgo, Panax ginseng, licorice, and others.

## ROUTE AND DOSAGE

❏ **Testicular Tumors**

■ **IV (Adults):** 25–30 mcg/kg once daily for 8–10 days *or* 25–50 mcg/kg every other day for up to 8 doses. May be repeated monthly.

❏ **Hypercalcemia/Hypercalciuria**

■ **IV (Adults):** 15–25 mcg/kg once daily for 3–4 days; may be repeated after 7 days or 1–3 times weekly.

## AVAILABILITY

■ *Powder for injection:* 2500 mcg/vial<sup>Rx</sup>.

TIME/ACTION PROFILE

|  | ONSET | PEAK | DURATION |
|---|---|---|---|
| IV (hematologic effects) | unknown | 7–10 days | 3–4 wk |
| IV (hypocalcemic effects) | 24–48 hr | 72 hr | 7–10 days |

# NURSING IMPLICATIONS

## ASSESSMENT

■ **General Info:** Monitor closely for bleeding (bleeding gums, bruising, petechiae; guaiac-test stools, urine, and emesis). May begin as epistaxis and progress to severe generalized or GI bleeding. May require blood transfusions, fresh-frozen plasma, vitamin K, or aminocaproic acid to control bleeding. Avoid IM injections and rectal temperatures. Apply pressure to venipuncture sites for 10 min.

❏ Monitor intake and output, appetite, and nutritional intake. Dehydration or volume depletion should be corrected before initiating plicamycin therapy. May cause nausea and vomiting, which usually occur 1–2 hr after therapy is initiated, persist 12–24 hr, and should be treated with prophylactic antiemetics. Adjust diet as tolerated to help maintain fluid and electrolyte balance and nutritional status.

❏ Assess for signs of infection (fever, chills, sore throat, cough, hoarseness, pain in lower

back or side, difficult or painful urination). Notify physician if these symptoms occur.

■ **Hypercalcemia:** Monitor symptoms of hypercalcemia (nausea, vomiting, anorexia, thirst, weakness, constipation, paralytic ileus, and bradycardia). Observe patient for evidence of hypocalcemia (paresthesia, muscle twitching, laryngospasm, colic, cardiac arrhythmias, and Chvostek's or Trousseau's sign).

■ *Lab Test Considerations:* Monitor CBC with differential, platelet count, prothrombin time, and bleeding time before and periodically throughout therapy. May cause thrombocytopenia, leukemia, and anemia. Notify physician if platelet count is <150,000/mm³, prothrombin time is elevated 4 or more sec above control, or leukocyte count is <4000/mm³.

❏ Monitor serum electrolytes before and daily during course of therapy. May cause hypocalcemia, hypokalemia, and hypophosphatemia. Correct electrolyte imbalances before beginning therapy. Calcium and phosphate levels may rebound after therapy.

❏ Monitor liver function studies (AST, ALT, LDH, bilirubin) and renal function studies (BUN, creatinine, urinalysis) before and periodically throughout therapy to detect hepatotoxicity and nephrotoxicity.

## POTENTIAL NURSING DIAGNOSES

■ Injury, risk for (Side Effects).
■ Infection, risk for (Side Effects).
■ Body image, disturbed (Side Effects).

## IMPLEMENTATION

■ **General:** Solution should be prepared in a biologic cabinet. Wear gloves, gown, and mask while handling medication. Discard equipment in designated containers.

❏ Ensure patency of the IV. If patient complains of discomfort at the IV site or if extravasation occurs, discontinue IV and restart at another site. Extravasation may cause irritation and cellulitis. Apply ice to site to prevent pain and swelling. If swelling occurs, application of moderate heat to site may help disperse medication and decrease discomfort.

■ **IV:** To reconstitute, add 4.9 ml of sterile water for injection to the 2.5-mg vial of plicamycin to yield a final concentration of 500 mcg/ml. Shake vial to dissolve drug. Use immediately after reconstitution. Discard unused portions.

■ **Direct IV:** May be administered undiluted IV push to decrease risk of extravasation.

■ *Rate:* Administer over 20–30 min.

■ **Intermittent Infusion:** Add to 1000 ml of D5W or 0.9% NaCl.

■ *Rate:* Infuse over 4–6 hr. Rapid infusion rate will increase incidence and severity of GI side effects.

■ **Y-Site Compatibility:** ◆ allopurinol ◆ amifostine ◆ aztreonam ◆ filgrastim ◆ melphalan ◆ piperacillin/tazobactam ◆ teniposide ◆ thiotepa ◆ vinorelbine.

## PATIENT/FAMILY TEACHING

❑ Advise patient to notify health care professional promptly if fever; chills; sore throat; signs of infection; bleeding gums; bruising; petechiae; or blood in urine, stool, or emesis occurs. Caution patient to avoid crowds and persons with known infections. Instruct patient to use soft toothbrush and electric razor. Patients should be cautioned not to drink alcoholic beverages or take products containing aspirin or NSAIDs.

❑ Instruct patient to notify health care professional if weakness, rash, persistent nausea or vomiting, or depression occurs.

❑ Instruct patient to inspect oral mucosa for redness and ulceration. If mouth sores occur, advise patient to use sponge brush and rinse mouth with water after eating and drinking. Topical medications may be used if pain interferes with eating. Stomatitis pain may require treatment with opioid analgesics.

❑ Advise patient that, although fertility may be decreased with plicamycin, contraception should be used during therapy because of potential teratogenic effects on the fetus.

❑ Instruct patient not to receive any vaccinations without advice of health care professional.

❑ Emphasize need for periodic lab tests to monitor for side effects.

## EVALUATION

**Effectiveness of therapy can be demonstrated by:** ■ Decrease in size and spread of malignant tissue ■ Normalization of elevated cal-

cium levels in hypercalcemia and hypercalciuria within 24–48 hr.

# polyethylene glycol
### (po-lee-**eth**-e-leen **glye**-kole)
MiraLax

### CLASSIFICATION(S):
**Therapeutic:** *laxatives*
**Pharmacologic:** *osmotics*

### Pregnancy Category C

## INDICATIONS

■ Treatment of occasional constipation.

## ACTION

■ Polyethylene glycol (PEG) in solution acts as an osmotic agent, drawing water into the lumen of the GI tract. **Therapeutic Effects:** ■ Evacuation of the GI tract without water or electrolyte imbalance.

## PHARMACOKINETICS

**Absorption:** Nonabsorbable.
**Distribution:** Unknown.
**Metabolism and Excretion:** Excreted in fecal contents.
**Half-life:** Unknown.

## CONTRAINDICATIONS AND PRECAUTIONS

**Contraindicated in:** ■ GI obstruction ■ Gastric retention ■ Toxic colitis ■ Megacolon.
**Use Cautiously in:** ■ Abdominal pain of uncertain cause, particularly if accompanied by fever ■ Pregnancy or children (safety not established).

## ADVERSE REACTIONS AND SIDE EFFECTS*

■ **GI:** abdominal bloating, cramping, flatulence, nausea.

## INTERACTIONS

**Drug-Drug:** ■ None significant.

## ROUTE AND DOSAGE

■ **PO (Adults):** 17 g (heaping tablespoon) in 8 oz of water; may be used for up to 2 wk.

## AVAILABILITY

■ *Powder:* in 14- and 26-oz container[Rx].

TIME/ACTION PROFILE (bowel movement)

| | ONSET | PEAK | DURATION |
|---|---|---|---|
| PO | unknown | 2–4 days | unknown |

## NURSING IMPLICATIONS

### ASSESSMENT

❑ Assess patient for abdominal distention, presence of bowel sounds, and usual pattern of bowel function.

❑ Assess color, consistency, and amount of stool produced.

### POTENTIAL NURSING DIAGNOSES

■ Constipation (Indications).
■ Diarrhea (Side Effects).

### IMPLEMENTATION

■ **PO:** Dissolve powder in 8 oz of water prior to administration.

### PATIENT/FAMILY TEACHING

❑ Inform patient that 2–4 days may be required to produce a bowel movement. PEG should not be used for more than 2 wk. Prolonged, frequent, or excessive use may result in electrolyte imbalance and laxative dependence.

❑ Advise patient to notify health care professional if unusual cramps, bloating, or diarrhea occurs.

### EVALUATION

**Effectiveness of therapy can be demonstrated by:** ■ A soft, formed bowel movement.

---

## polyethylene glycol/ electrolyte

(po-lee-**eth**-e-leen **glye**-kole/ e-**lek**-troe-lite)

Colovage, Colyte, GoLYTELY, {Klean-Prep}, NuLytely, OCL, Peglyte

### CLASSIFICATION(S):

**Therapeutic:** laxatives
**Pharmacologic:** osmotics

**Pregnancy Category C**

---

## INDICATIONS

■ Bowel cleansing in preparation for GI examination. **Unlabeled uses:** ■ Treatment of acute iron overdose in children.

## ACTION

■ Polyethylene glycol (PEG) in solution acts as an osmotic agent, drawing water into the lumen of the GI tract. **Therapeutic Effects:** ■ Evacuation of the GI tract without water or electrolyte imbalance.

## PHARMACOKINETICS

**Absorption:** Ions in the solution are nonabsorbable.

**Distribution:** Unknown.

**Metabolism and Excretion:** Solution is excreted in fecal contents.

**Half-life:** Unknown.

## CONTRAINDICATIONS AND PRECAUTIONS

**Contraindicated in:** ■ GI obstruction ■ Gastric retention ■ Toxic colitis ■ Megacolon.

**Use Cautiously in:** ■ Patients with absent or diminished gag reflex ■ Unconscious or semicomatose states, in which administration is via NG tube ■ History of ulcerative colitis (increased risk of hypoglycemia, dehydration, and hypokalemia) ■ Barium enema using double-contrast technique (may not allow proper barium coating of mucosa) ■ Abdominal pain of uncertain cause, particularly if accompanied by fever ■ Children (safety not established; children <2 yr more prone to hypoglycemia, dehydration, and hypokalemia).

## ADVERSE REACTIONS AND SIDE EFFECTS*

■ **GI:** abdominal fullness, diarrhea, bloating, cramps, nausea, vomiting ■ **Misc:** allergic reactions (rare).

## INTERACTIONS

**Drug-Drug:** ■ Interferes with the absorption of **orally administered medications** by decreasing transit time (do not administer within 1 hr of start of therapy).

---

{ } = Available in Canada only.
* CAPITALS indicates life-threatening; <u>underlines</u> indicate most frequent.

## ROUTE AND DOSAGE

■ **PO (Adults):** 240 ml q 10 min (up to 4 L) until fecal discharge appears clear and has no solid material; may be given through NG tube at 20–30 ml/min (up to 4 L).

■ **PO (Children ≥6 mo):** 25 ml/kg/hr until fecal discharge is clear and has no solid material; may also be given through a NG tube (unlabeled).

## AVAILABILITY

■ *Oral solution:* OCL—1500-ml 3-pack^Rx ■ *Powder for oral solution (regular, pineapple, citrus berry, lemon-lime, cherry flavor):* CoLyte—powder in bottles for reconstitution, GoLYTLEY—powder in packets and disposable jugs for reconstitution, NuLytely—powder in disposable jugs for reconstitution.

TIME/ACTION PROFILE

|    | ONSET | PEAK | DURATION |
|----|-------|------|----------|
| PO | 1 hr | unknown | 4 hr |

## NURSING IMPLICATIONS

### ASSESSMENT

❏ Assess patient for abdominal distention, presence of bowel sounds, and usual pattern of bowel function.

❏ Assess color, consistency, and amount of stool produced.

❏ Monitor semiconscious or unconscious patients closely for regurgitation when administering via NG tube.

### POTENTIAL NURSING DIAGNOSES

■ Diarrhea (Side Effects).

### IMPLEMENTATION

■ **General:** Do not add extra flavorings or additional ingredients to solution prior to administration.

❏ Patient should fast for 3–4 hr prior to administration and should never have solid food within 2 hr of administration.

❏ Patient should be allowed only clear liquids after administration.

❏ May be administered on the morning of the examination as long as time is allotted to drink solution (3 hr) and evacuate bowel (1 additional hr). For barium enema, administer solution early evening (6 PM) prior to

exam to allow proper mucosal coating by barium.

■ **PO:** Solution may be reconstituted with tap water. Shake vigorously until powder is dissolved.

❏ May be administered via NG tube at a rate of 20–30 ml/min.

### PATIENT/FAMILY TEACHING

❏ Instruct patient to drink 240 ml every 10 min until 4 L have been consumed or fecal discharge is clear and free of solid matter. Rapidly drinking each 240 ml is preferred over drinking small amounts continuously.

### EVALUATION

**Effectiveness of therapy can be demonstrated by:** ■ Diarrhea, which cleanses the bowel within 4 hr. The first bowel movement usually occurs within 1 hr of administration.

# POTASSIUM AND SODIUM PHOSPHATES

(po-**tas**-e-um/**soe**-dee-yum **foss**-fates)

**monobasic potassium and sodium phosphates**
K-Phos M.F., K-Phos Neutral, K-Phos No. 2

**potassium and sodium phosphates**
Neutra-Phos, Uro-KP Neutral

*CLASSIFICATION(S):*
*Therapeutic: antiurolithics, mineral and electrolyte replacements/supplements*

**Pregnancy Category C**

## INDICATIONS

■ Treatment and prevention of phosphate depletion in patients who are unable to ingest adequate dietary potassium (potassium and sodium phosphate) ■ Adjunct therapy of urinary tract infections with methenamine hippurate or mandelate (potassium and sodium phosphates or monobasic potassium phosphate) ■ Prevention of calcium urinary stones (potassium and sodium phosphates or monobasic potassium phosphate) ■ Phosphate salts of potassium may be used in hypokalemic patients with metabolic acidosis or coexisting phosphorus deficiency.

## ACTION

■ Phosphate is present in bone and is involved in energy transfer and carbohydrate metabolism ■ Serves as a buffer for the excretion of hydrogen ions by the kidneys ■ Dibasic potassium phosphate is converted in renal tubule to monobasic salt, resulting in urinary acidification, which is required for methenamine hippurate or mandelate to be active as urinary anti-infectives ■ Acidification of urine increases solubility of calcium, decreasing calcium stone formation. **Therapeutic Effects:** ■ Replacement of phosphorus in deficiency states ■ Urinary acidification ■ Increased efficacy of methenamine ■ Decreased formation of calcium urinary tract stones.

## PHARMACOKINETICS

**Absorption:** Well absorbed following oral administration. Vitamin D promotes GI absorption of phosphates.

**Distribution:** Phosphates enter extracellular fluids and are then actively transported to sites of action.

**Metabolism and Excretion:** Excreted mainly (>90%) by the kidneys.

**Half-life:** Unknown.

## CONTRAINDICATIONS AND PRECAUTIONS

**Contraindicated in:** ■ Hyperkalemia (potassium salts) ■ Hyperphosphatemia ■ Hypocalcemia ■ Severe renal impairment ■ Untreated Addison's disease (potassium salts) ■ Severe tissue trauma (potassium salts) ■ Hyperkalemic familial periodic paralysis (potassium salts).

**Use Cautiously in:** ■ Hyperparathyroidism ■ Cardiac disease ■ Hypernatremia (sodium phosphate only) ■ Hypertension (sodium phosphate only) ■ Renal impairment.

## ADVERSE REACTIONS AND SIDE EFFECTS*

Related to hyperphosphatemia, unless otherwise indicated. ■ **CNS:** confusion, listlessness, weakness ■ **CV:** ARRHYTHMIAS, CARDIAC ARREST, ECG changes (absent P waves, widening of the QRS complex with biphasic curve), hypotension; *hy-*

*perkalemia*—ARRHYTHMIAS, ECG changes (prolonged PR interval, ST segment depression, talltented T waves); *hypernatremia*—edema ■ **GI:** diarrhea, abdominal pain, nausea, vomiting ■ **F and E:** hyperkalemia, hypernatremia, hyperphosphatemia, hypocalcemia, hypomagnesemia ■ **Local:** irritation at IV site, phlebitis ■ **MS:** *hypocalcemia*—tremors; *hyperkalemia*—muscle cramps ■ **Neuro:** flaccid paralysis, heaviness of legs, paresthesias.

## INTERACTIONS

**Drug-Drug:** ■ Concurrent use of **potassium-sparing diuretics** or **ACE inhibitors** with potassium phosphates may result in hyperkalemia ■ Concurrent use of **corticosteroids** with sodium phosphate may result in hypernatremia ■ Concurrent administration of **calcium-, magnesium-,** or **aluminum-containing compounds** decreases absorption of phosphates by formation of insoluble complexes ■ **Vitamin D** enhances the absorption of phosphates.

**Drug-Food:** ■ **Oxalates** (in spinach and rhubarb) and **phytates** (in bran and whole grains) may decrease the absorption of phosphates by binding them in the GI tract.

## ROUTE AND DOSAGE

### ❏ Monobasic Potassium and Sodium Phosphates

■ **PO (Adults and Children >4 yr):** 250 mg (8 mmol) 4 times daily; may be increased to 250 mg (8 mmol) q 2 hr (not to exceed 2 g phosphorus/24 hr).

■ **PO (Children <4 yr):** 200 mg (6.4 mmol) 4 times daily.

### ❏ Potassium and Sodium Phosphates

■ **PO (Adults and Children >4 yr):** 250 mg (8 mmol) phosphorus 4 times daily.

■ **PO (Children <4 yr):** 200 mg (6.4 mmol) 4 times daily.

## AVAILABILITY

### ❏ Monobasic Potassium and Sodium Phosphates

■ *Tablets for oral solution:* 125.6 mg (4 mmol) phosphorus<sup>Rx</sup>, 250 mg (8 mmol) phosphorus<sup>Rx</sup>.

□ **Potassium and Sodium Phosphates**

■ *Capsules for oral solution:* 250 mg (8 mmol) phosphorus[Rx] ■ *Tablets for oral solution:* 250 mg (8 mmol) phosphorus[Rx] ■ *Powder for oral solution:* 250 mg (8 mmol)/75 ml when reconstituted[Rx].

TIME/ACTION PROFILE (effects on serum phosphate levels)

| | ONSET | PEAK | DURATION |
|---|---|---|---|
| PO | unknown | unknown | unknown |

# NURSING IMPLICATIONS

## ASSESSMENT

□ Assess patient for signs and symptoms of hypokalemia (weakness, fatigue, arrhythmias, presence of U waves on ECG, polyuria, polydipsia) and hypophosphatemia (anorexia, weakness, decreased reflexes, bone pain, confusion, blood dyscrasias) throughout therapy.

□ Monitor intake and output ratios and daily weight. Report significant discrepancies.

■ *Lab Test Considerations:* Monitor serum phosphate, potassium, sodium, and calcium levels prior to and periodically throughout therapy. Increased phosphate may cause hypocalcemia.

□ Monitor renal function studies prior to and periodically throughout therapy.

□ Monitor urinary pH in patients receiving potassium and sodium phosphate as a urinary acidifier.

## POTENTIAL NURSING DIAGNOSES

■ Nutrition, imbalanced: less than body requirements (Indications).

## IMPLEMENTATION

■ **PO:** Tablets should be dissolved in a full glass of water. Capsules should be opened and mixed thoroughly in $1/3$ cup of water each. Allow mixture to stand for 2–5 min to ensure it is fully dissolved. Solutions prepared by pharmacy should not be further diluted.

□ Medication should be administered after meals to minimize gastric irritation and laxative effect.

□ Do not administer simultaneously with antacids containing aluminum, magnesium, or calcium.

## PATIENT/FAMILY TEACHING

□ Explain to the patient the purpose of the medication and the need to take as directed. If a dose is missed, it should be taken as soon as remembered unless within 1 or 2 hr of the next dose. Explain that the tablets and capsules should not be swallowed whole. Tablets should be dissolved in water; capsules should be opened and the contents mixed in water.

□ Instruct patients in low-sodium diet (see Appendix Q).

□ Advise patient of the importance of maintaining a high fluid intake (drinking at least one 8-oz glass of water each hr) to prevent kidney stones.

□ Instruct the patient to promptly report diarrhea, weakness, fatigue, muscle cramps, unexplained weight gain, swelling of lower extremities, shortness of breath, unusual thirst, or tremors.

## EVALUATION

**Effectiveness of therapy can be demonstrated by:** ■ Prevention and correction of serum phosphate and potassium deficiencies ■ Maintenance of acid urine ■ Decreased urine calcium, which prevents formation of renal calculi.

High Alert

# POTASSIUM SUPPLEMENTS
(poe-**tass**-ee-um)

**potassium acetate**

**potassium bicarbonate**
K+Care ET, K-Electrolyte, K-Ide, Klor-Con/EF, K-Lyte, K-Vescent

**potassium bicarbonate/potassium chloride**
Klorvess, Klorvess Effervescent Granules, K-Lyte/Cl, {Neo-K}, {Potassium Sandoz}

**potassium bicarbonate/potassium citrate**
Effer-K, K-Lyte DS

## potassium chloride

{Apo-K}, Cena-K, Gen-K, K+ Care, K+ 10, {Kalium Durules}, Kaochlor, Kaochlor S-F, Kaon-Cl, Kay Ciel, KCl, K-Dur, K-Lease, {K-Long}, K-Lor, Klor-Con, Klorvess Liquid, Klotrix, K-Lyte/Cl Powder, K-Med, K-Norm, K-Sol, K-Tab, Micro-K, Micro-K ExtenCaps, Micro-LS, Potasalan, Roychlor, Rum-K, Slow-K, Ten-K

## potassium chloride/potassium bicarbonate/potassium citrate

Kaochlor Eff

## potassium gluconate

Kaon, Kaylixir, K-G Elixir, {Potassium-Rougier}

## potassium gluconate/potassium chloride

Kolyum

## potassium gluconate/potassium citrate

Twin-K

## trikates (potassium acetate/potassium bicarbonate/potassium citrate)

Tri-K

### CLASSIFICATION(S):

*Therapeutic: mineral and electrolyte replacements/supplements*

**Pregnancy Category C**

## INDICATIONS

■ **PO, IV:** Treatment/prevention of potassium depletion ■ **IV:** Arrhythmias due to digoxin toxicity.

## ACTION

■ Maintain acid-base balance, isotonicity, and electrophysiologic balance of the cell ■ Activator in many enzymatic reactions; essential to transmission of nerve impulses; contraction of cardiac, skeletal, and smooth muscle; gastric secretion; renal function; tissue synthesis; and carbohydrate metabolism. **Therapeutic Effects:** ■ Replacement ■ Prevention of deficiency.

## PHARMACOKINETICS

**Absorption:** Well absorbed following oral administration.

**Distribution:** Enters extracellular fluid; then actively transported into cells.

**Metabolism and Excretion:** Excreted by the kidneys.

**Half-life:** Unknown.

## CONTRAINDICATIONS AND PRECAUTIONS

**Contraindicated in:** ■ Hyperkalemia ■ Severe renal impairment ■ Untreated Addison's disease ■ Severe tissue trauma ■ Hyperkalemic familial periodic paralysis ■ Some products may contain tartrazine (FDC yellow dye #5) or alcohol; avoid using in patients with known hypersensitivity or intolerance ■ Potassium acetate injection contains aluminum, which may become toxic with prolonged use to high risk groups (renal impairment, premature neonates).

**Use Cautiously in:** ■ Cardiac disease ■ Renal impairment ■ Diabetes mellitus (liquids may contain sugar) ■ Hypomagnesemia (may make correction of hypokalemia more difficult) ■ GI hypomotility including dysphagia or esophageal compression from left atrial enlargement (tablets, capsules).

## ADVERSE REACTIONS AND SIDE EFFECTS*

■ **CNS:** confusion, restlessness, weakness ■ **CV:** ARRHYTHMIAS, ECG changes ■ **GI:** abdominal pain, diarrhea, flatulence, nausea, vomiting; *tablets, capsules only*—GI ulceration, stenotic lesions ■ **Local:** irritation at IV site ■ **Neuro:** paralysis, paresthesia.

## INTERACTIONS

**Drug-Drug:** ■ Use with **potassium-sparing diuretics** or **ACE inhibitors** or **angiotensin II receptor antagonists** may lead to hyperkalemia ■ **Anticholinergics** may ↑ GI mucosal lesions in patients taking wax-matrix potassium chloride preparations.

## ROUTE AND DOSAGE

Expressed as mEq of potassium. Potassium acetate contains 10.2 mEq/g; potassium bicarbonate contains 10 mEq potassium/g; potassium chloride contains 13.4 mEq potassium/g; potassium gluconate contains 4.3 mEq/g.

■ **PO (Adults):** *Prevention of deficiency*— 20 mEq/day; *treatment of depletion*—40–100 mEq/day; single dose should not exceed 20 mEq.

■ **PO (Children):** 2–3 mEq/kg/day or 20–40 mEq/m²/day in divided doses.

■ **IV (Adults):** *Serum potassium >2.5 mEq/ L*—Up to 200 mEq/day as an infusion (not to exceed 10 mEq/hr or a concentration of 40 mEq/L via peripheral line (up to 100 mEq/L have been used via central line [unlabeled]). *Serum potassium <2 mEq/L with symptoms*—Up to 400 mEq/day as an infusion (rate should generally not exceed 20 mEq/hr).

■ **IV (Children):** Up to 3 mEq/kg/day (40 mEq/m²/day) as an infusion.

## AVAILABILITY

❑ **Potassium Acetate**

■ *Concentrate for injection (contains aluminum):* 2 mEq/ml in 20-, 50-, and 100-ml vials$^{Rx}$, 40 mEq/ml in 50-ml vials$^{Rx}$.

❑ **Potassium Bicarbonate**

■ *Tablets for effervescent oral solution:* 25 mEq$^{Rx}$.

❑ **Potassium Bicarbonate/Potassium Chloride**

■ *Packets for effervescent oral solution:* 20 mEq/2.8-g packet$^{Rx}$ ■ *Tablets for effervescent oral solution:* {12 mEq$^{Rx}$}, 20 mEq$^{Rx}$, 25 mEq$^{Rx}$, 50 mEq$^{Rx}$.

❑ **Potassium Bicarbonate/Potassium Citrate**

■ *Tablets for effervescent oral solution:* 25 mEq$^{Rx}$, 50 mEq$^{Rx}$.

❑ **Potassium Chloride**

■ *Extended-release tablets:* 8 mEq$^{Rx}$, 10 mEq$^{Rx}$, 20 mEq$^{Rx}$ ■ Cost: 10 mEq $32.10/100, 20 mEq $58.46/100 ■ *Extended-release capsules:* 8 mEq$^{Rx}$, 10 mEq$^{Rx}$ ■ *Oral solution:* 10 mEq/15 ml$^{Rx}$, 20 mEq/15 ml$^{Rx}$, 30 mEq/15 ml$^{Rx}$, 40 mEq/15 ml$^{Rx}$ ■ *Powder/ packets for oral solution:* 15-mEq/1.2-g packet$^{Rx}$, 20-mEq/1.5-g packet$^{Rx}$, 25-mEq/1.8-g packet$^{Rx}$ ■ *Packets for oral suspension:* 20-mEq/1.5-g packet$^{Rx}$ ■ *Concentrate for injection:* 0.1 mEq/ml in 10-mEq ampules and vials$^{Rx}$, 0.2 mEq/ml in 10- and 20-mEq ampules and vials$^{Rx}$, 0.3 mEq/ml in 30-mEq ampules and vials$^{Rx}$, 0.4 mEq/ml in 20- and 40-mEq ampules and vials$^{Rx}$, 1.5 mEq/ml$^{Rx}$, 2 mEq/ ml$^{Rx}$, 3 mEq/ml$^{Rx}$ ■ *Solution for IV infusion:* 10 mEq/L in various dextrose and saline solutions in 250-, 500-, and 100-ml containers$^{Rx}$, 20 mEq/L in dextrose/saline/LRs in 250-, 500-, and 100-ml containers$^{Rx}$, 30 mEq/L in various dextrose and saline solutions in 250-, 500-, and 100-ml containers$^{Rx}$, 40 mEq/L in various dextrose and saline solutions in 250-, 500-, and 100-ml containers$^{Rx}$.

❑ **Potassium Chloride/Potassium Bicarbonate/Potassium Citrate**

■ *Tablets for effervescent oral solution:* 20 mEq$^{Rx}$.

❑ **Potassium Gluconate**

■ *Tablets:* 2 mEq$^{Rx}$, 5 mEq$^{Rx}$ ■ *Elixir:* 20 mEq/15 ml$^{Rx}$.

❑ **Potassium Gluconate/Potassium Chloride**

■ *Oral solution:* 20 mEq/15 ml$^{Rx}$ ■ *Powder for oral solution:* 20 mEq/5-g packet$^{Rx}$.

❑ **Potassium Gluconate/Potassium Citrate**

■ *Oral solution:* 20 mEq/15 ml$^{Rx}$.

❑ **Trikates (Potassium Acetate/Potassium Bicarbonate/Potassium Citrate)**

■ *Oral solution:* 15 mEq/5 ml$^{Rx}$.

TIME/ACTION PROFILE (increase in serum potassium levels)

| | ONSET | PEAK | DURATION |
|----|---------|---------------|---------|
| PO | unknown | 1–2 hr | unknown |
| IV | rapid | end of infu-sion | unknown |

# NURSING IMPLICATIONS

## ASSESSMENT

❑ Assess for signs and symptoms of hypokalemia (weakness, fatigue, U wave on ECG, arrhythmias, polyuria, polydipsia) and hyperkalemia (see Toxicity and Overdose).

❑ Monitor pulse, blood pressure, and ECG periodically during IV therapy.

- **Lab Test Considerations:** Monitor serum potassium before and periodically during therapy. Monitor renal function, serum bicarbonate, and pH. Determine serum magnesium level if patient has refractory hypokalemia; hypomagnesemia should be corrected to facilitate effectiveness of potassium replacement. Monitor serum chloride because hypochloremia may occur if replacing potassium without concurrent chloride.

- **Toxicity and Overdose:** Symptoms of toxicity are those of hyperkalemia (slow, irregular heartbeat; fatigue; muscle weakness; paresthesia; confusion; dyspnea; peaked T waves; depressed ST segments; prolonged QT segments; widened QRS complexes; loss of P waves; and cardiac arrhythmias).

  - Treatment includes discontinuation of potassium, administration of sodium bicarbonate to correct acidosis, dextrose and insulin to facilitate passage of potassium into cells, calcium salts to reverse ECG effects (in patients who are not receiving digoxin), sodium polystyrene used as an exchange resin, and/or dialysis for patient with impaired renal function.

## POTENTIAL NURSING DIAGNOSES

- Nutrition, imbalanced: less than body requirements (Indications).

## IMPLEMENTATION

- **High Alert:** Medication errors involving too rapid infusion or bolus IV administration of potassium chloride have resulted in fatalities. See IV administration guidelines below.

- **General:** Do not confuse K-Dur with Imdur (isosorbide mononitrate). Do not confuse Micro-K with micronase (glyburide).

  - For most purposes, potassium chloride should be used, except for renal tubular acidoses (hyperchloremic acidosis), in which other salts are more appropriate (potassium bicarbonate, potassium citrate, or potassium gluconate).

  - If hypokalemia is secondary to diuretic therapy, consideration should be given to decreasing the dose of diuretic, unless there is a history of significant arrhythmias or concurrent digitalis glycoside therapy.

- **PO:** Administer with or after meals to decrease GI irritation.

  - Use of tablets and capsules should be reserved for patients who cannot tolerate liquid preparations.

  - Dissolve effervescent tablets in 3–8 oz of cold water. Ensure that effervescent tablet is fully dissolved. Powders and solutions should be diluted in 3–8 oz of cold water or juice (do not use tomato juice if patient is on sodium restriction). Instruct patient to drink slowly over 5–10 min.

  - Tablets and capsules should be taken with a meal and full glass of water. Do not chew or crush enteric-coated or extended-release tablets or capsules. Micro-K ExtenCaps capsules can be opened and sprinkled on soft food (pudding, applesauce) and swallowed immediately with a glass of cool water or juice.

- **IV:** Assess for extravasation; severe pain and tissue necrosis may occur.

  - **High Alert:** Never administer potassium IV push or bolus.

  - ## Potassium Acetate

- **Continuous Infusion: High Alert:** Do not administer undiluted. Each single dose *must* be diluted and thoroughly mixed in 100–1000 ml of dextrose, saline, Ringer's or LR, dextrose/saline, dextrose/Ringer's, or LR combinations. Usually limited to 40 mEq/L via peripheral line (100 mEq/L via central line).

- **Rate: High Alert:** Infuse slowly, at a rate up to 10 mEq/hr on general care areas. Check hospital policy for maximum infusion rates.

  - ## Potassium Chloride

- **Continuous Infusion: High Alert:** Do not administer concentrations of ≥1.5 mEq/ml undiluted; fatalities have occurred. Concentrated products have black caps on vials or black stripes above constriction on ampules and are labeled with a warning about dilution requirement. Each single dose must be diluted and thoroughly mixed in 100–1000 ml of IV solution. Usually limited to 40 mEq/L via peripheral line (100 mEq/L via central line).

❑ Concentrations of 0.1 and 0.4 mEq/ml are intended for administration via calibrated infusion device and do not require dilution.

■ *Rate: High Alert:* Infuse slowly, at a rate up to 10 mEq/hr in general care areas. Check hospital policy for maximum infusion rates. Use an infusion pump.

■ **Solution Compatibility:** May be diluted in dextrose, saline, Ringer's solution, LR, dextrose/saline, dextrose/Ringer's solution, and dextrose/LR combinations. Commercially available premixed with many of the above IV solutions.

■ **Y-Site Compatibility:** ◆ acyclovir ◆ alatrofloxacin ◆ aldesleukin ◆ allopurinol ◆ amifostine ◆ aminophylline ◆ amiodarone ◆ ampicillin ◆ atropine ◆ aztreonam ◆ betamethasone ◆ calcium gluconate ◆ chlordiazepoxide ◆ chlorpromazine ◆ ciprofloxacin ◆ cisatracurium ◆ cladribine ◆ cyanocobalamin ◆ digoxin ◆ diltiazem ◆ diphenhydramine ◆ dobutamine ◆ docetaxel ◆ dopamine ◆ doxorubicin liposome ◆ droperidol ◆ edrophonium ◆ enalaprilat ◆ epinephrine ◆ esmolol ◆ conjugated estrogens ◆ ethacrynate sodium ◆ etoposide phosphate ◆ famotidine ◆ fentanyl ◆ filgrastim ◆ fludarabine ◆ fluorouracil ◆ furosemide ◆ gatifloxacin ◆ gemcitabine ◆ granisetron ◆ heparin ◆ hydralazine ◆ idarubicin ◆ inamrinone ◆ indomethacin ◆ insulin ◆ isoproterenol ◆ kanamycin ◆ labetalol ◆ lidocaine ◆ linezolid ◆ lorazepam ◆ magnesium sulfate ◆ melphalan ◆ menadiol ◆ meperidine ◆ methoxamine ◆ methylergonovine ◆ midazolam ◆ milrinone ◆ minocycline ◆ morphine ◆ neostigmine ◆ norepinephrine ◆ ondansetron ◆ oxacillin ◆ oxytocin ◆ paclitaxel ◆ penicillin G potassium ◆ pentazocine ◆ phytonadione ◆ piperacillin/tazobactam ◆ procainamide ◆ prochlorperazine ◆ propofol ◆ propranolol ◆ pyridostigmine ◆ remifentanil ◆ sargramostim ◆ scopolamine ◆ sodium bicarbonate ◆ succinylcholine ◆ tacrolimus ◆ teniposide ◆ theophylline ◆ thiotepa ◆ tirofiban ◆ trimethaphan ◆ trimethobenzamide ◆ vinorelbine ◆ warfarin ◆ zidovudine.

■ **Y-Site Incompatibility:** ◆ amphotericin B cholesteryl sulfate complex ◆ diazepam ◆ ergotamine tartrate ◆ phenytoin.

■ **Additive Compatibility:** ◆ calcium gluconate ◆ cimetidine ◆ lidocaine ◆ ranitidine ◆ sodium bicarbonate ◆ vitamin B complex with C.

## PATIENT/FAMILY TEACHING

❑ Explain to patient purpose of the medication and the need to take as directed, especially when concurrent digoxin or diuretics are taken. A missed dose should be taken as soon as remembered within 2 hr; if not, return to regular dose schedule. Do not double dose.

❑ Emphasize correct method of administration. GI irritation or ulceration may result from chewing enteric-coated tablets or insufficient dilution of liquid or powder forms.

❑ Some extended-release tablets are contained in a wax matrix that may be expelled in the stool. This occurrence is not significant.

❑ Instruct patient to avoid salt substitutes or low-salt milk or food unless approved by health care professional. Patient should be advised to read all labels to prevent excess potassium intake.

❑ Advise patient regarding sources of dietary potassium (see Appendix Q). Encourage compliance with recommended diet.

❑ Instruct patient to report dark, tarry, or bloody stools; weakness; unusual fatigue; or tingling of extremities. Notify health care professional if nausea, vomiting, diarrhea, or stomach discomfort persists. Dosage may require adjustment.

❑ Emphasize the importance of regular follow-up exams to monitor serum levels and progress.

## EVALUATION

**Effectiveness of therapy can be demonstrated by:** ■ Prevention and correction of serum potassium depletion ■ Cessation of arrhythmias caused by digoxin toxicity.

## pramipexole

(pra-mi-**pex**-ole)

Mirapex

### CLASSIFICATION(S):

**Therapeutic:** *antiparkinson agents*
**Pharmacologic:** *dopamine agonists*

**Pregnancy Category C**

## INDICATIONS

■ Management of idiopathic Parkinson's disease.

## ACTION

■ Stimulates dopamine receptors in the striatum of the brain. **Therapeutic Effects:** ■ Decreased tremor and rigidity in Parkinson's disease.

## PHARMACOKINETICS

**Absorption:** >90% absorbed following oral administration.

**Distribution:** Widely distributed.

**Metabolism and Excretion:** 90% excreted unchanged in urine.

**Half-life:** 8 hr (increased in geriatric patients and patients with renal impairment).

## CONTRAINDICATIONS AND PRECAUTIONS

**Contraindicated in:** ■ Hypersensitivity.

**Use Cautiously in:** ■ Geriatric patients (increased risk of hallucinations) ■ Renal impairment (increased dosing interval recommended if CCr <60 ml/min) ■ Pregnancy, lactation, or children (safety not established).

## ADVERSE REACTIONS AND SIDE EFFECTS*

■ **CNS:** SLEEP ATTACKS, amnesia, dizziness, drowsiness, hallucinations, weakness, abnormal dreams, confusion, dyskinesia, extrapyramidal syndrome, headache, insomnia ■ **CV:** postural hypotension ■ **GI:** constipation, dry mouth, dyspepsia, nausea, tooth disease ■ **GU:** urinary frequency ■ **MS:** leg cramps ■ **Neuro:** hypertonia, unsteadiness/falling.

## INTERACTIONS

**Drug-Drug:** ■ Concurrent **levodopa** increases the risk of hallucinations and dyskinesia ■ Effectiveness may be increased by **cimetidine** ■ Effectiveness may be decreased by **dopamine antagonists,** including **butyrophenones, metoclopramide, phenothiazines,** or **thioxanthenes.**

## ROUTE AND DOSAGE

■ **PO (Adults):** 0.125 mg 3 times daily initially; may be increased q 5–7 days (range 1.5–4.5 mg/day in 3 divided doses).

❑ **Renal Impairment**

■ **PO (Adults):** *CCr 35–59 ml/min*—0.125 mg twice daily initially, may be increased q 5–7 days up to 1.5 mg twice daily; *CCr 15–34 ml/min*—0.125 mg once daily initially, may be increased q 5–7 days up to 1.5 mg once daily.

## AVAILABILITY

■ *Tablets:* 0.125 mg$^{Rx}$, 0.25 mg$^{Rx}$, 0.5 mg$^{Rx}$, 1 mg$^{Rx}$, 1.5 mg$^{Rx}$ ■ Cost: 0.125 mg $47.75/90, 0.25 mg $90.54/90, 0.5 mg $177.66/90, 1 mg $177.66/90, 1.5 mg $177.66/90.

TIME/ACTION PROFILE (blood levels)

| | ONSET | PEAK | DURATION |
|---|---|---|---|
| PO | unknown | 2 hr | 8 hr |

# NURSING IMPLICATIONS

## ASSESSMENT

❑ Assess patient for signs and symptoms of Parkinson's disease (tremor, muscle weakness and rigidity, ataxia) before and throughout therapy.

❑ Assess patient for confusion or hallucinations. Notify physician or other health care professional if these occur.

❑ Monitor ECG and blood pressure frequently during dosage adjustment and periodically throughout therapy.

❑ Assess patient for drowsiness and sleep attacks. Drowsiness is a common side effect of pramipexole, but sleep attacks or episodes of falling asleep during activities that require active participation may occur without warning. Assess patient for concomitant medications that have sedating effects or may increase serum pramipexole levels (see Interactions). May require discontinuation of therapy.

## POTENTIAL NURSING DIAGNOSES

■ Mobility, impaired physical (Indications).

■ Injury, risk for (Indications, Side Effects).

## IMPLEMENTATION

■ **PO:** An attempt to reduce the dose of levodopa/carbidopa may be made cautiously during pramipexole therapy.

❑ Administer with meals to minimize nausea; usually resolves with continued therapy.

## PATIENT/FAMILY TEACHING

❑ Instruct patient to take medication exactly as directed. Missed doses should be taken as soon as remembered if it is not almost time for next dose. Do not double doses. Consult health care professional before reducing dose or discontinuing medication.

❑ May cause drowsiness and unexpected episodes of falling asleep. Caution patient to avoid driving or other activities requiring alertness until response to medication is known. Advise patient to notify health care professional if episodes of falling asleep occur.

❑ Advise patient to change position slowly to minimize orthostatic hypotension. May occur more frequently during initial therapy.

❑ Advise female patient to notify health care professional if pregnancy is planned or suspected or if currently breastfeeding or planning to breastfeed.

## EVALUATION

**Effectiveness of therapy can be demonstrated by:** ▪ Decreased tremor and rigidity in Parkinson's disease.

## pravastatin, See HMG-CoA REDUCTASE INHIBITORS.

## prazosin

(pra-zoe-sin)

Minipress

**CLASSIFICATION(S):**
**Therapeutic:** antihypertensives
**Pharmacologic:** peripherally acting antiadrenergics

**Pregnancy Category C**

## INDICATIONS

▪ Mild to moderate hypertension. **Unlabeled uses:** ▪ Management of urinary outflow obstruction in patients with benign prostatic hyperplasia.

## ACTION

▪ Dilates both arteries and veins by blocking postsynaptic alpha₁-adrenergic receptors ▪ Decreases contractions in smooth muscle of prostatic capsule. **Therapeutic Effects:** ▪ Lowering of blood pressure ▪ Decreased cardiac preload and afterload ▪ Decreased symptoms of prostatic hyperplasia (urinary urgency, urinary hesitancy, nocturia).

## PHARMACOKINETICS

**Absorption:** 60% absorbed following oral administration.
**Distribution:** Widely distributed.
**Protein Binding:** 97%.
**Metabolism and Excretion:** Extensively metabolized by the liver. Minimal (5–10%) renal excretion of unchanged drug.
**Half-life:** 2–3 hr.

## CONTRAINDICATIONS AND PRECAUTIONS

**Contraindicated in:** ▪ Hypersensitivity.
**Use Cautiously in:** ▪ Renal insufficiency (increased sensitivity to effects; dosage reduction may be required) ▪ Pregnancy, lactation, or children (safety not established) ▪ Angina pectoris ▪ When adding diuretics (reduce dose of prazosin).

## ADVERSE REACTIONS AND SIDE EFFECTS*

▪ **CNS:** dizziness, headache, weakness, drowsiness, mental depression, syncope ▪ **EENT:** blurred vision ▪ **CV:** first-dose orthostatic hypotension, palpitations, angina, edema ▪ **GI:** abdominal cramps, diarrhea, dry mouth, nausea, vomiting ▪ **GU:** impotence, priapism.

## INTERACTIONS

**Drug-Drug:** ▪ Additive hypotension with acute ingestion of **alcohol,** other **antihypertensives,** or **nitrates** ▪ Antihypertensive effects may be decreased by **NSAIDs.**

## ROUTE AND DOSAGE

❑ **Hypertension**
▪ **PO (Adults):** 1 mg 2–3 times daily (give first dose at bedtime) for initial 3 days of therapy, then increase gradually to maintenance dose of 6–15 mg/day in 2–3 divided doses (not to exceed 20–40 mg/day).
▪ **PO (Children):** 50–400 mcg (0.05–0.4 mg)/kg/day in 2–3 divided doses (not to exceed 7 mg/dose or 15 mg/day).

❑ **Benign Prostatic Hyperplasia**
▪ **PO (Adults):** 1–5 mg twice daily.

## AVAILABILITY (generic available)

■ *Capsules:* 1 mg$^{Rx}$, 2 mg$^{Rx}$, 5 mg$^{Rx}$ ■ Cost: *Minipress*—1 mg $44.16/100, 2 mg $34.60/ 60, 5 mg $62.87/60; *generic*—1 mg $23.51– $40.81/100, 2 mg $31.10–$56.82/100, 5 mg $53.16–$96.84/100 ■ *Tablets:* {1 mg$^{Rx}$}, {2 mg$^{Rx}$}, {5 mg$^{Rx}$} ■ Cost: 1 mg $8.07/30, 2 mg $11.81/30, 5 mg $60.50/100 ■ polythiazide (Minizide)$^{Rx}$. See Appendix B.

TIME/ACTION PROFILE (antihypertensive effects)

|  | ONSET | PEAK | DURATION |
|---|---|---|---|
| PO | 2 hr | 2–4 hr† | 10 hr |

†Following single dose; maximal antihypertensive effects occur after 3–4 wk of chronic dosing.

# NURSING IMPLICATIONS

## ASSESSMENT

■ **General Info:** Monitor intake and output ratios and daily weight and assess for edema daily, especially at beginning of therapy. Report significant weight gain or edema.

■ **Hypertension:** Monitor blood pressure and pulse frequently during initial dosage adjustment and periodically throughout therapy. Report significant changes.

❑ Monitor frequency of prescription refills to determine compliance.

■ **Benign Prostatic Hypertrophy:** Assess patient for urinary symptoms (retention, dribbling, hesitancy, urgency) periodically during therapy.

■ *Lab Test Considerations:* May cause elevated serum sodium levels.

❑ May cause increased vanillylmandelic acid (VMA) concentrations; false-positive results may occur in screening tests for pheochromocytoma.

## POTENTIAL NURSING DIAGNOSES

■ Injury, risk for (Side Effects).

■ Noncompliance (Patient/Family Teaching).

## IMPLEMENTATION

■ **General:** Following initial dose, patient may develop first-dose orthostatic hypotensive reaction, which most frequently occurs 30–90 min after initial dose and may be manifested by dizziness, weakness, and syncope. Observe patient closely during this period, and take precautions to prevent injury. The first dose may be given at bedtime to minimize this reaction.

❑ Commonly administered concurrently with a thiazide diuretic or a beta blockers for treatment of hypertension.

## PATIENT/FAMILY TEACHING

❑ Emphasize the importance of continuing to take this medication, even if feeling well. Instruct patient to take medication at the same time each day. If a dose is missed, take as soon as remembered unless almost time for next dose. Do not double doses.

❑ Encourage patient to comply with additional interventions for hypertension (weight reduction, low-sodium diet, smoking cessation, moderation of alcohol consumption, regular exercise, stress management).

❑ Instruct patient and family on proper technique for blood pressure monitoring. Advise them to check blood pressure at least weekly and to report significant changes.

❑ May cause drowsiness or dizziness. Advise patient to avoid driving or other activities requiring alertness until response to medication is known.

❑ Caution patient to change positions slowly to decrease orthostatic hypotension.

❑ Advise patient to consult health care professional before taking any OTC medications, especially cough, cold, or allergy remedies.

❑ Emphasize the importance of follow-up visits to determine effectiveness of therapy.

## EVALUATION

**Effectiveness of therapy can be demonstrated by:** ■ Decrease in blood pressure without appearance of side effects ■ Decrease in symptoms of prostatic hypertrophy.

## prednicarbate, See CORTICOSTEROIDS (TOPICAL/ LOCAL).

{ } = Available in Canada only.
*CAPITALS indicates life-threatening; underlines indicate most frequent.

**prednisolone, See CORTICOSTEROIDS (SYSTEMIC).**

**prednisone, See CORTICOSTEROIDS (SYSTEMIC).**

## procainamide
(proe-**kane**-ah-mide)
Procanbid, Promine, Pronestyl, Pronestyl-SR

**CLASSIFICATION(S):**
**Therapeutic:** antiarrhythmics (class IA)

**Pregnancy Category C**

### INDICATIONS
■ Treatment of a wide variety of ventricular and atrial arrhythmias, including: ▢ Atrial premature contractions ▢ Premature ventricular contractions ▢ Ventricular tachycardia ▢ Paroxysmal atrial tachycardia ■ Maintenance of normal sinus rhythm after conversion from atrial fibrillation or flutter.

### ACTION
■ Decreases myocardial excitability ■ Slows conduction velocity ■ May depress myocardial contractility. **Therapeutic Effects:** ■ Suppression of arrhythmias.

### PHARMACOKINETICS
**Absorption:** Well absorbed (75–90%) following oral and IM administration. Sustained-release oral preparation is more slowly absorbed.
**Distribution:** Rapidly and widely distributed.
**Metabolism and Excretion:** Converted by the liver to *N*-acetylprocainamide (NAPA), an active antiarrhythmic compound. Remainder (40–70%) excreted unchanged by the kidneys.
**Half-life:** 2.5–4.7 hr (NAPA—7 hr); prolonged in renal impairment.

### CONTRAINDICATIONS AND PRECAUTIONS
**Contraindicated in:** ■ Hypersensitivity ■ AV block ■ Myasthenia gravis ■ Hypersensitivity to tartrazine (FDC yellow dye #5; present in some oral products).

**Use Cautiously in:** ■ MI or cardiac glycoside toxicity ■ CHF, renal or hepatic insufficiency, geriatric patients (dosage reduction or increased dosing intervals recommended) ■ Pregnancy, lactation, or children (safety not established).

### ADVERSE REACTIONS AND SIDE EFFECTS*
■ **CNS:** SEIZURES, confusion, dizziness ■ **CV:** ASYSTOLE, HEART BLOCK, VENTRICULAR ARRHYTHMIAS, hypotension ■ **GI:** diarrhea, anorexia, bitter taste, nausea, vomiting ■ **Derm:** rashes ■ **Hemat:** AGRANULOCYTOSIS, eosinophilia, leukopenia, thrombocytopenia ■ **Misc:** chills, drug-induced systemic lupus syndrome, fever.

### INTERACTIONS
**Drug-Drug:** ■ May have additive or antagonistic effects with other **antiarrhythmics** ■ Additive neurologic toxicity (confusion, seizures) with **lidocaine** ■ **Antihypertensives** and **nitrates** may potentiate hypotensive effect ■ Potentiates **neuromuscular blocking agents** ■ May partially antagonize the therapeutic effects of **anticholinesterase agents** in myasthenia gravis ■ Increased risk of arrhythmias with **pimozide** ■ Additive anticholinergic effects with other **drugs possessing anticholinergic properties,** including **antihistamines, antidepressants, atropine, haloperidol,** and **phenothiazines** ■ Effects of procainamide may be increased by **cimetidine, quinidine,** or **trimethoprim.**

### ROUTE AND DOSAGE
■ **PO (Adults):** *Atrial arrhythmias*—1.25 g initially, then 750 mg 2 hr later, then 0.5–1 g q 2–3 hr followed by maintenance dosing of 0.5–1 g q 4–6 hr or 1 g q 12 hr as sustained-release tablets. *Ventricular arrhythmias*—50 mg/kg/day in divided doses q 3 hr or q 12 hr for sustained-release tablets. Lower doses/longer dosing intervals are recommended for geriatric patients or those with renal, hepatic, or cardiac insufficiency.
■ **PO (Children):** 12.5 mg/kg (375 mg/m$^2$) 4 times daily.
■ **IM (Adults):** 50 mg/kg/day in divided doses q 3–6 hr.
■ **IV (Adults):** 100 mg q 5 min until arrhythmia is abolished or 1000 mg have been given; wait at least 10 min until further dosing *or* loading infusion of 500–600 mg over 25–

30 min followed by maintenance infusion of 2–6 mg/min.

## AVAILABILITY

■ *Tablets:* 250 mg^{Rx}, 375 mg^{Rx}, 500 mg^{Rx} ■ *Sustained-release tablets:* 500 mg^{Rx}, 1000 mg^{Rx} ■ *Capsules:* 250 mg^{Rx}, 375 mg^{Rx}, 500 mg^{Rx} ■ *Injection:* 100 mg/ml in 10-ml vials^{Rx}, 500 mg/ml in 2-ml vials and 2- and 4-ml pre-filled syringes^{Rx}.

TIME/ACTION PROFILE (antiarrhythmic effects)

| | ONSET | PEAK | DURATION |
|---|---|---|---|
| PO | 30 min | 60–90 min | 3–4 hr |
| PO-ER | unknown | unknown | 6–12 hr |
| IV | immediate | 25–60 min | 3–4 hr |
| IM | 10–30 min | 15–60 min | 3–4 hr |

# NURSING IMPLICATIONS

## ASSESSMENT

❏ Monitor ECG, pulse, and blood pressure continuously throughout IV administration. Parameters should be monitored periodically during oral administration. IV administration is usually discontinued if any of the following occur: arrhythmia is resolved, QRS complex widens by 50%, PR interval is prolonged, blood pressure drops >15 mm Hg, or toxic side effects develop. Patient should remain supine throughout IV administration to minimize hypotension.

■ *Lab Test Considerations:* CBC should be monitored every 2 wk during the first 3 mo of therapy. May cause decreased leukocyte, neutrophil, and platelet counts. Therapy may be discontinued if leukopenia occurs. Blood counts usually return to normal within 1 mo of discontinuation of therapy.

❏ Monitor ANA periodically during prolonged therapy or if symptoms of lupus-like reaction occur. Therapy is discontinued if a steady increase in ANA titer occurs.

❏ May cause an increase in AST, ALT, alkaline phosphatase, LDH, bilirubin, and a positive Coombs' test result.

■ *Toxicity and Overdose:* Serum procainamide and N-acetylprocainamide levels may be monitored periodically during dosage ad-

justment. Therapeutic blood level of procainamide is 4–8 mcg/ml.

❏ Toxicity may occur with procainamide blood levels of 8–16 mcg/ml or greater.

❏ Signs of toxicity include confusion, dizziness, drowsiness, decreased urination, nausea, vomiting, and tachyarrhythmias.

## POTENTIAL NURSING DIAGNOSES

■ Cardiac output, decreased (Indications).

## IMPLEMENTATION

■ **General:** When converting from IV to oral dose regimen, allow 3–4 hr to elapse between last IV dose and administration of first oral dose.

■ **PO:** Administer with a full glass of water on an empty stomach either 1 hr before or 2 hr after meals for faster absorption. If GI irritation becomes a problem, may be administered with or immediately after meals. Tablets may be crushed and capsules opened and mixed with food or fluids for patients with difficulty swallowing. Do not break, crush, or chew sustained-release tablets (Procan SR, Pronestyl-SR). Wax matrix of sustained-release tablets may be found in stool but is not significant.

■ **IM:** Used only when oral and IV routes are not feasible.

■ **Direct IV:** Dilute each 100 mg with 10 ml of D5W or sterile water for injection.

■ *Rate:* Administer at a rate not to exceed 25–50 mg/min. Rapid administration may cause ventricular fibrillation or asystole.

■ **Intermittent Infusion:** Prepare IV infusion by adding 200 mg–1 g to 50–500 ml of D5W for a concentration of 2–4 mg/ml. Slight yellow color of solution will not alter potency; do not use when darker than light amber or if solution contains a precipitate.

■ *Rate:* Administer initial infusion over 30 min. Maintenance infusion should infuse at 2–6 mg/min to maintain control of arrhythmia. Use infusion pump to ensure accurate dosage.

■ **Y-Site Compatibility:** ◆ amiodarone ◆ famotidine ◆ heparin ◆ hydrocortisone sodium succinate ◆ potassium chloride ◆ ranitidine ◆ vitamin B complex with C.

■ **Y-Site Incompatibility:** ◆ milrinone.

## PATIENT/FAMILY TEACHING

❑ Instruct patient to take medication around the clock, exactly as directed, even if feeling well. If a dose is missed, take as soon as remembered within 2 hr (4 hr for sustained-release tablets); omit if remembered later. Do not double doses. Consult health care professional prior to discontinuing medication, because gradual reduction in dosage may be needed to prevent worsening of condition.

❑ Instruct patient or family member on how to take pulse. Advise patient to report changes in pulse rate or rhythm to health care professional.

❑ May cause dizziness. Caution patient to avoid driving or other activities requiring alertness until response to medication is known.

❑ Advise patient to notify health care professional immediately if signs of drug-induced lupus syndrome (fever, chills, joint pain or swelling, pain with breathing, skin rash), leukopenia (sore throat, mouth, or gums), or thrombocytopenia (unusual bleeding or bruising) occur. Medication may be discontinued if these occur.

❑ Caution patient not to take OTC medications with procainamide without consulting health care professional.

❑ Advise patient to inform health care professional of medication regimen prior to treatment or surgery.

❑ Advise patient to carry identification at all times describing disease process and medication regimen.

❑ Emphasize the importance of routine follow-up exams to monitor progress.

## EVALUATION

**Effectiveness of therapy can be demonstrated by:** ■ Resolution of cardiac arrhythmias without detrimental side effects.

---

**procaine penicillin G, See PENICILLINS.**

---

## prochlorperazine

(proe-klor-**pair**-a-zeen)
Compazine, {Stemetil}, Ultrazine

---

## INDICATIONS

■ Management of nausea and vomiting ■ Treatment of psychoses ■ Treatment of anxiety.

## ACTION

■ Alters the effects of dopamine in the CNS ■ Possesses significant anticholinergic and alpha-adrenergic blocking activity ■ Depresses the chemoreceptor trigger zone (CTZ) in the CNS. **Therapeutic Effects:** ■ Diminished nausea and vomiting ■ Diminished signs and symptoms of psychoses or anxiety.

## PHARMACOKINETICS

**Absorption:** Absorption from tablet is variable; may be better with oral liquid formulations. Well absorbed after IM administration.

**Distribution:** Widely distributed, high concentrations in the CNS. Crosses the placenta and probably enters breast milk.

**Protein Binding:** ≥90%.

**Metabolism and Excretion:** Highly metabolized by the liver and GI mucosa. Converted to some compounds with antipsychotic activity.

**Half-life:** Unknown.

## CONTRAINDICATIONS AND PRECAUTIONS

**Contraindicated in:** ■ Hypersensitivity ■ Cross-sensitivity with other phenothiazines may exist ■ Narrow-angle glaucoma ■ Bone marrow depression ■ Severe liver or cardiovascular disease ■ Hypersensitivity to bisulfites or benzyl alcohol (some parenteral products) ■ Children <2 yr or 9.1 kg.

**Use Cautiously in:** ■ Geriatric or debilitated patients (dosage reduction recommended) ■ Diabetes mellitus ■ Respiratory disease ■ Prostatic hypertrophy ■ CNS tumors ■ Epilepsy ■ Intestinal obstruction ■ Pregnancy or lactation (safety not established).

## ADVERSE REACTIONS AND SIDE EFFECTS*

■ **CNS:** NEUROLEPTIC MALIGNANT SYNDROME, extrapyramidal reactions, sedation, tardive dyskinesia

- **EENT:** <u>blurred vision</u>, <u>dry eyes</u>, lens opacities
- **CV:** ECG changes, hypotension, tachycardia ■
**GI:** <u>constipation</u>, <u>dry mouth</u>, anorexia, drug-induced hepatitis, ileus ■ **GU:** pink or reddish-brown discoloration of urine, urinary retention
- **Derm:** photosensitivity, pigment changes, rashes ■ **Endo:** galactorrhea ■ **Hemat:** AGRANULOCYTOSIS, leukopenia ■ **Metab:** hyperthermia ■ **Misc:** allergic reactions.

## INTERACTIONS

**Drug-Drug:** ■ Additive hypotension with **antihypertensives, nitrates,** or acute ingestion of **alcohol** ■ Additive CNS depression with other **CNS depressants,** including **alcohol, antidepressants, antihistamines, opioid analgesics, sedative/hypnotics,** or **general anesthetics** ■ Additive anticholinergic effects with other **drugs possessing anticholinergic properties,** including **antihistamines,** some **antidepressants, atropine, haloperidol,** and other **phenothiazines** ■ **Lithium** increases the risk of extrapyramidal reactions ■ May mask early signs of **lithium** toxicity ■ Increased risk of agranulocytosis with **antithyroid agents** ■ Decreases the beneficial effects of **levodopa** ■ **Antacids** may decrease absorption.

**Drug-Natural Products:** ■ Concomitant use of **kava, valerian, skullcap, chamomile,** or **hops** can increase CNS depression ■ Increased anticholinergic effects with **angel's trumpet, jimson weed,** and **scopolia.**

## ROUTE AND DOSAGE

Pediatric dose should not exceed 10 mg on the 1st day and then should not exceed 20 mg/day in children 2–5 yr or 25 mg/day in children 6–12 yr.

### ◻ Antiemetic

- **PO (Adults and Children ≥12 yr):** 5–10 mg 3–4 times daily; may also be given as 15–30 mg once daily *or* 10 mg twice daily as ER capsules (up to 40 mg/day).
- **PO (Children 18–39 kg):** 2.5 mg 3 times daily *or* 5 mg twice daily (not to exceed 15 mg/day).
- **PO (Children 14–17 kg):** 2.5 mg 2–3 times daily (not to exceed 10 mg/day).

- **PO (Children 9–13 kg):** 2.5 mg 1–2 times daily (not to exceed 7.5 mg/day).
- **IM (Adults and Children ≥12 yr):** 5–10 mg q 3–4 hr as needed. *Nausea/vomiting associated with surgery*—5–10 mg; may be repeated once.
- **IM (Children 2–12 yr):** 132 mcg (0.132 mg)/kg; usually only 1 dose is required.
- **IV (Adults and Children ≥12 yr):** 2.5–10 mg (not to exceed 40 mg/day). *Nausea/vomiting associated with surgery*—5–10 mg; may be repeated once.
- **Rect (Adults):** 25 mg twice daily.
- **Rect (Children 18–39 kg):** 2.5 mg 3 times daily or 5 mg twice daily (not to exceed 15 mg/day).
- **Rect (Children 14–17 kg):** 2.5 mg 2–3 times daily (not to exceed 10 mg/day).
- **Rect (Children 9–13 kg):** 2.5 mg 1–2 times daily (not to exceed 7.5 mg/day).

### ◻ Antipsychotic

- **PO (Adults and Children ≥12 yr):** 5–10 mg 3–4 times daily; may be increased q 2–3 days (up to 150 mg/day).
- **PO (Children 2–12 yr):** 2.5 mg 2–3 times daily.
- **IM (Adults):** 10–20 mg q 2–4 hr for up to 4 doses, then 10–20 mg q 4–6 hr (up to 200 mg/day).
- **IM (Children 2–12 yr):** 132 mcg (0.132 mg)/kg (not to exceed 10 mg/dose).
- **IV (Adults and Children ≥12 yr):** 2.5–10 mg (up to 40 mg/day).
- **Rect (Adults):** 10 mg 3–4 times daily; may be increased by 5–10 mg q 2–3 days as needed.

### ◻ Antianxiety

- **PO (Adults and Children ≥12 yr):** 5 mg 3–4 times daily (not to exceed 20 mg/day or longer than 12 wk); may also be given as 15 mg once daily or 10 mg twice daily as ER capsules.
- **IM (Adults and Children ≥12 yr):** 5–10 mg q 3–4 hr as needed (up to 40 mg/day).
- **IM (Children 2–12 yr):** 132 mcg (0.132 mg)/kg.
- **IV (Adults):** 2.5–10 mg (up to 40 mg/day).

## AVAILABILITY (generic available)

■ **Tablets:** 5 mg$^{Rx}$, 10 mg$^{Rx}$, 25 mg$^{Rx}$ ■ Cost: Compazine—10 mg $100.55/100; generic— $82.94/100 ■ **Syrup (fruit flavor):** 5 mg/5 ml (edisylate)$^{Rx}$, {5 mg/5 ml (mesylate)$^{Rx}$} ■ **Extended-release capsules:** 10 mg$^{Rx}$, 15 mg$^{Rx}$, 30 mg$^{Rx}$ ■ **Injection:** 5 mg/ml (edisylate)$^{Rx}$, {5 mg/ml (mesylate)$^{Rx}$} ■ **Suppositories:** 2.5 mg$^{Rx}$, 5 mg$^{Rx}$, 25 mg$^{Rx}$.

TIME/ACTION PROFILE (antiemetic effect)

|  | ONSET | PEAK | DURATION |
|---|---|---|---|
| PO | 30–40 min | unknown | 3–4 hr |
| PO-ER | 30–40 min | unknown | 10–12 hr |
| Rect | 60 min | unknown | 3–4 hr |
| IM | 10–20 min | 10–30 min | 3–4 hr |
| IV | rapid (min) | 10–30 min | 3–4 hr |

# NURSING IMPLICATIONS

## ASSESSMENT

■ **General Info:** Monitor blood pressure (sitting, standing, lying down), ECG, pulse, and respiratory rate before and frequently during the period of dosage adjustment. May cause Q-wave and T-wave changes in ECG.

❑ Assess patient for level of sedation after administration.

❑ Monitor patient for onset of akathisia (restlessness or desire to keep moving) and extrapyramidal side effects (*parkinsonian*—difficulty speaking or swallowing, loss of balance control, pill rolling, mask-like face, shuffling gait, rigidity, tremors; and *dystonic*—muscle spasms, twisting motions, twitching, inability to move eyes, weakness of arms or legs) every 2 mo during therapy and 8–12 wk after therapy has been discontinued. Report these symptoms; reduction in dosage or discontinuation may be necessary. Trihexyphenidyl or diphenhydramine may be used to control these symptoms.

❑ Monitor for tardive dyskinesia (uncontrolled rhythmic movement of mouth, face, and extremities; lip smacking or puckering; puffing of cheeks; uncontrolled chewing; rapid or worm-like movements of tongue). Report immediately; may be irreversible.

❑ Monitor for development of neuroleptic malignant syndrome (fever, respiratory distress, tachycardia, seizures, diaphoresis, hypertension or hypotension, pallor, tiredness, severe muscle stiffness, loss of bladder control).

Notify physician or other health care professional immediately if these symptoms occur.

■ **Antiemetic:** Assess patient for nausea and vomiting before and 30–60 min after administration.

■ **Antipsychotic:** Monitor patient's mental status (orientation to reality and behavior) before and periodically throughout therapy.

❑ Observe patient carefully when administering oral medication to ensure that medication is actually taken and not hoarded.

❑ Assess fluid intake and bowel function. Increased bulk and fluids in the diet may help minimize constipation.

■ **Anxiety:** Assess degree and manifestations of anxiety and mental status before and periodically during therapy.

■ **Lab Test Considerations:** CBC and liver function tests should be evaluated periodically throughout course of therapy. May cause blood dyscrasias, especially between wks 4 and 10 of therapy. Hepatotoxicity is more likely to occur between wks 2 and 4 of therapy. May recur if medication is restarted. Liver function abnormalities may require discontinuation of therapy.

❑ May cause false-positive or false-negative pregnancy test results and false-positive urine bilirubin test results.

❑ May cause increased serum prolactin levels and interfere with gonadorelin test results.

## POTENTIAL NURSING DIAGNOSES

■ Fluid volume, deficit (Indications).

■ Thought processes, disturbed (Indications).

## IMPLEMENTATION

■ **General:** Do not confuse prochlorperazine with chlorpromazine.

❑ To prevent contact dermatitis, avoid getting solution on hands.

❑ Phenothiazines should be discontinued 48 hr before and not resumed for 24 hr after myelography; they lower seizure threshold.

■ **PO:** Do not crush or chew extended-release capsules. Administer with food, milk, or a full glass of water to minimize gastric irritation.

❑ Dilute syrup in citrus or chocolate-flavored drinks.

❑ Do not open, crush, or chew extended-release capsules.

- **IM:** Do not inject subcut. Inject slowly, deep into well-developed muscle. Keep patient recumbent for at least 30 min after injection to minimize hypotensive effects. Slight yellow color will not alter potency. Do not administer solution that is markedly discolored or that contains a precipitate.
- **Direct IV:** Dilute to a concentration of 1 mg/ml.
- **Rate:** Administer at a rate of 1 mg/min; not to exceed 5 mg/min.
- **Intermittent Infusion:** Dilute 20 mg in up to 1 L dextrose, saline, Ringer's or LR, dextrose/saline, dextrose/Ringer's, or lactated Ringer's combinations.
- **Syringe Incompatibility:** Manufacturer does not recommend mixing prochlorperazine with other medications in syringe.
- **Y-Site Compatibility:** ◆ calcium gluconate ◆ cisatracurium ◆ cisplatin ◆ cyclophosphamide ◆ cytarabine ◆ doxorubicin ◆ doxorubicin liposome ◆ fluconazole ◆ gatifloxacin ◆ granisetron ◆ heparin ◆ hydrocortisone sodium succinate ◆ linezolid ◆ melphalan ◆ methotrexate ◆ ondansetron ◆ paclitaxel ◆ potassium chloride ◆ propofol ◆ remifentanil ◆ sargramostim ◆ sufentanil ◆ teniposide ◆ thiotepa ◆ topotecan ◆ vinorelbine ◆ vitamin B complex with C.
- **Y-Site Incompatibility:** ◆ aldesleukin ◆ allopurinol ◆ amphotericin B cholesteryl ◆ amifostine ◆ aztreonam ◆ cefepime ◆ filgrastim ◆ fludarabine ◆ foscarnet ◆ piperacillin/tazobactam.

## PATIENT/FAMILY TEACHING

- Instruct patient to take medication exactly as directed, not to skip doses or double up on missed doses. If a dose is missed, it should be taken as soon as remembered unless almost time for next dose. If more than 2 doses are scheduled each day, missed dose should be taken within about 1 hr of the ordered time. Abrupt withdrawal may lead to gastritis, nausea, vomiting, dizziness, headache, tachycardia, and insomnia.
- Inform patient of possibility of extrapyramidal symptoms and tardive dyskinesia. Instruct patient to report these symptoms immediately to health care professional.
- Advise patient to change positions slowly to minimize orthostatic hypotension.
- May cause drowsiness. Caution patient to avoid driving or other activities requiring alertness until response to medication is known.
- Caution patient to avoid taking alcohol or other CNS depressants concurrently with this medication.
- Advise patient to use sunscreen and protective clothing when exposed to the sun to prevent photosensitivity reactions. Extremes in temperature should also be avoided, because this drug impairs body temperature regulation.
- Instruct patient to use frequent mouth rinses, good oral hygiene, and sugarless gum or candy to minimize dry mouth. Consult health care professional if dry mouth continues for >2 wk.
- Advise patient not to take prochlorperazine within 2 hr of antacids or antidiarrheal medication.
- Advise patient that increasing bulk and fluids in the diet and exercise may help minimize the constipating effects of this medication.
- Inform patient that this medication may turn urine pink to reddish-brown.
- Advise patient to notify health care professional of medication regimen before treatment or surgery.
- Instruct patient to notify health care professional promptly if sore throat, fever, unusual bleeding or bruising, skin rashes, weakness, tremors, visual disturbances, dark-colored urine, or clay-colored stools are noted.
- Emphasize the importance of routine follow-up exams to monitor response to medication and detect side effects. Periodic ocular exams are indicated. Encourage continued participation in psychotherapy as ordered by health care professional.

## EVALUATION

**Effectiveness of therapy can be demonstrated by:** ■ Relief of nausea and vomiting ■ Decrease in excitable, paranoic, or withdrawn behavior when used as an antipsychotic ■ Decrease in feelings of anxiety.

## progesterone

(proe-**jess**-te-rone)

Crinone, Prochieve, Prometrium

### CLASSIFICATION(S):

*Therapeutic: hormones*
*Pharmacologic: progestins*

### Pregnancy Category D

### INDICATIONS

■ Secondary amenorrhea and abnormal uterine bleeding due to hormonal imbalance ■ **Prometrium:** Prevention of cell overgrowth in the uterine lining in postmenopausal women who have not had a hysterectomy (with estrogen) ■ Part of assisted reproductive technology (ART) in the management of infertility (4% and 8% vaginal gel). **Unlabeled uses:** ■ Corpus luteum dysfunction.

### ACTION

■ Produces: ■ Secretory changes in the endometrium ■ Increase in basal body temperature ■ Histologic changes in vaginal epithelium ■ Relaxation of uterine smooth muscle ■ Mammary alveolar tissue growth ■ Pituitary inhibition ■ Withdrawal bleeding in the presence of estrogen. **Therapeutic Effects:** ■ Restoration of hormonal balance with control of uterine bleeding ■ Successful outcome in assisted reproduction.

### PHARMACOKINETICS

**Absorption:** Micronization increases oral and vaginal absorption.

**Distribution:** Enters breast milk.

**Protein Binding:** ≥90%.

**Metabolism and Excretion:** Metabolized by the liver; 50–60% eliminated by kidneys; 10% eliminated in feces.

**Half-life:** Several minutes.

### CONTRAINDICATIONS AND PRECAUTIONS

**Contraindicated in:** ■ Hypersensitivity ■ Hypersensitivity to parabens orsesame oil (IM suspension only) ■ Thromboembolic disease ■ Cerebrovascular disease ■ Severe liver disease ■ Breast or genital cancer ■ Porphyria ■ Missed abortion ■ Pregnancy (except corpus luteum dysfunction).

**Use Cautiously in:** ■ History of liver disease ■ Renal disease ■ Cardiovascular disease ■ Seizure disorders ■ Mental depression.

### ADVERSE REACTIONS AND SIDE EFFECTS*

■ **CNS:** depression ■ **EENT:** retinal thrombosis ■ **CV:** PULMONARY EMBOLISM, THROMBOEMBOLISM, thrombophlebitis ■ **GI:** gingival bleeding, hepatitis ■ **GU:** cervical erosions ■ **Derm:** chloasma, melasma, rashes ■ **Endo:** amenorrhea, breakthrough bleeding, breast tenderness, changes in menstrual flow, galactorrhea, spotting ■ **F and E:** edema ■ **Local:** irritation or pain at IM injection site ■ **Misc:** allergic reactions including ANAPHYLAXIS and ANGIOEDEMA, weight gain, weight loss.

### INTERACTIONS

**Drug-Drug:** ■ May ↓ effectiveness of **bromocriptine** when used concurrently for galactorrhea and amenorrhea.

### ROUTE AND DOSAGE

■ **PO (Adults):** *Secondary amenorrhea—* 400 mg once daily in the evening for 10 days; *prevention of postmenopausal estrogen-induced endometrial hyperplasia—* 200 mg once daily at bedtime for 14 days on days 8–21 of a 28-day cycle or on days 12–25 of a 30-day cycle; if patient currently receives ≥1.25 mg/day of estrogen, then a daily of dose of 300 mg of progesterone as 100 mg 2 hr after breakfast and 200 mg at bedtime is used; further adjustments may be required.

■ **Vag (Adults):** *Secondary amenorrhea—* 45 mg (1 applicatorful of 4% gel) once every other day for up to 6 doses, may be increased to 90 mg (1 applicatorful of 8% gel) once every other day for up to 6 doses; *Corpus luteum insufficiency or assisted reproduction technology—* For luteal phase support: 90 mg (1 applicatorful of 8% gel) once daily; for *in vitro* fertilization: 90 mg (1 applicatorful of 8% gel) once daily beginning within 24 hr of embryo transfer and continued through day 30 post-transfer (if pregnancy occurs, treatment may be continued for up to 10–12 wk); *partial or complete ovarian failure—* 90 mg (1 applicatorful of 8% gel) twice daily while undergoing donor oocyte transfer (if pregnancy occurs, treatment may be continued for up to 10–12 wk).

- **IM (Adults):** *Secondary amenorrhea*— 100–150 mg (single dose) or 5–10 mg daily for 6–8 days given 8–10 days before expected menstrual period. *Dysfunctional uterine bleeding*—5–10 mg daily for 6 days. *Corpus luteum insufficiency*—12.5 mg/day at onset of ovulation for 2 wk; may continue until 11th wk of gestation (unlabeled).

## AVAILABILITY (generic available)

- ***Micronized capsules (Prometrium):*** 100 mg$^{Rx}$, 200 mg$^{Rx}$ ■ Cost: 100 mg $79.58/100, 200 mg $151.21/100 ■ ***Bioadhesive vaginal gel (Prochieve):*** 4%$^{Rx}$, 8%$^{Rx}$ ■ ***Micronized vaginal gel (Crinone):*** 4%$^{Rx}$, 8%$^{Rx}$ ■ ***Injection:*** 50 mg/ml in 10-ml vials$^{Rx}$.

TIME/ACTION PROFILE (blood levels)

|  | ONSET | PEAK | DURATION |
|---|---|---|---|
| PO | unknown | 2–4 hr | unknown |
| Vaginal | unknown | 34.8–55 hr | unknown |
| IM | unknown | 19.6–28 hr | unknown |

# NURSING IMPLICATIONS

## ASSESSMENT

- **General Info:** Blood pressure be monitored periodically during therapy.
- ◻ Monitor intake and output ratios and weekly weight. Report significant discrepancies or steady weight gain.
- **Amenorrhea:** Assess patient's usual menstrual history. Administration of drug usually begins 8–10 days before anticipated menstruation. Withdrawal bleeding usually occurs 48–72 hr after course of therapy. Therapy should be discontinued if menses occur during injection series.
- **Dysfunctional Bleeding:** Monitor pattern and amount of vaginal bleeding (pad count). Bleeding should end by sixth day of therapy. Therapy should be discontinued if menses occur during injection series.
- ***Lab Test Considerations:*** Monitor hepatic function before and periodically during therapy.
- ◻ May cause ↑ plasma amino acid and alkaline phosphatase levels.
- ◻ May ↓ pregnanediol excretion concentrations.

- ◻ May cause ↑ serum concentrations of LDL and ↓ concentrations of HDL.
- ◻ High doses may ↑ sodium and chloride excretion.
- ◻ May alter thyroid function test results.

## POTENTIAL NURSING DIAGNOSES

- Sexual dysfunction (Indications).

## IMPLEMENTATION

- **IM:** Shake vial before preparing IM dose. Administer deep IM. Rotate sites.
- **Vag:** Vaginal gel is administered with disposable applicator provided by manufacturer.
- ◻ If dose increase is required from 4% gel to 8% gel, doubling the volume of the 4% gel will not accomplish dose increase; changing to 8% gel is required.

## PATIENT/FAMILY TEACHING

- **General Info:** Advise patient to report signs and symptoms of fluid retention (swelling of ankles and feet, weight gain), thromboembolic disorders (pain, swelling, tenderness in extremities, headache, chest pain, blurred vision), mental depression, or hepatic dysfunction (yellowed skin or eyes, pruritus, dark urine, light-colored stools) to health care professional.
- ◻ Instruct patient to notify health care professional if change in vaginal bleeding pattern or spotting occurs.
- ◻ Instruct patient to stop taking medication and notify health care professional if pregnancy is suspected.
- ◻ Caution patient to use sunscreen and protective clothing to prevent photosensitivity reactions.
- ◻ Advise patient to notify health care professional of medication regimen before treatment or surgery.
- ◻ Emphasize the importance of routine follow-up physical exams, including blood pressure; breast, abdomen, and pelvic examinations; and Pap smears.
- **Vag:** Instruct patient not use vaginal gel concurrently with other vaginal agents. If these agents must be used concurrently, administer at least 6 hr before or after vaginal gel.

## EVALUATION

**Effectiveness of therapy can be demonstrated by:** ■ Development of normal cyclic menses ■ Successful outcome in assisted reproduction.

## promethazine

(proe-**meth**-a-zeen)

Anergan, Antinaus, {Histanil}, Pentazine, Phenazine, Phencen-50, Phenergan, Phenergan Fortis, Phenergan Plain, Phenerzine, Phenoject, Pro-50, Promacot, Pro-Med, Promet, Prorex, Prothazine, Shogan, V-Gan

### CLASSIFICATION(S):

**Therapeutic:** *antiemetics, antihistamines, sedative/hypnotics*
**Pharmacologic:** *phenothiazines*

### Pregnancy Category C

## INDICATIONS

■ Treatment of various allergic conditions and motion sickness ■ Preoperative sedation ■ Treatment and prevention of nausea and vomiting ■ Adjunct to anesthesia and analgesia.

## ACTION

■ Blocks the effects of histamine ■ Has inhibitory effect on the chemoreceptor trigger zone in the medulla, resulting in antiemetic properties ■ Alters the effects of dopamine in the CNS ■ Possesses significant anticholinergic activity ■ Produces CNS depression by indirectly decreased stimulation of the CNS reticular system. **Therapeutic Effects:** ■ Relief of symptoms of histamine excess usually seen in allergic conditions ■ Diminished nausea or vomiting ■ Sedation.

## PHARMACOKINETICS

**Absorption:** Well absorbed after oral and IM administration; rectal administration may be less reliable.

**Distribution:** Widely distributed; crosses the blood-brain barrier and the placenta.

**Protein Binding:** 65–90%.

**Metabolism and Excretion:** Metabolized by the liver.

**Half-life:** Unknown.

## CONTRAINDICATIONS AND PRECAUTIONS

**Contraindicated in:** ■ Hypersensitivity ■ Comatose patients ■ Prostatic hypertrophy ■ Bladder neck obstruction ■ Some products contain alcohol or bisulfites and should be avoided in patients with known intolerance ■ Narrow-angle glaucoma.

**Use Cautiously in:** ■ Hypertension ■ Sleep apnea ■ Epilepsy ■ Underlying bone marrow depression ■ Pregnancy (has been used safely during labor; avoid chronic use during pregnancy) ■ Lactation (safety not established; may cause drowsiness in infant).

## ADVERSE REACTIONS AND SIDE EFFECTS*

■ **CNS:** NEUROLEPTIC MALIGNANT SYNDROME, confusion, disorientation, sedation, dizziness, extrapyramidal reactions, fatigue, insomnia, nervousness ■ **EENT:** blurred vision, diplopia, tinnitus ■ **CV:** bradycardia, hypertension, hypotension, tachycardia ■ **GI:** constipation, drug-induced hepatitis, dry mouth ■ **Derm:** photosensitivity, rashes ■ **Hemat:** blood dyscrasias.

## INTERACTIONS

**Drug-Drug:** ■ Additive CNS depression with other **CNS depressants,** including **alcohol,** other **antihistamines, opioid analgesics,** and other **sedative/hypnotics** ■ Additive anticholinergic effects with other **drugs possessing anticholinergic properties,** including other **antihistamines, antidepressants, atropine, haloperidol,** other **phenothiazines, quinidine,** and **disopyramide** ■ Concurrent use with **MAO inhibitors** may result in increased sedation and anticholinergic side effects.

## ROUTE AND DOSAGE

❑ **Antihistamine**

■ **PO (Adults):** 25 mg at bedtime or 10–12.5 mg 4 times daily.

■ **PO (Children ≥2 yr):** 5–12.5 mg 3 times daily or 25 mg at bedtime.

■ **IM, IV, Rect (Adults):** 25 mg; may repeat in 2 hr.

■ **Rect (Children ≥2 yr):** 0.125 mg/kg (3.75 mg/m²) q 4–6 hr *or* 0.5 mg/kg (15 mg/m²) at bedtime; may also be given as 6.25–12.5 mg 3 times daily *or* 25 mg at bedtime.

- **Antivertigo (Motion Sickness)**
- **PO (Adults):** 25 mg 30–60 min before departure; may be repeated in 8–12 hr.
- **PO (Children ≥2 yr):** 10–25 mg or 0.5 mg/kg 30–60 min before departure; may be given twice daily.
- **Sedation**
- **PO, Rect, IM, IV (Adults):** 25–50 mg.
- **PO, Rect, IM (Children >2 yr):** 10–25 mg *or* 0.5–1.1 mg/kg.
- **Sedation during Labor**
- **IM, IV (Adults):** 50 mg in early labor; when labor is established, additional doses of 25–75 mg may be given 1–2 times at 4-hr intervals (24-hr dose should not exceed 100 mg).
- **Antiemetic**
- **PO, Rect, IM, IV (Adults):** 10–25 mg q 4 hr as needed; initial PO dose should be 25 mg.
- **PO, Rect, IM (Children ≥2 yr):** 0.25–0.5 mg/kg (7.5–15 mg/m²) q 4–6 hr *or* 10–25 mg q 4–6 hr.

## AVAILABILITY (generic available)

- **Tablets:** 10 mg$^{OTC}$, 12.5 mg$^{Rx}$, {12.5 mg$^{OTC}$}, 25 mg$^{Rx}$, {25 mg$^{OTC}$}, 50 mg$^{Rx}$, {50 mg$^{OTC}$} ■ Cost: *Phenergan*—25 mg $40.28/100; *generic*—$0.18/5 ■ **Syrup (cherry flavor):** 3.25 mg/120 ml$^{Rx}$, 6.25 mg/5 ml$^{Rx}$, {10 mg/5 ml$^{OTC}$}, 25 mg/5 ml$^{Rx}$ ■ Cost: *Phenergan*—$27.50/480 ml; *generic*—$4.50–$7.50/480 ml ■ **Injection:** 25 mg/ml in 1-ml ampules and 1- and 10-ml vials$^{Rx}$, 50 mg/ml in 1-ml ampules and 10-ml vials$^{Rx}$ ■ Cost: 25 mg/ml $20.00/1 ml, 50 mg/ml $25.00/1 ml ■ **Suppositories:** 2.5 mg$^{Rx}$, 5 mg$^{Rx}$, 25 mg$^{Rx}$ ■ Cost: 2.5 mg $31.16/12, 5 mg $34.61/12, 25 mg $42.83/12. ■ codeine, dextromethorphan, phenylephrine, and/or pseudoephedrine in a variety of cough and cold preparations$^{Rx}$. See Appendix B.

TIME/ACTION PROFILE (noted as antihistaminic effects; sedative effects last 2–8 hr)

|  | ONSET | PEAK | DURATION |
|---|---|---|---|
| PO, IM | 20 min | unknown | 4–12 hr |
| Rectal | 20 min | unknown | 4–12 hr |
| IV | 3–5 min | unknown | 4–12 hr |

# NURSING IMPLICATIONS

## ASSESSMENT

- **General Info:** Monitor blood pressure, pulse, and respiratory rate frequently in patients receiving IV doses.
- Assess patient for level of sedation after administration.
- Monitor patient for onset of extrapyramidal side effects (*akathisia*—restlessness; *dystonia*—muscle spasms and twisting motions; *pseudoparkinsonism*—mask-like face, rigidity, tremors, drooling, shuffling gait, dysphagia). Notify physician or other health care professional if these symptoms occur.
- **Allergy:** Assess allergy symptoms (rhinitis, conjunctivitis, hives) before and periodically throughout course of therapy.
- **Antiemetic:** Assess patient for nausea and vomiting before and after administration.
- **Lab Test Considerations:** May cause false-positive or false-negative pregnancy test results.
- CBC should be evaluated periodically during chronic therapy; blood dyscrasias may occur.
- May cause increased serum glucose.
- May cause false-negative results in skin tests using allergen extracts. Promethazine should be discontinued 72 hr before the test.

## POTENTIAL NURSING DIAGNOSES

- Fluid volume, deficit (Indications).
- Injury, risk for (Side Effects).

## IMPLEMENTATION

- **General:** When administering promethazine concurrently with opioid analgesics, supervise ambulation closely to prevent injury from increased sedation.
- **PO:** Administer with food, water, or milk to minimize GI irritation. Tablets may be crushed and mixed with food or fluids for patients with difficulty swallowing.
- **IM:** Administer deep into well-developed muscle. Subcut administration may cause tissue necrosis.
- **Direct IV:** Doses should not exceed a concentration of 25 mg/ml. Slight yellow color does not alter potency. Do not use if precipitate is present.

{ } = Available in Canada only.
*CAPITALS indicates life-threatening; underlines indicate most frequent.

■ **Rate:** Administer each 25 mg slowly, over at least 1 min. Rapid administration may produce a transient fall in blood pressure.

■ **Solution Compatibility:** ◆ dextrose ◆ saline ◆ Ringer's or LR ◆ dextrose/saline ◆ dextrose/Ringer's ◆ lactated Ringer's combinations.

■ **Syringe Compatibility:** ◆ atropine ◆ butorphanol ◆ cimetidine ◆ droperidol ◆ fentanyl ◆ glycopyrrolate ◆ hydromorphone ◆ meperidine ◆ metoclopramide ◆ midazolam ◆ pentazocine ◆ ranitidine ◆ scopolamine.

■ **Syringe Incompatibility:** ◆ heparin ◆ ketorolac ◆ pentobarbital ◆ thiopental.

■ **Y-Site Compatibility:** ◆ amifostine ◆ ztreonam ◆ ciprofloxacin ◆ cisatracurium ◆ cisplatin ◆ cyclophosphamide ◆ cytarabine ◆ doxorubicin ◆ filgrastim ◆ fluconazole ◆ fludarabine ◆ gatifloxacin ◆ linezolid ◆ melphalan ◆ ondansetron ◆ remifentanil ◆ sargramostim ◆ teniposide ◆ thiotepa ◆ vinorelbine.

■ **Y-Site Incompatibility:** ◆ aldesleukin ◆ amphotericin B cholesteryl ◆ cefepime ◆ cefoperazone ◆ cefotetan ◆ doxorubicin liposome ◆ foscarnet ◆ methotrexate ◆ piperacillin/tazobactam.

## PATIENT/FAMILY TEACHING

■ **General Info:** Review dosage schedule with patient. If medication is ordered regularly and a dose is missed, take as soon as remembered unless time for next dose.

❏ May cause drowsiness. Caution patient to avoid driving or other activities requiring alertness until response to medication is known.

❏ Advise patient that frequent mouth rinses, good oral hygiene, and sugarless gum or candy may decrease dry mouth. Health care professional should be notified if dry mouth persists >2 wk.

❏ Caution patient to use sunscreen and protective clothing to prevent photosensitivity reactions.

❏ Advise patient to change positions slowly to minimize orthostatic hypotension. Geriatric patients are at increased risk for this side effect.

❏ Caution patient to avoid concurrent use of alcohol and other CNS depressants with this medication.

❏ Instruct patient to notify health care professional if sore throat, fever, jaundice, or uncontrolled movements are noted.

■ **Motion Sickness:** When used as prophylaxis for motion sickness, advise patient to take medication at least 30 min and preferably 1–2 hr before exposure to conditions that may cause motion sickness.

## EVALUATION

**Effectiveness of therapy can be demonstrated by:** ■ Relief from allergic symptoms ■ Prevention of motion sickness ■ Sedation ■ Relief from nausea and vomiting.

## propafenone

(proe-**paff**-e-nown)
Rythmol

**CLASSIFICATION(S):**
**Therapeutic:** antiarrhythmics (class IC)

**Pregnancy Category C**

## INDICATIONS

■ Treatment of life-threatening ventricular arrhythmias, including ventricular tachycardia ■ Prolongs the time to recurrence of symptomatic paroxysmal atrial arrhythmias, including paroxysmal atrial fibrillation/flutter (PAF) and paroxysmal supraventricular tachycardia (PSVT).

## ACTION

■ Slows conduction in cardiac tissue by altering transport of ions across cell membranes. **Therapeutic Effects:** ■ Suppression of ventricular arrhythmias.

## PHARMACOKINETICS

**Absorption:** Although well absorbed following oral administration, undergoes rapid hepatic metabolism (bioavailability 3–11%).

**Distribution:** Widely distributed; crosses the placenta.

**Metabolism and Excretion:** Extensively metabolized by the liver (CYP 1A2, CYP2D6, and CYP3A4 enzyme systems), some metabolites have antiarrhythmic activity. >90% of patients are considered extensive metabolizers. Others metabolize propafenone more slowly.

**Half-life:** 2–10 hr in extensive metabolizers, 10–32 hr in slow metabolizers.

## CONTRAINDICATIONS AND PRECAUTIONS

**Contraindicated in:** ■ Hypersensitivity ■ Cardiogenic shock ■ Conduction disorders including sick sinus syndrome and AV block (without a pacemaker) ■ Bradycardia ■ Severe hypotension ■ Nonallergic bronchospasm ■ Electrolyte disturbances ■ Uncontrolled CHF.

**Use Cautiously in:** ■ Severe hepatic or renal impairment (dosage reduction may be necessary) ■ Geriatric patients (lower doses may be necessary) ■ Pregnancy, lactation, or children (safety not established).

## ADVERSE REACTIONS AND SIDE EFFECTS*

■ **CNS:** dizziness, shaking, weakness ■ **EENT:** blurred vision ■ **CV:** SUPRAVENTRICULAR ARRHYTHMIA, VENTRICULAR ARRHYTHMIAS, conduction disturbances, angina, bradycardia, hypotension ■ **GI:** altered taste, constipation, nausea, vomiting, diarrhea, dry mouth ■ **Derm:** rash ■ **MS:** joint pain.

## INTERACTIONS

**Drug-Drug:** ■ Any **inhibitors of the CYP1A2, CYP2D6, or CYP3A4 enzyme systems** may ↑ levels ■ ↑ serum **digoxin** levels by 35–85% ( ↓ dosage may be required) ■ ↑ blood levels of **metoprolol** and **propranolol** ( ↓ dosage may be required) ■ Concurrent use of **local anesthetics** may ↑ risk of CNS adverse reactions ■ ↑ effects of **warfarin** ( ↓ warfarin dose by 25–50%) ■ May ↑ **cyclosporine** through blood levels and risk of ne phrotoxicity ■ **Rifampin** may ↓ serum levels and effectiveness of propafenone.

## ROUTE AND DOSAGE

■ **PO (Adults):** 150 mg q 8 hr; may be gradually increased at 3–4-day intervals as required up to 300 mg q 8–12 hr.

## AVAILABILITY

■ *Tablets:* 150 mg$^{Rx}$, 225 mg$^{Rx}$, 300 mg$^{Rx}$.

TIME/ACTION PROFILE (antiarrhythmic effects)

| | ONSET | PEAK | DURATION |
|---|---|---|---|
| PO | hrs–days | 4–5 days† | hrs |

†Chronic dosing.

## NURSING IMPLICATIONS

### ASSESSMENT

❑ Monitor ECG or use Holter monitor prior to and periodically during therapy. May cause PR and QT prolongation.

❑ Monitor blood pressure and pulse periodically during therapy.

❑ Monitor intake and output ratios and daily weight. Assess patients for signs of CHF (peripheral edema, rales/crackles, dyspnea, weight gain, jugular venous distention). May require reduction or discontinuation of therapy.

■ *Lab Test Considerations:* May cause ↑ ANA titer, which is usually asymptomatic and reversible.

■ *Toxicity and Overdose:* Signs of toxicity include hypotension, excessive drowsiness, and decreased or abnormal heart rate. Notify physician or other health care professional if these signs occur.

### POTENTIAL NURSING DIAGNOSES

■ Cardiac output, decreased (Indications).

### IMPLEMENTATION

■ **PO:** Propafenone therapy should be initiated in a hospital with facilities for cardiac rhythm monitoring. Most serious proarrhythmic effects are seen in the first 2 wk of therapy.

❑ Previous antiarrhythmic therapy should be withdrawn 2–5 half-lives before starting propafenone.

❑ Dose adjustments should be at least 3–4 days apart because of the long half-life of propafenone.

❑ Correct pre-existing hypokalemia or hyperkalemia prior to instituting therapy.

### PATIENT/FAMILY TEACHING

❑ Instruct patient to take medication around the clock exactly as directed, even if feeling better. Take missed doses as soon as remembered if within 4 hr; omit if remembered later. Gradual dosage reduction may be necessary.

{ } = Available in Canada only.
*CAPITALS indicates life-threatening; underlines indicate most frequent.

- May cause dizziness. Caution patient to avoid driving and other activities requiring alertness until response to medication is known.
- Advise patient to notify health care professional of medication regimen prior to treatment or surgery.
- Instruct patient to notify health care professional if fever, sore throat, chills, or unusual bleeding or bruising occurs or if chest pain, shortness of breath, diaphoresis, palpitations, or visual changes become bothersome.
- Advise patient to carry identification describing disease process and medication regimen at all times.
- Emphasize the importance of follow-up exams to monitor progress.

## EVALUATION

**Effectiveness of therapy can be demonstrated by:** ■ Decrease in frequency of ventricular arrhythmias ■ Prolonged time to recurrence of symptomatic paroxysmal atrial arrhythmias, including paroxysmal atrial fibrillation/flutter and PSVT.

## propofol
(**proe**-poe-fol)
Diprivan, Disoprofol

**CLASSIFICATION(S):**
**Therapeutic:** general anesthetics

**Pregnancy Category B**

## INDICATIONS

■ Induction of general anesthesia ■ Maintenance of balanced anesthesia when used with other agents ■ Initiation and maintenance of monitored anesthesia care (MAC) ■ Sedation of intubated, mechanically ventilated patients in intensive care units (ICUs).

## ACTION

■ Short-acting hypnotic. Mechanism of action is unknown ■ Produces amnesia ■ Has no analgesic properties. **Therapeutic Effects:** ■ Induction and maintenance of anesthesia.

## PHARMACOKINETICS

**Absorption:** Administered IV only, resulting in complete absorption.

**Distribution:** Rapidly and widely distributed. Crosses the blood-brain barrier well; rapidly redistributed to other tissues. Crosses the placenta and enters breast milk.
**Protein Binding:** 95–99%.
**Metabolism and Excretion:** Rapidly metabolized by the liver.
**Half-life:** 3–12 hr (blood-brain equilibration half-life 2.9 min).

## CONTRAINDICATIONS AND PRECAUTIONS

**Contraindicated in:** ■ Hypersensitivity to propofol, soybean oil, egg lecithin, or glycerol ■ Labor and delivery.

**Use Cautiously in:** ■ Cardiovascular disease ■ Lipid disorders (emulsion may have detrimental effect) ■ Increased intracranial pressure ■ Cerebrovascular disorders ■ Geriatric (>60 yr), debilitated, or hypovolemic patients (lower induction and maintenance dosage reduction recommended) ■ Children <2 mos or lactation (safety not established).

## ADVERSE REACTIONS AND SIDE EFFECTS*

■ **CNS:** dizziness, headache ■ **Resp:** APNEA, cough ■ **CV:** bradycardia, hypotension, hypertension ■ **GI:** abdominal cramping, hiccups, nausea, vomiting ■ **Derm:** flushing ■ **Local:** burning, pain, stinging, coldness, numbness, tingling at IV site ■ **MS:** involuntary muscle movements, perioperative myoclonia ■ **Misc:** fever.

## INTERACTIONS

**Drug-Drug:** ■ Additive CNS and respiratory depression with **alcohol, antihistamines, opioid analgesics,** and **sedative/hypnotics** (dosage reduction may be required) ■ Increased risk of hypertriglyceridemia with **intravenous fat emulsion.**

## ROUTE AND DOSAGE

- **General Anesthesia**

- **IV (Adults <55 yr):** *Induction*—40 mg q 10 sec until induction achieved (2–2.5 mg/kg total). *Maintenance*—100–200 mcg/kg/min. Rates of 150–200 mcg/kg/min are usually required during first 10–15 min after induction, then decreased by 30–50% during first 30 min of maintenance. Rates of 50–100 mcg/kg/min are associated with optimal recovery time. May also be given intermittently in increments of 25–50 mg.

- **IV (Geriatric Patients, Cardiac patients, Debilitated Patients, or Hypovolemic Patients):** *Induction*—20 mg q 10 sec until induction achieved (1–1.5 mg/kg total). *Maintenance*—50–100 mcg/kg/min (dose in cardiac anesthesia ranges from 50–150 mcg/kg/min depending on concurrent use of opioid).

- **IV (Adults Undergoing Neurosurgical Procedures):** *Induction*—20 mg q 10 sec until induction achieved (1–2 mg/kg total). *Maintenance*—100–200 mcg/kg/min.

- **IV (Children ≥3 yr–16 yr):** *Induction*—2.5–3.5 mg/kg.

- **IV (Children 2 mos–16 yr):** *Maintenance*—125–300 mcg/kg/min (following first 30 min of maintenance, rate should be decreased if possible).

- **Monitored Anesthesia Care (MAC) Sedation**

- **IV (Adults <55 yr):** *Initiation*—100–150 mcg/kg/min infusion *or* 0.5 mg/kg as slow injection. *Maintenance*—25–75 mcg/kg/min infusion or incremental boluses of 10–20 mg.

- **IV (Geriatric Patients, Debilitated Patients, or ASA III/IV Patients):** *Initiation*—Use slower infusion or injection rates. *Maintenance*—20% less than the usual adult infusion dose; rapid/repeated bolus dosing should be avoided.

- **ICU Sedation**

- **IV (Adults):** 5 mcg/kg/min for a minimum of 5 min. Additional increments of 5–10 mcg/kg/min over 5–10 min may be given until desired response is obtained. (Range 5–50 mcg/kg/min.) Dose should be reassessed every 24 hr.

## AVAILABILITY (generic available)

- *Injection:* 10 mg/ml in 20-ml ampules, 50- and 100-ml infusion vials[Rx].

TIME/ACTION PROFILE (loss of consciousness)

| | ONSET | PEAK | DURATION† |
|---|---|---|---|
| IV | 40 sec | unknown | 3–5 min |

†Time to recovery is 8 min (up to 19 min if opioid analgesics have been used).

# NURSING IMPLICATIONS
## ASSESSMENT

- Assess respiratory status, pulse, and blood pressure continuously throughout propofol therapy. Frequently causes apnea lasting ≥60 sec. Maintain patent airway and adequate ventilation. Propofol should be used only by individuals experienced in endotracheal intubation, and equipment for this procedure should be readily available.

- Assess level of sedation and level of consciousness throughout and following administration.

- **Toxicity and Overdose:** If overdose occurs, monitor pulse, respiration, and blood pressure continuously. Maintain patent airway and assist ventilation as needed. If hypotension occurs, treatment includes IV fluids, repositioning, and vasopressors.

## POTENTIAL NURSING DIAGNOSES

- Breathing pattern, ineffective (Adverse Reactions).
- Injury, risk for (Side Effects).

## IMPLEMENTATION

- **General:** Do not confuse Diprivan (propofol) with Diflucan (fluconazole).
- Dose is titrated to patient response.
- Propofol has no effect on the pain threshold. Adequate analgesia should *always* be used when propofol is used as an adjunct to surgical procedures.
- **Direct IV:** Shake well before use. If diluted prior to administration, use only D5W and dilute to a concentration not less than 2 mg/ml. Solution is opaque, making detection of contaminants difficult. Do not use if separation of the emulsion is evident. Contains no preservatives; maintain sterile technique and administer immediately after preparation. Discard unused portions and IV lines at the end of procedure or within 6 hr. For ICU sedation, discard after 12 hr if administered directly from vial or after 6 hr if transferred to a syringe or other container.
- Aseptic technique is essential. Solution is capable of rapid growth of bacterial contaminants. Infections and subsequent deaths have been reported.

{ } = Available in Canada only.
*CAPITALS indicates life-threatening; underlines indicate most frequent.

❑ Frequently causes pain, burning, and stinging at injection site; use larger veins of the forearm, antecubital fossa, or a dedicated IV catheter. Lidocaine 10–20 mg IV may be administered prior to injection to minimize pain.

■ **Rate:** Administer over 3–5 min. Titrate to desired level of sedation.

■ **Continuous Infusion:** Intermittent/May be administered as an intermittent or continuous infusion (see Route and Dosage for rate). Administer via infusion pump to ensure accurate rate. Wake-up and assessment of CNS function should be done daily throughout maintenance to determine minimum dose required for sedation. Maintain a light level of sedation during these assessments; do not discontinue. Abrupt discontinuation may cause rapid awakening with anxiety, agitation, and resistance to mechanical ventilation.

■ **Solution Compatibility:** ◆ D5W ◆ LR ◆ D5/LR ◆ D5/0.45% NaCl ◆ D5/0.2% NaCl.

■ **Y-Site Compatibility:** ◆ acyclovir ◆ alfentanil ◆ ampicillin ◆ aztreonam ◆ bumetanide ◆ buprenorphine ◆ butorphanol ◆ calcium gluconate ◆ carboplatin ◆ cefazolin ◆ cefipime ◆ cefoperazone ◆ cefotaxime ◆ cefotetan ◆ cefoxitin ◆ ceftazidime ◆ ceftizoxime ◆ ceftriaxone ◆ cefuroxime ◆ chlorpromazine ◆ cimetidine ◆ cisplatin ◆ clindamycin ◆ cyclophosphamide ◆ cyclosporine ◆ cytarabine ◆ dexamethasone sodium phosphate ◆ diphenhydramine ◆ dobutamine ◆ dopamine ◆ doxycycline ◆ droperidol ◆ enalaprilat ◆ epinephrine ◆ esmolol ◆ famotidine ◆ fentanyl ◆ fluconazole ◆ fluorouracil ◆ furosemide ◆ ganciclovir ◆ glycopyrrolate ◆ granisetron ◆ haloperidol ◆ heparin ◆ hydrocortisone sodium succinate ◆ hydromorphone ◆ ifosfamide ◆ imipenem/cilastatin ◆ inamrinone ◆ insulin ◆ isoproterenol ◆ ketamine ◆ labetalol ◆ levorphanol ◆ lidocaine ◆ lorazepam ◆ magnesium sulfate ◆ mannitol ◆ meperidine ◆ milrinone ◆ nafcillin ◆ nalbuphine ◆ naloxone ◆ nitroglycerin ◆ nitroprusside ◆ norepinephrine ◆ ofloxacin ◆ paclitaxel ◆ pentobatbital ◆ phenobarbital ◆ piperacillin ◆ potassium chloride ◆ prochlorperazine ◆ propranolol ◆ ranitidine ◆ scopolamine ◆ sodium bicarbonate ◆ succinylcholine ◆ sufentanil ◆ ticarcillin ◆ ticarcillin/clavulanate ◆ vecuronium.

■ **Y-Site Incompatibility:** ◆ amikacin ◆ amphotericin ◆ atracurium ◆ bretylium ◆ blood ◆ calcium chloride ◆ ciprofloxacin ◆ diazepam ◆ digoxin ◆ doxorubicin ◆ gentamicin ◆ levofloxacin ◆ methotrexate ◆ methylprednisolone sodium succinate ◆ metoclopramide ◆ minocycline ◆ mitoxantrone ◆ netilmicin ◆ phenytoin ◆ plasma ◆ tobramycin ◆ verapamil.

■ **Additive Incompatibility:** Manufacturer does not recommend admixing propofol with other medications.

## PATIENT/FAMILY TEACHING

❑ Inform patient that this medication will decrease mental recall of the procedure.

❑ May cause drowsiness or dizziness. Advise patient to request assistance prior to ambulation and transfer and to avoid driving or other activities requiring alertness for 24 hr following administration.

❑ Advise patient to avoid alcohol or other CNS depressants without the advice of a health care professional for 24 hr following administration.

## EVALUATION

**Effectiveness of therapy can be demonstrated by:** ■ Induction and maintenance of anesthesia ❑ Amnesia ■ Sedation in mechanically ventilated patients in an intensive care setting.

# PROPOXYPHENE

**propoxyphene hydrochloride**
(pro-**pox**-i-feen hye-droe-**klor**-ide)
Darvon

**propoxyphene hydrochloride/aspirin/caffeine**
Darvon Compound-65

**propoxyphene napsylate**
(pro-**pox**-i-feen **nap**-si-late)
Darvon N

**propoxyphene napsylate/acetaminophen**
Darvocet-N, Propacet, Propoxyphene with APAP, Wygesic

**propoxyphene napsylate/aspirin**
{Darvon-N with ASA}

## propoxyphene/aspirin/caffeine
{Darvon-N Compound}, {692}

### CLASSIFICATION(S):
**Therapeutic:** *opioid analgesics*
**Pharmacologic:** *opioid agonists, opioid agonists/nonopioid analgesic combinations*

### Pregnancy Category C

See also Acetaminophen monograph and Salicylates monograph.

## INDICATIONS
■ Mild to moderate pain.

## ACTION
■ Binds to opiate receptors in the CNS ■ Alters the perception of and response to painful stimuli, while producing generalized CNS depression. **Therapeutic Effects:** ■ Decrease in mild to moderate pain.

## PHARMACOKINETICS
**Absorption:** Well absorbed following oral administration. Napsylate salt is more slowly absorbed.

**Distribution:** Widely distributed. Probably crosses the placenta. Enters breast milk in small amounts.

**Metabolism and Excretion:** Mostly metabolized by the liver. Some conversion to norpropoxyphene, a toxic metabolite. This metabolite accumulates in elderly patients and patients with decreased renal function.

**Half-life:** 6–12 hr.

## CONTRAINDICATIONS AND PRECAUTIONS
**Contraindicated in:** ■ Hypersensitivity ■ Pregnancy or lactation (avoid chronic use) ■ Children.

**Use Cautiously in:** ■ Head trauma ■ Increased intracranial pressure ■ Severe renal, hepatic, or pulmonary disease ■ Hypothyroidism ■ Adrenal insufficiency ■ Alcoholism ■ Geriatric or debilitated patients (dosage reduction recommended) ■ Undiagnosed abdominal pain ■ Prostatic hypertrophy ■ Lactation (has been used safely).

## ADVERSE REACTIONS AND SIDE EFFECTS*
■ **CNS:** dizziness, weakness, dysphoria, euphoria, headache, insomnia, paradoxical excitement, sedation ■ **EENT:** blurred vision ■ **CV:** hypotension ■ **GI:** nausea, abdominal pain, constipation, vomiting ■ **Derm:** rashes ■ **Misc:** physical dependence, psychological dependence, tolerance.

## INTERACTIONS
**Drug-Drug:** ■ Use with extreme caution in patients receiving **MAO inhibitors** (may result in unpredictable, severe, and potentially fatal reactions—decrease initial dose to 25% of usual dose) ■ Additive CNS depression with **alcohol, antidepressants,** and **sedative/hypnotics** ■ **Smoking** increases metabolism and may decrease analgesic effectiveness ■ Administration of **partial-antagonist opioid analgesics** may precipitate withdrawal in physically dependent patients ■ **Nalbuphine, buprenorphine,** or **pentazocine** may decrease analgesia.

**Drug-Natural Products:** ■ Concomitant use of **kava, valerian, skullcap, chamomile,** or **hops** can increase CNS depression.

## ROUTE AND DOSAGE
Consider cumulative effects of additional acetaminophen/aspirin; if toxic levels are exceeded, change to pure proxyphene product.
■ **PO (Adults):** 65 mg q 4 hr (hydrochloride—Darvon) or 100 mg q 4 hr (napsylate—Darvon-N) as needed (not to exceed 390 mg/day as hydrochloride or 600 mg/day as napsylate). 100 mg propoxyphene napsylate = 65 mg propoxyphene hydrochloride.

## AVAILABILITY (generic available)
❑ **Propoxyphene Hydrochloride**
■ *Capsules:* 65 mg^Rx ■ *Tablets:* {65 mg^Rx}.

❑ **Propoxyphene Napsylate**
■ *Capsules:* {100 mg^Rx} ■ *Tablets:* 50 mg^Rx, 100 mg^Rx ■ Cost: *Darvocet-N 100*—$70.27/ 100; *generic*—$10.99/100.

❑ **Propoxyphene Hydrochloride/Acetaminophen**
■ *Tablets:* propoxyphene 65 mg/acetaminophen 650 mg^Rx.

---

{ } = Available in Canada only.
*CAPITALS indicates life-threatening; underlines indicate most frequent.

❑ **Propoxyphene Napsylate/Acetamino-phen**

■ *Tablets:* propoxyphene 50 mg/acetaminophen 325 mg^Rx, propoxyphene 100 mg/acetaminophen 650 mg^Rx.

❑ **Propoxyphene Hydrochloride/Aspirin/Caffeine**

■ *Capsules:* propoxyphene 65 mg, aspirin 389 mg, caffeine 32.4 mg^Rx ■ *Tablets:* {propoxyphene 65 mg, aspirin 375 mg, caffeine 30 mg^Rx}.

❑ **Propoxyphene Napsylate/Aspirin**

■ *Tablets:* {propoxyphene 100 mg/aspirin 325 mg^Rx}.

❑ **Propoxyphene Napsylate/Aspirin/Caffeine**

■ *Tablets:* {propoxyphene 100 mg/aspirin 375 mg/caffeine 30 mg^Rx}.

TIME/ACTION PROFILE (analgesic effect)

| | ONSET | PEAK | DURATION |
|---|---|---|---|
| PO | 15–60 min | 2–3 hr | 4–6 hr |

# NURSING IMPLICATIONS

## ASSESSMENT

❑ Assess type, location, and intensity of pain prior to and 2 hr (peak) following administration. When titrating opioid doses, increases of 25–50% should be administered until there is either a 50% reduction in the patient's pain rating on a numeric or visual analogue scale or the patient reports satisfactory pain relief. A repeat dose can be safely administered at the time of the peak if previous dose is ineffective and side effects are minimal.

❑ An equianalgesic chart (see Appendix O) should be used when changing routes or when changing from one opioid to another.

❑ Prolonged, high-dose therapy may lead to physical and psychological dependence and tolerance. This should not prevent patient from receiving adequate analgesia. Most patients who receive propoxyphene for pain do not develop psychological dependence. Progressively higher doses or change to a stronger opioid may be required to relieve pain with long-term therapy.

❑ Assess blood pressure, pulse, and respirations before and periodically during administration. If respiratory rate is <10/min, assess level of sedation. Physical stimulation may be sufficient to prevent significant hypoventilation. Dose may need to be decreased by 25–50%. Initial drowsiness will diminish with continued use.

❑ Assess bowel function routinely. Prevention of constipation should be instituted with increased intake of fluids and bulk, and laxatives to minimize constipating effects. Stimulant laxatives should be administered routinely if opioid use exceeds 2–3 days, unless contraindicated.

■ *Lab Test Considerations:* May cause elevated serum amylase and lipase levels.

❑ May cause increased AST, ALT, serum alkaline phosphatase, LDH, and bilirubin concentrations.

■ *Toxicity and Overdose:* If an opioid antagonist is required to reverse respiratory depression or coma, naloxone (Narcan) is the antidote. Dilute the 0.4-mg ampule of naloxone in 10 ml of 0.9% NaCl and administer 0.5 ml (0.02 mg) by direct IV push every 2 min. For patients weighing <40 kg, dilute 0.1 mg of naloxone in 10 ml of 0.9% NaCl for a concentration of 10 mcg/ml and administer 0.5 mcg/kg every 2 min. Titrate dose to avoid withdrawal, seizures, and severe pain.

## POTENTIAL NURSING DIAGNOSES

■ Pain, acute (Indications).

■ Sensory perception, disturbed (visual, auditory) (Side Effects).

■ Injury, risk for (Side Effects).

## IMPLEMENTATION

■ **General:** Explain therapeutic value of medication prior to administration, to enhance the analgesic effect.

❑ Regularly administered doses may be more effective than prn administration. Analgesic is more effective if given before pain becomes severe.

❑ Coadministration with nonopioid analgesics may have additive analgesic effects and may permit lower opioid doses.

❑ Medication should be discontinued gradually after long-term use to prevent withdrawal symptoms.

- **PO:** Doses may be administered with food or milk to minimize GI irritation.

## PATIENT/FAMILY TEACHING

- Advise patient to take medication exactly as directed and not to take more than the recommended amount. Severe and permanent liver damage may result from prolonged use or high doses of acetaminophen. Renal damage may occur with prolonged use of acetaminophen or aspirin. Doses of nonopioid agents should not exceed the maximum recommended daily dose.
- Instruct patient on how and when to ask for pain medication.
- Medication may cause drowsiness or dizziness. Caution patient to avoid driving and other activities requiring alertness until response to the drug is known.
- Advise patient to change positions slowly to minimize orthostatic hypotension.
- Caution patient to avoid concurrent use of alcohol or other CNS depressants with this medication.
- Encourage patient to turn, cough, and breathe deeply every 2 hr to prevent atelectasis.
- Advise patient that good oral hygiene, frequent mouth rinses, and sugarless gum or candy may decrease dry mouth.

## EVALUATION

**Effectiveness of therapy can be demonstrated by:** ■ Decrease in severity of pain without a significant alteration in level of consciousness.

High Alert

# propranolol

(proe-**pran**-oh-lole)
{Apo-Propranolol}, {Betachron E-R}, Inderal, Inderal LA, InnoPran XL, {Novopranol}, {pms Propranolol}

## CLASSIFICATION(S):

**Therapeutic:** antianginals, antiarrhythmics (Class II), antihypertensives, vascular headache suppressants

**Pharmacologic:** beta blockers

**Pregnancy Category C**

## INDICATIONS

■ Management of hypertension ■ Management of angina pectoris ■ Management of arrhythmias ■ Prevention and management of MI ■ Also used to: □ Prevent vascular headaches □ Manage thyrotoxicosis □ Manage pheochromocytoma □ Treat essential tremors □ Manage hypertrophic cardiomyopathy. **Unlabeled uses:** ■ Also used to manage: □ Alcohol withdrawal □ Aggressive behavior □ Antipsychotic-associated akathisia □ Situational anxiety □ Esophageal varices.

## ACTION

■ Blocks stimulation of beta$_1$(myocardial) and beta$_2$(pulmonary, vascular, and uterine)-adrenergic receptor sites. **Therapeutic Effects:** ■ Decreased heart rate and blood pressure ■ Suppression of arrhythmias ■ Prevention of MI.

## PHARMACOKINETICS

**Absorption:** Well absorbed but undergoes extensive first-pass hepatic metabolism.
**Distribution:** Moderate CNS penetration. Crosses the placenta; enters breast milk.
**Protein Binding:** 93%.
**Metabolism and Excretion:** Almost completely metabolized by the liver.
**Half-life:** 3.4–6 hr.

## CONTRAINDICATIONS AND PRECAUTIONS

**Contraindicated in:** ■ Uncompensated CHF ■ Pulmonary edema ■ Cardiogenic shock ■ Bradycardia or heart block.
**Use Cautiously in:** ■ Renal impairment ■ Hepatic impairment ■ Geriatric patients (increased sensitivity to beta blockers; initial dosage reduction recommended) ■ Pulmonary disease (including asthma) ■ Diabetes mellitus (may mask signs of hypoglycemia) ■ Thyrotoxicosis (may mask symptoms) ■ Patients with a history of severe allergic reactions (intensity of reactions may be increased) ■ Children (increased risk of hypoglycemia especially during fasting, such as preoperatively, during prolonged exertion, or coexisting renal insufficiency) ■ Pregnancy, lactation, or children (safety not estab-

lished; all agents cross the placenta and may cause fetal/neonatal bradycardia, hypotension, hypoglycemia, or respiratory depression).

## ADVERSE REACTIONS AND SIDE EFFECTS*

■ **CNS:** fatigue, weakness, anxiety, dizziness, drowsiness, insomnia, memory loss, mental depression, mental status changes, nervousness, nightmares ■ **EENT:** blurred vision, dry eyes, nasal stuffiness ■ **Resp:** bronchospasm, wheezing ■ **CV:** ARRHYTHMIAS, BRADYCARDIA, CHF, PULMONARY EDEMA, orthostatic hypotension, peripheral vasoconstriction ■ **GI:** constipation, diarrhea, nausea ■ **GU:** impotence, decreased libido ■ **Derm:** itching, rashes ■ **Endo:** hyperglycemia, hypoglycemia (increased in children) ■ **MS:** arthralgia, back pain, muscle cramps ■ **Neuro:** paresthesia ■ **Misc:** drug-induced lupus syndrome.

## INTERACTIONS

**Drug-Drug:** ■ **General anesthesia, IV, phenytoin,** and **verapamil** may cause additive myocardial depression ■ Additive bradycardia may occur with **digoxin** ■ Additive hypotension may occur with other **antihypertensives,** acute ingestion of **alcohol,** or **nitrates** ■ Concurrent use with **amphetamines, cocaine, ephedrine, epinephrine, norepinephrine, phenylephrine,** or **pseudoephedrine** may result in unopposed alpha-adrenergic stimulation (excessive hypertension, bradycardia) ■ Concurrent **thyroid** administration may decrease effectiveness ■ May alter the effectiveness of **insulin** or **oral hypoglycemic agents** (dosage adjustments may be necessary) ■ May decrease the effectiveness of **beta-adrenergic bronchodilators** and **theophylline** ■ May decrease the beneficial beta cardiovascular effects of **dopamine** or **dobutamine** ■ Use cautiously within 14 days of **MAO inhibitor** therapy (may result in hypertension) ■ **Cimetidine** may increase blood levels and toxicity ■ Concurrent **NSAIDs** may decrease antihypertensive action ■ **Smoking** increases metabolism and decreases effects; smoking cessation may increase effects.

## ROUTE AND DOSAGE

■ **PO (Adults):** *Antianginal*—80–320 mg/day in 2–4 divided doses or once daily as extended/sustained-release capsules. *Antihypertensive*—40 mg twice daily initially; may be increased as needed (usual range 120–240 mg/day; doses up to 1 g/day have been used); *or* 80 mg once daily as extended/sus-

tained-release capsules, increased as needed up to 120 mg. *InnoPran XL* dosing form is designed to be given once daily at bedtime. *Antiarrhythmic*—10–30 mg 3–4 times daily. *Prevention of MI*—180–240 mg/day in divided doses. *Hypertrophic cardiomyopathy*—20–40 mg 3–4 times daily. *Adjunct therapy of pheochromocytoma*—20 mg 3 times daily to 40 mg 3–4 times daily concurrently with alpha-blocking therapy, started 3 days before surgery is planned. *Vascular headache prevention*—20 mg 4 times daily *or* 80 mg/day as extended/sustained-release capsules; may be increased as needed up to 240 mg/day. *Management of tremor*—40 mg twice daily; may be increased up to 120 mg/day (up to 320 mg have been used).

■ **PO (Children):** *Antihypertensive/antiarrhythmic*—0.5–1 mg/kg/day in 2–4 divided doses; may be increased as needed (usual range for maintenance dose is 2–4 mg/kg/day in 2 divided doses).

■ **IV (Adults):** *Antiarrhythmic*—1–3 mg; may be repeated after 2 min and again in 4 hr if needed.

■ **IV (Children):** *Antiarrhythmic*—10–100 mcg (0.01–0.1 mg)/kg (up to 1 mg/dose); may be repeated q 6–8 hr if needed.

## AVAILABILITY (generic available)

■ *Oral solution:* 4 mg/ml^Rx, 8 mg/ml^Rx, 80 mg/ml^Rx ■ *Tablets:* 10 mg^Rx, 20 mg^Rx, 40 mg^Rx, 60 mg^Rx, 90 mg^Rx, {120 mg^Rx} ■ *Sustained-release capsules:* 60 mg^Rx, 80 mg^Rx, 120 mg^Rx, 160 mg^Rx ■ *Extended-release capsules:* 60 mg^Rx, 80 mg^Rx, 120 mg^Rx, 160 mg^Rx ■ Cost: 60 mg $120.58/100, 80 mg $139.26/100, 120 mg $174.76/100, 160 mg $228.82/100 ■ *Injection:* 1 mg/ml^Rx ■ hydrochlorothiazide (Inderide^Rx, Inderide LA^Rx). See Appendix B.

TIME/ACTION PROFILE (cardiovascular effects)

| | ONSET | PEAK | DURATION |
|---|---|---|---|
| PO | 30 min | 60–90 min† | 6–12 hr |
| PO–ER | unknown | 6 hr | 24 hr |
| IV | immediate | 1 min | 4–6 hr |

†Following single dose, full effect not seen until several weeks of therapy.

## NURSING IMPLICATIONS

### ASSESSMENT

■ **General Info:** Monitor blood pressure and pulse frequently during dose adjustment period and periodically during therapy. Assess for orthostatic hypotension when assisting patient up from supine position.

❑ Patients receiving **propranolol IV** must have continuous ECG monitoring and may have pulmonary capillary wedge pressure (PCWP) or central venous pressure (CVP) monitoring during and for several hours after administration.

❑ Monitor intake and output ratios and daily weight. Assess patient routinely for evidence of fluid overload (peripheral edema, dyspnea, rales/crackles, fatigue, weight gain, jugular venous distention).

■ **Angina:** Assess frequency and characteristics of anginal attacks periodically during therapy.

■ **Vascular Headache Prophylaxis:** Assess frequency, severity, characteristics, and location of vascular headaches periodically during therapy.

■ *Lab Test Considerations:* May cause ↑ BUN, serum lipoprotein, potassium, triglyceride, and uric acid levels.

❑ May cause ↑ ANA titers.

❑ May cause ↓ or ↑ in blood glucose levels. In labile diabetic patients, hypoglycemia may be accompanied by precipitous ↑ of blood pressure.

■ *Toxicity and Overdose:* Monitor patients receiving beta blockers for signs of overdose (bradycardia, severe dizziness or fainting, severe drowsiness, dyspnea, bluish fingernails or palms, seizures). Notify physician or other health care professional immediately if these signs occur.

❑ Hypotension may be treated with modified Trendelenburg position and IV fluids unless contraindicated. Vasopressors (epinephrine, norepinephrine, dopamine, dobutamine) may also be used. Hypotension does not respond to beta agonists.

❑ Glucagon has been used to treat bradycardia and hypotension.

## POTENTIAL NURSING DIAGNOSES

■ Cardiac output, decreased (Side Effects).

■ Noncompliance (Patient/Family Teaching).

## IMPLEMENTATION

❑ *High Alert:* IV vasoactive medications are inherently dangerous. Oral and parenteral doses of *propranolol* are not interchangeable; IV dose is 1/10 the oral dose. Patient harm or fatalities have occurred when switching from oral to IV route. Before administering intravenously, have second practitioner independently check original order, dosage calculations, and infusion pump settings. Do not confuse propranolol with pravachol. Do not confuse Inderal (propranolol) with Adderall (amphetamine/dextroamphetamine).

■ **PO:** Take apical pulse prior to administering. If <50 bpm or if arrhythmia occurs, withhold medication and notify physician or other health care professional.

❑ Administer with meals or directly after eating to enhance absorption.

❑ Extended-release capsules should be swallowed whole; do not crush, open, or chew. *Propranolol tablets* may be crushed and mixed with food.

❑ Mix propranolol oral solution with liquid or semisolid food (water, juices, soda, applesauce, puddings). Make sure entire dose is taken. Rinse glass with more liquid to ensure all medication is taken. Do not store after mixing.

■ **Direct IV:** Administer undiluted or dilute each 1 mg in 10 ml of D5W for injection.

■ *Rate:* Administer over at least 1 min.

■ **Intermittent Infusion:** May also be diluted for infusion in 50 ml of 0.9% NaCl, D5W, D5/0.45% NaCl, D5/0.9% NaCl, or lactated Ringer's injection.

■ *Rate:* Infuse over 10–15 min.

■ **Syringe Compatibility:** ◆ inamrinone ◆ milrinone.

■ **Y-Site Compatibility:** ◆ alteplase ◆ gatifloxacin ◆ heparin ◆ hydrocortisone sodium succinate ◆ inamrinone ◆ linezolid ◆ meperidine ◆ milrinone ◆ morphine ◆ potassium chloride ◆ propofol ◆ tacrolimus ◆ vitamin B complex with vitamin C.

■ **Y-Site Incompatibility:** ◆ amphotericin B cholesteryl sulfate complex ◆ diazoxide.

## PATIENT/FAMILY TEACHING

- **General Info:** Instruct patient to take medication as directed, at the same time each day, even if feeling well; do not skip or double up on missed doses. Take missed doses as soon as possible up to 4 hr before next dose (8 hr with extended-release propranolol). Abrupt withdrawal may precipitate life-threatening arrhythmias, hypertension, or myocardial ischemia.
- ❏ Advise patient to make sure enough medication is available for weekends, holidays, and vacations. A written prescription may be kept in wallet in case of emergency.
- ❏ Teach patient and family how to check pulse daily and blood pressure biweekly. Advise patient to hold dose and contact health care professional if pulse is <50 bpm or blood pressure changes significantly.
- ❏ May cause drowsiness or dizziness. Caution patients to avoid driving or other activities that require alertness until response to the drug is known.
- ❏ Advise patients to change positions slowly to minimize orthostatic hypotension, especially during initiation of therapy or when dose is increased.
- ❏ Caution patient that this medication may increase sensitivity to cold.
- ❏ Instruct patient to consult health care professional before taking any OTC medications or herbal products, especially cold preparations, concurrently with this medication.
- ❏ Diabetic patients should closely monitor blood glucose, especially if weakness, malaise, irritability, or fatigue occurs. May mask tachycardia and increased blood pressure as signs of hypoglycemia, but dizziness and sweating may still occur.
- ❏ Advise patient to notify health care professional if slow pulse, difficulty breathing, wheezing, cold hands and feet, dizziness, light-headedness, confusion, depression, rash, fever, sore throat, unusual bleeding, or bruising occurs.
- ❏ Instruct patient to inform health care professional of medication regimen prior to treatment or surgery.
- ❏ Advise patient to carry identification describing disease process and medication regimen at all times.
- **Hypertension:** Reinforce the need to continue additional therapies for hypertension (weight loss, sodium restriction, stress reduction, regular exercise, moderation of alcohol consumption, and smoking cessation). Medication controls but does not cure hypertension.
- **Angina:** Caution patient to avoid overexertion with decrease in chest pain.
- **Vascular Headache Prophylaxis:** Caution patient that sharing this medication may be dangerous.

## EVALUATION

**Effectiveness of therapy can be demonstrated by:** ■ Decrease in blood pressure ■ Control of arrhythmias without appearance of detrimental side effects ■ Reduction in frquency of anginal attacks ❏ Increase in activity tolerance ■ Prevention of MI ■ Prevention of vascular headaches ■ Management of thyrotoxicosis ■ Managment of pheochromocytoma ■ Decrease in tremors ■ Management of hypertrophic cardiomyopathy.

## protamine sulfate
(**proe**-ta-meen)

*CLASSIFICATION(S):*
*Therapeutic:* antidotes
*Pharmacologic:* antiheparins

**Pregnancy Category C**

## INDICATIONS

■ Acute management of severe heparin overdosage ■ Used to neutralize heparin received during dialysis, cardiopulmonary bypass, and other procedures. **Unlabeled uses:** ■ Management of overdose of heparin-like compounds.

## ACTION

■ A strong base that forms a complex with heparin (an acid). **Therapeutic Effects:** ■ Inactivation of heparin.

## PHARMACOKINETICS

**Absorption:** Administered IV only, resulting in complete bioavailability.

**Distribution:** Unknown.

**Metabolism and Excretion:** Metabolic fate not known. Protamine-heparin complex eventually degrades.

**Half-life:** Unknown.

# CONTRAINDICATIONS AND PRECAUTIONS

**Contraindicated in:** ■ Hypersensitivity to protamine or fish ■ Avoid reconstitution with diluents containing benzyl alcohol if used in neonates.

**Use Cautiously in:** ■ Patients who have received previous protamine-containing insulin or vasectomized men (increased risk of hypersensitivity reactions) ■ Pregnancy, lactation, and children (safety not established).

# ADVERSE REACTIONS AND SIDE EFFECTS*

■ **Resp:** dyspnea ■ **CV:** bradycardia, hypertension, hypotension, pulmonary hypertension ■ **GI:** nausea, vomiting ■ **Derm:** flushing, warmth ■ **Hemat:** bleeding ■ **MS:** back pain ■ **Misc:** hypersensitivity reactions, including ANAPHYLAXIS, ANGIOEDEMA, and pulmonary edema.

# INTERACTIONS

**Drug-Drug:** ■ None significant.

# ROUTE AND DOSAGE

■ **IV (Adults and Children):** *Heparin overdose*—1 mg/100 units of heparin. If given >30 min after heparin, give 0.5 mg/100 units of heparin (not to exceed 100 mg/2 hr). Further doses should be determined by coagulation tests. *Enoxaparin overdose*—1 mg/ each mg of enoxaparin to be neutralized (unlabeled). *Dalteparin overdose*—1 mg/ 100 anti-Xa IU of dalteparin. If required, a second dose of 0.5 mg/100 anti-Xa IU of dalteparin may be given 2–4 hr later if laboratory assessment indicates need (unlabeled).

# AVAILABILITY (generic available)

■ *Injection:* 10 mg/ml in 5- and 25-ml ampules and 5-, 10-, and 25-ml vials^Rx.

TIME/ACTION PROFILE (reversal of heparin effect)

|  | ONSET | PEAK | DURATION |
|---|---|---|---|
| IV | 30 sec–1 min | unknown | 2 hr† |

†Depends on body temperature.

# NURSING IMPLICATIONS

## ASSESSMENT

❑ Assess for bleeding and hemorrhage throughout therapy. Hemorrhage may recur 8–9 hr after therapy because of rebound effects of heparin. Rebound may occur as late as 18 hr after therapy in patients heparinized for cardiopulmonary bypass.

❑ Assess for allergy to fish (salmon), previous reaction to or use of protamine insulin or protamine sulfate. Vasectomized and infertile men also have higher risk of hypersensitivity reaction.

❑ Observe patient for signs and symptoms of hypersensitivity reaction (hives, edema, coughing, wheezing). Keep epinephrine, an antihistamine, and resuscitative equipment close by in the event of anaphylaxis.

❑ Assess for hypovolemia before initiation of therapy. Failure to correct hypovolemia may result in cardiovascular collapse from peripheral vasodilating effects of protamine sulfate.

■ *Lab Test Considerations:* Monitor clotting factors, activated clotting time (ACT), activated partial thromboplastin time (aPTT), and thrombin time (TT) 5–15 min after therapy and again as necessary.

## POTENTIAL NURSING DIAGNOSES

■ Injury, risk for (Indications).
■ Tissue perfusion, ineffective (Indications).

## IMPLEMENTATION

■ **General:** Discontinue heparin infusion. In milder cases, overdosage may be treated by heparin withdrawal alone.

❑ In severe cases, fresh frozen plasma or whole blood may also be required to control bleeding.

❑ Dosage varies with type of heparin, route of heparin therapy, and amount of time elapsed since discontinuation of heparin.

❑ Do not administer >100 mg in 2 hr without rechecking clotting studies, as protamine sulfate has its own anticoagulant properties.

■ **IV:** Reconstitute 50-mg vial with 5 ml and 250-mg vial with 25 ml of sterile water for injection or bacteriostatic water for injection for a concentration of 10 mg/ml. Shake vig-

---

{ } = Available in Canada only.
*CAPITALS indicates life-threatening; underlines indicate most frequent.

orously. Solution reconstituted with sterile water for injection should be discarded after dose is withdrawn. Solution reconstituted with bacteriostatic water is stable for 24 hr when refrigerated.

■ **Direct IV:** May be administered undiluted.

■ **Rate:** May be administered by slow IV push over 1–3 min.

■ **Intermittent Infusion:** May be diluted in D5W or 0.9% NaCl.

■ **Rate:** Infuse no faster than 50 mg over 10 min. Rapid infusion rate may result in hypotension, bradycardia, flushing, or feeling of warmth. If these symptoms occur, stop infusion and notify physician.

## PATIENT/FAMILY TEACHING

❏ Explain purpose of the medication to patient. Instruct patient to report recurrent bleeding immediately.

❏ Advise patient to avoid activities that may result in bleeding (shaving, brushing teeth, receiving injections or rectal temperatures, or ambulating) until risk of hemorrhage has passed.

## EVALUATION

**Effectiveness of therapy can be demonstrated by:** ■ Control of bleeding ■ Normalization of clotting factors in heparinized patients.

# pseudoephedrine
## (soo-doe-e-**fed**-rin)

Afrin, Allermed, {Balminil Decongestant Syrup}, {Benylin Decongestant}, Cenafed, Children's Silfedrine, Children's Congestion Relief, Congestion Relief, Decofed, DeFed-60, Dorcol Children's Decongestant liquid, Drixoral Non-Drowsy Formula, Dynafed Pseudo, Efidac/24, {Eltor 120}, Genafed, Halofed, Mini Thin Pseudo, PediaCare Infants' Oral Decongestant Drops, Pediatric Nasal Decongestant, Pseudo, Pseudo-Gest, Seudotabs, Sinustop Pro, {Robidrine}, Sudafed, Sudafed 12 Hour, Sudex, Triaminic AM Decongestant Formula

## CLASSIFICATION(S):
**Therapeutic:** allergy, cold, and cough remedies, nasal drying agents/decongestants

### Pregnancy Category B

## INDICATIONS

■ Symptomatic management of nasal congestion associated with acute viral upper respiratory tract infections ■ Used in combination with antihistamines in the management of allergic conditions ■ Used to open obstructed eustachian tubes in chronic otic inflammation or infection.

## ACTION

■ Stimulates alpha- and beta-adrenergic receptors ■ Produces vasoconstriction in the respiratory tract mucosa (alpha-adrenergic stimulation) and possibly bronchodilation (beta$_2$-adrenergic stimulation). **Therapeutic Effects:** ■ Reduction of nasal congestion, hyperemia, and swelling in nasal passages.

## PHARMACOKINETICS

**Absorption:** Well absorbed after oral administration.

**Distribution:** Appears to enter the CSF; probably crosses the placenta and enters breast milk.

**Metabolism and Excretion:** Partially metabolized by the liver. 55–75% excreted unchanged by the kidneys (depends on urine pH).

**Half-life:** 7 hr (depends on urine pH).

## CONTRAINDICATIONS AND PRECAUTIONS

**Contraindicated in:** ■ Hypersensitivity to sympathomimetic amines ■ Hypertension, severe coronary artery disease ■ Concurrent MAO inhibitor therapy ■ Known alcohol intolerance (some liquid products).

**Use Cautiously in:** ■ Hyperthyroidism ■ Diabetes mellitus ■ Prostatic hypertrophy ■ Ischemic heart disease ■ Glaucoma ■ Pregnancy or lactation (safety not established).

## ADVERSE REACTIONS AND SIDE EFFECTS*

■ **CNS:** SEIZURES, anxiety, nervousness, dizziness, drowsiness, excitability, fear, hallucinations, headache, insomnia, restlessness, weakness ■ **Resp:** respiratory difficulty ■ **CV:** CARDIOVASCULAR

COLLAPSE, <u>palpitations</u>, hypertension, tachycardia ■ **GI:** <u>anorexia</u>, dry mouth ■ **GU:** dysuria.

## INTERACTIONS

**Drug-Drug:** ■Concurrent use with **MAO inhibitors** may cause hypertensive crisis ■ Additive adrenergic effects with other **adrenergics** ■ Concurrent use with **beta blockers** may result in hypertension or bradycardia ■ **Drugs that acidify the urine** may decrease effectiveness ■ **Drugs that alkalinize the urine (sodium bicarbonate, high-dose antacid therapy)** may intensify effectiveness.

**Drug-Food:** ■ Foods that acidify the urine may decrease effectiveness ■ Foods that alkalinize the urine may intensify effectiveness (see lists in Appendix Q).

## ROUTE AND DOSAGE

■ **PO (Adults and Children >12 yr):** 60 mg q 4–6 hr as needed (not to exceed 240 mg/day) *or* 120 mg of extended-release preparation q 12 hr *or* 240 mg extended-release preparation q 24 hr.

■ **PO (Children 6–12 yr):** 30 mg q 4–6 hr as needed (not to exceed 120 mg/day) *or* 4 mg/kg/day (125 mg/m²/day) in 4 divided doses.

■ **PO (Children 2–6 yr):** 15 mg q 4–6 hr (not to exceed 60 mg/day) *or* 4 mg/kg/day (125 mg/m²/day) in 4 divided doses.

■ **PO (Children 1–2 yr):** 7 drops (of 7.5 mg/0.8 ml solution)/kg q 4–6 hr (not to exceed 4 doses/24 hr).

■ **PO (Children 3–12 mo):** 3 drops (of 7.5 mg/0.8 ml solution)/kg q 4–6 hr (not to exceed 4 doses/24 hr).

## AVAILABILITY (generic available)

■ *Tablets:* 30 mg^OTC, 60 mg^OTC ■ Cost: 30 mg $4.93/100, 60 mg $8.44/100 ■ *Extended-release tablets:* 120 mg^OTC, 240 mg^OTC ■ *Capsules:* {60 mg^OTC} ■ *Extended-release capsules:* 120 mg^Rx, {240 mg^OTC} ■ *Syrup:* 30 mg/5 ml^OTC ■ *Oral solution (orange flavor):* 15 mg/5 ml^OTC, 30 mg/5 ml^OTC ■ *Drops (fruit flavor):* 7.5 mg/0.8 ml (0.8 ml = 1 dropperful)^OTC ■ antihistamines, acetaminophen, cough suppressants, and expectorants^OTC. See Appendix B.

TIME/ACTION PROFILE (decongestant effects)

| | ONSET | PEAK | DURATION |
|---|---|---|---|
| PO | 30 min | unknown | 4–8 hr |
| PO-ER | 60 min | unknown | 12 hr |

# NURSING IMPLICATIONS

## ASSESSMENT

❑ Assess congestion (nasal, sinus, eustachian tube) before and periodically throughout therapy.

❑ Monitor pulse and blood pressure before beginning therapy and periodically throughout therapy.

❑ Assess lung sounds and character of bronchial secretions. Maintain fluid intake of 1500–2000 ml/day to decrease viscosity of secretions.

## POTENTIAL NURSING DIAGNOSES

■ Airway clearance, ineffective (Indications).

## IMPLEMENTATION

■ **General:** Administer pseudoephedrine at least 2 hr before bedtime to minimize insomnia.

■ **PO:** Extended-release tablets and capsules should be swallowed whole; do not crush, break, or chew. Contents of the capsule can be mixed with jam or jelly and swallowed without chewing for patients with difficulty swallowing.

## PATIENT/FAMILY TEACHING

❑ Instruct patient to take medication exactly as directed and not to take more than recommended. If a dose is missed, take within 1 hr; if remembered later, omit. Do not double doses.

■ **Instruct patient to notify health care professional if nervousness, slow or fast heart rate, breathing difficulties, hallucinations, or seizures occur, because these symptoms may indicate overdosage.**

❑ Instruct patient to contact health care professional if symptoms do not improve within 7 days or if fever is present.

## EVALUATION

**Effectiveness of therapy can be demonstrated by:** ■ Decreased nasal, sinus, or eustachian tube congestion.

---

### psyllium

(**sill**-i-yum)

Alramucil, Cillium, Effer-Syllium, Fiberall, Fibrepur, Hydrocil, {Karacil}, Konsyl, Metamucil, Modane Bulk, Mylanta Natural Fiber Supplement, Naturacil Caramels, {Natural Source Fibre Laxative}, Perdiem, {Prodiem}, Pro-Lax, Reguloid Natural, Serutan, Siblin, Syllact, Vitalax, V-Lax

*CLASSIFICATION(S):*
*Therapeutic: laxatives*
*Pharmacologic: bulk-forming agents*

**Pregnancy Category UK**

---

### INDICATIONS

■ Management of simple or chronic constipation, particularly if associated with a low-fiber diet ■ Useful in situations in which straining should be avoided (after MI, rectal surgery, prolonged bed rest) ■ Used in the management of chronic watery diarrhea.

### ACTION

■ Combines with water in the intestinal contents to form an emollient gel or viscous solution that promotes peristalsis and reduces transit time. **Therapeutic Effects:** ■ Relief and prevention of constipation.

### PHARMACOKINETICS

**Absorption:** Not absorbed from the GI tract.
**Distribution:** No distribution occurs.
**Metabolism and Excretion:** Excreted in feces.
**Half-life:** Unknown.

### CONTRAINDICATIONS AND PRECAUTIONS

**Contraindicated in:** ■ Hypersensitivity ■ Abdominal pain, nausea, or vomiting (especially when associated with fever) ■ Serious adhesions ■ Dysphagia.

**Use Cautiously in:** ■ Some dosage forms contain sugar, aspartame, or excessive sodium and should be avoided in patients on restricted diets ■ Pregnancy and lactation (has been used safely).

### ADVERSE REACTIONS AND SIDE EFFECTS*

■ **Resp:** bronchospasm ■ **GI:** cramps, intestinal or esophageal obstruction, nausea, vomiting.

### INTERACTIONS

**Drug-Drug:** ■ May decrease the absorption of **warfarin, salicylates,** or **digoxins.**

### ROUTE AND DOSAGE

■ **PO (Adults):** 1–2 tsp/packet/wafer (3–6 g psyllium) in or with a full glass of liquid 2–3 times daily. Up to 30 g daily in divided doses.
■ **PO (Children >6 yr):** 1 tsp/packet/wafer (1.5–3 g psyllium) in or with 4–8 oz glass of liquid 2–3 times daily. Up to 15 g daily in divided doses.

### AVAILABILITY (generic available)

■ *Powder:* 3.3–3.5 g/dose or packet[OTC] ■ *Effervescent powder:* 3–3.5 g/dose or packet[OTC] ■ *Granules:* 2.5 g/dose[OTC] ■ *Wafers:* 3.4 g/dose[OTC].

TIME/ACTION PROFILE (laxative effect)

|    | ONSET | PEAK | DURATION |
|----|-------|------|----------|
| PO | 12–24 hr | 2–3 days | unknown |

## NURSING IMPLICATIONS

### ASSESSMENT

❑ Assess patient for abdominal distention, presence of bowel sounds, and usual pattern of bowel function.
❑ Assess color, consistency, and amount of stool produced.
■ *Lab Test Considerations:* May cause elevated blood glucose levels with prolonged use of preparations containing sugar.

### POTENTIAL NURSING DIAGNOSES

■ Constipation (Indications).

### IMPLEMENTATION

■ **General:** Packets are not standardized for volume, but each contains 3–3.5 g of psyllium.

■ **PO:** Administer with a full glass of water or juice, followed by an additional glass of liquid. Solution should be taken immediately after mixing; it will congeal. Do not administer without sufficient fluid and do not chew granules.

## PATIENT/FAMILY TEACHING

❑ Encourage patient to use other forms of bowel regulation, such as increasing bulk in the diet, increasing fluid intake, and increasing mobility. Normal bowel habits are individualized and may vary from 3 times/day to 3 times/wk.

❑ May be used for long-term management of chronic constipation.

❑ Instruct patients with cardiac disease to avoid straining during bowel movements (Valsalva maneuver).

❑ Advise patient not to use laxatives when abdominal pain, nausea, vomiting, or fever is present.

## EVALUATION

**Effectiveness of therapy can be demonstrated by:** ■ A soft, formed bowel movement, usually within 12–24 hr. May require 3 days of therapy for results.

---

# pyridostigmine

(peer-id-oh-**stig**-meen)

Mestinon, {Mestinon SR}, Mestinon Timespan, Regonol

**CLASSIFICATION(S):**
**Therapeutic:** antimyasthenics
**Pharmacologic:** cholinergics

**Pregnancy Category C**

## INDICATIONS

■ Used to increase muscle strength in the symptomatic treatment of myasthenia gravis ■ Reversal of nondepolarizing neuromuscular blocking agents ■ Prophylaxis of lethal effects of poisoning with the nerve agent soman.

## ACTION

■ Inhibits the breakdown of acetylcholine and prolongs its effects (anticholinesterase) ■ Effects include: ■ Miosis ■ Increased intestinal and skeletal muscle tone ■ Bronchial and ureteral constriction ■ Bradycardia ■ Increased salivation ■ Lacrimation ■ Sweating. **Therapeutic Effects:** ■ Improved muscular function in patients with myasthenia gravis ■ Reversal of paralysis from nondepolarizing neuromuscular blocking agents ■ Prevention of Soman nerve gas toxicity.

## PHARMACOKINETICS

**Absorption:** Poorly absorbed after oral administration, necessitating large oral doses compared with parenteral doses.
**Distribution:** Appears to cross the placenta.
**Metabolism and Excretion:** Metabolized by plasma cholinesterases and the liver.
**Half-life:** *PO*—3.7 hr; *IV*—1.9 hr.

## CONTRAINDICATIONS AND PRECAUTIONS

**Contraindicated in:** ■ Hypersensitivity to pyridostigmine or bromides ■ Mechanical obstruction of the GI or GU tract ■ Known alcohol intolerance (syrup only).
**Use Cautiously in:** ■ History of asthma ■ Ulcer disease ■ Cardiovascular disease ■ Epilepsy ■ Hyperthyroidism ■ Pregnancy or lactation (may cause uterine irritability after IV administration near term; 20% of newborns display transient muscle weakness).

## ADVERSE REACTIONS AND SIDE EFFECTS*

■ **CNS:** SEIZURES, dizziness, weakness ■ **EENT:** lacrimation, miosis ■ **Resp:** bronchospasm, excessive secretions ■ **CV:** bradycardia, hypotension ■ **GI:** abdominal cramps, diarrhea, excessive salivation, nausea, vomiting ■ **Derm:** sweating, rashes.

## INTERACTIONS

**Drug-Drug:** ■ Cholinergic effects may be antagonized by other **drugs possessing anticholinergic properties,** including **antihistamines, antidepressants, atropine, haloperidol, phenothiazines, procainamide, quinidine,** or **disopyramide** ■ Prolongs the

---

{ } = Available in Canada only.
*CAPITALS indicates life-threatening; underlines indicate most frequent.

action of **depolarizing muscle-relaxing agents** and **cholinesterase inhibitors (succinylcholine, decamethonium)** ▪ ↑ toxicity with other **cholinesterase inhibitors,** including **demecarium, echothiophate,** and **isoflurophate** ▪ Antimyasthenic effects may be ↓ by concurrent **guanadrel** or **guanethidine.**

## ROUTE AND DOSAGE

❑ **Myasthenia Gravis**

▪ **PO (Adults):** *Tablets/syrup*—30–60 mg q 3–4 hr initially; then adjusted as required; usual maintenance dose is 600 mg/day in divided doses (range 60–1500 mg/day). *Extended-release tablets*—180–540 mg 1–2 times daily (dosing interval should be at least 6 hr; may be associated with increased risk of cholinergic crisis; concurrent immediate-release products may be required).

▪ **PO (Children):** 7 mg/kg (200 mg/m²)/day in 5–6 divided doses.

▪ **IM, IV (Adults):** 2 mg (1/30 of oral dose); may be repeated q 2–3 hr. *During labor/delivery*—1 mg before second stage of labor is complete.

▪ **IM (Neonates Born to Myasthenic Mothers):** 50–150 mcg/kg q 4–6 hr.

❑ **Antidote for Nondepolarizing Neuromuscular Blocking Agents**

▪ **IV (Adults):** 10–20 mg; pretreat with 0.6–1.2 mg atropine IV.

❑ **Prevention of Soman Nerve Gas Effects**

▪ **PO (Adults):** 30 mg every 8 hr before exposure, stopped on exposure to gas.

## AVAILABILITY (generic available)

▪ *Tablets:* 30 mg^Rx, 60 mg^Rx ▪ *Extended-release tablets:* 180 mg^Rx ▪ *Syrup:* 60 mg/5 ml^Rx ▪ *Injection:* 5 mg/ml in 2-ml ampules and 5-ml vials^Rx.

TIME/ACTION PROFILE (cholinergic effects)

| | ONSET | PEAK | DURATION |
|---|---|---|---|
| PO | 30–35 min | unknown | 3–6 hr |
| PO-SR | 30–60 min | unknown | 6–12 hr |
| IM | 15 min | unknown | 2–4 hr |
| IV | 2–5 min | unknown | 2–3 hr |

## NURSING IMPLICATIONS

### ASSESSMENT

▪ **General Info:** Assess pulse, respiratory rate, and blood pressure before administration. Report significant changes in heart rate.

▪ **Myasthenia Gravis:** Assess neuromuscular status, including vital capacity, ptosis, diplopia, chewing, swallowing, hand grasp, and gait before administering and at peak effect. Patients with myasthenia gravis may be advised to keep a daily record of their condition and the effects of this medication.

❑ Assess patient for overdosage, underdosage, or resistance. Both have similar symptoms (muscle weakness, dyspnea, dysphagia), but symptoms of overdosage usually occur within 1 hr of administration, whereas symptoms of underdosage occur ≥3 hr after administration. Overdosage (cholinergic crisis) symptoms may also include increased respiratory secretions and saliva, bradycardia, nausea, vomiting, cramping, diarrhea, and diaphoresis. A Tensilon test (edrophonium chloride) may be used to differentiate between overdosage and underdosage.

▪ **Antidote to Nondepolarizing Neuromuscular Blocking Agents:** Monitor reversal of effect of neuromuscular blocking agents with a peripheral nerve stimulator. Recovery usually occurs consecutively in the following muscles: diaphragm, intercostal muscles, muscles of the glottis, abdominal muscles, limb muscles, muscles of mastication, and levator muscles of eyelids. Closely observe patient for residual muscle weakness and respiratory distress throughout the recovery period. Maintain airway patency and ventilation until recovery of normal respirations occurs.

▪ *Toxicity and Overdose:* Atropine is the antidote.

### POTENTIAL NURSING DIAGNOSES

▪ Mobility, impaired physical (Indications).

▪ Breathing pattern, ineffective (Indications).

### IMPLEMENTATION

▪ **General:** For patients who have difficulty chewing, pyridostigmine may be administered 30 min before meals.

❑ Oral dose is not interchangeable with IV dose. Parenteral form is 30 times more potent.

□ When used as an antidote to nondepolarizing neuromuscular blocking agents, atropine may be ordered before or currently with large doses of pyridostigmine to prevent or to treat bradycardia and other side effects.

■ **PO:** Administer with food or milk to minimize side effects. Extended-release tablets should be swallowed whole; do not crush, break, or chew. Regular tablets or syrup may be administered with extended-release tablets for optimum control of symptoms. Mottled appearance of sustained-release tablet does not affect potency.

■ **Direct IV:** Administer undiluted. Do not add to IV solutions. May be given through Y-site of infusion of D5W, 0.9% NaCl, LR, D5/Ringer's solution, or D5/LR.

■ *Rate:* For myasthenia gravis, administer each 0.5 mg over 1 min. For reversal of nondepolarizing neuromuscular blocking agents, administer each 5 mg over 1 min.

■ **Syringe Compatibility:** ◆ glycopyrrolate.

■ **Y-Site Compatibility:** ◆ heparin ◆ hydrocortisone sodium succinate ◆ potassium chloride ◆ vitamin B complex with C.

## PATIENT/FAMILY TEACHING

□ Instruct patient to take medication as directed. Do not skip or double up on missed doses. Patients with a history of dysphagia should have a nonelectric or battery-operated back-up alarm clock to remind them of exact dose time. Patients with dysphagia may not be able to swallow medication if the dose is not taken exactly on time. Taking dose late may result in myasthenic crisis. Taking dose early may result in cholinergic crisis. Patients with myasthenia gravis must continue this regimen as a life-long therapy.

□ Advise patient to carry identification describing disease and medication regimen at all times.

□ Instruct patient to space activities to avoid fatigue.

## EVALUATION

**Effectiveness of therapy can be demonstrated by:** ■ Relief of ptosis and diplopia; improved chewing, swallowing, extremity strength, and breathing without the appearance of cholinergic symptoms ■ Reversal of nondepo-larizing neuromuscular blocking agents in general anesthesia ■ Prevention of Soman nerve gas toxicity.

# pyridoxine
(peer-i-**dox**-een)
Beesix, Doxine, Nestrex, Pyri, Rodex, Vitabee 6, vitamin B$_6$

## CLASSIFICATION(S):
**Therapeutic:** *vitamins*
**Pharmacologic:** *water soluble vitamins*

## Pregnancy Category A

## INDICATIONS

■ Treatment and prevention of pyridoxine deficiency (may be associated with poor nutritional status or chronic debilitating illnesses) ■ Treatment and prevention of neuropathy, which may develop from isoniazid, penicillamine, or hydralazine therapy ■ Management of isoniazid overdose >10 g.

## ACTION

■ Required for amino acid, carbohydrate, and lipid metabolism ■ Used in the transport of amino acids, formation of neurotransmitters, and synthesis of heme. **Therapeutic Effects:** ■ Prevention of pyridoxine deficiency ■ Prevention or reversal of neuropathy associated with hydralazine, penicillamine, or isoniazid therapy.

## PHARMACOKINETICS

**Absorption:** Well absorbed from the GI tract.
**Distribution:** Stored in liver, muscle, and brain. Crosses the placenta and enters breast milk.
**Metabolism and Excretion:** Converted in RBCs to pyridoxal phosphate and another active metabolite. Amounts in excess of requirements are excreted unchanged by the kidneys.
**Half-life:** 15–20 days.

## CONTRAINDICATIONS AND PRECAUTIONS

**Contraindicated in:** ■ No known contraindications.

---

**Use Cautiously in:** ■ Parkinson's disease (treatment with levodopa only) ■ Pregnancy (chronic ingestion of large doses may produce pyridoxine-dependency syndrome in newborn).

## ADVERSE REACTIONS AND SIDE EFFECTS*

Adverse reactions listed are seen with excessive doses only. ■ **Neuro:** sensory neuropathy ■ **Misc:** pyridoxine-dependency syndrome.

## INTERACTIONS

**Drug-Drug:** ■ Interferes with the therapeutic response to **levodopa** ■ Requirements are increased by **isoniazid, hydralazine, chloramphenicol, penicillamine, estrogens,** and **immunosuppressants.**

## ROUTE AND DOSAGE

❑ **Prevention of Deficiency**

■ **PO (Adults and Children >10 yr):** 1.4–2.2 mg/day (larger doses required with cycloserine, ethionamide, hydralazine, immunosuppressants, isoniazid, penicillamine, and estrogen-containing oral contraceptives).

■ **PO (Children 4–10 yr):** 1.1–1.4 mg/day (larger doses required with cycloserine, ethionamide, hydralazine, immunosuppressants, isoniazid, and penicillamine).

■ **PO (Children birth–3 yr):** 0.3–1 mg/day (larger doses required with cycloserine, ethionamide, hydralazine, immunosuppressants, isoniazid, and penicillamine).

❑ **Treatment of Deficiency**

■ **PO, IM, IV (Adults and Children):** Must be individualized.

❑ **Pyridoxine-Dependency Syndrome**

■ **IM, IV (Adults and Children):** 30–600 mg/day.

❑ **Isoniazid Overdose (>10 g)**

■ **IM, IV (Adults):** Amount in mg equal to amount of isoniazid ingested given as 4 g IV, then 1 g IM q 30 min.

## AVAILABILITY (generic available)

■ **Tablets:** 10 mg^OTC, 25 mg^OTC, 50 mg^OTC, 100 mg^OTC, 200 mg^OTC, 250 mg^OTC, 500 mg^OTC ■ **Extended-release tablets:** 100 mg^OTC, 200 mg^OTC, 500 mg^OTC ■ **Extended-release capsules:** 150 mg^OTC ■ **Injection:** 100 mg/ml in 10- and 30-ml vials^Rx ■Cost: 100 mg/ml $5.50/10 ml ■ vitamins, minerals, and trace elements in a variety of multivitamin preparations^OTC.

| | ONSET | PEAK | DURATION |
|---|---|---|---|
| PO, IM, IV | unknown | unknown | unknown |

# NURSING IMPLICATIONS

## ASSESSMENT

❑ Assess patient for signs of vitamin $B_6$ deficiency (anemia, dermatitis, cheilosis, irritability, seizures, nausea, and vomiting) before and periodically throughout therapy. Institute seizure precautions in pyridoxine-dependent infants.

■ **Lab Test Considerations:** May cause false elevations in urobilinogen concentrations.

## POTENTIAL NURSING DIAGNOSES

■ Nutrition, imbalanced: less than body requirements (Indications).

## IMPLEMENTATION

■ **General:** Because of infrequency of single B-vitamin deficiencies, combinations are commonly administered.

❑ Administration of parenteral vitamin $B_6$ is limited to patients who are NPO or who have nausea and vomiting or malabsorption syndromes.

❑ Protect parenteral solution from light; decomposition will occur.

■ **PO:** Extended-release capsules and tablets should be swallowed whole, without crushing, breaking, or chewing. For patients unable to swallow capsule, contents of capsules may be mixed with jam or jelly.

■ **IM:** Rotate sites; burning or stinging at site may occur.

■ **IV:** May be administered direct IV or as infusion in standard IV solutions.

❑ Pyridoxine-dependent seizures should cease within 2–3 min of IV administration.

■ **Rate:** Infusion rates of 15–30 min and up to 3 hr have been used.

■ **Additive Incompatibility:** ◆ alkaline solutions ◆ riboflavin.

## PATIENT/FAMILY TEACHING

❑ Instruct patient to take medication as directed. If a dose is missed, it may be omitted because an extended period of time is required to become deficient in vitamin $B_6$.

❏ Encourage patient to comply with diet recommended by health care professional. Explain that the best source of vitamins is a well-balanced diet with foods from the four basic food groups. Foods high in vitamin $B_6$ include bananas, whole-grain cereals, potatoes, lima beans, and meats.

❏ Patients self-medicating with vitamin supplements should be cautioned not to exceed RDA. The effectiveness of megadoses for treatment of various medical conditions is unproved and may cause side effects, such as unsteady gait, numbness in feet, and difficulty with hand coordination.

❏ Emphasize the importance of follow-up exams to evaluate progress.

## EVALUATION

**Effectiveness of therapy can be demonstrated by:** ▪ Decrease in the symptoms of vitamin $B_6$ deficiency.

# quetiapine

(kwet-**eye**-a-peen)

Seroquel

## CLASSIFICATION(S):

**Therapeutic:** antipsychotics

**Pregnancy Category C**

## INDICATIONS

■ Management of the symptoms of schizophrenia.

## ACTION

■ Probably acts by serving as an antagonist of dopamine and serotonin ■ Also antagonizes histamine $H_1$ receptors and alpha$_1$-adrenergic receptors. **Therapeutic Effects:** ■ Decreased manifestations of psychoses.

## PHARMACOKINETICS

**Absorption:** Well absorbed after oral administration.

**Distribution:** Widely distributed.

**Metabolism and Excretion:** Extensively metabolized by the liver (mostly by P450 CYP3A4 enyzme system); <1% excreted unchanged in the urine.

**Half-life:** 6 hr.

## CONTRAINDICATIONS AND PRECAUTIONS

**Contraindicated in:** ■ Hypersensitivity ■ Lactation.

**Use Cautiously in:** ■ Cardiovascular disease, cerebrovascular disease, dehydration or hypovolemia (increased risk of hypotension) ■ History of seizures, Alzheimer's dementia, or age ≥65 yr ■ Hepatic impairment (dosage reduction may be necessary) ■ Hypothyroidism (may be exacerbated) ■ History of suicide attempt ■ Pregnancy or children (safety not established).

## ADVERSE REACTIONS AND SIDE EFFECTS*

■ **CNS:** NEUROLEPTIC MALIGNANT SYNDROME, SEIZURES, dizziness, cognitive impairment, extrapyramidal symptoms, sedation, tardive dyskinesia ■ **EENT:** ear pain, rhinitis ■ **Resp:** cough, dyspnea, pharyngitis ■ **CV:** palpitations, peripheral edema, postural hypotension ■ **GI:** anorexia, constipation, dry mouth, dyspepsia ■ **Derm:** sweating ■ **Hemat:** leukopenia ■ **Metab:** weight gain ■ **Misc:** flu-like syndrome.

## INTERACTIONS

**Drug-Drug:** ■ Additive CNS depression may occur with **alcohol, antihistamines, opioid analgesics,** and **sedative/hypnotics** ■ Increased risk of hypotension with acute ingestion of **alcohol** or **antihypertensives** ■ **Phenytoin** and **thioridazine** increase clearance and decrease effectiveness of quetiapine (dosage adjustment may be necessary); similar effects may occur with **carbamazepine, barbiturates, rifampin,** or **corticosteroids** ■ Effects may be increased by **ketoconazole, itraconazole, fluconazole,** or **erythromycin,** as well as by other **agents that inhibit the cytochrome P450 CYP3A4 enzyme.**

## ROUTE AND DOSAGE

■ **PO (Adults):** 25 mg twice daily initially, increased by 25–50 mg 2–3 times daily over 3 days, up to 300–400 mg/day in 2–3 divided doses by the 4th day (not to exceed 800 mg/day).

## AVAILABILITY

■ **Tablets:** 25 mg$^{Rx}$, 100 mg$^{Rx}$, 200 mg$^{Rx}$, 300 mg$^{Rx}$ ■ Cost: 25 mg $147.26/100, 100 mg $268.01/100, 200 mg $505.61/100, 300 mg $433.14/60.

TIME/ACTION PROFILE (antipsychotic effects)

|  | ONSET | PEAK | DURATION |
|---|---|---|---|
| PO | unknown | unknown | 8–12 hr |

# NURSING IMPLICATIONS

## ASSESSMENT

❏ Monitor patient's mental status (delusions, hallucinations, and behavior) before and periodically throughout therapy.

❏ Monitor mood changes. Assess for suicidal tendencies, especially during early therapy. Restrict amount of drug available to patient.

❏ Monitor blood pressure (sitting, standing, lying) and pulse before and frequently dur-

{ } = Available in Canada only.
*CAPITALS indicates life-threatening; underlines indicate most frequent.

ing initial dosage titration. If hypotension occurs during dose titration, return to the previous dose.

❏ Observe patient carefully when administering medication to ensure that medication is actually swallowed and not hoarded.

❏ Monitor patient for onset of extrapyramidal side effects (*akathisia*—restlessness; *dystonia*—muscle spasms and twisting motions; or *pseudoparkinsonism*—mask-like faces, rigidity, tremors, drooling, shuffling gait, dysphagia). Report these symptoms; reduction of dosage or discontinuation of medication may be necessary. Trihexyphenidyl or diphenhydramine may be used to control these symptoms.

❏ Monitor for tardive dyskinesia (involuntary rhythmic movement of mouth, face, and extremities). Report immediately; may be irreversible.

❏ Monitor for development of neuroleptic malignant syndrome (fever, respiratory distress, tachycardia, seizures, diaphoresis, hypertension or hypotension, pallor, tiredness). Notify physician or other health care professional immediately if these symptoms occur.

■ *Lab Test Considerations:* May cause asymptomatic increases in AST and ALT.

❏ May also cause anemia, thrombocytopenia, leukocytosis, and leukopenia.

❏ May cause increased total cholesterol and triglycerides.

## POTENTIAL NURSING DIAGNOSES

■ Violence, for self-directed (Indications).

■ Thought processes, disturbed (Indications).

■ Injury, risk for (Side Effects).

## IMPLEMENTATION

■ **General:** Do not confuse Seroquel (quetiapine) with Serzone (nefazodone). If therapy is reinstituted after an interval of ≥1 wk off, follow initial titration schedule.

■ **PO:** May be administered without regard to food.

## PATIENT/FAMILY TEACHING

❏ Instruct patient to take medication exactly as directed.

❏ Inform patient of the possibility of extrapyramidal symptoms. Instruct patient to report these symptoms immediately to health care professional.

❏ Advise patient to change positions slowly to minimize orthostatic hypotension.

❏ May cause drowsiness. Caution patient to avoid driving or other activities requiring alertness until response to medication is known.

❏ Advise patient that extremes in temperature should be avoided because this drug impairs body temperature regulation.

❏ Caution patient to avoid concurrent use of alcohol, other CNS depressants, and OTC medications without consulting health care professional.

❏ Advise female patients to notify health care professional if pregnancy is planned or suspected or if they are breastfeeding or planning to breastfeed.

❏ Advise patient to notify health care professional of medication regimen before treatment or surgery.

❏ Instruct patient to notify health care professional promptly of sore throat, fever, unusual bleeding or bruising, or rash.

❏ Emphasize the need for continued follow-up for psychotherapy and monitoring for side effects. Ophthalmologic exams should be performed before and every 6 mo during therapy.

## EVALUATION

**Effectiveness of therapy can be demonstrated by:** ■ Decrease in excited, paranoic, or withdrawn behavior.

# quinapril, See ANGIOTENSIN-CONVERTING ENZYME (ACE) INHIBITORS.

# QUINIDINE

(**kwin**-i-deen)

### quinidine gluconate
Quinaglute Dura-Tabs, Quinalan, {Quinate}

### quinidine sulfate
{Apo-Quinidine}, Cin-Quin, {Novoquinidin}, Quinidex Extentabs, Quinora

## CLASSIFICATION(S):

**Therapeutic:** antiarrhythmics (class IA)

## Pregnancy Category C

## INDICATIONS

■ Management of a wide variety of atrial and ventricular arrhythmias, including: ❑ Atrial premature contractions ❑ Premature ventricular contractions ❑ Ventricular tachycardia ❑ Paroxysmal atrial tachycardia ❑ Maintenance of normal sinus rhythm after conversion from atrial fibrillation or flutter. **Unlabeled uses:** ■ Treatment of malaria (IV gluconate only).

## ACTION

■ Decrease myocardial excitability ■ Slow conduction velocity. **Therapeutic Effects:** ■ Suppression of arrhythmias.

## PHARMACOKINETICS

**Absorption:** Well absorbed from the GI tract and IM sites. Extended-release quinidine sulfate (Quinidex Extentabs) or gluconate (Quinaglute, Quinalan) oral preparations are absorbed more slowly following oral administration.

**Distribution:** Widely distributed. Cross the placenta; enter breast milk.

**Metabolism and Excretion:** Metabolized by the liver; 10–30% excreted unchanged by the kidneys.

**Half-life:** 6–8 hr (increased in CHF or severe liver impairment).

## CONTRAINDICATIONS AND PRECAUTIONS

**Contraindicated in:** ■ Hypersensitivity ■ Conduction defects ■ Digoxin toxicity.

**Use Cautiously in:** ■ CHF or severe liver disease (dosage reduction recommended) ■ Hypokalemia or hypomagnesemia (increases the risk of $QT_c$ prolongation) ■ Pregnancy, lactation, or children (safety not established; extended-release preparations should not be used in children).

## ADVERSE REACTIONS AND SIDE EFFECTS*

■ **CNS:** dizziness, headache, syncope ■ **EENT:** blurred vision, diplopia, mydriasis, photophobia, tinnitus ■ **CV:** HYPOTENSION, arrhythmias, tachycardia ■ **GI:** anorexia, cramping, diarrhea, nausea, bitter taste, drug-induced hepatitis ■ **Derm:** rashes ■ **Hemat:** hemolytic anemia, thrombocytopenia ■ **Misc:** fever.

## INTERACTIONS

**Drug-Drug:** ■ Increases serum **digoxin** levels and may cause toxicity (dosage reduction recommended) ■ **Amiodarone** increases quinidine levels and risk of toxicity ■ **Phenytoin, phenobarbital,** or **rifampin** may increase metabolism and decrease effectiveness ■ **Cimetidine, diltiazem,** and **verapamil** decrease metabolism and may increase blood levels ■ Excretion is delayed and effects increased by **carbonic anhydrase inhibitors** and **thiazide diuretics** ■ Potentiates **neuromuscular blocking agents** and **warfarin** ■ Additive hypotension with **antihypertensives, nitrates,** and acute ingestion of **alcohol** ■ May increase **procainamide, propafenone,** or **tricyclic antidepressant** levels and risk of toxicity ■ May antagonize **anticholinesterase therapy** in patients with myasthenia gravis ■ **Drugs that alkalinize the urine,** including high-dose **antacid** therapy or **sodium bicarbonate,** increase blood levels and the risk of toxicity ■ Additive anticholinergic effects may occur with **agents having anticholinergic properties** (including **antihistamines, tricyclic antidepressants**) ■ Increased risk of arrhythmias with **pimozide.**

**Drug-Food:** ■ **Grapefruit juice** increases serum levels and effect ■ **Foods that alkalinize the urine** (see Appendix Q) may increase serum quinidine levels and the risk of toxicity.

## ROUTE AND DOSAGE

❑ **Quinidine Gluconate (62% Quinidine)**

■ **PO (Adults):** 324–660 mg q 6–12 hr as extended-release tablets, 325–650 mg q 6 hr if not extended release.

■ **IM (Adults):** 600 mg initially, followed by 400 mg as often as q 2 hr.

■ **IV (Adults):** *Antiarrhythmic*—Infuse at 16 mg/min until arrhythmia is suppressed, QRS complex widens, bradycardia or hypotension occurs.

❑ **Quinidine Sulfate (83% Quinidine)**

■ **PO (Adults):** *Paroxysmal supraventricular tachycardia*—400–600 mg q 2–3 hr until arrhythmia is terminated. *Conversion of atrial fibrillation*—200 mg q 2–3 hr for 5–8 doses; dosage may be increased at daily intervals if necessary. *Premature atrial/ventricular contractions*—200–300 mg q 6–8 hr or 300–600 mg of extended-release preparation every 8–12 hr maintenance (not to exceed 4 g/day).

■ **PO (Children):** 6 mg/kg or 180 mg/m² 5 times daily.

## AVAILABILITY (generic available)

❑ **Quinidine Gluconate**

■ *Tablets:* {325 mg^Rx} ■ *Extended-release tablets:* 324 mg^Rx, 330 mg^Rx ■ *Injection:* 80 mg/ml in 10-ml vials^Rx.

❑ **Quinidine Sulfate**

■ *Tablets:* 100 mg^Rx, 200 mg^Rx, 300 mg^Rx ■ *Extended-release tablets:* 300 mg^Rx ■ *Capsules:* 200 mg^Rx, 300 mg^Rx.

TIME/ACTION PROFILE (antiarrhythmic effects)

| | ONSET | PEAK | DURATION |
|---|---|---|---|
| PO (sulfate) | 30 min | 1–1.5 hr | 6–8 hr |
| PO (sulfate-ER) | unknown | 4 hr | 8–12 hr |
| PO (gluconate) | unknown | 3–4 hr | 6–8 hr |
| IM | 30 min | 30–90 min | 6–8 hr |
| IV | 1–5 min | rapid | 6–8 hr |

# NURSING IMPLICATIONS

## ASSESSMENT

❑ Monitor ECG, pulse, and blood pressure continuously throughout IV administration and periodically during oral administration. IV administration is usually discontinued if any of the following occur: arrhythmia is resolved, QRS complex widens by 50%, PR or QT intervals are prolonged, or frequent ventricular ectopic beats or tachycardia develops. Patient should remain supine throughout IV administration to minimize hypotension.

■ *Lab Test Considerations:* Hepatic and renal function, CBC, and serum potassium levels should be periodically monitored during prolonged therapy.

■ *Toxicity and Overdose:* Serum quinidine levels may be monitored periodically during dosage adjustment. Therapeutic serum concentrations are 2–6 mcg/ml. Toxic effects usually occur at concentrations >8 mcg/ml.

❑ Signs and symptoms of toxicity or cinchonism include tinnitus, hearing loss, visual disturbances, headache, nausea, and dizziness. These may occur after a single dose.

❑ Cardiac signs of toxicity include QRS widening, cardiac asystole, ventricular ectopic beats, idioventricular rhythms (ventricular tachycardia, ventricular fibrillation), paradoxical tachycardia, and arterial embolism.

## POTENTIAL NURSING DIAGNOSES

■ Cardiac output, decreased (Indications).

## IMPLEMENTATION

■ **General:** Do not confuse quinidine with quinine.

❑ A test dose of a single 200-mg quinidine sulfate tablet or 200 mg IM quinidine gluconate may be administered prior to quinidine therapy to check for intolerance.

❑ Higher doses may be required to correct atrial arrhythmias than are required for ventricular arrhythmias.

■ **PO:** Administer with a full glass of water on an empty stomach either 1 hr before or 2 hr after meals for faster absorption. If GI irritation becomes a problem, may be administered with or immediately after meals. Extended-release preparations (Quinaglute Dura-Tabs, Quinidex Extentabs, Quinalan) should be swallowed whole; do not break, crush, or chew.

■ **IV:** Use only clear, colorless solution.

■ **Intermittent Infusion:** Dilute 800 mg of quinidine gluconate (10 ml) in 50 ml of D5W for injection for a concentration of 16 mg/ml. Solution is stable for 24 hr at room temperature or 48 hr if refrigerated.

■ *Rate:* Administer quinidine gluconate at a rate not to exceed 1 ml/min. Administer via infusion pump to ensure accurate dose. Rapid administration may cause peripheral vascular collapse and severe hypotension.

■ **Y-Site Compatibility:** ◆ diazepam ◆ milrinone.

■ **Y-Site Incompatibility:** ◆ furosemide.

## PATIENT/FAMILY TEACHING

❏ Instruct patient to take medication around the clock, exactly as directed, even if feeling well. If a dose is missed, take as soon as remembered if within 2 hr; if remembered later, omit. Do not double doses.

❏ Instruct patient or family member on how to take pulse. Advise patient to report changes in pulse rate or rhythm to health care professional.

❏ May cause dizziness or blurred vision. Caution patient to avoid driving or other activities requiring alertness until response to medication is known.

❏ Inform patient that quinidine may cause increased sensitivity to light. Dark glasses may minimize this effect.

❏ Advise patient to inform health care professional of medication regimen prior to treatment or surgery.

❏ Instruct patient not to take OTC medications with quinidine without consulting health care professional.

❏ Advise patient to consult health care professional if symptoms of cinchonism, rash, or dyspnea occur or if diarrhea is severe or persistent.

❏ Advise patient to carry identification at all times describing disease process and medication regimen.

❏ Emphasize the importance of routine follow-up exams to monitor progress.

## EVALUATION

**Effectiveness of therapy can be demonstrated by:** ■ Resolution of cardiac arrhythmias without detrimental side effects.

---

## quinine

(**kwi**-nine)

### CLASSIFICATION(S):

**Therapeutic:** antimalarials

### Pregnancy Category X

---

## INDICATIONS

■ Combination with other agents in the treatment of chloroquine-resistant malaria. **Unlabeled uses:** ■ Prophylaxis and treatment of nocturnal recumbency leg cramps, including those associated with arthritis, diabetes, varicose veins, thrombophlebitis, arteriosclerosis, and static foot deformities.

## ACTION

■ Disrupts metabolism of the erythrocytic phase of *Plasmodium falciparum* ■ Increases the refractory period of skeletal muscle, increases the distribution of calcium within muscle fibers, decreases the excitability of motor end-plate regions, resulting in decreased response to repetitive nerve stimulation and acetylcholine. **Therapeutic Effects:** ■ Death of *P. falciparum* ■ Decreased severity of leg cramps.

## PHARMACOKINETICS

**Absorption:** Rapidly and almost completely (80%) absorbed following oral administration.

**Distribution:** Varies with condition and patient; does not enter CSF well. Crosses the placenta and enters breast milk.

**Protein Binding:** >90% in patients with cerebral malaria, pregnant women and children, 85–90% in patients with uncomplicated malaria, 70% in healthy adults.

**Metabolism and Excretion:** >80% metabolized by the liver; metabolites have less activity than quinine; metabolites excreted in urine. 20% excreted unchanged in urine. Excretion increased in acidic urine.

**Half-life:** 11 hr (increased in patients with malaria).

## CONTRAINDICATIONS AND PRECAUTIONS

**Contraindicated in:** ■ Hypersensitivity ■ Pregnancy or lactation.

**Use Cautiously in:** ■ Recurrent or interrupted malaria therapy ■ History of arrhythmias, especially QT prolongation ■ G6PD deficiency ■ Hypoglycemia ■ Myasthenia gravis ■ History of thrombocytopenic purpura.

## ADVERSE REACTIONS AND SIDE EFFECTS*

■ **GI:** abdominal cramps/pain, diarrhea, nausea, vomiting, hepatotoxicity ■ **Derm:** rash ■ **Endo:** hypoglycemia ■ **Hemat:** bleeding, blood dyscrasias ■ **Misc:** cinchonism, hypersensitivity reactions including fever and HEMOLYTIC UREMIC SYNDROME.

## INTERACTIONS

**Drug-Drug:** ■ **Antacids** may delay/decrease absorption ■ **Cimetidine** decreases metabolism and may increase effects ■ **Rifampin** and **rifabutin** increase metabolism and may decrease effects ■ May increase the effects of **neuromuscular blocking agents** ■ May increase serum **digoxin** levels ■ May increase the risk of hemolytic, ototoxic, or neurotoxic reactions when used concurrently with **agents sharing these toxicities** ■ Concurrent use with **quinidine** may increase the risk of adverse cardiovascular reactions ■ May increase the risk of bleeding with **warfarin** ■ Concurrent use with **mefloquine** increases the risk of seizures and adverse cardiovascular reactions.

## ROUTE AND DOSAGE

■ **PO (Adults):** *Malaria*—600–650 mg q 8 hr for 3 days (7 days in southeast Asia) with tetracycline or doxycycline or sulfadoxine/pyramethamine or clindamycin; *leg cramps (unlabeled)*—200–300 mg at bedtime, if needed an additional 200–300 mg may be given with supper.

■ **PO (Children):** 8.3 mg/kg q 8 hr for 3 days (7 days in southeast Asia) with tetracycline or doxycycline (if child is over 8 yr) or sulfadoxine/pyramethamine or clindamycin.

## AVAILABILITY

■ *Capsules:* 200 mg$^{Rx}$, 300 mg$^{Rx}$, 325 mg$^{Rx}$ ■ Cost: 325 mg $5.15–$8.28/30 ■ *Tablets:* 260 mg$^{Rx}$, 325 mg$^{Rx}$ ■ Cost: 260 mg $14.50/100, 325 mg $18.82/100.

TIME/ACTION PROFILE (antimalarial blood levels)

| | ONSET | PEAK | DURATION |
|---|---|---|---|
| PO | unknown | 3.2–5.9 hr | 8 hr |

## NURSING IMPLICATIONS

### ASSESSMENT

■ **Malaria:** Assess patient for improvement in signs and symptoms of condition daily throughout therapy.

■ **Nocturnal recumbency leg cramps:** Assess frequency and severity of nocturnal leg cramps. If cramps do not occur for several consecutive nights, may be discontinued to determine whether continued use is required.

■ *Lab Test Considerations:* May cause elevated urinary 17-ketogenic steroids when metyrapone or Zimmerman method is used.

■ *Toxicity and Overdose:* Plasma quinine levels of >10 mcg/ml may cause tinnitus and impaired hearing.

❑ Signs of toxicity or cinchonism include tinnitus, headache, nausea, and slightly disturbed vision; usually disappear rapidly upon discontinuing quinine.

### POTENTIAL NURSING DIAGNOSES

■ Infection, risk for (Indications).
■ Pain, chronic (Indications).

### IMPLEMENTATION

■ **PO:** Administer with or after meals to minimize GI distress. Aluminum-containing antacids will decrease and delay absorption; avoid concurrent use.

### PATIENT/FAMILY TEACHING

❑ Instruct patient to take medication exactly as directed and continue full course of therapy, even if feeling better. Missed doses should be taken as soon as remembered, unless almost time for the next dose. Do not double doses or take more than recommended.

❑ Review methods of minimizing exposure to mosquitoes with patients receiving chloroquine prophylactically (use insect repellent, wear long-sleeved shirt and long trousers, use screen or netting).

❑ Quinine may cause visual changes. Caution patient to avoid driving or other activities requiring alertness until response to medication is known.

❑ May cause diarrhea, nausea, stomach cramps or pain, vomiting, or ringing in the ears. Advise patient to notify health care professional promptly if these become pronounced.

▫ Advise patient to stop quinine and notify health care professional of any evidence of allergy (flushing, itching, rash, fever, stomach pain, difficult breathing, ringing in the ears, visual problems).

## EVALUATION

**Effectiveness of therapy can be demonstrated by:** ■ Prevention of or improvement in signs and symptoms of malaria ■ Decrease in frequency and severity of nocturnal redundancy leg cramps.

---

# quinupristin/dalfopristin
(kwin-oo-**pris**-tin/dal-foe-**pris**-tin)
Synercid

**CLASSIFICATION(S):**
**Therapeutic:** anti-infectives
**Pharmacologic:** streptogramins

**Pregnancy Category B**

---

## INDICATIONS

■ Treatment of serious or life-threatening infections associated with vancomycin-resistant *Enterococcus faecium* (VREF) ■ Complicated skin/skin structure infections caused by *Staphylococcus aureus* (methicillin-susceptible) or *Streptococcus pyogenes.*

## ACTION

■ Quinupristin inhibits the late phase of protein synthesis at the level of the bacterial ribosome; dalfopristin inhibits the early phase. **Therapeutic Effects:** ■ Bacteriostatic effect against susceptible organisms. **Spectrum:** ■ Active against vancomycin-resistant and multidrug-resistant strains of *E. faecium, S. aureus* (methicillin-susceptible), and *S. pyogenes.* ■ Not active against *E. faecalis.*

## PHARMACOKINETICS

**Absorption:** IV administration results in complete bioavailability.
**Distribution:** Unknown.
**Protein Binding:** Moderate.

**Metabolism and Excretion:** Both are converted to compounds with additional anti-infective activity; parent drugs and metabolites are mostly excreted in feces (75–77%); 15% of quinupristin and 17% of dalfopristin excreted in urine.
**Half-life:** *Quinupristin*—0.85 hr; *dalfopristin*—0.7 hr.

## CONTRAINDICATIONS AND PRECAUTIONS

**Contraindicated in:** ■ Hypersensitivity.

**Use Cautiously in:** ■ Concurrent use of other drugs metabolized by the cytochrome P450 3A4 enzyme system (serious interactions may occur; see Drug-Drug Interactions) ■ Hepatic impairment (dosage adjustment may be necessary) ■ Patients with a history of GI disease, especially colitis ■ Pregnancy, lactation, or children <16 yr (safety not established).

## ADVERSE REACTIONS AND SIDE EFFECTS*

■ **CNS:** headache ■ **CV:** thrombophlebitis ■ **GI:** PSEUDOMEMBRANOUS COLITIS, diarrhea, nausea, vomiting ■ **Derm:** pruritus, rash ■ **Local:** edema/inflammation/pain at infusion site, infusion site reactions ■ **Misc:** allergic reactions including ANAPHYLAXIS, pain.

## INTERACTIONS

**Drug-Drug:** ■ Inhibits the cytochrome P450 3A4 drug metabolizing enzyme system; inhibits metabolism of **cyclosporine, midazolam,** and **nifedipine** and increases the risk of toxicity (careful monitoring required) ■ Similar effects may be expected with concurrent use of **delavirdine, nevirapine, indinavir, ritonavir, vinca alkaloids, docetaxel, paclitaxel, diazepam, verapamil, diltiazem, HMG CoA reductase inhibitors, tacrolimus, methylprednisolone, carbamazepine, quinidine, lidocaine,** and **disopyramide.**

## ROUTE AND DOSAGE

■ **IV (Adults):** *Vancomycin-resistant E. faecium*—7.5 mg/kg q 8 hr for at least 7 days; *complicated skin/skin structure infections*—7.5 mg/kg q 12 hr for at least 7 days.

## AVAILABILITY

■ *Powder for injection:* 500 mg (150 mg quinuprostin and 350 mg dalfopristin in 10-ml vials)[Rx].

TIME/ACTION PROFILE

|    | ONSET | PEAK | DURATION |
|----|-------|------|----------|
| IV | rapid | end of infu-<br>sion | 8–12 hr |

## NURSING IMPLICATIONS

### ASSESSMENT

❏ Assess patient for infection (vital signs; appearance of wound, sputum, urine, and stool; WBC) at beginning of and throughout therapy.

❏ Obtain specimens for culture and sensitivity before initiating therapy. First dose may be given before receiving results.

❏ Monitor patient for pain or inflammation at the infusion site frequently throughout infusion. Increasing the volume of diluent from 250 ml to 500 ml or 750 ml or infusing via a peripherally inserted central catheter or central venous catheter may be required.

❏ Observe patient for signs and symptoms of anaphylaxis (rash, pruritus, laryngeal edema, wheezing). Discontinue drug and notify physician or other health care professional immediately if these problems occur. Keep epinephrine, an antihistamine, and resuscitation equipment close by in case of an anaphylactic reaction.

❏ Assess patient for myalgia and arthralgia after infusion. May be severe. Reducing dose frequency to every 12 hr may decrease pain. Symptoms usually resolve upon discontinuation of medication.

■ *Lab Test Considerations:* May cause elevated serum total bilirubin concentrations.

## POTENTIAL NURSING DIAGNOSES

■ Infection, risk for (Indications, Side Effects).

■ Diarrhea (Adverse Reactions).

## IMPLEMENTATION

■ **Intermittent Infusion:** Reconstitute by slowly adding 5 ml of D5W or sterile water for injection for a concentration of 100 mg/ml. Gently swirl vial to mix. Avoid shaking to prevent foam formation. Allow solution to sit until all foam has disappeared. Solution should be clear. Dilute further by adding dose of constituted solution to 250 ml of D5W (100 ml can be used for central line infusion). Diluted solution is stable for 5 hr at room temperature or 54 hr if refrigerated.

■ *Rate:* Administer over 60 min using an infusion control device. Flush line before and after infusion with D5W. Do not use 0.9% NaCl or heparin.

■ **Y-Site Compatibility:** ◆ aztreonam ◆ ciprofloxacin ◆ fluconazole ◆ haloperidol ◆ metoclopramide ◆ potassium chloride.

■ **Additive Incompatibility:** Do not admix with other solutions of medications.

■ **Solution Incompatibility:** 0.9% NaCl.

## PATIENT/FAMILY TEACHING

❏ Instruct patient to notify health care professional if fever and diarrhea develop, especially if stool contains blood, pus, or mucus. Advise patient not to treat diarrhea without consulting health care professional.

## EVALUATION

**Effectiveness of therapy can be demonstrated by:** ■ Resolution of signs and symptoms of infection. Length of time for complete resolution depends on the organism and site of infection.

# rabeprazole

(ra-**bep**-ra-zole)

Aciphex

## CLASSIFICATION(S):

**Therapeutic:** antiulcer agents
**Pharmacologic:** proton-pump inhibitors

## Pregnancy Category B

## INDICATIONS

■ Gastroesophageal reflux disease (GERD) ■ Duodenal ulcers (including combination therapy with clarithromycin and amoxicillin to eradicate *h. pylori* and prevent recurrence) ■ Pathological hypersecretory conditions, including Zollinger-Ellison syndrome.

## ACTION

■ Binds to an enzyme in the presence of acidic gastric pH, preventing the final transport of hydrogen ions into the gastric lumen. **Therapeutic Effects:** ■ Diminished accumulation of acid in the gastric lumen, with lessened acid reflux ■ Healing of duodenal ulcers and esophagitis ■ Decreased acid secretion in hypersecretory conditions.

## PHARMACOKINETICS

**Absorption:** Delayed-release tablet is designed to allow rabeprazole, which is not stable in gastric acid, to pass through the stomach intact. Subsequently 52% is absorbed after oral administration.

**Distribution:** Unknown.

**Protein Binding:** 96.3%.

**Metabolism and Excretion:** Mostly metabolized by the liver (hepatic cytochrome P450 3A and 2C19 enzyme systems); 10% excreted in feces; remainder excreted in urine as inactive metabolites.

**Half-life:** 1–2 hr.

## CONTRAINDICATIONS AND PRECAUTIONS

**Contraindicated in:** ■ Hypersensitivity to rabeprazole or related drugs (benzimidazoles).

**Use Cautiously in:** ■ Severe hepatic impairment (dosage reduction may be necessary) ■ Pregnancy, lactation, or children (breastfeeding not recommended; use in pregnancy only if needed; safety not established).

## ADVERSE REACTIONS AND SIDE EFFECTS*

■ **CNS:** dizziness, headache, malaise ■ **GI:** abdominal pain, constipation, diarrhea, nausea ■ **Derm:** photosensitivity, rash ■ **MS:** neck pain ■ **Misc:** allergic reactions, chills, fever.

## INTERACTIONS

**Drug-Drug:** ■ Rabeprazole is metabolized by the CYP450 enzyme system and may interact with other drugs metabolized by this system ■ ↓ blood levels of **ketoconazole** ■ ↑ blood levels of **digoxin** ■ May alter the effects of **drugs whose absorption is pH dependent** ■ May increase the risk of bleeding with **warfarin** (monitor INR/PT).

## ROUTE AND DOSAGE

■ **PO (Adults):** *GERD, duodenal ulcers*—20 mg once daily *prevention of duodenal ulcer recurrence*—20 mg twice daily for 7 days with amoxicillin 1000 mg twice daily for 7 days and clarithromycin 500 mg twice daily for 7 days; *hypersecretory conditions*—60 mg once daily initially, may be adjusted as needed and continued as necessary; doses up to 100 mg daily or 60 mg twice daily have been used.

## AVAILABILITY

■ *Delayed-release tablets:* 20 mg^Rx ■Cost: 20 mg $117.60/30.

TIME/ACTION PROFILE (acid suppression)

| | ONSET | PEAK | DURATION |
|---|---|---|---|
| PO | within 1 hr | unknown | 24 hr† |

†Suppression continues to increase over the first week of therapy.

# NURSING IMPLICATIONS

## ASSESSMENT

❑ Assess patient routinely for epigastric or abdominal pain and frank or occult blood in the stool, emesis, or gastric aspirate.

■ *Lab Test Considerations:* Monitor CBC with differential periodically during therapy.

## POTENTIAL NURSING DIAGNOSES

■ Pain, acute (Indications).

## IMPLEMENTATION

■ **PO:** Administer doses before meals, preferably in the morning. Tablets should be swallowed whole; do not crush, break, or chew.

## PATIENT/FAMILY TEACHING

❑ Instruct patient to take medication as directed for the full course of therapy, even if feeling better. Take missed doses as soon as remembered but not if almost time for next dose. Do not double doses.

❑ May cause occasional drowsiness or dizziness. Caution patient to avoid driving or other activities requiring alertness until response to medication is known.

❑ Advise patient to avoid alcohol, products containing aspirin or NSAIDs, and foods that may cause an increase in GI irritation.

❑ Caution patients to wear sunscreen and protective clothing to prevent photosensitivity reactions.

❑ Advise patient to report onset of black, tarry stools; diarrhea; abdominal pain; or persistent headache to health care professional promptly.

## EVALUATION

**Effectiveness of therapy can be demonstrated by:** ■ Decrease in abdominal pain or prevention of gastric irritation and bleeding. Healing of duodenal ulcers can be seen on x-ray examination or endoscopy ■ Decrease in symptoms of GERD. Therapy is continued for 4–8 wk after initial episode.

---

# raloxifene

(ra-**lox**-i-feen)
Evista

## CLASSIFICATION(S):

***Therapeutic:*** *bone resorption inhibitors*
***Pharmacologic:*** *selective estrogen receptor modulators*

**Pregnancy Category X**

---

## INDICATIONS

■ Treatment and prevention of osteoporosis in postmenopausal women.

## ACTION

■ Binds to estrogen receptors, producing estrogen-like effects on bone, resulting in reduced resorption of bone and decreased bone turnover. **Therapeutic Effects:** ■ Prevention of osteoporosis in patients at risk.

## PHARMACOKINETICS

**Absorption:** Although well absorbed (>60%), after oral administration, extensive first-pass metabolism results in 2% bioavailability.

**Distribution:** Highly bound to plasma proteins; remainder of distribution unknown.

**Protein Binding:** Highly bound to plasma proteins.

**Metabolism and Excretion:** Extensively metabolized by the liver; undergoes enterohepatic cycling; excreted primarily in feces.

**Half-life:** 27.7 hr.

## CONTRAINDICATIONS AND PRECAUTIONS

**Contraindicated in:** ■ Hypersensitivity ■ History of thromboembolic events ■ Women with childbearing potential ■ Pregnancy, lactation, or children.

**Use Cautiously in:** ■ Potential immobilization (increased risk of thromboembolic events).

## ADVERSE REACTIONS AND SIDE EFFECTS*

■ **MS:** leg cramps ■ **Misc:** hot flashes.

## INTERACTIONS

**Drug-Drug:** ■ **Cholestyramine** decreases absorption (avoid concurrent use) ■ May alter effects of **warfarin** and other **highly protein-bound drugs** ■ Concurrent systemic **estrogen** therapy is not recommended.

## ROUTE AND DOSAGE

■ **PO (Adults):** 60 mg once daily.

## AVAILABILITY

■ *Tablets:* 60 mg$^{Rx}$ ■ Cost: $66.36/30 tablets.

TIME/ACTION PROFILE (effects on bone turnover)

| | ONSET | PEAK | DURATION |
|---|---|---|---|
| PO | unknown | 3 mo | unknown |

## NURSING IMPLICATIONS

### ASSESSMENT

❑ Assess patient for bone mineral density with x-ray, serum, and urine bone turnover markers (bone-specific alkaline phosphatase, osteocalcin, and collagen breakdown products) before and periodically during therapy.

■ *Lab Test Considerations:* May cause increased apolipoprotein A-I and reduced serum total cholesterol, LDL cholesterol, fibrinogen, apolipoprotein B, and lipoprotein.

❑ May cause increased hormone-binding globulin (sex steroid-binding globulin, thyroxine-binding globulin, corticosteroid-binding globulin) with increases in total hormone concentrations.

❑ May cause small decreases in serum total calcium, inorganic phosphate, total protein, and albumin.

❑ May also cause slight decrease in platelet count.

### POTENTIAL NURSING DIAGNOSES

■ Injury, risk for (Indications).

### IMPLEMENTATION

■ **PO:** May be administered without regard to meals.

❑ Calcium supplementation should be added to diet if daily intake is inadequate.

### PATIENT/FAMILY TEACHING

❑ Instruct patient to take raloxifene as directed. Discuss the importance of adequate calcium and vitamin D intake or supplementation. Advise patient to discontinue smoking and alcohol consumption.

❑ Emphasize the importance of regular weight-bearing exercise. Advise patient that raloxifene should be discontinued at least 72 hr before and during prolonged immobilization (recovery from surgery, prolonged bedrest). Instruct patient to avoid prolonged restrictions of movement during travel because of the increased risk of venous thrombosis.

❑ Advise patient that raloxifene will not reduce hot flashes or flushes associated with estrogen deficiency and may cause hot flashes.

❑ Advise patient that raloxifene may have teratogenic effects. Instruct patient to notify health care provider immediately if pregnancy is planned or suspected.

❑ Instruct patient to read the patient package insert when initiating therapy and again with each prescription refill.

### EVALUATION

**Effectiveness of therapy can be demonstrated by:** ■ Prevention of osteoporosis in postmenopausal women.

## ramipril, See ANGIOTENSIN-CONVERTING ENZYME (ACE) INHIBITORS.

## ranitidine, See HISTAMINE H₂ ANTAGONISTS.

## ranitidine bismuth citrate, See HISTAMINE H₂ ANTAGONISTS.

## rasburicase

(ras-**byoor**-i-case)
Elitek

**CLASSIFICATION(S):**
*Therapeutic:* antigout agents, antihyperuricemics
*Pharmacologic:* enzymes

**Pregnancy Category C**

### INDICATIONS

■ Initial management of increased uric acid levels in children with leukemia, lymphoma or other malignancies who are being treated with antineoplastics which are expected to produce hyperuricemia.

## ACTION

■ An enzyme which promotes the conversion of uric acid to allantoin, an inactive, water-soluble compound ■ Produced by recombinant DNA technology. **Therapeutic Effects:** ■ Decreased sequelae of hyperuricemia (nephropathy, arthropathy).

## PHARMACOKINETICS

**Absorption:** IV administration results in complete bioavailability.

**Distribution:** Unknown.

**Metabolism and Excretion:** Unknown.

**Half-life:** 18 hr.

## CONTRAINDICATIONS AND PRECAUTIONS

**Contraindicated in:** ■ G6–PD deficiency ■ Previous allergic reaction, hemolysis or methemoglobinemia from rasburicase ■ Lactation.

**Use Cautiously in:** ■ Pregnancy (use only if clearly needed).

## ADVERSE REACTIONS AND SIDE EFFECTS*

■ **CNS:** headache ■ **Resp:** respiratory distress ■ **GI:** abdominal pain, constipation, diarrhea, nausea, vomiting, mucositis ■ **Derm:** rash ■ **Hemat:** HEMOLYSIS, METHEMOGLOBINEMIA, neutropenia ■ **Misc:** hypersensitivity reactions including ANAPHYLAXIS, fever, sepsis.

## INTERACTIONS

**Drug-Drug:** ■ None known.

## ROUTE AND DOSAGE

■ **IV (Children):** 0.15 or 0.2 mg/kg daily as a single dose for 5 days.

## AVAILABILITY

■ *lyophilized powder for reconstitution:* 1.5 mg/vial in cartons of 3 vials with specific diluent<sup>Rx</sup>.

TIME/ACTION PROFILE (decrease in uric acid))

|    | ONSET | PEAK    | DURATION |
|----|-------|---------|----------|
| IV | rapid | unknown | 4–24 hr  |

## NURSING IMPLICATIONS

### ASSESSMENT

❑ Monitor patients for signs of allergic reactions and anaphylaxis (chest pain, dyspnea, hypotension, urticaria). If these signs occur, rasburicase should be immediately and permanently discontinued.

■ *Lab Test Considerations:* Monitor patients for hemolysis. Patients at higher risk for G6PD deficiency (patients of African American or Mediterranean ancestry) should be screened prior to therapy. If hemolysis occurs, discontinue and do not restart rasburicase.

❑ Monitor patients for methemoglobinemia. Discontinue rasburicase and do not restart in patients who develop methemoglobinemia.

❑ May cause spuriously low uric acid levels in blood samples left at room temperature. Collect blood for uric acid levels in pre-chilled tubes containing heparin and immediately immerse and maintain in an ice water bath. Uric acid must be analyzed in plasma. Plasma samples must be assayed within 4 hr of collection.

### POTENTIAL NURSING DIAGNOSES

■ Knowledge, deficient, related to medication regimen (Patient/Family Teaching).

### IMPLEMENTATION

■ **General:** Chemotherapy is initiated 4–24 hr after first dose of rasburicase.

■ **Intermittent Infusion:** Determine number of vials of rasburicase needed based on patient's weight and dose/kg. Reconstitute in diluent provided. Add 1 ml of diluent provided to each vial and mix by swirling very gently. Do not shake or vortex. Solution should be clear and colorless. Do not use solutions that are discolored or contain particulate matter. Remove dose from reconstituted vials and inject into infusion bag of 0.9% NaCl for a final total volume of 50 ml. Administer within 24 hr of reconstitution. Store reconstituted or diluted solution in refrigerator for up to 24 hr.

■ *Rate:* Administer over 30 min. Do not administer as a bolus.

■ **Y-Site Incompatibility:** Infuse through a separate line. Do not use a filter with infusion. If separate line is not possible, flush line with at least 15 ml of 0.9% NaCl prior to rasburicase infusion.

## PATIENT/FAMILY TEACHING

❑ Inform patient and family of purpose of rasburicase infusion.

## EVALUATION

**Effectiveness of therapy can be demonstrated by:** ■ Decrease in plasma uric acid levels in pediatric patients receiving antineoplastics expected to result in tumor lysis and subsequent elevation of plasma uric acid levels.

## repaglinide
(re-**pag**-gli-nide)
Gluconorm, Prandin

**CLASSIFICATION(S):**
**Therapeutic:** antidiabetics
**Pharmacologic:** meglitinides

**Pregnancy Category C**

## INDICATIONS

■ Type 2 diabetes mellitus, with diet and exercise; may be used with metformin, rosiglitazone, or pioglitazone.

## ACTION

■ Stimulates the release of insulin from pancreatic beta cells by closing potassium channels, which results in the opening of calcium channels in beta cells. This is followed by release of insulin. **Therapeutic Effects:** ■ Lowering of blood glucose levels.

## PHARMACOKINETICS

**Absorption:** Well absorbed (56%) following oral administration.

**Distribution:** Unknown.

**Protein Binding:** >98%.

**Metabolism and Excretion:** Mostly metabolized by the liver; metabolites are excreted primarily in feces.

**Half-life:** 1 hr.

## CONTRAINDICATIONS AND PRECAUTIONS

**Contraindicated in:** ■ Hypersensitivity ■ Lactation ■ Diabetic ketoacidosis ■ Insulin-dependent diabetes.

**Use Cautiously in:** ■ Impaired liver function (longer dosing intervals may be necessary) ■ Severe renal impairment (dosage reduction recommended) ■ Pregnancy and children (safety not established; insulin recommended to control diabetes during pregnancy).

## ADVERSE REACTIONS AND SIDE EFFECTS*

■ **CV:** angina, chest pain ■ **Endo:** HYPOGLYCEMIA, hyperglycemia.

## INTERACTIONS

**Drug-Drug:** ■ **Ketoconazole, miconazole,** and **erythromycin** may ↓ metabolism and ↑ risk of hypoglycemia ■ Effects may also be ↑ by **NSAIDs, hormonal contraceptives, simvastatin, sulfonamides, chloramphenicol, warfarin, probenecid, MAO inhibitors,** and **beta blockers** ■ Effects may be ↓ by **corticosteroids, phenothiazines, thyroid preparations, estrogens, hormonal contraceptives, phenytoin, nicotinic acid, sympathomimetics, isoniazid,** and **calcium channel blockers.**

**Drug-Natural Products:** ■ **Glucosamine** may worsen blood glucose control ■ **Fenugreek, chromium,** and **coenzyme Q-10** may produce ↑ hypoglycemic effects.

## ROUTE AND DOSAGE

■ **PO (Adults):** 0.5–4 mg taken before meals (not to exceed 16 mg/day).

❑ **Renal Impairment**

■ **PO (Adults):** *Severe renal impairment—* start with 0.5 mg/day and titrate carefully.

## AVAILABILITY

■**Tablets:** 0.5 mg$^{Rx}$, 1 mg$^{Rx}$, 2 mg$^{Rx}$ ■Cost: 0.5 mg $92.96/100, 1 mg $92.96/100, 2 mg $92.96/100.

TIME/ACTION PROFILE

|  | ONSET | PEAK | DURATION |
| --- | --- | --- | --- |
| PO | within 30 min | 60–90 min | <4 hr |

# NURSING IMPLICATIONS

## ASSESSMENT

❑ Observe patient for signs and symptoms of hypoglycemic reactions (abdominal pain, sweating, hunger, weakness, dizziness, headache, tremor, tachycardia, anxiety). Hypoglycemia may be difficult to recognize in geriatric patients and in patients taking beta blockers. Hypoglycemia is more likely to occur with insufficient caloric intake, following intense prolonged exercise, or when alcohol or more than one hypoglycemic agent is used.

■ *Lab Test Considerations:* Monitor fasting serum glucose and glycosylated hemoglobin periodically during therapy to evaluate effectiveness.

## POTENTIAL NURSING DIAGNOSES

■ Nutrition, imbalanced: more than body requirements (Indications).

■ Noncompliance (Patient/Family Teaching).

## IMPLEMENTATION

■ **General:** Patients stabilized on a diabetic regimen who are exposed to stress, fever, trauma, infection, or surgery may require administration of insulin. Withhold repaglinide and reinstitute after resolution of acute episode.

❑ Repaglinide therapy should be temporarily discontinued from patients requiring surgery involving restricted intake of food and fluids.

❑ There is no fixed dose of repaglinide. Dose is based on periodic monitoring of blood glucose and long-term response is based on glycolysated hemoglobin levels. If adequate response is not achieved, metformin may be added to regimen. If combination therapy is unsuccessful, oral hypoglycemic therapy may need to be discontinued and replaced with insulin.

❑ When replacing other oral hypoglycemic agents, repaglinide may be started on the day following discontinuation of the other agent. Monitor blood glucose closely. Discontinua-

tion of long-acting oral hypoglycemics may require monitoring for a week or more.

❑ Short-term repaglinide therapy may be used for patients well controlled with diet experiencing transient loss of control.

■ **PO:** Administer up to 30 min before meals. Patients who skip a meal or add an extra meal should skip or add a dose, respectively, for that meal.

## PATIENT/FAMILY TEACHING

❑ Instruct patient to take repaglinide before each meal, exactly as directed.

❑ Explain to patient that repaglinide helps control hyperglycemia but does not cure diabetes. Therapy is usually long term.

❑ Encourage patient to follow prescribed diet, medication, and exercise regimen to prevent hyperglycemic or hypoglycemic episodes.

❑ Review signs of hypoglycemia and hyperglycemia with patient. If hypoglycemia occurs, advise patient to take a glass of orange juice or 2–3 tsp of sugar, honey, or corn syrup dissolved in water, and notify health care professional.

❑ Instruct patient in proper testing of blood glucose. These tests should be monitored closely during periods of stress or illness and a health care professional notified if significant changes occur.

❑ Caution patient to avoid taking other prescription or OTC medications, herbal products, or alcohol during repaglinide therapy without consulting health care professional.

❑ Insulin is the recommended method of controlling blood glucose during pregnancy. Counsel female patients to use a form of contraception other than oral contraceptives and to notify health care professional promptly if pregnancy is planned or suspected.

❑ Advise patient to inform health care professional of medication regimen prior to treatment or surgery.

❑ Advise patient to carry a form of sugar (sugar packets, candy) and identification describing disease process and medication regimen at all times.

❑ Emphasize the importance of routine follow-up exams and regular testing of blood glucose and glycosylated hemoglobin.

## EVALUATION

**Effectiveness of therapy can be demonstrated by:** ■ Control of blood glucose levels without the appearance of hypoglycemic or hyperglycemic episodes.

## reteplase, See THROMBOLYTIC AGENTS.

## Rh$_o$(D) IMMUNE GLOBULIN

(arr aych oh dee im-**yoon** glob-yoo-lin)

**Rh$_o$(D) immune globulin standard dose IM**

BayRho-D Full Dose, Gamulin Rh, HypRho-D, Rhesonativ, RhoGAM

**Rh$_o$(D) globulin microdose IM**

BayRho-D Mini Dose, HypRho-D Mini-Dose, MICRhoGAM, Mini-Gamulin R

**Rh$_o$(D) globulin IV**

WinRho SD, WinRho SDF

*CLASSIFICATION(S):*
*Therapeutic: vaccines/immunizing agents*
*Pharmacologic: immune globulins*

Pregnancy Category C

## INDICATIONS

■ **IM, IV:** Administered to Rh$_o$(D)-negative patients who have been exposed to Rh$_o$(D)-positive blood by: ❑ Delivering an Rh$_o$(D)-positive infant ❑ Miscarrying or aborting an Rh$_o$(D)-positive fetus ❑ Having amniocentesis or intra-abdominal trauma while carrying an Rh$_o$(D)-positive fetus ❑ Following accidental transfusion of Rh$_o$(D)-positive blood to an Rh$_o$(D)-negative patient ■ **IV:** Management of immune thrombocytopenic purpura (ITP).

## ACTION

■ Prevent production of anti-Rh$_o$(D) antibodies in Rh$_o$(D)-negative patients who were exposed to Rh$_o$(D)-positive blood ■ Increase platelet counts in patients with ITP. **Therapeutic Effects:** ■ Prevention of antibody response and hemolytic disease of the newborn (erythroblastosis fetalis) in future pregnancies of women who have conceived an Rh$_o$(D)-positive fetus ■ Prevention of Rh$_o$(D) sensitization following transfusion accident ■ Decreased bleeding in patients with ITP.

## PHARMACOKINETICS

**Absorption:** Well absorbed from IM sites.

**Distribution:** Unknown.

**Metabolism and Excretion:** Unknown.

**Half-life:** *IM*—30 days; *IV*—24 days.

## CONTRAINDICATIONS AND PRECAUTIONS

**Contraindicated in:** ■ Rh$_o$(D)- or Du-positive patients ■ Patients previously sensitized to Rh$_o$(D) or Du.

**Use Cautiously in:** ■ Patients with previous hypersensitivity reactions to immune globulins or thimerosal (IM product) ■ ITP patients with pre-existing anemia (decreased dose if Hgb <10 g/dl).

## ADVERSE REACTIONS AND SIDE EFFECTS*

■ **Hemat:** *ITP*—anemia, introvascular hemolysis (D-positive patients with ITP only) ■ **Local:** pain at IM site ■ **Misc:** fever.

## INTERACTIONS

**Drug-Drug:** ■ May decrease antibody response to some **live-virus vaccines (measles, mumps, rubella).**

## ROUTE AND DOSAGE

❑ **Rh$_o$ (D) Immune Globulin (for IM use only)**

**Following Delivery**

■ **IM (Adults):** 1 vial standard dose (300 mcg) within 72 hr of delivery.

**Before Delivery**

■ **IM (Adults):** 1 vial standard dose (300 mcg) at 26–28 wk.

## Termination of Pregnancy (<13 wk Gestation)

■ **IM (Adults):** 1 vial of microdose (50 mcg) within 72 hr.

## Termination of Pregnancy (>13 wk Gestation)

■ **IM (Adults):** 1 vial standard dose (300 mcg) within 72 hr.

## Large Fetal-Maternal Hemorrhage

■ **IM (Adults):** Packed RBC volume of hemorrhage/15 = number of vials of standard dose (300 mcg) preparation (round to next whole number of vials).

## Transfusion Accident

■ **IM (Adults):** (Volume of Rh-positive blood administered × Hct of donor blood)/15 = number of vials of standard dose (300 mcg) preparation (round to next whole number of vials).

## ❑ Rh$_o$(D) Immune Globulin IV (for IM or IV Use)

### Following Delivery

■ **IM, IV (Adults):** 600 IU (120 mcg) within 72 hr of delivery.

### Prior to Delivery

■ **IM, IV (Adults):** 1500 IU (300 mcg) of Rh$_o$(D) immune globulin IV at 28 wk; if initiated earlier in pregnancy, repeat q 12 wk.

■ **IM, IV (Adults):** 600 IU (120 mcg) within 72 hr.

### Following Amniocentesis <34 wk or Chorionic Villus Sampling

■ **IM, IV (Adults):** 1500 IU (300 mcg) within 72 hr; repeat q 12 wk during pregnancy.

### Large Fetal-Maternal Hemorrhage/Transfusion Accident

■ **IM (Adults):** 6000 IU (1200 mcg) q 12 hr until total dose is given (total dose determined by amount of blood loss/hemorrhage).

■ **IV (Adults):** 3000 IU (600 mcg) q 8 hr until total dose is given (total dose determined by amount of blood loss/hemorrhage).

### Immune Thrombocytopenic Purpura (ITP)

■ **IV (Adults and Children):** 50 mcg (250 IU)/kg initially (if Hgb <10g/dl, decrease dose to 25–40 mcg [125–200 IU]/kg); fur-

ther dosing/frequency determined by clinical response (range 25–60 mcg [125–300 IU]/kg). Each dose may be given as a single dose or in 2 divided doses on separate days.

## AVAILABILITY

### ❑ Rh$_o$(D) Immune Globulin (for IM Use)

■ *Injection:* 50 mcg/vial (microdose)$^{Rx}$, 300 mcg/vial (standard dose)$^{Rx}$.

### ❑ Rh$_o$(D) Immune Globulin Intravenous (for IM or IV Use)

■ *Injection:* 600 IU (120 mcg)/vial$^{Rx}$, 1500 IU (300 mcg)/vial$^{Rx}$, 5000 IU (1000 mcg)/vial$^{Rx}$.

TIME/ACTION PROFILE (blood levels)

| | ONSET | PEAK | DURATION |
|---|---|---|---|
| IM | rapid | 5–10 days | unknown |
| IV† | unknown | 2 hr | unknown |

†When given for ITP, platelet counts start to rise in 1–2 days, peak after 5–7 days, and last for 30 days.

# NURSING IMPLICATIONS

## ASSESSMENT

■ **IV:** Assess vital signs periodically during therapy in patients receiving Rh$_o$(D) IG IV.

■ **ITP:** Monitor patient for signs and symptoms of intravascular hemolysis (back pain, shaking chills, hemoglobinuria [IVH]), anemia, and renal insufficiency. If transfusions are required, use Rh$_o$(D) negative packed red blood cells to prevent exacerbation of IVH.

■ *Lab Test Considerations: Pregnancy:* Type and cross-match of mother and newborn's cord blood must be performed to determine need for medication. Mother must be Rh$_o$(D)-negative and Du-negative. Infant must be Rh$_o$(D)-positive. If there is doubt regarding infant's blood type or if father is Rh$_o$(D)-positive, medication should be given.

❑ An infant born to a woman treated with Rh$_o$(D) immune globulin antepartum may have a weakly positive direct Coombs' test result on cord or infant blood.

❑ *ITP:* Monitor platelet counts, RBC counts, hemoglobin, and reticulocyte levels to determine effectiveness of therapy.

## POTENTIAL NURSING DIAGNOSES

■ Knowledge, deficient, related to medication regimen (Patient/Family Teaching).

## IMPLEMENTATION

- **General:** Do not give to infant, to $Rh_o(D)$-positive individual, or to $Rh_o(D)$-negative individual previously sensitized to the $Rh_o(D)$ antigen. However, there is no more risk than when given to a woman who is not sensitized. When in doubt, administer $Rh_o(D)$ immune globulin. Do not confuse IM and IV formulations. Rh immune globulin for IV administration is labelled 'Rh Immune Globulin Intravenous.' Rh Immune Globulin Intravenous may be given IM; however, Rh Immune Globulin (microdose and standard dose) is for IM use only and cannot be given IV.
- **IM:** Reconstitute $Rh_o(D)$ immune globulin IV for IM use immediately before use with 1.25 ml of 0.9% NaCl. Inject diluent onto inside wall of vial and wet pellet by gently swirling until dissolved. Do not shake.
- ☐ Administer into the deltoid muscle. Dose should be given within 3 hr but may be given up to 72 hr after delivery, miscarriage, abortion, or transfusion.
- **Direct IV:** Reconstitute $Rh_o(D)$ immune globulin IV for IV administration immediately before use with 2.5 ml of 0.9% NaCl. Inject diluent onto inside wall of vial and wet pellet by gently swirling until dissolved. Do not shake.
- *Rate:* Administer over 3–5 min.

## PATIENT/FAMILY TEACHING

- **Pregnancy:** Explain to patient that the purpose of this medication is to protect future $Rh_o(D)$-positive infants.
- **ITP:** Explain purpose of medication to patient.

## EVALUATION

**Effectiveness of therapy can be demonstrated by:** ■ Prevention of erythroblastosis fetalis in future $Rh_o(D)$-positive infants ■ Prevention of $Rh_o(D)$ sensitization following transfusion accident ■ Decreased bleeding episodes in patients with ITP.

---

# ribavirin

(rye-ba-**vye**-rin)
Copegus, Rebetol, Virazole

---

## CLASSIFICATION(S):
*Therapeutic:* antivirals
*Pharmacologic:* nucleoside analogues

**Pregnancy Category X**

## INDICATIONS

■ **Inhaln:** Treatment of severe lower respiratory tract infections caused by the respiratory syncytial virus (RSV) in infants and young children ■ **PO:** *Rebetol*—with interferon alfa-2b (*Intron A*) or peginterferon alfa-2b (*PEG-Intron*) in the treatment of chronic hepatitis C who have failed previous therapy ■ **PO:** *Copegus*—with peginterferon alfa-2a (Pegasys) in the treatment of chronic hepatitis C who have failed previous therapy. **Unlabeled uses:** ■ Early (within 24 hr of symptoms) secondary treatment of influenza A or B in young adults.

## ACTION

■ Inhibits viral DNA and RNA synthesis and subsequent replication ■ Must be phosphorylated intracellularly to be active. **Therapeutic Effects:** ■ **Inhaln:** Virustatic action ■ **PO:** Decreased progression and sequelae of chronic hepatitis C.

## PHARMACOKINETICS

**Absorption:** Systemic absorption occurs following nasal and oral inhalation. Rapidly and extensively absorbed following oral administration, but undergoes first-pass hepatic metabolism (64% bioavailability).

**Distribution:** 70% of inhaled drug is deposited in the respiratory tract. Appears to concentrate in the respiratory tract and red blood cells. Enters breast milk.

**Metabolism and Excretion:** Eliminated from the respiratory tract by distribution across membranes, macrophages, and ciliary motion. Metabolized primarily by the liver; metabolites are renally excreted.

**Half-life:** *Inhaln*—9.5 hr (40 days in RBCs); *oral*—43.6 hr (single dose); 12 days (multiple dose).

---

## CONTRAINDICATIONS AND PRECAUTIONS

**Contraindicated in:** ■ Hypersensitivity ■ **Inhalation:** Patients receiving mechanically assisted ventilation ■ **Oral:** Pregnancy or lactation ■ Male partners of pregnant patients ■ CCr <50 ml/min ■ Significant/unstable cardiovascular disease ■ Hemoglobinopathies ■ Autoimmune hepatitis or hepatic decompensation before/ during treatment (for combined therapy with interferon alfa-2b) ■ Concurrent use of didanosine, stavudine or zidovudine.

**Use Cautiously in:** ■ **Oral:** Sarcoidosis (may exacerbate condition ■ Anemia (dosage reduction/discontinuation may be required) ■ Any pre-existing cardiac disease ■ Patients with childbearing potential.

## ADVERSE REACTIONS AND SIDE EFFECTS*

Inhalation ■ **CNS:** dizziness, faintness ■ **EENT:** blurred vision, conjunctivitis, erythema of the eyelids, ocular irritation, photosensitivity ■ **CV:** CARDIAC ARREST , hypotension ■ **Derm:** rash ■ **Hemat:** reticulocytosis. *Oral* (may reflect combination with interferon) ■ **CNS:** emotional lability ( ↑ in children), fatigue ( ↓ in children), impaired concentration ( ↓ in children), insomnia ( ↓ in children), irritability ( ↓ in children) ■ **Resp:** dyspnea( ↓ in children) ■ **GI:** anorexia ( ↑ in children), dyspepsia ( ↓ in children), vomiting ( ↑ in children) ■ **Hemat:** hemolytic anemia ■ **Derm:** pruritus ( ↓ in children) ■ **MS:** arthralgia ( ↓ in children) ■ **Misc:** fever ( ↑ in children).

## INTERACTIONS

**Drug-Drug:** ■ **Oral:** May ↓ the antiretroviral action of **stavidine** and **zidovudine** ■ May ↑ hematologic toxicity of **zidovudine** ■ May ↑ blood levels and risk of toxicity of **didanosine**.

## ROUTE AND DOSAGE

■ **Inhaln (Infants and Young Children):** 300 ml of 20 mg/ml solution delivered via mist for 12–18 hr/day.

❏ **Rebetol (with interferon alfa-2b or peginterferon alfa-2b)**

■ **PO (Adults >75 kg):** 600 mg in the morning, then 600 mg in the evening for 6 mo.

■ **PO (Adults ≤75 kg and children >61 kg):** 400 mg in the morning, then 600 mg in the evening for 6 mo.

■ **PO (Children 50–61 kg):** 400 mg in the morning and evening.

■ **PO (Children 37–49 kg):** 200 mg in the morning and 400 mg in the evening.

■ **PO (Children 25–36 kg):** 200 mg in the morning and evening.

❏ **Copegus—viral genotype 1 or 4 (with peginterferon alfa-2a)**

■ **PO (Adults ≥75 kg):** 600 mg twice daily for 48 wk

■ **PO (Adults <75 kg):** 500 mg twice daily for 48 wk

❏ **Copegus-viral genotype 2 or 4 (with peginterferon alfa-2a)**

■ **PO (Adults):** 400 mg twice daily for 24 wk

## AVAILABILITY

■ *Powder for reconstitution for aerosol use:* 6 g/vial<sup>Rx</sup> ■ *Capsules (Rebetol):* 200 mg<sup>Rx</sup> ■ *Tablets (Copegus):* 200 mg<sup>Rx</sup> ■ Rebetrol with interferon alfa-2b (Intron A) as combination therapy for chronic hepatitis C (Rebetron). See Appendix B. *Copegus* is intended for combined therapy with pegylated interferon alfa-2a (*Pegasys*).

TIME/ACTION PROFILE (blood levels)

| | ONSET | PEAK | DURATION |
|---|---|---|---|
| Inhaln | unknown | end of inhaln | unknown |
| PO | unknown | 1.7–3 hr | 12 hr |

# NURSING IMPLICATIONS

## ASSESSMENT

■ **RSV:** Assess patient for infection (vital signs, sputum, WBC) at beginning of and during therapy.

❏ Obtain specimens for culture and sensitivity prior to initiating therapy. First dose may be given before receiving results.

❏ Assess respiratory (lung sounds, quality and rate of respirations) and fluid status prior to and frequently throughout therapy.

■ **Chronic Hepatitis C:** Monitor symptoms of hepatitis during therapy.

❏ Assess patient for signs of depression during therapy.

❏ Assess patient for cardiovascular disorders (pulse, blood pressure, chest pain). May cause myocardial infarction.

◻ Assess patients for signs of colitis (abdominal pain, bloody diarrhea, fever) and pancreatitis (nausea, vomiting, abdominal pain) during therapy. Discontinue therapy if these occur; may be fatal.

◻ Assess pulmonary status (lung sounds, respirations) periodically during therapy. May require discontinuation.

■ *Lab Test Considerations:* **Chronic Hepatitis C:** Monitor CBC with differential and platelet count prior to initiation, at week 2, and week 4, and regularly during therapy. If hemoglobin <10 g/dl in patients with no history of cardiac disease or ↓ more than 2 g/dl in any 4 wk treatment period in patients with history of stable cardiac disease, decrease ribavirin dose to 600 mg (200 mg in AM and 400 mg in PM). If hemoglobin <8.5 g/dl in patients with no history of cardiac disease or <12 g/dl despite dose reduction in patients with history of stable cardiac disease, discontinue combination therapy permanently.

◻ Monitor liver function tests and thyroid stimulating hormone prior to and periodically during therapy.

◻ Monitor pregnancy tests prior to, monthly during and for 6 mo following discontinuation of therapy in women of childbearing age. Ribavarin should be started following a negative pregnancy test.

◻ May cause ↑ serum bilirubin and uric acid levels.

## POTENTIAL NURSING DIAGNOSES

■ Infection, risk for (Indications, Side Effects).
■ Gas exchange, impaired (Indications).

## IMPLEMENTATION

**Inhaln:** Infants requiring assisted ventilation should be suctioned every 1–2 hr and pulmonary pressures monitored every 2–4 hr.

◻ Ribavirin treatment should begin within the first 3 days of RSV infection to be effective.

◻ Ribavirin aerosol should be administered using the Viratek SPAG model SPAG-2 only. Do not administer via other aerosol-generating devices. Usually administered using an infant oxygen hood attached to the SPAG-2 aerosol generator. Administration by face mask may be used if the oxygen hood cannot be used.

◻ Reconstitute ribavirin 6-g vial with preservative-free sterile water for injection or inhalation. Transfer to clean, sterilized Erlenmeyer flask of the SPAG-2 reservoir and dilute to a final volume of 300 ml. This recommended concentration (20 mg/ml) in the reservoir provides a concentration of aerosol ribavirin of 190 mcg/liter of air over a 12-hr period. Solution should be discarded and replaced every 24 hr.

◻ Aerosol treatments should be administered continuously 12–18 hr/day for 3–7 days.

■ **PO:** Administer with food. Capsules should be swallowed whole; do not open, crush, or chew.

## PATIENT/FAMILY TEACHING

■ **RSV:** Explain the purpose and route of treatment to the patient and parents.

◻ Inform patient and parents that ribavirin may cause blurred vision and photosensitivity.

■ **Chronic Hepatitis C:** Instruct patient to take ribavirin for the full course of therapy. Emphasize the importance of routine lab test to monitor for side effects.

◻ Inform patient about teratogenic effects of ribavirin. Instruct women with childbearing potential, and men, to use 2 forms of effective contraception during and for at least 6 mo following conclusion of therapy. Men must use a condom.

◻ May cause dizziness. Caution patient to avoid driving or other activities requiring alertness until response to medication is known.

◻ Inform patient that ribavarin may not reduce the risk of transmission of HCV to others or prevent cirrhosis, liver failure, or liver cancer.

## EVALUATION

**Clinical response to therapy can be evaluated by:** ■ Resolution of the signs and symptoms of RSV ■ Decreased progression and sequelae of chronic hepatitis C.

## rifabutin

(riff-a-**byoo**-tin)

Mycobutin

---

## INDICATIONS

■ Prevention of disseminated *Mycobacterium avium* complex (MAC) disease in patients with advanced HIV infection. **Unlabeled uses:** ■ Treatment of *Helicobacter pylori* ulcer disease which has failed on other regimens (with pantoprazole and amoxicillin).

## ACTION

■ Appears to inhibit DNA-dependent RNA polymerase in susceptible organisms. **Therapeutic Effects:** ■ Antimycobacterial action against susceptible organisms. **Spectrum:** ■ Active against *M. avium* and most strains of *M. tuberculosis.*

## PHARMACOKINETICS

**Absorption:** Well absorbed following oral administration (50–85%). Absorption is decreased in HIV-positive patients (20%).

**Distribution:** Widely distributed to body tissues and fluids.

**Metabolism and Excretion:** Mostly metabolized by the liver; <5% excreted unchanged by the kidneys.

**Half-life:** 45 hr.

## CONTRAINDICATIONS AND PRECAUTIONS

**Contraindicated in:** ■ Hypersensitivity. Cross-sensitivity with other rifamycins (rifampin) may occur ■ Active tuberculosis ■ Concurrent ritonavir or delavirdine.

**Use Cautiously in:** ■ Pregnancy, lactation, or children (safety not established).

## ADVERSE REACTIONS AND SIDE EFFECTS*

■ **EENT:** brown-orange discoloration of tears, ocular disturbances ■ **Resp:** dyspnea ■ **CV:** chest pain, chest pressure ■ **GI:** brown-orange discoloration of saliva, altered taste, drug-induced hepatitis ■ **GU:** brown-orange discoloration of urine ■ **Derm:** rash, skin discoloration ■ **Hemat:** hemolysis, neutropenia, thrombocytopenia ■ **MS:** arthralgia, myositis ■ **Misc:** brown-orange discoloration of body fluids, flu-like syndrome.

## INTERACTIONS

**Drug-Drug:** ■ Increases metabolism and may decrease the effectiveness of other drugs, including **amprenavir, efavirenz, indinavir, nelfinavir, nevirapine, saquinavir** (dosage adjustment may be necessary), **delavirdine,** (concurrent use should be avoided), **corticosteroids, disopyramide, quinidine, opioid analgesics, oral hypoglycemic agents, warfarin, estrogens, estrogen-containing contraceptives, phenytoin, verapamil, fluconazole, quinidine, tocainide, theophylline, zidovudine,** and **chloramphenicol** ■ **Ritonavir** increases blood levels of rifabutin (concurrent use is contraindicated), similar effects occur with **efavirenz** and **nevirapine.**

## ROUTE AND DOSAGE

■ **PO (Adults):** 300 mg once daily. If GI upset occurs, may give as 150 mg twice daily with food. *H. pylori*—300 mg/day (unlabeled).

## AVAILABILITY

■ *Capsules:* 150 mg^Rx.

TIME/ACTION PROFILE (blood levels)

|    | ONSET | PEAK | DURATION |
|----|-------|------|----------|
| PO | rapid | 2–4 hr | 24 hr |

# NURSING IMPLICATIONS

## ASSESSMENT

❑ Monitor patient for signs of active tuberculosis (purified protein derivative [PPD], chest x-ray, sputum culture, blood culture, urine culture, biopsy of suspicious lymph nodes) prior to and throughout therapy. Rifabutin must not be administered to patients with active tuberculosis.

■ *Lab Test Considerations:* Monitor CBC periodically throughout therapy. May cause neutropenia and thrombocytopenia.

## POTENTIAL NURSING DIAGNOSES

■ Infection, risk for (Indications).
■ Noncompliance (Patient/Family Teaching).

## IMPLEMENTATION

■ **General:** Do not confuse rifabutin with rifampin.
■ **PO:** May be administered without regard to meals. High-fat meals slow rate but not extent of absorption. May be mixed with foods

such as applesauce. If GI upset occurs, administer with food.

## PATIENT/FAMILY TEACHING

❑ Advise patient to take medication exactly as directed. Do not skip doses or double up on missed doses. Emphasize the importance of continuing therapy even if asymptomatic.

❑ Advise patient to notify health care professional promptly if signs and symptoms of neutropenia (sore throat, fever, signs of infection), thrombocytopenia (unusual bleeding or bruising), or hepatitis (yellow eyes and skin, nausea, vomiting, anorexia, unusual tiredness, weakness) occur.

❑ Caution patient to avoid the use of alcohol during this therapy, because this may increase the risk of hepatotoxicity.

❑ Instruct patient to report symptoms of myositis (myalgia, arthralgia) or uveitis (intraocular inflammation) to health care professional promptly.

❑ Inform patient that saliva, sputum, sweat, tears, urine, and feces may become red-orange to red-brown and that soft contact lenses may become permanently discolored.

❑ Advise patient that this medication has teratogenic properties and may decrease the effectiveness of oral contraceptives. Counsel patient to use a nonhormonal form of contraception throughout therapy.

❑ Emphasize the importance of regular follow-up exams to monitor progress and to check for side effects.

## EVALUATION

**Effectiveness of therapy can be demonstrated by:** ■ Prevention of disseminated MAC in patients with advanced HIV infection.

# rifampin

(rif-**am**-pin)

Rifadin, Rimactane, {Rofact}

*CLASSIFICATION(S):*
*Therapeutic: antituberculars*
*Pharmacologic: rifamycins*

**Pregnancy Category C**

## INDICATIONS

■ Active tuberculosis (with other agents) ■ Elimination of meningococcal carriers. **Unlabeled uses:** ■ Prevention of disease caused by *Haemophilus influenzae* type B in close contacts.

## ACTION

■ Inhibits RNA synthesis by blocking RNA transcription in susceptible organisms. **Therapeutic Effects:** ■ Bactericidal action against susceptible organisms. **Spectrum:** ■ Broad spectrum notable for activity against: ❑*Mycobacterium* spp ❑*Staphylococcus aureus* ❑*H. influenzae* ❑ *Legionella pneumophila* ❑ *Neisseria meningitidis.*

## PHARMACOKINETICS

**Absorption:** Well absorbed following oral administration.

**Distribution:** Widely distributed; enters CSF. Crosses placenta; enters breast milk.

**Metabolism and Excretion:** Mostly metabolized by the liver; 60% eliminated in feces via biliary elimination.

**Half-life:** 3 hr.

## CONTRAINDICATIONS AND PRECAUTIONS

**Contraindicated in:** ■ Hypersensitivity ■ Concurrent indinavir, nelfinavir, pyrazinamide, or saquinavir.

**Use Cautiously in:** ■ History of liver disease ■ Concurrent use of other hepatotoxic agents ■ Pregnancy or lactation.

## ADVERSE REACTIONS AND SIDE EFFECTS*

■ CNS: ataxia, confusion, drowsiness, fatigue, headache, weakness ■ EENT: red discoloration of tears ■ GI: abdominal pain, diarrhea, flatulence, heartburn, nausea, vomiting, drug-induced hepatitis, red discoloration of saliva ■ GU: red discoloration of urine ■ Hemat: hemolytic anemia, thrombocytopenia ■ MS: arthralgia, myalgia ■ Misc: red discoloration of all body fluids, flu-like syndrome.

## INTERACTIONS

**Drug-Drug:** ■ ↑ risk of hepatotoxicity with other **hepatotoxic agents**, including **alcohol, ketoconazole isoniazid, pyrazinamide**

(concurrent use with **pyrazinamide** may result in potentially fatal hepatotoxicity and should be avoided) ▪ Rifampin significantly ↓ blood levels of **delavirdine, indinavir, nelfinavir,** and **saquinavir**; concurrent use is contraindicated ▪ Rifampin stimulates liver enzymes, which may ↑ metabolism and ↓ effectiveness of other drugs, including **ritonavir, nevirapine,** and **efavirenz** (dosage adjustment may be necessary), **corticosteroids, disopyramide, quinidine, opioid analgesics, oral hypoglycemic agents, warfarin, estrogens, phenytoin, verapamil, fluconazole, ketoconazole, itraconazole, quinidine, tocainide, theophylline, chloramphenicol,** and **hormonal contraceptive agents**

## ROUTE AND DOSAGE

❑ **Tuberculosis**

▪ **PO, IV (Adults):** 600 mg/day or 10 mg/kg/day (up to 600 mg/day) single dose; may also be given 2–3 times weekly.

▪ **PO, IV (Children):** 10–20 mg/kg/day single dose (not to exceed 600 mg/day); may also be given 2–3 times weekly.

❑ **Asymptomatic Carriers of Meningococcus**

▪ **PO, IV (Adults):** 600 mg q 12 hr for 2 days.

▪ **PO, IV (Children ≥1 mo):** 10 mg/kg q 12 hr for 2 days.

▪ **PO (Infants <1 mo):** 5 mg/kg q 12 hr for 2 days.

❑ **Prevention of** *H. influenzae* **Type B Infection**

▪ **PO (Adults):** 600 mg/day for 4 days.

▪ **PO (Children):** 20 mg/kg/day for 4 days.

## AVAILABILITY (generic available)

▪ *Capsules:* 150 mg[Rx], 300 mg[Rx] ▪ Cost: 150 mg $40.23/30, 300 mg $57.02/30 ▪ *Powder for injection:* 600 mg/vial[Rx] ▪ isoniazid (Rifamate)[Rx]; isoniazid and pyrazinamide (Rifater)[Rx]. See Appendix B.

TIME/ACTION PROFILE (blood levels)

| | ONSET | PEAK | DURATION |
|---|---|---|---|
| PO | rapid | 2–4 hr | 12–24 hr |
| IV | rapid | end of infusion | 12–24 hr |

# NURSING IMPLICATIONS

## ASSESSMENT

❑ Perform mycobacterial studies and susceptibility tests prior to and periodically during therapy to detect possible resistance.

❑ Assess lung sounds and character and amount of sputum periodically during therapy.

▪ *Lab Test Considerations:* Evaluate renal function, CBC, and urinalysis periodically and during therapy.

❑ Monitor hepatic function at least monthly during therapy. May cause ↑ BUN, AST, ALT, and serum alkaline phosphatase, bilirubin, and uric acid concentrations.

❑ May cause false-positive direct Coombs' test results. May interfere with folic acid and vitamin B assays.

❑ May interfere with dexamethasone suppression test results; discontinue rifampin 15 days prior to test.

❑ May interfere with methods for determining serum folate and vitamin B levels and with urine tests based on color reaction.

❑ May delay hepatic uptake and excretion of sulfobromophthalein (SBP) during SBP uptake and excretion tests; perform test prior to daily dose of rifampin.

## POTENTIAL NURSING DIAGNOSES

▪ Infection, risk for (Indications).

▪ Noncompliance (Patient/Family Teaching).

## IMPLEMENTATION

▪ **General:** Do not confuse rifampin with rifabutin.

▪ **PO:** Administer medication on an empty stomach at least 1 hr before or 2 hr after meals with a full glass (240 ml) of water. If GI irritation becomes a problem, may be administered with food. Antacids may also be taken 1 hr prior to administration. Capsules may be opened and contents mixed with applesauce or jelly for patients with difficulty swallowing.

❑ Pharmacist can compound a syrup for patients unable to swallow solids.

▪ **Intermittent Infusion:** Reconstitute 600-mg vial with 10 ml of sterile water for injection and swirl gently to dissolve completely. Dilute further in 500 ml or 100 ml of D5W or 0.9% NaCl. Solution is stable for 24 hr at room temperature; however, manufacturer recommends administration within 4 hr to prevent precipitation.

- **Rate:** Administer solutions diluted in 500 ml over 3 hr and solutions diluted in 100 ml over 30 min.
- **Additive Incompatibility:** Do not admix with other solutions or medications.

## PATIENT/FAMILY TEACHING

- Advise patient to take medication once daily (unless biweekly regimens are used), as directed, and not to skip doses or double up on missed doses. Emphasize the importance of continuing therapy even after symptoms have subsided. Length of therapy for tuberculosis depends on regimen being used and underlying disease states. Patients on short-term prophylactic therapy should also be advised of the importance of compliance with therapy.
- Advise patient to notify health care professional promptly if signs and symptoms of hepatitis (yellow eyes and skin, nausea, vomiting, anorexia, unusual tiredness, weakness) or of thrombocytopenia (unusual bleeding or bruising) occur.
- Caution patient to avoid the use of alcohol during this therapy, because this may increase the risk of hepatotoxicity.
- Instruct patient to report the occurrence of flu-like symptoms (fever, chills, myalgia, headache) promptly.
- Rifampin may occasionally cause drowsiness. Caution patient to avoid driving or other activities requiring alertness until response to medication is known.
- Inform patient that saliva, sputum, sweat, tears, urine, and feces may become red-or-ange to red-brown and that soft contact lenses may become permanently discolored.
- Advise patient that this medication has teratogenic properties and may decrease the effectiveness of oral contraceptives. Counsel patient to use a nonhormonal form of contraception throughout therapy.
- Emphasize the importance of regular follow-up exams to monitor progress and to check for side effects.

## EVALUATION

**Effectiveness of therapy can be demonstrated by:** ■ Decreased fever and night sweats ◻ Diminished cough and sputum production ◻ Negative sputum cultures ◻ Increased appetite ◻ Weight gain ◻ Reduced fatigue ◻ Sense of well-being in patients with tuberculosis ■ Prevention of meningococcal meningitis ■ Prevention of *H. influenzae* type B infection. Prophylactic course is usually short-term.

# rifapentine

(rif-a-**pen**-teen)
Priftin

**CLASSIFICATION(S):**
**Therapeutic:** *agents for amyotrophic lateral sclerosis, antituberculars*

**Pregnancy Category C**

## INDICATIONS

■ Treatment of pulmonary tuberculosis ◻ Must be used in combination with other agents.

## ACTION

■ Inhibits DNA-dependent RNA polymerase. **Therapeutic Effects:** ■ Bactericidal action against intracellular and extracellular susceptible strains of *Mycobacterium tuberculosis*.

## PHARMACOKINETICS

**Absorption:** 70% absorbed following oral administration.

**Distribution:** Widely distributed in body tissues and fluids.

**Protein Binding:** *Rifapentine*—97.7%; *desacetyl rifapentine*—93.2%.

**Metabolism and Excretion:** Mostly metabolized by the liver; 17% excreted by the kidneys; some conversion to another active compound (25-desacetyl rifapentine).

**Half-life:** 13 hr (rifapentine and desacetyl rifapentine).

## CONTRAINDICATIONS AND PRECAUTIONS

**Contraindicated in:** ■ Hypersensitivity to rifapentine or other rifamycins (rifampin or rifabutin).
**Use Cautiously in:** ■ History of liver disease ■ Pregnancy, lactation, or children <12 yr (safety not established).
**Exercise Extreme Caution in:** ■ Concurrent protease inhibitor therapy.

## ADVERSE REACTIONS AND SIDE EFFECTS*

■ **CNS:** dizziness, headache ■ **Resp:** hemoptysis ■ **CV:** hypertension ■ **GI:** PSEUDOMEMBRANOUS COLITIS, anorexia, diarrhea, dyspepsia, increased liver enzymes, nausea, vomiting ■ **GU:** hematuria, proteinuria, pyuria, urinary casts ■ **Derm:** acne, pruritus, rash ■ **Hemat:** anemia, leukopenia, lymphopenia, neutropenia, thrombocytosis ■ **MS:** arthralgia ■ **Misc:** pain.

## INTERACTIONS

**Drug-Drug:** ■ Increases metabolism and may decrease activity of **phenytoin, disopyramide, mexiletine, quinidine, tocainide, chloramphenicol, clarithromycin, dapsone, doxycycline, fluoroquinolones, warfarin, fluconazole, itraconazole, ketoconazole,** some **sedative/hypnotics (benzodiazepines** and **barbiturates),** some **beta blockers,** some **calcium channel blockers, corticosteroids, digoxin, clofibrate, hormonal contraceptives, haloperidol, protease inhibitors (indinavir, ritonavir, nelfinavir, saquinavir), sulfonylurea oral hypoglycemic agents, cyclosporine, tacrolimus, levothyroxine,** some **opioids, progestins, quinine, reverse transcriptase inhibitors (delavirdine, zidovudine), sildenafil, theophylline,** and some **reverse transcriptase inhibitors,** and **tricyclic antidepressants**; dosage adjustments may be necessary ■ **Antacids** decrease absorption.
**Drug-Food:** ■ Food increases absorption.

## ROUTE AND DOSAGE

Must be used in combination with other antituberculars.

■ **PO (Adults):** *Intensive phase*—600 mg twice weekly (not less than 72 hr between doses) for 2 months; *continuation phase*—600 mg once weekly for 4 months.

## AVAILABILITY

■ *Tablets:* 150 mg^Rx.

TIME/ACTION PROFILE (blood levels)

|    | ONSET | PEAK | DURATION |
|----|-------|------|----------|
| PO | unknown | 5–6 hr | unknown |

# NURSING IMPLICATIONS

## ASSESSMENT

❑ Mycobacterial studies and susceptibility tests should be performed prior to and periodically throughout therapy to detect possible resistance.
❑ Assess lung sounds and character and amount of sputum periodically throughout therapy.
■ *Lab Test Considerations:* Assess hepatic enzymes, bilirubin, CBC, and platelet count prior to therapy. Monitor at least monthly, especially in relation to adverse reactions. Patients with liver disease or abnormal liver tests should have liver tests (especially AST and ALT) monitored every 2–4 weeks. Signs of worsening disease may require discontinuation.
❑ May interfere with methods for determining serum folate and vitamin B levels and with urine tests based on color reaction.
❑ Hyperuricemia is common during intensive phase, especially when combined with pyrazinamide.

## POTENTIAL NURSING DIAGNOSES

■ Infection, risk for (Indications).
■ Noncompliance (Patient/Family Teaching).

## IMPLEMENTATION

■ **General:** Rifapentine is not administered alone. When used with isoniazid, pyridoxine (vitamin B) is administered concurrently in patients who are malnourished, predisposed to neuropathy (patients with alcoholism or diabetes), or adolescents to prevent neuropathy.
■ **PO:** May be administered with food to minimize nausea, vomiting, or GI upset.
❑ Antacids should not be administered within 1 hr before or 2 hr after rifapentine.

## PATIENT/FAMILY TEACHING

❑ Advise patient to take medication exactly as directed; not to skip doses or double up on missed doses of daily companion medications. Emphasize the importance of continuing therapy even after symptoms have subsided. Length of therapy for tuberculosis depends on regimen being used and underlying disease states.

❑ Advise patient to notify health care professional promptly if fever, malaise, darkened urine, yellow eyes and skin, nausea, vomiting, anorexia, or pain or swelling of joints occur.

❑ Instruct patient to notify health care professional if fever and diarrhea develop, especially if stool contains blood, pus, or mucus. Advise patient not to treat diarrhea without consulting health care professional.

❑ Caution patient to avoid the use of alcohol during this therapy, because this may increase the risk of hepatotoxicity.

❑ Rifapentine may occasionally cause dizziness. Caution patient to avoid driving or other activities requiring alertness until response to medication is known.

❑ Inform patient that saliva, sputum, teeth, tongue, sweat, tears, CSF, urine, and feces may become red-orange, and that soft contact lenses may become permanently discolored.

❑ Advise patient that this medication has teratogenic properties and may decrease the effectiveness of oral contraceptives. Counsel patient to use a nonhormonal form of contraception throughout therapy.

❑ Emphasize the importance of regular follow-up exams to monitor progress and to check for side effects.

## EVALUATION

**Effectiveness of therapy can be demonstrated by:** ■ Decreased fever and night sweats ❑ Diminished cough and sputum production ❑ Negative sputum cultures ❑ Increased appetite ❑ Weight gain ❑ Reduced fatigue ❑ Increased sense of well-being in patients with tuberculosis.

## risedronate
(riss-**ed**-roe-nate)
Actonel

### CLASSIFICATION(S):
**Therapeutic:** bone resorption inhibitors
**Pharmacologic:** biphosphonates
**Pregnancy Category C**

## INDICATIONS
■ Prevention and treatment of postmenopausal and corticosteroid-induced osteoporosis ■ Management of Paget's disease of bone in patients who ❑ have a serum alkaline phosphatase level of at least twice normal ❑ have symptoms ❑ are at risk for complications.

## ACTION
■ Inhibits bone resorption by binding to bone hydroxyapatite, which inhibits osteoclast activity. **Therapeutic Effects:** ■ Reversal of the progression of osteoporosis with decreased fractures and other sequelae ■ Reduced bone turnover and resorption; normalization of serum alkaline phosphatase with reduced complications of Paget's disease.

## PHARMACOKINETICS
**Absorption:** Rapidly but poorly absorbed following oral administration (0.63% bioavailability).
**Distribution:** 60% of absorbed dose distributes to bone.
**Metabolism and Excretion:** 40% of absorbed dose is excreted unchanged by kidneys; unabsorbed drug is excreted in feces.
**Half-life:** Initial—1.5 hr; terminal—220 hr (reflects dissociation from bone).

## CONTRAINDICATIONS AND PRECAUTIONS
**Contraindicated in:** ■ Hypersensitivity ■ Hypocalcemia ■ Lactation ■ Severe renal impairment (CCr <30 ml/min).
**Use Cautiously in:** ■ History of upper GI disorders ■ Other disturbances of bone or mineral metabolism (correct abnormalities before initiating therapy) ■ Dietary deficiencies (supplemental vitamin D and calcium may be required) ■ Pregnancy or children (safety not established; use in pregnancy only if potential benefit justifies potential risks).

## ADVERSE REACTIONS AND SIDE EFFECTS*

■ **CNS:** weakness ■ **EENT:** amblyopia, conjunctivitis, dry eyes, eye pain/inflammation, tinnitus ■ **CV:** chest pain, edema ■ **GI:** abdominal pain, diarrhea, belching, colitis, constipation, dysphagia, esophagitis, esophageal ulcer, gastric ulcer, nausea ■ **Derm:** rash ■ **MS:** arthralgia, bone pain, leg cramps, myasthenia ■ **Misc:** flu-like syndrome.

## INTERACTIONS

**Drug-Drug:** ■ Concurrent use with **NSAIDs** or **aspirin** ↑ risk of GI irritation ■ Absorption is ↓ by **calcium supplements** or **antacids**. **Drug-Food:** ■ Food decreases absorption (administer at least 30 min before breakfast).

## ROUTE AND DOSAGE

■ **PO (Adults):** *Osteoporosis*—5 mg once daily; taken 30 min before breakfast *or* 35 mg once weekly; *Paget's disease*—30 mg once daily for 2 mo; taken 30 min before breakfast. Retreatment may be considered after 2 mo off therapy.

## AVAILABILITY

■ *Tablets:* 5 mg$^{Rx}$, 30 mg$^{Rx}$, 35 mg$^{Rx}$.

TIME/ACTION PROFILE (effects on serum alkaline phosphatase)

|    | ONSET | PEAK | DURATION |
|----|-------|------|----------|
| PO | within days | 30 days | up to 16 mo |

# NURSING IMPLICATIONS

## ASSESSMENT

■ **Osteoporosis:** Assess patients via bone density study for low bone mass before and periodically during therapy.
■ **Paget's disease:** Assess for symptoms of Paget's disease (bone pain, headache, decreased visual and auditory acuity, increased skull size).
■ *Lab Test Considerations: Osteoporosis:* Assess serum calcium before and periodically during therapy. Hypocalcemia and vitamin D deficiency should be treated before initiating alendronate therapy. May cause mild, transient ↑ of calcium and phosphate. *Paget's disease:* Monitor alkaline phosphatase prior to and periodically during therapy to monitor effectiveness of therapy.

## POTENTIAL NURSING DIAGNOSES

■ Injury, risk for (Indications).

## IMPLEMENTATION

■ **PO:** Administer first thing in the morning with 6–8 oz of plain water, 30 min prior to other medications, beverages, or food.
❏ Calcium-, magnesium-, or aluminum-containing agents may interfere with absorption of risedronate and should be taken at a different time of day with food.

## PATIENT/FAMILY TEACHING

❏ Instruct patient on the importance of taking exactly as directed, first thing in the morning, 30 min prior to other medications, beverages, or food. Waiting longer than 30 min will improve absorption. Risedronate should be taken with 6–8 oz of plain water (mineral water, orange juice, coffee, and other beverages decrease absorption). If a dose is missed, skip dose and resume the next morning; do not double doses or take later in the day. Do not discontinue without consulting health care professional.
❏ Caution patients to remain upright for 30 min following dose to facilitate passage to stomach and minimize risk of esophageal irritation.
❏ Advise patient to eat a balanced diet and consult health care professional about the need for supplemental calcium and vitamin D.
❏ Encourage patient to participate in regular exercise and to modify behaviors that increase the risk of osteoporosis (stop smoking, reduce alcohol consumption).
❏ Advise female patients to notify health care professional if pregnancy is planned or suspected or if she is nursing.

## EVALUATION

**Effectiveness of therapy can be demonstrated by:** ■ Reversal of the progression of osteoporosis with decreased fractures and other sequelae ■ Decrease in serum alkaline phosphatase and the progression of Paget's disease.

# risperidone
(riss-**per**-i-done)
Risperdal, Risperdal M-TAB

## CLASSIFICATION(S):
**Therapeutic:** antipsychotics

**Pregnancy Category C**

## INDICATIONS

- Schizophrenia (treatment and prevention of relapse).

## ACTION

- May act by antagonizing dopamine and serotonin in the CNS. **Therapeutic Effects:** ■ Decreased symptoms of psychoses.

## PHARMACOKINETICS

**Absorption:** Well absorbed (70%) after oral administration.
**Distribution:** Unknown.
**Metabolism and Excretion:** Extensively metabolized by the liver. Metabolism is genetically determined; extensive metabolizers (most patients) convert risperidone to 9-hydroxyrisperidone rapidly. Poor metabolizers (6–8% of whites) convert it more slowly. The 9-hydroxyrisperidone is an antipsychotic compound. Risperidone and its active metabolite are renally eliminated.
**Half-life:** *Extensive metabolizers*—3 hr for risperidone, 21 hr for 9-hydroxyrisperidone. *Poor metabolizers*—20 hr for risperidone and 30 hr for 9-hydroxyrisperidone.

## CONTRAINDICATIONS AND PRECAUTIONS

**Contraindicated in:** ■ Hypersensitivity.
**Use Cautiously in:** ■ Geriatric or debilitated patients, patients with renal or hepatic impairment (initial dosage reduction recommended) ■ Geriatric patients (may ↑ risk of stroke in elderly patients with dementia-related psychoses) ■ Underlying cardiovascular disease (may be more prone to arrhythmias and hypotension) ■ History of seizures ■ History of suicide attempt or drug abuse ■ Pregnancy, lactation, or children (safety not established).

## ADVERSE REACTIONS AND SIDE EFFECTS*

■ **CNS:** NEUROLEPTIC MALIGNANT SYNDROME, aggressive behavior, dizziness, extrapyramidal reactions, headache, increased dreams, increased sleep duration, insomnia, sedation, fatigue, impaired temperature regulation, nervousness, tardive dyskinesia ■ **EENT:** pharyngitis, rhinitis, visual disturbances ■ **Resp:** cough, dyspnea, rhinitis ■ **CV:** arrhythmias, orthostatic hypotension, tachycardia ■ **GI:** constipation, diarrhea, dry mouth, nausea, abdominal pain, anorexia, dyspepsia, increased salivation, vomiting ■ **GU:** decreased libido, dysmenorrhea/menorrhagia, difficulty urinating, polyuria ■ **Derm:** itching/skin rash, dry skin, increased pigmentation, increased sweating, photosensitivity, seborrhea ■ **Endo:** galactorrhea ■ **MS:** arthralgia, back pain ■ **Misc:** weight gain, weight loss, polydipsia.

## INTERACTIONS

**Drug-Drug:** ■ May ↓ the antiparkinsonian effects of **levodopa** or other **dopamine agonists** ■ **Carbamazepine** ↑ metabolism and may ↓ effectiveness ■ **Clozapine** ↓ metabolism and may ↑ effects of risperidone ■ **Fluoxetine** ↑ blood levels and may ↑ effects ■ ↑ CNS depression may occur with other **CNS depressants,** including **alcohol, antihistamines, sedative/hypnotics,** or **opioid analgesics.**

## ROUTE AND DOSAGE

- **PO (Adults):** 1 mg twice daily, increased by 3rd day to 3 mg twice daily. Further increments may be made at weekly intervals by 1 mg twice daily (usual range, 4–6 mg/day; not to exceed 16 mg/day). May also be given as a single daily dose after initial titration.
- **PO (Geriatric Patients or Debilitated Patients):** Start with 0.5 mg twice daily; increase by 0.5 mg twice daily, up to 1.5 mg twice daily; then increase at weekly intervals if necessary. May also be given as a single daily dose after initial titration.
- ❑ **Renal/Hepatic Impairment**
- **PO (Adults):** Start with 0.5 mg twice daily; increase by 0.5 mg twice daily, up to 1.5 mg twice daily; then increase at weekly intervals if necessary. May also be given as a single daily dose after initial titration.

## AVAILABILITY

- *Tablets:* 0.25 mgRx, 0.5 mgRx, 1 mgRx, 2 mgRx, 3 mgRx, 4 mgRx ■Cost: 0.25 mg $167.27/

60, 0.5 mg $167.27/60, 1 mg $167.27/60, 2 mg $278.40/60, 3 mg $328.70/60, 4 mg $433.25/60 ■ *Orally disintegrating tablets:* 0.5 mg$^{Rx}$, 1 mg$^{Rx}$, 2 mg$^{Rx}$ ■ Cost: 0.25 mg $167.27/60, 0.5 mg 167.27/60, 1 mg $167.27/60, 2 mg $278.40/60, 3 mg $328.70/60, 4 mg $433.25/60 ■ *Oral solution:* 1 mg/ml in 30-ml and 100-ml bottles$^{Rx}$ ■ Cost: 30 ml $103.20.

TIME/ACTION PROFILE (clinical effects)

| | ONSET | PEAK | DURATION |
|---|---|---|---|
| PO | 1–2 wk | unknown | up to 6 wk† |

†After discontinuation.

## NURSING IMPLICATIONS

### ASSESSMENT

❑ Monitor patient's mental status (delusions, hallucinations, and behavior) before and periodically during therapy.

❑ Monitor mood changes. Assess for suicidal tendencies, especially during early therapy. Restrict amount of drug available to patient.

❑ Monitor blood pressure (sitting, standing, lying down) and pulse before and frequently during initial dosage titration. May cause prolonged QT interval, tachycardia, and orthostatic hypotension. If hypotension occurs, dose may need to be decreased.

❑ Observe patient when administering medication to ensure that medication is actually swallowed and not hoarded.

❑ Monitor patient for onset of extrapyramidal side effects (*akathisia*—restlessness; *dystonia*—muscle spasms and twisting motions; or *pseudoparkinsonism*—mask-like face, rigidity, tremors, drooling, shuffling gait, dysphagia). Report these symptoms; reduction of dosage or discontinuation of medication may be necessary. Trihexyphenidyl or diphenhydramine may be used to control these symptoms.

❑ Monitor for tardive dyskinesia (involuntary rhythmic movement of mouth, face, and extremities). Report immediately; may be irreversible.

❑ Monitor for development of neuroleptic malignant syndrome (fever, respiratory distress, tachycardia, seizures, diaphoresis, hypertension or hypotension, pallor, tiredness). Notify physician or other health care professional immediately if these symptoms occur.

■ *Lab Test Considerations:* May cause ↑ serum prolactin levels.

❑ May cause ↑ AST and ALT.

❑ May also cause anemia, thrombocytopenia, leukocytosis, and leukopenia.

### POTENTIAL NURSING DIAGNOSES

■ Violence, for self-directed (Indications).

■ Thought processes, disturbed (Indications).

■ Injury, risk for (Side Effects).

### IMPLEMENTATION

■ **General:** Do not confuse risperidone with reserpine.

❑ When switching from other antipsychotics, discontinue previous agents when starting risperidone and minimize the period of overlapping antipsychotic agents.

❑ If therapy is reinstituted after an interval off risperidone, follow initial 3-day titration schedule.

■ **PO:** For orally disintegrating tablets, blister pack by pealing back foil to expose tablet; do not try to push tablet through foil. Use dry hands to remove tablet from blister and immediately place entire tablet on tongue. Tablets disintegrate in mouth within seconds and can be swallowed with or without liquid. Do not attempt to split or chew tablet. Do not try to store tablets once removed from blister.

### PATIENT/FAMILY TEACHING

❑ Instruct patient to take medication exactly as directed.

❑ Inform patient of the possibility of extrapyramidal symptoms. Instruct patient to report these symptoms immediately to health care professional.

❑ Advise patient to change positions slowly to minimize orthostatic hypotension.

❑ May cause drowsiness. Caution patient to avoid driving or other activities requiring alertness until response to medication is known.

❑ Advise patient to use sunscreen and protective clothing when exposed to the sun to prevent photosensitivity reactions. Extremes in temperature should also be avoided; this drug impairs body temperature regulation.

❑ Caution patient to avoid concurrent use of alcohol, other CNS depressants, and OTC medications or herbal products without consulting health care professional.

□ Advise female patients to notify health care professional if pregnancy is planned or suspected or if they are breastfeeding or planning to breastfeed.

□ Advise patient to notify health care professional of medication regimen before treatment or surgery.

□ Instruct patient to notify health care professional promptly if sore throat, fever, unusual bleeding or bruising, rash, or tremors occur.

□ Emphasize the need for continued follow-up for psychotherapy and monitoring for side effects.

## EVALUATION

**Effectiveness of therapy can be demonstrated by:** ■ Decrease in excited, paranoic, or withdrawn behavior.

## ritonavir

(ri-**toe**-na-veer)

Norvir

### CLASSIFICATION(S):

**Therapeutic:** antiretrovirals
**Pharmacologic:** protease inhibitors

### Pregnancy Category B

## INDICATIONS

■ HIV infection (with other antiretrovirals).

## ACTION

■ Inhibits the action of HIV protease and prevents the cleavage of viral polyproteins. **Therapeutic Effects:** ■ Increased CD4 cell counts and decreased viral load with subsequent slowed progression of HIV infection and its sequelae.

## PHARMACOKINETICS

**Absorption:** Appears to be well absorbed after oral administration.
**Distribution:** Poor CNS penetration.
**Protein Binding:** 98–99%.
**Metabolism and Excretion:** Highly metabolized by the liver (by P450 CYP3A and CYP2D6 enzymes); one metabolite has antiretroviral activity; 3.5% excreted unchanged in urine.

**Half-life:** 3–5 hr.

## CONTRAINDICATIONS AND PRECAUTIONS

**Contraindicated in:** ■ Hypersensitivity ■ Concurrent use of alprazolam, amiodarone, bupropion, clorazepate, clozapine, diazepam, dihydroergotamine, encainide, ergotamine, estazolam, flecainide, flurazepam, meperidine, midazolam, pimozide, piroxicam, propafenone, propoxyphene, quinidine, rifabutin, triazolam, or zolpidem ■ Hypersensitivity or intolerance to alcohol or castor oil (present in capsules and liquid).

**Use Cautiously in:** ■ Impaired hepatic function, history of hepatitis ■ Diabetes mellitus ■ Hemophilia (increased risk of bleeding) ■ Pregnancy, lactation, or children <12 yr (safety not established; breast feeding not recommended in HIV-infected patients).

## ADVERSE REACTIONS AND SIDE EFFECTS*

■ **CNS:** SEIZURES, abnormal thinking, weakness, dizziness, headache, malaise, somnolence, syncope ■ **EENT:** pharyngitis, throat irritation ■ **Resp:** ANGIOEDEMA, bronchospasm ■ **CV:** orthostatic hypotension, vasodilation ■ **GI:** abdominal pain, altered taste, anorexia, diarrhea, nausea, vomiting, constipation, dyspepsia, flatulence ■ **GU:** renal insufficiency ■ **Derm:** rash, skin eruptions, sweating, urticaria ■ **Endo:** hyperglycemia ■ **F and E:** dehydration ■ **Metab:** hyperlipidemia ■ **MS:** increased creatine phosphokinase, myalgia ■ **Neuro:** circumoral paresthesia, peripheral paresthesia ■ **Misc:** hypersensitivity reactions including STEVENS-JOHNSON SYNDROME and ANAPHYLAXIS, fat redistribution, fever.

## INTERACTIONS

**Drug-Drug:** ■ Produces large ↑ in blood levels and effects of **amiodarone, bupropion, clozapine, encainide, flecainide, meperidine, piroxicam, propafenone, propoxyphene, quinidine,** and **rifabutin**; because of the increased risk of serious arrhythmias, hematologic toxicity, or seizures, these agents should not be used with ritonavir ■ Ergot toxicity may occur with concurrent use of **ergotamine** or **dihydroergotamine**; concurrent use should be avoided ■ Should not be used with **pimozide** ■ ↑ blood levels and the risk of excessive sedation and/or respiratory depression from **alprazolam, clorazepate, diazepam, estazolam, flurazepam, midazolam, triazolam,** and **zolpidem;** concurrent use should be avoided ■ May also increase blood levels and effects of some **opioid analgesics** (alfentanil, fentanyl, hydrocodone, oxycodone), **tramadol;** some **NSAIDs** (diclofenac, ibuprofen, indomethacin); some **antiarrhythmics** (disopyramide, lidocaine, mexiletine); some **anti-infectives** (clarithromycin, erythromycin); many **antidepressants** (amitriptyline, clomipramine, desipramine, imipramine, maprotiline, nortriptyline, nefazodone, sertraline, trazodone, fluoxetine, paroxetine, venlafaxine); some **antiemetics** (dronabinol, ondansetron); some **beta blockers** (metoprolol, pindolol, propranolol, timolol); many **calcium channel blockers** (amlodipine, diltiazem, felodipine, isradipine, nicardipine, nifedipine, nimodipine, nisoldipine, verapamil); some **antineoplastics** (etoposides, paclitaxel, tamoxifen, vinblastine, vincristine); some **corticosteroids** (dexamethasone, prednisone), most **HMG CoA reductase inhibitors;** some **immunosuppressants** (cyclosporine, tacrolimus); some **antipsychotics** (chlorpromazine, haloperidol, perphenazine, risperidone, thioridazine); and also **quinidine, saquinavir, methamphetamine,** and **warfarin.** Dosage ↓ may be necessary ■ ↓ blood levels and effects of **hormonal contraceptives, zidovudine, sulfamethoxazole,** and **theophylline;** dosage alteration or alternative therapy may be necessary ■ Levels may be ↑ by **clarithromycin** or **fluoxetine.**

**Drug-Natural Products:** ■ St. John's wort decreases levels and may promote resistance.

**Drug-Food:** ■ **Food** ↑ absorption.

## ROUTE AND DOSAGE

- **PO (Adults):** 300 mg twice daily for 1 day, then 400 mg twice daily for 3 days, then 500 mg twice daily for 1 day, then 600 mg twice daily as maintenance.
- **PO (Children):** 250 mg/m² twice daily initially; increase by 50 mg/m² twice daily q 2–3 days up to 400 mg/m² twice daily (if unable to get up to 400 mg/m² twice daily, additional antiretroviral therapy is required).

## AVAILABILITY

■ **Capsules:** 100 mg^Rx ■ **Oral solution:** 600 mg/7.5 ml (80 mg/ml) in 240-ml bottles^Rx.

TIME/ACTION PROFILE (blood levels)

|  | ONSET | PEAK | DURATION |
|---|---|---|---|
| PO | rapid | 4 hr* | 12 hr |

*Nonfasting.

## NURSING IMPLICATIONS

### ASSESSMENT

❑ Assess patient for change in severity of HIV symptoms and for symptoms of opportunistic infections during therapy.

■ **Lab Test Considerations:** Monitor viral load and CD4 counts regularly during therapy.

❑ May cause hyperglycemia.

❑ May cause ↑ serum AST, ALT, GGT, total bilirubin, CPK, triglycerides, and uric acid concentrations.

### POTENTIAL NURSING DIAGNOSES

■ Infection, risk for (Indications).

■ Noncompliance (Patient/Family Teaching).

### IMPLEMENTATION

- **General:** Do not confuse with Retrovir (zidovudine).
- **PO:** Administer with a meal or light snack.
- ❑ Oral powder may be mixed with chocolate milk, Ensure, or Advera within 1 hr of dosing to improve taste. Capsules should be stored in the refrigerator and protected from light. Use calibrated oral dosing syringe for oral solution. Oral solution does not require refrigeration if used within 30 days and stored below 77°F in the original container. Keep cap tightly closed.
- ❑ If nausea occurs on dose of 600 mg twice daily, may titrate by 300 mg twice daily for 1 day, then 400 mg twice daily for 2 days, then 500 mg twice daily for 1 day, then 600 mg twice daily thereafter.
- ❑ Patients initiating concurrent therapy with nucleoside analogues may have less GI intolerance by initiating ritonavir for 2 wk and then adding the nucleoside analogue.

## PATIENT/FAMILY TEACHING

❑ Emphasize the importance of taking ritonavir exactly as directed, at evenly spaced times throughout day. Do not take more than prescribed amount and do not stop taking without consulting health care professional. Take missed doses as soon as remembered; do not double doses.

❑ Instruct patient that ritonavir should not be shared with others.

❑ Advise patient to avoid taking other medications, prescription or OTC, without consulting health care professional.

❑ Inform patient that ritonavir does not cure AIDS or prevent associated or opportunistic infections. Ritonavir does not reduce the risk of transmission of HIV to others through sexual contact or blood contamination. Caution patient to use a condom during sexual contact and to avoid sharing needles or donating blood to prevent spreading the AIDS virus to others. Advise patient that the long-term effects of ritonavir are unknown at this time.

❑ Inform patient that ritonavir may cause hyperglycemia. Advise patient to notify health care professional if increased thirst or hunger; unexplained weight loss; increased urination; fatigue; or dry, itchy skin occurs.

❑ Advise patients taking oral contraceptives to use a nonhormonal method of birth control during ritonavir therapy.

❑ Inform patient that redistribution and accumulation of body fat may occur, causing central obesity, dorsocervical fat enlargement (buffalo hump), peripheral wasting, breast enlargement, and cushingoid appearance. The cause and long-term effects are not known.

❑ Emphasize the importance of regular follow-up exams and blood counts to determine progress and monitor for side effects.

## EVALUATION

**Effectiveness of therapy can be demonstrated by:** ■ Delayed progression of AIDS and decreased opportunistic infections in patients with HIV ■ Decrease in viral load and improvement in CD4 cell counts.

# rituximab
(ri-**tux**-i-mab)
Rituxan

### CLASSIFICATION(S):
**Therapeutic:** antineoplastics
**Pharmacologic:** monoclonal antibodies

### Pregnancy Category C

## INDICATIONS

■ Treatment of low-grade or follicular, CD20-positive, B-cell non-Hodgkin's lymphoma.

## ACTION

■ Binds to the CD20 antigen on the surface of lymphoma cells, preventing the activation process for cell cycle initiation and differentiation. **Therapeutic Effects:** ■ Death of lymphoma cells.

## PHARMACOKINETICS

**Absorption:** IV administration results in complete bioavailability.
**Distribution:** Binds specifically to CD20 binding sites on lymphoma cells.
**Metabolism and Excretion:** Unknown.
**Half-life:** 59.8–174 hr (depending on tumor burden).

## CONTRAINDICATIONS AND PRECAUTIONS

**Contraindicated in:** ■ Hypersensitivity to murine (mouse) proteins ■ Pregnancy or lactation.
**Use Cautiously in:** ■ Pre-existing bone marrow depression ■ Children (safety not established).

## ADVERSE REACTIONS AND SIDE EFFECTS*

■ **CNS:** headache ■ **Resp:** bronchospasm, cough, dyspnea ■ **CV:** ARRHYTHMIAS, hypotension, peripheral edema ■ **GI:** abdominal pain, altered taste, dyspepsia ■ **Derm:** MUCOCUTANEOUS SKIN REACTIONS, flushing, urticaria ■ **Endo:** hyperglycemia ■ **F and E:** hypocalcemia ■ **Hemat:** ANEMIA, NEUTROPENIA, THROMBOCYTOPENIA ■ **MS:** arthralgia, back pain ■ **Misc:** allergic reactions including ANAPHY-

LAXIS and ANGIOEDEMA, INFUSION REACTIONS, TUMOR LYSIS SYNDROME, fever/chills/rigors (infusion related).

## INTERACTIONS

**Drug-Drug:** ■ None known.

## ROUTE AND DOSAGE

■ **IV (Adults):** 375 mg/m$^2$ once weekly for 4–8 doses.

## AVAILABILITY

■ *Solution for injection (requires dilution):* 10 mg/ml in 100 mg and 500-mg vials$^{Rx}$.

TIME/ACTION PROFILE (B-cell depletion)

| | ONSET | PEAK | DURATION |
|---|---|---|---|
| IV | within 14 days | 3–4 wk | 6–9 mo† |

†Duration of depletion after 4 wk of treatment.

## NURSING IMPLICATIONS

### ASSESSMENT

❑ Monitor patient for fever, chills/rigors, nausea, urticaria, fatigue, headache, pruritus, bronchospasm, dyspnea, sensation of tongue or throat swelling, rhinitis, vomiting, hypotension, flushing, and pain at disease sites. These infusion-related events occur frequently within 30 min–2 hr of beginning first infusion and may resolve with slowing or discontinuing infusion and treatment with IV saline, diphenhydramine, and acetaminophen. Patients with increased risk (females, patients with pulmonary infiltrates, chronic lymphocytic leukemia, or mantle cell leukemia) may have more severe reactions, which may be fatal. Signs of severe reactions include hypotension, angioedema, hypoxia, or bronchospasm and may require interruption of infusion. May result in pulmonary infiltrates, adult respiratory distress syndrome, MI, ventricular fibrillation, and cardiogenic shock. Monitor closely. Incidence decreases with subsequent infusions.

❑ Monitor patient for tumor lysis syndrome due to rapid reduction in tumor volume (acute renal failure, hyperkalemia, hypocalcemia, hyperuricemia, or hypophosphatasemia) usually occurring 12–24 hr after first infusion. Risks are higher in patients with greater tumor burden; may be fatal. Correct electrolyte abnormalities, monitor renal

function and fluid balance, and administer supportive care, including dialysis, as indicated.

❑ Assess patient for hypersensitivity reactions (hypotension, bronchospasm, angioedema) during administration. May respond to decrease in infusion rate. Premedication with diphenhydramine and acetaminophen is recommended. Treatment includes diphenhydramine, acetaminophen, bronchodilators, or IV saline as indicated. Epinephrine, antihistamines, and corticosteroids should be readily available in the event of a severe reaction. If severe reactions occur, discontinue infusion; may be resumed at 50% of the rate when symptoms have resolved completely.

❑ Monitor ECG during and immediately after infusion in patients with pre-existing cardiac conditions (arrhythmias, angina) or patients who have developed arrhythmias during previous infusions of rituximab. Life-threatening arrhythmias may occur.

■ *Lab Test Considerations:* Monitor CBC and platelet count regularly during therapy and frequently in patients with blood dyscrasias. May cause anemia, thrombocytopenia, or neutropenia.

❑ Frequently causes B-cell depletion with an associated decrease in serum immunoglobulins in a minority of patients; does not appear to cause an increased incidence of infection.

## POTENTIAL NURSING DIAGNOSES

■ Infection, risk for (Side Effects).

## IMPLEMENTATION

■ **General:** Transient hypotension may occur during infusion; antihypertensive medications may be held for 12 hr before infusion.

■ **Intermittent Infusion:** Dilute to a concentration of 1–4 mg/ml with 0.9% NaCl or D5W. Gently invert bag to mix. Solution is clear and colorless; do not administer solutions that are discolored or contain particulate matter. Discard unused portion remaining in vial. Solution is stable for 12 hr at room temperature and for 24 hr if refrigerated.

■ *Rate:* Do not administer as an IV push or bolus.

❑ *First infusion:* Administer at an initial rate of 50 mg/hr. If hypersensitivity or infusion-related events do not occur, rate may be escalated in 50 mg/hr increments every 30 min to a maximum of 400 mg/hr.

❑ *Subsequent infusions:* May be administered at an initial rate of 100 mg/hr and increased by 100-mg/hr increments at 30 min intervals to a maximum of 400 mg/hr.

■ **Additive Incompatibility:** Do not admix with other medications.

## PATIENT/FAMILY TEACHING

❑ Inform patient of the purpose of the medication.

❑ Advise patient to report infusion-related events or symptoms of hypersensitivity reactions immediately.

❑ Instruct patient to notify health care professional promptly if fever; chills; cough; hoarseness; sore throat; signs of infection; lower back or side pain; painful or difficult urination; bleeding gums; bruising; petechiae; blood in stools, urine, or emesis; increased fatigue; dyspnea; or orthostatic hypotension occurs. Caution patient to avoid crowds and persons with known infections. Instruct patient to use soft toothbrush and electric razor and to avoid falls. Caution patient not to drink alcoholic beverages or take medication containing aspirin or NSAIDs; may precipitate gastric bleeding.

❑ Instruct patient to use contraception throughout therapy.

## EVALUATION

**Effectiveness of therapy can be demonstrated by:** ■ Decrease in spread of malignancy.

## rivastigmine

(rye-va-**stig**-meen)

Exelon

### *CLASSIFICATION(S):*

***Therapeutic:*** *anti-Alzheimer's agents*
***Pharmacologic:*** *cholinergics (cholinesterase inhibitors)*

**Pregnancy Category B**

## INDICATIONS

■ Managment of mild to moderate dementia associated with Alzheimer's disease.

## ACTION

■ Enhances cholinergic function by reversible inhibition of cholinesterase ■ Does not alter the course of the disease. **Therapeutic Effects:** ■ Decreased dementia (temporary) associated with Alzheimer's disease.

## PHARMACOKINETICS

**Absorption:** Well absorbed following oral administration.

**Distribution:** Widely distributed.

**Metabolism and Excretion:** Rapidly and extensively metabolized by the liver; metabolites are excreted by the kidneys.

**Half-life:** 1.5 hr.

## CONTRAINDICATIONS AND PRECAUTIONS

**Contraindicated in:** ■ Hypersensitivity to rivastigmine or other carbamates.

**Use Cautiously in:** ■ History of asthma or obstructive pulmonary disease ■ History of GI bleeding ■ Sick sinus syndrome or other supraventricular cardiac conduction abnormalities ■ Pregnancy, lactation, or children (safety not established).

## ADVERSE REACTIONS AND SIDE EFFECTS*

■ **CNS:** <u>weakness</u>, dizziness, drowsiness, headache ■ **CV:** edema, heart failure, hypotension ■ **GI:** <u>anorexia</u>, dyspepsia, <u>nausea</u>, <u>vomiting</u>, abdominal pain, flatulence ■ **Neuro:** tremor ■ **Misc:** fever, weight loss.

## INTERACTIONS

**Drug-Drug:** ■ **Nicotine** use may increase metabolism and decrease blood levels.

## ROUTE AND DOSAGE

■ **PO (Adults):** 1.5 mg twice daily initially; after at least 2 weeks, dose may be increased to 3 mg twice daily. Further increments may be made at 2-week intervals up to 6 mg twice daily.

## AVAILABILITY

■ *Capsules:* 1.5 mg, 3 mg, 4.5 mg, 6 mg ■
*Oral Solution:* 2 mg/ml in 120-ml bottle.

TIME/ACTION PROFILE (improvement in dementia)

| | ONSET | PEAK | DURATION |
|---|---|---|---|
| PO | within 2 wk | up to 12 wk | unknown |

## NURSING IMPLICATIONS

### ASSESSMENT

❑ Assess cognitive function (memory, attention, reasoning, language, ability to perform simple tasks) periodically throughout therapy.
❑ Monitor patient for nausea, vomiting, anorexia, and weight loss. Notify health care professional if these side effects occur.

### POTENTIAL NURSING DIAGNOSES

■ Thought processes, disturbed (Indications).
■ Nutrition, imbalanced: less than body requirements (Side Effects).

### IMPLEMENTATION

■ **General:** Rivastigmine oral solution and capsules may be interchanged at equal doses.
■ **PO:** Administer in the morning and evening with food.
❑ Oral solution may be administered directly from syringe provided or mixed with a small glass of water, cold fruit juice, or soda. Mixture should be stirred prior to drinking. Ensure patient drinks entire mixture. Oral solution is stable for 4 hours at room temperature when mixed with cold fruit juice or soda. Do not mix with other solutions.

### PATIENT/FAMILY TEACHING

❑ Emphasize the importance of taking rivastigmine at regular intervals as directed.
❑ Explain to patient and caregiver how to use oral dosing syringe provided with oral solution. Remove syringe from protective case and push down and twist child resistant closure to open bottle. Insert syringe into opening in white stopper in bottle. Hold the syringe and pull plunger to the level corresponding to the prescribed dose. Before removing syringe from bottle, push out larger bubbles (small bubbles will not alter dose) by moving plunger up and down a few times.

After large bubbles are gone, move plunger to level of dose. Remove syringe from bottle.
❑ Caution patient and caregiver that rivastigmine may cause dizziness.
❑ Advise patient and caregiver to notify health care professional if nausea, vomiting, anorexia, or weight loss occur.
❑ Advise patient and caregiver to notify health care professional of medication regimen prior to treatment or surgery.

### EVALUATION

**Clinical response to therapy can be evaluated by:** ■ Temporary improvement in cognitive function (memory, attention, reasoning, language, ability to perform simple tasks) in patients with Alzheimer's disease.

# rizatriptan

(riz-a-**trip**-tan)
Maxalt, Maxalt-MLT

## CLASSIFICATION(S):

*Therapeutic: vascular headache suppressants*
*Pharmacologic: 5 HT$_1$ agonists*

### Pregnancy Category C

### INDICATIONS

■ Acute treatment of migraine headache.

### ACTION

■ Acts as an agonist at specific 5-HT$_1$ receptor sites in intracranial blood vessels and sensory trigeminal nerves. **Therapeutic Effects:** ■ Cranial vessel vasoconstriction with associated decrease in release of neuropeptides and resultant decrease in migraine headache.

### PHARMACOKINETICS

**Absorption:** Completely absorbed after oral administration, but first-pass metabolism results in 45% bioavailability.

**Distribution:** Unknown.

**Metabolism and Excretion:** Primarily metabolized by monoamine oxidase-A (MAO-A); minor conversion to an active compound; 14% excreted unchanged in urine.

**Half-life:** 2–3 hr.

## CONTRAINDICATIONS AND PRECAUTIONS

**Contraindicated in:** ■ Hypersensitivity ■ Ischemic or vasospastic cardiovascular, cerebrovascular, or peripheral vascular syndromes ■ History of significant cardiovascular disease ■ Uncontrolled hypertension ■ Should not be used within 24 hr of other 5-HT₁ agonists or ergot-type compounds (dihydroergotamine) ■ Basilar or hemiplegic migraine ■ Concurrent MAO-A inhibitor therapy or within 2 wk of discontinuing MAO-A inhibitor therapy ■ Phenylketonuria (orally disintegrating tablet contains aspartame).

**Use Cautiously in:** ■ Severe renal impairment, especially in patients on dialysis ■ Moderate hepatic impairment ■ Pregnancy, lactation, or children <18 yr (safety not established).

**Exercise Extreme Caution in:** ■ Cardiovascular risk factors (hypertension, hypercholesterolemia, cigarette smoking, obesity, diabetes, strong family history, menopausal women or men >40 yr); use only if cardiovascular status has been evaluated and determined to be safe and first dose is administered under supervision.

## ADVERSE REACTIONS AND SIDE EFFECTS*

■ **CNS:** dizziness, drowsiness, weakness ■ **CV:** CORONARY ARTERY VASOSPASM, MI, VENTRICULAR FIBRILLATION, VENTRICULAR TACHYCARDIA, chest pain, myocardial ischemia ■ **GI:** dry mouth, nausea ■ **Misc:** hypersensitivity reactions including ANGIOEDEMA, toxic epidermal necrolysis, pain.

## INTERACTIONS

**Drug-Drug:** ■ Concurrent use with **MAO-A inhibitors** ↑ blood levels and adverse reactions (concurrent use or use within 2 wk or MAO inhibitor is contraindicated) ■ Concurrent use with other **5-HT agonists** or **ergot-type compounds (dihydroergotamine)** may result in ↑ vasoactive properties (avoid use within 24 hr of each other) ■ **Propranolol** ↑ blood levels and risk of adverse reactions (dosage reduction recommended) ■ Concurrent use with **SSRI antidepressants** may result in weakness, hyperreflexia, and incoordination.

**Drug-Natural Products:** ■ Increased risk of serotinergic side effects including serotonin syndrome with **St. John's wort** and **SAMe.**

## ROUTE AND DOSAGE

■ **PO (Adults):** 5–10 mg (use 5-mg dose in patients receiving propranolol); may be repeated in 2 hr; not to exceed 3 doses/24 hr. Dose is same for both types of tablets.

## AVAILABILITY

■ **Tablets:** 5 mgᴿˣ, 10 mgᴿˣ ■ Cost: 5 mg $93.11/6; 10 mg $93.11/6 ■ *Orally disintegrating tablets (Maxalt-MLT):* 5 mgᴿˣ, 10 mgᴿˣ ■ Cost: 5 mg $93.11/6; 10 mg $93.11/6.

TIME/ACTION PROFILE (blood levels)

|    | ONSET | PEAK | DURATION |
|----|-------|------|----------|
| PO | 30 min | 1–1.5 hr | unknown |

# NURSING IMPLICATIONS

## ASSESSMENT

❏ Assess pain location, character, intensity, and duration and associated symptoms (photophobia, phonophobia, nausea, vomiting) during migraine attack.

## POTENTIAL NURSING DIAGNOSES

■ Pain, acute (Indications).

## IMPLEMENTATION

■ **PO:** Tablets should be swallowed whole with liquid.

❏ Orally disintegrating tablets should be left in the package until use. Remove from the blister pouch. Do not push tablet through the blister; peel open the blister pack with dry hands and place tablet on tongue. Tablet will dissolve rapidly and be swallowed with saliva. No liquid is needed to take the orally disintegrating tablet.

## PATIENT/FAMILY TEACHING

❏ Inform patient that rizatriptan should be used only during a migraine attack. It is meant to be used for relief of migraine attacks but not to prevent or reduce the number of attacks.

- Instruct patient to administer rizatriptan as soon as symptoms of a migraine attack appear, but it may be administered at any time during an attack. If migraine symptoms return, a second dose may be used. Allow at least 2 hr between doses, and do not use more than 30 mg in any 24-hr period.
- If first dose does not relieve headache, additional rizatriptan doses are not likely to be effective; notify health care professional.
- Caution patient not to take rizatriptan within 24 hr of other vascular headache suppressants.
- Advise patient that lying down in a darkened room after rizatriptan administration may further help relieve headache.
- Caution patient not to use rizatriptan if she is pregnant, suspects she is pregnant, plans to become pregnant, or is breastfeeding. Adequate contraception should be used during therapy.
- Advise patient to notify health care professional before next dose of rizatriptan if pain or tightness in the chest occurs during use. If pain is severe or does not subside, notify health care professional immediately. If feelings of tingling, heat, flushing, heaviness, pressure, drowsiness, dizziness, tiredness, or sickness develop, discuss with health care professional at next visit.
- May cause dizziness or drowsiness. Caution patient to avoid driving or other activities requiring alertness until response to medication is known.
- Advise patient to avoid alcohol, which aggravates headaches, during rizatriptan use.

## EVALUATION

**Effectiveness of therapy can be demonstrated by:** ■ Relief of migraine attack.

---

# rofecoxib

(roe-fe-**kox**-ib)

Vioxx

## CLASSIFICATION(S):

**Therapeutic:** *nonsteroidal anti-inflammatory agents, nonopioid analgesics*
**Pharmacologic:** *COX-2 inhibitors*

**Pregnancy Category C**

## INDICATIONS

■ Osteoarthritis and rheumatoid arthritis (decreases symptoms) ■ Acute pain in adults ■ Primary dysmenorrhea.

## ACTION

■ Inhibits the enzyme cyclo-oxygenase-2 (COX-2). This enzyme is required for the synthesis of prostaglandins ■ Has analgesic, antipyretic, and anti-inflammatory properties ■ Does not inhibit COX-1 and may produce less GI damage than other NSAIDs. **Therapeutic Effects:** ■ Decreased pain and inflammation.

## PHARMACOKINETICS

**Absorption:** 93% absorbed following oral administration.
**Distribution:** Unknown.
**Metabolism and Excretion:** Mostly metabolized by the liver; 14% excreted unchanged in feces; <1% excreted unchanged in urine.
**Half-life:** 17 hr.

## CONTRAINDICATIONS AND PRECAUTIONS

**Contraindicated in:** ■ Hypersensitivity ■ Cross-sensitivity may occur with other NSAIDs, including aspirin ■ History of asthma, urticaria, or allergic-type reactions to aspirin or other NSAIDs ■ Advanced renal disease (may precipitate acute renal failure in patients with renal insufficiency) ■ Moderate to severe hepatic impairment ■ Lactation ■ Should not be used in late pregnancy (may cause premature closure of the ductus arteriosus).
**Use Cautiously in:** ■ Elderly or debilitated patients (use lowest dose) ■ History of cardiovascular disease ■ Pregnancy or children <18 yr (safety not established; use not recommended late in pregnancy).
**Exercise Extreme Caution in:** ■ Prior history of ulcer disease or GI bleeding.

## ADVERSE REACTIONS AND SIDE EFFECTS*

■ **CNS:** aseptic meningitis, fatigue ■ **CV:** CARDIO-VASCULAR THROBOTIC EVENTS , hypertension, lower extremity edema ■ **GI:** GI BLEEDING , nausea ■ **Hemat:** anemia ■ **Misc:** allergic reactions including ANAPHYLAXIS .

## INTERACTIONS

**Drug-Drug:** ■ May ↓ the effectiveness of **diuretics** or **antihypertensives** ■ Concurrent use of **aspirin** may ↑ risk of GI bleeding ▪ ↑ serum **lithium** levels ▪ May ↑ **methotrexate** levels and the risk of toxicity ▪ **Rifampin** ↓ rofecoxib levels (initiate therapy at 25 mg/day for osteoarthritis) ▪ May ↑ effects of **warfarin.**

### ROUTE AND DOSAGE

❏ **Osteoarthritis**

▪ **PO (Adults):** 12.5 mg once daily initially; may be increased if needed to 25 mg once daily.

❏ **Acute Pain/Primary Dysmenorrhea**

▪ **PO (Adults):** 50 mg once daily initially for up to 5 days.

### AVAILABILITY

▪*Tablets:* 12.5 mg$^{Rx}$, 25 mg$^{Rx}$, 50 mg$^{Rx}$ ▪Cost: 12.5 mg $264.18/100, 25 mg $264.18/100, 50 mg $385.81/100 ▪ *Oral suspension (strawberry flavored):* 12.5 mg/5 ml$^{Rx}$, 25 mg/5 ml$^{Rx}$ ▪ Cost: $117.71/150-ml bottle.

TIME/ACTION PROFILE (analgesia)

|  | ONSET | PEAK | DURATION |
|---|---|---|---|
| PO | within 45 min | 2–3 hr | up to 24 hr |

## NURSING IMPLICATIONS

### ASSESSMENT

▪ **General Info:** Patients who have asthma, aspirin-induced allergy, and nasal polyps are at increased risk for developing hypersensitivity reactions. Assess for rhinitis, asthma, and urticaria.

▪ **Pain:** Assess pain (note type, location, and intensity) prior to and 2–3 hr following administration.

▪ **Arthritis:** Assess patient's range of motion, degree of swelling, and pain in affected joints before and periodically during therapy.

▪ *Lab Test Considerations:* Rofecoxib has no effect on bleeding time.

### POTENTIAL NURSING DIAGNOSES

▪ Pain, acute (Indications).

▪ Mobility, impaired physical (Indications).

### IMPLEMENTATION

▪ **General:** To minimize the risk of adverse GI effects, the lowest effective dose should be used for the shortest time possible. Administration in higher than recommended doses does not provide increased effectiveness but may cause increased side effects.

❏ Doses of rofecoxib 12.5 and 25 mg are comparable to ibuprofen 800 mg tid and diclofenac 50 mg tid for signs and symptoms of osteoarthritis, and rofecoxib 50 mg is comparable to naproxen sodium 550 mg for acute pain.

❏ Coadministration with opioid analgesics may have additive analgesic effects and may permit lower opioid doses.

▪ **PO:** May be administered without regard to food.

❏ Shake oral suspension before administering.

▪ **Dysmenorrhea:** Administer as soon as possible after the onset of menses. Prophylactic treatment has not been shown to be effective.

### PATIENT/FAMILY TEACHING

❏ Advise patients to take this medication with a full glass of water and to remain in an upright position for 15–30 min after administration.

❏ Instruct patient to take medication as directed. Take missed doses as soon as remembered but not if almost time for next dose. Do not double doses.

❏ May occasionally cause dizziness. Caution patient to avoid driving or other activities requiring alertness until response to medication is known.

❏ Caution patient to avoid the concurrent use of alcohol, aspirin, acetaminophen, or other OTC medications or herbal products without consulting health care professional.

❏ Advise patient to inform health care professional of medication regimen prior to treatment or surgery.

❏ Caution patient that use of an NSAID with 3 or more glasses of alcohol per day may increase the risk of GI bleeding.

❏ Advise patient to consult health care professional promptly if abdominal pain or black tarry stools occur. GI toxicity can occur at any time, without warning. Patient should

---

{ } = Available in Canada only.
*CAPITALS indicates life-threatening; <u>underlines</u> indicate most frequent.

also notify health care professional if rash, weight gain, edema, nausea, fatigue, lethargy, itching, jaundice, upper right quadrant tenderness, or influenza-like syndrome (chills, fever, muscle aches, pain) occur.

## EVALUATION

**Effectiveness of therapy can be demonstrated by:** ■ Decrease in severity of pain ■ Improved joint mobility.

---

# ropinirole
(roe-**pin**-i-role)
Requip

### CLASSIFICATION(S):
**Therapeutic:** antiparkinson agents
**Pharmacologic:** dopamine agonists

### Pregnancy Category C

---

## INDICATIONS

■ Management of signs and symptoms of idiopathic Parkinson's disease.

## ACTION

■ Stimulates dopamine receptors in the brain. **Therapeutic Effects:** ■ Decreased tremor and rigidity in Parkinson's disease.

## PHARMACOKINETICS

**Absorption:** 55% absorbed following oral administration.

**Distribution:** Widely distributed.

**Metabolism and Excretion:** Extensively metabolized by the liver (by cytochrome P450 CYP1A2 enzyme system); <10% excreted unchanged in urine.

**Half-life:** 6 hr.

## CONTRAINDICATIONS AND PRECAUTIONS

**Contraindicated in:** ■ Hypersensitivity.

**Use Cautiously in:** ■ Geriatric patients (increased risk of hallucinations in patients >65 yr) ■ Hepatic impairment (slower titration may be required) ■ Severe cardiovascular disease ■ Pregnancy, lactation, or children (safety not established; may inhibit lactation).

## ADVERSE REACTIONS AND SIDE EFFECTS*

■ **CNS:** SLEEP ATTACKS, dizziness, syncope, confusion, drowsiness, fatigue, hallucinations, headache, increased dyskinesia, weakness ■ **EENT:** abnormal vision ■ **CV:** orthostatic hypotension, peripheral edema ■ **GI:** constipation, dry mouth, dyspepsia, nausea, vomiting ■ **Derm:** increased sweating.

## INTERACTIONS

**Drug-Drug:** ■ **Drugs that alter the activity of cytochrome P450 CYP1A2 enzyme system** may affect the activity of ropinirole ■ Effects may be increased by **estrogens** ■ Effects may be decreased by **phenothiazines, butyrophenones, thioxanthenes,** or **metoclopramide** ■ May increase the effects of **levodopa** (may allow dosage reduction of levodopa).

## ROUTE AND DOSAGE

■ **PO (Adults):** 0.25 mg 3 times daily for 1 wk, then 0.5 mg 3 times daily for 1 wk, then 0.75 mg 3 times daily for 1 wk, then 1 mg 3 times daily for 1 wk; then may increase by 1.5 mg/day every wk, up to 9 mg/day; then may increase by up to 3 mg/day every wk up to 24 mg/day.

## AVAILABILITY

■ **Tablets:** 0.25 mg$^{Rx}$, 0.5 mg$^{Rx}$, 1 mg$^{Rx}$, 2 mg$^{Rx}$, 4 mg$^{Rx}$, 5 mg$^{Rx}$ ■ Cost: 0.25 mg $29.20/30, 0.5 mg $97.30/100, 1 mg $29.20/30, 2 mg $29.20/30, 4 mg $194.60/30, 5 mg $194.60/30.

TIME/ACTION PROFILE

|  | ONSET | PEAK | DURATION |
|----|---------|---------|----------|
| PO | unknown | unknown | 8 hr |

# NURSING IMPLICATIONS

## ASSESSMENT

❑ Assess patient for signs and symptoms of Parkinson's disease (tremor, muscle weakness and rigidity, ataxic gait) prior to and throughout therapy.

❑ Assess blood pressure periodically throughout therapy.

❑ Assess patient for drowsiness and sleep attacks. Drowsiness is a common side effect of ropinirole, but sleep attacks or episodes of falling asleep during activities that require active participation may occur without warning. Assess patient for concomitant medications that have sedating effects or may increase serum ropinirole levels (see Interactions). May require discontinuation of therapy.

■ **Lab Test Considerations:** May cause elevated BUN.

## POTENTIAL NURSING DIAGNOSES

■ Mobility, impaired physical (Indications).
■ Injury, risk for (Indications, Side Effects).

## IMPLEMENTATION

■ **PO:** May be administered with or without food. Administration with food may decrease nausea.

## PATIENT/FAMILY TEACHING

❑ Instruct patient to take medication exactly as directed. Missed doses should be taken as soon as possible, but not if almost time for next dose. Do not double doses.

❑ Caution patient to change positions slowly to minimize orthostatic hypotension.

❑ May cause drowsiness and unexpected episodes of falling asleep. Caution patient to avoid driving or other activities requiring alertness until response to medication is known. Advise patient to notify health care professional if episodes of falling asleep occur.

❑ Advise patient to avoid alcohol and other CNS depressants concurrently with ropinirole.

❑ Advise patient that increasing fluids, sugarless gum or candy, ice, or saliva substitutes may help minimize dry mouth. Consult health care professional if dry mouth continues for >2 wk.

## EVALUATION

**Effectiveness of therapy can be demonstrated by:** ■ Decreased tremor and rigidity in Parkinson's disease.

---

**ropivacaine, See EPIDURAL LOCAL ANESTHETICS.**

---

# rosiglitazone
(roe-zi-**glit**-a-zone)
Avandia

**CLASSIFICATION(S):**
**Therapeutic:** antidiabetics
**Pharmacologic:** thiazolidinediones

**Pregnancy Category C**

## INDICATIONS

■ Used as an adjunct to diet and exercise in the management of type 2 diabetes mellitus; may be used with metformin sulfonylureas or insulin.

## ACTION

■ Improves sensitivity to insulin by acting as an agonist at receptor sites involved in insulin responsiveness and subsequent glucose production and utilization ■ Requires insulin for activity. **Therapeutic Effects:** ■ Decreased insulin resistance, resulting in glycemic control without hypoglycemia.

## PHARMACOKINETICS

**Absorption:** Well absorbed (99%) following oral administration.
**Distribution:** Unknown.
**Protein Binding:** 99.8% bound to plasma proteins.
**Metabolism and Excretion:** Entirely metabolized by the liver.
**Half-life:** 3.2–3.6 hr (increased in liver disease).

## CONTRAINDICATIONS AND PRECAUTIONS

**Contraindicated in:** ■ Hypersensitivity ■ Pregnancy or lactation (not recommended for use during pregnancy or lactation; insulin should be used) ■ Children <18 yr or type 1 diabetes (requires insulin for activity) ■ Diabetic ketoacidosis ■ Clinical evidence of active liver disease or increased ALT (>2.5 times upper limit of normal).

**Use Cautiously in:** ■ Edema ■ CHF (avoid use in moderate to severe CHF unless benefits outweigh risks) ■ Concurrent use with insulin (may increase risk of adverse cardiovascular reactions) ■ Hepatic impairment ■ Women with childbearing potential (may restore ovulation and risk of pregnancy).

## ADVERSE REACTIONS AND SIDE EFFECTS*

■ **CV:** CHF, edema ■ **Hemat:** anemia ■ **Metab:** increased total cholesterol, LDL and HDL, weight gain.

## INTERACTIONS

**Drug-Drug:** ■ None known.
**Drug-Natural Products:** ■ **Glucosamine** may worsen blood glucose control ■ **Fenugreek, chromium,** and **coenzyme Q-10** may produce additive hypoglycemic effects.

## ROUTE AND DOSAGE

■ **PO (Adults):** 4 mg as a single dose once daily or 2 mg twice daily; after 12 weeks, may be increased if necessary to 8 mg once daily or 4 mg twice daily.

## AVAILABILITY

■ *Tablets:* 2 mg$^{Rx}$, 4 mg$^{Rx}$, 8 mg$^{Rx}$ ■ Cost: 2 mg $115.09/60, 4 mg $153.65/60, 8 mg $473.84/100.

TIME/ACTION PROFILE (effects on blood glucose)

| | ONSET | PEAK | DURATION |
|---|---|---|---|
| PO | unknown | unknown | 12–24 hr |

# NURSING IMPLICATIONS

## ASSESSMENT

❑ Observe patient taking current insulin for signs and symptoms of hypoglycemia (sweating, hunger, weakness, dizziness, tremor, tachycardia, anxiety).
❑ Assess patient for edema and signs of CHF (dyspnea, rales/crackles, peripheral edema, weight gain, jugular venous distension). May require discontinuation of rosiglitazone.
■ *Lab Test Considerations:* Monitor serum glucose and glycosylated hemoglobin periodically during therapy to evaluate effectiveness.
❑ Monitor CBC with differential periodically during therapy. May cause ↓ in hemoglobin, hematocrit, and WBC, usually during the first 4–8 wk of therapy; then levels stabilize.
❑ Monitor AST and ALT every 2 months during the first 12 months of therapy and periodi-

cally thereafter or if jaundice or symptoms of hepatic dysfunction occur. May cause irreversible ↑ in AST and ALT or hepatic failure (rare). If ALT increases to >3 times the upper limit of normal, recheck ALT promptly. Discontinue rosiglitazone if ALT remains >3 times normal.
❑ May cause ↑ in total cholesterol, LDL, and HDL and ↓ in free fatty acids.

## POTENTIAL NURSING DIAGNOSES

■ Nutrition, imbalanced: more than body requirements (Indications).

## IMPLEMENTATION

■ **General:** Patients stabilized on a diabetic regimen who are exposed to stress, fever, trauma, infection, or surgery may require administration of insulin.
■ **PO:** May be administered with or without meals.

## PATIENT/FAMILY TEACHING

❑ Instruct patient to take medication exactly as directed. If dose for 1 day is missed, do not double dose the next day.
❑ Explain to patient that this medication controls hyperglycemia but does not cure diabetes. Therapy is long term.
❑ Review signs of hypoglycemia and hyperglycemia with patient. If hypoglycemia occurs, advise patient to take a glass of orange juice or 2–3 tsp of sugar, honey, or corn syrup dissolved in water and notify health care professional.
❑ Encourage patient to follow prescribed diet, medication, and exercise regimen to prevent hypoglycemic or hyperglycemic episodes.
❑ Instruct patient in proper testing of serum glucose and ketones. These tests should be closely monitored during periods of stress or illness and health care professional notified if significant changes occur.
❑ Advise patient to notify health care professional immediately if signs of hepatic dysfunction (nausea, vomiting, abdominal pain, fatigue, anorexia, dark urine, jaundice) or CHF occur.
❑ Insulin is the preferred method of controlling blood glucose during pregnancy. Counsel female patients that higher doses of oral contraceptives or a form of contraception other than oral contraceptives may be required and to notify health care professional

promptly if pregnancy is planned or suspected.

❏ Advise patient to inform health care professional of medication regimen prior to treatment or surgery.

❏ Advise patient to carry a form of sugar (sugar packets, candy) and identification describing disease process and medication regimen at all times.

❏ Emphasize the importance of routine follow-up exams.

## EVALUATION

**Effectiveness of therapy can be demonstrated by:** ▪ Control of blood glucose levels.

## rosuvastatin, See HMG-CoA REDUCTASE INHIBITORS.

# SALICYLATES

## aspirin

(**as**-pir-in)

acetylsalicylic acid, Acuprin, {Apo-ASA}, {Apo-ASEN}, {Arthrinol}, {Arthrisin}, {Artria S.R.}, ASA, Aspergum, Aspir-Low, Aspirtab, {Astrin}, Bayer Aspirin, Bayer Timed-Release Arthritic Pain Formula, {Coryphen}, Easprin, Ecotrin, 8-Hour Bayer Timed-Release, Empirin, {Entrophen}, Halfprin, {Headache Tablets}, Healthprin, Norwich Aspirin, {Novasen}, {PMS-ASA}, Sloprin, St. Joseph Adult Chewable Aspirin, Therapy Bayer, ZORprin

## choline salicylate

(**koe**-leen sal-**i**-sil-ate)

Arthropan

## choline and magnesium salicylates

(**koe**-leen mag-**neez**-ee-um sal-**i**-sil-ates)

CMT, Tricosal, Trilisate

## magnesium salicylate

(mag-**neez**-ee-um sal-**i**-sil-ate)

{Doan's Backache Pills}, Doan's Regular Strength Tablets, Magan, Mobidin

## salsalate

(**sal**-sa-late)

Amigesic, Anaflex, Disalcid, Marthritic, Mono-Gesic, Salflex, Salgesic, Salsitab

## sodium salicylate

(**soe**-dee-yum sal-**i**-sil-ate)

{Dodd's Extra Strength}, {Dodd's Pills}, {Gin Pain Pills}

## CLASSIFICATION(S):

*Therapeutic:* antipyretics, nonopioid analgesics
*Pharmacologic:* salicylates

**Pregnancy Category D (aspirin–first trimester), C (magnesium salicylate, salsalate–first trimester)**

## INDICATIONS

■ Inflammatory disorders including: ❏ Rheumatoid arthritis ❏ Osteoarthritis ■ Mild to moderate pain ■ Fever ■ **Aspirin:** Prophylaxis of transient ischemic attacks and MI.

## ACTION

■ Produce analgesia and reduce inflammation and fever by inhibiting the production of prostaglandins ■ **Aspirin Only:** Decreases platelet aggregation. **Therapeutic Effects:** ■ Analgesia ■ Reduction of inflammation ■ Reduction of fever ■ **Aspirin:** Decreased incidence of transient ischemic attacks and MI.

## PHARMACOKINETICS

**Absorption:** *Aspirin*—Well absorbed from the upper small intestine; absorption from enteric-coated preparations may be unreliable; rectal absorption is slow and variable. *Choline and magnesium salicylates*—Well absorbed after oral administration. *Salsalate*—Splits into 2 molecules of salicylic acid after oral administration; absorbed in the small intestine.

**Distribution:** All salicylates are rapidly and widely distributed; cross the placenta and enter breast milk.

**Metabolism and Excretion:** Extensively metabolized by the liver; inactive metabolites excreted by the kidneys. Amount excreted unchanged by the kidneys depends on urine pH; as pH increases, amount excreted unchanged increases from 2–3% up to 80%.

**Half-life:** 2–3 hr for low doses; up to 15–30 hr with larger doses because of saturation of liver metabolism.

{ } = Available in Canada only.
*CAPITALS indicates life-threatening; <u>underlines</u> indicate most frequent.

## CONTRAINDICATIONS AND PRECAUTIONS

**Contraindicated in:** ▪ Hypersensitivity to aspirin, tartrazine (FDC yellow dye #5), or other salicylates ▪ Cross-sensitivity with other NSAIDs may exist (less with nonaspirin salicylates) ▪ Bleeding disorders or thrombocytopenia (more important with aspirin) ▪ Children or adolescents with viral infections (may increase the risk of Reye's syndrome).

**Use Cautiously in:** ▪ History of GI bleeding or ulcer disease ▪ Chronic alcohol use/abuse ▪ Severe renal disease (magnesium toxicity may occur with magnesium salicylate) ▪ Severe hepatic disease ▪ Geriatric patients (increased risk of adverse reactions; more sensitive to toxic levels) ▪ Pregnancy; salicylates may have adverse effects on fetus and mother and in general should be avoided during pregnancy, especially during the 3rd trimester ▪ Lactation (safety not established).

## ADVERSE REACTIONS AND SIDE EFFECTS*

▪ **EENT:** hearing loss, tinnitus ▪ **GI:** GI BLEEDING, dyspepsia, epigastric distress, heartburn, nausea, abdominal pain, anorexia, hepatotoxicity, vomiting ▪ **Hemat:** *aspirin*—anemia, hemolysis, increased bleeding time ▪ **Misc:** allergic reactions including ANAPHYLAXIS and LARYNGEAL EDEMA, noncardiogenic pulmonary edema.

## INTERACTIONS

**Drug-Drug:** ▪ **Aspirin:** May ↑ the risk of bleeding with **warfarin, heparin, heparin-like agents, thrombolytic agents, ticlopidine, clopidogrel, tirofiban,** or **eptifibatide,** although these agents are frequently used safely in combination and in sequence ▪ **Ibuprofen:** may negate the cardioprotective antiplatelet effects of low-dose aspirin ▪ **Aspirin:** May ↑ risk of bleeding with **cefoperazone, cefotetan, valproic acid,** or **plicamycin** ▪ **All salicylates:** May ↑ activity of **penicillins, phenytoin, methotrexate, valproic acid, oral hypoglycemic agents,** and **sulfonamides** ▪ May ↓ beneficial effects of **probenecid** or **sulfinpyrazone** ▪ **Corticosteroids** may ↓ serum salicylate levels ▪ **Urinary acidification** ↑ reabsorption and may ↑ serum salicylate levels ▪ **Alkalinization of the urine** or the ingestion of large amounts of **antacids** ↑ excretion and ↓ serum salicylate levels ▪ May blunt the therapeutic response to **diuret-**ics, antihypertensives, or some **NSAIDs** ▪ ↑ risk of GI irritation with **NSAIDs** ▪ ↑ risk of ototoxicity with **vancomycin.**

**Drug-Natural Products:** ▪ Aspirin: ↑ anticoagulant effect and bleeding risk with **anise, arnica, chamomile, clove, fenugreek, feverfew, garlic, ginger, ginkgo, Panax ginseng, licorice,** and others.

**Drug-Food:** ▪ **Foods capable of acidifying the urine** (see Appendix Q) may ↑ serum salicylate levels.

## ROUTE AND DOSAGE

### ❑ Aspirin for Pain/Fever

▪ **PO, Rect (Adults):** 325–500 mg q 3 hr or 325–650 mg q 4 hr or 650–1000 mg q 6 hr (not to exceed 4 g/day). *Extended-release tablets*—650 mg q 8 hr or 800 mg q 12 hr.
▪ **PO, Rect (Children 2–11 yr):** 65 mg/kg/day (1.5 g/m²/day) in 4–6 divided doses.

### ❑ Aspirin for Inflammation

▪ **PO (Adults):** 2.4 g/day initially; increased to maintenance dose of 3.6–5.4 g/day in divided doses (up to 7.8 g/day for acute rheumatic fever).
▪ **PO (Children):** 80–100 mg/kg/day in divided doses (up to 130 mg/kg/day for acute rheumatic fever).

### ❑ Aspirin for Prevention of Transient Ischemic Attacks

▪ **PO (Adults):** 1–1.3 g daily in 2–4 divided doses (doses as low as 325 mg/day may be used in patients who are intolerant of the higher dose).

### ❑ Aspirin for Prevention of Myocardial Infarction

▪ **PO (Adults):** 300–325 mg/day (doses as low as 80 mg/day may be effective).

### ❑ Aspirin for Kawasaki Disease

▪ **PO (Children):** 80–120 mg/kg/day in 4 divided doses initially; may be followed by maintenance dose of 3–8 mg/kg/day as a single dose for up to 8 wk.

### ❑ Choline Salicylate

435 mg of choline salicylate is equivalent to 325 mg of aspirin.

▪ **PO (Adults):** *Analgesic/antipyretic*—435–669 mg (¹/₂–³/₄ tsp) q 3 hr or 425–870 mg (¹/₂–1 tsp) q 4 hr or 870–1305 mg (1–1¹/₂ tsp) q 6 hr as needed. *Anti-inflammatory*—4.8–7.2 g/day in divided doses.

- **PO (Children):** *Pain/fever*—2 g/m²/day in 4–6 divided doses. *Inflammation*—107–133 mg/kg/day in 4–6 divided doses (up to 174 mg/kg).
- ❏ **Magnesium Salicylate**
- **PO (Adults):** 303.7 mg q 4 hr or 467 mg q 6 hr.
- ❏ **Choline and Magnesium Salicylates**

5 ml of liquid equivalent to 500 mg salicylate or 650 mg of aspirin. Tablet strength expressed in mg of salicylate: 500-mg tablet equivalent to 650 mg of aspirin, 750-mg tablet equivalent to 975 mg of aspirin, 1000-mg tablet equivalent to 1.3 g of aspirin.

- **PO (Adults):** *Analgesic/antipyretic*—2–3 g of salicylate/day in 2–3 divided doses. *Anti-inflammatory*—3 g/day at bedtime or in 2–3 divided doses.
- **PO (Children >37 kg):** 2.2 g of salicylate/day in 2 divided doses.
- **PO (Children <37 kg):** 50 mg of salicylate/kg/day in 2 divided doses.

❏ **Salsalate**

- **PO (Adults):** 1 g 3 times daily initially; further titration may be required.

❏ **Sodium Salicylate**

- **PO (Adults):** *Pain/fever*—325–650 mg q 4 hr. *Inflammation*—3.6–5.4 g/day in divided doses.
- **PO (Children):** *Pain/fever*—1.5 g/m²/day in 4–6 divided doses. *Inflammation*—80–100 mg/kg/day in 4–6 divided doses.

## AVAILABILITY

❏ **Aspirin**

- **Tablets:** 81 mgᴼᵀᶜ, 162.5 mgᴼᵀᶜ, 325 mgᴼᵀᶜ, 500 mgᴼᵀᶜ, 650 mgᴼᵀᶜ, {975 mgᴼᵀᶜ} ■ **Chewable tablets:** {80 mgᴼᵀᶜ}, 81 mgᴼᵀᶜ ■ **Chewing gum:** 227 mgᴼᵀᶜ ■ **Dispersible tablets:** 325 mgᴼᵀᶜ, 500 mgᴼᵀᶜ ■ **Enteric-coated (delayed-release) tablets:** 80 mgᴼᵀᶜ, 165 mgᴼᵀᶜ, {300 mgᴼᵀᶜ}, 325 mgᴼᵀᶜ, 500 mgᴼᵀᶜ, {600 mgᴼᵀᶜ}, 650 mgᴼᵀᶜ, 975 mgᴼᵀᶜ ■ **Extended-release tablets:** {325 mgᴼᵀᶜ}, 650 mgᴼᵀᶜ, 800 mgᴿˣ ■ **Delayed-release capsules:** {325 mgᴼᵀᶜ}, {500 mgᴼᵀᶜ} ■ **Suppositories:** 60 mgᴼᵀᶜ, 120 mgᴼᵀᶜ, 125 mgᴼᵀᶜ, 130 mgᴼᵀᶜ, {150 mgᴼᵀᶜ}, {160 mgᴼᵀᶜ}, 195 mgᴼᵀᶜ, 200 mgᴼᵀᶜ, 300 mgᴼᵀᶜ, {320 mgᴼᵀᶜ}, 325 mgᴼᵀᶜ, 600 mgᴼᵀᶜ, {640 mgᴼᵀᶜ}, 650 mgᴼᵀᶜ, 1.2 gᴼᵀᶜ ■ antihistamines, decongestants, cough suppressantsᴼᵀᶜ, and opioidsᴿˣ. See Appendix B.

❏ **Choline Salicylate**

- **Oral solution:** 870 mg/5 mlᴼᵀᶜ.

❏ **Magnesium Salicylate**

- **Tablets:** 325 mgᴼᵀᶜ, 500 mgᴼᵀᶜ, 545 mgᴿˣ, 600 mgᴿˣ.

❏ **Choline and Magnesium Salicylates (listed as salicylate content)**

- **Tablets:** 500 mgᴿˣ, 750 mgᴿˣ, 1000 mgᴿˣ ■ **Liquid:** 500 mg/5 mlᴿˣ.

❏ **Salsalate**

- **Tablets:** 500 mgᴿˣ, 750 mgᴿˣ ■ Cost: *Disalcid*—500 mg $22.90/20, 750 mg $41.87/30; *generic*—500 mg $32.74/100, 750 mg $41.04/100 ■ **Capsules:** 500 mgᴿˣ.

❏ **Sodium Salicylate**

- **Tablets:** 325 mgᴼᵀᶜ, 650 mgᴼᵀᶜ ■ **Delayed-release tablets:** 324 mgᴼᵀᶜ, 325 mgᴼᵀᶜ, 650 mgᴼᵀᶜ.

TIME/ACTION PROFILE (analgesia/fever reduction†)

| | ONSET | PEAK | DURATION |
|---|---|---|---|
| Aspirin–PO | 5–30 min | 1–3 hr | 3–6 hr |
| Aspirin–PO-ER | 5–30 min | 2–4 hr | 8–12 hr |
| Aspirin–Rect | 1–2 hr | 4–5 hr | 7 hr |
| All other salicylates–PO | 5–30 min | 1–3 hr | 3–6 hr |

†Antirheumatic effect may take 2–3 wk of chronic dosing.

## NURSING IMPLICATIONS
### ASSESSMENT

- **General Info:** Patients who have asthma, allergies, and nasal polyps or who are allergic to tartrazine are at an increased risk for developing hypersensitivity reactions.
- **Pain:** Assess pain and limitation of movement; note type, location, and intensity before and at the peak (see Time/Action Profile) after administration.
- **Fever:** Assess fever and note associated signs (diaphoresis, tachycardia, malaise, chills).

{ } = Available in Canada only.
*CAPITALS indicates life-threatening; underlines indicate most frequent.

■ *Lab Test Considerations:* Monitor hepatic function before antirheumatic therapy and if symptoms of hepatotoxicity occur; more likely in patients, especially children, with rheumatic fever, systemic lupus erythematosus, juvenile arthritis, or pre-existing hepatic disease. May cause ↑ serum AST, ALT, and alkaline phosphatase, especially when plasma concentrations exceed 25 mg/100 ml. May return to normal despite continued use or dose reduction. If severe abnormalities or active liver disease occurs, discontinue and use with caution in future.

❑ Monitor serum salicylate levels periodically with prolonged high-dose therapy to determine dose, safety, and efficacy, especially in children with Kawasaki disease.

❑ May alter results of serum uric acid, urine vanillylmandelic acid (VMA), protirelin-induced thyroid-stimulating hormone (TSH), urine hydroxyindoleacetic acid (5-HIAA) determinations, and radionuclide thyroid imaging.

❑ May cause ↓ serum potassium and cholesterol concentrations.

❑ *Aspirin:* In addition to the above lab tests, aspirin prolongs bleeding time for 4–7 days and, in large doses, may cause prolonged prothrombin time. Monitor hematocrit periodically in prolonged high-dose therapy to assess for GI blood loss.

■ *Toxicity and Overdose:* Monitor patient for the onset of tinnitus, headache, hyperventilation, agitation, mental confusion, lethargy, diarrhea, and sweating. If these symptoms appear, withhold medication and notify physician or other health care professional immediately.

## POTENTIAL NURSING DIAGNOSES

■ Pain, acute (Indications).
■ Mobility, impaired physical (Indications).

## IMPLEMENTATION

■ **PO:** Administer after meals or with food or an antacid to minimize gastric irritation. Food slows but does not alter the total amount absorbed.

❑ Do not crush or chew enteric-coated tablets. Do not take antacids within 1–2 hr of enteric-coated tablets. Chewable tablets may be chewed, dissolved in liquid, or swallowed whole. Some extended-release tablets may be broken or crumbled but must not be ground

up before swallowing. See manufacturer's prescribing information for individual products.

## PATIENT/FAMILY TEACHING

■ **General Info:** Instruct patient to take salicylates with a full glass of water and to remain in an upright position for 15–30 min after administration.

❑ Advise patient to report tinnitus; unusual bleeding of gums; bruising; black, tarry stools; or fever lasting longer than 3 days.

❑ Caution patient to avoid concurrent use of alcohol with this medication to minimize possible gastric irritation; 3 or more glasses of alcohol per day may increase the risk of GI bleeding. Caution patient to avoid taking concurrently with acetaminophen or NSAIDs for more than a few days, unless directed by health care professional to prevent analgesic nephropathy.

❑ Teach patients on a sodium-restricted diet to avoid effervescent tablets or buffered-aspirin preparations.

❑ Tablets with an acetic (vinegar-like) odor should be discarded.

❑ Advise patients on long-term therapy to inform health care professional of medication regimen before surgery. Aspirin may need to be withheld for 1 wk before surgery.

❑ Centers for Disease Control and Prevention warns against giving aspirin to children or adolescents with varicella (chickenpox) or influenza-like or viral illnesses because of a possible association with Reye's syndrome.

■ **Transient Ischemic Attacks or MI:** Advise patients receiving aspirin prophylactically to take only prescribed dosage. Increasing the dosage has not been found to provide additional benefits.

## EVALUATION

**Effectiveness of therapy can be demonstrated by:** ■ Relief of mild to moderate discomfort ■ Increased ease of joint movement. May take 2–3 wk for maximum effectiveness ■ Reduction of fever ■ Prevention of transient ischemic attacks ■ Prevention of MI.

## salmeterol

(sal-**me**-te-role)
Serevent

## INDICATIONS

■ Long-term control of reversible airway obstruction due to asthma and for maintenance treatment of asthma and prevention of bronchospasm ■ Prevention of exercise-induced asthma ■ Maintenance treatment to prevent bronchospasm in COPD including chronic bronchitis and emphysema.

## ACTION

■ Produces accumulation of cyclic adenosine monophosphate (cAMP) at beta$_2$-adrenergic receptors ■ Relatively specific for beta (pulmonary) receptors. **Therapeutic Effects:** ■ Bronchodilation.

## PHARMACOKINETICS

**Absorption:** Minimal systemic absorption follows inhalation.

**Distribution:** Action is primarily local.

**Metabolism and Excretion:** Unknown.

**Half-life:** 5.5 hr.

## CONTRAINDICATIONS AND PRECAUTIONS

**Contraindicated in:** ■ Hypersensitivity ■ Acute attack of asthma (onset of action is delayed).

**Use Cautiously in:** ■ Cardiovascular disease (including angina and hypertension) ■ Diabetes ■ Glaucoma ■ Hyperthyroidism ■ Pheochromocytoma ■ Excessive use (may lead to tolerance and paradoxical bronchospasm) ■ Pregnancy, lactation, or children <4 yr (dry powder inhalation may be used in children 4–12 yr; aerosol inhalation may be used in children >12 yr; may inhibit contractions during labor).

## ADVERSE REACTIONS AND SIDE EFFECTS*

■ **CNS:** <u>headache</u>, nervousness ■ **CV:** palpitations, tachycardia ■ **GI:** abdominal pain, diarrhea, nausea ■ **MS:** muscle cramps/soreness ■ **Neuro:** trembling.

## INTERACTIONS

**Drug-Drug:** ■ Beta blockers may ↓ therapeutic effects of salmeterol.

**Drug-Natural Products:** ■ Use with caffeine-containing herbs (**cola nut, guarana, mate, tea, coffee**) ↑ stimulant effect.

## ROUTE AND DOSAGE

■ **Inhaln (Adults and Children ≥12 yr):** 50 mcg (one inhalation as dry powder) twice daily (approximately 12 hr apart); *exercise-induced bronchospasm*—50 mcg (one inhalation as dry powder) 30–60 min before exercise.

■ **Inhaln (Children 4–12 yr):** 50 mcg (as dry powder) twice daily (approximately 12 hr apart); *exercise-induced bronchospasm*—50 mcg (as dry powder) 30–60 min before exercise.

## AVAILABILITY

■ *Powder for inhalation:* 50 mcg/blister$^{Rx}$ ■ Cost: inhaler with 28 blisters $49.60, inhaler with 60 blisters $80.02. ■ fluticasone (Advair Diskus, see Appendix B).

TIME/ACTION PROFILE (bronchodilation)

| | ONSET | PEAK | DURATION |
|---|---|---|---|
| Inhalation | 10–25 min | 3–4 hr | 12 hr† |

†9 hr in adolescents.

# NURSING IMPLICATIONS

## ASSESSMENT

❑ Assess lung sounds, pulse, and blood pressure before administration and periodically during therapy.

❑ Monitor pulmonary function tests before initiating therapy and periodically during course to determine effectiveness.

❑ Observe for paradoxical bronchospasm (wheezing, dyspnea, tightness in chest) and hypersensitivity reaction (rash; urticaria; swelling of the face, lips, or eyelids). Frequently occurs with first use of new canister or vial. If condition occurs, withhold medication and notify physician or other health care professional immediately.

■ **Lab Test Considerations:** May cause ↑ serum glucose concentrations; occurs rarely with recommended doses and is more pronounced with frequent use of high doses.

❑ May cause ↓ serum potassium concentrations, which are usually transient and dose related; rarely occurs at recommended doses and is more pronounced with frequent use of high doses.

■ **Toxicity and Overdose:** Symptoms of overdose include persistent agitation, chest pain or discomfort, decreased blood pressure, dizziness, hyperglycemia, hypokalemia, seizures, tachyarrhythmias, persistent trembling, and vomiting.

❑ Treatment includes discontinuing salmeterol and other beta-adrenergic agonists and providing symptomatic, supportive therapy. Cardioselective beta blockers are used cautiously because they may induce bronchospasm.

## POTENTIAL NURSING DIAGNOSES

■ Airway clearance, ineffective (Indications).

## IMPLEMENTATION

■ **General:** Do not confuse salmeterol with Salbutamol (albuterol).

■ **Inhaln:** Once removed from foil overwrap, discard discus when every blister has been used or 6 wk have passed, whichever comes first.

❑ Do not use a spacer with powder for inhalation.

## PATIENT/FAMILY TEACHING

❑ Instruct patient on proper technique for use of powder for inhalation and advise patient to take salmeterol as directed. Do not use more than the prescribed dose. If a regularly scheduled dose is missed, use as soon as possible and resume regular schedule. Do not double doses. If symptoms occur before next dose is due, use a rapid-acting inhaled bronchodilator.

❑ Instruct patient using *powder for inhalation* never to exhale into discus device and always to hold device in a level horizontal position. Mouthpiece should be kept dry; never wash.

❑ Caution patient not to use salmeterol to treat acute symptoms. A rapid-acting inhaled beta-adrenergic bronchodilator should be used for relief of acute asthma attacks.

❑ Advise patients on chronic therapy not to use additional salmeterol to prevent exercise-induced bronchospasm. Patients using salmeterol for prevention of exercise-induced bronchospasm should not use additional doses of salmeterol for 12 hr after prophylactic administration.

❑ Advise patient to notify health care professional immediately if difficulty in breathing persists after use of salmeterol, if condition worsens, if more inhalations of rapid-acting bronchodilator than usual are needed to relieve an acute attack, or if using 4 or more inhalations of a rapid-acting bronchodilator for 2 or more consecutive days or more than 1 canister in an 8-wk period.

❑ Salmeterol is often used with inhaled corticosteroids and is not a substitute for corticosteroids or adrenergic bronchodilators. Advise patients using inhalation or systemic corticosteroids to consult health care professional before stopping or reducing therapy.

❑ Emphasize the importance of regular follow-up exams to determine progress during therapy.

## EVALUATION

**Effectiveness of therapy can be demonstrated by:** ■ Prevention of bronchospasm or reduction of frequency of acute asthma attacks in patients with chronic asthma ■ Prevention of exercise-induced asthma.

# saquinavir

(sa-**kwin**-a-vir)

Fortovase, Invirase

## CLASSIFICATION(S):

**Therapeutic:** antiretrovirals
**Pharmacologic:** protease inhibitors

### Pregnancy Category B

## INDICATIONS

■ HIV infection (with other antiretrovirals).

## ACTION

■ Inhibits the action of HIV protease and prevents the cleavage of viral polyproteins. **Therapeutic Effects:** ■ Slowing of the progression of HIV infection and its sequelae ■ Increased CD4 cell counts and decreased viral load.

## PHARMACOKINETICS

**Absorption:** Incompletely absorbed after oral administration; rapidly undergoes extensive first-pass hepatic metabolism. Absorption of Invirase and Fortovase is not the same; products are not interchangeable.
**Distribution:** Distributes into tissues, but CNS penetration is poor.
**Protein Binding:** 98%.
**Metabolism and Excretion:** Mostly metabolized by the liver. <1% excreted unchanged in urine.
**Half-life:** 13 hr.

## CONTRAINDICATIONS AND PRECAUTIONS

**Contraindicated in:** ■ Hypersensitivity ■ Concurrent dihydroergotamine (or other ergot derivatives), midazolam, rifabutin, rifampin, lovastatin, simvastatin, and triazolam ■ Lactation.
**Use Cautiously in:** ■ Diabetes mellitus (may exacerbate hyperglycemia; hyperglycemia may progress to ketoacidosis) ■ Hemophilia (increased risk of bleeding) ■ Hepatic impairment (may exacerbate liver dysfunction caused by hepatitis B or C or other causes) ■ Pregnancy or children <16 yr (safety not established).

## ADVERSE REACTIONS AND SIDE EFFECTS*

■ **CNS:** SEIZURES, confusion, headache, mental depression, psychic disorders, weakness ■ **CV:** thrombophlebitis ■ **GI:** abdominal discomfort, diarrhea, increased liver enzymes, jaundice, nausea ■ **Derm:** photosensitivity, severe cutaneous reactions ■ **Endo:** hyperglycemia ■ **Hemat:** acute myeloblastic leukemia, hemolytic anemia, thrombocytopenia ■ **Neuro:** ataxia ■ **Misc:** STEVENS-JOHNSON SYNDROME.

## INTERACTIONS

**Drug-Drug:** ■ **Rifampin** and **rifabutin** significantly ↓ saquinavir levels; concurrent use is contraindicated ■ **Dihydroergotamine** and **ergotamine** ( ↑ risk of vasoconstriction); **midazolam** and **triazolam** ( ↑ CNS depression); **lovastatin** and **simvastatin** ( ↑ risk of myopathy); concurrent use is contraindicated ■ Coadministration with **clarithromycin** significantly ↑ saquinavir levels and ↓ clarithromycin levels ■ Saquinavir levels are also signifi-

cantly ↑ by **indinavir, delavirdine, nelfinavir, ritonavir,** and **ketoconazole** (dosage adjustments may be necessary) ■ **Carbamazepine, phenobarbital, phenytoin, nevirapine,** and **dexamethasone** may ↓ saquinavir levels.
**Drug-Natural Products:** ■ **St. John's wort** ↓ levels and effectiveness; may promote development of drug resistance.
**Drug-Food:** ■ **Grapefruit juice** ↑ serum levels and effects ■ **Food** significantly increases ↑ the absorption of saquinavir. **Garlic** can significantly ↓ levels.

## ROUTE AND DOSAGE

❑ **Invirase**
■ **PO (Adults):** 600 mg 3 times daily within 2 hr of a meal.

❑ **Fortovase**
■ **PO (Adults):** 1200 mg 3 times daily within 2 hr of a meal.

## AVAILABILITY

❑ **Invirase**
■ *Capsules:* 200 mg^Rx.

❑ **Fortovase**
■ *Soft gelatin capsules:* 200 mg^Rx.

TIME/ACTION PROFILE (blood levels)

| | ONSET | PEAK | DURATION |
|---|---|---|---|
| PO | unknown | unknown | 8 hr |

## NURSING IMPLICATIONS

### ASSESSMENT

❑ Assess patient for change in severity of symptoms of HIV and for symptoms of opportunistic infections during therapy.
■ *Lab Test Considerations:* Monitor viral load and CD4 count regularly during therapy.
❑ May cause hyperglycemia, which may result in diabetic ketoacidosis.
❑ Monitor hematologic and hepatic function before and periodically during therapy. May cause anemia, thrombocytopenia, and ↑ liver enzymes.

## POTENTIAL NURSING DIAGNOSES

■ Infection, risk for (Indications, Side Effects).

## IMPLEMENTATION

■ **PO:** Administer within 2 hr after a full meal to increase effectiveness. Taking without food causes decreased blood concentrations and may result in no antiviral activity.

❑ Capsules are stable until expiration date if refrigerated or for 3 mo when brought to room temperature.

## PATIENT/FAMILY TEACHING

❑ Instruct patient to take saquinavir as directed at the same time each day, within 2 hr after a full meal. Take missed doses as soon as possible if not almost time for next dose; do not double doses. Do not discontinue without consulting health care professional. Changes from Invirase to Fortovase should be made under supervision of health care professional.

❑ Instruct patient that saquinavir should not be shared with others.

❑ Inform patient that saquinavir does not cure HIV or prevent associated or opportunistic infections. Saquinavir does not reduce the risk of transmission of HIV to others through sexual contact or blood contamination. Caution patient to use a condom during sexual contact and to avoid sharing needles or donating blood to prevent spreading HIV to others. Advise patient that the long-term effects of saquinavir are unknown at this time.

❑ Advise patient not to take other medications, prescription or OTC, or herbal products concurrently without consulting health care professional.

❑ Inform patient that saquinavir may cause hyperglycemia. Advise patient to notify health care professional if increased thirst or hunger; unexplained weight loss; increased urination; fatigue; or dry, itchy skin occurs. Rare but serious bullous skin eruptions with polyarthritis may also occur.

❑ Inform patient that long-term effects of saquinavir are unknown at this time.

❑ Emphasize the importance of regular follow-up exams and blood tests to determine progress and monitor for side effects.

## EVALUATION

**Effectiveness of therapy can be demonstrated by:** ■ Slowing of the progression of HIV infection and its sequelae ■ Decrease in viral load and improvement in CD4 cell counts.

# sargramostim

(sar-**gram**-oh-stim)
Leukine, rHu GM-CSF (recombinant human granulocyte/macrophage colony-stimulating factor)

## CLASSIFICATION(S):

**Therapeutic:** colony-stimulating factors
**Pharmacologic:** biologic response modifiers

### Pregnancy Category C

## INDICATIONS

■ Acceleration of bone marrow recovery after: ❑ Autologous bone marrow transplantation in patients with non-Hodgkin's lymphoma, acute lymphoblastic leukemia, or Hodgkin's disease ❑ Allogenic bone marrow transplantation from HLA-matched donors ■ Management of bone marrow transplant failure or engraftment delay ■ After induction chemotherapy for acute myelogenous leukemia (AML) in patients ≥55 yr ■ Mobilization and after transplant of autologous peripheral blood progenitor cells (PBPCs); increases harvest by leukapheresis.

## ACTION

■ Consists of a glycoprotein produced by recombinant DNA technique that is capable of binding to and stimulating the production, division, differentiation, and activation of granulocytes and macrophages. **Therapeutic Effects:** ■ Accelerated recovery of bone marrow after autologous bone marrow transplantation, resulting in decreased risk of infection and other complications.

## PHARMACOKINETICS

**Absorption:** After IV administration, absorption is essentially complete. Well absorbed after subcut administration.

**Distribution:** Unknown.

**Metabolism and Excretion:** Unknown.

**Half-life:** Unknown.

## CONTRAINDICATIONS AND PRECAUTIONS

**Contraindicated in:** ■ Presence of ≥10% leukemic myeloid blast cells in bone marrow or peripheral blood ■ Hypersensitivity to granulocyte macrophage colony-stimulating factor (GM-CSF), yeast products, or additives (mannitol, tromethamine, or sucrose) ■ Products containing benzyl alcohol should not be used in newborns.

**Use Cautiously in:** ■ Pre-existing fluid retention, CHF, or pulmonary infiltrates ■ Pre-existing cardiac disease ■ Myeloid malignancies ■ Previous extensive radiation or chemotherapy (response may be limited) ■ Pregnancy (use only if clearly needed) ■ Lactation or children (safety not established).

## ADVERSE REACTIONS AND SIDE EFFECTS*

■ **CNS:** headache, malaise, weakness ■ **Resp:** dyspnea ■ **CV:** pericardial effusion, peripheral edema, transient supraventricular tachycardia ■ **GI:** diarrhea ■ **Derm:** itching, rash ■ **MS:** arthralgia, bone pain, myalgia ■ **Misc:** chills, fever, first-dose reaction.

## INTERACTIONS

**Drug-Drug:** ■ **Lithium** or **corticosteroids** may potentiate myeloproliferative effects of sargramostim (concurrent use should be undertaken cautiously).

## ROUTE AND DOSAGE

❏ **After Bone Marrow Transplantation**

■ **IV (Adults):** 250 mcg/m²/day for 21 days.

❏ **Failure/Delay of Engraftment after Bone Marrow Transplantation**

■ **IV (Adults):** 250 mcg/m²/day for 14 days; may be repeated after a 7-day rest between courses; if results are inadequate, a 3rd course at 500 mcg/m²/day for 14 days may be given after a 7-day rest.

❏ **After Chemotherapy for AML**

■ **IV (Adults):** 250 mcg/m²/day started around day 11 or 4 days after induction if day 10 bone marrow is hypoplastic with <5% blast cells and continued until absolute neutrophil count (ANC) >1500 cells/mm³ for 3 consecutive days (not to exceed 42 days); if adverse reactions occur, decrease dose by 50% or temporarily discontinue.

❏ **Mobilization of PBPCs**

■ **IV, Subcut (Adults):** 250 mcg/m²/day continued throughout collection of PBPCs.

❏ **After PBPC Transplantation**

■ **IV, Subcut (Adults):** 250 mcg/m²/day continued until ANC >1500 cells/mm³ for 3 consecutive days.

## AVAILABILITY

■ *Powder for injection:* 250 mcg/vial^Rx, 500 mcg/vial^Rx.

TIME/ACTION PROFILE (noted as effects on blood counts)

| | ONSET | PEAK | DURATION |
|---|---|---|---|
| Subcut, IV | rapid | unknown | 3–7 days |

# NURSING IMPLICATIONS

## ASSESSMENT

❏ Monitor heart rate, blood pressure, and respiratory status during and immediately after infusion. If dyspnea develops, slow infusion rate by half. Reassess; medication may need to be discontinued. Assess for peripheral edema daily throughout therapy. Capillary leak syndrome (swelling of feet or lower legs, sudden weight gain, dyspnea) and pleural or pericardial effusion may occur, usually at doses >32 mcg/kg/day.

❏ Monitor for first-dose reaction (flushing, hypotension, syncope, weakness). Does not recur with first dose of each course but may occur with first dose of more than 1 course.

❏ Assess patient for fever daily during therapy. Usually mild and dose related and resolves with discontinuation or administration of antipyretics.

❏ Assess patient for arthralgias and myalgias, usually in lower extremities, which tend to occur when granulocyte counts are returning to normal. May also cause mild to moderate bone pain, possibly from bone marrow expansion. Usually occurs over a 1–3-day period before myeloid recovery and occurs in the sternum, spine, pelvis, and long bones. Treat with analgesics.

---

{ } = Available in Canada only.
*CAPITALS indicates life-threatening; underlines indicate most frequent.

■ *Lab Test Considerations:* Obtain a CBC with differential and platelet count before chemotherapy and twice weekly during therapy to avoid leukocytosis. Monitor ANC; may increase rapidly. If ANC >20,000/mm³ or 10,000/mm³ after the nadir has occurred or if platelet count >500,000/mm³, interrupt administration and reduce dose by half or discontinue. Excessive blood levels usually return to baseline 3–7 days after discontinuation of therapy. If blast cells appear, sargramostim should be discontinued.

❏ Monitor renal and hepatic function before and biweekly throughout therapy in patients with renal or hepatic dysfunction. May cause increased BUN, creatinine, and hepatic enzymes.

❏ May cause decreased serum albumin concentrations.

**POTENTIAL NURSING DIAGNOSES**

■ Infection, risk for (Indications).

**IMPLEMENTATION**

■ **General:** Do not confuse Leukine (sargramostim) with leukeran (chlorambucil) or leucovorin.

❏ Administer 2–4 hr after bone marrow transplant and no earlier than 24 hr after cytotoxic chemotherapy or 12 hr after last dose of radiotherapy.

❏ Refrigerate but do not freeze powder, reconstituted solution, or diluted solution. Reconstitute with 1 ml of sterile water without preservatives injected toward side of vial. Swirl gently to avoid foaming. Do not shake. Solution should be clear and colorless. Discard if left at room temperature for >6 hr. Vial is for 1-time use only.

■ **Intermittent Infusion:**

■ **Subcut:** Administer reconstituted solution without further dilution.

❏ Dilute in 0.9% NaCl. If final concentration is <10 mcg/ml, add a final concentration of 0.1% human albumin to 0.9% NaCl before addition of sargramostim to prevent absorption of the components of the drug delivery system. Do not administer with an in-line filter.

■ *Rate:* Usually infused over 2–4 hr. Has been administered over 30–60 min, over 5–12 hr, and as a continuous infusion over 24 hr.

❏ *After bone marrow transplantation or failure of engraftment:* Administer over 2 hr.

❏ *Chemotherapy for AML:* Administer over 4 hr.

❏ *Mobilization of PBPCs or PBPC transplant:* Administer as a continuous infusion over 24 hr.

■ **Y-Site Compatibility:** ◆ amikacin ◆ aminophylline ◆ aztreonam ◆ bleomycin ◆ butorphanol ◆ calcium gluconate ◆ carboplatin ◆ carmustine ◆ cefazolin ◆ cefepime ◆ cefotaxime ◆ cefotetan ◆ ceftizoxime ◆ ceftriaxone ◆ cefuroxime ◆ cimetidine ◆ cisplatin ◆ clindamycin ◆ cyclophosphamide ◆ cyclosporine ◆ cytarabine ◆ dacarbazine ◆ dactinomycin ◆ dexamethasone sodium phosphate ◆ diphenhydramine ◆ dopamine ◆ doxorubicin ◆ doxycycline ◆ droperidol ◆ etoposide ◆ famotidine ◆ fentanyl ◆ floxuridine ◆ fluconazole ◆ fluorouracil ◆ furosemide ◆ gentamicin ◆ heparin ◆ idarubicin ◆ ifosfamide ◆ immune globulin ◆ magnesium sulfate ◆ mannitol ◆ mechlorethamine ◆ meperidine ◆ mesna ◆ methotrexate ◆ metoclopramide ◆ metronidazole ◆ mezlocillin ◆ miconazole ◆ minocycline ◆ mitoxantrone ◆ netilmicin ◆ pentostatin ◆ piperacillin/tazobactam ◆ potassium chloride ◆ prochlorperazine ◆ promethazine ◆ ranitidine ◆ teniposide ◆ ticarcillin ◆ ticarcillin/clavulanate ◆ trimethoprim/sulfamethoxazole ◆ vinblastine ◆ vincristine ◆ zidovudine.

■ **Y-Site Incompatibility:** ◆ acyclovir ◆ ampicillin ◆ ampicillin/sulbactam ◆ cefonicid ◆ cefoperazone ◆ chlorpromazine ◆ ganciclovir ◆ haloperidol ◆ hydrocortisone ◆ hydromorphone ◆ imipenem/cilastatin ◆ lorazepam ◆ methylprednisolone sodium succinate ◆ mitomycin ◆ morphine ◆ nalbuphine ◆ ondansetron ◆ piperacillin ◆ sodium bicarbonate ◆ tobramycin.

■ **Additive Incompatibility:** Do not admix with other medications.

**PATIENT/FAMILY TEACHING**

❏ Instruct patient to notify nurse or physician if dyspnea or palpitations occur.

**EVALUATION**

**Effectiveness of therapy can be demonstrated by:** ■ Acceleration of bone marrow recovery and decreased incidence of infection in patients after autologous and allogenic bone marrow transplantation, bone marrow transplant failure or engraftment delay, chemotherapy for AML, and PBPC transplantation.

# scopolamine

(scoe-**pol**-a-meen)

Isopto Hyoscine, Transderm-Scp, {Transderm-V}

## CLASSIFICATION(S):

**Therapeutic:** antiemetics

**Pharmacologic:** anticholinergics

## Pregnancy Category C

## INDICATIONS

■ **Transdermal:** Prevention of motion sickness ■ Management of nausea and vomiting associated with opioid analgesia or general anesthesia ■ **IM, IV, Subcut:** Preoperatively to produce amnesia and to decrease salivation and excessive respiratory secretions.

## ACTION

■ Inhibits the muscarinic activity of acetylcholine ■ Corrects the imbalance of acetylcholine and norepinephrine in the CNS, which may be responsible for motion sickness. **Therapeutic Effects:** ■ Reduction of nausea and vomiting ■ Preoperative amnesia and decreased secretions.

## PHARMACOKINETICS

**Absorption:** Well absorbed following IM, subcut, and transdermal administration.

**Distribution:** Crosses the placenta and blood-brain barrier.

**Metabolism and Excretion:** Mostly metabolized by the liver.

**Half-life:** 8 hr.

## CONTRAINDICATIONS AND PRECAUTIONS

**Contraindicated in:** ■ Hypersensitivity ■ Hypersensitivity to bromides (injection only) ■ Narrow-angle glaucoma ■ Acute hemorrhage ■ Tachycardia secondary to cardiac insufficiency or thyrotoxicosis.

**Use Cautiously in:** ■ Geriatric patients, infants, and children (increased risk of adverse reactions) ■ Possible intestinal obstruction ■ Prostatic hypertrophy ■ Chronic renal, hepatic, pulmonary, or cardiac disease ■ Pregnancy or lactation (safety not established).

## ADVERSE REACTIONS AND SIDE EFFECTS*

■ **CNS:** drowsiness, confusion ■ **EENT:** blurred vision, mydriasis, photophobia ■ **CV:** tachycardia, palpitations ■ **GI:** dry mouth, constipation ■ **GU:** urinary hesitancy, urinary retention ■ **Derm:** decreased sweating.

## INTERACTIONS

**Drug-Drug:** ■ Additive anticholinergic effects with **antihistamines, antidepressants, quinidine,** or **disopyramide** ■ Additive CNS depression with **alcohol, antidepressants, antihistamines, opioid analgesics,** or **sedative/hypnotics** ■ May alter the absorption of other **orally administered drugs** by slowing motility of the GI tract ■ May increase GI mucosal lesions in patients taking oral **wax-matrix potassium chloride preparations.**

**Drug-Natural Products:** ■ Increased anticholinergic effects with **angel's trumpet, jimson weed,** and **scopolia.**

## ROUTE AND DOSAGE

■ **Transdermal (Adults):** 1.5 mg Transderm-Scp system delivers 1 mg over 72 hr; for motion sickness, apply 4 hr prior to travel (US product).

■ **IM, IV, Subcut (Adults):** *Antiemetic/anticholinergic* 0.3–0.6 mg; *antisecretory effect*—0.2–0.6 mg; *amnestic effect*—0.32–0.65 mg; *sedation*—0.6 mg 3–4 times daily.

■ **IM, IV, Subcut (Children):** *Antiemetic/anticholinergic*—6 mcg/kg or 0.2 mg/m$^2$.

■ **IM (Children 8–12 yr):** *Antisecretory*—0.3 mg.

■ **IM (Children 3–8 yr):** *Antisecretory*—0.2 mg.

■ **IM (Children 7 mo–3 yr):** *Antisecretory*—0.15 mg.

■ **IM (Children 4–7 mo):** *Antisecretory*—0.1 mg.

## AVAILABILITY (generic available)

■ *Transdermal therapeutic system:* Transderm-Scop—1.5 mg scopolamine/patch releases 0.5 mg scopolaine over 3 days in packs of 4 units[Rx], {Transderm-V—1.5 mg scopolamine/patch releases 1 mg scopolamine over 3 days[Rx]} ■ Cost: *Transderm-Scop*—$18.48/4 ■

*Injection:* 0.3 mg/ml in 1-ml vials$^{Rx}$, 0.4 mg/ml in 0.5-ml ampules and 1-ml vials$^{Rx}$, 0.86 mg/ml in 0.5-ml ampules$^{Rx}$, 1 mg/ml in 1-ml vials$^{Rx}$.

TIME/ACTION PROFILE (antiemetic, sedative properties)

|  | ONSET | PEAK | DURATION |
|---|---|---|---|
| PO, IM, subcut | 30 min | 1 hr | 4–6 hr |
| IV | 10 min | 1 hr | 2–4 hr |
| Transdermal | 4 hr | unknown | 72 hr |

## NURSING IMPLICATIONS

### ASSESSMENT

- **General Info:** Assess patient for signs of urinary retention periodically throughout therapy.
- Monitor heart rate periodically throughout parenteral therapy.
- Assess patient for pain prior to administration. Scopolamine may act as a stimulant in the presence of pain, producing delirium if used without morphine or meperidine.
- **Antiemetic:** Assess patient for nausea and vomiting periodically during therapy.

### POTENTIAL NURSING DIAGNOSES

- Oral mucous membrane, impaired (Indications, Side Effects).
- Injury, risk for (Side Effects).

### IMPLEMENTATION

- **Direct IV:** Scopolamine should be diluted with sterile water for injection prior to IV administration. Inject slowly.
- **Syringe Compatibility:** ◆ benzquinamide ◆ butorphanol ◆ chlorpromazine ◆ cimetidine ◆ diphenhydramine ◆ droperidol ◆ fentanyl ◆ hydromorphone ◆ meperidine ◆ metoclopramide ◆ midazolam ◆ morphine ◆ nalbuphine ◆ pentazocine ◆ pentobarbital ◆ perphenazine ◆ prochlorperazine ◆ promethazine ◆ ranitidine ◆ sufentanil ◆ thiopental.
- **Y-Site Compatibility:** ◆ heparin ◆ hydrocortisone sodium succinate ◆ potassium chloride ◆ sufentanil ◆ vitamin B complex with C.

### PATIENT/FAMILY TEACHING

- **General Info:** Instruct patient to take medication exactly as directed. If a dose is missed, take as soon as remembered. Do not double doses.
- Medication may cause drowsiness or blurred vision. Caution patient to avoid driving or other activities requiring alertness until response to medication is known.
- Patient should use caution when exercising and in hot weather; overheating may result in heatstroke.
- Advise patient to avoid concurrent use of alcohol and other CNS depressants with this medication.
- Inform patient that frequent mouth rinses, good oral hygiene, and sugarless gum or candy may minimize dry mouth.
- **Transdermal:** Instruct patient on application of transdermal patches. Apply at least 4 hr (US product) before exposure to travel to prevent motion sickness. Wash hands and dry thoroughly before and after application. Apply to hairless, clean, dry area behind ear; avoid areas with cuts or irritation. Apply pressure over system to ensure contact with skin. System is effective for 3 days. If system becomes dislodged, replace with a new system on another site behind the ear. System is waterproof and not affected by bathing or showering.
- Instruct patient to remove patch and notify health care professional immediately if symptoms of acute narrow-angle glaucoma (pain or reddening of the eyes with pupil dilation) occur.
- Caution patients engaging in underwater sports of potentially distorting effects of scopolamine.

### EVALUATION

**Effectiveness of therapy can be demonstrated by:** ■ Decrease in salivation and respiratory secretion preoperatively ■ Postoperative amnesia ■ Prevention of motion sickness ■ Prevention and treatment of opioid- or anesthesia-induced nausea and vomiting.

## selegiline

(se-**le**-ji-leen)

Apo-Selegiline, Carbex, Eldepryl, Gen-Selegiline, Nu-Selegiline, {Novo-Selegiline}, SD-Deprenyl

## INDICATIONS

■ Management of Parkinson's disease (with levodopa or levodopa/carbidopa) in patients who fail to respond to levodopa/carbidopa alone.

## ACTION

■ Following conversion by MAO to its active form, selegiline inactivates MAO by irreversibly binding to it at type B (brain) sites ■ Inactivation of MAO leads to increased amounts of dopamine available in the CNS. **Therapeutic Effects:** ■ Increased response to levodopa/dopamine therapy in Parkinson's disease.

## PHARMACOKINETICS

**Absorption:** Appears to be well absorbed following oral administration.

**Distribution:** Widely distributed.

**Metabolism and Excretion:** Metabolism involves some conversion to amphetamine and methamphetamine. 45% excreted in urine as metabolites.

**Half-life:** Unknown.

## CONTRAINDICATIONS AND PRECAUTIONS

**Contraindicated in:** ■ Hypersensitivity ■ Concurrent meperidine or opioid analgesic therapy (possible fatal reactions) ■ Concurrent use of SSRIs or tricyclic antidepressants.

**Use Cautiously in:** ■ Doses >10 mg/day (increased risk of hypertensive reactions with tyramine-containing foods and some medications) ■ History of peptic ulcer disease.

## ADVERSE REACTIONS AND SIDE EFFECTS*

■ **CNS:** confusion, dizziness, fainting, hallucinations, insomnia, vivid dreams ■ **GI:** <u>nausea</u>, abdominal pain, dry mouth.

## INTERACTIONS

**Drug-Drug:** ■ Concurrent use with **meperidine** or other **opioid analgesics** may possibly result in a potentially fatal reaction (excitation, sweating, rigidity, and hypertension; or hypotension and coma) ■ Serotonin syndrome (confusion, agitation, hyperpyrexia, hypertension, seizures) may occur with concurrent use of **nefazodone** or **SSRI antidepressants** (fluoxetine should be discontinued 5 wk prior to selegiline, venlafaxine should be discontinued 7 days before selegiline; other agents should be discontinued 2 wk before selegiline). Selegiline should be discontinued 2 wk before SSRIs are initiated ■ Concurrent use with **tricyclic antidepressants** may result in asystole, diaphoresis, hypertension, syncope, behavioral changes, altered consciousness, hyperpyrexia, tremors, muscle rigidity, and seizures (avoid concurrent use; discontinue selegiline 2 wk before initiating tricyclic antidepressant therapy) ■ May initially ↑ risk of side effects of **levodopa/carbidopa** (dosage of levodopa/carbidopa may need to be ↓ by 10–30%).

**Drug-Food:** ■ Doses >10 mg/day may produce hypertensive reactions with **tyramine-containing foods** (see Appendix Q).

## ROUTE AND DOSAGE

■ **PO (Adults):** 5 mg bid, with breakfast and lunch (some patients may require further dividing of doses—2.5 mg 4 times daily).

## AVAILABILITY (generic available)

■ *Capsules:* 5 mg$^{Rx}$ ■ *Tablets:* 5 mg$^{Rx}$.

TIME/ACTION PROFILE (onset of beneficial effects in Parkinson's disease)

|    | ONSET | PEAK | DURATION |
|----|-------|------|----------|
| PO | 2–3 days | unknown | unknown |

## NURSING IMPLICATIONS

### ASSESSMENT

❑ Assess patient for signs and symptoms of Parkinson's disease (tremor, muscle weakness and rigidity, ataxic gait) prior to and during therapy.
❑ Assess blood pressure periodically during therapy.

## POTENTIAL NURSING DIAGNOSES

- Mobility, impaired physical (Indications).
- Injury, risk for (Indications, Side Effects).

## IMPLEMENTATION

- **General:** Do not confuse selegiline with sertraline.
- An attempt to reduce the dose of levodopa/carbidopa by 10–30% may be made after 2–3 days of selegiline therapy.
- **PO:** Administer 5-mg tablet with breakfast and lunch.

## PATIENT/FAMILY TEACHING

- Instruct patient to take medication as directed. Take missed doses as soon as possible, but not if late afternoon or evening or almost time for next dose. Do not double doses. Caution patient that taking more than the prescribed dose may increase side effects and place patient at risk for hypertensive crisis if foods containing tyramine are consumed (see Appendix Q).
- Advise patients taking selegiline ≥20 mg/day to avoid large amounts of tyramine-containing foods (see Appendix Q), alcoholic beverages, large quantities of caffeine-containing beverages, or OTC or herbal cough or cold medications.
- Inform patient and family of the signs and symptoms of MAO inhibitor–induced hypertensive crisis (severe headache, chest pain, nausea, vomiting, photosensitivity, enlarged pupils). Advise patient to notify health care professional immediately if severe headache or any other unusual symptom occurs.
- Caution patient to change positions slowly to minimize orthostatic hypotension.
- Advise patient that increasing fluids, sugarless gum or candy, ice, or saliva substitutes may help minimize dry mouth. Consult health care professional if dry mouth continues for >2 wk.

## EVALUATION

**Effectiveness of therapy can be demonstrated by:** ■ Improved response to levodopa/carbidopa in patients with Parkinson's disease.

## sennosides
(**sen**-oh-sides)

Black-Draught, Ex-Lax, Ex-Lax Chocolated, Fletchers' Castoria, Maximum Relief Ex-Lax, Sena-Gen, Senexon, Senokot, SenokotXTRA

*CLASSIFICATION(S):*
*Therapeutic: laxatives*
*Pharmacologic: stimulant laxatives*

**Pregnancy Category C**

## INDICATIONS

- Treatment of constipation, particularly when associated with: □ Slow transit time □ Constipating drugs □ Irritable or spastic bowel syndrome □ Neurologic constipation.

## ACTION

- Active components of senna (sennosides) alter water and electrolyte transport in the large intestine, resulting in accumulation of water and increased peristalsis. **Therapeutic Effects:** ■ Laxative action.

## PHARMACOKINETICS

**Absorption:** Minimally absorbed following oral administration.

**Distribution:** Unknown.

**Metabolism and Excretion:** Unknown.

**Half-life:** Unknown.

## CONTRAINDICATIONS AND PRECAUTIONS

**Contraindicated in:** ■ Hypersensitivity ■ Abdominal pain of unknown cause, especially if associated with fever ■ Rectal fissures ■ Ulcerated hemorrhoids ■ Known alcohol intolerance (some liquid products).

**Use Cautiously in:** ■ Chronic use (may lead to laxative dependence) ■ Possible intestinal obstruction ■ Pregnancy or lactation (safety not established; may be used safely during breastfeeding).

## ADVERSE REACTIONS AND SIDE EFFECTS*

■ **GI:** <u>cramping</u>, <u>diarrhea</u>, nausea ■ **GU:** pink-red or brown-black discoloration of urine ■ **F and E:** electrolyte abnormalities (chronic use or dependence) ■ **Misc:** laxative dependence.

## INTERACTIONS

**Drug-Drug:** ■ May decrease absorption of other **orally administered drugs** because of decreased transit time.

## ROUTE AND DOSAGE

Larger doses have been used to treat/prevent opioid-induced constipation. Consult labeling of individual OTC products for more speceific dosing information.

■ **PO (Adults and Children >12 yr):** 12–50 mg 1–2 times daily.
■ **PO (Children 6–12 yr):** 6–25 mg 1–2 times daily.
■ **PO (Children 2–6 yr):** 3–12.5 mg 1–2 times daily.

## AVAILABILITY (generic available)

Noted as sennoside content.

■ *Tablets:* 6 mg$^{OTC}$, 8.6 mg$^{OTC}$, 15 mg$^{OTC}$, 17 mg$^{OTC}$, 25 mg$^{OTC}$ ■ *Granules:* 15 mg/5 ml$^{OTC}$, 20 mg/5 ml$^{OTC}$ ■ *Syrup:* 8.8 mg/5 ml$^{OTC}$ ■ *Liquid:* 25 mg/15 ml$^{OTC}$, 33.3 mg/ml senna concentrate$^{OTC}$ ■ psyllium and docusate$^{OTC}$. See Appendix B.

TIME/ACTION PROFILE (laxative effect)

| | ONSET | PEAK | DURATION |
|---|---|---|---|
| PO | 6–12 hr† | unknown | 3–4 days |

†May take as long as 24 hr.

# NURSING IMPLICATIONS

## ASSESSMENT

❑ Assess patient for abdominal distention, presence of bowel sounds, and usual pattern of bowel function.
❑ Assess color, consistency, and amount of stool produced.

## POTENTIAL NURSING DIAGNOSES

■ Constipation (Indications).
■ Diarrhea (Side Effects).

## IMPLEMENTATION

■ **PO:** Take with a full glass of water. Administer at bedtime for evacuation 6–12 hr later. Administer on an empty stomach for more rapid results.

❑ Shake oral solution well before administering.
❑ Granules should be dissolved or mixed in water or other liquid before administration.

## PATIENT/FAMILY TEACHING

❑ Advise patient that laxatives should be used only for short-term therapy. Long-term therapy may cause electrolyte imbalance and dependence.
❑ Encourage patient to use other forms of bowel regulation, such as increasing bulk in the diet, increasing fluid intake, and increasing mobility. Normal bowel habits are individualized and may vary from 3 times/day to 3 times/wk.
❑ Inform patient that this medication may cause a change in urine color to pink, red, violet, yellow, or brown.
❑ Instruct patients with cardiac disease to avoid straining during bowel movements (Valsalva maneuver).
❑ Advise patient not to use laxatives when abdominal pain, nausea, vomiting, or fever is present.

## EVALUATION

**Effectiveness of therapy can be demonstrated by:** ■ A soft, formed bowel movement

# sertraline

(**ser**-tra-leen)
Zoloft

**CLASSIFICATION(S):**
*Therapeutic: antidepressants*
*Pharmacologic: selective serotonin reuptake inhibitors (SSRIs)*

**Pregnancy Category B**

## INDICATIONS

■ Management of the following (in conjunction with psychotherapy): ❑ Depression ❑ Panic disorder ❑ OCD ❑ Post-traumatic stress disorder (PTSD) ❑ Social anxiety disorder ❑ Premenstrual dysphoric disorder.

## ACTION

■ Inhibits neuronal uptake of serotonin in the CNS, thus potentiating the activity of serotonin. Has little effect on norepinephrine or dopamine. **Therapeutic Effects:** ■ Antidepressant action ■ Decreased incidence of panic attacks ■ Decreased obsessive and compulsive behavior ■ Decreased feelings of intense fear, helplessness, or horror ■ Decreased social anxiety ■ Decrease in premenstrual dysphoria.

## PHARMACOKINETICS

**Absorption:** Appears to be well absorbed after oral administration.
**Distribution:** Extensively distributed throughout body tissues.
**Protein Binding:** 98%.
**Metabolism and Excretion:** Extensively metabolized by the liver; one metabolite has some antidepressant activity; 14% excreted unchanged in feces.
**Half-life:** 24 hr.

## CONTRAINDICATIONS AND PRECAUTIONS

**Contraindicated in:** ■ Hypersensitivity ■ Concurrent MAO inhibitor therapy (may result in serious, potentially fatal reactions) ■ Concurrent pimozide ■ Oral concentrate contains alcohol and should be avoided in patients with known intolerance.
**Use Cautiously in:** ■ Severe hepatic or renal impairment ■ Patients with a history of mania ■ Patients at risk of suicide ■ Pregnancy or lactation ■ Children (increased incidence of adverse CNS reactions).

## ADVERSE REACTIONS AND SIDE EFFECTS*

■ **CNS:** <u>dizziness</u>, <u>drowsiness</u>, <u>fatigue</u>, <u>headache</u>, <u>insomnia</u>, agitation, anxiety, confusion, emotional lability, impaired concentration, manic reaction, nervousness, weakness, yawning ■ **EENT:** pharyngitis, rhinitis, tinnitus, visual abnormalities ■ **CV:** chest pain, palpitations ■ **GI:** <u>diarrhea</u>, <u>dry mouth</u>, <u>nausea</u>, abdominal pain, altered taste, anorexia, constipation, dyspepsia, flatulence, increased appetite, vomiting ■ **GU:** <u>sexual dysfunction</u>, menstrual disorders, urinary disorders, urinary frequency ■ **Derm:** <u>increased sweating</u>, hot flashes, rash ■ **MS:** back pain, myalgia ■ **Neuro:** <u>tremor</u>, hypertonia, hypoesthesia, paresthesia, twitching ■ **Misc:** fever, thirst.

## INTERACTIONS

**Drug-Drug:** ■ Serious, potentially fatal reactions (hyperthermia, rigidity, myoclonus, autonomic instability, with fluctuating vital signs and extreme agitation, which may proceed to delirium and coma) may occur with concurrent **MAO inhibitors.** MAO inhibitors should be stopped at least 14 days before sertraline therapy. Sertraline should be stopped at least 14 days before MAO inhibitor therapy ■ May ↑ **pimozide** levels and the risk of potentially life-threatening cardiovascular reactions ■ May ↑ sensitivity to **adrenergics** and ↑ the risk of serotonin syndrome ■ Concurrent use with **alcohol** is not recommended ■ May ↑ levels/effects of **warfarin, phenytoin, tricyclic antidepressants,** some **benzodiazepines (alprazolam), clozapine,** or **tolbutamide** ■ **Cimetidine** ↑ blood levels and effects.
**Drug-Natural Products:** ■ ↑ risk of serotonergic side effects including serotonin syndrome with **St. John's wort** and **SAMe.**

## ROUTE AND DOSAGE

❑ **Depression/OCD**
■ **PO (Adults):** 50 mg/day as a single dose in the morning or evening initially; after several weeks may be increased at weekly intervals up to 200 mg/day, depending on response.
■ **PO (Children 13–17 yr):** *OCD*—50 mg once daily.
■ **PO (Children 6–12 yr):** *OCD*—25 mg once daily.

❑ **Panic Disorder**
■ **PO (Adults):** 25 mg/day initially, may increase after 1 wk to 50 mg/day.

❑ **PTSD**
■ **PO (Adults):** 25 mg once daily for 7 days, then increase to 50 mg once daily; may then be increased if needed at intervals of at least 7 days (range 50–200 mg once daily).

❑ **Social Anxiety Disorder**
■ **PO (Adults):** 25 mg once daily initially, then 50 mg once daily; may be increased at weekly intervals up to 200 mg/day.

❑ **Premenstrual Dysphoric Disorder**
■ **PO (Adults):** 50 mg/day initially either daily or daily during luteal phase of cycle. Daily dosing may be titrated upward in 50 mg increments at the beginning of a cycle. In luteal phase-only dosing a 50 mg/day titra-

tion step for three days at the beginning of each luteal phase dosing period should be used (range 50–150 mg/day).

## AVAILABILITY

■ *Tablets:* 25 mg$^{Rx}$, 50 mg$^{Rx}$, 100 mg$^{Rx}$ ■ Cost: *Zoloft*—25 mg $126.04/50, 50 mg $252.08/100, 100 mg $252.08/100 ■ *Capsules:* {50 mg$^{Rx}$}, {100 mg$^{Rx}$} ■ *Oral concentrate (12% alcohol):* 20 mg/ml$^{Rx}$.

TIME/ACTION PROFILE (antidepressant effect)

|    | ONSET | PEAK | DURATION |
|----|-------|------|----------|
| PO | within 2–4 wk | unknown | unknown |

# NURSING IMPLICATIONS

## ASSESSMENT

■ **General Info:** Monitor appetite and nutritional intake. Weigh weekly. Notify physician or other health care professional of continued weight loss. Adjust diet as tolerated to support nutritional status.

■ **Depression:** Monitor mood changes. Inform physician or other health care professional if patient demonstrates significant increase in anxiety, nervousness, or insomnia.

❏ Assess for suicidal tendencies, especially during early therapy. Restrict amount of drug available to patient.

■ **OCD:** Assess patient for frequency of obsessive-compulsive behaviors. Note degree to which these thoughts and behaviors interfere with daily functioning.

■ **Panic Attacks:** Assess frequency and severity of panic attacks.

■ **PTSD:** Assess patient for feelings of fear, helplessness, and horror. Determine effect on social and occupational functioning.

■ **Social Anxiety Disorder:** Assess patient for symptoms of social anxiety disorder (blushing, sweating, trembling, tachycardia during interactions with new people, people in authority, or groups) periodically during therapy.

■ **Premenstrual Dysphoric Disorder:** Assess patient for symptoms of premenstrual dysphoric disorder (feeling angry, tense, or tired; crying easily, feeling sad or hopeless; arguing with family or friends for no reason; difficulty sleeping or paying attention; feeling out of control or unable to cope; having cramping, bloating, food craving, or breast tenderness) periodically during therapy.

## POTENTIAL NURSING DIAGNOSES

■ Coping, ineffective (Indications).

■ Injury, risk for (Side Effects).

## IMPLEMENTATION

■ **General:** Do not confuse sertraline with selegiline.

❏ Periodically reassess dose and continued need for therapy.

■ **PO:** Administer as a single dose in the morning or evening.

## PATIENT/FAMILY TEACHING

❏ Instruct patient to take sertraline as directed. Take missed doses as soon as possible and return to regular dosing schedule. Do not double doses.

❏ May cause drowsiness or dizziness. Caution patient to avoid driving and other activities requiring alertness until response to the drug is known.

❏ Advise patient to avoid alcohol or other CNS depressant drugs during therapy and to consult with health care professional before taking other medications with sertraline.

❏ Inform patient that frequent mouth rinses, good oral hygiene, and sugarless gum or candy may minimize dry mouth. If dry mouth persists for more than 2 wk, consult health care professional regarding use of saliva substitute.

❏ Advise patient to wear sunscreen and protective clothing to prevent photosensitivity reactions.

❏ Instruct female patient to inform health care professional if pregnancy is planned or suspected or if she is breastfeeding.

❏ Advise patient to notify health care professional if headache, weakness, nausea, anorexia, anxiety, or insomnia persists.

❏ Emphasize the importance of follow-up exams to monitor progress. Encourage patient participation in psychotherapy.

## EVALUATION

**Effectiveness of therapy can be demonstrated by:** ■ Increased sense of well-being ❑ Renewed interest in surroundings. May require 1–4 wk of therapy to obtain antidepressant effects ■ Decrease in obsessive-compulsive behaviors ■ Decrease in frequency and severity of panic attacks ■ Decrease in symptoms of PTSD ■ Decrease in social anxiety disorder ■ Decrease in symptoms of premenstrual dysphoric disorder.

---

## sevelamer

(se-**vel**-a-mer)

Renagel

**CLASSIFICATION(S):**
**Therapeutic:** electrolyte modifiers
**Pharmacologic:** phosphate binders

**Pregnancy Category C**

---

## INDICATIONS

■ Reduction of serum phosphate levels in patients with hyperphosphatemia associated with end-stage renal disease.

## ACTION

■ A polymer that binds phosphate in the GI tract, preventing its absorption. **Therapeutic Effects:** ■ Decreased serum phosphate levels and reduction in the consequences of hyperphosphatemia (ectopic calcification, secondary hyperparathyroidism with osteitis fibrosa).

## PHARMACOKINETICS

**Absorption:** Not absorbed; action is local (in GI tract).
**Distribution:** Unknown.
**Metabolism and Excretion:** Eliminated in feces.
**Half-life:** Unknown.

## CONTRAINDICATIONS AND PRECAUTIONS

**Contraindicated in:** ■ Hypersensitivity ■ Hypophosphatemia ■ Bowel obstruction.
**Use Cautiously in:** ■ Dysphagia, swallowing disorders, severe GI motility disorders, or major GI tract surgery ■ Pregnancy, lactation, or children (safety not established).

## ADVERSE REACTIONS AND SIDE EFFECTS*

■ **GI:** diarrhea, dyspepsia, vomiting, constipation, flatulence, nausea.

## INTERACTIONS

**Drug-Drug:** ■ Concurrent **anticonvulsants** or **antiarrhythmics** (sevelamer may affect absorption; administer 1 hr before or 3 hr after) ■ May decrease absorption of other drugs and decrease effectiveness, especially **drugs whose efficacy is dependent on tightly controlled blood levels.**

## ROUTE AND DOSAGE

■ **PO (Adults):** 800–1600 mg with each meal.

## AVAILABILITY

■ *Capsules:* 403 mg (anhydrous)[Rx] ■ *Tablets:* 400 mg[Rx], 800 mg[Rx].

TIME/ACTION PROFILE (decrease in serum phosphate levels)

|  | ONSET | PEAK | DURATION |
|----|----|----|----|
| PO | 5 days | 2 wks | unknown |

# NURSING IMPLICATIONS

## ASSESSMENT

❑ Assess patient for GI side effects periodically throughout therapy.
■ *Lab Test Considerations:* Monitor serum phosphorous, calcium, bicarbonate, and chloride levels periodically throughout therapy.

## POTENTIAL NURSING DIAGNOSES

■ Knowledge, deficient, related to medication regimen (Patient/Family Teaching).

## IMPLEMENTATION

■ **General:** Doses of concurrent medications, especially antiarrhythmics, should be spaced at least 1 hr before or 3 hr after sevelamer.
■ **PO:** Administer with meals. Do not chew or take capsules apart; contents expand in water.

## PATIENT/FAMILY TEACHING

❑ Instruct patient to take sevelamer with meals as directed and to adhere to prescribed diet. Do not open or chew capsules.

❏ Caution patient to space concurrent medications at least 1 hr before or 3 hr after sevelamer.

❏ Advise patient to notify health care professional if GI effects are severe or prolonged.

### EVALUATION

**Effectiveness of therapy can be demonstrated by:** ■ Decrease in serum phosphorous concentration to ≤6 mg/dl. Dosage adjustment is based on serum phosphorous concentrations.

---

### sildenafil

(sil-**den**-a-fil)

Viagra

**CLASSIFICATION(S):**

**Therapeutic:** anti-impotence agents
**Pharmacologic:** phosphodiesterase type 5 inhibitors

**Pregnancy Category B**

---

### INDICATIONS

■ Treatment of erectile dysfunction.

### ACTION

■ Enhances the effects of nitric oxide released during sexual stimulation. Nitric oxide activates the enzyme guanylate cyclase, which produces increased levels of cyclic guanosine monophosphate (cGMP). cGMP produces smooth muscle relaxation of the corpus cavernosum, which promotes increased blood flow and subsequent erection. Sildenafil inhibits the enzyme phosphodiesterase type 5 (PDE5), PDE5 inactivates cGMP. **Therapeutic Effects:** ■ Enhanced blood flow to the corpus cavernosum and erection sufficient to allow sexual intercourse ■ Requires sexual stimulation.

### PHARMACOKINETICS

**Absorption:** Rapidly absorbed (40%) after oral administration.

**Distribution:** Widely distributed to tissues; negligible amount in semen.

**Protein Binding:** 96%.

**Metabolism and Excretion:** Mostly metabolized by the liver (by P450 3A4 enzyme system); one metabolite is active and accounts for 20% of drug effect. Metabolites excreted mostly (80%) in feces; 13% excreted in urine.

**Half-life:** 4 hr (for sildenafil and active metabolite).

### CONTRAINDICATIONS AND PRECAUTIONS

**Contraindicated in:** ■ Hypersensitivity ■ Concurrent organic nitrate therapy (nitroglycerin, isosorbide mononitrate, isosorbide dinitrate) ■ Newborns, women, children.

**Use Cautiously in:** ■ Serious underlying cardiovascular disease (including history of MI, stroke, or serious arrhythmia within 6 mo); cardiac failure, or coronary artery disease with unstable angina ■ History of CHF, coronary artery disease, uncontrolled hypertension or hypotension ■ Concurrent treatment with antihypertensives or glipizide ■ Geriatric patients (>65 yr), renal impairment (CCr 30 ml/min, hepatic impairment; all result in increased blood levels and dosage reduction is required) ■ Anatomic penile deformity (angulation, cavernosal fibrosis, Peyronie's disease) ■ Conditions associated with priapism (sickle cell anemia, multiple myeloma, leukemia) ■ Bleeding disorders or active peptic ulceration ■ Resting hypotension (BP <90/50 mmHg) or hypertension (BP >170/110 mmHg) ■ Retinitis pigmentosa ■ Concurrent erythromycin, saquinavir, ketoconazole, or itraconazole (dosage reduction recommended).

### ADVERSE REACTIONS AND SIDE EFFECTS*

■ **CNS:** <u>headache</u>, dizziness ■ **EENT:** abnormal vision (color tinge to vision, increased sensitivity to light, blurred vision), nasal congestion ■ **CV:** MI, SUDDEN DEATH, CARDIOVASCULAR COLLAPSE ■ **GI:** diarrhea, dyspepsia ■ **GU:** priapism, urinary tract infection ■ **Derm:** <u>flushing</u>, rash.

### INTERACTIONS

**Drug-Drug:** ■ Increases the risk of hypotension with **nitrates** in any form; concurrent use is contraindicated because of the risk of serious and potentially fatal hypotension ■ Blood levels and effects may be increased by **enzyme in-**

---

hibitors including **cimetidine, erythromycin, ketoconazole, nelfinavir, indinavir, ritonavir, saquinavir, itraconazole** (initial dose should be decreased to 25 mg) ▪ Increased risk of hypotension with **antihypertensives** ▪ Use cautiously with **glipizide.**

## ROUTE AND DOSAGE

▪ **PO (Adults):** 50 mg taken 1 hr before sexual activity (range 25–100 mg taken 30 min–4 hr before sexual activity); not more than once daily.

▪ **PO (Geriatric Patients ≥65 yr or with concurrent enzyme inhibitors):** 25 mg taken 1 hr before sexual activity (range 25–100 mg taken 30 min–4 hr before sexual activity); not more than once daily.

▫ **Renal/Hepatic Impairment**

▪ **PO (Adults):** 25 mg taken 1 hr before sexual activity (range 25–100 mg taken 30 min–4 hr before sexual activity); not more than once daily.

## AVAILABILITY

▪ *Tablets:* 25 mg$^{Rx}$, 50 mg$^{Rx}$, 100 mg$^{Rx}$ ▪ Cost: 25 mg $272.60/30, 50 mg $272.60/30, 100 mg $272.60/30.

TIME/ACTION PROFILE (ability to produce erection)

| | ONSET | PEAK | DURATION |
|---|---|---|---|
| PO | within 1 hr | unknown | up to 4 hr |

## NURSING IMPLICATIONS

### ASSESSMENT

▫ Determine erectile dysfunction before administration. Sildenafil has no effect in the absence of sexual stimulation.

### POTENTIAL NURSING DIAGNOSES

▪ Sexual dysfunction (Indications).

### IMPLEMENTATION

▪ **PO:** Dose is usually administered 1 hr before sexual activity. May be administered 30 min to 4 hr before sexual activity.

### PATIENT/FAMILY TEACHING

▫ Instruct patient to take sildenafil approximately 1 hr before sexual activity and not more than once per day.

▫ Advise patient that sildenafil is not indicated for use in women.

▫ Caution patient not to take sildenafil concurrently with nitrates.

▫ Instruct patient to notify health care professional promptly if erection lasts longer than 4 hr.

▫ Inform patient that sildenafil offers no protection against sexually transmitted diseases. Counsel patient that protection against sexually transmitted diseases and HIV infection should be considered.

### EVALUATION

**Effectiveness of therapy can be demonstrated by:** ▪ Male erection sufficient to allow intercourse.

## simethicone

(si-**meth**-i-kone)

Degas, Extra Strength Gas-X, {Extra Strength Maalox GRF Gas Relief Formula}, Flatulex, Gas-X, Genasyme, {Maalox GRF Gas Relief Formula}, Maximum Strength Mylanta Gas, Mylanta Gas, Mylicon, {Ovol}, {Ovol-40}, Phazyme

**CLASSIFICATION(S):**
**Therapeutic:** *antiflatulents*

**Pregnancy Category UK**

### INDICATIONS

▪ Relief of painful symptoms of excess gas in the GI tract that may occur postoperatively or as a consequence of: ▫ Air swallowing ▫ Dyspepsia ▫ Peptic ulcer ▫ Diverticulitis.

### ACTION

▪ Causes the coalescence of gas bubbles ▪ Does not prevent the formation of gas. **Therapeutic Effects:** ▪ Passage of gas through the GI tract by belching or passing flatus.

### PHARMACOKINETICS

**Absorption:** No systemic absorption occurs.
**Distribution:** Not systemically distributed.
**Metabolism and Excretion:** Excreted unchanged in the feces.
**Half-life:** Unknown.

## CONTRAINDICATIONS AND PRECAUTIONS

**Contraindicated in:** ▪ Not recommended for infant colic.

**Use Cautiously in:** ▪ Abdominal pain of unknown cause, especially when accompanied by fever ▪ Has been used safely during pregnancy and lactation.

## ADVERSE REACTIONS AND SIDE EFFECTS*

None significant.

## INTERACTIONS

**Drug-Drug:** ▪ None significant.

## ROUTE AND DOSAGE

- ▪ **PO (Adults):** 40–125 mg qid, after meals and at bedtime (up to 500 mg/day).
- ▪ **PO (Children 2–12 yr):** 40 mg 4 times daily.
- ▪ **PO (Children <2 yr):** 20 mg 4 times daily (up to 240 mg/day).

## AVAILABILITY (generic available)

▪ *Chewable tablets:* 40 mg^OTC, 80 mg^OTC, 125 mg^OTC, 150 mg^OTC ▪ Cost: 80 mg $2.99/100, 125 mg $5.02/100 ▪ *Tablets:* 60 mg^OTC, 80 mg^OTC, 95 mg^OTC ▪ *Capsules:* {95 mg^OTC}, 125 mg^OTC ▪ *Drops:* 40 mg/0.6 ml^OTC, {40 mg/1 ml^OTC}, {95 mg/1.425 ml^OTC} ▪ Cost: 40 mg/0.6 ml $91.80/12/30 ml/12 ▪ antacids^OTC. See Appendix B.

TIME/ACTION PROFILE (antiflatulent effect)

|     | ONSET | PEAK | DURATION |
|-----|-------|------|----------|
| PO  | immediate | unknown | 3 hr |

# NURSING IMPLICATIONS

## ASSESSMENT

- ❑ Assess patient for abdominal pain, distention, and bowel sounds prior to and periodically throughout course of therapy. Frequency of belching and passage of flatus should also be assessed.

## POTENTIAL NURSING DIAGNOSES

- ▪ Pain, acute (Indications).

## IMPLEMENTATION

- ▪ **PO:** Administer after meals and at bedtime for best results. Shake liquid preparations well prior to administration. Chewable tablets should be chewed thoroughly before swallowing, for faster and more complete results.
- ❑ Drops can be mixed with 30 ml of cool water, infant formula, or other liquid as directed. Shake well before using.

## PATIENT/FAMILY TEACHING

- ❑ Explain to patient the importance of diet and exercise in the prevention of gas. Also explain that this medication does not prevent the formation of gas.
- ❑ Advise patient to notify health care professional if symptoms are persistent.

## EVALUATION

**Effectiveness of therapy can be demonstrated by:** ▪ Decrease in abdominal distention and discomfort.

## simvastatin, See HMG-CoA REDUCTASE INHIBITORS.

## sirolimus

(sir-**oh**-li-mus)

Rapamune

*CLASSIFICATION(S):*

*Therapeutic: immunosuppressants*

**Pregnancy Category C**

## INDICATIONS

▪ Prevention of organ rejection in allogenic kidney transplantation (concurrently with corticosteroids and cyclosporine) ▪ Sirolimus is also eluted from the Cypher coronary stent used in angioplasty procedures.

## ACTION

▪ Inhibits T-lymphocyte activation/proliferation, which occurs as a response to antigenic and cytokine stimulation; antibody production is also inhibited. **Therapeutic Effects:** ▪ Decreased incidence and severity of organ rejection.

## PHARMACOKINETICS

**Absorption:** Rapidly absorbed following oral administration (14% bioavailability).

**Distribution:** Concentrates in erythrocytes; distributes to heart, intestines, kidneys, liver, lungs, muscle, spleen, and testes in high concentrations.

**Protein Binding:** 92%.

**Metabolism and Excretion:** Extensively metabolized (some metabolism by P450 3A4 system); 91% excreted in feces.

**Half-life:** 62 hr.

## CONTRAINDICATIONS AND PRECAUTIONS

**Contraindicated in:** ■ Hypersensitivity ■ Alcohol intolerance/sensitivity (solution contains ethanol) ■ Concurrent ketoconazole or grapefruit juice ■ Severe hepatic impairment ■ Pregnancy and lactation.

**Use Cautiously in:** ■ Mild to moderate hepatic impairment ■ Women with childbearing potential ■ Children <13 yr (safety not established).

## ADVERSE REACTIONS AND SIDE EFFECTS*

Reflects combined therapy with corticosteroids and cyclosporine. ■ **CNS:** <u>insomnia</u> ■ **Resp:** interstitial lung disease ■ **CV:** edema, hypotension ■ **GI:** hepatic toxicity ■ **GU:** renal impairment ■ **Derm:** <u>acne</u>, <u>rash</u>, thrombocytopenic purpura ■ **F and E:** hypokalemia ■ **Hemat:** <u>leukopenia</u>, <u>thrombocytopenia</u>, anemia ■ **Metab:** <u>hyperlipidemia</u> ■ **MS:** <u>arthralgias</u> ■ **Neuro:** <u>tremor</u> ■ **Misc:** ↑ risk of infection, ↑ risk of lymphoma, ↑ risk of lymphocele, mucosal herpes simplex infections, ↓ wound healing.

## INTERACTIONS

**Drug-Drug:** ■ **Cyclosporine** greatly ↑ blood levels (administer sirolimus 4 hr after cyclosporine) ■ **Ketoconazole** significantly ↑ blood levels (concurrent use is contraindicated ■ Blood levels are also ↑ by **diltiazem** (monitor sirolimus levels and adjust dose as necessary) and may be ↑ by **nicardipine, verapamil, clotrimazole, fluconazole, itraconazole, clarithromycin, erythromycin, troleandomycin, metoclopramide, cimetidine, danazol,** and **protease inhibitor antiretrovirals** ■ **Rifampin** ↑ metabolism and

significantly ↓ blood levels (consider alternative therapy) ■ Blood levels may also be ↓ by **carbamazepine, phenobarbital, phenytoin, rifabutin,** and **rifapentine** ■ Risk of renal impairment may be ↑ by concurrent use of other **nephrotoxic agents** ■ Concurrent use with tacrolimus and corticosteroids in lung transplantation may ↑ risk of anastamotic dehiscence; fatalities have been reported (not approved for this use) ■ Concurrent use with tacrolimus and corticosteroids in liver transplantation may ↑ risk of hepatic artery thrombosis; fatalities have been reported (not approved for this use) ■ May ↓ antibody response to and ↑ risk of adverse reactions to **live-virus vaccines.**

**Drug-Natural Products:** ■ Concomitant use with **echinacea** and **melatonin** may interfere with immunosuppression ■ **St. John's wort** may ↑ blood levels and the risk of toxicity.

**Drug-Food:** ■ **Grapefruit juice** ↓ CYP3A4 metabolism and ↑ levels; do not use as a diluent and avoid concurrent ingestion.

## ROUTE AND DOSAGE

■ **PO (Adults and Children ≥13 yr):** 6-mg loading dose, followed by 2 mg/day maintenance dose. *Dosing following cyclosprine withdrawal*—Patients at low to moderate risk for rejection after transplantation may be withdrawn from cyclosporine over 4–8 wk beginning 2–4 mo after transplant. Thereafter, sirolimus dose should be titrated upward to maintain a whole blood trough level of 12–14 ng/ml. Clinical assessment should also be used to gauge dose. Dose changes can be made at 7–14 day intervals. The following formula may also be used: sirolimus maintenance dose = current dose x (target concentration/current concentration). If a large increase is needed, a loading dose may be given and blood levels reassessed 3–4 days later. Loading dose may be calculated by the following formula: sirolimus loading dose = 3 x (new maintenance dose-current maintenance dose). Loading doses >40 mg should be spread over 2 days.

■ **PO (Adults and Children ≥13 yr and <40 kg):** 3 mg/m$^2$ loading dose, followed by 1 mg/m$^2$/day maintenance dose. *See adjustments above for doses following cyclosporine withdrawal.*

❑ **Hepatic Impairment**

- **PO (Adults and Children ≥13 yr and <40 kg):** Decrease maintenance dose by 33%; loading dose is unchanged.

## AVAILABILITY

- *Tablet:* 1 mg$^{Rx}$, 2 mg$^{Rx}$  ■ *Oral solution:* 1 mg/ml with syringe adapter in 60- and 150-ml bottles and 1-, 2-, and 5-ml unit of use pouches$^{Rx}$.

TIME/ACTION PROFILE (blood levels)

| | ONSET | PEAK | DURATION |
|---|---|---|---|
| PO | rapid | 1–2 hr | 24 hr |

## NURSING IMPLICATIONS

### ASSESSMENT

- Monitor blood pressure closely during therapy. Hypertension is a common complication of sirolimus therapy and should be treated.
- **Lab Test Considerations:** Monitor sirolimus blood levels in patients likely to have altered drug metabolism, patients ≥13 yr who weigh <40 kg, patients with hepatic impairment, and during concurrent administration of drugs that may interact with sirolimus. Trough concentrations of ≥15 ng/ml are associated with an ↑ in adverse effects.
- Monitor patients for hyperlipidemia. May require additional interventions to treat hyperlipidemia.
- May cause anemia, leukopenia, thrombocytopenia, and hypokalemia.

### POTENTIAL NURSING DIAGNOSES

- Infection, risk for (Adverse Reactions).

### IMPLEMENTATION

- **General:** Therapy with sirolimus should be started as soon as possible post-transplant. Concurrent therapy with cyclosporine and corticosteroids is recommended. Sirolimus should be taken 4 hr after cyclosporine (MODIFIED, Neoral).
- Sirolimus should be ordered only by physicians skilled in immunosuppressive therapy, with the staff and facilities to manage renal transplant patients.
- Antimicrobial prophylaxis for *Pneumocystis carinii* pneumonia for 1 year and for cytomegalovirus protection for 3 months post-transplant are recommended.
- **PO:** Administer consistently with or without food. Do not administer with or mix with grapefruit juice.
- To dilute from bottle, use amber oral dose syringe to withdraw prescribed amount. Empty sirolimus from syringe into a glass or plastic container holding at least 2 oz (60 ml) of water or orange juice; do not use other liquids. Stir vigorously and drink at once. Refill container with at least 4 oz of additional liquid, stir vigorously, and drink at once.
- If using the pouch, empty entire contents of pouch into at least 2 oz of water or orange juice; do not use other liquids. Stir vigorously and drink at once. Refill container with at least 4 oz of additional liquid, stir vigorously, and drink at once.
- Store bottles and pouches in refrigerator. Solution may develop a slight haze when refrigerated; allow to stand at room temperature and shake gently until haze disappears. Sirolimus may remain in syringe at room temperature or refrigerated for up to 24 hr. Discard syringe after 1 use.

### PATIENT/FAMILY TEACHING

- Instruct patient to take sirolimus at the same time each day, as directed. Do not skip or double up on missed doses. Do not discontinue medication without advice of health care professional.
- Reinforce the need for lifelong therapy to prevent transplant rejection. Review symptoms of rejection for transplanted organ and stress need to notify health care professional immediately if they occur.
- Emphasize the importance of repeated lab tests during sirolimus therapy.
- Advise patient of the risk of taking sirolimus during pregnancy. Caution women of childbearing years to use effective contraception prior to, during, and for 12 weeks following therapy.

### EVALUATION

**Effectiveness of therapy can be demonstrated by:** ■ Prevention of transplanted kidney rejection.

---

{ } = Available in Canada only.
*CAPITALS indicates life-threatening; underlines indicate most frequent.

# sodium bicarbonate

(**soe**-dee-um bye-**kar**-boe-nate)
Baking Soda, Bell-Ans, Citrocarbonate, Neut, Soda Mint

## CLASSIFICATION(S):
**Therapeutic:** antiulcer agents
**Pharmacologic:** alkalinizing agents

## Pregnancy Category C

## INDICATIONS

■ **PO, IV:** Management of metabolic acidosis ■ **PO, IV:** Used to alkalinize urine and promote excretion of certain drugs in overdosage situations (phenobarbital, aspirin) ■ **PO:** Antacid.

## ACTION

■ Acts as an alkalinizing agent by releasing bicarbonate ions ■ Following oral administration, releases bicarbonate, which is capable of neutralizing gastric acid. **Therapeutic Effects:** ■ Alkalinization ■ Neutralization of gastric acid.

## PHARMACOKINETICS

**Absorption:** Following oral administration, excess bicarbonate is absorbed and results in metabolic alkalosis and alkaline urine.

**Distribution:** Widely distributed into extracellular fluid.

**Metabolism and Excretion:** Sodium and bicarbonate are excreted by the kidneys.

**Half-life:** Unknown.

## CONTRAINDICATIONS AND PRECAUTIONS

**Contraindicated in:** ■ Metabolic or respiratory alkalosis ■ Hypocalcemia ■ Excessive chloride loss ■ As an antidote following ingestion of strong mineral acids ■ Patients on sodium-restricted diets (oral use as an antacid only) ■ Renal failure (oral use as an antacid only) ■ Severe abdominal pain of unknown cause, especially if associated with fever (oral use as an antacid only).

**Use Cautiously in:** ■ CHF ■ Renal insufficiency ■ Concurrent corticosteroid therapy ■ Children with diabetic ketoacidosis (may increase the risk of cerebral edema) ■ Chronic use as an antacid (may cause metabolic alkalosis and possible sodium overload).

## ADVERSE REACTIONS AND SIDE EFFECTS*

■ **CV:** edema ■ **GI:** *PO*—flatulence, gastric distention ■ **F and E:** <u>metabolic alkalosis</u>, hypernatremia, hypocalcemia, hypokalemia, sodium and water retention ■ **Local:** irritation at IV site ■ **Neuro:** tetany.

## INTERACTIONS

**Drug-Drug:** ■ Following oral administration, may decrease the absorption of **ketoconazole** ■ Concurrent use with **calcium-containing antacids** may lead to milk-alkali syndrome ■ Urinary alkalinization may result in decreased **salicylate** or **barbiturate** blood levels; increased blood levels of **quinidine, mexiletine, flecainide,** or **amphetamines**; increased risk of crystalluria from **fluoroquinolones**; decreased effectiveness of **methenamine** ■ May negate the protective effects of **enteric-coated products** (do not administer within 1–2 hr of each other).

## ROUTE AND DOSAGE

Contains 12 mEq of sodium/g.

❏ **Alkalinization of Urine**

■ **PO (Adults):** 48 mEq (4 g) initially. Then 12–24 mEq (1–2 g) q 4 hr (up to 48 mEq q 4 hr) or 1 tsp of powder q 4 hr as needed.

■ **PO (Children):** 1–10 mEq/kg (12–120 mg/kg) per day in divided doses.

■ **IV (Adults and Children):** 2–5 mEq/kg as a 4–8 hr infusion.

❏ **Antacid**

■ **PO (Adults):** *Tablets/powder*—325 mg–2 g 1–4 times daily or ½ tsp q 2 hr as needed. *Effervescent powder*—3.9–10 g in water after meals; patients >60 yr should receive 1.9–3.9 g after meals.

■ **PO (Children 6–12 yr):** 520 mg; may repeat in 30 min.

❏ **Systemic Alkalinization/Cardiac Arrest**

■ **IV (Adults and Children):** *Cardiac arrest/urgent situations*—1 mEq/kg; may repeat 0.5 mEq/kg q 10 min. *Less urgent situations*—2–5 mEq/kg as a 4–8 hr infusion.

## AVAILABILITY (generic available)

■ *Oral powder:* (20.9 mEq Na/½ tsp) in 120-, 240-, 480-, and 2400-g containers<sup>OTC</sup> ■ *Tablets:* 325 mg (3.9 mEq Na/tablet)<sup>OTC</sup>, {500 mg (6.0 mEq Na/tablet<sup>OTC</sup>}, 520 mg (6.2 mEq Na/

tablet)<sup>OTC</sup>, 650 mg (7.7 mEq Na/tablet)<sup>OTC</sup> ■ *Solution for injection:* 4.2% (0.5 mEq/ml) in 2.5-, 5-, and 10-ml prefilled syringes<sup>Rx</sup>, 5% (0.6 mEq/ml) in 500-ml containers<sup>Rx</sup>, 7.5% (0.9 mEq/ml) in 50-ml vials and prefilled syringes and 200-ml vials<sup>Rx</sup>, 8.4% (1 mEq/ml) in 10- and 50-ml vials and prefilled syringes<sup>Rx</sup> ■ *Neutralizing additive solution for injection:* 4% (0.48 mEq/ml) in 5-ml vials<sup>Rx</sup>, 4.2% (0.5 mEq/ml) in 6-ml vials<sup>Rx</sup>.

TIME/ACTION PROFILE (PO = antacid effect; IV = alkalinization)

| | ONSET | PEAK | DURATION |
|---|---|---|---|
| PO | immediate | 30 min | 1–3 hr |
| IV | immediate | rapid | unknown |

# NURSING IMPLICATIONS

## ASSESSMENT

■ **IV:** Assess fluid balance (intake and output, daily weight, edema, lung sounds) throughout therapy. Report symptoms of fluid overload (hypertension, edema, dyspnea, rales/crackles, frothy sputum) if they occur.

❑ Assess patient for signs of acidosis (disorientation, headache, weakness, dyspnea, hyperventilation), alkalosis (confusion, irritability, paresthesia, tetany, altered breathing pattern), hypernatremia (edema, weight gain, hypertension, tachycardia, fever, flushed skin, mental irritability), or hypokalemia (weakness, fatigue, U wave on ECG, arrhythmias, polyuria, polydipsia) throughout therapy.

❑ Observe IV site closely. Avoid extravasation, as tissue irritation or cellulitis may occur. If infiltration occurs, confer with physician or other health care professional regarding warm compresses and infiltration of site with lidocaine or hyaluronidase.

■ **Antacid:** Assess patient for epigastric or abdominal pain and frank or occult blood in the stool, emesis, or gastric aspirate.

■ *Lab Test Considerations:* Monitor serum sodium, potassium, calcium, bicarbonate concentrations, serum osmolarity, acid-base balance, and renal function prior to and periodically throughout therapy.

❑ Arterial blood gases (ABGs) should be obtained frequently in emergency situations and during parenteral therapy.

❑ Monitor urine pH frequently when used for urinary alkalinization.

❑ Antagonizes effects of pentagastrin and histamine during gastric acid secretion test. Avoid administration during the 24 hr preceding the test.

## POTENTIAL NURSING DIAGNOSES

■ Gas exchange, impaired (Indications).
■ Fluid volume, excess (Side Effects).

## IMPLEMENTATION

■ **General:** This medication may cause premature dissolution of enteric-coated tablets in the stomach.

■ **PO:** Tablets must be taken with a full glass of water.

❑ When used in treatment of peptic ulcers, may be administered 1 and 3 hr after meals and at bedtime.

■ **Direct IV:** Administer direct IV push in arrest situation. Use premeasured ampules or prefilled syringes to ensure accurate dosage. Doses should be based on ABG results. Dose may be repeated every 10 min.

■ *Rate:* May be administered by rapid bolus.

❑ Flush IV line before and after administration to prevent incompatible medications used in arrest management from precipitating.

■ **Continuous Infusion:** May be diluted in dextrose, saline, and dextrose/saline combinations.

■ *Rate:* May be administered over 4–8 hr.

■ **Y-Site Compatibility:** ◆ acyclovir ◆ amifostine ◆ asparaginase ◆ aztreonam ◆ cefepime ◆ ceftriaxone ◆ cladribine ◆ cyclophosphamide ◆ cytarabine ◆ daunorubicin ◆ docetaxel ◆ doxorubicin ◆ etoposide ◆ famotidine ◆ filgrastim ◆ fludarabine ◆ gemcitabine ◆ granisetron ◆ heparin ◆ ifosfamide ◆ indomethacin ◆ insulin ◆ melphalan ◆ mesna ◆ methylprednisolone ◆ milrinone ◆ morphine ◆ paclitaxel ◆ piperacillin/tazobactam ◆ potassium chloride ◆ propofol ◆ remifentanil ◆ tacrolimus ◆ teniposide ◆ thiotepa ◆ tolazoline ◆ vancomycin ◆ vitamin B complex with C.

■ **Y-Site Incompatibility:** ✦ alatrofloxacin ✦ allopurinol ✦ amiodarone ✦ amphotericin B cholesteryl sulfate complex ✦ calcium chloride ✦ doxorubicin liposome ✦ gatifloxacin ✦ idarubicin ✦ imipenem/cilastatin ✦ inamrinone ✦ leucovorin calcium ✦ levofloxacin ✦ linezolid ✦ midazolam ✦ nalbuphine ✦ ondansetron ✦ oxacillin ✦ sargramostim ✦ verapamil ✦ vincristine ✦ vinorelbine.

■ **Solution Incompatibility:** Do not add to Ringer's solution, LR, or Ionosol products, as compatibility varies with concentration.

## PATIENT/FAMILY TEACHING

■ **General Info:** Instruct patient to take medication as directed. A missed dose should be taken as soon as remembered unless almost time for next dose.

❑ Review symptoms of electrolyte imbalance with patients on chronic therapy; instruct patient to notify health care professional if these symptoms occur.

❑ Advise patient not to take milk products concurrently with this medication. Renal calculi or hypercalcemia (milk-alkali syndrome) may result.

❑ Emphasize the importance of regular follow-up examinations to monitor serum electrolyte levels and acid-base balance and to monitor progress.

■ **Antacid:** Advise patient to avoid routine use of sodium bicarbonate for indigestion. Dyspepsia that persists >2 wk should be evaluated by a health care professional.

❑ Advise patient on sodium-restricted diet to avoid use of baking soda as a home remedy for indigestion.

❑ Instruct patient to notify health care professional if indigestion is accompanied by chest pain, difficulty breathing, or diaphoresis or if stools become dark and tarry.

## EVALUATION

**Effectiveness of therapy can be demonstrated by:** ■ Increase in urinary pH ■ Clinical improvement of acidosis ■ Enhanced excretion of selected overdoses and poisonings ■ Decreased gastric discomfort.

**High Alert**

## sodium chloride (iv/oral)
(**soe**-dee-um **klor**-ide)

Slo-Salt

### CLASSIFICATION(S):
***Therapeutic:*** *mineral and electrolyte replacements/supplements*

### Pregnancy Category C

## INDICATIONS

■ **IV:** Hydration and provision of NaCl in deficiency states ■ Maintenance of fluid and electrolyte status in situations in which losses may be excessive (excess diuresis or severe salt restriction) ■ 0.45% ("half-normal saline") solution is most commonly used for hydration and the treatment of hyperosmolar diabetes (hypotonic) ■ 0.9% ("normal saline") solution is used for: ❑ Replacement ❑ Treatment of metabolic alkalosis ❑ A priming fluid for hemodialysis ❑ To begin and end blood transfusions ■ Small volumes of 0.9% NaCl (preservative-free or bacteriostatic) are used to reconstitute or dilute other medications ■ Hypertonic solution (3%, 5%) may be required in situations in which rapid replacement of sodium is necessary: ❑ Hyponatremia ❑ Hypochloremia ❑ Renal failure ❑ Heart failure ■ **PO:** Prevention of or management of volume depletion due to salt restriction or heat prostration when excessive sweating occurs during exposures to high temperatures ■ **Irrigating Solutions:** 0.9% and 0.45% may be used as irrigating solutions ■ **Concentrated sodium chloride:** Used as an additive to parenteral fluid therapy in very specific situations.

## ACTION

■ Sodium is a major cation in extracellular fluid and helps maintain water distribution, fluid and electrolyte balance, acid-base equilibrium, and osmotic pressure ■ Chloride is the major anion in extracellular fluid and is involved in maintaining acid-base balance. Solutions of NaCl resemble extracellular fluid ■ Reduces corneal edema by an osmotic effect. **Therapeutic Effects:** ■ **IV, PO:** Replacement in deficiency states and maintenance of homeostasis.

## PHARMACOKINETICS

**Absorption:** Well absorbed following oral administration. Replacement solutions of NaCl are administered IV only.

**Distribution:** Rapidly and widely distributed.

**Metabolism and Excretion:** Excreted primarily by the kidneys.

**Half-life:** Unknown.

## CONTRAINDICATIONS AND PRECAUTIONS

**Contraindicated in:** ■ **IV solution:** ❑ Hypertonic (3%, 5%) solutions should not be used in patients with elevated, slightly decreased, or normal serum sodium ❑ Fluid retention or hypernatremia.

**Use Cautiously in:** ■ **IV:** Patients prone to metabolic, acid-base, or fluid and electrolyte abnormalities, including: ❑ Geriatric patients ❑ Those with nasogastric suctioning ❑ Vomiting ❑ Diarrhea ❑ Diuretic therapy ❑ Glucocorticoid therapy ❑ Fistulas ❑ CHF ❑ Severe renal failure ❑ Severe liver diseases (additional electrolytes may be required) ■ NaCl preserved with benzyl alcohol should not be used in neonates ■ **PO:** Inadequate hydration (water and other electrolytes must be replaced).

## ADVERSE REACTIONS AND SIDE EFFECTS*

Seen primarily during PO and IV use. ■ **CV:** CHF, PULMONARY EDEMA, edema ■ **F and E:** hypernatremia, hypervolemia, hypokalemia ■ **Local:** *IV*— extravasation, irritation at IV site.

## INTERACTIONS

**Drug-Drug:** ■ Excessive amounts of NaCl may partially antagonize the effects of **antihypertensives** ■ Use with **corticosteroids** may result in excess sodium retention.

## ROUTE AND DOSAGE

■ **IV (Adults):** *0.9% NaCl (isotonic)*—1 L (contains 150 mEq sodium/L), rate and amount determined by condition being treated. *0.45% NaCl (hypotonic)*—1–2 L (contains 75 mEq sodium/L), rate and amount determined by condition being treated. *3%, 5% NaCl (hypertonic)*—100 ml over 1 hr (3% contains 50 mEq sodium per 100 ml; 5% contains 83.3 mEq sodium per 100 ml).

■ **PO (Adults):** 1–2 g 3 times daily.

## AVAILABILITY (generic available)

■ *IV solutions:* 0.45%^Rx, 0.9%^Rx, 3%^Rx, 5%^Rx ■ *Diluents:* 0.9%^Rx ■ *Concentrate for dilution:* 14.6%^Rx, 23.4%^Rx ■ *Tablets:* 650 mg^OTC

■ potassium (Slo-Salt-K), dextrose, electrolytes^Rx.

TIME/ACTION PROFILE (various clinical effects†)

| | ONSET | PEAK | DURATION |
|---|---|---|---|
| PO | unknown | unknown | unknown |
| IV | rapid (min) | end of infusion | unknown |

†PO, IV = electrolyte effects.

## NURSING IMPLICATIONS

### ASSESSMENT

❑ Assess fluid balance (intake and output, daily weight, edema, lung sounds) throughout therapy.

❑ Assess patient for symptoms of hyponatremia (headache, tachycardia, lassitude, dry mucous membranes, nausea, vomiting, muscle cramps) or hypernatremia (edema, weight gain, hypertension, tachycardia, fever, flushed skin, mental irritability) throughout therapy. Sodium is measured in relation to its concentration to fluid in the body, and symptoms may change based on patient's hydration status.

■ *Lab Test Considerations:* Monitor serum sodium, potassium, bicarbonate, and chloride concentrations and acid-base balance periodically for patients receiving prolonged therapy with sodium chloride.

❑ Monitor serum osmolarity in patients receiving hypertonic saline solutions.

### POTENTIAL NURSING DIAGNOSES

■ Fluid volume, deficit (Indications).
■ Fluid volume, excess (Side Effects).

### IMPLEMENTATION

❑ *High Alert:* Accidental administration of hypertonic sodium chloride solutions (greater than 0.9%) have resulted in serious electrolyte imbalances. Do not confuse vials of concentrated sodium chloride (23.4%) with vials of sodium chloride flush solution (0.9%).

■ **General:** Dosage of NaCl depends on patient's age, weight, condition, fluid and electrolyte balance, and acid-base balance.

❏ Do not administer bacteriostatic NaCl containing benzyl alcohol as a preservative to neonates. This should not be used to reconstitute or to dilute solutions or to flush intravascular catheters in neonates.

❏ Infusion of 0.45% NaCl is hypotonic, 0.9% NaCl is isotonic, and 3% and 5% NaCl are hypertonic.

■ **Intermittent Infusion:** Administer 3% or 5% NaCl via a large vein and prevent infiltration. After the first 100 ml, sodium, chloride, and bicarbonate concentrations should be re-evaluated to determine the need for further administration.

■ *Rate:* Rate of hypertonic NaCl solutions should not exceed 100 ml/hr.

■ **Solution Compatibility:** ◆ D5W ◆ D10W ◆ Ringer's and lactated Ringer's injection ◆ dextrose/Ringer's solution combinations ◆ dextrose/LR combinations ◆ dextrose/saline combinations ◆ ⅙ M sodium lactate.

## PATIENT/FAMILY TEACHING

❏ Explain to patient the purpose of the infusion.

❏ Advise patients at risk for dehydration due to exposure to extreme temperatures when and how to take NaCL tablets. Inform patients that undigested tablets may be passed in the stool; oral electrolyte solutions are preferable.

## EVALUATION

**Effectiveness of therapy can be demonstrated by:** ■ Prevention or correction of dehydration ■ Normalization of serum sodium and chloride levels ■ Prevention of heat prostration during exposure to high temperatures.

---

# sodium citrate and citric acid

**(soe**-dee-um **sye**-trate and **sit**-rik **as**-id)

Bicitra, Oracit, {PMS-Dicitrate}, Shohl's Solution modified

### CLASSIFICATION(S):

**Therapeutic:** *antiurolithics, mineral and electrolyte replacements/supplements*
**Pharmacologic:** *alkalinizing agents*

**Pregnancy Category C**

## INDICATIONS

■ Management of chronic metabolic acidosis associated with chronic renal insufficiency or renal tubular acidosis ■ Alkalinization of urine ■ Prevention of cystine and urate urinary calculi ■ Prevention of aspiration pneumonitis during surgical procedures ■ Used as a neutralizing buffer.

## ACTION

■ Converted to bicarbonate in the body, resulting in increased blood pH ■ As bicarbonate is renally excreted, urine is also alkalinized, increasing the solubility of cystine and uric acid ■ Neutralizes gastric acid. **Therapeutic Effects:** ■ Provision of bicarbonate in metabolic acidosis ■ Alkalinization of the urine ■ Prevention of cystine and urate urinary calculi ■ Prevention of aspiration pneumonitis.

## PHARMACOKINETICS

**Absorption:** Well absorbed following oral administration.

**Distribution:** Rapidly and widely distributed.

**Metabolism and Excretion:** Rapidly oxidized to bicarbonate, which is excreted primarily by the kidneys. Small amounts (<5%) excreted unchanged by the lungs.

**Half-life:** Unknown.

## CONTRAINDICATIONS AND PRECAUTIONS

**Contraindicated in:** ■ Severe renal insufficiency ■ Severe sodium restriction ■ CHF, untreated hypertension, edema, or toxemia of pregnancy.

**Use Cautiously in:** ■ Pregnancy or lactation (safety not established).

## ADVERSE REACTIONS AND SIDE EFFECTS*

■ **GI:** diarrhea ■ **F and E:** fluid overload, hypernatremia (severe renal impairment), hypocalcemia, metabolic alkalosis (large doses only) ■ **MS:** tetany.

## INTERACTIONS

**Drug-Drug:** ■ May partially antagonize the effects of **antihypertensives** ■ Urinary alkalinization may result in decreased **salicylate** or **barbiturate** blood levels or increased blood levels of **quinidine, flecainide**, or **amphetamines.**

## ROUTE AND DOSAGE

Adjust dosage according to urine pH. Contains 1 mEq sodium and 1 mEq bicarbonate/ml solution.

❑ **Alkalinizer**

■ **PO (Adults):** 10–30 ml solution diluted in water qid.

■ **PO (Children):** 5–15 ml solution diluted in water qid.

❑ **Antiurolithic**

■ **PO (Adults):** 10–30 ml solution diluted in water qid.

❑ **Neutralizing Buffer**

■ **PO (Adults):** 15–30 ml solution diluted in 15–30 ml of water.

## AVAILABILITY

■ *Oral solution:* 500 mg sodium citrate/334 mg citric acid/5 ml (Bicitra, PMS-Dicitrate)[Rx], 490 mg sodium citrate/640 mg citric acid/5 ml (Oracit)[Rx].

TIME/ACTION PROFILE (effects on serum pH)

| | ONSET | PEAK | DURATION |
|---|---|---|---|
| PO | rapid (min–hr) | unknown | 4–6 hr |

## NURSING IMPLICATIONS

### ASSESSMENT

❑ Assess patient for signs of alkalosis (confusion, irritability, paresthesia, tetany, altered breathing pattern) or hypernatremia (edema, weight gain, hypertension, tachycardia, fever, flushed skin, mental irritability) throughout therapy.

❑ Monitor patients with renal dysfunction for fluid overload (discrepancy in intake and output, weight gain, edema, rales/crackles, and hypertension).

■ *Lab Test Considerations:* Prior to and every 4 mo throughout chronic therapy, monitor hematocrit, hemoglobin, electrolytes, pH, creatinine, urinalysis, and 24-hr urine for citrate.

❑ Monitor urine pH if used to alkalinize urine.

## POTENTIAL NURSING DIAGNOSES

■ Knowledge, deficient, related to medication regimen (Patient/Family Teaching).

## IMPLEMENTATION

■ **PO:** Solution is more palatable if chilled. Administer with 30–90 ml of chilled water. Administer 30 min after meals or as bedtime snack to minimize saline laxative effect.

❑ When used as preanesthetic, administer 15–30 ml of sodium citrate with 15–30 ml of chilled water.

## PATIENT/FAMILY TEACHING

❑ Instruct patient to take as directed. Missed doses should be taken within 2 hr. Do not double doses.

❑ Instruct patients receiving chronic sodium citrate on correct method of monitoring urine pH, maintenance of alkaline urine, and the need to increase fluid intake to 3000 ml/day. When treatment is discontinued, pH begins to fall toward pretreatment levels.

❑ Advise patients receiving long-term therapy on need to avoid salty foods.

## EVALUATION

**Effectiveness of therapy can be demonstrated by:** ■ Correction of metabolic acidosis ■ Maintenance of alkaline urine with resulting decreased stone formation ■ Buffering the pH of gastric secretions, thereby preventing aspiration pneumonitis associated with intubation and anesthesia.

# sodium polystyrene sulfonate

(**soe**-dee-um po-lee-**stye**-reen **sul**-fon-ate)

Kayexalate, {K-Exit}, {PMS-Sodium Polystyrene Sulfonate}, SPS

### CLASSIFICATION(S):

*Therapeutic:* hypokalemics, electrolyte modifiers
*Pharmacologic:* cationic exchange resins

**Pregnancy Category C**

## INDICATIONS

■ Mild to moderate hyperkalemia (if severe, more immediate measures such as sodium bicarbonate IV, calcium, or glucose/insulin infusion should be instituted).

## ACTION

■ Exchanges sodium ions for potassium ions in the intestine (each 1 g is exchanged for 0.5–1 mEq potassium). **Therapeutic Effects:** ■ Reduction of serum potassium levels.

## PHARMACOKINETICS

**Absorption:** Distributed throughout the intestine but is nonabsorbable.

**Distribution:** Not distributed.

**Metabolism and Excretion:** Eliminated in the feces.

**Half-life:** Unknown.

## CONTRAINDICATIONS AND PRECAUTIONS

**Contraindicated in:** ■ Life-threatening hyperkalemia (other, more immediate measures should be instituted) ■ Hypersensitivity to saccharin or parabens (some products) ■ Ileus ■ Known alcohol intolerance (suspension only).

**Use Cautiously in:** ■ Geriatric patients ■ CHF, hypertension, edema ■ Sodium restriction ■ Constipation.

## ADVERSE REACTIONS AND SIDE EFFECTS*

■ **GI:** constipation, fecal impaction, anorexia, gastric irritation, nausea, vomiting ■ **F and E:** hypocalcemia, hypokalemia, sodium retention.

## INTERACTIONS

**Drug-Drug:** ■ Administration with **calcium** or **magnesium-containing antacids** may decrease resin-exchanging ability and increase risk of systemic alkalosis ■ Hypokalemia may enhance **digoxin** toxicity.

## ROUTE AND DOSAGE

4 level tsp = 15 g (4.1 mEq sodium/g).

■ **PO (Adults):** 15 g 1–4 times daily in water or sorbitol (up to 40 g 4 times daily).

■ **Rect (Adults):** 25–100 g as a retention enema; repeat as needed.

■ **PO, Rect (Children):** 1 g/kg/dose.

## AVAILABILITY (generic available)

■ **Suspension:** {15 g sodium polystyrene sulfonate with 20 g sorbitol/60 ml$^{Rx}$, 15 g sodium polystyrene sulfonate with 14.1 g sorbitol/60 ml$^{Rx}$} ■ **Powder:** {15 g/4 level tsp$^{Rx}$}.

TIME/ACTION PROFILE (decrease in serum potassium)

|        | ONSET   | PEAK    | DURATION |
|--------|---------|---------|----------|
| PO     | 2–12 hr | unknown | 6–24 hr  |
| Rectal | 2–12 hr | unknown | 4–6 hr   |

# NURSING IMPLICATIONS

## ASSESSMENT

❑ Monitor response of symptoms of hyperkalemia (fatigue, muscle weakness, paresthesia, confusion, dyspnea, peaked T waves, depressed ST segments, prolonged QT segments, widened QRS complexes, loss of P waves, and cardiac arrhythmias). Assess for development of hypokalemia (weakness, fatigue, arrhythmias, flat or inverted T waves, prominent U waves).

❑ Monitor intake and output ratios and daily weight. Assess for symptoms of fluid overload (dyspnea, rales/crackles, jugular venous distention, peripheral edema). Concurrent low-sodium diet may be ordered for patients with CHF (see Appendix Q).

❑ In patients receiving concurrent digoxin, assess for symptoms of digitalis toxicity (anorexia, nausea, vomiting, visual disturbances, arrhythmias).

❑ Assess abdomen and note character and frequency of stools. Concurrent sorbitol or laxatives may be ordered to prevent constipation or impaction. Some products contain sorbitol to prevent constipation. Patient should ideally have 1–2 watery stools each day during course of therapy.

■ *Lab Test Considerations:* Monitor serum potassium daily during therapy. Notify physician or other health care professional when potassium decreases to 4–5 mEq/L.

❑ Monitor renal function and electrolytes (especially sodium, calcium, bicarbonate, and magnesium) prior to and periodically throughout therapy.

## POTENTIAL NURSING DIAGNOSES

■ Constipation (Side Effects).

## IMPLEMENTATION

- **General:** Solution is stable for 24 hr when refrigerated.
- ❑ Consult physician or other health care professional regarding discontinuation of medications that may increase serum potassium (angiotensin-converting enzyme inhibitors, potassium-sparing diuretics, potassium supplements, salt substitutes).
- **PO:** An osmotic laxative (sorbitol) is usually administered concurrently to prevent constipation.
- ❑ For oral administration, add prescribed amount of powder to 3–4 ml water/g of powder. Shake well. Syrup may be ordered to improve palatability. Resin cookie or candy recipes are available; discuss with pharmacist or dictitian.
- **Retention Enema:** Precede retention enema with cleansing enema. Administer solution via rectal tube or 28-French Foley catheter with 30-ml balloon. Insert tube at least 20 cm and tape in place.
- ❑ For retention enema, add powder to 100 ml of prescribed solution (usually sorbitol or 20% dextrose in water). Shake well to dissolve powder thoroughly; should be of liquid consistency. Position patient on left side and elevate hips on pillow if solution begins to leak. Follow administration of medication with additional 50–100 ml of diluent to ensure administration of complete dose. Encourage patient to retain enema as long as possible, at least 30–60 min.
- ❑ After retention period, irrigate colon with 1–2 L of non–sodium-containing solution. Y-connector with tubing may be attached to Foley or rectal tube; cleansing solution is administered through one port of the Y and allowed to drain by gravity through the other port.

## PATIENT/FAMILY TEACHING

- ❑ Explain purpose and method of administration of medication to patient.
- ❑ Inform patient of need for frequent lab tests to monitor effectiveness.

## EVALUATION

**Effectiveness of therapy can be demonstrated by:** ■ Normalization of serum potassium levels.

## sodium salicylate, See SALICYLATES.

## somatrem, See GROWTH HORMONES.

## somatropin, See GROWTH HORMONES.

## sotalol

(**soe**-ta-lole)
Betapace, Betapace AF, {Sotacor}

### CLASSIFICATION(S):

**Therapeutic:** antiarrhythmics (classes II and III)
**Pharmacologic:** beta blockers

**Pregnancy Category B**

## INDICATIONS

■ Management of life-threatening ventricular arrhythmias ■ **Betapace AF:** Maintenance of normal sinus rhythm in patients with highly symptomatic atrial fibrillation/atrial flutter (AFIB/AFL) who are currently in sinus rhythm.

## ACTION

■ Blocks stimulation of beta$_1$ (myocardial) and beta$_2$ (pulmonary, vascular, and uterine) -adrenergic receptor sites. **Therapeutic Effects:** ■ Suppression of arrhythmias.

## PHARMACOKINETICS

**Absorption:** Well absorbed following oral administration.
**Distribution:** Crosses the placenta; enters breast milk.
**Metabolism and Excretion:** Elimination is mostly renal.

{ } = Available in Canada only.
*CAPITALS indicates life-threatening; underlines indicate most frequent.

**Half-life:** 12 hr (increased in renal impairment).

## CONTRAINDICATIONS AND PRECAUTIONS

**Contraindicated in:** ■ Hypersensitivity ■ Uncompensated CHF ■ Pulmonary edema ■ Asthma ■ Cardiogenic shock ■ Congenital or acquired long QT syndromes ■ Sinus bradycardia, 2nd- and 3rd-degree AV block (unless a functioning pacemaker is present) ■ CCr <40 ml/min in patients who are being treated with Betapace AF

**Use Cautiously in:** ■ Renal impairment (increased dosing interval recommended if CCr ≤60 ml/min for patients with ventricular arrhythmias) ■ Hepatic impairment ■ Hypokalemia (increased risk of serious arrhythmias) ■ Geriatric patients (increased sensitivity to beta blockers; initial dosage reduction recommended) ■ Other pulmonary pathology ■ Diabetes mellitus (may mask signs of hypoglycemia) ■ Thyrotoxicosis (may mask symptoms) ■ Patients with a history of severe allergic reactions (intensity of reactions may be increased) ■ Pregnancy, lactation, or children (safety not established; may cause fetal/neonatal bradycardia, hypotension, hypoglycemia, or respiratory depression).

## ADVERSE REACTIONS AND SIDE EFFECTS*

■ **CNS:** fatigue, weakness, anxiety, dizziness, drowsiness, insomnia, memory loss, mental depression, mental status changes, nervousness, nightmares ■ **EENT:** blurred vision, dry eyes, nasal stuffiness ■ **Resp:** bronchospasm, wheezing ■ **CV:** ARRHYTHMIAS, BRADYCARDIA, CHF, PULMONARY EDEMA, orthostatic hypotension, peripheral vasoconstriction ■ **GI:** constipation, diarrhea, nausea ■ **GU:** impotence, decreased libido ■ **Derm:** itching, rashes ■ **Endo:** hyperglycemia, hypoglycemia ■ **MS:** arthralgia, back pain, muscle cramps ■ **Neuro:** paresthesia ■ **Misc:** drug-induced lupus syndrome.

## INTERACTIONS

**Drug-Drug:** ■ Concurrent use with other **class 1A antiarrhythmics** is not recommended due to increased risk of arrhythmias ■ **General anesthesia, IV phenytoin,** and **verapamil** may cause additive myocardial depression ■ Concurrent use with other **calcium channel blockers** may increase the risk of adverse cardiovascular reactions ■ Additive bradycardia may occur with **digoxin** ■ Additive hypotension may occur with other **antihypertensives,** acute ingestion of **alcohol,** or **nitrates** ■ Concurrent use with **amphetamines, cocaine, ephedrine, epinephrine, norepinephrine, phenylephrine,** or **pseudoephedrine** may result in unopposed alpha-adrenergic stimulation (excessive hypertension, bradycardia) ■ Concurrent **thyroid** administration may decrease effectiveness ■ May alter the effectiveness of **insulin** or **oral hypoglycemic agents** (dosage adjustments may be necessary) ■ May decrease the effectiveness of **beta-adrenergic bronchodilators** and **theophylline** ■ May decrease the beneficial beta₁ cardiovascular effects of **dopamine** or **dobutamine** ■ Discontinuation of **clonidine** in patients receiving sotalol may result in excessive rebound hypertension ■ Use cautiously within 14 days of **MAO inhibitors** (may result in hypertension).

## ROUTE AND DOSAGE

❏ **Ventricular Arrhythmias**
■ **PO (Adults):** 80 mg twice daily; may be gradually increased (usual maintenance dose is 160–320 mg/day in 2–3 divided doses; some patients may require up to 480–640 mg/day).

❏ **Renal Impairment**
■ **PO (Adults):** *CCr 30–59 ml/min*—initial dose of 80 mg, with subsequent doses given q 24 hr; *CCr <10 ml/min–29 ml/min*—initial dose of 80 mg, with subsequent doses given q 36–48 hr.

❏ **Atrial Fibrillation/Atrial Flutter**
■ **PO (Adults):** 80 mg twice daily, may be increased during careful monitoring to 120 mg twice daily if necessary.

❏ **Renal Impairment**
■ **PO (Adults):** *CCr 40–60 ml/min*—80 mg once daily.

## AVAILABILITY (generic available)

■ *Tablets:* 80 mg^Rx, 120 mg^Rx, 160 mg^Rx, 240 mg^Rx ■ Cost: 80 mg $211.80/100, 120 mg $282.72/100, 160 mg $353.42/100, 240 mg $459.45/100 ■ *Tablets (Betapace AF):* 80 mg^Rx, 120 mg^Rx, 160 mg^Rx.

TIME/ACTION PROFILE (antiarrhythmic effects)

|  | ONSET | PEAK | DURATION |
| --- | --- | --- | --- |
| PO | hrs | 2–3 days | 8–12 hr |

# NURSING IMPLICATIONS

## ASSESSMENT

■ **General Info:** Monitor blood pressure and pulse frequently during dosage adjustment period and periodically throughout therapy. Assess for orthostatic hypotension when assisting patient up from supine position.
❑ Monitor intake and output ratios and daily weight. Assess patient routinely for evidence of fluid overload (peripheral edema, dyspnea, rales/crackles, fatigue, weight gain, jugular venous distention).

■ **Lab Test Considerations:** May cause increased BUN, serum lipoprotein, potassium, triglyceride, and uric acid levels.
❑ May cause increased ANA titers.
❑ May cause increase in blood glucose levels.

■ **Toxicity and Overdose:** Monitor patients receiving beta blockers for signs of overdose (bradycardia, severe dizziness or fainting, severe drowsiness, dyspnea, bluish fingernails or palms, seizures). Notify physician or other health care professional immediately if these signs occur.
❑ Glucagon has been used to treat bradycardia and hypotension.

## POTENTIAL NURSING DIAGNOSES

■ Cardiac output, decreased (Side Effects).
■ Noncompliance (Patient/Family Teaching).

## IMPLEMENTATION

■ **General:** Patients should be hospitalized and monitored for arrhythmias during initiation of therapy and dose increases.
❑ Do not substitute Betapace for Betapace AF. Make sure patients transfered from Betapace to Betapace AF have enough Betapace AF upon leaving the hospital to allow for uninterrupted therapy until Betapace AF prescription can be filled.

■ **PO:** Take apical pulse prior to administering. If <50 bpm or if arrhythmia occurs, withhold medication and notify physician or other health care professional.
❑ Administer on an empty stomach, 1 hr before or 2 hr after meals. Administration with food, especially milk or milk products, reduces absorption by approximately 20%.

❑ Avoid administering antacids containing aluminum or magnesium within 2 hr before administration of sotalol.

## PATIENT/FAMILY TEACHING

❑ Instruct patient to take medication exactly as directed, at the same time each day, even if feeling well; do not skip or double up on missed doses. If a dose is missed, it should be taken as soon as possible up to 8 hr before next dose. Abrupt withdrawal may precipitate life-threatening arrhythmias, hypertension, or myocardial ischemia.

❑ Advise patient to make sure enough medication is available for weekends, holidays, and vacations. A written prescription may be kept in wallet in case of emergency.

❑ Teach patient and family how to check pulse and blood pressure. Instruct them to check pulse daily and blood pressure biweekly. Advise patient to hold dose and contact physician or other health care professional if pulse is <50 bpm or if blood pressure changes significantly.

❑ May cause drowsiness or dizziness. Caution patients to avoid driving or other activities that require alertness until response to the drug is known.

❑ Advise patients to change positions slowly to minimize orthostatic hypotension, especially during initiation of therapy or when dose is increased.

❑ Caution patient that this medication may increase sensitivity to cold.

❑ Instruct patient to consult health care professional before taking any OTC medications, especially cold preparations, concurrently with this medication.

❑ Diabetic patients should closely monitor blood glucose, especially if weakness, malaise, irritability, or fatigue occurs. Medication may mask tachycardia and increased blood pressure as signs of hypoglycemia, but dizziness and sweating may still occur.

❑ Advise patient to notify health care professional if slow pulse, difficulty breathing, wheezing, cold hands and feet, dizziness, confusion, depression, rash, fever, sore throat, unusual bleeding, or bruising occurs.

{ } = Available in Canada only.
*CAPITALS indicates life-threatening; underlines indicate most frequent.

□ Instruct patient to inform health care professional of medication regimen prior to treatment or surgery.

□ Advise patient to carry identification describing disease process and medication regimen at all times.

## EVALUATION

**Effectiveness of therapy can be demonstrated by:** ■ Control of arrhythmias without appearance of detrimental side effects.

---

## sparfloxacin, See FLUOROQUINOLONES.

---

## spironolactone, See DIURETICS (POTASSIUM-SPARING).

---

## stavudine

(**stav**-yoo-deen)

d4T, Zerit, Zerit XR

### CLASSIFICATION(S):

**Therapeutic:** antiretrovirals
**Pharmacologic:** nucleoside reverse transcriptase inhibitors

### Pregnancy Category C

## INDICATIONS

■ HIV infection unresponsive or intolerant to conventional therapy.

## ACTION

■ Converted intracellularly to stavudine triphosphate, which inhibits viral DNA synthesis and replication. **Therapeutic Effects:** ■ Virustatic action against HIV ■ Decreased viral load and increased cell count ■ Not curative, but may slow progression of HIV infection and decrease the incidence and severity of its sequelae.

## PHARMACOKINETICS

**Absorption:** Well absorbed after oral administration (78–80% bioavailability). XR formulation produces less fluctuation in levels.

**Distribution:** Crosses the blood-brain barrier; enters RBCs and plasma equally.

**Metabolism and Excretion:** Converted intracellularly to stavudine triphosphate, which is

the active drug; 40% excreted unchanged in urine; 50% nonrenally eliminated.

**Half-life:** *Adults*—1–1.6 hr; *children*—0.9–1.1 hr; *adults with renal impairment*—4.8 hr; *intracellular half-life*—3.5 hr.

## CONTRAINDICATIONS AND PRECAUTIONS

**Contraindicated in:** ■ Hypersensitivity.

**Use Cautiously in:** ■ Patients with a history of alcohol abuse ■ Patients with a history of liver disease or hepatic impairment ■ Renal impairment (dosage reduction and/or increased dosing interval recommended if CCr <50 ml/min) ■ History of peripheral neuropathy ■ Pregnancy or lactation (safety not established; breastfeeding should be avoided by HIV-infected mothers because of transmission of the virus in breast milk; concurrent use with didanosine during pregnancy may increase the risk of fetal lactic acidosis).

## ADVERSE REACTIONS AND SIDE EFFECTS*

■ **CNS:** headache, insomnia, weakness ■ **GI:** HEPATIC TOXICITY, PANCREATITIS, anorexia, diarrhea ■ **F and E:** LACTIC ACIDOSIS ■ **Hemat:** anemia ■ **MS:** arthralgia, myalgia ■ **Neuro:** peripheral neuropathy.

## INTERACTIONS

**Drug-Drug:** ■ Use cautiously with **drugs causing peripheral neuropathy** (**chloramphenicol, cisplatin, dapsone, didanosine, ethambutol, ethionamide, hydralazine, isoniazid, lithium, metronidazole, nitrofurantoin, phenytoin, vincristine,** or **zalcitabine**) ■ Concurrent use with **didanosine** may ↑ risk of pancreatitis ■ Concurrent use with **zidovudine** is not recommended because of possible antiretroviral antagonism.

## ROUTE AND DOSAGE

■ **PO (Adults ≥60 kg):** 40 mg twice daily *or* 100 mg once daily as XR capsules.

■ **PO (Adults <60 kg):** 30 mg twice daily *or* 75 mg once daily as XR capsules.

■ **PO (Children at least 14 days old and <30 kg):** 1 mg/kg every 12 hr (not to exceed 40 mg q 12 hr).

■ **PO (Infants birth–13 days):** 0.5 mg/kg every 12 hr.

□ **Renal Impairment**

- **PO (Adults ≥60 kg):** *CCr 26–50 ml/ min*—20 mg q 12 hr; *CCr 10–25 ml/ min*—20 mg q 24 hr.
- **PO (Adults <60 kg):** *CCr 26–50 ml/ min*—15 mg q 12 hr; *CCr 10–25 ml/ min*—15 mg q 24 hr.

## AVAILABILITY

- *Capsules:* 15 mg<sup>Rx</sup>, 20 mg<sup>Rx</sup>, 30 mg<sup>Rx</sup>, 40 mg<sup>Rx</sup> ■ *Powder for oral solution (fruit flavored):* 1 mg/ml (after reconstitution) in 200–ml bottle<sup>Rx</sup> ■ *Extended-release capsules:* 37.5 mg<sup>Rx</sup>, 50 mg<sup>Rx</sup>, 75 mg<sup>Rx</sup>, 100 mg<sup>Rx</sup>.

TIME/ACTION PROFILE (blood levels)

|  | ONSET | PEAK | DURATION |
|---|---|---|---|
| PO | unknown | 0.5–1.5 hr | 12 hr |
| PO-XR | unknown | 3 hr | 24 hr |

## NURSING IMPLICATIONS

### ASSESSMENT

- ❏ Assess patient for change in severity of symptoms of HIV infection and for symptoms of opportunistic infection during therapy.
- ❏ Monitor patient for signs and symptoms of peripheral neuropathy (tingling, burning, numbness, or pain in hands or feet); may be difficult to differentiate from peripheral neuropathy of severe HIV disease or lactic acidosis. May resolve if stavudine therapy is discontinued promptly or may temporarily worsen after discontinuation of therapy. If symptoms resolve completely, stavudine therapy may resume at 50% of the regular dose.
- ❏ Assess patient for signs of pancreatitis (nausea, vomiting, abdominal pain) periodically throughout therapy. Occurs rarely, but may require discontinuation of therapy.
- ■ *Lab Test Considerations:* Monitor viral load CD4 counts before and regularly during therapy.
- ❏ Monitor liver function. May cause ↑ levels of AST, ALT, and alkaline phosphatase, which usually resolve after interruption of therapy. Lactic acidosis may occur with hepatic toxicity causing hepatic steatosis; may be fatal, especially in women.

- ❏ May cause ↑ serum amylase and lipase levels.

## POTENTIAL NURSING DIAGNOSES

- ■ Infection, risk for (Indications).

## IMPLEMENTATION

- ■ **PO:** May be administered without regard to food.
- ❏ Shake solution vigorously before administration. Keep refrigerated; discard unused portion after 30 days.
- ❏ XR capsules can be opened and mixed with 2 tbsp of yogurt or applesauce. Entire contents should be swallowed immediately. Advise patient not to chew or crush beads while swallowing.

## PATIENT/FAMILY TEACHING

- ❏ Instruct patient to take stavudine as directed. Emphasize the importance of compliance with full course of therapy, not taking more than the prescribed amount, and not discontinuing without consulting health care professional. Take missed doses as soon as possible unless almost time for next dose. Do not double doses. Caution patient not to share medication with others.
- ❏ Inform patient that stavudine does not cure HIV disease and does not reduce the risk of transmission of HIV to others through sexual contact or blood contamination. Caution patient to avoid sexual contact or to use a condom, and to avoid sharing needles or donating blood to prevent spreading HIV to others.
- ❏ Instruct patient to notify health care professional promptly if signs of lactic acidosis (unexplained weight loss, abdominal discomfort, nausea, vomiting, fatigue, dyspnea, motor weakness), peripheral neuropathy, or pancreatitis occur.
- ❏ Advise patient not to take other OTC or prescription medications without consulting health care professional.
- ❏ Emphasize the importance of regular follow-up exams and blood tests to determine progress and monitor for side effects.

{ } = Available in Canada only.
*CAPITALS indicates life-threatening; underlines indicate most frequent.

**EVALUATION**

**Effectiveness of therapy can be demonstrated by:** ▪ Decrease in viral load and improvement in CD4 counts in patients with advanced HIV infection.

**streptokinase, See THROMBOLYTIC AGENTS.**

**streptomycin, See AMINOGLYCOSIDES.**

**sulconazole, See ANTIFUNGALS (TOPICAL).**

**sulfasalazine**

(sul-fa-**sal**-a-zeen)

Azulfidine, Azulfidine EN-tabs, {PMS-Sulfasalazine}, {Salazopyrin}, {S.A.S.}

**CLASSIFICATION(S):**
**Therapeutic:** *antirheumatics (DMARD), gastrointestinal anti-inflammatories*

**Pregnancy Category B**

**INDICATIONS**

▪ Inflammatory bowel diseases including: ❑ Ulcerative colitis ❑ Proctitis ❑ Proctosigmoiditis ▪ Rheumatoid arthritis unresponsive or intolerant to salicylates and/or NSAIDs.

**ACTION**

▪ Locally acting anti-inflammatory action in the colon, where activity is probably a result of inhibition of prostaglandin synthesis. **Therapeutic Effects:** ▪ Reduction in the symptoms of inflammatory bowel disease.

**PHARMACOKINETICS**

**Absorption:** 10–15% absorbed after oral administration.
**Distribution:** Widely distributed; crosses the placenta and enters breast milk.
**Protein Binding:** 99%.

**Metabolism and Excretion:** Split by intestinal bacteria into sulfapyridine and 5-aminosalicylic acid. Some absorbed sulfasalazine is excreted by bile back into intestines; 15% excreted unchanged by the kidneys. Sulfapyridine also excreted mostly by the kidneys.
**Half-life:** 6 hr.

**CONTRAINDICATIONS AND PRECAUTIONS**

**Contraindicated in:** ▪ Hypersensitivity reactions to sulfonamides, salicylates, or sulfasalazine ▪ Cross-sensitivity with furosemide, sulfonylurea hypoglycemic agents, or carbonic anhydrase inhibitors may exist ▪ G6PD deficiency ▪ Hypersensitivity to bisulfites (mesalamine enema only) ▪ Urinary tract or intestinal obstruction ▪ Porphyria ▪ Children <2 yr.

**Use Cautiously in:** ▪ Severe hepatic or renal impairment ▪ Renal impairment ▪ History of porphyria ▪ Pregnancy (has been used safely) ▪ Lactation (safety not established).

**ADVERSE REACTIONS AND SIDE EFFECTS\***

▪ **CNS:** <u>headache</u> ▪ **Resp:** pneumonitis ▪ **GI:** <u>anorexia</u>, <u>diarrhea</u>, <u>nausea</u>, <u>vomiting</u>, drug-induced hepatitis ▪ **GU:** crystalluria, oligospermia, orange-yellow discoloration of urine ▪ **Derm:** <u>rashes</u>, exfoliative dermatitis, photosensitivity, yellow discoloration ▪ **Hemat:** AGRANULOCYTOSIS, APLASTIC ANEMIA, blood dyscrasias, eosinophilia, megaloblastic anemia, thrombocytopenia ▪ **Neuro:** peripheral neuropathy ▪ **Misc:** *hypersensitivity reactions including*—SERUM SICKNESS and STEVENS-JOHNSON SYNDROME, <u>fever</u>.

**INTERACTIONS**

**Drug-Drug:** ▪ May ↑ action/risk of toxicity from **oral hypoglycemic agents, phenytoin, methotrexate, zidovudine,** or **warfarin** ▪ ↑ risk of drug-induced hepatitis with other **hepatotoxic agents** ▪ ↑ risk of crystalluria with **methenamine** ▪ May ↓ metabolism and increase effects/toxicity of **mercaptopurine** or **thioguanine.**

**Drug-Food:** ▪ May decrease **iron** and **folic acid** absorption.

**ROUTE AND DOSAGE**

❑ **Inflammatory Bowel Disease**

▪ **PO (Adults):** *Inflammatory bowel disease*—1 g q 6–8 hr (may start with 500 mg q 6–12 hr), followed by maintenance dose of 500 mg q 6 hr.

- **PO (Children >2 yr):** *Initial*—6.7–10 mg/kg q 4 hr *or* 10–15 mg/kg q 6 hr *or* 13.3–20 mg/kg q 8 hr. *Maintenance*—7.5 mg/kg q 6 hr (not to exceed 2 g/day).

□ **Rheumatoid Arthritis**

- **PO (Adults):** 500 mg–1 g/day (as delayed-release tablets) for 1 wk, then increase by 500 mg/day q wk up to 2 g/day in 2 divided doses; if no benefit seen after 12 wk, increase to 3 g/day in 2 divided doses.

- **PO (Children ≥6 yr):** 30–50 mg/kg/day in 2 divided doses (as delayed-release tablets); initiate therapy at 1/4–1/3 of planned maintenance dose and increase q 7 days until maintenance dose is reached (not to exceed 2 g/day).

## AVAILABILITY (generic available)

■ *Tablets:* 500 mg$^{Rx}$ ■ Cost: *generic*—$33.38/100 ■ *Delayed-release (enteric-coated) tablets (Azulfidine EN-tabs):* 500 mg$^{Rx}$ ■ Cost: *Azulfidine*—$39.99/100 ■ *Oral suspension:* {250 mg/5 ml$^{Rx}$} ■ *Rectal suspension:* {3 g$^{Rx}$}.

TIME/ACTION PROFILE (blood levels)

| | ONSET | PEAK | DURATION |
|---|---|---|---|
| PO | 1 hr | 1.5–6 hr | 6–12 hr |

## NURSING IMPLICATIONS

### ASSESSMENT

- **General Info:** Assess patient for allergy to sulfonamides and salicylates. Therapy should be discontinued if rash or fever occurs.
- □ Monitor intake and output ratios. Fluid intake should be sufficient to maintain a urine output of at least 1200–1500 ml daily to prevent crystalluria and stone formation.
- **Inflammatory Bowel Disease:** Assess abdominal pain and frequency, quantity, and consistency of stools at the beginning of and during therapy.
- **Rheumatoid Arthritis:** Assess range of motion and degree of swelling and pain in affected joints before and periodically during therapy.

- *Lab Test Considerations:* Monitor urinalysis, BUN, and serum creatinine before and periodically during therapy. May cause crystalluria and urinary cell calculi formation. Monitor CBC before and every 3–6 mo during prolonged therapy. Discontinue sulfasalazine if blood dyscrasias occur.

## POTENTIAL NURSING DIAGNOSES

- Pain, acute (Indications).
- Diarrhea (Indications).

## IMPLEMENTATION

- **General:** Do not confuse sulfasalazine with sulfisoxazole.
- □ Varying dosing regimens of sulfasalazine may be used to minimize GI side effects.
- **PO:** Administer after meals or with food to minimize GI irritation, with a full glass of water. Do not crush or chew enteric-coated tablets. Shake oral suspension well before administration. Use a calibrated measuring device to measure liquid preparations.
- **Rect:** Patient should empty bowel before administration of rectal dose forms.
- □ Administer 60-ml retention enema once daily at bedtime. Solution should be retained for approximately 8 hr. Before administration of *rectal suspension,* shake bottle well and remove the protective cap. Have patient lie on left side with the lower leg extended and the upper leg flexed for support or place the patient in knee-chest position. Gently insert the applicator tip into the rectum, pointing toward the umbilicus. Squeeze the bottle steadily to discharge most of the preparation.

## PATIENT/FAMILY TEACHING

- □ Instruct patient on the correct method of administration. Advise patient to take medication as directed, even if feeling better. Take missed doses as soon as remembered unless almost time for next dose.
- □ May cause dizziness. Caution patient to avoid driving or other activities that require alertness until response to medication is known.
- □ Advise patient to notify health care professional if skin rash, sore throat, fever, mouth sores, unusual bleeding or bruising, wheezing, fever, or hives occur.

{ } = Available in Canada only.
*CAPITALS indicates life-threatening; underlines indicate most frequent.

❏ Caution patient to use sunscreen and protective clothing to prevent photosensitivity reactions.

❏ Inform patient that this medication may cause orange-yellow discoloration of urine and skin, which is not significant. May permanently stain contact lenses yellow.

❏ Instruct patient to notify health care professional if symptoms worsen or do not improve. If symptoms of acute intolerance (cramping, acute abdominal pain, bloody diarrhea, fever, headache, rash) occur, discontinue therapy and notify health care professional immediately.

❏ Inform patient that proctoscopy and sigmoidoscopy may be required periodically during treatment to determine response.

❏ Instruct patient to notify health care professional if symptoms do not improve after 1–2 mo of therapy.

■ **Rect:** Instruct patient to use *rectal suspension* at bedtime and retain suspension all night for best results.

## EVALUATION

**Clinical response to therapy can be evaluated by:** ■ Decrease in diarrhea and abdominal pain ■ Return to normal bowel pattern in patients with inflammatory bowel disease. Effects may be seen within 3–21 days. The usual course of therapy is 3–6 wk ■ Maintenance of remission in patients with inflammatory bowel disease ■ Decrease in pain and inflammation, and increase in mobility in patients with rheumatoid arthritis.

---

# sulindac
(**soo**-lin-dak)
{Apo-Sulin}, Clinoril, {Novo-Sundac}

### CLASSIFICATION(S):
***Therapeutic:*** *antirheumatics, nonsteroidal anti-inflammatory agents*

**Pregnancy Category UK**

---

## INDICATIONS

■ Management of inflammatory disorders, including: ❏ Rheumatoid arthritis ❏ Osteoarthritis ❏ Acute gouty arthritis ❏ Bursitis.

## ACTION

■ Inhibits prostaglandin synthesis. **Therapeutic Effects:** ■ Suppression of pain and inflammation.

## PHARMACOKINETICS

**Absorption:** Well absorbed from the GI tract after oral administration.
**Distribution:** Unknown. Enters breast milk in small amounts.
**Metabolism and Excretion:** Converted by the liver to active drug. Minimal amounts excreted unchanged by the kidneys.
**Half-life:** 7.8 hr (16.4 hr for active metabolite).

## CONTRAINDICATIONS AND PRECAUTIONS

**Contraindicated in:** ■ Hypersensitivity ■ Cross-sensitivity may occur with other NSAIDs, including aspirin ■ Active GI bleeding or ulcer disease.
**Use Cautiously in:** ■ Severe cardiovascular, renal, or hepatic disease (dosage modification recommended) ■ History of ulcer disease ■ Pregnancy, lactation, or children (use not recommended).

## ADVERSE REACTIONS AND SIDE EFFECTS*

■ **CNS:** dizziness, headache, drowsiness ■ **EENT:** blurred vision, tinnitus ■ **CV:** edema ■ **GI:** GI BLEEDING, DRUG-INDUCED HEPATITIS, constipation, diarrhea, discomfort, dyspepsia, nausea, vomiting, anorexia, flatulence, pancreatitis ■ **GU:** renal failure ■ **Derm:** rashes, photosensitivity ■ **Hemat:** blood dyscrasias, prolonged bleeding time ■ **Misc:** allergic reactions including ANAPHYLAXIS and HYPERSENSITIVITY SYNDROME.

## INTERACTIONS

**Drug-Drug:** ■ Concurrent use of **aspirin** may decrease effectiveness ■ Increased risk of bleeding with **anticoagulants, thrombolytic agents, tirofiban, eptifibatide, clopidogrel, ticlopidine, cefoperazone, cefotetan, valproic acid,** or **plicamycin** ■ Additive adverse GI side effects with **aspirin, corticosteroids,** and other **NSAIDs** ■ May decrease response to **antihypertensives** or **diuretics** ■ May increase serum levels and risk of toxicity from **lithium** ■ May increase the risk of hematologic toxicity from **antineoplastics** or **radiation therapy** ■ Increased risk of adverse renal effects with **gold compounds, cyclosporine,** or chronic use of **acetaminophen** ■ **Antacids** decrease blood levels and decrease effectiveness of sulindac ■ Increased risk of photosensitivity reactions with other **photosensitizing medications** ■ Increased risk of hypoglycemia with **insulins** or **oral hypoglycemic agents** ■ Should not be used concurrently with **dimethyl sulfoxide** because of increased risk of peripheral neuropathy and decreased levels of sulindac and its metabolite.

## ROUTE AND DOSAGE

■ **PO (Adults):** 150–200 mg bid (not to exceed 400 mg/day).

## AVAILABILITY (generic available)

■ *Tablets:* 150 mg$^{Rx}$, 200 mg$^{Rx}$ ■ Cost: *Clinoril*—150 mg $85.72/100, 200 mg $111.49/100; *generic*—150 mg $85.72/100, 200 mg $111.49/100.

TIME/ACTION PROFILE

|  | ONSET | PEAK | DURATION |
|---|---|---|---|
| PO (analgesic) | 1–2 days | unknown | 12 hr |
| PO (anti-inflammatory) | few days–1 wk | 2 wk or more | unknown |

## NURSING IMPLICATIONS

### ASSESSMENT

❑ Patients who have asthma, aspirin-induced allergy, and nasal polyps are at increased risk for developing hypersensitivity reactions. Monitor for rhinitis, asthma, and urticaria.
❑ Assess pain and range of movement before and after 1–2 wk of therapy.
■ *Lab Test Considerations:* BUN, serum creatinine, CBC, and liver function tests should be evaluated periodically in patients receiving prolonged therapy.
❑ Serum potassium, glucose, alkaline phosphatase, AST, and ALT may show increased levels.
❑ Bleeding time may be prolonged for 1 day after discontinuation of therapy.

### POTENTIAL NURSING DIAGNOSES

■ Pain, acute (Indications).

■ Mobility, impaired physical (Indications).

## IMPLEMENTATION

■ **General:** Do not confuse Clinoril (sulindac) with Clozaril (clozapine).
❑ Administration in higher than recommended doses does not provide increased effectiveness but may cause increased side effects.
■ **PO:** May be administered with food, milk, or antacids to decrease GI irritation. Food slows but does not reduce the extent of absorption. Tablets may be crushed and mixed with fluids or food.

## PATIENT/FAMILY TEACHING

❑ Advise patient to take this medication with a full glass of water and to remain in an upright position for 15–30 min after administration.
❑ Instruct patient to take medication exactly as directed. If a dose is missed, it should be taken as soon as remembered but not if almost time for the next dose. Do not double doses.
❑ May cause dizziness. Advise patient to avoid driving or other activities requiring alertness until response to the medication is known.
❑ Caution patient to avoid the concurrent use of alcohol, aspirin, NSAIDs, acetaminophen, or other OTC medications without consulting health care professional.
❑ Advise patient to inform health care professional of medication regimen before treatment or surgery.
❑ Advise patient to inform health care professional if pregnancy is planned or suspected.
❑ Advise patient to use sunscreen and protective clothing to prevent photosensitivity reactions.
❑ Advise patient to consult health care professional if rash, itching, visual disturbances, tinnitus, weight gain, edema, black stools, persistent headache, or influenza-like syndrome (chills, fever, muscle aches, pain) occurs.

### EVALUATION

**Effectiveness of therapy can be demonstrated by:** ■ Decreased pain and improved joint mobility. Partial arthritic relief may be seen within 7 days, but maximum effectiveness may require 2–3 wk of continuous therapy. Patients who do not respond to one NSAID may respond to another.

## sumatriptan

(soo-ma-**trip**-tan)

Imitrex

### CLASSIFICATION(S):

**Therapeutic:** vascular headache suppressants

**Pharmacologic:** 5 $HT_1$ agonists

### Pregnancy Category C

## INDICATIONS

■ Acute treatment of migraine attacks ■ **Subcut:** Acute treatment of cluster headache episodes.

## ACTION

■ Acts as a selective agonist of 5-$HT_1$ at specific vascular serotonin receptor sites, causing vasoconstriction in large intracranial arteries. **Therapeutic Effects:** ■ Relief of acute attacks of migraine.

## PHARMACOKINETICS

**Absorption:** Well absorbed (97%) after subcut administration. Absorption after oral administration is incomplete and significant amounts undergo substantial hepatic metabolism, resulting in poor bioavailability (14%). Well absorbed after intranasal administration.

**Distribution:** Does not cross the blood-brain barrier. Remainder of distribution not known.

**Metabolism and Excretion:** Mostly metabolized (80%) by the liver.

**Half-life:** 2 hr.

## CONTRAINDICATIONS AND PRECAUTIONS

**Contraindicated in:** ■ Hypersensitivity ■ Patients with ischemic heart disease or signs and symptoms of ischemic heart disease, Prinzmetal's angina, or uncontrolled hypertension ■ Concurrent MAO inhibitor therapy ■ Elderly patients (excessive risk of cardiovascular complications).

**Use Cautiously in:** ■ Patients with childbearing potential ■ Pregnancy, lactation, or children <18 yr (safety not established).

**Exercise Extreme Caution in:** ■ Cardiovascular risk factors (hypertension, hypercholesterolemia, smoking, obesity, diabetes, family history, menopausal women or men >40 yr); use only if cardiovascular status has been evaluated and determined to be safe and first dose is administered under supervision.

## ADVERSE REACTIONS AND SIDE EFFECTS*

All adverse reactions are less common after oral administration. ■ **CNS:** dizziness, vertigo, anxiety, drowsiness, fatigue, feeling of heaviness, feeling of tightness, headache, malaise, strange feeling, tight feeling in head, weakness ■ **EENT:** alterations in vision, nasal sinus discomfort, throat discomfort ■ **CV:** MI, angina, chest pressure, chest tightness, coronary vasospasm, ECG changes, transient hypertension ■ **GI:** abdominal discomfort, dysphagia ■ **Derm:** tingling, warm sensation, burning sensation, cool sensation, flushing ■ **Local:** injection site reaction ■ **MS:** jaw discomfort, muscle cramps, myalgia, neck pain, neck stiffness ■ **Neuro:** numbness.

## INTERACTIONS

**Drug-Drug:** ■ The risk of vasospastic reactions may be increased by concurrent use of **ergotamine** or **dihydroergotamine** (avoid within 24 hr of each other) ■ Concurrent use with **lithium, MAO inhibitors** (do not use within 2 wk of discontinuing MAO inhibitor), or **SSRI antidepressants** (may cause weakness, hyperreflexia, and incoordination).

**Drug-Natural Products:** ■ Increased risk of serotinergic side effects including serotonin syndrome with **St. John's wort** and **SAMe.**

## ROUTE AND DOSAGE

- **PO (Adults):** 25 mg initially; if response is inadequate at 2 hr, up to 100 mg may be given (initial doses of 25–50 mg may be more effective than 25 mg). If headache recurs, doses may be repeated q 2 hr (not to exceed 300 mg/day). If PO therapy is to follow subcut injection, additional PO sumatriptan may be taken q 2 hr (not to exceed 200 mg/day).

- **Subcut (Adults):** 6 mg; may repeat after 1 hr (not to exceed 12 mg in 24 hr).

- **Intranasal (Adults):** Single dose of 5, 10, or 20 mg in one nostril; may be repeated in

2 hr, not to exceed 40 mg/24 hr or treatment of >5 episodes/mo.

❏ **Hepatic Impairment**

■ **PO (Adults):** 25 mg initially; if response is inadequate at 2 hr, up to 50 mg may be given (initial doses of 25–50 mg may be more effective than 25 mg). If headache recurs, doses may be repeated q 2 hr (not to exceed 300 mg/day). If PO therapy is to follow sub-cut injection, additional PO sumatriptan may be taken q 2 hr (not to exceed 200 mg/day); no single oral dose should exceed 50 mg.

## AVAILABILITY

■ *Tablets:* 25 mg$^{Rx}$, 50 mg$^{Rx}$, {100 mg$^{Rx}$} ■ Cost: 25 mg $151.26/9, 50 mg $144.06/9, 100 mg $144.06/9 ■ *Injection:* 6 mg/0.5-ml pre-filled syringes$^{Rx}$, 0.6 mg/0.5-ml vials$^{Rx}$, SELF-dose injection kit (containing 2 prefilled syringes and instructions)$^{Rx}$ ■ Cost: $103.62/2 prefilled syringes ■ *Nasal spray:* 5 mg in 100 mcl-unit dose spray device (package of 6)$^{Rx}$, 20 mg in 100 mcl-unit dose spray device (package of 6)$^{Rx}$ ■ Cost: 5 mg $131.09/6, 20 mg $131.09/6.

TIME/ACTION PROFILE (relief of migraine)

| | ONSET | PEAK | DURATION |
|---|---|---|---|
| PO | within 30 min | 2–4 hr | up to 24 hr |
| Subcut | 30 min | up to 2 hr | up to 24 hr |
| Nasal | within 60 min | 2 hr | unknown |

# NURSING IMPLICATIONS

## ASSESSMENT

❏ Assess pain location, intensity, duration, and associated symptoms (photophobia, phonophobia, nausea, vomiting) during migraine attack.

❏ Give initial subcut under observation to patients with potential for coronary artery disease including postmenopausal women, men >40 years, patients with risk factors for coronary artery disease such as hypertension, hypercholesterolemia, obesity, diabetes, smoking, or family history. Monitor blood pressure before and for 1 hr after initial injection. If angina occurs, monitor ECG for ischemic changes.

## POTENTIAL NURSING DIAGNOSES

■ Pain, acute (Indications).

## IMPLEMENTATION

■ **General:** Do not confuse sumatriptan with zolmitriptan.

■ **PO:** Tablets should be swallowed whole; do not crush, break, or chew. Tablets are film-coated to prevent contact with tablet contents, which have an unpleasant taste and may cause nausea and vomiting.

■ **Subcut:** Administer as a single injection just below the skin.

■ **Intranasal:** 10-mg dose may be administered as 2 sprays of 5 mg in one nostril or 1 spray in each nostril.

## PATIENT/FAMILY TEACHING

■ **General Info:** Inform patient that sumatriptan should be used only during a migraine attack. It is meant to be used for relief of migraine attacks but not to prevent or reduce the number of attacks.

❏ Instruct patient to administer sumatriptan as soon as symptoms of a migraine attack appear, but it may be administered at any time during an attack. If migraine symptoms return, a 2nd injection may be used. Allow at least 1 hr between doses, and do not use more than 2 injections in any 24-hr period.

❏ Advise patient that lying down in a darkened room after sumatriptan administration may further help relieve headache.

❏ Caution patient not to use sumatriptan if she is pregnant, suspects that she is pregnant, or plans to become pregnant. Adequate contraception should be used during therapy.

❏ Advise patient to notify health care professional before next dose of sumatriptan if pain or tightness in the chest occurs during use. If pain is severe or does not subside, notify health care professional immediately. If wheezing; heart throbbing; swelling of eyelids, face, or lips; skin rash; skin lumps; or hives occur, notify health care professional immediately and do not take more sumatriptan without approval of health care professional. Additional sumatriptan doses are not likely to be effective and alternative medications, as previously discussed with health

---

{ } = Available in Canada only.
*CAPITALS indicates life-threatening; underlines indicate most frequent.

care professional, may be used. If usual dose fails to relieve 3 consecutive headaches or if frequency and/or severity increases, notify health care professional. If feelings of tingling, heat, flushing, heaviness, pressure, drowsiness, dizziness, tiredness, or sickness develop, discuss with health care professional at next visit.

❏ Sumatriptan may cause dizziness or drowsiness. Caution patient to avoid driving or other activities requiring alertness until response to medication is known.

❏ Advise patient to avoid alcohol, which aggravates headaches, during sumatriptan use.

■ **Subcut:** Instruct patient on the proper technique for loading, administering, and discarding the autoinjector. Patient information pamphlet is provided. Instructional video is available from the manufacturer.

❏ Inform patient that pain or redness at the injection site usually lasts less than 1 hr.

■ **Intranasal:** Instruct patient in proper technique for intranasal administration. Usual dose is a single spray in one nostril. If headache returns, a 2nd dose may be administered in ≥2 hr. Do not administer 2nd dose if no relief was provided by 1st dose without consulting health care professional.

### EVALUATION

**Effectiveness of therapy can be demonstrated by:**   ■ Relief of migraine attack.

# tacrine

## (tak-rin)
Cognex

### CLASSIFICATION(S):
**Therapeutic:** anti-Alzheimer's agents
**Pharmacologic:** cholinergics (cholinesterase inhibitors)

### Pregnancy Category C

## INDICATIONS
■ Mild to moderate dementia associated with Alzheimer's disease.

## ACTION
■ Increases levels of acetylcholine in the CNS by inhibiting its breakdown. **Therapeutic Effects:** ■ Improved cognitive function in patients with mild to moderate Alzheimer's disease. Does not affect the course of the disease.

## PHARMACOKINETICS
**Absorption:** Rapidly absorbed following oral administration, although bioavailability is low (17%).

**Distribution:** Unknown.

**Metabolism and Excretion:** Highly metabolized by the liver (mostly by the P450 enzyme system).

**Half-life:** 2–4 hr.

## CONTRAINDICATIONS AND PRECAUTIONS
**Contraindicated in:** ■ Hypersensitivity to tacrine or other acridines ■ Jaundice associated with previous courses of tacrine therapy.

**Use Cautiously in:** ■ Patients with a history or risk of GI bleeding, including current therapy with NSAIDs.

## ADVERSE REACTIONS AND SIDE EFFECTS*
■ **CNS:** dizziness, headache ■ **CV:** bradycardia ■ **GI:** GI BLEEDING, anorexia, diarrhea, drug-induced hepatitis, dyspepsia, nausea, vomiting.

## INTERACTIONS
**Drug-Drug:** ■ Metabolized by the cytochrome P450 enzyme system; levels and effects may be altered by other drugs which increase/inhibit this system or drugs that may compete for this metabolic pathway ■ Increases **theophylline** levels and risk of toxicity (blood level monitoring recommended; dosage reduction may be required) ■ Potentiates the effects of **succinylcholine** (increases neuromuscular blockade) during anesthesia; also potentiates the effects of other **cholinesterase inhibitors** ■ May potentiate the action of **cholinergics (bethanechol)** ■ **Fluvoxamine** significantly increases blood levels and the risk of adverse reactions ■ **Cigarette smoking** decreases blood levels of tacrine ■ **Cimetidine** increases tacrine levels ■ May interfere with the action of **anticholinergics** ■ Concurrent use of **NSAIDs** may increase the risk of GI bleeding.

**Drug-Food:** ■ **Food** decreases absorption of tacrine by 30–40%.

## ROUTE AND DOSAGE
■ **PO (Adults):** 10 mg 4 times daily for 4 wk. If ALT remains unchanged, increase dose to 20 mg 4 times daily. Further increments may be made at 4-wk intervals as tolerated, up to 160 mg/day.

## AVAILABILITY
■ *Capsules:* 10 mg$^{Rx}$, 20 mg$^{Rx}$, 30 mg$^{Rx}$, 40 mg$^{Rx}$ ■ Cost: 10 mg $147.01/120, 20 mg $147.01/120, 30 mg $147.01/120, 40 mg $147.01/120.

TIME/ACTION PROFILE (improvement in cognitive function)

| | ONSET | PEAK | DURATION |
|---|---|---|---|
| PO | within 6 wk | 18–24 wk | unknown |

# NURSING IMPLICATIONS

## ASSESSMENT
❑ Assess cognitive function (memory, attention, reasoning, language, ability to perform simple tasks) periodically throughout therapy.
❑ Monitor heart rate periodically during therapy. May cause bradycardia.

■ *Lab Test Considerations:* May cause ALT elevations; monitor levels every other wk for the first 16 wk of therapy, monthly for 2 mo, and then every 3 mo throughout therapy. Biweekly monitoring should be resumed for at least 6 wk after any dose increase. If ALT levels are <3 times the upper limit of normal, continue dose titration; if levels are >3 to <5 times the upper limit of normal, decrease the dose of tacrine by 40 mg/day and resume dose titration when ALT returns to normal. Tacrine should be discontinued if ALT levels are >5 times the upper limit of normal. Levels usually return to normal 4–6 wk after discontinuation of therapy.

❑ Tacrine should be permanently discontinued and a new trial should not be attempted in patients with clinical jaundice and a total bilirubin >3 mg/dl.

## POTENTIAL NURSING DIAGNOSES

■ Thought processes, disturbed (Indications).
■ Injury, risk for (Indications).

## IMPLEMENTATION

■ **PO:** Administer at regular intervals between meals on an empty stomach. If GI upset occurs, may be administered with meals; however, plasma levels may be reduced by 30–40%.

❑ Tacrine capsules may be dissolved in any aqueous solution for patients with difficulty swallowing (orange juice best masks the bitter taste). Place intact capsule in liquid to avoid loss of medication by spillage.

## PATIENT/FAMILY TEACHING

❑ Emphasize the importance of taking tacrine at regular intervals as directed. If a dose is missed, take as soon as possible unless within 2 hr of next dose; do not double doses or discontinue without consulting health care professional. Abrupt discontinuation of doses >80 mg/day may cause a decline in cognitive function and behavioral disturbances.

❑ Caution patient and caregiver that tacrine may cause dizziness, unsteadiness, and clumsiness.

❑ Advise patient and caregiver to notify health care professional if nausea, vomiting, diarrhea, rash, jaundice, or changes in the color of the stool occur or if new symptoms occur or previously noted symptoms increase in severity.

❑ Advise patient to notify health care professional of medication regimen prior to treatment or surgery.

## EVALUATION

**Clinical response to therapy can be evaluated by:** ■ Improvement in cognitive function (memory, attention, reasoning, language, ability to perform simple tasks) in patients with Alzheimer's disease.

# TACROLIMUS

**tacrolimus (oral, IV)**
(ta-**kroe**-li-mus)
Prograf

**tacrolimus (topical)**
Protopic

**CLASSIFICATION(S):**
*Therapeutic: immunosuppressants*

**Pregnancy Category C**

## INDICATIONS

■ **PO, IV:** Prevention of organ rejection in patients who have undergone allogenic liver transplantation (used concurrently with corticosteroids). ■ **Topical:** Management of moderate to severe atopic dermatitis in patients who do not respond to or cannot tolerate alternative, conventional therapies. **Unlabeled uses:** ■ Prevention of rejection of other types of organ transplantation ■ Autoimmune diseases ■ Severe recalcitrant psoriasis.

## ACTION

■ Inhibits T-lymphocyte activation. **Therapeutic Effects:** ■ Prevention of transplanted organ rejection.

## PHARMACOKINETICS

**Absorption:** Absorption following oral administration is variable (bioavailability ranges from 14.4–21.8%); minimal amounts absorbed following topical use.

**Distribution:** Crosses the placenta and enters breast milk.

**Protein Binding:** 75–99%.

**Metabolism and Excretion:** 99% metabolized by the liver.

**Half-life:** *Liver transplant patients*—11.7 hr; *healthy volunteers*—21.2 hr.

## CONTRAINDICATIONS AND PRECAUTIONS

**Contraindicated in:** ■ Hypersensitivity to tacrolimus or to castor oil (a component in the injection) ■ Concurrent use with cyclosporine should be avoided ■ Breastfeeding should be avoided.

**Use Cautiously in:** ■ Renal or hepatic impairment (dosage reduction may be required; if oliguria occurs, wait 48 hr before initiating tacrolimus) ■ Children (higher end of dosing range required to maintain adequate blood levels) ■ Pregnancy (hyperkalemia and renal impairment may occur in the newborn; use only if benefit to mother justifies risk to the fetus) ■ topical: superficial skin infections.

## ADVERSE REACTIONS AND SIDE EFFECTS*

Noted primarily for PO and IV use ■ **CNS:** SEIZURES, headache, insomnia, tremor, abnormal dreams, agitation, anxiety, confusion, dizziness, emotional lability, mental depression, hallucinations, psychoses, somnolence ■ **EENT:** abnormal vision, amblyopia, rhinitis, sinusitis, tinnitus, voice change ■ **Resp:** asthma, bronchitis, cough, pharyngitis, pneumonia, pulmonary edema ■ **CV:** ascites, hypertension, peripheral edema ■ **GI:** GI BLEEDING, abdominal pain, anorexia, diarrhea, nausea, vomiting, cholangitis, cholestatic jaundice, dyspepsia, dysphagia, flatulence, increased appetite, increased liver function studies, oral thrush, peritonitis ■ **GU:** nephrotoxicity, urinary tract infection ■ **Derm:** pruritus, rash, alopecia, herpes simplex, hirsutism, photosensitivity, sweating ■ **Endo:** hyperglycemia ■ **F and E:** hyperkalemia, hypomagnesemia, acidosis, alkalosis, hyperlipidemia, hyperphosphatemia, hyperuricemia, hypocalcemia, hypokalemia, hyponatremia, hypophosphatemia ■ **Hemat:** anemia, lymphocytosis, thrombocytopenia, coagulation defects, leukopenia ■ **Local:** *topical*—burning, stinging, soreness ■ **MS:** arthralgia, hypertonia, leg cramps, muscle spasm, myalgia, myasthenia, osteoporosis ■ **Neuro:** paresthesia, neuropathy ■ **Misc:** allergic reactions including ANAPHYLAXIS, general-

ized pain, abnormal healing, chills, fever, increased risk of lymphoma.

## INTERACTIONS

Noted primarily for PO and IV use, but should be considered for topical use.

**Drug-Drug:** ■ Risk of nephrotoxicity is increased by concurrent use of **aminoglycosides, amphotericin B, cisplatin,** or **cyclosporine** (allow 24 hr to pass after stopping cyclosporine before starting tacrolimus) ■ Concurrent use of **potassium-sparing diuretics** or **ACE inhibitors** increases the risk of hyperkalemia ■ The following drugs increase tacrolimus blood levels: **azole antifungals, bromocriptine, calcium channel blockers, cimetidine, clarithromycin, cyclosporine, danazol, erythromycin, methylprednisolone,** and **metoclopramide** ■ **Phenobarbital, phenytoin, carbamazepine,** and **rifamycins** may decrease tacrolimus blood levels ■ **Vaccinations** may be less effective if given concurrently with tacrolimus (avoid use of live-virus vaccines).

**Drug-Natural Products:** ■ Concomitant use with **astragalus, echinacea,** and **melatonin** may interfere with immunosuppression.

**Drug-Food:** ■ **Food** decreases the rate and extent of GI absorption ■ **Grapefruit juice** increases absorption.

## ROUTE AND DOSAGE

■ **PO (Adults):** 0.075–0.15 mg/kg q 12 hr.
■ **PO (Children):** Start therapy at 0.15 mg/kg q 12 hr.
■ **IV (Adults):** 0.05–0.1 mg/kg/day as a continuous infusion.
■ **IV (Children):** 0.1 mg/kg/day as a continuous infusion.
■ **Topical (Adults):** Apply 0.03% or 0.1% ointment twice daily, continue for one week following resolution of atopic dermatitis.
■ **Topical (Children ≥2–15 yr):** Apply 0.03% ointment twice daily, continue for one week following resolution of atopic dermatitis.

## AVAILABILITY

■ *Capsules:* 1 mg$^{Rx}$, 5 mg$^{Rx}$ ■ *Injection:* 5 mg/ml in 1-ml ampules$^{Rx}$ ■ *Ointment:*

---

{ } = Available in Canada only.
*CAPITALS indicates life-threatening; underlines indicate most frequent.

0.03%$^{Rx}$ in 30- and 60-g tubes, 0.1% in 30- and 60-g tubes.

TIME/ACTION PROFILE (immunosuppression)

| | ONSET | PEAK | DURATION |
|---|---|---|---|
| PO | rapid | 1.3–3.2 hr* | 12 hr |
| IV | rapid | unknown | 8–12 hr |
| topical† | unknown | 1–2 wk | unknown |

*Blood level.
†Improvement in atopic dermatitis.

## NURSING IMPLICATIONS

### ASSESSMENT

- **Prevention of Organ Rejection:** Monitor blood pressure closely during therapy. Hypertension is a common complication of tacrolimus therapy and should be treated.

- ◻ Observe patients receiving IV tacrolimus for the development of anaphylaxis (rash, pruritus, laryngeal edema, wheezing) for at least 30 min and frequently thereafter. If signs develop, stop infusion and initiate treatment.

- **Atopic Dermatitis:** Assess skin lesions prior to and periodically during therapy.

- **Lab Test Considerations:** Tacrolimus blood level monitoring may be helpful in the evaluation of rejection and toxicity, dose adjustments, and assessment of compliance. Tacrolimus whole blood concentrations measured with enzyme-linked immunosorbent assay (ELISA) were the most variable during the 1st wk post-transplantation. After the 1st wk, median trough blood concentrations ranged from 9.8–19.4 ng/ml.

- ◻ Monitor serum creatinine, potassium, and glucose closely. Elevated serum creatinine and decreased urine output may indicate nephrotoxicity. May cause hyperglycemia; may require insulin therapy.

- ◻ May also cause hyperuricemia, hypokalemia, hypomagnesemia, acidosis, alkalosis, hyperlipidemia, hyperphosphatemia, hypophosphatemia, hypocalcemia, and hyponatremia.

- ◻ Monitor CBC and platelet count. May cause anemia, lymphocytosis, and thrombocytopenia.

- **Toxicity and Overdose:** Tremor and headache have been associated with high whole blood concentrations of tacrolimus and may respond to dose adjustment.

## POTENTIAL NURSING DIAGNOSES
- Infection, risk for (Adverse Reactions).

## IMPLEMENTATION

- **General:** Therapy with tacrolimus should be started no sooner than 6 hr post-transplantation. Concurrent therapy with corticosteroids is recommended in the early postoperative period.

- ◻ Oral therapy is preferred because of the risk of anaphylactic reactions with IV tacrolimus. IV therapy should be replaced with oral therapy as soon as possible.

- ◻ Adults should be started at the lower end of the dose range; children require and tolerate higher doses and should be started at upper end of dosing range.

- **PO:** Oral doses can be initiated 8–12 hr after discontinuation of IV doses.

- **Continuous Infusion:** Dilute in 0.9% NaCl or D5W for a concentration of 0.004–0.02 mg/ml prior to use. May be stored in polyethylene or glass containers for 24 hr following dilution. Do not store in PVC containers.

- **Rate:** Administer daily dose as a continuous infusion over 24 hr.

- **Y-Site Compatibility:** ◆ acyclovir ◆ aminophylline ◆ amphotericin B ◆ ampicillin ◆ ampicillin/sulbactam ◆ benztropine ◆ calcium gluconate ◆ cefazolin ◆ cefotetan ◆ ceftazidime ◆ ceftriaxone ◆ cefuroxime ◆ chloramphenicol ◆ cimetidine ◆ ciprofloxacin ◆ clindamycin ◆ digoxin ◆ diphenhydramine ◆ dobutamine ◆ dopamine ◆ doxycycline ◆ erythromycin lactobionate ◆ esmolol ◆ fluconazole ◆ furosemide ◆ ganciclovir ◆ gentamicin ◆ haloperidol ◆ heparin ◆ hydrocortisone sodium succinate ◆ hydromorphone ◆ imipenem/cilastatin ◆ insulin ◆ isoproterenol ◆ leucovorin ◆ lorazepam ◆ methylprednisolone ◆ metoclopramide ◆ metronidazole ◆ multivitamins ◆ nitroprusside ◆ nitroglycerin ◆ oxacillin ◆ penicillin G potassium ◆ perphenazine ◆ phenytoin ◆ piperacillin ◆ potassium ◆ propranolol ◆ ranitidine ◆ sodium bicarbonate ◆ tobramycin ◆ trimethoprim/sulfamethoxazole ◆ vancomycin.

## PATIENT/FAMILY TEACHING
- ◻ Instruct patient to take tacrolimus at the same time each day, as directed. Do not skip or double up on missed doses. Do not discontinue medication without advice of health care professional.

❑ Reinforce the need for lifelong therapy to prevent transplant rejection. Review symptoms of rejection for transplanted organ and stress need to notify health care professional immediately if they occur.

❑ Emphasize the importance of repeated lab tests during tacrolimus therapy.

❑ Advise patient to avoid eating raw oysters or other shellfish; make sure they are fully cooked before eating.

❑ Instruct patient to avoid exposure to chicken pox, measles, mumps, and rubella. If exposed, see health care professional for prophylactic therapy.

❑ Advise patient of the risk of taking tacrolimus during pregnancy.

❑ Inform patient of the risk of lymphoma with tacrolimus therapy.

## EVALUATION

**Effectiveness of therapy can be demonstrated by:** ■ Prevention of transplanted liver rejection ■ Management of atopic dermatitis.

## tamoxifen

(ta-**mox**-i-fen)

{Alpha-Tamoxifen}, {Med Tamoxifen}, Nolvadex, {Nolvadex-D}, {Novo-Tamoxifen}, {Tamofen}, {Tamone}, {Tamoplex}

### CLASSIFICATION(S):

**Therapeutic:** antineoplastics
**Pharmacologic:** antiestrogens

### Pregnancy Category D

## INDICATIONS

■ Adjuvant therapy of breast cancer after surgery and radiation (delays recurrence) ■ Palliative or adjunctive treatment of advanced breast cancer ■ Prevention of breast cancer in high-risk patients ■ Treatment of ductal carcinoma *in situ* following breast surgery and radiation ■ McCune-Albright syndrome with precocious puberty in girls 2–10 yr.

## ACTION

■ Competes with estrogen for binding sites in breast and other tissues ■ Reduces DNA synthesis and estrogen response. **Therapeutic Effects:** ■ Suppression of tumor growth ■ Reduced incidence of breast cancer in high-risk patients ■ Delayed puberty in McCune-Albright syndrome.

## PHARMACOKINETICS

**Absorption:** Absorbed after oral administration.

**Distribution:** Widely distributed.

**Metabolism and Excretion:** Mostly metabolized by the liver. Slowly eliminated in the feces. Minimal amounts excreted in the urine.

**Half-life:** 7 days.

## CONTRAINDICATIONS AND PRECAUTIONS

**Contraindicated in:** ■ Hypersensitivity ■ Concurrent warfarin therapy with history of deep vein thrombosis (patients at high risk for breast cancer only) ■ Pregnancy or lactation.

**Use Cautiously in:** ■ Decreased bone marrow reserve ■ Women with childbearing potential.

## ADVERSE REACTIONS AND SIDE EFFECTS*

■ **CNS:** confusion, depression, headache, weakness ■ **EENT:** blurred vision ■ **CV:** PULMONARY EMBOLISM STROKE edema ■ **GI:** nausea, vomiting ■ **GU:** UTERINE MALIGNANCIES vaginal bleeding ■ **F and E:** hypercalcemia ■ **Hemat:** leukopenia, thrombocytopenia ■ **Metab:** hot flashes ■ **MS:** bone pain ■ **Misc:** tumor flare.

## INTERACTIONS

**Drug-Drug:** ■ Estrogens and aminoglutethimide may ↓ effectiveness of concurrently administered tamoxifen ■ Blood levels are ↑ by bromocriptine ■ May ↑ the anticoagulant effect of warfarin ■ Risk of thromboembolic events is ↑ by concurrent use of other antineoplastics.

## ROUTE AND DOSAGE

❑ **Treatment of Breast Cancer**
■ **PO (Adults):** 10–20 mg twice daily; doses of 20 mg/day may be taken as a single dose.

❏ **Prevention of Breast Cancer/Ductal Carcinoma** *in situ*

▪ **PO (Adults):** 20 mg once daily for 5 yr.

❏ **McCune-Albright Syndrome**

▪ **PO (Children (girls) 2–10 yr):** 20 mg once daily for up to one year.

## AVAILABILITY (generic available)

▪ *Tablets:* 10 mg$^{Rx}$, 20 mg$^{Rx}$ ▪ Cost: *Nolvadex*—10 mg $118.51/60, 20 mg $118.51/30; *generic*—10 mg $118.51/60 ▪ *Enteric-coated tablets:* {20 mg$^{Rx}$}.

TIME/ACTION PROFILE (tumor response)

| | ONSET | PEAK | DURATION |
|---|---|---|---|
| PO | 4–10 wk | several mo | several wk |

# NURSING IMPLICATIONS

## ASSESSMENT

❏ Assess for an increase in bone or tumor pain. Confer with physician or other health care professional regarding analgesics. This transient pain usually resolves despite continued therapy.

▪ *Lab Test Considerations:* Monitor CBC, platelets, and calcium levels before and during therapy. May cause transient hypercalcemia in patients with metastases to the bone. An estrogen receptor assay should be assessed before initiation of therapy.

❏ Monitor serum cholesterol and triglyceride concentrations in patients with pre-existing hyperlipidemia. May cause ↑ concentrations.

❏ Monitor hepatic function tests and thyroxine (T$_4$) periodically during therapy. May cause ↑ serum hepatic enzyme and thyroxine concentrations.

❏ Gynecologic examinations should be performed regularly; may cause variations in Papanicolaou and vaginal smears.

## POTENTIAL NURSING DIAGNOSES

▪ Knowledge, deficient, related to medication regimen (Patient/Family Teaching).

## IMPLEMENTATION

▪ **PO:** Administer with food or fluids if GI irritation becomes a problem. Consult physician or other health care professional if patient vomits shortly after administration of medication to determine need for repeat dose.

❏ Do not crush, break, chew, or administer an antacid within 1–2 hr of enteric-coated tablet.

## PATIENT/FAMILY TEACHING

❏ Instruct patient to take medication as directed. If a dose is missed, it should be omitted.

❏ If skin lesions are present, inform patient that lesions may temporarily increase in size and number and may have increased erythema.

❏ Advise patient to report bone pain to health care professional promptly. This pain may be severe. Inform patient that this may be an indication of the drug's effectiveness and will resolve over time. Analgesics should be ordered to control pain.

❏ Instruct patient to monitor weight weekly. Weight gain or peripheral edema should be reported to health care professional.

❏ This medication may induce ovulation and may have teratogenic properties. Advise patient to use a nonhormonal method of contraception during and for 1 mo after the therapy.

❏ Advise patient that medication may cause hot flashes. Notify health care professional if these become bothersome.

❏ Instruct patient to notify health care professional promptly if pain or swelling of legs, shortness of breath, weakness, sleepiness, confusion, nausea, vomiting, weight gain, dizziness, headache, loss of appetite, or blurred vision occurs. Patient should also report menstrual irregularities, vaginal bleeding, pelvic pain, or pressure.

## EVALUATION

**Effectiveness of therapy can be demonstrated by:** ▪ Decrease in the size or spread of breast cancer. Observable effects of therapy may not be seen for 4–10 wk after initiation ▪ Delayed puberty in McCune-Albright syndrome.

# tamsulosin

(tam-**soo**-loe-sin)

Flomax

*CLASSIFICATION(S):*
*Therapeutic: none assigned*

**Pharmacologic:** *peripherally acting antiadrenergics*

**Pregnancy Category B**

## INDICATIONS

■ Management of outflow obstruction in male patients with prostatic hyperplasia.

## ACTION

■ Decreases contractions in smooth muscle of the prostatic capsule by preferentially binding to alpha$_1$-adrenergic receptors. **Therapeutic Effects:** ■ Decreased symptoms of prostatic hyperplasia (urinary urgency, hesitancy, nocturia).

## PHARMACOKINETICS

**Absorption:** Slowly absorbed after oral administration.
**Distribution:** Widely distributed.
**Protein Binding:** 94–99%.
**Metabolism and Excretion:** Extensively metabolized by the liver; <10% excreted unchanged in urine.
**Half-life:** 14 hr.

## CONTRAINDICATIONS AND PRECAUTIONS

**Contraindicated in:** ■ Hypersensitivity.
**Use Cautiously in:** ■ Patients at risk for prostate carcinoma (symptoms may be similar).

## ADVERSE REACTIONS AND SIDE EFFECTS*

■ **CNS:** <u>dizziness</u>, <u>headache</u> ■ **EENT:** rhinitis ■ **CV:** orthostatic hypotension ■ **GU:** retrograde/diminished ejaculation.

## INTERACTIONS

**Drug-Drug:** ■ **Cimetidine** may increase blood levels and the risk of toxicity ■ Increased risk of hypotension with other peripherally acting antiadrenergics (**doxazosin, prazosin, terazosin**); concurrent use should be avoided.

## ROUTE AND DOSAGE

■ **PO (Adults):** 0.4 mg once daily after a meal; may be increased after 2–4 wk to 0.8 mg/day.

## AVAILABILITY

■ **Capsules:** 0.4 mg$^{Rx}$ ■ Cost:$172.97/100.

TIME/ACTION PROFILE (increase in urine flow)

| | ONSET | PEAK | DURATION |
|---|---|---|---|
| PO | unknown | 2 wk | unknown |

# NURSING IMPLICATIONS

## ASSESSMENT

❑ Assess patient for symptoms of prostatic hyperplasia (urinary hesitancy, feeling of incomplete bladder emptying, interruption of urinary stream, impairment of size and force of urinary stream, terminal urinary dribbling, straining to start flow, dysuria, urgency) before and periodically throughout therapy.
❑ Assess patient for first-dose orthostatic hypotension and syncope. Incidence may be dose related. Observe patient closely during this period and take precautions to prevent injury.
❑ Monitor intake and output ratios and daily weight, and assess for edema daily, especially at beginning of therapy. Report weight gain or edema.

## POTENTIAL NURSING DIAGNOSES

■ Injury, risk for (Side Effects).
■ Urinary elimination, impaired (Indications).

## IMPLEMENTATION

■ **General:** Do not confuse Flomax (tamsulosin) with Fosamax (alendronate) or Volmax (albuterol).
■ **PO:** Administer daily dose 30 min after the same meal each day.
❑ If dose is interrupted for several days at either the 0.4-mg or 0.8-mg dose, restart therapy with the 0.4-mg/day dose.

## PATIENT/FAMILY TEACHING

❑ Emphasize the importance of continuing to take this medication, even if feeling well. Instruct patient to take medication at the same time each day. If a dose is missed, take as soon as remembered unless almost time for next dose. Do not double doses.

❑ May cause dizziness. Advise patient to avoid driving or other activities requiring alertness until response to medication is known.

❑ Caution patient to change positions slowly to minimize orthostatic hypotension.

❑ Advise patient to consult health care professional before taking any cough, cold, or allergy remedies.

❑ Emphasize the importance of follow-up visits to determine effectiveness of therapy.

### EVALUATION

**Effectiveness of therapy can be demonstrated by:** ■Decrease in urinary symptoms of benign prostatic hyperplasia.

## tegaserod
(te-**gas**-er-od)
Zelnorm

### CLASSIFICATION(S):
**Therapeutic:** anti-irritable bowel syndrome agents
**Pharmacologic:** 5 HT₄ agonists

### Pregnancy Category B

### INDICATIONS

■ Short-term treatment of irritable bowel syndrome (IBS) in women whose primary symptom is constipation.

### ACTION

■ Acts as a partial agonist of 5–hydroxytryptamine (5–HT, serotonin) at the 5–HT$_4$ receptor site. Agonist activity causes the release of other neurotransmitters and results in increased peristalsis, increased intestinal secretion, and decreased visceral sensitivity. **Therapeutic Effects:** ■ Decreased constipation as a chronic symptom of IBS.

### PHARMACOKINETICS

**Absorption:** 10% absorbed following oral administration.
**Distribution:** Extensively distributed to tissues.
**Protein Binding:** 98% bound to plasma proteins.
**Metabolism and Excretion:** 66% excreted unchanged in feces; remainder is metabolized in the GI tract and by the liver. Metabolites are renally excreted.

**Half-life:** 11 hr.

### CONTRAINDICATIONS AND PRECAUTIONS

**Contraindicated in:** ■ Hypersensitivity ■ Moderate to severe hepatic impairment ■ Severe renal impairment ■ History of bowel obstruction, gallbladder disease, sphincter of Oddi dysfunction, or intra-abdominal adhesions ■ Concurrent or frequent diarrhea ■ New or worsening abdominal pain.

**Use Cautiously in:** ■ Mild hepatic impairment ■ Pregnancy, lactation, or children <18 yr (safety not established).

### ADVERSE REACTIONS AND SIDE EFFECTS*

■ **CNS:** headache ■ **GI:** diarrhea.

### INTERACTIONS

**Drug-Drug:** ■ None known.

### ROUTE AND DOSAGE

■ **PO (Adults):** *Females*—6 mg twice daily before meals for 4–6 wk; if response is favorable, may be used for additional 4–6 wk.

### AVAILABILITY

■ *Tablets:* 2 mg$^{Rx}$, 6 mg$^{Rx}$.

TIME/ACTION PROFILE

| | ONSET | PEAK | DURATION |
|---|---|---|---|
| PO | unknown | 1 hr† | 1–2wk‡ |

†Blood levels.
‡Return of symptoms following discontinuation.

## NURSING IMPLICATIONS

### ASSESSMENT

❑ Assess patient for symptoms of IBS (abdominal pain or discomfort, bloating, constipation).

### POTENTIAL NURSING DIAGNOSES

■ Constipation (Indications).
■ Diarrhea (Adverse Reactions).

### IMPLEMENTATION

■ **PO:** Administer twice daily shortly before meals.

### PATIENT/FAMILY TEACHING

❑ Instruct patient to take tegaserod exactly as directed. Missed doses should be omitted; do not double dose. Take next dose as scheduled. Medication increases the movement of stool through the bowels, but does not cure IBS. If tegaserod is stopped, IBS symptoms may return within 1–2 wk.

❏ Caution patient to notify health care professional prior to taking other Rx or OTC medications or herbal products concurrently with tegaserod.

❏ Advise patient to notify health care professional if pregnancy is planned or suspected, or if breastfeeding an infant.

## EVALUATION

**Effectiveness of therapy can be demonstrated by:** ■ Decrease in abdominal pain/discomfort, bloating, and constipation.

---

## telmisartan, See ANGIOTENSIN II RECEPTOR ANTAGONISTS.

---

## temazepam

(tem-**az**-a-pam)
Restoril

### CLASSIFICATION(S):

**Therapeutic:** sedative/hypnotics
**Pharmacologic:** benzodiazepines

### Schedule IV

### Pregnancy Category X

## INDICATIONS

■ Short-term management of insomnia.

## ACTION

■ Acts at many levels in the CNS, producing generalized depression ■ Effects may be mediated by GABA, an inhibitory neurotransmitter. **Therapeutic Effects:** ■ Relief of insomnia.

## PHARMACOKINETICS

**Absorption:** Well absorbed after oral administration.

**Distribution:** Widely distributed; crosses blood-brain barrier. Probably crosses the placenta and enters breast milk. Accumulation of drug occurs with chronic dosing.

**Protein Binding:** 96%.

**Metabolism and Excretion:** Metabolized by the liver.

**Half-life:** 10–20 hr.

## CONTRAINDICATIONS AND PRECAUTIONS

**Contraindicated in:** ■ Hypersensitivity ■ Cross-sensitivity with other benzodiazepines may exist ■ Pre-existing CNS depression ■ Severe uncontrolled pain ■ Narrow-angle glaucoma ■ Pregnancy or lactation.

**Use Cautiously in:** ■ Pre-existing hepatic dysfunction ■ History of suicide attempt or drug addiction ■ Geriatric or debilitated patients (dosage reduction recommended).

## ADVERSE REACTIONS AND SIDE EFFECTS*

■ **CNS:** <u>hangover</u>, dizziness, drowsiness, lethargy, paradoxic excitation ■ **EENT:** blurred vision ■ **GI:** constipation, diarrhea, nausea, vomiting ■ **Derm:** rashes ■ **Misc:** physical dependence, psychological dependence, tolerance.

## INTERACTIONS

**Drug-Drug:** ■ Additive CNS depression with **alcohol, antidepressants, antihistamines, opioid analgesics,** and other **sedative/hypnotics** ■ May decrease efficacy of **levodopa** ■ **Rifampin** or **smoking** increases metabolism and may decrease effectiveness of temazepam ■ **Probenecid** may prolong the effects of temazepam ■ Sedative effects may be antagonized by **theophylline.**

**Drug-Natural Products:** ■ Concomitant use of **kava, valerian, skullcap, chamomile,** or **hops** can increase CNS depression.

## ROUTE AND DOSAGE

■ **PO (Adults):** 15–30 mg at bedtime initially if needed; some patients may require only 7.5 mg.

■ **PO (Geriatric Patients or Debilitated Patients):** 7.5 mg at bedtime.

## AVAILABILITY (generic available)

■ *Capsules:* 7.5 mg$^{Rx}$, 15 mg$^{Rx}$, 30 mg$^{Rx}$ ■ Cost: *Restoril*—7.5 mg $78.38/100, 15 mg

$87.64/100, 30 mg $98.01/100; *generic*—7.5 mg $53.39/100, 15 mg $62.75/100, 30 mg $59.84/100.

TIME/ACTION PROFILE (sedation)

| | ONSET | PEAK | DURATION |
|---|---|---|---|
| PO | 30 min | 2–3 hr | 6–8 hr |

## NURSING IMPLICATIONS

### ASSESSMENT

❏ Assess sleep patterns before and periodically throughout course of therapy.
❏ Prolonged high-dose therapy may lead to psychological or physical dependence. Restrict amount of drug available to patient, especially if patient is depressed or suicidal or has a history of addiction.

### POTENTIAL NURSING DIAGNOSES

■ Sleep pattern disturbed (Indications).
■ Injury, risk for (Side Effects).

### IMPLEMENTATION

■ **General:** Do not confuse temazepam with flurazepam.
❏ Supervise ambulation and transfer of patients after administration. Remove cigarettes. Side rails should be raised and call bell within reach at all times.
■ **PO:** Administer with food if GI irritation becomes a problem.

### PATIENT/FAMILY TEACHING

❏ Instruct patient to take temazepam exactly as directed. Discuss the importance of preparing environment for sleep (dark room, quiet, avoidance of nicotine and caffeine). If less effective after a few weeks, consult health care professional; do not increase dose.
❏ May cause daytime drowsiness or dizziness. Caution patient to avoid driving or other activities requiring alertness until response to medication is known.
❏ Advise patient to avoid the use of alcohol and other CNS depressants and to consult health care professional before using OTC preparations that contain antihistamines or alcohol.
❏ Advise patient to inform health care professional if pregnancy is planned or suspected.
❏ Emphasize the importance of follow-up appointments to monitor progress.

### EVALUATION

**Effectiveness of therapy can be demonstrated by:** ■ Improvement in sleep habits, which may not be noticeable until the 3rd day of therapy.

## tenecteplase, See THROMBOLYTIC AGENTS.

## tenofovir disoproxil fumarate
(te-**noe**-fo-veer die-**so**-prox-ill fume-**uh**-rate)
Viread

### CLASSIFICATION(S):
**Therapeutic:** *antiretrovirals*
**Pharmacologic:** *nucleoside reverse transcriptase inhibitors*

**Pregnancy Category B**

### INDICATIONS

■ HIV infection (with other antiretrovirals).

### ACTION

■ Active drug (tenofovir) is phosphorylated intracellularly; tenofovir diphosphate inhibits HIV reverse transcriptase resulting in disruption of DNA synthesis. **Therapeutic Effects:** ■ Slowed progression of HIV infection and decreased occurrence of sequelae ■ Increases CDT cell count and decreases viral load.

### PHARMACOKINETICS

**Absorption:** Tenofovir disoproxil fumarate is a prodrug, which is split into tenofovir, the active component.

**Distribution:** Absorption is enhanced by food.

**Metabolism and Excretion:** 70–80% excreted unchanged in urine by glomerular filtration and active tubular secretion.

**Half-life:** Unknown.

### CONTRAINDICATIONS AND PRECAUTIONS

**Contraindicated in:** ■ Hypersensitivity ■ Lactation (HIV-infected women should not breastfeed).

**Use Cautiously in:** ■ Obesity, women, prolonged nucleoside exposure (may be risk factors for lactic acidosis/hepatomegaly) ■ Renal impairment (use cautiously if CCr <60 ml/min) ■ Pregnancy (has been used safely) ■ Children (safety not established).

## ADVERSE REACTIONS AND SIDE EFFECTS*

■ **CNS:** headache, weakness ■ **GI:** HEPATOMEGALY (with steatosis), <u>nausea</u>, abdominal pain, anorexia, diarrhea, vomiting, flatulence ■ **GU:** renal impairment ■ **F and E:** LACTIC ACIDOSIS hypophosphatemia.

## INTERACTIONS

**Drug-Drug:** ■ Concurrent use with **didanosine** results in ↑ blood levels of didanosine (tenofovir should be given 2 hours before or 1 hour after didanosine) ■ Blood levels may be ↑ by **cidofovir, acyclovir, ganciclovir,** or **valganciclovir** ■ Risk of renal toxicity ↑ by other **nephrotoxic agents** ■ Combination therapy with **atazanavir** may lead to ↓ virologic response and possible resistance to atazanavir (small amounts of **ritonavir** may be added to boost blood levels) ■ Combination therapy with **abacavir** and **lamivudine** may also lead to virologic nonresponse and should be avoided.

## ROUTE AND DOSAGE

■ **PO (Adults):** 300 mg once daily.

## AVAILABILITY

■ *Tablets:* 300 mg^Rx.

TIME/ACTION PROFILE (blood levels)

| | ONSET | PEAK | DURATION |
|---|---|---|---|
| PO | unknown | 2 hr* | 24 hr |

*When taken with food.

## NURSING IMPLICATIONS

### ASSESSMENT

❑ Monitor patient for change in severity of HIV symptoms and for symptoms of opportunistic infection before and during therapy.

■ *Lab Test Considerations:* Monitor viral load and CD4 count before and routinely during therapy to determine response.

❑ May cause ↑ AST, ALT, alkaline phosphatase, creatine kinase, amylase, and triglyceride concentrations. Lactic acidosis may occur with hepatic toxicity causing hepatic steatosis; may be fatal, especially in women.

❑ May cause hypophosphatemia in patients with renal impairment.

❑ May cause hyperglycemia and glucosuria.

## POTENTIAL NURSING DIAGNOSES

■ Infection, risk for (Indications, Side Effects).

■ Injury, risk for (Side Effects).

## IMPLEMENTATION

■ **General:** When tenofovir is administered concomitantly with didanosine, administer tenofovir 2 hr before or 1 hr after didanosine.

■ **PO:** Administer once daily with a meal.

## PATIENT/FAMILY TEACHING

❑ Instruct patient on the importance of taking tenofovir as directed, even if feeling better. Do not take more than prescribed amount and do not stop taking without consulting health care professional. Take missed doses as soon as remembered; do not double doses. Caution patient not to share or trade this medication with others.

❑ Inform patient that tenofovir may cause hyperglycemia. Advise patient to notify health care professional if increased thirst or hunger; unexplained weight loss; increased urination; fatigue; or dry, itchy skin occurs.

❑ Advise patient to avoid taking other medications (prescription, OTC, or herbal products), without consulting health care professional.

❑ Caution patient to avoid crowds and persons with known infections.

❑ Inform patient that tenofovir does not cure AIDS and does not reduce the risk of transmission of HIV to others through sexual contact or blood contamination. Caution patient to use a condom and avoid sharing needles or donating blood to prevent spreading HIV to others.

❑ Inform patient that changes in body fat distribution (increased fat in upper back and neck, breast, and trunk, and loss of fat from

legs, arms, and face) may occur, but may not be related to drug therapy.
- ❑ Emphasize the importance of regular exams to monitor for side effects.

### EVALUATION
**Effectiveness of therapy can be demonstrated by:** ▪ Decreased incidence of opportunistic infection and slowed progression of HIV infection.

---

## terazosin
(ter-**ay**-zoe-sin)
Hytrin

**CLASSIFICATION(S):**
**Therapeutic:** *antihypertensives*
**Pharmacologic:** *peripherally acting antiadrenergics*

**Pregnancy Category C**

---

### INDICATIONS
▪ Mild to moderate hypertension (alone or with other agents) ▪ Urinary outflow obstruction in patients with prostatic hyperplasia.

### ACTION
▪ Dilates both arteries and veins by blocking postsynaptic alpha₁-adrenergic receptors ▪ Decreases contractions in smooth muscle of the prostatic capsule. **Therapeutic Effects:** ▪ Lowering of blood pressure ▪ Decreased symptoms of prostatic hyperplasia (urinary urgency, hesitancy, nocturia).

### PHARMACOKINETICS
**Absorption:** Well absorbed after oral administration.
**Distribution:** Unknown.
**Metabolism and Excretion:** 50% metabolized by the liver. 10% excreted unchanged by the kidneys. 20% excreted unchanged in feces. 40% eliminated in bile.
**Half-life:** 12 hr.

### CONTRAINDICATIONS AND PRECAUTIONS
**Contraindicated in:** ▪ Hypersensitivity.
**Use Cautiously in:** ▪ Deyhdration, volume or sodium depletion, increased risk of hypoten-

sion ▪ Pregnancy, lactation, or children (safety not established).

### ADVERSE REACTIONS AND SIDE EFFECTS*
▪ **CNS:** <u>dizziness</u>, <u>headache</u>, <u>weakness</u>, drowsiness, nervousness ▪ **EENT:** <u>nasal congestion</u>, blurred vision, conjunctivitis, sinusitis ▪ **Resp:** dyspnea ▪ **CV:** <u>first-dose orthostatic hypotension</u>, arrhythmias, chest pain, palpitations, peripheral edema, tachycardia ▪ **GI:** <u>nausea</u>, abdominal pain, diarrhea, dry mouth, vomiting ▪ **GU:** impotence, urinary frequency ▪ **Derm:** pruritus ▪ **Metab:** weight gain ▪ **MS:** arthralgia, back pain, extremity pain ▪ **Neuro:** paresthesia ▪ **Misc:** fever.

### INTERACTIONS
**Drug-Drug:** ▪ ↑ hypotension with other **antihypertensives,** acute ingestion of **alcohol,** or **nitrates** ▪ **NSAIDs, sympathomimetics,** or **estrogens** may ↓ effects of antihypertensive therapy.

### ROUTE AND DOSAGE
The first dose should be taken at bedtime.

❑ **Hypertension**
▪ **PO (Adults):** 1 mg initially, then slowly increase up to 5 mg/day (usual range 1–5 mg/day); may be given as single dose or in 2 divided doses (not to exceed 20 mg/day).

❑ **Benign Prostatic Hyperplasia**
▪ **PO (Adults):** 1 mg at bedtime; gradually may be increased up to 5–10 mg/day.

### AVAILABILITY (generic available)
▪ **Tablets:** 1 mg^Rx, 2 mg^Rx, 5 mg^Rx, 10 mg^Rx ▪ Cost: 1 mg $203.90/100, 2 mg $203.90/100, 5 mg $203.90/100, 10 mg $203.90/100.

TIME/ACTION PROFILE

|  | ONSET† | PEAK‡ | DURATION† |
|---|---|---|---|
| PO-hypertension | 15 min | 6–8 wk | 24 hr |
| PO-prostatic hyperplasia | 2–6 wk | unknown | unknown |

†After single dose.
‡After multiple oral dosing.

## NURSING IMPLICATIONS

### ASSESSMENT

- **General Info:** Monitor blood pressure (lying and standing) and pulse frequently during initial dose adjustment and periodically during therapy. Notify physician or other health care professional of significant changes.
- Assess patient for first-dose orthostatic reaction and syncope. May occur 30 min–2 hr after initial dose and occasionally thereafter. Incidence may be dose related. Volume-depleted or sodium-restricted patients may be more sensitive to this effect.
- Monitor intake and output ratios and daily weight; assess for edema daily, especially at beginning of therapy.
- **Hypertension:** Monitor frequency of prescription refills to determine adherence.
- **Benign Prostatic Hyperplasia:** Assess patient for symptoms of prostatic hyperplasia (urinary hesitancy, feeling of incomplete bladder emptying, interruption of urinary stream, impairment of size and force of urinary stream, terminal urinary dribbling, straining to start flow, dysuria, urgency) before and periodically during therapy.
- Rule out prostatic carcinoma before therapy; symptoms are similar.

### POTENTIAL NURSING DIAGNOSES

- Injury, risk for (Side Effects).
- Noncompliance (Patient/Family Teaching).

### IMPLEMENTATION

- **General:** May be used in combination with diuretics or beta blockers to minimize sodium and water retention. If these are added to terazosin therapy, reduce dose of terazosin initially and titrate to effect.
- **PO:** Administer daily dose at bedtime. If necessary, dose may be increased to twice daily.

### PATIENT/FAMILY TEACHING

- **General Info:** Instruct patient to take medication at the same time each day. Take missed doses as soon as remembered. If not remembered until next day, omit; do not double doses.

- Advise patient to weigh self twice weekly and assess feet and ankles for fluid retention.
- May cause dizziness or drowsiness. Advise patient to avoid driving or other activities requiring alertness until response to the medication is known.
- Caution patient to avoid sudden changes in position to decrease orthostatic hypotension. Alcohol, CNS depressants, standing for long periods, hot showers, and exercising in hot weather should be avoided because of enhanced orthostatic effects.
- Advise patient to consult health care professional before taking any cough, cold, or allergy remedies.
- Instruct patient to notify health care professional of medication regimen before any surgery.
- Advise patient to notify health care professional if frequent dizziness, fainting, or swelling of feet or lower legs occurs.
- Emphasize the importance of follow-up exams to evaluate effectiveness of medication.
- **Hypertension:** Emphasize the importance of continuing to take this medication as directed, even if feeling well. Medication controls but does not cure hypertension.
- Encourage patient to comply with additional interventions for hypertension (weight reduction, low-sodium diet, smoking cessation, moderation of alcohol consumption, regular exercise, and stress management).
- Instruct patient and family on proper technique for blood pressure monitoring. Advise them to check blood pressure at least weekly and to report significant changes.

### EVALUATION

**Effectiveness of therapy can be demonstrated by:** ■ Decrease in blood pressure without appearance of side effects ■ Decreased symptoms of prostatic hyperplasia. May require 2–6 wk of therapy before effects are noticeable.

## terbinafine
(ter-**bi**-na-feen)
Lamisil

---

## INDICATIONS

■ Onychomycosis (fungal nail infection).

## ACTION

■ Interferes with fungal cell wall synthesis (ergosterol biosynthesis) by inhibiting the enzyme squalene epoxidase. **Therapeutic Effects:** ■ Fungal cell death. **Spectrum:** ■ Active against dermatophytes and other fungi.

## PHARMACOKINETICS

**Absorption:** 70–80% absorbed after oral administration.
**Distribution:** Extensively distributed; penetrates dermis and epidermis; concentrates in stratum corneum, hair, scalp, and nails. Enters breast milk.
**Protein Binding:** 99%.
**Metabolism and Excretion:** Extensively metabolized by the liver.
**Half-life:** *Plasma*—22 days; longer from skin and nails.

## CONTRAINDICATIONS AND PRECAUTIONS

**Contraindicated in:** ■ Hypersensitivity ■ Chronic or active liver disease ■ CHF of left ventricular dysfunction.
**Use Cautiously in:** ■ History of alcoholism ■ Renal impairment (dosage reduction recommended for CCr <50 ml/min) ■ Pregnancy, lactation, or children (safety not established).

## ADVERSE REACTIONS AND SIDE EFFECTS*

■ **CV:** CHF ■ **GI:** HEPATOTOXICITY, anorexia, diarrhea, nausea, stomach pain, vomiting, altered taste, drug-induced hepatitis, taste disturbance ■ **Derm:** TOXIC EPIDERMAL NECROLYSIS, itching, rash ■ **Hemat:** neutropenia, pancytopenia ■ **Misc:** STEVENS-JOHNSON SYNDROME.

## INTERACTIONS

**Drug-Drug:** ■ **Alcohol** or other **hepatotoxic agents** may increase the risk of hepatotoxicity ■ **Rifampin** and other **drugs that induce he-**patic drug-metabolizing enzymes may decrease effectiveness ■ **Cimetidine** and other **drugs that inhibit hepatic drug-metabolizing enzymes** may increase effectiveness.
**Drug-Natural Products:** ■ Increased **caffeine** levels and side effects with caffeine-containing herbs (**cola nut, guarana, mate, tea, coffee**).

## ROUTE AND DOSAGE

■ **PO (Adults):** 250 mg once daily for 6 wk for fingernail infection or 12 wk for toenail infection.

## AVAILABILITY

■ *Tablets:* 250 mg^Rx ■ Cost: $229.61/30.

TIME/ACTION PROFILE (antifungal tissue levels)

|  | ONSET | PEAK | DURATION |
|------|---------------|------------|--------------|
| PO | several days | days–wks | several wks |

# NURSING IMPLICATIONS

## ASSESSMENT

❑ Assess patient for signs and symptoms of infection (nail beds) before and periodically throughout therapy.
❑ Specimens for culture should be taken before instituting therapy. Therapy may be started before results are obtained.
■ *Lab Test Considerations:* CBC should be monitored in patients receiving therapy for >6 wk. Discontinue if abnormal values occur.
❑ Monitor AST and ALT prior to, and periodically throughout, therapy. Terbinafine should be discontinued if symptomatic elevations occur.
❑ If signs of secondary infection occur, monitor neutrophil count. If <1000/mm³, discontinue treatment.
❑ May cause decrease in absolute lymphocyte count.
❑ Monitor serum potassium. May cause hypokalemia.

## POTENTIAL NURSING DIAGNOSES

■ Infection, risk for (Indications).
■ Noncompliance (Patient/Family Teaching).

## IMPLEMENTATION

- **General:** Do not confuse with lamotrigine (Lamictal).
- **PO:** May be administered without regard to food.

## PATIENT/FAMILY TEACHING

- Instruct patient to take medication exactly as directed, for the full course of therapy, even if feeling better. Doses should be taken at the same time each day.
- Instruct patient to notify health care professional immediately if signs and symptoms of liver dysfunction (unusual fatigue, anorexia, nausea, vomiting, upper right abdominal pain, jaundice, dark urine, or pale stools) occur. Terbinafine should be discontinued.
- Advise patient to consult health care professional before taking any Rx or OTC medications concurrently with terbinafine.

## EVALUATION

**Effectiveness of therapy can be demonstrated by:** ■ Resolution of clinical and laboratory indications of fungal nail infections. Inadequate period of treatment may lead to recurrence of active infection.

## terbutaline

(ter-**byoo**-ta-leen)
Brethaire, Bricanyl

*CLASSIFICATION(S):*
*Therapeutic:* bronchodilators
*Pharmacologic:* adrenergics

**Pregnancy Category B**

## INDICATIONS

■ Management of reversible airway disease due to asthma or COPD; inhalation and subcut used for short-term control and oral agent as long-term control. **Unlabeled uses:** ■ Management of preterm labor (tocolytic).

## ACTION

■ Results in the accumulation of cyclic adenosine monophosphate (cAMP) at beta-adrenergic receptors ■ Produces bronchodilation ■ Inhibits the release of mediators of immediate hypersensitivity reactions from mast cells ■ Relatively selective for beta$_2$(pulmonary)-adrenergic receptor sites, with less effect on beta$_1$(cardiac)-adrenergic receptors. **Therapeutic Effects:** ■ Bronchodilation.

## PHARMACOKINETICS

**Absorption:** 35–50% absorbed following oral administration but rapidly undergoes first-pass metabolism. Well absorbed following subcut administration. Minimal absorption occurs following inhalation.

**Distribution:** Enters breast milk.

**Metabolism and Excretion:** Partially metabolized by the liver; 60% excreted unchanged by the kidneys following subcut administration.

**Half-life:** Unknown.

## CONTRAINDICATIONS AND PRECAUTIONS

**Contraindicated in:** ■ Hypersensitivity to adrenergic amines ■ Known hypersensitivity or intolerance to fluorocarbons (inhalation only).

**Use Cautiously in:** ■ Cardiac disease ■ Hypertension ■ Hyperthyroidism ■ Diabetes ■ Glaucoma ■ Geriatric patients (more susceptible to adverse reactions; may require dosage reduction) ■ Excessive use may lead to tolerance and paradoxical bronchospasm (inhaler) ■ Pregnancy (near term), lactation, and children <2 yr (safety not established).

## ADVERSE REACTIONS AND SIDE EFFECTS*

■ **CNS:** nervousness, restlessness, tremor, headache, insomnia ■ **Resp:** PARADOXICAL BRONCHOSPASM (excessive use of inhalers) ■ **CV:** angina, arrhythmias, hypertension, tachycardia ■ **GI:** nausea, vomiting ■ **Endo:** hyperglycemia.

## INTERACTIONS

**Drug-Drug:** ■ Concurrent use with other **adrenergics** (sympathomimetic) will have additive adrenergic side effects ■ Use with **MAO inhibitors** may lead to hypertensive crisis ■ **Beta blockers** may negate therapeutic effect.

**Drug-Natural Products:** ■ Use with caffeine-containing herbs (**cola nut, guarana, mate, tea, coffee**) increases stimulant effect.

## ROUTE AND DOSAGE

■ **PO (Adults and Children >15 yr):** *Bronchodilation*—2.5–5 mg 3 times daily, given q 6 hr (not to exceed 15 mg/24 hr). *Tocolysis*—2.5 mg q 4–6 hr until delivery (unlabeled).

■ **PO (Children 12–15 yr):** 2.5 mg 3 times daily (given q 6 hr).

■ **Inhaln (Adults and Children ≥12 yr):** 2 inhalations (200 mcg/spray) q 4–6 hr.

■ **Subcut (Adults):** *Bronchodilation*—250 mcg; may repeat in 15–30 min (not to exceed 500 mcg/4 hr). *Tocolysis*—250 mcg q 1 hr until contractions stop (unlabeled).

■ **IV (Adults):** *Tocolysis*—10 mcg/min infusion; increase by 5 mcg/min q 10 min until contractions stop (not to exceed 80 mcg/min). After contractions have stopped for 30 min, decrease infusion rate to lowest effective amount and maintain for 4–8 hr (unlabeled).

## AVAILABILITY (generic available)

■ *Tablets:* 2.5 mg$^{Rx}$, 5 mg$^{Rx}$ ■ *Injection:* 1 mg/ml$^{Rx}$ ■ *Inhalation aerosol:* 200 mcg/spray (≥300 inhalations/10.5-g canister)$^{Rx}$, {500 mcg/spray$^{Rx}$}.

TIME/ACTION PROFILE (bronchodilation)

|        | ONSET          | PEAK              | DURATION |
|--------|----------------|-------------------|----------|
| PO     | within 60–120 min | within 2–3 hr   | 4–8 hr   |
| Inhaln | 5–30 min       | 1–2 hr            | 3–6 hr   |
| Subcut | within 15 min  | within 0.5–1 hr   | 1.5–4 hr |

## NURSING IMPLICATIONS

### ASSESSMENT

■ **Bronchodilator:** Assess lung sounds, respiratory pattern, pulse, and blood pressure before administration and during peak of medication. Note amount, color, and character of sputum produced, and notify physician or other health care professional of abnormal findings.

❑ Monitor pulmonary function tests before initiating therapy and periodically throughout course to determine effectiveness of medication.

❑ Observe for paradoxical bronchospasm (wheezing). If condition occurs, withhold medication and notify physician or other health care professional immediately.

❑ Observe patient for drug tolerance and rebound bronchospasm. Patients requiring more than 3 inhalation treatments in 24 hr should be under close supervision. If minimal or no relief is seen after 3–5 inhalation treatments within 6–12 hr, further treatment with aerosol alone is not recommended.

■ **Preterm Labor:** Monitor maternal pulse and blood pressure, frequency and duration of contractions, and fetal heart rate. Notify physician or other health care professional if contractions persist or increase in frequency or duration or if symptoms of maternal or fetal distress occur. Maternal side effects include tachycardia, palpitations, tremor, anxiety, and headache.

❑ Assess maternal respiratory status for symptoms of pulmonary edema (increased rate, dyspnea, rales/crackles, frothy sputum).

❑ Monitor mother and neonate for symptoms of hypoglycemia (anxiety; chills; cold sweats; confusion; cool, pale skin; difficulty in concentration; drowsiness; excessive hunger; headache; irritability; nausea; nervousness; rapid pulse; shakiness; unusual tiredness; or weakness) and mother for hypokalemia (weakness, fatigue, U wave on ECG, arrhythmias).

■ *Lab Test Considerations:* May cause transient decrease in serum potassium concentrations with higher than recommended doses.

❑ Monitor maternal serum glucose and electrolytes. May cause hypokalemia and hypoglycemia. Monitor neonate's serum glucose, because hypoglycemia may also occur in neonates.

■ *Toxicity and Overdose:* Symptoms of overdose include persistent agitation, chest pain or discomfort, decreased blood pressure, dizziness, hyperglycemia, hypokalemia, seizures, tachyarrhythmias, persistent trembling, and vomiting.

❑ Treatment includes discontinuing beta-adrenergic agonists and symptomatic, supportive therapy. Cardioselective beta blockers are used cautiously, because they may induce bronchospasm.

## POTENTIAL NURSING DIAGNOSES

■ Airway clearance, ineffective (Indications).

## IMPLEMENTATION

- **PO:** Administer with meals to minimize gastric irritation.

- ❏ Tablet may be crushed and mixed with food or fluids for patients with difficulty swallowing.

- **Subcut:** Administer subcut injections in lateral deltoid area. Do not use solution if discolored.

- **Continuous Infusion:** May be diluted in D5W, 0.9% NaCl, or 0.45% NaCl.

- **Rate**Use infusion pump to ensure accurate dosage. Begin infusion at 10 mcg/min. Increase dosage by 5 mcg every 10 min until contractions cease. Maximum dose is 80 mcg/min. Begin to taper dose in 5-mcg decrements after a 30–60 min contraction-free period is attained. Switch to oral dosage form after patient is contraction-free 4–8 hr on the lowest effective dose.

- **Y-Site Compatibility:** ◆ insulin.

## PATIENT/FAMILY TEACHING

- **General Info:** Instruct patient to take medication exactly as directed. If on a scheduled dosing regimen, take a missed dose as soon as possible; space remaining doses at regular intervals. Do not double doses. Caution patient not to exceed recommended dose; may cause adverse effects, paradoxical bronchospasm, or loss of effectiveness of medication.

- ❏ Instruct patient to contact health care professional immediately if shortness of breath is not relieved by medication or is accompanied by diaphoresis, dizziness, palpitations, or chest pain.

- ❏ Advise patient to consult health care professional before taking any OTC medications or alcoholic beverages concurrently with this therapy. Caution patient also to avoid smoking and other respiratory irritants.

- **Inhaln:** Review correct administration technique with patient. See Appendix F for administration with metered-dose inhaler. Wait 1–5 min before administering next dose. Mouthpiece should be washed after each use.

- ❏ Do not spray inhaler near eyes.

- ❏ Instruct patient to save inhaler; refill canisters may be available.

- ❏ Advise patients to use bronchodilator first if using other inhalation medications, and allow 15 min to elapse before administering other inhalant medications, unless otherwise directed.

- ❏ Advise patient to rinse mouth with water after each inhalation dose to minimize dry mouth.

- ❏ Advise patient to maintain adequate fluid intake (2000–3000 ml/day) to help liquefy tenacious secretions.

- ❏ Advise patient to consult health care professional if respiratory symptoms are not relieved or worsen after treatment or if chest pain, headache, severe dizziness, palpitations, nervousness, or weakness occurs.

- ❏ Instruct patient to notify health care professional if contents of one canister are used up in less than 2 wk.

- **Preterm Labor:** Health care professional should be notified immediately if labor resumes or if significant side effects occur.

## EVALUATION

**Effectiveness of therapy can be demonstrated by:** ■ Prevention or relief of bronchospasm ■ Increase in ease of breathing ■ Control of preterm labor in a fetus of 20–36 wk gestational age.

# terconazole, See ANTIFUNGALS (VAGINAL).

# teriparatide
(ter-i-**par**-a-tide)
Forteo

### CLASSIFICATION(S):
**Therapeutic:** hormones
**Pharmacologic:** parathyroid hormones (rDNA origin)

### Pregnancy Category C

## INDICATIONS

■ Treatment of osteoporosis in postmenopausal women at high risk for fractures ■ To increase bone mass in men with osteoporosis at high risk for fracture ■ Most useful for those have failed or are intolerant to other osteoporosis therapies.

## ACTION

■ Regulates calcium and phosphate metabolism in bone and kidney by binding to specific cell receptors; stimulates osteoblastic activity ■ Increases serum calcium and decreases serum phosphorus. **Therapeutic Effects:** ■ Increased bone mineral density with reduced risk of fractures.

## PHARMACOKINETICS

**Absorption:** Extensively absorbed after subcut administration.

**Distribution:** Unknown.

**Metabolism and Excretion:** Metabolized by the liver; metabolites renally excreted.

**Half-life:** 1 hr (after subcut use).

## CONTRAINDICATIONS AND PRECAUTIONS

**Contraindicated in:** ■ Hypersensitivity ■ Paget's disease of the bone or other metabolic bone disease ■ Unexplained ↑ alkaline phosphatase ■ Pediatric or young adult patients ■ Previous radiation therapy, history of bone metastases, or skeletal malignancy ■ Pre-existing hypercalcemia ■ Pregnancy or lactation.

**Use Cautiously in:** ■ Concurrent **digoxin**.

## ADVERSE REACTIONS AND SIDE EFFECTS*

■ **CV:** orthostatic hypotension.

## INTERACTIONS

**Drug-Drug:** ■ Transient hypercalcemia may increase the risk of **digoxin** toxicity.

## ROUTE AND DOSAGE

■ **Subcut (Adults):** 20 mcg once daily.

## AVAILABILITY

■ *Pre-filled pen delivery device (FORTEO pen):* delivers 20 mcg/day[Rx].

TIME/ACTION PROFILE (effects on serum calcium)

| | ONSET | PEAK | DURATION |
|---|---|---|---|
| Subcut | 2 hr | 4–6 hr | 16–24 hr |

## NURSING IMPLICATIONS

### ASSESSMENT

❑ Assess patient for bone mineral density before and periodically during therapy.

■ *Lab Test Considerations:* Effects increase serum calcium and decrease serum phosphorus. Maximum effect is within 4–6 hr. By 16-hr post-dose, serum calcium has returned to near baseline. If hypercalcemia persists, discontinue teriperatide and evaluate cause of hypercalcemia.

❑ May asymptomatically increase serum uric acid concentrations.

### POTENTIAL NURSING DIAGNOSES

■ Injury, risk for (Indications).

### IMPLEMENTATION

■ **General:** Use of teriparatide should not continue more than 2 yr.

■ **Subcut:** Administer subcut into thigh or abdominal wall once daily. May be administered at any time of day without regard to food. Solution should be clear and colorless. Do not use if solid particles appear, or if solution is cloudy or colored. Store pen in the refrigerator; do not freeze or use if it has been frozen. Minimize time out of refrigerator; use immediately and return to refrigerator. *Forteo* pen can be used for up to 28 days after the first injection. After the 28-day use period, discard the *Forteo* pen, even if it still contains some unused solution.

### PATIENT/FAMILY TEACHING

❑ Advise patient to administer medication at same time each day. If a dose is missed, administer as soon as remembered that day. Do not take more than one injection/day.

❑ Instruct patient on proper administration technique and disposal of needles. Patient should read *Medication Guide* and *User Manual* before starting therapy and re-read them each time prescription is refilled. User manual can be found at www.forteo.com/control/pen_user_manual. Caution patient to throw pen away after 28–day use period and not to share their pen with other patients.

❑ Advise patient to administer at same time each day. If a dose is missed, administer as soon as remembered that day. Do not take more than one injection/day.

❑ Discuss the importance of other treatments for osteoporosis (supplemental calcium and/or vitamin D, weight-bearing exercise, modification of behavioral factors such as smoking and/or alcohol consumption).

❑ May cause orthostatic hypotension during first several doses. Caution patient to administer medication in a lying or sitting position. If light-headedness or palpitations occur, lie down until symptoms resolve. Notify health care professional if symptoms persist or worsen.

❑ Instruct patient to notify health care professional if persistent symptoms of hypercalcemia (nausea, vomiting, constipation, lethargy, muscle weakness) occur.

❑ Emphasize the importance of follow-up tests for bone mineral density.

### EVALUATION

**Effectiveness of therapy can be demonstrated by:** ■ Increased bone mineral density with reduced risk of fractures.

# TESTOSTERONE

(tess-**toss**-te-rone)

**testosterone base**

Andro, Histerone, {Malogen}, Testamone, Testaqua, Testoject

**testosterone buccal system, mucoadhesive**

Striant

**testosterone cypionate**

Andro-Cyp, Andronate, depAndro, Depotest, Depo-Testosterone, Duratest, T-Cypionate, Testa-C, Testred, Testoject-LA, Virilon IM

**testosterone enanthate**

Andro LA, Andropository, Andryl, Delatest, Delatestryl, Everone, {Malogex}, Testone LA, Testrin-PA

**testosterone propionate**

{Malogen}, Testex

**testosterone transdermal**

Androderm, Androgel, Testim, Testoderm

### CLASSIFICATION(S):

**Therapeutic:** hormones
**Pharmacologic:** androgens

**Schedule III**

**Pregnancy Category X**

### INDICATIONS

■ Hypogonadism in androgen-deficient men ■ Delayed puberty in men ■ Androgen-responsive breast cancer (palliative).

### ACTION

■ Responsible for the normal growth and development of male sex organs ■ Maintenance of male secondary sex characteristics: ■ Growth and maturation of the prostate, seminal vesicles, penis, scrotum ■ Development of male hair distribution ■ Vocal cord thickening ■ Alterations in body musculature and fat distribution. **Therapeutic Effects:** ■ Correction of hormone deficiency in male hypogonadism ■ Initiation of male puberty ■ Suppression of tumor growth in some forms of breast cancer.

### PHARMACOKINETICS

**Absorption:** Well absorbed from IM sites. Cypionate, propionate, and enanthate salts are absorbed slowly. Well absorbed through skin (scrotal skin is 5–30 times more permeable than other sites) and buccal mucosa.

**Distribution:** Probably crosses the placenta and enters breast milk.

**Metabolism and Excretion:** Metabolized by the liver. Absorption from buccal mucosa bypasses initial liver metabolism.

**Half-life:** Base—10–100 min; cypionate—8 days.

### CONTRAINDICATIONS AND PRECAUTIONS

**Contraindicated in:** ■ Hypersensitivity ■ Pregnancy and lactation ■ Male patients with breast or prostate cancer ■ Hypercalcemia ■ Severe liver, renal, or cardiac disease ■ Some products contain tartrazine and should be avoided in patients with known hypersensitivity.

**Use Cautiously in:** ■ Diabetes mellitus ■ Coronary artery disease ■ Geriatric patients ( ↑ risk of prostatic hyperplasia/carcinoma) ■ History of liver disease ■ Prepubertal males.

## ADVERSE REACTIONS AND SIDE EFFECTS*

■ **EENT:** deepening of voice ■ **CV:** edema ■ **GI:** changes in appetite, drug-induced hepatitis, nausea, vomiting ■ **GU:** bladder irritability, menstrual irregularities, prostatic enlargement ■ **Endo:** *women*—change in libido, clitoral enlargement, decreased breast size; *men*—acne, facial hair, gynecomastia, impotence, oligospermia, priapism ■ **F and E:** hypercalcemia ■ **Local:** chronic skin irritation (transdermal), pain at injection site ■ **Misc:** gum pain/irritation (buccal system).

## INTERACTIONS

**Drug-Drug:** ■ ↓ and may ↑ action of **warfarin, oral hypoglycemic agents,** and **corticosteroids** ■ May ↑ effect of **insulin** ■ ↑ risk of hepatotoxicity with other **hepatotoxic agents** ■ Concurrent use with **corticosteroids** may ↑ risk of edema formation.

## ROUTE AND DOSAGE

◘ **Replacement Therapy**
■ **IM (Adults):** 25–50 mg 2–3 times/wk (base or propionate) *or* 50–400 mg q 2–4 wk (enanthate or cypionate).
■ **Transdermal (Adults):** *Testoderm*—4–6 mg applied q 22–24 hr. *Androderm*—5 mg applied q 24 hr; *Androgel, Testim*—5 g (contains 50 mg) applied once daily, if needed may be increased to 10 g (100 mg).
■ **Buccal (Adults):** 30 mg twice daily.

◘ **Delayed Male Puberty**
■ **IM (Children >12 yr):** Up to 100 mg/mo for up to 6 mo.

◘ **Palliative Management of Breast Cancer**
■ **IM (Adults):** 50–100 mg 3 times/wk (propionate or base) *or* 200–400 mg q 2–4 wk (cypionate or enanthate).

## AVAILABILITY (generic available)

■ ***Sterile testosterone suspension for injection (base):*** 25 mg/ml in 10-ml vials[Rx], 50 mg/ml in 10- and 30-ml vials[Rx], 100 mg/ml in 10-ml vials[Rx] ■ ***Testosterone cypionate injection (in oil):*** 100 mg/ml in 10-ml vials[Rx], 200 mg/ml in 1- and 10-ml vials[Rx] ■ ***Testosterone enanthate injection (in oil):*** 100 mg/ml in 10-ml vials[Rx], 200 mg/ml in 5- and 10-ml vials and 1-ml prefilled syringes[Rx] ■ ***Testosterone propionate injection (in oil):*** 100 mg/ml in 10-ml vials[Rx] ■ ***Testosterone transdermal patches:*** Testoderm—4 mg/ day in packages of 30[Rx], 6 mg/day in packages of 30[Rx], Androderm—2.5 mg/day in packages of 60[Rx]; 5 mg/day in packages of 60[Rx] ■ ***Testosterone gel 1% (Androgel):*** 2.5-g unit of use packets[Rx], 5-g unit of use packets ■ ***Testosterone gel 1% (Testim):*** 5-g unit of use tubes in boxes of 30[Rx] ■ ***Testosterone buccal, mucoadhesive:*** 30 mg/system in blister packs of 10 systems/pack ■ estradiol[Rx]. See Appendix B.

TIME/ACTION PROFILE (androgenic effects†)

| | ONSET | PEAK | DURATION |
|---|---|---|---|
| IM—base | unknown | unknown | 1–3 days |
| IM—cypion- ate, enant- hate | unknown | unknown | 2–4 wk |
| IM—propio- nate | unknown | unknown | 1–3 days |
| Buccal | unknown | 10–12 hr | 12 hr |
| Transdermal | unknown | 2–4 hr‡ | 2 hr§ |

†Response is highly variable among individuals; may take months.
‡Plasma testosterone levels following applications of patch (plateaus after 3–4 wk).
§Following patch removal.

# NURSING IMPLICATIONS

## ASSESSMENT

■ **General Info:** Monitor intake and output ratios, weigh patient twice weekly, and assess patient for edema. Report significant changes indicative of fluid retention.

■ **Men:** Monitor for precocious puberty in boys (acne, darkening of skin, development of male secondary sex characteristics—increase in penis size, frequent erections, growth of body hair). Bone age determinations should be measured every 6 mo to determine rate of bone maturation and effects on epiphyseal closure.

◘ Monitor for breast enlargement, persistent erections, and increased urge to urinate in men. Monitor for difficulty urinating in elderly men, because prostate enlargement may occur.

- **Women:** Assess for virilism (deepening of voice, unusual hair growth or loss, clitoral enlargement, acne, menstrual irregularity).
- In women with metastatic breast cancer, monitor for symptoms of hypercalcemia (nausea, vomiting, constipation, lethargy, loss of muscle tone, thirst, polyuria).
- *Lab Test Considerations:*Monitor hemoglobin and hematocrit periodically during therapy; may cause polycythemia.
- Monitor hepatic function tests and serum cholesterol levels periodically during therapy. May cause ↑ serum AST and bilirubin, ↑ or ↓ cholesterol levels, and suppression of clotting factors II, V, VII, and X.
- Monitor serum and urine calcium levels and serum alkaline phosphatase concentrations in metastatic cancer.
- May alter results of fasting blood glucose, glucose tolerance tests, thyroid function tests, and metyrapone tests. Increased creatine and CCr may last up to 2 wk following discontinuation of therapy. Serum chloride, potassium, phosphate, and sodium levels may be ↑.
- May cause increased levels in 24-hr urine tests for 17-ketosteroid concentrations.
- May cause decreased corticosteroid-binding globulin and sex steroid–binding globulin; free hormone concentrations remain unchanged. May also cause reduced follicle-stimulating hormone (FSH), luteinizing hormone (LH), sperm count, and hamster ova penetration test (HOPT).
- *Transdermal:* Monitor prostatic acid phosphatase and prostatic-specific antigen at regular intervals during therapy with transdermal patch. Serum testosterone determinations should be measured 2–4 hr after patch application, after 3–4 wk use.
- LH and serum ALT should be measured every 6 mo during gender change androgen therapy to monitor success and side effects.

## POTENTIAL NURSING DIAGNOSES

- Sexual dysfunction (Indications, Side Effects).

## IMPLEMENTATION

- **General:** Do not confuse testaderm (testosterone) with estraderm (estradiol). Do not confuse Virilon (testosterone) with Verelan (verapamil).
- Range-of-motion exercises should be done with all bedridden patients to prevent mobilization of calcium from the bone.
- **IM:** Administer IM deep into gluteal muscle. Crystals may form at low temperatures; warming and shaking vial will redissolve crystals. Use of a wet syringe or needle will cause a cloudy solution but will not affect potency. **Transdermal:** Apply patch(es) to clean, dry, hairless skin. Skin may be dry-shaved; do not use chemical depilatories. May be reapplied after bathing, showering, or swimming. *Testoderm* is applied to skin of scrotum. *Androderm* is applied to skin of back, abdomen, upper arms, or thighs.
- If skin irritation occurs, apply a small amount of OTC topical hydrocortisone cream after system removal or a small amount of 0.1% triamcinolone cream[Rx] may be applied to the skin under the central drug reservoir of the Androderm system without affecting the absorption of testosterone. Ointment formulations should not be used for pretreatment because they may significantly reduce testosterone absorption.
- **Gel:** Apply gel once daily, preferably in the morning, to clean dry intact skin of shoulders and upper arms or abdomen. **Buccal:** Apply to gum region twice daily (about 12 hr apart), rotating sides with each dose.

## PATIENT/FAMILY TEACHING

- **General Info:** Advise patient to report the following signs and symptoms promptly: in male patients, priapism (sustained and often painful erections) or gynecomastia; in female patients, virilism (which may be reversible if medication is stopped as soon as changes are noticed), hypercalcemia (nausea, vomiting, constipation, and weakness), edema (unexpected weight gain, swelling of feet), hepatitis (yellowing of skin or eyes and abdominal pain), or unusual bleeding or bruising.

- ❑ Explain rationale for prohibition of use for increasing athletic performance. Testosterone is neither safe nor effective for this use and has a potential risk of serious side effects.
- ❑ Instruct patient to notify health care professional immediately if pregnancy is planned or suspected.
- ❑ Advise diabetic patients to monitor blood closely for alterations in blood glucose concentrations.
- ❑ Emphasize the importance of regular follow-up physical exams, lab tests, and x-ray exams to monitor progress.
- ❑ Radiologic bone age determinations should be evaluated every 6 mo in prepubertal children to determine rate of bone maturation and effects on epiphyseal centers.
- ■ **Transdermal:** Advise patient to notify health care professional if female sexual partner develops mild virilization.
- ■ **Buccal:** Instruct patient to place the rounded side surface of the buccal system in a comfortable position just above incisor tooth, and hold firmly in place with a finger over the lip and against the product for 30 seconds to ensure adhesion. Buccal system is designed to stay in position until removed; if it fails to adhere to the gum or falls off during the 12-hr dosing interval, remove old system and apply a new one. If the buccal system falls out of place within 4 hr prior to next dose, apply new system and leave in place until time of next regularly scheduled dosing.
- ❑ Advise patient to avoid dislodging buccal system and to check on placement after toothbrushing, use of mouthwash, eating, or drinking. Do not chew or swallow buccal system. To remove, slide system downwards from gum toward tooth to avoid scratching the gum.

## EVALUATION

**Effectiveness of therapy can be demonstrated by:** ■ Resolution of the signs of androgen deficiency without side effects. Therapy is usually limited to 3–6 mo followed by bone growth or maturation determinations ■ Decrease in the size and spread of breast malignancy in postmenopausal women. In antineoplastic therapy, response may require 3 mo of therapy; if signs of disease progression appear, therapy should be discontinued.

## TETRACYCLINES

**doxycycline**

(dox-i-**sye**-kleen)

Adoxa, {Apo-Doxy}, Doryx, Doxy, Doxy Caps, {Doxycin}, Monodox, {Novodoxylin}, Periostat, Vibramycin, Vibra-Tabs

**minocycline**

(min-oh-**sye**-kleen)

Arestin, Dyancin, Minocin, Vectrin

**tetracycline**

(te-tra-**sye**-kleen)

Achromycin, Actisite, {Apo-Tetra}, {Novotetra}, {Nu-Tetra}, Panmycin, Robitet, Sumycin, Tetracap, Tetracyn, Tetralan

### CLASSIFICATION(S):
**Therapeutic:** anti-infectives
**Pharmacologic:** tetracyclines

**Pregnancy Category D**

### INDICATIONS

■ Treatment of various infections caused by unusual organisms, including: ❑ *Mycoplasma* ❑ *Chlamydia* ❑ *Rickettsia* ❑ *Borrelia burgdorferi* ■ Treatment of gonorrhea and syphilis in penicillin-allergic patients ■ Prevention of exacerbations of chronic bronchitis ■ Treatment of anthrax (doxycycline only) ■ Treatment of acne ■ Minocycline microspheres (Arestin), tetracycline fiber (Actisite), and low-dose doxycycline (Periostat) are used in the adjunctive management of periodontitis.

### ACTION

■ Inhibits bacterial protein synthesis at the level of the 30S bacterial ribosome ■ Low-dose products used in the management of periodontitis inhibit collagenase. **Therapeutic Effects:** ■ Bacteriostatic action against susceptible bacteria ■ Decreased complications of periodontitis. **Spectrum:** ■ Includes activity against some gram-positive pathogens: ❑ *Bacillus anthracis* ❑ *Clostridium perfringens* ❑ *Clostridium tetani* ❑ *Listeria monocytogenes* ❑ *Nocardia* ❑ *Propionibacterium acnes* ❑ *Actinomyces israelii* ■ Active against some gram-negative pathogens:

❏ *Haemophilus influenzae* ❏ *Legionella pneumophila* ❏ *Yersinia enterocolitica* ❏ *Yersinia pestis* ❏ *Neisseria gonorrhoeae* ❏ *Neisseria meningitidis* ■ Also active against several other pathogens, including: ❏ *Mycoplasma* ❏ *Treponema pallidum* ❏ *Chlamydia* ❏ *Rickettsia* ❏ *B. burgdorferi.*

## PHARMACOKINETICS

**Absorption:** *Tetracycline*—60–80% absorbed following oral administration. *Doxycycline, minocycline*—well absorbed from the GI tract.

**Distribution:** Widely distributed, some penetration into CSF; crosses the placenta and enters breast milk.

**Metabolism and Excretion:** *Doxycycline*—20–40% excreted unchanged by the urine; some inactivation in the intestine and some enterohepatic circulation with excretion in bile and feces. *Minocycline*—5–20% excreted unchanged by the urine; some metabolism by the liver with enterohepatic circulation and excretion in bile and feces. *Tetracycline*—Excreted mostly unchanged by the kidneys.

**Half-life:** *Doxycycline*—14–17 hr (increased in severe renal impairment). *Minocycline*—11–26 hr. *Tetracycline*—6–12 hr.

## CONTRAINDICATIONS AND PRECAUTIONS

**Contraindicated in:** ■ Hypersensitivity ■ Some products contain alcohol or bisulfites and should be avoided in patients with known hypersensitivity or intolerance ■ Pregnancy (risk of permanent staining of teeth in infant if used during last half of pregnancy) ■ Lactation ■ Can be used in children and pregnant and lactating women for the treatment of anthrax (doxycycline only).

**Use Cautiously in:** ■ Cachectic or debilitated patients ■ Renal disease ■ Hepatic impairment (doxycycline, minocycline) ■ Nephrogenic diabetes insipidus.

## ADVERSE REACTIONS AND SIDE EFFECTS*

■ **CNS:** benign intracranial hypertension (higher in children); *minocycline* dizziness ■ **EENT:** *minocycline*— vestibular reactions ■ **GI:** diarrhea, nausea, vomiting, esophagitis, hepatotox-icity, pancreatitis ■ **Derm:** photosensitivity, rashes; *minocycline*—pigmentation of skin and mucous membranes ■ **Hemat:** blood dyscrasias ■ **Local:** *doxycycline, minocycline*—phlebitis at IV site ■ **Misc:** hypersensitivity reactions, superinfection.

## INTERACTIONS

**Drug-Drug:** ■ May ↑ effect of **warfarin** ■ May ↓ effectiveness of **estrogen-containing hormonal contraceptives** ■ **Antacids, calcium, iron,** and **magnesium** form insoluble compounds (chelates) and ↓ absorption of tetracyclines; effect is least with doxycycline ■ **Sucralfate** may bind to tetracycline and ↓ its absorption from the GI tract ■ **Cholestyramine** or **colestipol** ↓ oral absorption of tetracyclines ■ **Adsorbent antidiarrheals** may ↓ absorption ■ **Barbiturates, carbamazepine,** or **phenytoin** may ↓ activity of doxycycline.

**Drug-Food:** ■ **Calcium** in foods or **dairy products** ↓ absorption by forming insoluble compounds (chelates); this effect is minimal with doxycycline.

## ROUTE AND DOSAGE

### ❏Doxycycline

■ **PO (Adults and Children >45 kg):** *Most infections*—100 mg q 12 hr on the 1st day, then 100–200 mg once daily or 50–100 mg q 12 hr. *Gonorrhea*—100 mg q 12 hr for 7 days or 300 mg followed 1 hr later by another 300-mg dose. *Malaria prophylaxis*—100 mg once daily. *Lyme disease*—100 mg twice daily *Periodontitis*—20 mg twice daily. *Anthrax*—100 mg twice daily for 60 days.

■ **PO (Children ≤45 kg):** 2.2 mg/kg q 12 hr on the 1st day, then 2.2–4.4 mg/kg/day given once daily or 1.1–2.2 mg/kg q 12 hr. *Anthrax*—2.2 mg/kg twice daily for 60 days.

■ **IV (Adults and Children >45 kg):** 200 mg once daily or 100 mg q 12 hr on the 1st day, then 100–200 mg once daily or 50–100 mg q 12 hr. *Anthrax*—100 mg q 12 hr change to oral when appropriate, for 60 days.

■ **IV (Children ≤45 kg):** 4.4 mg/kg once daily or 2.2 mg/kg q 12 hr on the 1st day, then 2.2–4.4 mg/kg/day given once daily or 1.1–2.2 mg/kg q 12 hr. *Anthrax*—100 mg q

12 hr change to oral when appropriate, for 60 days.

□ **Minocycline**

■ **PO (Adults):** 100–200 mg initially, then 100 mg q 12 hr or 50 mg q 6 hr. *Acne*—50 mg 1–3 times daily.

■ **Subgingival (Adults):** *periodontitis*—variable amounts inserted into periodontal pocket

■ **PO (Children ≥8 yr):** 4 mg/kg initially, then 2 mg/kg q 12 hr.

■ **IV (Adults):** 200 mg initially, then 100 mg q 12 hr (up to 400 mg/day).

■ **IV (Children ≥8 yr):** 4 mg/kg initially, then 2 mg/kg q 12 hr.

□ **Tetracycline**

■ **PO (Adults):** 250–500 mg q 6 hr or 500 mg–1 g q 12 hr. *Chronic treatment of acne*—500 mg–2 g/day for 3 wk, then decrease to 125 mg–1 g/day.

■ **Subgingival (Adults):** *periodontitis*—variable length of fiber inserted into periodontal pocket

■ **PO (Children ≥8 yr):** 6.25–12.5 mg/kg q 6 hr or 12.5–25 mg/kg q 12 hr.

## AVAILABILITY

□ **Doxycycline**

■ *Tablets:* 100 mg$^{Rx}$ ■ Cost: *Vibra-Tabs*— $217.48/50; *generic*—$12.50/50 ■ *Capsules:* 50 mg$^{Rx}$, 100 mg$^{Rx}$ ■ *Oral suspension (raspberry flavor):* 25 mg/5 ml in 60 ml bottles ■ *Syrup (apple-raspberry flavor):* 50 mg/5 ml in 473 ml bottles ■ *Lyophilized powder for injection (requires reconsititution):* 100 mg vials$^{Rx}$, 200 mg vials$^{Rx}$.

□ **Minocycline**

■ *Capsules:* 50 mg$^{Rx}$, 75 mg$^{Rx}$, 100 mg$^{Rx}$ ■ *Pellet-filled capsules (Minocin):* 50 mg$^{Rx}$, 100 mg$^{Rx}$ ■ *Oral suspension (custard flavor):* 50 mg/5ml$^{Rx}$ ■ *Sustained-release microspheres:* 1 mg$^{Rx}$.

□ **Tetracycline**

■ *Capsules:* 250 mg$^{Rx}$, 500 mg$^{Rx}$ ■ *Oral suspension:* 125 mg/5ml in 473–ml bottles$^{Rx}$ ■ *Fiber:* 12.7 mg/23 cm$^{Rx}$.

## TIME/ACTION PROFILE (blood levels)

| | ONSET | PEAK | DURATION |
|---|---|---|---|
| Doxycycline-PO | 1–2 hr | 1.5–4 hr | 12 hr |
| Doxycycline-IV | rapid | end of infu-sion | 12 hr |
| Minocycline-PO | rapid | 2–3 hr | 6–12 hr |
| Minocycline-IV | rapid | end of infu-sion | 6–12 hr |
| Tetracycline-PO | 1–2 hr | 2–4 hr | 6–12 hr |

# NURSING IMPLICATIONS

## ASSESSMENT

□ Assess patient for infection (vital signs; appearance of wound, sputum, urine, and stool; WBC) at beginning of and throughout therapy.

□ Obtain specimens for culture and sensitivity before initiating therapy. First dose may be given before receiving results.

■ **IV:** Assess IV site frequently; may cause thrombophlebitis.

■ *Lab Test Considerations:* Monitor renal and hepatic functions and CBC periodically during long-term therapy.

□ May cause ↑ AST, ALT, serum alkaline phosphatase, bilirubin, and amylase concentrations. Tetracyclines, except doxycycline, may cause ↑ serum BUN.

□ May cause false ↑ in urinary catecholamine levels.

## POTENTIAL NURSING DIAGNOSES

■ Infection, risk for (Indications, Side Effects).

■ Noncompliance (Patient/Family Teaching).

## IMPLEMENTATION

■ **General:** May cause yellow-brown discoloration and softening of teeth and bones if administered prenatally or during early childhood. Not recommended for children under 8 yr of age or during pregnancy or lactation unless used for the treatment of anthrax.

■ **PO:** Administer around the clock. Administer at least 1 hr before or 2 hr after meals. *Doxycycline and minocycline* may be taken with food or milk if GI irritation occurs. Administer with a full glass of liquid and at least 1 hr before going to bed to avoid esophageal ulceration. Use calibrated measuring device for liquid preparations. Shake liquid preparations well. Do not administer within 1–3 hr of other medications.

❑ Avoid administration of calcium, antacids, magnesium-containing medications, sodium bicarbonate, or iron supplements within 1–3 hr of oral tetracyclines.

## ❑Doxycycline

■ **PO:** To prepare doses for infants and children exposed to anthrax place one 100 mg tablet in a small bowl and crush to a fine powder with a metal spoon, leaving no large pieces. Add 4 level teaspoons of lowfat milk, lowfat chocolate milk, regular chocolate milk, chocolate pudding, or an apple juice and sugar mixture made by combining 4 teaspoons of sugar and 4 teaspoons of apple juice. Mix food or drink and doxycycline powder until powder dissolves. Mixture is stable in a covered container for 24 hrs if refrigerated (if made with milk or pudding) or at room temperature (if made with juice). Number of teaspoons to administer/dose is based on child's weight (0–12.5 lbs—$^1/_2$ tsp; 12.5–25 lbs—1 tsp; 25–37.5 lbs—$1^1/_2$ tsp; 37.5–50 lbs—2 tsp; 50–62.5 lbs—$2^1/_2$ tsp; 62.5–75 lbs—3 tsp; 75–87.5 lbs—$3^1/_2$ tsp; 87.5–100 lbs—4 tsp).

■ **Intermittent Infusion:** Dilute each 100 mg with 10 ml of sterile water or 0.9% NaCl for injection. Dilute further in 100–1000 ml of 0.9% NaCl, D5W, D5/LR, Ringer's, or LR. Solution is stable for 12 hr at room temperature and 72 hr if refrigerated. If diluted with D5/LR or LR, administer within 6 hr. Protect solution from direct sunlight. Concentrations of less than 1 mcg/ml or greater than 1 mg/ml are not recommended.

■ *Rate:*Administer over a minimum of 1–4 hr. Avoid rapid administration. Avoid extravasation.

■**Y-Site Compatibility:** ◆ acyclovir ◆ amifostine ◆ amiodarone ◆ aztreonam ◆ cisatracurium ◆ cyclophosphamide ◆ diltiazem ◆ docetaxel ◆ etoposide phosphate ◆ filgrastim ◆ fludarabine ◆ gemcitabine ◆ granisetron ◆ hydromorphone ◆ linezolid ◆ magnesium ◆ melphalan ◆ meperidine ◆ morphine ◆ ondansetron ◆ perphenazine ◆ propofol ◆ remifentanil ◆ sargramostim ◆ tacrolimus ◆ teniposide ◆ theophylline ◆ thiotepa ◆ vinorelbine.

■**Y-Site Incompatibility:** ◆ allopurinol ◆ heparin ◆ piperacillin/tazobactam.

## ❑Minocycline

■ **Intermittent Infusion:** Dilute each 100 mg with 5–10 ml of sterile water for injection. Dilute further in 500–1000 ml of 0.9% NaCl, D5W, D5/0.9% NaCl, Ringer's or LR. Solution is stable for 24 hr at room temperature.

■ *Rate:*Administer over 6 hr immediately following dilution. Avoid rapid infusions. May cause thrombophlebitis; avoid extravasation.

■**Y-Site Compatibility:** ◆ aztreonam ◆ cisatracurium ◆ cyclophosphamide ◆ docetaxel ◆ etoposide phosphate ◆ filgrastim ◆ fludarabine ◆ gemcitabine ◆ granisetron ◆ heparin ◆ hydrocortisone sodium succinate ◆ linezolid ◆ magnesium sulfate ◆ melphalan ◆ perphenazine ◆ potassium chloride ◆ remifentanil ◆ sargramostim ◆ teniposide ◆ vinorelbine ◆ vitamin B complex with C.

■**Y-Site Incompatibility:** ◆ allopurinol ◆ amifostine ◆ hydromorphone ◆ meperidine ◆ morphine ◆ piperacillin/tazobactam ◆ propofol ◆ thiotepa.

## PATIENT/FAMILY TEACHING

■ **General Info:** Instruct patient to take medication around the clock and to finish the drug completely as directed, even if feeling better. Take missed doses as soon as possible unless it is almost time for next dose; do not double doses. Advise patient that sharing of this medication may be dangerous.

❑ Advise patient to avoid taking milk or other dairy products concurrently with *tetracycline*. Also avoid taking antacids, calcium, magnesium-containing medications, sodium bicarbonate, and iron supplements within 1–3 hr of oral tetracyclines.

❑ Advise female patient to use a nonhormonal method of contraception while taking tetracyclines and until next menstrual period.

❑ *Minocycline* commonly causes dizziness or unsteadiness. Caution patient to avoid driving or other activities requiring alertness until response to medication is known. Notify health care professional if these symptoms occur.

❑ Caution patient to use sunscreen and protective clothing to prevent photosensitivity reactions.

❑ Advise patient to report the signs of superinfection (black, furry overgrowth on the tongue, vaginal itching or discharge, loose or foul-smelling stools). Skin rash, pruritus, and urticaria should also be reported.

❑ Instruct patient to notify health care professional of medication regimen before treatment or surgery.

❑ Instruct patient to notify health care professional if symptoms do not improve within a few days for systemic preparations.

❑ Caution patient to discard outdated or decomposed tetracyclines; they may be toxic.

## EVALUATION

**Clinical response to therapy can be evaluated by:** ■ Resolution of the signs and symptoms of infection. Length of time for complete resolution depends on the organism and site of infection ■ Decrease in acne lesions ■ Treatment of inhalation anthrax (post exposure) or treatment of cutaneous anthrax.

## theophylline, See BRONCHODILATORS (XANTHINES).

## thiamine

**(thye**-a-min)
{Betaxin}, {Bewon}, Biamine, vitamin B1

**CLASSIFICATION(S):**
**Therapeutic:** *vitamins*
**Pharmacologic:** *water soluble vitamins*

**Pregnancy Category A**

## INDICATIONS

■ Treatment of thiamine deficiencies (beriberi) ■ Prevention of Wernicke's encephalopathy ■ Dietary supplement in patients with GI disease, alcoholism, or cirrhosis.

## ACTION

■ Required for carbohydrate metabolism. **Therapeutic Effects:** ■ Replacement in deficiency states.

## PHARMACOKINETICS

**Absorption:** Well absorbed from the GI tract by an active process. Excessive amounts are not absorbed completely. Also well absorbed from IM sites.

**Distribution:** Widely distributed. Enters breast milk.

**Metabolism and Excretion:** Metabolized by the liver. Excess amounts are excreted unchanged by the kidneys.

**Half-life:** Unknown.

## CONTRAINDICATIONS AND PRECAUTIONS

**Contraindicated in:** ■ Hypersensitivity ■ Known alcohol intolerance or bisulfite hypersensitivity (elixir only).

**Use Cautiously in:** ■ Wernicke's encephalopathy (condition may be worsened unless thiamine is administered before glucose).

## ADVERSE REACTIONS AND SIDE EFFECTS*

Adverse reactions and side effects are extremely rare and are usually associated with IV administration or extremely large doses. ■ **CNS:** restlessness, weakness ■ **EENT:** tightness of the throat ■ **Resp:** pulmonary edema, respiratory distress ■ **CV:** VASCULAR COLLAPSE , hypotension, vasodilation ■ **GI:** GI bleeding, nausea ■ **Derm:** cyanosis, pruritus, sweating, tingling, urticaria, warmth ■ **Misc:** ANGIOEDEMA .

## INTERACTIONS

**Drug-Drug:** ■ None significant.

## ROUTE AND DOSAGE

❑ **Thiamine Deficiency (Beriberi)**
■ **PO (Adults):** 5–10 mg 3 times daily.
■ **PO (Children):** 10–50 mg/day in divided doses.
■ **IM, IV (Adults):** 5–100 mg 3 times daily.
■ **IM, IV (Children):** 10–25 mg/day.

❑ **Dietary Supplement**
■ **PO (Adults):** 1–1.6 mg/day.
■ **PO (Children 4–10 yr):** 0.9–1 mg/day.
■ **PO (Children birth–3 yr):** 0.3–0.7 mg/day.

## AVAILABILITY (generic available)

■ *Tablets:* 5 mg^OTC, 10 mg^OTC, 25 mg^OTC, 50 mg^OTC, 100 mg^OTC, 250 mg^OTC, 500 mg^OTC ■ *Elixir:* {250 mcg/5 ml^OTC} ■ *Injection:* 100 mg/ml in 1-ml ampules and prefilled syringes and 1-, 2-, 10-, and 30-ml vials$^{Rx}$ ■ other vitamins, minerals, and trace elements in multi-vitamin preparations$^{OTC}$.

TIME/ACTION PROFILE (time for symptoms of deficiency—edema and heart failure—to resolve†)

| | ONSET | PEAK | DURATION |
|---|---|---|---|
| PO, IM, IV | hr | days | days–wks |

†Confusion and psychosis take longer to respond.

## NURSING IMPLICATIONS

### ASSESSMENT

❏ Assess patient for signs and symptoms of thiamine deficiency (anorexia, GI distress, irritability, palpitations, tachycardia, edema, paresthesia, muscle weakness and pain, depression, memory loss, confusion, psychosis, visual disturbances, elevated serum pyruvic acid levels).

❏ Assess patient's nutritional status (diet, weight) prior to and throughout therapy.

❏ Monitor patients receiving IV thiamine for anaphylaxis (wheezing, urticaria, edema).

■ *Lab Test Considerations:* May interfere with certain methods of testing serum theophylline, uric acid, and urobilinogen concentrations.

### POTENTIAL NURSING DIAGNOSES

■ Nutrition, imbalanced: less than body requirements (Indications).

### IMPLEMENTATION

■ **General:** Because of infrequency of single B-vitamin deficiencies, combinations are commonly administered.

■ **IM, IV:** Parenteral administration is reserved for patients in whom oral administration is not feasible.

■ **IM:** Administration may cause tenderness and induration at injection site. Cool compresses may decrease discomfort.

■ **IV:** Sensitivity reactions and death have occurred from IV administration. An intradermal test dose is recommended in patients with suspected sensitivity. Monitor site for erythema and induration.

■ **Direct IV:** Administer undiluted.

■ *Rate:*Administer at a rate of 100 mg over 5 min.

■ **Continuous Infusion:** May be diluted in dextrose/Ringer's or LR combinations, dextrose/saline combinations, D5W, D10W, Ringer's and LR injection, 0.9% NaCl, or 0.45% NaCl and is usually administered with other vitamins.

■**Y-Site Compatibility:** ◆ famotidine.

■**Additive Incompatibility:** ◆ solutions with neutral or alkaline pH, such as carbonates, bicarbonates, citrates, and acetates.

### PATIENT/FAMILY TEACHING

❏ Encourage patient to comply with dietary recommendations of health care professional. Explain that the best source of vitamins is a well-balanced diet with foods from the four basic food groups.

❏ Teach patient that foods high in thiamine include cereals (whole grain and enriched), meats (especially pork), and fresh vegetables; loss is variable during cooking.

❏ Caution patients self-medicating with vitamin supplements not to exceed RDA. The effectiveness of megadoses of vitamins for treatment of various medical conditions is unproved and may cause side effects.

### EVALUATION

**Effectiveness of therapy can be demonstrated by:** ■ Prevention of or decrease in the signs and symptoms of vitamin B deficiency ❏ Decrease in the symptoms of neuritis, ocular signs, ataxia, edema, and heart failure may be seen within hours of administration and may disappear within a few days ❏ Confusion and psychosis may take longer to respond and may persist if nerve damage has occurred.

# thioridazine

(thye-oh-**rid**-a-zeen)

{Apo-Thioridazine}, Mellaril, Mellaril-S, {Novo-Ridazine}, {PMS Thioridazine}

## CLASSIFICATION(S):

*Therapeutic: antipsychotics*

---

{ } = Available in Canada only.
*CAPITALS indicates life-threatening; underlines indicate most frequent.

*Pharmacologic: phenothiazines*

**Pregnancy Category C**

## INDICATIONS

■ Management of schizophrenia in patients who do not have an acceptable response to treatment with conventional therapy.

## ACTION

■ Alters the effects of dopamine in the CNS ■ Possesses significant anticholinergic and alpha-adrenergic blocking activity. **Therapeutic Effects:** ■ Diminished signs and symptoms of psychoses.

## PHARMACOKINETICS

**Absorption:** Absorption from tablets is variable; may be better with oral liquid formulations.

**Distribution:** Widely distributed, high concentrations in the CNS. Crosses the placenta and enters breast milk.

**Protein Binding:** ≥90%.

**Metabolism and Excretion:** Highly metabolized by the liver and GI mucosa.

**Half-life:** 21–24 hr.

## CONTRAINDICATIONS AND PRECAUTIONS

**Contraindicated in:** ■ Hypersensitivity ■ Cross-sensitivity with other phenothiazines may exist ■ Narrow-angle glaucoma ■ Bone marrow depression ■ Severe liver or cardiovascular disease ■ Known alcohol intolerance (concentrate only) ■ Concurrent fluvoxamine, propranolol, pindolol, fluoxetine, other agents known to inhibit the CYP450 2D6 enzyme, or agents known to prolong the QTc interval (risk of life-threatening arrhythmias) ■ Hypokalemia (correct prior to use) ■ QTc interval >450 msec.

**Use Cautiously in:** ■ Geriatric or debilitated patients ■ Diabetes mellitus ■ Patients with risk factors for electrolyte imbalance (dehydration, diuretic therapy) ■ Respiratory disease ■ Prostatic hypertrophy ■ CNS tumors ■ Epilepsy ■ Intestinal obstruction ■ Pregnancy or lactation (safety not established).

## ADVERSE REACTIONS AND SIDE EFFECTS*

■ **CNS:** NEUROLEPTIC MALIGNANT SYNDROME, sedation, extrapyramidal reactions, tardive dyskinesia ■ **EENT:** blurred vision, dry eyes, lens opacities, pigmentary retinopathy (high doses) ■ **CV:** ARRHYTHMIAS, QTC PROLONGATION, hypotension, tachycardia ■ **GI:** constipation, dry mouth, anorexia, drug-induced hepatitis, ileus ■ **GU:** urinary retention ■ **Derm:** photosensitivity, pigment changes, rashes ■ **Endo:** galactorrhea ■ **Hemat:** AGRANULOCYTOSIS, leukopenia ■ **Metab:** hyperthermia ■ **Misc:** allergic reactions.

## INTERACTIONS

**Drug-Drug:** ■ Concurrent **fluvoxamine, propranolol, pindolol, fluoxetine,** other **agents known to inhibit the CYP450 2D6 enzyme,** or **agents known to prolong the QTc interval** (risk of life-threatening arrhythmias) ■ **Diuretics** increase the risk of electrolyte imbalance and arrhythmias ■ Additive hypotension with other **antihypertensives, nitrates,** and acute ingestion of **alcohol** ■ Additive CNS depression with other **CNS depressants,** including **alcohol, antihistamines, opioid analgesics, sedative/hypnotics,** and **general anesthetics** ■ Additive anticholinergic effects with other **drugs possessing anticholinergic properties,** including **antihistamines, antidepressants, atropine, haloperidol,** other **phenothiazines,** and **disopyramide** ■ **Lithium** decreases blood levels of thioridazine ■ Thioridazine may mask early signs of **lithium** toxicity and increase the risk of extrapyramidal reactions ■ Increased risk of agranulocytosis with **antithyroid agents** ■ Concurrent use with **epinephrine** may result in severe hypotension and tachycardia ■ May decrease the effectiveness of **levodopa.**

## ROUTE AND DOSAGE

■ **PO (Adults and Children >12 yr):** 50–100 mg tid initially; may be gradually increased to a maintenance dose of up to 800 mg/day.

■ **PO (Children):** 0.5 mg/kg/day in divided doses initially; may be gradually increased to a maintenance dose of up to 3 mg/kg/day.

## AVAILABILITY (generic available)

■ *Tablets:* 10 mg$^{Rx}$, 15 mg$^{Rx}$, 25 mg$^{Rx}$, 50 mg$^{Rx}$, 100 mg$^{Rx}$, 150 mg$^{Rx}$, 200 mg$^{Rx}$ ■ Cost: *Mellaril*—10 mg $38.42/100, 15 mg $45.29/100, 25 mg $54.05/100, 50 mg $65.62/100, 100 mg $77.05/100, 150 mg $101.38/100, 200 mg $115.47/100; *generic*—10 mg $12.04/100, 25 mg $21.09/100, 50 mg $23.97/100, 100 mg $31.34/100 ■ *Oral suspension:* {10 mg/5 ml$^{Rx}$}, 25 mg/5 ml$^{Rx}$, 100 mg/5 ml$^{Rx}$ ■

*Concentrated oral solution:* 30 mg/ml$^{Rx}$, 100 mg/ml$^{Rx}$.

TIME/ACTION PROFILE (antipsychotic effects)

| | ONSET | PEAK | DURATION |
|---|---|---|---|
| PO | unknown | unknown | 8–12 hr |

## NURSING IMPLICATIONS

### ASSESSMENT

❑ Assess mental status (orientation, mood, behavior) and degree of anxiety before and periodically throughout therapy.

❑ Monitor blood pressure (sitting, standing, lying), ECG, pulse, and respiratory rate before and frequently during the period of dosage adjustment. May cause Q-wave and T-wave changes in ECG.

❑ Observe patient carefully when administering medication to ensure that medication is actually taken and not hoarded.

❑ Assess patient for level of sedation after administration.

❑ Monitor intake and output ratios and daily weight. Report significant discrepancies.

❑ Monitor patient for onset of akathisia (restlessness or desire to keep moving) and extrapyramidal side effects (*parkinsonian*—difficulty speaking or swallowing, loss of balance control, pill rolling, mask-like face, shuffling gait, rigidity, tremors; and *dystonic*—muscle spasms, twisting motions, twitching, inability to move eyes, weakness of arms or legs) every 2 mo during therapy and 8–12 wk after therapy has been discontinued. Report these symptoms; reduction in dosage or discontinuation of medication may be necessary. Trihexyphenidyl or diphenhydramine may be used to control these symptoms.

❑ Monitor for tardive dyskinesia (uncontrolled rhythmic movement of mouth, face, and extremities; lip smacking or puckering; puffing of cheeks; uncontrolled chewing; rapid or worm-like movements of tongue). Report immediately; may be irreversible.

❑ Monitor for development of neuroleptic malignant syndrome (fever, respiratory distress, tachycardia, seizures, diaphoresis, hypertension or hypotension, pallor, tiredness, severe muscle stiffness, loss of bladder control). Notify physician or other health care professional immediately if these symptoms occur.

■ *Lab Test Considerations:* CBC, liver function tests, and ocular examinations should be evaluated periodically throughout therapy. May cause decreased hematocrit, hemoglobin, leukocytes, granulocytes, platelets. May cause elevated bilirubin, AST, ALT, and alkaline phosphatase. Agranulocytosis occurs between 4–10 wk of therapy with recovery 1–2 wk after discontinuation. May recur if medication is restarted. Liver function abnormalities may require discontinuation of therapy.

❑ May cause false-positive or false-negative pregnancy test results and false-positive urine bilirubin test results.

❑ May cause increased serum prolactin levels, thereby interfering with gonadorelin test results.

### POTENTIAL NURSING DIAGNOSES

■ Coping, ineffective (Indications).

■ Thought processes, disturbed (Indications).

### IMPLEMENTATION

■ **General:** To prevent contact dermatitis, avoid getting liquid preparations on hands, and wash hands thoroughly if spillage occurs.

❑ Phenothiazines should be discontinued 48 hr before and not resumed for 24 hr after myelography, as they lower the seizure threshold.

■ **PO:** Administer with food, milk, or full glass of water to minimize gastric irritation.

❑ Dilute concentrate in 120 ml of distilled or acidified tap water or fruit juice just before administration.

### PATIENT/FAMILY TEACHING

❑ Advise patient to take medication exactly as directed and not to skip doses or double up on missed doses. If a dose is missed, it should be taken as soon as remembered unless almost time for the next dose. If more than 2 doses a day are ordered, the missed dose should be taken within 1 hr of the scheduled time or omitted. Abrupt withdrawal may lead to gastritis, nausea, vomiting, dizziness, headache, tachycardia, and insomnia.

❑ Inform patient of possibility of extrapyramidal symptoms and tardive dyskinesia. Instruct patient to report these symptoms immediately to health care professional.

❑ Advise patient to change positions slowly to minimize orthostatic hypotension.

❑ May cause drowsiness. Caution patient to avoid driving or other activities requiring alertness until response to medication is known.

❑ Advise patient to use sunscreen and protective clothing when exposed to the sun. Exposed surfaces may develop a blue-gray pigmentation, which may fade after discontinuation of the medication. Extremes in temperature should also be avoided, as this drug impairs body temperature regulation.

❑ Instruct patient to use frequent mouth rinses, good oral hygiene, and sugarless gum or candy to minimize dry mouth. Consult health care professional if dry mouth continues for >2 wk.

❑ Advise patient that increasing activity and bulk and fluids in the diet helps minimize the constipating effects of this medication.

❑ Caution patient to avoid taking alcohol or other CNS depressants concurrently with this medication.

❑ Advise patient not to take thioridazine within 2 hr of antacids or antidiarrheal medication.

❑ Inform patient that this medication may turn urine pink to reddish brown.

❑ Advise patient to notify health care professional of medication regimen before treatment or surgery.

❑ Instruct patient to notify health care professional promptly if sore throat, fever, unusual bleeding or bruising, rash, weakness, tremors, visual disturbances, dark-colored urine, or clay-colored stools occur.

❑ Emphasize the importance of routine follow-up exams to monitor response to medication and to detect side effects. Periodic ocular exams are indicated. Encourage continued participation in psychotherapy.

## EVALUATION

**Effectiveness of therapy can be demonstrated by:** ■ Decrease in excitable, paranoic, or withdrawn behavior ■ Decrease in anxiety associated with depression ■ Improvement in severe behavioral problems in children.

High Alert

# THROMBOLYTIC AGENTS

## alteplase

(**al**-te-plase)

Activase, {Activase rt-PA}, {Lysatec rt-PA}, Cathflo Activase, tissue plasminogen activator, t-PA

## anistreplase

(an-**eye**-strep-lase)

anisoylated plasminogen–streptokinase activator complex, APSAC, Eminase

## reteplase

(**re**-te-plase)

Retavase

## streptokinase

(strep-toe-**kye**-nase)

Kabbikinase, Streptase

## tenecteplase

(te-**nek**-te-plase)

TNKase

## urokinase

(yoor-oh-**kye**-nase)

Abbokinase

## *CLASSIFICATION(S):*

***Therapeutic:*** *thrombolytics*
***Pharmacologic:*** *plasminogen activators*

**Pregnancy Category B (urokinase), C (alteplase, anistreplase, reteplase, streptokinase, tenecteplase)**

## INDICATIONS

■Acute coronary thrombosis (MI) ■ **Streptokinase, urokinase:** Massive pulmonary emboli ■ **Alteplase:** Acute ischemic stroke ■ **Streptokinase:** Deep vein thrombosis or arterial thromboembolism ■ **Alteplase:** Occluded central venous access devices.

## ACTION

■ Convert plasminogen to plasmin, which is then able to degrade fibrin present in clots. Alteplase, reteplase, and urokinase directly activate plasminogen. Anistreplase and streptokinase combine with plasminogen to form activator complexes, which then convert plasminogen to plasmin. **Therapeutic Effects:** ■ Lysis of thrombi in coronary arteries, with preservation of ventricular function ■ Lysis of pulmonary emboli or deep vein thrombosis ■ Decreased neurologic sequelae of stroke ■ Clearing of clots in cannulae/catheters (alteplase).

## PHARMACOKINETICS

**Absorption:** After IV administration, absorption is essentially complete. Intracoronary administration or administration into occluded catheters or cannulae has a more localized effect.

**Distribution:** Streptokinase appears to cross the placenta minimally, if at all. Remainder of distribution for streptokinase or other agents is not known.

**Metabolism and Excretion:** *Alteplase*—Rapidly metabolized by the liver. *Anistreplase*—Inactivated by binding to plasmin inactivators. *Reteplase*—Cleared primarily by the liver and kidneys. *Streptokinase*—Rapidly cleared from circulation. *Tenecteplase*—Mostly metabolized by the liver.

**Half-life:** *Alteplase*—35 min; *anistreplase*—70–120 min; *reteplase*—13–16 min; *streptokinase activator complex*—23 min; *Tenecteplase initial phase*—20–24 min; *tenecteplase terminal phase*—90–130 min; *urokinase*—up to 20 min.

## CONTRAINDICATIONS AND PRECAUTIONS

**Contraindicated in:** ■ Active internal bleeding ■ History of cerebrovascular accident, recent CNS trauma or surgery, neoplasm, or arteriovenous malformation ■ Severe uncontrolled hypertension ■ Known bleeding tendencies ■ Hypersensitivity; cross-sensitivity with anistreplase and streptokinase may occur.

**Use Cautiously in:** ■ Recent (within 10 days) major surgery, trauma, GI or GU bleeding ■ Left heart thrombus ■ Severe hepatic or renal disease ■ Hemorrhagic ophthalmic conditions ■ Septic phlebitis ■ Previous puncture of a noncompressible vessel ■ Subacute bacterial endocarditis or acute pericarditis ■ Recent streptococcal infection or previous therapy with anistreplase or streptokinase (from 5 days–6 mo); may produce resistance because of antibody formation; increased dosage requirements may be encountered (anistreplase and streptokinase only) ■ Geriatric patients (>75 yr; increased risk of intracranial bleeding) ■ Pregnancy, lactation, or children (safety not established).

**Exercise Extreme Caution in:** ■ Patients receiving warfarin therapy ■ Early postpartum period (10 days).

## ADVERSE REACTIONS AND SIDE EFFECTS*

■ **CNS:** INTRACRANIAL HEMORRHAGE , headache ■ **EENT:** epistaxis, gingival bleeding; *streptokinase*—periorbital edema ■ **Resp:** bronchospasm, hemoptysis ■ **CV:** reperfusion arrhythmias, hypotension ■ **GI:** GI BLEEDING , RETROPERITONEAL BLEEDING ■ **GU:** GU TRACT BLEEDING ■ **Derm:** ecchymoses, flushing, urticaria ■ **Hemat:** BLEEDING ■**Local:** hemorrhage at injection sites, phlebitis at IV site ■ **MS:** musculoskeletal pain ■ **Misc:** allergic reactions including ANAPHYLAXIS , fever.

## INTERACTIONS

**Drug-Drug:** ■ **Aspirin,** other **NSAIDs, warfarin, heparin** and **heparin-like agents, abciximab, eptifibatide, tirofiban, clopidogrel, ticlopidine,** or **dipyridamole**—concurrent use ↑ risk of bleeding, although these agents are frequently used together or in sequence ■ Risk of bleeding ↑ by concurrent use of **cefotetan, cefoperazone, plicamycin,** or **valproic acid** ■ Effects may be ↓ by **antifibrinolytic agents,** including **aminocaproic acid, aprotinin,** or **tranexamic acid.**

**Drug-Natural Products:** ■ ↑ anticoagulant effect and bleeding risk with **anise, arnica, chamomile, clove, dong quai, fenugreek, feverfew, garlic, ginger, ginkgo, Panax ginseng, licorice,** and others.

## ROUTE AND DOSAGE

### ❏Alteplase

#### Myocardial Infarction (Accelerated or Front-Loading Regimen)

- **IV (Adults):** 15 mg initially, then 0.75 mg/kg (up to 50 mg) over 30 min, then 0.5 mg/kg (up to 35 mg) over next 60 min; usually accompanied by heparin therapy.

#### Myocardial Infarction (Standard Regimen)

- **IV (Adults >65 kg):** 60 mg over 1st hr (6–10 mg given as a bolus over first 1–2 min), 20 mg over the 2nd hr, and 20 mg over the 3rd hr for a total dose of 100 mg.
- **IV (Adults <65 kg):** 0.75 mg/kg over 1st hr (0.075–0.125 mg/kg given as a bolus over first 1–2 min), 0.25 mg/kg over the 2nd hr, and 0.25 mg/kg over the 3rd hr for a total dose of 1.25 mg/kg (not to exceed 100 mg total).

#### Pulmonary Embolism

- **IV (Adults):** 100 mg over 2 hr; follow with heparin.

#### Acute Ischemic Stroke

- **IV (Adults):** 0.9 mg/kg (not to exceed 90 mg), given as an infusion over 1 hr, with 10% of the dose given as a bolus over the 1st min.

#### Occluded Venous Access Devices

- **IV (Adults and Children >30 kg):** 2 mg/2 ml instilled into occluded catheter; if unsuccessful, may repeat once after 2 hr.
- **IV (Children 10–30 kg):** 110% of the lumen volume (not to exceed 2 mg in 2 ml) instilled into occluded catheter; if unsuccessful, may repeat once after 2 hr.

### ❏Anistreplase

- **IV (Adults):** 30 units over 2–5 min.

### ❏Reteplase

- **IV (Adults):** 10 units, followed 30 min later by an additional 10 units.

### ❏Streptokinase

#### Myocardial Infarction

- **IV (Adults):** 1.5 million IU.
- **Intracoronary (Adults):** 20,000 IU bolus followed by 2000 IU/min infusion for 60 min (140,000 IU total dose).

### Deep Vein Thrombosis, Pulmonary Emboli, Arterial Emboli, or Thromboses

- **IV (Adults):** 250,000 IU loading dose, followed by 100,000 IU/hr for 24 hr for pulmonary emboli, 72 hr for recurrent pulmonary emboli or deep vein thrombosis.

### ❏Tenecteplase

- **IV (Adults <60 kg):** 30 mg.
- **IV (Adults ≥60 kg and <70 kg):** 35 mg.
- **IV (Adults ≥70 kg and <80 kg):** 40 mg.
- **IV (Adults ≥80 kg and <90 kg):** 45 mg.
- **IV (Adults ≥90 kg):** 50 mg.

### ❏Urokinase

#### Pulmonary Emboli

- **IV (Adults):** 4400 IU/kg loading dose, followed by 4400 IU/kg/hr for 12 hr.

## AVAILABILITY

### ❏Alteplase

- ***Powder for injection:*** 2 mg vial$^{Rx}$, 20 mg/vial$^{Rx}$, 50 mg/vial$^{Rx}$ ■ Cost2 mg $75.00/vial, 50 mg $1375.00/vial.

### ❏Anistreplase

- ***Powder for injection:*** 30 units/vial$^{Rx}$.

### ❏Reteplase

- ***Powder for injection:*** 10.8 units (18.8 mg)/vial$^{Rx}$.

### ❏Streptokinase

- ***Powder for injection:*** 250,000 IU/vial$^{Rx}$, 600,000 IU/vial$^{Rx}$, 750,000 IU/vial$^{Rx}$, 1,500,000 IU/vial$^{Rx}$.

### ❏Tenecteplase

- ***Powder for injection:*** 50 mg/vial with 10 ml syringe and TwinPak Dual Cannula Device and 10 ml vial of sterile water for injection$^{Rx}$.

### ❏Urokinase

- ***Powder for injection:*** 250,000 IU/vial$^{Rx}$.

TIME/ACTION PROFILE (fibrinolysis)

| | ONSET | PEAK† | DURATION |
|---|---|---|---|
| Alteplase IV | unknown | 20 min–2 hr (45 min avg) | unknown |
| Anistreplase IV | unknown | 45 min | 6 hr‡ |
| Reteplase IV | rapid | within 2 hr | 48 hr |
| Streptokinase IV | immediate | rapid | 4 hr (up to 12 hr) |

| Tenecteplase rapid IV | unknown | unknown | |
| Urokinase IV immediate | rapid | up to 12 hr | |

†Reperfusion of myocardium generally occurs 20 min–2 hr after start of IV dosing (average 45 min).

‡Systemic hyperfibrinolytic state may persist for 2 days.

## NURSING IMPLICATIONS

### ASSESSMENT

- **General Info:** Begin therapy as soon as possible after the onset of symptoms.

- ❏ Monitor vital signs, including temperature, continuously for coronary thrombosis and at least every 4 hr during therapy for other indications. Do not use lower extremities to monitor blood pressure. Notify physician if systolic BP >180 mm Hg or diastolic BP >110 mm Hg. Tenecteplase should not be given if hypertension is uncontrolled. Inform physician if hypotension occurs. Hypotension may result from the drug, hemorrhage, or cardiogenic shock.

- ❏ Assess patient carefully for bleeding every 15 min during the 1st hr of therapy, every 15–30 min during the next 8 hr, and at least every 4 hr for the duration of therapy. Frank bleeding may occur from sites of invasive procedures or from body orifices. Internal bleeding may also occur (decreased neurologic status; abdominal pain with coffee-grounds emesis or black, tarry stools; hematuria; joint pain). If uncontrolled bleeding occurs, stop medication and notify physician immediately.

- ❏ Inquire about previous reaction to anistreplase or streptokinase therapy. Assess patient for hypersensitivity reaction (rash, dyspnea, fever, changes in facial color, swelling around the eyes, wheezing). If these occur, inform physician promptly. Keep epinephrine, an antihistamine, and resuscitation equipment close by in the event of an anaphylactic reaction.

- ❏ Inquire about recent streptococcal infection. *Anistreplase* and *streptokinase* may be less effective if administered between 5 days and 6 mo of a streptococcal infection.

- ❏ Assess neurologic status throughout therapy. Altered sensorium or neurologic changes may be indicative of intracranial bleeding.

- ■ **Coronary Thrombosis:** Monitor ECG continuously. Notify physician if significant arrhythmias occur. IV lidocaine or procainamide (Pronestyl) may be ordered prophylactically. Monitor cardiac enzymes. Radionuclide myocardial scanning and/or coronary angiography may be ordered 7–10 days after therapy to monitor effectiveness of therapy.

- ❏ Assess intensity, character, location, and radiation of chest pain. Note presence of associated symptoms (nausea, vomiting, diaphoresis). Administer analgesics as directed. Notify physician if chest pain is unrelieved or recurs.

- ❏ Monitor heart sounds and breath sounds frequently. Inform physician if signs of CHF occur (rales/crackles, dyspnea, $S_3$ heart sound, jugular venous distention, relieved CVP).

- ■ **Pulmonary Embolism:** Monitor pulse, blood pressure, hemodynamics, and respiratory status (rate, degree of dyspnea, ABGs).

- ■ **Deep Vein Thrombosis/Acute Arterial Occlusion:** Observe extremities and palpate pulses of affected extremities every hour. Notify physician immediately if circulatory impairment occurs. Computerized tomography, impedance plethysmography, quantitative Doppler effect determination, and/or angiography or venography may be used to determine restoration of blood flow and duration of therapy; however, repeated venograms are not recommended.

- ■ **Cannula/Catheter Occlusion:** Monitor ability to aspirate blood as indicator of patency. Ensure that patient exhales and holds breath when connecting and disconnecting IV syringe to prevent air embolism.

- ■ **Acute Ischemic Stroke:** Assess neurologic status. Determine time of onset of stroke symptoms. Alteplase must be administered within 3 hr of onset.

- ■ *Lab Test Considerations:* Hematocrit, hemoglobin, platelet count, fibrin/fibrin degradation product (FDP/fdp) titer, fibrinogen concentration, prothrombin time, thrombin time, and activated partial thromboplastin time may be evaluated before and frequently during therapy. Bleeding time may be as-

---

{ } = Available in Canada only.
*CAPITALS indicates life-threatening; underlines indicate most frequent.

sessed before therapy if patient has received platelet aggregation inhibitors.

❑ Obtain type and crossmatch and have blood available at all times in case of hemorrhage.

❑ Stools should be tested for occult blood loss and urine for hematuria periodically during therapy.

■ *Toxicity and Overdose: High Alert:* If local bleeding occurs, apply pressure to site. If severe or internal bleeding occurs, discontinue infusion. Clotting factors and/or blood volume may be restored through infusions of whole blood, packed RBCs, fresh frozen plasma, or cryoprecipitate. Do not administer dextran; it has antiplatelet activity. Aminocaproic acid (Amicar) may be used as an antidote.

## POTENTIAL NURSING DIAGNOSES

■ Tissue perfusion, ineffective (Indications).

■ Injury, risk for (Side Effects).

## IMPLEMENTATION

❑ *High Alert:* Overdosage and under-dosage of thrombolytic medications have resulted in patient harm or death. Have second practitioner independently check original order, dosage calculations, and infusion pump settings. Do not confuse the abbreviation *t-PA* for alteplase (Activase) with the abbreviation *TNK t-PA* for tenecteplase (TNKase). Clarify orders that contain either of these abbreviations. Do not begin systemic anticoagulation with heparin until 8 hours after the completion of thrombolytic therapy.

■ **General:** Thrombolytic agents should be used only in settings in which hematologic function and clinical response can be adequately monitored.

❑ Starting two IV lines before therapy is recommended: one for the thrombolytic agent, the other for any additional infusions.

❑ Avoid invasive procedures, such as IM injections or arterial punctures, with this therapy. If such procedures must be performed, apply pressure to all arterial and venous puncture sites for at least 30 min. Avoid venipunctures at noncompressible sites (jugular vein, subclavian site).

❑ Acetaminophen may be ordered to control fever.

## ⌐Alteplase

■ **Intermittent Infusion:** Vials are packaged with sterile water for injection (without preservatives) to be used as diluent. Do not use bacteriostatic water for injection. Reconstitute 20-mg vials with 20-ml and 50-mg vials with 50 ml using an 18-gauge needle. Avoid excess agitation during dilution; swirl or invert gently to mix. Solution may foam upon reconstitution. Bubbles will resolve upon standing a few min. Solution will be clear to pale yellow. Stable for 8 hr at room temperature. May be administered as reconstituted (1 mg/ml) or may be further diluted immediately before use in an equal amount of 0.9% NaCl or D5W.

■ *Rate:* Flush line with 20–30 ml of saline at completion of infusion to ensure entire dose is received.

❑ Standard dose for *MI* is administered over 3 hr.

❑ For *pulmonary embolism,* administer over 2 hr.

❑ For *acute ischemic stroke,* administer 10% of total dose IV bolus over 1 min, with the remaining dose infused over 60 min.

■ **Y-Site Compatibility:** ♦ lidocaine ♦ metoprolol ♦ propranolol.

■ **Y-Site Incompatibility:** ♦ dobutamine ♦ dopamine ♦ heparin ♦ nitroglycerin.

■ **Cathflo Activase:** Reconstitute by withdrawing 2.2 ml of sterile water (provided) and injecting into Cathflo Activase vial, directing diluent into powder for a concentration of 1 mg/ml. Allow slight foaming to dissipate by letting vial stand undisturbed. Do not use bacteriostatic water. Mix by gently swirling to dissolve; complete dissolution should occur within 3 min. Do not shake. Solution should be colorless to pale yellow. Use solution within 8 hr.

❑ Withdraw 2.0 ml of reconstituted solution and instill into occluded catheter. After 30 min dwell time, attempt to aspirate blood. If catheter remains occluded, allow 120 min dwell time. If catheter function is not restored after one dose, second dose may be instilled. If catheter function is restored, aspirate 4–5 ml of blood to remove Cathflo Activase and residual clot. Gently irrigate catheter with 0.9% NaCl.

□ **Anistreplase**

■ **Direct IV:** Reconstitute with 5 ml of sterile water for injection (direct to sides of vial) and swirl gently; do not shake to minimize foaming. Do not dilute further. Use reconstituted solution within 30 min of preparation.

■ *Rate:* Administer via IV line or vein over 2–5 min.

■ **Y-Site Incompatibility:** Do not admix or administer via Y-site injection with any other medications.

□ **Reteplase**

■ **Direct IV:** Reconstitute using diluent, needle, syringe, and dispensing pin provided. Reconstitute only with sterile water for injection without preservatives. Solution is colorless. Do not administer solutions that are discolored or contain a precipitate. Slight foaming may occur; allow vial to stand undisturbed for several min to dissipate bubbles. Reconstitute immediately before use. Stable for 4 hr at room temperature.

■ *Rate:* Administer each bolus over 2 min into an IV line containing D5W; flush line before and after bolus.

■ **Y-Site Incompatibility:** ◆ heparin ◆ No other medication should be infused or injected into line used for reteplase.

□ **Streptokinase**

■ **Intracoronary:** Dilute 250,000 IU vial to a total volume of 125 ml with 0.9% NaCl or D5W. Administer 20,000 IU (10 ml) via bolus injection.

■ *Rate:* Intracoronary bolus is administered over 15 sec–2 min.

■ **Intermittent Infusion:** Reconstitute with 5 ml of 0.9% NaCl or D5W (direct to sides of vial) and swirl gently; do not shake. Dilute further with 0.9% NaCl for a total volume of 45–500 ml (45 ml for MI, 90 ml for deep vein thrombosis or pulmonary embolism). Solution is slightly yellow in color. Administer through 0.8-micron pore–size filter. Use reconstituted solution within 24 hr.

■ *Rate:* Administer dose for MI within 60 min.

□ Intracoronary bolus should be followed by an intracoronary maintenance infusion of 2000 IU/min for 60 min.

□ Loading dose for *deep vein thrombosis* or *pulmonary embolism* is administered over 30 min, followed by an infusion of 100,000 IU/hr.

□ Use infusion pump to ensure accurate dose.

■ **Y-Site Compatibility:** ◆ dobutamine ◆ dopamine ◆ heparin ◆ lidocaine ◆ nitroglycerin.

■ **Additive Incompatibility:** Do not admix with any other medication.

■ **Cannula/Catheter Clearance:** Dilute 250,000 IU in 2 ml of 0.9% NaCl or D5W.

■ *Rate:* Administer slowly, over 25–35 min, into each occluded limb of cannula, and then clamp for at least 2 hr. Aspirate contents carefully and flush lines with 0.9% NaCl.

□ **Tenecteplase**

■ **Intermittent Infusion:** Vials are packaged with sterile water for injection (without preservatives) to be used as diluent. Do not use bacteriostatic water for injection. Do not discard shield assembly. To reconstitute aseptically withdraw 10 ml of diluent and inject into the tenectplase vial, directing the stream into the powder. Slight foaming may occur; large bubbles will dissipate if left standing undisturbed for several minutes. Swirl gently until contents are completely dissolved; do not shake. Solution containing 5 mg/ml is clear and colorless to pale yellow. Withdraw dose from reconstituted vial with the syringe and discard unused portion. Once dose is in syringe, stand the shield vertically on a flat surface (with green side down) and passively recap the red hub cannula. Remove the entire shield assembly, including the red hub cannula, by twisting counter clockwise. Shield assembly also contains the clear-ended blunt plastic cannula; retain for split septum IV access. Reconstitute immediately before use. May be refrigerated and administered within 8 hrs.

■ *Rate:* Administer as a single IV bolus over 5 seconds.

■ **Y-Site Incompatibility:** Precipate forms in line when administered with dextrose-containing solutions. Flush line with saline-containing solution prior to and following administration of tenecteplase.

■ **Additive Incompatibility:** Do not admix.

### ▫Urokinase

■ **Intermittent Infusion:** Reconstitute each 250,000 IU vial with 5 ml of sterile water for injection without preservatives (direct to sides of vial) and swirl gently; do not shake. Solution is light straw colored. Do not administer solutions that are discolored or contain a precipitate. Use reconstituted solution immediately after preparation. Infuse through a 0.45-micron filter.

❏ For *pulmonary embolism*, dilute the reconstituted solution further with 190 ml of 0.9% NaCl or D5W.

■ *Rate:* For *pulmonary embolism*, administer loading dose over 10 min and follow with infusion of 4400 IU/kg/hr for 12 hr.

❏ Administer via infusion pump to ensure accurate dosage.

### PATIENT/FAMILY TEACHING

❏ Explain purpose of medication and the need for close monitoring to patient and family. Instruct patient to report hypersensitivity reactions (rash, dyspnea) and bleeding or bruising.

❏ Explain need for bedrest and minimal handling during therapy to avoid injury. Avoid all unnecessary procedures such as shaving and vigorous tooth brushing.

### EVALUATION

**Effectiveness of therapy can be demonstrated by:** ■ Lysis of thrombi and restoration of blood flow ■ Prevention of neurologic sequelae in acute ischemic stroke ■ Cannula or catheter patency.

## THYROID PREPARATIONS

### levothyroxine

### (lee-voe-thye-**rox**-een)

{Eltroxin}, Levo-T, Levothroid, Levoxyl, Novothrox, {PMS-Levothyroxine Sodium}, Synthroid, $T_4$, Unithroid

### liothyronine

### (lye-oh-**thye**-roe-neen)

Cytomel, l-triiodothyronine, $T_3$, Triostat

### liotrix

### (**lye**-oh-trix)

$T_3/T_4$, Thyrolar

### thyroid

### (**thye**-royd)

Armour thyroid, Thyrar, Thyroid Strong, Westhroid

### CLASSIFICATION(S):

**Therapeutic:** hormones
**Pharmacologic:** thyroid preparations

### Pregnancy Category A

## INDICATIONS

■ Replacement/substitution in diminished or absent thyroid function ■ Thyroid cancer (some forms).

## ACTION

■ Principal effect is increasing metabolic rate of body tissues: ■ Promote gluconeogenesis ■ Increase utilization and mobilization of glycogen stores ■ Stimulate protein synthesis ■ Promote cell growth and differentiation ■ Aid in the development of the brain and CNS ■ Contain $T_3$ (triiodothyronine) and $T_4$ (thyroxine) activity. **Therapeutic Effects:** ■ Replacement in deficiency states with restoration of normal hormonal balance ■ Suppression of thyrotropin-dependent thyroid cancers.

## PHARMACOKINETICS

**Absorption:** Levothyroxine is variably (50–80%) absorbed from the GI tract. Liothyronine and thyroid hormone are well absorbed.

**Distribution:** Distributed into most body tissues. Thyroid hormones do not readily cross the placenta; minimal amounts enter breast milk.

**Metabolism and Excretion:** Metabolized by the liver and other tissues. Thyroid hormone undergoes enterohepatic recirculation and is excreted in the feces via the bile.

**Half-life:** $T_3$ *(liothyronine)*—1–2 days; $T_4$ *(thyroxine)*—6–7 days.

## CONTRAINDICATIONS AND PRECAUTIONS

**Contraindicated in:** ■ Hypersensitivity ■ Recent MI ■ Thyrotoxicosis ■ Known alcohol intolerance (liothyronine injection only) ▪ Hypersensitivity to beef (Thyrar product).

**Use Cautiously in:** ▪ Cardiovascular disease (initiate therapy with lower doses) ▪ Severe renal insufficiency ▪ Uncorrected adrenocortical disorders ▪ Geriatric and myxedematous patients (extremely sensitive to thyroid hormones—initial dosage should be markedly reduced).

## ADVERSE REACTIONS AND SIDE EFFECTS*

Seen mostly with excessive doses. ▪ **CNS:** <u>insomnia</u>, <u>irritability</u>, <u>nervousness</u>, headache ▪ **CV:** CARDIOVASCULAR COLLAPSE, <u>arrhythmias</u>, <u>tachycardia</u>, angina pectoris, hypotension, increased blood pressure, increased cardiac output ▪ **GI:** cramps, diarrhea, vomiting ▪ **Derm:** hair loss (in children), increased sweating ▪ **Endo:** hyperthyroidism, menstrual irregularities ▪ **Metab:** <u>weight loss</u>, heat intolerance ▪ **MS:** accelerated bone maturation in children.

## INTERACTIONS

**Drug-Drug:** ▪ **Bile acid sequestrants** ↓ absorption of orally administered thyroid preparations ▪ May alter the effectiveness of **warfarin** ▪ May ↑ requirement for **insulin** or **oral hypoglycemic agents** in diabetics ▪ Concurrent **estrogen** therapy may ↑ thyroid replacement requirements ▪ ↑ cardiovascular effects with **adrenergics** (sympathomimetics) ▪ May ↓ response to **beta blockers.**

## ROUTE AND DOSAGE

Each 1 gr = 60 mg and is equivalent to 100 mcg or less of levothyroxine ($T_4$) or 25 mcg of liothyronine ($T_3$).

### ▫ Levothyroxine

▪ **PO (Adults):** *Hypothyroidism*—50 mcg as a single dose initially; may be increased q 2–3 wk; usual maintenance dose is 75–125 mcg/day (1.5 mcg/kg/day). *Severe hypothyroidism*—12.5–25 mcg/day; may increase q 2–4 wk by 25 mcg/day; usual maintenance dose is 75–125 mcg/day (1.5 mcg/kg/day).

▪ **PO (Geriatric Patients and Patients with Increased Sensitivity to Thyroid Hormones):** 12.5–25 mcg as a single dose initially; may be increased q 6–8 wk wk; usual maintenance dose is 75 mcg/day.

▪ **PO (Children >10 yr):** 2–3 mcg/kg/day (up to 150–200 mcg/day).

▪ **PO (Children 6–10 yr):** 4–5 mcg/kg/day (100–150 mcg/day).

▪ **PO (Children 1–5 yr):** 3–5 mcg/kg/day (75–100 mcg/day).

▪ **PO (Children 6–12 mo):** 5–6 mcg/kg/day (50–75 mcg/day).

▪ **PO (Infants <6 mo):** 5–6 mcg/kg/day (25–50 mcg/day).

▪ **PO (Infants <2000 g or Infants at Risk for Cardiac Failure):** 25 mcg/day; may be increased after 4–6 wk to 50 mcg.

▪ **IM, IV (Adults):** *Hypothyroidism*—50–100 mcg/day as a single dose. *Myxedema coma/stupor*—200–500 mcg IV; additional 100–300 mcg may be given on 2nd day, followed by daily administration of smaller doses.

▪ **IM, IV (Children):** *Hypothyroidism*—50% of the calculated oral dose.

### ▫ Liothyronine

▪ **PO (Adults):** *Mild hypothyroidism*—25 mcg once daily; may increase by 12.5–25 mcg/day q 1–2 wk intervals; usual maintenance dose is 25–50 mcg/day. *Myxedema*—2.5–5 mcg once daily initially; increase by 5–10 mcg/day q 1–2 wk up to 25 mcg/day, then increase by 12.5–25 mcg/day; usual maintenance dose is 25–50 mcg/day. *Simple goiter*—5 mcg once daily initially; increase by 5–10 mcg/day q 1–2 wk up to 25 mcg/day, then increase by 12.5–25 mcg/day q wk until desired effect is obtained; usual maintenance dose is 50–100 mcg/day. *$T_3$ suppression test*—75–100 mcg daily for 7 days. Radioactive $^{131}$I is administered before and after 7-day course.

▪ **PO (Geriatric Patients or Patients with Cardiovascular Disease):** 5 mcg/day initially; increase by not more than 5 mcg/day q 2 wk.

▪ **IV (Adults):** *Myxedema coma/precoma*—25–50 mcg initially (if cardiovascular disease is present, initial dose should be 10–20 mcg). Additional doses may be given to a total of at least 65 mcg/day (not to exceed 100 mcg/day). Doses should be at least 4 hr but not more than 12 hr apart.

---

## ◻Liotrix

Contains T₄ and T₃ in a ratio of 4:1.

- **PO (Adults):** *Hypothyroidism*—Start with 50 mcg levothyroxine/12.5 mcg liothyronine; increase by 50 mcg levothyroxine/12.5 mcg liothyronine q mo until desired effect is obtained; usual maintenance dose is 50–100 mcg levothyroxine/12.5–25 mcg liothyronine daily. *Myxedema/hypothyroidism with cardiovascular disease*—12.5 mcg levothyroxine/3.1 mcg liothyronine/day; increase by 12.5 mcg levothyroxine/3.1 mcg liothyronine q 2–3 wk until desired effect is obtained.
- **PO (Geriatric Patients):** 12.5–25 mcg levothyroxine/3.1–6.2 mcg liothyronine/day; increase by 12.5–25 mcg levothyroxine/3.1–6.2 mcg liothyronine q 6–8 wk until desired effect is obtained.

## ◻Thyroid

- **PO (Adults and Children):** *Hypothyroidism*—60 mg/day; increase q mo by 30 mg; usual maintenance dose is 60–120 mg/day. *Myxedema/hypothyroidism with cardiovascular disease*—15 mg/day initially; increase by 30 mg/day q 2 wk, then may increase by 30–60 mg q 2 wk; usual maintenance dose is 60–120 mg/day.
- **PO (Geriatric Patients):** 7.5–15 mg/day initially; may double dose q 6–8 wk until desired effect is obtained.

## AVAILABILITY

### ◻Levothyroxine

- **Tablets:** 25 mcg^Rx, 50 mcg^Rx, 75 mcg^Rx, 88 mcg^Rx, 100 mcg^Rx, 112 mcg^Rx, 125 mcg^Rx, 137 mcg^Rx, 150 mcg^Rx, 175 mcg^Rx, 200 mcg^Rx, 300 mcg^Rx ▪ Cost:*Levoxyl*—50 mcg $24.89/100, 100 mcg $28.34/100, 150 mcg $33.96/100 ▪ *Powder for injection:* 200 mcg/vial in 6- and 10-ml vials^Rx, 500 mcg/vial in 6- and 10-ml vials^Rx.

### ◻Liothyronine

- **Tablets:** 5 mcg^Rx, 25 mcg^Rx, 50 mcg^Rx ▪ *Injection:* 10 mcg/ml in 1-ml vials^Rx.

### ◻Liotrix

- **Tablets:** 12.5 mcg levothyroxine/3.1 mcg liothyronine^Rx, 25 mcg levothyroxine/6.25 mcg liothyronine^Rx, 50 mcg levothyroxine/12.5 mcg liothyronine^Rx, 100 mcg levothyroxine/25 mcg liothyronine^Rx, 150 mcg levothyroxine/37.5 mcg liothyronine^Rx.

### ◻Thyroid

- **Tablets (regular):** 15 mg^Rx, 30 mg^Rx, 60 mg^Rx, 90 mg^Rx, 120 mg^Rx, 180 mg^Rx, 240 mg^Rx, 300 mg^Rx ▪ Cost:15 mg $10.96/100, 30 mg $12.88/100, 60 mg $14.28/100, 90 mg $22.57/100, 120 mg $26.44/100, 180 mg $41.95/100.

TIME/ACTION PROFILE (effects on thyroid function tests)

| | ONSET | PEAK | DURATION |
|---|---|---|---|
| Levothyroxine PO | unknown | 1–3 wk | 1–3 wk |
| Levothyroxine IV | 6–8 hr | 24 hr | unknown |
| Liothyronine PO | unknown | 24–72 hr | 72 hr |
| Liothyronine IV | unknown | unknown | unknown |
| Thyroid PO | days–wks | 1–3 wk | days–wks |

# NURSING IMPLICATIONS

## ASSESSMENT

- **General Info:** Assess apical pulse and blood pressure prior to and periodically during therapy. Assess for tachyarrhythmias and chest pain.
- **Children:** Monitor height, weight, and psychomotor development.
- **Lab Test Considerations**Monitor thyroid function studies prior to and during therapy.
- ◻ Monitor blood and urine glucose in diabetic patients. Insulin or oral hypoglycemic dose may need to be increased.
- **Toxicity and Overdose**Overdose is manifested as hyperthyroidism (tachycardia, chest pain, nervousness, insomnia, diaphoresis, tremors, weight loss). Usual treatment is to withhold dose for 2–6 days. Acute overdose is treated by induction of emesis or gastric lavage, followed by activated charcoal. Sympathetic overstimulation may be controlled by antiadrenergic drugs (beta blockers), such as propranolol. Oxygen and supportive measures to control symptoms such as fever are also used.

## POTENTIAL NURSING DIAGNOSES

- Knowledge, deficient, related to medication regimen (Patient/Family Teaching).

## IMPLEMENTATION

- **General:** Administer as a single dose, preferably before breakfast to prevent insomnia.

- Initial dose is low, especially in geriatric and cardiac patients. Dose is increased gradually, based on thyroid function tests. Side effects occur more rapidly with liothyronine because of its rapid onset of effect.

□ **Levothyroxine**

- **Direct IV:** Dilute the 200-mcg and 500-mcg vials with 2 or 5 ml, respectively, of 0.9% NaCl without preservatives (diluent usually provided), for a concentration of 100 mcg/ml. Shake well to dissolve completely. Administer solution immediately after preparation; discard unused portion.

- **Rate:** Administer at a rate of 100 mcg over 1 min. Do not add to IV infusions; may be administered through Y-tubing.

□ **Liothyronine**

- **IV:** Liothyronine injection is for IV use only. Do not give IM or subcut. Administer doses at least 4 hr and not more than 12 hr apart. Base doses on continuous monitoring of patient and response to therapy.

- Resume PO therapy as soon as patient is stable and able to take PO medication. When switching to PO therapy, discontinue IV liothyronine and initiate PO at low dose, increasing gradually according to patient's response.

- **Direct IV:** May be administered undiluted.
- **Rate:** Administer as a bolus.

**PATIENT/FAMILY TEACHING**

- **General Info:** Instruct patient to take medication as directed at the same time each day. Take missed doses as soon as remembered unless almost time for next dose. If more than 2–3 doses are missed, notify health care professional. Do not discontinue without consulting health care professional.

- Instruct patient and family on correct technique for checking pulse. Dose should be withheld and health care professional notified if resting pulse >100 bpm.

- Explain to patient that medication does not cure hypothyroidism; it provides a thyroid hormone. Therapy is lifelong.

- Caution patient not to change brands of thyroid preparations, as this may affect drug bioavailability.

- Advise patient to notify health care professional if headache, nervousness, diarrhea, excessive sweating, heat intolerance, chest pain, increased pulse rate, palpitations, weight loss >2 lb/wk, or any unusual symptoms occur.

- Caution patient to avoid taking other medications concurrently with thyroid preparations unless instructed by health care professional.

- Instruct patient to inform health care professional of thyroid therapy.

- Emphasize importance of follow-up exams to monitor effectiveness of therapy. Thyroid function tests are performed at least yearly.

- **Children:** Discuss with parents the need for routine follow-up studies to ensure correct development. Inform patient that partial hair loss may be experienced by children on thyroid therapy. This is usually temporary.

**EVALUATION**

**Clinical response to therapy can be evaluated by:** ■ Resolution of symptoms of hypothyroidism. Response includes: □ Diuresis □ Weight loss □ Increased sense of well-being □ Increased energy, pulse rate, appetite, psychomotor activity □ Normalization of skin texture and hair □ Correction of constipation □ Increased $T_3$ and $T_4$ levels ■ In children, effectiveness of therapy is determined by: □ Appropriate physical and psychomotor development.

# tiagabine
(tye-**a**-ga-been)
Gabatril

**CLASSIFICATION(S):**
**Therapeutic:** anticonvulsants

**Pregnancy Category C**

**INDICATIONS**

- Adjunctive treatment of partial seizures.

**ACTION**

- Enhances the activity of gamma-aminobutyric acid, an inhibitory neurotransmitter. **Therapeutic Effects:** ■ Decreased frequency of seizures.

## PHARMACOKINETICS

**Absorption:** 90% absorbed following oral administration.
**Distribution:** Unknown.
**Protein Binding:** 96%.
**Metabolism and Excretion:** Mostly metabolized by the liver; 2% excreted unchanged in urine.
**Half-life:** *Without enzyme-inducing antiepileptic drugs*—7–9 hr; *with enzyme-inducing antiepileptic drugs*—4–7 hr.

## CONTRAINDICATIONS AND PRECAUTIONS

**Contraindicated in:** ■ Hypersensitivity.

**Use Cautiously in:** ■ Hepatic impairment (decreased dose/increased interval may be necessary) ■ Patients receiving concurrent non–enzyme-inducing antiepileptic drug therapy such as valproates (may require lower doses and/or slower titration) ■ Pregnancy, lactation, or children <12 yr (safety not established).

## ADVERSE REACTIONS AND SIDE EFFECTS*

■ **CNS:** <u>DIZZINESS</u> drowsiness, <u>nervousness</u>, <u>weakness</u>, cognitive impairment, confusion, difficulty concentrating, hallucinations, headache, mental depression, personality disorder ■ **EENT:** abnormal vision, ear pain, tinnitus ■ **Resp:** dyspnea, epistaxis ■ **CV:** chest pain, edema, hypertension, palpitations, syncope, tachycardia ■ **GI:** abdominal pain, gingivitis, nausea, stomatitis ■ **GU:** dysmenorrhea, dysuria, metrorrhagia, urinary incontinence ■ **Derm:** alopecia, dry skin, rash, sweating ■ **Metab:** weight gain, weight loss ■ **MS:** arthralgia, neck pain ■ **Neuro:** ataxia, tremors ■ **Misc:** allergic reactions, chills, lymphadenopathy.

## INTERACTIONS

**Drug-Drug:** ■ **Carbamazepine, phenytoin, primidone,** and **phenobarbital** induce metabolism and decrease blood levels; although concurrent therapy is usually necessary, adjustments may be required when altering regimens.

## ROUTE AND DOSAGE

■ **PO (Adults >18 yr):** 4 mg once daily initially for 1 wk; may increase by 4–8 mg/day at weekly intervals, up to 56 mg/day in 2–4 divided doses.
■ **PO (Children 12–18 yr):** 4 mg once daily initially for 1 wk; may increase by 4 mg/day after 1 wk, then may increase by 4–8 mg/day at weekly intervals, up to 32 mg/day in 2–4 divided doses.

## AVAILABILITY

■ *Tablets:* 2 mg$^{Rx}$, 4 mg$^{Rx}$, 12 mg$^{Rx}$, 16 mg$^{Rx}$, 20 mg$^{Rx}$ ■ Cost:4 mg $110.26/100, 12 mg $146.91/100, 16 mg $195.89/100, 20 mg $244.86/100.

TIME/ACTION PROFILE (blood levels)

| | ONSET | PEAK | DURATION |
|---|---|---|---|
| PO | unknown | 45 min | unknown |

# NURSING IMPLICATIONS

## ASSESSMENT

❑ Assess location, duration, and characteristics of seizure activity.
❑ Assess mental status. May cause impaired concentration, speech or language problems, confusion, fatigue, and drowsiness. Symptoms may decrease with dose reduction or discontinuation.
  ■ *Toxicity and Overdose:*Therapeutic serum levels have not been determined. However, levels may be monitored prior to and following changes in the therapeutic regimen.

## POTENTIAL NURSING DIAGNOSES

■ Injury, risk for (Side Effects).

## IMPLEMENTATION

■ **General:** Do not confuse tiagabine with tizanidine.
■ **PO:** Administer with food.
❑ Tiagabine should be discontinued gradually. Abrupt discontinuation may cause increase in seizure frequency.

## PATIENT/FAMILY TEACHING

❑ Instruct patient to take medication exactly as directed. If a dose is missed, take as soon as possible unless almost time for next dose. Do not double doses. Do not discontinue abruptly; may cause increase in frequency of seizures.
❑ Advise patient to notify health care professional immediately if frequency of seizures increases.
❑ May cause dizziness. Caution patient to avoid driving or activities requiring alertness until

response to medication is known. Do not resume driving until physician gives clearance based on control of seizure disorder.

❏ Advise patient to notify health care professional if pregnancy is planned or suspected or if patient intends to breastfeed or is breastfeeding.

❏ Instruct patient to notify health care professional of medication regimen prior to treatment or surgery.

❏ Advise patient to carry identification describing disease process and medication regimen at all times.

## EVALUATION
**Effectiveness of therapy can be demonstrated by:** ■ Decrease in the frequency or cessation of seizures.

---

## ticarcillin
(tye-kar-**sil**-in)
Ticar

## ticarcillin/clavulanate
(tye-kar-**sil**-in/klav-yoo-**la**-nate)
Timentin

### CLASSIFICATION(S):
**Therapeutic:** anti-infectives
**Pharmacologic:** extended spectrum penicillins

### Pregnancy Category B

---

## INDICATIONS
■ Treatment of: ❏ Skin and skin structure infections ❏ Bone and joint infections ❏ Septicemia ❏ Respiratory tract infections ❏ Intra-abdominal, gynecologic, and urinary tract infections.

## ACTION
■ Binds to bacterial cell wall membrane, causing cell death ■ Addition of clavulanate enhances resistance to beta-lactamase, an enzyme that can inactivate penicillins. **Therapeutic Effects:** ■ Bactericidal action. **Spectrum:** ■ Similar to penicillin but extended to include several gram-negative aerobic pathogens, notably: ❏ *Pseudomonas aeruginosa* ❏ *Escherichia coli* ❏

*Proteus mirabilis* ❏ *Providencia rettgeri* ■ Active against some anaerobic bacteria, including bacteroides.

## PHARMACOKINETICS
**Absorption:** Ticarcillin is well absorbed following IM administration.

**Distribution:** Widely distributed. Enters CSF well when meninges are inflamed. Crosses the placenta; enters breast milk in low concentrations.

**Metabolism and Excretion:** 10% of ticarcillin is metabolized by the liver; 90% excreted unchanged by the kidneys. Clavulanate is metabolized by the liver.

**Half-life:** *Ticarcillin*—0.9–1.3 hr (increased in renal impairment); *clavulanate*—1.1–1.5 hr.

## CONTRAINDICATIONS AND PRECAUTIONS
**Contraindicated in:** ■ Hypersensitivity to penicillins (cross-sensitivity with cephalosporins may occur).

**Use Cautiously in:** ■ Renal impairment (dosage reduction and/or increased interval required if CCr <60 ml/min) ■ Pregnancy and lactation (safety not established) ■ Severe liver disease.

## ADVERSE REACTIONS AND SIDE EFFECTS*
■ **CNS:** SEIZURES (high doses), confusion, lethargy ■ **CV:** CHF, arrhythmias ■ **GI:** PSEUDOMEMBRANOUS COLITIS, diarrhea, nausea ■ **GU:** hematuria (children only) ■ **Derm:** rashes, urticaria ■ **F and E:** hypokalemia, hypernatremia ■ **Hemat:** bleeding, blood dyscrasias, increased bleeding time ■ **Local:** phlebitis ■ **Metab:** metabolic alkalosis ■ **Misc:** hypersensitivity reactions including ANAPHYLAXIS, superinfection.

## INTERACTIONS
**Drug-Drug:** ■ **Probenecid** decreases renal excretion and increases blood levels ■ May alter excretion of **lithium** ■ **Potassium-losing diuretics, amphotericin B,** or **corticosteroids** may increase the risk of hypokalemia ■ Hypokalemia increases the risk of **digoxin** toxicity.

---

## ROUTE AND DOSAGE

Ticarcillin contains 5.2 mEq sodium/g; ticarcillin/clavulanate contains 4.75–6.2 mEq sodium/g ticarcillin and 0.15 mEq potassium/100 mg clavulanate.

### ▢Ticarcillin

■ **IV (Adults and Children >40 kg):** *Most infections*—3 g q 4 hr *or* 4 g q 6 hr (150–300 mg/kg/day in divided doses; not to exceed 24 g/day). *Complicated urinary tract infections*—3 g q 6 hr IV. *Uncomplicated urinary tract infections*—1 g q 6 hr IM/IV.

■ **IV (Children <40 kg):** *Most infections*—33.3–50 mg/kg q 4 hr *or* 50–75 mg/kg q 6 hr IV. *Complicated urinary tract infections*—25–33.3 mg/kg q 4 hr *or* 37.5–50 mg/kg q 6 hr IV. *Uncomplicated urinary tract infections*—12.5–25 mg/kg q 6 hr *or* 16.7–33.3 mg/kg q 8 hr IM/IV.

■ **IM, IV (Neonates ≥2 kg):** 75 mg/kg q 8 hr for the first 7 days of life, then 75 mg/kg q 6 hr.

■ **IM, IV (Neonates <2 kg):** 75 mg/kg q 12 hr for the first 7 days of life, then 75 mg/kg q 8 hr.

### ▢Ticarcillin/Clavulanate

3 g ticarcillin plus 100 mg clavulanate labeled as 3.1 g combined potency.

■ **IV (Adults and Children ≥60 kg):** 3.1 g q 4–6 hr.

■ **IV (Adults <60 kg):** 33.3–50 mg/kg ticarcillin plus 1.1–1.7 mg/kg clavulanate q 4 hr *or* 50–75 mg/kg ticarcillin plus 1.7–2.5 mg clavulanate q 6 hr.

■ **IV (Children ≥3 mo–<60 kg):** 50 mg ticarcillin/kg plus 1.7 mg clavulanate/kg q 4–6 hr. *Children with cystic fibrosis*—up to 350–450 mg ticarcillin/kg plus 11.7–17 mg clavulanate/kg daily in divided doses.

## AVAILABILITY

### ▢Ticarcillin

■ *Powder for injection:* 1 g/vial[Rx], 3 g/vial[Rx], 6 g/vial[Rx], 20 g/vial[Rx], 30 g/vial[Rx].

### ▢Ticarcillin/Clavulanate

■ *Powder for injection:* 3.1 g/vials and piggyback bottles[Rx] ■ *Solution for injection:* 3.1-g premixed 100-ml bottles[Rx].

## TIME/ACTION PROFILE (blood levels)

|       | ONSET | PEAK | DURATION |
|-------|-------|------|----------|
| IM    | rapid | 30–75 min | 4–6 hr |
| IV    | rapid | end of infusion | 4–6 hr |

# NURSING IMPLICATIONS

## ASSESSMENT

❑ Assess patient for infection (vital signs; appearance of wound, sputum, urine, and stool; WBC) at beginning of and throughout therapy.

❑ Obtain a history before initiating therapy to determine use of and reactions to penicillins or cephalosporins. Persons with a negative history of penicillin sensitivity may still have an allergic response.

❑ Obtain specimens for culture and sensitivity before initiating therapy. First dose may be given before receiving results.

❑ Observe patient for signs and symptoms of anaphylaxis (rash, pruritus, laryngeal edema, wheezing). Discontinue drug and notify physician immediately if these problems occur. Keep epinephrine, an antihistamine, and resuscitation equipment close by in case of anaphylactic reaction.

■ *Lab Test Considerations:*Renal and hepatic function, CBC, serum potassium, and bleeding times should be evaluated prior to and routinely throughout therapy.

❑ May cause false-positive urine protein testing and increased BUN, creatinine, AST, ALT, serum bilirubin, alkaline phosphatase, LDH, and uric acid levels. May also cause increased bleeding time.

❑ May cause hypernatremia and hypokalemia with high doses.

## POTENTIAL NURSING DIAGNOSES

■ Infection, risk for (Indications, Side Effects).

## IMPLEMENTATION

■ **IM:** Reconstitute with 2 ml of sterile or bacteriostatic water for injection or 1% lidocaine hydrochloride injection (without epinephrine) to each 1-g vial for a concentration of 1 g/2.5 ml.

❑ Inject deep into a well-muscled mass to minimize discomfort, and massage well. IM injections should not exceed 2 g at each site. Do not administer ticarcillin/clavulanate IM.

- **IV:** Change IV sites every 48 hr to prevent phlebitis.

❑ **Ticarcillin**

- **Direct IV:** Add at least 4 ml of sterile water for injection to each 1-g vial. Further dilute to at least 20 ml with 0.9% NaCl, D5W, Ringer's or LR. Solution is stable for 48 hr at room temperature, 14 days if refrigerated.
- *Rate:* Administer as slowly as possible to minimize vein irritation. Do not administer concentrations >50 mg/ml.
- **Intermittent Infusion:** Dilute further for a concentration of 10–100 mg/ml.
- *Rate:* Administer over 30 min–2 hr, 10–20 min in neonates.

- **Y-Site Compatibility:** ◆ acyclovir ◆ amifostine ◆ aztreonam ◆ cyclophosphamide ◆ diltiazem ◆ famotidine ◆ filgrastim ◆ fludarabine ◆ gatifloxacin ◆ hydromorphone ◆ insulin ◆ linezolid ◆ magnesium sulfate ◆ melphalan ◆ meperidine ◆ morphine ◆ ondansetron ◆ perphenazine ◆ sargramostim ◆ teniposide ◆ theophylline ◆ thiotepa ◆ verapamil ◆ vinorelbine.

- **Y-Site Incompatibility:** ◆ fluconazole. If aminoglycosides and penicillins must be administered concurrently, administer in separate sites at least 1 hr apart.

❑ **Ticarcillin/Clavulanate**

- **Intermittent Infusion:** Add 13 ml of sterile water or 0.9% NaCl for injection to each 3.1-g vial, to provide a concentration of ticarcillin 200 mg/ml and clavulanic acid 6.7 mg/ml. Further dilute in 0.9% NaCl, D5W, or Ringer's or LR. Stable for 6 hr at room temperature, 72 hr if refrigerated.
- *Rate:* Administer over 30 min via Y-site or direct IV.

- **Y-Site Compatibility:** ◆ amifostine ◆ aztreonam ◆ cefepime ◆ cyclophosphamide ◆ diltiazem ◆ famotidine ◆ filgrastim ◆ fludarabine ◆ foscarnet ◆ gatifloxacin ◆ granisetron ◆ heparin ◆ insulin ◆ melphalan ◆ meperidine ◆ morphine ◆ ondansetron ◆ perphenazine ◆ sargramostim ◆ teniposide ◆ theophylline ◆ thiotepa ◆ vinorelbine.

- **Y-Site Incompatibility:** If aminoglycosides and penicillins must be administered concur-

rently, administer in separate sites at least 1 hr apart. ◆ alatrofloxacin.

## PATIENT/FAMILY TEACHING

- ❑ Advise patient to report signs of superinfection (black, furry overgrowth on the tongue; vaginal itching or discharge; loose or foul-smelling stools) and allergy.
- ❑ Caution patient to notify health care professional if fever and diarrhea occur, especially if stool contains blood, pus, or mucus. Advise patient not to treat diarrhea without consulting health care professional. May occur up to several weeks after discontinuation of medication.

## EVALUATION

**Clinical response to therapy can be evaluated by:** ■ Resolution of the signs and symptoms of infection. Length of time for complete resolution depends on the organism and site of infection.

## ticlopidine
(tye-**cloe**-pi-deen)
Ticlid

*CLASSIFICATION(S):*
***Therapeutic:*** *antiplatelet agents*
***Pharmacologic:*** *platelet aggregation inhibitors*

**Pregnancy Category B**

## INDICATIONS

■ Prevention of stroke in patients who have had a completed thrombotic stroke or precursors to stroke and are unable to tolerate aspirin. **Unlabeled uses:** ■ Prevention of early restenosis in intracoronary stents.

## ACTION

■ Inhibits platelet aggregation by altering the function of platelet membranes ■ Prolongs bleeding time. **Therapeutic Effects:** ■ Decreased incidence of stroke in high-risk patients.

## PHARMACOKINETICS

**Absorption:** >80% absorbed after oral administration.

**Distribution:** Unknown.

**Protein Binding:** 98%.

**Metabolism and Excretion:** Extensively metabolized by the liver; minimal excretion of unchanged drug by the kidneys.

**Half-life:** *Single dose*—12.6 hr; *multiple dosing*—4–5 days.

## CONTRAINDICATIONS AND PRECAUTIONS

**Contraindicated in:** ■ Hypersensitivity ■ Bleeding disorders ■ Active bleeding ■ Severe liver disease.

**Use Cautiously in:** ■ Risk of bleeding (trauma, surgery, history of ulcer disease) ■ Renal or hepatic impairment (dosage adjustments may be necessary) ■ Geriatric patients (increased sensitivity) ■ Pregnancy, lactation, or children <18 yr (safety not established).

## ADVERSE REACTIONS AND SIDE EFFECTS*

■ **CNS:** dizziness, headache, weakness ■ **EENT:** epistaxis, tinnitus ■ **GI:** diarrhea, abnormal liver function tests, anorexia, GI fullness, GI pain, nausea, vomiting ■ **GU:** hematuria ■ **Derm:** rashes, ecchymoses, pruritus, urticaria ■ **Hemat:** AGRANULOCYTOSIS APLASTIC ANEMIA INTRACEREBRAL BLEEDING NEUTROPENIA bleeding, thrombocytopenia ■ **Metab:** hypercholesterolemia, hypertriglyceridemia.

## INTERACTIONS

**Drug-Drug:** ■ **Aspirin** potentiates the effect of ticlopidine on platelets (concurrent use not recommended) ■ Increased risk of bleeding with **heparins, warfarin, tirofiban, eptifibatide, clopidogrel,** or **thrombolytic agents** ■ **Cimetidine** decreases metabolism of ticlopidine and may increase the risk of toxicity ■ Ticlopidine decreases metabolism of **theophylline** and increases the risk of toxicity.

**Drug-Food:** ■ Absorption of ticlopidine is increased by taking with **food.**

## ROUTE AND DOSAGE

■ **PO (Adults):** 250 mg bid with food.

## AVAILABILITY

■ *Tablets:* 250 mg$^{Rx}$ ■ Cost: $64.10/30.

TIME/ACTION PROFILE (effect on platelet function)

| | ONSET | PEAK | DURATION |
|---|---|---|---|
| PO | within 4 days | 8–11 days | 2 wk |

# NURSING IMPLICATIONS

## ASSESSMENT

❏ Assess patient for symptoms of stroke periodically throughout therapy.

■ *Lab Test Considerations:* Monitor bleeding time throughout therapy. Prolonged bleeding time (2–5 times the normal limit), which is time- and dose-dependent, is expected.

❏ Monitor CBC with differential and platelet count every 2 wk from the 2nd wk to the end of the 3rd mo of therapy; more frequently if absolute neutrophil count (ANC) is declining or <30% of baseline. If neutropenia occurs, ticlopidine should be discontinued. Neutrophil counts usually return to normal within 1–3 wk of discontinuation of therapy. After the first 3 mo of therapy, CBCs need to be obtained only for patients with signs and symptoms of infection.

❏ May cause thrombocytopenia, usually within 3–12 wk of initiation of therapy. If platelet count is <80,000/mm³, discontinue ticlopidine.

❏ May cause increased serum total cholesterol and triglyceride levels. Levels usually increase 8–10% within the first mo and persist at that level.

❏ May cause elevated alkaline phosphatase, bilirubin, AST, and ALT levels during the first 4 mo of therapy.

■ *Toxicity and Overdose:* Prolonged bleeding time is normalized within 2 hr after administration of IV methylprednisolone. May also use platelet transfusions to reverse effects of ticlopidine on bleeding time.

## POTENTIAL NURSING DIAGNOSES

■ Injury, risk for (Indications, Side Effects).

## IMPLEMENTATION

■ **PO:** Administer with food or immediately after eating to minimize GI discomfort and increase absorption.

## PATIENT/FAMILY TEACHING

❑ Instruct patient to take medication exactly as directed. Missed doses should be taken as soon as possible unless almost time for next dose; do not double doses.

❑ Advise patient to notify health care professional promptly if fever, chills, sore throat, unusual bleeding or bruising, severe or persistent diarrhea, skin rash, jaundice, dark-colored urine, or light-colored stools occur.

❑ Advise patient to notify health care professional of medication regimen before treatment or surgery. Medication may need to be discontinued 10–14 days before surgery.

❑ Emphasize the importance of routine lab tests during the first 3 mo of therapy to monitor for side effects.

## EVALUATION

**Effectiveness of therapy can be demonstrated by:** ■ Prevention of stroke.

---

## tiludronate

(tye-**loo**-droe-nate)

Skelid

### CLASSIFICATION(S):

**Therapeutic:** bone resorption inhibitors

**Pharmacologic:** biphosphonates

**Pregnancy Category C**

---

## INDICATIONS

■ Management of Paget's disease of the bone in patients with: ❑ Serum alkaline phosphatase ≥2 times the upper limit of normal ❑ Symptoms ❑ Risk for complications.

## ACTION

■ Inhibits resorption of bone by inhibiting osteoclast activity. **Therapeutic Effects:** ■ Decreased progression of Paget's disease.

## PHARMACOKINETICS

**Absorption:** Rapidly but poorly absorbed following oral administration (6% bioavailability).
**Distribution:** Distributes to bone and soft tissue; subsequently is slowly released from bone.

**Protein Binding:** 90% protein binding.
**Metabolism and Excretion:** Excreted mostly in urine.
**Half-life:** 150 hr.

## CONTRAINDICATIONS AND PRECAUTIONS

**Contraindicated in:** ■ Hypersensitivity ■ Severe renal impairment (CCr <30 ml/min).
**Use Cautiously in:** ■ Pregnancy, lactation, or children <18 yr (safety not established).

## ADVERSE REACTIONS AND SIDE EFFECTS*

■ **CNS:** anxiety, drowsiness, fatigue, insomnia, nervousness, syncope, vertigo, weakness ■ **EENT:** cataracts, conjunctivitis, glaucoma, pharyngitis, rhinitis, sinusitis ■ **Resp:** bronchitis ■ **CV:** chest pain, dependent edema, hypertension, peripheral edema ■ **GI:** abdominal pain, anorexia, constipation, diarrhea, dry mouth, dysphagia, esophageal ulcer, esophagitis, flatulence, gastric ulcer, gastritis, nausea, tooth disorder, vomiting ■ **GU:** urinary tract infection ■ **Derm:** flushing, increased sweating, pruritus, rash, skin disorder ■ **Endo:** hyperparathyroidism ■ **F and E:** hypocalcemia ■ **MS:** arthrosis, involuntary muscle contractions, pathological fractures ■ **Neuro:** paresthesia ■ **Misc:** infection.

## INTERACTIONS

**Drug-Drug:** ■ Absorption is decreased by concurrent administration of **calcium supplements, aspirin,** or **aluminum-** or **magnesium-containing antacids** ■ Bioavailability is increased by concurrent administration of **indomethacin.**
**Drug-Food:** ■ **Food** decreases absorption.

## ROUTE AND DOSAGE

■ **PO (Adults):** 400 mg/day taken with 8 oz of plain water only, for 3 mo.

## AVAILABILITY

■ **Tablets:** 400 mg^Rx ■ Cost: $420.89/56.

TIME/ACTION PROFILE (blood levels)

| | ONSET | PEAK | DURATION |
|---|---|---|---|
| PO | unknown | within 2 hr | unknown |

# NURSING IMPLICATIONS

## ASSESSMENT

■ **Paget's Disease:** Assess for symptoms of Paget's disease (bone pain, headache, decreased visual and auditory acuity, increased skull size).

■ *Lab Test Considerations:*Monitor alkaline phosphatase prior to and periodically during therapy. Tiludronate is indicated for patients with alkaline phosphatase 2 times the upper limit of normal.

## POTENTIAL NURSING DIAGNOSES

■ Injury, risk for (Indications).

## IMPLEMENTATION

■ **PO:** Administer first thing in the morning with 6–8 oz plain water 30 min prior to other medications, beverages, or food.

❑ Calcium supplements, aspirin, or indomethacin should not be taken for 2 hr before or 2 hr after tiludronate; antacids should not be taken for at least 2 hr following tiludronate.

## PATIENT/FAMILY TEACHING

❑ Instruct patient on the importance of taking exactly as directed, first thing in the morning, 30 min prior to other medications, beverages, or food. Waiting longer than 30 min will improve absorption. Tiludronate should be taken with 6–8 oz plain water (mineral water, orange juice, coffee, and other beverages decrease absorption). If a dose is missed, skip dose and resume the next morning; do not double doses or take later in the day. Do not discontinue without consulting health care professional.

❑ Caution patients to remain upright for 30 min following dose to facilitate passage to stomach and minimize risk of esophageal irritation.

❑ Advise patient to eat a balanced diet and consult health care professional about the need for supplemental calcium and vitamin D.

❑ Encourage patient to participate in regular exercise and to modify behaviors that increase the risk of osteoporosis (stop smoking, reduce alcohol consumption).

❑ Advise female patient to notify health care professional if pregnancy is planned or suspected or if she is nursing.

## EVALUATION

**Effectiveness of therapy can be demonstrated by:** ■ Decrease in the progression of Paget's disease.

## timolol†

(tim-oh-lole)
{Apo-Timol}, Blocadren, {Novo-Timol}

### CLASSIFICATION(S):

*Therapeutic: antihypertensives, vascular headache suppressants*
*Pharmacologic: beta blockers*

### Pregnancy Category C

†For ophthalmic use, see Appendix C.

## INDICATIONS

■ Hypertension(alone or with other agents) ■ Prevention of MI ■ Prevention of migraine headaches. **Unlabeled uses:** ■ Ventricular arrhythmias ■ Essential tremor ■ Anxiety.

## ACTION

■ Blocks stimulation of beta$_1$(myocardial)- and beta$_2$(pulmonary, vascular, and uterine)-adrenergic receptor sites. **Therapeutic Effects:** ■ Decreased heart rate and blood pressure ■ Prevention of MI ■ Decreased frequency of migraine headache.

## PHARMACOKINETICS

**Absorption:** Well absorbed after oral administration.

**Distribution:** Enters breast milk.

**Metabolism and Excretion:** Extensively metabolized by the liver.

**Half-life:** 3–4 hr.

## CONTRAINDICATIONS AND PRECAUTIONS

**Contraindicated in:** ■ Uncompensated CHF ■ Pulmonary edema ■ Cardiogenic shock ■ Bradycardia or heart block.

**Use Cautiously in:** ■ Renal impairment ■ Hepatic impairment ■ Geriatric patients (increased sensitivity to beta blockers; initial dosage reduction recommended, consider age-related decrease in body mass, renal/hepatic/cardiac function) ■ Pulmonary disease (including asthma) ■ Diabetes mellitus (may mask signs of hypoglycemia) ■ Thyrotoxicosis (may mask symptoms) ■ Patients with a history of severe allergic reactions (intensity of reactions may be increased) ■ Pregnancy, lactation, or children (safety not established; all agents cross the placenta and may cause fetal/neonatal bradycardia, hypotension, hypoglycemia, or respiratory depression).

## ADVERSE REACTIONS AND SIDE EFFECTS*

■ **CNS:** <u>fatigue</u>, <u>weakness</u>, anxiety, depression, dizziness, drowsiness, insomnia, memory loss, mental status changes, nervousness, nightmares ■ **EENT:** blurred vision, dry eyes, nasal stuffiness ■ **Resp:** bronchospasm, wheezing ■ **CV:** ARRHYTHMIAS, BRADYCARDIA, CHF, PULMONARY EDEMA, orthostatic hypotension, peripheral vasoconstriction ■ **GI:** constipation, diarrhea, nausea ■ **GU:** <u>impotence</u>, decreased libido ■ **Derm:** itching, rashes ■ **Endo:** hyperglycemia, hypoglycemia ■ **MS:** arthralgia, back pain, muscle cramps ■ **Neuro:** paresthesia ■ **Misc:** ANAPHYLAXIS (rare).

## INTERACTIONS

**Drug-Drug:** ■ **General anesthesia, IV phenytoin,** and **verapamil** may ↑ myocardial depression ■ ↑ bradycardia may occur with **digoxin** ■ ↑ hypotension may occur with other **antihypertensives,** acute ingestion of **alcohol,** or **nitrates** ■ Concurrent use with **amphetamines, cocaine, ephedrine, epinephrine, norepinephrine, phenylephrine,** or **pseudoephedrine** may result in unopposed alpha-adrenergic stimulation (excessive hypertension, bradycardia) ■ Concurrent **thyroid** administration may ↓ effectiveness ■ May alter the effectiveness of **insulins** or **oral antidiabetics** (dosage adjustments may be necessary) ■ May ↓ effectiveness of **bronchodilators** and **theophylline** ■ May ↓ beneficial cardiovascular effects of **dopamine** or **dobutamine** ■ Use cautiously within 14 days of **MAO inhibitor** therapy (may result in hypertension) ■ **Cimetidine** may ↑ toxicity ■ Concurrent **NSAIDs** may ↓ antihypertensive action.

## ROUTE AND DOSAGE

■ **PO (Adults):** *Antihypertensive*—10 mg twice daily initially; may be increased q 7

days as needed (usual maintenance dose is 10–20 mg twice daily; up to 60 mg/day). *Prevention of MI*—10 mg twice daily, starting 1–4 wk after MI. *Prevention of vascular headache*—10 mg twice daily initially, may be given as a single daily dose; may be increased up to 10 mg in the morning and 20 mg in the evening.

## AVAILABILITY (generic available)

■ *Tablets:* 5 mg^Rx, 10 mg^Rx, 20 mg^Rx.

TIME/ACTION PROFILE (cardiovascular effects)

| | ONSET | PEAK | DURATION |
|---|---|---|---|
| PO | unknown | 1–2 hr* | 12–24 hr |

*After single dose, full effect is not seen until several weeks of therapy.

## NURSING IMPLICATIONS

### ASSESSMENT

■ **General Info:** Monitor blood pressure and pulse frequently during dose adjustment period and periodically during therapy. Assess for orthostatic hypotension when assisting patient up from supine position.
❑ Monitor intake and output ratios and daily weight. Assess patient routinely for evidence of fluid overload (peripheral edema, dyspnea, rales/crackles, fatigue, weight gain, jugular venous distention).
■ **Hypertension:** Monitor frequency of prescription refills to determine adherence.
■ **Vascular Headache Prophylaxis:** Assess frequency, severity, characteristics, and location of vascular headaches periodically during therapy.
■ *Lab Test Considerations:* May cause ↑ BUN, serum lipoprotein, potassium, triglyceride, and uric acid levels.
❑ May cause ↑ ANA titers.
❑ May cause ↑ in blood glucose levels.
■ *Toxicity and Overdose:* Monitor patients receiving beta blockers for signs of overdose (bradycardia, severe dizziness or fainting, severe drowsiness, dyspnea, bluish fingernails or palms, seizures). Notify physician or other health care provider immediately if these signs occur.

{ } = Available in Canada only.
*CAPITALS indicates life-threatening; <u>underlines</u> indicate most frequent.

❑ Glucagon has been used to treat bradycardia and hypotension.

## POTENTIAL NURSING DIAGNOSES

■ Cardiac output, decreased (Side Effects).
■ Noncompliance (Patient/Family Teaching).

## IMPLEMENTATION

■ **PO:** Take apical pulse before administering. If <50 bpm or if arrhythmia occurs, withhold medication and notify physician or other health care professional.
❑ May be administered with food or on an empty stomach.
❑ Tablets may be crushed and mixed with food.

## PATIENT/FAMILY TEACHING

■ **General Info:** Instruct patient to take medication as directed, at the same time each day, even if feeling well; do not skip or double up on missed doses. Take missed doses as soon as possible up to 4 hr before next dose. Abrupt withdrawal may precipitate life-threatening arrhythmias, hypertension, or myocardial ischemia.
❑ Advise patient to make sure that enough medication is available for weekends, holidays, and vacations. A written prescription may be kept in wallet in case of emergency.
❑ Teach patient and family how to check pulse daily and blood pressure biweekly. Advise patient to hold dose and contact health care professional if pulse is <50 bpm or blood pressure changes significantly.
❑ May cause drowsiness or dizziness. Caution patients to avoid driving or other activities that require alertness until response to the drug is known.
❑ Advise patients to change positions slowly to minimize orthostatic hypotension, especially during initiation of therapy or when dose is increased.
❑ Caution patient that this medication may increase sensitivity to cold.
❑ Instruct patient to consult health care professional before taking any OTC medications or herbal products, especially cold preparations, concurrently with this medication.
❑ Patients with diabetes should closely monitor blood glucose, especially if weakness, malaise, irritability, or fatigue occurs. Medication may mask tachycardia and increased blood pressure as signs of hypoglycemia, but dizziness and sweating may still occur.

❑ Advise patient to notify health care professional if slow pulse, difficulty breathing, wheezing, cold hands and feet, dizziness, confusion, depression, rash, fever, sore throat, unusual bleeding, or bruising occurs.
❑ Instruct patient to inform health care professional of medication regimen before treatment or surgery.
❑ Advise patient to carry identification describing disease process and medication regimen at all times.
■ **Hypertension:** Reinforce the need to continue additional therapies for hypertension (weight loss, sodium restriction, stress reduction, regular exercise, moderation of alcohol consumption, and smoking cessation). Medication controls but does not cure hypertension.
■ **Vascular Headache Prophylaxis:** Caution patient that sharing this medication may be dangerous.

## EVALUATION

**Effectiveness of therapy can be demonstrated by:** ■ Decrease in blood pressure ■ Prevention of MI ■ Prevention of vascular headaches.

---

**tinzaparin, See HEPARINS (LOW MOLECULAR WEIGHT)/ HEPARINOIDS.**

---

**tioconazole, See ANTIFUNGALS (VAGINAL).**

---

**High Alert**

**tirofiban**
(tye-roe-**fye**-ban)
Aggrastat

**CLASSIFICATION(S):**
**Therapeutic:** antiplatelet agents
**Pharmacologic:** glycoprotein IIb/IIIa inhibitors

**Pregnancy Category B**

## INDICATIONS

■ Treatment of acute coronary syndrome (unstable angina/non–Q-wave MI), including patients who will be managed medically and those who will undergo percutaneous transluminal angioplasty (PCTA) or atherectomy ■ Used concurrently with aspirin and heparin.

## ACTION

■ Decreases platelet aggregation by reversibly antagonizing the binding of fibrinogen to the glycoprotein IIb/IIIa binding site on platelet surfaces. **Therapeutic Effects:** ■ Inhibition of platelet aggregation resulting in decreased incidence of new MI, death, or refractory ischemia with the need for repeat cardiac procedures.

## PHARMACOKINETICS

**Absorption:** IV administration results in complete bioavailability.

**Distribution:** Unknown.

**Metabolism and Excretion:** Excreted mostly unchanged by the kidneys (65%); 25% excreted unchanged in feces.

**Half-life:** 2 hr.

## CONTRAINDICATIONS AND PRECAUTIONS

**Contraindicated in:** ■ Hypersensitivity ■ Active internal bleeding or history of bleeding within previous 30 days ■ History of intracranial hemorrhage, intracranial neoplasm, arteriovenous malformation or aneurysm ■ History of thrombocytopenia during previous tirofiban therapy ■ History of hemorrhagic stroke or other stroke within 30 days ■ Major surgical procedure or severe physical trauma within 30 days ■ History, symptoms, or other findings associated with aortic aneurysm ■ Severe hypertension (systolic BP >180 mmHg and/or diastolic BP >110 mmHg) ■ Concurrent use of other glycoprotein IIb/IIIa receptor antagonists ■ Acute pericarditis ■ Lactation.

**Use Cautiously in:** ■ Platelet count <150,000/mm³ ■ Hemorrhagic retinopathy ■ Female patients and geriatric patients (increased risk of bleeding) ■ Severe renal insufficiency (decrease rate of infusion by 50% if CCr <30 ml/min) ■ Pregnancy or children (safety not established; use in pregnancy only if clearly needed).

## ADVERSE REACTIONS AND SIDE EFFECTS*

Noted for patients receiving heparin and aspirin in addition to tirofiban. ■ **CNS:** dizziness, headache ■ **CV:** bradycardia, coronary dissection, edema, vasovagal reaction ■ **GI:** nausea ■ **Derm:** hives, rash ■ **Hemat:** BLEEDING, thrombocytopenia ■ **MS:** leg pain ■ **Misc:** fever, hypersensitivity reactions, pelvic pain, sweating.

## INTERACTIONS

**Drug-Drug:** ■ **Aspirin**, other **NSAIDs**, **warfarin**, **heparin** and **heparin-like agents**, **abciximab**, **eptifibatide**, **clopidogrel**, **ticlopidine**, or **dipyridamole**—concurrent use may increase the risk of bleeding, although these agents are frequently used together or in sequence ■ Risk of bleeding may be increased by concurrent use of **cefotetan**, **cefoperazone**, **plicamycin**, or **valproic acid**.

**Drug-Natural Products:** ■ Increased anticoagulant effect and bleeding risk with **anise**, **arnica**, **chamomile**, **clove**, **dong quai**, **fenugreek**, **feverfew**, **garlic**, **ginger**, **ginkgo**, **Panax ginseng**, **licorice**, and others.

## ROUTE AND DOSAGE

■ **IV (Adults):** 0.4 mcg/kg/min for 30 min, then 0.1 mcg/kg/min, continued throughout angiography and for 12–24 hr after angioplasty or atherectomy.

■

❑ **Renal Impairment**

■ **IV (Adults):** *CCr <30 ml/min*—0.2 mcg/kg/min for 30 min, then 0.05 mcg/kg/min, continued throughout angiography and for 12–24 hr after angioplasty or atherectomy.

## AVAILABILITY

■ *Concentrated solution for IV infusion (dilute before use):* 12.5 mg/50 ml (250 mcg/ml) in 50-ml vials^Rx ■ *Premixed solution for infusion:* 25 mg/500 ml (50 mcg/ml) in 500-ml single-dose containers^Rx.

TIME/ACTION PROFILE (effects on platelet function)

| | ONSET | PEAK | DURATION |
|---|---|---|---|
| IV | rapid | 30 min† | brief‡ |

†>90% inhibition of platelet aggregation at end of initial 30-min infusion.

‡Inhibition is reversible following cessation of infusion.

## NURSING IMPLICATIONS

### ASSESSMENT

❏ Assess patient for bleeding. Most common is oozing from the arterial access site for cardiac catheterization. Arterial and venous punctures, IM injections, and use of urinary catheters, nasotracheal intubation, and nasogastric tubes should be minimized. Noncompressible sites for IV access should be avoided. If bleeding cannot be controlled with pressure, discontinue tirofiban and heparin immediately.

❏ During vascular access, avoid puncturing posterior wall of femoral artery. Maintain bedrest with head of bed elevated 30° and affected limb restrained in a straight position while the vascular sheath is in place. Heparin should be discontinued for 3–4 hr and activated clotting time (ACT) <180 sec or activated partial thromboplastin time (aPTT) <45 sec prior to pulling the sheath. Use compressive techniques to obtain hemostasis and monitor closely. Sheath hemostasis should be maintained for >4 hr before discharge from the hospital.

❏ Monitor for signs of thrombocytopenia (chills, low-grade fever) during therapy.

■ **Lab Test Considerations:** Assess hemoglobin, hematocrit, and platelet count prior to tirofiban therapy, within 6 hr following loading infusion, and at least daily during therapy (more frequently if evidence of significant decline). May cause decreased hemoglobin and hematocrit.

❏ If platelet count decreases to <90,000/mm³, perform additional platelet counts to rule out pseudothrombocytopenia. If thrombocytopenia is confirmed, tirofiban and heparin should be discontinued and condition monitored and treated.

❏ To monitor unfractionated heparin, assess aPTT 6 hr after the start of heparin infusion. Adjust heparin to maintain aPTT at approximately 2 times control.

❏ May cause presence of urine and fecal occult blood.

### POTENTIAL NURSING DIAGNOSES

■ Tissue perfusion, ineffective (Indications).

### IMPLEMENTATION

❏ **High Alert:** Use of antiplatelet medications has resulted in patient harm and/or death from internal hemorrhage or intracranial bleeding. Have second practitioner independently check original order, dosage calculations, and infusion pump settings.

■ **General:** Most patients receive heparin and aspirin concurrently with tirofiban.

❏ Do not administer solutions that are discolored or contain particulate matter. Discard unused portion.

■ **Intermittent Infusion:** Tirofiban injection must be diluted to same strength as tirofiban injection premixed. Withdraw and discard 100 ml from a 500-ml bag of 0.9% NaCl or D5W and replace volume with 100 ml of tirofiban from two 50-ml vials or withdraw and discard 50 ml from a 250-ml bag of 0.9% NaCl or D5W and replace volume with 50 ml of tirofiban for a concentration of 50 mcg/ml. Mix well prior to administration.

❏ Tirofiban injection premix is supplied in *IntraVia* containers. To open, tear off dust cover. Plastic may be opaque, but opacity will diminish gradually. Check for leaks by squeezing inner bag firmly; discard if leak is found. Do not add other drugs or remove solution directly from bag with syringe. Do not use plastic containers in series connections; may result in air embolism. Discard unused solution 24 hr following start of infusion.

■ **Rate:** Rate is based on patient weight. Administer at an initial rate of 0.4 mcg/kg/min for 30 min; then continue at 0.1 mcg/kg/min.

■ **Y-Site Compatibility:** ◆ heparin.

■ **Y-Site Incompatibility:** ◆ diazepam.

### PATIENT/FAMILY TEACHING

❏ Inform patient of the purpose of tirofiban.

❏ Instruct patient to notify health care professional immediately if any bleeding is noted.

### EVALUATION

**Effectiveness of therapy can be demonstrated by:** ■ Inhibition of platelet aggregation resulting in decreased incidence of new MI, death, or refractory ischemia with the need for repeat cardiac procedures.

## tizanidine
(tye-**zan**-i-deen)
Zanaflex

## INDICATIONS

■ Increased muscle tone associated with spasticity due to multiple sclerosis or spinal cord injury.

## ACTION

■ Acts as an agonist at central alpha-adrenergic receptor sites ■ Reduces spasticity by increasing presynaptic inhibition of motor neurons. **Therapeutic Effects:** ■ Decreased spasticity, allowing better function.

## PHARMACOKINETICS

**Absorption:** Completely absorbed after oral administration but rapidly metabolized, resulting in 40% bioavailability.
**Distribution:** Widely distributed.
**Metabolism and Excretion:** 95% metabolized by the liver.
**Half-life:** 2.5 hr.

## CONTRAINDICATIONS AND PRECAUTIONS

**Contraindicated in:** ■ Hypersensitivity.
**Use Cautiously in:** ■ Renal impairment ■ Geriatric patients ■ Concurrent antihypertensive therapy ■ Pregnancy, lactation, or children (safety not established).
**Exercise Extreme Caution in:** ■ Impaired hepatic function.

## ADVERSE REACTIONS AND SIDE EFFECTS*

■ **CNS:** <u>anxiety</u>, <u>depression</u>, <u>dizziness</u>, <u>sedation</u>, <u>weakness</u>, dyskinesia, hallucinations, nervousness ■ **EENT:** blurred vision, pharyngitis, rhinitis ■ **CV:** <u>hypotension</u>, bradycardia ■ **GI:** <u>abdominal pain</u>, <u>diarrhea</u>, <u>dry mouth</u>, <u>dyspepsia</u>, constipation, hepatocellular injury, increased liver enzymes, vomiting ■ **GU:** urinary frequency ■ **Derm:** <u>rash</u>, <u>skin ulcers</u>, <u>sweating</u> ■ **MS:** <u>back pain</u>, <u>myasthenia</u>, <u>paresthesia</u> ■ **Misc:** <u>fever</u>, speech disorder.

## INTERACTIONS

**Drug-Drug:** ■ Blood levels and effects ↑ by concurrent use of **hormonal contraceptives** or **alcohol** ■ ↑ risk of hypotension with **alpha₂-adrenergic agonist antihypertensives** (avoid concurrent use) ■ ↑ CNS depression may occur with **alcohol** or other **CNS depressants** including some **antidepressants, sedative/hypnotics, antihistamines,** and **opioid analgesics.**

## ROUTE AND DOSAGE

■ **PO (Adults):** 4 mg q 6–8 hr initially (no more than 3 doses/24 hr); increase by 2–4 mg/dose up to 8 mg/dose or 24 mg/day (not to exceed 36 mg/day). Some patients may tolerate twice-daily dosing.

## AVAILABILITY (generic available)

■ ***Tablets:*** 2 mg^Rx, 4 mg^Rx ■ Cost: 2 mg $203.66/150, 4 mg $203.66/150 ■ ***Capsules:*** 2 mg^Rx, 4 mg^Rx, 6 mg^Rx.

TIME/ACTION PROFILE (reduced muscle tone)

|     | ONSET   | PEAK   | DURATION |
|-----|---------|--------|----------|
| PO  | unknown | 1–2 hr | 3–6 hr   |

# NURSING IMPLICATIONS

## ASSESSMENT

❑ Assess muscle spasticity before and periodically during therapy.
❑ Monitor blood pressure and pulse, especially during dose titration. May cause orthostatic hypotension, bradycardia, dizziness, and, rarely, syncope. Effects are usually dose related.
❑ Observe patient for drowsiness, dizziness, and asthenia. A change in dose may alleviate these problems.
■ *Lab Test Considerations:* Monitor liver function tests before and at 1, 3, and 6 mo of therapy. May cause ↑ in serum glucose, alkaline phosphatase, AST, and ALT levels.

## POTENTIAL NURSING DIAGNOSES

■ Mobility, impaired physical (Indications).
■ Injury, risk for (Adverse Reactions).

## IMPLEMENTATION

- **General:** Do not confuse tizanidine with tiagibine.
- Doses should be titrated carefully to prevent side effects.
- **PO:** May be taken without regard to meals.

## PATIENT/FAMILY TEACHING

- Instruct patient to take tizanidine as directed. Tizanidine may need to be discontinued gradually.
- May cause dizziness and drowsiness. Advise patient to avoid driving or other activities requiring alertness until response to drug is known.
- Instruct patient to change positions slowly to minimize orthostatic hypotension.
- Advise patient to avoid concurrent use of alcohol or other CNS depressants while taking this medication.

## EVALUATION

**Effectiveness of therapy can be demonstrated by:** ■ Decrease in muscle spasticity with an increased ability to perform activities of daily living.

---

# tobramycin, See AMINOGLYCOSIDES.

---

# tolcapone

(**tole**-ka-pone)

Tasmar

## CLASSIFICATION(S):

**Therapeutic:** antiparkinson agents
**Pharmacologic:** catechol-O-methyltransferase inhibitors

## Pregnancy Category C

## INDICATIONS

■ Management of Parkinson's disease with carbidopa/levodopa in patients without severe movement abnormalities who do not respond to other treatment.

## ACTION

■ Acts as a selective and reversible inhibitor of the enzyme catechol-O-methyltransferase ■ Inhibition of this enzyme prevents the breakdown of levodopa, greatly increasing its availability to the CNS. **Therapeutic Effects:** ■ Prolongs duration of response to levodopa without end-of-dose motor fluctuations ■ Decreased signs and symptoms of Parkinson's disease.

## PHARMACOKINETICS

**Absorption:** Rapidly absorbed following oral administration with 65% bioavailability.

**Distribution:** Unknown.

**Protein Binding:** >99% bound to plasma proteins.

**Metabolism and Excretion:** Mostly metabolized by the liver; <0.5% excreted unchanged in urine.

**Half-life:** 2–3 hr.

## CONTRAINDICATIONS AND PRECAUTIONS

**Contraindicated in:** ■ Hypersensitivity ■ Concurrent MAO inhibitor therapy ■ Clinical evidence of liver disease.

**Use Cautiously in:** ■ Severe renal impairment (safety not established if CCr <25 ml/min) ■ Pregnancy or lactation (safety not established).

## ADVERSE REACTIONS AND SIDE EFFECTS*

■ **CNS:** <u>headache</u>, <u>sleep disorder</u>, hallucinations, syncope ■ **CV:** orthostatic hypotension ■ **GI:** HEPATOTOXICITY <u>constipation</u>, <u>diarrhea</u>, anorexia, elevated liver enzymes, nausea, vomiting ■ **GU:** hematuria, yellow discoloration of urine ■ **Derm:** increased sweating ■ **Neuro:** <u>dyskinesia</u>, <u>dystonia</u>.

## INTERACTIONS

**Drug-Drug:** ■ Concurrent use with **MAO inhibitors** is not recommended; both agents inhibit the metabolic pathways of catecholamines ■ May increase the effects of **methyldopa, apomorphine, dobutamine,** or **isoproterenol**; dosage reduction may be necessary ■ Increases the bioavailability of **levodopa** by two-fold; this is a desired effect.

## ROUTE AND DOSAGE

- **PO (Adults):** 100 mg 3 times daily; may be cautiously increased to 200 mg 3 times daily if benefit is justified.

## AVAILABILITY

- **Tablets:** 100 mg$^{Rx}$, 200 mg$^{Rx}$.

**Half-life:** *Tolterodine*—1.9–3.7 hr; *5-hydroxymethyltolterodine*—2.9–3.1 hr.

## CONTRAINDICATIONS AND PRECAUTIONS

**Contraindicated in:** ■ Urinary retention ■ Gastric retention ■ Uncontrolled narrow-angle glaucoma ■ Lactation.

**Use Cautiously in:** ■ GI obstructive disorders, including pyloric stenosis (increased risk of gastric retention) ■ Significant bladder outflow obstruction (increased risk of urinary retention) ■ Controlled narrow-angle glaucoma ■ Significant hepatic impairment (lower doses recommended) ■ Impaired renal function ■ Pregnancy (safe use not established; use only if potential maternal benefit justifies potential risk to fetus) ■ Children (safety not established).

## ADVERSE REACTIONS AND SIDE EFFECTS*

■ **CNS:** headache, dizziness ■ **EENT:** blurred vision, dry eyes ■ **GI:** dry mouth, constipation, dyspepsia.

## INTERACTIONS

**Drug-Drug:** ■ **Erythromycin, clarithromycin, ketoconazole, itraconazole,** and **miconazole** may inhibit metabolism and increase effects of tolterodine.

## ROUTE AND DOSAGE

■ **PO (Adults):** 2 mg twice daily as tablets; may be lowered depending on response *or* 2–4 mg once daily as extended-release capsules.
■ **PO (Adults with impaired hepatic function or concurrent enzyme inhibitors):** 1 mg twice daily.

## AVAILABILITY

■ *Tablets:* 1 mg$^{Rx}$, 2 mg$^{Rx}$ ■ Cost: 1 mg $75.60/60, 2 mg $77.58/60 ■ *Extended-release capsules:* 2 mg$^{Rx}$, 4 mg$^{Rx}$.

TIME/ACTION PROFILE (effects on bladder function)

| | ONSET | PEAK | DURATION |
|---|---|---|---|
| PO | unknown | unknown | 12 hr |

## NURSING IMPLICATIONS

### ASSESSMENT

❑ Assess patient for urinary urgency, frequency, and urge incontinence periodically throughout therapy.

### POTENTIAL NURSING DIAGNOSES

■ Urinary elimination, impaired (Indications).
■ Urinary retention (Indications).

### IMPLEMENTATION

■ **PO:** Administer without regard to food.
❑ Extended-release capsules should be swallowed whole; do not open or chew.

### PATIENT/FAMILY TEACHING

❑ Instruct patient to take tolterodine exactly as directed.
❑ May cause dizziness and blurred vision. Caution patient to avoid driving or other activities requiring alertness until response to medication is known.

### EVALUATION

**Effectiveness of therapy can be demonstrated by:** ■ Decreased urinary frequency, urgency, and urge incontinence.

---

## topiramate
(toe-**peer**-i-mate)
Topamax

**CLASSIFICATION(S):**
*Therapeutic: anticonvulsants*

**Pregnancy Category C**

---

### INDICATIONS

■ Adjunctive therapy of seizures including ❑ partial-onset ❑ primary generalized tonic-clonic ❑ seizures due to Lennox-Gastaut syndrome.

### ACTION

■ Action may be due to: ■ Blockade of sodium channels in neurons ■ Enhancement of gamma-aminobutyrate, an inhibitory neurotransmitter ■ Prevention of activation of excitatory receptors. **Therapeutic Effects:** ■ Decreased incidence of seizures.

TIME/ACTION PROFILE (blood levels)

| | ONSET | PEAK | DURATION |
|---|---|---|---|
| PO | unknown | 1.7 hr | 8 hr |

## NURSING IMPLICATIONS

### ASSESSMENT

- Assess patient for signs and symptoms of Parkinson's disease (tremor, muscle weakness and rigidity, ataxic gait) prior to and throughout therapy.
- Assess blood pressure periodically throughout therapy.
- **Lab Test Considerations:** Monitor liver function tests monthly during the first 3 mo of therapy and every 6 wk for the next 6 wk of treatment. Tolcapone should be discontinued if liver function tests reach 5 times the upper limit of normal or if jaundice occurs.

### POTENTIAL NURSING DIAGNOSES

- Mobility, impaired physical (Indications).
- Injury, risk for (Indications, Side Effects).

### IMPLEMENTATION

- **PO:** Administer first dose of the day of tolcapone together with carbidopa/levodopa. Administer subsequent doses 6 and 12 hr later.
- May be administered without regard to food.

### PATIENT/FAMILY TEACHING

- Instruct patient to take medication exactly as directed. Caution patient not to discontinue medication without consulting health care professional. Abrupt discontinuation or rapid dose reduction may result in neuroleptic malignant syndrome (elevated temperature, muscular rigidity, altered consciousness).
- Caution patient to make position changes slowly to minimize orthostatic hypotension, especially at the beginning of therapy.
- May affect mental and/or motor performance. Caution patient to avoid driving or other activities requiring alertness until response to medication is known.
- Advise patient to avoid taking alcohol or other CNS depressants concurrently with tolcapone.
- Inform patient and caregiver that hallucinations, nausea, dyskinesia, or dystonia may occur during tolcapone therapy.
- Advise patient to notify health care professional if pregnancy is planned or suspected.
- Instruct patient to notify health care professional if persistent diarrhea occurs.

### EVALUATION

**Effectiveness of therapy can be demonstrated by:** ■ Decrease in signs and symptoms of Parkinson's disease.

## tolnaftate, See ANTIFUNGALS (TOPICAL).

## tolterodine

(tol-**ter**-oh-deen)

Detrol, Detrol LA

### CLASSIFICATION(S):

**Therapeutic:** urinary tract antispasmodics
**Pharmacologic:** anticholinergics

**Pregnancy Category C**

### INDICATIONS

■ Treatment of overactive bladder function that results in urinary frequency, urgency, or urge incontinence.

### ACTION

■ Acts as a competitive muscarinic receptor antagonist resulting in inhibition of cholinergically mediated bladder contraction. **Therapeutic Effects:** ■ Decreased urinary frequency, urgency, and urge incontinence.

### PHARMACOKINETICS

**Absorption:** Well absorbed (77%) following oral administration.
**Distribution:** Unknown.
**Protein Binding:** 96.3%.
**Metabolism and Excretion:** Extensively metabolized by the liver; one metabolite (5-hydroxymethyltolterodine) is active; other metabolites are excreted in urine.

## PHARMACOKINETICS

**Absorption:** Well absorbed (80%) after oral administration.
**Distribution:** Unknown.
**Metabolism and Excretion:** 70% excreted unchanged in urine.
**Half-life:** 21 hr.

## CONTRAINDICATIONS AND PRECAUTIONS

**Contraindicated in:** ■ Hypersensitivity.
**Use Cautiously in:** ■ Renal impairment (dosage reduction recommended if CCr <70 ml/min/1.73 m²) ■ Hepatic impairment ■ Children (more prone to oligohydrosis and hyperthermia) ■ Dehydration ■ Pregnancy, lactation, or children <2 yr (safety not established).

## ADVERSE REACTIONS AND SIDE EFFECTS*

■ **CNS:** INCREASED SEIZURES, dizziness, drowsiness, fatigue, impaired concentration/memory, nervousness, psychomotor slowing, speech problems, aggressive reaction, agitation, anxiety, confusion, depression, malaise, mood problems ■ **EENT:** abnormal vision, diplopia, nystagmus, acute myopia, secondary angle closure glaucoma ■ **GI:** nausea, abdominal pain, anorexia, constipation, dry mouth ■ **GU:** kidney stones ■ **Derm:** ↓ sweating (in children) ■ **Hemat:** leukopenia ■ **Metab:** weight loss, hyperthermia (↑ in children) ■ **Neuro:** ataxia, paresthesia, tremor ■ **Misc:** SUICIDE ATTEMPT, fever.

## INTERACTIONS

**Drug-Drug:** ■ Blood levels and effects may be ↓ by **phenytoin, carbamazepine**, or **valproic acid** ■ May ↑ blood levels and effects of **phenytoin** ■ May ↓ blood levels and effects of **hormonal contraceptives** or **valproic acid** ■ ↑ risk of CNS depression with **alcohol** or other **CNS depressants** ■ Carbonic anhydrase inhibitors (**acetazolamide**) may ↑ risk of kidney stones.

## ROUTE AND DOSAGE

■ **PO (Adults and children ≥17 yr):** 25–50 mg/day initially, gradually increased by 25–50 mg weekly up to 200 mg twice daily (not to exceed 1600 mg/day).

---

_topiramate_

2 ... based ... ₋17 yr): 5–9 mg/kg ... increase ... titiate with 25 mg (or less 1–3 mg/kg/... nightly for 7 days then should be base... rvals in increments of ...ded doses; titration
□ **Renal Impairment** ...ical outcome.
■ **PO (Adults):** CCr<70 mb ... usual dose. ...−50% of the

## AVAILABILITY

■ **Sprinkle capsules:** 15 mg$^{Rx}$, 25 mg$^{Rx}$, ... mg$^{Rx}$ ■ Cost: 15 mg $78.66/60, 25 mg $95.08/60 ■ **Tablets:** 25 mg$^{Rx}$, 100 mg$^{Rx}$, 200 mg$^{Rx}$ ■ Cost: 25 mg $83.17/60, 100 mg $194.99/60, 200 mg $228.28/60.

TIME/ACTION PROFILE (blood levels†)

| | ONSET | PEAK | DURATION |
|---|---|---|---|
| PO | unknown | 2 hr | 12 hr |

†After single dose.

## NURSING IMPLICATIONS

### ASSESSMENT

□ Assess location, duration, and characteristics of seizure activity.
■ **Lab Test Considerations:** Monitor CBC with differential and platelet count before therapy to determine baseline levels and periodically during therapy. Frequently causes anemia.
□ Hepatic function should be monitored periodically throughout therapy. May cause ↑ AST and ALT levels.

### POTENTIAL NURSING DIAGNOSES

■ Injury, risk for (Indications, Side Effects).

### IMPLEMENTATION

■ **General:** Implement seizure precautions.
■ **PO:** May be administered without regard to meals.
□ Do not break tablets because of bitter taste.
□ Contents of the sprinkle capsules can be sprinkled on a small amount (teaspoon) of soft food, such as applesauce, custard, ice cream, oatmeal, pudding, or yogurt. To open, hold the capsule upright so that you can read the word "TOP." Carefully twist off

...potecan It may be ...clear portion ...portion of the best to do this ...be pouring the food onto ...ire contents of the sprinkles. Spri... Be sure the patient capsule onto spoonful of the sprinkle/ swallows the...ately without chewing. food mixtur...s immediately to make sure Follow with ...re is swallowed. Never store a all of the...rd mixture for use at another sprinkl...
ti...

## PATIENT/FAMILY TEACHING

- Instruct patient to take topiramate exactly as directed. Take missed doses as soon as possible but not just before next dose; do not double doses. Notify health care professional if more than 1 dose is missed. Medication should be gradually discontinued to prevent seizures and status epilepticus.
- May cause decreased sweating and increased body temperature. Advise patients, especially parents of pediatric patients, to provide adequate hydration and monitoring, especially during hot weather.
- May cause dizziness, drowsiness, confusion, and difficulty concentrating. Caution patients to avoid driving or other activities requiring alertness until response to medication is known.
- Advise patient to maintain a fluid intake of 2000–3000 ml of fluid/day to prevent the formation of kidney stones.
- Instruct patient to notify health care professional immediately if periorbital pain or blurred vision occurs. Medication should be discontinued if ocular symptoms occur. May lead to permanent loss of vision.
- Caution patient to make position changes slowly to minimize orthostatic hypotension.
- Advise patient not to take alcohol or other CNS depressants concurrently with this medication.
- Advise patient to use a nonhormonal form of contraception while taking topiramate.
- Instruct patient to notify health care professional of medication regimen before treatment or surgery.
- Advise patient to use sunscreen and wear protective clothing to prevent photosensitivity reactions.

- Advise patient to carry identification describing disease and medication regimen at all times.

## EVALUATION

**Clinical response to therapy can be evaluated by:** ■ Absence or reduction of seizure activity.

# topotecan
(toe-poe-**tee**-kan)
Hycamtin

**CLASSIFICATION(S):**
*Therapeutic: antineoplastics*
*Pharmacologic: enzyme inhibitors*

**Pregnancy Category D**

## INDICATIONS

■ Metastatic ovarian cancer that has not responded to previous chemotherapy ■ Small cell lung cancer unresponsive to first-line therapy.

## ACTION

■ Interferes with DNA synthesis by inhibiting the enzyme topoisomerase. **Therapeutic Effects:** ■ Death of rapidly replicating cells, particularly malignant ones.

## PHARMACOKINETICS

**Absorption:** IV administration results in complete bioavailability.

**Distribution:** Unknown.

**Metabolism and Excretion:** 30% excreted in urine; small amounts metabolized by the liver.

**Half-life:** 2–3 hr.

## CONTRAINDICATIONS AND PRECAUTIONS

**Contraindicated in:** ■ Hypersensitivity ■ Pregnancy or lactation ■ Pre-existing severe myelosuppression.

**Use Cautiously in:** ■ Impaired renal function (reduce dose if CCr <40 ml/min) ■ Platelet count <25,000 cells/mm³ (reduce dose) ■ Patients with childbearing potential.

## ADVERSE REACTIONS AND SIDE EFFECTS*

■ **CNS:** headache, fatigue, weakness ■ **Resp:** dyspnea ■ **GI:** abdominal pain, diarrhea, nausea, vomiting, anorexia, constipation, increased liver enzymes, stomatitis ■ **Derm:** alopecia ■ **Hemat:** anemia, leukopenia, thrombocytopenia ■ **MS:** arthralgia.

## INTERACTIONS

**Drug-Drug:** ■ Neutropenia is prolonged by concurrent use of **filgrastim** (do not use until day 6; 24 hr following completion of topotecan) ■ ↑ myelosuppression with other **antineoplastics** (especially **cisplatin**) or **radiation therapy** ■ May ↓ antibody response to and ↑ risk of adverse reactions from **live virus vaccines.**

## ROUTE AND DOSAGE

■ **IV (Adults):** 1.5 mg/m²/day for 5 days starting on day 1 of a 21-day course.

❑ **Renal Impairment**
■ **IV (Adults):** *CCr 20–39 ml/min*—0.75 mg/m²/day for 5 days starting on day 1 of a 21-day course.

## AVAILABILITY

■*Lyophilized powder for injection:* 4 mg/vial^Rx.

TIME/ACTION PROFILE (effects on WBCs)

| | ONSET | PEAK | DURATION |
|----|-------|------|----------|
| IV | within days | 11 days | 7 days |

# NURSING IMPLICATIONS

## ASSESSMENT

❑ Monitor vital signs frequently during administration.

❑ Monitor for bone marrow depression. Assess for bleeding (bleeding gums, bruising, petechiae; guaiac stools, urine, and emesis) and avoid IM injections and taking rectal temperatures if platelet count is low. Apply pressure to venipuncture sites for 10 min. Assess for signs of infection during neutropenia. Anemia may occur. Monitor for increased fatigue, dyspnea, and orthostatic hypotension.

❑ Nausea and vomiting are common. Prevment with antiemetics should be considered.

❑ Assess IV site frequently for extravasation, which causes mild local erythema and bruising.

■ *Lab Test Considerations:* Monitor CBC with differential and platelet count prior to administration and frequently during therapy. Baseline neutrophil count of ≥1500 cells/mm³ and platelet count of ≥100,000 cells/mm³ are required before first dose. The nadir of neutropenia occurs in 11 days, with a duration of 7 days. The nadir of thrombocytopenia occurs in 15 days, with a duration of 5 days. The nadir of anemia occurs in 15 days. Subsequent doses should not be administered until neutrophils recover to >1000 cells/mm³, platelets recover to >100,000 cells/mm³, and hemoglobin levels recover to 9.0 mg/dl. If severe neutropenia occurs during any course, subsequent doses should be reduced by 0.25 mg/m² or filgrastim may be administered following the subsequent course of therapy starting on day 6, 24 hr after the completion of topotecan.

❑ Monitor liver function. May cause transient ↑ in AST, ALT, and bilirubin concentrations.

## POTENTIAL NURSING DIAGNOSES

■ Infection, risk for (Adverse Reactions).

## IMPLEMENTATION

❑ *High Alert:* Fatalities have occurred with chemotherapeutic agents. Before administering, clarify all ambiguous orders; double check single, daily, and course-of-therapy dose limits; have second practitioner independently double check original order, dose calculations, and infusion pump settings.

■ **General:** Solution should be prepared in a biologic cabinet. Wear gloves, gown, and mask while handling IV medication. Discard IV equipment in specially designated containers.

■ **Intermittent Infusion:** Reconstitute each vial with 4 ml of sterile water for injection. Dilute further in 0.9% NaCl or D5W. Use solution immediately after preparing. Solution is yellow to yellow-green. Solution is stable for 24 hr at room temperature.

■ *Rate:* Administer dose over 30 min.

■ **Y-Site Compatibility:** ◆ carboplatin ◆ cimetidine ◆ cisplatin ◆ cyclophosphamide ◆ doxorubicin ◆ etoposide ◆ gemcitabine ◆ granisetron ◆ ifosfamide ◆ methylprednisolone ◆ metoclopramide ◆ ondansetron ◆ paclitaxel ◆ prochlorperazine ◆ vincristine.

■ **Y-Site Incompatibility:** ◆ fluorouracil ◆ mitomycin.

■ **Additive Incompatibility:** Information unavailable. Do not admix with other solutions or medications.

## PATIENT/FAMILY TEACHING

❑ Instruct patient to notify health care professional if fever; chills; sore throat; signs of infection; bleeding gums; bruising; petechiae; blood in urine, stool, or emesis occurs. Caution patient to avoid crowds and persons with known infections. Instruct patient to use soft toothbrush and electric razor. Patient should be cautioned not to drink alcoholic beverages or take products containing aspirin or NSAIDs.

❑ Discuss with patient the possibility of hair loss. Explore methods of coping.

❑ Advise patient that this medication may have teratogenic effects. Contraception should be used during therapy.

❑ Instruct patient not to receive any vaccinations without advice of health care professional.

❑ Emphasize the need for periodic lab tests to monitor for side effects.

## EVALUATION

**Effectiveness of therapy can be demonstrated by:** ■ Decrease in size and spread of malignancy.

## toremifene
(**tore**-em-i-feen)
Fareston

*CLASSIFICATION(S):*
*Therapeutic: antineoplastics*
*Pharmacologic: antiestrogens*

**Pregnancy Category D**

## INDICATIONS

■ Management of metastatic breast cancer in postmenopausal women with estrogen receptor–positive or unknown tumors.

## ACTION

■ Exerts antiestrogenic effects by competing for estrogen-binding sites found in breast cancers. **Therapeutic Effects:** ■ Regression of breast cancer.

## PHARMACOKINETICS

**Absorption:** Well absorbed following oral administration.
**Distribution:** Widely distributed; 99% bound to plasma proteins.
**Protein Binding:** 99.5%.
**Metabolism and Excretion:** Extensively metabolized; undergoes enterohepatic circulation.
**Half-life:** 5 days.

## CONTRAINDICATIONS AND PRECAUTIONS

**Contraindicated in:** ■ Hypersensitivity ■ Pregnancy or lactation ■ History of thromboembolic disease.

**Use Cautiously in:** ■ Bone metastases (increased risk of hypercalcemia) ■ Pre-existing endometrial hyperplasia (long-term treatment should be avoided).

## ADVERSE REACTIONS AND SIDE EFFECTS*

■ **CNS:** depression, dizziness, headache, lethargy ■ **EENT:** blurred vision, cataracts, corneal keratopathy, dry eyes, glaucoma ■ **CV:** CHF, MI, PULMONARY EMBOLISM, angina, arrhythmias, edema, thrombophlebitis ■ **GI:** nausea, elevated liver enzymes, vomiting ■ **GU:** vaginal discharge, vaginal bleeding ■ **Derm:** sweating ■ **F and E:** hypercalcemia ■ **Hemat:** anemia ■ **Misc:** hot flashes, tumor flare.

## INTERACTIONS

**Drug-Drug:** ■ Concurrent use of **agents that decrease urinary excretion of calcium (thiazide diuretics )** may increase the risk of hypercalcemia ■ May increase the effect of **warfarin**.

## ROUTE AND DOSAGE

■ **PO (Adults):** 60 mg once daily.

## AVAILABILITY

■ *Tablets:* 60 mg$^{Rx}$.

TIME/ACTION PROFILE (blood levels)

| | ONSET | PEAK | DURATION |
|---|---|---|---|
| PO | unknown | 3 hr | 4–6 wk† |

†Steady-state blood levels occur after 4–6 wk.

## NURSING IMPLICATIONS

### ASSESSMENT

❏ Assess for an increase in bone or tumor pain. Confer with physician or other health care professional regarding analgesics. This transient pain usually resolves despite continued therapy.

❏ Gynecologic examinations should be done regularly; may cause variations in Papanicolaou and vaginal smears.

■ *Lab Test Considerations:* Monitor CBC, platelets, and calcium levels prior to and throughout therapy. May cause transient hypercalcemia in patients with metastases to bone. An estrogen receptor assay should be assessed prior to initiation of therapy.

❏ Monitor hepatic function tests periodically during therapy. May cause elevated serum AST, alkaline phosphatase, and bilirubin concentrations.

### POTENTIAL NURSING DIAGNOSES

■ Pain, acute (Adverse Reactions).

### IMPLEMENTATION

■ **PO:** Administer once daily.

### PATIENT/FAMILY TEACHING

❏ Instruct patient to take medication exactly as directed. If a dose is missed, it should be omitted.

❏ Advise patient to report bone pain to health care professional promptly. This pain may be severe. Inform patient that this may be an indication of the drug's effectiveness and will resolve over time. Analgesics should be ordered to control pain.

❏ This medication may induce ovulation and may have teratogenic properties. Advise patient to use a nonhormonal method of contraception during and for 1 mo after course of therapy.

❏ Advise patient that medication may cause hot flashes. Notify health care professional if these become bothersome.

❏ Instruct patient to notify health care professional promptly if pain or swelling of legs, shortness of breath, weakness, sleepiness, confusion, nausea, vomiting, dizziness, headache, loss of appetite, or blurred vision occurs. Patient should also report menstrual irregularities, vaginal bleeding, pelvic pain or pressure.

### EVALUATION

**Effectiveness of therapy can be demonstrated by:** ■ Decrease in the size or spread of breast cancer.

---

## torsemide

**(tore**-se-mide)
Demadex

### CLASSIFICATION(S):
**Therapeutic:** *antihypertensives*
**Pharmacologic:** *loop diuretics*

### Pregnancy Category B

### INDICATIONS

■ Edema due to: ❏ CHF ❏ Hepatic or renal disease ■ Treatment of hypertension.

### ACTION

■ Inhibits the reabsorption of sodium and chloride from the loop of Henle and distal renal tubule ■ Increases renal excretion of water, sodium, chloride, magnesium, hydrogen, and calcium ■ May have renal and peripheral vasodilatory effects ■ Effectiveness persists in impaired renal function. **Therapeutic Effects:** ■ Diuresis and subsequent mobilization of excess fluid (edema, pleural effusions) ■ Decreased blood pressure.

### PHARMACOKINETICS

**Absorption:** 80% absorbed after oral administration.
**Distribution:** Unknown.

**Protein Binding:** ≥97%.
**Metabolism and Excretion:** 80% metabolized by liver, 20% excreted in urine.
**Half-life:** 3.5 hr.

## CONTRAINDICATIONS AND PRECAUTIONS

**Contraindicated in:** ■ Hypersensitivity ■ Cross-sensitivity with thiazides and sulfonamides may occur ■ Pre-existing electrolyte imbalance, hepatic coma, or anuria.

**Use Cautiously in:** ■ Severe liver disease (may precipitate hepatic coma; concurrent use with potassium-sparing diuretics may be necessary) ■ Electrolyte depletion ■ Geriatric patients (difficulty assessing hearing status; increased risk of hypotension) ■ Diabetes mellitus ■ Increasing azotemia ■ Pregnancy, lactation, or children <18 yr (safety not established).

## ADVERSE REACTIONS AND SIDE EFFECTS*

■ **CNS:** dizziness, encephalopathy, headache, insomnia, nervousness ■ **EENT:** hearing loss, tinnitus ■ **CV:** hypotension ■ **GI:** constipation, diarrhea, dry mouth, dyspepsia, nausea, vomiting ■ **GU:** excessive urination ■ **Derm:** photosensitivity, rashes ■ **Endo:** hyperglycemia ■ **F and E:** dehydration, hypochloremia, hypokalemia, hypomagnesemia, hyponatremia, hypovolemia, metabolic alkalosis ■ **Metab:** hyperglycemia, hyperuricemia ■ **MS:** arthralgia (increased with torsemide), muscle cramps, myalgia ■ **Misc:** increased BUN.

## INTERACTIONS

**Drug-Drug:** ■ ↑ hypotension with **antihypertensives, nitrates,** or acute ingestion of **alcohol** ■ ↑ risk of hypokalemia with other **diuretics, piperacillin, amphotericin B, stimulant laxatives,** and **corticosteroids** ■ Hypokalemia may ↑ risk of **digoxin** toxicity ■ ↓ **lithium** excretion, may cause toxicity ■ ↑ risk of ototoxicity with **aminoglycosides** ■ May ↑ the effectiveness of **warfarin, thrombolytic agents,** or **anticoagulants.**

## ROUTE AND DOSAGE

■ **PO, IV (Adults):** *CHF*—10–20 mg once daily. *Chronic renal failure*—20 mg once daily; dose may be doubled until desired effect is obtained (up to 200 mg). *Hepatic cirrhosis*—5–10 mg once daily (with aldosterone antagonist or potassium-sparing di-

uretic); dose may be doubled until desired effect is obtained (up to 40 mg). *Hypertension*—5 mg once daily, may be increased to 10 mg once daily after 4–6 wk (if still not effective, add another agent).

## AVAILABILITY

■ *Tablets:* 5 mg^Rx, 10 mg^Rx, 20 mg^Rx, 100 mg^Rx ■Cost: *Demadex*—5 mg $65.14/100, 10 mg $72.18/100, 20 mg $84.31/100, 100 mg $312.40/100 ■ *Injection:* 10 mg/ml^Rx ■ Cost: 10 mg/ml $50.66/2 ml.

TIME/ACTION PROFILE (diuretic effect)

|    | ONSET | PEAK | DURATION |
|----|-------|------|----------|
| PO | within 60 min | 60–120 min | 6–8 hr |
| IV | within 10 min | within 60 min | 6–8 hr |

# NURSING IMPLICATIONS

## ASSESSMENT

❑ Assess fluid status during therapy. Monitor daily weight, intake and output ratios, amount and location of edema, lung sounds, skin turgor, and mucous membranes. Notify physician or other health care provider if thirst, dry mouth, lethargy, weakness, hypotension, or oliguria occurs.

❑ Monitor blood pressure and pulse before and during administration. Monitor frequency of prescription refills to determine compliance in patients treated for hypertension.

❑ Assess patients receiving digitalis glycosides for anorexia, nausea, vomiting, muscle cramps, paresthesia, and confusion. Patients taking digoxin are at increased risk of digoxin toxicity due to potassium-depleting effect of the diuretic. Potassium supplements or potassium-sparing diuretics may be used concurrently to prevent hypokalemia.

❑ Assess patient for tinnitus and hearing loss. Audiometry is recommended for patients receiving prolonged high-dose IV therapy. Hearing loss is most common following rapid or high-dose IV administration in patients with decreased renal function or those taking other ototoxic drugs.

❑ Assess for allergy to sulfonamides.

■ *Lab Test Considerations:* Monitor electrolytes, renal and hepatic function, serum glucose, and uric acid levels prior to and periodically during therapy. May cause ↓

serum potassium, calcium, and magnesium concentrations. May also cause ↑ BUN, serum glucose, creatinine, and uric acid levels.

❑ May cause ↑ in total plasma cholesterol and lipids during initial therapy. Those elevations usually return to normal with chronic therapy.

## POTENTIAL NURSING DIAGNOSES

■ Fluid volume, excess (Indications).

■ Fluid volume, risk for deficit (Side Effects).

## IMPLEMENTATION

■ **General:** Administer medication in the morning to prevent disruption of sleep cycle.

❑ IV is preferred over IM for parenteral administration.

■ **PO:** Administer orally with food or milk to minimize gastric irritation.

■ **Direct IV:** Administer undiluted. Do not administer if solution is discolored or contains particulate matter.

■ *Rate:* Administer slowly over 2 min.

❑ May also be administered as a continuous infusion.

■ **Syringe Incompatibility:** Information unavailable. Do not mix with other drugs or solutions.

## PATIENT/FAMILY TEACHING

■ **General Info:** Instruct patient to take torsemide as directed. Take missed doses as soon as possible; do not double doses.

❑ Caution patient to make position changes slowly to minimize orthostatic hypotension. Caution patient that the use of alcohol, exercise during hot weather, or standing for long periods during therapy may enhance orthostatic hypotension.

❑ Instruct patient to consult health care professional regarding a diet high in potassium (see Appendix Q).

❑ Advise patient to consult health care professional before taking OTC medication or herbal products concurrently with this therapy.

❑ Instruct patient to notify health care professional of medication regimen prior to treatment or surgery.

❑ Caution patient to use sunscreen and protective clothing to prevent photosensitivity reactions.

❑ Advise patient to contact health care professional immediately if muscle weakness, cramps, nausea, dizziness, numbness, or tingling of extremities occurs.

❑ Advise diabetic patients to monitor blood glucose closely; may cause increased blood glucose levels.

❑ Emphasize the importance of routine follow-up examinations.

■ **Hypertension:** Advise patients on antihypertensive regimen to continue taking medication even if feeling better. Torsemide controls but does not cure hypertension.

❑ Reinforce the need to continue additional therapies for hypertension (weight loss, exercise, restricted sodium intake, stress reduction, regular exercise, moderation of alcohol consumption, cessation of smoking).

## EVALUATION

**Effectiveness of therapy can be demonstrated by:** ■ Decrease in edema ❑ Decrease in abdominal girth ❑ Increase in urinary output ■ Decrease in blood pressure ■ Decrease in serum calcium when used to manage hypercalcemia.

---

# tramadol
(**tra**-ma-dol)
Ultram

*CLASSIFICATION(S):*
*Therapeutic: analgesics (centrally acting)*

**Pregnancy Category C**

---

## INDICATIONS

■ Moderate to moderately severe pain.

## ACTION

■ Binds to mu-opioid receptors ■ Inhibits reuptake of serotonin and norepinephrine in the CNS. **Therapeutic Effects:** ■ Decreased pain.

## PHARMACOKINETICS

**Absorption:** 75% absorbed after oral administration.

**Distribution:** Crosses the placenta; enters breast milk.

**Metabolism and Excretion:** Mostly metabolized by the liver; one metabolite has analgesic activity; 30% is excreted unchanged in urine.

**Half-life:** *Tramadol*—5–9 hr; *active metabolite*—5–9 hr (both are increased in renal or hepatic impairment).

## CONTRAINDICATIONS AND PRECAUTIONS

**Contraindicated in:** ■ Hypersensitivity ■ Cross-sensitivity with opioids may occur ■ Patients who are acutely intoxicated with alcohol, sedative/hypnotics, centrally acting analgesics, opioid analgesics, or psychotropic agents ■ Patients who are physically dependent on opioid analgesics (may precipitate withdrawal) ■ Not recommended for use during pregnancy or lactation.

**Use Cautiously in:** ■ Geriatric patients (not to exceed 300 mg/day in patients >75 yr) ■ Patients with a history of epilepsy or risk factors for seizures ■ Renal impairment (increased dosing interval recommended if CCr <30 ml/min) ■ Hepatic impairment (increased interval recommended in patients with cirrhosis) ■ Patients receiving MAO inhibitors or CNS depressants ■ Increased intracranial pressure or head trauma ■ Acute abdomen (may preclude accurate clinical assessment) ■ Patients with a history of opioid dependence or who have recently received large doses of opioids ■ Children <16 yr (safety not established).

## ADVERSE REACTIONS AND SIDE EFFECTS*

■ **CNS:** SEIZURES, dizziness, headache, somnolence, anxiety, CNS stimulation, confusion, coordination disturbance, euphoria, malaise, nervousness, sleep disorder, weakness ■ **EENT:** visual disturbances ■ **CV:** vasodilation ■ **GI:** constipation, nausea, abdominal pain, anorexia, diarrhea, dry mouth, dyspepsia, flatulence, vomiting ■ **GU:** menopausal symptoms, urinary retention/frequency ■ **Derm:** pruritus, sweating ■ **Neuro:** hypertonia ■ **Misc:** physical dependence, psychological dependence, tolerance.

## INTERACTIONS

**Drug-Drug:** ■ ↑ risk of CNS depression when used concurrently with other **CNS depressants,** including **alcohol, antihistamines, sedative/hypnotics, opioid analgesics, anesthetics,** or **psychotropic agents** ■ ↑ risk of seizures with high doses of **penicillins** or **cephalosporins, phenothiazines, opioid analgesics,** or **antidepressants** ■ **Carbamazepine** ↑ metabolism and ↓ effectiveness of tramadol (increased doses may be required) ■ Use cautiously in patients who are receiving **MAO inhibitors** ( ↑ risk of adverse reactions) ■ Effectiveness may be altered by concurrent **quinidine.**

**Drug-Natural Products:** ■ Concomitant use of **kava, valerian,** or **chamomile** can ↑ CNS depression.

## ROUTE AND DOSAGE

■ **PO (Adults):** *Rapid titration*—50–100 mg q 4–6 hr (not to exceed 400 mg/day or 300 mg in patients >75 yr). *Gradual titration*—25 mg/day initially, increase by 25 mg/day every 3 days to 100 mg/day, then increase by 50 mg/day every 3 days up to 200 mg/day.

❑ **Renal Impairment**

■ **PO (Adults):** *CCr <30 ml/min*—increase dosing to q 12 hr (not to exceed 200 mg/day).

❑ **Hepatic Impairment**

■ **PO (Adults):** 50 mg q 12 hr.

## AVAILABILITY (generic available)

■ *Tablets:* 50 mg$^{Rx}$ ■ Cost: $85.25/100 ■ acetaminophen (Ultracet). See Appendix B.

TIME/ACTION PROFILE (analgesia)

| | ONSET | PEAK | DURATION |
|---|---|---|---|
| PO | 1 hr | 2–3 hr | 4–6 hr |

# NURSING IMPLICATIONS

## ASSESSMENT

❑ Assess type, location, and intensity of pain before and 2–3 hr (peak) after administration.

❑ Assess blood pressure and respiratory rate before and periodically during administration. Respiratory depression has not occurred with recommended doses.

- ❑ Assess bowel function routinely. Prevention of constipation should be instituted with increased intake of fluids and bulk and with laxatives to minimize constipating effects.
- ❑ Assess previous analgesic history. Tramadol is not recommended for patients dependent on opioids or who have previously received opioids for more than 1 wk; may cause opioid withdrawal symptoms.
- ❑ Prolonged use may lead to physical and psychological dependence and tolerance, although these may be milder than with opioids. This should not prevent patient from receiving adequate analgesia. Most patients who receive tramadol for pain do not develop psychological dependence. If tolerance develops, changing to an opioid agonist may be required to relieve pain.
- ❑ Monitor patient for seizures. May occur within recommended dose range. Risk is increased with higher doses and in patients taking antidepressants (SSRIs, tricyclics, or MAO inhibitors), opioid analgesics, or other drugs that decrease the seizure threshold.
- ■ *Lab Test Considerations:* May cause ↑ serum creatinine, elevated liver enzymes, decreased hemoglobin, and proteinuria.
- ■ *Toxicity and Overdose:* Overdose may cause respiratory depression and seizures. Naloxone (Narcan) may reverse some, but not all, of the symptoms of overdose. Treatment should be symptomatic and supportive. Maintain adequate respiratory exchange. Hemodialysis is not helpful because it removes only a small portion of administered dose. Seizures may be managed with barbiturates or benzodiazepines; naloxone increases risk of seizures.

## POTENTIAL NURSING DIAGNOSES

- ■ Pain, acute (Indications).
- ■ Injury, risk for (Side Effects).

## IMPLEMENTATION

- ■ **General:** Do not confuse tramadol with Toradol (ketorolac).
- ❑ Tramadol is considered to provide more analgesia than codeine 60 mg but less than combined aspirin 650 mg/codeine 60 mg for acute postoperative pain.

- ❑ For chronic pain, daily doses of 250 mg of tramadol provide pain relief similar to that of 5 doses/day of acetaminophen 300 mg/codeine 30 mg, 5 doses/day of aspirin 325 mg/codeine 30 mg, or 2–3 doses/day of acetaminophen 500 mg/oxycodone 5 mg.
- ❑ Explain therapeutic value of medication before administration to enhance the analgesic effect.
- ❑ Regularly administered doses may be more effective than prn administration. Analgesic is more effective if given before pain becomes severe.
- ❑ Tramadol should be discontinued gradually after long-term use to prevent withdrawal symptoms.
- ■ **PO:** Tramadol may be administered without regard to meals.

## PATIENT/FAMILY TEACHING

- ❑ Instruct patient on how and when to ask for pain medication.
- ❑ May cause dizziness and drowsiness. Caution patient to avoid driving or other activities requiring alertness until response to medication is known.
- ❑ Advise patient to change positions slowly to minimize orthostatic hypotension.
- ❑ Caution patient to avoid concurrent use of alcohol or other CNS depressants with this medication.
- ❑ Encourage patient to turn, cough, and breathe deeply every 2 hr to prevent atelectasis.

## EVALUATION

**Effectiveness of therapy can be demonstrated by:** ■ Decrease in severity of pain without a significant alteration in level of consciousness or respiratory status.

---

**trandolapril, See ANGIOTENSIN-CONVERTING ENZYME (ACE) INHIBITORS.**

---

**tranylcypromine, See MONOAMINE OXIDASE (MAO) INHIBITORS.**

---

| High Alert |

## trastuzumab

(traz-**too**-zoo-mab)

Herceptin

### CLASSIFICATION(S):

**Therapeutic:** antineoplastics

**Pharmacologic:** monoclonal antibodies

### Pregnancy Category B

## INDICATIONS

■ Metastatic breast cancer alone or with paclitaxel for tumors that display overexpression of the human epidermal growth factor receptor 2 (HER2) protein.

## ACTION

■ A monoclonal antibody that binds to HER2 sites in breast cancer tissue and inhibits proliferation of cells that overexpress HER2 protein. **Therapeutic Effects:** ■ Regression of breast cancer and metastases.

## PHARMACOKINETICS

**Absorption:** IV administration results in complete bioavailability.

**Distribution:** Binds to HER2 proteins.

**Metabolism and Excretion:** Unknown.

**Half-life:** 10-mg dose—1.7 days; 500-mg dose—12 days.

## CONTRAINDICATIONS AND PRECAUTIONS

**Contraindicated in:** ■ None known.

**Use Cautiously in:** ■ Pre-existing pulmonary conditions ■ Hypersensitivity to trastuzumab, Chinese hamster ovary cell proteins, or other components of the product ■ Hypersensitivity to benzyl alcohol (use sterile water for injection instead of bacteriostatic water, which accompanies the vial) ■ Geriatric patients (may have increased risk of cardiac dysfunction) ■ Pregnancy (use only if clearly needed) ■ Lactation (use not recommended) ■ Children (safety not established).

**Exercise Extreme Caution in:** ■ Patients with pre-existing cardiac dysfunction.

## ADVERSE REACTIONS AND SIDE EFFECTS*

■ **CNS:** dizziness, headache, insomnia, weakness, depression ■ **Resp:** dyspnea, increased cough, pharyngitis, rhinitis, sinusitis ■ **CV:** CHF, tachycardia ■ **GI:** abdominal pain, anorexia, diarrhea, nausea, vomiting ■ **Derm:** rash, acne, herpes simplex ■ **F and E:** edema ■ **Hemat:** anemia, leukopenia ■ **MS:** back pain, arthralgia, bone pain ■ **Neuro:** neuropathy, paresthesia, peripheral neuritis ■ **Misc:** HYPERSENSITIVITY REACTIONS, chills, fever, infection, pain, allergic reactions, flu-like syndrome.

## INTERACTIONS

**Drug-Drug:** ■ Concurrent **anthracycline** (**daunorubicin, doxorubicin,** or **idarubicin**) therapy may ↑ risk of cardiotoxicity ■ Blood levels are ↑ by concurrent **paclitaxel**.

## ROUTE AND DOSAGE

■ **IV (Adults):** 4 mg/kg initially followed by 2 mg/kg weekly.

## AVAILABILITY

■ *Lyophilized powder for injection:* 440 mg/vial with 30 ml bacteriostatic water for injection (contains benzyl alcohol)[Rx].

TIME/ACTION PROFILE (blood levels)

|    | ONSET | PEAK | DURATION |
|----|-------|------|----------|
| IV | unknown | unknown | unknown |

# NURSING IMPLICATIONS

## ASSESSMENT

❑ Assess for infusion-related symptoms (chills, fever) following initial infusion. May be treated with acetaminophen, diphenhydramine, and meperidine. Rarely requires discontinuation.

❑ Assess for signs and symptoms of cardiac dysfunction (dyspnea, increased cough, paroxysmal nocturnal dyspnea, peripheral edema, $S_3$ gallop, reduced ejection fraction) frequently during therapy. Baseline cardiac assessment of history, physical exam, and one or more of: ECG, echocardiogram, and multiple gated acquisition (MUGA) scan. CHF associated with trastuzumab may be severe, resulting in cardiac failure, death, and stroke. Trastuzumab should be discontinued upon the development of significant CHF.

❑ Monitor patient for signs of pulmonary hypersensitivity reactions (dyspnea, pulmonary infiltrates, pleural effusion, noncardiogenic pulmonary edema, pulmonary insufficiency, hypoxia, acute respiratory distress syndrome). Patients with symptomatic pulmonary disease or extensive lung tumor involvement are at increased risk. Infusion should be discontinued if severe symptoms occur.

■ *Lab Test Considerations:* HER2 protein overexpression is used to determine whether treatment with trastuzumab is indicated. HER2 protein overexpression is detected by HercepTest™ (IHC assay) and PathVysion™ (FISH assay).

❑ May cause anemia and leukopenia.

## POTENTIAL NURSING DIAGNOSES

■ Diarrhea (Adverse Reactions).
■ Infection, risk for (Adverse Reactions).

## IMPLEMENTATION

❑ *High Alert:* Fatalities have occurred with chemotherapeutic agents. Before administering, clarify all ambiguous orders; double check single, daily, and course-of-therapy dose limits; have second practitioner independently double check original order, dose calculations and infusion pump settings.

■ **General:** May be administered in the outpatient setting.

■ **Intermittent Infusion:** Dilute each vial with 20 ml of bacteriostatic water for injection, directing the stream of diluent into lyophilized cake of trastuzumab, resulting in a multidose solution containing 21 mg/ml. Swirl the vial gently; do not shake. May foam slightly; allow the vial to stand undisturbed for 5 min. Solution should be clear to slightly opalescent and colorless to pale yellow, without particulate matter. Label vial immediately in the area marked "Do not use after" with the date 28 days from the date of reconstitution. Stable for 24 hr at room temperature or 28 days if refrigerated. If patient is allergic to benzyl alcohol, use sterile water for injection for reconstitution. Use immediately and discard any unused portion. Calculate to volume required for the desired dose, withdraw, and add it to an infusion containing 250 ml of 0.9% NaCl. Invert bag gently to mix.

■ *Rate:* Infuse the 4 mg/kg loading dose over 90 min and the weekly 2 mg/kg dose over 30 min if the loading dose was well tolerated. Do not administer as an IV push or bolus.

■ **Additive Incompatibility:** Do not dilute trastuzumab with or add to solutions containing dextrose. Do not mix or dilute with other drugs.

## PATIENT/FAMILY TEACHING

❑ Instruct patient to notify health care professional promptly if symptoms of CHF, fever, sore throat, signs of infection, lower back or side pain, or difficult or painful urination occur. Caution patient to avoid crowds and persons with known infections.

❑ Advise patient not to receive any vaccinations without advice of health care professional.

## EVALUATION

**Effectiveness of therapy can be demonstrated by:** ■ Regression of breast cancer and metastases.

## trazodone
(**traz**-oh-done)
Desyrel, Trialodine, Trazon

*CLASSIFICATION(S):*
*Therapeutic: antidepressants*
**Pregnancy Category C**

## INDICATIONS

■ Treatment of major depression often in conjunction with psychotherapy. **Unlabeled uses:** ■ Management of insomnia and chronic pain syndromes, including diabetic neuropathy.

## ACTION

■ Alters the effects of serotonin in the CNS. **Therapeutic Effects:** ■ Antidepressant action, which may develop only over several weeks.

## PHARMACOKINETICS

**Absorption:** Well absorbed after oral administration.
**Distribution:** Widely distributed.
**Protein Binding:** 89–95%.

**Metabolism and Excretion:** Extensively metabolized by the liver; minimal excretion of unchanged drug by the kidneys.
**Half-life:** 5–9 hr.

## CONTRAINDICATIONS AND PRECAUTIONS

**Contraindicated in:** ■ Hypersensitivity ■ Recovery period after MI ■ Concurrent electroconvulsive therapy.

**Use Cautiously in:** ■ Cardiovascular disease ■ Suicidal behavior ■ Severe hepatic or renal disease (dosage reduction recommended) ■ Geriatric patients (initial dosage reduction recommended) ■ Pregnancy, lactation, or children (safety not established).

## ADVERSE REACTIONS AND SIDE EFFECTS*

■ **CNS:** drowsiness, confusion, dizziness, fatigue, hallucinations, headache, insomnia, nightmares, slurred speech, syncope, weakness ■ **EENT:** blurred vision, tinnitus ■ **CV:** hypotension, arrhythmias, chest pain, hypertension, palpitations, tachycardia ■ **GI:** dry mouth, altered taste, constipation, diarrhea, excess salivation, flatulence, nausea, vomiting ■ **GU:** hematuria, impotence, priapism, urinary frequency ■ **Derm:** rashes ■ **Hemat:** anemia, leukopenia ■ **MS:** myalgia ■ **Neuro:** tremor.

## INTERACTIONS

**Drug-Drug:** ■ May increase **digoxin** or **phenytoin** serum levels ■ Additive CNS depression with other **CNS depressants,** including **alcohol, opioid analgesics,** and **sedative/hypnotics** ■ Additive hypotension with **antihypertensives,** acute ingestion of **alcohol,** or **nitrates** ■ Concurrent use with **fluoxetine** increases levels and risk of toxicity from trazodone.

**Drug-Natural Products:** ■ Concomitant use of **kava, valerian, skullcap, chamomile,** or **hops** can increase CNS depression ■ Increased risk of serotinergic side effects including serotonin syndrome with **St. John's wort** and **SAMe.**

## ROUTE AND DOSAGE

■ **PO (Adults):** *Depression*—150 mg/day in 3 divided doses; increase by 50 mg/day q 3–4 days until desired response (not to exceed 400 mg/day in outpatients or 600 mg/day in

hospitalized patients). *Insomnia*—25–100 mg at bedtime.

■ **PO (Geriatric Patients):** 75 mg/day in divided doses initially; may be increased q 3–4 days.

■ **PO (Children 6–18 yr):** 1.5–2 mg/kg/day in divided doses. May be increased q 3–4 days up to 6 mg/kg/day.

## AVAILABILITY (generic available)

■ *Tablets:* 50 mg$^{Rx}$, 100 mg$^{Rx}$, 150 mg$^{Rx}$, 300 mg$^{Rx}$ ■ Cost: *Desyrel*—50 mg $176.15/100, 100 mg $307.81/100, 150 mg $285.07/100, 300 mg $507.38/100; *generic*—50 mg $41.73/100, 100 mg $70.18/100, 150 mg $146.92/100, 300 mg $426.52/100.

TIME/ACTION PROFILE (antidepressant effect)

|    | ONSET | PEAK | DURATION |
|----|-------|------|----------|
| PO | 1–2 wk | 2–4 wk | wks |

# NURSING IMPLICATIONS

## ASSESSMENT

■ **General Info:** Monitor blood pressure and pulse rate before and during initial therapy. Patients with pre-existing cardiac disease should have ECGs monitored before and periodically during therapy to detect arrhythmias.

■ **Depression:** Assess mental status and mood changes frequently. Assess for suicidal tendencies, especially during early therapy. Restrict amount of drug available to patient.

■ **Pain:** Assess location, duration, intensity, and characteristics of pain before and periodically during therapy.

■ *Lab Test Considerations:* Assess CBC and renal and hepatic function before and periodically during therapy. Slight, clinically insignificant decrease in leukocyte and neutrophil counts may occur.

## POTENTIAL NURSING DIAGNOSES

■ Coping, ineffective (Indications).

## IMPLEMENTATION

■ **PO:** Administer with or immediately after meals to minimize side effects (nausea, dizziness) and allow maximum absorption of trazodone. A larger portion of the total daily dose may be given at bedtime to decrease daytime drowsiness and dizziness.

**PATIENT/FAMILY TEACHING**

❏ Instruct patient to take medication exactly as directed. If a dose is missed, take as soon as remembered. Do not take if within 4 hr of next scheduled dose; do not double doses. Consult health care professional before discontinuing medication; gradual dosage reduction is necessary to prevent aggravation of condition.

❏ May cause drowsiness and blurred vision. Caution patient to avoid driving and other activities requiring alertness until response to drug is known.

❏ Caution patient to change positions slowly to minimize orthostatic hypotension.

❏ Advise patient to avoid concurrent use of alcohol or other CNS depressant drugs.

❏ Inform patient that frequent rinses, good oral hygiene, and sugarless candy or gum may diminish dry mouth. Health care professional should be notified if this persists >2 wk. An increase in fluid intake, fiber, and exercise may prevent constipation.

❏ Advise patient to notify health care professional of medication regimen before treatment or surgery.

❏ Instruct patient to notify health care professional if priapism, irregular heartbeat, fainting, confusion, skin rash, or tremors occur or if dry mouth, nausea and vomiting, dizziness, headache, muscle aches, constipation, or diarrhea becomes pronounced.

❏ Emphasize the importance of follow-up exams to evaluate progress.

**EVALUATION**

**Effectiveness of therapy can be demonstrated by:** ■ Resolution of depression ❏ Increased sense of well-being ❏ Renewed interest in surroundings ❏ Increased appetite ❏ Improved energy level ❏ Improved sleep ■ Decrease in severity of pain in chronic pain syndromes. Therapeutic effects are usually seen within 1 wk, although 4 wk may be required to obtain significant therapeutic results.

**triamcinolone, See CORTICOSTEROIDS (INHALATION), CORTICOSTEROIDS (NASAL), CORTICOSTEROIDS (SYSTEMIC), CORTICOSTEROIDS (TOPICAL/ LOCAL).**

**triamterene, See DIURETICS (POTASSIUM-SPARING).**

# triazolam

(trye-**az**-oh-lam)

{Apo-Triazo}, {Gen-Triazolam}, Halcion, {Novo-Triolam}, {Nu-Triazo}

**CLASSIFICATION(S):**
**Therapeutic:** sedative/hypnotics
**Pharmacologic:** benzodiazepines

**Schedule IV**

**Pregnancy Category X**

**INDICATIONS**

■ Short-term management of insomnia.

**ACTION**

■ Acts at many levels in the CNS, producing generalized depression ■ Effects may be mediated by GABA, an inhibitory neurotransmitter. **Therapeutic Effects:** ■ Relief of insomnia.

**PHARMACOKINETICS**

**Absorption:** Well absorbed following oral administration.
**Distribution:** Widely distributed, crosses blood-brain barrier. Probably crosses the placenta and enters breast milk.
**Protein Binding:** 89%.
**Metabolism and Excretion:** Metabolized by the liver.
**Half-life:** 1.6–5.4 hr.

**CONTRAINDICATIONS AND PRECAUTIONS**

**Contraindicated in:** ■ Hypersensitivity ■ Cross-sensitivity with other benzodiazepines may occur ■ Pre-existing CNS depression ■ Uncontrolled severe pain ■ Pregnancy, lactation, or children.

**Use Cautiously in:** ■ Pre-existing hepatic dysfunction (dosage reduction recommended) ■ History of suicide attempt or drug addiction ■ Geriatric or debilitated patients (initial dosage reduction recommended).

## ADVERSE REACTIONS AND SIDE EFFECTS*

■ **CNS:** dizziness, excessive sedation, hangover, headache, anterograde amnesia, confusion, lethargy, mental depression, paradoxical excitation ■ **EENT:** blurred vision ■ **GI:** constipation, diarrhea, nausea, vomiting ■ **Derm:** rashes ■ **Misc:** physical dependence, psychological dependence, tolerance.

## INTERACTIONS

**Drug-Drug:** ■ Cimetidine, erythromycin, fluconazole, itraconazole, ketoconazole, indinavir, nelfinavir, ritonavir, or saquinavir may decrease metabolism and enhance actions of triazolam; combination should be avoided ■ Additive CNS depression with alcohol, antidepressants, antihistamines, and opioid analgesics ■ May decrease effectiveness of levodopa ■ May increase toxicity of zidovudine ■ Isoniazid may decrease excretion and increase effects of triazolam ■ Sedative effects may be decreased by theophylline.

**Drug-Natural Products:** ■ Concomitant use of kava, valerian, skullcap, chamomile, or hops can increase CNS depression.

**Drug-Food:** ■ Grapefruit juice significantly increases blood levels and effects.

## ROUTE AND DOSAGE

■ **PO (Adults):** 125–250 mcg (up to 500 mcg) at bedtime.

■ **PO (Geriatric Patients or Debilitated Patients):** 125 mcg at bedtime initially; may be increased as needed.

## AVAILABILITY (generic available)

■ *Tablets:* 125 mcg[Rx], 250 mcg[Rx] ■ Cost: *generic*—0.125 mg $67.30/100, 0.25 mg $72.30/100; *Halcion*—0.125 mg $102.00/100, 0.25 mg $111.54/100.

**TIME/ACTION PROFILE** (sedation)

| | ONSET | PEAK | DURATION |
|---|---|---|---|
| PO | 15–30 min | 6–8 hr | unknown |

# NURSING IMPLICATIONS

## ASSESSMENT

❑ Assess sleep patterns prior to and periodically throughout therapy.

❑ Prolonged high-dose therapy may lead to psychological or physical dependence. Restrict the amount of drug available to patient, especially if patient is depressed, suicidal, or has a history of addiction.

## POTENTIAL NURSING DIAGNOSES

■ Sleep pattern disturbed (Indications).

■ Injury, risk for (Side Effects).

## IMPLEMENTATION

■ **General:** Supervise ambulation and transfer of patients following administration. Remove cigarettes. Side rails should be raised and call bell within reach at all times.

■ **PO:** Administer with food if GI irritation becomes a problem.

## PATIENT/FAMILY TEACHING

❑ Instruct patient to take triazolam exactly as directed. Discuss the importance of preparing environment for sleep (dark room, quiet, avoidance of nicotine and caffeine). If less effective after a few weeks, consult health care professional; do not increase dose.

❑ May cause daytime drowsiness or dizziness. Caution patient to avoid driving or other activities requiring alertness until response to medication is known.

❑ Advise patient to avoid the use of alcohol and other CNS depressants and to consult health care professional prior to using OTC preparations that contain antihistamines or alcohol.

❑ Advise patient to inform health care professional if pregnancy is planned or suspected or if confusion, depression, or persistent headaches occur. Instruct family or caregiver to notify health care professional if personality changes occur.

❑ Instruct patient to notify health care professional if an increase in daytime anxiety occurs. May occur after as few as 10 days of therapy. May require discontinuation of triazolam.

❏ Emphasize the importance of follow-up appointments to monitor progress.

## EVALUATION

**Effectiveness of therapy can be demonstrated by:** ▪ Improvement in sleep patterns, which may not be noticeable until the 3rd day of therapy.

## tricalcium phosphate, See CALCIUM SALTS.

## trimethoprim

(trye-**meth**-oh-prim)

Primsol, Proloprim, Trimpex

### CLASSIFICATION(S):
*Therapeutic:* anti-infectives
*Pharmacologic:* folate antagonists

### Pregnancy Category C

## INDICATIONS

▪ Treatment of uncomplicated urinary tract infections ▪ Treatment of umcomplicated otitis media in children. **Unlabeled uses:** ▪ Prophylaxis of chronic recurrent urinary tract infections ▪ Treatment of head lice ▪ With dapsone in the management of mild to moderate *Pneumocystis carinii* pneumonia (PCP).

## ACTION

▪ Interferes with bacterial folic acid synthesis. **Therapeutic Effects:** ▪ Bactericidal action against susceptible organisms. **Spectrum:** ▪ Some gram-positive pathogens, including: ❏ *Streptococcus pneumoniae* ❏ Group A beta-hemolytic streptococci ❏ Some staphylococci and *Enterococcus* ▪ Gram-negative spectrum includes the following *Enterobacteriaceae:* ❏ *Acinetobacter* ❏ *Citrobacter* ❏ *Enterobacter* ❏ *Escherichia coli* ❏ *Haemophilus influenzae* ❏ *Klebsiella pneumoniae* ❏ *Proteus mirabilis* ❏ *Salmonella* ❏ *Shigella* ▪ Other strains of *Proteus*, some *Providencia*, some *Serratia*, and *P. carinii* are also susceptible.

## PHARMACOKINETICS

**Absorption:** Well absorbed following oral administration.

**Distribution:** Widely distributed. Crosses the placenta and is distributed into breast milk in high concentrations.

**Metabolism and Excretion:** 80% excreted unchanged in the urine; 20% metabolized by the liver.

**Half-life:** 8–11 hr (increased in renal impairment).

## CONTRAINDICATIONS AND PRECAUTIONS

**Contraindicated in:** ▪ Hypersensitivity ▪ Megaloblastic anemia secondary to folate deficiency.
**Use Cautiously in:** ▪ Renal impairment (dosage reduction required if CCr ≤30 ml/min) ▪ Debilitated patients ▪ Severe hepatic impairment ▪ Folate deficiency ▪ Pregnancy, lactation, or children <12 yr (safety as a single agent not established).

## ADVERSE REACTIONS AND SIDE EFFECTS*

▪ **GI:** <u>altered taste</u>, <u>epigastric discomfort</u>, <u>glossitis</u>, <u>nausea</u>, <u>vomiting</u>, drug-induced hepatitis ▪ **Derm:** <u>pruritus</u>, <u>rash</u> ▪ **Hemat:** megaloblastic anemia, neutropenia, thrombocytopenia ▪ **Misc:** fever.

## INTERACTIONS

**Drug-Drug:** ▪ Increased risk of folate deficiency when used with **phenytoin** or **methotrexate** ▪ Increased risk of bone marrow depression when used with **antineoplastics** or **radiation therapy** ▪ **Rifampin** may decrease effectiveness by increasing elimination.

## ROUTE AND DOSAGE

❏ **Treatment of Urinary Tract Infections**
▪ **PO (Adults and Children ≥12 yr):** 100 mg q 12 hr or 200 mg as a single daily dose.

❏ **Treatment of Otitis Media**
▪ **PO (Children >6 mo):** 5 mg/kg q 12 hr.

❏ **Prophylaxis of Chronic Urinary Tract Infections**
▪ **PO (Adults):** 100 mg/day as a single dose (unlabeled).

❏ *Pneumocystis carinii* **Pneumonia**

■ **PO (Adults):** 20 mg/kg/day with 100 mg dapsone daily for 21 days (unlabeled).

❏ **Renal Impairment**

■ **PO (Adults):** *CCr 15–30 ml/min*—50 mg q 12 hr (for urinary tract infections).

## AVAILABILITY (generic available)

■ *Tablets:* 100 mg$^{Rx}$, 200 mg$^{Rx}$ ■ *Oral solution (alcohol- and dye-free) (bubblegum flavor):* 50 mg/5 ml in 473-ml bottles$^{Rx}$ ■ sulfamethoxazole$^{Rx}$. See Trimethoprim/Sulfamethoxazole monograph.

TIME/ACTION PROFILE (blood levels)

|    | ONSET | PEAK | DURATION |
|----|-------|------|----------|
| PO | rapid | 1–4 hr | 12–24 hr |

# NURSING IMPLICATIONS

## ASSESSMENT

❏ Assess patient for urinary tract infection (fever, cloudy urine, frequency, urgency, pain and burning on urination) or other signs of infection at beginning of and throughout therapy.

❏ Obtain specimens for culture and sensitivity prior to initiating therapy. First dose may be given before receiving results.

❏ Monitor intake and output ratios. Fluid intake should be sufficient to maintain urine output of at least 1200–1500 ml daily.

■ *Lab Test Considerations:* May produce elevated serum bilirubin, creatinine, BUN, AST, and ALT.

❏ Monitor CBC and urinalysis periodically throughout therapy. Therapy should be discontinued if blood dyscrasias occur.

## POTENTIAL NURSING DIAGNOSES

■ Infection, risk for (Indications, Side Effects).

## IMPLEMENTATION

■ **PO:** Administer on an empty stomach, at least 1 hr before or 2 hr after meals, with a full glass of water. May be administered with food if GI irritation occurs.

## PATIENT/FAMILY TEACHING

❏ Instruct patient to take medication and to finish medication completely as directed, even if feeling better. If a dose is missed, it should be taken as soon as remembered, with subsequent doses spaced evenly apart. Advise patient that sharing of this medication may be dangerous.

❏ Advise patient to notify health care professional if skin rash, sore throat, fever, mouth sores, or unusual bleeding or bruising occurs. Leucovorin (folinic acid) may be administered if folic acid deficiency occurs.

❏ Instruct patient to notify health care professional if symptoms do not improve.

❏ Emphasize the importance of routine follow-up exams to evaluate progress.

## EVALUATION

**Clinical response to therapy can be evaluated by:** ■ Resolution of the signs and symptoms of infection. Therapy is usually required for 10–14 days for resolution of urinary tract infection ■ Decreased incidence of urinary tract infections during prophylactic therapy.

---

# trimethoprim/sulfamethoxazole

(trye-**meth**-oh-prim/sul-fa-meth-**ox**-a-zole)

{Apo-Sulfatrim}, {Apo-Sulfatrim DS}, Bactrim, Bactrim DS, Cofatrim, Cotrim, Cotrim DS, {Novo-Trimel}, {Novo-Trimel DS}, {Nu-Cotrimox}, {Nu-Cotrimox DS}, {Roubac}, Septra, Septra DS, SMZ/TMP, Sulfatrim, Sulfatrim DS, TMP/SMX, TMP/SMZ

## CLASSIFICATION(S):

*Therapeutic: anti-infectives, antiprotozoals*
*Pharmacologic: folate antagonists, sulfonamides*

## Pregnancy Category C

## INDICATIONS

■ Treatment of: ❏ Bronchitis ❏ *Shigella* enteritis ❏ Otitis media ❏ *Pneumocystis carinii* pneumonia (PCP) ❏ Urinary tract infections ❏ Traveler's diarrhea ■ Prevention of PCP in HIV-positive patients. **Unlabeled uses:** ■ Biliary tract infections, osteomyelitis, burn and wound infections, chlamydial infections, endocarditis, gonorrhea, intra-abdominal infections, nocardiosis, rheumatic fever prophylaxis, sinusitis, eradication of meningococcal carriers, prophylaxis of urinary tract infections, and an alternative agent in the treatment of chancroid ■ Prevention of bacterial infections in immunosuppressed patients.

### ACTION

■ Combination inhibits the metabolism of folic acid in bacteria at two different points. **Therapeutic Effects:** ■ Bactericidal action against susceptible bacteria. **Spectrum:** ■ Active against many strains of gram-positive aerobic pathogens including: ❑ *Streptococcus pneumoniae* ❑ *Staphylococcus aureus* ❑ Group A beta-hemolytic streptococci ❑ *Nocardia* ❑ *Enterococcus* ■ Has activity against many aerobic gram-negative pathogens, such as: ❑ *Acinetobacter* ❑ *Enterobacter* ❑ *Klebsiella pneumoniae* ❑ *Escherichia coli* ❑ *Proteus mirabilis* ❑ *Shigella* ❑ *Haemophilus influenzae*, including ampicillin-resistant strains ■ *P. carinii* (a protozoa) ■ Not active against *Pseudomonas aeruginosa*.

### PHARMACOKINETICS

**Absorption:** Well absorbed from the GI tract. **Distribution:** Widely distributed. Crosses the blood-brain barrier and placenta and enters breast milk.
**Metabolism and Excretion:** Some metabolism by the liver (20%); remainder excreted unchanged by the kidneys.
**Half-life:** *Trimethoprim*—8–11 hr; *sulfamethoxazole*—7–12 hr.

### CONTRAINDICATIONS AND PRECAUTIONS

**Contraindicated in:** ■ Hypersensitivity to sulfonamides or trimethoprim ■ Megaloblastic anemia secondary to folate deficiency ■ Severe renal impairment ■ Pregnancy, lactation, or children <2 mo.
**Use Cautiously in:** ■ Impaired hepatic or renal function (dosage reduction required if CCr <30 ml/min) ■ HIV-positive patients (increased incidence of adverse reactions).

### ADVERSE REACTIONS AND SIDE EFFECTS*

■ **CNS:** fatigue, hallucinations, headache, insomnia, mental depression ■ **GI:** HEPATIC NECROSIS, nausea, vomiting, diarrhea, stomatitis ■ **GU:** crystalluria ■ **Derm:** TOXIC EPIDERMAL NECROLYSIS,

rashes, photosensitivity ■ **Hemat:** AGRANULOCYTOSIS, APLASTIC ANEMIA, hemolytic anemia, leukopenia, megaloblastic anemia, thrombocytopenia ■ **Local:** phlebitis at IV site ■ **Misc:** allergic reactions including ERYTHEMA MULTIFORME, STEVENS-JOHNSON SYNDROME, fever.

### INTERACTIONS

**Drug-Drug:** ■ May ↑ half-life, ↓ clearance, and exaggerate folic acid deficiency caused by **phenytoin** ■ May ↑ effects of **sulfonylurea oral antidiabetics** and **warfarin** ■ May ↑ toxicity of **methotrexate** ■ ↑ risk of thrombocytopenia from **thiazide diuretics** ( ↑ in geriatric patients) ■ ↓ efficacy of **cyclosporine** and ↑ risk of nephrotoxicity.

### ROUTE AND DOSAGE

(TMP = trimethoprim; SMZ = sulfamethoxazole)

❑ **Bacterial Infections**

■ **PO (Adults and Children ≥40 kg):** 160 mg TMP/800 mg SMZ q 12 hr.
■ **PO (Children >2):** 4–6 mg/kg TMP/20–30 mg/kg SMZ q 12 hr.
■ **IV (Adults and Children >2 mo):** 2–2.5 mg/kg TMP/10–12.5 mg/kg SMZ q 6 hr *or* 2.7–3.3 mg/kg TMP/13.3–16.7 mg/kg SMZ q 8 hr *or* 4–5 mg/kg TMP/20–25 mg/kg SMZ q 12 hr.

❑ *P. carinii* **Pneumonia (Treatment)**

■ **PO (Adults and Children >2 mo):** 3.75–5 mg/kg TMP/18.75–25 mg SMZ q 6 hr.
■ **IV (Adults and Children >2 mo):** 3.75–5 mg/kg TMP/18.75–25 mg SMZ q 6 hr *or* 5–6.7 mg/kg TMP/25–33.3 mg SMZ q 8 hr.

❑ *P. carinii* **Pneumonia (Prevention)**

■ **PO (Adults):** 160 mg TMP/800 mg SMZ daily (may also be given 3 times weekly).
■ **PO (Children >1 mo):** 75 mg/m² TMP/325 mg/m² SMZ q 12 hr on 3 consecutive days/wk (not to exceed 320 mg TMP/1600 mg SMZ per day).

### AVAILABILITY (generic available)

■ *Tablets:* {20 mg TMP/100 mg SMZ^Rx}, 80 mg TMP/400 mg SMZ^Rx, 160 mg TMP/800 mg SMZ^Rx ■ Cost: *Bactrim*—80 mg TMP/400 mg SMZ $89.48/100 ■ *Suspension (cherry,*

---

*grape flavors):* 40 mg TMP/200 mg SMZ per 5 ml<sup>Rx</sup> ▪ *Injection:* 80 mg TMP/400 mg SMZ per 5 ml in 5-, 10-, 20-, and 30-ml vials<sup>Rx</sup>.

TIME/ACTION PROFILE (blood levels)

| | ONSET | PEAK | DURATION |
|---|---|---|---|
| PO | rapid | 2–4 hr | 6–12 hr |
| IV | rapid | end of infusion | 6–12 hr |

## NURSING IMPLICATIONS

### ASSESSMENT

❏ Assess for infection (vital signs; appearance of wound, sputum, urine, and stool; WBC) at beginning of and during therapy.

❏ Obtain specimens for culture and sensitivity before initiating therapy. First dose may be given before receiving results.

❏ Inspect IV site frequently. Phlebitis is common.

❏ Assess patient for allergy to sulfonamides.

❏ Monitor intake and output ratios. Fluid intake should be sufficient to maintain a urine output of at least 1200–1500 ml daily to prevent crystalluria and stone formation.

▪ *Lab Test Considerations:* Monitor CBC and urinalysis periodically during therapy.

❏ May produce ↑ serum bilirubin, creatinine, and alkaline phosphatase.

### POTENTIAL NURSING DIAGNOSES

▪ Infection, risk for (Indications, Side Effects).

▪ Noncompliance (Patient/Family Teaching).

### IMPLEMENTATION

▪ **General:** Do not confuse DS (double-strength) formulations with single-strength formulations.

❏ Do not administer medication IM.

▪ **PO:** Administer around the clock with a full glass of water. Use calibrated measuring device for liquid preparations.

▪ **Intermittent Infusion:** Dilute each 5-ml ampule with 100–125 ml of D5W. May reduce diluent to 75 ml if fluid restriction is required. Do not use if solution is cloudy or contains a precipitate. Solution is stable for 6 hr in standard dilution and 2 hr in fluid-restricted dilution at room temperature. Do not refrigerate.

▪ *Rate:* Infuse over 60–90 min. Do not administer rapidly or by bolus injection.

▪ **Y-Site Compatibility:** ◆ acyclovir ◆ aldesleukin ◆ allopurinol ◆ amifostine ◆ amphotericin B cholesteryl sulfate ◆ atracurium ◆ aztreonam ◆ cefepime ◆ cyclophosphamide ◆ diltiazem ◆ docetaxel ◆ doxorubicin liposome ◆ enalaprilat ◆ esmolol ◆ etoposide phosphate ◆ filgrastim ◆ fludarabine ◆ gatifloxacin ◆ gemcitabine ◆ granisetron ◆ hydromorphone ◆ labetalol ◆ lorazepam ◆ magnesium sulfate ◆ melphalan ◆ meperidine ◆ morphine ◆ pancuronium ◆ perphenazine ◆ piperacillin/tazobactam ◆ remifentanil ◆ sargramostim ◆ tacrolimus ◆ teniposide ◆ thiotepa ◆ vecuronium ◆ zidovudine.

▪ **Y-Site Incompatibility:** ◆ fluconazole ◆ midazolam ◆ vinorelbine.

▪ **Additive Incompatibility:** Manufacturer recommends that no other medication or solution be admixed with trimethoprim/sulfamethoxazole.

## PATIENT/FAMILY TEACHING

❏ Instruct patient to take medication around the clock and to finish drug completely as directed, even if feeling well. Take missed doses as soon as remembered unless almost time for next dose. Advise patient that sharing of this medication may be dangerous.

❏ Caution patient to use sunscreen and protective clothing to prevent photosensitivity reactions.

❏ Advise patient to notify health care professional if skin rash, sore throat, fever, mouth sores, or unusual bleeding or bruising occurs.

❏ Instruct patient to notify health care professional if symptoms do not improve within a few days.

❏ Emphasize importance of regular follow-up exams to monitor blood counts in patients on prolonged therapy.

▪ **Home Care Issues:** Instruct family or caregiver on dilution, rate, and administration of drug and proper care of IV equipment.

### EVALUATION

**Clinical response to therapy can be evaluated by:** ▪ Resolution of the signs and symptoms of infection. Length of time for complete resolution depends on organism and site of infection ▪ Resolution of symptoms of traveler's diarrhea ▪ Prevention of PCP in patients with HIV.

# triptorelin

(trip-to-**rel**-in)

Trelstar Depot

**CLASSIFICATION(S):**
**Therapeutic:** antineoplastics
**Pharmacologic:** hormones

**Pregnancy Category X**

## INDICATIONS

■ Palliative treatment of advanced prostate cancer when orchiectomy or estrogen administration are contraindicated or unacceptable.

## ACTION

■ A synthetic analog of luteinizing hormone-releasing hormone (LHRH). Initially causes a transient increase in testosterone; however, with continuous administration, testosterone levels are decreased. Reduces gonadotropins, testosterone, and estradiol. **Therapeutic Effects:** ■ Decreased testosterone levels and resultant decrease in spread of prostate cancer.

## PHARMACOKINETICS

**Absorption:** Well absorbed following IM administration.
**Distribution:** Unknown.
**Metabolism and Excretion:** Unknown.
**Half-life:** 3 hr.

## CONTRAINDICATIONS AND PRECAUTIONS

**Contraindicated in:** ■ Hypersensitivity to triptorelin or similar agents ■ Pregnancy, lactation, or children.
**Use Cautiously in:** ■ Metastatic vertebral lesions and/or upper or lower urinary tract obstruction (symptoms may transiently worsen following initiation of therapy) ■ Renal or hepatic impairment (may need dosage adjustment).

## ADVERSE REACTIONS AND SIDE EFFECTS*

■ **CNS:** dizziness, emotional lability, fatigue, headache, insomnia ■ **CV:** hypertension ■ **GI:** diarrhea, vomiting ■ **GU:** impotence, urinary

retention, urinary tract infection ■ **Derm:** pruritus ■ **Hemat:** anemia ■ **Local:** injection site pain ■ **MS:** musculoskeletal pain ■ **Misc:** allergic reactions including ANAPHYLAXIS and ANGIOEDEMA.

## INTERACTIONS

**Drug-Drug:** ■ Concurrent use of **hyperprolactinemic drugs** should be avoided (may decrease number of drug receptor sites).

## ROUTE AND DOSAGE

■ **IM (Adults):** 3.75 mg monthly.

## AVAILABILITY

■ **Suspension for IM injection (Depot):** 3.75 mg/vial^Rx.

TIME/ACTION PROFILE (effects on hormone levels)

| | ONSET | PEAK | DURATION |
|---|---|---|---|
| IM | Unknown | 1 hr† | 4 wk |

†Blood level of triptorelin.

# NURSING IMPLICATIONS

## ASSESSMENT

❏ Assess patient for symptoms of prostate cancer prior to and throughout therapy. Symptoms may worsen or onset of new symptoms (bone pain, neuropathy, hematuria, urethral or bladder outlet obstruction) may occur during first few weeks of treatment.
❏ Monitor patient for signs and symptoms of anaphylaxis (dyspnea, rash, laryngeal edema) following each dose. Have diphenhydramine, epinephrine, and resuscitation equipment readily available.
■ **Lab Test Considerations:** Monitor response by measuring serum testosterone and prostate-specific antigen levels periodically during therapy.

## POTENTIAL NURSING DIAGNOSES

■ Knowledge, deficient, related to medication regimen (Patient/Family Teaching).

## IMPLEMENTATION

■ **General:** Triptorelin must be administered under the supervision of a physician.

■ **IM:** Reconstitute by withdrawing 2 ml of sterile water for injection into a syringe with a 20-gauge needle and inject into vial. Shake well to obtain a uniform suspension and thoroughly disperse particles. Suspension will appear milky. Withdraw entire contents of reconstituted suspension and inject immediately. Discard suspension if not used immediately after reconstitution.

❏ Rotate injection sites periodically.

## PATIENT/FAMILY TEACHING

❏ Explain the purpose of triptorelin to patient and family.

❏ May cause dizziness. Caution patient not to drive or other activities requiring alertness until response to medication is known.

❏ Emphasize the importance of routine examinations to monitor for side effects and assess response.

## EVALUATION

**Clinical response to therapy can be evaluated by:** ■ Decreased testosterone levels and resultant decrease in spread of prostate cancer.

**trovafloxacin, See FLUOROQUINOLONES.**

## urokinase, See THROMBOLYTIC AGENTS.

## valacyclovir

(val-ay-**sye**-kloe-veer)
Valtrex

*CLASSIFICATION(S):*
*Therapeutic: antivirals*

**Pregnancy Category B**

### INDICATIONS

■ Treatment of herpes zoster (shingles) ■ Treatment/suppression of genital herpes ■ Reduction of transmission of genital herpes ■ Treatment of herpes labialis (cold sores).

### ACTION

■ Rapidly converted to acyclovir. Acyclovir interferes with viral DNA synthesis. **Therapeutic Effects:** ■ Inhibited viral replication, decreased viral shedding, reduced time to healing of lesions ■ Reduced transmission of genital herpes.

### PHARMACOKINETICS

**Absorption:** 54% bioavailable as acyclovir after oral administration of valacyclovir.

**Distribution:** CSF concentrations of acyclovir are 50% of plasma concentrations. Acyclovir crosses placenta; enters breast milk.

**Metabolism and Excretion:** Rapidly converted to acyclovir via intestinal/hepatic metabolism.

**Half-life:** 2.5–3.3 hr; up to 14 hr in renal impairment (acyclovir).

### CONTRAINDICATIONS AND PRECAUTIONS

**Contraindicated in:** ■ Hypersensitivity to valacyclovir or acyclovir.

**Use Cautiously in:** ■ Renal impairment (dosage reduction/increased dosing interval recommended if CCr <50 ml/min) ■ Geriatric patients (dosage reduction may be necessary) ■ Pregnancy, lactation, or children (safety not established).

### ADVERSE REACTIONS AND SIDE EFFECTS*

■ **CNS:** <u>headache</u>, dizziness, weakness ■ **GI:** <u>nausea</u>, abdominal pain, anorexia, constipation, diarrhea ■ **Hemat:** THROMBOTIC THROMBOCYTOPENIC PURPURA/HEMOLYTIC UREMIC SYNDROME (very high doses in immunosuppressed patients).

### INTERACTIONS

**Drug-Drug:** ■ **Probenecid** and **cimetidine** ↑ blood levels; significant only in renal impairment.

### ROUTE AND DOSAGE

❏ **Herpes Zoster**
■ **PO (Adults):** 1 g 3 times daily for 7 days.

❏ **Genital Herpes**
■ **PO (Adults):** *Initial treatment*—1 g twice daily for 10 days. *Recurrence*—500 mg twice daily for 3 days. *Suppression of recurrence*—1 g once daily or 500 mg once daily in patients experiencing <10 recurrences/yr. *Suppression of recurrence in HIV-infected patients*—500 mg q 12 hr. *Reduction of transmission*—500 mg once daily for source partner.

❏ **Herpes Labialis**
■ **PO (Adults):** 2 g then 2 g 12 hr later.

❏ **Renal Impairment**
■ **PO (Adults):** *CCr 30–49 ml/min*—1 g q 12 hr for herpes zoster treatment, no reduction required for treatment of genital herpes;1 g then 1 g 12 hr later for herpes labialis. *CCr 10–29 ml/min*—1 g q 24 hr for initial treatment of genital herpes, 500 mg q 24 hr for treatment of recurrent episodes of genital herpes, 500 mg q 48 hr for suppression of genital herpes in patients with 9 or fewer recurrences/yr, 500 mg q 24 hr for suppression of genital herpes in patients with ≥10 recurrences/yr or HIV-infected patients, 1 g q 24 hr for treatment of herpes zoster; 500 mg then 500 mg 12 hr later for herpes labialis. *CCr <10 ml/min*—500 mg q 24 hr for initial treatment of genital herpes, 500 mg q 24 hr for treatment of recurrent episodes of genital herpes, 500 mg q 48 hr for suppression of genital herpes in patients with 9 or fewer recurrences/yr, 500

mg q 24 hr for suppression of genital herpes in patients with ≥10 recurrences/yr or HIV-infected patients, 500 mg q 24 hr for treatment of herpes zoster; single 500 mg dose for herpes labialis.

## AVAILABILITY

■ *Tablets:* 500 mg$^{Rx}$, 1 g$^{Rx}$ ■ Cost: 500 mg $151.86/42, 1 g $103.24/20.

TIME/ACTION PROFILE (blood levels†)

| | ONSET | PEAK | DURATION |
|---|---|---|---|
| PO | unknown | 1.5–2.5 hr | 8–24 hr |

†Acyclovir.

# NURSING IMPLICATIONS

## ASSESSMENT

❑ Assess lesions before and daily during therapy.
❑ Monitor patient for signs of thrombotic thrombocytic purpura/hemolytic uremic syndrome (thrombocytopenia, microangiopathic hemolytic anemia, neurologic findings, renal dysfunction, fever). Requires prompt treatment; may be fatal.

## POTENTIAL NURSING DIAGNOSES

■ Skin integrity, risk for impaired (Indications).
■ Infection, risk for (Indications, Patient/Family Teaching).

## IMPLEMENTATION

■ **PO:** May be administered without regard to meals.
■ **Herpes Zoster:** Implement valacyclovir therapy as soon as possible after the onset of signs or symptoms of herpes zoster; most effective if started within 48 hr of the onset of zoster rash. Efficacy of treatment started >72 hr after rash onset is unknown.
■ **Genital Herpes and Herpes Labialis:** Implement treatment for genital herpes as soon as possible after onset of symptoms.

## PATIENT/FAMILY TEACHING

■ **General Info:** Instruct patient to take valacyclovir exactly as directed for the full course of therapy. If a dose is missed, take as soon as remembered if not just before next dose.
■ **Herpes Zoster:** Inform patient that valacyclovir does not prevent the spread of infec-

tion to others. Precautions should be taken around others who have not had chickenpox or varicella vaccine, or are immunosuppressed, until all lesions have crusted.
■ **Genital Herpesand Herpes Labialis:** Inform patient that valacyclovir does not prevent the spread of herpes labialis to others. Advise patient to avoid contact with lesions while lesions or symptoms are present. Valacyclovir prevents transmission of genital herpes to others. Advise patient to practice safe sex (avoid sexual intercourse when lesions are present and wear a condom made of latex or polyurethane during sexual contact).

## EVALUATION

**Effectiveness of therapy can be demonstrated by:** ■ Decrease in time to full crusting, loss of vesicles, loss of ulcers, and development of crusts in patients with acute herpes zoster (shingles) ■ Decrease in time to full crusting, loss of vesicles, loss of ulcers, and development of crusts in patients with genital herpes ■ Decrease in frequency of outbreaks in patients with genital herpes ■ Decrease in time to full crusting, loss of vesicles, loss of ulcers, and development of crusts in patients with herpes labialis. Decrease in transmission of genital herpes.

# valdecoxib
(val-de-**cox**-ib)
Bextra

## CLASSIFICATION(S):

*Therapeutic:* nonsteroidal anti-inflammatory agents, nonopioid analgesics
*Pharmacologic:* COX-2 inhibitors

**Pregnancy Category C**

## INDICATIONS

■ Osteoarthritis ■ Adult rheumatoid arthritis ■ Primary dysmenorrhea.

## ACTION

■ Inhibits the enzyme cyclo-oxygenase-2 (COX-2). This enzyme is required for the synthesis of prostaglandins ■ Has analgesic, anti-inflammatory and antipyretic properties ■ Does not inhibit COX-1 and may produce less GI damage than other NSAIDs. **Therapeutic Effects:** ■ Decreased pain and inflammation caused by arthritis ■ Decreased pain due to dysmenorrhea.

## PHARMACOKINETICS

**Absorption:** Well absorbed (83%) following oral administration.

**Distribution:** Preferentially partitions into erythrocytes; remainder of distibution unknown.

**Metabolism and Excretion:** Mostly metabolized by the hepatic P450 enzymes (3A4 and 2C9) and other metabolic processes; <5% excreted unchanged in urine. One metabolite has COX-2 inhibitory properties.

**Half-life:** 8–11 hr.

## CONTRAINDICATIONS AND PRECAUTIONS

**Contraindicated in:** ■ Hypersensitivity ■ History of allergy to sulfas/sulfonamides ■ Cross-sensitivity may exist with other NSAIDs, including aspirin ■ History of asthma, urticaria or allergic-type reactions to aspirin or other NSAIDs including the aspirin triad (asthma, nasal polyps, and severe hypersensitivity reactions to aspirin) ■ Advanced renal disease ■ Lactation ■ Should not be used late in pregnancy (may cause premature closure of the ductus arteriosus).

**Use Cautiously in:** ■ Elderly patients, patients who smoke, patients receiving corticosteroids, anticoagulants or prolonged NSAID therapy, chronic alcoholism, old age or poor general health (may increase risk of GI bleeding) ■ Dehydration (rehydrate prior to therapy) ■ Mild-to-moderate renal impairment, CHF, hepatic impairment, concurrent diuretics or ACE inhibitors, or elderly patients (increased risk of deterioration in renal function) ■ Children <18 yr (safety not established).

**Exercise Extreme Caution in:** ■ Prior history of ulcer disease or GI bleeding.

## ADVERSE REACTIONS AND SIDE EFFECTS*

■ **CNS:** increased blood pressure ■ **CV:** edema ■ **F and E:** fluid retention ■ **GI:** GI BLEEDING, abdominal pain ■ **Derm:** rash ■ **Hemat:** anemia

■ **Misc:** allergic reactions including ANAPHYLACTOID REACTIONS, ANAPHYLAXIS, ANGIOEDEMA, STEVENS-JOHNSON SYNDROME.

## INTERACTIONS

**Drug-Drug:** ■ Does not inhibit the cardioprotective effect of low-dose **aspirin** ■ ↑ risk of GI bleeding with **aspirin, corticosteroids,** or other **NSAIDs** ■ May ↓ response to **furosemide, thiazide diuretics, ACE inhibitors,** and other **antihypertensives** ■ ↓ clearance and may ↑ levels of **lithium** (lithium serum level monitoring recommended) ■ Blood levels of valdecoxib are ↑ by **ketoconazole** and **itraconazole**.

## ROUTE AND DOSAGE

■ **PO (Adults):** *Osteoarthritis/rheumatoid arthritis*—10 mg once daily; *dysmenorrhea*—20 mg twice daily.

## AVAILABILITY

■ **Tablets:** 10 mg$^{Rx}$, 20 mg$^{Rx}$ ■ Cost: 10 mg $291.50/100, 20 mg $291.50/100.

TIME/ACTION PROFILE (analgesia)

| | ONSET | PEAK | DURATION |
|---|---|---|---|
| PO | within 1 hr | 3 hr | up to 12 hr |

# NURSING IMPLICATIONS

## ASSESSMENT

■ **General Info:** Patients who have asthma, aspirin-induced allergy, and nasal polyps are at increased risk for developing hypersensitivity reactions. Assess for rhinitis, asthma, and urticaria.

■ **Pain:** Assess pain (note type, location, and intensity) prior to and 2–3 hr following administration.

■ **Arthritis:** Assess patient's range of motion, degree of swelling, and pain in affected joints before and periodically during therapy.

■ **Lab Test Considerations:** Valdecoxib does not affect platelet count, prothrombin time (PT), partial thromboplastin time (PTT), and does not appear to inhibit platelet aggregation.

❑ Monitor hemoglobin and hematocrit in patients receiving prolonged valdecoxib therapy if signs or symptoms of anemia occur.

## POTENTIAL NURSING DIAGNOSES

■ Pain, acute (Indications).

■ Mobility, impaired physical (Indications).

## IMPLEMENTATION

■ **PO:** May be administered without regard to food.

■ **Dysmenorrhea:** Administer as soon as possible after the onset of menses. Prophylactic treatment has not been shown to be effective.

## PATIENT/FAMILY TEACHING

❑ Advise patients to take this medication with a full glass of water and to remain in an upright position for 15–30 min after administration.

❑ Instruct patient to take medication as directed. Take missed doses as soon as remembered but not if almost time for next dose. Do not double doses.

❑ Caution patient to avoid the concurrent use of alcohol, aspirin, acetaminophen, other OTC medications, or herbal products without consulting health care professional.

❑ Advise patient to inform health care professional of medication regimen prior to treatment or surgery.

❑ Caution patient that use of an NSAID with 3 or more glasses of alcohol per day may increase the risk of GI bleeding.

❑ Advise patient to consult health care professional promptly if abdominal pain or black tarry stools occur. GI toxicity can occur at any time, without warning. Patient should also notify health care professional if rash, weight gain, edema, nausea, fatigue, lethargy, itching, jaundice, upper right quadrant tenderness, or influenza-like syndrome (chills, fever, muscle aches, pain) occur.

## EVALUATION

**Effectiveness of therapy can be demonstrated by:** ■ Decrease in severity of pain ■ Improved joint mobility.

---

## valganciclovir

(val-gan-**sye**-kloe-veer)

Valcyte

---

**CLASSIFICATION(S):**
**Therapeutic:** antivirals

**Pregnancy Category C**

## INDICATIONS

■ Treatment of cytomegalovirus (CMV) retinitis in patients with AIDS.

## ACTION

■ Valganciclovir is a prodrug which is rapidly converted to ganciclovir by intestinal and hepatic enzymes. CMV virus converts ganciclovir to its active form (ganciclovir phosphate) inside host cell, where it inhibits viral DNA polymerase. **Therapeutic Effects:** ■ Antiviral effect directed preferentially against CMV-infected cells.

## PHARMACOKINETICS

**Absorption:** 59.4% absorbed following oral administration, rapidly converted to ganciclovir.

**Distribution:** Unknown.

**Metabolism and Excretion:** Rapidly converted to ganciclovir; ganciclovir is mostly excreted by the kidneys.

**Half-life:** 4.1 hr (intracellular half-life of ganciclovir phosphate is 18 hr).

## CONTRAINDICATIONS AND PRECAUTIONS

**Contraindicated in:** ■ Hypersensitivity to valganciclovir or ganciclovir ■ Pregnancy or planned pregnancy ■ Lactation ■ Hemodialysis.

**Use Cautiously in:** ■ Renal impairment (dosage reduction recommended if CCR <60 ml/min) ■ Pre-existing bone marrow depression ■ Previous or concurrent myelosuppressive drug therapy or radiation therapy ■ Geriatric patients (age-related decrease in renal function requires dosage reduction) ■ Children (safety not established).

## ADVERSE REACTIONS AND SIDE EFFECTS*

■ **CNS:** SEIZURES, headache, insomnia, agitation, confusion, dizziness, hallucinations, psychosis, sedation ■ **GI:** abdominal pain, diarrhea, nausea, vomiting ■ **GU:** renal impairment ■ **Hemat:** NEUTROPENIA, THROMBOCYTOPENIA, anemia, aplastic anemia, bone marrow depression, pancytopenia ■ **Neuro:** ataxia, paresthesia, peripheral neuropathy ▪ **Misc:** <u>fever</u>, hypersensitivity reactions, infections.

## INTERACTIONS

**Drug-Drug:** ▪ Increase risk of hematologic toxicity with **zidovudine** ▪ Blood levels and effects may be increased by **probenecid** ▪ Patients with renal impairment may experience accumulation of metabolites of **mycophenolate** and valganciclovir ▪ Increases blood levels and risk of toxicity from **didanosine**.

**Drug-Food:** ▪ Food enhances absorption.

## ROUTE AND DOSAGE

▪ **PO (Adults):** *Induction*—900 mg twice daily for 21 days; *maintenance treatment or patients with inactive CMV retinitis*—900 mg once daily.

❏ **Renal Impairment**
▪ **CCr 40–59 ml/min: (Adults):** *Induction*—450 mg twice daily for 21 days; *maintenance treatment or patients with inactive CMV retinitis*—450 mg once daily.

❏ **Renal Impairment**
▪ **CCr 25–39 ml/min: (Adults):** *Induction*—450 mg once daily for 21 days; *maintenance treatment or patients with inactive CMV retinitis*—450 mg every two days.

❏ **Renal Impairment**
▪ **CCr 10–24 ml/min: (Adults):** *Induction*—450 mg every two days for 21 days; *maintenance treatment or patients with inactive CMV retinitis*—450 mg twice weekly.

## AVAILABILITY

▪ **Tablets:** 450 mg.

TIME/ACTION PROFILE (ganciclovir blood levels)

| | ONSET | PEAK | DURATION |
|----|-------|------|----------|
| PO | rapid | 2 hr | 12–24 hr |

# NURSING IMPLICATIONS

## ASSESSMENT

❏ Diagnosis of CMV retinitis should be determined by ophthalmoscopy prior to treatment with ganciclovir.

❏ Culture for CMV (urine, blood, throat) may be taken prior to administration. However, a negative CMV culture does not rule out CMV retinitis. If symptoms do not respond after several weeks, resistance to ganciclovir may have occurred. Ophthalmologic exams should be performed weekly during induction and every 2 wk during maintenance or more frequently if the macula or optic nerve is threatened. Progression of CMV retinitis may occur during or following ganciclovir treatment.

❏ Assess for signs of infection (fever, chills, cough, hoarseness, lower back or side pain, sore throat, difficult or painful urination). Notify physician or other health care professional if these symptoms occur.

❏ Assess for bleeding (bleeding gums, bruising, pete-
chiae, or guaiac stools, urine, and emesis). Avoid IM injections and taking rectal temperatures. Apply pressure to venipuncture sites for 10 min.

▪ *Lab Test Considerations:* May cause granulocytopenia, anemia, and thrombocytopenia. Monitor neutrophil and platelet count closely throughout therapy. Do not administer if ANC <500/mm$^3$, platelet count <25,000/mm$^3$, or hemoglobin <8 g/dl. Recovery begins within 3–7 days of discontinuation of therapy.

❏ Monitor BUN and serum creatinine at least once every 2 wk throughout therapy. May cause elevations in serum creatinine.

## POTENTIAL NURSING DIAGNOSES

▪ Infection, risk for (Indications, Patient/Family Teaching).

## IMPLEMENTATION

▪ **General:** Valganciclovir and ganciclovir are not interchangeable. Do not substitute.

❏ Valganciclovir tablets should be handled carefully. Do not break or crush. May be potentially teratogenic; avoid direct contact with broken or crushed tablets. If contact with the skin or mucous membranes occurs, wash thoroughly with soap and water and rinse eyes thoroughly with plain water.

▪ **PO:** Administer capsules with food.

## PATIENT/FAMILY TEACHING

◻ Instruct patient to take valganciclovir with food, exactly as directed.

◻ Inform patient that valganciclovir is not a cure for CMV retinitis. Progression of retinitis may continue in immunocompromised patients during and following therapy. Advise patients to have regular ophthalmic exams at least every 4–6 wk. Duration of therapy for CMV prevention is based on the duration and degree of immunosuppression.

◻ May cause seizures, sedation, dizziness, ataxia, and/or confusion. Caution patient not to drive or do other activities requiring alertness until response to medication is known.

◻ Advise patient to notify health care professional if fever; chills; sore throat; other signs of infection; bleeding gums; bruising; petechiae; or blood in urine, stool, or emesis occurs. Caution patient to avoid crowds and persons with known infections. Instruct patient to use soft toothbrush and electric razor. Patient should be cautioned not to drink alcoholic beverages or take products containing aspirin or NSAIDs.

◻ Advise patient that valganciclovir may have teratogenic effects. Women should use a nonhormonal and men a barrier method of contraception during and for at least 90 days following therapy.

◻ Caution patient to use sunscreen and protective clothing to prevent photosensitivity reactions.

◻ Emphasize the importance of frequent follow-up exams to monitor blood counts.

## EVALUATION

**Effectiveness of therapy can be demonstrated by:** ■ Management of the symptoms of CMV retinitis in patients with AIDS.

# VALPROATES

### divalproex sodium

(dye-val-**proe**-ex **soe**-dee-um)
Depakote, Depakote ER, {Epival}

### valproate sodium

(val-**proe**-ate **soe**-dee-um)
Depacon

### valproic acid

(val-**proe**-ik **as**-id)
Depakene

### CLASSIFICATION(S):

*Therapeutic: anticonvulsants, vascular headache suppressants*

**Pregnancy Category D**

## INDICATIONS

■ Simple and complex absence seizures ■ Partial seizures with complex symptomatology ■ **Divalproex only:** ◻ Manic episodes associated with bipolar disorder (delayed-release only) ◻ Prevention of migraine headache (delayed and extended release). **Unlabeled uses:** ■ IV: Treatment of migraine headache.

## ACTION

■ Increase levels of GABA, an inhibitory neurotransmitter in the CNS. **Therapeutic Effects:** ■ Suppression of absence seizures ■ Decreased manic behavior ■ Decreased frequency of migraine headaches.

## PHARMACOKINETICS

**Absorption:** Well absorbed following oral administration; divalproex is enteric-coated, and absorption is delayed. ER form produces lower blood levels. IV administration results in complete bioavailability.

**Distribution:** Rapidly distributed into plasma and extracellular water. Cross blood-brain barrier and placenta; enter breast milk.

**Protein Binding:** 90–95%.

**Metabolism and Excretion:** Mostly metabolized by the liver; minimal amounts excreted unchanged in urine.

**Half-life:** 5–20 hr.

## CONTRAINDICATIONS AND PRECAUTIONS

**Contraindicated in:** ■ Hypersensitivity ■ Hepatic impairment ■ Some products contain tartrazine; avoid in patients with known hypersensitivity ■ Known/suspected urea cycle disorders (may result in fatal hyperammonemic encephalopathy).

**Use Cautiously in:** ■ Bleeding disorders ■ History of liver disease ■ Organic brain disease ■ Bone marrow depression ■ Renal impairment ■ Children (increased risk of hepatotoxicity) ■

Pregnancy and lactation (safety not established).

## ADVERSE REACTIONS AND SIDE EFFECTS*

■ **CNS:** confusion, dizziness, headache, sedation ■ **EENT:** visual disturbances ■ **GI:** HEPATOTOXICITY, indigestion, nausea, vomiting, anorexia, constipation, diarrhea, hypersalivation, increased appetite, pancreatitis ■ **Derm:** rashes ■ **Hemat:** leukopenia, prolonged bleeding time, thrombocytopenia ■ **Metab:** hyperammonemia ■ **Neuro:** ataxia, paresthesia.

## INTERACTIONS

**Drug-Drug:** ■ ↑ risk of bleeding with **antiplatelet agents** (including **aspirin, NSAIDs, tirofiban, eptifibatide,** and **abciximab**), **cefoperazone, ccfotctan, heparins** and **thrombolytic agents,** or **warfarin** ■ ↓ metabolism of **barbiturates** and **primidone,** ↑ risk of toxicity ■ Blood levels and toxicity may be ↑ by **carbamazepine, cimetidine, erythromycin,** or **felbamate** ■ ↑ CNS depression with other **CNS depressants,** including **alcohol, antihistamines, antidepressants, opioid analgesics, MAO inhibitors,** and **sedative/hypnotics** ■ ↑ doses of **salicylates** (in children) increase the effects of valproic acid ■ May ↑ or ↓ effects and toxicity of **phenytoin** ■ **MAO inhibitors** and other **antidepressants** may ↓ seizure threshold and ↓ effectiveness of valproates ■ **Carbamazepine, rifampin,** or **lamotrigine** may ↓ valproic acid blood levels ■ Valproic acid may ↑ toxicity of **carbamazepine, ethosuximide, lamotrigine,** or **zidovudine.**

## ROUTE AND DOSAGE

Doses expressed in mg of valproic acid.

❑ **Anticonvulsant**

■ **PO (Adults and children >10 yr):** *Single-agent therapy*—Initial dose of 5–15 mg/kg/ day; increase by 5–10 mg/kg/day weekly until therapeutic levels are reached (not to exceed 60 mg/kg/day); when daily dosage exceeds 250 mg, give in 2 divided doses. *Polytherapy*—Initial dose of 10–30 mg/kg/day; increase by 5–10 mg/kg/day weekly until therapeutic levels are reached (not to exceed

60 mg/kg/day); when daily dosage exceeds 250 mg, give in 2 divided doses.

■ **PO (Children):** *Single-agent therapy*—Initial dose of 15–45 mg/kg/day; increase by 5–10 mg/kg/day weekly until therapeutic levels are reached. *Polytherapy*—Initial dose of 30–100 mg/kg/day.

■ **IV (Adults and Children):** Give same daily dose as was given orally; if daily dose >250 mg, give in divided doses q 6 hr. In patients with no detectable levels, may be given as a one-time infusion of 1000 mg.

❑ **Antimanic**

■ **PO (Adults):** *Divalproex*—750 mg/day in divided doses initially, titrated rapidly to desired clinical effect or trough plasma levels of 50–125 mcg/ml (not to exceed 60 mg/kg/ day).

❑ **Migraine Prevention**

■ **PO (Adults):** *Divalproex*—250 mg twice daily (up to 1000 mg/day) as delayed-release tablets (Depakote) *or* 500 mg once daily initially as extended-release tablets (Depakote ER), increased after one week to 1000 mg once daily.

## AVAILABILITY

❑ **Valproic Acid**

■ *Capsules:* 250 mg$^{Rx}$, {500 mg$^{Rx}$} ■ *Syrup:* 250 mg/5 ml$^{Rx}$.

❑ **Valproate Sodium**

■ *Injection:* 100 mg/ml in 5-ml vials$^{Rx}$.

❑ **Divalproex Sodium**

■ *Delayed-release tablets (Depakote):* 125 mg$^{Rx}$, 250 mg$^{Rx}$, 500 mg$^{Rx}$ ■ Cost: 125 mg $50.15/100, 250 mg $98.48/100, 500 mg $181.63/100 ■ *Capsules-sprinkle:* 125 mg$^{Rx}$ ■ *Extended-release tablets (Depakote ER):* 250 mg$^{Rx}$, 500 mg$^{Rx}$.

TIME/ACTION PROFILE (onset = anticonvulsant effect; peak = blood levels)

| | ONSET | PEAK | DURATION |
|---|---|---|---|
| PO—liquid | 2–4 days | 15–120 min | 6–24 hr |
| PO—capsules | 2–4 days | 1–4 hr | 6–24 hr |

| PO—delayed-release products | 2–4 days | 3–5 hr | 12–24 hr |
| PO—extended-release products | 2–4 days | 7–14 hr | 24 hr |
| IV | 2–4 days | end of infusion | 6–24 hr |

## NURSING IMPLICATIONS

### ASSESSMENT

- **Seizures:** Assess location, duration, and characteristics of seizure activity. Institute seizure precautions.
- **Bipolar Disorder:** Assess mood, ideation, and behavior frequently.
- **Migraine Prophylaxis:** Monitor frequency of migraine headaches.
- **Lab Test Considerations:** Monitor CBC, platelet count, and bleeding time prior to and periodically during therapy. May cause leukopenia and thrombocytopenia.
- ❏ Monitor hepatic function (LDH, AST, ALT, and bilirubin) and serum ammonia concentrations prior to and periodically during therapy. May cause hepatotoxicity; monitor closely, especially during initial 6 mo of therapy; fatalities have occurred. Therapy should be discontinued if hyperammonemia occurs.
- ❏ May interfere with accuracy of thyroid function tests and decrease response to metyrapone tests.
- ❏ May cause false-positive results in urine ketone tests.
- **Toxicity and Overdose:** Therapeutic serum levels range from 50–100 mcg/ml. Doses are gradually ↑ until a predose serum concentration of at least 50 mcg/ml is reached. However, a good correlation among daily dose, serum level, and therapeutic effects has not been established. Patients receiving near the maximum recommended 60 mg/kg/day should be monitored for toxicity.

### POTENTIAL NURSING DIAGNOSES

- Injury, risk for (Indications).

### IMPLEMENTATION

- **General:** Do not confuse Depakote ER and regular dose forms; available in same strengths. Depakote ER produces lower blood levels than Depakote dosing forms. If switching from Depakote to Depakote ER, increase dose by 8-20%.
- ❏ Single daily doses are usually administered at bedtime because of sedation.
- **PO:** Administer with or immediately after meals to minimize GI irritation. Tell patient to swallow extended-release and delayed-release tablets whole, not to break or chew them, because this will cause irritation of the mouth or throat. Do not administer tablets with milk, to prevent premature dissolution. Delayed-release divalproex sodium may cause less GI irritation than valproic acid capsules.
- ❏ Shake liquid preparations well before pouring. Use calibrated measuring device to ensure accurate dosage. Syrup may be mixed with food or other liquids to improve taste.
- ❏ Sprinkle capsules may be swallowed whole or opened and entire capsule contents sprinkled on a teaspoonful of soft, cool food (applesauce, pudding). Tell patient to swallow drug/food mixture immediately, not to chew it. Do not store for future use.
- ❏ To convert from valproic acid to divalproex sodium, initiate divalproex sodium at same total daily dose and dosing schedule as valproic acid. Once patient is stabilized on divalproex sodium, attempt administration 2–3 times daily.
- **Intermittent Infusion:** May be diluted in D5W, 0.9% NaCl, or LR. Solution is stable for 24 hr at room temperature.
- **Rate:** Infuse over 60 min (≤20 mg/min). Rapid infusion may cause increased side effects. Has been given as a one-time infusion of 1000 mg over 5-10 min @ 3 mg/kg/min up to 15 mg/kg in patients with no detectable levels.

### PATIENT/FAMILY TEACHING

- ❏ Instruct patient to take medication as directed. If a dose is missed on a once-a-day schedule, take as soon as remembered that day. If on a multiple-dose schedule, take it within 6 hr of the scheduled time, then space remaining doses throughout the remainder of the day. Abrupt withdrawal may lead to status epilepticus.
- ❏ May cause drowsiness or dizziness. Caution patient to avoid driving or other activities requiring alertness until effects of medication are known. Tell patient not to resume driving

until physician gives clearance based on control of seizure disorder.

❑ Caution patient to avoid taking alcohol, CNS depressants, OTC medications, or herbal products concurrently with valproates without consulting health care professional.

❑ Instruct patient to notify health care professional of medication regimen prior to treatment or surgery.

❑ Advise patient to carry identification at all times describing medication regimen.

❑ Advise patient to notify health care professional if anorexia, abdominal pain, severe nausea and vomiting, yellow skin or eyes, fever, sore throat, malaise, weakness, facial edema, lethargy, unusual bleeding or bruising, pregnancy, or loss of seizure control occurs. Children <2 yr of age are especially at risk for fatal hepatotoxicity.

❑ Emphasize the importance of routine exams to monitor progress.

## EVALUATION

**Effectiveness of therapy can be demonstrated by:** ■ Decrease in or cessation of seizures without excessive sedation ■ Decreased incidence of mood swings in patients with bipolar disorders ■ Decreased frequency of migraine headaches.

---

## valsartan, See ANGIOTENSIN II RECEPTOR ANTAGONISTS.

---

# vancomycin

(van-koe-**mye**-sin)

Lyphocin, Vancocin, Vancoled

*CLASSIFICATION(S):*

*Therapeutic: anti-infectives*

**Pregnancy Category C**

## INDICATIONS

■ **IV:** Treatment of potentially life-threatening infections when less toxic anti-infectives are contraindicated. Particularly useful in staphylococcal infections, including: ❑ Endocarditis ❑ Osteomyelitis ❑ Pneumonia ❑ Septicemia ❑ Soft-tissue infections in patients who have allergies to penicillin or its derivatives or when sensitivity testing demonstrates resistance to methicillin ■ **PO:** Treatment of pseudomembranous colitis due to *Clostridium difficile* ■ **IV:** Part of endocarditis prophylaxis in high-risk patients who are allergic to penicillin.

## ACTION

■ Binds to bacterial cell wall, resulting in cell death. **Therapeutic Effects:** ■ Bactericidal action against susceptible organisms. **Spectrum:** ■ Active against gram-positive pathogens, including: ❑ Staphylococci (including methicillin-resistant strains of *Staphylococcus aureus*) ❑ Group A beta-hemolytic streptococci ❑ *Streptococcus pneumoniae* ❑ *Corynebacterium* ❑ *Clostridium* ❑ *Enterococcus faecalis* ❑ *Enterococcus faecium.*

## PHARMACOKINETICS

**Absorption:** Poorly absorbed from the GI tract.

**Distribution:** Widely distributed. Some penetration (20–30%) of CSF; crosses placenta.

**Metabolism and Excretion:** Oral doses excreted primarily in the feces; IV vancomycin eliminated almost entirely by the kidneys.

**Half-life:** 6 hr (increased in renal impairment).

## CONTRAINDICATIONS AND PRECAUTIONS

**Contraindicated in:** ■ Hypersensitivity.

**Use Cautiously in:** ■ Renal impairment (dosage reduction required if CCr ≤80 ml/min) ■ Hearing impairment ■ Intestinal obstruction or inflammation (increased systemic absorption when given orally) ■ Pregnancy and lactation (safety not established).

## ADVERSE REACTIONS AND SIDE EFFECTS*

■ **EENT:** ototoxicity ■ **CV:** hypotension ■ **GI:** nausea, vomiting ■ **GU:** nephrotoxicity ■ **Derm:** rashes ■ **Hemat:** eosinophilia, leukopenia ■ **Local:** phlebitis ■ **MS:** back and neck pain ■ **Misc:** hypersensitivity reactions including ANAPHYLAXIS, chills, fever, "red man" syndrome, superinfection.

## INTERACTIONS

**Drug-Drug:** ■ May cause additive ototoxicity and nephrotoxicity with other **ototoxic** and **nephrotoxic drugs** (**aspirin, aminoglycosides, cyclosporine, cisplatin, loop diuretics**) ■ May enhance neuromuscular blockade from **nondepolarizing neuromuscular blocking agents** ■ Increased risk of histamine flush when used with **general anesthetics** in children.

## ROUTE AND DOSAGE

❏ **Serious Systemic Infections**

■ **IV (Adults):** 500 mg (7.5 mg/kg) q 6 hr *or* 1 g (15 mg/kg) q 12 hr (up to 3–4 g/day).

■ **IV (Children >1 mo):** 10 mg/kg q 6 hr *or* 20 mg/kg q 12 hr.

■ **IV (Neonates 1 wk–1 mo):** 15 mg/kg initially, then 10 mg/kg q 8 hr.

■ **IV (Neonates <1 wk):** 15 mg/kg initially, then 10 mg/kg q 12 hr.

❏ **Endocarditis Prophylaxis in Penicillin-Allergic Patients**

■ **IV (Adults and Adolescents):** 1-g single dose 1-hr preprocedure.

■ **IV (Children):** 20-mg/kg single dose 1-hr preprocedure.

❏ **Pseudomembranous Colitis**

■ **PO (Adults):** 125–500 mg q 6 hr.

■ **PO (Children):** 10 mg/kg q 6 hr (up to 125 mg/dose; not to exceed 2 g/day).

❏ **Renal Impairment**

■ **IV (Adults):** An initial loading dose of 750 mg–1 g (not less than 15 mg/kg); serum level monitoring is optimal for choosing maintenance dosage in patients with renal impairment; these guidelines may be helpful. *CCr 50–80 ml/min*—1 g q 1–3 days; *CCr 10–50 ml/min*—1 g q 3–7 days; *CCr <10 ml/min*—1 g q 7–14 days.

## AVAILABILITY (generic available)

■ *Capsules:* 125 mg$^{Rx}$, 250 mg$^{Rx}$ ■ *Oral solution:* 250 mg/5 ml$^{Rx}$, 500 mg/6 ml$^{Rx}$ ■ *Injection:* 500-mg, 1-, 5-, 10-g vials$^{Rx}$.

TIME/ACTION PROFILE (blood levels)

| | ONSET | PEAK | DURATION |
|---|---|---|---|
| IV | rapid | end of infusion | 12–24 hr |

## NURSING IMPLICATIONS

### ASSESSMENT

❏ Assess patient for infection (vital signs; appearance of wound, sputum, urine, and stool; WBC) at beginning of and throughout therapy.

❏ Obtain specimens for culture and sensitivity prior to initiating therapy. First dose may be given before receiving results.

❏ Monitor IV site closely. Vancomycin is irritating to tissues and causes necrosis and severe pain with extravasation. Rotate infusion site.

❏ Monitor blood pressure throughout IV infusion.

❏ Evaluate eighth cranial nerve function by audiometry and serum vancomycin levels prior to and throughout therapy in patients with borderline renal function or those >60 yr of age. Prompt recognition and intervention are essential in preventing permanent damage.

❏ Monitor intake and output ratios and daily weight. Cloudy or pink urine may be a sign of nephrotoxicity.

❏ Assess patient for signs of superinfection (black, furry overgrowth on tongue; vaginal itching or discharge; loose or foul-smelling stools). Report occurrence.

■ **Pseudomembranous Colitis:** Assess bowel status (bowel sounds, frequency and consistency of stools, presence of blood in stools) throughout therapy.

■ *Lab Test Considerations:* Monitor for casts, albumin, or cells in the urine or decreased specific gravity, CBC, and renal function periodically throughout course of therapy.

❏ May cause increased BUN levels.

■ *Toxicity and Overdose:* Peak serum vancomycin levels should not exceed 25 mcg/ml. Trough concentrations should not exceed 5–10 mcg/ml.

### POTENTIAL NURSING DIAGNOSES

■ Infection, risk for (Indications).

■ Sensory perception, disturbed (auditory) (Side Effects).

### IMPLEMENTATION

■ **PO:** Use calibrated measuring device for liquid preparations. IV dosage form may be diluted in 30 ml of water for oral or nasogastric tube administration. Resulting solution has bitter, unpleasant taste. Stable for 14 days if refrigerated.

■ **Intermittent Infusion:** Dilute each 500-mg vial with 10 ml of sterile water for injection. Dilute further with 100–200 ml of 0.9% NaCl, D5W, D10W, or LR. Solution is stable for 14 days after initial reconstitution if refrigerated. After further dilution, solution is stable for 96 hr if refrigerated.

■ *Rate:* Administer over at least 60 min. Do not administer rapidly or as a bolus, to minimize risk of thrombophlebitis, hypotension, and "red man (neck)" syndrome (sudden, severe hypotension; flushing and/or maculopapular rash of face, neck, chest, and upper extremities). Thrombophlebitis can be minimized by using dilute solutions of 2.5–5 mg/ml and rotating sites.

■ **Continuous Infusion:** Should be used only if intermittent infusion is not feasible.

■ *Rate:* May also be prepared with 1–2 g in sufficient volume to infuse over 24 hr.

■ **Y-Site Compatibility:** ◆ acyclovir ◆ alatrofloxacin ◆ allopurinol ◆ amifostine ◆ amiodarone ◆ atracurium ◆ cisatracurium ◆ clarithromycin ◆ cyclophosphamide ◆ diltiazem ◆ docetaxel ◆ doxorubicin liposome ◆ enalaprilat ◆ esmolol ◆ etoposide ◆ filgrastim ◆ fluconazole ◆ fludarabine ◆ gemcitabine ◆ granisetron ◆ hydromorphone ◆ insulin ◆ labetalol ◆ levofloxacin ◆ linezolid ◆ lorazepam ◆ magnesium sulfate ◆ melphalan ◆ meperidine ◆ meropenem ◆ midazolam ◆ morphine ◆ ondansetron ◆ paclitaxel ◆ pancuronium ◆ perphenazine ◆ propofol ◆ remifentanil ◆ sodium bicarbonate ◆ tacrolimus ◆ teniposide ◆ theophylline ◆ thiotepa ◆ tolazoline ◆ vecuronium ◆ vinorelbine ◆ zidovudine.

■ **Y-Site Incompatibility:** ◆ albumin ◆ albumin ◆ amphotericin B cholesteryl sulfate ◆ cefepime ◆ gatifloxacin ◆ heparin ◆ idarubicin ◆ piperacillin/tazobactam.

## PATIENT/FAMILY TEACHING

❑ Advise patients on oral vancomycin to take exactly as directed. Tell patients that missed doses should be taken as soon as remembered unless almost time for next dose; do not double dose.

❑ Instruct patient to report signs of hypersensitivity, tinnitus, vertigo, or hearing loss.

❑ Advise patient to notify health care professional if no improvement is seen in a few days.

❑ Patients with a history of rheumatic heart disease or valve replacement need to be taught importance of using antimicrobial prophylaxis prior to invasive dental or medical procedures.

## EVALUATION

**Clinical response to therapy can be evaluated by:** ■ Resolution of signs and symptoms of infection. Length of time for complete resolution depends on organism and site of infection ■ Endocarditis prophylaxis.

---

# vasopressin

(vay-soe-**press**-in)

Pitressin, {Pressyn}

### CLASSIFICATION(S):

*Therapeutic: hormones*

*Pharmacologic: antidiuretic hormones*

### Pregnancy Category C

## INDICATIONS

■ Central diabetes insipidus due to deficient antidiuretic hormone. **Unlabeled uses:** ■ Management of pulseless VF/VT unresponsive to initial shocks (ACLS guidlines).

## ACTION

■ Alters the permeability of the renal collecting ducts, allowing reabsorption of water ■ Directly stimulates musculature of GI tract ■ In high doses acts as a nonadrenergic peripheral vasoconstrictor. **Therapeutic Effects:** ■ Decreased urine output and increased urine osmolality in diabetes insipidus.

## PHARMACOKINETICS

**Absorption:** IM absorption may be unpredictable.

**Distribution:** Widely distributed throughout extracellular fluid.

**Metabolism and Excretion:** Rapidly degraded by the liver and kidneys; <5% excreted unchanged by the kidneys.

**Half-life:** 10–20 min.

## CONTRAINDICATIONS AND PRECAUTIONS

**Contraindicated in:** ■ Chronic renal failure with increased BUN ■ Hypersensitivity to beef or pork proteins.

**Use Cautiously in:** ■ Perioperative polyuria (increased sensitivity to vasopressin) ■ Comatose patients ■ Seizures ■ Migraine headaches ■ Asthma ■ Heart failure ■ Cardiovascular disease ■ Geriatric patients and children (increased sensitivity to vasopressin) ■ Renal impairment.

## ADVERSE REACTIONS AND SIDE EFFECTS*

■ **CNS:** dizziness, "pounding" sensation in head ■ **CV:** MI, angina, chest pain ■ **GI:** abdominal cramps, belching, diarrhea, flatulence, heartburn, nausea, vomiting ■ **Derm:** paleness, perioral blanching, sweating ■ **Neuro:** trembling ■ **Misc:** allergic reactions, fever, water intoxication (higher doses).

## INTERACTIONS

**Drug-Drug:** ■ Antidiuretic effect may be decreased by concurrent administration of **alcohol, lithium, demeclocycline, heparin,** or **norepinephrine** ■ Antidiuretic effect may be increased by concurrent administration of **carbamazepine, chlorpropamide, clofibrate, tricyclic antidepressants,** or **fludrocortisone** ■ Vasopressor effect may be increased by concurrent administration of **ganglionic blocking agents.**

## ROUTE AND DOSAGE

■ **IM, Subcut (Adults):** 5–10 units 2–4 times daily.

■ **IM, Subcut (Children):** 2.5–10 units 2–4 times daily.

■ **IV (Adults):** *Pulseless VF/VT (ACLS guidelines)* 40 units as a single dose (unlabeled).

## AVAILABILITY (generic available)

■ *Injection:* 20 units/ml in 0.5- and 1-ml ampules and vials[Rx].

### TIME/ACTION PROFILE (antidiuretic effect)

| | ONSET | PEAK | DURATION |
|---|---|---|---|
| IM, subcut | unknown | unknown | 2–8 hr |

## NURSING IMPLICATIONS

### ASSESSMENT

■ **General Info:** Monitor ECG periodically throughout therapy and continuously throughout cardiopulmonary resuscitation.

■ **Diabetes Insipidus:** Monitor urine osmolality and urine volume frequently to determine effects of medication. Assess patient for symptoms of dehydration (excessive thirst, dry skin and mucous membranes, tachycardia, poor skin turgor). Weigh patient daily, monitor intake and output, and assess for edema.

■ *Lab Test Considerations:* Monitor urine specific gravity throughout course of therapy.

❑ Monitor serum electrolyte concentrations periodically throughout therapy.

■ *Toxicity and Overdose:* Signs and symptoms of water intoxication include confusion, drowsiness, headache, weight gain, difficulty urinating, seizures, and coma.

❑ Treatment of overdose includes water restriction and temporary discontinuation of vasopressin until polyuria occurs. If symptoms are severe, administration of mannitol, hypertonic dextrose, urea, and/or furosemide may be used.

### POTENTIAL NURSING DIAGNOSES

■ Fluid volume, deficit (Indications).

■ Fluid volume, excess (Adverse Reactions).

### IMPLEMENTATION

■ **General:** Do not confuse Pitressin (vasopressin) with Pitocin (oxytocin).

❑ Aqueous vasopressin injection may be administered subcut or IM for diabetes insipidus.

❑ Administer 1–2 glasses of water at the time of administration to minimize side effects (blanching of skin, abdominal cramps, nausea).

■ **Direct IV:** Administer as a single IV push dose during cardiac arrest.

## PATIENT/FAMILY TEACHING

❑ Instruct patient to take medication exactly as directed. Caution patient not to use more than prescribed amount. Take missed doses as soon as remembered, unless almost time for next dose.

❑ Advise patient to drink 1–2 glasses of water at time of administration to minimize side effects (blanching of skin, abdominal cramps, nausea). Inform patient that these side effects are not serious and usually disappear in a few minutes.

❑ Caution patient to avoid concurrent use of alcohol while taking vasopressin.

❑ Patients with diabetes insipidus should carry identification at all times describing disease process and medication regimen.

## EVALUATION

**Effectiveness of therapy can be demonstrated by:** ■ Decrease in urine volume ❑ Relief of polydipsia ❑ Increased urine osmolality in patients with central diabetes insipidus.

---

## venlafaxine

(ven-la-**fax**-een)

Effexor, Effexor XR

### CLASSIFICATION(S):

**Therapeutic:** antidepressants, anti-anxiety agents

**Pregnancy Category C**

## INDICATIONS

■ Major depressive illness or relapse, often in conjunction with psychotherapy ■ Generalized anxiety disorder (Effexor XR only) ■ Social anxiety disorder (Effexor XR only). **Unlabeled uses:** ■ Premenstrual dysphoric disorder (PMDD).

## ACTION

■ Inhibits serotonin and norepinephrine reuptake in the CNS. **Therapeutic Effects:** ■ Decrease in depressive symptomatology, with fewer relapses/recurrences ■ Decreased anxiety.

## PHARMACOKINETICS

**Absorption:** 92–100% absorbed after oral administration.

**Distribution:** Extensive distribution into body tissues.

**Metabolism and Excretion:** Extensively metabolized on 1st pass through the liver. One metabolite, O-desmethylvenlafaxine (ODV), has antidepressant activity; 5% of venlafaxine is excreted unchanged in urine; 30% of the active metabolite is excreted in urine.

**Half-life:** *Venlafaxine*—3–5 hr; *ODV*—9–11 hr (both are increased in hepatic/renal impairment).

## CONTRAINDICATIONS AND PRECAUTIONS

**Contraindicated in:** ■ Hypersensitivity ■ Concurrent MAO inhibitor therapy.

**Use Cautiously in:** ■ Cardiovascular disease, including hypertension ■ Hepatic impairment (↓ dose recommended) ■ Impaired renal function (↓ dose recommended) ■ History of seizures or neurologic impairment ■ History of mania ■ History of drug abuse ■ Pregnancy, lactation, or children <18 yr (use only if clearly required during pregnancy; safety not established).

## ADVERSE REACTIONS AND SIDE EFFECTS*

■ **CNS:** SEIZURES, abnormal dreams, anxiety, dizziness, headache, insomnia, nervousness, weakness, abnormal thinking, agitation, confusion, depersonalization, drowsiness, emotional lability, worsening depression ■ **EENT:** rhinitis, visual disturbances, tinnitus ■ **CV:** chest pain, hypertension, palpitations, tachycardia ■ **GI:** abdominal pain, altered taste, anorexia, constipation, diarrhea, dry mouth, dyspepsia, nausea, vomiting, weight loss ■ **GU:** sexual dysfunction, urinary frequency, urinary retention ■ **Derm:** ecchymoses, itching, photosensitivity, skin rash ■ **Neuro:** paresthesia, twitching ■ **Misc:** chills, yawning.

## INTERACTIONS

**Drug-Drug:** ■ Concurrent use with **MAO inhibitors** may result in serious, potentially fatal reactions (wait at least 2 wk after stopping MAO inhibitor before initiating venlafaxine; wait at least 1 wk after stopping venlafaxine before starting MAO inhibitors) ■ Concurrent use with **alcohol** or other **CNS depressants,** including **sedative/hypnotics, antihistamines,** and **opioid analgesics,** in depressed patients is not recommended ■ ↑ risk of serotonin syndrome with **trazodone sibutramine** and **sumatriptan** ■ **Lithium** may have ↑ serotonergic effects with venlafaxine; use cautiously in patients receiving venlafaxine ■ ↑ blood levels and may ↑ effects of **desipramine** and **haloperidol** ■ **Cimetidine** may ↑ the effects of venlafaxine (may be more pronounced in geriatric patients, those with hepatic or renal impairment, or those with pre-existing hypertension).

**Drug-Natural Products:** ■ Concomitant use of **kava, valerian, skullcap, chamomile,** or **hops** can ↑ CNS depression ■ ↑ risk of serotinergic side effects including serotonin syndrome with **St. John's wort** and **SAMe.**

## ROUTE AND DOSAGE

■ **PO (Adults):** *Tablets*—75 mg/day in 2–3 divided doses; may increase by up to 75 mg/day every 4 days, up to 225 mg/day (not to exceed 375 mg/day in 3 divided doses); *Extended-release (XR) capsules*—75 mg once daily (some patients may be started at 37.5 mg once daily) for 4–7 days; doses may then be increased at intervals of not less than 4 days up to 225 mg/day.

❏ **Hepatic Impairment**
■ **PO (Adults):** Decrease daily dose by 50% in patients with moderate hepatic impairment.

❏ **Renal Impairment**
■ **PO (Adults):** *Mild to moderate renal impairment*—Daily dose should be decreased by 25–50%.

## AVAILABILITY

■ *Tablets:* 25 mg$^{Rx}$, 37.5 mg$^{Rx}$, 50 mg$^{Rx}$, 75 mg$^{Rx}$, 100 mg$^{Rx}$ ■ Cost: 25 mg $137.88/100, 37.5 mg $142.00/100, 50 mg $146.22/100, 75 mg $155.05/100, 100 mg $164.32/100 ■ *Extended-release capsules:* 37.5 mg$^{Rx}$, 75 mg$^{Rx}$, 150 mg$^{Rx}$ ■ Cost: 37.5 mg $233.56/100, 75 mg $261.63/100, 150 mg $285.00/100.

TIME/ACTION PROFILE (antidepressant action)

| | ONSET | PEAK | DURATION |
|---|---|---|---|
| PO | within 2 wk | 2–4 wk | unknown |

## NURSING IMPLICATIONS

### ASSESSMENT

❏ Assess mental status and mood changes. Inform physician or other health care professional if patient demonstrates significant increase in anxiety, nervousness, or insomnia.

❏ Assess suicidal tendencies, especially in early therapy. Restrict amount of drug available to patient.

❏ Monitor blood pressure before and periodically during therapy. Sustained hypertension may be dose related; decrease dose or discontinue therapy if this occurs.

❏ Monitor appetite and nutritional intake. Weigh weekly. Report continued weight loss. Adjust diet as tolerated to support nutritional status.

■ *Lab Test Considerations:* Monitor CBC with differential and platelet count periodically during therapy. May cause anemia, leukocytosis, leukopenia, thrombocytopenia, basophilia, and eosinophilia.

❏ May cause an ↑ in serum alkaline phosphatase, bilirubin, AST, ALT, BUN, and creatinine.

❏ May also cause ↑ serum cholesterol.

❏ May cause electrolyte abnormalities (hyperglycemia or hypoglycemia, hyperkalemia or hypokalemia, hyperuricemia, hyperphosphatemia or hypophosphatemia, and hyponatremia).

### POTENTIAL NURSING DIAGNOSES

■ Coping, ineffective (Indications).
■ Injury, risk for (Side Effects).

### IMPLEMENTATION

■ **PO:** Administer venlafaxine with food.
❏ Extended-release capsules should be swallowed whole; do not crush, break, or chew.
❏ Extended-release capsules may also be opened and contents sprinkled on a spoonful of applesauce. Take immediately and follow with a glass of water. Do not store mixture for later use.

### PATIENT/FAMILY TEACHING

❏ Instruct patient to take medication exactly as directed at the same time each day. Take missed doses as soon as possible unless almost time for next dose. Do not double doses or discontinue abruptly. Patients taking

venlafaxine for >6 wk should have dose gradually decreased before discontinuation.
- ❑ May cause drowsiness or dizziness. Caution patient to avoid driving or other activities requiring alertness until response to the drug is known.
- ❑ Caution patient to avoid taking alcohol or other CNS-depressant drugs during therapy and not to take other Rx, OTC, or herbal products without consulting health care professional.
- ❑ Instruct female patients to inform health care professional if pregnancy is planned or suspected or if breastfeeding.
- ❑ Instruct patient to notify health care professional if signs of allergy (rash, hives) occur.
- ❑ Emphasize the importance of follow-up exams to monitor progress. Encourage patient participation in psychotherapy.

## EVALUATION

**Effectiveness of therapy can be demonstrated by:** ■ Increased sense of well-being ❑ Renewed interest in surroundings. Need for therapy should be periodically reassessed. Therapy is usually continued for several months ■ Decreased anxiety.

# verapamil
(ver-**ap**-a-mil)
Apo-Verap, Calan, Calan SR, Covera-HS, Isoptin, Isoptin SR, {Novo-Veramil}, {Nu-Verap}, Verelan, Verelan PM

## CLASSIFICATION(S):
**Therapeutic:** *antianginals, antiarrhythmics (class IV), antihypertensives, vascular headache suppressants*
**Pharmacologic:** *calcium channel blockers*

## Pregnancy Category C

## INDICATIONS

■ Management of hypertension, angina pectoris, and/or vasospastic (Prinzmetal's) angina ■ Management of supraventricular arrhythmias and rapid ventricular rates in atrial flutter or fibrillation. **Unlabeled uses:** ■ Prevention of migraine headache ■ Management of cardiomyopathy.

## ACTION

■ Inhibits the transport of calcium into myocardial and vascular smooth muscle cells, resulting in inhibition of excitation-contraction coupling and subsequent contraction ■ Decreases SA and AV conduction and prolongs AV node refractory period in conduction tissue. **Therapeutic Effects:** ■ Systemic vasodilation resulting in decreased blood pressure ■ Coronary vasodilation resulting in decreased frequency and severity of attacks of angina ■ Suppression of ventricular tachyarrhythmias.

## PHARMACOKINETICS

**Absorption:** 90% absorbed after oral administration, but much is rapidly metabolized, resulting in bioavailability of 20–25%.

**Distribution:** Small amounts enter breast milk.

**Protein Binding:** 90%.

**Metabolism and Excretion:** Mostly metabolized by the liver.

**Half-life:** 4.5–12 hr.

## CONTRAINDICATIONS AND PRECAUTIONS

**Contraindicated in:** ■ Hypersensitivity ■ Sick sinus syndrome ■ 2nd- or 3rd-degree AV block (unless an artificial pacemaker is in place) ■ BP <90 mmHg ■ CHF, severe ventricular dysfunction, or cardiogenic shock, unless associated with supraventricular tachyarrhythmias ■ Concurrent IV beta blocker therapy.

**Use Cautiously in:** ■ Severe hepatic impairment (dosage reduction recommended for most agents) ■ Geriatric patients (dosage reduction/slower IV infusion rates recommended for most agents; increased risk of hypotension) ■ History of serious ventricular arrhythmias or CHF ■ Pregnancy or lactation (safety not established; verapamil is approved for use in children).

## ADVERSE REACTIONS AND SIDE EFFECTS*

■ **CNS:** abnormal dreams, anxiety, confusion, dizziness/lightheadedness, drowsiness, headache, jitteriness, nervousness, psychiatric disturbances, weakness ■ **EENT:** blurred vision, disturbed equilibrium, epistaxis, tinnitus ■ **Resp:** cough, dyspnea, shortness of breath ■ **CV:** ARRHYTHMIAS, CHF, bradycardia, chest pain, hypotension, palpitations, peripheral edema, syncope, tachycardia ■ **GI:** abnormal liver function studies, anorexia, constipation, diarrhea, dry mouth, dysgeusia, dyspepsia, nausea, vomiting ■ **GU:** dysuria, nocturia, polyuria, sexual dysfunction, urinary frequency ■ **Derm:** dermatitis, erythema multiforme, flushing, increased sweating, photosensitivity, pruritus/urticaria, rash ■ **Endo:** gynecomastia, hyperglycemia ■ **Hemat:** anemia, leukopenia, thrombocytopenia ■ **Metab:** weight gain ■ **MS:** joint stiffness, muscle cramps ■ **Neuro:** paresthesia, tremor ■ **Misc:** STEVENS-JOHNSON SYNDROME, gingival hyperplasia.

## INTERACTIONS

**Drug-Drug:** ■ Additive hypotension may occur when used concurrently with **fentanyl,** other **antihypertensives, nitrates,** acute ingestion of **alcohol,** or **quinidine** ■ Antihypertensive effects may be decreased by concurrent use of **NSAIDs** ■ Serum **digoxin** levels may be increased ■ Concurrent use with **beta blockers, digoxin, disopyramide,** or **phenytoin** may result in bradycardia, conduction defects, or CHF ■ May decrease the metabolism of and increase the risk of toxicity from **cyclosporine, prazosin, quinidine,** or **carbamazepine** ■ May decrease the effectiveness of **rifampin** ■ Increases the muscle-paralyzing effects of **nondepolarizing neuromuscular-blocking agents** ■ Effectiveness may be decreased by coadministration with **vitamin D compounds** and **calcium** ■ May alter serum **lithium** levels.

**Drug-Natural Products:** ■ Increased **caffeine** levels with caffeine-containing herbs (**cola nut, guarana, mate, tea, coffee**).

**Drug-Food:** ■ **Grapefruit juice** increases serum levels and effect.

## ROUTE AND DOSAGE

■ **PO (Adults):** 80–120 mg 3 times daily, increased as needed. *Patients with poor ventricular function, hepatic impairment, or geriatric patients*—40 mg 3 times daily initially. *Extended-release preparations*—120–240 mg/day as a single dose; may be increased as needed (range 240–480 mg/day).

■ **PO (Children up to 15 yr):** 4–8 mg/kg/day in divided doses.

■ **IV (Adults):** 5–10 mg (75–150 mcg/kg); may repeat with 10 mg (150 mcg/kg) after 15–30 min.

■ **IV (Children 1–15 yr):** 2–5 mg (100–300 mcg/kg); may repeat after 30 min (initial dose not to exceed 5 mg; repeat dose not to exceed 10 mg).

■ **IV (Children <1 yr):** 0.75–2 mg (100–200 mcg/kg); may repeat after 30 min.

## AVAILABILITY (generic available)

■ *Tablets:* 40 mg<sup>Rx</sup>, 80 mg<sup>Rx</sup>, 120 mg<sup>Rx</sup> ■ *Extended-release tablets:* 120 mg<sup>Rx</sup>, 180 mg<sup>Rx</sup>, 240 mg<sup>Rx</sup> ■ *Extended-release capsules:* 100 mg<sup>Rx</sup>, 200 mg<sup>Rx</sup>, 240 mg<sup>Rx</sup>, 300 mg<sup>Rx</sup> ■ Cost: *Verelan*—120 mg $134.25/100, 180 mg $145.24/100, 240 mg $199.10/100, 360 mg $218.41/100 ■ *Injection:* 2.5 mg/m<sup>Rx</sup> in 2- and 4-ml vials, ampules, and syringes ■ trandolapril (Tarka<sup>Rx</sup>); see Appendix B.

TIME/ACTION PROFILE (cardiovascular effects)

|        | ONSET     | PEAK         | DURATION |
|--------|-----------|--------------|----------|
| PO     | 1–2 hr    | 30–90 min†   | 3–7 hr   |
| PO-ER  | unknown   | 5–7 hr       | 24 hr    |
| IV     | 1–5 min‡  | 3–5 min      | 2 hr‡    |

†Single dose; effects from multiple doses may not be evident for 24–48 hr.

‡Antiarrhythmic effects; hemodynamic effects begin 3–5 min after injection and persist for 10–20 min.

# NURSING IMPLICATIONS

## ASSESSMENT

■ **General Info:** Monitor blood pressure and pulse before therapy, during dosage titration, and periodically throughout therapy. Monitor ECG periodically during prolonged therapy. Verapamil may cause prolonged PR interval.

❑ Monitor intake and output ratios and daily weight. Assess for signs of CHF (peripheral edema, rales/crackles, dyspnea, weight gain, jugular venous distention).

❑ Patients receiving digoxin concurrently with calcium channel blockers should have routine serum digoxin levels and be monitored for signs and symptoms of digoxin toxicity.

- **Angina:** Assess location, duration, intensity, and precipitating factors of patient's anginal pain.
- **Arrhythmias:** Monitor ECG continuously during administration. Notify physician promptly if bradycardia or prolonged hypotension occurs. Emergency equipment and medication should be available. Monitor blood pressure and pulse before and frequently during administration.
- *Lab Test Considerations:* Total serum calcium concentrations are not affected by calcium channel blockers.
- ❑ Monitor serum potassium periodically. Hypokalemia increases the risk of arrhythmias and should be corrected.
- ❑ Monitor renal and hepatic functions periodically during long-term therapy. May cause increase in hepatic enzymes after several days of therapy, which return to normal on discontinuation of therapy.

## POTENTIAL NURSING DIAGNOSES

- Cardiac output, decreased (Indications).
- Pain, acute (Indications).

## IMPLEMENTATION

- **General:** Do not confuse verapamil with Virilon (testosterone). Do not confuse Covera (verapamil) with Provera (medroxyprogesterone).
- **PO:** Administer verapamil with meals or milk to minimize gastric irritation.
- ❑ Do not open, crush, break, or chew sustained-release capsules or tablets. Empty tablets that appear in stool are not significant.
- **IV:** Patients should remain recumbent for at least 1 hr after IV administration to minimize hypotensive effects.
- **Direct IV:** Administer IV undiluted through Y-site over 2 min for each single dose. Administer over 3 min in geriatric patients.
- **Syringe Compatibility:** ◆ heparin ◆ inamrinone ◆ milrinone.
- **Y-Site Compatibility:** ◆ ciprofloxacin ◆ dobutamine ◆ dopamine ◆ famotidine ◆ gatifloxacin ◆ hydralazine ◆ inamrinone ◆ linezolid ◆

meperidine ◆ milrinone ◆ penicillin G potassium ◆ piperacillin ◆ ticarcillin.

- **Y-Site Incompatibility:** ◆ albumin ◆ amphotericin B cholesteryl sulfate ◆ ampicillin ◆ mezlocillin ◆ nafcillin ◆ oxacillin ◆ sodium bicarbonate.

## PATIENT/FAMILY TEACHING

- **General Info:** Advise patient to take medication exactly as directed, even if feeling well. If a dose is missed, take as soon as possible unless almost time for next dose; do not double doses. May need to be discontinued gradually.
- ❑ Instruct patient on correct technique for monitoring pulse. Instruct patient to contact health care professional if heart rate is <50 bpm.
- ❑ Caution patient to change positions slowly to minimize orthostatic hypotension.
- ❑ May cause drowsiness or dizziness. Advise patient to avoid driving or other activities requiring alertness until response to the medication is known.
- ❑ Instruct patient on importance of maintaining good dental hygiene and seeing dentist frequently for teeth cleaning to prevent tenderness, bleeding, and gingival hyperplasia (gum enlargement).
- ❑ Instruct patient to avoid concurrent use of alcohol or OTC medications, especially cold preparations, without consulting health care professional.
- ❑ Advise patient to notify health care professional if irregular heartbeats, dyspnea, swelling of hands and feet, pronounced dizziness, nausea, constipation, or hypotension occurs or if headache is severe or persistent.
- ❑ Caution patient to wear protective clothing and use sunscreen to prevent photosensitivity reactions.
- **Angina:** Instruct patient on concurrent nitrate or beta-blocker therapy to continue taking both medications as directed and use SL nitroglycerin as needed for anginal attacks.
- ❑ Advise patient to contact health care professional if chest pain does not improve, worsens after therapy, or occurs with diaphoresis; if shortness of breath occurs; or if severe, persistent headache occurs.

{ } = Available in Canada only.
*CAPITALS indicates life-threatening; underlines indicate most frequent.

❑ Caution patient to discuss exercise restrictions with health care professional before exertion.

■ **Hypertension:** Encourage patient to comply with other interventions for hypertension (weight reduction, low-sodium diet, smoking cessation, moderation of alcohol consumption, regular exercise, and stress management). Medication controls but does not cure hypertension.

❑ Instruct patient and family in proper technique for monitoring blood pressure. Advise patient to take blood pressure weekly and to report significant changes to health care professional.

## EVALUATION

**Effectiveness of therapy can be demonstrated by:** ■ Decrease in blood pressure ■ Decrease in frequency and severity of anginal attacks ❑ Decrease in need for nitrate therapy ❑ Increase in activity tolerance and sense of well-being ■ Suppression and prevention of atrial tachyarrhythmias.

---

**High Alert**

## vinblastine

(vin-**blass**-teen)

Velban, {Velbe}

*CLASSIFICATION(S):*

***Therapeutic:*** *antineoplastics*

***Pharmacologic:*** *vinca alkaloids*

**Pregnancy Category D**

---

## INDICATIONS

■ Combination chemotherapy of: ❑ Lymphomas ❑ Nonseminomatous testicular carcinoma ❑ Advanced breast cancer ❑ Other tumors.

## ACTION

■ Binds to proteins of mitotic spindle, causing metaphase arrest. Cell replication is stopped as a result (cell cycle–specific for M phase). **Therapeutic Effects:** ■ Death of rapidly replicating cells, particularly malignant ones ■ Has immunosuppressive properties.

## PHARMACOKINETICS

**Absorption:** Administered IV only, resulting in complete bioavailability.

**Distribution:** Does not cross the blood-brain barrier well.

**Metabolism and Excretion:** Converted by the liver to an active antineoplastic compound; excreted in the feces via biliary excretion, some renal elimination.

**Half-life:** 24 hr.

## CONTRAINDICATIONS AND PRECAUTIONS

**Contraindicated in:** ■ Hypersensitivity ■ Pregnancy or lactation.

**Use Cautiously in:** ■ Patients with childbearing potential ■ Infections ■ Decreased bone marrow reserve ■ Other chronic debilitating illnesses ■ Patients with impaired hepatic function (decrease dose by 50% if serum bilirubin >3 mg/dl).

## ADVERSE REACTIONS AND SIDE EFFECTS*

■ **CNS:** SEIZURES, mental depression, neurotoxicity, weakness ■ **Resp:** BRONCHOSPASM ■ **GI:** nausea, vomiting, anorexia, constipation, diarrhea, stomatitis ■ **GU:** gonadal suppression ■ **Derm:** alopecia, dermatitis, vesiculation ■ **Endo:** syndrome of inappropriate antidiuretic hormone (SIADH) ■ **Hemat:** anemia, leukopenia, thrombocytopenia ■ **Local:** phlebitis at IV site ■ **Metab:** hyperuricemia ■ **Neuro:** neuritis, paresthesia, peripheral neuropathy.

## INTERACTIONS

**Drug-Drug:** ■ Additive bone marrow depression with other **antineoplastics** or **radiation therapy** ■ Bronchospasm may occur in patients who have been previously treated with **mitomycin** ■ May decrease antibody response to **live-virus vaccines** and increase the risk of adverse reactions ■ May decrease serum **phenytoin** levels.

## ROUTE AND DOSAGE

Doses may vary greatly, depending on tumor, schedule, condition of patient, and blood counts.

■ **IV (Adults):** *Initial*—3.7 mg/m² (100 mcg/kg), single dose; increase weekly as tolerated by 1.8 mg/m² (50 mcg/kg) to maximum of 18.5 mg/m² (usual dose is 5.5–7.4 mg/m²). *Maintenance*—10 mg 1–2 times/mo or one increment less than last dose q 7–14 days.

■ **IV (Children):** *Initial*—2.5 mg/m², single dose; increase weekly as tolerated by 1.25

mg/m² to maximum of 7.5 mg/m². *Maintenance*—one increment less than last dose q 7 days.

## AVAILABILITY (generic available)

■ *Solution for injection:* 1 mg/ml in 10-ml vials^Rx ■ *Powder for injection:* 10 mg/vial^Rx.

TIME/ACTION PROFILE (effects on white blood cell counts)

| | ONSET | PEAK | DURATION |
|---|---|---|---|
| IV | 5–7 days | 10 days | 7–14 days |

# NURSING IMPLICATIONS

## ASSESSMENT

❑ Monitor blood pressure, pulse, and respiratory rate during course of therapy. Notify physician immediately if respiratory distress occurs. Bronchospasm can be life-threatening and may occur at time of infusion or several hours to weeks later.

❑ Monitor for bone marrow depression. Assess for bleeding (bleeding gums, bruising, petechiae, guaiac stools, urine, and emesis) and avoid IM injections and taking rectal temperatures if platelet count is low. Apply pressure to venipuncture sites for 10 min. Assess for signs of infection during neutropenia. Anemia may occur. Monitor for increased fatigue, dyspnea, and orthostatic hypotension.

❑ May cause nausea and vomiting. Monitor intake and output, appetite, and nutritional intake. Prophylactic antiemetics may be used. Adjust diet as tolerated.

❑ Assess injection site frequently for redness, irritation, or inflammation. If extravasation occurs, infusion must be stopped and restarted elsewhere to avoid damage to subcut tissue. Standard treatment includes infiltration with hyaluronidase and application of heat.

❑ Monitor for symptoms of gout (increased uric acid, joint pain, edema). Encourage patient to drink at least 2 L of fluid per day. Allopurinol or alkalinization of urine may be used to decrease uric acid levels.

■ *Lab Test Considerations:* Monitor CBC prior to and routinely throughout therapy. If

WBC <2000, subsequent doses are usually withheld until WBC is ≥4000. The nadir of leukopenia occurs in 5–10 days and recovery usually occurs 7–14 days later. Thrombocytopenia may also occur in patients who have received radiation or other chemotherapy agents.

❑ Monitor liver function studies (AST, ALT, LDH, bilirubin) and renal function studies (BUN, creatinine) prior to and periodically throughout therapy.

❑ May cause increased uric acid. Monitor periodically during therapy.

## POTENTIAL NURSING DIAGNOSES

■ Infection, risk for (Adverse Reactions).

■ Nutrition, imbalanced: less than body requirements (Adverse Reactions).

## IMPLEMENTATION

❑ *High Alert:* Fatalities have occurred with chemotherapeutic agents. Before administering, clarify all ambiguous orders; double check single, daily, and course-of-therapy dose limits; have second practitioner independently double check original order, dose calculations, and infusion pump settings. Do not administer subcut, IM, or intrathecally (IT). IT administration is fatal. Vinblastine must be dispensed in an overwrap stating, "For IV use only." Overwrap should remain in place until immediately before administration. Do not confuse vinblastine with vincristine.

■ **General:** Solution should be prepared in a biologic cabinet. Wear gloves, gown, and mask while handling medication. Discard IV equipment in specially designated containers.

❑ Do not inject into extremities with impaired circulation; may cause thrombophlebitis.

■ **Direct IV:** Dilute each 10 mg with 10 ml of 0.9% NaCl for injection with phenol or benzyl alcohol for a concentration of 1 mg/ml. Solution is clear. Reconstituted medication is stable for 28 days if refrigerated.

■ *Rate:* Administer each single dose over 1 min through Y-site injection of a free-flowing infusion of 0.9% NaCl or D5W.

■ **Intermittent Infusion:** Dilution in large volumes (100–250 ml) or prolonged infusion (≥30 min) increases chance of vein irritation and extravasation.

■ **Syringe Compatibility:** ◆ bleomycin ◆ cisplatin ◆ cyclophosphamide ◆ droperidol ◆ fluorouracil ◆ leucovorin calcium ◆ methotrexate ◆ metoclopramide ◆ mitomycin ◆ vincristine.

■ **Y-Site Compatibility:** ◆ amifostine ◆ aztreonam ◆ bleomycin ◆ cefepime ◆ cisplatin ◆ cyclophosphamide ◆ doxorubicin ◆ droperidol ◆ filgrastim ◆ fludarabine ◆ fluorouracil ◆ gatifloxacin ◆ heparin ◆ leucovorin calcium ◆ melphalan ◆ methotrexate ◆ metoclopramide ◆ mitomycin ◆ ondansetron ◆ paclitaxel ◆ piperacillin/tazobactam ◆ sargramostim ◆ teniposide ◆ thiotepa ◆ vincristine ◆ vinorelbine.

■ **Y-Site Incompatibility:** ◆ furosemide.

## PATIENT/FAMILY TEACHING

❑ Advise patient to notify health care professional if fever; chills; sore throat; signs of infection; bleeding gums; bruising; petechiae; or blood in urine, stool, or emesis occurs. Caution patient to avoid crowds and persons with known infections. Instruct patient to use soft toothbrush and electric razor. Caution patient not to drink alcoholic beverages or take products containing aspirin or NSAIDs.

❑ Instruct patient to inspect oral mucosa for redness and ulceration. Advise patient that, if ulceration occurs, to avoid spicy foods, use sponge brush, and rinse mouth with water after eating and drinking. Topical agents may be used if mouth pain interferes with eating. Stomatitis pain may require treatment with opioid analgesics.

❑ Instruct patient to report symptoms of neurotoxicity (paresthesia, pain, difficulty walking, persistent constipation).

❑ Advise patient that jaw pain, pain in organs containing tumor tissue, nausea, and vomiting may occur. Avoid constipation and report other adverse reactions.

❑ Advise patient that this medication may have teratogenic effects. Contraception should be used during and for at least 2 mo after therapy is concluded.

❑ Discuss with patient the possibility of hair loss. Explore coping strategies.

❑ Instruct patient not to receive any vaccinations without advice of health care professional.

❑ Emphasize need for periodic lab tests to monitor for side effects.

## EVALUATION

**Effectiveness of therapy can be demonstrated by:** ■ Regression of malignancy without the appearance of detrimental side effects.

**High Alert**

# vincristine

(vin-**kriss**-teen)
Oncovin, Vincasar PFS

*CLASSIFICATION(S):*
*Therapeutic:* antineoplastics
*Pharmacologic:* vinca alkaloids

**Pregnancy Category D**

## INDICATIONS

■ Used alone and in combination with other treatment modalities (antineoplastics, surgery, or radiation therapy) in treatment of: ❑ Hodgkin's disease ❑ Leukemias ❑ Neuroblastoma ❑ Malignant lymphomas ❑ Rhabdomyosarcoma ❑ Wilms' tumor ❑ Other tumors.

## ACTION

■ Binds to proteins of mitotic spindle, causing metaphase arrest ■ Cell replication is stopped as a result (cell cycle–specific for M phase) ■ Has little or no effect on bone marrow. **Therapeutic Effects:** ■ Death of rapidly replicating cells, particularly malignant ones ■ Has immunosuppressive properties.

## PHARMACOKINETICS

**Absorption:** Administered IV only, resulting in complete bioavailability.
**Distribution:** Rapidly and widely distributed; extensively bound to tissues.
**Metabolism and Excretion:** Metabolized by the liver and eliminated in the feces via biliary excretion.
**Half-life:** 10.5–37.5 hr.

## CONTRAINDICATIONS AND PRECAUTIONS

**Contraindicated in:** ■ Hypersensitivity ■ Pregnancy or lactation.
**Use Cautiously in:** ■ Patients with childbearing potential ■ Infections ■ Decreased bone

marrow reserve ■ Other chronic debilitating illnesses ■ Hepatic impairment (50% dosage reduction recommended if serum bilirubin >3 mg/dl).

## ADVERSE REACTIONS AND SIDE EFFECTS*

■ **CNS:** agitation, insomnia, mental depression, mental status changes ■ **EENT:** cortical blindness, diplopia ■ **Resp:** bronchospasm ■ **GI:** nausea, vomiting, abdominal cramps, anorexia, constipation, ileus, stomatitis ■ **GU:** gonadal suppression, nocturia, oliguria, urinary retention ■ **Derm:** alopecia ■ **Endo:** syndrome of inappropriate antidiuretic hormone (SIADH) ■ **Hemat:** anemia, leukopenia, thrombocytopenia (mild and brief) ■ **Local:** phlebitis at IV site, tissue necrosis (from extravasation) ■ **Metab:** hyperuricemia ■ **Neuro:** ascending peripheral neuropathy.

## INTERACTIONS

**Drug-Drug:** ■ Bronchospasm may occur in patients who have been previously treated with **mitomycin** ■ **L-asparaginase** may decrease hepatic metabolism of vincristine (give vincristine 12–24 hr prior to asparaginase) ■ May decrease antibody response to **live-virus vaccines** and increase the risk of adverse reactions.

## ROUTE AND DOSAGE

Many other protocols are used.

■ **IV (Adults):** 10–30 mcg/kg (0.4–1.4 mg/m²); may repeat weekly (not to exceed 2 mg/dose).

■ **IV (Children >10 kg):** 1.5–2 mg/m² single dose; may repeat weekly.

■ **IV (Children <10 kg):** 50 mcg/kg single dose; may repeat weekly.

## AVAILABILITY (generic available)

■ **Solution for injection:** 1 mg/ml in 1-, 2-, 5-ml vials^Rx ■ Cost: $43.23/1 ml, $86.46/2 ml ■ **Powder for injection:** 5 mg/vial^Rx.

TIME/ACTION PROFILE (effects on blood counts†)

| | ONSET | PEAK | DURATION |
|---|---|---|---|
| IV | unknown | 4 days | 7 days |

†Usually mild.

## NURSING IMPLICATIONS

### ASSESSMENT

❑ Monitor blood pressure, pulse, and respiratory rate during course of therapy. Report significant changes.

❑ Monitor neurologic status. Assess for paresthesia (numbness, tingling, pain), loss of deep tendon reflexes (Achilles reflex is usually first involved), weakness (wrist drop or footdrop, gait disturbances), cranial nerve palsies (jaw pain, hoarseness, ptosis, visual changes), autonomic dysfunction (ileus, difficulty voiding, orthostatic hypotension, impaired sweating), and CNS dysfunction (decreased level of consciousness, agitation, hallucinations). Notify physician if these symptoms develop, as they may persist for months.

❑ Monitor intake and output ratios and daily weight; report significant discrepancies. Decreased urine output with concurrent hyponatremia may indicate SIADH, which usually responds to fluid restriction.

❑ Assess infusion site frequently for redness, irritation, or inflammation. If extravasation occurs, infusion must be stopped and restarted elsewhere to avoid damage to subcut tissue. Cellulitis and discomfort may be minimized by infiltration with hyaluronidase and application of moderate heat or by application of cold compresses.

❑ Assess nutritional status. An antiemetic may be used to minimize nausea and vomiting.

❑ Monitor for symptoms of gout (increased uric acid, joint pain, edema). Encourage patient to drink at least 2 liters of fluid per day. Allopurinol or alkalinization of urine may be used to decrease uric acid levels.

■ **Lab Test Considerations:** Monitor CBC prior to and periodically throughout therapy. May cause slight leukopenia 4 days after therapy, which resolves within 7 days. Platelet count may increase or decrease.

❑ Monitor liver function studies (AST, ALT, LDH, bilirubin) and renal function studies (BUN, creatinine) prior to and periodically throughout therapy.

❑ May cause increased uric acid. Monitor periodically during therapy.

{ } = Available in Canada only.
*CAPITALS indicates life-threatening; underlines indicate most frequent.

## POTENTIAL NURSING DIAGNOSES

■ Injury, risk for (Adverse Reactions).

■ Nutrition, imbalanced: less than body requirements (Adverse Reactions).

## IMPLEMENTATION

❑ **High Alert:** Fatalities have occurred with chemotherapeutic agents. Before administering, clarify all ambiguous orders; double check single, daily, and course-of-therapy dose limits; have second practitioner independently double check original order, dose calculations, and infusion pump settings. Do not administer subcut, IM, or intrathecally (IT). IT administration is fatal. Vincristine must be dispensed in an overwrap stating "For IV use only." Overwrap should remain in place until immediately before administration. Do not confuse vincristine with vinblastine.

■ **General:** Solution should be prepared in a biologic cabinet. Wear gloves, gown, and mask while handling medication. Discard IV equipment in specially designated containers (see Appendix M).

■ **Direct IV:** Reconstitute by adding 5 ml of sterile water for injection to each vial for a concentration of 1 mg/ml. Administer undiluted.

■ **Rate:** Administer each dose direct IV push over 1 min through Y-site injection of a free-flowing infusion of 0.9% NaCl or D5W.

■ **Syringe Compatibility:** ◆ bleomycin ◆ cisplatin ◆ cyclophosphamide ◆ doxapram ◆ doxorubicin ◆ droperidol ◆ fluorouracil ◆ heparin ◆ leucovorin calcium ◆ methotrexate ◆ metoclopramide ◆ mitomycin ◆ vinblastine.

■ **Syringe Incompatibility:** ◆ furosemide.

■ **Y-Site Compatibility:** ◆ allopurinol ◆ amifostine ◆ aztreonam ◆ bleomycin ◆ cisplatin ◆ cyclophosphamide ◆ doxorubicin ◆ droperidol ◆ filgrastim ◆ fludarabine ◆ fluorouracil ◆ gatifloxacin ◆ granisetron ◆ heparin ◆ leucovorin calcium ◆ linezolid ◆ melphalan ◆ methotrexate ◆ metoclopramide ◆ mitomycin ◆ ondansetron ◆ paclitaxel ◆ piperacillin/tazobactam ◆ sargramostim ◆ teniposide ◆ thiotepa ◆ topotecan ◆ vinblastine ◆ vinorelbine.

■ **Y-Site Incompatibility:** ◆ cefepime ◆ furosemide ◆ idarubicin ◆ sodium bicarbonate.

## PATIENT/FAMILY TEACHING

❑ Instruct patient to notify health care professional immediately if redness, swelling, or pain at injection site occurs.

❑ Instruct patient to report symptoms of neurotoxicity (paresthesia, pain, difficulty walking, persistent constipation). Inform patient that increased fluid intake, dietary fiber, and exercise may minimize constipation. Stool softeners or laxatives may be used. Patient should inform health care professional if severe constipation or abdominal discomfort occurs, as this may be a sign of neuropathy.

❑ Advise patient to notify health care professional if fever; chills; sore throat; signs of infection; bleeding gums; bruising; petechiae; blood in urine, stool, or emesis; or mouth sores occur. Caution patient to avoid crowds and persons with known infections.

❑ Advise patient that this medication may have teratogenic effects. Contraception should be used during and for at least 2 mo after therapy is concluded.

❑ Discuss with patient the possibility of hair loss. Explore coping strategies.

❑ Instruct patient not to receive any vaccinations without advice of health care professional.

❑ Emphasize need for periodic lab tests to monitor for side effects.

## EVALUATION

**Effectiveness of therapy can be demonstrated by:** ■ Regression of malignancy without the appearance of detrimental side effects.

---

High Alert

## vinorelbine

(vine-oh-**rel**-been)

Navelbine

**CLASSIFICATION(S):**
**Therapeutic:** antineoplastics
**Pharmacologic:** vinca alkaloids

**Pregnancy Category D**

## INDICATIONS

■ Inoperable non–small-cell cancer of the lung in ambulatory patients (alone or with cisplatin).

## ACTION

- Binds to a protein (tubulin) of cellular microtubules, where it interferes with microtubule assembly. Cell replication is stopped as a result (cell cycle–specific for M phase). **Therapeutic Effects:** ■ Death of rapidly replicating cells, particularly malignant ones.

## PHARMACOKINETICS

**Absorption:** IV administration results in complete bioavailability.

**Distribution:** Highly bound to platelets and lymphocytes.

**Metabolism and Excretion:** Mostly metabolized by the liver. At least one metabolite is active. Large amounts eliminated in feces; 11% excreted unchanged by the kidneys.

**Half-life:** 28–44 hr.

## CONTRAINDICATIONS AND PRECAUTIONS

**Contraindicated in:** ■ Hypersensitivity ■ Pregnancy or lactation ■ Active infections ■ Decreased bone marrow reserve ■ Other chronic debilitating illnesses.

**Use Cautiously in:** ■ Patients with childbearing potential ■ Impaired hepatic function (dosage reduction recommended if total bilirubin >2 mg/dl) ■ Debilitated patients (increased risk of hyponatremia) ■ Granulocytopenic patients (temporarily discontinue or reduce dose) ■ Children (safe use not established).

## ADVERSE REACTIONS AND SIDE EFFECTS*

■ **CNS:** fatigue ■ **Resp:** shortness of breath ■ **CV:** chest pain ■ **GI:** constipation, nausea, abdominal pain, anorexia, diarrhea, transient increase in liver enzymes, vomiting ■ **Derm:** alopecia, rashes ■ **F and E:** hyponatremia ■ **Hemat:** anemia, neutropenia, thrombocytopenia ■ **Local:** irritation at IV site, skin reactions, phlebitis ■ **MS:** arthralgia, back pain, jaw pain, myalgia ■ **Neuro:** neurotoxicity ■ **Misc:** pain in tumor-containing tissue.

## INTERACTIONS

**Drug-Drug:** ■ ↑ bone marrow depression with other **antineoplastics** or **radiation therapy** ■ Concurrent use with **cisplatin** ↑ risk and severity of bone marrow depression ■ Concurrent use with **mitomycin** or **chest radiation** ↑ risk of pulmonary reactions.

## ROUTE AND DOSAGE

- **IV (Adults):** 30 mg/m² once weekly.
- ❑ **Hepatic Impairment**
- **IV (Adults):** *Total bilirubin 2.1–3 mg/dl*—15 mg/m² once weekly; *total bilirubin ≥3 mg/dl*—7.5 mg/m² once weekly.

## AVAILABILITY (generic available)

■ *Injection:* 10 mg/ml^Rx ■ Cost: $104.58/1 ml, $522.58/5 ml.

TIME/ACTION PROFILE (effect on WBCs)

|    | ONSET   | PEAK       | DURATION   |
|----|---------|------------|------------|
| IV | unknown | 7–10 days  | 7–15 days  |

# NURSING IMPLICATIONS

## ASSESSMENT

- ❑ Monitor blood pressure, pulse, and respiratory rate during therapy. Note significant changes. Acute shortness of breath and severe bronchospasm may occur infrequently shortly after administration. Treatment with corticosteroids, bronchodilators, and supplemental oxygen may be required, especially in patients with a history of pulmonary disease.
- ❑ Assess frequently for signs of infection (sore throat, temperature, cough, mental status changes), especially when nadir of granulocytopenia is expected.
- ❑ Monitor neurologic status. Assess for paresthesia (numbness, tingling, pain), loss of deep tendon reflexes (Achilles reflex is usually first involved), weakness (wrist drop or footdrop, gait disturbances), cranial nerve palsies (jaw pain, hoarseness, ptosis, visual changes), autonomic dysfunction (constipation, ileus, difficulty voiding, orthostatic hypotension, impaired sweating), and CNS dysfunction (decreased level of consciousness, agitation, hallucinations). These symptoms may persist for months. The incidence of neurotoxicity associated with vinorelbine is less than that of other vinca alkaloids.
- ❑ Monitor intake and output and daily weight for significant discrepancies.

❑ Assess nutritional status. Mild to moderate nausea is common. An antiemetic may be used to minimize nausea and vomiting.

❑ Monitor for symptoms of gout (increased uric acid, joint pain, edema). Encourage patient to drink at least 2 L of fluid/day. Allopurinol and alkalinization of urine may decrease uric acid levels.

■ **Lab Test Considerations:** Monitor CBC prior to each dose and routinely during therapy. The nadir of granulocytopenia usually occurs 7–10 days after vinorelbine administration and recovery usually follows within 7–15 days. If granulocyte count is <1500/ mm$^3$, dosage reduction or temporary interruption of vinorelbine may be warranted. If repeated episodes of fever and/or sepsis occur during granulocytopenia, future dosage of vinorelbine should be modified. May also cause mild to moderate anemia. Thrombocytopenia rarely occurs.

❑ Monitor liver function studies (AST, ALT, LDH, bilirubin) and renal function studies (BUN, creatinine) prior to and periodically during therapy. May cause ↑ uric acid; monitor periodically during therapy.

## POTENTIAL NURSING DIAGNOSES

■ Injury, risk for (Adverse Reactions).
■ Infection, risk for (Adverse Reactions).

## IMPLEMENTATION

❑ **High Alert:** Fatalities have occurred with chemotherapeutic agents. Before administering, clarify all ambiguous orders; double check single, daily, and course-of-therapy dose limits; have second practitioner independently double check original order, dose calculations, and infusion pump settings.

■ **General:** Solution should be prepared in a biologic cabinet. Wear gloves, gown, and mask while handling medication. Discard IV equipment in specially designated containers.

❑ Assess infusion site frequently for redness, irritation, or inflammation. Vinorelbine is a vesicant. If extravasation occurs, infusion must be stopped and restarted elsewhere to avoid damage to subcut tissue. Treatment of extravasation includes application of warm compresses applied over the area immediately for 30–60 min, then alternating on/off every 15 min for 1 day to increase systemic absorption of the drug. Hyaluronidase 150 units diluted in 1–2 ml of 0.9% NaCl, 1 ml

for each ml extravasated, should be injected through existing IV cannula or subcut if the needle has been removed to enhance absorption and dispersion of the extravasated drug.

■ **Direct IV:** Dilute vinorelbine to a concentration of 1.5–3 mg/ml with 0.9% NaCl or D5W.

■ **Rate:** Infuse over 6–10 min into Y-site closest to bag of a free-flowing IV or into a central line.

❑ Flush vein with at least 75–125 ml of 0.9% NaCl or D5W administered over 10 min or more following administration of vinorelbine.

■ **Intermittent Infusion:** Dilute vinorelbine to a concentration of 0.5–2 mg/ml with 0.9% NaCl, D5W, 0.45% NaCl, D5/0.45% NaCl, Ringer's, or lactated Ringer's injection. Solution should be colorless to pale yellow. Do not administer solutions that are discolored or contain particulate matter. Diluted solution is stable for 24 hr at room temperature.

■ **Rate:** Infuse over 6–10 min into Y-site closest to bag of a free-flowing IV or into a central line.

❑ Flush vein with at least 75–125 ml of 0.9% NaCl or D5W administered over 10 min or more following administration of vinorelbine.

■ **Y-Site Compatibility:** amikacin ◆ aztreonam ◆ bleomycin ◆ bumetanide ◆ buprenorphine ◆ butorphanol ◆ calcium gluconate ◆ carboplatin ◆ carmustine ◆ cefotaxime ◆ ceftazidime ◆ ceftizoxime ◆ chlorpromazine ◆ cimetidine ◆ cisplatin ◆ clindamycin ◆ cyclophosphamide ◆ cytarabine ◆ dacarbazine ◆ dactinomycin ◆ daunorubicin ◆ dexamethasone sodium phosphate ◆ diphenhydramine ◆ doxorubicin ◆ doxorubicin liposome ◆ doxycycline ◆ droperidol ◆ enalaprilat ◆ etoposide ◆ famotidine ◆ floxuridine ◆ fluconazole ◆ fludarabine ◆ gatifloxacin ◆ gemcitabine ◆ gentamicin ◆ granisetron ◆ haloperidol ◆ hydrocortisone ◆ hydromorphone ◆ idarubicin ◆ ifosfamide ◆ imipenem/cilastatin ◆ lorazepam ◆ mannitol ◆ mechlorethamine ◆ melphalan ◆ meperidine ◆ mesna ◆ methotrexate ◆ metoclopramide ◆ metronidazole ◆ minocycline ◆ mitoxantrone ◆ morphine ◆ nalbuphine ◆ netilmicin ◆ ondansetron ◆ plicamycin ◆ streptozocin ◆ teniposide ◆ ticarcillin ◆ ticarcillin/clavulanate ◆ tobramycin ◆ vancomycin ◆ vinblastine ◆ vincristine ◆ zidovudine.

■ **Y-Site Incompatibility:** ◆ acyclovir ◆ allopurinol ◆ aminophylline ◆ amphotericin B ◆ amphotericin B cholesteryl sulfate ◆ ampicillin ◆ cefazolin ◆ cefoperazone ◆ cefotetan ◆ ceftriaxone ◆ cefuroxime ◆ fluorouracil ◆ furosemide ◆ ganciclovir ◆ methylprednisolone ◆ mitomycin ◆ piperacillin ◆ sodium bicarbonate ◆ thiotepa ◆ trimethoprim/sulfamethoxazole.

## PATIENT/FAMILY TEACHING

❏ Instruct patient to report symptoms of neurotoxicity (paresthesia, pain, difficulty walking, persistent constipation).

❏ Inform patient that increased fluid intake, dietary fiber, and exercise may minimize constipation. Stool softeners or laxatives may be necessary. Patient should be advised to report severe constipation or abdominal discomfort, as this may be a sign of ileus, which may occur as a consequence of neuropathy.

❏ Advise patient to notify health care professional if fever; chills; sore throat; signs of infection; bleeding gums; bruising; petechiae; blood in urine, stool, or emesis; or mouth sores occur.

❏ Caution patient to avoid crowds and persons with known infections.

❏ Advise patient that this medication may have teratogenic effects. Contraception should be used during and for at least 2 mo after therapy is concluded.

❏ Discuss with patient the possibility of hair loss and explore coping strategies.

❏ Instruct patient not to receive any vaccinations without advice of health care professional.

❏ Emphasize the need for periodic lab tests to monitor for side effects.

## EVALUATION

**Effectiveness of therapy can be demonstrated by:** ■ Decrease in the size or spread of malignancy without detrimental side effects.

# VITAMIN B$_{12}$ PREPARATIONS

## cyanocobalamin
## (sye-an-oh-koe-**bal**-a-min)

{Anacobin}, {Bedoz}, Big Shot B-12, Cobex, Cobolin-M, Crystamine, Crysti-1000, Cyanoject, Cyomin, Ener-B, Nascobal, Neuroforte-R, Primabalt, Rubesol-1000, Rubramin PC, Shovite, Vibal, Vitabee-12

## hydroxocobalamin
## (hye-drox-oh-koe-**bal**-a-min)

Alphamin, Hydrobexan, Hydro Cobex, Hydro-Crysti-12, Hydroxy-Cobal, LA-12, Vibal LA

### CLASSIFICATION(S):
**Therapeutic:** antianemics, vitamins
**Pharmacologic:** water soluble vitamins

### Pregnancy Category C

## INDICATIONS

■ Vitamin B$_{12}$ deficiency ■ Pernicious anemia (parenteral products only) ■ Part of the Schilling test (diagnostic).

## ACTION

■ Necessary coenzyme for metabolic processes, including fat and carbohydrate metabolism and protein synthesis ■ Required for RBC formation. **Therapeutic Effects:** ■ Corrects manifestations of pernicious anemia (megaloblastic indices, GI lesions, and neurologic damage) ■ Prevents vitamin B$_{12}$ deficiency.

## PHARMACOKINETICS

**Absorption:** GI Absorption requires intrinsic factor and calcium (only 5 mcg/day may be absorbed); well absorbed after IM, subcut, and nasal administration.

**Distribution:** Stored in the liver; crosses placenta; enters breast milk.

**Metabolism and Excretion:** Excess amounts excreted unchanged in urine.

**Half-life:** 6 days (400 days in liver).

## CONTRAINDICATIONS AND PRECAUTIONS

**Contraindicated in:** ■ Hypersensitivity ■ Hereditary optic nerve atrophy (accelerates nerve damage) ■ Avoid using preparations containing benzyl alcohol in premature infants (associated with fatal "gasping syndrome").

**Use Cautiously in:** ■ Cardiac disease ■ Uremia, folic acid deficiency, concurrent infection, iron deficiency (response to B$_{12}$ will be impaired).

## ADVERSE REACTIONS AND SIDE EFFECTS*

■ **CV:** peripheral vascular thrombosis ■ **GI:** diarrhea ■ **Derm:** itching, swelling of the body, urticaria ■ **F and E:** hypokalemia ■ **Local:** pain at IM site ■ **Misc:** hypersensitivity reactions including ANAPHYLAXIS.

## INTERACTIONS

**Drug-Drug:** ■ **Chloramphenicol** and **antineoplastics** may decrease the hematologic response to vitamin B$_{12}$ ■ **Aminoglycosides, colchicine, extended-release potassium supplements, aminosalicylic acid, anticonvulsants, cimetidine,** excess intake of **alcohol,** or **vitamin C** may decrease oral absorption/effectiveness of vitamin B$_{12}$.

## ROUTE AND DOSAGE

❑ **Cyanocobalamin**

■ **PO (Adults and Children):** Amount depends on degree of deficiency; up to 1000 mcg/day.

■ **IM, Subcut (Adults):** 30–100 mcg/day for 6–7 days; then 100–200 mcg/month. (Doses up to 1000 mcg have been used.) "Flushing" dose for Schilling test is 1000 mcg.

■ **IM, Subcut (Children):** 30–50 mcg/day for 14 or more days; then 100 mcg/month. (Doses up to 1000 mcg have been used.) "Flushing" dose for Schilling test is 1000 mcg.

■ **Intranasal (Adults):** 500 mcg (one spray in one nostril) once weekly.

❑ **Hydroxocobalamin Deficiency**

■ **IM, Subcut (Adults):** 30–50 mcg/day for 5–10 days; then 100–200 mcg monthly. "Flushing" dose for Schilling test is 1000 mcg.

■ **IM, Subcut (Children):** 30–50 mcg/day for 5–10 days; then 100 mcg monthly.

## AVAILABILITY

❑ **Cyanocobalamin**

■ **Tablets:** {25 mcg$^{OTC}$}, {50 mcg$^{OTC}$}, {100 mcg$^{OTC}$}, {250 mcg$^{OTC}$}, 500 mcg$^{OTC}$, 1000 mcg$^{OTC}$, 5000 mcg$^{OTC}$ ■ **Extended-release tablets:**

{100 mcg$^{OTC}$}, {200 mcg$^{OTC}$}, 500 mcg$^{OTC}$, 1000 mcg$^{OTC}$ ■ **Lozenges:** 100 mcg$^{OTC}$, 250 mcg$^{OTC}$, 500 mcg$^{OTC}$ ■ **Nasal gel:** 500 mcg/spray (8 sprays/bottle)$^{Rx}$ ■ **Injection:** 100 mcg/ml in 30-ml vials$^{Rx}$, 1000 mcg/ml in 10- and 30-ml vials$^{Rx}$.

❑ **Hydroxocobalamin**

■ **Injection:** 1000 mcg/ml in 30-ml vials$^{Rx}$.

TIME/ACTION PROFILE (reticulocytosis)

| | ONSET | PEAK | DURATION |
|---|---|---|---|
| Cyanocobalamin IM, subcut, nasal | unknown | 3–10 days | unknown |
| Hydroxocobalamin IM, subcut | unknown | 3–10 days | unknown |

# NURSING IMPLICATIONS

## ASSESSMENT

❑ Assess patient for signs of vitamin B$_{12}$ deficiency (pallor; neuropathy; psychosis; red, inflamed tongue) before and periodically during therapy.

■ **Lab Test Considerations:** Monitor plasma folic acid levels, reticulocyte count, and plasma vitamin B$_{12}$ levels before and between the 5th and 7th days of therapy. Patients receiving vitamin B$_{12}$ for megaloblastic anemia should have serum potassium level evaluated for hypokalemia during the first 48 hr of treatment. Patients with pernicious anemia should be monitored every 5–6 mo.

## POTENTIAL NURSING DIAGNOSES

■ Nutrition, imbalanced: less than body requirements (Indications).

■ Activity intolerance (Indications).

## IMPLEMENTATION

■ **General:** Usually administered in combination with other vitamins; solitary vitamin B$_{12}$ deficiencies are rare.

❑ Administration of vitamin B$_{12}$ by the oral route is useful only for nutritional deficiencies. Patients with small-bowel disease, malabsorption syndrome, or gastric or ileal resections require parenteral administration.

■ **PO:** Administer with meals to increase absorption.

- ❑ May be mixed with fruit juices. Administer immediately after mixing; ascorbic acid alters stability.
- ■ **IV:** IV route is not recommended; however, small amounts of cyanocobalamin may be admixed in TPN solutions.
- ■ **Y-Site Compatibility:** ◆ heparin ◆ hydrocortisone sodium succinate ◆ potassium chloride ◆ vitamin B complex with C.
- ■ **Additive Compatibility:** ◆ 0.45% NaCl ◆ 0.9% NaCl ◆ ascorbic acid ◆ D5W ◆ D10W ◆ dextrose/Ringer's or lactated Ringer's combinations ◆ dextrose/saline combinations ◆ Ringer's or LR ◆ vitamin B complex with C.
- ■ **Solution Compatibility:** ◆ 0.45% NaCl ◆ 0.9% NaCl ◆ ascorbic acid ◆ D5W ◆ D10W ◆ dextrose/Ringer's or lactated Ringer's combinations ◆ dextrose/saline combinations ◆ Ringer's or LR ◆ vitamin B complex with C.
- ■ **Intranasal:** Dose should not be administered within 1 hr of hot food or fluids.

## PATIENT/FAMILY TEACHING

- ■ **General Info:** Encourage patient to comply with diet recommendations of health care professional. Explain that the best source of vitamins is a well-balanced diet with foods from the four basic food groups.
- ❑ Foods high in vitamin $B_{12}$ include meats, seafood, egg yolk, and fermented cheeses; few vitamins are lost with ordinary cooking.
- ❑ Patients self-medicating with vitamin supplements should be cautioned not to exceed RDA. Effectiveness of megadoses for treatment of various medical conditions is unproved and may cause side effects.
- ❑ Inform patients of the lifelong need for vitamin $B_{12}$ replacement after gastrectomy or ileal resection.
- ❑ Emphasize the importance of follow-up exams to evaluate progress.
- ■ **Intranasal:** Instruct patient in proper administration technique. Unit must be primed with 3 strokes if not used for 18 hr or longer. Advise patient to clear nose, then place tip approximately 1 in. into nostril and press pump once, firmly and quickly. After dose, remove unit from nose and massage dosed nostril gently for a few seconds. Vial delivers 8 doses.

## EVALUATION

**Effectiveness of therapy can be demonstrated by:** ■ Resolution of the symptoms of vitamin $B_{12}$ deficiency ❑ Increase in reticulocyte count ■ Improvement in manifestations of pernicious anemia.

# VITAMIN D COMPOUNDS

**calcifediol**

(kal-si-fe-**dye**-ole)

Calderol

**calcitriol**

(kal-si-**trye**-ole)

1,25-dihydroxycholecalciferol, Calcijex, Rocaltrol, vitamin $D_3$

**dihydrotachysterol**

(dye-hye-droh-tak-**iss**-ter-ole)

DHT, Hytakerol

**doxercalciferol**

(**dox**-er-**kal**-si-fe-role)

{Hectorol}

**ergocalciferol**

(er-goe-kal-**sif**-e-role)

Calciferol, Deltalin, Drisdol, {Ostoforte}, {Radiostol}, vitamin $D_2$

**paricalcitol**

(par-i-**kal**-si-tole)

Zemplar

## CLASSIFICATION(S):

**Therapeutic:** *vitamins*

**Pharmacologic:** *fat-soluble vitamins*

**Pregnancy Category A (Vitamin D in RDA doses), B (doxercalciferol), C (calcifediol, calcitriol, dihydrotachysterol, ergocalciderol, paracalcitol)**

## INDICATIONS

■ **Calcifediol:** Treatment/management of metabolic bone disease and treatment of hypocalcemia in hemodialysis patients ■ **Calcitriol:** Management of hypocalcemia in chronic renal failure patients ■ Treatment of hypoparathyroidism or pseudohypoparathyroidism ■ Management of secondary hyperparathyroidism and metabolic bone disease in predialysis patients with moderate to severe renal insufficiency (CCr 15–55 ml/min) ■ **Dihydrotachysterol:** Treatment of hypophosphatemia ■ Treatment of hypocalcemia ■ Prevention and treatment of rickets ■ Prevention and treatment of vitamin D deficiency ■ Prevention and treatment of postoperative and idiopathic tetany ■ **Doxercaliciferol:** Reduction of elevated intact parathyroid hormone (iPTH) levels in the management of secondary hyperparathyroidism in patients undergoing chronic renal dialysis ■ **Ergocalciferol:** Prophylaxis and treatment of vitamin D deficiency ■ Treatment of hypophosphatemia or hypocalcemia ■ Treatment of osteodystrophy ■ Treatment of osteomalacia secondary to chronic anticonvulsant therapy ■ Treatment of rickets ■ **Paricalcitol:** Prevention and treatment of secondary hyperparathyroidism due to chronic renal failure.

## ACTION

■ Dihydrotachysterol and ergocalciferol are inactive forms of vitamin D; activation occurs in the liver and kidneys. Calcifediol requires activation by the kidneys. Calcitriol is the active form. ■ Vitamin D ❏ Promotes the absorption of calcium and phosphorus ❏ Regulates calcium homeostasis in conjunction with parathyroid hormone and calcitonin. **Therapeutic Effects:** ■ Treatment and prevention of deficiency states, particularly bone manifestations ■ Improved calcium and phosphorous homeostasis in patients with chronic renal failure.

## PHARMACOKINETICS

**Absorption:** *Calcifediol, calcitriol*—Well absorbed following oral administration. *Dihydrotachysterol, ergocalciferol*—Well absorbed in an inactive form. *Doxercaliferol*—Doxercalciferol is a prodrug which is well absorbed following oral administration. *Paricalcitol*—IV administration results in complete bioavailability.

**Distribution:** Stored in the liver and other fatty tissues; calcitriol crosses the placenta.

**Metabolism and Excretion:** *Calcitriol*—Undergoes enterohepatic recycling and is excreted mostly in bile. *Dihydrotachysterol, ergocalciferol*—Converted to active form by sunlight, the liver, and the kidneys. Calcifediol is activated to vitamin D in the liver and kidneys. *Doxercalciferol*—Converted by the liver to 1,25–(OH)$_2$D$_2$ (the major metabolite) and 1,24–dihydroxyvitamin D$_2$ (the minor metabolite). *Paricalcitol*—mostly metabolized by the liver and excreted via hepatobiliary elimination.

**Half-life:** *Calcitriol*—3–8 hr. *Doxercalciferol metabolites*—*1,25–(OH)$_2$D$_2$*—32–37 hr (up to 96 hr). *Paricalcitol*—15 hr.

## CONTRAINDICATIONS AND PRECAUTIONS

**Contraindicated in:** ■ Hypersensitivity ■ Hypercalcemia/hyperphosphatemia ■ Vitamin D toxicity ■ Lactation (large doses) ■ **Doxercalciferol:** Concurrent use of magnesium-containing antacids or other vitamin D supplements.

**Use Cautiously in:** ■ Sarcoidosis ■ Hyperparathyroidism ■ Patients receiving digitalis glycosides ■ Pregnancy (larger doses; safety not established).

## ADVERSE REACTIONS AND SIDE EFFECTS*

Seen primarily as manifestations of toxicity (hypercalcemia). ■ **CNS:** headache, somnolence, weakness; *doxercalciferol*—dizziness, malaise, sleep disorder ■ **EENT:** conjunctivitis, photophobia, rhinorrhea ■ **Resp:** *doxercalciferol*—dyspnea ■ **CV:** arrhythmias, hypertension; *doxercalciferol*—bradycardia; *paricalcitol*—edema, palpitations ■ **GI:** anorexia, constipation, dry mouth, metallic taste, nausea, polydipsia, vomiting, weight loss ■ **GU:** albuminuria, decreased libido, nocturia, polyuria ■ **Derm:** pruritus ■ **Endo:** *doxercalciferol*—oversuppression of PTH ■ **F and E:** hypercalcemia; *doxercalciferol*—hypercalcuria, hyperphosphatemia ■ **Metab:** hyperthermia ■ **MS:** bone pain, muscle pain; *doxercalciferol*—adynamic bone disease, arthralgia; *paricalcitol*—metastatic calcification ■ **Misc:** *paricalcitol*—allergic reactions, chills, fever.

## INTERACTIONS

**Drug-Drug:** ■ **Cholestyramine, colestipol,** or **mineral oil** decreases absorption of vitamin D analogues ■ Use with **thiazide diuretics** in patients with hypoparathyroidism may result in hypercalcemia ■ **Corticosteroids** decrease the effectiveness of vitamin D analogues ■ Use with **digoxin** increases the risk of arrhythmias ■ Vitamin D requirements are increased by **phenytoin** and other **hydantoin anticonvulsants, sucralfate, barbiturates,** and **primidone** ■ Use with caution in patients receiving **magnesium-containing antacids** or **calcium-containing drugs** ■ Concurrent use of **magnesium-containing antacids** (may lead to hypermagnesemia) ■ Concurrent use of other **Vitamin D supplements** (increases risk of hypercalcemia) ■ **Agents that induce liver enzymes (phenobarbital)** and **agents that inhibit liver enzymes (phenytoin)** may alter requirements for doxercalciferol.

**Drug-Food:** ■ Ingestion of **foods high in calcium content** (see Appendix Q) may lead to hypercalcemia.

## ROUTE AND DOSAGE

### ❑ Calcifediol

■ **PO (Adults):** 20–100 mcg/day or 20–200 mcg/day on alternate days; increase dose at 4 wk intervals, or 300–350 mcg/week, administered daily or on alternate days.

### ❑ Calcitriol

■ **PO (Adults):** *Hypocalcemia during chronic dialysis*—0.25 mcg/day or every other day (may require 0.5–1 mcg/day). *Hypoparathyroidism*—0.25–2.0 mcg/day. *Renal osteodystrophy*—0.25 mcg every other day– 3 mcg/day (larger doses have been used). *Predialysis patients*—0.25 mcg/day (up to 0.5 mcg/day).

■ **PO (Children):** *Hypocalcemia during chronic dialysis*—0.25–2 mcg/day. *Hypoparathyroidism*—0.04–0.08 mcg/kg/day. *Renal osteodystrophy*—0.014–0.041 mcg/kg/day. Children with liver disease may require larger initial doses. *Predialysis patients*—0.25 mcg/day (up to 0.5 mcg/day).

■ **PO (Children <3 yr):** *Predialysis patients*—1015 ng/kg/day.

■ **IV (Adults):** *Initial*—0.5 mcg (0.01 mcg/kg) 3 times weekly. May be increased by 0.25–0.5 mcg/dose at 2- to 4-wk intervals. *Maintenance*—0.5–3.0 mcg 3 times weekly (0.01–0.05 mcg/kg 3 times weekly).

### ❑ Dihydrotachysterol

■ **PO (Adults):** *Hypocalcemic tetany*—0.75– 2.5 mg/day for 3 days initially; then 0.25/ week–1 mg/day. *Hypoparathyroidism/pseudohypoparathyroidism*—0.75–2.5 mg/day initially for several days; then 0.2–1 mg/day (up to 1.5 mg/day). *Renal osteodystrophy*—0.1–0.25 mg/day initially; then 0.2–1 mg/day.

■ **PO (Children):** *Hypoparathyroidism/pseudohypoparathyroidism*—1–5 mg/day for 4 days; then 0.5–1.5 mg/day.

### ❑ Doxercalciferol

■ **PO (Adults):** 10 mcg 3 times weekly (at dialysis); dose may be adjusted at 8-wk intervals based on laboratory assessment.

■ **IV (Adults):** 4 mcg 3 times weekly (at the end of dialysis); dose may be adjusted at 8-wk intervals (not to exceed 18 mcg/dose).

### ❑ Ergocalciferol

■ **PO (Adults):** *Vitamin D deficiency*—Depends on degree of deficiency. *Vitamin D-resistant rickets*—12,000–150,000 units/day. *Vitamin D-dependent rickets*—10,000–60,000 units/day (up to 150,000 units/day). *Familial hypophosphatemia*—50,000–100,000 units/day. *Osteomalacia from anticonvulsants*—1000–4000 units/day. *Hypoparathyroidism*—50,000–150,000 units/day.

■ **PO (Children):** *Vitamin D deficiency*—Depends on degree of deficiency. *Vitamin D–dependent rickets*—3000–10,000 units/day (up to 50,000 units/day). *Osteomalacia from anticonvulsants*—1000 units/day. *Hypoparathyroidism*—50,000–200,000 units/day.

■ **IM (Adults and Children):** *Malabsorption*—10,000 units/day.

■ **IV (Adults and Children):** As part of TPN, amount determined by need on an individual basis.

### ❑ Paricalcitol

■ **IV (Adults):** 0.04–0.1 mcg/kg no more frequently than every other day at any time during dialysis (up to 0.24 mcg/kg has been used); dosage increments of 2–4 mcg may be made at 2–4 wk intervals.

## AVAILABILITY

❑ **Calcifediol**

■ *Capsules:* 20 mcg$^{Rx}$, 50 mcg$^{Rx}$.

❑ **Calcitriol**

■ *Capsules:* 0.25 mcg$^{Rx}$, 0.5 mcg$^{Rx}$ ■ *Oral solution:* 1 mcg/ml in 15-ml bottle$^{Rx}$ ■ *Injection:* 1 mcg/ml in 1-ml ampules$^{Rx}$, 2 mcg/ml in 1-ml ampules$^{Rx}$.

❑ **Dihydrotachysterol**

■ *Tablets:* 0.125 mg$^{Rx}$, 0.2 mg$^{Rx}$, 0.4 mg$^{Rx}$ ■ *Capsules:* 0.125 mg$^{Rx}$ ■ *Oral solution:* 0.2 mg/ml in 30-ml bottles$^{Rx}$.

❑ **Doxercalciferol**

■ *Capsules:* 2.5 mcg$^{Rx}$ ■ *Solution for injection:* 2 mcg/ml ampules$^{Rx}$, 4 mcg/2 ml ampules$^{Rx}$.

❑ **Ergocalciferol**

■ *Liquid:* 8000 units/ml in 60-ml bottles$^{Rx, \, OTC}$ ■ *Capsules:* 50,000 units$^{Rx}$ ■ *Tablets:* 50,000 units$^{Rx}$ ■ *Injection:* 500,000 units/ml in 1-ml ampules$^{Rx}$.

❑ **Paricalcitol**

■ *Solution for injection:* 5 mcg/ml in 1- and 2-ml vials$^{Rx}$.

TIME/ACTION PROFILE (effects on serum calcium)

| | ONSET | PEAK | DURATION |
|---|---|---|---|
| Calcitriol-PO | 2–6 hr | 2–6 hr | 3–5 days |
| Calcitriol-IV | unknown | unknown | unknown |
| Dihydrota-chysterol-PO | several hr | 1–up to 9 wk | 2 wk |
| Doxercalci-ferol PO | unknown | 8 wk | 1 wk |
| Ergocalcifer-ol-PO | 12–24 hr† | unkown | up to 6 mo |
| Paricalitol IV | unknown | up to 2 wk | unknown |

†Therapeutic effect may take 10–14 days.

# NURSING IMPLICATIONS

## ASSESSMENT

❑ Assess for symptoms of vitamin deficiency prior to and periodically during therapy.
❑ Assess patient for bone pain and weakness prior to and during therapy.
❑ Observe patient carefully for evidence of hypocalcemia (paresthesia, muscle twitching, laryngospasm, colic, cardiac arrhythmias, and Chvostek's or Trousseau's sign). Protect symptomatic patient by raising and padding side rails; keep bed in low position.

■ **Children:** Monitor height and weight; growth arrest may occur in prolonged high-dose therapy.
■ **Rickets/Osteomalacia:** Assess patient for bone pain and weakness prior to and during therapy.
■ *Lab Test Considerations:* Serum ionized calcium concentrations should be drawn weekly during initial therapy.
❑ Monitor BUN, serum creatinine, alkaline phosphatase, parathyroid hormone levels, urinary calcium/creatinine ratio, 24-hr urinary calcium periodically.
❑ Monitor serum phosphorus levels prior to and periodically during therapy. Serum phosphorus must be controlled prior to initiating calcitriol. Aluminum carbonate or aluminum hydroxide is used for this purpose in dialysis patients.
❑ A ↓ in alkaline phosphatase levels may signal onset of hypercalcemia. Overdose is associated with a serum calcium times phosphate (Ca × P) level of >70 and ↑ BUN, AST, and ALT.
❑ May cause false ↑ cholesterol levels.
■ *Toxicity and Overdose:* Toxicity is manifested as hypercalcemia, hypercalciuria, and hyperphosphatemia. Assess patient for appearance of nausea, vomiting, anorexia, weakness, constipation, headache, bone pain, and metallic taste. Later symptoms include polyuria, polydipsia, photophobia, rhinorrhea, pruritus, and cardiac arrhythmias. Notify physician or other health care professional immediately if these signs of hypervitaminosis D occur. Treatment usually consists of discontinuation of calcitriol, a low-calcium diet, use of low-calcium dialysate in peritoneal dialysis patients, and administration of a laxative. IV hydration and loop diuretics may be ordered to increase urinary excretion of calcium. Hemodialysis may also be used.

## POTENTIAL NURSING DIAGNOSES

■ Nutrition, imbalanced: less than body requirements (Indications).

## IMPLEMENTATION

■ **General:** Do not confuse Calciferol (ergocalciferol) with calcitriol.

❑ Because solitary vitamin deficiencies are rare, combinations are commonly administered.

■ **PO:** May be administered without regard to meals. Measure solution accurately with calibrated dropper provided by manufacturer. May be mixed with juice, cereal, or food, or dropped directly into mouth.

■ **IM:** *Ergocalciferol* injection is oil-based; avoid IV administration.

■ **Direct IV:** Administer *calcitriol* by rapid injection through the catheter at the end of a hemodialysis period.

**PATIENT/FAMILY TEACHING**

❑ Advise patient to take medication as directed. Take missed doses as soon as remembered that day, unless almost time for next dose; do not double up on doses.

❑ Review diet modifications with patient. See Appendix Q for foods high in calcium and vitamin D. Renal patients must still consider renal failure diet in food selection. Health care professional may order concurrent calcium supplement.

❑ Encourage patient to comply with dietary recommendations of health care professional. Explain that the best source of vitamins is a well-balanced diet with foods from the 4 basic food groups and the importance of sunlight exposure. See Appendix Q for foods high in vitamin D.

❑ Patients self-medicating with vitamin supplements should be cautioned not to exceed RDA. The effectiveness of megadoses for treatment of various medical conditions is unproved and may cause side effects.

❑ Advise patient to avoid concurrent use of antacids containing magnesium.

❑ Review symptoms of overdosage and instruct patient to report these promptly to health care professional.

❑ Emphasize the importance of follow-up exams to evaluate progress.

**EVALUATION**

**Effectiveness of therapy can be demonstrated by:** ■ Normalization of serum calcium and parathyroid hormone levels ■ Decreased bone pain and weakness in patients with renal osteodystrophy ■ Improvement in symptoms of vitamin D–resistant rickets.

# vitamin E
(**vye**-ta-min E)
alpha tocopherol, Amino-Opti-E, Aquasol E, E-200, E-400, E-1000, E-Complex-600, E-Vitamin, Liqui-E, Pheryl-E, Vita Plus E, {Webber Vitamin E}

*CLASSIFICATION(S):*
*Therapeutic: vitamins*
*Pharmacologic: fat-soluble vitamins*

**Pregnancy Category A (doses within RDA), C (doses >RDA)**

**INDICATIONS**

■ **PO:** Used as a dietary supplement ■ Used in low-birth-weight infants to prevent and treat hemolysis due to vitamin E deficiency ■ **Topical:** Treatment of irritated, chapped, or dry skin. **Unlabeled uses:** ■ Prevention of coronary artery disease.

**ACTION**

■ Prevents the oxidation (antioxidant) of other substances ■ Protects RBC membranes against hemolysis, especially in low-birth-weight neonates. **Therapeutic Effects:** ■ Prevention and treatment of deficiency in high-risk patients.

**PHARMACOKINETICS**

**Absorption:** 20–80% absorbed following oral administration. Absorption requires fat and bile salts.

**Distribution:** Widely distributed, stored in adipose tissue (4-yr supply).

**Metabolism and Excretion:** Metabolized by the liver, excreted in bile.

**Half-life:** Unknown.

**CONTRAINDICATIONS AND PRECAUTIONS**

**Contraindicated in:** ■ Hypersensitivity to ingredients in preparations (parabens, propylene, glycol).

**Use Cautiously in:** ■ Anemia due to iron deficiency ■ Low-birth-weight infants (oral administration may cause necrotizing enterocolitis) ■ Vitamin K deficiency (may increase risk of bleeding).

## ADVERSE REACTIONS AND SIDE EFFECTS*

Seen primarily with large doses over long periods of time. ■ **CNS:** fatigue, headache, weakness ■ **EENT:** blurred vision ■ **GI:** NECROTIZING ENTEROCOLITIS (oral administration in low-birth-weight infants), cramps, diarrhea, nausea ■ **Derm:** rash ■ **Endo:** gonadal dysfunction.

## INTERACTIONS

**Drug-Drug:** ■ **Cholestyramine, colestipol, orlistat, mineral oil,** and **sucralfate** decrease absorption ■ May decrease hematologic response to **iron supplements** ■ May increase the risk of bleeding with **warfarin.**

**Drug-Natural Products:** ■ Increased bleeding risk with **anise, arnica, chamomile, clove, dong quai, fenugreek, feverfew, garlic, ginger, ginkgo, Panax ginseng, licorice,** and others.

## ROUTE AND DOSAGE

Other dosing regimens may be used.

■ **PO (Adults and Children):** Determined by nutritional intake or degree of deficiency.

■ **Topical (Adults and Children):** Apply to affected areas as needed.

## AVAILABILITY

■ *Capsules:* 100 units^OTC, 200 units^OTC, 400 units^OTC, 600 units^OTC, {800 units^OTC}, 1000 units^OTC ■ *Oral solution:* 26.6 units/ml^OTC, 50 units/ml^OTC, 77 units/ml^OTC ■ *Tablets:* 100 units^OTC, 200 units^OTC, 400 units^OTC, 500 units^OTC, 800 units^OTC ■ *Chewable tablets:* 400 units^OTC ■ *Ointment*^OTC ■ *Cream*^OTC ■ *Lotion*^OTC ■ *Oil*^OTC.

TIME/ACTION PROFILE

| | ONSET | PEAK | DURATION |
|---|---|---|---|
| PO | unknown | unknown | unknown |

# NURSING IMPLICATIONS

## ASSESSMENT

❑ Assess patient for signs of vitamin E deficiency (*neonates*—irritability, edema, hemoly-

tic anemia, creatinuria; *adults/children [rare]*—muscle weakness, ceroid deposits, anemia, creatinuria) prior to and periodically throughout therapy.

❑ Assess nutritional status through 24-hr diet recall. Determine frequency of consumption of vitamin E–rich foods.

■ *Lab Test Considerations:* Large doses may increase cholesterol, triglyceride, and CPK levels.

## POTENTIAL NURSING DIAGNOSES

■ Nutrition, imbalanced: less than body requirements (Indications).

## IMPLEMENTATION

■ **PO:** Administer with or after meals.

❑ Chewable tablets should be chewed well or crushed before swallowing. Solution may be dropped directly into mouth or mixed with cereal, fruit juice, or other food. Use calibrated dropper supplied by manufacturer to measure solution accurately.

## PATIENT/FAMILY TEACHING

❑ Instruct patient to take medication as directed. If a dose is missed, it should be omitted, because fat-soluble vitamins are stored in the body for long periods.

❑ Encourage patient to comply with diet recommendations of health care professional. Explain that the best source of vitamins is a well-balanced diet with foods from the four basic food groups.

❑ Foods high in vitamin E include vegetable oils, wheat germ, whole-grain cereals, egg yolk, and liver. Vitamin E content is not markedly affected by cooking.

❑ Patients self-medicating with vitamin supplements should be cautioned not to exceed RDA. The effectiveness of megadoses for treatment of various medical conditions is unproved, and this may cause side effects and toxicity.

❑ Review symptoms of overdosage (blurred vision, flu-like symptoms, headache, breast enlargement). Instruct patient to report these promptly to health care professional.

❑ Mineral oil may interfere with the absorption of fat-soluble vitamins and should not be used concurrently.

## EVALUATION

**Effectiveness of therapy can be demonstrated by:** ■ Prevention of or decrease in the symptoms of vitamin E deficiency ■ Control of dry or chapped skin.

# voriconazole

(vor-i-**kon**-a-zole)

VFEND

*CLASSIFICATION(S):*
*Therapeutic: antifungals*

**Pregnancy Category D**

## INDICATIONS

■ Invasive apergillosis and other serious systemic fungal infections unresponsive or intolerant to other treatment.

## ACTION

■ Inhibits fungal ergosterol synthesis leading to production of abnormal fungal cell wall. **Therapeutic Effects:** ■ Antifungal activity.

## PHARMACOKINETICS

**Absorption:** Well absorbed following oral administration (96%); IV administration results in complete bioavailability.

**Distribution:** Extensive tissue distribution.

**Metabolism and Excretion:** Highly metabolized by the hepatic P450 enzymes (CYP2C19, CYP2C9, CYP3A4); <2% excreted unchanged in urine. Much individual variation in metabolism; metabolites are inactive.

**Half-life:** Dose-dependent; increased in hepatic impairment.

## CONTRAINDICATIONS AND PRECAUTIONS

**Contraindicated in:** ■ Concurrent use of rifampin, carbamazepine, phenobarbital, mephobarbital (decrease antifungal activity) ■ Concurrent use of sirolimus, pimozide, quinidine, ergotamine, and dihydroergotamine (increased risk of toxicity of these agents) ■ Tablets contain lactose and should be avoided in patients with galactose intolerance, Lapp lactase deficiency, or glucose-galactose malabsorption.

**Use Cautiously in:** ■ Mild to moderate liver disease (Child-Pugh Class A and B); maintenance dose reduction recommended ■ Renal impairment (CCr <50 ml/min); use only if justified by risk/benefit assessment (IV form should be avoided, use oral form only) ■ Pregnancy or lactation (use only if benefits justify risk) ■ Children <12 yr (safety not established).

## ADVERSE REACTIONS AND SIDE EFFECTS*

■ **CNS:** dizziness, hallucinations, headache ■ **EENT:** visual disturbances, eye hemorrhage ■ **CV:** changes in blood pressure, tachycardia, peripheral edema, tachycardia ■ **GI:** HEPATOTOXICITY, abdominal pain, diarrhea, nausea, vomiting ■ **Derm:** photosensitivity, rash ■ **F and E:** hypokalemia, Hypomagnesemia ■ **Misc:** allergic reactions including STEVENS-JOHNSON SYNDROME, chills, fever, infusion reactions.

## INTERACTIONS

**Drug-Drug:** ■ **Carbamazepine, mephobarbital, phenobarbital,** and **rifampin** ↑ metabolism and ↓ antifungal activity of voriconazole; concurrent use is contraindicated ■ ↓ metabolism and ↑ risk of toxicity from **dihydroergotamine, ergotamine, pimozide, quinidine,** and **sirolimus**; concurrent use is contraindicated ■ ↓ metabolism and ↑ risk of toxicity from **cyclosporine, HMG-CoA reductase inhibitors,** some **benzodiazepines (alprazolam, midazolam, triazolam),** some **calcium channel blockers, sulfonlyureas (glipizide, glyburide, tolbutamine),** **tacrolimus, warfarin, vinca alkaloids (vincristine, vinblastine);** careful monitoring required during concurrent use ■ **Phenytoin** ↑ metabolism and ↓ antifungal activity of voriconazole; voriconazole ↑ **phenytoin** levels and may cause toxicity; careful monitoring required during concurrent use ■ ↑ blood levels of **omeprazole;** ↓ omeprazole dose by 50% during concurrent use. Similar effects may occur with other **proton-pump inhibitors** ■ May ↓ metabolism and ↑ blood levels and effects of **protease-inhibitor antiretrovirals** and **non-nucleoside reverse transcriptase inhibitor antiretrovirals;** frequent monitoring recommended ■ **Non-nucleoside reverse transcriptase inhibitor antiretrovirals;** may induce or inhibit the metabolism of voriconazole; frequent monitoring recommended.

## ROUTE AND DOSAGE

■ **IV (Adults and children >12 yr):** *Loading dose—*6 mg/kg every 12 hour for 2 doses, followed by *maintenance dosing—*4 mg/kg every 12 hours. IV then switched to oral dosing when possible. If intolerance occurs, dose may be decreased to 3 mg/kg every 12 hr. If phenytoin is coadministered, increase maintenance dose to 5 mg/kg every 12 hr.

■ **PO (Adults and children >12 yr and >40 kg):** (following IV loading dose) 200 mg every 12 hr; may be increased to 300 mg every 12 hr if response if inadequate. If phenytoin is coadministered, increase maintenance dose to 400 mg every 12 hr.

■ **PO (Adults and children >12 yr and <40 kg):** (following IV loading dose) 100 mg every 12 hr; may be increased to 150 mg every 12 hr if response is inadequate. If phenytoin is coadministered, increase maintenance dose to 200 mg every 12 hr.

❏ **Hepatic Impairment**

■ **IV (Adults and Children >12 yr):** Use standard loading dose; decrease maintenance dose by 50%.

## AVAILABILITY

■ *Tablets:* 50 mg^Rx, 200 mg^Rx ■ *Powder for injection (requires reconstitution):* 200 mg/vial^Rx.

TIME/ACTION PROFILE (blood levels)

|    | ONSET | PEAK | DURATION |
|----|-------|------|----------|
| PO | rapid | 1–2 hr | 12 hr |
| IV | rapid | end of infusion | 12 hr |

## NURSING IMPLICATIONS

### ASSESSMENT

❏ Obtain specimens for culture and histopathology prior to therapy to isolate and identify organism. Therapy may be started before results are received.

❏ Monitor visual function including visual acuity, visual field, and color perception in patients receiving more than 28 days of therapy. Vision usually returns to normal within 14 days after discontinuation of therapy.

❏ Monitor for allergic reactions during infusion of voriconazole (flushing, fever, sweating, tachycardia, chest tightness, dyspnea, faintness, nausea, pruritus, rash). Symptoms occur immediately upon start of infusion. May require discontinuation.

■ *Lab Test Considerations:* Monitor liver function tests prior to and during therapy. If abnormal liver function tests occur, monitor for development of severe hepatic injury. Discontinue therapy if clinical signs and symptoms of liver disease develop.

❏ Monitor renal function (serum creatinine) during therapy.

### POTENTIAL NURSING DIAGNOSES

■ Infection, risk for (Indications).

### IMPLEMENTATION

■ **General:** Once patient can tolerate oral medication, PO voriconazole may be used.

■ **PO:** Administer 1 hr before or 1 hr after a meal.

■ **Intermittent Infusion:** Reconstitute voriconazole with 19 ml of sterile water for injection for a volume of 20 ml with a concentration of 10 mg/ml. Discard vial if vacuum does not pull diluent into vial. Shake vial until all powder is dissolved. Solution should be clear without particulate matter. Dilute further with 0.9% NaCl, LR, D5/LR, D5/0.45% NaCl, D5W, D5/20 mEq potassium chloride, 0.45% NaCl, or D5/0.9% NaCl by calculating volume of 10 mg/ml concentrate required for patient dose. Withdraw and discard equal volume of diluent from infusion bag. Concentration in bag after adding voriconazole should be not <0.5 mg/ml and not >5 mg/ml. Withdraw required volume of voriconazole concentrate from appropriate number of vials and add to infusion bag. Use reconstituted solution within 24 hr. Discard partially used vials.

■ *Rate:* Infuse over 1–2 hr at a rate not to exceed 3 mg/kg/hr.

■ **Y-Site Incompatibility:** Do not infuse with other drugs including parenteral nutrition, blood products, or other medications.

### PATIENT/FAMILY TEACHING

❏ May cause blurred vision, photophobia, and dizziness. Caution patient to avoid driving and other activities requiring alertness until response to medication is known. Also advise patient to avoid driving at night during voriconazole therapy

❏ Advise patient to avoid direct sunlight during voriconazole therapy.

### EVALUATION

Effectiveness of therapy can be demonstrated by: ■ Resolution of fungal infections.

## High Alert

# warfarin
(**war**-fa-rin)
Coumadin, {Warfilone}

## CLASSIFICATION(S):
**Therapeutic:** anticoagulants
**Pharmacologic:** coumarins

## Pregnancy Category X

## INDICATIONS
■ Prophylaxis and treatment of: ❑ Venous thrombosis ❑ Pulmonary embolism ❑ Atrial fibrillation with embolization ■ Management of myocardial infarction ❑ Decreases risk of death ❑ Decreases risk of subsequent MI ❑ Decreases risk of future thromboembolic events ■ Prevention of thrombus formation and embolization after prosthetic valve placement.

## ACTION
■ Interferes with hepatic synthesis of vitamin K-dependent clotting factors (II, VII, IX, and X). **Therapeutic Effects:** ■ Prevention of thromboembolic events.

## PHARMACOKINETICS
**Absorption:** Well absorbed from the GI tract after oral administration.
**Distribution:** Crosses the placenta but does not enter breast milk.
**Protein Binding:** 99%.
**Metabolism and Excretion:** Metabolized by the liver.
**Half-life:** 0.5–3 days.

## CONTRAINDICATIONS AND PRECAUTIONS
**Contraindicated in:** ■ Uncontrolled bleeding ■ Open wounds ■ Active ulcer disease ■ Recent brain, eye, or spinal cord injury or surgery ■ Severe liver disease ■ Uncontrolled hypertension ■ Pregnancy.
**Use Cautiously in:** ■ Malignancy ■ Patients with history of ulcer or liver disease ■ History of poor compliance ■ Women with childbearing potential.

## ADVERSE REACTIONS AND SIDE EFFECTS*
■ **GI:** cramps, nausea ■ **Derm:** dermal necrosis ■ **Hemat:** BLEEDING ■ **Misc:** fever.

## INTERACTIONS
**Drug-Drug:** ■ Abciximab, androgens, capecitabine, cefoperazone, cefotetan, chloral hydrate, chloramphenicol, clopidogrel, disulfiram, fluconazole, fluoroquinolones, itraconazole, metronidazole (including vaginal use), plicamycin, thrombolytic agents, eptifibatide, tirofiban, ticlopidine, sulfonamides, quinidine, quinine, NSAIDs, valproates, and aspirin may increase the response to warfarin and increase the risk of bleeding ■ Chronic use of acetaminophen may increase the risk of bleeding ■ Alcohol, barbiturates, and hormonal contraceptives containing estrogen may decrease the anticoagulant response to warfarin ■ Many other drugs may affect the activity of warfarin.
**Drug-Natural Products:** ■ St. John's wort decreases effect ■ Increased bleeding risk with anise, arnica, chamomile, clove, dong quai, fenugreek, feverfew, garlic, ginger, ginkgo, Panax ginseng, licorice, and others.
**Drug-Food:** ■ Ingestion of large quantities of foods high in vitamin K content (see list in Appendix Q) may antagonize the anticoagulant effect of warfarin.

## ROUTE AND DOSAGE
■ **PO, IV (Adults):** 2.5–10 mg/day for 2–4 days; then adjust daily dose by results of prothrombin time or international normalized ratio (INR). Initiate therapy with lower doses in geriatric or debilitated patients.

## AVAILABILITY (generic available)
■ *Tablets:* 1 mg^Rx, 2 mg^Rx, 2.5 mg^Rx, 3 mg^Rx, 4 mg^Rx, 5 mg^Rx, 6 mg^Rx, 7.5 mg^Rx, 10 mg^Rx ■ Cost: *Coumadin*—5 mg $71.35/100; *generic*—5 mg $63.68/100 ■ *Injection:* 5 mg/vial^Rx.

TIME/ACTION PROFILE (effects on coagulation tests)

|  | ONSET | PEAK | DURATION |
|---|---|---|---|
| PO, IV | several hr | 0.5–3 days | 2–5 days |

{ } = Available in Canada only.
* CAPITALS indicates life-threatening; <u>underlines</u> indicate most frequent.

# NURSING IMPLICATIONS

## ASSESSMENT

❑ Assess patient for signs of bleeding and hemorrhage (bleeding gums; nosebleed; unusual bruising; tarry, black stools; hematuria; fall in hematocrit or blood pressure; guaiac-positive stools, urine, or nasogastric aspirate).

❑ Assess patient for evidence of additional or increased thrombosis. Symptoms depend on area of involvement.

■ *Lab Test Considerations:* PT and other clotting factors should be monitored frequently during therapy. Therapeutic PT ranges from 1.3–1.5 times greater than control. May also be reported as INR, a standardized system that provides a common basis for communicating and interpreting PT results. PT values of 1.3–1.5 times the control are equivalent to INR values of 2–3 times the control value. PT of 1.5–2 or INR of 3–4.5 may be used for patients with high risk of embolization.

❑ Hepatic function and CBC should be monitored before and periodically throughout therapy.

❑ Stool and urine should be monitored for occult blood before and periodically throughout therapy.

■ *Toxicity and Overdose:* Withholding 1 or more doses of medication is usually sufficient if PT is excessively prolonged or if minor bleeding occurs. If overdose occurs or anticoagulation needs to be immediately reversed, the antidote is vitamin K (phytonadione, AquaMEPHYTON). Administration of whole blood or plasma also may be required in severe bleeding because of the delayed onset of vitamin K.

## POTENTIAL NURSING DIAGNOSES

■ Tissue perfusion, ineffective (Indications).

■ Injury, risk for (Side Effects).

## IMPLEMENTATION

❑ *High Alert:* Medication errors involving anticoagulants have resulted in serious harm and death from internal or intracranial bleeding. Before administering, evaluate recent INR or PT results and have second practitioner independently check original order.

■ **General:** Because of the large number of medications capable of significantly altering warfarin's effects, careful monitoring is recommended when new agents are started or other agents are discontinued. Interactive potential should be evaluated for all new medications (Rx, OTC, and natural products).

❑ Administer medication at same time each day.

■ **PO:** Medication requires 3–5 days to reach effective levels. It is usually begun while patient is still on heparin.

❑ Do not interchange brands; potencies may not be equivalent.

■ **Direct IV:** Reconstitute with 2.7 ml of sterile water for injection. Do not use solutions that are discolored or contain particulate matter. Stable for 4 hr at room temperature.

■ *Rate:* Administer as low bolus injection over 1–2 min into a peripheral vein.

■ **Y-Site Compatibility:** ◆ cefazolin ◆ ceftriaxone ◆ dopamine ◆ heparin ◆ lidocaine ◆ morphine ◆ nitroglycerine ◆ potassium chloride ◆ ranitidine.

■ **Y-Site Incompatibility:** ◆ aminophylline ◆ bretylium ◆ ceftazidime ◆ cimetidine ◆ ciprofloxacin ◆ dobutamine ◆ esmolol ◆ gentamicin ◆ labetalol ◆ metronidazole ◆ vancomycin.

## PATIENT/FAMILY TEACHING

❑ Instruct patient to take medication exactly as directed. If a dose is missed, tell patient to take it as soon as remembered that day. Patient should not double doses. Health care professional should be informed of missed doses at time of checkup or lab tests.

❑ Review foods high in vitamin K (see Appendix Q). Patient should have consistent limited intake of these foods, as vitamin K is the antidote for warfarin, and alternating intake of these foods will cause PT levels to fluctuate.

❑ Caution patient to avoid IM injections and activities leading to injury. Instruct patient to use a soft toothbrush, not to floss, and to shave with an electric razor during warfarin therapy. Advise patient that venipunctures and injection sites require application of pressure to prevent bleeding or hematoma formation.

❑ Advise patient to report any symptoms of unusual bleeding or bruising (bleeding gums; nosebleed; black, tarry stools; hematuria; excessive menstrual flow). Notify health care professional if these occur.

- *High Alert:* Instruct patient not to drink alcohol or take OTC medications, especially those containing aspirin or NSAIDs, or to start or stop any new medications during warfarin therapy without advice of health care professional.
- *High Alert:* Emphasize the importance of frequent lab tests to monitor coagulation factors.
- Instruct patient to carry identification describing medication regimen at all times and to inform all health care personnel caring for patient on anticoagulant therapy before lab tests, treatment, or surgery.

## EVALUATION

**Clinical response to therapy can be evaluated by:** ■ Prolonged PT (1.3–2.0 times the control; may vary with indication) or INR of 2–4.5 without signs of hemorrhage.

# zaleplon

(za-**lep**-lon)

Sonata

**CLASSIFICATION(S):**
*Therapeutic: sedative/hypnotics*

**Schedule IV**

**Pregnancy Category C**

## INDICATIONS

■ Short-term management of insomnia in patients unable to get at least 4 hours of sleep; especially useful in sleep initiation disorders.

## ACTION

■ Produces CNS depression by binding to GABA receptors in the CNS ■ Has no analgesic properties. **Therapeutic Effects:** ■ Sedation and induction of sleep.

## PHARMACOKINETICS

**Absorption:** Rapidly absorbed following oral administration.

**Distribution:** Enters breast milk.

**Metabolism and Excretion:** Extensively metabolized in the liver (mostly by aldehyde oxidase and some by CYP 450 3A4 enzymes).

**Half-life:** Unknown.

## CONTRAINDICATIONS AND PRECAUTIONS

**Contraindicated in:** ■ Hypersensitivity ■ Not recommended for use during pregnancy, lactation, or in patients with severe hepatic impairment.

**Use Cautiously in:** ■ Mild to moderate hepatic impairment, age ≥65 yr or weight ≤50 kg or concurrent cimetidine therapy (initiate therapy at lowest dose) ■ Impaired respiratory function ■ History of suicide attempt ■ Children <18 yr (safety not established).

## ADVERSE REACTIONS AND SIDE EFFECTS*

■ **CNS:** amnesia, anxiety, depersonalization, dizziness, drowsiness, hallucinations, headache, impaired memory (briefly following dose), impaired psychomotor function (briefly following dose), malaise, vertigo, weakness ■ **EENT:** abnormal vision, ear pain, epistaxis, hearing sensitivity, ocular pain, altered sense of smell ■ **CV:** peripheral edema ■ **GI:** abdominal pain, anorexia, colitis, dyspepsia, nausea ■ **GU:** dysmenorrhea ■ **Derm:** photosensitivity ■ **Neuro:** hyperesthesia, paresthesia, tremor ■ **Misc:** fever.

## INTERACTIONS

**Drug-Drug:** ■ **Cimetidine** decreases metabolism and increases effects (initiate therapy at a lower dose) ■ Additive CNS depression with other **CNS depressants** including **alcohol, antihistamines, opioid analgesics,** other **sedative/hypnotics, phenothiazines,** and **tricyclic antidepressants** ■ Effects may be decreased by drugs that induce the CYP 450 3A4 enzyme system including **rifampin, phenytoin, carbamazepine,** and **phenobarbital**.

**Drug-Natural Products:** ■ Concomitant use of **kava, valerian, skullcap, chamomile,** or **hops** can increase CNS depression.

**Drug-Food:** ■ Concurrent ingestion of a **high-fat meal** slows the rate of absorption.

## ROUTE AND DOSAGE

■ **PO (Adults <65 yr):** 10 mg (range 5–20 mg) at bedtime.

■ **PO (Geriatric Patients or Patients <50 kg):** Initiate therapy at 5 mg at bedtime (not to exceed 10 mg at bedtime).

❏ **Hepatic Impairment**

■ **PO (Adults):** Initiate therapy at 5 mg at bedtime (not to exceed 10 mg at bedtime).

## AVAILABILITY

■ ***Capsules:*** 5 mg$^{Rx}$, 10 mg$^{Rx}$ ■ Cost: 5 mg $181.60/100, 10 mg $223.38/100.

TIME/ACTION PROFILE

|    | ONSET | PEAK | DURATION |
|----|-------|------|----------|
| PO | within minutes | unknown | 3–4 hr |

# NURSING IMPLICATIONS

## ASSESSMENT

❏ Assess mental status, sleep patterns, and potential for abuse prior to administering this medication. Prolonged use of >7–10 days may lead to physical and psychological dependence. Limit amount of drug available to the patient.

□ Assess alertness at time of peak effect. Notify physician or other health care professional if desired sedation does not occur.

□ Assess patient for pain. Medicate as needed. Untreated pain decreases sedative effects.

## POTENTIAL NURSING DIAGNOSES

■ Sleep pattern disturbed (Indications).

■ Injury, risk for (Side Effects).

## IMPLEMENTATION

■ **General:** Before administering, reduce external stimuli and provide comfort measures to increase effectiveness of medication.

□ Protect patient from injury. Supervise ambulation and transfer of patients after administration. Remove cigarettes. Side rails should be raised and call bell within reach at all times.

■ **PO:** Tablets should be swallowed whole with full glass of water immediately before bedtime or after going to bed and experiencing difficulty falling asleep. Do not administer with or immediately after a high-fat or heavy meal.

## PATIENT/FAMILY TEACHING

□ Instruct patient to take zaleplon exactly as directed. Do not take more than the amount prescribed because of the habit-forming potential. Not recommended for use longer than 7–10 days. Rebound insomnia (1–2 nights) may occur when stopped. If used for 2 wk or longer, abrupt withdrawal may result in dysphoria, insomnia, abdominal or muscle cramps, vomiting, sweating, tremors, and seizures.

□ Because of rapid onset, advise patient to go to bed immediately after taking zaleplon.

□ May cause daytime drowsiness or dizziness. Advise patient to avoid driving or other activities requiring alertness until response to this medication is known.

□ Inform patient that amnesia may occur, but can be avoided if zaleplon is only taken when patient is able to get >4 hr sleep.

□ Caution patient to avoid concurrent use of alcohol or other CNS depressants.

## EVALUATION

**Effectiveness of therapy can be demonstrated by:** ■ Relief of insomnia.

## zanamivir

(za-**na**-mi-veer)

Relenza

### CLASSIFICATION(S):

**Therapeutic:** antivirals

**Pharmacologic:** neuramidase inhibitors

### Pregnancy Category C

## INDICATIONS

■ Treatment of uncomplicated acute illness caused by influenza virus in adults and children ≥7 yr who have been symptomatic no more than 2 days.

## ACTION

■ Inhibits the enzyme neuramidase, which may alter virus particle aggregation and release. **Therapeutic Effects:** ■ Reduced duration of flu-related symptoms.

## PHARMACOKINETICS

**Absorption:** 4–17% of inhaled dose is systemically absorbed.

**Distribution:** Unknown.

**Protein Binding:** <10%.

**Metabolism and Excretion:** Mainly excreted by kidneys as unchanged drug; unabsorbed drug is excreted in feces.

**Half-life:** 2.5–5.1 hr.

## CONTRAINDICATIONS AND PRECAUTIONS

**Contraindicated in:** ■ Hypersensitivity.

**Use Cautiously in:** ■ Chronic obstructive pulmonary disease or asthma (increased risk of decreased lung function and/or bronchospasm) ■ Pregnancy, lactation, or children <12 yr (safety not established).

## ADVERSE REACTIONS AND SIDE EFFECTS*

■ **Resp:** bronchospasm.

## INTERACTIONS

**Drug-Drug:** ■ None noted.

## ROUTE AND DOSAGE

■ **Inhaln (Adults and children ≥7 yr):** 2 inhalations of 5 mg each for a total dose of 10 mg twice daily for 5 days via the DISK-HALER inhalation device.

## AVAILABILITY

■ *Powder for inhalation:* 5 mg/blister^Rx ■ Cost: $44.40/20.

TIME/ACTION PROFILE (blood levels)

| | ONSET | PEAK | DURATION |
|---|---|---|---|
| Inhalation | rapid | 1–2 hr | 12 hr |

## NURSING IMPLICATIONS

### ASSESSMENT

❑ Assess patient for signs and symptoms of influenza (fever, headache, myalgia, cough, sore throat) before administration. Determine duration of symptoms. Indicated for patients who have been symptomatic for up to 2 days.

### POTENTIAL NURSING DIAGNOSES

■ Infection, risk for (Indications).

### IMPLEMENTATION

**Inhaln:** Administer 2 doses on the first day of treatment whenever possible; must have at least 2 hours between doses. Doses should be administered 12 hr apart on subsequent days.

### PATIENT/FAMILY TEACHING

❑ Instruct patient to use zanamivir exactly as directed and to finish entire 5-day course, even if feeling better.

❑ Instruct patient in the use of the DISKHALER. Patient should read the accompanying Patient Instructions for Use.

❑ Advise patients that zanamivir is not a substitute for a flu shot. Patients should receive annual flu shot according to immunization guidelines.

❑ Patients with a history of asthma should be advised to have a fast-acting inhaled bronchodilator available in case of bronchospasm following zanamivir administration. If using bronchodilator and zanamivir concurrently, administer bronchodilator first.

## EVALUATION

**Clinical response to therapy can be evaluated by:** ■ Decrease in signs and symptoms of influenza (fever, headache, myalgia, cough, sore throat).

## zidovudine

(zye-**doe**-vue-deen)

{Apo-Zidovudine}, azidothymidine, AZT, {Novo-AZT}, Retrovir

### CLASSIFICATION(S):

**Therapeutic:** antiretrovirals
**Pharmacologic:** nucleoside reverse transcriptase inhibitors

### Pregnancy Category C

### INDICATIONS

■ HIV infection (with other antiretrovirals) ■ Reduction of maternal/fetal transmission of HIV.

### ACTION

■ Following intracellular conversion to its active form, inhibits viral RNA synthesis by inhibiting the enzyme DNA polymerase (reverse transcriptase) ■ Prevents viral replication. **Therapeutic Effects:** ■ Virustatic action against selected retroviruses ■ Slowed progression and decreased sequelae of HIV infection ■ Decreased viral load and improved CD4 cell counts ■ Decreased transmission of HIV to infants born to HIV-infected mothers.

### PHARMACOKINETICS

**Absorption:** Well absorbed following oral administration.

**Distribution:** Widely distributed; enters the CNS. Crosses the placenta.

**Metabolism and Excretion:** Mostly (75%) metabolized by the liver; 15–20% excreted unchanged by the kidneys.

**Half-life:** 1 hr.

### CONTRAINDICATIONS AND PRECAUTIONS

**Contraindicated in:** ■ Hypersensitivity ■ Lactation.

**Use Cautiously in:** ■ Decreased bone marrow reserve (dosage reduction required for anemia or granulocytopenia) ■ Severe hepatic or renal disease (dosage modification may be required).

## ADVERSE REACTIONS AND SIDE EFFECTS*

■ **CNS:** SEIZURES, headache, weakness, anxiety, confusion, decreased mental acuity, dizziness, insomnia, mental depression, restlessness, syncope ■ **GI:** abdominal pain, diarrhea, nausea, anorexia, drug-induced hepatitis, dyspepsia, oral mucosa pigmentation, vomiting ■ **Derm:** nail pigmentation ■ **Endo:** gynecomastia ■ **Hemat:** anemia, granulocytopenia, pure red-cell aplasia, thrombocytosis ■ **MS:** back pain, myopathy ■ **Neuro:** tremor.

## INTERACTIONS

**Drug-Drug:** ■ ↑ bone marrow depression with other **agents having bone marrow–depressing properties,** antineoplastics, **radiation therapy,** or **ganciclovir** ■ ↑ neurotoxicity may occur with **acyclovir** ■ Toxicity may be ↑ by concurrent administration of **probenecid** or **fluconazole** ■ Zidovudine levels are ↓ by **clarithromycin.**

## ROUTE AND DOSAGE

❑ **Management of HIV Infection**
■ **PO (Adults and Children >13 yr):** 100 mg q 4 hr while awake or 200 mg 3 times daily or 300 mg twice daily (depends on combination and clinical situation).
■ **PO (Children 3 mo–12 yr):** 90–180 mg/m² every 6 hr (not to exceed 200 mg q 6 hr).
■ **IV (Adults and Children >12 yr):** 1 mg/kg infused over 1 hr q 4 hr. Change to oral therapy as soon as possible.
■ **IV (Children):** 120 mg/m² q 6 hr (not to exceed 160 mg/dose).

❑ **Prevention of Maternal/Fetal Transmission of HIV Infection**
■ **PO (Adults >14 wk Pregnant):** 100 mg 5 times daily until onset of labor.
■ **IV (Adults during Labor and Delivery):** 2 mg/kg over 1 hr, then continuous infusion of 1 mg/kg/hr until umbilical cord is clamped.
■ **IV (Infants):** 1.5 mg/kg q 6 hr until able to take PO.
■ **PO (Infants):** 2 mg/kg q 6 hr, started within 12 hr of birth and continued for 6 wk.

## AVAILABILITY

■ **Capsules:** 100 mg^Rx, 300 mg^Rx ■ Cost: 100 mg $196.94/100 ■ **Oral syrup:** 50 mg/5 ml^Rx ■ Cost: $47.27/240 ml ■ **Injection:** 200 mg/20 ml^Rx ■ Cost: $213.04/10 vials ■ lamivudine (Combivir^Rx; see Appendix B).

TIME/ACTION PROFILE (blood levels)

|  | ONSET | PEAK | DURATION |
|---|---|---|---|
| PO | unknown | 0.5–1.5 hr | 4 hr |
| IV | rapid | end of infusion | 4 hr |

## NURSING IMPLICATIONS

### ASSESSMENT

❑ Assess patient for change in severity of symptoms of HIV and for symptoms of opportunistic infections during therapy.
■ **Lab Test Considerations:** Monitor viral load and CD4 counts prior to and periodically during therapy.
❑ Monitor CBC every 2 wk during the first 8 wk of therapy in patients with advanced HIV disease, and decrease to every 4 wk after the first 2 mo if zidovudine is well tolerated or monthly during the first 3 mo and every 3 mo thereafter unless indicated in patients who are asymptomatic or have early symptoms. Commonly causes granulocytopenia and anemia. Anemia may occur 2–4 wk after initiation of therapy. Anemia may respond to epoetin administration (see epoetin monograph). Granulocytopenia usually occurs after 6–8 wk of therapy. Consider dose reduction, discontinuation of therapy, or blood transfusions if hemoglobin is <7.5 g/dl or reduction of >25% from baseline and/or granulocyte count is <750/mm³ or reduction of >50% from baseline. Treatment with sargramostim may be necessary (see sargramostim monograph). Therapy may be gradually resumed when bone marrow recovery is evident.

### POTENTIAL NURSING DIAGNOSES

■ Infection, risk for (Indications, Side Effects).

### IMPLEMENTATION

■ **General:** Do not confuse Retonavir (zidovudine) with Ritonavir.
❑ Administer doses around the clock.

- **IV:** Patient should receive the IV infusion only until oral therapy can be administered.
- **Intermittent Infusion:** Remove the calculated dose from the vial and dilute with D5W or 0.9% NaCl for concentration of <4 mg/ml. Do not use solutions that are discolored. Stable for 8 hr at room temperature or 24 hr if refrigerated.
- *Rate:* Infuse at a constant rate over 1 hr. Avoid rapid infusion or bolus injection.
- **Y-Site Compatibility:** ◆ acyclovir ◆ allopurinol ◆ amifostine ◆ amikacin ◆ amphotericin B ◆ amphotericin B cholesteryl sulfate ◆ aztreonam ◆ cefepime ◆ ceftazidine ◆ ceftriaxone ◆ cimetidine ◆ cisatracurium ◆ clindamycin ◆ dobutamine ◆ docetaxel ◆ dopamine ◆ doxorubicin liposome ◆ erythromycin lactobionate ◆ etoposide phosphate ◆ filgrastim ◆ fluconazole ◆ fludarabine ◆ gatifloxacin ◆ gemcitabine ◆ gentamicin ◆ granisetron ◆ heparin ◆ imipenem/cilastatin ◆ linezolid ◆ lorazepam ◆ melphalan ◆ metoclopramide ◆ morphine ◆ nafcillin ◆ ondansetron ◆ oxacillin ◆ paclitaxel ◆ pentamidine ◆ phenylephrine ◆ piperacillin ◆ piperacillin/tazbactam ◆ potassium chloride ◆ ranitidine ◆ remifentanil ◆ sargramostim ◆ teniposide ◆ thiotepa ◆ tobramycin ◆ trimethoprim/sulfamethoxazole ◆ trimetrexate ◆ vancomycin ◆ vinorelbine.
- **Additive Incompatibility:** blood products or protein solutions.

## PATIENT/FAMILY TEACHING

- ❏ Instruct patient to take zidovudine as directed, around the clock, even if sleep is interrupted. Emphasize the importance of compliance with therapy, not taking more than prescribed amount, and not discontinuing without consulting health care professional. Take missed doses as soon as remembered unless almost time for next dose; do not double doses. Inform patient that long-term effects of zidovudine are unknown at this time.
- ❏ Instruct patient that zidovudine should not be shared with others.
- ❏ Zidovudine may cause dizziness or fainting. Caution patient to avoid driving or other activities requiring alertness until response to medication is known.
- ❏ Inform patient that zidovudine does not cure HIV and does not reduce the risk of transmission of HIV to others through sexual contact or blood contamination. Caution patient to use a condom during sexual contact and avoid sharing needles or donating blood to prevent spreading the AIDS virus to others.
- ❏ Instruct patient to notify health care professional promptly if fever, sore throat, or signs of infection occur. Caution patient to avoid crowds and persons with known infections. Instruct patient to use soft toothbrush, to use caution when using toothpicks or dental floss, and to have dental work done prior to therapy or deferred until blood counts return to normal. Patient should also notify health care professional if shortness of breath, muscle aches, symptoms of hepatitis or pancreatitis, or other unexpected reactions occur.
- ❏ Advise patient to avoid taking any RX or OTC medications or herbal products without consulting health care professional.
- ❏ Emphasize the importance of regular follow-up exams and blood counts to determine progress and monitor for side effects.

## EVALUATION

**Effectiveness of therapy can be demonstrated by:** ■ Decrease in viral load and increase in CD4 counts in patients with HIV ■ Delayed progression of AIDS and decreased opportunistic infections in patients with HIV.

---

# ziprasidone

(zi-**pra**-si-done)
Geodon

### CLASSIFICATION(S):
*Therapeutic:* antipsychotics
*Pharmacologic:* piperazine derivatives

### Pregnancy Category C

## INDICATIONS

- Schizophrenia; IM form is reserved for control of acutely agitated patients.

## ACTION

- Effects probably mediated by antagonism of dopamine type 2 (D2) and serotonin type 2 (5-

HT$_2$). Also antagonizes $\alpha_2$ adrenergic receptors. **Therapeutic Effects:** ▪ Dimished schizophrenic behavior.

## PHARMACOKINETICS

**Absorption:** 60% absorbed following oral administration; 100% absorbed from IM sites.

**Distribution:** Unknown.

**Protein Binding:** 99%; potential for drug interactions due to drug displacement is minimal.

**Metabolism and Excretion:** 99% metabolized by the liver; <1% excreted unchanged in urine.

**Half-life:** *PO*—7 hr; *IM*—2–5 hr.

## CONTRAINDICATIONS AND PRECAUTIONS

**Contraindicated in:** ▪ Hypersensitivity ▪ History of QT prolongation (persistent QTc measurements >500 msec), arrhythmias, recent MI or uncompensated heart failure ▪ Concurrent use of other drugs known to prolong the QT interval including quinidine, dofetilide, sotalol, other class Ia and III antiarrhythmics, pimozide, sotalol, thioridazine, mesoridazine, chlorpromazine, floquine, pentamadine, arsenic trioxide, halofantrine, mefloquine, dolasetron, tacrolimus, droperidol, gatifloxacin, moxifloxacin, and sparfloxacin ▪ Hypokalemia or hypomagnesemia ▪ Lactation.

**Use Cautiously in:** ▪ Concurrent diuretic therapy or diarrhea (may increase the risk of hypotension, hypokalemia, or hypomagnesemia) ▪ Patients with significant hepatic impairment ▪ History of cardiovascular or cerebrovascular disease ▪ Hypotension, concurrent antihypertensive therapy, dehydration, or hypovolemia (may ↑ risk of orthostatic hypotension) ▪ Alzheimer's dementia or age >65 yr (may ↑ risk of seizures) ▪ Patients at risk for aspiration pneumonia ▪ History of suicide attempt ▪ Geriatric patients (consider initiating therapy at lower dose) ▪ Pregnancy (use only if potential benefit outweighs potential risk to the fetus) ▪ Children <18 yr (safety not established).

## ADVERSE REACTIONS AND SIDE EFFECTS*

▪ **CNS:** NEUROLEPTIC MALIGNANT SYNDROME, seizures, dizziness, drowsiness, restlessness, extrapyramidal reactions, syncope, tardive dyskinesia ▪ **Resp:** cough/runny nose ▪ **CV:** PROLONGED QT INTERVAL, orthostatic hypotension ▪ **GI:** constipation, diarrhea, nausea, dysphagia ▪ **Derm:** rash, urticaria.

## INTERACTIONS

**Drug-Drug:** ▪ Concurrent use of **quinidine, dofetilide, sotalol, other class Ia and III antiarrhythmics, pimozide, thioridazine, mesoridazine, chlorpromazine, floquine, pentamadine, arsenic trioxide, halofantrine, mefloquine, dolasetron, tacrolimus, droperidol, gatifloxacin, moxifloxacin,** and **sparfloxacin** or other agents that prolong the QT interval may result in potentially life-threatening adverse drug reactions and is contraindicated. ▪ Additive CNS depression may occur with **alcohol, antidepressants, antihistamines, opioid analgesics,** or **sedative/hypnotics** ▪ Blood levels and effectiveness may be ↓ by **carbamazepine** ▪ Blood levels and effects may be ↑ by **ketoconazole.**

## ROUTE AND DOSAGE

▪ **PO (Adults):** 20 mg twice daily initially; dose increments may be made at 2-day intervals up to 80 mg twice daily.

▪ **IM (Adults):** 10–20 mg as needed up to 40 mg/day; may be given as 10 mg every 2 hr or 20 mg every 4 hr.

## AVAILABILITY

▪ *Capsules:* 20 mg$^{Rx}$, 40 mg$^{Rx}$, 60 mg$^{Rx}$, 80 mg$^{Rx}$ ▪ *Lyophilized powder for injection (requires reconstitution):* 20 mg/vial$^{Rx}$.

TIME/ACTION PROFILE (blood levels)

| | ONSET | PEAK | DURATION |
|---|---|---|---|
| PO | within hours | 1–3 days† | Unknown |
| IM | rapid | 60 min | Unknown |

†steady state achieved following continuous use.

## NURSING IMPLICATIONS

### ASSESSMENT

❑ Monitor patient's mental status (delusions, hallucinations, and behavior) prior to, and periodically during therapy.

❑ Monitor blood pressure (sitting, standing, lying) and pulse rate prior to and frequently during initial dosage titration. Patients found to have persistent QTc measurements of >500 msec should have ziprasidone discontinued. Patients who experience dizziness, paliptations, or syncope may require further evaluation (i.e., Holter monitoring).

- Assess patient for rash during therapy. May be treated with antihistamines or corticosteroids. Usually resolves upon discontinuation of ziprasidone. Medication should be discontinued if no alternative etiology for rash is found.

- Observe patient carefully when administering medication to ensure medication is actually taken and not hoarded.

- Monitor patient for onset of akathisia (restlessness or desire to keep moving) and extrapyramidal side effects (*parkinsonian*— difficulty speaking or swallowing, loss of balance control, pill rolling, mask-like face, shuffling gait, rigidity, tremors and dystonic muscle spasms, twisting motions, twitching, inability to move eyes, weakness of arms or legs) every 2 mo during therapy and 8–12 wk after therapy has been discontinued. Notify physician or other health care professional if these symptoms occur, as reduction in dose or discontinuation of medication may be necessary. Trihexyphenidyl or diphenhydramine may be used to control these symptoms.

- Although not yet reported for ziprasidone, monitor for possible tardive dyskinesia (uncontrolled rhythmic movement of mouth, face, and extremities, lip smacking or puckering, puffing of cheeks, uncontrolled chewing, rapid or worm-like movements of tongue). Report these symptoms immediately; may be irreversible.

- Monitor frequency and consistency of bowel movements. Increasing bulk and fluids in the diet may help to minimize constipation.

- Ziprasidone lowers the seizure threshold. Institute seizure precautions for patients with history of seizure disorder.

- Monitor for development of neuroleptic malignant syndrome (fever, respiratory distress, tachycardia, seizures, diaphoresis, hypertension or hypotension, pallor, tiredness). Notify physician immediately if these symptoms occur.

- **Lab Test Considerations:** Monitor serum potassium and magnesium prior to and periodically during therapy. Patients with low potassium or magnesium should have levels treated and check prior to resuming therapy.

## POTENTIAL NURSING DIAGNOSES

- Violence, risk for other-directed (Indications).
- Thought processes, disturbed (Indications).
- Injury, risk for (Side Effects).

## IMPLEMENTATION

- **General:** Dosage adjustments should be made at intervals of no less than 2 days. Usually patients should be observed for several weeks before dose titration.
- Patients on parenteral therapy should be converted to oral doses as soon as possible.
- **PO:** Administer capsules with food or milk to decrease gastric irritation. Capsules should be swallowed whole; do not open.

## PATIENT/FAMILY TEACHING

- Instruct patient to take medication as directed. Do not discontinue medication without discussing with health care professional, even if feeling well. Patients on long-term therapy may need to discontinue gradually.
- Inform patient of possibility of extrapyramidal symptoms. Instruct patient to report these symptoms immediately.
- Advise patient to change positions slowly to minimize orthostatic hypotension.
- May cause seizures and drowsiness. Caution patient to avoid driving or other activities requiring alertness until response to medication is known.
- Caution patient to avoid concurrent use of alcohol, other CNS depressants, OTC medications, and herbal/alternative products without consulting health care professional.
- Advise patient to notify health care professional of medication regimen prior to treatment or surgery.
- Instruct patient to notify health care professional promptly if dizziness, loss of consciousness, or palpitations occur or if pregnancy is planned or suspected.
- Advise patient of need for continued medical follow-up for psychotherapy, eye exams, and laboratory tests.

## EVALUATION

**Effectiveness of therapy can be demonstrated by:** ■ Diminished schizophrenic behaviors (hearing voices, seeing things, sensing things that are not there, mistaken beliefs, unusual suspiciousness, becoming withdrawn from family and friends).

# zoledronic acid

(zoe-led-**dron**-ic **as**-id)
Zometa

## CLASSIFICATION(S):

*Therapeutic: bone resorption inhibitors, electrolyte modifiers, hypocalcemics*
*Pharmacologic: biphosphonates*

## Pregnancy Category C

## INDICATIONS

■ Hypercalcemia of malignancy ■ Multiple myeloma and metastatic bone lesions from solid tumors.

## ACTION

■ Inhibits bone resorption ■ Inhibits increased osteoclast activity and skeletal calcium release induced by tumors. **Therapeutic Effects:** ■ Decreased serum calcium.

## PHARMACOKINETICS

**Absorption:** IV administration results in complete bioavailability.
**Distribution:** Unknown.
**Metabolism and Excretion:** Mostly excreted unchanged by the kidneys.
**Half-life:** 167 hr.

## CONTRAINDICATIONS AND PRECAUTIONS

**Contraindicated in:** ■ Hypersensitivity to zoledronic acid or other biphosphonates.
**Use Cautiously in:** ■ Renal impairment (if serum creatinine ≥4.5 use only if potential benefits outweigh risks of further deterioration in renal function) ■ History of aspirin-induced asthma ■ Concurrent use of loop diuretics or dehydration (correct deficits prior to use) ■ Pregnancy, lactation, or children (safety not established).

## ADVERSE REACTIONS AND SIDE EFFECTS*

■ **CNS:** agitation, anxiety, confusion, insomnia ■ **EENT:** conjunctivitis ■ **CV:** hypotension, chest pain, leg edema ■ **GI:** abdominal pain, constipation, diarrhea, nausea, vomiting, dysphagia ■ **GU:** renal failure ■ **Derm:** pruritus, rash ■ **F and E:** hypophosphatemia, hypocalcemia, hypokalemia, hypomagnesemia ■ **Hemat:** anemia ■ **MS:** skeletal pain ■ **Misc:** fever, flu-like syndrome.

## INTERACTIONS

**Drug-Drug:** ■ Concurrent use of **loop diuretics** or **aminoglycosides** ↑ risk of hypocalcemia.

## ROUTE AND DOSAGE

■ **IV (Adults):** *Hypercalcemia of malignancy*—4 mg, may be repeated after 7 days; *Multiple myeloma and bone metastases from solid tumors*—4 mg every 3–4 wk (has been used for up to 15 mo).

## AVAILABILITY

■ *Powder for reconstitution for IV infusion:* 4 mg/vial^Rx.

TIME/ACTION PROFILE (effect on serum calcium)

| | ONSET | PEAK | DURATION |
|---|---|---|---|
| IV | within 4 days | 4-7 days | 30 days |

# NURSING IMPLICATIONS

## ASSESSMENT

❑ Monitor symptoms of hypercalcemia (nausea, vomiting, anorexia, weakness, constipation, thirst, cardiac arrhythmias).
❑ Observe for evidence of hypocalcemia (paresthesia, muscle twitching, laryngospasm, Chvostek's or Trousseau's sign).
❑ Monitor intake and output ratios. Vigorous saline hydration should be initiated promptly and a urine output of 2 L/day should be maintained during therapy. Patients should be adequately hydrated, but avoid overhydration. Do not use diuretics prior to treatment of hypovolemia.
■ *Lab Test Considerations:* Monitor renal function during therapy. Patients with a normal serum creatinine prior to treatment, who develop an increase of 0.5 mg/dL within 2

wks of next dose should have next dose withheld until serum creatinine is within 10% of
baseline value. Patients with an abnormal
serum creatinine prior to treatment who
have an increase of 1.0 mg/dL within 2 wks
of next dose should have next dose withheld
until serum creatinine is within 10% of baseline value.

❏ Assess serum calcium, phosphate, and magnesium before and periodically during therapy. If hypocalcemia, hypophosphatemia, or
hypomagnesemia occur, temporary supplementation may be required.

❏ Monitor CBC with differential and hemoglobin and hematocrit closely during therapy.

## POTENTIAL NURSING DIAGNOSES

■ Injury, risk for (Indications).

## IMPLEMENTATION

■ **General:** Vigorous saline hydration alone
may be sufficient to treat mild, asymptomatic
hypercalcemia. Adequate rehydration is required prior to administration.

❏ Patients on long term therapy should have
500 mg or oral calcium and a multivitamin
with 400 units of vitamin D each day.

■ **Intermittent Infusion:** Reconstitute by
adding 5 ml of sterile water for infection to
each vial for a solution containing 4 mg of
zoledronic acid. Medication must be completely dissolved prior to withdrawal of solution. Do not administer solution that is discolored or contains particulate matter. Dilute
4 mg dose further with 100 ml of 0.9% NaCl
or D5W. If not used immediately, may be
refrigerated for up to 24 hr.

■ *Rate:* Administer as a single infusion of not
more than 4 mg and over at least 15 min.
Rapid infusions increase risk of renal deterioration and renal failure.

■ **Y-Site Incompatibility:** Do not mix with
solutions containing calcium, such as Lactated Ringer's solution. Administer as a single
infusion in a line separate from all other
drugs.

## PATIENT/FAMILY TEACHING

❏ Explain the purpose of zoledronic acid to
patient.

❏ Advise patients of the importance of adequate
hydration.

❏ Emphasize the importance of lab tests to
monitor progress.

## EVALUATION

**Effectiveness of therapy can be demon-
strated by:** ■ Decrease in serum calcium.

## zolmitriptan

(zole-mi-**trip**-tan)
Zomig, Zomig- ZMT

### CLASSIFICATION(S):

**Therapeutic:** *vascular headache
suppressants*
**Pharmacologic:** *5 HT₁ agonists*

### Pregnancy Category C

## INDICATIONS

■ Acute treatment of migraine headache.

## ACTION

■ Acts as an agonist at specific 5-HT₁receptor
sites in intracranial blood vessels and sensory
trigeminal nerves. **Therapeutic Effects:** ■ Cranial vessel vasoconstriction with resultant decrease in migraine headache.

## PHARMACOKINETICS

**Absorption:** Well absorbed (40%) following
oral administration.
**Distribution:** Unknown.
**Metabolism and Excretion:** Mostly metabolized by the liver; some conversion to metabolites that are more active than zolmitriptan. 8%
excreted unchanged in urine.
**Half-life:** 3 hr (for zolmitriptan and active
metabolite).

## CONTRAINDICATIONS AND PRECAUTIONS

**Contraindicated in:** ■ Hypersensitivity ■ Significant underlying heart disease (including ischemic heart disease, history of MI, coronary
artery vasospasm, uncontrolled hypertension) ■
Concurrent (or within 24 hr) use of other 5-HT
agonists, ergotamine, or ergot-type medications

■ Concurrent (or within 2 wk) use of MAO inhibitors ■ Hemiplegic or basilar migraine ■ Symptomatic Wolff-Parkinson-White syndrome or other arrhythmias.

**Use Cautiously in:** ■ Cardiovascular risk factors (hypertension, hypercholesterolemia, cigarette smoking, obesity, diabetes, strong family history, menopausal females or males >40 yr [use only if cardiovascular status has been evaluated and determined to be safe and first dose is administered under supervision]) ■ Hepatic impairment (use lower doses) ■ Pregnancy, lactation, or children (safety not established).

## ADVERSE REACTIONS AND SIDE EFFECTS*

■ **CNS:** dizziness, drowsiness, vertigo, weakness ■ **EENT:** throat pain/tightness/pressure ■ **CV:** chest pain/pressure/tightness/heaviness, hypertension, palpitations ■ **GI:** dry mouth, dyspepsia, dysphagia, nausea ■ **Derm:** sweating, warm/cold sensation ■ **MS:** myalgia, myasthenia ■ **Neuro:** hypesthesia, paresthesia ■ **Misc:** feeling of heaviness, pain.

## INTERACTIONS

**Drug-Drug:** ■ Because of increased risk of cerebral vasospasm, avoid concurrent use of other **5-HT agonists (naratriptan, sumatriptan, rizatriptan)** and/or **ergot-type preparations (dihydroergotamine)** ■ Concurrent use of **MAO inhibitors** increases blood level and risk of toxicity (avoid use within 2 wk of MAO inhibitors) ■ Blood levels may be increased by **hormonal contraceptives** ■ May increase the risk of adverse reactions with **SSRI antidepressants** ■ **Cimetidine** increases half-life of zolmitriptan and its active metabolite ■ Concurrent use with **SSRI antidepressants** may result in weakness, hyperreflexia and incoordination.

**Drug-Natural Products:** ■ Increased risk of serotinergic side effects including serotonin syndrome with **St. John's wort** and **SAMe**.

## ROUTE AND DOSAGE

■ **PO (Adults):** 2.5 mg or less initially; if headache returns, dose may be repeated after 2 hr (not to exceed 10 mg/24 hr).

## AVAILABILITY

■ *Tablets:* 2.5 mg^Rx, 5 mg^Rx ■ *Orally disintegrating tablets:* 2.5 mg^Rx, 5 mg^Rx.

TIME/ACTION PROFILE (relief of headache)

| | ONSET | PEAK | DURATION |
|---|---|---|---|
| PO | unknown | 2 hr | unknown |

# NURSING IMPLICATIONS

## ASSESSMENT

❑ Assess pain location, intensity, duration, and associated symptoms (photophobia, phonophobia, nausea, vomiting) during migraine attack.

## POTENTIAL NURSING DIAGNOSES

■ Pain, acute (Indications).

## IMPLEMENTATION

■ **General:** Do not confuse zolmitriptan with sumatriptan.

■ **PO:** Initial dose is 2.5 mg. Lower doses can be achieved by breaking 2.5-mg tablet.

❑ Orally disintegrating tablets should be left in the package until use. Remove from the blister pouch. Do not push tablet through the blister; peel open the blister pack with dry hands and place tablet on tongue. Tablet will dissolve rapidly and be swallowed with saliva. No liquid is needed to take the orally disintegrating tablet.

## PATIENT/FAMILY TEACHING

■ **General Info:** Inform patient that zolmitriptan should be used only during a migraine attack. It is meant to be used to relieve migraine attack but not to prevent or reduce the number of attacks.

❑ Instruct patient to administer zolmitriptan as soon as symptoms appear, but it may be administered any time during an attack. If migraine symptoms return, a second dose may be used. Allow at least 2 hr between doses, and do not use more than 10 mg in any 24-hr period.

❑ If dose does not relieve headache, additional zolmitriptan doses are not likely to be effective; notify health care professional.

❑ Advise patient that lying down in a darkened room following zolmitriptan administration may further help relieve headache.

❑ Caution patient not to use zolmitriptan if she is pregnant, suspects she is pregnant, plans to become pregnant, or is breastfeeding. Adequate contraception should be used during therapy.

❑ May cause dizziness or drowsiness. Caution patient to avoid driving or other activities requiring alertness until response to medication is known.

❑ Advise patient to notify health care professional prior to next dose of zolmitriptan if pain or tightness in the chest occurs during use. If pain is severe or does not subside, notify health care professional immediately. If wheezing; heart throbbing; swelling of eyelids, face, or lips; skin rash; skin lumps; or hives occur, notify health care professional immediately and do not take more zolmitriptan without approval of health care professional. If feelings of tingling, heat, flushing, heaviness, pressure, drowsiness, dizziness, tiredness, or sickness develop, discuss with health care professional at next visit.

❑ Advise patient to avoid alcohol, which aggravates headaches, during zolmitriptan use.

## EVALUATION

**Effectiveness of therapy can be demonstrated by:** ■ Relief of migraine attack.

---

## zolpidem
(**zole**-pi-dem)
Ambien

*CLASSIFICATION(S):*
*Therapeutic:* sedative/hypnotics

**Pregnancy Category B**

---

## INDICATIONS

■ Insomnia.

## ACTION

■ Produces CNS depression by binding to GABA receptors ■ Has no analgesic properties. **Therapeutic Effects:** ■ Sedation and induction of sleep.

## PHARMACOKINETICS

**Absorption:** Rapidly absorbed following oral administration.

**Distribution:** Minimal amounts enter breast milk; remainder of distribution not known.

**Metabolism and Excretion:** Converted to inactive metabolites, which are excreted by the kidneys.

**Half-life:** 2.5–2.6 hr (increased in geriatric patients and patients with hepatic impairment).

## CONTRAINDICATIONS AND PRECAUTIONS

**Contraindicated in:** ■ Hypersensitivity ■ Sleep apnea.

**Use Cautiously in:** ■ History of previous psychiatric illness, suicide attempt, drug or alcohol abuse ■ Geriatric patients and patients with impaired hepatic function (initial dosage reduction recommended) ■ Patients with pulmonary disease ■ Pregnancy, lactation, or children (safety not established).

## ADVERSE REACTIONS AND SIDE EFFECTS*

■ **CNS:** amnesia, daytime drowsiness, dizziness, "drugged" feeling ■ **GI:** diarrhea, nausea, vomiting ■ **Misc:** hypersensitivity reactions, physical dependence, psychological dependence, tolerance.

## INTERACTIONS

**Drug-Drug:** ■ ↑ CNS depression may with **sedative/hypnotics, alcohol, phenothiazines, tricyclic antidepressants, opioid analgesics,** or **antihistamines**.

**Drug-Natural Products:** ■ Concomitant use of **kava, valerian** or **chamomile** can ↑ CNS depression.

**Drug-Food:** ■ **Food** ↓ and delays absorption.

## ROUTE AND DOSAGE

■ **PO (Adults):** 10 mg at bedtime.

■ **PO (Geriatric Patients, Debilitated Patients, or Patients with Hepatic Impairment):** 5 mg at bedtime initially; may be increased to 10 mg.

## AVAILABILITY (generic available)

■ *Tablets:* 5 mg$^{Rx}$, 10 mg$^{Rx}$ ■ Cost: 5 mg $207.56/100, 10 mg $255.30/100.

TIME/ACTION PROFILE (sedation)

| | ONSET | PEAK | DURATION |
|---|---|---|---|
| PO | rapid | 30 min–2 hr | 6–8 hr |

## NURSING IMPLICATIONS

### ASSESSMENT

❑ Assess mental status, sleep patterns, and potential for abuse prior to administration. Prolonged use of >7–10 days may lead to physical and psychological dependence. Limit amount of drug available to the patient.

❑ Assess alertness at time of peak effect. Notify physician or other health care professional if desired sedation does not occur.

❑ Assess patient for pain. Medicate as needed. Untreated pain decreases sedative effects.

### POTENTIAL NURSING DIAGNOSES

■ Sleep pattern disturbed (Indications).

■ Injury, risk for (Side Effects).

### IMPLEMENTATION

■ **General:** Before administering, reduce external stimuli and provide comfort measures to increase effectiveness of medication.

❑ Protect patient from injury. Raise bed side rails. Assist with ambulation. Take patient's cigarettes.

■ **PO:** Tablets should be swallowed whole with full glass of water. For faster onset of sleep, do not administer with or immediately after a meal.

### PATIENT/FAMILY TEACHING

❑ Instruct patient to take zolpidem as directed. Do not take more than the amount prescribed because of the habit-forming potential. Not recommended for use longer than 7–10 days. If used for 2 wk or longer, abrupt withdrawal may result in fatigue, nausea, flushing, light-headedness, uncontrolled crying, vomiting, GI upset, panic attack, or nervousness.

❑ Because of rapid onset, advise patient to go to bed immediately after taking zolpidem.

❑ May cause daytime drowsiness or dizziness. Advise patient to avoid driving or other activities requiring alertness until response to this medication is known.

❑ Caution patient to avoid concurrent use of alcohol or other CNS depressants.

## EVALUATION

Effectiveness of therapy can be demonstrated by: ■ Relief of insomnia.

---

# zonisamide
(zoe-**niss**-a-mide)
Zonegran

## CLASSIFICATION(S):
**Therapeutic:** anticonvulsants
**Pharmacologic:** sulfonamides

## Pregnancy Category C

---

### INDICATIONS

■ Partial seizures in adults.

### ACTION

■ Raises the threshold for seizures and reduces duration of seizures probably by action on sodium and calcium channels. **Therapeutic Effects:** ■ Decreased frequency of partial seizures.

### PHARMACOKINETICS

**Absorption:** Well absorbed following oral administration.

**Distribution:** Binds extensively to red blood cells.

**Metabolism and Excretion:** Mostly metabolized by the liver; 35% excreted unchanged in urine. Some metabolism occurs via CYP3A4 enzyme system.

**Half-life:** 63 hr (plasma).

### CONTRAINDICATIONS AND PRECAUTIONS

**Contraindicated in:** ■ Hypersensitivity to zonisamide or sulfonamides.

**Use Cautiously in:** ■ Hepatic or renal disease (may require slower titration/more frequent monitoring) ■ Pregnancy or lactation (use only if potential benefit justifies risk to fetus/infant) ■ Children ≤16 yr (safety not established; increased risk of oligohydrosis/hyperthermia).

### ADVERSE REACTIONS AND SIDE EFFECTS*

■ **CNS:** <u>drowsiness</u>, <u>fatigue</u>, agitation/irritability, depression, dizziness, psychomotor slowing, psychosis, weakness ■ **EENT:** amblyopia, tinnitus ■ **Resp:** cough, pharyngitis ■ **GI:** anorexia, nausea, vomiting ■ **GU:** kidney stones ■ **Derm:** oligohydrosis ( ↑ in children), rash ■ **Metab:** hyperthermia ( ↑ in children) ■ **Neuro:** abnormal gait, hyperasthesia, incoordination, tremor ■ **Misc:** ALLERGIC REACTIONS INCLUDING STEVENS-JOHNSON SYNDROME.

## INTERACTIONS

**Drug-Drug:** ■ **Drugs that induce or inhibit CYP3A4** may alter blood levels and effects of zonisamide ■ Blood levels and effects may be ↓ by **phenytoin, carbamzepine, phenobarbital,** or **valproate.**

## ROUTE AND DOSAGE

■ **PO (Adults and Children >16 yr):** 100 mg once daily initially for 2 wk, then increase to 200 mg daily for 2 wk; with subsequent increments of 100 mg made at 2-wk intervals as required (range 100–600 mg/day).

## AVAILABILITY

■ *Capsules:* 100 mg.

TIME/ACTION PROFILE (blood levels†)

|  | ONSET | PEAK | DURATION |
|---|---|---|---|
| PO | unknown | 2–6 hr | 24 hr |

†Requires 2 weeks of dosing to achieve steady-state blood levels.

## NURSING IMPLICATIONS

### ASSESSMENT

❏ Monitor frequency, duration, and characteristics of seizures.

❏ Monitor patient frequently for development of skin rash. Unexplained rash may require discontinuation of therapy.

❏ Assess patient for allergy to sulfa drugs.

■ *Lab Test Considerations:* Monitor renal function periodically during therapy. May cause ↑ creatinine and BUN.

❏ May cause ↑ in serum alkaline phosphatase.

## POTENTIAL NURSING DIAGNOSES

■ Injury, risk for (Adverse Reactions).

## IMPLEMENTATION

■ **PO:** May be administered with or without meals. Capsules should be swallowed whole.

## PATIENT/FAMILY TEACHING

❏ Instruct patient to take zonisamide as directed, even if feeling well. Consult health care professional if a dose is missed. Do not discontinue abruptly without consulting health care professional; may cause seizures.

❏ Instruct patient to contact health care professional immediately if skin rash occurs or seizures worsen. Patient should also contact health care professional if a child taking zonisamide is not sweating as usual, with or without a fever, or if they develop fever, sore throat, oral ulcers, easy bruising, depression, unusual thoughts, speech or language problems.

❏ May cause drowsiness. Caution patient to avoid driving or other activities requiring alertness until cleared by physician and effects of medication are known.

❏ Advise patient to increase fluid intake to at least 6–8 glasses of water/day to minimize risk of kidney stones. Instruct patient to contact health care professional if symptoms of kidney stones (sudden back pain, abdominal pain, blood in urine) occur.

❏ Instruct patient to consult health care professional prior to taking other prescription or OTC medications or herbal/alternative preparations.

❏ May have teratogenic effects. Advise women of childbearing age to use effective contraception throughout therapy. Instruct patient to notify health care professional if pregnancy is planned or suspected or if planning to breastfeed.

## EVALUATION

**Effectiveness of therapy can be demonstrated by:** ■ Decrease in frequency and duration of partial seizures.

# APPENDICES

# APPENDIX A
# Recent Drug Approvals

To view full-text monographs of drugs that have been recently released from the FDA or to learn about changes to dosage forms, please visit www.DrugGuide.com.

| Generic Name (Brand Name) Classification(s) Pregnancy Category Schedule | Indications | Adverse Reactions and Side Effects* | Route and Dosage | Contraindications and Precautions | Drug-Drug Interactions |
|---|---|---|---|---|---|
| **abarelix** (Plenaxis) **Therapeutic:** *antineoplastics* **Pharmacologic:** *GnRH antagonists* Pregnancy Category X | Advanced prostate cancer when LHRH agonists are inappropriate or surgical castration is refused and there is risk of neurologic compromise from metastatic disease, ureteral/bladder obstruction due to local/metastatic disease or severe metastatic bone pain unresponsive to adequate opioid analgesia. | **CNS:** dizziness, fatigue, headache, sleep disturbances ■ **CV:** peripheral edema, prolonged QTc interval ■ **GI:** constipation, diarrhea, nausea, increased transaminases ■ **GU:** dysuria, urinary frequency ■ **Derm:** hot flushes ■ **Endo:** breast enlargement/nipple tenderness ■ **MS:** back pain ■ **Misc:** allergic reactions, decreased bone mineral density. | **IM (Adults):** 100 mg on Day 1, 15, and 29 and then every 4 wk thereafter. | **Contraindicated in:** Hypersensitivity. Adult females or children. **Use Cautiously in:** Patients with pre-existing QTc prolongation or concurrent use of Class IA antiarrhythmics (amiodarone, sotalol). Weight >225 pounds (decreased effectiveness over time). | None noted. |
| **botulism immune globulin IV** (BabyBIG) **Therapeutic:** *vaccines/ immunizing agents* **Pharmacologic:** *immune globulins* | Treatment of patients <1 yr old with infant botulism due to toxin type A or B. | **Derm:** rash ■ **Misc:** allergic reactions including anaphylaxis. | **IV (Children):** 50 mg/kg single dose. | **Contraindicated in:** Severe reaction to immunoglobulin preparations. **Use Cautiously in:** Renal disease or concurrent illness associated with renal impairment. | May interfere with immune response to live-virus vaccines (defer for 5 mo following use). |

| Generic Name (Brand Name) Classification(s) Pregnancy Category Schedule | Indications | Adverse Reactions and Side Effects | Route and Dosage | Contraindications and Precautions | Drug-Drug Interactions |
|---|---|---|---|---|---|
| **daptomycin** (Cubicin) *Therapeutic: anti-infectives* *Pharmacologic: cyclic lipopeptide antibacterial agents* Pregnancy Category B | Complicated skin and skin structure infections caused by aerobic Gram-positive bacteria. | **CNS:** dizziness ■ **Resp:** dyspnea ■ **CV:** hypertension, hypotension ■ **GI:** PSEUDO-MEMBRANOUS COLITIS, constipation, diarrhea, nausea, vomiting, ↑ liver function tests ■ **GI:** renal failure ■ **Hemat:** anemia ■ **Local:** injection site reactions ■ **MS:** ↑ CPK ■ **Misc:** fever. | **IV (Adults):** 4 mg/kg every 24 hr. *Renal/ Hepatic Impairment* **IV (Adults):** CCr <30 ml/ min—4 mg/kg every 48 hr. | **Contraindicated in:** Hypersensitivity. **Use Cautiously in:** CCr <30 ml/min (dosage reduction required). Geriatric patients (may have ↓ clinical response with ↑ risk of adverse reactions). Pregnancy (use only if clearly needed). Lactation. Children <18 yr (safety not established). | Tobramycin ↑ blood levels. Concurrent HMG-CoA reductase inhibitors may ↑ the risk of myopathy. |
| **efalizumab** (Raptiva) *Therapeutic: antipsoriatics* *Pharmacologic: monoclonal antibodies* Pregnancy Category C | Chronic moderate to severe plaque psoriasis. | **GI:** nausea ■ **Hemat:** thrombocytopenia ■ **MS:** arthralgia, arthritis ■ **Misc:** first dose reaction complex, chills, fever, infection, malignancy, worsening psoriasis. | **Subcut (Adults):** 0.7-mg/kg conditioning dose, followed by 1 mg/kg weekly thereafter (not to exceed 200 mg/dose). | **Contraindicated in:** Hypersensitivity, active untreated infections, lactation. **Use Cautiously in:** History of chronic /recurrent infection, thrombocytopenia, pregnancy (use only if clearly needed), children (safety not established). | May decrease the antibody response to and increase the risk of adverse reactions from vaccines and immunizations (avoid administration during treatment). |
| **memantine** (Namenda) *Therapeutic: anti-Alzheimer's agents* *Pharmacologic:* Pregnancy Category B | Moderate to severe Alzheimer's dementia. | **CNS:** dizziness, fatigue, headache ■ **CV:** hypertension ■ **Derm:** rash ■ **GU:** urinary frequency ■ **Hemat:** anemia. | **PO (Adults):** 5 mg once daily initially, increased at weekly intervals to 10 mg/ day (5 mg twice daily), then 15 mg/ day (5 mg once daily, 10 mg once daily as separate doses), then to target dose of 20 mg/day (as 10 mg twice daily). | **Contraindicated in:** Severe renal impairment. **Use Cautiously in:** Moderate renal impairment (consider ↓ dose). Concurrent use of other NMDA antagonists (amantadine, rimantadine, ketamine, dextromethorphan). Concurrent use of drugs or diets that cause alkaline urine. Pregnancy, lactation, or children (safety not established). Conditions that ↑ urine pH including severe urinary tract infections or renal tubular acidosis (lead to ↓ excretion and ↑ levels). | Medications that ↑ urine pH lead to ↓ excretion and ↑ blood levels (carbonic anhydrase inhibitors, sodium bicarbonate). |

| Generic Name (Brand Name) Classification(s) Pregnancy Category Schedule | Indications | Adverse Reactions and Side Effects* | Route and Dosage | Contraindications and Precautions | Drug-Drug Interactions |
|---|---|---|---|---|---|
| miglustat (Zavesca) *Therapeutic: none assigned* *Pharmacologic: enzyme inhibitors (D-glucose analogue)* Pregnancy Category X | Mild to moderate type 1 Gaucher's disease, when enzyme replacement therapy is not an option. | **CNS:** headache ■ **GI:** abdominal pain, diarrhea, flatulence, nausea, anorexia, dyspepsia ■ **GI:** ↓ male fertility ■ **Hemat:** thrombocytopenia ■ **Metab:** weight loss ■ **Neuro:** paresthesia, peripheral neuropathy, tremor. | **PO (Adults):** 100 mg three times daily at regular intervals. *Renal/Hepatic Impairment* **PO (Adults):** *CCr 50–70 ml/min*—100 mg twice daily; *CCr 30–50 ml/min*— 100 mg once daily. | **Contraindicated in:** Hypersensitivity. Pregnancy or lactation. Severe renal impairment (<30 ml/min). **Use Cautiously in:** Mild to moderate renal impairment (dosage alteration recommended if CCr <70 ml/min). Geriatric patients (consider age related decrease in body mass, cardiac, renal and hepatic function, other chronic illnesses, and concurrent drug therapies). Children <18 yr (safety not established). | ↑ clearance of imiglucerase (should not be used concurrently). |
| pemetrexed (Alimta) *Therapeutic: antineoplastics* *Pharmacologic: folate antagonists* Pregnancy Category D | Malignant pleural mesothelioma (with cisplatin). | **CNS:** fatigue, chest pain ■ **Derm:** desquamation/rash ■ **GI:** anorexia, diarrhea, nausea, vomiting, constipation, esophagitis ■ **GU:** renal toxicity ■ **Hemat:** MYELOSUPPRESSION ■ **Neuro:** neuropathy ■ **Resp:** dyspnea. | **IV (Adults):** 500 mg/m²on day 1 of each 21-day cycle (requires concurrent dexamethasone to decrease dermatologic toxicity and folic acid supplementation to decrease hematologic and renal toxicity). Dose modification required for renal/hepatic/impairment and myelosuppression. | **Contraindicated in:** Hypersensitivity, CCr <45 ml/min, lactation, pregnancy, severe hepatic impairment. **Use Cautiously in:** Mild/moderate hepatic impairment, children (safety not established), renal impairment. | Blood levels and risk of toxicity are increased by NSAIDs. |

| Generic Name (Brand Name) Classification(s) Pregnancy Category Schedule | Indications | Adverse Reactions and Side Effects' | Route and Dosage | Contraindications and Precautions | Drug-Drug Interactions |
|---|---|---|---|---|---|
| **Prussian blue, insoluble** (ferric [III] hexacyanoferrate [II], Radiogardase) *Therapeutic: antidotes* *Pharmacologic: chelating agents* Pregnancy Category C | Known/suspected internal contamination with thallium or radioactive cesium. | **GI:** constipation ■ **F and E:** hypokalemia. | **PO (Adults):** 3 g three times daily **PO (Children 2–12):** 1 g three times a day. | **Contraindicated in:** No known contraindications. **Use Cautiously in:** Hepatic impairment, decreased GI motility. | May bind some therapeutic drugs and nutrients. |
| **tadalafil** (Cialis) *Therapeutic: anti-impotence agents* *Pharmacologic: phosphodiesterase type 5 inhibitors* Pregnancy Category B | Erectile dysfunction. | **CNS:** headache ■ **EENT:** nasal congestion ■ **CV:** hypotension ■ **GI:** dyspepsia ■ **GU:** priapism ■ **Derm:** flushing ■ **MS:** back pain, limb pain, myalgia. | Renal/hepatic disease (dose alteration required) **PO (Adults):** 10 mg prior to sexual activity (range 5–20 mg; not to exceed one dose/24 hr); *concurrent use of CYP3A4 inhibitors including itraconazole, ketoconazole and ritonavir*—single dose should not exceed 10 mg in any 72 h period. | **Contraindicated in:** Hypersensitivity. Concurrent use of nitrates, nitric oxide donors, alpha adrenergic blockers (except tamsulosin 0.4 mg once daily). Unstable angina, recent history of stroke, life-threatening heart failure within 6 mo, uncontrolled hypertension, arrhythmias, stroke within 6 mo, or MI within 90 days. Any other cardiovascular pathology including known hereditary degenerative retinal disorders. Severe hepatic impairment. Congenital or acquired QT prolongation or concurrent use of Class IA or III antiarrhythmics. Women, children, or newborns. **Use Cautiously in:** Left ventricular outflow obstruction. Penile deformity. Underlying conditions predisposing to priapism including sickle cell anemia, multiple myeloma, or leukemia. Bleeding disorders or active peptic ulcer disease. Strong inhibitors of the CYP 3A4 enzyme system. Geriatric patients (may have ↑ sensitivity to effects). | Concurrent use of nitrates or alpha adrenergic blockers may cause serious, life threatening hypotension and is contraindicated except for tamsulosin 0.4 mg once daily. ↑ risk of hypotension with acute ingestion of alcohol. Strong inhibitors of CYP3A4 including ritonavir, ketoconazole, itraconazole ↑ effects and the risk of adverse reactions (dosage adjustments recommended) Similar effects may be expected of other inhibitors of CY3A4. |

| Generic Name (Brand Name) Classification(s) Pregnancy Category Schedule | Indications | Adverse Reactions and Side Effects | Route and Dosage | Contraindications and Precautions | Drug-Drug Interactions |
|---|---|---|---|---|---|
| **tiotropium** (Spiriva) *Therapeutic: allergy, cold, and cough remedies, bronchodilators* ***Pharmacologic:*** *anticholinergics* Pregnancy Category C | A long-term maintenance treatment of bronchospasm due to COPD including chronic bronchitis and emphysema. | **CV:** tachycardia ■ **EENT:** blurred vision, glaucoma ■ **GI:** dry mouth, constipation ■ **GU:** urinary difficulty, urinary retention ■ **Resp:** paradoxical bronchospasm. | **Inhaln (Adults):** 18 mcg (one dry powder capsule) once daily via HandiHaler device. | **Contraindicated in:** Concurrent use of other anticholinergic agents. **Use Cautiously in:** Narrow-angle glaucoma. Prostatic hyperplasia or bladder neck obstruction, moderate to severe renal impairment, pregnancy, lactation, or children (safety not established). | None noted; avoid concurrent use of other anticholinergics, due to possible additive effects. |
| **sertaconazole** (Ertaczo) *Therapeutic: antifungals (topical)* Pregnancy Category C | Topical treatment of tinea pedis. | **Derm:** local irritation. | **Topical (Adults):** Apply 2% cream twice daily for 4 wk. | **Contraindicated in:** Hypersensitivity. **Use Cautiously in:** Pregnancy (use only if clearly needed), lactation, and children <12 yr (safety not established). | None noted. |

| Generic Name (Brand Name) Classification(s) Pregnancy Category Schedule | Indications | Adverse Reactions and Side Effects* | Route and Dosage | Contraindications and Precautions | Drug-Drug Interactions |
|---|---|---|---|---|---|
| **vardenafil** (Levitra) *Therapeutic: anti-impotence agents* *Pharmacologic: phosphodiesterase type 5 inhibitors* Pregnancy Category C | Erectile dysfunction. | **CNS:** headache, dizziness ■ **EENT:** rhinitis, sinusitis ■ **GI:** dyspepsia, nausea ■ **GU:** priapism ■ **Derm:** flushing ■ **Misc:** flu syndrome. | Renal/hepatic disease (dose alteration required) **PO (Adults):** 10 mg taken 1 hr prior to sexual activity (range 5–20 mg; not to exceed one dose/24 hr); *concurrent use of ritonavir*—single dose should not exceed 2.5 mg in any 72 h period; *concurrent use of indinavir, ketoconazole 400 mg daily or itraconazole 400 mg daily*—single dose should not exceed 2.5 mg/ 24 hr; *concurrent use of ketoconazole or itraconazole 200 mg daily or erythromycin*—single dose should not exceed 5 mg/24 hr. | **Contraindicated in:** Hypersensitivity. Concurrent use of nitrates, nitric oxide donors, alpha adrenergic blockers. Unstable angina, recent history of stroke, life-threatening arrhythmias, CHF or MI within 6 mo. End-stage renal disease requiring dialysis. Known hereditary degenerative retinal disorders. Severe hepatic impairment (Child-Pugh C). Congenital or acquired QT prolongation or concurrent use of Class IA or III antiarrhythmics. Women, children, or newborns. **Use Cautiously in:** Other serious underlying cardiovascular disease or left ventricular outflow obstruction. Penile deformity. Underlying conditions predisposing to priapism including sickle cell anemia, multiple myeloma, or leukemia. Bleeding disorders or active peptic ulcer diseases. Strong inhibitors of the CYP3A4 enzyme system. | Concurrent use of nitrates or alpha adrenergic blockers may cause serious, life-threatening hypotension and is contraindicated. Concurrent use of Class IA antiarrhythmics (such as quinidne or procainamide) or Class III antiarrhythmics (such as amiodarone or sotalol) ↑ risk of serious arrhythmias and should be avoided. Strong inhibitors of CYP3A4 including ritonavir, indinavir, ketoconazole, and itraconazole ↑ effects and the risk of adverse reactions (dosage adjustments recommended). Concurrent use of moderate inhibitors of CYP2C including erythromycin may also ↑ effects. ↑ risk of hypotension with antihypertensives and acute ingestion of alcohol. |

# NEW DOSAGE FORMS

| Generic Name (Brand Name) | New Dosage Form |
|---|---|
| **acetylcysteine, injection** (Acetadote) | 20% solution for intravenous use. |
| **amlodipine/atorvastatin** (Caduet) | 5/10 5 mg amlodipine/10 mg atorvastatin. |
| | 10/10 10 mg amlodipine/10 mg atorvastatin. |
| | 5/20 5 mg amlodipine/20 mg atorvastatin. |
| | 10/20 10 mg amlodipine/20 mg atorvastatin. |
| | 5/40 5 mg amlodipine/40 mg atorvastatin. |
| | 10/40 10 mg amlodipine/40 mg atorvastatin. |
| | 5/80 5 mg amlodipine/80 mg atorvastatin. |
| | 10/80 10 mg amlodipine/80 mg atorvastatin. |
| **aripiprazole** (Abilify) | 5 mg tablet. |
| **baclofen orally-disintegrating tablet** (Kemstro) | 10 mg tablets. |
| | 20 mg tablets. |
| **cephalex in tablets for oral suspension** (Panixine, DisperDose) | 125 mg (prepares a 125 mg/5 ml dose). |
| | 250 mg (prepares a 250 mg/5 ml dose). |
| **esmolol double strength injection** (Brevibloc) | 20 mg/ml |
| **estradiol topical emulsion** (Estrasorb) | Each 1.74 g pouch contains 4.35 mg/pouch (daily dose is 2 pouches). |
| **estradiol/levonrogestrel combination transdermal patch** (Climara Pro) | Releases 0.045 mg estradiol and 0.015 mg levonorgestral/day. |
| **metformin oral solution** (Riomet) | 100 mg/ml. |
| **risperidone long-acting injection** (Risperdal Consta) | 25, 37.5, and 50 mg dose pack with 2-ml diluent. |
| **zolmitripan nasal spray** (Zomig) | 5 mg single use nasal spray units in boxes of 6. |
| **zonisamide capsules** (Zonegran) | 25 mg capsule. |
| | 50 mg capsule. |

## NEW INDICATIONS

| Generic Name (Brand Name) | New Indications | Dose |
|---|---|---|
| eplerenone (Inspra) | Congestive heart failure (to improve survival of CHF patients after myocardial infarction). | **PO (Adults):** 25 mg once daily, increase to 50 mg once daily within 4 wks. |
| escitalopram (Lexapro) | Generalized anxiety disorder. | **PO (Adults):** 10 mg once daily, may be increased after 1 wk to 20 mg once daily. |
| paroxetine (Paxil) | Premenstrual Dysphoric Disorder. | **PO (Adults):** 12.5 mg/day initially, may be increased after 1 wk to 25 mg/day. |
| voriconazole (Vfend) | Esophageal candidiasis. | **PO (Adults ≥40 kg):** 200 mg every 12 hr. **PO (Adults <40 kg):** 100 mg every 12 hr. |

## DISCONTINUED DRUGS

| Generic Name (Brand Name) | Reason for Discontinuation |
|---|---|
| ardeparin (Normiflo) | Other agents available. |
| bepridil (Vascor) | Other agents available. |
| cefamandole (Mandole) | Other anti-infectives available. |
| cefixime (Suprax) | Other anti-infectives available. |
| danaparoid (Orgaran) | Other agents available. |

| | |
|---|---|
| **ephedra**<br>(in numerous over-the-counter products) | Unreasonable risk of cardiovascular adverse reactions. |
| **halofantrine**<br>(Halfan) | Other agents available. |
| **hyaluronidase**<br>(Wydase) | No longer used. |
| **methysergide**<br>(Sansert) | Safer agents available. |
| **valrubicin**<br>(Valstar) | No longer used. |

*CAPITALS indicate life-threatening; underlines indicate most frequent.

# Combination Drugs

**Note:** The drugs listed in this section are in alphabetical order according to trade names. If the trade name does not specify dosage form, the dosage form is either a tablet or capsule. Following each trade name are the generic names and doses of the active ingredients contained in each preparation. For information on these drugs, look up each generic name in the combination. For inert ingredients, see drug label. **Rx** signifies that a physician's prescription is required; **otc** signifies 'over-the-counter' or nonprescription medication.

*A-200 Shampoo*—0.33% pyrethrins/4% piperonyl butoxide **(otc)**

*Accuretic 10/12.5*—quinapril 10 mg/hydrochlorothiazide 12.5 mg **(Rx)**

*Accuretic 20/12.5*—quinapril 20 mg/hydrochlorothiazide 12.5 mg **(Rx)**

*Accuretic 20/25*—quinapril 20 mg/hydrochlorothiazide 25 mg **(Rx)**

*Acid-X*—acetaminophen 500 mg/calcium carbonate 250 mg **(otc)**

*Actagen-C Cough Syrup*—triprolidine 1.25 mg/pseudoephedrine 30 mg/codeine 10 mg/5 ml **(Rx)**

*Actagen syrup*—triprolidine 1.25 mg/pseudoephedrine 30 mg/5 ml **(otc)**

*Actagen tablets*—triprolidine 2.5 mg/pseudoephedrine 60 mg **(otc)**

*Actifed*—pseudoephedrine 60 mg/triprolidine 2.5 mg **(otc)**

*Actifed with codeine*—pseudoephedrine 30 mg/triprolidine 1.25 mg/codeine 10 mg **(Rx)**

*Actifed with codeine Cough Syrup*—pseudoephedrine 30 mg/triprolidine 1.25 mg/codeine 10 mg/5 ml **(Rx)**

*Actifed Cold and Allergy*—pseudoephedrine 60 mg/triprolidine 2.5 mg **(Rx)**

*Actifed Cold and Sinus Maximum Strength Tablets*—chlorpheniramine 2 mg/pseudoephedrine 30 mg/acetaminophen 500 mg **(otc)**

*Actifed Syrup*—triprolidine 1.25 mg/pseudoephedrine 30 mg/5 ml **(otc)**

*Activella Tablets*—estradiol 1 mg/norethindrone 0.5 mg **(Rx)**

*Adderall 5 mg*—dextroamphetamine sulfate 1.25 mg/dextroamphetamine saccharate 1.25 mg/dextroamphetamine aspartate 1.25 mg/amphetamine sulfate 1.25 mg **(Rx)**

*Adderall 10 mg*—dextroamphetamine sulfate 2.5 mg/dextroamphetamine saccharate 2.5 mg/dextroamphetamine aspartate 2.5 mg/amphetamine sulfate 2.5 mg **(Rx)**

*Adderall 20 mg*—dextroamphetamine sulfate 5 mg/dextroamphetamine saccharate 5 mg/dextroamphetamine aspartate 5 mg/amphetamine sulfate 5 mg **(Rx)**

*Adderall 30 mg*—dextroamphetamine sulfate 7.5 mg/dextroamphetamine saccharate 7.5 mg/dextroamphetamine aspartate 7.5 mg/amphetamine sulfate 7.5 mg **(Rx)**

*Adderall XR 10 mg*—dextroamphetamine saccinarate 2.5 mg/dextroamphetamine sulfate 2.5 mg/amphetamine aspartate 2.5 mg/amphetamine sulfate 2.5 mg **(Rx)**

*Adderall XR 20 mg*—dextroamphetamine saccharate 5 mg/dextroamphetamine sulfate 5 mg/amphetamine aspartate 5 mg/amphetamine sulfate 5 mg **(Rx)**

*Adderall XR 30 mg*—dextroamphetamine saccharate 7.5 mg/dextroamphetamine sulfate 7.5 mg/amphetamine aspartate 7.5 mg/amphetamine sulfate 7.5 mg **(Rx)**

*Advair Diskus 100*—fluticasone 100 mcg/salmeterol 50 mcg **(Rx)**

*Advair Diskus 250*—fluticasone 250 mcg/salmeterol 50 mcg **(Rx)**

*Advair Diskus 500*—fluticasone 500 mcg/salmeterol 50 mcg **(Rx)**

*Advicor 500*—niacin 500 mg/lovastatin 20 mg **(Rx)**

*Advicor 750*—niacin 750 mg/lovastatin 20 mg **(Rx)**

*Advicor 1000*—niacin 1000 mg/lovastatin 20 mg **(Rx)**

*Advil Cold & Sinus*—pseudoephedrine 30 mg/ibuprofen 200 mg **(otc)**

*Aggrenox*—aspirin 25 mg/extended-release dipyridamole 200 mg **(Rx)**

*AK-Cide Ophthalmic Suspension/Ointment*—0.5% prednisolone acetate/10% sulfacetamide sodium **(Rx)**

*Aldactazide 25/25*—hydrochlorothiazide 25 mg/spironolactone 25 mg **(Rx)**

*Aldactazide 50/50*—hydrochlorothiazide 50 mg/spironolactone 50 mg **(Rx)**

*Aldoclor-150*—methyldopa 250 mg/chlorothiazide 150 mg **(Rx)**

*Aldoclor-250*—methyldopa 250 mg/chlorothiazide 250 mg **(Rx)**

*Aldoril-15*—hydrochlorothiazide 15 mg/methyldopa 250 mg **(Rx)**

*Aldoril-25*—hydrochlorothiazide 25 mg/methyldopa 250 mg **(Rx)**

*Aleve Cold & Sinus*—naproxen 220 mg/extended-release pseudoephedrine 120 mg **(otc)**

*Alka-Seltzer Effervescent, Original*—citric acid 1000 mg/sodium bicarbonate 1916 mg/aspirin 325 mg **(otc)**

*Alka-Seltzer Plus Cold & Cough*—pseudoephedrine 30 mg/chlorpheniramine 2 mg/dextromethorphan 10 mg/acetaminophen 325 mg **(otc)**

*Alka-Seltzer Plus Cold & Cough Liqui-Gels*—dextromethorphan 10 mg/pseudoephedrine 30 mg/chlorpheniramine 2 mg/acctaminophen 325 mg **(otc)**

*Alka-Seltzer Plus Cold Liqui-Gels*—pseudoephedrine 30 mg/chlorpheniramine 2 mg/acetaminophen 325 mg **(otc)**

*Alka-Seltzer Plus Night-Time Cold*—phenylephrine HCl 5 mg/doxylamine 6.25 mg/dextromethorphan 10 mg **(otc)**

*Alka-Seltzer Plus Night-Time Cold Liqui-Gels*—doxylamine 6.25 mg/dextromethorphan 10 mg/pseudoephedrine 30 mg/acetaminophen 250 mg **(otc)**

*Alka-Seltzer Plus Cold and Sinus*—pseudoephedrine 30 mg/acetaminophen 325 mg **(otc)**

*Allegra-D*—fexofenadine 60 mg/pseudoephedrine 120 mg **(Rx)**

*Allercon Tablets*—triprolidine 2.5 mg/pseudoephrine 60 mg **(otc)**

*Allerest Maximum Strength*—pseudoephedrine 30 mg/chlorpheniramine 2 mg **(otc)**

*Allerest Allergy and Sinus Relief Maximum Strength*—pseudoephedrine 30 mg/acetaminophen 325 mg **(otc)**

*Allerfrim Syrup*—triprolidine 1.25 mg/pseudoephrine 30 mg/5ml **(otc)**

*Allerfrim Tablets*—triprolidine 2.5 mg/pseudoephrine 60 mg **(otc)**

*All-Nite Cold Formula Liquid*—(per 5 ml) pseudoephedrine 10 mg/doxylamine 1.25 mg/dextromethorphan 5 mg/acetaminophen 167 mg **(otc)**

*Alor 5/500*—hydrocodone 5 mg/aspirin 500 mg **(Rx)**

*Amaphen*—acetaminophen 325 mg/butalbital 50 mg/caffeine 40 mg **(Rx)**

*Ambenyl Cough Syrup*—(per 5 ml) codeine 10 mg/bromodiphenhydramine 12.5 mg/5% alcohol **(Rx)**

*Anacin*—aspirin 400 mg/caffeine 32 mg **(otc)**

*Anacin Maximum Strength*—aspirin 500 mg/caffeine 32 mg **(otc)**

*Anacin PM (Aspirin Free)*—diphenhydramine 25 mg/acetaminophen 500 mg **(otc)**

*Anaplex HD Syrup*—(per 5 ml) hydrocodone 1.7 mg/phenylephrine 5 mg/chlorpheniramine 2 mg **(Rx)**

*Anaplex Liquid*—(per 5 ml) chlorpheniramine 2 mg/pseudoephedrine 30 mg **(Rx)**

*Anatuss LA*—pseudoephedrine 120 mg/guaifenesin 400 mg **(Rx)**

*Anexsia 5/500*—hydrocodone 5 mg/acetaminophen 500 mg **(Rx)**

*Anexsia 7.5/650*—hydrocodone 7.5 mg/acetaminophen 650 mg **(Rx)**

*Apresazide 25/25*—hydralazine 25 mg/hydrochlorothiazide 25 mg **(Rx)**

*Apresazide 50/50*—hydralazine 50 mg/hydrochlorothiazide 50 mg **(Rx)**

*Apri*—desogestrel 0.15 mg/ethinyl estradiol 30 mcg **(Rx)**

*Arthritis Pain Formula*—aspirin 500 mg/aluminum hydroxide 27 mg/magnesium hydroxide 100 mg **(otc)**

*Arthrotec*—diclofenac 50 or 75 mg/misoprostol 200 mcg **(Rx)**

*Ascriptin A/D*—aspirin 325 mg/aluminum hydroxide 75 mg/magnesium hydroxide 75 mg/calcium carbonate 75 mg **(otc)**

*Aspirin-Free Bayer Select Allergy Sinus*—pseudoephedrine 30 mg/chlorpheniramine 2 mg/acetaminophen 500 mg **(otc)**

*Aspirin-Free Excedrin*—acetaminophen 500 mg **(otc)**

*Aspirin-Free Excedrin Dual*—acetaminophen 500 mg/calcium carbonate 111 mg/magnesium carbonate 64 mg/magnesium oxide 30 mg **(otc)**

*Atacand HCT 16*—candesartan 16 mg/hydrochlorothiazide 12.5 mg **(Rx)**

*Atacand HCT 32*—candesartan 32 mg/hydrochlorothiazide 12.5 mg **(Rx)**

*Augmentin 250*—amoxicillin 250 mg/clavulanic acid 125 mg **(Rx)**

*Augmentin 500*—amoxicillin 500 mg/clavulanic acid 125 mg **(Rx)**

*Augmentin 875*—amoxicillin 875 mg/clavulanic acid 125 mg **(Rx)**

*Augmentin 125 Chewable*—amoxicillin 125 mg/clavulanic acid 31.25 mg **(Rx)**

*Augmentin 200 Chewable*—amoxicillin 200 mg/clavulanic acid 28.5 mg **(Rx)**

*Augmentin 250 Chewable*—amoxicillin 250 mg/clavulanic acid 62.5 mg **(Rx)**

*Augmentin 400 Chewable*—amoxicillin 400 mg/clavulanic acid 57 mg **(Rx)**

*Augmentin 125 mg/5 ml Suspension*—(per 5 ml) amoxicillin 125 mg/clavulanic acid 31.25 mg **(Rx)**

*Augmentin 200 mg/5 ml Suspension*—(per 5 ml) amoxicillin 200 mg/clavulanic acid 28.5 mg **(Rx)**

*Augmentin 250 mg/5 ml Suspension*—(per 5 ml) amoxicillin 250 mg/clavulanic acid 62.5 mg **(Rx)**

*Augmentin 400 mg/5 ml Suspension*—(per 5 ml) amoxicillin 400 mg/clavulanic acid 57 mg **(Rx)**

*Auralgan Otic Solution*—5.4% antipyrine/1.4% benzocaine **(Rx)**

*Avalide*—hydrochlorothiazide 12.5 mg/irbesartan 150 mg **(Rx)**

*Avalide 300*—hydrochlorothiazide 12.5 mg/irbesartan 300 mg **(Rx)**

*Avandamet 1*—rosiglitazone 1 mg/metformin 500 mg **(Rx)**

*Avandamet 2*—rosiglitazone 2 mg/metformin 500 mg **(Rx)**

*Avandamet 4*—rosiglitazone 4 mg/metformin 500 mg **(Rx)**

*B & O Supprettes No. 15A Supps*—belladonna extract 15 mg/opium 30 mg **(Rx)**

*B & O Supprettes No. 16A Supps*—belladonna extract 16.2 mg/opium 60 mg **(Rx)**

*Bactrim*—trimethoprim 80 mg/sulfamethoxazole 400 mg **(Rx)**

*Bactrim DS*—trimethoprim 160 mg/sulfamethoxazole 800 mg **(Rx)**

*Bactrim I.V. For Injection*—(per 5 ml) trimethoprim 80 mg/sulfamethoxazole 400 mg **(Rx)**

*Bancap HC*—acetaminophen 500 mg/hydrocodone 5 mg **(Rx)**

*Bayer Plus, Extra Strength*—aspirin 500 mg buffered with: calcium carbonate/magnesium carbonate, magnesium oxide **(otc)**

*Bayer Select Chest Cold*—dextromethorphan 15 mg/acetaminophen 500 mg **(otc)**

*Bayer Select Flu Relief*—acetaminophen 500 mg/pseudoephedrine 30 mg/dextromethorphan 15 mg/chlorpheniramine 2 mg **(otc)**

*Bayer Select Head Cold*—pseudoephedrine 30 mg/acetaminophen 500 mg **(otc)**

*Bayer Select Maximum Strength Headache*—acetaminophen 500 mg/caffeine 65 mg **(otc)**

*Bayer Select Maximum Strength Menstrual*—acetaminophen 500 mg/pamabrom 25 mg **(otc)**

*Bayer Select Maximum Strength Night Time Pain Relief*—acetaminophen 500 mg/diphenhydramine 25 mg **(otc)**

*Bayer Select Maximum Strength Sinus Pain Relief*—acetaminophen 500 mg/pseudoephedrine 30 mg **(otc)**

*Bayer Select Night Time Cold*—acetaminophen 500 mg/pseudoephedrine 30 mg/dextromethorphan 15 mg/triprolidine 1.25 mg **(otc)**

*Bayer Women's Aspirin plus Calcium*—aspirin 81 mg/calcium carbonate 300 mg **(otc)**

*Bellatal*—phenobarbital 16.2 mg/hyoscyamine sulfate 0.1037 mg/atropine sulfate 0.0194 mg/scopolamine hydrobromide 0.0065 mg **(Rx)**

*Bellergal-S*—ergotamine 0.6 mg/phenobarbital 40 mg/l-alkaloids of belladonna 0.2 mg **(Rx)**

*Bel-Phen-Ergot-SR*—phenobarbital 40 mg/ergotamine tartrate 0.6 mg/l-alkaloids of belladonna 0.2 mg **(Rx)**

*Benadryl Allergy Decongestant Liquid*—(per 5 ml) diphenhydramine 12.5 mg/pseudoephedrine 30 mg **(otc)**

*Benadryl Allergy/Sinus Headache Caplets*—diphenhydramine 12.5 mg/pseudoephedrine 30 mg/acetaminophen 500 mg **(otc)**

*Benadryl Decongestant Allergy*—pseudoephedrine 60 mg/diphenhydramine 25 mg **(otc)**

*Benylin Expectorant Liquid*—(per 5 ml) guaifenesin 100 mg/dextromethorphan 5 mg/5% alcohol **(otc)**

*Benylin Multi-Symptom Liquid*—(per 5 ml) dextromethorphan 5 mg/pseudoephedrine 15 mg/guaifenesin 100 mg **(otc)**

*Benzamycin*—benzoyl peroxide 5%/erythromycin 3% **(Rx)**

*BenzaClin*—clindamycin 1%/benzoyl peroxide 5% topical **(Rx)**

*Bicitra Solution*—(per 5 ml) sodium citrate 500 mg/citric acid 334 mg **(Rx)**

*Bion Tears Ophthalmic Solution*—0.1% dextran 70/0.3% hydroxypropyl methylcellulose 2910 **(otc)**

*Blephamide Ophthalmic Suspension/Ointment*—0.2% prednisolone/10% sodium sulfacetamide **(Rx)**

*Bromfed Capsules*—brompheniramine 12 mg/pseudoephedrine 120 mg **(Rx)**

*Bromfed Tablets*—pseudoephedrine 60 mg/brompheniramine 4 mg **(Rx)**

*Bromfenex*—brompheniramine 12 mg/pseudoephedrine 120 mg **(Rx)**

*Bromfenex PD*—brompheniramine 6 mg/pseudoephedrine 60 mg **(Rx)**

*Bromo Seltzer*—(effervescent granules) sodium bicarbonate 2781 mg/acetaminophen 325 mg/citric acid 2224 mg **(otc)**

*Bronkaid Dual Action*—ephedrine 25 mg/guaifenesin 400 mg **(otc)**

*Brontex*—codeine 10 mg/guaifenesin 300 mg **(Rx)**

*Bufferin*—aspirin 325 mg/calcium carbonate 158 mg/magnesium oxide 63 mg/magnesium carbonate 34 mg **(otc)**

*Bufferin AF Nite Time*—acetaminophen 500 mg/diphenhydramine 38 mg **(otc)**

*Butibel*—belladonna extract 15 mg/butabarbital 15 mg **(Rx)**

*Cafatine-PB*—ergotamine 1 mg/caffeine 100 mg/l-alkaloids of belladonna 0.125 mg/sodium pentobarbital 30 mg **(Rx)**

*Cafergot*—ergotamine 1 mg/caffeine 100 mg **(Rx)**

*Cafergot Suppositories*—ergotamine 2 mg/caffeine 100 mg **(Rx)**

*Caladryl Lotion*—1% diphenhydramine/8% calamine and camphor/2% alcohol **(otc)**

*Calcet*—elemental calcium 152.8 mg/vitamin D 100 IU **(otc)**

*Caltrate 600+D*—vitamin D 200 IU/calcium 600 mg **(otc)**

*Cama Arthritis Pain Reliever*—aspirin 500 mg/magnesium oxide 150 mg/aluminum hydroxide 125 mg **(otc)**

*Capozide 25/15*—captopril 25 mg/hydrochlorothiazide 15 mg **(Rx)**

*Capozide 25/25*—captopril 25 mg/hydrochlorothiazide 25 mg **(Rx)**

*Capozide 50/15*—captopril 50 mg/hydrochlorothiazide 15 mg **(Rx)**

*Capozide 50/25*—captopril 50 mg/hydrochlorothiazide 25 mg **(Rx)**

*Cardec DM Syrup*—(per 5 ml) pseudoephedrine 60 mg/carbinoxamine 4 mg/dextromethorphan 15 mg **(Rx)**

*Cenafed Plus Tablets*—triprolidine 2.5 mg/pseudoephrine 60 mg **(otc)**

*Cetacaine Topical*—14% benzocaine/2% tetracaine/0.5% benzalkonium chloride/0.005% cetyl dimethyl ethyl ammonium bromide **(Rx)**

*Cetapred Ophthalmic Ointment*—0.25% prednisolone/10% sodium sulfacetamide **(Rx)**

*Cheracol Cough Syrup*—(per 5 ml) codeine 10 mg/guaifenesin 100 mg **(Rx)**

*Children's Advil Cold*—(per 5 ml) ibuprofen 100 mg/pseudoephedrine 15 mg **(otc)**

*Children's Cepacol Liquid*—(per 5 ml) acetaminophen 160 mg/pseudoephedrine 15 mg **(otc)**

*Chlor-Trimeton 4 Hour Relief*—pseudoephedrine 60 mg/chlorpheniramine 4 mg **(otc)**

*Chlor-Trimeton 12 Hour Relief*—pseudoephedrine 120 mg/chlorpheniramine 8 mg **(otc)**

*Chromagen*—ferrous fumarate 66 mg/vitamin $B_{12}$ 10 mcg/vitamin C 250 mg/intrinsic factor 100 mg **(Rx)**

*Ciprodex Otic*—ciprofloxacin 0.3% dexamethasone 0.1% **(Rx)**

*Cipro HC Otic*—(per ml otic) ciprofloxacin 2 mg/hydrocortisone 10 mg **(Rx)**

*Claritin-D 12 Hour*—loratadine 5 mg/pseudoephedrine 120 mg **(Rx)**

*Claritin-D 24-Hour*—loratadine 10 mg/pseudoephedrine 240 mg **(Rx)**

*Clindex*—chlordiazepoxide 5 mg/clidinium 2.5 mg **(Rx)**

*Clomycin Ointment*—bacitracin 400 units/neomycin sulfate (equiv. to 3.5 g neomycin base)/polymyxin B sulfate 5000 units/lidocaine 40 mg **(otc)**

*Co-Apap*—pseudoephedrine 30 mg/chlorpheniramine 2 mg/dextromethorphan 15 mg/acetaminophen 325 mg **(otc)**

*Co-Gesic*—acetaminophen 500 mg/hydrocodone 5 mg **(Rx)**

*Codiclear DH Syrup*—(per 5 ml) hydrocodone 5 mg/guaifenesin 100 mg **(Rx)**

*Codimal*—pseudoephedrine 30 mg/chlorpheniramine 2 mg/acetaminophen 325 mg **(otc)**

*Codimal DH Syrup*—(per 5 ml) hydrocodone 1.66 mg/phenylephrine 5 mg/pyrilamine 8.33 mg **(Rx)**

*Codimal DM Syrup*—(per 5 ml) phenylephrine 5 mg/pyrilamine 8.33 mg/dextromethorphan 10 mg **(otc)**

*Codimal-L.A.*—chlorpheniramine 8 mg/pseudoephedrine 120 mg **(Rx)**

*Codimal PH Syrup*—(per 5 ml) codeine 10 mg/phenylephrine 5 mg/pyrilamine 8.33 mg **(Rx)**

*ColBenemid*—colchicine 0.5 mg/probenecid 500 mg **(Rx)**

*Coldrine*—pseudoephedrine 30 mg/acetaminophen 500 mg **(otc)**

*Col-Probenecid*—probenecid 500 mg/colchicine 0.5 mg **(Rx)**

*Coly-Mycin S Otic Suspension*—1% hydrocortisone/neomycin base 3.3 mg/ml/colistin 3 mg/ml/0.05% thonzonium bromide **(Rx)**

*CombiPatch 0.05/0.14*—estradiol 0.05 mg/day/norethindrone 0.14 mg/day **(Rx)**

*CombiPatch 0.05/0.25*—estradiol 0.05 mg/day/norethindrone 0.25 mg/day **(Rx)**

*Combipres Tablets 0.1*—chlorthalidone 15 mg/clonidine 0.1 mg **(Rx)**

*Combipres Tablets 0.2*—chlorthalidone 15 mg/clonidine 0.2 mg **(Rx)**

*Combipres Tablets 0.3*—chlorthalidone 15 mg/clonidine 0.3 mg **(Rx)**

*Combivent*—(per actuation) ipratropium bromide 18 mcg/albuterol 103 mcg **(Rx)**

*Combivir*—lamivudine 150 mg/zidovudine 300 mg **(Rx)**

*Comtrex Allergy-Sinus*—chlorpheniramine 2 mg/acetaminophen 500 mg/pseudoephedrine 30 mg **(otc)**

*Comtrex Liquid*—(per 5 ml) chlorpheniramine 0.67 mg/acetaminophen 108.3 mg/dextromethorphan 3.3 mg/pseudoephedrine 10 mg **(otc)**

***Comtrex Maximum Strength Caplets***—acetaminophen 500 mg/pseudoephedrine 30 mg/chlorpheniramine 2 mg/dextromethorphan 15 mg **(otc)**

***Comtrex Maximum Strength Multi-Symptom Cold & Flu Relief***—pseudoephedrine 30 mg/dextromethorphan 15 mg/chlorpheniramine 2 mg/acetaminophen 500 mg **(otc)**

***Comtrex Maximum Strength Non-Drowsy Caplets***—acetaminophen 500 mg/pseudoephedrine 30 mg/dextromethorphan 15 mg **(otc)**

***Congess SR***—guaifenesin 250 mg/pseudoephedrine 120 mg **(Rx)**

***Congestac***—guaifenesin 400 mg/pseudoephedrine 60 mg **(otc)**

***Contac Cough & Chest Cold Liquid***—(per 5 ml) pseudoephedrine 15 mg/dextromethorphan 5 mg/guaifenesin 50 mg/acetaminophen 125 mg **(otc)**

***Contac Cough & Sore Throat Liquid***—(per 5 ml) dextromethorphan 5 mg/acetaminophen 125 mg **(otc)**

***Contac Day Allergy/Sinus***—pseudoephedrine 60 mg/acetaminophen 650 mg **(otc)**

***Contac Day Cold and Flu***—pseudoephedrine 60 mg/dextromethorphan 30 mg/acetaminophen 650 mg **(otc)**

***Contac Non-Drowsy Maximum Strength 12 Hour***—psuedoephedrine 120 mg **(Rx)**

***Contac Night Allergy Sinus***—pseudoephedrine 60 mg/diphenhydramine 50 mg/acetaminophen 650 mg **(otc)**

***Contac Night Cold and Flu Caplets***—pseudoephedrine 60 mg/diphenhydramine 50 mg/acetaminophen 650 mg **(otc)**

***Contac Severe Cold and Flu Nighttime Liquid***—(per 5 ml) pseudoephedrine 10 mg/chlorpheniramine 0.67 mg/dextromethorphan 5 mg/acetaminophen 167 mg/18.5% alcohol **(otc)**

***Coricidin D***—pseudoephedrine 30 mg/chlorpheniramine 2 mg/acetaminophen 325 mg **(otc)**

***Coricidin HBP Chest Congestion and Cough***—dextromethorphan 10 mg/guaifenesin 200 mg

***Coricidin HBP Cold and Flu***—acetaminophen 325 mg/chlorpheniramine 2 mg **(otc)**

***Coricidin HBP Cough and Cold***—chlorpheniramine 4 mg/dextromethorphan 30 mg **(otc)**

***Coricidin HBP Maximum Strength Flu***—acetaminophen 500 mg/chlorpheniramine 2 mg/dextromethorphan 15 mg **(otc)**

***Cortisporin Ophthalmic (Ointment/Suspension)/Otic (Solution/Suspension)***—0.35% neomycin base/polymyxin B 10,000 units/ml/1% hydrocortisone **(Rx)**

***Cortisporin Topical Cream***—0.5% neomycin sulfate/polymyxin B 10,000 units/0.5% hydrocortisone **(Rx)**

***Cortisporin Topical Ointment***—0.5% neomycin sulfate/bacitracin 400 units/polymyxin B 5000 units/1% hydrocortisone **(Rx)**

***Corzide 40/5***—nadolol 40 mg/bendroflumethiazide 5 mg **(Rx)**

***Corzide 80/5***—nadolol 80 mg/bendroflumethiazide 5 mg **(Rx)**

***Cosopt***—dorzolamide 2 %/timolol 0.5 % ophthalmic **(Rx)**

***Cough-X***—dextromethorphan 5 mg/benzocaine 2 mg **(otc)**

***Creon***—lipase 8000 units/amylase 30,000 units/protease 13,000 units/pancreatin 300 mg **(Rx)**

***Cyclomydril Ophthalmic Solution***—0.2% cyclopentolate/1% phenylephrine **(Rx)**

***Dallergy Caplets***—chlorpheniramine 8 mg/phenylephrine 20 mg/methscopolamine 2.5 mg **(Rx)**

***Dallergy-JR Capsules***—pseudoephedrine 60 mg bromphenerimine 6 mg

***Dallergy extended release***—phenylephrine 20 mg/chlorpheniramine 12 mg/methscopolamine 2.5 mg

***Dallergy Syrup***—(per 5 ml) chlorpheniramine 2 mg/phenylephrine 10 mg/methscopolamine 0.625 mg **(Rx)**

***Dallergy Tablets***—chlorpheniramine 4 mg/phenylephrine 10 mg/methscopolamine 1.25 mg **(Rx)**

***Damason-P***—hydrocodone 5 mg/aspirin 500 mg **(Rx)**

***Darvocet-N 100***—propoxyphene-N 100 mg/acetaminophen 650 mg **(Rx)**

***Darvon Compound-65***—propoxyphene 65 mg/aspirin 389 mg/caffeine 32.4 mg **(Rx)**

***Deconamine***—pseudoephedrine 60 mg/chlorpheniramine 4 mg **(Rx)**

***Deconamine CX***—hydrocodone 5 mg/pseudoephedrine 30 mg/guaifenesin 300 mg **(Rx)**

***Deconamine SR***—pseudoephedrine 120 mg/chlorpheniramine 8 mg **(Rx)**

***Deconamine Syrup***—(per 5 ml) pseudoephedrine 30 mg/chlorpheniramine 2 mg **(Rx)**

***Defen-LA***—pseudoephedrine 60 mg/guaifenesin 600 mg **(Rx)**

***Demi-Regroton***—chlorthalidone 25 mg/reserpine 0.125 mg **(Rx)**

***Demulen 1/35***—ethinyl estradiol 35 mcg/ethynodiol diacetate 1 mg **(Rx)**

***Demulen 1/50***—ethinyl estradiol 50 mcg/ethynodiol diacetate 1 mg **(Rx)**

***Desogen***—ethinyl estradiol 30 mcg/desogestrel 0.15 mg **(Rx)**

***Dexacidin Ophthalmic Ointment/Suspension***—(per g/per ml) 0.1% dexamethasone/0.35% neomycin base/polymyxin B 10,000 units **(Rx)**

***Dexasporin Ophthalmic Ointment***—(per g) 0.1% dexamethasone/0.35% neomycin base/polymyxin B 10,000 units **(Rx)**

***DHC Plus***—dihydro codeine 16 mg/acetaminophen 356.4 mg/caffeine 30 mg **(Rx)**

***Dialose Plus***—docusate sodium 100 mg/casanthranol 30 mg **(otc)**

***Di-Gel, Advanced Formula***—magnesium hydroxide 128 mg/calcium carbonate 280 mg/simethicone 20 mg **(otc)**

***Di-Gel Liquid***—(per 5 ml) aluminum hydroxide 200 mg/magnesium hydroxide 200 mg/simethicone 20 mg **(otc)**

***Dihistine DH Liquid***—(per 5 ml) pseudoephedrine 30 mg/chlorpheniramine 2 mg/codeine 10 mg **(Rx)**

***Dilaudid Cough Syrup***—(per 5 ml) guaifenesin 100 mg/hydromorphone 1 mg/5% alcohol **(Rx)**

***Dilor-G***—dyphylline 200 mg/guaifenesin 200 mg **(Rx)**

***Dimetane Decongestant***—brompheniramine 4 mg/phenylephrine 10 mg **(otc)**

***Dimetane-DX Cough Syrup***—(per 5 ml) brompheniramine 2 mg/pseudoephedrine 30 mg/dextromethorphan 10 mg **(Rx)**

***Dimetapp DM Elixir***—(per 5 ml) pseudoephedrine 5 mg/brompheniramine 2 mg/dextromethorphan 10 mg **(otc)**

***Dimetapp Elixir***—(per 5 ml) pseudoephedrine 15 mg/brompheniramine 2 mg **(otc)**

***Dimetapp Sinus***—pseudoephedrine 30 mg/ibuprofen 200 mg **(otc)**

***Diovan 80 HCT***—valsartan 80 mg/hydrochlorothide 12.5 mg **(Rx)**

***Diovan160 HCT***—valsartan 160 mg/hydrochlorothide 12.5 mg **(Rx)**

***Diovan HCT 160/25***—Valsartan 160 mg/Hydrochlorothiazide 25 mg **(Rx)**

***Diphtheria and Tetanus Toxoids, Adsorbed (Pediatric)***—(per 0.5 ml) 6.6 Lf units diphtheria/5 Lf units tetanus (Connaught); 12.5 Lf units diphtheria/5 Lf units tetanus (Lederle-Praxis); 7.5 Lf units diphtheria/7.5 Lf units tetanus (Massachusetts Public Health Biologic Labs); 10 Lf units diphtheria/5 Lf units tetanus (Wyeth-Ayerst) **(Rx)**

***Diphtheria and Tetanus Toxoids, Adsorbed (Adult)***—(per 0.5 ml) 2 Lf units diphtheria/5 Lf units tetanus (Connaught); 2 Lf units diphtheria/5 Lf units tetanus (Lederle-Praxis); 2 Lf units diphtheria/2 Lf units tetanus (Massachusetts Public Health Biologic Labs); 26.6 Lf units diphtheria/5 Lf units tetanus (Connaught); 12.5 Lf units diphtheria/5 Lf units tetanus (Lederle-Praxis); 7.5 Lf units diphtheria/7.5 Lf units tetanus (Massachusetts Public Health Biologic Labs); 10 Lf units diphtheria/5 Lf units tetanus (Wyeth-Ayerst); 6.6 Lf units diphtheria/5 Lf units tetanus (Connaught); 12.5 Lf units diphtheria/5 Lf units tetanus (Lederle-Praxis); 7.5 Lf units diphtheria/7.5 Lf units tetanus (Massachusetts Public Health Biologic Labs); 10 Lf units diphtheria/5 Lf units tetanus (Wyeth-Ayerst) **(Rx)**

***Diutensin-R***—methyclothiazide 2.5 mg/reserpine 0.1 mg **(Rx)**

***Doan's PM Extra Strength***—magnesium salicylate 500 mg/diphenhydramine 25 mg **(otc)**

***Dolacet***—hydrocodone 5 mg/acetaminophen 500 mg **(Rx)**

***Donnatal***—phenobarbital 16.2 mg/hyoscyamine 0.1037 mg/atropine 0.0194 mg/scopolamine 0.0065 mg **(Rx)**

***Donnatal Elixir***—(per 5 ml) phenobarbital 16.2 mg/hyoscyamine 0.1037 mg/atropine 0.0194 mg/scopolamine 0.0065 mg/23% alcohol **(Rx)**

***Donnatal Extentabs***—phenobarbital 48.6 mg/hyoscyamine 0.3111 mg/atropine 0.0582 mg/scopolamine 0.0195 mg **(Rx)**

***Donnazyme***—pancreatin 500 mg/lipase 1000 units/protease 12,500 units/amylase 12,500 units **(Rx)**

***Dorcol Children's Cold Formula Liquid***—(per 5 ml) pseudoephedrine 15 mg/chlorpheniramine 1 mg **(otc)**

***Doxidan***—docusate calcium 60 mg/casantranol 30 mg **(otc)**

***Dristan Cold***—pseudoephedrine 30 mg/acetaminophen 500 mg **(otc)**

***Dristan Cold Maximum Strength Caplets***—pseudoephedrine 30 mg/brompheniramine 2 mg/acetaminophen 500 mg **(otc)**

***Dristan Cold Multi-Symptom Formula***—acetaminophen 325 mg/phenylephrine 5 mg/chlorpheniramine 2 mg **(otc)**

***Dristan Sinus***—pseudoephedrine 30 mg/ibuprofen 200 mg **(otc)**

***Drixoral Cold & Allergy***—pseudoephedrine 120 mg/dexbrompheniramine 6 mg **(otc)**

***Drixoral Cold & Flu***—pseudoephedrine 60 mg/dexbrompheniramine 3 mg/acetaminophen 500 mg **(otc)**

***Drixoral Nasal Decongestant***—pseudoephedrine 120 mg **(otc)**

***Duac Topical Gel***—clindamycin 1%/benzoyl peroxide 5% **(Rx)**

***DuoNeb***—(per 3 ml) albuterol sulfate 3 mg/ipratroprium bromide 0.5 mg inhalation solution **(Rx)**

***Dura-Vent/DA***—phenylephrine 20 mg/chlorpheniramine 8 mg/methscopolamine 2.5 mg **(Rx)**

***Dyazide***—hydrochlorothiazide 25 mg/triamterene 37.5 mg **(Rx)**

***Dynafed Asthma Relief***—ephedrine 25 mg/guaifenesin 200 mg **(otc)**

***Dynafed Plus Maximum Strength***—pseudoephedrine 30 mg/acetaminophen 500 mg **(otc)**

***Dyphylline-GG Elixir***—(per 5 ml) dyphylline 100 mg/guaifenesin 100 mg **(Rx)**

***Elase Ointment***—(per g) fibrinolysin 1 unit/desoxyribonuclease 666.6 units **(Rx)**

***Elixophyllin-GG Liquid***—(per 15 ml) guaifenesin 100 mg/theophylline 100 mg **(Rx)**

***EMLA Cream and Anesthetic Disc***—lidocaine 2.5 mg/prilocaine 2.5 mg **(Rx)**

***Empirin w/codeine No. 3***—aspirin 325 mg/codeine phosphate 30 mg **(Rx)**

***Empirin w/codeine No. 4***—aspirin 325 mg/codeine phosphate 60 mg **(Rx)**

***Enduronyl***—methyclothiazide 5 mg/deserpidine 0.25 mg **(Rx)**

***Entex PSE***—pseudoephedrine 120 mg/guaifenesin 600 mg **(Rx)**

***Epifoam Aerosol Foam***—1% hydrocortisone/1% pramoxine **(Rx)**

***E-Pilo-1 Ophthalmic Solution***—1% epinephrine bitartrate/1% pilocarpine **(Rx)**

***E-Pilo-2 Ophthalmic Solution***—1% epinephrine bitartrate/2% pilocarpine **(Rx)**

***E-Pilo-4 Ophthalmic Solution***—1% epinephrine bitartrate/4% pilocarpine **(Rx)**

***E-Pilo-6 Ophthalmic Solution***—1% epinephrine bitartrate/6% pilocarpine **(Rx)**

***Eryzole oral suspension***—(per 5 ml) erythromycin 200 mg/sulfisoxazole 600 mg **(Rx)**

***Esgic-Plus***—butalbital 50 mg/acetaminophen 500 mg/caffeine 40 mg **(Rx)**

***Esimil***—guanethidine 10 mg/hydrochlorothiazide 25 mg **(Rx)**

***Estratest***—esterified estrogens 1.25 mg/methyltestosterone 2.5 mg **(Rx)**

***Estratest HS***—esterified estrogens 0.625 mg/methyltestosterone 1.25 mg **(Rx)**

***Etrafon***—perphenazine 2 mg/amitriptyline 25 mg **(Rx)**

***Etrafon-Forte***—perphenazine 4 mg/amitriptyline 25 mg **(Rx)**

*Excedrin Quick Tabs*—acetaminophen 500 mg/caffeine 65 mg
*Excedrin Tension Headache*—acetaminophen 500 mg/caffeine 65 mg
*Excedrin Migraine*—aspirin 250 mg/acetaminophen 250 mg/caffeine 65 mg **(otc)**
*Excedrin P.M.*—acetaminophen 500 mg/diphenhydramine citrate 38 mg **(otc)**
*Excedrin P.M. Liquigels*—acetaminophen 500 mg/diphenhydramine 25 mg **(otc)**
*Excedrin Sinus Extra Strength*—pseudoephedrine 30 mg/acetaminophen 500 mg **(otc)**
*Fansidar*—sulfidoxine 500 mg/pyrimethamine 25 mg **(Rx)**
*Fedahist*—pseudoephedrine 60 mg/chlorpheniramine 4 mg **(otc)**
*Fedahist Expectorant Syrup*—(per 5 ml) guaifenesin 200 mg/pseudoephedrine 20 mg **(otc)**
*Fedahist Gyrocaps*—pseudoephedrine 65 mg/chlorpheniramine 10 mg **(Rx)**
*Fedahist Timecaps*—pseudoephedrine 120 mg/chlorpheniramine 8 mg **(Rx)**
*Feen-A-Mint Pills*—bisacodyl 5 mg **(otc)**
*Fem-1*—acetaminophen 500 mg/pamabrom 25 mg **(otc)**
*Fembrt 1/5*—norethindrone 1 mg/ethinyl estradiol 5 mcg **(Rx)**
*Ferro-Sequels*—docusate sodium 100 mg/ferrous fumarate 150 mg **(otc)**
*Fioricet*—acetaminophen 325 mg/caffeine 40 mg/butalbital 50 mg **(Rx)**
*Fioricet w/codeine*—acetaminophen 325 mg/caffeine 40 mg/butalbital 50 mg/codeine 30 mg **(Rx)**
*Fiorinal*—aspirin 325 mg/caffeine 40 mg/butalbital 50 mg **(Rx)**
*Fiorinal w/codeine*—aspirin 325 mg/caffeine 40 mg/butalbital 50 mg/codeine 30 mg **(Rx)**
*FML-S Ophthalmic Suspension*—0.1% fluorometholone/10% sulfacetamide **(Rx)**
*Gas-Ban*—calcium carbonate 300 mg/simethicone 40 mg **(otc)**
*Gas-Ban DS Liquid*—(per 5 ml) aluminum hydroxide 400 mg/magnesium hydroxide 400 mg/simethicone 40 mg **(otc)**
*Gaviscon*—magnesium trisilicate 20 mg/aluminum hydroxide 80 mg **(otc)**
*Gaviscon Liquid*—(per 5 ml) aluminum hydroxide 31.7 mg/magnesium carbonate 119.3 mg **(otc)**
*Gelusil*—aluminum hydroxide 200 mg/magnesium hydroxide 200 mg/simethicone 25 mg **(otc)**
*Genac Tablets*—triprolidine 2.5 mg/pseudoephrine 60 mg **(otc)**
*Genatuss DM Syrup*—(per 5 ml) guaifenesin 100 mg/dextromethorphan 10 mg **(otc)**
*Glucovance 1.25*—glyburide 1.25 mg/metformin 500 mg **(Rx)**
*Glucovance 2.5*—glyburide 2.5 mg/metformin 500 mg **(Rx)**
*Glucovance 5*—glyburide 5 mg/metformin 500 mg **(Rx)**
*Granulex Aerosol*—(per 0.82 ml) trypsin 0.1 mg/Balsam Peru 72.5 mg/castor oil 650 mg **(Rx)**
*Guaifenex PSE 60*—pseudoephedrine 60 mg/guaifenesin 600 mg **(Rx)**
*Guaifenex PSE 120*—pseudoephedrine 120 mg/guaifenesin 600 mg **(Rx)**
*Guaituss AC*—(per 5 ml) codeine 10 mg/guaifenesin 100 mg **(Rx)**
*Haley's M-O Liquid*—(per 15 ml) magnesium hydroxide 900 mg/mineral oil 3.75 ml **(otc)**
*Halotussin-DM Sugar-Free Liquid*—(per 5 ml) guaifenesin 100 mg/dextromethorphan 10 mg **(otc)**
*Helidac*—bismuth subsalicylate 262.4-mg tablets plus metronidazole 250-mg tablets plus tetracycline 500-mg capsules in a compliance package **(Rx)**
*Humalog Mix 50/50*—insulin lispro protamine 50%/insulin lispro [rDNA origin] 50% **(Rx)**
*Humalog Mix 75/25*—insulin lispro protamine 75%/insulin lispro [rDNA origin] 25% **(Rx)**
*Humibid DM Pediatric*—dextromethorphan 15 mg/guaifenesin 300 mg **(Rx)**
*Humibid DM Tablets*—dextromethorphan 30 mg/guaifenesin 600 mg **(Rx)**
*HycoClear Tuss*—(per 5 ml) hydrocodone 5 mg/guaifenesin 100 mg **(Rx)**
*Hycodan*—hydrocodone 5 mg/homatropine 1.5 mg **(Rx)**
*Hycodan Syrup*—(per 5 ml) hydrocodone 5 mg/homatropine 1.5 mg **(otc)**

*Hycomine Compound*—chlorpheniramine 2 mg/acetaminophen 250 mg/phenylephrine 10 mg/ hydrocodone 5 mg/caffeine 30 mg **(Rx)**

*Hycomine Syrup*—(per 5 ml) hydrocodone 5 mg/phenylpropanolamine 25 mg **(Rx)**

*Hycotuss Expectorant*—(per 5 ml) guaifenesin 100 mg/hydrocodone 5 mg/10% alcohol **(Rx)**

*Hydrocet*—hydrocodone 5 mg/acetaminophen 500 mg **(Rx)**

*Hydrogesic*—hydrocodone 5 mg/acetaminophen 500 mg **(Rx)**

*Hydropres-50*—hydrochlorothiazide 50 mg/reserpine 0.125 mg **(Rx)**

*Hydro-Serp*—hydrochlorothiazide 50 mg/reserpine 0.125 mg **(Rx)**

*Hydroserpine #1*—hydrochlorothiazide 25 mg/reserpine 0.125 mg **(Rx)**

*Hyzaar*—losartan potassium 50 mg/hydrochlorothiazide 12.5 mg **(Rx)**

*Hyzaar*—losartan potassium 100 mg/hydrochlorothiazide 25 mg **(Rx)**

*Imodium Advanced*—loperamide 2 mg/simethicone 125 mg **(otc)**

*Inderide 40/25*—propranolol 40 mg/hydrochlorothiazide 25 mg **(Rx)**

*Innovar*—(per 1 ml) droperidol 2.5 mg/fentanyl 0.05 mg **(Rx)**

*Iofed*—brompheniramine 12 mg/pseudoephedrine 120 mg **(Rx)**

*Iofed PD*—brompheniramine 6 mg/pseudoephedrine 60 mg **(Rx)**

*Kaletra capsules*—lopinavir 133.3 mg/ritonavir 33.3 mg **(Rx)**

*Kaletra solution*—(per ml) lopinavir 80 mg/ritonavir 20 mg **(Rx)**

*Lactinex*—mixed culture of *Lactobacillus acidophilus* and *L. bulgaricus* **(otc)**

*Levlite*—levonorgestrel 0.100 mg/ethinyl estradiol 20 mcg **(Rx)**

*Levsin-PB Drops*—(per ml) hyoscyamine 0.125 mg/phenobarbital 15 mg/5% alcohol **(Rx)**

*Levsin w/Phenobarbital*—hyoscyamine 0.125 mg/phenobarbital 15 mg **(Rx)**

*Lexxel*—enalapril 5 mg/felodipine 5 mg **(Rx)**

*Lexxel*—enalapril 5 mg/felodipine 2.5 mg **(Rx)**

*Librax*—chlordiazepoxide 5 mg/clidinium 2.5 mg **(Rx)**

*Lida-Mantle-HC Cream*—0.5% hydrocortisone/3% lidocaine **(Rx)**

*Limbitrol DS 10-25*—chlordiazepoxide 10 mg/amitriptyline 25 mg **(Rx)**

*Lobac*—salicylamide 200 mg/phenyltoloxamine 20 mg/acetaminophen 300 mg **(Rx)**

*Loestrin Fe 1/20*—norethindrone acetate 1 mg/ethinyl estradiol 20 mcg per tablet with 7 tablets of ferrous fumarate 75 mg per container **(Rx)**

*Loestrin Fe 1.5/30*—norethindrone acetate 1.5 mg/ethinyl estradiol 30 mcg **(Rx)**

*Lomotil*—diphenoxylate 2.5 mg/atropine 0.025 mg **(Rx)**

*Lomotil Liquid*—(per 5 ml) diphenoxylate 2.5 mg/atropine 0.025 mg **(Rx)**

*Lo/Ovral*—ethinyl estradiol 30 mcg/norgestrel 0.3 mg **(Rx)**

*Lopressor HCT 50/25*—metoprolol 50 mg/hydrochlorothiazide 25 mg **(Rx)**

*Lopressor HCT 100/25*—metoprolol 100 mg/hydrochlorothiazide 25 mg **(Rx)**

*Lopressor HCT 100/50*—metoprolol 100 mg/hydrochlorothiazide 50 mg **(Rx)**

*Lorcet-HD*—hydrocodone 10 mg/acetaminophen 500 mg **(Rx)**

*Lorcet Plus*—hydrocodone 7.5 mg/acetaminophen 650 mg **(Rx)**

*Lorcet 10/650*—acetaminophen 650 mg/hydrocodone 10 mg **(Rx)**

*Lortab 2.5/500*—hydrocodone 2.5 mg/acetaminophen 500 mg **(Rx)**

*Lortab 5/500*—hydrocodone 5 mg/acetaminophen 500 mg **(Rx)**

*Lortab 7.5/500*—hydrocodone 7.5 mg/acetaminophen 500 mg **(Rx)**

*Lortab 10/500*—hydrocodone 10 mg/acetaminophen 500 mg **(Rx)**

*Lortab ASA*—aspirin 500 mg/hydrocodone 5 mg **(Rx)**

*Lortab Elixir*—(per 5 ml) hydrocodone 2.5 mg/acetaminophen 167 mg **(Rx)**

*[Losec 1-2-3 A]*—omeprazole 20 mg (14 doses), clarithromycin 500 mg (14 doses), amoxicillin 1 g (14 doses) in a convenience package **(Rx)**

*[Losec 1-2-3 M]*—omeprazole 20 mg (14 doses), clarithromycin 250 mg (14 doses), metronidazole 500 mg (14 doses) in a convenience package **(Rx)**

*Lotensin HCT 5/6.25*—benazepril 5 mg/hydrochlorothiazide 6.25 mg **(Rx)**

*Lotensin HCT 10/12.5*—benazepril 10 mg/hydrochlorothiazide 12.5 mg **(Rx)**

*Lotensin HCT 20/12.5*—benazepril 20 mg/hydrochlorothiazide 12.5 mg **(Rx)**

*Lotensin HCT 20/25*—benazepril 20 mg/hydrochlorothiazide 25 mg **(Rx)**

*Lotrel 2.5/10*—amlodipine 2.5 mg/benazepril 10 mg **(Rx)**

*Lotrel 5/10*—amlodipine 5 mg/benazepril 10 mg **(Rx)**

*Lotrel 5/20*—amlodipine 5 mg/benazepril 20 mg **(Rx)**

*Lotrel 10/20*—amlodipine 10 mg/benazepril 20 mg **(Rx)**

*Lotrisone Topical*—0.05% betamethasone/1% clotrimazole **(Rx)**

*Lufyllin-EPG Elixir*—(per 5 ml) ephedrine 24 mg/dyphylline 150 mg/guaifenesin 300 mg/phenobarbital 24 mg **(Rx)**

*Lufyllin-GG*—dyphylline 200 mg/guaifenesin 200 mg **(Rx)**

*Lunelle Monthly Contraceptive Injection*—(per 0.5 ml) medroxyprogesterone acetate 25 mg/ethinyl estradiol 5 mg **(Rx)**

*M-M-R II*—mixture of 3 viruses: measles/mumps/rubella **(Rx)**

*Maalox*—aluminum hydroxide 200 mg/magnesium hydroxide 200 mg **(otc)**

*Maalox Plus*—aluminum hydroxide 200 mg/magnesium hydroxide 200 mg/simethicone 25 mg **(otc)**

*Maalox Plus Extra Strength Suspension*—(per 5 ml) aluminum hydroxide 500 mg/magnesium hydroxide 450 mg/simethicone 40 mg **(otc)**

*Maalox Suspension*—(per 5 ml) aluminum hydroxide 225 mg/magnesium hydroxide 200 mg **(otc)**

*Malarone*—atovaquone 250 mg/proguanil 100 mg **(Rx)**

*Malarone Pediatric*—atovaquone 62.5 mg/proguanil 25 mg **(Rx)**

*Mapap Cold Formula*—acetaminophen 325 mg/chlorpheniramine 2 mg/pseudoephedrine 30 mg/dextromethorphan 15 mg **(otc)**

*Marax*—ephedrine 25 mg/theophylline 130 mg/hydroxyzine 10 mg **(Rx)**

*Maxitrol Ophthalmic Suspension/Ointment*—0.35% neomycin base/0.1% dexamethasone/polymyxin B 10,000 U/ml **(Rx)**

*Maxzide*—hydrochlorothiazide 50 mg/triamterene 75 mg **(Rx)**

*Maxzide-25MG*—hydrochlorothiazide 25 mg/triamterene 37.5 mg **(Rx)**

*Medi-Flu-Liquid*—(per 5 ml) pseudoephedrine 10 mg/chlorpheniramine 0.67 mg/dextromethorphan 5 mg/acetaminophen 167 mg/18.5% alcohol **(otc)**

*Mepergan Fortis*—meperidine 50 mg/promethazine 25 mg **(Rx)**

*Metaglip 250*—glipizide 2.5 mg/metformin 250 mg **(Rx)**

*Metaglip 2.5*—glipizide 2.5 mg/metformin 500 mg **(Rx)**

*Metaglip 5*—glipizide 5 mg/metformin 500 mg **(Rx)**

*Metimyd Ophthalmic Suspension/Ointment*—0.5% prednisolone/10% sodium sulfacetamide **(Rx)**

*Micardis HCT 40*—telmesartan 40 mg/hydrochlorothiazide 12.5 mg **(Rx)**

*Micardis HCT 80*—telmesartan 80 mg/hydrochlorothiazide 12.5 mg **(Rx)**

*Microgestin Fe 1/20*—norethindrone acetate 1 mg/ethinyl estradiol 20 mcg per tablet with 7 tablets of ferrous fumarate 75 mg per container **(Rx)**

*Microgestin Fe 1.5/30*—norethindrone acetate 1.5 mg/ethinyl estradiol 30 mcg per tablet with 7 tablets of ferrous fumarate 75 mg per container **(Rx)**

*Midol Maximum Strength Multi-Symptom Menstrual Gelcaps*—acetaminophen 500 mg/pyrilamine 15 mg/caffeine 60 mg **(otc)**

*Midol PM*—acetaminophen 500 mg/diphenhydramine 25 mg **(otc)**

*Midol PMS Maximum Strength Caplets*—acetaminophen 500 mg/pyrilamine 15 mg/pamabrom 25 mg **(otc)**

**Midol, Teen**—acetaminophen 400 mg/pamabrom 25 mg **(otc)**

**Midrin**—isometheptene 65 mg/acetaminophen 325 mg/dichloralphenazone 100 mg **(Rx)**

**Minizide 1**—prazosin 1 mg/polythiazide 0.5 mg **(Rx)**

**Minizide 2**—prazosin 2 mg/polythiazide 0.5 mg **(Rx)**

**Minizide 5**—prazosin 5 mg/polythiazide 0.5 mg **(Rx)**

**Moduretic**—hydrochlorothiazide 50 mg/amiloride 5 mg **(Rx)**

**Monopril-HCT 10**—fosinopril 10 mg/hydrochlorothiazine 12.5 mg **(Rx)**

**Monopril-HCT 20**—fosinopril 20 mg/hydrochlorothiazine 12.5 mg **(Rx)**

**Motrin Children's Cold Suspension**—(per 5 ml) ibuprofen 100 mg/pseudoephedrine 15 mg **(otc)**

**Motrin Sinus Headache**—pseudoephedrine 30 mg/ibuprofen 200 mg **(otc)**

**Murocoll-2 Ophthalmic Drops**—0.3% scopolamine/10% phenylephrine **(Rx)**

**Mycolog II Topical**—0.1% triamcinolone acetonide/nystatin 100,000 units/g **(Rx)**

**Mylanta**—aluminum hydroxide 200 mg/magnesium hydroxide 200 mg/simethicone 20 mg **(otc)**

**Mylanta Double Strength Liquid**—(per 5 ml) aluminum hydroxide 400 mg/magnesium hydroxide 400 mg/simethicone 40 mg **(otc)**

**Mylanta Gelcaps**—calcium carbonate 311 mg/magnesium carbonate 232 mg **(otc)**

**Naphcon-A Ophthalmic Solution**—0.25% naphazoline/0.3% pheniramine **(otc)**

**Nasatab LA**—guaifenesin 500 mg/pseudoephedrine 120 mg **(Rx)**

**NeoDecadron Ophthalmic Ointment**—0.35% neomycin/0.05% dexamethasone **(Rx)**

**NeoDecadron Ophthalmic Solution**—0.35% neomycin/0.1% dexamethasone **(Rx)**

**NeoDecadron Topical**—0.5% neomycin sulfate/0.1% dexamethasone **(Rx)**

**Neosporin Cream**—(per g) polymyxin B 10,000 units/neomycin 3.5 mg **(otc)**

**Neosporin G.U. Irrigant**—(per ml) neomycin 40 mg/polymyxin B 200,000 units **(Rx)**

**Neosporin Ophthalmic Ointment**—(per g) polymyxin B 10,000 units/neomycin 3.5 mg/bacitracin 400 units **(Rx)**

**Neosporin Ophthalmic Solution**—(per ml) polymyxin B 10,000 units/neomycin 1.75 mg/gramicidin 0.025 mg **(Rx)**

**Neosporin Plus Cream**—(per g) polymyxin B 10,000 units/neomycin 3.5 mg/lidocaine 40 mg **(otc)**

**Neosporin Topical Ointment**—(per g) neomycin 3.5 mg/bacitracin zinc 400 units/polymyxin B 5000 units **(otc)**

**Niferex-150 Forte**—ferrous sulfate 150 mg/vitamin B12 25 mcg/folic acid 1 mg **(Rx)**

**Norco 5/325**—hydrocodone 5 mg/acetaminophen 325 mg **(Rx)**

**Norco**—hydrocodone 10 mg/acetaminophen 325 mg **(Rx)**

**Norgesic**—orphenadrine 25 mg/caffeine 30 mg/aspirin 385 mg **(Rx)**

**Norgesic Forte**—orphenadrine 50 mg/caffeine 60 mg/aspirin 770 mg **(Rx)**

**Novacet Lotion**—10% sodium sulfacetamide/5% sulfur **(Rx)**

**Novafed A**—chlorpheniramine 8 mg/pseudoephedrine 120 mg **(Rx)**

**NuLytely**—PEG 3350 420 g/sodium bicarbonate 5.72 g/sodium chloride 11.2 g/potassium chloride 1.48 g **(Rx)**

**Numby Stuff Topical Solution**—lidocaine 2%/epinephrine 1:100,000 **(Rx)**

**NyQuil Nighttime Cold/Flu Medicine Liquid**—(per 5 ml) pseudoephedrine 10 mg/doxylamine 1.25 mg/dextromethorphan 5 mg/acetaminophen 167 mg/25% alcohol (may contain tartrazine) **(otc)**

**Octicair Otic Suspension**—1% hydrocortisone/neomycin 5 mg/ml/polymyxin B 10,000 units/ml **(Rx)**

**Opcon-A Ophthalmic Solution**—0.027% naphazoline/0.315% pheniramine **(otc)**

**Ornex**—pseudoephedrine 30 mg/acetaminophen 500 mg **(otc)**

**Ornex No Drowsiness**—pseudoephedrine 30 mg/acetaminophen 325 mg **(otc)**

*Orphengesic*—orphenadrine 25 mg/aspirin 385 mg/caffeine 30 mg **(Rx)**
*Orphengesic forte*—orphenadrine 50 mg/aspirin 770 mg/caffeine 60 mg **(Rx)**
*Ortho-cept*—ethinyl estradiol 30 mcg/desogestrel 0.15 mg **(Rx)**
*Ortho-cyclen*—ethinyl estradiol 35 mcg/norgestimate 0.25 mg **(Rx)**
*Ortho-Prefest*—estradiol 1 mg 15 tablets and estradiol 1 mg/norgestimate 0.09 mg 15 tablets in a 30-tablet blister package **(Rx)**
*Otocort Otic Suspension*—1% hydrocortisone/neomycin 5 mg/ml/polymyxin B 10,000 units/ml **(Rx)**
*Ovcon-50*—ethyinyl estradiol 50 mcg/norethindrone 1 mg **(Rx)**
*P-V-Tussin*—guaifenesin 200 mg/hydrocodone 5 mg/phenindamine 25 mg **(Rx)**
*Pain-X Topical*—0.05% capsaicin/5% menthol/4% camphor **(otc)**
*Pamprin Maximum Pain Relief*—acetaminophen 250 mg/pamabrom 25 mg/magnesium salicylate 250 mg **(otc)**
*Pamprin Multi-Symptom*—acetaminophen 500 mg/pamabrom 25 mg/pyrilamine 15 mg **(otc)**
*Pamprin Nighttime*—acetamnophen 650 mg/diphehydramine 50 mg
*Panacet 5/500*—hydrocodone 5 mg/acetaminophen 500 mg **(Rx)**
*Panasal 5/500*—hydrocodone 5 mg/aspirin 500 mg **(Rx)**
*Pancrease*—lipase 4500 units/amylase 20,000 units/protease 25,000 units **(Rx)**
*Pediacare Cold-Allergy Chewable*—pseudoephedrine 15 mg/chlorpheniramine 1 mg **(otc)**
*Pediacare Children's Multisymptom Cold*—(per 5 ml) pseudoephedrine 15 mg/chlorpheniramine 1 mg/dextromethorphan 5 mg **(otc)**
*Pediacare NightRest Cough-Cold Liquid*—(per 5 ml) pseudoephedrine 15 mg/chlorpheniramine 1 mg/dextromethorphan 7.5 mg **(otc)**
*Pediarix*—(per 0.5 ml) diptheria toxoid 25 Lf/tetanus toxoid inactivated 10 Lf/pertussis toxin, inactivated 25 mcg/filamentous hemagglutinin 25 mcg/pertactin 8 mcg/hepatitis B surface antigen 10 mcg/Type 1 poliovirus 40 D-antigen units/Type 2 poliovirus 8 D-antigen unite/Type 3 poliovirus 32 D-antigen units
*Pediazole Suspension*—(per 5 ml) erythromycin 200 mg/sulfisoxazole 600 mg **(Rx)**
*Pepcid Complete*—Calcium carbonate 800 mg/magnesium hydroxide 165 mg/famotidine 10 mg **(otc)**
*Percocet 2.5/325*—oxycodone 2.5 mg/acetaminophen 325 mg **(Rx)**
*Percocet 5/325*—oxycodone 5 mg/acetaminophen 325 mg **(Rx)**
*Percocet 7.5/325*—oxycodone 7.5 mg/acetaminophen 325 mg **(Rx)**
*Percocet 7.5/500*—oxycodone 7.5 mg/acetaminophen 500 mg **(Rx)**
*Percocet 10/325*—oxycodone 10 mg/acetaminophen 325 mg **(Rx)**
*Percocet 10/650*—oxycodone 10 mg/acetaminophen 650 mg **(Rx)**
*Percodan*—oxycodone 4.88 mg/aspirin 325 mg **(Rx)**
*Percogesic*—phenyltoloxamine 30 mg/acetaminophen 325 mg **(otc)**
*Perdiem Granules*—(per teaspoonful) senna 0.74 g/psyllium 3.25 g/sodium 1.8 mg/potassium 35.5 mg **(otc)**
*Peri-Colace*—docusate sodium 100 mg/casanthranol 30 mg **(otc)**
*Peri-Colace Syrup*—(per 15 ml) docusate sodium 60 mg/casanthranol 30 mg **(otc)**
*Phenerbel-S*—phenobarbital 40 mg/ergotamine tartrate 0.6 mg/l-alkaloids of belladonna 0.2 mg **(Rx)**
*Phenergan VC Syrup*—(per 5 ml) phenylephrine 5 mg/promethazine 6.25 mg **(Rx)**
*Phenergan VC w/codeine Syrup*—(per 5 ml) phenylephrine 5 mg/promethazine 6.25 mg/codeine 10 mg **(Rx)**
*Phenergan w/codeine Syrup*—(per 5 ml) promethazine 6.25 mg/codeine 10 mg **(Rx)**
*Phillips' Laxative Gelcaps*—docusate 100 mg **(otc)**

***Polaramine Expectorant Liquid***—(per 5 ml) guaifenesin 100 mg/dexchlorpheniramine 2 mg/pseudoephedrine 20 mg/7.5% alcohol **(Rx)**

***Polycitra Syrup***—(per 5 ml) potassium citrate 550 mg/sodium citrate 500 mg/citric acid 334 mg **(Rx)**

***Poly-Histine Elixir***—(per 5 ml) pheniramine 4 mg/pyrilamine 4 mg/phenyltoloxamine 4 mg/4% alcohol **(Rx)**

***Polysporin Ophthalmic Ointment***—(per g) polymyxin B 10,000 units/bacitracin 500 units **(Rx)**

***Polysporin Topical Ointment***—(per g) polymyxin B 10,000 units/bacitracin 500 units **(otc)**

***Polytrim Ophthalmic Solution***—(per ml) polymyxin B 10,000 units/trimethoprim 1 mg **(Rx)**

***Pravagard PAC 81/20***—aspirin (buffered) 81 mg (10 tablets) plus pravastatin 20 mg (10 tablets) in a compliance package **(Rx)**

***Pravagard PAC 81/40***—aspirin (buffered) 81 mg (10 tablets) plus pravastatin 40 mg (10 tablets) in a compliance package **(Rx)**

***Pravagard PAC 81/80***—aspirin (buffered) 81 mg (10 tablets) plus pravastatin 80 mg (10 tablets) in a compliance package **(Rx)**

***Pravagard PAC 325/20***—aspirin (buffered) 325 mg (10 tablets) plus pravastatin 20 mg (10 tablets) in a compliance package **(Rx)**

***Pravagard PAC 325/40***—aspirin (buffered) 325 mg (10 tablets) plus pravastatin 40 mg (10 tablets) in a compliance package **(Rx)**

***Pravagard PAC 325/80***—aspirin (buffered) 325 mg (10 tablets) plus pravastatin 80 mg (10 tablets) in a compliance package **(Rx)**

***Premphase***—conjugated estrogens 0.625 mg/medroxyprogesterone 5 mg (14 tablets) plus conjugated estrogens 0.625 mg (14 tablets) in a compliance package **(Rx)**

***Prempro 0.625/2.5***—conjugated estrogens 0.625 mg/medroxyprogesterone 2.5 mg (28 tablets) in a compliance package **(Rx)**

***Prempro 0.625/5***—conjugated estrogens 0.625 mg/medroxyprogesterone 5 mg (28 tablets) in a compliance package **(Rx)**

***Premsyn PMS***—acetaminophen 500 mg/pamabrom 25 mg/pyrilamine 15 mg **(otc)**

***Prevpac***—amoxicillin 500 mg capsules/clarithromycin 500 mg tablets/lansoprazole 30 mg capsules in a compliance package **(Rx)**

***Primatene***—ephedrine 12.5 mg/guaifenesin 200 mg **(otc)**

***Primaxin 250 mg I.V. For Injection***—imipenem 250 mg/cilastatin sodium 250 mg **(Rx)**

***Primaxin 500 mg I.V. For Injection***—imipenem 500 mg/cilastatin sodium 500 mg **(Rx)**

***Prinzide 10-12.5***—lisinopril 10 mg/hydrochlorothiazide 12.5 mg **(Rx)**

***Prinzide 20-12.5***—lisinopril 20 mg/hydrochlorothiazide 12.5 mg **(Rx)**

***Prinzide 20-25***—lisinopril 20 mg/hydrochlorothiazide 25 mg **(Rx)**

***Proben-C***—colchicine 0.5 mg/probenecid 500 mg **(Rx)**

***Proctofoam-HC Aerosol Foam***—1% hydrocortisone/1% pramoxine **(Rx)**

***Propacet 100***—propoxyphene-N 100 mg/acetaminophen 650 mg **(Rx)**

***Pseudo-Chlor***—pseudoephedrine 120 mg/chlorpheniramine 8 mg **(Rx)**

***Pseudo-Gest Plus***—pseudoephedrine 60 mg/chlorpheniramine 4 mg **(otc)**

***Quadrinal***—ephedrine 24 mg/theophylline 65 mg/potassium iodide 320 mg/phenobarbital 24 mg **(Rx)**

***Quelidrine Cough Syrup***—(per 5 ml) dextromethorphan 10 mg/phenylephrine 5 mg/ephedrine 5 mg/chlorpheniramine 2 mg/ammonium chloride 40 mg/ipecac 0.005 ml **(otc)**

***Quibron-300***—guaifenesin 180 mg/theophylline 300 mg **(Rx)**

***R&C Shampoo***—0.3% pyrethrins/3% piperonyl butoxide **(otc)**

***Rauzide***—bendroflumethiazide 4 mg/powdered rauwolfia serpentina 50 mg **(Rx)**

***Rebetron***—interferon alfa-2b (Intron A)/oral ribavirin (Rebetrol) 200 mg **(Rx)**

*Regulace*—docusate sodium 100 mg/casanthranol 30 mg **(otc)**
*Renese-R*—polythiazide 2 mg/reserpine 0.25 mg **(Rx)**
*Respahist*—pseudoephedrine 60 mg/brompheniramine 6 mg **(Rx)**
*Respaire-60*—guaifenesin 200 mg/pseudoephedrine 60 mg **(Rx)**
*RID Mousse*—pyrethrins 0.33%/piperonyl butoxide 4% **(otc)**
*RID Shampoo*—pyrethrins 0.3%/piperonyl butoxide 3% **(otc)**
*Rifamate*—isoniazid 150 mg/rifampin 300 mg **(Rx)**
*Rifater*—rifampin 120 mg/isoniazid 50 mg/pyrazinamide 300 mg **(Rx)**
*Riopan Plus Suspension*—(per 5 ml) magaldrate 540 mg/simethicone 40 mg **(otc)**
*Robaxisal*—aspirin 325 mg/methocarbamol 400 mg **(Rx)**
*Robitussin A-C Syrup*—(per 5 ml) codeine 10 mg/guaifenesin 100 mg/3.5% alcohol **(Rx)**
*Robitussin Cold & Cough Liqui-Gels*—pseudoephedrine 30 mg/guaifenesin 200 mg/dextro-
   methorphan 10 mg **(otc)**
*Robitussin-DAC Syrup*—(per 5 ml) codeine 10 mg/guaifenesin 100 mg/pseudoephedrine 30
   mg/1.4% alcohol **(Rx)**
*Robitussin-DM Liquid*—(per 5 ml) guaifenesin 100 mg/dextromethorphan 10 mg **(otc)**
*Robitussin Maximum Strength Cough and Cold Syrup*—dextromethorphan 15 mg/pseu-
   doephedrine 30 mg **(otc)**
*Robitussin Night Relief Liquid*—dextromethorphan 5 mg/pyrilamine 8.3 mg/pseudoephed-
   rine 10 mg/acetaminophen 108.3 mg **(otc)**
*Robitussin Pediatric Cough & Cold Liquid*—(per 5 ml) pseudoephedrine 15 mg/dextrome-
   thorphan 7.5 mg **(otc)**
*Robitussin-PE Syrup*—guaifenesin 100 mg/pseudoephedrine 30 mg/1.4% alcohol **(otc)**
*Robitussin Severe Congestion Liqui-Gels*—guaifenesin 200 mg/pseudoephedrine 30 mg
   **(otc)**
*Rolaids Calcium Rich*—magnesium hydroxide 80 mg/calcium carbonate 412 mg **(otc)**
*Rondec*—pseudoephedrine 60 mg/carbinoxamine 4 mg **(Rx)**
*Rondec DM Drops*—(per 1 ml) pseudoephedrine 25 mg/carbinoxamine 2 mg/dextromethor-
   phan 4 mg **(Rx)**
*Rondec DM Syrup*—(per 5 ml) pseudoephedrine 60 mg/carbinoxamine 4 mg/dextromethor-
   phan 15 mg **(Rx)**
*Rondec Oral Drops*—(per 1 ml) pseudoephedrine 25 mg/carbinoxamine 2 mg **(Rx)**
*Roxicet*—oxycodone 5 mg/acetaminophen 325 mg **(Rx)**
*Roxicet Oral Solution*—(per 5 ml) acetaminophen 325 mg/oxycodone 5 mg **(Rx)**
*Roxicet 5/500*—oxycodone 5 mg/acetaminophen 500 mg **(Rx)**
*Ru-Tuss DE*—pseudoephedrine 120 mg/guaifenesin 600 mg **(Rx)**
*Ru-Tuss Expectorant Liquid*—(per 5 ml) guaifenesin 100 mg/pseudoephedrine 30 mg/dex-
   tromethorphan 10 mg/10% alcohol **(otc)**
*Ru-Tuss w/Hydrocodone Liquid*—(per 5 ml) hydrocodone 1.7 mg/phenylephrine 5 mg/pyri-
   lamine 3.3 mg/pheniramine 3.3 mg/phenylpropanolamine 3.3 mg/5% alcohol **(Rx)**
*Ryna-C Liquid*—(per 5 ml) pseudoephedrine 30 mg/chlorpheniramine 2 mg/codeine 10 mg
   **(Rx)**
*Ryna Liquid*—(per 5 ml) pseudoephedrine 30 mg/chlorpheniramine 2 mg **(otc)**
*Rynatan*—phenylephrine 25 mg/chlorpheniramine 8 mg/pyrilamine 25 mg **(Rx)**
*Rynatan Pediatric Suspension*—(per 5 ml) phenylephrine 5 mg/chlorpheniramine 2 mg/
   pyrilamine 12.5 mg **(Rx)**
*Rynatuss*—ephedrine 10 mg/carbetapentane 60 mg/chlorpheniramine 5 mg/phenylephrine 10
   mg **(Rx)**
*Salutensin*—reserpine 0.125 mg/hydroflumethiazide 50 mg **(Rx)**
*Salutensin-Demi*—reserpine 0.125 mg/hydroflumethiazide 25 mg **(Rx)**

***Scot-Tussin DM Liquid***—(per 5 ml) chlorpheniramine 2 mg/dextromethorphan 15 mg **(otc)**
***Scot-Tussin Original 5-Action Liquid***—phenylephrine 4.2 mg/pheniramine 13.3 mg/sodium citrate 83.3 mg/sodium salicylate 83.3 mg/caffeine citrate 25 mg **(otc)**
***Sedapap-10***—acetaminophen 650 mg/butalbital 50 mg **(Rx)**
***Semprex-D***—acrivastine 8 mg/pseudoephedrine 60 mg **(Rx)**
***Senokot-S***—standardized senna concentrate 187 mg/docusate sodium 50 mg **(otc)**
***Septra***—trimethoprim 80 mg/sulfamethoxazole 400 mg **(Rx)**
***Septra DS***—trimethoprim 160 mg/sulfamethoxazole 800 mg **(Rx)**
***Septra I.V. For Injection***—(per 5 ml) trimethoprim 80 mg/sulfamethoxazole 400 mg **(Rx)**
***Septra Suspension***—(per 5 ml) trimethoprim 40 mg/sulfamethoxazole 200 mg **(Rx)**
***Ser-Ap-Es***—hydralazine 25 mg/hydrochlorothiazide 15 mg/reserpine 0.1 mg **(Rx)**
***Silafed Syrup***—(per 5 ml) pseudoephedrine 30 mg/triprolidine 1.25 mg **(otc)**
***Silaminic Cold Syrup***—(per 5 ml) phenylpropanolamine 12.5 mg/chlorpheniramine 2 mg **(otc)**
***Sinarest Extra Strength***—pseudoephedrine 30 mg/chlorpheniramine 2 mg/acetaminophen 500 mg **(otc)**
***Sinarest No Drowsiness***—pseudoephedrine 30 mg/acetaminophen 500 mg **(otc)**
***Sinarest Sinus***—pseudoephedrine 30 mg/chlorpheniramine 2 mg/acetaminophen 325 mg **(otc)**
***Sine-Aid IB***—pseudoephedrine 30 mg/ibuprofen 200 mg **(otc)**
***Sine-Aid Maximum Strength***—pseudoephedrine 30 mg/acetaminophen 500 mg **(otc)**
***Sinemet 10/100***—carbidopa 10 mg/levodopa 100 mg **(Rx)**
***Sinemet 25/100***—carbidopa 25 mg/levodopa 100 mg **(Rx)**
***Sinemet 25/250***—carbidopa 25 mg/levodopa 250 mg **(Rx)**
***Sinemet CR 25-100***—carbidopa 25 mg/levodopa 100 mg **(Rx)**
***Sinemet CR 50-200***—carbidopa 50 mg/levodopa 200 mg **(Rx)**
***Sine-Off Maximum Strength No Drowsiness Formula Caplets***—pseudoephedrine 30 mg/acetaminophen 500
***Sine-Off Sinus Medicine***—pseudoephedrine 30 mg/chlorpheniramine 2 mg/acetaminophen 500 mg **(otc)**
***Sinutab Maximum Strength Sinus Allergy***—acetaminophen 500 mg/chlorpheniramine 2 mg/pseudoephedrine 30 mg **(otc)**
***Sinutab Maximum Strength Without Drowsiness***—pseudoephedrine 30 mg/acetaminophen 500 mg **(otc)**
***Sinutab Non-Drying***—pseudoephedrine 30 mg/guaifenesin 200 mg **(otc)**
***Slo-Phyllin GG***—guaifenesin 90 mg/theophylline 150 mg **(Rx)**
***Slow-Salt-K***—Sodium chloride 410 mg/potassium chloride 150 mg **(Rx)**
***Solage***—mequinol 2%/tretinoin 0.01% topical **(Rx)**
***Soma Compound***—aspirin 325 mg/carisoprodol 200 mg **(Rx)**
***Spec-T Lozenge***—dextromethorphan 10 mg/benzocaine 10 mg **(otc)**
***Stalevo 50***—carbidopa 12.5 mg/entacapone 200 mg/levodopa 50 mg **(Rx)**
***Stalevo 100***—carbidopa 25 mg/entacapone 200 mg/levodopa 100 mg **(Rx)**
***Stalevo 150***—carbidopa 37.5 mg/entacapone 200 mg/levodopa 150 mg **(Rx)**
***Suboxone N2***—Buprenorphine 2 mg/naloxone 0.5 mg **(Rx)**
***Suboxone N8***—Buprenorphine 8 mg/naloxone 2 mg **(Rx)**
***Sudafed Cold & Cough Liquicaps***—pseudoephedrine 30 mg/dextromethorphan 10 mg/guaifenesin 100 mg/acetaminophen 250 mg **(otc)**
***Sudafed Cold & Sinus***—pseudoephedrine 30 mg/acetaminophen 325 mg **(otc)**
***Sudafed Cold & Allergy***—pseudoephedrine 60 mg/chlorpheniramine 4 mg **(otc)**
***Sudafed Plus***—pseudoephedrine 60 mg/chlorpheniramine 4 mg **(otc)**
***Sudafed Severe Cold***—pseudoephedrine 30 mg/dextromethorphan 15 mg **(otc)**

*Sudafed Sinus Maximum Strength*—pseudoephedrine 30 mg/acetaminophen 500 mg **(otc)**
*Sudal 60/500*—pseudoephedrine 60 mg/guaifenesin 500 mg **(Rx)**
*Sudal 120/600*—pseudoephedrine 120 mg/guaifenesin 600 mg **(Rx)**
*Sultrin Triple Sulfa Vaginal Cream*—3.42% sulfathiazole/2.86% sulfacetamide/3.7% sulfabenzamide **(Rx)**
*Sultrin Triple Sulfa Vaginal Tablets*—sulfathiazole 172.5 mg/sulfacetamide 143.75 mg/sulfabenzamide 184 mg/urea **(Rx)**
*Symbyax 6/25*—olanzapine 6 mg/fluoxetine 25 mg **(Rx)**
*Symbyax 6/50*—olanzapine 6 mg/fluoxetine 50 mg **(Rx)**
*Symbyax 12/25*—olanzapine 12 mg/fluoxetine 25 mg **(Rx)**
*Symbyax 12/50*—olanzapine 12 mg/fluoxetine 50 mg **(Rx)**
*Synalgos-DC*—aspirin 356.4 mg/caffeine 30 mg/dihydrocodeine 16 mg **(Rx)**
*Synercid*—(per 10 ml) quinupristin 150 mg/dalfopristin 350 mg **(Rx)**
*Talacen*—acetaminophen 650 mg/pentazocine 25 mg **(Rx)**
*Talwin Compound*—aspirin 325 mg/pentazocine 12.5 mg **(Rx)**
*Talwin NX*—pentazocine 50 mg/naloxone 0.5 mg **(Rx)**
*Tarka 182*—trandolapril 2 mg (immediate release)/verapamil 180 mg (sustained release) **(Rx)**
*Tarka 241*—trandolapril 1 mg (immediate release)/verapamil 240 mg (sustained release) **(Rx)**
*Tarka 242*—trandolapril 2 mg (immediate release)/verapamil 240 mg (sustained release) **(Rx)**
*Tarka 244*—trandolapril 4 mg (immediate release)/verapamil 240 mg (sustained release) **(Rx)**
*Tavist Allergy/Sinus/Headache*—clemastine fumarate 0.335 mg/pseudoephedrine hydrochloride 30 mg/acetaminophen 500 mg **(otc)**
*Tavist Sinus*—acetaminophen 500 mg/pseudoephedrine 30 mg **(otc)**
*Teczem*—enalapril 5 mg (extended release)/diltiazem 180 mg (extended release) **(Rx)**
*Tedrigen*—ephedrine 22.5 mg/theophylline 120 mg/phenobarbital 7.5 mg **(Rx)**
*Teen Midol*—see *Midol, Teen*
*Tegrin-LT Shampoo*—0.33% pyrethrins/3.15% piperonyl butoxide **(otc)**
*Tenoretic 50*—chlorthalidone 25 mg/atenolol 50 mg **(Rx)**
*Tenoretic 100*—chlorthalidone 25 mg/atenolol 100 mg **(Rx)**
*Terra-Cortril Ophthalmic Suspension*—1.5% hydrocortisone acetate/0.5% oxytetracycline **(Rx)**
*Terramycin with Polymyxin B Sulfate Ophthalmic Ointment*—(per g) polymyxin B 10,000 units/oxytetracycline 5 mg **(Rx)**
*T-Gesic*—hydrocodone 5 mg/acetaminophen 500 mg **(Rx)**
*Theodrine*—ephedrine 22.5 mg/theophylline 120 mg **(otc)**
*Thera-Flu, Flu & Cold Medicine Powder*—(per packet) pseudoephedrine 60 mg/chlorpheniramine 4 mg/acetaminophen 650 mg **(otc)**
*Thera-Flu, Flu, Cold & Cough Powder*—(per pack) pseudoephedrine 60 mg/chlorpheniramine 4 mg/dextromethorphan 20 mg/acetaminophen 650 mg **(otc)**
*Thera-Flu NightTime Powder*—(per pack) pseudoephedrine 60 mg/chlorpheniramine 4 mg/dextromethorphan 30 mg/acetaminophen 1000 mg **(otc)**
*Thera-Flu Non-Drowsy Flu, Cold & Cough Maximum Strength Powder*—(per pack) pseudoephedrine 60 mg/dextromethorphan 30 mg/acetaminophen 1000 mg **(otc)**
*Thera-Flu Non-Drowsy Formula Maximum Strength Caplets*—pseudoephedrine 30 mg/dextromethorphan 15 mg/acetaminophen 500 mg **(otc)**
*Timentin for Injection*—(3.1-g vials) ticarcillin 3 g/clavulanic acid 0.1 g **(Rx)**
*Timolide 10-25*—timolol 10 mg/hydrochlorothiazide 25 mg **(Rx)**
*Titralac Plus*—calcium carbonate 420 mg/simethicone 21 mg **(otc)**
*TobraDex Ophthalmic Suspension/Ointment*—0.1% dexamethasone/0.3% tobramycin **(Rx)**

*Triacin-C Cough Syrup*—(per 5 ml) codeine 10 mg/pseudoephedrine 30 mg/triprolidine 1.25 mg **(Rx)**

*Tri-Hydroserpine*—hydralazine 25 mg/hydrochlorothiazide 15 mg/reserpine 0.1 mg **(Rx)**

*Tri-Levlen*
   *Phase I*—levonorgestrel 0.05 mg/ethinyl estradiol 30 mcg **(Rx)**
   *Phase II*—levonorgestrel 0.075 mg/ethinyl estradiol 40 mcg **(Rx)**
   *Phase III*—levonorgestrel 0.125 mg/ethinyl estradiol 30 mcg **(Rx)**

*Triaminic AM Cough & Decongestant Formula Liquid*—(per 5 ml) pseudoephedrine 15 mg/dextromethorphan 7.5 mg **(otc)**

*Triaminic Nite Light Liquid*—(per 5 ml) pseudoephedrine 15 mg/chlorpheniramine 1 mg/dextromethorphan 7.5 mg **(otc)**

*Triaminic Sore Throat Formula Liquid*—(per 5 ml) pseudoephedrine 15 mg/dextromethorphan 7.5 mg/acetaminophen 160 mg **(otc)**

*Triavil 2-10*—perphenazine 2 mg/amitriptyline 10 mg **(Rx)**

*Triavil 2-25*—perphenazine 2 mg/amitriptyline 25 mg **(Rx)**

*Triavil 4-10*—perphenazine 4 mg/amitriptyline 10 mg **(Rx)**

*Triavil 4-25*—perphenazine 4 mg/amitriptyline 25 mg **(Rx)**

*Triavil 4-50*—perphenazine 4 mg/amitriptyline 50 mg **(Rx)**

*Tri-Luma*—fluocinolone 0.01%/hydroquinone 4%/tretinoin 0.05% **(Rx)**

*Trinalin Repetabs*—azatadine maleate 1 mg/pseudoephedrine 120 mg **(Rx)**

*Triphasil*
   *Phase I*—levonorgestrel 0.05 mg/ethinyl estradiol 30 mcg **(Rx)**
   *Phase II*—levonorgestrel 0.075 mg/ethinyl estradiol 40 mcg **(Rx)**
   *Phase III*—levonorgestrel 0.125 mg/ethinyl estradiol 30 mcg **(Rx)**

*Triple Antibiotic Ophthalmic Ointment*—(per g) polymyxin B 10,000 units/neomycin 3.5 mg/bacitracin 400 units **(Rx)**

*Tripolidine/pseudoephedrine Syrup (generic)*—triprolidine 1.25 mg/pseudoephrine 30 mg/5 ml **(otc)**

*Tripolidine/pseudoephedrine Tablets (generic)*—triprolidine 2.5 mg/pseudoephrine 60 mg **(otc)**

*Trizivir*—abacavir 300 mg/lamivudine 150 mg/zidovudine 300 mg **(Rx)**

*Tuinal 100 mg*—amobarbital 50 mg/secobarbital 50 mg **(Rx)**

*Tusibron-DM Syrup*—(per 5 ml) guaifenesin 100 mg/dextromethorphan 15 mg **(otc)**

*Tussionex Pennkinetic Suspension*—(per 5 ml) chlorpheniramine 8 mg/hydrocodone 10 mg (as polistirex) **(Rx)**

*Tussi-Organidin NR Liquid*—(per 5 ml) codeine 10 mg/guaifenesin 100 mg **(Rx)**

*Tussi-Organidin DM NR Liquid*—(per 5 ml) guaifenesin 100 mg/dextromethorphan 10 mg **(Rx)**

*Twinrix*—hepatitis A vaccine, inactivated not less than 720 enzyme-linked immunosorbent assay units/hepatitis B vaccine [recombinant] 20 mcg per ml **(Rx)**

*Tylenol Allergy Sinus, Maximum Strength Gelcaps*—acetaminophen 500 mg/chlorpheniramine 2 mg/pseudoephedrine 30 mg **(otc)**

*Tylenol Children's Cold*—acetaminophen 80 mg/chlorpheniramine 0.5 mg/pseudoephedrine 7.5 mg **(otc)**

*Tylenol Children's Cold Liquid*—(per 5 ml) acetaminophen 160 mg/chlorpheniramine 1 mg/pseudoephedrine 15 mg **(otc)**

*Tylenol Children's Cold Multi-Symptom Plus Cough Liquid*—(per 5 ml) acetaminophen 160 mg/dextromethorphan 5 mg/chlorpheniramine 1 mg/pseudoephedrine 15 mg **(otc)**

*Tylenol Children's Cold Plus Cough Chewable*—acetaminophen 80 mg/pseudoephedrine 7.5 mg/dextromethorphan 2.5 mg/chlorpheniramine 0.5 mg **(otc)**

***Tylenol Cold Multi-Symptom***—acetaminophen 325 mg/chlorpheniramine 2 mg/pseudoephedrine 30 mg/dextromethorphan 15 mg **(otc)**

***Tylenol Cold No Drowsiness***—acetaminophen 325 mg/pseudoephedrine 30 mg/dextromethorphan 15 mg **(otc)**

***Tylenol Flu Maximum Strength Gelcaps***—dextromethorphan 15 mg/pseudoephedrine 30 mg/acetaminophen 500 mg **(otc)**

***Tylenol Flu NightTime Maximum Strength Gelcaps***—pseudoephedrine 30 mg/chlorpheniramine 2 mg/acetaminophen 500 mg **(otc)**

***Tylenol Flu NightTime Maximum Strength Powder***—pseudoephedrine 60 mg/diphenhydramine 50 mg/acetaminophen 1000 mg **(otc)**

***Tylenol Headache Plus, Extra Strength***—acetaminophen 500 mg/calcium carbonate 250 mg **(otc)**

***Tylenol Multi-Symptom Cough Liquid***—(per 5 ml) dextromethorphan 10 mg/acetaminophen 216.7 mg/5% alcohol **(otc)**

***Tylenol Multi-Symptom Cough w/Decongestant Liquid***—(per 5 ml) dextromethorphan 10 mg/acetaminophen 200 mg/pseudoephedrine 20 mg **(otc)**

***Tylenol Multi-Symptom Hot Medication***—(per pack) acetaminophen 650 mg/chlorpheniramine 4 mg/pseudoephedrine 60 mg/dextromethorphan 30 mg **(otc)**

***Tylenol PM, Extra Strength***—acetaminophen 500 mg/diphenhydramine 25 mg **(otc)**

***Tylenol Severe Allergy***—diphenhydramine 12.5 mg/acetaminophen 500 mg **(otc)**

***Tylenol Sinus Maximum Strength***—pseudoephedrine 30 mg/acetaminophen 500 mg **(otc)**

***Tylenol w/codeine Elixir***—(per 5 ml) codeine 12 mg/acetaminophen 120 mg **(Rx)**

***Tylenol w/codeine No. 2***—acetaminophen 300 mg/codeine 15 mg **(Rx)**

***Tylenol w/codeine No. 3***—acetaminophen 300 mg/codeine 30 mg **(Rx)**

***Tylenol w/codeine No. 4***—acetaminophen 300 mg/codeine 60 mg **(Rx)**

***Tylox***—oxycodone 5 mg/acetaminophen 500 mg **(Rx)**

***Tyrodone Liquid***—(per 5 ml) hydrocodone 5 mg/pseudoephedrine 60 mg/5% alcohol **(Rx)**

***Ultracet***—tramadol 37.5 mg/acetaminophen 325 mg **(Rx)**

***Unasyn for Injection 1.5 g***—ampicillin 1 g/sulbactam 0.5 g **(Rx)**

***Unasyn for Injection 3 g***—ampicillin 2 g/sulbactam 1 g **(Rx)**

***Uniretic***—moexipril 7.5 mg/hydrochlorothiazide 12.5 mg or moexipril 15 mg/hydrochlorothiazide 25 mg **(Rx)**

***Unituss HC Syrup***—(per 5 ml) hydrocodone 2.5 mg/phenylephrine 5 mg/chlorpheniramine 2 mg **(Rx)**

***Urised***—methenamine 40.8 mg/phenyl salicylate 18.1 mg/atropine 0.03 mg/hyoscyamine 0.3 mg/benzoic acid 4.5 mg/methylene blue 5.4 mg **(Rx)**

***Vanquish***—aspirin 227 mg/acetaminophen 194 mg/caffeine 33 mg **(otc)**

***Vaseretic 5-12.5***—enalapril 5 mg/hydrochlorothiazide 12.5 mg **(Rx)**

***Vaseretic 10-25***—enalapril 10 mg/hydrochlorothiazide 25 mg **(Rx)**

***Vasocidin Ophthalmic Ointment***—0.5% prednisolone/10% sulfacetamide **(Rx)**

***Vasocidin Ophthalmic Solution***—0.25% prednisolone/10% sulfacetamide **(Rx)**

***Vasocon-A Ophthalmic Solution***—0.05% naphazoline/0.5% antazoline **(Rx)**

***Vicks 44D Cough & Head Congestion Liquid***—(per 5 ml) dextromethorphan 10 mg/pseudoephedrine 20 mg **(otc)**

***Vicks 44E Liquid***—(per 5 ml) dextromethorphan 6.7 mg/guaifenesin 66.7 mg **(otc)**

***Vicks 44M Cold, Flu,& Cough LiquiCaps***—dextromethorphan 10 mg/pseudoephedrine 30 mg/chlorpheniramine 2 mg/acetaminophen 250 mg **(otc)**

***Vicks 44 Non-Drowsy Cold & Cough LiquiCaps***—dextromethorphan 30 mg/pseudoephedrine 60 mg **(otc)**

*Vicks Children's NyQuil Nighttime Cough/Cold Liquid*—(per 5 ml) pseudoephedrine 10 mg/chlorpheniramine 0.67 mg/dextromethorphan 5 mg **(otc)**

*Vicks DayQuil Liquid*—(per 5 ml) dextromethorphan 3.3 mg/pseudoephedrine 10 mg/acetaminophen 108.3 mg/guaifenesin 33.3 mg **(otc)**

*Vicks DayQuil Sinus Pressure & Pain Relief*—pseudoephedrine 30 mg/acetaminophen 500 mg **(otc)**

*Vicks NyQuil Liquicaps*—pseudoephedrine 30 mg/doxylamine 6.25 mg/dextromethorphan 10 mg/acetaminophen 250 mg **(otc)**

*Vicks NyQuil Multi-Symptom Cold Flu Relief Liquid*—(per 5 ml) pseudoephedrine 10 mg/doxylamine 2.1 mg/dextromethorphan 5 mg/acetaminophen 167 mg **(otc)**

*Vicks Pediatric Formula 44e Liquid*—(per 5 ml) dextromethorphan 3.3 mg/guaifenesin 33.3 mg **(otc)**

*Vicks Pediatric Formula 44m Multi-Symptom Cough & Cold Liquid*—(per 5 ml) pseudoephedrine 10 mg/chlorpheniramine 0.67 mg/dextromethorphan 5 mg **(otc)**

*Vicodin*—acetaminophen 500 mg/hydrocodone 5 mg **(Rx)**

*Vicodin ES*—hydrocodone 7.5 mg/acetaminophen 750 mg **(Rx)**

*Vicodin HP*—hydrocodone 10 mg/acetaminophen 660 mg **(Rx)**

*VicodinTuss*—(per 5 ml) hydrocodone 5 mg/guaifenesin 100 mg **(Rx, C-III)**

*Vicoprofen*—hydrocodone 7.5 mg/ibuprofen 200 mg **(Rx)**

*Wigraine Suppositories*—ergotamine 2 mg/caffeine 100 mg **(Rx)**

*Yasmin 28*—drosperinone 3 mg/ethinyl estradiol 30 mcg **(Rx)**

*Zestoretic 10/12.5*—lisinopril 10 mg/hydrochlorothiazide 12.5 mg **(Rx)**

*Zestoretic 20/12.5*—lisinopril 20 mg/hydrochlorothiazide 12.5 mg **(Rx)**

*Zestoretic 20/25*—lisinopril 20 mg/hydrochlorothiazide 25 mg **(Rx)**

*Ziac 2.5 mg*—bisoprolol 2.5 mg/hydrochlorothiazide 6.25 mg **(Rx)**

*Ziac 5 mg*—bisoprolol 5 mg/hydrochlorothiazide 6.25 mg **(Rx)**

*Ziac 10 mg*—bisoprolol 10 mg/hydrochlorothiazide 6.25 mg **(Rx)**

*Ziks Cream*—methyl salicylate 12%/menthol 1%/capsaicin 0.025% **(otc)**

*Zotrim*—phenazopyridine 200 mg/sulfamethoxazole 160 mg/I trimethoprim 800 mg **(Rx)**

*Zydone*—hydrocodone 5 mg/acetaminophen 500 mg **(Rx)**

*Zyrtec-D*—cetirizine 5 mg/pseudoephedrine 120 mg **(Rx)**

# APPENDIX C
# Ophthalmic Medications

General Info: See Appendix F for administration techniques for ophthalmic agents.
Consult health care professional regarding;
Concurrent use of contact lenses (medication or additives may be absorbed by the lens).
Concurrent administration of other ophthalmic agents (order and spacing may be important).

## Alpha-Adrenergic Blocker

Uses: Reverses mydriasis from phenylephrine or tropicamide.
Cautions: Avoid using in conditions in which miosis is undesirable; not to be used more than once weekly.

| Generic Name (Brand Name) [Canadian Brand Name] | Dose | Notes |
|---|---|---|
| dapiprazole (Rev-Eyes) | Adults: 1 drop followed after 5 min by another drop | ▪ Administer immediately following retinal exam ▪ ADRs* : blurred vision, irritation, corneal edema, punctate keratitis |

## Anesthetics

Uses: Provide brief local anesthesia to allow measurement of intraocular pressure, removal of foreign bodies, or other superficial procedures.
Cautions: Repeated use may result in increased risk of CNS and cardiovascular toxicity; cross-sensitivity with some local anesthetics may occur.

| Generic Name (Brand Name) [Canadian Brand Name] | Dose | Notes |
|---|---|---|
| proparacaine (AK-Taine, Alcaine, Ocu-Caine, Ophthaine, Ophthetic, Spectro-Caine) [Diocane] | Adults and children: 1–2 drops of 0.5% solution (single dose) | ▪ Does not interact with ophthalmic cholinesterase inhibitors ▪ ADRs: ophthalmic—irritation; systemic—irregular heartbeat, CNS depression, CNS stimulation |
| tetracaine (Pontocaine) [Minims Tetracaine] | Adults: 1–2 drops of 0.5–1% solution (single dose) | ▪ May interact with ophthalmic cholinesterase inhibitors, resulting in increased duration of action and risk of toxicity ▪ ADRs: ophthalmic—irritation; systemic—irregular heartbeat, CNS depression, CNS stimulation |

Antihistamines

Uses: Various forms of allergic conjunctivitis.

Generic Name (Brand Name) {Canadian Brand Name}	Dose	Notes
azelastine (Optivar)	Adults: 1 drop of 0.5 mg/ml solution into each affected eye twice daily	■ ADRs: transient burning/stinging, headache, bitter taste
emedastine (Emadine)	Adults: 1 drop in affected eye up to 4 times daily	■ ADRs: headache, drowsiness, malaise, local irritation
levocabastine (Livostin)	Adults: 1 drop of 0.05% solution 4 times daily	■ ADRs: mild transient stinging, burning, headache, lid edema, drowsiness, dry mouth, nausea
olopatadine (Patanol)	Adults and children ≥3 yr: 1–2 drops of 0.1% solution twice daily (given 6–8 hr apart)	■ Small amounts are absorbed; excreted in urine ■ ADRs: headache, conjunctival irritation

Anti-infectives / Antifungals / Antivirals

Uses: Localized superficial ophthalmic infections.
Cautions: Small amounts may be absorbed and result in hypersensitivity reactions.

Generic Name (Brand Name) {Canadian Brand Name}	Dose	Notes
chloramphenicol (AK-Chlor, Chlorofair, Chloroptic, Clorachol, Econochlor, I-Chlor, Ocu-Chlor, Ophthochlor, Spectro-Chlor) {Fenicol, Ophtho-Chloram, Pentamycetin}	Adults and children: 1 drop of solution or thin strip of ointment q 1–4 hr	■ May rarely cause systemic hematologic toxicity if used chronically and in excessive doses
ciprofloxacin (Ciloxan)	Adult: *bacterial conjunctivitis*—1 drop in each eye q 2 hr while awake for 48 hr, then q 4 hr while awake for 5 days; *corneal ulcers*—1 drop in affected eye q 15 min for 6 hr, then q 30 min while awake for rest of day, then q 1 hr while awake for next 24 hr, then q 4 hr while awake until re-epithelialization occurs or ribbon of ophthalmic ointment 3 times daily for 2 days, then twice daily for 5 days.	■ May cause harmless white crystalline precipitate that resolves over time ■ ADRs: altered taste, systemic allergic reactions, photophobia, discomfort

| Generic Name (Brand Name) {Canadian Brand Name} | Dose | Notes |
|---|---|---|
| erythromycin (Ilotycin) | Adults and children: *treatment of infections*—thin strip up to 6 times daily<br>Infants: *prophylaxis of ophthalmia neonatorum*—thin strip in each eye as a single dose | ■ ADRs: irritation |
| gatifloxacin (Zymar) | Adults and children >1 yr: 1 drop of 0.3% soln q 2 hr while awake for two days, then 4 times daily for 5 more days | ■ ADRs: irritation, headache, reduced visual acuity, taste disturbance. |
| gentamicin (Garamycin, Genoptic, Gentacidin, Gentafair, Gentak, Gentrasul, Ocu-Mycin, Spectro-Genta) {Alcomicin} | Adults and children: 1 drop of solution q 1–4 hr or thin strip of ointment q 8–12 hr | ■ ADRs: irritation, burning, stinging, blurred vision (ointment) |
| levofloxacin (Quixin) | Adults: 1–2 drops of 0.5% solution in each affected eye every 2 h while awake for 2 days (up to 8 times/day); then every 4 h for 5 more days (up to 4 times/day) | ■ ADRs: altered taste, systemic allergic reactions, photophobia |
| moxifloxacin (Vigamox) | Adults and Children >1 yr: 1 drop of 0.5% solution into affected eye 3 times daily for 7 days. | ■ ADRs: irritation, decreased visual acuity |
| norfloxacin (Chibroxin) | Adults and children ≥1 yr: 1 drop 4 times daily while awake (up to q 2 hr while awake) | ■ ADRs: altered taste, systemic allergic reactions, photophobia |
| ofloxacin (Ocuflox) | Adults and children ≥1 yr: 1 drop q 2–4 hr while awake for 2 days, then 4 times daily for up to 5 more days | ■ ADRs: altered taste, systemic allergic reactions, photophobia |
| sulfacetamide (AK-Sulf, Bleph, Isopto Cetamide, I-Sulfacet, Ocu-Sul, Ocusulf, Sodium Sulamyd, Spectro-Sulf, Sulf, Sulfair, Sulfamide, Sulten) {Sulfex} | Adults: 1 drop of solution q 1–3 hr while awake (less frequently at night) or thin strip of ointment 4 times daily and at bedtime | ■ Cross-sensitivity with other sulfonamides (including thiazides) may occur<br>■ ADRs: local irritation |
| tobramycin (Tobrex) | Adults and children >2 yr: 1 drop of solution q 1–4 hr depending on severity of infection or thin strip of ointment q 8–12 hr | ■ ADRs: irritation, burning, stinging, blurred vision (ointment)<br>■ Ointment may retard corneal wound healing<br>■ Avoid wearing contact lenses during use |

## Antifungal

| Generic Name (Brand Name) {Canadian Brand Name} | Dose | Notes |
|---|---|---|
| natamycin (Natacyn) | Adults: 1 drop q 1–6 hr, depending on severity of infection | ■ ADRs: irritation, swelling, chemosis |

## Antivirals

| Generic Name (Brand Name) {Canadian Brand Name} | Dose | Notes |
|---|---|---|
| trifluridine (Viroptic) | Adults and children ≥6 yr: 1 drop q 2 hr (up to 9 drops/day) while awake until cornea re-epithelializes, then 1 drop q 4 hr (at least 5 times daily) for up to 7 days | ■ ADRs: burning, stinging; keratopathy rarely |
| vidarabine (Vira-A) | Adults and children: thin strip of ointment q 3 hr (5 times daily) until cornea is re-epithelialized, then twice daily for up to 7 days | ■ ADRs: irritation, hypersensitivity |

**Artificial Tears/Ocular Lubricants** (sterile buffered isotonic solutions/ointments)

**Uses:** Artificial tears—keep the eyes moist with isotonic solutions and wetting agents in the management of dry eyes due to lack of tears; also provide lubrication for artificial eyes. Ocular lubricants—provide lubrication and protection in a variety of conditions including exposure keratitis, decreased corneal sensitivity, corneal erosions, keratitis sicca, during/following ocular surgery or removal of a foreign body.

| Generic Name (Brand Name) {Canadian Brand Name} | Dose | Notes |
|---|---|---|
| Artificial tears (Adsorbotear, Akwa Tears, Aquasite, Artifical Tears Plus, Cellufresh, Celluvisc, Comfort Tears, Dakrina, Dry Eye Therapy, Dry Eyes Duratears Naturale, Dwelle, Eye-Lube-A, Genteal Lubricant Eye Gel, HypoTears, HypoTears PF, Isopto Alkaline, Isopto Plain, Just Tears, Lacril, Lacri-Lube NP, Lacri-Lube S.O.P., Lacrisert, Liquifilm Forte, Liquifilm Tears, LubriTears, Moisture Drops, Murine Solution, Murocel, Nature's Tears, Nu-Tears, Nu-Tears II, Nutra Tear, Paralube, Refresh, Refresh PM, Tear Drop, TearGard, Teargen, Tearisol, Tears Naturale, Tears Naturale Free, Tears Naturale II, Tears Plus, Tears Renewed, Ultra Tears, Vit-A-Drops, Viva-Drops) | Adults and children: 1–2 drops 3–4 times daily or 1 insert (Lacrisert) 1–2 times daily<br><br>Ocular lubricants<br>Adults and children: small amount instilled into conjunctiva several times daily | ■ May alter effects of other concurrently administered ophthalmic medications<br>■ ADRs: photophobia, lid edema stinging (insert only), temporarily blurred vision, eye discomfort |

**Beta Blockers**

**Uses:** Management of chronic open-angle glaucoma and other forms of ocular hypertension (decreases the formation of aqueous humor).
**Cautions:** Systemic absorption is minimal but may occur. Systemic absorption may result in additive adverse cardiovascular effects (bradycardia, hypotension), especially when used with other cardiovascular agents (antihypertensives, antiarrhythmics). Other systemic adverse reactions may occur, including bronchospasm or delirium (geriatric patients). Concurrent use with ophthalmic epinephrine may decrease effectiveness.

| Generic Name (Brand Name) {Canadian Brand Name} | Dose | Notes |
|---|---|---|

| | Dose | |
|---|---|---|
| betaxolol (Betoptic, Betoptic S) | Adults: 1 drop of 0.5% solution twice daily or 1 drop of 0.25% suspension twice daily | ▪ ADRs: conjunctivitis, decreased visual acuity, ocular burning, rashes (may be less likely than others to cause bronchospasm if systemically absorbed) |
| carteolol (Ocupress) | Adults: 1 drop of 1% solution twice daily | ▪ ADRs: bronchospasm, conjunctivitis, decreased visual acuity, ocular burning, rashes (may be less likely than others to cause bradycardia if systemically absorbed) |
| levobetaxolol (Betaxon) | Adults: 1 drop of 0.5% suspension twice daily | ▪ ADRs: transient ophthalmic discomfort, blurred vision |
| levobunolol (AKBeta, Betagan) | Adults: 1 drop of 0.25% solution 1–2 times daily or 1 drop of 0.5% solution once daily | ▪ ADRs: conjunctivitis, decreased visual acuity, ocular burning, rashes |
| metipranolol (OptiPranolol) | Adults: 1 drop of 0.3% solution twice daily | ▪ ADRs: conjunctivitis, decreased visual acuity, ocular burning, rashes<br>▪ Lasts up to 24 hr<br>▪ Can be used safely with pilocarpine, epinephrine, and acetazolamide |
| timolol (Betimol, Timoptic, Timoptic-XE) {Apo-Timop} | Adults and children ≥10 yr: 0.25% or 0.5% solution—1 drop 1–2 times daily; 0.25% or 0.5% gel-forming solution—1 drop once daily<br>Children <10 yr: 1 drop 0.25% solution 1–2 times daily | ▪ ADRs: conjunctivitis, decreased visual acuity, ocular burning, rashes<br>▪ Lasts up to 24 hr |

**Carbonic Anhydrase Inhibitor**

**Uses:** Management of open-angle glaucoma or other forms of ocular hypertension (decreases formation of aqueous humor).
**Cautions:** May exacerbate kidney stones; should not be used in patients with CCr <30 ml/min.

| Generic Name<br>(Brand Name) {Canadian Brand Name} | Dose | Notes |
|---|---|---|
| brinzolamide (Azopt) | Adults: 1 drop of 1% suspension into each affected eye three times daily | ▪ ADRs: burning, stinging, unusual taste |
| dorzolamide (Trusopt) | Adults: 1 drop 3 times daily | ▪ ADRs: bitter taste, cross-sensitivity with sulfonamides, ocular irritation or allergy |

**Cholinergics** (direct-acting)

**Uses:** Treatment of open-angle glaucoma (facilitates the outflow of aqueous humor); also used to facilitate miosis after ophthalmic surgery or before examination (to counteract mydriatics).
**Cautions:** Conditions in which pupillary constriction should be avoided. If significant systemic absorption occurs, bronchospasm, sweating, increased urination, and salivation may occur.

| Generic Name (Brand Name) [Canadian Brand Name] | Dose | Notes |
|---|---|---|
| carbachol (Carboptic, Isopto Carbachol) | Adults and children: 1 drop of 0.75–3% solution 1–3 times daily | ■ ADRs: blurred vision, altered vision, stinging, eye pain |
| pilocarpine (Adsorbocarpine, Akarpine, Isopto Carpine, Ocu-Carpine, Ocusert Pilo, Pilocar, Pilopine, Piloptic, Pilostat) [Miocarpine, Spersacarpine] | Adults and children: glaucoma—1 drop of 1–4% solution 2–4 times daily (may be given more frequently for acute angle-closure glaucoma) or 1 ocular insert weekly or 1/2-in. strip of 4% gel at bedtime; counteracting mydriatic sympathomimetics—1 drop of 1% solution (may be repeated prior to surgery) | ■ Use 1% or less solution in infants<br>■ ADRs: blurred vision, altered vision, stinging, eye pain, headache, browache |

**Cholinergics** (cholinesterase inhibitors)

**Uses:** Management of glaucoma not controlled with short-acting miotics or other agents; also used in varying doses for accommodative esotropia (diagnosis and treatment).
**Cautions:** Enhance neuromuscular blockade from succinylcholine; intensify the actions of cocaine and some other local anesthetics; additive toxicity with antimyasthenics, anticholinergics, and cholinesterase inhibitors (including some pesticides). Use cautiously in patients with history or risk of retinal detachment.

| Generic Name (Brand Name) [Canadian Brand Name] | Dose | Notes |
|---|---|---|
| demecarium (Humorsol) | Adults: 1 drop 1–2 times daily | ■ Avoid use during pregnancy<br>■ ADRs: blurred vision, change in vision, browache, miosis, eyelid twitching, watering eyes |
| echothiophate (Phospholine Iodide) | Adults: 1 drop 1–2 times daily | ■ May cause hyperactivity in patients with Down syndrome<br>■ ADRs: blurred vision, change in vision, browache, miosis, eyelid twitching, watering eyes<br>■ Irreversible cholinesterase inhibitor |
| isoflurophate (Floropryl) | Adults: thin strip of ointment once every 3 days, 3 times daily | ■ Avoid use during pregnancy<br>■ ADRs: blurred vision, change in vision, browache, miosis, eyelid twitching, watering eyes |
| physostigmine (Eserine Salicylate, Isopto Eserin) | Adults and children: 1 drop of 0.25–0.5% solution up to 4 times daily or 1 cm of 0.25% ointment 1–3 times daily | ■ ADRs: blurred vision (ointment), change in vision, browache, miosis, eyelid twitching, watering eyes |

**Corticosteroids**

**Uses:** Management of inflammatory eye conditions including allergic conjunctivitis, nonspecific superficial keratitis, infectious conjunctivitis (with anti-infectives); management of corneal injury; suppression of graft rejection following keratoplasty; prevention of postoperative inflammation.
**Cautions:** Infectious ocular processes (avoid in herpes simplex keratitis), especially fungal and viral ocular infections (may mask symptoms); diabetes; glaucoma.

| Generic Name (Brand Name) [Canadian Brand Name] | Dose | Notes |
|---|---|---|
| dexamethasone (AK-Dex, Decadron, Maxidex) [Diodex, PMS Dexamethasone, RO-Dexasone, Spersadex] | Adults and children: 1–2 drops of solution 4–6 times daily (up to q 1 hr) or thin strip of ointment 3–4 times daily initially | ■ As condition improves, decrease frequency of administration<br>■ ADRs: blurred vision (ointment), corneal thinning, increased intraocular pressure, irritation |
| fluorometholone (FML, Flarex, Fluor-Op) | 1–2 drops 4 times daily (up to 1–2 drops q 1 hr) as suspension or thin strip of ointment 1–3 times daily (up to q 4 hr) initially | ■ As condition improves, decrease frequency of administration<br>■ ADRs: blurred vision (ointment), corneal thinning, increased intraocular pressure, irritation |
| loteprednol (Alrex, Lotemax) | Adults: 1 drop of 0.2% suspension (Alrex) 4 times daily or 1–2 drops 4 times daily of 0.5% suspension (lotemax); up to 1 drop every hour | ■ 0.2% suspension used for seasonal allergic conjunctivitis<br>■ 0.5% suspension used for steroid-responsive inflammatory conditions and postoperatively |
| medrysone (HMS) | Adults and children: 1 drop of 1% suspension up to q 4 hr initially | ■ As condition improves, decrease frequency of administration<br>■ ADRs: corneal thinning, increased intraocular pressure, irritation |
| prednisolone (AK-Pred, Econopred, Inflamase, Pred Mild) | Adults and children: 1–2 drops of 0.12–1% solution/suspension 2–6 times daily (up to q 1 hr) initially | ■ As condition improves, decrease frequency of administration<br>■ ADRs: corneal thinning, increased intraocular pressure, irritation |
| rimexolone (Vexol) | Adults and children: 1–2 drops of 1% suspension q 6 hr (up to q 1 hr) initially | ■ As condition improves, decrease frequency of administration<br>■ ADRs: corneal thinning, increased intraocular pressure, irritation |

## Cycloplegic Mydriatics

**Uses:** Preparation for cycloplegic refraction; management of uveitis (not tropicamide).
**Cautions:** Use cautiously in patients with a history of glaucoma; systemic absorption may cause anticholinergic effects such as confusion, unusual behavior, flushing, hallucinations, slurred speech, drowsiness, swollen stomach (infants), tachycardia, dry mouth.

| Generic Name (Brand Name) [Canadian Brand Name] | Dose | Notes |
|---|---|---|

| Generic Name (Brand Name) [Canadian Brand Name] | Dose | Notes |
|---|---|---|
| atropine (Atropair, Atropisol, Atrosulf, Isopto Atropine, I-Tropine, Ocu-Tropine) | Children: cycloplegic refraction (solution)—1 drop twice daily for 1-3 days prior to refraction (use 0.125% solution in children <1 yr, 0.25% solution for children 1-5 yr, 0.25% solution for children >5 yr with blue irides, 0.5-1% for children >5 yr with dark irides; cycloplegic refraction (ointment)—0.3 cm of 0.5% ointment in children <2 yr with blue irides, 1% ointment in children <2 yr with dark irides or children >2 yr 3 times daily for 1-3 days prior to refraction; uveitis—1 drop of 0.125-1% solution 1-3 times daily. Adults: uveitis—1 drop of 1% solution 1-2 times daily (up to 4 times daily) or 0.3-0.5 cm of 1% ointment 1-2 times daily | ■ Cycloplegic refraction in children only (too long-acting to use in adults); treatment of uveitis ■ Avoid using in children who have had a prior serious reaction to atropine ■ Effects on accommodation may last 6 days; mydriasis may last 12 days ■ ADRs: irritation, blurred vision, photophobia |
| cyclopentolate (AK-Pentolate, Cyclogyl, I-Pentolate, Cyclopentolate, Ocu-Pentolate, Pentolair, Spectro-Pentolate) {Minims} | Adults: 1 drop of 0.5-2% solution; may repeat in 5-10 min. Children: 1 drop of 0.5-2% solution; may be followed 5-10 min later by 1 drop of 0.5-1% solution. Premature and small infants: 1 drop of 0.5% solution single dose | ■ Peak of cycloplegia is within 25-75 min and lasts 6-24 hr ■ Peak of mydriasis is within 30-60 min and may last several days ■ ADRs: irritation, blurred vision, photophobia |
| homatropine (Isopto Homatropine, Spectro-Homatropine) {Minims Homatropine} | Adults and children: cycloplegic refraction—1 drop of 2-5% solution, may repeat in 5-10 min for 2-3 more doses; uveitis—1 drop of 2-5% solution 2-3 times daily (up to q 3-4 hr in adults) | ■ Cycloplegia and mydriasis may persist for 24-72 hr ■ ADRs: irritation, blurred vision, photophobia |
| scopolamine (Isopto Hyoscine) | Adults and children: cycloplegic refraction—1 drop of 0.25% solution (repeat twice daily for 2 days in children); uveitis—1 drop of 0.25% solution up to 4 times daily | ■ Shorter duration than atropine, but mydriasis and cycloplegia may persist for 3-7 days ■ ADRs: irritation, blurred vision, photophobia |
| tropicamide (Mydriacyl, Mydriafair, Ocu-Tropic, Opticyl, Spectro-Cyl, Tropicacyl) {Minims Tropicamide} | Adults and children: 1 drop of 0.5-1% solution | ■ Stronger solution/repeated dosing may be required in patients with dark irides ■ Peak effect occurs in 20-40 min ■ Cycloplegia lasts 2-6 hr; mydriasis lasts up to 7 hr ■ ADRs: irritation, blurred vision, photophobia |

### Immunomodulators

**Uses:** To increase tear production when the cause of dry eye is inflammation secondary to keratoconjunctivitis sicca.
**Cautions:** Tear production is not increased during concurrent use of ophthalmic NSAIDs or punctal plugs.

| Generic Name (Brand Name) [Canadian Brand Name] | Dose | Notes |
|---|---|---|
| cyclosporine (Restasis) | Adults: 1 drop of 0.05% ophthalmic emulsion in each eye twice daily | ■ ADRs: irritation, blurred vision ■ Emulsion should be inverted to obtain uniform opaque appearance prior to use |

**Mast Cell Stabilizers**

**Uses:** Vernal keratoconjunctivitis.
**Cautions:** Require several days of treatment before effects are seen.

| Generic Name (Brand Name) {Canadian Brand Name} | Dose | Notes |
|---|---|---|
| cromolyn (Crolom) {Opticrom} | Adults and children ≥4 yr: 1 drop of 4% solution 4-6 times daily | ▪ ADRs: chemosis, irritation<br>▪ Do not wear contact lenses concurrently |
| ketotifen (Zaditor) | Adults: 1 drop of 0.025% solution to affected eye q 8-12 hr | ▪ ADRs: conjuctival injection, headaches, rhinitis |
| lodoxamide (Alomide) | Adults and children ≥2 yr: 1 drop of 0.1% solution 4 times daily for up to 3 mo | ▪ ADRs: blurred vision, foreign body sensation, irritation |
| nedocromil (Alocril) | Adults and children >3 yr: 1-2 drops of 2% solution in each eye twice daily throughout period of exposure | ▪ Avoid concurrent use of contact lenses<br>▪ ADRs: headache, ocular burning, unpleaseant taste, nasal congestion |
| Pemirolast (Alamast) | Adults: 1-2 drops of 0.1% solution in each affected eye 4 times daily | ▪ ADRs: discomfort, dry eyes, foreign body sensation<br>▪ Symptoms may improve within a few days, but optimal response may take up to 4 wk |

**Nonsteroidal Anti-inflammatory Drugs**

**Uses:** Management of inflammation following surgery (diclofenac, ketorolac), allergic conjunctivitis (ketorolac), inhibition of perioperative miosis (flurbiprofen, suprofen).
**Cautions:** Cross-sensitivity with systemic NSAIDs may occur; concurrent use of anticoagulants, other NSAIDs, thrombolytics, some cephalosporins, and valproates may increase the risk of bleeding.

| Generic Name (Brand Name) {Canadian Brand Name} | Dose | Notes |
|---|---|---|
| diclofenac (Voltaren) | Adults: 1 drop of 0.1% solution 4 times daily for up to 6 wk | ▪ Do not wear hydrocel contact lenses concurrently<br>▪ ADRs: irritation, allergic reactions |
| flurbiprofen (Ocufen) | Adults: 1 drop of 0.03% solution q 30 min, beginning 2 hr prior to surgery (4 drops total) | ▪ ADRs: irritation, allergic reactions |

| | | |
|---|---|---|
| ketorolac (Acular, Acular LS) | Adults and children >3 yr: *Allergic conjunctivitis*—1 drop of 0.5% solution 4 times daily (Acular); *Postoperative*—1 drop of 0.4% solution 4 times daily in operated eye as needed for up to 4 days after corneal refractive surgery. | ■ ADRs: irritation, allergic reactions |
| suprofen (Profenal) | Adults: 2 drops of 1% solution given 3 hr, 2 hr, and 1 hr before surgery or 2 drops q 4 hr while awake on day prior to surgery | ■ ADRs: irritation, allergic reactions |

## Ocular Decongestants/Vasoconstrictors

**Uses:** Decrease ocular congestion due to irritation by vasoconstricting conjunctival blood vessels; stronger solutions have mydriatic effects.
**Cautions:** Systemic absorption may result in adverse cardiovascular effects; excessive/prolonged use may produce rebound hyperemia; use caution in patients at risk for acute angle-closure glaucoma; cardiovascular effects may be exaggerated by MAO inhibitors and dose adjustment may be required within 21 days of MAO inhibitors; increased risk of arrhythmias with inhalation anesthetics.

| Generic Name (Brand Name) {Canadian Brand Name} | Dose | Notes |
|---|---|---|
| naphazoline (Albalon, Allerest, Allergy Drops, Clear Eyes Lubricating Eye Redness Reliever, Comfort Eye Drops, Degest 2, Estivin II, Nafazair, Naphcon, Ocu-Zoline, VasoClear, Vasocon) {AK-Con} | Adults: 1 drop of 0.012% solution 4 times daily as needed or 1 drop of 0.1% solution q 3–4 hr as needed | ■ ADRs: ophthalmic—rebound hyperemia; systemic—dizziness, headache, nausea, sweating, weakness |
| oxymetazoline (OcuClear, Visine LR) | Adults and children >6 yr: 1 drop of 0.025% solution q 6 hr as needed | ■ ADRs: ophthalmic—rebound hyperemia; systemic—headache, insomnia, nervousness, tachycardia |
| phenylephrine (AK-Dilate, AK-Nefrin, Dilatair, I-Phrine, Isopto Frin, Mydfrin, Ocu-Phrin, Prefrin) {Minims Phenylephrine, Spersaphrine} | Adults: decongestant—1 drop of 0.12% solution q 3–4 hr as needed; mydriasis—2.5 or 10% solution up to 3 times daily Children: mydriasis—2.5% solution up to 3 times daily | ■ ADRs: ophthalmic—blurred vision, browache, irritation; systemic—dizziness, tachycardia, hypertension, paleness, sweating, trembling |
| tetrahydrozoline (Collyrium Fresh, Eyesine, Geneye, Mallazine, Murine Plus, Optigene 3, Tetrazine, Visine) | Adults: 1–2 drops of 0.05% solution up to 4 times daily | ■ ADRs: ophthalmic—irritation; systemic—tachycardia, hypertension |

## Osmotics

**Uses:** Decreases superficial edema of the cornea prior to examination.

| Generic Name (Brand Name) {Canadian Brand Name} | Dose | Notes |
|---|---|---|
| glycerin (Ophthalgan) | Adults: 1–2 drops prior to exam | ■ Avoid using in patients with hypersensitivity to chlorobutanol |

## Prostaglandin Agonist

**Uses:** Management of glaucoma or lowering of intraocular pressure (increases outflow of aqueous humor).

**Cautions:** May change eye color to brown; will form precipitate with thimerosal-containing products; can be used with other agents to lower intraocular pressure.

| Generic Name<br>(Brand Name) {Canadian Brand Name} | Dose | Notes |
|---|---|---|
| bimatoprost (Lumigan) | Adults: 1 drop 0.03% solution in each affected eye once daily in the evening | ■ ADRs: local irritation, foreign body sensation, increased eyelash growth, increased brown pigmentation |
| latanoprost (Xalatan) | Adults: 1 drop once daily | ■ ADRs: local irritation, foreign body sensation |
| travoprost (Travatan) | Adults: 1 drop 0.004% solution in each affected eye once daily in the evening | ■ ADRs: local irritation, foreign body sensation, increased eyelash growth, increased brown pigmentation in iris |
| unoprostone (Rescula) | Adults: 1 drop 0.15% solution in each affected eye twice daily | ■ ADRs: local irritation, foreign body sensation, increased eyelash growth, increased brown pigmentation |

## Sympathomimetics

**Uses:** Management of glaucoma (lowers intraocular pressure by decreasing formation of aqueous humor).

**Cautions:** Systemic absorption may result in adverse cardiovascular and CNS reactions (especially in patients with cardiovascular disease); avoid use in patients predisposed to acute angle-closure glaucoma.

| Generic Name<br>(Brand Name) {Canadian Brand Name} | Dose | Notes |
|---|---|---|
| apraclonidine (Iopidine) | Adults: glaucoma—1-2 drops of 0.5% solution 3 times daily; preoperative use—1 drop of 1% solution 1 hr prior to surgery | ■ A selective alpha-adrenergic agonist<br>■ ADRs: ophthalmic—irritation, mydriasis; systemic—allergic reactions, arrhythmias, bradycardia, drowsiness, dry nose, fainting, headache, nervousness, weakness<br>■ Monitor pulse and blood pressure<br>■ Avoid concurrent use with MAO inhibitors |

brimonidine (Alphagan)

Adults: 1 drop 3 times daily (8 hr apart)

- A selective alpha-adrenergic agonist
- ADRs: ophthalmic—irritation; systemic—drowsiness, dizziness, dry mouth, headache, weakness, muscular pain
- Avoid concurrent use with MAO inhibitors
- Tricyclic antidepressants may decrease effectiveness; additive CNS depression may occur with other CNS depressants; additive adverse cardiovascular effects with other cardiovascular agents

dipivefrin (Propine)

Adults: 1 drop q 12 hr

- Converted to epinephrine in the eye
- ADRs: ophthalmic—local irritation, macular edema (aphakic patients); systemic—arrhythmias, hypertension
- Wait 15 min before inserting soft contact lenses

epinephrine (Epifrin, Epinal, Eppy/N, Glaucon)

Adults: 1 drop of 1–2% solution 1–2 times daily

- Increased risk of arrhythmias with inhalation anesthetics
- ADRs: headache, local irritation
- Cardiovascular effects may be exaggerated by MAO inhibitors; dose adjustment may be required within 21 days of MAO inhibitors

*ADRs = adverse reactions.

# APPENDIX D
## Additional Drugs

| Generic Name<br>(Brand Name)<br>[Canadian name]<br>Classification(s)<br>Schedule<br>Pregnancy Category | Indications | Adverse Reactions and Side Effects | Route and Dosage |
|---|---|---|---|
| **acetazolamide**<br>(AK-Zol, Dazamide, Diamox, Diamox Sequels, Storzolamide) {Acetazolam, Apo-Acetazolamide}<br>*Therapeutic:* anticonvulsants, antiglaucoma agents, diuretics, ocular hypotensive agents<br>*Pharmacologic:* carbonic anhydrase inhibitors<br>Pregnancy Category C | Lowering of intraocular pressure in the treatment of glaucoma. Management of acute altitude sickness. **Unlabeled uses:** Prevention of renal calculi composed of uric acid or cystine. | **CNS:** depression, tiredness, weakness, drowsiness ■ **EENT:** transient nearsightedness ■ **GI:** anorexia, metallic taste, nausea, vomiting ■ **GU:** crystalluria, renal calculi ■ **Derm:** rashes ■ **Endo:** hyperglycemia ■ **F and E:** hyperchloremic acidosis, hypokalemia ■ **Hemat:** APLASTIC ANEMIA, HEMOLYTIC ANEMIA, LEUKOPENIA ■ **Metab:** weight loss, hyperuricemia ■ **Neuro:** paresthesias ■ **Misc:** allergic reactions. | **PO (Adults):** *Glaucoma*—250–1000 mg/day in 1–4 divided doses (up to 250 mg q 4 hr) or 500-mg extended-release capsules twice daily. *Epilepsy*—4–30 mg/kg/day in 1–4 divided doses (range 375 mg–1g/day). *Altitude sickness*—250 mg 2–4 times daily started 24–48 hr before ascent, continued for 48 hr or longer to control symptoms. *Antiurolithic*—250 mg at bedtime.<br>**PO (Children):** *Glaucoma*—8–30 mg/kg (300–900 mg/m²)/day in 3 divided doses (usual range 10–15 mg/kg/day). *Epilepsy*—4–30 mg/kg/day in 1–4 divided doses.<br>**IM, IV (Adults):** 250–500 mg, may repeat in 2–4 hr.<br>**IM, IV (Children):** 5–10 mg/kg q 6 hr. |

**Contraindicated in:** Hypersensitivity or cross-sensitivity with sulfonamides may occur. Avoid during first trimester of pregnancy. Concurrent use with ophthalmic carbonic anhydrase inhibitors (brinzolamide, dorzolamide) is not recommended. **Use Cautiously in:** Chronic respiratory disease. Renal or hepatic disease. Electrolyte abnormalities. Diabetes mellitus. Second or third trimester of pregnancy or lactation (safety not established).

| Generic Name (Brand Name) {Canadian name} Classification(s) Schedule Pregnancy Category | Indications | Adverse Reactions and Side Effects | Route and Dosage |
|---|---|---|---|
| **activated charcoal** (Acta-Char Liquid-A, Actidose-Aqua, CharcoAid 2000, Insta-Char, Insta-Char Aqueous Suspension, Liqui-Char, SuperChar Aqueous) {Aqueous Charcodote, Charac-50, Charcodote} *Therapeutic: antidotes* *Pharmacologic: adsorbents* Pregnancy Category C | Acute management of many oral poisonings following emesis/lavage. | **GI:** black stools, constipation, diarrhea, vomiting. | Antidote **PO (Adults):** 25–100 g (may be repeated q 4–6 hr). **PO (Children 1–12 yr):** 25–50 g (may be repeated q 4–6 hr). **PO (Children <1 yr):** 1 g/kg (may be repeated q 4–6 hr). |

**Contraindicated in:** No known contraindications. **Use Cautiously in:** Poisonings due to cyanide, corrosives, ethanol, methanol, petroleum distillates, organic solvents, mineral acids, or iron. Endoscopic examination (observation will be obscured).

| **aldesleukin** (interleukin-2, IL-2, Proleukin) *Therapeutic: antineoplastics* *Pharmacologic: interleukins* Pregnancy Category C | Management of metastatic renal cell carcinoma. | **Resp:** APNEA, RESPIRATORY FAILURE, dyspnea, pulmonary congestion, pulmonary edema, hemoptysis, pleural effusion, pneumothorax, tachypnea, wheezing ■ **CV:** CARDIAC ARREST, CHF, MI, STROKE, arrhythmias, hypotension, tachycardia, myocardial ischemia, pericardial effusion, thrombosis ■ **GI:** BOWEL PERFORATION, diarrhea, jaundice, nausea, stomatitis, vomiting, ascites, hepatomegaly ■ **GU:** oliguria/anuria, proteinuria, dysuria, hematuria, renal failure ■ **Derm:** EXFOLIATIVE DERMATITIS, pruritus ■ **F and E:** acidosis, hypocalcemia, hypokalemia, hypomagnesemia, hypophosphatemia, alkalosis, hyperkalemia, hyperuricemia, hyponatremia ■ **Hemat:** anemia, coagulation disorders, leukopenia, thrombocytopenia, eosinophilia, leukocytosis ■ **Misc:** CAPILLARY LEAK SYNDROME, chills, fever, weight gain, weight loss. | **IV (Adults):** 600,000 IU/kg (0.037 mg/kg) every 8 hr for 14 doses. Cycle is repeated once after a 9-day rest period to a total of 28 doses. After a rest period of 7 wk, patients who have had a beneficial response may be evaluated for additional courses. |

**Contraindicated in:** Hypersensitivity to aldesleukin or mannitol. Cross-sensitivity to *Escherichia coli*–derived proteins may occur. Patients with any history of cardiac or pulmonary disease as assessed by abnormal thallium stress testing or abnormal pulmonary function testing. Patients who have experienced any of the following toxicities during previous courses of aldesleukin—sustained ventricular tachycardia (≥5 beats), angina pectoris or MI as indicated by ECG changes, respiratory problems requiring more than 72 hr of intubation, pericardial tamponade, renal toxicity requiring more than 72 hr of dialysis, CNS dysfunction consisting of more than 48 hr of coma or psychosis, intractable seizures, bowel perforation or ischemia, GI bleeding requiring surgical intervention. Patients who have had allograft organ transplantation (increased risk of rejection). **Use Cautiously in:** Patients with a history of cardiovascular, respiratory, hepatic, or renal disease. Patients with a history of seizures or suspected CNS metastases (symptoms may be exaggerated and seizures may occur). Patients with child-bearing potential. Pregnancy, lactation, or children <18 yr (safety not established).

| Generic Name (Brand Name) [Canadian name] Classification(s) Schedule Pregnancy Category | Indications | Adverse Reactions and Side Effects | Route and Dosage |
|---|---|---|---|
| **alemtuzumab** (Campath) ***Therapeutic:*** *antineoplastics* ***Pharmacologic:*** *monoclonal antibodies* Pregnancy Category C | Treatment of B-cell chronic lymphocytic leukemia in patients who have been treated with alkylating agents and in which fludarabine therapy has failed. | **CNS:** depression, dizziness, drowsiness, fatigue, headache, weakness ■ **Resp:** bronchospasm, cough, dyspnea ■ **CV:** hypertension, hypotension, tachycardia ■ **GI:** abdominal pain, anorexia, constipation, stomatitis ■ **Derm:** rash, sweating ■ **F and E:** edema ■ **Hemat:** NEUTROPENIA, PANCYTOPENIA/MARROW HYPOPLASIA, anemia, lymphopenia, thrombocytopenia ■ **MS:** back pain, skeletal pain ■ **Misc:** infusion-related events, infection, sepsis. | **IV (Adults):** 3 mg/day initially, as tolerated increase dose to 10 mg/day and then 30 mg/day given three times weekly for up to 12 weeks; single doses should not exceed 30 mg or more than 90 mg/wk. |
| **Contraindicated in:** Hypersensitivity. Systemic infections. Underlying immunodeficiency, including HIV infection. | | | |
| **alitretinoin** (Panretin) ***Therapeutic:*** *antineoplastics* ***Pharmacologic:*** *retinoids* Pregnancy Category D | Topical treatment of cutaneous lesions from AIDS-related Kaposi's sarcoma (KS). | **Local:** <u>pain</u>, pruritus, <u>rash</u>, edema, exfoliative, dermatitis, paresthesia. | **Topical (Adults):** Apply generous coating twice daily to KS lesions initially; application may be increased to 3–4 times daily. |
| **Contraindicated in:** Hypersensitivity to retinoids. Pregnancy or lactation. **Use Cautiously in:** Patients with childbearing potential. Children (safety not established). | | | |
| **altretamine** (Hexalen, hexamethylmelamine) [Hexastat] ***Therapeutic:*** *antineoplastics* Pregnancy Category D | Management of ovarian cancer unresponsive to treatment with other agents. | **CNS:** SEIZURES, fatigue ■ **GI:** nausea, vomiting, anorexia, hepatic toxicity ■ **GU:** gonadal suppression, renal toxicity ■ **Derm:** alopecia, pruritus, skin rash ■ **Endo:** gonadal suppression ■ **Hemat:** anemia, leukopenia, thrombocytopenia ■ **Neuro:** <u>peripheral neuropathy</u>. | **PO (Adults):** 65 mg/m² 4 times daily (after meals and at bedtime) for 14 or 21 days of each 28-day cycle. Dosage reduction to 50 mg/m² 4 times daily (after meals and at bedtime) recommended after 14 or more days' rest for any of the following: GI intolerance, severe bone marrow depression, or progressive neurologic toxicity. |
| **Contraindicated in:** Hypersensitivity. Pregnancy or lactation. **Use Cautiously in:** Pre-existing neurologic diseases. Patients with childbearing potential. Infections. Decreased bone marrow reserve. Other chronic debilitating illnesses. Children (safety not established). | | | |
| **aminolevulinic acid** (Levulan Kerastick) ***Therapeutic:*** *none assigned* ***Pharmacologic:*** *photosensitizers* Pregnancy Category C | Treatment of nonhyperkeratotic actinic keratoses of the face and scalp in conjunction with blue light illumination using the BLU-U Blue Light Photodynamic Therapy Illuminator. | **Local:** burning, edema, pruritus, stinging, oozing, scaling, ulceration. | **Topical (Adults):** One application via the Kerastick system (contains 354 mg of aminolevulinic acid), followed 14–18 hr later by blue light illumination. |

| Generic Name (Brand Name) [Canadian name] Classification(s) Schedule Pregnancy Category | Indications | Adverse Reactions and Side Effects | Route and Dosage |
|---|---|---|---|
| **Contraindicated in:** Hypersensitivity. History of cutaneous photosensitization. Porphyria. Hypersensitivity to porphyrins. Pregnancy or lactation. **Use Cautiously in:** Other photodermatoses. Acquired or inherited coagulation defects. Concurrent warfarin therapy. | | | |
| **amoxapine** (Asendin) *Therapeutic:* antidepressants Pregnancy Category C | Treatment of depression accompanied by anxiety, often used in conjunction with psychotherapy. | **CNS:** NEUROLEPTIC MALIGNANT SYNDROME, fatigue, sedation, extrapyramidal reactions, tardive dyskinesia ■ **EENT:** blurred vision, dry eyes, dry mouth ■ **CV:** ARRHYTHMIAS, hypotension, ECG changes ■ **GI:** constipation, increased appetite, paralytic ileus ■ **GU:** testicular swelling, urinary retention ■ **Derm:** photosensitivity, rash ■ **Endo:** gynecomastia, sexual dysfunction ■ **Hemat:** blood dyscrasias ■ **Misc:** fever, weight gain. | **PO (Adults):** 50 mg 2–3 times daily, increase to 100 mg 2–3 times daily by end of 1 week (not to exceed 300 mg daily in outpatients, 600 mg daily in divided doses in hospitalized patients). Once optimal dose is achieved, may be given as a single bedtime dose; no single dose to exceed 300 mg. **PO (Geriatric Patients):** 25 mg 2–3 times daily, may be increased to 50 mg 2–3 times daily (not >300 mg/day). |
| **Contraindicated in:** Narrow-angle glaucoma. Pregnancy, and lactation. **Use Cautiously in:** Geriatric patients (dosage reduction required). Pre-existing cardiovascular disease. Prostatic hypertrophy (increased susceptibility to urinary retention). History of seizures (threshold may be lowered). Children <16 yr (safety not established). | | | |
| **arsenic trioxide** (Trisenox) *Therapeutic:* antineoplastics *Pharmacologic:* heavy metals Pregnancy Category D | Induction of remission and consolidation in patients with acute promyelocytic leukemia (APL) who do not respond to or tolerate retinoid and anthracycline chemotherapy and whose disease is associated with the presence of the t(15;17) translocation or PML/RAR-alpha gene expression. | **CNS:** fatigue, headache, insomnia, weakness ■ **Resp:** hypoxia, dyspnea, pleural effusion ■ **CV:** QT PROLONGATION, COMPLETE AV BLOCK, atrial arrhythmias ■ **GI:** abdominal pain, constipation, increased liver enzymes ■ **GU:** renal failure ■ **Derm:** dermatitis ■ **Endo:** hyperglycemia, hypoglycemia ■ **F and E:** acidosis, hypocalcemia, hyperkalemia, hypokalemia, hypomagnesemia ■ **Hemat:** NEUTROPENIA, APL DIFFERENTIATION SYNDROME, DISSEMINATED INTRAVASCULAR COAGULATION, THROMBOCYTOPENIA, hyperleukocytosis, anemia, leukocytosis ■ **MS:** back pain, arthralgia, bone pain, neck pain, limb pain, myalgia ■ **Misc:** allergic reactions, fever, infection/sepsis. | **IV (Adults and Children ≥5 yr):** *Induction*—0.15 mg/kg/day until bone marrow remission (not to exceed 60 doses); *consolidation*—starting 3–6 wks after completion of induction: 0.15 mg/kg/day for 25 doses over a period of 5 weeks. |
| **Contraindicated in:** Hypersensitivity to arsenic. Pregnancy, lactation, or children <5 yr. **Use Cautiously in:** Renal impairment. **Exercise Extreme Caution in:** Pre-existing electrolyte abnormalities (correct prior to administration); concurrent use of drugs known to prolong QT interval, concurrent use of potassium-wasting diuretics or amphotericin. | | | |

| Generic Name (Brand Name) {Canadian name} Classification(s) Schedule Pregnancy Category | Indications | Adverse Reactions and Side Effects | Route and Dosage |
|---|---|---|---|
| **ascorbic acid** (Ascorbicap, Cebid, Cecon, Cecore-500, Cemill, Cenolate, Cetane, Cevalin, Cevi-Bid, Flavorcee, Mega-C/A Plus, Ortho/CS, Sunkist) {Apo-C} *Therapeutic: vitamins* *Pharmacologic: water soluble vitamins* Pregnancy Category C | Treatment and prevention of vitamin C deficiency (scurvy) with dietary supplementation. Supplemental therapy in some GI diseases during long-term parenteral nutrition or chronic hemodialysis. States of increased requirements such as: pregnancy, lactation, stress, hyperthyroidism, trauma, burns, infancy. **Unlabeled uses:** Prevention of the common cold. | **CNS:** drowsiness, fatigue, headache, insomnia ■ **GI:** cramps, diarrhea, heartburn, nausea, vomiting ■ **Derm:** flushing ■ **GU:** kidney stones ■ **Hemat:** deep vein thrombosis, hemolysis (in G6PD deficiency), sickle cell crisis ■ **Local:** pain at subcut or IM sites. | **PO (Adults):** *Scurvy*—500 mg/day for at least 14 days. *Prevention of deficiency*—50–100 mg/day. **PO (Children):** *Scurvy*—100–300 mg/day for at least 14 days. *Prevention of deficiency*—30–45 mg/day. **IM (Adults):** *Scurvy*—100–500 mg/day for at least 14 days. **IM (Children):** *Scurvy*—100–300 mg/day for at least 14 days. **IV (Adults and Children):** *Prevention of deficiency*—determined by need. |

**Contraindicated in:** Tartrazine hypersensitivity (some products contain tartrazine—FDC yellow dye #5). **Use Cautiously in:** Recurrent kidney stones. Avoid chronic use of large doses in pregnant women.

| | | | |
|---|---|---|---|
| **atovaquone** (Mepron) *Therapeutic: antiprotozoals* Pregnancy Category C | Treatment of mild to moderate *Pneumocystis carinii* pneumonia (PCP) in patients who are unable to tolerate trimethoprim/sulfamethoxazole. Prophylaxis of *PCP*. | **CNS:** headache, insomnia ■ **Resp:** cough ■ **GI:** diarrhea, nausea, vomiting ■ **Derm:** rash ■ **Misc:** fever. | Treatment **PO (Adults):** 750 mg twice daily for 21 days. **PO (Children):** 40 mg/kg/day (unlabeled). **PO (Adults and Adolescents 13–16 yr):** 1500 mg once daily. |

**Contraindicated in:** Hypersensitivity. **Use Cautiously in:** Decreased hepatic, renal, or cardiac function (dosage modification may be necessary). GI disorders (absorption may be limited). Pregnancy, lactation, or children (safety not established).

| | | | |
|---|---|---|---|
| **azatadine** (Optimine) *Therapeutic: allergy, cold, and cough remedies* *Pharmacologic: antihistamines* Pregnancy Category B | Symptomatic relief of allergic symptoms (rhinitis, urticaria) caused by histamine release. | **CNS:** dizziness, sedation, excitation, headache, seizures ■ **EENT:** tinnitus, blurred vision, nasal stuffiness ■ **Resp:** thickened bronchial secretions, wheezing ■ **CV:** hypertension, arrhythmias, chest tightness, hypotension, palpitations, tachycardia ■ **GI:** epigastric distress, anorexia, constipation, diarrhea, dry mouth, vomiting ■ **GU:** early menses, urinary hesitancy, urinary retention ■ **Derm:** sweating ■ **Hemat:** anemia, thrombocytopenia. | **PO (Adults and Children >12 yr):** 1–2 mg twice daily. **PO (Children >12 yr):** 1 mg twice daily as needed. |

| Generic Name [Brand Name] {Canadian name} Classification(s) Schedule Pregnancy Category | Indications | Adverse Reactions and Side Effects | Route and Dosage |
|---|---|---|---|
| **Contraindicated in:** Hypersensitivity. Acute attacks of asthma. Lactation (avoid use). **Use Cautiously in:** Narrow-angle glaucoma. Liver disease. Geriatric patients (more susceptible to adverse reactions). Hyperthyroidism. Hypertension. Pregnancy or children <12 yr (safety not established). | | | |
| **becaplermin** (Regranex) ***Therapeutic:** wound/ulcer/ decubiti healing agents* ***Pharmacologic:** platelet-derived growth factors* Pregnancy Category C | Treatment of lower extremity diabetic neuropathic ulcers extending to subcut tissue or beyond and having adequate blood supply. | **Derm:** erythematous rash at application site. | **Topical (Adults):** Length of gel *in inches* from 15- or 7.5-g tube = length × width of ulcer area × 0.6; from the 2-g tube = length × width of ulcer area × 1.3. Length of gel *in centimeters* from 15- or 7.5-g tube = length × width of ulcer area ÷ 4; from the 2-g tube = length × width of ulcer area ÷ 2; for 12 hr each day. |
| **Contraindicated in:** Known hypersensitivity to becaplermin or parabens. Known neoplasm at site of application. Wounds that close by primary intention. **Use Cautiously in:** Pregnancy, lactation, or children <16 yr (safety not established). | | | |
| **bromocriptine** (Parlodel) {Alti-Bromocriptine, Apo-Bromocriptine} ***Therapeutic:** antiparkinson agents* ***Pharmacologic:** dopamine agonists* Pregnancy Category B | Adjunct to levodopa in the treatment of parkinsonism. Treatment of hyperprolactinemia (amenorrhea/galactorrhea), including associated female infertility. Treatment of acromegaly. **Unlabeled uses:** Management of pituitary prolactinomas. Management of neuroleptic malignant syndrome. | **CNS:** dizziness, confusion, drowsiness, hallucinations, headache, insomnia, nightmares ■ **EENT:** burning eyes, nasal stuffiness, visual disturbances ■ **Resp:** effusions, pulmonary infiltrates ■ **CV:** MI, hypotension ■ **GI:** nausea, abdominal pain, anorexia, dry mouth, metallic taste, vomiting ■ **Derm:** urticaria ■ **MS:** leg cramps ■ **Misc:** digital vasospasm (acromegaly only). | Parkinsonism<br>**PO (Adults):** 1.25 mg 1–2 times daily, increased by 2.5 mg/day in 2–4 wk intervals (range is 2.5–100 mg/day in divided doses; up to 40 mg/day have been used).<br>Hyperprolactinemia<br>**PO (Adults):** 1.25–2.5 mg/day initially, may be gradually increased q 3–7 days up to 2.5 mg 2–3 times daily.<br>Acromegaly<br>**PO (Adults):** 1.25–2.5 mg/day for 3 days, increase by 1.25–2.5 mg q 3–7 days until optimal response is obtained (usual range 10–30 mg/day; up to 100 mg/day).<br>Pituitary Adenomas<br>**PO (Adults):** 1.25 mg 2–3 times daily, may be increased over several weeks (range 2.5–20 mg/day).<br>Neuroleptic Malignant Syndrome (Unlabeled)<br>**PO (Adults):** 5 mg once daily initially, dosage increased as required up to 20 mg/day. |
| **Contraindicated in:** Hypersensitivity to bromocriptine, ergot alkaloids, or bisulfites (capsules only). Severe cardiovascular disease or peripheral vascular disease. Lactation. **Use Cautiously in:** Cardiac disease. Mental disturbances. May restore fertility (additional contraception may be required if pregnancy is undesirable). Severe liver impairment (dosage reduction required). Pregnancy and children <15 yr (safety not established). | | | |

| Generic Name (Brand Name) [Canadian name] Classification(s) Schedule Pregnancy Category | Indications | Adverse Reactions and Side Effects | Route and Dosage |
|---|---|---|---|
| **brompheniramine** (Bromfenac, Dimetapp Allergy, Nasahist B) {Dimetane} *Therapeutic: allergy, cold, and cough remedies, antihistamines* Pregnancy Category B | Symptomatic relief of allergic symptoms (rhinitis, urticaria) caused by histamine release. Severe allergic or hypersensitivity reactions, including anaphylaxis and transfusion reactions. | **CNS:** drowsiness, sedation, dizziness, excitation (in children) ■ **EENT:** blurred vision ■ **CV:** hypertension, arrhythmias, hypotension, palpitations ■ **GI:** dry mouth, constipation, obstruction ■ **GU:** retention, urinary hesitancy ■ **Derm:** sweating ■ **Misc:** hypersensitivity reaction (IV use) | **PO (Adults and Children ≥12 yr):** 4 mg q 4–6 hr daily as needed (not to exceed 24 mg/day). **PO (Children 6–12 yr):** 2 mg q 4–6 hr as needed (not to exceed 12 mg/day). **PO (Children 2–6 yr):** 1 mg q 4–6 hr as needed (not to exceed 6 mg/day). **Subcut, IM, IV (Adults):** 10 mg q 8–12 hr as needed (not to exceed 40 mg/day). **Subcut, IM, IV (Children):** 125 mcg (0.125 mg)/kg or 3.75 mg/m² 3–4 times daily as needed. |

**Contraindicated in:** Hypersensitivity. Acute attacks of asthma. Lactation (avoid use). Known alcohol intolerance (some elixirs). **Use Cautiously in:** Narrow-angle glaucoma. Liver disease. Geriatric patients (more susceptible to adverse reactions; use lower initial dose). Pregnancy (safety not established).

| | | | |
|---|---|---|---|
| **cevimeline** (Evoxac) *Therapeutic: xerostomia therapy adjuncts* *Pharmacologic: cholinergics, muscarinic agonists, sialagogues* Pregnancy Category UK | Treatment of the symptoms of dry mouth associated with Sjögren's syndrome. | **CNS:** coughing ■ **EENT:** rhinitis, visual disturbances ■ **GI:** nausea, diarrhea, excessive salivation ■ **Derm:** excessive sweating, hot flashes. | **PO (Adults):** 30 mg three times daily. |

**Contraindicated in:** Hypersensitivity. When miosis is undesirable (acute iritis, narrow angle glaucoma). Lactation. **Use Cautiously in:** Cardiovascular disease including angina pectoris or history of MI. Pulmonary disease including asthma, chronic bronchitis, or chronic obstructive pulmonary disease. Nephrolithiasis or cholelithiasis. Geriatric patients. Pregnancy (use only if potential benefit justifies potential risk to the fetus). Children (safety not established).

| | | | |
|---|---|---|---|
| **chlorambucil** (Leukeran) *Therapeutic: antineoplastics, immunosuppressants* *Pharmacologic: alkylating agents* Pregnancy Category D | Management of chronic lymphocytic leukemia, malignant lymphoma, and Hodgkin's disease (alone and in combination with other agents). | **Resp:** pulmonary fibrosis ■ **GI:** nausea, stomatitis (rare), vomiting ■ **GU:** decreased sperm count, sterility ■ **Derm:** alopecia (rare), dermatitis, rash ■ **Hemat:** LEUKOPENIA, anemia, thrombocytopenia ■ **Metab:** hyperuricemia ■ **Misc:** allergic reactions, risk of second malignancy. | **PO (Adults):** 0.1–0.2 mg/kg/day (3–6 mg/m²/day) (usual range 4–10 mg/day as a single dose or in divided doses), then adjust dose on basis of blood counts; *or* 0.4 mg/kg (12 mg/m²) twice weekly, increased by 0.1 mg/kg (3 mg/m²) q 2 wk, then adjusted as necessary. **PO (Geriatric Patients):** Initial dose should not be more than 2–4 mg/day. **PO (Children):** 0.1–0.2 mg/kg/day (4.5 mg/m²/day) single dose or in divided doses. |

| Generic Name (Brand Name) [Canadian name] Classification(s) Schedule | | | |
|---|---|---|---|
| **Pregnancy Category** | **Indications** | **Adverse Reactions and Side Effects** | **Route and Dosage** |

**Contraindicated in:** Hypersensitivity. Previous resistance. Pregnancy or lactation. **Use Cautiously in:** Infection. Other chronic debilitating diseases. Geriatric patients (more sensitive to effects). Patients with childbearing potential.

| | | | |
|---|---|---|---|
| **chlorpromazine** (Thorazine, Thor-Prom) [Chlorpromanyl, Largactil, Novo-Chlorpromazine] *Therapeutic:* *antiemetics,* *antipsychotics* *Pharmacologic:* *phenothi-* *azines* Pregnancy Category UK | Acute and chronic psychoses, particularly when accompanied by increased psychomotor activity. Nausea and vomiting. Intractable hiccups. Preoperative sedation. Treatment of acute intermittent porphyria. **Unlabeled uses:** Vascular headache. | **CNS:** NEUROLEPTIC MALIGNANT SYNDROME, sedation, extrapyramidal reactions, tardive dyskinesia ■ **EENT:** blurred vision, dry eyes, lens opacities ■ **CV:** hypotension (increased with IM, IV), tachycardia ■ **GI:** constipation, dry mouth, anorexia, hepatitis, ileus ■ **GU:** urinary retention ■ **Derm:** photosensitivity, pigment changes, rashes ■ **Endo:** galactorrhea ■ **Hemat:** AGRANULOCYTOSIS, leukopenia ■ **Metab:** hyperthermia ■ **Misc:** allergic reactions. | **PO (Adults):** *Psychoses*—10–25 mg 2–4 times daily; may increase every 3–4 days (usual dose is 200 mg/day; up to 1 g/day) *or* 30–300 mg 1–3 times daily as extended-release capsules. *Nausea and vomiting*—10–25 mg q 4 hr as needed. *Preoperative sedation*—25–50 mg 2–3 hr before surgery. *Hiccups/porphyria*—25–50 mg 3–4 times daily. **PO (Children):** *Psychoses/nausea and vomiting*—0.55 mg/kg (15 mg/m²) q 4–6 hr as needed. *Preoperative sedation*—0.55 mg/kg (15 mg/m²) 2–3 hr before surgery. **Rect (Adults):** *Nausea/vomiting*—50–100 mg q 6–8 hr as needed. **Rect (Children >6 mo):** 1 mg/kg q 6–8 hr as needed. **IM (Adults):** *Severe psychoses*—25–50 mg initially, may be repeated in 1 hr; increase to maximum of 400 mg q 3–12 hr if needed (up to 1 g/day). *Nausea/vomiting*—25 mg initially, may repeat with 25–50 mg q 3–4 hr as needed. *Nausea/vomiting during surgery*—12.5 mg, may be repeated in 30 min as needed. *Preoperative sedation*—12.5–25 mg 1–2 hr prior to surgery. *Hiccups/tetanus*—25–50 mg 3–4 times daily. *Porphyria*—25 mg q 6–8 hr until patient can take PO. **IM (Children >6 mo):** *Psychoses/nausea and vomiting*—0.55 mg/kg (15 mg/m²) q 6–8 hr (not to exceed 40 mg/day in children 6 mo—5 yr, or 75 mg/day in children 5–12 yr). *Nausea/vomiting during surgery*—0.275 mg/kg, may repeat in 30 min as needed. *Preoperative sedation*—0.55 mg/kg 1–2 hr prior to surgery. *Tetanus*—0.55 mg/kg q 6–8 hr. **IV (Adults):** *Nausea/vomiting during surgery*—up to 25 mg. *Hiccups/tetanus*—25–50 mg. *Porphyria*—25 mg q 8 hr. **IV (Children):** *Nausea/vomiting during surgery*—0.275 mg/kg. *Tetanus*—0.55 mg/kg. |

| Generic Name (Brand Name) [Canadian name] Classification(s) Schedule Pregnancy Category | Indications | Adverse Reactions and Side Effects | Route and Dosage |
|---|---|---|---|
| **Contraindicated in:** Hypersensitivity to sulfites (injectable) or benzyl alcohol (sustained-release capsules). Cross-sensitivity with other phenothiazines may occur. Narrow-angle glaucoma. Bone marrow depression. Severe liver/cardiovascular disease. Concurrent pimozide use. **Use Cautiously in:** Geriatric/debilitated patients (decrease initial dose). Children with acute illnesses infections, gastroenteritis or dehydration (increased risk of extrapyramidal reactions). Diabetes. Respiratory disease. Prostatic hypertrophy. CNS tumors. Epilepsy. Intestinal obstruction. Pregnancy or lactation (safety not established). | | | |
| **clomipramine** (Anafranil) ***Therapeutic:*** *antiobsessive agents* ***Pharmacologic:*** *tricyclic antidepressants* Pregnancy Category C | Management of OCD. **Unlabeled uses:** Treatment of depression. | **CNS:** SEIZURES, lethargy, sedation, weakness, aggressive behavior ■ **EENT:** blurred vision, dry eyes, dry mouth, vestibular disorder ■ **CV:** ARRHYTHMIAS, ECG changes, orthostatic hypotension ■ **GI:** constipation, nausea, vomiting, eructation ■ **GU:** male sexual dysfunction, urinary retention ■ **Derm:** dry skin, photosensitivity ■ **Endo:** gynecomastia ■ **Hemat:** anemia ■ **MS:** muscle weakness ■ **Neuro:** extrapyramidal reactions ■ **Misc:** hyperthermia, weight gain. | **PO (Adults):** *Antiobsessive*—25 mg/day, increased over 2-wk period to 100 mg/day in divided doses. May be further increased over several weeks up to 250–300 mg/day in divided doses. Once stabilizing dose is reached, entire daily dose may be given at bedtime. *Antidepressant*—25 mg 3 times daily, may be increased as needed (unlabeled). **PO (Geriatric Patients):** 20–30 mg/day initially, may be increased as needed. **PO (Children >10–17 yr):** 25 mg/day initially, increased over 2-wk period to 3 mg/kg/day or 100 mg/day (whichever is smaller) in divided doses. May be further increased to 3 mg/kg/day or 200 mg/day (whichever is smaller) in divided doses. Once stabilizing dose is reached, entire daily dose may be given at bedtime. |
| **Contraindicated in:** Hypersensitivity. Narrow-angle glaucoma. Recent myocardial infarction. Concurrent MAO inhibitor or clonidine use (avoid if possible). Pregnancy or lactation. **Use Cautiously in:** History of seizures (threshold may be lowered). Geriatric patients. Patients with pre-existing cardiovascular disease. Older men with prostatic hypertrophy (may be more susceptible to urinary retention). Hyperthyroidism (increased risk of arrhythmias). Children <10 yr (safety not established). | | | |
| **cytomegalovirus immune globulin** (CMVIG, CytoGam) ***Therapeutic:*** *vaccines/immunizing agents* ***Pharmacologic:*** *immune globulins* Pregnancy Category C | Prevention of cytomegalovirus (CMV) disease associated with transplantation of kidney, lung, liver, pancreas, or heart (if transplant is other than kidney from CMV-positive donors to CMV-negative recipient, then concurrent ganciclovir should be considered). | **Resp:** wheezing ■ **CV:** hypotension ■ **GI:** nausea, vomiting ■ **Derm:** flushing ■ **MS:** back pain, muscle cramps ■ **Misc:** allergic reactions including chills, fever, ANAPHYLAXIS. | Kidney Transplant **IV (Adults):** 150 mg/kg within 72 hr of transplantation, followed by 100 mg/kg after 2, 4, 6, and 8 wk, then 50 mg/kg at 12 and 16 wk. Liver, Pancreas, Lung, or Heart Transplant **IV (Adults):** 150 mg/kg within 72 hr of transplantation, and at 2, 4, 6, and 8 wk after transplant, then 100 mg/kg after at 12 and 16 wk. |
| **Contraindicated in:** Hypersensitivity to immune globulins or albumin. Selective IgA deficiency. **Use Cautiously in:** Pregnancy or lactation (safety not established). | | | |

| Generic Name [Brand Name] {Canadian name} Classification(s) Schedule Pregnancy Category | Indications | Adverse Reactions and Side Effects | Route and Dosage |
|---|---|---|---|
| **danazol** (Danocrine) {Cyclomen} *Therapeutic: hormones* *Pharmacologic: androgens* Pregnancy Category X | Treatment of moderate endometriosis that is unresponsive to conventional therapy. Palliative therapy of fibrocystic breast disease. Prophylaxis of hereditary angioedema. | **CNS:** =emotional lability ■ **EENT:** deepening of voice ■ **CV:** edema ■ **GI:** hepatitis (cholestatic jaundice) ■ **GU:** amenorrhea, clitoral enlargement, testicular atrophy ■ **Derm:** acne, hirsutism, oiliness ■ **Endo:** amenorrhea, anovulation, decreased breast size (women), decreased libido ■ **Metab:** weight gain. | **PO (Adults and Adolescents):** *Endometriosis*—400 mg twice daily (for milder cases may initiate therapy with 100–200 mg twice daily). *Fibrocystic breast disease*—50–200 mg twice daily. *Hereditary angioedema*—200 mg 2–3 times daily. Attempt to decrease dosage by 50% or less q 1–3 mo. If acute attack occurs, increase dose by up to 200 mg/day. |

**Contraindicated in:** Hypersensitivity. Male patients with breast or prostate cancer. Hypercalcemia. Severe hepatic, renal, or cardiac disease. Pregnancy or lactation. **Use Cautiously in:** Previous history of liver disease. History of porphyria. Coronary artery disease. Prepubertal boys.

| | | | |
|---|---|---|---|
| **deferoxamine** (Desferal) *Therapeutic: antidotes* *Pharmacologic: heavy metal antagonists* Pregnancy Category C | Acute toxic iron ingestion. Secondary iron overload syndromes associated with multiple transfusion therapy. | **EENT:** blurred vision, cataracts, ototoxicity ■ **CV:** hypotension, tachycardia ■ **GI:** abdominal pain, diarrhea ■ **GU:** red urine ■ **Derm:** erythema, flushing, urticaria ■ **Local:** induration at injection site, pain at injection site ■ **MS:** leg cramps ■ **Misc:** allergic reactions, fever, shock after rapid IV administration. | Acute Iron Ingestion **IM, IV (Adults and Children ≥3 yr):** 1 g (20 mg/kg or 600 mg/m²), then 500 mg (10 mg/kg or 300 mg/m²) q 4 hr for 2 doses. Additional doses of 500 mg (10 mg/kg or 300 mg/m²) q 4–12 hr may be needed (not to exceed 6 g/24 hr). Chronic Iron Overload **IM, IV (Adults and Children ≥3 yr):** 500 mg–1 g daily; additional doses of 2 g should be given IV for each unit of blood transfused. **Subcut (Adults and Children ≥3 yr):** 1–2 g/day (20–40 mg/kg/day) infused over 8–24 hr. |

**Contraindicated in:** Severe renal disease. Anuria. Early pregnancy or childbearing potential (however, may be used safely in pregnant patients with moderate-to-severe acute iron intoxication). **Use Cautiously in:** Children <3 yr (safety not established).

| | | | |
|---|---|---|---|
| **dexrazoxane** (Zinecard) *Therapeutic: cardioprotective agents* Pregnancy Category C | Reducing incidence and severity of cardiomyopathy from doxorubicin in women with metastatic breast cancer who have already received a cumulative dose of doxorubicin >300 mg/m². | **Hemat:** myelosuppression ■ **Local:** pain at injection site. | **IV (Adults):** 10 mg of dexrazoxane/1 mg doxorubicin. |

**Contraindicated in:** Any other type of chemotherapy except other anthracyclines (doxorubicin-like agents). **Use Cautiously in:** Pregnancy, lactation, or children (safety not established).

| Generic Name (Brand Name) {Canadian name} Classification(s) Schedule | Indications | Adverse Reactions and Side Effects | Route and Dosage |
|---|---|---|---|
| **docosanol** (Abreva) *Therapeutic: antivirals (topical)* Pregnancy Category B | Treatment of recurrent orofacial herpes simplex (cold sores, fever blisters). | All local reactions occured at site of application ■ **Local:** acne, skin, itching, rash. | **Topical (Adults and Children ≥ 12 yr):** Apply small amount 5 times daily to sores on lips or face until healed. |

**Contraindicated in:** Hypersensitivity to docosanol or any other components of the formulation (benzyl alcohol, mineral oil, propylene glycol or sucrose). **Use Cautiously in:** Children <12 yr (safety not established). Pregnancy (use only if clearly needed).

| | | | |
|---|---|---|---|
| **eflornithine (topical)** (Vaniqa) *Therapeutic: facial hair removers (topical)* Pregnancy Category C | Reduction of unwanted facial hair in women. | **Local:** burning, rash, stinging, tingling. | **Topical (Adults):** Apply a thin layer to affected areas of the face and adjacent involved areas under the chin and rub in thoroughly. Do not wash for 4 hr following application. Use twice daily at least 8 hr apart. |

**Contraindicated in:** Hypersensitivity. **Use Cautiously in:** Pregnancy, lactation, or children <12 yr (safety not established).

| | | | |
|---|---|---|---|
| **ethambutol** (Myambutol) [Etibi] *Therapeutic: antituberculars* Pregnancy Category C | Active tuberculosis or other mycobacterial diseases (with at least one other drug). | **CNS:** confusion, dizziness, hallucinations, headache, malaise ■ **EENT:** optic neuritis ■ **GI:** HEPATITIS, abdominal pain, anorexia, nausea, vomiting ■ **Metab:** hyperuricemia ■ **MS:** joint pain ■ **Neuro:** peripheral neuritis ■ **Misc:** anaphylactoid reactions, fever. | **PO (Adults and Children >13 yr):** 15–25 mg/kg/day (maximum 2.5 g/day) *or* 50 mg/kg (up to 2.5 g) twice weekly *or* 25–30 mg/kg (up to 2.5 g) 3 times weekly. |

**Contraindicated in:** Hypersensitivity. Optic neuritis. **Use Cautiously in:** Renal and severe hepatic impairment (dosage reduction required). Children <13 yr (safety not established). Pregnancy (although safety not established, ethambutol has been used with isoniazid in pregnant women without adverse effects on the fetus). Lactation.

| Generic Name (Brand Name) [Canadian name] Classification(s) Schedule Pregnancy Category | Indications | Adverse Reactions and Side Effects | Route and Dosage |
|---|---|---|---|
| **flecainide** (Tambocor) **Therapeutic:** *antiarrhyth-mics (class IC)* Pregnancy Category C | Life-threatening ventricular ar-rhythmias, including ventricu-lar tachycardia. Supraventric-ular tachyarrhythmias includ-ing .Paroxysmal supraventric-ular tachycardia (PSVT). Par-oxysmal atrial fibrillation/flut-ter (PAF). | **CNS:** dizziness, anxiety, fatigue, headache, mental depression ■ **EENT:** blurred vision, visual disturbances ■ **CV:** ARRHYTHMIAS, CHEST PAIN, CHF ■ **GI:** anorexia, constipation, drug-induced hepatitis, nausea, stomach pain, vomiting ■ **Derm:** rashes ■ **Neuro:** tremor. | Ventricular Tachycardia **PO (Adults):** 100 mg q 12 hr initially, increased by 50 mg bid until response is obtained or maximum total daily dose of 400 mg is reached. Some patients may require q 8 hr dosing. Renal/Hepatic Impairment **PO (Adults):** *CCr <35 ml/min*—100 mg once a day or 50 mg q 12 hr initially; further dosing on the basis of frequent blood level moni-toring. PSVT/PAF **PO (Adults):** 50 mg q 12 hr initially, increased by 50 mg bid until re-sponse is obtained or maximum total daily dose of 300 mg is reached. Some patients may require q 8 hr dosing. |

**Contraindicated in:** Hypersensitivity. Cardiogenic shock. **Use Cautiously in:** CHF (dosage reduction may be required). Pre-existing sinus node dysfunction or 2nd- or 3rd-degree heart block (without a pacemaker). Renal impairment (dosage reduction required if CCr <35 ml/min). Pregnancy, lactation, or children (safety not established).

| **flurbiprofen\*** (Ansaid) [Apo-Flurbiprofen, Froben, Novo-Flurprofen, Nu-Flurbiprofen] **Therapeutic:** *antirheumat-ics, nonsteroidal anti-in-flammatory agents* Pregnancy Category B (first trimester) | **PO:** Inflammatory disorders in-cluding: Rheumatoid arthritis. Osteoarthritis. **Unlabeled uses:** Nonopioid analgesic. Antidysmenorrheal. | **CNS:** dizziness, drowsiness, headache, insomnia, mental depression, psychic disturbances ■ **EENT:** blurred vision, corneal opacities, tinnitus ■ **CV:** changes in blood pressure, edema, palpitations ■ **GI:** GI BLEED-ING, abdominal pain, heartburn, nausea, bloated feeling, constipation, diarrhea, drug-induced hepatitis, stomatitis ■ **GI:** incontinence ■ **Derm:** increased sweating, rashes ■ **Hemat:** *PO*— blood dyscrasias, prolonged bleeding time ■ **MS:** myalgia ■ **Misc:** allergic reactions in-cluding anaphylaxis, STEVENS-JOHNSON SYNDROME, chills, fever. | **PO (Adults):** *Anti-inflammatory*—200–300 mg daily in 2–4 divid-ed doses (not to exceed 300 mg/day or 100 mg/dose). *Non-opioid analgesic/antidysmenorrheal*—50 mg q 4–6 hr as needed (unla-beled). |

**Contraindicated in:** Hypersensitivity. Cross-sensitivity may exist with other NSAIDs, including aspirin. Active GI bleeding or ulcer disease. **Use Cautiously in:** Severe cardiovascular, renal, or hepatic disease. History of ulcer disease. Diabetes mellitus. Bleeding disorders. Pregnancy (not recommended for use during second half of pregnancy). Lactation, or children (safety not established).

| Generic Name (Brand Name) [Canadian name] Classification(s) Schedule Pregnancy Category | Indications | Adverse Reactions and Side Effects | Route and Dosage |
|---|---|---|---|
| **fluvoxamine** (Luvox) *Therapeutic: antidepressants, antiobsessive agents* *Pharmacologic: selective serotonin reuptake inhibitors (SSRIs)* Pregnancy Category C | Obsessive-compulsive disorder. **Unlabeled uses:** Depression. | **CNS:** dizziness, drowsiness, headache, insomnia, nervousness, weakness, agitation, anxiety, apathy, emotional lability, manic reactions, mental depression, psychotic reactions, syncope ■ **EENT:** sinusitis ■ **Resp:** cough, dyspnea ■ **CV:** edema, hypertension, palpitations, postural hypotension, tachycardia, vasodilation ■ **GI:** constipation, diarrhea, dry mouth, dyspepsia, nausea, anorexia, dysphagia, elevated liver enzymes, flatulence, vomiting ■ **GI:** decreased libido/sexual dysfunction ■ **Derm:** excessive sweating ■ **Metab:** weight gain, weight loss ■ **MS:** hypertonia, myoclonus/twitching ■ **Neuro:** hypokinesia/hyperkinesia, tremor ■ **Misc:** allergic reactions, chills, flu-like symptoms, tooth disorder/caries, yawning. | **PO (Adults):** *Initial dose*—50 mg daily at bedtime; increase by 50 mg q 4–7 days until desired effect is achieved. If daily dose >100 mg, give in two equally divided doses or give a larger dose at bedtime (not to exceed 300 mg/day). *Maintenance dose*—Make periodic adjustments to maintain lowest possible dose to control symptoms. **PO (Children 8–17 yr):** 25 mg at bedtime, may increase by 25 mg/day q 4–7 days (not to exceed 200 mg/day; daily doses >50 mg should be given in divided doses with a larger dose at bedtime). **Renal/Hepatic Impairment** **PO (Adults):** 25 mg daily at bedtime initially, slower titration and longer dosing intervals should be used. |

**Contraindicated in:** Hypersensitivity to fluvoxamine or other SSRIs. Concurrent MAO inhibitor therapy. **Use Cautiously in:** Geriatric patients or patients with impaired hepatic function (lower initial dose and slower dosage titration recommended). Pregnancy, lactation, or children <18 yr (safety not established).

| | | | |
|---|---|---|---|
| **gemtuzumab ozogamicin** (Mylotarg) *Therapeutic: antineoplastics* *Pharmacologic: monoclonal antibodies, antitumor antibiotics* Pregnancy Category D | Treatment of patients with CD33 positive acute myeloid leukemia in first relapse who are ≥60 years old and who are not considered to be candidates for cytotoxic chemotherapy. | **CNS:** headache ■ **Resp:** dyspnea, hypoxia ■ **CV:** hypotension, hypertension. **GI:** mucositis, nausea, vomiting, hepatotoxicity ■ **Derm:** rash ■ **Endo:** hyperglycemia ■ **F and E:** hypokalemia ■ **Hemat:** NEUTROPENIA, anemia, bleeding, thrombocytopenia ■ **Misc:** chills, fever, post-infusion reaction, allergic reactions, infection, tumor lysis syndrome. | **IV (Adults ≥60 yr):** 9 mg/m² as a 2-hr infusion followed by a second dose 14 days later. |

**Contraindicated in:** Hypersensitivity. Pregnancy. Lactation. **Use Cautiously in:** Patients with hepatic impairment. Children (safety not established).

| Generic Name (Brand Name) {Canadian name} Classification(s) Schedule Pregnancy Category | Indications | Adverse Reactions and Side Effects | Route and Dosage |
|---|---|---|---|
| **goserelin** (Zoladex) *Therapeutic: antineoplastics, hormones* *Pharmacologic: gonadotropin-releasing hormones* Pregnancy Category D (breast cancer), X (endometriosis) | Prostate cancer in patients who cannot tolerate orchiectomy or estrogen therapy (palliative). With flutamide and radiation therapy in the treatment of locally confined stage T2b-T4 (stage B2-C) prostate cancer. Advanced breast cancer in peri- and postmenopausal women (palliative). Endometriosis. Produces thinning of the endometrium before endometrial ablation for dysfunctional uterine bleeding. | **CNS:** headache, anxiety, depression, dizziness, fatigue, insomnia, weakness ■ **Resp:** dyspnea ■ **CV:** CEREBROVASCULAR ACCIDENT, MYOCARDIAL INFARCTION, vasodilation, chest pain, hypertension, palpitations ■ **GI:** anorexia, constipation, diarrhea, nausea, ulcer, vomiting ■ **GU:** renal insufficiency, urinary obstruction ■ **Derm:** sweating, rashes ■ **Endo:** decreased libido, impotence, breast tenderness, infertility, ovarian cysts, ovarian hyperstimulation syndrome (with gonadotropins) ■ **F and E:** peripheral edema ■ **Hemat:** anemia ■ **Metab:** gout, hyperglycemia, ↑ lipids ■ **MS:** ↑ bone pain, arthralgia, ↓ bone density ■ **Misc:** hot flashes, chills, fever, weight gain. | **Subcut (Adults):** 3.6 mg every 4 wk or 10.8 mg q 12 wk. *Endometrial thinning*—1 or 2 depots given 4 wk apart; if 1 depot used, surgery is performed at 4 wk; if 2 depots used, surgery is performed 2–4 wk after 2nd depot. |

**Contraindicated in:** Hypersensitivity. Undiagnosed vaginal bleeding. Pregnancy or lactation. **Use Cautiously in:** Lactation, or children <18 yr (safety not established).

| | | | |
|---|---|---|---|
| **guanabenz** (Wytensin) *Therapeutic: antihypertensives* *Pharmacologic: centrally acting antiadrenergics* Pregnancy Category C | Management of hypertension. | **CNS:** dizziness, drowsiness, weakness, headache, irritability, nervousness ■ **EENT:** blurred vision, dry eyes, miosis, nasal congestion ■ **Resp:** dyspnea ■ **CV:** arrhythmias, bradycardia, chest pain, edema, hypotension, palpitations ■ **GI:** dry mouth, abdominal pain, abnormal taste, anorexia, constipation, diarrhea, nausea, vomiting ■ **GU:** impotence, urinary frequency ■ **Derm:** pruritus, rashes, sweating ■ **End:** gynecomastia ■ **MS:** backache, painful extremities ■ **Misc:** withdrawal phenomenon. | **PO (Adults):** 4 mg bid; may increase q 1–2 wk in 4–8-mg increments (range 8–16 mg/day; not to exceed 32 mg/day). |

**Contraindicated in:** Hypersensitivity. **Use Cautiously in:** Serious cardiac or cerebrovascular disease, renal or hepatic insufficiency. Geriatric patients (more prone to adverse reactions). Pregnancy, lactation, or children <12 yr (safety not established).

| Generic Name<br>(Brand Name)<br>[Canadian name]<br>Classification(s)<br>Schedule<br>Pregnancy Category | Indications | Adverse Reactions and Side Effects | Route and Dosage |
|---|---|---|---|
| **guanadrel**<br>(Hylorel)<br>***Therapeutic:*** *antihypertensives*<br>***Pharmacologic:*** *peripherally acting antiadrenergics*<br>Pregnancy Category B | Moderate to severe hypertension (with at least one other agent, usually a diuretic). | **CNS:** confusion, dizziness, drowsiness, fainting, fatigue, headaches, anxiety, depression, sleep disturbances ■ **EENT:** nasal stuffiness, visual disturbances ■ **Resp:** cough, shortness of breath ■ **CV:** chest pain, edema, orthostatic hypotension, palpitations ■ **GI:** anorexia, constipation, diarrhea, dry mouth, gas pain, indigestion, abdominal pain, nausea ■ **GU:** ejaculation disturbances, impotence, nocturia, urinary frequency ■ **MS:** aching limbs, leg cramps ■ **Neuro:** paresthesia. | **PO (Adults):** 5 mg bid, increased weekly or monthly as needed (range 20–75 mg/day in 2–4 divided doses).<br>**Renal/Hepatic Impairment**<br>**PO (Adults):** *CCr 30—60 ml/min*—5 mg q 24 hr initially, dosage may be adjusted at 7-day intervals; *CCr <30 ml/min*—5 mg q 48 hr initially, dosage may be adjusted at 14-day intervals. |

**Contraindicated in:** Hypersensitivity. CHF. Pheochromocytoma. Lactation. **Use Cautiously in:** Asthma. Cardiovascular or cerebrovascular insufficiency. Peptic ulcer disease. Patients with renal failure (increased dosing interval recommended if CCr <60 ml/min). Geriatric patients. Pregnancy, lactation, or children <18 yr (safety not established).

| | | | |
|---|---|---|---|
| **hydroxyurea**<br>(Droxia, Hydrea, Mylocel)<br>***Therapeutic:*** *antineoplastics*<br>***Pharmacologic:*** *antimetabolites*<br>Pregnancy Category D | Treatment of head and neck carcinoma. Treatment of ovarian carcinoma. Treatment of resistant chronic myelogenous leukemia. Treatment of melanoma. Reduction of painful crises in sickle cell anemia and decreased need for transfusions in adult patients with a history of recurrent moderate to severe crises (at least 3 in the preceding yr). **Unlabeled uses:** Used as part of antiretroviral therapy in patients with HIV infection. | **CNS:** drowsiness (large doses) ■ **GI:** anorexia, diarrhea, nausea, vomiting, constipation, hepatitis, stomatitis ■ **GU:** dysuria, infertility, renal tubular dysfunction ■ **Derm:** alopecia, exacerbation of post-radiation erythema, erythema, pruritus, rashes ■ **Hemat:** leukopenia, anemia, thrombocytopenia ■ **Metab:** hyperuricemia ■ **Misc:** chills, fever, malaise. | Head and Neck Cancer, Ovarian Cancer, Malignant Melanoma<br>**PO (Adults):** 60–80 mg/kg (2–3 g/m²) as a single daily dose q 3 days or 20–30 mg/kg/day as a single dose. Therapy should be initiated 7 days prior to radiation and continued.<br>Resistant Chronic Myelogenous Leukemia<br>**PO (Adults):** 20–30 mg/kg/day in 1–2 divided doses.<br>Sickle Cell Anemia<br>**PO (Adults and Children):** 15 mg/kg/day as a single dose, may increase by 5 mg/kg/day q 12 wks up to 35 mg/kg/day. |

**Contraindicated in:** Hypersensitivity. Pregnancy or lactation. Some products contain tartrazine (FDC yellow dye #5) and should be avoided in patients with known hypersensitivity. **Use Cautiously in:** Patients with childbearing potential. Renal impairment (close monitoring of hematologic parameters recommended, dosage reduction may be necessary). Hepatic impairment (close monitoring of hematologic parameters recommended). Active infections. Decreased bone marrow reserve. Other chronic debilitating illness. Geriatric patients (may be more sensitive to effects, lower doses may be required). Obese patients or patients with edema (dose should be determined using ideal body weight).

| Generic Name (Brand Name) [Canadian name] Classification(s) Schedule Pregnancy Category | Indications | Adverse Reactions and Side Effects | Route and Dosage |
|---|---|---|---|
| **kaolin/pectin** (Kao-Spen, Kapectolin) {Donnagel-MB} *Therapeutic:* antidiarrheals *Pharmacologic:* adsorbents Pregnancy Category C | Adjunctive therapy in the treatment of mild to moderate diarrhea. | **GI:** constipation. | Kaolin/pectin suspension contains 5.2–6 g kaolin/30 ml and 130–260 mg pectin/30 ml. **PO (Adults):** 60–120 ml after each loose stool. **PO (Children ≥12 yr):** 45–60 ml after each loose stool. **PO (Children 6–12 yr):** 30–60 ml after each loose stool. **PO (Children 3–6 yr):** 15–30 ml after each loose stool. |

**Contraindicated in:** Severe abdominal pain of unknown cause, especially when associated with fever. Children <3 yr. Some products contain alcohol and should be avoided in patients with known intolerance. **Use Cautiously in:** Geriatric patients (>60 yr). Diarrhea continuing >48 hr (health care professional should be consulted).

| | | | |
|---|---|---|---|
| **mebendazole** (Vermox) *Therapeutic:* antihelmintics Pregnancy Category C | Treatment of: Whipworm (trichuriasis). Pinworm (enterobiasis). Roundworm (ascariasis). Hookworm (uncinariasis). infections. | Most side effects and adverse reactions are seen with high-dose therapy only ■ **CNS:** SEIZURES (rare), dizziness, headache ■ **EENT:** tinnitus ■ **GI:** abdominal pain, diarrhea, increased liver enzymes (high dose, long-term therapy), nausea, vomiting ■ **Derm:** rash, urticaria ■ **Hemat:** agranulocytosis, reversible myelosuppression (leukopenia, thrombocytopenia) ■ **Neuro:** numbness ■ **Misc:** fever. | Enterobiasis **PO (Adults and Children >2 yr):** 100 mg as a single dose; repeat in 2–3 wk. Trichuriasis, Ascariasis, Hookworm, or Mixed Infections **PO (Adults and Children >2 yr):** 100 mg twice daily for 3 days. If not cured in 2–3 wk, a 2nd course is given. |

**Contraindicated in:** Hypersensitivity. **Use Cautiously in:** Impaired liver function. Crohn's ileitis. Ulcerative colitis. Pregnancy, lactation, or children <2 yr (safety not established; may be used in first trimester only if benefit justifies potential risk to fetus).

| | | | |
|---|---|---|---|
| **mechlorethamine** (Mustargen, nitrogen mustard) *Therapeutic:* antineoplastics *Pharmacologic:* alkylating agents Pregnancy Category D | Part of combination therapy of Hodgkin's disease and malignant lymphomas. Used palliatively in: Bronchogenic carcinoma Leukemias. Administered into cavities (pleural, peritoneal) to prevent reaccumulation of malignant effusions. | **CNS:** SEIZURES, drowsiness, headache, vertigo, weakness ■ **GI:** nausea, vomiting, anorexia, diarrhea ■ **GU:** infertility ■ **Derm:** rashes, alopecia ■ **Hemat:** LEUKOPENIA, THROMBOCYTOPENIA, anemia ■ **Local:** tissue necrosis, phlebitis at IV site ■ **Metab:** hyperuricemia ■ **Misc:** reactivation of herpes zoster. | **IV (Adults and Children):** 0.4 mg/kg as single dose or divided over 2–4 days (not to exceed 0.2–0.3 mg/kg in patients who have received previous chemotherapy or radiation therapy); *as part of MOPP regimen for Hodgkin's lymphoma in adults*—6 mg/m² on days 1 and 8 of 28-day cycle; doses in subsequent cycles are determined by blood counts. **Intracavitary: (Adults):** 0.4 mg/kg. **Intrapericardial: (Adults):** 0.2 mg/kg. |

**Contraindicated in:** Hypersensitivity. Pregnancy. Lactation. **Use Cautiously in:** Infections. Decreased bone marrow reserve. Previous radiotherapy or chemotherapy (dosage reduction required). Obesity or severe edema (dosage should be based on ideal dry body weight). Geriatric patients or patients with chronic debilitating illnesses. Patients with childbearing potential.

| Generic Name (Brand Name) {Canadian name} Classification(s) Schedule Pregnancy Category | Indications | Adverse Reactions and Side Effects | Route and Dosage |
|---|---|---|---|
| **meprobamate** (Equanil, Miltown) {Apo-Meprobamate} *Therapeutic: antianxiety agents, sedative/hypnotics* *Pharmacologic: carbamates* Schedule IV Pregnancy Category D | Anxiety disorders (provides sedation). | **CNS:** drowsiness ■ **EENT:** blurred vision ■ **CV:** hypotension ■ **GI:** anorexia, diarrhea, nausea, vomiting ■ **Derm:** pruritus, rashes, urticaria ■ **Neuro:** ataxia ■ **Misc:** hypersensitivity reactions, physical dependence, psychological dependence, tolerance. | **PO (Adults):** 400 mg 3–4 times daily or 600 mg twice daily. *Extended-release capsules*—400–800 mg twice daily (not to exceed 2400 mg/day). **PO (Children 6–12 yr):** 100–200 mg 2–3 times daily. *Extended-release capsules*—200 mg twice daily. |

**Contraindicated in:** Hypersensitivity. Comatose patients or those with pre-existing CNS depression. Uncontrolled severe pain. Pregnancy and lactation. **Use Cautiously in:** Hepatic dysfunction or severe renal impairment. History of suicide attempt or drug abuse. Geriatric patients (dosage reduction suggested).

| **mexiletine** (Mexitil) *Therapeutic: antiarrhythmics (class IB)* Pregnancy Category C | Prophylaxis/treatment of serious ventricular arrhythmias, including VT and PVCs. **Unlabeled uses:** Management of chronic neuropathic pain. | **CNS:** dizziness, nervousness, confusion, fatigue, headache, sleep disorder ■ **EENT:** blurred vision, tinnitus ■ **Resp:** dyspnea ■ **CV:** ARRHYTHMIAS, chest pain, edema, palpitations ■ **GI:** HEPATIC NECROSIS, heartburn, nausea, vomiting ■ **Derm:** rashes ■ **Hemat:** blood dyscrasias ■ **Neuro:** tremor, coordination difficulties, paresthesia. | **PO (Adults):** 400-mg loading dose initially, then 200 mg 8 hr later, then 200–400 mg q 8 hr; dosage alterations of 50–100 mg may be made q 2–3 days. If controlled on ≤300 mg q 8 hr, can give same daily dose at 12-hr intervals (not to exceed 1200 mg/day). Some patients may require q 6-hr dosing. |

**Contraindicated in:** Hypersensitivity. Cardiogenic shock. 2nd- or 3rd-degree heart block (if a pacemaker has not been inserted). Lactation. **Use Cautiously in:** Sinus node or intraventricular conduction abnormalities. Hypotension. CHF. Severe hepatic impairment (dosage reduction suggested). Pregnancy or children (safety not established).

| **minoxidil (systemic)** (Loniten) *Therapeutic: antihypertensives* *Pharmacologic: vasodilators* Pregnancy Category C | Severe symptomatic hypertension or hypertension associated with end-organ damage that has failed to respond to combinations of more conventional therapy. | **CNS:** headache ■ **Resp:** PULMONARY EDEMA ■ **CV:** CHF, ECG changes (alteration in T waves), tachycardia, angina, pericardial effusion ■ **GI:** nausea ■ **Derm:** hypertrichosis, pigment changes, rashes ■ **Endo:** gynecomastia, menstrual irregularities ■ **F and E:** sodium and water retention ■ **Misc:** intermittent claudication. | **PO (Adults and Children >12 yr):** *Hypertension*—5 mg once daily or in 2 divided doses; may double at 3-day intervals; usual range 10–40 mg/day (for rapid control with careful monitoring, doses may be adjusted q 6 hr; up to 100 mg/day have been used). **PO (Children <12 yr):** *Hypertension*—0.2 mg/kg/day (5 mg maximum) as a single dose or 2 divided doses; may be gradually increased at 3-day intervals in increments of 50–100% until response is obtained; usual range 0.25–1 mg/kg/day (for rapid control, doses may be adjusted q 6 hr; not to exceed 50 mg/day). |

**Contraindicated in:** Hypersensitivity. Pheochromocytoma. Patients currently receiving guanethidine. **Use Cautiously in:** Recent MI. Severe renal impairment (can be used in moderate renal impairment). Geriatric patients (may be more sensitive to effects; consider age-related decline in body mass, hepatic/renal/cardiovascular function). Pregnancy or lactation (safety not established).

| Generic Name (Brand Name) [Canadian name] Classification(s) Schedule Pregnancy Category | Indications | Adverse Reactions and Side Effects | Route and Dosage |
|---|---|---|---|
| **orlistat** (Xenical) **Therapeutic: weight control agents** **Pharmacologic: lipase inhibitors** Pregnancy Category B | Obesity management (weight loss and maintenance) when used in conjunction with a reduced-calorie diet in patients with an initial BMI $\geq$30 kg/m² or $\geq$27 kg/m² in the presence of additional risk factors (diabetes, hypertension, hyperlipidemia). Reduces the risk of weight regain after prior loss. | With initial use; incidence decreases with prolonged use ■ **GI:** fecal urgency, flatus with discharge, increased defecation, oily evacuation, oily spotting, fecal incontinence. | **PO (Adults):** 120 mg three times daily with each meal containing fat. |
| **Contraindicated in:** Hypersensitivity. Chronic malabsorption syndrome or cholestasis. Pregnancy or lactation. **Use Cautiously in:** Children (safety not established). | | | |
| **pemoline** (Cylert, PemADD, PemADD CT) **Therapeutic: central nervous system stimulants** Schedule IV Pregnancy Category B | Adjunct in the management of ADHD in children >6 yr (not considered first-line treatment). **Unlabeled uses:** Treatment of fatigue or mental depression. Treatment of schizophrenia. As a stimulant in geriatric patients. | **CNS:** SEIZURES, insomnia, dizziness, dyskinetic movements, headache, irritability, mental depression, nervousness (increased doses) ■ **CV:** tachycardia (increased doses) ■ **GI:** HEPATIC FAILURE, anorexia, drug-induced hepatitis ■ **Derm:** rash, sweating ■ **Metab:** weight loss ■ **Misc:** fever. | **PO (Children >6 yr):** 37.5 mg initially as single morning dose; may be increased by 18.75 mg at weekly intervals until optimum response is achieved (range 56.25–75 mg/day, not to exceed 112.5 mg/day). |
| **Contraindicated in:** Hypersensitivity. Liver disease. **Use Cautiously in:** Renal impairment. Unstable emotional status or psychoses. History of seizure disorders. Tics. Pregnancy or lactation (safety not established). | | | |
| **penciclovir** (Denavir) **Therapeutic: antivirals (topical)** Pregnancy Category B | Recurrent herpes labialis (cold sores). | **CNS:** headache ■ **Local:** application site reactions. | **PO (Adults):** Apply 1% cream q 2 hr for 4 days while awake. |
| **Contraindicated in:** Hypersensitivity to penciclovir or other components of the formulation. **Use Cautiously in:** Pregnancy, lactation, or children (safety not established). | | | |

| Generic Name (Brand Name) [Canadian name] Classification(s) Schedule Pregnancy Category | Indications | Adverse Reactions and Side Effects | Route and Dosage |
|---|---|---|---|
| **penicillamine** (Cuprimine, Depen) *Therapeutic: antidotes, antirheumatics (DMARD), antiurolithics* *Pharmacologic: chelating agents* Pregnancy Category D | Progressive rheumatoid arthritis resistant to conventional therapy. Management of copper deposition in Wilson's disease. Management of recurrent cystine calculi. **Unlabeled uses:** Adjunct in the treatment of heavy metal poisoning. | **EENT:** blurred vision, eye pain ■ **Resp:** coughing, shortness of breath, wheezing ■ **GI:** altered taste, anorexia, cholestatic jaundice, diarrhea, drug-induced pancreatitis, dyspepsia, epigastric pain, hepatic dysfunction, nausea, oral ulceration, vomiting ■ **GU:** proteinuria ■ **Derm:** pemphigus, ecchymoses, hives, itching, rashes, wrinkling ■ **Hemat:** APLASTIC ANEMIA, anemia, eosinophilia, leukopenia, thrombocytopenia, thrombocytosis ■ **MS:** arthralgia, migratory polyarthritis ■ **Neuro:** myasthenia gravis syndrome ■ **Misc:** GOODPASTURE'S SYNDROME (GLOMERULONEPHRITIS AND INTRA-ALVEOLAR HEMORRHAGE), allergic reactions, fever, lymphadenopathy, systemic lupus erythematosus–like syndrome. | **PO (Adults):** *Antirheumatic*—125–250 mg/day as a single dose; may be slowly increased up to 1.5 g/day. *Chelating agent (Wilson's disease)*—250 mg qid. *Antiurolithic*—500 mg 4 times daily. **PO (Children >6 mo):** *Chelating agent (Wilson's disease)*—250 mg/day as a single dose; older children may receive the adult dose. *Antiurolithic*—7.5 mg/kg 4 times daily. |

**Contraindicated in:** Hypersensitivity. Cross-sensitivity with penicillin may exist. Patients currently receiving gold salts, antimalarials, antineoplastics, oxyphenbutazone, or phenylbutazone. Concurrent use of iron supplements. Pregnancy (penicillamine should be avoided in pregnant patients with rheumatoid arthritis or cystinuria). Lactation. **Use Cautiously in:** Renal impairment (increased risk of adverse renal reactions in patients with rheumatoid arthritis). History of aplastic anemia due to penicillamine. Patients requiring surgery (may impair wound healing). Geriatric patients (increased risk of hematologic toxicity; dosage reduction recommended). Pregnancy (for patients with Wilson's disease, limit daily dose to <1 g. If cesarean section is planned, decrease daily dose to 250 mg for last 6 wk of pregnancy and until incision is healed).

| | | | |
|---|---|---|---|
| **pentazocine** (Talwin, Talwin NX) *Therapeutic: opioid analgesics* *Pharmacologic: opioid agonists/antagonists* Schedule IV Pregnancy Category C | Moderate to severe pain. Also used for: analgesia during labor; sedation prior to surgery; supplementation in balanced anesthesia. | **CNS:** dizziness, euphoria, hallucinations, headache, sedation, confusion, dysphoria, floating feeling, unusual dreams ■ **EENT:** blurred vision, diplopia, miosis (high doses) ■ **CV:** hypertension, hypotension, palpitations ■ **GI:** nausea, constipation, dry mouth, ileus, vomiting ■ **GU:** urinary retention ■ **Derm:** clammy feeling, sweating ■ **Local:** severe tissue damage at subcut sites ■ **Misc:** physical dependence, psychological dependence, tolerance. | **PO (Adults):** 50–100 mg q 3–4 hr (not to exceed 600 mg/day). **Subcut, IV, IM (Adults):** 30 mg q 3–4 hr (not to exceed 30 mg/dose IV or 60 mg/dose IM or subcut; not to exceed 360 mg/day subcut, IV, or IM). *Obstetrical use*—20 mg IV or 30 mg IM when contractions become regular, may repeat q 2–3 hr for 2–3 doses. |

**Contraindicated in:** Hypersensitivity. Patients who are physically dependent on opioids (may precipitate withdrawal). **Use Cautiously in:** Head trauma. History of drug abuse. Increased intracranial pressure. Severe renal, hepatic, or pulmonary disease. Hypothyroidism. Adrenal insufficiency. Alcoholism. Geriatric, debilitated patients, or patients with severe liver impairment (dosage reduction recommended). Undiagnosed abdominal pain. Prostatic hypertrophy. Patients who have recently received opioid agonists. Pregnancy (has been used during labor but may cause respiratory depression in the newborn). Lactation, or children (safety not established).

| Generic Name (Brand Name) [Canadian name] Classification(s) Pregnancy Category | Indications | Adverse Reactions and Side Effects | Route and Dosage |
|---|---|---|---|
| **pentobarbital** (Nembutal) [Novopentobarb, Nova Rectal] *Therapeutic: anticonvulsants, sedative/hypnotics* *Pharmacologic: barbiturates* Schedule II (oral and parenteral) III (rectal) Pregnancy Category D | Hypnotic agent (short-term). Preoperative sedation and other situations in which sedation is required. Treatment of seizures. **Unlabeled uses:** **IV:** Induction of coma in selected patients with cerebral ischemia and management of increased intracranial pressure (high doses). | **CNS:** drowsiness, hangover, lethargy, delirium, excitation, mental depression, vertigo **Resp:** respiratory depression; *IV*— LARYNGOSPASM, bronchospasm **CV:** *IV*— hypotension **GI:** constipation, diarrhea, nausea, vomiting **Derm:** rashes, urticaria **Local:** phlebitis at IV site **MS:** arthralgia, myalgia, neuralgia **Misc:** hypersensitivity reactions including angioedema and serum sickness, physical dependence, psychological dependence. | **PO (Adults):** *Sedative*—20 mg 3–4 times daily. *Hypnotic/preoperative sedative*—100 mg. **PO (Children):** *Sedative*—2–6 mg/kg/day. *Preoperative sedative*—2–6 mg/kg (up to 100 mg/dose). **IM (Adults):** *Hypnotic/preoperative sedative*—150–200 mg. **IM (Children):** *Sedative*—2–6 mg/kg/day in divided doses. *Preoperative sedative*—2–6 mg/kg (up to 100 mg/dose). **IV (Adults):** *Hypnotic/anticonvulsant*—100 mg initially; additional small doses may be given q min up to 500 mg total. *Induction of coma*—5–7 mg/kg, then 3–4 mg/kg q 3–4 hr dose adjusted by serum level (unlabeled). **IV (Children):** *Hypnotic/anticonvulsant*—50 mg; additional, smaller doses may be given q min. **Rect (Adults):** *Sedative*—30 mg 2–4 times daily. *Hypnotic*—120–200 mg at bedtime. **Rect (Children):** *Sedative*—2 mg/kg (60 mg/m²) 3 times daily. **Rect (Children 12–14 yr):** *Preoperative sedative/hypnotic*—60–120 mg. **Rect (Children 5–12 yr):** *Preoperative sedative/hypnotic*—60 mg. **Rect (Children 1–4 yr):** *Preoperative sedative/hypnotic*—30–60 mg. **Rect (Children 2 mo–1 yr):** *Preoperative sedative/hypnotic*—30 mg. |

**Contraindicated in:** Hypersensitivity. Some products contain tartrazine, alcohol, or propylene glycol and should be avoided in patients with known hypersensitivity or intolerance. Comatose patients or those with pre-existing CNS depression (unless used to induce coma). Uncontrolled severe pain. Pregnancy or lactation. **Use Cautiously in:** Hepatic dysfunction. Severe renal impairment. Patients who may be suicidal or who may have been addicted to drugs previously. Geriatric or debilitated patients (initial dosage reduction recommended). Hypnotic use should be short-term (chronic use may lead to dependence).

| Generic Name (Brand Name) {Canadian name} Classification(s) Schedule Pregnancy Category | Indications | Adverse Reactions and Side Effects | Route and Dosage |
|---|---|---|---|
| **phentermine** (Adipex-P, Banobese, Fastin, Ionamin, Obi-Nix, OBY-CAP, Phentercot, Phentride, T-Diet, Teramine, Zantryl) ***Therapeutic:*** *weight control agents* ***Pharmacologic:*** *appetite suppressants* Schedule IV Pregnancy Category UK | Short-term treatment of obesity in conjunction with other interventions (dietary restriction, exercise); used to produce and maintain weight loss in patients with a BMI $\geq$30 kg/m$^2$ or $\geq$27 kg/m$^2$ in the presence of other risk factors (diabetes, hypertension, hyperlipidemia). | **CNS:** CNS stimulation, confusion, dizziness, dysphoria, euphoria, headache, insomnia, mental depression, restlessness ■ **EENT:** blurred vision ■ **CV:** hypertension, palpitations, tachycardia ■ **GI:** constipation, diarrhea, dry mouth, nausea, unpleasant taste, vomiting ■ **GU:** changes in libido, impotence. | **PO (Adults):** *Phentermine hydrochloride tablets or capsules*—8 mg 3 times daily or 15–37.5 mg once daily; *Phentermine resin complex capsules*—15–30 mg once daily. |

**Contraindicated in:** Hypersensitivity or known intolerance to sympathomimetic amines. Cardiovascular disease. Hyperthyroidism. Moderate to severe hypertension. History of drug abuse. Agitation. Glaucoma. Concurrent or recent (within 14 days). MAO inhibitor therapy. Concurrent SSRI antidepressants. **Use Cautiously in:** Mild hypertension. Diabetes mellitus. Pregnancy, lactation, or children <12 yr (safety not established).

| | | | |
|---|---|---|---|
| **polycarbophil** (Bulk Forming Fiber Laxative, Equalactin, Fiberall, FiberCon, Fiber-Lax, Konsyl Fiber, Mitrolan) ***Therapeutic:*** *antidiarrheals, laxatives* ***Pharmacologic:*** *bulk-forming agents* Pregnancy Category UK | Treatment of constipation or diarrhea that may be associated with diverticulosis or irritable bowel syndrome. | **GI:** abdominal fullness. | **PO (Adults):** 1 g 1–4 times daily or as needed (not to exceed 6 g/24 hr); for severe diarrhea, may repeat q 30 min. **PO (Children 6–12 yr):** 500 mg 1–3 times daily or as needed (not to exceed 3 g/24 hr); for severe diarrhea, may repeat q 30 min. **PO (Children 2–6 yr):** 500 mg 1–2 times daily or as needed (not to exceed 1.5 g/24 hr); for severe diarrhea, may repeat q 30 min. |

**Contraindicated in:** Hypersensitivity. Abdominal pain. Nausea or vomiting (especially when associated with fever or other signs of acute abdomen). Serious intra-abdominal adhesions. Dysphagia. **Use Cautiously in:** Pregnancy or lactation (has been used safely).

| Generic Name (Brand Name) [Canadian name] Classification(s) Pregnancy Category | Indications | Adverse Reactions and Side Effects | Route and Dosage |
|---|---|---|---|
| **POTASSIUM PHOSPHATES** monobasic potassium phosphate (K-Phos Original) potassium phosphates (Neutra-Phos-K) potassium phosphate *Therapeutic: antiurolitics, mineral and electrolyte replacements/supplements* Pregnancy Category C | Treatment and prevention of phosphate depletion in patients who are unable to ingest adequate dietary potassium. Adjunct therapy of urinary tract infections with methenamine hippurate or mandelate (potassium and sodium phosphates or monobasic potassium phosphate). Prevention of calcium urinary stones (potassium and sodium phosphates or monobasic potassium phosphate). Phosphate salts of potassium may be used in hypokalemic patients with metabolic acidosis or coexisting phosphorus deficiency. | Related to hyperphosphatemia, unless otherwise indicated ■ **CNS:** confusion, listlessness, weakness ■ **CV:** ARRHYTHMIAS, CARDIAC ARREST, ECG changes (absent P waves, widening of the QRS complex with biphasic curve), hypotension; *hyperkalemia*— ARRHYTHMIAS, ECG changes (prolonged PR interval, ST segment depression, tall-tented T waves) ■ **GI:** diarrhea, abdominal pain, nausea, vomiting ■ **F and E:** hyperkalemia, hyperphosphatemia, hypocalcemia, hypomagnesemia ■ **Local:** irritation at IV site, phlebitis ■ **MS:** *hyperkalemia*—muscle cramps; *hypercalcemia*—tremors ■ **Neuro:** flaccid paralysis, heaviness of legs, paresthesias. | *Monobasic Potassium Phosphate* **PO (Adults and Children >4 yr):** 1 g (7.4 mmol) in water 4 times daily. **PO (Children <4 yr):** 200 mg (6.4 mmol) in water 4 times daily. *Potassium Phosphates* **PO (Adults and Children >4 yr):** 1.45 g (8 mmol) 4 times daily. **PO (Children <4 yr):** 200 mg (6.4 mmol) phosphorus 4 times daily. **IV (Adults):** 10 mmol phosphorus/day as an infusion. **IV (Infants):** 1.5–2 mmol phosphorus/day as an infusion. |

**Contraindicated in:** Hyperkalemia. Hyperphosphatemia. Hypocalcemia. Severe renal impairment. Untreated Addison's disease. Severe tissue trauma. Hyperkalemic familial periodic paralysis. **Use Cautiously in:** Hyperparathyroidism. Cardiac disease. Renal impairment.

| | | | |
|---|---|---|---|
| **probenecid** (Probalan) [Benuryl] *Therapeutic: antigout agents, uricosurics* Pregnancy Category B | Prevention of recurrences of gouty arthritis. Treatment of hyperuricemia secondary to thiazide therapy. Used to increase and prolong serum levels of penicillin and related anti-infectives. | **CNS:** headache, dizziness ■ **GI:** nausea, vomiting, abdominal pain, diarrhea, drug-induced hepatitis, sore gums ■ **GU:** uric acid stones, urinary frequency ■ **Derm:** flushing, rashes ■ **Hemat:** APLASTIC ANEMIA, anemia. | **PO (Adults and Children >50 kg):** *Hyperuricemia*—250 mg bid for 1 wk; increase to 500 mg twice daily, then may increase by 500 mg/day every 4 wk (not to exceed 3 g/day). *Augmentation of penicillin/cephalosporins*—500 mg 4 times daily. *Single-dose therapy of gonorrhea*—1 g with amoxicillin or penicillin. **PO (Children 2–14 yr and ≤50 kg):** 25 mg/kg (700 mg/m²) initially, then 10 mg/kg (300 mg/m²) 4 times daily. |

**Contraindicated in:** Hypersensitivity. Chronic high-dose salicylate therapy. Children <2 yr. **Use Cautiously in:** Peptic ulcer. Blood dyscrasias. Uric acid kidney stones. Renal impairment (dosage reduction recommended; may not be effective if CCr ≤30 ml/min). Pregnancy or lactation (has been used safely during pregnancy; safety during lactation not established).

| Generic Name (Brand Name) {Canadian name} Classification(s) Schedule Pregnancy Category | Indications | Adverse Reactions and Side Effects | Route and Dosage |
|---|---|---|---|
| procarbazine (Matulane) {Natulan} *Therapeutic:* antineoplastics *Pharmacologic:* alkylating agents Pregnancy Category D | Treatment of Hodgkin's disease (with other treatment modalities). **Unlabeled uses:** Other lymphomas. Brain and lung tumors. Multiple myeloma. Malignant melanoma. Polycythemia vera. | **CNS:** SEIZURES, confusion, dizziness, drowsiness, hallucinations, headache, mania, mental depression, nightmares, psychosis, syncope, tremor ■ **EENT:** nystagmus, photophobia, retinal hemorrhage ■ **Resp:** cough, pleural effusions ■ **CV:** edema, hypotension, tachycardia ■ **GI:** nausea, vomiting, anorexia, diarrhea, dry mouth, dysphagia, hepatic dysfunction, stomatitis ■ **GU:** gonadal suppression ■ **Derm:** alopecia, photosensitivity, pruritus, rashes ■ **Endo:** gynecomastia ■ **Hemat:** anemia, leukopenia, thrombocytopenia ■ **Neuro:** neuropathy, paresthesia ■ **Misc:** ascites, secondary malignancy. | **PO (Adults):** 2–4 mg/kg/day as a single dose or in divided doses for 1 wk, then 4–6 mg/kg/day until response is obtained; then maintenance dose of 1–2 mg/kg/day. Dosage should be rounded off to the nearest 50 mg. **PO (Children):** 50 mg/m²/day for 7 days, then 100 mg/m²/day, maintenance dose of 50 mg/m²/day. |

**Contraindicated in:** Hypersensitivity. Pregnancy or lactation. Alcoholism. Severe renal or liver impairment. Pheochromocytoma. CHF. **Use Cautiously in:** Patients with childbearing potential. Infections. Decreased bone marrow reserve. Other chronic debilitating illnesses. Headaches. Psychiatric illness. Liver impairment. Cardiovascular disease.

| | | | |
|---|---|---|---|
| propantheline (Pro-Banthine) {Probanthel} *Therapeutic:* antiulcer agents *Pharmacologic:* anticholinergics, antimuscarinics Pregnancy Category C | Adjunctive therapy in the treatment of peptic ulcer disease. **Unlabeled uses:** Antisecretory or antispasmodic agent. | **CNS:** confusion, dizziness, drowsiness, excitement ■ **EENT:** blurred vision, mydriasis, photophobia ■ **CV:** tachycardia, orthostatic hypotension, palpitations ■ **GI:** constipation, dry mouth ■ **GU:** urinary hesitancy, urinary retention ■ **Derm:** rash ■ **Misc:** decreased sweating. | **PO (Adults):** 15 mg 3 times daily, 30 mg at bedtime. **PO (Geriatric Patients, Patients with Mild Symptoms, or Small Stature):** 7.5 mg 3–4 times daily. **PO (Children):** 0.375 mg/kg (10 mg/m²) 4 times daily. |

**Contraindicated in:** Hypersensitivity. Narrow-angle glaucoma. Tachycardia secondary to cardiac insufficiency or thyrotoxicosis. Myasthenia gravis. **Use Cautiously in:** Geriatric patients or patients of small stature (dosage reduction required). Prostatic hypertrophy. Chronic renal, cardiac, or pulmonary disease. Patients who may have intra-abdominal infections. Pregnancy, lactation, or children (safety not established).

| | | | |
|---|---|---|---|
| propylthiouracil (PTU) {Propyl-Thyracil} *Therapeutic:* antithyroid agents Pregnancy Category D | Palliative treatment of hyperthyroidism. Adjunct in the control of hyperthyroidism in preparation for thyroidectomy or radioactive iodine therapy. | **CNS:** drowsiness, headache, vertigo ■ **GI:** nausea, vomiting, diarrhea, drug-induced hepatitis, loss of taste ■ **Derm:** rash, skin discoloration, urticaria ■ **Endo:** hypothyroidism ■ **Hemat:** AGRANULOCYTOSIS, leukopenia, thrombocytopenia ■ **MS:** arthralgia ■ **Misc:** fever, lymphadenopathy, parotitis. | **PO (Adults):** *Thyrotoxic crisis*—200–400 mg q 4 hr during the first 24 hr. *Hyperthyroidism*—300–900 mg once daily or in 2–4 divided doses initially (up to 1.2 g/day); maintenance dose 50–600 mg/day once daily or in 2–4 divided doses. **PO (Children >10 yr):** 50–300 mg/day given once daily or in 2–4 divided doses. **PO (Children 6–10 yr):** 50–150 mg/day given once daily or in 2–4 divided doses. **PO (Neonates):** 10 mg/kg/day in divided doses. |

| Generic Name (Brand Name) [Canadian name] Classification(s) Pregnancy Category | Indications | Adverse Reactions and Side Effects | Route and Dosage |
|---|---|---|---|
| **pyrazinamide** ([PMS Pyrazinamide, Tebrazid]) *Therapeutic: antitubercular* Pregnancy Category C | Used in combination with other agents in the treatment of active tuberculosis. | **GI:** HEPATOTOXICITY, anorexia, diarrhea, nausea, vomiting ■ **GU:** dysuria ■ **Derm:** acne, itching, photosensitivity, skin rash ■ **Hemat:** anemia, thrombocytopenia ■ **Metab:** hyperuricemia ■ **MS:** arthralgia, gouty arthritis. | **PO (Adults and Children):** 15–30 mg/kg/day as a single dose. Up to 60 mg/kg/day has been used in isoniazid-resistant tuberculosis (not to exceed 2 g/day as a single dose or 3 g/day in divided doses). May also be given as 50–70 mg/kg 2–3 times weekly (not to exceed 2 g/dose on daily regimen, 3 g/dose for 3-times-weekly regimen, or 4 g/dose for twice-weekly regimen). *Patients with HIV*—20–30 mg/kg/day for first 2 mo of therapy; further dosing depends on regimen employed. |

**Contraindicated in:** Hypersensitivity. **Use Cautiously in:** Decreased bone marrow reserve. Pregnancy (may be used safely; however, fetus may develop thyroid problems). Lactation (safety not established).

| | | | |
|---|---|---|---|
| **pyrimethamine** (Daraprim) *Therapeutic: antimalarials, antiprotozoals* Pregnancy Category C | Used in combination with other antimalarials in the treatment of chloroquine-resistant malaria. Used in combination with a sulfonamide in the treatment of toxoplasmosis. **Unlabeled uses:** Used in combination with other agents (sulfonamides, dapsone) in the treatment of *Pneumocystis carinii* pneumonia. | **CNS:** SEIZURES (high doses), headache, insomnia, light-headedness, malaise, mental depression ■ **Resp:** dry throat, pulmonary eosinophilia ■ **CV:** ARRHYTHMIAS (large doses) ■ **GI:** atrophic glossitis (high doses), anorexia, diarrhea, nausea ■ **GU:** hematuria ■ **Derm:** abnormal pigmentation, dermatitis ■ **Hemat:** megaloblastic anemia (high doses), pancytopenia, thrombocytopenia ■ **Misc:** fever. | Treatment of Malaria **PO (Adults and Children >10 yr):** 50 mg/day for for 2 days, then 25 mg once weekly in combination with other agents. **PO (Children 4–10 yr):** 25 mg daily for 2 days, then 12.5 mg once weekly in combination with other agents. Toxoplasmosis **PO (Adults):** 50–200 mg/day for 1–2 days, followed by 25–50 mg/day for 2–6 wk; given with a sulfonamide. **PO (Children):** 1 mg/kg/day for 1–3 days, then 0.5 mg/kg/day for 4–6 wk; given with a sulfonamide. Toxoplasmosis in AIDS Patients **PO (Adults):** 100–200 mg/day for 1–2 days, followed by 50–100 mg/day for 3–6 wk, then 25–50 mg/day for life; given with clindamycin or sulfadiazine. |

**Contraindicated in:** Hypersensitivity. Cross-sensitivity with ethionamide, isoniazid, niacin, or nicotinic acid may exist. Severe liver impairment. Concurrent use with rifampin. **Use Cautiously in:** Gout. Diabetes mellitus. Acute intermittent porphyria. Pregnancy (safety not established).

**Contraindicated in:** Hypersensitivity. First 14–16 wk of pregnancy. Megaloblastic anemia caused by folate deficiency. Concurrent folate antagonist therapy (because of risk of megaloblastic anemia). **Use Cautiously in:** History of seizures (high doses). Underlying anemia or bone marrow depression. Impaired liver function (G6PD deficiency). Pregnancy >16 wk (may require concurrent leucovorin). Lactation (large doses to mother may cause folic acid deficiency in infant).

| Generic Name (Brand Name) [Canadian name] Classification(s) Schedule Pregnancy Category | Indications | Adverse Reactions and Side Effects | Route and Dosage |
|---|---|---|---|
| **riboflavin** (vitamin B₂) *Therapeutic: vitamins* *Pharmacologic: water soluble vitamins* Pregnancy Category A | Treatment and prevention of riboflavin deficiency, which may be associated with poor nutritional status or chronic debilitating illnesses. | **GI:** yellow discoloration of urine (large doses only). | Treatment of Deficiency **PO (Adults):** 5–10 mg/day. |

**Contraindicated in:** No known contraindications. **Use Cautiously in:** No known precautions.

| | | | |
|---|---|---|---|
| **sibutramine** (Meridia) *Therapeutic: weight control agents* *Pharmacologic: appetite suppressants* Schedule IV Pregnancy Category C | Treatment of obesity in patients with body mass index ≥30 kg/m² (or ≥27 kg/m²) in patients with diabetes, hypertension, or other risk factors) in conjunction with other interventions (dietary restriction, exercise); used to produce and maintain weight loss. | **CNS:** SEIZURES, headache, insomnia, CNS stimulation, dizziness, drowsiness, emotional lability, nervousness ■ **EENT:** laryngitis/pharyngitis, rhinitis, sinusitis ■ **CV:** hypertension, palpitations, tachycardia, vasodilation ■ **GI:** anorexia, constipation, dry mouth, altered taste, dyspepsia, increased appetite, nausea ■ **GU:** dysmenorrhea ■ **Derm:** increased sweating, rash. | **PO (Adults):** 10 mg once daily; may be increased to 15 mg/day after 4 wk. Patients who do not tolerate an initial dose of 10 mg/day may be started on 5 mg/day. |

**Contraindicated in:** Hypersensitivity. Anorexia nervosa. Concurrent use of other centrally acting appetite suppressants, MAO inhibitors, SSRIs, sumatriptan, naratriptan, zolmitriptan, dihydroergotamine, dextromethorphan, meperidine, pentazocine, fentanyl, lithium, or tryptophan. Organic causes of obesity (untreated hypothyroidism). Severe hepatic/renal impairment. Uncontrolled/poorly controlled hypertension. History of coronary artery disease, CHF, arrhythmias, or stroke. Excessive consumption of alcohol. Pregnancy or lactation. **Use Cautiously in:** History of seizures. Narrow-angle glaucoma. Geriatric patients. Children <16 yr (safety not established).

| | | | |
|---|---|---|---|
| **sodium phosphate** *Therapeutic: mineral and electrolyte replacements/ supplements* *Pharmacologic: phosphate supplements* Pregnancy Category C | Treatment and prevention of phosphate depletion in patients who are unable to ingest adequate dietary phosphates. | Related to hyperphosphatemia, unless otherwise indicated ■ **CNS:** confusion, listlessness, weakness ■ **Resp:** *hypernatremia*—shortness of breath ■ **CV:** ARRHYTHMIAS, CARDIAC ARREST, ECG changes (absent P waves, widening of the QRS complex with biphasic curve), hypotension; *hypernatremia*—edema ■ **GI:** diarrhea, abdominal pain, nausea, vomiting ■ **F and E:** hyperkalemia, hypernatremia, hyperphosphatemia, hypocalcemia, hypomagnesemia ■ **Local:** irritation at IV site, phlebitis ■ **MS:** *hypocalcemia*—tremors ■ **Neuro:** flaccid paralysis, heaviness of legs, paresthesias of extremities. | **IV (Adults):** 12–15 mM phosphorus/liter of parenteral nutrition. **IV (Neonates):** 1.5–2 mM/kg/day (infused as part of parenteral nutrition). |

**Contraindicated in:** Hyperphosphatemia. Hypocalcemia. Severe renal impairment. **Use Cautiously in:** Hyperparathyroidism. Cardiac disease. Hypernatremia. Hypertension.

| Generic Name (Brand Name) [Canadian name] Classification(s) Schedule Pregnancy Category | Indications | Adverse Reactions and Side Effects | Route and Dosage |
|---|---|---|---|
| **succimer** (Chemet) ***Therapeutic:*** *antidotes* ***Pharmacologic:*** *chelating agents* Pregnancy Category C | Treatment of lead poisoning in children with blood lead levels >45 mcg/dl. | **CNS:** dizziness, drowsiness, headache ■ **EENT:** cloudy film in eye, otitis media, plugged ears, watery eyes ■ **Resp:** cough, nasal congestion, rhinorrhea, sore throat ■ **CV:** arrhythmias ■ **GI:** nausea, vomiting, abdominal cramps, anorexia, diarrhea, elevated liver function tests, hemorrhoidal symptoms, metallic taste ■ **GU:** oliguria, proteinuria, voiding difficulty ■ **Derm:** mucocutaneous eruptions, pruritus, rashes ■ **Hemat:** eosinophilia, thrombocytosis ■ **MS:** back, rib, flank pain, leg pain ■ **Neuro:** paresthesia, sensorimotor neuropathy ■ **Misc:** chills, fever, flu-like syndrome, moniliasis. | **PO (Adults and Children):** 10 mg/kg (350 mg/m²) q 8 hr for 5 days, then reduce to 10 mg/kg (350 mg/m²) q 12 hr for 2 more wk. Repeated courses should follow a 2-wk rest period. |

**Contraindicated in:** Hypersensitivity or allergy to succimer. Lactation (should be discouraged during succimer therapy). **Use Cautiously in:** Renal failure (chelates are not dialyzable). Children (increased risk of bradyarrhythmias). Children with skeletal muscle myopathy (more prone to rare, but serious, adverse reactions. Geriatric patients (use lower doses to adjust for decreased renal, hepatic, and cardiac function). Pregnancy or children <1 yr (safety not established).

| | | | |
|---|---|---|---|
| **sucralfate** (Carafate) {Sulcrate} ***Therapeutic:*** *antiulcer agents* ***Pharmacologic:*** *GI protectants* Pregnancy Category B | Short-term management of duodenal ulcers. Maintenance (preventive) therapy of duodenal ulcers. **Unlabeled uses:** Management of gastric ulcer or gastroesophageal reflux. Prevention of gastric mucosal injury caused by high-dose aspirin or other NSAIDs in patients with rheumatoid arthritis or in high-stress situations (e.g., intensive care unit). **Suspension:** Mucositis/stomatitis/oral ulceration with various etiologies. | **CNS:** dizziness, drowsiness ■ **GI:** constipation, diarrhea, dry mouth, gastric discomfort, indigestion, nausea ■ **Derm:** pruritus, rashes. | Treatment of Ulcers **PO (Adults):** 1 g qid, 1 hr before meals and at bedtime; or 2 g twice daily, on waking and at bedtime. Prevention of Ulcers **PO (Adults):** 1 g twice daily, 1 hr before a meal. Gastroesophageal Reflux **PO (Adults):** 1 g qid, 1 hr before meals and at bedtime (unlabeled). **PO (Children):** 500 mg qid, 1 hr before meals and at bedtime (unlabeled). |

**Contraindicated in:** Hypersensitivity. **Use Cautiously in:** Children (safety not established).

| Generic Name (Brand Name) [Canadian name] Classification(s) Schedule Pregnancy Category | Indications | Adverse Reactions and Side Effects | Route and Dosage |
|---|---|---|---|
| **temozolomide** (Temodar) **Therapeutic:** *antineoplastics* **Pharmacologic:** *alkylating agents* Pregnancy Category D | Refractory anaplastic astrocytoma progressing despite treatment with a nitrosurea and procarbazine. | **CNS:** SEIZURES, fatigue, headache, abnormal coordination, anxiety, depression, dizziness, drowsiness, mental status changes, weakness ■ **EENT:** abnormal vision, diplopia ■ **Resp:** cough ■ **CV:** peripheral edema ■ **GI:** nausea, vomiting, abdominal pain, anorexia, constipation, diarrhea, dysphagia ■ **Derm:** pruritus, rash ■ **Endo:** adrenal hypercorticism ■ **Hemat:** leukopenia, thrombocytopenia, anemia ■ **Metab:** increased weight ■ **MS:** abnormal gait, back pain ■ **Neuro:** hemiparesis, myalgia ■ **Misc:** breast pain (women), fever. | **PO (Adults):** 150 mg/m²/day for 5 consecutive days of each 28-day treatment cycle; doses adjusted on the basis of blood counts. |

**Contraindicated in:** Hypersensitivity to temozolomide or dacarbazine (DTIC). Pregnancy or lactation. **Use Cautiously in:** Severe hepatic or renal impairment. Geriatric patients and women (increased risk of myelosuppression). Active infection. Decreased bone marrow reserve. Other chronic debilitating illness. Patients with childbearing potential. Children (safety not established).

| | | | |
|---|---|---|---|
| **thalidomide** (Thalomid) **Therapeutic:** *immunosuppressants* Pregnancy Category X | Cutaneous manifestations of moderate to severe erythema nodosum leprosum (ENL). Prevention (maintenance) and suppression of recurrent ENL. **Unlabeled uses:** Behcet's syndrome. HIV-associated wasting syndrome. Aphthous stomatitis (including HIV associated). Crohn's disease. | **CNS:** dizziness, drowsiness ■ **CV:** bradycardia, edema, orthostatic hypotension ■ **GI:** constipation ■ **Derm:** rash, photosensitivity ■ **Hemat:** neutropenia ■ **Neuro:** peripheral neuropathy ■ **Misc:** SEVERE BIRTH DEFECTS, hypersensitivity reactions, increased HIV viral load. | **PO (Adults ≥50 kg):** 100–300 mg/day initially; up to 400 mg/day has been used, depending on previous response. Every 3–6 mo attempts should be made to taper and discontinue in decrements of 50 mg q 2–4 wk. **PO (Adults <50 kg):** 100 mg/day initially; up to 400 mg/day has been used, depending on previous response. Every 3–6 mo attempts should be made to taper and discontinue in decrements of 50 mg q 2–4 wk. |

**Contraindicated in:** Pregnancy. Women with childbearing potential (unless specific conditions are met). Sexually mature men (unless specific conditions are met). Lactation. Hypersensitivity. **Use Cautiously in:** Children <12 yr (safety not established).

| | | | |
|---|---|---|---|
| **thiethylperazine** (Norzine, Torecan) **Therapeutic:** *antiemetics* **Pharmacologic:** *phenothiazines* Pregnancy Category UK | Management of nausea and vomiting. | **CNS:** NEUROLEPTIC MALIGNANT SYNDROME, sedation, cerebral vascular spasm, extrapyramidal reactions, headache, restlessness, tardive dyskinesia ■ **EENT:** dry eyes, blurred vision, lens opacities, tinnitus ■ **CV:** hypotension (following IM use), peripheral edema ■ **GI:** constipation, dry mouth, altered taste, anorexia, drug-induced hepatitis, ileus ■ **GU:** urinary retention ■ **Derm:** photosensitivity, pigment changes, rashes ■ **Endo:** galactorrhea ■ **Hemat:** AGRANULOCYTOSIS, leukopenia ■ **Metab:** hyperthermia ■ **Neuro:** trigeminal neuralgia ■ **Misc:** allergic reactions. | **PO, IM (Adults):** 10 mg 1–3 times daily. |

| Generic Name (Brand Name) [Canadian name] Classification(s) Schedule Pregnancy Category | Indications | Adverse Reactions and Side Effects | Route and Dosage |
|---|---|---|---|
| **Contraindicated in:** Hypersensitivity. Hypersensitivity to aspirin or tartrazine (tablets). Cross-sensitivity with other phenothiazines may occur. Narrow-angle glaucoma. Bone marrow depression. Severe liver or cardiovascular disease. Pregnancy. **Use Cautiously in:** Geriatric or debilitated patients (dosage reduction recommended). Diabetes mellitus. Respiratory disease. Prostatic hypertrophy. CNS tumors. Epilepsy. Intestinal obstruction. Children <12 yr or lactation (safety not established). | | | |
| **tocainide** (Tonocard) **Therapeutic:** *antiarrhythmics (class IB)* Pregnancy Category C | Life-threatening ventricular arrhythmias, including multifocal and unifocal premature ventricular contractions and ventricular tachycardia. | **CNS:** SEIZURES, changes in mood, drowsiness, hallucinations, headache, restlessness, tremor, coma, dizziness, mental depression, paranoia ■ **EENT:** blurred vision, thirst, tinnitus ■ **Resp:** PULMONARY FIBROSIS, pneumonia ■ **CV:** SINUS ARREST, CHF, arrhythmias, bradycardia, hypotension, palpitations, tachycardia, angina, conduction disturbances, hypertension ■ **GI:** anorexia, diarrhea, nausea, vomiting, abdominal discomfort, constipation, drug-induced hepatitis, dyspepsia, dysphagia ■ **GU:** urinary retention ■ **Derm:** alopecia, flushing, rashes, sweating ■ **Hemat:** AGRANULOCYTOSIS, leukopenia, neutropenia, thrombocytopenia ■ **MS:** arthralgia, myalgia ■ **Neuro:** myasthenia gravis, numbness. | **PO (Adults):** 400 mg q 8 hr initially; usual maintenance dose 1.2–1.8 g/day in divided doses q 8–12 hr. |
| **Contraindicated in:** Hypersensitivity. Advanced heart block. **Use Cautiously in:** CHF. Geriatric patients or hepatic or renal impairment (dosage reduction recommended). Pregnancy, lactation, or children (safety not established). | | | |
| **tolmetin** (Tolectin, Tolectin DS) [Novo-Tolmetin] **Therapeutic:** *antirheumatics, nonsteroidal anti-inflammatory agents* Pregnancy Category UK | Management of inflammatory disorders including Rheumatoid arthritis. Juvenile rheumatoid arthritis Osteoarthritis. | **CNS:** dizziness, headache, drowsiness, mental depression, sleep disturbances ■ **EENT:** tinnitus, visual disturbances ■ **CV:** edema, hypertension ■ **GI:** DRUG-INDUCED HEPATITIS, GI BLEEDING, diarrhea, discomfort, dyspepsia, nausea, vomiting, constipation, flatulence ■ **GU:** renal failure ■ **Derm:** rashes ■ **Hemat:** prolonged bleeding time ■ **MS:** muscle weakness ■ **Misc:** allergic reactions including anaphylaxis. | **PO (Adults):** 400 mg 3 times daily initially, followed by maintenance dose of 600–1800 mg/day in 3–4 divided doses (not to exceed 2000 mg/day). **PO (Children >2 yr):** 20 mg/kg/day in 3–4 divided doses initially, followed by maintenance dose of 15–30 mg/kg/day in 3–4 divided doses. |
| **Contraindicated in:** Hypersensitivity. Cross-sensitivity may exist with other NSAIDs, including aspirin. Active GI bleeding or ulcer disease. **Use Cautiously in:** Severe cardiovascular, renal, or hepatic disease. History of ulcer disease. Severe hepatic or renal impairment (dosage reduction recommended). Pregnancy and lactation (safety not established; avoid use during 2nd and 3rd trimesters). | | | |

| Generic Name (Brand Name) [Canadian name] Classification(s) Schedule Pregnancy Category | Indications | Adverse Reactions and Side Effects | Route and Dosage |
|---|---|---|---|
| **trifluoperazine** (Stelazine) {Apo-Trifluoperazine, Novo-Flurazine, PMS-Trifluoperazine, Solazine, Terfluzine} **Therapeutic:** *antipsychotics* **Pharmacologic:** *phenothiazines* Pregnancy Category C | Treatment of acute and chronic psychoses. Adjunct in the management of anxiety when safer agents are contraindicated. | **CNS:** NEUROLEPTIC MALIGNANT SYNDROME, extrapyramidal reactions, sedation, tardive dyskinesia ■ **EENT:** dry eyes, blurred vision, lens opacities ■ **CV:** hypotension, tachycardia ■ **GI:** constipation, anorexia, dry mouth, hepatitis, ileus ■ **GU:** urinary retention ■ **Derm:** photosensitivity, pigment changes, rashes ■ **Endo:** galactorrhea ■ **Hemat:** AGRANULOCYTOSIS, leukopenia ■ **Metab:** hyperthermia ■ **Misc:** allergic reactions. | **PO (Adults):** *Psychoses*—2–5 mg 1–2 times daily (up to 40 mg/day). *Anxiety*—1–2 mg bid (not to exceed 6 mg/day or treatment longer than 12 wk). **PO (Children 6–12 yr):** 1 mg once or twice daily (up to 15 mg/day). **IM (Adults):** 1–2 mg q 4–6 hr (up to 10 mg/day). **IM (Children):** 1 mg once or twice daily. |

**Contraindicated in:** Hypersensitivity. Cross-sensitivity with other phenothiazines may exist. Hypersensitivity to bisulfites (oral concentrate only). Narrow-angle glaucoma. Bone marrow depression. Severe liver or cardiovascular disease. **Use Cautiously in:** Geriatric or debilitated patients (dosage reduction recommended). Pregnancy or lactation (safety not established; may cause adverse effects in the newborn). Diabetes mellitus. Respiratory disease. Prostatic hypertrophy. CNS tumors. Epilepsy. Intestinal obstruction. Pregnancy or lactation (safety not established; may cause adverse effects in the newborn).

| | | | |
|---|---|---|---|
| **trihexyphenidyl** (Artane, Trihexane, Trihexy) {Apo-Trihex, PMS-Trihexyphenidyl} **Therapeutic:** *antiparkinson agents* **Pharmacologic:** *anticholinergics* Pregnancy Category C | Adjunct in the management of parkinsonian syndrome of many causes, including drug-induced parkinsonism. | **CNS:** dizziness, nervousness, confusion, drowsiness, headache, psychoses, weakness ■ **EENT:** blurred vision, mydriasis ■ **CV:** orthostatic hypotension, tachycardia ■ **GI:** dry mouth, nausea, constipation, vomiting ■ **GU:** urinary hesitancy, urinary retention ■ **Derm:** decreased sweating. | **PO (Adults):** 1–2 mg/day initially; increase by 2 mg q 3–5 days. Usual maintenance dose is 6–10 mg/day in 3 divided doses (up to 15 mg/day). Extended-release (Artane Sequels) preparations may be given q 12 hr after daily dose has been determined using conventional tablets or liquid. |

**Contraindicated in:** Hypersensitivity. Narrow-angle glaucoma. Acute hemorrhage. Tachycardia secondary to cardiac insufficiency. Thyrotoxicosis. Known alcohol intolerance (elixir only). **Use Cautiously in:** Geriatric and very young patients (increased risk of adverse reactions). Intestinal obstruction or infection. Prostatic hypertrophy. Chronic renal, hepatic, pulmonary, or cardiac disease. Pregnancy, lactation, or children (safety not established).

| Generic Name (Brand Name) [Canadian name] Classification(s) Schedule Pregnancy Category | Indications | Adverse Reactions and Side Effects | Route and Dosage |
|---|---|---|---|
| **trimethobenzamide** (Arrestin, Benzacot, Brogan, Stemetic, Tebamide, Tegamide, T-Gen, Ticon, Tigan, Tiject-20, Triban, Tribenzagan, Trimazide) *Therapeutic: antiemetics* *Pharmacologic: anticholinergics* Pregnancy Category C | Mild to moderate nausea and vomiting. | **CNS:** COMA, SEIZURES, drowsiness, depression, extrapyramidal reactions ■ **CV:** hypotension ■ **GI:** diarrhea, hepatitis ■ **Derm:** rashes ■ **Hemat:** blood dyscrasias ■ **Local:** pain, rectal irritation (suppositories), burning at IM injection site, redness at IM injection site, stinging at IM injection site. | **PO (Adults):** 250 mg 3–4 times daily. **PO (Children 15–45 kg):** 100–200 mg 3–4 times daily as needed or 15 mg/kg/day in 3–4 divided doses. **IM, Rect (Adults):** 200 mg 3–4 times daily as needed. **Rect (Children 15–45 kg):** 100–200 mg 3–4 times daily as needed. **Rect (Children <15 kg):** 100 mg 3–4 times daily as needed. |
| **Contraindicated in:** Hypersensitivity. Hypersensitivity to benzocaine (suppositories only). Premature or newborn infants. **Use Cautiously in:** Children who may have a viral illness (may increase risk of Reye's syndrome). Pregnancy or lactation (safety not established). | | | |
| **verteporfin** (Visudyne) *Therapeutic: none assigned* *Pharmacologic: photodynamic agents* Pregnancy Category C | Treatment of age-related macular degeneration in patients with predominantly classic subfoveal choroidal neovascularization. | **CNS:** headache, weakness ■ **EENT:** visual disturbances, cataracts, conjunctivitis/conjunctival injection, dry eyes, ocular itching, severe vision loss, subconjunctival/subretinal/vitreous hemorrhage ■ **Derm:** photosensitivity ■ **Local:** injection site reactions including extravasation and rashes ■ **MS:** back pain (during infusion) ■ **Misc:** fever, flu-like syndrome. | **IV (Adults):** 6 mg/m² infused over 10 min, followed by appropriate laser light delivery initiated 15 min after the start of the infusion. |
| **Contraindicated in:** Hypersensitivity. Porphyria. Exposure to direct sunlight. **Use Cautiously in:** Moderate/severe hepatic impairment. Pregnancy, lactation, or children (safety not established). | | | |
| **zafirlukast** (Accolate) *Therapeutic: antiasthmatics, bronchodilators* *Pharmacologic: leukotriene antagonists* Pregnancy Category B | Long-term control agent in the management of asthma. | **CNS:** headache, dizziness, weakness ■ **GI:** abdominal pain, diarrhea, drug-induced hepatitis (females), dyspepsia, nausea, vomiting ■ **MS:** arthralgia, back pain, myalgia ■ **Misc:** CHURG-STRAUSS SYNDROME, fever, infection (geriatric patients), pain. | **PO (Adults and Children ≥12 yr):** 20 mg twice daily. **PO (Children 7–11 yr):** 10 mg twice daily. |
| **Contraindicated in:** Hypersensitivity. Lactation. **Use Cautiously in:** Acute attacks of asthma. Patients >55 yr (increased risk of infection). Geriatric patients ≥65 yr or patients with hepatic impairment (may need lower doses). Pregnancy or children <7 yr (safety not established). | | | |

| Generic Name (Brand Name) [Canadian name] Classification(s) Schedule Pregnancy Category | Indications | Adverse Reactions and Side Effects | Route and Dosage |
|---|---|---|---|
| **zalcitabine** (ddC, dideoxycytidine, HIVID) *Therapeutic: antiretrovirals* *Pharmacologic: nucleoside reverse transcriptase inhibitors* Pregnancy Category C | Management of HIV infection in combination with other antiretrovirals. | **CNS:** confusion, dizziness, fatigue, headache, impaired concentration ■ **EENT:** pharyngitis ■ **CV:** CARDIOMYOPATHY, CHF, chest pain ■ **GI:** PANCREATITIS/HEPATOMEGALY/STEATOSIS, oral ulcers, abdominal pain, anorexia, diarrhea, dysphagia, esophageal ulcerations, increased liver enzymes, nausea, vomiting ■ **Derm:** dermatitis, pruritus, rash ■ **F and E:** LACTIC ACIDOSIS ■ **Hemat:** leukopenia, neutropenia ■ **MS:** arthralgia, myalgia ■ **Neuro:** peripheral neuropathy ■ **Misc:** hypersensitivity reactions, weight loss. | **PO (Adults):** 0.75 mg q 8 hr. *Renal/Hepatic Impairment* **PO (Adults):** *CCr 10–40 ml/min*—0.75 mg q 12 hr; *CCr <10 ml/min*—0.75 mg q 24 hr. |

**Contraindicated in:** Hypersensitivity. **Use Cautiously in:** Patients with renal impairment (dosage modification recommended if CCr is <40 ml/min). Patients with any signs of peripheral neuropathy (zalcitabine should be briefly discontinued and restarted at 50% of the previous dose if improvement occurs). Dosage modification may be required for other concurrent toxicities including hematologic toxicity and toxicity from other therapies. Pre-existing liver disease, including hepatitis B or history of alcohol abuse (increased risk of drug-induced liver function abnormalities). History of pancreatitis or hypertriglyceridemia. History of cardiomyopathy or CHF. Safe use in pregnancy, lactation, or children has not been established.

| | | | |
|---|---|---|---|
| **zileuton** (Zyflo) *Therapeutic: bronchodilators* *Pharmacologic: leukotriene antagonists* Pregnancy Category C | Long-term control agent in the management of asthma. | **CNS:** headache, dizziness, insomnia, malaise, nervousness, somnolence, weakness ■ **EENT:** conjunctivitis ■ **CV:** chest pain ■ **GI:** abdominal pain, constipation, dyspepsia, flatulence, increased liver enzymes, nausea, vomiting ■ **GU:** urinary tract infection, vaginitis ■ **Derm:** pruritus ■ **MS:** arthralgia, myalgia, neck pain ■ **Neuro:** hypertonia ■ **Misc:** fever, lymphadenopathy. | **PO (Adults and Children ≥12 yr):** 600 mg 4 times daily. |

**Contraindicated in:** Hypersensitivity. Active liver disease or transaminases ≥3 times upper limit of normal. **Use Cautiously in:** Acute attacks of asthma. History of liver disease or alcohol consumption. Pregnancy, lactation, or children <12 yr (safety not established).

| Generic Name (Brand Name) {Canadian name} Classification(s) Schedule Pregnancy Category | Indications | Adverse Reactions and Side Effects | Route and Dosage |
|---|---|---|---|
| **zinc sulfate** (Orazinc, Verazinc, Zinc 220, Zincate, Zinkaps) {PMS Egozinc} *Therapeutic: mineral and electrolyte replacements/ supplements* *Pharmacologic: trace metals* Pregnancy Category C (parenteral) | Replacement and supplementation therapy in patients who are at risk for zinc deficiency, including patients on long-term parenteral nutrition. **Unlabeled uses:** Management of impaired wound healing due to zinc deficiency. | **GI:** gastric irritation (oral use only), nausea, vomiting. | RDA = 15 mg. Doses expressed in mg of elemental zinc unless otherwise noted. Zinc sulfate contains 23% zinc. Deficiency **PO (Adults):** *Prevention of deficiency*—15–19 mg/day; *treatment of deficiency*—must be individualized; based on degree of deficiency. IV Nutritional Supplementation—Metabolically Stable Patients **IV (Adults):** 2.5–4 mg/day; up to 12 mg/day in patients with excessive losses. **IV (Infants and Children ≤5 yr):** 100 mcg/kg/day. **IV (Infants up to 3 kg):** 300 mcg/kg/day. |

**Contraindicated in:** Hypersensitivity or allergy to any components in formulation. Pregnancy or lactation (supplemental amounts >RDA for pregnant or lactating patients). Preparations containing benzyl alcohol should not be used in neonates. **Use Cautiously in:** Renal failure.

*See Appendix C for ophthalmic use.

# Natural/Herbal Products

The following monographs introduce some commonly used natural products. Because the amounts of active ingredients in these agents are not standardized or currently subject to FDA guidelines for medicines, *Davis's Drug Guide for Nurses*, although respectful of patients' right to choose from a variety of therapeutic options, does not endorse their routine use unless supervised by a knowledgeable health care professional. Users should take into account the possibility of adverse reactions and interactions and consider the relative lack of data supporting widespread use of these products. Doses are poorly standardized, and individuals are advised to read package labels carefully to ensure safe and efficacious use.

## arnica

### (ar-ni-cuh)

*OTHER NAME(S):*
leopard's bane, mountain tobacco, mountain snuff, wolf's bane

*CLASSIFICATION(S):*
*Therapeutic: anti-infectives*

## COMMON USES

■ Topical treatment of insect bites, bruises, acne, boils, sprains, muscle, and joint pain.

## ACTION

■ Polysaccharides in arnica may produce a slight anti-inflammatory and analgesic effect. Some antibacterial effects are seen, in addition to a counterirritant effect, which may aid in wound healing.

## PHARMACOKINETICS

**Absorption:** Systemic absorption may occur following topical application to broken skin.
**Distribution:** Unknown.
**Metabolism and Excretion:** Unknown.
**Half-life:** Unknown.

## CONTRAINDICATIONS AND PRECAUTIONS

**Contraindicated in:** ■ Not for oral use (except in highly diluted homeopathic preparations). Do not apply to open wounds ■ Arnica allergy ■ Avoid use on broken skin.

## ADVERSE REACTIONS AND SIDE EFFECTS*

■ **Derm:** edematous dermatitis with pustules (chronic treatment of damaged skin), eczema (prolonged use) ■ **Misc:** local allergic reactions.

## INTERACTIONS

**Natural Product-Drug:** ■ Alcohol-containing preparations may interact with **disulfuram** and **metronidazole** ■ Potential for reduced effectiveness of **antihypertensives** has been noted.

## ROUTE AND COMMONLY USED DOSES

■ **Topical (Adults):** *Topical*—rub or massage arnica tincture, cream, or gel onto injured area, only if skin isn't broken; *compress*—dilute 1 tablespoon of arnica tincture in 1/2 L water. Wet a gauze pad with solution and apply to affected area for 15 minutes. For use in poultices, dilute tincture 3 to 10 times with water.

## AVAILABILITY

■ *Cream, tincture, salve, ointment, gel, and oil^orc ■ Topical (preparations should contain not more than 20-25% arnica tincture or 15% arnica oil)^orc ■ Homeopathic preparations^orc.*

TIME/ACTION PROFILE

| | ONSET | PEAK | DURATION |
|---|---|---|---|
| Topical | unknown | unknown | unknown |

# NURSING IMPLICATIONS

## ASSESSMENT

❑ Inspect skin for breaks prior to application to ensure arnica is applied only to an intact surface. Note the size, character, and location of affected area prior to application of arnica.

❑ After application, assess the affected area for signs of allergic response.

■ *Toxicity and Overdose:* ■ Systemic absorption may result in nausea, vomiting, organ damage, hypertension, cardiotoxicity, arrhythmias, muscular weakness, collapse, vertigo, renal dysfunction, coma, and death. If ingested orally, induce emesis and gastric lavage to remove undigested contents. Supportive care may be necessary. Do not take orally or apply to nonintact skin to avoid systemic absorption.

## POTENTIAL NURSING DIAGNOSES

■ Pain, acute (Indications).

## IMPLEMENTATION

❑ Clean skin with a nonalcohol containing cleanser prior to applying arnica. Apply topically to affected area, or site of injury ensuring skin is intact.

❑ Do not take orally or apply to an open wound because of potential for systemic absorption with toxicity.

❑ Avoid prolonged topical use because of potential for allergic hypersensitiviy reaction.

## PATIENT/FAMILY TEACHING

❑ Teach patients to inspect the affected area for breaks in the skin and not to apply arnica to any areas where the skin is broken.

❑ Warn patients that use on nonintact skin and oral ingestion may cause life-threatening toxicity.

❑ Inform patients that although the German Commission E has found this herbal supplement to be an effective anti-inflammatory, analgesic, and antibacterial agent, FDA has classified arnica as an **unsafe herb.**

❑ Advise patients that arnica should only be used for short period of time in the treatment of minor aches and pains associated with local muscle, joint, or skin pain. Prolonged use may cause allergic/hypersensitivity reactions to develop.

❑ Instruct patients taking antihypertensive agents to avoid concurrent use of arnica.

## EVALUATION

**Effectiveness of therapy can be demonstrated by:** ■ Relief of, or improvement in, minor aches and pains associated with muscle or joint overuse, or sprains and/or local skin irritation from insect bites, bruises, boils, or acne.

---

# black cohosh
## (blak**coe**-hosh)

### OTHER NAME(S):
baneberry, black snakeroot, bugbane, rattle root, rattleweed, squawroot

### CLASSIFICATION(S):
**Therapeutic:** *none assigned*

Do not confuse black cohosh with blue or white cohosh.

---

## COMMON USES

■ Management of menopausal symptoms ■ Premenstrual discomfort ■ Dysmenorrhea.

## ACTION

■ Therapeutic effects are produced by glycosides isolated from the fresh or dried rhizome with attached roots ■ Mechanism of action is unclear. **Therapeutic Effects:** ■ May decrease symptoms of menopause, including hot flashes, sweating, sleep disturbance, and anxiety. Has no effect on vaginal epithelium. Black cohosh may be safe in women with a history of breast and other estrogen-sensitive cancers, but more study is needed.

## PHARMACOKINETICS

**Absorption:** Unknown.

**Distribution:** Unknown.

**Metabolism and Excretion:** Unknown.

**Half-life:** Unknown.

## CONTRAINDICATIONS AND PRECAUTIONS

**Contraindicated in:** ■ Pregnancy and lactation.

---

*CAPITALS indicates life-threatening; <u>underlines</u> indicate most frequent.

**Use Cautiously in:** ■ Not studied in combination with hormonal therapies ■ Not studied in patients with hormone-dependent cancers (e.g., breast, endometrial, ovarian cancer) ■ Longer than 6 mo use ■ Alcohol containing preparations should be used cautiously in patients with known intolerance or liver disease.

## ADVERSE REACTIONS AND SIDE EFFECTS*

■ **Neuro:** SEIZURES (in combination with evening primrose and chasteberry) ■ **GI:** GI upset.

## INTERACTIONS

**Natural Product-Drug:** ■ Unknown effects when combined with hormone replacement therapy and **antiestrogens** (e.g., **tamoxifen**) ■ **Alcohol** -containing preparations may interact with **disulfuram** and **metronidazole** ■ May precipitate hypotension when used in combination with **antihypertensives**.

## ROUTE AND COMMONLY USED DOSES

■ **PO (Adults):** *Tablets (Remifemin®)*—20 mg bid. *Liquid extract*—0.3–2.0 ml bid-tid. *Tincture*—2–4 ml bid–tid. *Dried rhizome*—0.3–2 g tid. Do not use for more than 6 mo.

## AVAILABILITY

■ *Alone or in combination with other herbal medicinals^{OTC}* ■ *Tablets^{OTC} (Remifemin® 20 mg [best studied black cohosh product])* ■ *Liquid extract^{OTC} (1:1 in 90% alcohol)* ■ *Tincture^{OTC} (1:10 in 60% alcohol)* ■ *Dried rhizome.*

TIME/ACTION PROFILE

|    | ONSET | PEAK | DURATION |
|----|-------|------|----------|
| PO | unknown | unknown | unknown |

# NURSING IMPLICATIONS

## ASSESSMENT

❏ Assess frequency and severity of menopausal symptoms.
❏ Monitor blood pressure for patients on antihypertensive drugs because it may increase effects of drugs and cause hypotension.
❏ Assess for nausea and vomiting.
❏ Assess for history of seizures, liver disease, and alcohol intake

❏ Assess patients with irregular periods for pregnancy prior to taking this drug because large doses of black cohosh may induce a miscarriage.

## POTENTIAL NURSING DIAGNOSES

■ Sleep deprivation (Indications).
■ Knowledge, deficient, related to medication regimen.

## IMPLEMENTATION

❏ Administration with food may help to minimize nausea.

## PATIENT/FAMILY TEACHING

❏ Instruct patient that this herbal supplement should not be taken if pregnant because it may induce a miscarriage.
❏ Tell patient that if she suspects she is pregnant to stop taking the medication and to contact her healthcare provider.
❏ May potentiate antihypertensive drugs with consequent hypotension. Warn patients on antihypertensive drugs not to take this herbal supplement without consulting their health care provider.
❏ Patients with seizures, liver dysfunction, excessive alcohol intake, cancer, or other medical problems should be advised to consult their health care provider prior to initiating self-therapy with this herb.
❏ If nausea becomes a problem, advise patients to take herbal supplement on a full stomach.
❏ Advise patient that this herbal supplement should not be taken with other estrogen replacements without seeking the advice of her health care provider.
❏ Emphasize the importance of continued medical supervision for Pap smears, mammograms, pelvic examinations, and blood pressure monitoring at the intervals indicated by health care provider.

## EVALUATION

**Clinical response to therapy can be evaluated by:** ■ Resolution of menopausal vasomotor symptoms.

## chondroitin

(konn-**droy**-tinn)

*OTHER NAME(S):*
chondroitin sulfate

*CLASSIFICATION(S):*
*Therapeutic: nonopioid analgesics*

### COMMON USES
- Osteoarthritis.

### ACTION
- May serve as a building block of articular cartilage

### PHARMACOKINETICS
**Absorption:** Unknown.
**Distribution:** Unknown.
**Metabolism and Excretion:** Unknown.
**Half-life:** Unknown.

### CONTRAINDICATIONS AND PRECAUTIONS
**Contraindicated in:** ■ Pregnancy and lactation.

### ADVERSE REACTIONS AND SIDE EFFECTS*
■ **GI:** heartburn, nausea, diarrhea ■ **Hemat:** bleeding (antiplatelet effect) ■ **Misc:** allergic reactions.

### INTERACTIONS
**Natural Product-Drug:** ■ Use of chondroitin with **anticoagulant** and **antiplatelet** drugs, **thrombolytics**, **NSAIDs**, some **cephalosporins**, **plicamycin** and **valproates** may increase risk of bleeding.
**Natural Product-Natural Product:** ■ Herbs with anticoagulant or antiplatelet properties may increase bleeding risk when combined with chondroitin, including: **anise**, **arnica**, **chamomile**, **clove**, **dong quai**, **fenugreek**, **feverfew**, **ginger**, **ginkgo**, **Panax ginseng**, **licorice**, and others.

### ROUTE AND COMMONLY USED DOSES
■ **PO (Adults):** 200–400 mg 2–3 times daily.

### AVAILABILITY
■ *Tablets^{OTC}* ■ *Capsules^{OTC}*.

TIME/ACTION PROFILE

| | ONSET | PEAK | DURATION |
|---|---|---|---|
| PO | unknown | unknown | unknown |

## NURSING IMPLICATIONS

### ASSESSMENT
- ❑ Evaluate drug profile before starting therapy with this herbal supplement. If the patient is taking anticoagulants or antiplatelet drugs, avoid use of this herb.
- ❑ Monitor pain (type, location, and intensity) and range of motion on an ongoing basis as an indicator of drug efficacy.
- ❑ Evaluate gastric discomfort and instruct patient to seek out the advice of a health care provider if persistent gastric discomfort occurs.
- ❑ Assess for signs of bleeding and discontinue herbal supplement promptly and seek out healthcare provider for follow up.

### POTENTIAL NURSING DIAGNOSES
- Pain, acute (Indications).
- Mobility, impaired physical (Indications).
- Knowledge, deficient, related to medication regimen (Patient/Family Teaching)

### IMPLEMENTATION
- ❑ Take with food.

### PATIENT/FAMILY TEACHING
- ❑ Advise patients that this herbal supplement is usually taken with glucosamine.
- ❑ Caution patients who take aspirin or NSAIDs or other nonprescription medications not to take this herbal supplement without conferring with their health care provider.
- ❑ Warn women taking this herbal supplement to stop it if they suspect they are pregnant, and not to use it if they are breastfeeding.
- ❑ Instruct patients that this medication works by building up cartilage and that this requires that the medication be taken consistently over a period of time. It is not recommended as a supplemental pain medication.

### EVALUATION
**Clinical response to therapy can be evaluated by:** ■ Improvement in pain and range of

*CAPITALS indicates life-threatening; <u>underlines</u> indicate most frequent.

motion ■ Reduced need for supplemental or breakthrough pain medication.

*Crataegus Species*, see **HAWTHORN.**

## dong quai
### (donkwi)

**OTHER NAME(S):**
Angelica sinensis, Chinese Angelica, Dang Gui, Danggui, Dong Qua, Ligustilides, Phytoestrogen, Tang Kuei, Tan Kue Bai Zhi

**CLASSIFICATION(S):**
*Therapeutic: none assigned*

### COMMON USES
■ Menstrual cramps, menstrual irregularity, menopausal symptoms.

### ACTION
■ May have vasodilating and antispasmodic properties ■ Binds to estrogen receptors

### PHARMACOKINETICS
**Absorption:** Unknown.
**Distribution:** Unknown.
**Metabolism and Excretion:** Unknown.
**Half-life:** Unknown.

### CONTRAINDICATIONS AND PRECAUTIONS
**Contraindicated in:** ■ Pregnancy and lactation.

### ADVERSE REACTIONS AND SIDE EFFECTS*
■ **Derm:** photosensitivity ■ **Misc:** Some constituents are carcinogenic and mutagenic.

### INTERACTIONS
**Natural Product-Drug:** ■ **Alcohol**-containing preparations may interact with **disulfuram** and **metronidazole** ■ Use of dong quai with **anticoagulant** and **antiplatelet** drugs, **thrombolytics, NSAIDs,** some **cephalosporins, plicamycin,** and **valproates** may increase risk of bleeding.

### ROUTE AND COMMONLY USED DOSES
■ **PO (Adults):** *Bulk herb*—3–4 g per day in divided doses with meals; *extract*—1 ml (20–40 drops) three times daily.

### AVAILABILITY
■ *Bulk herb^(OTC)* ■ *Extract^(OTC).*

TIME/ACTION PROFILE

|    | ONSET | PEAK | DURATION |
|----|-------|------|----------|
| PO | unknown | unknown | unknown |

## NURSING IMPLICATIONS

### ASSESSMENT
❑ Assess pain and menstrual patterns prior to and following menstrual cycle to determine effectiveness of this herbal supplement.
❑ Assess for pregnancy prior to recommending use of the herbal supplement and warn women not to take this herb if pregnancy is suspected.
❑ Assess medication profile including prescription and over-the-counter use of products such as aspirin and ibuprofen-based products to treat menstrual pain.

### POTENTIAL NURSING DIAGNOSES
■ Pain, acute (Indications).
■ Knowledge, deficient, related to medication regimen (Patient/Family Teaching).

### IMPLEMENTATION
❑ Take with meals.

### PATIENT/FAMILY TEACHING
❑ Warn patients not to take this medication if pregnant or breastfeeding.
❑ Inform patients to avoid use of aspirin or other NSAIDs concurrently because of the risk of bleeding.
❑ Notify patients that there are no studies supporting the use of this herbal supplement for treatment of menopausal symptoms.
❑ Tell patients to consult their health care provider if taking prescription medications before taking Dong Quai.
❑ Discontinue the herbal supplement if diarrhea or excessive bleeding occurs and contact a health care provider if symptoms do not resolve.

❏ Instruct patients that photosensitivity may occur and to wear sun screen and protective clothing if sun exposure is anticipated.

## EVALUATION

**Clinical response to therapy can be evaluated by:** ■ Reduction in menstrual pain and cramping and regular periods with normal flow.

---

## echinacea (Echinacea Purpurea)

(ek-i-**nay**-sha)

### OTHER NAME(S):

American coneflower, black sampson, black susans, purple coneflower, red sunflower, rudbeckia, sampson root

### CLASSIFICATION(S):

*Therapeutic: anti-infectives, antipyretics*

---

## COMMON USES

■ Bacterial and viral infections ■ Prevention and treatment of colds, coughs, flu, and bronchitis ■ Fevers ■ Wounds and burns ■ Inflammation of the mouth and pharynx ■ Urinary tract infections.

## ACTION

■ Medicinal parts derived from the roots, leaves, or whole plant of perennial herb (Echinacea) ■ *Echinacea purpurea herba* has been reported to promote wound healing, which may be due to an increase in white blood cells, spleen cells, and increased activity of granulocytes, as well as an increase in helper T cells and cytokines ■ *E. purpurea radix* has been shown to have antibacterial, antiviral, anti-inflammatory, and immune-modulating effects. **Therapeutic Effects:** ■ Resolution respiratory and urinary tract infections ■ Decreased duration and intensity of common cold ■ Improved wound healing ■ Stimulates phagocytosis; inhibits action of hyaluronidase (secreted by bacteria), which helps bacteria gain access to healthy cells ■ Externally, has antifungal and bacteriostatic properties.

## PHARMACOKINETICS

**Absorption:** Unknown.
**Distribution:** Unknown.
**Metabolism and Excretion:** Unknown.
**Half-life:** Unknown.

## CONTRAINDICATIONS AND PRECAUTIONS

**Contraindicated in:** ■ Multiple sclerosis, leukosis, collagenoses, AIDS, tuberculosis, autoimmune diseases ■ Hypersensitivity and crosssensitivity in patients allergic to plants in Asteraceae/Compositae plant family (daisies, chrysanthemums, marigolds, etc.) ■ Pregnancy and lactation.

**Use Cautiously in:** ■ Diabetes ■ Tinctures should be used cautiously in alcoholics or patients with liver disease ■ Do not take longer than 8 wk—may suppress immune function.

## ADVERSE REACTIONS AND SIDE EFFECTS*

■ **CNS:** dizziness, fatigue, headache, somnolence ■ **EENT:** tingling sensation on tongue, sore throat ■ **GI:** nausea, vomiting ■ **Derm:** allergic reaction ■ **Misc:** fever.

## INTERACTIONS

**Natural Product-Drug:** ■ May possibly interfere with **immunosuppressants** because of its immunostimulant activity ■ **Anabolic steroids**, **methotrexate**, or **ketoconazole** may interact with echinacea.

## ROUTE AND COMMONLY USED DOSES

■ **PO (Adults):** *Fluid extract*—1–2 ml tid; solid form (6.5:1)—300 mg tid. Should not be used for more than 8 wk at a time. *Tea*—1/2 tsp comminuted drug, steeped and strained after 10 min, 1 cup several times daily. *Echinacea purpuren herb juice*—6-9 ml/day.
■ **Topical (Adults):** *Ointment, lotion, tincture used externally*—1.5–7.5 ml tincture, 2–5 g dried root.

## AVAILABILITY

■ *Capsules^{OTC}:* 300 mg ■ *Dried Root^{OTC}:* The dried root can be steeped and strained in boiling water and taken as a tea ■ *Liquid extract^{OTC}:* 1:1 in 45% alcohol ■ *Tincture^{OTC}:* 1:5 in 45% alcohol ■ *Blended teas^{OTC}* ■ *Echinacea purpuren herb juice^{OTC}*.

---

*CAPITALS indicates life-threatening; <u>underlines</u> indicate most frequent.

TIME/ACTION PROFILE

|    | ONSET | PEAK | DURATION |
|----|-------|------|----------|
| PO | unknown | unknown | unknown |

## NURSING IMPLICATIONS

### ASSESSMENT

❑ Assess wound for size, appearance, and drainage prior to the start of and periodically during therapy.

❑ Assess frequency of common mild illnesses (such as a cold) in response to use of this herb.

### POTENTIAL NURSING DIAGNOSES

■ Skin integrity, impaired (Indications).

■ Knowledge, deficient, related to medication regimen.

### IMPLEMENTATION

❑ Tinctures may contain significant concentrations of alcohol and may not be suitable for children, alcoholics, patients with liver disease, or those taking disulfiram, metronidazole, some cephalosporins, or sulfonylurea oral antidiabetic agents.

❑ Prolonged use of this agent may cause overstimulation of the immune system, and use beyond 8 wk is not recommended. Therapy of 10–14 days is usually considered sufficient.

❑ May be taken without regard to food.

### PATIENT/FAMILY TEACHING

❑ Herb is more effective for treatment than prevention of colds. Take at first sign of symptoms.

❑ Advise patient to seek immediate treatment for an illness that does not improve after taking this herb.

❑ Instruct patient that the usual course of therapy is 10–14 days and 8 wk is the maximum.

❑ Inform patient that use of this herb is not recommended in severe illnesses (e.g., AIDS, tuberculosis) or autoimmune diseases (e.g., multiple sclerosis, collagen diseases, etc.).

❑ Caution patient that prolonged use of this herb may result in overstimulation of the immune system, possibly with subsequent immunosuppression.

❑ Warn pregnant or breastfeeding women not to use this herb.

❑ Instruct patient to consult health care professional before taking any prescription or OTC medications concurrently with echinacea.

❑ Keep tincture in a dark bottle away from sunlight. Should be taken several times a day.

❑ Store herb in airtight container away from sunlight.

### EVALUATION

**Clinical response to therapy can be evaluated by:** ■ Improved wound healing ■ Infrequent common illnesses ■ Illnesses of shorter duration and less severity.

## feverfew
## (fee-vurr fyoo)

### OTHER NAME(S):
Altamisa, Bachelor's Button, Chrysanthemum parethenium, Featerfoiul, Featherfew, Featherfoil, Flirtwort Midsummer Daisy, Pyrethrum parthenium, Santa Maria, Tanaceti parthenii, Wild chamomile, Wild quinine

### CLASSIFICATION(S):
**Therapeutic:** vascular headache suppressants

### COMMON USES

■ **PO:** Migraine headache prophylaxis.

### ACTION

■ The sesquiterpene lactone, parthenolide, may provide feverfew's migraine prophylaxis effects
■ Feverfew may also have antiplatelet and vasodilatory effects and block prostaglandin synthesis

### PHARMACOKINETICS

**Absorption:** Unknown.

**Distribution:** Unknown.

**Metabolism and Excretion:** Unknown.

**Half-life:** Unknown.

## CONTRAINDICATIONS AND PRECAUTIONS

**Contraindicated in:** ■ Pregnancy and lactation ■ Feverfew hypersensitivity or allergy to Asteraceae/Compositae family plants, including ragweed, chrysanthemums, daisies, and marigolds ■ Ineffective for treating or aborting migraines. **Use Cautiously in:** ■ Use >4 months (safety and efficacy not established).

## ADVERSE REACTIONS AND SIDE EFFECTS*

■ **CNS:** "Post-Feverfew Syndrome" (anxiety, headache, insomnia, muscle aches) ■ **CV:** *with long-term use*—tachycardia ■ **GI:** nausea, vomiting, diarrhea, mouth ulceration, and soreness ■ **Derm:** contact dermatitis.

## INTERACTIONS

**Natural Product-Drug:** ■ Use of feverfew with **anticoagulant** and **antiplatelet** drugs, **thrombolytics, NSAIDs,** some **cephalosporins, plicamycin** and **valproates** may increase risk of bleeding ■ Concomitant use with **NSAIDs** may also reduce feverfew effectiveness. **Natural Product-Natural Product:** ■ Use with **anise, arnica, chamomile, clove, dong quai, fenugreek, garlic, ginger, gingko, licorice** and **Panax ginseng** may increase anticoagulant potential of feverfew.

## ROUTE AND COMMONLY USED DOSES

■ **PO (Adults):** 50–100 mg feverfew extract daily (standardized to 0.2–0.35% parthenolide) or 50–125 mg freeze-dried leaf daily with or after food.

## AVAILABILITY

■ *Feverfew extract^OTC:* standardized to 0.2-0.35% parthenolide ■ *Freash leaf^OTC* ■ *Freeze-dried leaf^OTC.*

TIME/ACTION PROFILE

| | ONSET | PEAK | DURATION |
|---|---|---|---|
| PO | 2–4 mo | unknown | unknown |

# NURSING IMPLICATIONS

## ASSESSMENT

❏ Monitor frequency, intensity, and duration of migraine headaches prior to and during ongoing therapy.

❏ Assess for mouth ulcers or skin ulcerations during therapy.

## POTENTIAL NURSING DIAGNOSES

■ Pain, acute (Indications).

■ Knowledge, deficient, related to medication regimen (Patient/Family Teaching).

## IMPLEMENTATION

❏ Take with food or on a full stomach.

## PATIENT/FAMILY TEACHING

❏ Instruct patients to take this medication on a consistent basis to prevent migraine headaches. This herbal supplement is not for treatment of migraines.

❏ Warn patients about mouth ulcers and sores and that if this occurs to seek the advice of a healthcare professional. Encourage proper oral hygiene.

❏ Advise patients not to abruptly stop this product because of the possibility of post-feverfew syndrome. Tell patients that anxiety, headache, insomnia, and muscle aches may indicate withdrawal. Feverfew should be gradually tapered.

❏ Review dietary and medication profile of patient to identify potential interactions. Instruct patient about other herbs that may interact with feverfew.

❏ Counsel patients on anticoagulants not to take feverfew except as directed by their healthcare provider

❏ Advise patients to avoid using NSAIDs as this may reduce the effectiveness of feverfew.

❏ Instruct patients to look for signs of bleeding such as unusual bruising or inability to clot after a cut and to seek the advice of a healthcare professional if this occurs.

❏ Inform patients that feverfew should reduce the number of migraines and severity of symptoms but that duration of the migraine may not be affected.

## EVALUATION

**Clinical response to therapy can be evaluated by:** ■ Reduction in the frequency and severity of migraine headaches.

*CAPITALS indicates life-threatening; underlines indicate most frequent.

## garlic
(gar-lik)

*OTHER NAME(S):*
Alli sativa bulbus, Allium sativum

*CLASSIFICATION(S):*
*Therapeutic:* lipid-lowering agents

### COMMON USES

■ **PO:** Hypertension, hyperlipidemia, cardiovascular disease prevention ■ **Topical:** Dermal fungal infections.

### ACTION

■ May have HMG-CoA inhibitor properties in lowering cholesterol, but less effectively than statin drugs; vasodilatory and antiplatelet properties

### PHARMACOKINETICS

**Absorption:** Garlic oil is well absorbed.
**Distribution:** Unknown.
**Metabolism and Excretion:** Kidney and lungs.
**Half-life:** Unknown.

### CONTRAINDICATIONS AND PRECAUTIONS

**Contraindicated in:** ■ Bleeding disorders. Discontinue use 1-2 weeks prior to surgery. **Use Cautiously in:** ■ Diabetes, gastrointestinal infection or inflammation.

### ADVERSE REACTIONS AND SIDE EFFECTS*

■ **CNS:** dizziness ■ **GI:** Irritation of the mouth, esophagus, and stomach, nausea, vomiting ■ **Derm:** Contact dermatitis and other allergic reactions (asthma, rash, anaphylaxis [rare]), Diaphoresis ■ **Hemat:** Chronic use or excessive dosage may lead to decreased hemoglobin production and lysis of RBCs.

### INTERACTIONS

**Natural Product-Drug:** ■ Use of garlic with **anticoagulants, antiplatelet agents,** and **thrombolytic agents** may increase risk of bleeding.
**Natural Product-Natural Product:** ■ Herbs with anticoagulant or antiplatelet properties may increase bleeding risk when combined with garlic, including: **angelica, anise, asafoetida, bogbean, boldo, capsicum, celery, chamomile, clove, danshen, dong quai, fenugreek, feverfew, ginger, ginkgo, Panax ginseng, horse chestnut, horseradish, licorice, meadowsweet, prickly ash, onion, papain, passionflower, poplar, quassia, red clover, turmeric, wild carrot, wild lettuce, willow,** and others.

### ROUTE AND COMMONLY USED DOSES

■ **PO (Adults):** 200–400 mg tid of standardized garlic powder extract with 1.3% allin. *Fresh garlic*—1–7 cloves per day.

### AVAILABILITY

■ *Capsules^{OTC}* ■ *Tablets^{OTC}* ■ *Fresh garlic^{OTC}*.

TIME/ACTION PROFILE

|    | ONSET | PEAK | DURATION |
|----|-------|------|----------|
| PO | 4–25 wk | unknown | unknown |

## NURSING IMPLICATIONS

### ASSESSMENT

❑ Elicit from patients their usual dietary intake especially in regard to fat consumption.
❑ Assess patient's reason for using this herbal remedy and knowledge about hyperlipidemia.
❑ Ascertain the amount of garlic the patient consumes on a regular basis.

### POTENTIAL NURSING DIAGNOSES

■ Knowledge, deficient, related to medication regimen (Patient/Family Teaching).
■ Noncompliance (Patient/Family Teaching).

### IMPLEMENTATION

❑ Take orally as a tea, capsule, or tablet.
❑ Do not exceed recommended dosage.

### PATIENT/FAMILY TEACHING

❑ Instruct patients about the need to follow a healthy diet (low in fat and high in vegetables and fruits) in conjunction with garlic. Other lipid-reducing strategies, such as exercise and smoking cessation, should also be employed.
❑ Inform patients that there are other more effective agents for lipid reduction available.

❑ Emphasize the need for follow up exams with a healthcare provider to assess effectiveness of the regimen.

❑ Warn patients about the potential for bleeding and not to take this herbal remedy without notifying their healthcare provider if they are on other medications. Instruct patients undergoing elective surgery to stop using garlic 2 weeks prior to surgery and to notify the surgeon that they are taking garlic in the event of emergent surgery.

❑ Notify patients that allergies may occur and to discontinue use if symptoms develop.

## EVALUATION

**Clinical response to therapy can be evaluated by:** ■ Normalization of lipid profile ■ Prevention of cardiac disease.

## ginger (Zingiber Officinale)
(jin-jer)

*OTHER NAME(S):*

Calicut, cochin, gengibre, ginger root, Ingwerwurzel, ingwer, Jamaica ginger, jenjibre, zenzero, zingiber

*CLASSIFICATION(S):*
*Therapeutic: antiemetics*

## COMMON USES

■ Prevention and treatment of nausea and vomiting associated with motion sickness, loss of appetite, pregnancy, surgery, and chemotherapy ■ Prevention of postoperative nausea and vomiting ■ May be used for dyspepsia, flatulence, relief of joint pain in rheumatoid arthritis, cramping, and diarrhea ■ Tonic (toning/strengthening agent) in gout, gas, respiratory infections, anti-inflammatory, stimulant (tones the gut, increases saliva and gastric juices, acts as anticoagulant, decreases blood cholesterol).

## ACTION

■ Antiemetic effect due to increasing GI motility and transport; may act on serotonin receptors ■ Shown to be hypoglycemic, hypotensive or hypertensive, and positive inotropic agent ■ Inhibits prostaglandins and platelets, lowers cholesterol, and improves appetite and digestion.

**Therapeutic Effects:** ■ Decreased nausea and vomiting due to motion sickness, surgery, and chemotherapy ■ Decreased joint pain and improvement of joint motion in rheumatoid arthritis ■ Antioxidant.

## PHARMACOKINETICS

**Absorption:** Unknown.
**Distribution:** Unknown.
**Metabolism and Excretion:** Unknown.
**Half-life:** Unknown.

## CONTRAINDICATIONS AND PRECAUTIONS

**Contraindicated in:** ■ Pregnancy and lactation (if using large amounts) ■ Gallstones.
**Use Cautiously in:** ■ Patients with increased risk of bleeding ■ Diabetes ■ Anticoagulant therapy ■ Cardiovascular disease.

## ADVERSE REACTIONS AND SIDE EFFECTS*

■ **GI:** minor heartburn ■ **Derm:** dermatitis.

## INTERACTIONS

**Natural Product-Drug:** ■ May increase risk of bleeding when used with **anticoagulants, antiplatelet agents**, and **thrombolytic agents**.
**Natural Product-Natural Product:** ■ May theoretically increase risk of bleeding when used with other **herbs** that have anticoagulant or antiplatelet activities.

## ROUTE AND COMMONLY USED DOSES

■ **PO (Adults):** *Motion sickness*—1000 mg ginger taken 30 min–4 hr before travel. *Surgery*—1000 mg ginger taken 1 hr before induction or anesthesia. *Chemotherapy-induced nausea*—2–4 g/day. Up to 2 g freshly powdered drug has been used as an antiemetic (not to exceed 4 g/day). Whole root rhizome*—0.25–1 g for other illnesses. Tea*—pour 150 ml boiling water over 0.5–1 g of ginger and strain after 5 min. *Tincture*—0.25-3 ml.

## AVAILABILITY

■ *Alone or in combination with other herbal medicinals^{OTC}* ■ *Dried powdered root^{OTC}* ■ *Syrup^{OTC}* ■ *Tincture^{OTC}* ■ *Tablets^{OTC}* ■ *Capsules (≥550 mg)^{OTC}* ■ *Spice^{OTC}* ■ *Tea^{OTC}*.

*CAPITALS indicates life-threatening; underlines indicate most frequent.

TIME/ACTION PROFILE

|  | ONSET | PEAK | DURATION |
|---|---|---|---|
| PO | unknown | unknown | unknown |

## NURSING IMPLICATIONS

### ASSESSMENT

- Assess patient for nausea, vomiting, abdominal distention, and pain prior to and after administration of the herb when used as an antiemetic agent.
- Assess pain, swelling, and range of motion in affected joints prior to and after administration when used in the treatment of arthritis.
- Assess patient for epigastric pain prior to and after administration when used as a gastroprotective agent.
- Monitor blood pressure in patients with cardiovascular disease including hypertension.

### POTENTIAL NURSING DIAGNOSES

- Pain, acute (Indications).
- Knowledge, deficient, related to medication regimen (Patient/Family Teaching).

### IMPLEMENTATION

- Administer ginger prior to situations where nausea or vomiting is anticipated (e.g., motion sickness).
- Dosage form and strengths vary with each disease state. Ensure that proper formulation and dosage are administered for the indicated use.
- Give to increase peristalsis.

### PATIENT/FAMILY TEACHING

- Instruct patients receiving anticoagulants not to take this herb without the advice of health care professional (increased risk of bleeding).
- Tell patient to stop the herb immediately if palpitations occur and contact health care professional.
- Advise patient to observe for easy bruising or other signs of bleeding. If they occur, stop the herb immediately and contact health care professional.
- Warn patients with a history of gallbladder disease to use this herb only under the supervision of health care professional.
- Instruct patient to consult health care professional before taking any prescription or OTC medications concurrently with ginger.
- Herb is meant to be used as a tonic, not for long-term use.

### EVALUATION

**Clinical response to therapy can be evaluated by:** ▪ Prevention of nausea and vomiting ▪ Relief of epigastric pain ▪ Improved joint mobility and relief of pain.

## ginkgo

## (ging-ko)

### OTHER NAME(S):

Bai guo ye, fossil tree, ginkgo folium, Japanese silver apricot, kew tree, maidenhair-tree, yinhsing

### CLASSIFICATION(S):

**Therapeutic:** antiplatelet agents, central nervous system stimulants

### COMMON USES

▪ Symptomatic relief of organic brain dysfunction (dementia syndromes, short-term memory deficits, inability to concentrate, depression) ▪ Intermittent claudication ▪ Vertigo and tinnitus of vascular origin ▪ Improvement of peripheral circulation ▪ Sexual dysfunction.

### ACTION

▪ Improves tolerance to hypoxia, especially in cerebral tissue ▪ Inhibits development of cerebral edema and accelerates its regression ▪ Improves memory, blood flow (microcirculation), compensation of disequilibrium, and rheological properties of blood ▪ Inactivates toxic oxygen radicals ▪ Antagonizes platelet-activating factor ▪ Interferes with bronchoconstriction and phagocyte chemotaxis. **Therapeutic Effects:** ▪ Symptomatic relief of dementia syndromes ▪ Inhibits arterial spasm, decreases capillary fragility and blood viscosity ▪ Improves venous tone, relaxes vascular smooth muscle.

### PHARMACOKINETICS

**Absorption:** 70–100% absorption.
**Distribution:** Unknown.
**Metabolism and Excretion:** Unknown.

**Half-life:** Unknown.

## CONTRAINDICATIONS AND PRECAUTIONS

**Contraindicated in:** ■ Hypersensitivity ■ Pregnancy and lactation.
**Use Cautiously in:** ■ Bleeding disorders ■ Children ■ Diabetes ■ Epilepsy.

## ADVERSE REACTIONS AND SIDE EFFECTS*

■ **CNS:** CEREBRAL BLEEDING, dizziness, headache, vertigo, seizure ■ **CV:** palpitations ■ **GI:** flatulence, stomach upset ■ **Derm:** allergic skin reaction ■ **Hemat:** bleeding ■ **Misc:** hypersensitivity reactions.

## INTERACTIONS

**Natural Product-Drug:** ■ Theoretically may potentiate effects of **anticoagulants, thrombolytics, antiplatelet agents,** and **MAO inhibitors** ■ May also increase the risk of bleeding with some **cephalosporins, valproic acid,** and **NSAIDs.**
**Natural Product-Natural Product:** ■ May increase risk of bleeding when used with other **herbs** with antiplatelet effects (including **angelica, arnica, chamomile, feverfew, garlic, ginger,** and **licorice**).

## ROUTE AND COMMONLY USED DOSES

### Organic Brain Syndromes

■ **PO (Adults):** 120–240 mg ginkgo leaf extract daily in 2 or 3 doses.

### Sexual Dysfunction

■ **PO (Adults):** 60 mg BID ginkgo leaf extract.

### Intermittent Claudication

■ **PO (Adults):** 120–240 mg ginkgo leaf extract daily in 2 or 3 doses.

### Vertigo and Tinnitus

■ **PO (Adults):** 120–160 mg ginkgo leaf extract daily in 2 or 3 doses.

## AVAILABILITY

■ *Ginkgo leaf extract (acetone/water):* 22–27% flavonoid glycosides, 5–7% terpene lactones, 2.6–3.2% bilobalide, <5 ppm of ginkgolic acids.

## TIME/ACTION PROFILE

| | ONSET | PEAK | DURATION |
|---|---|---|---|
| PO | unknown | unknown | unknown |

# NURSING IMPLICATIONS

## ASSESSMENT

❏ Exclude other treatable causes of dementia prior to instituting treatment with ginkgo.
❏ Assess cognitive function (memory, attention, reasoning, language, ability to perform simple tasks) periodically throughout therapy.
❏ Assess frequency, duration, and severity of muscle cramps (claudication) experienced by the patient prior to and periodically throughout therapy.
❏ Assess for headache and neurosystem changes (thromboembolism).

## POTENTIAL NURSING DIAGNOSES

■ Thought processes, disturbed (Indications).
■ Pain, acute (Indications).
■ Knowledge, deficient, related to medication regimen (Patient/Family Teaching).

## IMPLEMENTATION

❏ Start dose at 120 mg per day and increase as needed to minimize side effects.
❏ Administration for a minimum of 6–8 wk of 80 mg (tid) (not <6 wk) is required to determine response.
❏ May be administered without regard to food.
❏ Use of dried leaf preparations in the form of a tea is not recommended because of insufficient quantity of active ingredients.
❏ Take this herb at the same time daily.
❏ Keep this herb out of the reach of children as seizures may occur with increased doses of ginkgo seeds.

## PATIENT/FAMILY TEACHING

❏ Advise patient to observe for easy bruising and other signs of bleeding and report to health care professional if they occur.
❏ Caution patient to keep this herb out of the reach of children because ingestion has been associated with seizures.
❏ Warn patient to avoid handling the pulp or seed coats because of the risk of contact

*CAPITALS indicates life-threatening; <u>underlines</u> indicate most frequent.

dermatitis. Wash skin under free-flowing water promptly if contact does occur.

❑ Instruct patient not to exceed recommended doses because large doses may result in toxicity (restlessness, diarrhea, nausea and vomiting, headache).

❑ Notify patients receiving anticoagulant or antiplatelet therapy not to take this medication without approval of health care professional and frequent monitoring.

❑ Instruct patient to consult health care professional before taking any prescription or OTC medications concurrently with ginkgo.

## EVALUATION

**Clinical response to therapy can be evaluated by:** ■ Improvement in walking distances pain-free ■ Improvement in tinnitus and vertigo ■ Improvement in short-term memory, attention span, and ability to perform simple tasks ■ Improvement in sexual function.

---

## ginseng (Panax Ginseng)

### (jin-seng)

**OTHER NAME(S):**
American ginseng, Chinese ginseng, Korean ginseng

**CLASSIFICATION(S):**
**Therapeutic:** none assigned

---

## COMMON USES

■ Improving physical and mental stamina ■ General tonic to energize during times of fatigue and inability to concentrate ■ Sedative, sleep aid, antidepressant ■ Diabetes ■ Enhanced sexual performance/aphrodisiac ■ Increased longevity, treatment of cancer ■ Adjunctive treatment of cancer ■ Increased immune response ■ Increased appetite.

## ACTION

■ Main active ingredient is ginsenoside from the dried root ■ Serves as CNS stimulant and depressant ■ Enhances immune function ■ Interferes with platelet aggregation and coagulation ■ Has analgesic, anti-inflammatory, and estrogen-like effects. **Therapeutic Effects:** ■ Improves mental and physical ability ■ May improve appetite, memory, sleep pattern ■ May

reduce fasting blood glucose level in diabetic patients.

## PHARMACOKINETICS

**Absorption:** Unknown.
**Distribution:** Unknown.
**Metabolism and Excretion:** Unknown.
**Half-life:** Unknown.

## CONTRAINDICATIONS AND PRECAUTIONS

**Contraindicated in:** ■ Pregnancy (androgenization of fetus) ■ Lactation ■ Manic-depressive disorders and psychosis ■ Hypertension ■ Asthma ■ Infection ■ Fever ■ Hormone-sensitive cancers.

**Use Cautiously in:** ■ Cardiovascular disease ■ Diabetics (may have hypoglycemic effects) ■ Patients receiving anticoagulants ■ Bleeding disorders.

## ADVERSE REACTIONS AND SIDE EFFECTS*

■ **CNS:** agitation, depression, dizziness, euphoria, headaches, insomnia, nervousness ■ **CV:** hypertension, tachycardia ■ **GI:** diarrhea ■ **GU:** amenorrhea, vaginal bleeding ■ **Derm:** skin eruptions ■ **Endo:** estrogen-like effects ■ **Misc:** fever, mastalgia, STEVENS-JOHNSON SYNDROME.

## INTERACTIONS

**Natural Product-Drug:** ■ May decrease anticoagulant activity of **warfarin** ■ May interfere with **MAO inhibitors** treatment and cause headache, tremulousness, and manic episodes ■ Use with caution when taking **estrogens**.

**Natural Product-Natural Product:** ■ May increase risk of bleeding when used with **herbs** that have antiplatelet or anticoagulant activities.

**Natural Product-Food:** ■ May potentiate effects of **caffeine** in **coffee** or **tea** and CNS stimulant effects of **mate**.

## ROUTE AND COMMONLY USED DOSES

■ **PO (Adults):** *Capsule*—200–600 mg/day; *extract*—100–300 mg 3 times daily; *crude root*—1–2 g/day; *infusion—tea*—1–2 g root daily (1/2 tbsp/cup water) up to 3 times daily (P. ginseng tea bag usually contains 1500 mg of ginseng root). Do not use for longer than 3 months.

## AVAILABILITY (generic available)

■ *Root powder*^*OTC* ■ *Extract in alcohol*^*OTC* ■ *Capsules*^*OTC*: 100 mg, 250 mg, 500 mg ■ *Tea bags*^*OTC*.

### TIME/ACTION PROFILE

|  | ONSET | PEAK | DURATION |
|---|---|---|---|
| PO | unknown | unknown | unknown |

## NURSING IMPLICATIONS

### ASSESSMENT

❏ Assess level of energy, attention span, and fatigue person is experiencing prior to initiating and periodically throughout the course of therapy.

❏ Assess appetite; sleep duration; and perceived quality, emotional lability, and work efficiency prior to and during therapy.

❏ Patients with chronic medical problems should not use this herb without the advice of health care professional.

❏ Assess for ginseng toxicity (nervousness, insomnia, palpitations, and diarrhea).

❏ Monitor patients with diabetes more frequently for hypoglycemia until response to the agent is ascertained.

❏ Assess for the development of ginseng abuse syndrome (occurs when large doses of the herb are taken concomitantly with other psychomotor stimulants such as coffee and tea. May present as diarrhea, hypertension, restlessness, insomnia, skin eruptions, depression, appetite suppression, euphoria, and edema).

### POTENTIAL NURSING DIAGNOSES

■ Energy field, disturbed (Indications).

■ Sleep pattern disturbed (Indications).

■ Knowledge, deficient, related to medication regimen (Patient/Family Teaching).

### IMPLEMENTATION

❏ May be taken without regard to food.

❏ Take at the same time daily and do not increase dose above the recommended amount because of potential toxic effects.

### PATIENT/FAMILY TEACHING

❏ Warn patients with cardiovascular disease, hypertension or hypotension, or on steroid therapy to avoid the use of this herb.

❏ Warn pregnant or breastfeeding women not to use this herb.

❏ Instruct patient in the symptoms of ginseng toxicity and to reduce dose or stop use of the herb if they occur.

❏ Inform patient to limit the amount of caffeine consumed.

❏ Advise patients with diabetes to monitor blood sugar levels until response to this agent is known.

❏ Tell patient that the recommended course of therapy is 3 wk. A repeated course is feasible. Do not use for longer than 3 months.

❏ Teach patient about the signs and symptoms of hepatitis and to stop use of the herb and promptly contact health care professional if they occur. (This herb is hepatoprotectant at low doses, but hepatodestructive at high doses.)

❏ Caution patient not to exceed recommended doses because of potential side effects and toxicity.

❏ If diarrhea develops, stop herb.

❏ Instruct patient to consult health care professional before taking any prescription or OTC medications concurrently with ginseng.

### EVALUATION

**Clinical response to therapy can be evaluated by:** ■ Improved energy level and sense of well-being ■ Improved quality of sleep ■ Improved concentration and work efficiency ■ Improved appetite ■ May need to take for several weeks before seeing results.

## glucosamine
(glew-**kos**-ah-meen)

*OTHER NAME(S):*
2-amino-2-deoxyglucose sulfate

*CLASSIFICATION(S):*
*Therapeutic: antirheumatics*

## COMMON USES

■ Osteoarthritis.

---

*CAPITALS indicates life-threatening; <u>underlines</u> indicate most frequent.

## ACTION

■ May stop or slow osteoarthritis progression by stimulating cartilage and synovial tissue metabolism

## PHARMACOKINETICS

**Absorption:** 0.9% absorbed.
**Distribution:** Unknown.
**Metabolism and Excretion:** 74% eliminated via first-pass metabolism.
**Half-life:** Unknown.

## CONTRAINDICATIONS AND PRECAUTIONS

**Contraindicated in:** ■ Shellfish allergy (glucosamine is often derived from marine exoskeletons) ■ Pregnancy and lactation.
**Use Cautiously in:** ■ Diabetes (may worsen glycemic control).

## ADVERSE REACTIONS AND SIDE EFFECTS*

■ **GI:** nausea, heartburn, diarrhea, constipation.

## INTERACTIONS

**Natural Product-Drug:** ■ May antagonize the effects of **antidiabetics**.
**Natural Product-Natural Product:** ■ None known.

## ROUTE AND COMMONLY USED DOSES

■ **PO (Adults):** 500 mg three times daily.

## AVAILABILITY

■ *Tablets^{OTC}* ■ *Capsules^{OTC}*.

TIME/ACTION PROFILE

| | ONSET | PEAK | DURATION |
|---|---|---|---|
| PO | unknown | unknown | unknown |

# NURSING IMPLICATIONS

## ASSESSMENT

❑ Evaluate for shellfish allergy prior to initiating therapy.
❑ Monitor pain (type, location, and intensity) and range of motion on an ongoing basis as an indicator of drug efficacy.
❑ Assess glucose levels via home monitoring device for patients with diabetes until response is ascertained.

❑ Evaluate gastric discomfort and instruct patient to seek out the advice of a health care provider if persistent gastric discomfort occurs.
❑ Assess bowel function and symptomatically treat constipation with improved fluid intake and bulk in diet and bulk laxatives if necessary.

## POTENTIAL NURSING DIAGNOSES

■ Pain, acute (Indications).
■ Mobility, impaired physical (Indications).
■ Knowledge, deficient, related to medication regimen (Patient/Family Teaching).

## IMPLEMENTATION

❑ Take prior to meals.

## PATIENT/FAMILY TEACHING

❑ Warn patients with a shellfish allergy that this herbal supplement should not be used.
❑ Instruct patients that the effects of this drug come from stimulating cartilage and synovial tissue metabolism and that the supplement must be taken on a regular basis to achieve benefit. It should not be used as an intermittent pain medication.
❑ Contact a health care provider if gastric discomfort develops and persists.
❑ Caution diabetics to monitor glucose values to ascertain impact on glycemic control.

## EVALUATION

**Clinical response to therapy can be evaluated by:** ■ Improvement in pain and range of motion.

---

### hawthorne (Crataegus Species)

(**haw**-thorn)

### CLASSIFICATION(S):
*Therapeutic: antihypertensives, inotropics*

## COMMON USES

■ Hypertension ■ Mild to moderate CHF ■ Angina ■ Spasmolytic ■ Sedative.

## ACTION

■ Active compounds in hawthorn include flavonoids and procyanidins ■ Increase coronary blood flow ■ Positive inotropic and chronotropic effects because of increased permeability to calcium and inhibition of phosphodiesterase. **Therapeutic Effects:** ■ Increased cardiac output ■ Decreased blood pressure, myocardial workload, and oxygen consumption.

## PHARMACOKINETICS

**Absorption:** Unknown.
**Distribution:** Unknown.
**Metabolism and Excretion:** Unknown.
**Half-life:** Unknown.

## CONTRAINDICATIONS AND PRECAUTIONS

**Contraindicated in:** ■ Pregnancy (potential uterine activity) ■ Lactation.
**Use Cautiously in:** ■ Concurrent use with ACE inhibitors and digoxin ■ Do not discontinue use abruptly.

## ADVERSE REACTIONS AND SIDE EFFECTS*

■ **CNS:** agitation, dizziness, fatigue, headache, sedation (high dose), sleeplessness, sweating ■ **CV:** hypotension (high dose), palpitations ■ **GI:** nausea.

## INTERACTIONS

**Natural Product-Drug:** ■ May potentiate effect of **digoxin** and other **cardioactive** drugs ■ Concurrent use with **theophylline, caffeine, epinephrine**, and other **cardioactive** drugs may potentiate adverse cardiovascular effects ■ May cause additive CNS depression when used with other **CNS depressants**.
**Natural Product-Natural Product:** ■ Additive effect with other cardiac glycoside–containing herbs (**digitalis leaf, black helle-bore, oleander leaf**, and others) ■ Additive effect with other cardioactive herbs (**devil's claw, fenugreek**, and others).

## ROUTE AND COMMONLY USED DOSES

■ **PO (Adults):** 5 g of drug or 160–900 mg extract daily. *Hawthorn fluid extract (1:1 in 25% alcohol)*—0.5–1 ml tid; *hawthorn fruit tincture (1:5 in 45% alcohol)*—1–2 ml tid; *dried hawthorn berries*—300–1000 mg tid.

## AVAILABILITY (generic available)

■ *Dried fruit^OTC* ■ *Liquid extract of the fruit or leaf^OTC* ■ *Tincture of the fruit or leaf^OTC.*

TIME/ACTION PROFILE

| | ONSET | PEAK | DURATION |
|---|---|---|---|
| PO | unknown | 6-8 wk | unknown |

## NURSING IMPLICATIONS

### ASSESSMENT

❏ Auscultate lung sounds for signs of heart failure (rales, crackles, wheezing).
❏ Assess weight daily and look for signs of fluid overload (swelling of ankles, shortness of breath, sleeping with multiple pillows).
❏ Assess blood pressure periodically throughout therapy.
❏ Assess pulse for rate and regularity of rhythm.

### POTENTIAL NURSING DIAGNOSES

■ Cardiac output, decreased (Indications).
■ Knowledge, deficient, related to medication regimen (Patient/Family Teaching).

### IMPLEMENTATION

❏ Administered as 2–3 divided doses daily at the same time.
❏ May be taken without regard to food.

### PATIENT/FAMILY TEACHING

❏ Advise patients that there are other proven therapies available for treatment of heart failure. These therapies should be employed prior to initiating treatment with hawthorn.
❏ Tell patient not to take hawthorn without the advice of health care professional.
❏ Instruct patients in the symptoms of a heart attack (pain in the region of the heart, jaw, arm, or upper abdomen; sweating; chest tightness) and heart failure (shortness of breath, chest tightness, dizziness, sweating) and to promptly contact health care professional if they occur.
❏ Advise patient to report weight gain or persistent swelling of the feet to health care professional.
❏ Warn patients who self-medicate to consult health care professional if there is no im-

*CAPITALS indicates life-threatening; underlines indicate most frequent.

provement in symptoms in 6–8 wk. Effects may not be seen for 3 mo.

□ Teach patient to make position changes slowly to minimize the risk of orthostatic hypotension.

□ Caution patient not to combine with other cardiac and BP medications unless under supervision of health care professional because of possible additive effects.

□ This herb may cause drowsiness. Patients should avoid driving or other activities that require mental alertness until response to herb is known.

□ Avoid alcohol and other CNS depressants while taking hawthorn unless under supervision of health care professional.

□ Profuse sweating and dehydration under extreme heat may increase the BP-lowering properties of hawthorn, leading to severe hypotension. Warn patients to avoid exertion in hot weather to minimize the risk of side effects.

□ Instruct patients that hawthorn helps control the symptoms of heart failure but does not cure the disease. Lifestyle changes (salt restriction, weight management, exercise as tolerated, adherence to medication regimens) still need to be followed.

□ Although hawthorn has been studied in Europe for management of heart failure, there are no conclusive studies to recommend use of this herb.

□ Instruct patient to consult health care professional before taking any prescription or OTC medications concurrently with hawthorn.

### EVALUATION

**Clinical response to therapy can be evaluated by:** ■ Decrease in symptoms of CHF ■ Improved cardiac output as evidenced by improved activity tolerance.

---

*Hypericum Perforatum*, see **St. John's wort**

---

### kava-kava (Piper Methysticum)
(**ka**-va**ka**-va)

---

**OTHER NAME(S):**
Ava pepper, intoxicating pepper, kew, tonga, wurzelstock

**CLASSIFICATION(S):**
**Therapeutic:** *antianxiety agents, sedative/hypnotics*

### COMMON USES

■ Anxiety, stress, restlessness, insomnia ■ Mild muscle aches and pains ■ Menstrual cramps and PMS.

### ACTION

■ Alters the limbic system modulation of emotional processes ■ Shown to have centrally acting skeletal muscle relaxant properties activated. **Therapeutic Effects:** ■ Relief of anxiety ■ Sedation.

### PHARMACOKINETICS

**Absorption:** Peak plasma level occurs about 1.8 hr after an oral dose.

**Distribution:** Enters breast milk.

**Metabolism and Excretion:** Elimination occurs primarily by renal excretion (both unchanged and metabolites) and in the feces. Metabolized by the liver (reduction or demethylation).

**Half-life:** Approximately 9 hr.

### CONTRAINDICATIONS AND PRECAUTIONS

**Contraindicated in:** ■ Pregnancy (may affect uterine tone) and lactation ■ Patients with endogenous depression (may increase risk of suicide) ■ Children under 12 yr of age ■ Hepatitis or other liver disease.

**Use Cautiously in:** ■ Concurrent use of other hepatotoxic agents ■ Should not be used for more 3 mo to prevent psychological addiction.

### ADVERSE REACTIONS AND SIDE EFFECTS*

■ **CNS:** dizziness, headache, drowsiness, sensory disturbances ■ **EENT:** Pupil dilation, red eyes, visual accommodation disorders ■ **GI:** HEPATIC TOXICITY (rare), gastrointestinal complaints ■ **Derm:** allergic skin reactions, yellow discoloration of skin, pellagroid dermopathy ■ **Hemat:** decreased lymphocytes, decreased platelets ▪**Metab:** weight loss (long term, high dose) ▪ **Neuro:** ataxia, muscle weakness.

## INTERACTIONS

**Natural Product-Drug:** ▪ Additive effect when used with **alprazolam** ▪ Potentiates effect of **CNS depressants** (**ethanol, barbiturates, benzodiazepines, opioid analgesics**) ▪ Has decreased the effectiveness of **levodopa** in few cases ▪ Theoretically, may have additive effects with **antiplatelet agents.**

**Natural Product-Natural Product:** ▪ Theoretically, may have additive sedative effects when used with other **herbs** with sedative properties.

## ROUTE AND COMMONLY USED DOSES

▪ **PO (Adults):** *Antianxiety*—50–75 kavalactones 3 times daily; *insomnia*—180–210 mg kavalactones. Typically taken as a tea by simmering the root in boiling water and then straining.

## AVAILABILITY (generic available)

▪*Dried root extracts (alcohol or acetone based) containing 30–70% kavapyrones.*

TIME/ACTION PROFILE

|    | ONSET | PEAK | DURATION |
|----|-------|------|----------|
| PO | 1.8 hr | unknown | 8 hr |

# NURSING IMPLICATIONS

## ASSESSMENT

❏ Assess muscle spasm, associated pain, and limitations of movement prior to and periodically throughout therapy.

❏ Assess degree of anxiety and level of sedation (visual disturbances and changes in motor reflexes are side effects) prior to and periodically throughout therapy.

❏ Assess sleep patterns and level of sedation upon arising.

❏ Prolonged use may lead to depression of platelet and lymphocyte counts.

## POTENTIAL NURSING DIAGNOSES

▪ Anxiety (Indications).

▪ Mobility, impaired physical (Adverse Reactions).

▪ Injury, risk for (Side Effects).

## IMPLEMENTATION

❏ Prepared as a drink from pulverized roots, tablets, capsules, or extract.

## PATIENT/FAMILY TEACHING

❏ Inform patient that significant, serious side effects may occur with prolonged use. Use for longer than 1 mo is not recommended without supervision of health care professional.

❏ Caution patient to not use alcohol or other CNS depressants while taking this herb because the combination potentiates the herb's sedative effect.

❏ Advise patients that driving a car or performing other activities requiring mental alertness should be avoided until response to therapy is determined.

❏ Warn patients to stop use of the herb immediately if shortness of breath or signs of liver disease (yellowing of the skin or whites of the eyes, brown urine, nausea, vomiting, light-colored stools, unusual tiredness, weakness, stomach or abdominal pain, loss of appetite) occur and contact health care professional.

❏ Advise patients who have liver disease or liver problems, or persons who are taking drug products that can affect the liver, to consult health care professional before using kava-containing supplements.

❏ Inform patient that although there is no evidence of physiological dependence, the risk of psychological dependence still exists.

❏ Counsel pregnant and breastfeeding women not to use this herb.

❏ Instruct patient to consult health care professional before taking any prescription or OTC medications concurrently with kava-kava.

## EVALUATION

**Clinical response to therapy can be evaluated by:** ▪ Decrease in anxiety level ▪ Decrease in muscle spasms ▪ Relief of insomnia.

---

**milk thistle**

(milk**this**-ul)

*OTHER NAME(S):*

Holy thistle, Lady's thistle, Mary Thistle, Silymarin

---

*CAPITALS indicates life-threatening; <u>underlines</u> indicate most frequent.

---

*CLASSIFICATION(S):*
*Therapeutic:* antidotes

---

## COMMON USES

■ Cirrhosis, chronic hepatitis, gallstones, psoriasis, liver cleansing and detoxification, treatment of liver toxicity due to alcohol, Amanita mushroom poisoning (European IV formulation), and chemicals.

## ACTION

■ The active component, silymarin, has antioxidant and hepatoprotectant actions. Silymarin helps prevent toxin penetration and stimulates hepatocyte regeneration.

## PHARMACOKINETICS

**Absorption:** 23–47% absorbed after oral administration.
**Distribution:** Unknown.
**Metabolism and Excretion:** Hepatic metabolism by cytochrome P450 3A4.
**Half-life:** 6 hr.

## CONTRAINDICATIONS AND PRECAUTIONS

**Contraindicated in:** ■ Pregnancy and lactation (insufficient information available) ■ Allergy to chamomile, ragweed, asters, chrysanthemums and other members of the family Compositae

## ADVERSE REACTIONS AND SIDE EFFECTS*

■ **GI:** Laxative effect ■ **Misc:** Allergic reactions.

## INTERACTIONS

**Natural Product-Drug:** ■ In vitro, milk thistle extract inhibited the drug-metabolizing enzyme **cytochrome P450 3A4.** Interactions have not been reported in humans, but milk thistle should be used cautiously with other drugs metabolized by 3A4, such as **cyclosporin, carbamazepine, HMG-CoA inhibitors, ketoconazole,** and **alprazolam.**
**Natural Product-Natural Product:** ■ None known.

## ROUTE AND COMMONLY USED DOSES

■ **PO (Adults):** *Extract (70%)*—200–400 mg/d; *Dried fruit/seed*—12–15 g/day; *Tea*—3–4 times daily 30 minutes before meals. Tea is not recommended as silymarin is not sufficiently water-soluble.

## AVAILABILITY

■ *Capsules^{OTC}* ■ *Tablets^{OTC}* ■ *Crude drug^{OTC}* ■ *Tea^{OTC}* ■ *Extract^{OTC}.*

### TIME/ACTION PROFILE

|    | ONSET | PEAK | DURATION |
|----|-------|------|----------|
| PO | 5–30 days or more | unknown | unknown |

# NURSING IMPLICATIONS

## ASSESSMENT

❑ Assess patients for signs of liver failure such as jaundice, mental status changes, abdominal distention (ascites), and generalized edema.
❑ Monitor liver function tests periodically throughout therapy.
❑ Evaluate consistency and frequency of bowel movements.

## POTENTIAL NURSING DIAGNOSES

■ Knowledge, deficient, related to medication regimen (Patient/Family Teaching).

## IMPLEMENTATION

❑ Orally as an extract, capsule, tablets, or as a dried fruit as a single daily dose or divided into three doses.
❑ Tea is not recommended as Milk Thistle is not water-soluble.

## PATIENT/FAMILY TEACHING

❑ Instruct patients in the symptoms of liver failure and to report worsening symptomatology promptly to their healthcare provider.
❑ Emphasize the need for blood tests to monitor liver function tests.
❑ Advise patients to abstain from alcohol and to follow a diet consistent with the liver or gall bladder disease being treated.

## EVALUATION

**Clinical response to therapy can be evaluated by:** ■ Normalization of liver function tests ■ Reduction in jaundice, abdominal distention, fatigue, and other symptoms associated with liver disease.

*Panax Ginseng*, see ginseng.

*Piper Methysticum*, see kava-kava.

## SAMe
## (sam-ee)

*OTHER NAME(S):*
Ademetionine, S-adenosylmethionine,

*CLASSIFICATION(S):*
*Therapeutic: antidepressants*

**Pregnancy Category UK**

### COMMON USES

■ Treatment of depression ■ Has also been used to manage: ■ osteoarthritis ■ fibromyalgia ■ liver disease ■ migraine headaches

### ACTION

■ May aid in the production, activation, and metabolism of various amines, phospholipids, hormones, and neurotransmitters. **Therapeutic Effects:** ■ Decreased depression.

### PHARMACOKINETICS

**Absorption:** Rapidly and extensively metabolized following oral administration.
**Distribution:** Unknown.
**Metabolism and Excretion:** Actively metabolized by the liver.
**Half-life:** 100 min.

### CONTRAINDICATIONS AND PRECAUTIONS

**Contraindicated in:** ■ Hypersensitivity ■ Bipolar disorder.
**Use Cautiously in:** ■ Pregnancy, lactation, or children (safety not established)

### ADVERSE REACTIONS AND SIDE EFFECTS*

■ **CNS:** agitation, manic reactions (in patients with bipolar disorder) ■ **GI:** vomiting, diarrhea, flatulence.

### INTERACTIONS

**Natural Product-Drug:** ■ Avoid use with other **antidepressants** (additive serotinergic effects may occur) ■ Should not be used concurrently with **MAO inhibitors**. Avoid use of SAMe within 2 wk of using a **MAO inhibitor**.

### ROUTE AND COMMONLY USED DOSES

■ **PO (Adults):** *Depression*—200 mg once or twice daily, adjusted upward over 2 wk (range 400–1600 mg/day); *liver disorders*—1600 mg/day; *osteoarthritis*—200 mg tid.

### AVAILABILITY

■ *Tablets:* 100 mg, 200 mg, 400 mg$^{OTC}$.

TIME/ACTION PROFILE (antidepressant action)

| | ONSET | PEAK | DURATION |
|---|---|---|---|
| PO (depression) | 1–2 wk | unknown | unknown |
| PO (osteoarthritis) | 30 days | unknown | unknown |

## NURSING IMPLICATIONS

### ASSESSMENT

❏ Assess mental status for symptoms of depression prior to and periodically during therapy; advise patients with depression to be evaluated by a health care professional.
❏ Assess symptoms of pain and fatigue prior to and periodically during therapy.

### POTENTIAL NURSING DIAGNOSES

■ Coping, ineffective (Indications).
■ Knowledge, deficient, related to medication regimen (Patient/Family Teaching).

### IMPLEMENTATION

■ **General:** ■ Only enteric-coated formulations are recommended due to bioavailability problems.
■ **PO:** ■ Initial dose should be 200 mg once or twice daily to minimize GI disturbances. Dosage may be adjusted upward over 1–2 wk depending on response and tolerance.

### PATIENT/FAMILY TEACHING

❏ Instruct patient to take SAMe according to directions.

*CAPITALS indicates life-threatening; underlines indicate most frequent.

❏ The SAMe bufanedisulfonate salt may be preferable due to greater stability.

## EVALUATION

**Clinical response to therapy can be evaluated by:** ■ Decrease in symptoms of depression.

---

## saw palmetto

### OTHER NAME(S):
American Dwarf Palm Tree, Cabbage Palm, Ju-Zhong, Palmier Nain, Sabal, Sabal Fructus, Saw Palmetto Berry, Serenoa repens

### CLASSIFICATION(S):
**Therapeutic:** *none assigned*

## COMMON USES

■ Benign prostatic hypertrophy (BPH) ■ Prostate cancer (in combination with 7 other herbs as PC-SPES).

## ACTION

■ Antiandrogenic, antiinflammatory and antiproliferative properties in prostate tissue result in improvement in BPH symptoms such as frequent urination, hesitancy, urgency, and nocturia ■ Comparable in efficacy to finasteride but may be less effective than prazosin

## PHARMACOKINETICS

**Absorption:** Unknown.
**Distribution:** Unknown.
**Metabolism and Excretion:** Unknown.
**Half-life:** Unknown.

## CONTRAINDICATIONS AND PRECAUTIONS

**Contraindicated in:** ■ Pregnancy and lactation.

## ADVERSE REACTIONS AND SIDE EFFECTS*

■ **CNS:** dizziness ■ **GI:** nausea, vomiting, constipation, and diarrhea.

## INTERACTIONS

**Natural Product-Drug:** ■ Hormonal action may interfere with other hormonal therapies (**testosterone, hormonal contraceptives**).

## ROUTE AND COMMONLY USED DOSES

■ **PO (Adults):** *Lipophilic extract (80–90% fatty acids)*—160 mg twice daily or 320 mg once daily. *Whole berries*—1–2 grams daily. *Liquid extract*—0.6–1.5 ml daily. *Tea (efficacy is questionable due to lipophilicity of active constituents)*—1 cup three times daily. Tea is prepared by steeping 0.5–1 g dried berry in 150 ml boiling water for 5–10 minutes.

## AVAILABILITY

■ *Lipophilic extract (80-90% fatty acids)$^{OTC}$* ■ *Whole berries$^{OTC}$* ■ *Liquid extract$^{OTC}$*.

TIME/ACTION PROFILE

|  | ONSET | PEAK | DURATION |
|---|---|---|---|
| PO | 1–2 mos | unknown | 48 wk (longest studied treatment duration) |

---

# NURSING IMPLICATIONS

## ASSESSMENT

❏ Assess patient for symptoms of benign prostatic hypertrophy (BPH) (urinary hesitancy, feeling of incomplete bladder emptying, interruption in urinary stream, impairment in size and force of urinary stream, terminal urinary dribbling, straining to start flow, dysuria, urgency) before and periodically throughout therapy.

❏ Rectal exams prior to and periodically throughout therapy to assess prostate size are recommended.

## POTENTIAL NURSING DIAGNOSES

■ Urinary elimination, impaired (Indications).
■ Knowledge, deficient, related to medication regimen (Patient/Family Teaching).

## IMPLEMENTATION

❏ Take on a full stomach to minimize GI effects.

## PATIENT/FAMILY TEACHING

❏ Advise patients to start therapy with this herbal supplement only after evaluation by a health care provider who will provide continued follow-up care.

❑ Inform patients that saw palmetto does not alter the size of the prostate but still should relieve the symptoms associated with BPH.

❑ Tell patients that taking this herbal supplement with food should reduce the GI effects and make it easier to tolerate.

## EVALUATION

**Clinical response to therapy can be evaluated by:** ■ Decrease in urinary symptoms of BPH.

---

### St. John's wort (Hypericum Perforatum)

(sayntjonzwort)

**OTHER NAME(S):**
Amber, Goatweed, Hardhay, Klamath weed, Tipton weed

**CLASSIFICATION(S):**
*Therapeutic: antidepressants*

---

## COMMON USES

■**PO:** Management of mild to moderate depression ■ **Topical:** Inflammation of the skin, blunt injury, wounds, and burns ■ Other uses are for capillary strengthening, decreasing uterine bleeding, and reducing tumor size.

## ACTION

■ Derived from *Hypericum perforatum*; the active component is *hypericin* ■ **PO:** ■ Antidepressant action my be due to ability to inhibit reuptake of serotonin and other neurotransmitters ■ **Topical:** Anti-inflammatory, antifungal, antiviral, and antibacterial properties. **Therapeutic Effects:** ■ **PO:** ■ Decreased signs and symptoms of depression ■ **Topical:** Decreased inflammation of burns or other wounds.

## PHARMACOKINETICS

**Absorption:** Unknown.

**Distribution:** Unknown.

**Metabolism and Excretion:** Unknown.

**Half-life:** *Hypericum constituents*—24.8–26.5 hr.

## CONTRAINDICATIONS AND PRECAUTIONS

**Contraindicated in:** ■ Pregnancy, lactation, or children.

**Use Cautiously in:** ■ History of phototoxicity ■ History of suicide attempt, moderate to severe depression, or psychosis.

## ADVERSE REACTIONS AND SIDE EFFECTS*

■ **CNS:** dizziness, restlessness, sleep disturbances ■ **CV:** hypertension ■ **GI:** abdominal pain, bloating, constipation, dry mouth, feeling of fullness, flatulence, nausea, vomiting ■ **Derm:** allergic skin reactions (hives, itching, skin rash), phototoxicity.

## INTERACTIONS

**Natural Product-Drug:** ■ Concurrent use with **alcohol** or other **antidepressants** (including **SSRIs** and **MAO inhibitors**) may increase the risk of adverse CNS reactions ■ Use with **MAO Inhibitors** could result in serotonin syndrome ■ Avoid use of St. John's Wort and **MAO Inhibitors** within 2 wk of each other.

## ROUTE AND COMMONLY USED DOSES

■ **PO (Adults):** *Depression*—300 mg of St. John's Wort standardized to 0.3% hypericum 3 times daily.

■ **Topical (Adults):** 0.2–1 mg total hypericin daily.

## AVAILABILITY

❑ **Preparations for Oral Use**
■ *Dried herb^{orc}* ■ *Dried (hydroalcoholic) extract^{orc}* ■ *Oil^{orc}* ■ *Tincture^{orc}*.

❑ **Preparations for Topical Application**
■ *Liquid^{orc}* ■ *Semisolid^{orc}*.

TIME/ACTION PROFILE

| | ONSET | PEAK | DURATION |
|---|---|---|---|
| PO | 10–14 days | within 4–6 wk | unknown |

## NURSING IMPLICATIONS

### ASSESSMENT

■ **Depression:** ■ Assess patient for depression periodically throughout therapy.

■ **Inflammation:** ■ Assess skin or skin lesions periodically throughout therapy.

## POTENTIAL NURSING DIAGNOSES

■ Coping, ineffective (Indications).

■ Anxiety (Indications).

■ Knowledge, deficient, related to medication regimen (Patient/Family Teaching).

## IMPLEMENTATION

■ **PO:** ■ Tea can be prepared by mixing 2-4 dried herbs in 150 ml of boiling water and steeping for 10 min.

## PATIENT/FAMILY TEACHING

❑ Instruct patient to take St. John's wort as directed.

❑ Patients with depression should be evaluated by health care professional. Standard therapy may be of greater benefit for moderate to severe depression.

❑ Advise patient to notify health care professional of medication regimen prior to treatment or surgery.

❑ Caution patients to avoid sun exposure and use protective sunscreen to reduce the risk of photosensitivity reactions.

❑ Inform patient that St. John's wort is usually taken for a period of 4–6 wk. If no improvement is seen, another therapy should be considered.

❑ Inform patient to purchase herbs from a reputable source and that products and their contents vary among different manufacturers.

❑ Warn patient not to use alcohol while taking St. John's wort.

❑ Warn patients that St. John's wort may reduce the therapeutic effectiveness of several drugs.

❑ May potentiate effect of sedatives and side effects of other antidepressants. Do not take within 2 wk of MAO Inhibitor therapy

❑ Instruct patient to consult healthcare professional before taking any prescription or OTC medications concurrently with St. John's wort.

## EVALUATION

**Clinical response to therapy can be evaluated by:** ■ Decrease in signs and symptoms of depression or anxiety ■ Improvement in skin inflammation.

## valerian
### (vuh-lare-ee-en)

### OTHER NAME(S):
Amantilla, All-Heal, Baldrian, Baldrianwurzel, Belgium Valerian, Common Valerian, Fragrant Valerian, Garden Heliotrope, Garden Valerian, Indian Valerian, Mexican Valerian, Pacific Valerian, Valeriana, Valeriana officinalis, Valerianae radix, Valeriana rhizome, Valeriane

### CLASSIFICATION(S):
**Therapeutic:** antianxiety agents, sedative/hypnotics

## COMMON USES

■ Insomnia ■ Anxiety

## ACTION

■ May increase concentrations of the inhibitory CNS transmitter GABA

## PHARMACOKINETICS

**Absorption:** Unknown.

**Distribution:** Unknown.

**Metabolism and Excretion:** Unknown.

**Half-life:** Unknown.

## CONTRAINDICATIONS AND PRECAUTIONS

**Contraindicated in:** ■ Pregnancy and lactation.

## ADVERSE REACTIONS AND SIDE EFFECTS*

■ **CNS:** drowsiness, headache ■ **Misc:** Benzodiazepine-like withdrawal symptoms with discontinuation after long-term use.

## INTERACTIONS

**Natural Product-Drug:** ■ Additive CNS depression with **alcohol, antihistamines, sedative hypnotics,** and other **CNS depressants** ■ Alcohol-containing preparations may interact with **disulfuram** and **metronidazole.**

## ROUTE AND COMMONLY USED DOSES

■ **PO (Adults):** *Tea*—1 cup tea 1–5 times daily. Tea is made by steeping 2–3 g root in

150 ml boiling water for 5–10 min then straining. *Tincture*—1–3 mL 1–5 times daily. *Extract*—400–900 mg up to 2 hours before bedtime or 450 mg three times daily.

## AVAILABILITY

■ *Capsules*<sup>OTC</sup> ■ *Extract*<sup>OTC</sup> ■ *Tea*<sup>OTC</sup> ■ *Tincture*<sup>OTC</sup>.

TIME/ACTION PROFILE

|  | ONSET | PEAK | DURATION |
|---|---|---|---|
| PO | 30–60 min | 2 hr | unknown |

## NURSING IMPLICATIONS

### ASSESSMENT

- ❏ Assess degree of anxiety and level of sedation prior to and periodically throughout therapy.
- ❏ Assess sleep patterns.
- ❏ Assess response in the elderly population where drowsiness and loss of balance may pose a significant risk for injury.

### POTENTIAL NURSING DIAGNOSES

- ■ Anxiety (Indications).
- ■ Injury, risk for (Side Effects).

### IMPLEMENTATION

- ❏ Take one to two hours before bedtime if used for nighttime hypnotic.

- ❏ Administer orally three to five times daily to control anxiety.

### PATIENT/FAMILY TEACHING

- ❏ Warn patients to avoid use of other medications or herbals that have a sedative effect, as the combination will increase drowsiness and sedation.
- ❏ Inform patients not to take this herbal supplement if pregnant or breastfeeding.
- ❏ Counsel patients to avoid activities requiring mental alertness until response to this supplement is known.
- ❏ Notify patients that dependence with withdrawal symptoms may develop with prolonged use.
- ❏ Instruct patients to avoid consuming alcohol while taking this herbal supplement.
- ❏ Encourage patients to eliminate stimulants such as caffeine and to provide an environment that promotes restful sleep.

### EVALUATION

**Clinical response to therapy can be evaluated by:** ■ Decreased anxiety level ■ Improvement in sleep with a feeling of restfulness without drowsiness upon awakening.

*Zingiber Officinale*, see **ginger**.

# Medication Administration Techniques

## Subcutaneous Injection Sites

## Administration of Ophthalmic Medications

For instillation of ophthalmic solutions, instruct patient to lie down or tilt head back and look at ceiling. Pull down on lower lid, creating a small pocket, and instill solution into pocket. With systemically acting drugs, apply pressure to the inner canthus for 1–2 min to minimize systemic absorption. Instruct patient to gently close eye. Wait 5 min before instilling second drop or any other ophthalmic solutions.

For instillation of ophthalmic ointment, instruct patient to hold tube in hand for several minutes to warm. Squeeze a small amount of ointment (1/4–1/2 in.) inside lower lid. Instruct patient to close eye gently and roll eyeball around in all directions with eye closed. Wait 10 min before instilling any other ophthalmic ointments.

Do not touch cap or tip of container to eye, fingers, or any surface.

## Administration of Medications with Metered-Dose Inhalers

Instruct patient on the proper use of the metered-dose inhaler. There are 3 methods of using a metered-dose inhaler. Shake inhaler well. (1) Take a drink of water to moisten the throat; place the inhaler mouthpiece 2 finger-widths away from mouth; tilt head back slightly. While activating the inhaler, take a slow, deep breath for 3–5 sec; hold the breath for 10 sec; and breathe out slowly. (2) Exhale and close lips firmly around mouthpiece. Administer during second half of inhalation, and hold breath for as long as possible to ensure deep instillation of medication. (3) Use of spacer. Consult health care professional to determine method desired prior to instruction.

Allow 1–2 min between inhalations. Rinse mouth with water or mouthwash after each use to minimize dry mouth and hoarseness. Wash inhalation assembly at least daily in warm running water.

For use of dry powder inhalers, turn head away from inhaler and exhale (do not blow into inhaler). Do not shake. Close mouth tightly around the mouthpiece of the inhaler and inhale rapidly.

**Steps for Using Your Inhaler** *
1. Remove the cap and hold inhaler upright.
2. Shake the inhaler.
3. Tilt your head back slightly and breathe out slowly.
4. Position the inhaler in one of the following ways (A or B is optimal, but C is acceptable for those who have difficulty with A or B. C is required for breath-activated inhalers):

A. Open mouth with inhaler 1 to 2 inches away.

B. Use space/holding chamber (this is recommended especially for young children and for people using corticosteroids).

C. In the mouth. Do not use for corticosteroids.

D. NOTE: Inhaled dry powder capsules require a different inhalation technique. To use a dry powder inhaler, it is important to close the mouth tightly around the mouthpiece of the inhaler and to inhale rapidly.

5. Press down on the inhaler to release medication as you start to breathe in slowly.
6. Breathe in slowly (3 to 5 seconds).
7. Hold your breath for 10 seconds to allow the medicine to reach deeply into your lungs.
8. Repeat puff as directed. Waiting 1 minute between puffs may permit second puff to penetrate your lungs better.
9. Spacers/holding chambers are useful for all patients. They are particularly recommended for young children and older adults and for use with inhaled corticosteroids. Avoid common inhaler mistakes. Follow these inhaler tips:

- Breathe out before pressing your inhaler.
- Inhale slowly.
- Breathe in through your mouth, not your nose.
- Press down on your inhaler at the start of inhalation (or within the first second of inhalation).
- Keep inhaling as you press down on inhaler.
- Press your inhaler only once while you are inhaling (one breath for each puff).
- Make sure you breathe in evenly and deeply.
- If you are using a short-acting bronchodilator inhaler and a corticosteroid inhaler, use the bronchodilator first, and allow 5 minutes to elapse before using the corticosteroid.

Other inhalers have become available in addition to the one illustrated here. Different types of inhalers may require different techniques.

## Administration of Medications by Nebulizer

Administer in a location where patient can sit comfortably for 10–15 min. Plug in compressor. Mix medication as directed, or empty unit-dose vials into nebulizer. Do not mix different types of medications without checking with health care professional. Assemble mask or mouthpiece and

*Source: Expert Panel Report 2: Guidelines for the Diagnosis and Management of Asthma. National Asthma Education and Prevention Program, National Heart, Lung, and Blood Institute, 1997.

connect tubing to port on compressor. Have patient sit in a comfortable upright position. Make sure that mask fits properly over nose and mouth and that mist does not flow into eyes, or put mouthpiece into mouth. Turn on compressor. Instruct patient to take slow deep breaths. If possible, patient should hold breath for 10 sec before slowly exhaling. Continue this process until medication chamber is empty. Wash mask in hot soapy water; rinse well and allow to air dry before next use.

## Administration of Nasal Sprays

Clear nasal passages of secretions prior to use. If nasal passages are blocked, use a decongestant immediately prior to use to ensure adequate penetration of the spray. Keep head upright. Breathe in through nose during administration. Sniff hard for a few minutes after administration.

## Intramuscular Injection Sites

### Deltoid site

### Ventrogluteal site

### Dorsogluteal site

### Vastus lateralis site

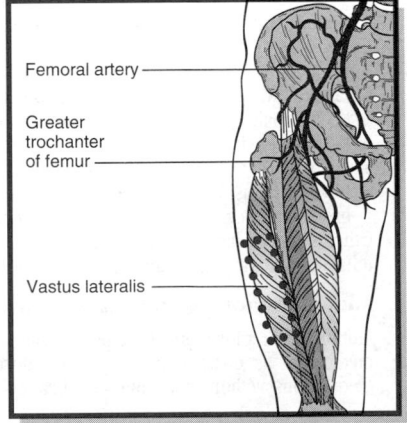

# Formulas Helpful for Calculating Doses

### Ratio and Proportion

A ratio is the same as a fraction and can be expressed as a fraction (1/2) or in the algebraic form (1:2). This relationship is stated as *one is to two*.

A proportion is an equation of equal fractions or ratios.

$$\frac{1}{2} = \frac{4}{8}$$

To calculate doses, begin each proportion with the two known values, for example, 15 grains = 1 gram (known equivalent) or 10 milligrams = 2 milliliters (dosage available) on one side of the equation. Next, make certain that the units of measure on the opposite side of the equation are the same as the units of the known values and are placed on the same level of the equation.

Problem A:
$$\frac{15 \text{ gr}}{1 \text{ g}} = \frac{10 \text{ gr}}{x \text{ g}}$$

Problem B:
$$\frac{10 \text{ mg}}{2 \text{ ml}} = \frac{5 \text{ mg}}{x \text{ ml}}$$

Once the proportion is set up correctly, cross-multiply the opposing values of the proportion.

Problem A:
$$\frac{15 \text{ gr}}{1 \text{ gr}} \bowtie \frac{10 \text{ gr}}{x \text{ g}}$$

$$15x = 10$$

Problem B:
$$\frac{10 \text{ mg}}{2 \text{ ml}} \bowtie \frac{5 \text{ mg}}{x \text{ ml}}$$

$$10x = 10$$

Next, divide each side of the equation by the number with the $x$ to determine the answer. Then, add the unit of measure corresponding to $x$ in the original equation.

Problem A:
$$\frac{15x}{15} = \frac{10}{15}$$

$$x = \frac{2}{3} \text{ or } 0.6 \text{ g}$$

Problem B:
$$\frac{10x}{10} = \frac{10}{10}$$

$$x = 1 \text{ ml}$$

### Calculation of IV Drip Rate

To calculate the drip rate for an intravenous infusion, 3 values are needed:

I. The amount of solution and corresponding time for infusion. May be ordered as:

$$1000 \text{ ml over } 8 \text{ hr}$$

or

$$125 \text{ ml/hr}$$

II. The equivalent in time to convert hours to minutes.

$$1 \text{ hr} = 60 \text{ min}$$

III. The drop factor or number of drops that equal 1 ml of fluid. (This information can be found on the IV tubing box.)

$$10 \text{ gtt} = 1 \text{ ml}$$

Set up the problem by placing each of the 3 values in a proportion.

$$\frac{125 \text{ ml}}{1 \text{ hr}} \times \frac{1 \text{ hr}}{60 \text{ min}} \times \frac{10 \text{ gtt}}{1 \text{ ml}}$$

Numbers and units of measure can be canceled out from the upper and lower levels of this equation.

The numbers cancel, leaving:

$$\frac{125 \text{ ml}}{1 \text{ hr}} \times \frac{1 \text{ hr}}{\cancel{60}^{} \text{ min}} \times \frac{\cancel{10}^{1} \text{ gtt}}{1 \text{ ml}}$$

The units cancel, leaving:

$$\frac{125 \text{ ml}}{1 \text{ hr}} \times \frac{1 \text{ hr}}{6 \text{ min}} \times \frac{1 \text{ gtt}}{1 \text{ ml}}$$

Next, multiply each level across and divide the numerator by the denominator for the answer.

$$\frac{125 \text{ ml}}{1 \text{ hr}} \times \frac{1 \text{ hr}}{6 \text{ min}} \times \frac{1 \text{ gtt}}{1 \text{ ml}} = \frac{125 \text{ gtt}}{6 \text{ min}}$$

$$125 \div 6 = 20.8 \text{ or } 21 \text{ gtt/min}$$

### Calculation of Creatinine Clearance (CCr) in Adults from Serum Creatinine

$$\text{Men: CCr} = \frac{\text{weight (kg)} \times (140 - \text{age})}{72 \times \text{serum creatinine (mg/dl)}}$$

Women: CCr = 0.85 × calculation for men

### Calculation of Ideal Body Weight (kg) in Adults

$$\text{Men} = 50 \text{ kg} + 2.3 \text{ kg (each inch} >5 \text{ ft)}$$

$$\text{Women} = 45.5 \text{ kg} + 2.3 \text{ kg (each inch} >5 \text{ ft)}$$

## Calculation of Body Surface Area (BSA) in Adults and Children

*Dubois method:*

SA (cm$^2$) = wt (kg)$^{0.425}$ × ht (cm)$^{0.725}$ × 71.84

SA (m$^2$) K × $\sqrt[3]{\text{wt}^2 \text{ (kg)}}$ (common K value 0.1 for toddlers, 0.103 for neonates)

*Simplified method:*

$$\text{BSA (m}^2) = \sqrt{\frac{\text{ht (cm)} \times \text{wt (kg)}}{3600}}$$

## Body Mass Index

$$\text{BMI} = \text{wt (kg)} \div \text{ht (m}^2)$$

# Body Surface Area Nomograms

## ESTIMATING BODY SURFACE AREA IN CHILDREN

For pediatric patients of average size, body surface area may be estimated with the scale on the left. Match weight to corresponding surface area. For other pediatric patients, use the scale on the right. Lay a straightedge on the correct height and weight points for your patient, and observe the point where it intersects on the surface area scale at center.

**FOR CHILDREN OF NORMAL HEIGHT AND WEIGHT**

**NOMOGRAM FOR OTHER CHILDREN**

Reproduced from *Nelson Textbook of Pediatrics*, 16th edition. Courtesy W.B. Saunders Co., Philadelphia. PA.

## ESTIMATING BODY SURFACE AREA IN ADULTS

Use a straightedge to connect the patient's height in the left-hand column to weight in the right-hand column. The intersection of this line with the center scale estimates the body surface area.

| HEIGHT | BODY SURFACE AREA | WEIGHT |
|---|---|---|
| cm 200 ⎯ 79 inch | ⎯ 2.80 m² | kg 150 ⎯ 330 lb |
| 78 | | 145 ⎯ 320 |
| 195 ⎯ 77 | ⎯ 2.70 | 140 ⎯ 310 |
| 76 | | 135 ⎯ 300 |
| 190 ⎯ 75 | ⎯ 2.60 | 130 ⎯ 290 |
| 74 | ⎯ 2.50 | 280 |
| 185 ⎯ 73 | | 125 ⎯ 270 |
| 72 | ⎯ 2.40 | 120 ⎯ 260 |
| 180 ⎯ 71 | | 115 ⎯ 250 |
| 70 | ⎯ 2.30 | 110 ⎯ 240 |
| 175 ⎯ 69 | ⎯ 2.20 | 105 ⎯ 230 |
| 68 | | 100 ⎯ 220 |
| 170 ⎯ 67 | ⎯ 2.10 | |
| 66 | | 95 ⎯ 210 |
| 165 ⎯ 65 | ⎯ 2.00 | 90 ⎯ 200 |
| 64 | ⎯ 1.95 | |
| 160 ⎯ 63 | ⎯ 1.90 | 85 ⎯ 190 |
| 62 | ⎯ 1.85 | 180 |
| 155 ⎯ 61 | ⎯ 1.80 | 80 ⎯ 170 |
| 60 | ⎯ 1.75 | |
| 150 ⎯ 59 | ⎯ 1.70 | 75 ⎯ 160 |
| 58 | ⎯ 1.65 | 70 ⎯ 150 |
| 145 ⎯ 57 | ⎯ 1.60 | |
| 56 | ⎯ 1.55 | 65 ⎯ 140 |
| 140 ⎯ 55 | ⎯ 1.50 | |
| 54 | ⎯ 1.45 | 60 ⎯ 130 |
| 135 ⎯ 53 | ⎯ 1.40 | |
| 52 | ⎯ 1.35 | 55 ⎯ 120 |
| 130 ⎯ 51 | ⎯ 1.30 | |
| 50 | ⎯ 1.25 | 50 ⎯ 110 |
| 125 ⎯ 49 | | 105 |
| 48 | ⎯ 1.20 | 45 ⎯ 100 |
| 120 ⎯ 47 | ⎯ 1.15 | 95 |
| 46 | ⎯ 1.10 | 40 ⎯ 90 |
| 115 ⎯ 45 | | 85 |
| 44 | ⎯ 1.05 | |
| 110 ⎯ 43 | ⎯ 1.00 | 80 |
| 42 | ⎯ 0.95 | 35 ⎯ 75 |
| 105 ⎯ 41 | ⎯ 0.90 | 70 |
| 40 | | |
| cm 100 ⎯ 39 in | ⎯ 0.86 m² | kg 30 ⎯ 66 lb |

Reproduced from Lenter, C. (ed.) *Geigy Scientific Tables*, 8th edition. Courtesy CIBA-GEIGY, Basel Switzerland.

# Normal Values of Common Laboratory Tests

## SERUM TESTS

| HEMATOLOGIC | MEN | WOMEN |
|---|---|---|
| Hemoglobin | 13.5–18 g/dl | 12–16 g/dl |
| Hematocrit | 40–54% | 38–47% |
| Red blood cells (RBC) | 4.6–6.2 million/mm$^3$ | 4.2–5.4 million/mm$^3$ |
| Mean corpuscular volume (MCV) | 76–100 (micrometer)$^3$ | 76–100 (micrometer)$^3$ |
| Mean corpuscular hemoglobin (MCH) | 27–33 picogram | 27–33 picogram |
| Mean corpuscular hemoglobin concentration (MCHC) | 33–37 g/dl | 33–37 g/dl |
| Erythrocyte sedimentation rate (ESR) | ≤20 mm/hr | ≤30 mm/hr |
| Leukocytes (WBC) | 5000–10,000/mm$^3$ | 5000–10,000/mm$^3$ |
| Neutrophils | 54–75% (3000–7500/mm$^3$) | 54–75% (3000–7500/mm$^3$) |
| Bands | 3–8% (150–700/mm$^3$) | 3–8% (150–700/mm$^3$) |
| Eosinophils | 1–4% (50–400/mm$^3$) | 1–4% (50–400/mm$^3$) |
| Basophils | 0–1% (25–100/mm$^3$) | 0–1% (25–100/mm$^3$) |
| Monocytes | 2–8% (100–500/mm$^3$) | 2–8% (100–500/mm$^3$) |
| Lymphocytes | 25–40% (1500–4500/mm$^3$) | 25–40% (1500–4500/mm$^3$) |
| T lymphocytes | 60–80% of lymphocytes | 60–80% of lymphocytes |
| B lymphocytes | 10–20% of lymphocytes | 10–20% of lymphocytes |
| Platelets | 150,000–450,000/mm$^3$ | 150,000–450,000/mm$^3$ |
| Prothrombin time (PT) | 9.6–11.8 sec | 9.5–11.3 sec |
| Partial thromboplastin time (PTT) | 30–45 sec | 30–45 sec |
| Bleeding time (duke) | 1–3 min | 1–3 min |
| (ivy) | 3–6 min | 3–6 min |
| (template) | 3–6 min | 3–6 min |
| Clotting time (Lee-White) | 4–8 min | 4–8 min |

| CHEMISTRY | MEN | WOMEN |
|---|---|---|
| Sodium | 135–145 mEq/L | 135–145 mEq/L |
| Potassium | 3.5–5.0 mEq/L | 3.5–5.0 mEq/L |
| Chloride | 95–105 mEq/L | 95–105 mEq/L |
| Bicarbonate (HCO$_3$) | 19–25 mEq/L | 19–25 mEq/L |
| Total calcium | 9–11 mg/dl or 4.5–5.5 mEq/L | 9–11 mg/dl or 4.5–5.5 mEq/L |
| Ionized calcium | 4.2–5.4 mg/dl or 2.1–2.6 mEq/L | 4.2–5.4 mg/dl or 2.1–2.6 mEq/L |
| Phosphorus/phosphate | 2.4–4.7 mg/dl | 2.4–4.7 mg/dl |
| Magnesium | 1.8–3.0 mg/dl or 1.5–2.5 mEq/L | 1.8–3.0 mg/dl or 1.5–2.5 mEq/L |
| Glucose | 70–110 mg/dl | 70–110 mg/dl |
| Osmolality | 285–310 mOsm/kg | 285–310 mOsm/kg |
| Ammonia (NH$_3$) | 10–80 mcg/dl | 10–80 mcg/dl |
| Amylase | ≤130 U/L | ≤130 U/L |
| Creatine phosphokinase total (CK, CPK) | <150 U/L | <150 U/L |
| Creatine kinase isoenzymes, MB fraction | >5% in MI | >5% in MI |
| Lactic dehydrogenase (LDH) | 50–150 U/L | 50–150 U/L |
| Protein, total | 6–8 g/d | 6–8 g/d |
| Albumin | 4–6 g/dl | 4–6 g/dl |

| HEPATIC | MEN | WOMEN |
|---|---|---|
| AST | 8–46 U/L | 7–34 U/L |
| ALT | 10–30 IU/ml | 10–30 IU/ml |
| Total bilirubin | 0.3–1.2 mg/dl | 0.3–1.2 mg/dl |
| Conjugated bilirubin | 0.0–0.2 mg/dl | 0.0–0.2 mg/dl |
| Unconjugated (indirect) bilirubin | 0.2–0.8 mg/dl | 0.2–0.8 mg/dl |
| Alkaline phosphatase | 20–90 U/L | 20–90 U/L |

| RENAL | MEN | WOMEN |
|---|---|---|
| BUN | 6–20 mg/dl | 6–20 mg/dl |
| Creatinine | 0.6–1.3 mg/dl | 0.5–1.0 mg/dl |
| Uric acid | 4.0–8.5 mg/dl | 2.7–7.3 mg/dl |

| ARTERIAL BLOOD GASES | MEN | WOMEN |
|---|---|---|
| pH | 7.35–7.45 | 7.35–7.45 |
| $Po_2$ | 80–100 mmHg | 80–100 mmHg |
| $Pco_2$ | 35–45 mmHg | 35–45 mmHg |
| $O_2$ saturation | 95–97% | 95–97% |
| Base excess | +2–(−2) | +2–(−2) |
| Bicarbonate ($HCO_3^-$) | 22–26 mEq/L | 22–26 mEq/L |

**URINE TESTS**

| URINE | MEN | WOMEN |
|---|---|---|
| pH | 4.5–8.0 | 4.5–8.0 |
| Specific gravity | 1.010–1.025 | 1.010–1.025 |

# COMMONLY USED ABBREVIATIONS

| | |
|---|---|
| ABGs | arterial blood gases |
| ac | before meals |
| ACE | angiotensin-converting enzyme |
| ADH | antidiuretic hormone |
| A-G ratio | albumin-globulin ratio |
| AHF | antihemolytic factor |
| ALT | alanine aminotransferase |
| ANA | antinuclear antibodies |
| ANC | absolute neutrophil count |
| AST | aspartate aminotransferase |
| ATP | adenosine triphosphate |
| AV | atrioventricular |
| bid | two times a day |
| BMI | body mass index |
| BP | blood pressure |
| bpm | beats per minute |
| BSA | body surface area |
| BUN | blood urea nitrogen |
| cap | capsule |
| CBC | complete blood count |
| CCr | creatinine clearance |
| CNS | central nervous system |
| CPK | creatine phosphokinase |
| CR | controlled-release |
| CSF | colony-stimulating factor; cerebrospinal fluid |
| CT | computed tomography |
| CV | cardiovascular |
| CVP | central venous pressure |
| D5/LR | 5% dextrose and lactated Ringer's solution |
| D5/0.9% NaCl | 5% dextrose and 0.9% NaCl; 5% dextrose and normal saline |
| D5/0.25% NaCl | 5% dextrose and 0.25% NaCl; 5% dextrose and quarter normal saline |
| D5/0.45% NaCl | 5% dextrose and 0.45% NaCl; 5% dextrose and half normal saline |
| D5W | 5% dextrose in water |
| D10W | 10% dextrose in water |
| Derm | dermatologic |
| dl | deciliter |
| DMARD | disease-modifying antirheumatic drug |
| DNA | deoxyribonucleic acid |
| DVT | deep vein thrombosis |
| ECG | electrocardiogram |
| EENT | eye, ear, nose, and throat |
| Endo | endocrine |
| ER | extended-release |
| ESRD | end-stage renal disease |
| F and E | fluid and electrolyte |
| g | gram(s) |
| GABA | gamma-aminobutyric acid |
| GERD | gastroesophageal reflux disease |
| GFR | glomerular filtration rate |
| GI | gastrointestinal |
| G6PD | glucose-6-phosphate dehydrogenase |
| gt(t) | drop(s) |
| GTT | glucose tolerance test |
| GU | genitourinary |
| Hb A$_{1c}$ | hemoglobin A$_{1c}$, glycosylated hemoglobin |
| HDL | high-density lipoproteins |
| Hemat | hematologic |
| hr(s) | hour(s) |
| HRT | hormone replacement therapy |
| IA | intra-articular |
| IL | intralesional |
| IM | intramuscular |
| Inhaln | inhalation |
| INR | international normalized ratio |
| IPPB | intermittent positive-pressure breathing |
| IS | intrasynovial |

| | | | |
|---|---|---|---|
| **IT** | intrathecal | **pc** | after meals |
| **IV** | intravenous | **PCA** | patient-controlled analgesia |
| **K** | potassium | | |
| **KCl** | potassium chloride | **PO** | by mouth, orally |
| **kg** | kilogram | **prn** | as needed |
| **L** | liter | **PT** | prothrombin time |
| **LA** | long-acting | **PTT** | partial thromboplastin time |
| **LDH** | lactic dehydrogenase | | |
| **LDL** | low-density lipoproteins | **PVC** | premature ventricular contraction |
| **LR** | lactated Ringer's solution | | |
| **M** | molar | **q** | every |
| **MAO** | monoamine oxidase | **qid** | four times a day |
| **mcg** | microgram(s) | **q 2 hr** | every 2 hours |
| **MDI** | metered dose inhaler | **q 3 hr** | every 3 hours |
| **mEq** | milliequivalent | **q 4 hr** | every 4 hours |
| **Metab** | metabolic | **RBC** | red blood cell count |
| **mg** | milligram(s) | **Rect** | rectally or rectal |
| **min(s)** | minute(s) | **REM** | rapid eye movement |
| **Misc** | miscellaneous | **Resp** | respiratory |
| **ml** | milliliter(s) | **RTU** | ready to use |
| **mM** | millimole | **Rx** | prescription |
| **MRI** | magnetic resonance imaging | **SA** | sinoatrial |
| | | **subcut** | subcutaneous |
| **MS** | musculoskeletal | **sec(s)** | second(s) |
| **MUGA** | multiple-gated (image) acquisition (analysis) | **SL** | sublingual |
| | | **SR** | sustained-release |
| | | **SSRI(s)** | selective serotonin reuptake inhibitor(s) |
| **Na** | sodium | | |
| **NaCl** | sodium chloride | **stat** | immediately |
| **0.9% NaCl** | 0.9% sodium chloride, normal saline | **supp** | suppository |
| | | **tab** | tablet |
| **Neuro** | neurologic | **tbs** | tablespoon(s) |
| **NPO** | nothing by mouth | **tid** | three times a day |
| **NS** | sodium chloride, normal saline (0.9% NaCl) | **Top** | topically or topical |
| | | **tsp** | teaspoon(s) |
| | | **UK** | unknown |
| **NSAIDs** | nonsteroidal anti-inflammatory drugs | **Vag** | vaginal |
| | | **VFib** | ventricular fibrillation |
| **OCD** | obsessive-compulsive disorder | **VLDL** | very low-density lipoproteins |
| | | | |
| **Oint** | ointment | **VT** | ventricular tachycardia |
| **Ophth** | ophthalmic | **WBC** | white blood cell count |
| **OTC** | over-the-counter | **wk(s)** | week(s) |
| | | **yr(s)** | year(s) |

# Routine Pediatric and Adult Immunizations

## ROUTINE PEDIATRIC IMMUNIZATIONS

| GENERIC NAME (BRAND NAMES) | ROUTE AND DOSAGE | CONTRAINDICATIONS AND PRECAUTIONS | ADVERSE REACTIONS/SIDE EFFECTS | NOTES |
|---|---|---|---|---|
| DTaP diphtheria toxoid, tetanus toxoid, and acellular pertussis vaccine (Daptacel, Infanrix, Tripedia) | 0.5 ml IM at 2, 4, 6, and 15–18 mo; booster at 4–6 yr. | Acute infection, immunosuppressive therapy, previous CNS damage or convulsions. | Redness, tenderness, induration at site; fever; malaise; myalgia; urticaria; hypotension; neurologic reactions; allergic reactions (all less than with DTwP). | Individual components may be given as separate injections if unusual reactions occur. Tetanus and diphtheria toxoids (Td) should be given at 11–12 yr if at least 5 yr has elapsed since last dose of DTaP and then every 10 yr. |
| Polio vaccine, inactivated (IPV, IPOL, Poliovax) | 0.5 ml subcut at 2, 4, and 6–18 mo with a booster at 4–6 yr. | Hypersensitivity to neomycin, streptomycin, or polymyxin B; acute febrile illness. | Erythema, induration, pain at injection site; fever. | Oral polio vaccine (OPV) is no longer recommended for use in the United States. |
| Measles, mumps, and rubella vaccines (M-M-R II) | Single dose 0.5 ml subcut at 12–15 mo with a booster at 4–6 yr or 11–12 yr. | Allergy to egg, gelatin, or neomycin; active infection; immunosuppression. | Burning, stinging, pain at injection site; arthritis/arthralgia (40%); fever; encephalitis; allergic reactions. | If unusual reactions occur, individual components may be given as separate injections. |
| Hemophilus b conjugate vaccine (PedvaxHIB, ActHIB, HibTITER)* | 0.5 ml IM at 2, 4, and 6 mo (6 mo dose not needed for PedvaxHIB), with a booster at 12–15 mo. | If co-administered with other immunizations, consider contraindications of all products. | Induration, erythema, tenderness at injection site; fever. | |
| Hepatitis B vaccine (Engerix-B, Recombivax HB) | 10 mcg IM Engerix-B or 5 mcg IM Recombivax HB 1st dose at 0–2 mo, 2nd dose at 1–4 mo, and 3rd dose at 6–18 mo (1st and 2nd dose about 1 mo apart). Dose is same for patients up to 20 yr old. | Hypersensitivity to yeast. | Local soreness. | Children who have not been vaccinated as infants should complete the series by 12 yr. |

| GENERIC NAME (BRAND NAMES) | ROUTE AND DOSAGE | CONTRAINDICATIONS AND PRECAUTIONS | ADVERSE REACTIONS/SIDE EFFECTS | NOTES |
|---|---|---|---|---|
| | *Infants born to HBsAg-positive mothers:* Administer 0.5 ml of hepatitis B immune globulin within 12 hours of birth and 1st dose of 5 mcg Recombivax or 10 mcg of Engerix B IM and 2nd dose at 1–2 mo, 3rd dose at 6 mo. *Children up to 10 yr:* 2.5 mcg Recombivax HB or 10 mcg Engerix-B IM as 3-dose series; 2nd dose 1 mo after 1st dose, 3rd dose 4 mo after 1st dose, and 2 mo after 2nd dose. *Children up to 11–19 yr:* 5 mcg Recombivax HB or 10 mcg Engerix-B as 3-dose series; 2nd dose 1 mo after 1st dose, 3rd dose 4 mo after 1st dose, and 2 mo after 2nd dose. In children 11–15 yr, may also be given as two doses of 10 mcg/ml (Recombivax HB) 4–6 mo apart. | | | |
| Varicella vaccine (Varivax) | 0.5 ml IM single dose any time after 1st birthday; those without a history of chickenpox should be vaccinated at the 11–12 yr visit; children around age 13 yr should receive 2 doses 1 mo apart. | Allergy to gelatin or neomycin; active infection; immunosuppression, including HIV. | Local soreness, fever. | Given to children who have not been vaccinated or have not had chickenpox. Salicylates should be avoided for 6 wk following vaccination. |

| GENERIC NAME (BRAND NAMES) | ROUTE AND DOSAGE | CONTRAINDICATIONS AND PRECAUTIONS | ADVERSE REACTIONS/SIDE EFFECTS | NOTES |
|---|---|---|---|---|
| Hepatitis A vaccine (Havrix, Vaqta) | *Children 2–18 yr:* 0.5 ml IM (pediatric formulation), repeated 6–12 mo later (pediatric dose form). | Acute febrile illness. | Local reactions, headache. | Recommended for children in areas with high rates of hepatitis A and other high-risk groups. |
| Pneumococcal 7-valent conjugate vaccine (Prevnar) | *Infants:* 0.5 ml IM for 4 doses at 2, 4, 6, and 12–15 mo. *Older infants and children starting at 7–11 mo of age:* Three doses of 0.5 ml IM, 2 doses at least 4 wk apart, 3rd dose after 1 yr birthday. *Starting at 12–23 mo of age:* Two doses of 0.5 ml IM at least 2 mo apart. *Starting 2–6 yr:* Single dose 0.5 ml IM. | Hypersensitivity to all components including diphtheria toxoid; moderate to severe febrile illness; thrombocytopenia or coagulation disorder. Use cautiously in patients receiving anticoagulants; safe use in children <6 wk not established. | Erythema induration, tenderness, nodule formation at injection site, fever. | Antineoplastics, corticosteroids, radiation therapy, and immunosuppressants decrease antibody response; product is a suspension, shake before use. |

| GENERIC NAME (BRAND NAMES) | ROUTE AND DOSAGE | CONTRAINDICATIONS AND PRECAUTIONS | ADVERSE REACTIONS/SIDE EFFECTS | NOTES |
|---|---|---|---|---|
| Influenza vaccine *injection:* (Fluvirin, Fuzone); *intranasal:* (FluMist) | *Injection: Children 6–35 mo:* 0.25 ml IM 1–2 doses (2 doses at least one mo apart for initial season) followed by single dose annually. *Children 3–8 yr:* 0.5 ml IM 1–2 doses (2 doses at least one mo apart for initial season) followed by single dose annually. *Children ≥9 yr:* 0.5 ml IM single dose annually. *Nasal: Children 5–8 yr:* If not previously immunized with Flu- Mist—2 doses of 0.5 ml intranasally (given as one 0.25 ml dose in each nostril) at least 2 mo apart, then one dose annually. If previously immunized with FluMist, 1 dose of 0.5 ml intranasally (given as one 0.25-ml dose in each nostril) annually. *Children ≥9 yr:* 1 dose of 0.5 ml intranasally (given as one 0.25-ml dose in each nostril) annually. | Hypersensitivity to eggs/egg products. Hypersensitivity to thimerosal (injection only). Fluvirin should be used in children >4 yr only. Avoid use in patients with acute neurologic compromise. FluMist should be avoided in patients receiving salicylates or who are immunocompromised. | *Injection:* local soreness, fever myalgia, possible neurologic toxicity. *Intranasal:* upper respiratory congestion, malaise. | Immunosupression may decrease antibody response to injection and increase the risk of viral transmission with intranasal route. |

*Available in varying concentrations.

## Nursing Implications:

### Assessment

Assess previous immunization history and history of hypersensitivity.

Assess patient for history of asthma or reactive airway disease. Patients with positive history should not receive FluMist.

### Potential Nursing Diagnoses

Infection, risk for (Indications).

Knowledge, deficient, related to medication regimen (Patient/Family Teaching).

### Implementation

■ Measles, mumps, and rubella vaccine; trivalent oral poliovirus vaccine; and diphtheria toxoid, tetanus toxoid, and pertussis vaccine may be given concomitantly.

■ Do not administer FluMist concurrently with other vaccines, or in patients who have received a live virus vaccine within 1 mo or an inactivated vaccine within 2 wks of vaccination.

■ Administer each immunization by appropriate route:

■ PO: Polio (Orimune)

■ Subcut: measles, mumps, rubella, polio (IPOl, Poliovax)

■ IM: diphtheria, tetanus toxoid, pertussis.

■ Intranasal: FluMist.

### Patient/Family Teaching

■ Inform parent of potential and reportable side effects of immunization. Physician should be notified if patient develops fever higher than 39.4°C (103°F); difficulty breathing; hives; itching; swelling of eyes, face, or inside of nose; sudden, severe tiredness or weakness; or convulsions.

■ Review next scheduled immunization with parent.

### Evaluation

**Effectiveness of therapy can be demonstrated by:** Prevention of diseases through active immunity.

## ROUTINE ADULT IMMUNIZATIONS

| GENERIC NAME (BRAND NAMES) | INDICATIONS | DOSAGE/ROUTE | CONTRAINDICATIONS | ADVERSE REACTIONS/SIDE EFFECTS |
|---|---|---|---|---|
| Hepatitis A vaccine (Havrix, Vaqta)† | High-risk patients, some health care workers, food handlers, clotting disorders, travel to endemic areas, chronic liver disease. | 1 ml IM, followed by 1 ml IM 6–12 mo later (adult dose form). | Hypersensitivity to alum or 2-phenoxyethanol. | Local soreness, headache. |
| Hepatitis B vaccine (Engerix-B, Recombivax HB) | High-risk patients, health care workers, all unvaccinated adolescents. | 3 doses of 1 ml IM, given at 0, 1, and 4–6 mo. | Anaphylactic allergy to yeast. | Local soreness. |
| Influenza vaccine (*Injection:* Fluzone, Fluvirin); *nasal:* (FluMist) | All adults | *Injection:* 0.5 ml IM annually. *Intranasal for adults <50 yr:* Single 0.5 ml dose given as 0.25 ml in each nostril annually. | Hypersensitivity to eggs/egg products. Hypersensitivity to thimerosal (injection only). Avoid use in patients with acute neurologic compromise. Flu-Mist should be avoided in patients receiving salicylates or who are immunocompromised. | *Injection:* local soreness, fever myalgia, possible neurologic toxicity. *Intranasal:* upper respiratory congestion, malaise. Immunosuppression may decrease antibody response to injection and increase the risk of viral transmission with intranasal route. |
| Measles, mumps, and rubella vaccines (M-M-R II) | Adults with unreliable history MMR illness or immunization, occupational exposure. | 0.5 ml subcut, single dose in those with unreliable history, 2 doses one mo apart for those with occupational exposure. | Allergy to egg, gelatin, or neomycin; active infection; immunosuppression; pregnancy; also avoid becoming pregnant for 4 wk after immunization. | Burning, stinging, pain at injection site; arthritis/arthralgia; fever; encephalitis; allergic reactions. |
| Pneumococcal vaccine, polyvalent (Pneumovax 23, Pnu-Imune 23) | Everyone >65 yr, high-risk patients with chronic illnesses including HIV and other high-risk patients. | 0.5 ml IM, high-risk patients (asplenics) should have a booster after 6 yr. | Safety in first trimester of pregnancy not established. | Local soreness. |
| Tetanus-diphtheria (Adult Td) | All adults. | *Unimmunized:* 2 doses 0.5 ml IM 1–2 mo apart, then a 3rd dose 6–12 mo later; *immunized:* booster every 10 yr. | Neurologic or severe hypersensitivity reaction to prior dose. | Local pain and swelling. |

| GENERIC NAME (BRAND NAMES) | INDICATIONS | DOSAGE/ROUTE | CONTRAINDICATIONS | ADVERSE REACTIONS/SIDE EFFECTS |
|---|---|---|---|---|
| Varicella vaccine (Varivax) | Any adult without a history of chickenpox or herpes zoster. | 0.5 ml subcut; repeated 4–8 wk later. | Allergy to gelatin or neomycin; active infection; immunosuppression including HIV; pregnancy; family history of immunodeficiency; blood/blood product in past 5 mo. | Salicylates should be avoided for 6 wk following vaccination. |

†Less commonly used vaccines are not included.

SOURCE: Adapted from the recommendations of the National Immunization Program: http://www.cdc.gov/nip.

# Food and Drug Administration Pregnancy Categories

## Category A

Adequate, well-controlled studies in pregnant women have not shown an increased risk of fetal abnormalities.

## Category B

Animal studies have revealed no evidence of harm to the fetus, however, there are no adequate and well-controlled studies in pregnant women. **or** Animal studies have shown an adverse effect, but adequate and well-controlled studies in pregnant women have failed to demonstrate a risk to the fetus.

## Category C

Animal studies have shown an adverse effect and there are no adequate and well-controlled studies in pregnant women. **or** No animal studies have been conducted and there are no adequate and well-controlled studies in pregnant women.

## Category D

Studies, adequate well-controlled or observational, in pregnant women have demonstrated a risk to the fetus. However, the benefits of therapy may outweigh the potential risk.

## Category X

Studies, adequate well-controlled or observational, in animals or pregnant women have demonstrated positive evidence of fetal abnormalities. The use of the product is contraindicated in women who are or may become pregnant.

# Recommendations for the Safe Handling of Hazardous Drugs*

## Introduction/Categorization

This is a summary of the revised Occupational Safety and Health Administration Guidelines for the Safe Handling of Hazardous Drugs. Previous guidelines referred to Safe Handling of *Cytotoxic* Drugs. The revised guidelines use the term *Hazardous* Drugs (HDs) in order to include other drugs (such as some antivirals, hormones) that also display toxic, carcinogenic, mutagenic, and/or teratogenic potential. These agents may also cause irritation to the skin, eyes, and mucous membranes and ulceration and necrosis of tissue. The toxicity of HDs dictates that the exposure of health care personnel to these drugs in any setting should be minimized. At the same time, the requirement for maintenance of aseptic conditions for most agents must be satisfied.

Some substances are also identified as hazardous waste pharmaceuticals as part of the Resource Conservation and Recovery Act (RCRA) of the Environmental Protection Agency. Epinephrine, nitroglycerin, and warfarin are such products.

## HDs as Occupational Risks

Exposure to HDs should be minimized because they bind to genetic material and may affect cellular protein synthesis. HDs also may not be able to differentiate between cancerous and normal cells. These risks have been documented in animal and human studies.

The primary potential routes of exposure during preparation and administration are via inhalation of dusts or aerosols, dermal absorption, and ingestion. Potential exposure to hazardous drugs may occur at many points in the handling of these agents. These sources of exposure have been documented by studies demonstrating the presence of HDs or their metabolites in the blood or urine of workers who handle them, in overt toxicity to organ systems in these workers, or in reproductive abnormalities. Deleterious effects may be increased if workers also smoke cigarettes.

## Preparation Areas

In large specialized institutions, HDs are usually prepared in the pharmacy. However, in many small hospitals, clinics, and physicians' offices, HDs are routinely prepared in uncontrolled settings. The risk of exposure is greatest for nurses who work in outpatient settings. During the preparation of HDs for administration, even when great care is taken, splattering, spraying, and aerosolization may occur during needle withdrawal from vials, during drug transfer, during opening of ampules, and during expulsion of air from syringes. Although horizontal-airflow workbenches provide an aseptic area for preparation of HDs, they increase exposure to HDs by personnel in the work area. As a result, horizontal Biologic Safety Cabinets (BSCs) should not be used in preparation areas. Risk of exposure is also increased by smoking, drinking, applying cosmetics, or eating in areas where HDs are prepared, stored, or administered.

Other activities that increase exposure during administration should also be prohibited. These include clipping needles and crushing syringes. Excreta from patients receiving HDs may contain

---

*Controlling occupational exposure to hazardous drugs. Am J Health Syst Pharm 1996; 53:1669-1685.

potentially damaging concentrations of HDs and/or their metabolites; unprotected handling should be avoided. When materials contaminated in any way with HDs are to be handled, the use of properly labeled, sealed, and covered containers by trained personnel is required. Additional procedures are required where contamination with blood or body fluids has occurred.

## Prevention of Employee Exposure

Each setting should have a written HD safety and health plan. This plan should be easily accessible and include the following:

- Procedures that safeguard safety and health of workers exposed to HDs
- Criteria for measures designed to reduce HD exposure
- Presence of ventilation equipment and its maintenance
- Provision of information and training
- Procedures for handling investigational HDs
- Provision of medical care for employees exposed to HDs
- Designation of specific employees responsible for implementation of the HD safety and health plan

## Preparation of HDs

Where allowable, specified HD-handling areas should be designated in a restricted, centralized location. Activities known to increase exposure should be prohibited in this area. The posting in the work area of guidelines for handling spills and emergencies is recommended. Under optimal conditions, preparation of HDs should take place in a Class II, Type B, or Class III BSC (with venting to the outside) that undergoes routine maintenance and decontamination. If a BSC is not available, personnel preparing HDs should wear a respirator with a high-efficiency filter until a BSC is available. Full face coverage or partial face coverage with splash goggles should be used with the respirator.

Personnel handling HDs should wear personal protective equipment (PPE). Double latex gloving is generally recommended. Gloves should be changed hourly or more frequently if damaged or contaminated. Protective gowns should also be worn and should be tucked into gloves at the wrist (inner glove under cuff, outer glove over cuff). Employees should be trained in the proper removal of PPE. Chemical-barrier face and eye protection should be used near splashes, sprays, or aerosols. Eyewash facilities should be available. All PPEs should be disposed of properly or, when appropriate, cleaned for reuse.

When working with HDs, a disposable plastic-backed paper liner should be placed in the BCS and changed routinely. Syringes and IV sets with Luer-Lok fittings should be used for preparation of HDs. Syringe size should be compatible with volume required. Excess solution should be discarded in a covered disposable container; a covered "sharps" container should also be available. All HDs and materials should be disposed of in clearly labeled bags.

Aseptic technique should be used in a manner consistent with working in a BSC. PPEs should be donned prior to work and necessary equipment placed in the BSC. All syringes and IV bags must be labeled with a distinctive warning label in addition to standard labeling. Needles must be disposed of in "sharps" containers (crushing, clipping, or capping is prohibited). Extremes in pressure generated in vials should be avoided. Multi-use dispensing pins or venting devices may be preferable to needles alone for this purpose. The remainder of the procedure involving vials or ampules should be performed to minimize spraying or dripping. Once prepared, bags or bottles should be wiped with moist gauze; entry ports should be swabbed with alcohol and capped. The entire unit should be packaged in a sealed plastic bag placed inside a secure container. Nonliquid doses should be counted, compounded, or handled inside a BSC using equipment designated for that purpose only.

## Administration of HDs

The same PPEs should be worn as for preparation (gown, gloves, splash goggles). A respirator should be worn while administering aerosolized drugs. In addition to PPE the following equipment may be packaged for use during administration: gauze for cleanup, alcohol wipes, disposable plastic-backed absorbent liner, puncture-resistant container (for needles/syringes), resealable plastic bag with warning label and other accessory warning labels.

The following work practices should be employed:

- Hands should be washed before donning gloves and after gloves are removed. Contaminated equipment should be replaced immediately and disposed of properly.
- All infusion pumps and IV sets should have Luer-Lok fittings and be inspected frequently for leakage. Disposable plastic-backed absorbent liner should be placed under tubing; sterile gauze should cover IV push sites and connection sites should be taped.
- Priming/air expelling should take place in the BSC; if not, priming should be done with a nondrug solution or a backflow closed system should be used. Vented systems should not be used.
- Syringes, IV bottles, bags, and pumps should be wiped clean with gauze. Needles and syringes should be placed in a puncture-resistant container and then into an HD disposal bag. Administration sets should be disposed of intact. Waste bags should follow HD disposal requirements, and unused drugs should be returned to the pharmacy. PPE should be properly disposed of and reusable materials washed for future use.
- Spill and emergency skin and eye decontamination kits and other materials should be readily available in areas where HDs are administered.
- If splashing is a possibility, PPE should be used during administration of oral HDs.
- Investigational HDs should be administered only by experienced personnel.

These procedures should be observed as closely as possible in the home care environment. Patients and caregivers should have ready access to providers and emergency protocols.

Aerosolized drugs require controls to prevent exposure to individuals in the vicinity of drug administration. Specific isolation and ventilation techniques may be used.

## Caring for Patients Receiving HDs

Universal precautions should be observed to prevent contact with any potentially infectious/hazardous materials. Gowns and gloves should be worn by personnel for 48 hr following administration and replaced if contamination occurs. If splashing is possible, eye protection should be worn. Contaminated linens should be bagged separately and prewashed before being washed with other laundry. Laundry personnel should wear gowns/gloves when handling contaminated linens. Reusable items should be washed twice with detergent by personnel wearing gowns and double gloves.

Disposed equipment must be specially bagged and labeled. Needles/syringes/breakable items contaminated with blood or other potentially infectious materials must be disposed of in a "sharps" container. Such disposal containers should be readily available in patient care areas and sealed and replaced routinely. Care should be taken to avoid exterior contamination of all waste containers; if this occurs, the contaminated container should be placed inside another uncontaminated container. HD waste must be disposed of separately from other waste in accordance with applicable regulations.

Spills should be cleaned up by properly protected personnel, using the facility's procedure. The area of spill should be identified and reported.

If contamination of personnel occurs, the following should be performed:

- Immediately remove gloves/gown.
- Immediately cleanse the affected skin with soap and water.

- Flood affected eye at eyewash fountain or flush with water or isotonic eyewash for at least 15 min.
- Obtain medical attention and follow protocols for specific exposure.
- Document exposure.

Small spills (less than 5 ml or 5 g) should be cleaned up by personnel in gowns, gloves, splash protectors, and a respirator, if necessary. Liquids may be mopped up with absorbent gauze, solids with damp gauze, followed by three washings of the area with detergent followed by water. Broken fragments should be picked up with a scoop and properly disposed of.

Large spill areas should be isolated. Absorbent sheets or spill-control pads should be used. Damp cloths should be used if a powder is spilled. Spills greater than 150 ml (or 1 vial) in a BSC necessitate decontamination of the BSC. If the filter of the BSC is contaminated, the unit should be sealed until maintenance can be performed by experienced personnel.

Spill kits should be readily available in areas where HDs are handled. The kit should include splash goggles, 2 pairs of gloves, utility gloves, gown, 2 sheets of absorbent material, spill-control pillows (2 sizes), "sharps" container, and 2 large HD disposal bags.

## Medical Surveillance

Personnel who work with HDs should be routinely monitored to prevent occupational injury and disease. This should include examination before employment, routinely during employment, following acute exposure, and upon termination of employment. Special consideration should be given to reproductive issues. Employers must develop and maintain hazard communication programs and provide information about HDs. Employees must be informed of the risks of working with HDs. Training must be provided to minimize exposure. Records of such programs must be maintained by the institution.

# Schedules of Controlled Substances

Classes or schedules are determined by the Drug Enforcement Agency (DEA), an arm of the United States Justice Department, and are based on the potential for abuse and dependence liability (physical and psychological) of the medication. Some states may have stricter prescription regulations. Physicians, dentists, podiatrists, and veterinarians may prescribe controlled substances. Nurse practitioners and physician's assistants may prescribe controlled substances with certain limitations.

## Schedule I (C-I)

Potential for abuse is so high as to be unacceptable. May be used for research with appropriate limitations. Examples are LSD and heroin.

## Schedule II (C-II)

High potential for abuse and extreme liability for physical and psychological dependence (amphetamines, opioid analgesics, dronabinol, certain barbiturates). Outpatient prescriptions must be in writing. In emergencies, telephone orders may be acceptable if a written prescription is provided within 72 hr. No refills are allowed.

### Schedule II Drugs Included in *Davis's Drug Guide for Nurses:*

**amphetamine**
**codeine** (single entity; solid dosage form or injectable)
**dexmethylphenidate**
**dextroamphetamine**
**droperidol**
**fentanyl**
**hydromorphone**

**meperidine**
**methadone**
**methylphenidate**
**morphine**
**oxycodone** (alone and in combination with nonopioid analgesics)
**pentobarbital** (oral and parenteral)

## Schedule III (C-III)

Intermediate potential for abuse (less than C-II) and intermediate liability for physical and psychological dependence (certain nonbarbiturate sedatives, certain nonamphetamine CNS stimulants, and limited dosages of certain opioid analgesics). Outpatient prescriptions can be refilled 5 times within 6 mo from date of issue if authorized by prescriber. Telephone orders are acceptable.

### Schedule III Drugs Included in *Davis's Drug Guide for Nurses:*

**butalbital compound** (in combination with nonopioid analgesics)
**codeine** (in combination with nonopioid analgesics; solid oral dosage forms)

**hydrocodone** (in combination with nonopioid analgesics)
**nandrolone decanoate**
**pentobarbital** (rectal)
**testosterone transdermal**

## Schedule IV (C-IV)

Less abuse potential than Schedule III with minimal liability for physical or psychological dependence (certain sedative/hypnotics, certain antianxiety agents, some barbiturates, benzodiazepines, chloral hydrate, pentazocine, and propoxyphene). Outpatient prescriptions can be refilled 6 times within 6 mo from date of issue if authorized by prescriber. Telephone orders are acceptable.

**Schedule IV Drugs Included in** *Davis's Drug Guide for Nurses:*

alprazolam
butorphanol
chloral hydrate
chlordiazepoxide
clonazepam
clorazepate
codeine (elixir or oral suspension with acetaminophen)
diazepam
difenoxin/atropine
flurazepam
lorazepam
meprobamate

midazolam
oxazepam
pemoline
pentazocine
phenobarbital
phentermine
propoxyphene
sibutramine
temazepam
triazolam
zaleplon
zolpidem

## Schedule V (C-V)

Minimal abuse potential. Number of outpatient refills determined by prescriber. Some products (cough suppressants with small amounts of codeine, antidiarrheals containing paregoric) may be available without prescription to patients >18 yr of age.

**Schedule V Drugs Included in** *Davis's Drug Guide for Nurses:*

buprenorphine
diphenoxylate/atropine

# APPENDIX O
# Equianalgesic Dosing Guidelines

## Opioid Analgesics Starting Oral Dose Commonly Used for Severe Pain

| Name | Equianalgesic Dose | | Starting Oral Dose | | Comments | Precautions and Contraindications |
|------|------|------|------|------|------|------|
| | Oral* | Parenteral† | Adults | Children | | |
| **a. Morphine-like agonists (mu agonists)** | | | | | | |
| *morphine*off | 30 mg | 10 mg | 15–30 mg | 0.3 mg/kg | Standard of comparison for opioid analgesics. Sustained release preparations (MS Contin, OramorphSR) release over 8–12 hours. Other formulations (Kadian and Avinza) last 12–24 hours. Generic sustained release morphine preparations are now available. | For all opioids, caution in patients with impaired ventilation, bronchial asthma, increased intracranial pressure, liver failure. |
| *hydromorphone*off *(Dilaudid)* | 7.5 mg | 1.5 mg | 4–8 mg | 0.06 mg/kg | Slightly shorter duration than morphine. | |
| *oxycodone*off | 20 mg | — | 10–20 mg | 0.3 mg/kg | Good oral potency, long plasma half-life (24–36 hours). | |
| *methadone*off | 10 mg | 5 mg | 5–10 mg | 0.2 mg/kg | | |
| *levorphanol*off *(Levodromoran)* | 4 mg (acute) 1 mg (chronic) | 2 mg (acute) 1 mg (chronic) | 2–4 mg | 0.04 mg/kg | Long plasma half-life (12–16 hours, but may be as long as 90–120 hrs after one week of dosing). | Accumulates on days 2 and 3. Use with caution in older adults. |
| *oxymorphone*off *(Numorphan)* | — | 1 mg | — | — | 5 mg rectal suppository ~ 5 mg morphine parenteral. | Like parenteral morphine. |

Accumulates with repeated dosing, requiring decreases in dose size and frequency, especially on days 2–5. Use with caution in older adults.

| Name | Equianalgesic Dose | | Starting Oral Dose | | Comments | Precautions and Contraindications |
|---|---|---|---|---|---|---|
| | Oral[*] | Parenteral[†] | Adults | Children | | |
| *meperidine*off (*Demerol*) | 300 mg | 75 mg | Not Recommended | | Slightly shorter acting than morphine accumulates with repetitive dosing causing CNS excitation; avoid in children with impaired renal function or who are receiving monoamine oxidase inhibitors.[‡] | Use with caution. Normeperidine (toxic metabolite) accumulates with repetitive dosing causing CNS excitation and a high risk of seizure. Avoid in children, renal impairment and patients on monoamine oxidase inhibitors.[‡] |
| **b. Mixed agonists–antagonists (kappa agonists)** | | | | | | |
| *nalbuphine*off (*Nubain*) | — | 10 mg | — | — | Not available orally, not scheduled under Controlled Substances Act. | Incidence of psychotomimetic effects lower than with pentazocine; may precipitate withdrawal in opioid-dependent patients. |
| *butorphanol*off (*Stadol*) | — | 2 mg | — | — | Like nalbuphine. Also available in nasal spray. | Like nalbuphine. |
| *pentazocine*off (*Talwin*) | 50 mg | 30 mg | — | — | Lower abuse liability than morphine; does not produce psychotomimetic effects. Sublingual tablets now available both plain and with naloxone for opioid-dependent patient management for specially certified physicians. These tablets are not approved as analgesics. | |
| **c. Partial agonist** | | | | | | |
| *buprenorphine*off (*Buprenex*) | — | 0.4 mg | — | — | | May precipitate withdrawal in narcotic-dependent patients; not readily reversed by naloxone; avoid in labor. |

*Starting dose should be lower for older adults.

†These are standard parenteral doses for acute pain in adults and can also be used to convert doses for IV infusions and repeated small IV boluses. For single IV boluses, use half the IM dose. IV doses for children >6 mos. = parenteral equianalgesic dose times weight (kg)/100.

‡Irritating to tissues with repeated IM injections.

Modified from *American Pain Society, Principles of Analgesic Use in the Treatment of Acute Pain and Cancer Pain*, ed.5. American Pain Society, 2003.

**Guidelines for Patient-Controlled Intravenous Opioid Administration for Adults with Acute Pain**

| Drug[§] | Usual Starting Dose After Loading | Usual Dose Range | Usual Lockout (minutes) | Usual Lockout Range (minutes) |
|---|---|---|---|---|
| Morphine (1 mg/mL) | 1 mg | 0.5–2.5 mg | 8 | 5–10 |
| Hydromorphone (0.2 mg/mL) | 0.2 mg | 0.05–0.4 mg | 8 | 5–10 |
| Fentanyl (50 mcg/mL) | 10 mcg | 10–50 mcg | 6 | 5–8 |

§Standard concentrations for most PCA machines are listed in parentheses.
Modified from *American Pain Society, Principles of Analgesic Use in the Treatment of Acute Pain and Cancer Pain*, ed.5. American Pain Society, 2003.

## FENTANYL TRANSDERMAL DOSE BASED ON DAILY MORPHINE DOSE[¶]

| ORAL 24-HR MORPHINE (mg/day) | IM 24-HR MORPHINE (mg/day) | FENTANYL TRANSDERMAL (mcg/hr) |
|---|---|---|
| 45–134 | 8–22 | 25 |
| 135–224 | 23–37 | 50 |
| 225–314 | 38–52 | 75 |
| 315–404 | 53–67 | 100 |
| 405–494 | 68–82 | 125 |
| 495–584 | 83–97 | 150 |
| 585–674 | 98–112 | 175 |
| 675–764 | 113–127 | 200 |
| 765–854 | 128–142 | 225 |
| 855–944 | 143–157 | 250 |
| 945–1034 | 158–172 | 275 |
| 1035–1124 | 173–187 | 300 |

¶A 10-mg IM or 60-mg oral dose of morphine every 4 hr for 24 hr (total of 60 mg/day IM or 360 mg/day oral) was considered approximately equivalent to fentanyl transdermal 100 mcg/hr.

# APPENDIX P

# Syringe Compatibility Chart

**KEY**

- C = Compatible
- L = Compatible for a limited period
- I = Incompatible
- * = Conflicting data
- − = Data unavailable
- ■ = Identical drug

## Syringe Compatibility

| Drug | 1. atropine | 2. benzquinamide | 3. buprenorphine | 4. butorphanol | 5. chlorpromazine | 6. diazepam | 7. diphenhydramine | 8. droperidol | 9. glycopyrrolate | 10. hydromorphone | 11. hydroxyzine | 12. meperidine | 13. metoclopramide | 14. midazolam | 15. morphine | 16. nalbuphine | 17. pentazocine | 18. pentobarbital | 19. prochlorperazine | 20. promethazine | 21. scopolamine |
|---|---|---|---|---|---|---|---|---|---|---|---|---|---|---|---|---|---|---|---|---|---|
| 1. atropine | ■ | C | − | L | L | − | L | L | C | L | L | L | L | L | L | C | L | * | L | L | L |
| 2. benzquinamide | C | ■ | − | − | − | I | − | − | C | − | C | C | − | L | C | − | C | I | − | − | C |
| 3. buprenorphine | − | − | ■ | − | − | − | − | − | − | − | − | − | L | − | − | − | − | − | − | − | − |
| 4. butorphanol | L | − | − | ■ | L | − | L | L | − | − | C | L | L | L | L | L | − | L | I | L | L |
| 5. chlorpromazine | L | − | − | L | ■ | − | L | L | C | L | L | L | L | L | L | L | − | L | I | L | L |
| 6. diazepam | − | I | − | − | − | ■ | − | − | I | − | − | − | − | − | − | I | − | − | − | − | − |
| 7. diphenhydramine | L | − | − | L | L | − | ■ | L | C | L | L | L | L | L | L | C | L | I | L | L | L |
| 8. droperidol | L | − | − | L | L | − | L | ■ | C | − | L | L | L | L | L | C | L | I | L | L | L |
| 9. glycopyrrolate | C | C | − | − | C | I | C | C | ■ | C | C | C | − | L | C | C | I | I | C | C | C |
| 10. hydromorphone | L | − | − | − | L | − | L | − | C | ■ | L | − | − | L | − | − | L | L | * | L | L |
| 11. hydroxyzine | L | C | − | C | L | − | L | L | C | L | ■ | L | L | L | L | C | L | I | L | L | L |
| 12. meperidine | L | C | − | L | L | − | L | L | C | − | L | ■ | L | L | I | − | L | I | L | L | L |
| 13. metoclopramide | L | − | − | L | L | − | L | L | − | − | L | L | ■ | L | * | − | L | − | L | L | L |
| 14. midazolam | L | L | L | L | L | − | L | L | L | L | L | L | L | ■ | L | * | L | − | I | I | L |
| 15. morphine | L | C | − | L | L | − | L | L | C | − | L | I | * | * | ■ | − | L | * | * | * | L |
| 16. nalbuphine | C | − | − | − | − | I | C | C | C | − | C | − | − | L | − | ■ | − | I | C | * | C |
| 17. pentazocine | L | C | − | L | L | − | L | L | I | L | L | L | L | − | L | − | ■ | I | L | L | L |
| 18. pentobarbital | * | I | − | I | I | − | I | I | I | L | I | I | − | I | * | I | I | ■ | I | I | L |
| 19. prochlorperazine | L | − | − | L | L | − | L | L | C | * | L | L | L | I | * | C | L | I | ■ | L | L |
| 20. promethazine | L | − | − | L | L | − | L | L | C | L | L | L | L | L | * | * | L | I | L | ■ | L |
| 21. scopolamine | L | C | − | L | L | − | L | L | C | L | L | L | L | L | L | C | L | L | L | L | ■ |

# Food Sources for Specific Nutrients

## Potassium-Rich Foods

apricots
avocados
bananas
broccoli
cantaloupe
dried fruits
grapefruit
honey dew

kiwi
lima beans
meats
dried peas and beans
nuts
oranges
peaches
plantains (white and sweet)

potatoes
prunes
rhubarb
spinach
sunflower seeds
tomatoes
winter squash

## Sodium-Rich Foods

baking mixes (pancakes, muffins)
barbecue sauce
buttermilk
butter/margarine
canned chili
canned seafood
canned soups

canned spaghetti sauce
cured meats
dry onion soup mix
"fast" foods
frozen dinners
macaroni and cheese
microwave dinners
Parmesan cheese

pickles
potato salad
pretzels, potato chips
salad dressings (prepared)
salt
sauerkraut
tomato ketchup

## Calcium-Rich Foods

bok choy
broccoli
canned salmon/sardines
clams

cream soups
milk and dairy products
molasses (blackstrap)
oysters

refried beans
spinach
tofu
turnip greens

## Vitamin K-Rich Foods

asparagus
beans
broccoli
brussel sprouts
cabbage

cauliflower
collards
green tea
kale
milk

mustard greens
spinach
swiss chard
turnips
yogurt

## Low-Sodium Foods

baked or broiled poultry
canned pumpkin
cooked turnips
egg yolk
fresh vegetables
fruit

grits (not instant)
honey
jams and jellies
lean meats
low-calorie mayonnaise
macaroons

potatoes
puffed wheat and rice
red kidney and lima beans
sherbet
unsalted nuts
whiskey

## Foods That Acidify Urine

cheeses
corn
cranberries
eggs
fish

grains (breads and cereals)
lentils
meats
nuts (Brazil, filberts, walnuts)
pasta

plums
poultry
prunes
rice

## Foods That Alkalinize Urine

all fruits except cranberries,
   prunes, plums

all vegetables (except corn)
milk

nuts (almonds, chestnuts)

## Foods Containing Tyramine

aged cheeses (blue, Boursault,
   brick, Brie, Camembert,
   cheddar, Emmentaler,
   Gruyère, mozzarella, Parmesan, Romano, Roquefort,
   Stilton, Swiss)
American processed cheese
avocados (especially over-ripe)
bananas
bean curd
beer and ale

caffeine-containing beverages
   (coffee, tea, colas)
caviar
chocolate
distilled spirits
fermented sausage (bologna, sa-
   lami, pepperoni, summer
   sausage)
liver
meats prepared with tenderizer
miso soup
over-ripe fruit

peanuts
raisins
raspberries
red wine (especially Chianti)
sauerkraut
sherry
shrimp paste
smoked or pickled fish
soy sauce
vermouth
yeasts
yogurt

## Iron-Rich Foods

cereals
clams
dried beans and peas

dried fruit
leafy green vegetables
lean red meats

molasses (blackstrap)
organ meats

## Vitamin D-Rich Foods

canned salmon, sardines, tuna
cereals

fish
fish liver oils

fortified milk
nonfat dry milk

# Insulins and Insulin Therapy

Most insulins used today are recombinant DNA human insulins. Produced through genetic engineering, synthetic human insulin is "manufactured" by yeast or nonpathogenic *E. coli*. In recent years, pharmaceutical companies have developed several new types and formulations of insulin.

Insulins differ in how quickly they are absorbed, the time and length of peak activity, and overall duration. There are 4 kinds of insulins: rapid-acting, short-acting, intermediate-acting, and long-acting. Onset, peak, and duration of action should always be considered approximate and may vary according to individual factors, which may include injection site, blood supply, concurrent illnesses, lifestyle, and exercise level. These factors can vary from patient to patient and can vary in any patient from day to day.

## Rapid-Acting Insulins

Rapid-acting insulins are analogs of regular insulin. An analog is a chemical structure similar to another but different in one component. Insulin lispro (Humalog) and insulin aspart (Novolog) are two rapid-acting insulin analogs currently available. The amino acid sequence of lispro is identical to human insulin except that the positions of lysine and proline are reversed through recombinant technology, hence the name lispro. In insulin aspart, the amino acid proline has been replaced by aspartic acid, and therefore gets its name from this biochemical switch. These chemical changes allow the insulin analogs to enter the bloodstream more rapidly—as quickly as within 10 minutes of subcutaneous injection. This closely mimics the body's own insulin response and allows greater flexibility in eating schedules for diabetic patients. Insulin lispro (Humalog) or insulin aspart (Novolog) should be injected immediately before a meal to control postprandial hypergylcemia. The peak time for rapid acting insulins is 0.5–3 hours and the duration is 3–5 hours. Also, because these insulins leave the bloodstream quickly, there is less chance of hypoglycemia several hours after the meal. Rapid-acting insulin solutions are clear.

## Short-Acting Insulin

Short-acting insulin is regular insulin and is also given before meals to control postprandial hypergylcemia. Regular insulin is available commercially as Humulin R (a synthetic human insulin), Iletin II Regular (animal insulin derived from pork), and Novolin R (synthetic human insulin). The onset of regular insulin is 0.5–1 hour; its peak activity occurs 2–3 hours after subcutaneous injection and its duration of action is 6–8 hours. This time/action profile makes rigid meal scheduling necessary, as the patient must estimate that a meal will occur within 45 minutes of injection. Short-acting insulin solutions are clear. Regular insulin is the only insulin that can be given intravenously.

## Intermediate-Acting Insulins

In intermediate-acting insulins, protamine is combined with insulin to form a suspension that is more slowly absorbed and has a different time/action profile. It is given to control blood glucose levels when the patient is not eating. For intermediate-acting insulins, action starts between 1 and 4 hours after injecting. Peak activity occurs between 6 and 12 hours. Duration of action lasts 24–28 hours. Commercially, intermediate-acting insulins are available as Humulin N and Humulin L. The "N" stands for NPH (neutral protamine Hagedorn) and the "L" stands for lente, which means slowly in Latin. Both are synthetic insulins made by Lilly. Lente insulin has a slower onset, more delayed peak, and longer duration of action than NPH. Iletin II NPH (derived from pork pancreas and made by Lilly) and Novolin N (synthetic human insulin made by Novo Nordisk) are also available. The addition of protamine causes the cloudy appearance of intermediate-acting insulins and results in the formulation being a suspension rather than a solution. This is why these insulins must be gently mixed before administering. Intermediate-acting insulins can be mixed with short- or rapid-acting insulins to provide both basal and bolus coverage.

## Long-Acting Insulins

Long acting insulins have the most delayed onset and the longest duration of all insulins. The most commonly used products include ultralente (Humulin U, made by Lilly) and insulin glargine (Lantus, made by Aventis). Peaks are not as prominent in long-acting insulins. In fact, insulin glargine has no real peak action because it forms slowly dissolving crystals in the subcutaneous tissue after injection. The onset of action of insulin glargine is 1 hour after subcutaneous injection. Full activity occurs within 4 to 5 hours and remains constant for 24 hours. Ultralente differs somewhat in its time action profile, most notably in that onset of action begins in 6 hours and duration may last as long as 36 hours. Even though insulin glargine is a clear solution, it cannot be diluted or mixed with any other insulin or solution. Mixing insulin glargine with other insulin products can unpredictably alter the onset of action and time to peak effect. If bolus insulin is to be given at the same time as insulin glargine, two separate syringes and injection sites must be used.

## Combination Insulins

Various combinations of premixed insulins are available, containing fixed proportions of two different insulins, usually a short- and an intermediate-acting insulin. Typically, the intermediate-acting insulin makes up 70% to 75% of the mixture, with rapid- or short- acting insulin making up the remainder. Onset, peak, and duration vary according to each specific product. Brand names of these products include Humulin 70/30 (70% NPH, 30% regular), Humalog Mix 75/25 (75% insulin lispro protamine suspension and 25% insulin lispro), and Novolin 70/30 (70% NPH, 30% regular), or Novolog 70/30 (70% insulin aspart protamine suspension and 20% insulin aspart).

## Insulin Therapy

The goal of therapy for diabetic patients is to provide insulin coverage that most closely resembles endogenous insulin production and results in the best glycemic control without hypoglycemia. Although daytime control of hyperglycemia may be accomplished with bolus doses of rapid-acting insulin analogs, elevations in fasting glucose may remain a problem. If fasting blood glucose levels remain elevated, the basal insulin dose (intermediate- or long-acting) may have to be adjusted.

# BIBLIOGRAPHY

Acute Pain Management Guideline Panel: Acute Pain Management in Adults: Operative Procedures. Quick Reference Guide for Clinicians. Agency for Health Care Policy and Research, Public Health Service, US Department of Health and Human Services, Rockville, MD, 1992.

American Hospital Formulary Service: Drug Information 2000. American Society of Hospital Pharmacists, Bethesda, MD, 2002.

American Pain Society: Principles of Analgesic Use in the Treatment of Acute Pain and Cancer Pain, ed 4. American Pain Society, Skokie, IL, 1999.

Blumenthal, M, et al: The Complete German Commission E Monographs: Therapeutic Guide to Herbal Medicines. Integrative Medical Communications, Boston, 1998.

Cancer Chemotherapy Guidelines. Recommendations for the Management of Vesicant Extravasation, Hypersensitivity, and Anaphylaxis. Oncology Nursing Society, Pittsburgh, PA, 1996.

Cavanaugh, BM: Nurse's Manual of Laboratory and Diagnostic Tests, ed 3. F.A. Davis, Philadelphia, 1999.

Drug Facts and Comparisons. Facts and Comparisons, a Wolters Kluwer Company, St. Louis, 2002.

Expert Panel Report 2: Guidelines for the Diagnosis and Management of Asthma. National Asthma Education and Prevention Program, National Heart, Lung, and Blood Institute, 1997.

Fetrow, CW and Avila, JR: Professional's Handbook of Complementary & Alternative Medicines. Springhouse Corporation, Springhouse, PA, 1999.

Jellin, JM, Batz, F, and Hitchens, K: Pharmacist's Letter/Prescriber's Letter Natural Medicines Comprehensive Database. Therapeutic Research Faculty, Stockton, CA, 1999.

Jonas, WB, and Levin, JS (eds): Essentials of Complementary and Alternative Medicine. Lippincott Williams & Wilkins, a Wolters Kluwer Company, Baltimore and Philadelphia, 1999.

Kuhn, MA, Winston, D: Herbal Therapy and Supplements: A Scientific and Traditional Approach. Lippincott, Philadelphia, 2000.

Mahan, LK, Escott-Stump, S: Krause's Food, Nutrition, and Diet Therapy, ed 9. W.B. Saunders, Philadelphia, 1996.

McCaffery, M, and Pasero, C: Pain: Clinical Manual, ed 2. Mosby-Yearbook, St Louis, 1999.

PDR for Herbal Medicines. Medical Economics Company, Montvale, NJ, 1998.

Phelps, SJ, and Cochran, EB: Guidelines for Administration of Intravenous Medications to Pediatric Patients, ed 4. American Society of Hospital Pharmacists, Bethesda, MD, 1993.

Physicians' Desk Reference (PDR). Medical Economics Company, Montvale, NJ, 2002.

Trissel, LA: Handbook on Injectable Drugs, ed 11. American Society of Hospital Pharmacists, Bethesda, MD, 2002.

Trissel, LA: Supplement to Handbook on Injectable Drugs, ed 11. American Society of Hospital Pharmacists, Bethesda, MD, 2001.

USP Dispensing Information (USP-DI): Advice for the Patient, Volume II, ed 20. United States Pharmacopeial Convention, Rockville, MD, 2002.

USP Dispensing Information (USP-DI): Drug Information for the Health Care Professional, Volume 1, ed 20. Micromedex, Rockville, MD, 2002.

http://www.fda.gov/cder/drug/

---

COMPREHENSIVE INDEX

---

*Entries for **generic** names appear in **boldface type**, trade names appear in regular type, CLASSIFICATIONS appear in BOLDFACE SMALL CAPS, Combination Drugs appear in *italics*, and herbal products are preceded by a leaf icon (❧). A "C" and a **boldface** page number following a generic name identify the page in the "Classification" section on which that drug is listed.

*Entries for **generic** names appear in **boldface type,** trade names appear in regular type, CLASSIFICATIONS appear in BOLDFACE SMALL CAPS, Combination Drugs appear in *italics,* and herbal products are preceded by a leaf icon (❦). A "C" and a **boldface** page number following a generic name identify the page in the "Classification" section on which that drug is listed.

*Entries for **generic** names appear in **boldface type,** trade names appear in regular type, CLASSIFICATIONS appear in **BOLDFACE SMALL CAPS,** Combination Drugs appear in *italics,* and herbal products are preceded by a leaf icon (✿). A "C" and a **boldface** page number following a generic name identify the page in the "Classification" section on which that drug is listed.

*Entries for **generic** names appear in **boldface type,** trade names appear in regular type, CLASSIFICATIONS appear in **BOLDFACE SMALL CAPS,** Combination Drugs appear in *italics,* and herbal products are preceded by a leaf icon (♣). A "C" and a **boldface** page number following a generic name identify the page in the "Classification" section on which that drug is listed.

C
O
M
P
R
E
H
E
N
S
I
V
E

I
N
D
E
X

*Entries for **generic** names appear in **boldface type,** trade names appear in regular type, CLASSIFICATIONS appear in BOLDFACE SMALL CAPS, Combination Drugs appear in *italics,* and herbal products are preceded by a leaf icon (✤). A "C" and a **boldface** page number following a generic name identify the page in the "Classification" section on which that drug is listed.

*Entries for **generic** names appear in **boldface type**, trade names appear in regular type, CLASSIFICATIONS appear in BOLDFACE SMALL CAPS, Combination Drugs appear in *italics*, and herbal products are preceded by a leaf icon (✿). A "C" and a **boldface** page number following a generic name identify the page in the "Classification" section on which that drug is listed.

C
O
M
P
R
E
H
E
N
S
I
V
E

I
N
D
E
X

*Entries for **generic** names appear in **boldface type,** trade names appear in regular type, CLASSIFICATIONS appear in BOLDFACE SMALL CAPS, Combination Drugs appear in *italics*, and herbal products are preceded by a leaf icon (♣). A "C" and a **boldface** page number following a generic name identify the page in the "Classification" section on which that drug is listed.

*Entries for **generic** names appear in **boldface type**, trade names appear in regular type, CLASSIFICATIONS appear in BOLDFACE SMALL CAPS, Combination Drugs appear in *italics*, and herbal products are preceded by a leaf icon (♣). A "C" and a **boldface** page number following a generic name identify the page in the "Classification" section on which that drug is listed.

*Entries for **generic** names appear in **boldface type**, trade names appear in regular type, CLASSIFICATIONS appear in BOLDFACE SMALL CAPS, Combination Drugs appear in *italics*, and herbal products are preceded by a leaf icon (✿). A "C" and a **boldface** page number following a generic name identify the page in the "Classification" section on which that drug is listed.

# Measurement Conversion Table

**Metric System Equivalents**

1 gram (g) = 1000 milligrams (mg)
1000 grams = 1 kilogram (kg)
.001 milligram = 1 microgram (mcg)
1 liter (L) = 1000 milliliters (ml)
1 milliliter = 1 cubic centimeter (cc)
1 meter = 100 centimeters (cm)
1 meter = 1000 millimeters (mm)

**Conversion Equivalents**

*Volume*

1 milliliter = 15 minims (M) = 15 drops (gtt)
5 milliliters = 1 fluidram (ℨ) = 1 teaspoon (tsp)
15 milliliters = 4 fluidrams = 1 tablespoon (T)
30 milliliters = 1 ounce (oz) = 2 tablespoons
500 milliliters = 1 pint (pt)
1000 milliliters = 1 quart (qt)

*Weight*

1 kilogram = 2.2 pound (lb)
1 gram (g) = 1000 milligrams = 15 grains (gr)
0.6 gram = 600 milligrams = 10 grains
0.5 gram = 500 milligrams = 7.5 grains
0.3 gram = 300 milligrams = 5 grains
0.06 gram = 60 milligrams = 1 grain

*Length*

2.5 centimeters = 1 inch

**Centigrade/Fahrenheit Conversions**

$C = (F - 32) \times \frac{5}{9}$
$F = (C \times \frac{9}{5}) + 32$

(cm)
1
2
3
4
5
6
7
8
9
10
11
12
13
14
15

PUPIL SCALE mm
1  2  3  4  5  6  7  8

# Minimal System Requirements

## PC
CPU: Pentium II PC, 200 MHz
OS: Windows 9x/ME/NT/2000/XP
8x CD–ROM Drive
20Mb Hard disk space
32Mb RAM
800 x 600 monitor with thousands of colors
Requires Internet Explorer 5.0 or greater
Requires Adobe Acrobat 5.0

## LICENSE AGREEMENT

1. F. A. Davis ("FAD") grants the purchaser of the *Student Resource Kit to Accompany: Davis's Drug Guide for Nurses, Edition 9,* limited license for the program on the enclosed disk ("Software"). FAD retains complete copyright to the Software and associated content.

2. Licensee has nonexclusive right to use this copy of the Software on one computer on one screen at one location. Any other use is forbidden.

3. Licensee may physically transfer the Software from one computer to another, provided that it is used on only one computer at any one time. Except for the initial loading of the Software on a hard disk or for archival or backup purposes. Licensee may not copy, electronically transfer, or otherwise distribute copies.

4. This License Agreement automatically terminates if Licensee fails to comply with any term of this Agreement.

5. SOFTWARE UPDATES. Updated versions of the Software may be created or issued by FAD from time to time. At its sole option, FAD may make such updates available to the Licensee or authorized transferees who have returned the registration card, paid the update fee, and returned the original CD-ROM to FAD.

## LIMITED WARRANTY AND DISCLAIMER

FAD warrants that the disk on which the Software is furnished will be free from defects for sixty (60) days from the date of delivery to you by FAD or FAD's authorized representative or distributor. Your receipt shall be evidence of the date of delivery. The Software and accompanying materials are provided "as is" without warranty of any kind. The complete risk as to quality and performance of a nonwarranted program is with you.

FAD makes no warranty that the Software will meet your requirements or that Software operation will be uninterrupted or error free or that Software defects are correctable. No oral or written information or advice given by FAD, its dealers, distributors, agents, or employees shall create warranty or in any way increase the scope of this limited warranty.

REMEDIES. FAD's entire liability and your exclusive remedy shall be limited to replacing the defective media if returned to FAD (at your expense) accompanied by dated proof of purchase satisfactory to FAD not later than one week after the end of the warranty period, provided you have first received a Return Authorization by calling or writing FAD in advance. The maximum liability of FAD and its licensors shall be the purchase price of the software. In no event shall FAD and its licensors be liable to you or any other person for any direct, indirect, incidental, consequential, special, exemplary or punitive damages for tort, contract, strict liability or other theory arising out of the use of, or inability to use, the software.

ENTIRE AGREEMENT. This Agreement contains the entire understanding of the parties hereto relating to the subject matter hereof and supersedes all prior representations or agreements.

GOVERNING LAW. This Agreement and Limited Warranty are governed by the laws of the State of Pennsylvania. All warranty matters should be addressed to:
F. A. Davis, Publishers, 1915 Arch Street, Philadelphia, PA 19103